SIXTEENTH EDITION

MATERNITY NURSING

Family, Newborn, and Women's Health Care

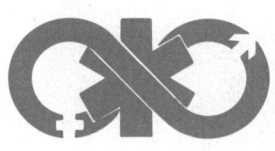

We have chosen the signs for woman, man, birth, and infinity for our logo. As woman and man combine their corporal and spiritual energy in the drama of birth, new beings are brought into existence which have, in turn, their own energy and existence. We know from principles of physics that once matter and energy exist they can never be destroyed, although their forms may change. Hence, once an individual's substance and energy are created, they exist infinitely. Indeed, the phenomenon of birth is the most awe-inspiring and dramatic episode of a lifetime and beyond.

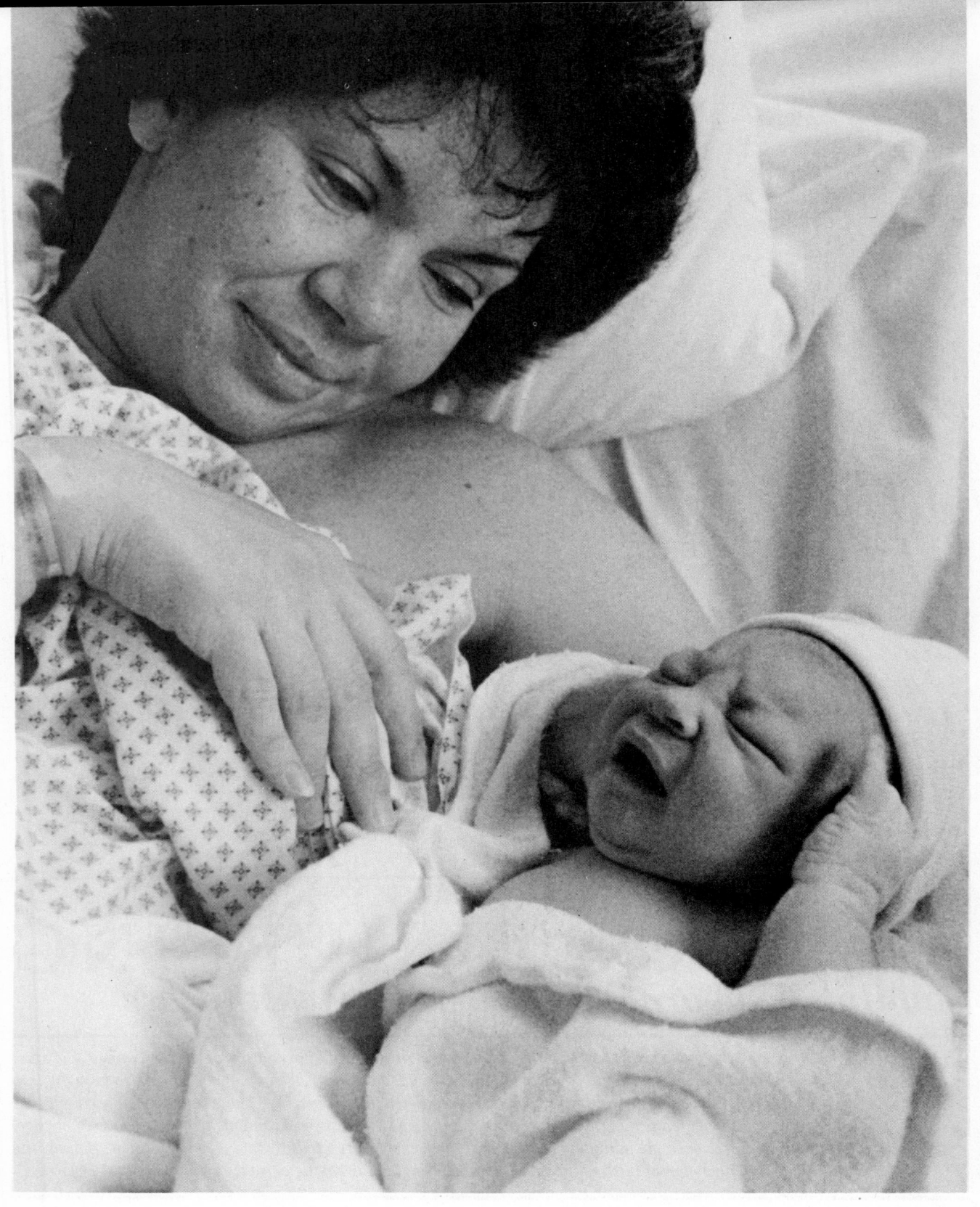

J. B. Lippincott Company   *Philadelphia*

London   Mexico City   New York
St. Louis   São Paulo   Sydney

Sharon J. Reeder

R.N., Ph.D., F.A.A.N.

Professor of Nursing and Associate Dean,
School of Nursing,
University of California,
Los Angeles, California

Leonide L. Martin

R.N., M.S., Dr. P.H.

Professor,
Department of Nursing;
Director,
Family Nurse Practitioner Program,
Sonoma State University,
Rohnert Park, California

SIXTEENTH EDITION

MATERNITY NURSING

Family, Newborn, and Women's Health Care

Sponsoring Editor: Paul R. Hill
Developmental Editor: Eleanor Faven
Senior Manuscript Editor: Shirley Kuhn
Indexer: Julie Schwager
Art Director: Tracy Baldwin

Design Coordinator: Anne O'Donnell
Production Manager: J. Corey Gray
Senior Production Coordinator: Charlene
   Catlett Squibb
Compositor: Tapsco, Inc.
Printer/Binder: Murray Printing

16th Edition

Library of Congress Cataloging-in-Publication Data

Reeder, Sharon J.
   Maternity nursing.

Includes bibliographies and index.
   1. Obstetrical nursing.   I. Martin, Leonide L.
II. Title.   [DNLM: 1. Gynecology—nurses' instruction.
2. Obstetrical Nursing.   3. Perinatology—nurses'
instruction. WY 157 R325m]
RG951.Z3   1987   618.2   86–21484
ISBN 0-397-54578-9

The authors and publisher have exerted every effort to ensure that drug selection and dosage set forth in this text are in accord with current recommendations and practice at the time of publication. However, in view of ongoing research, changes in government regulations, and the constant flow of information relating to drug therapy and drug reactions, the reader is urged to check the package insert for each drug for any change in indications and dosage and for added warnings and precautions. This is particularly important when the recommended agent is a new or infrequently employed drug.

*The 16th edition of **Maternity Nursing: Family, Newborn, and Women's Health Care** is dedicated to the future of nursing with all the challenges and excitement its practitioners will face.*

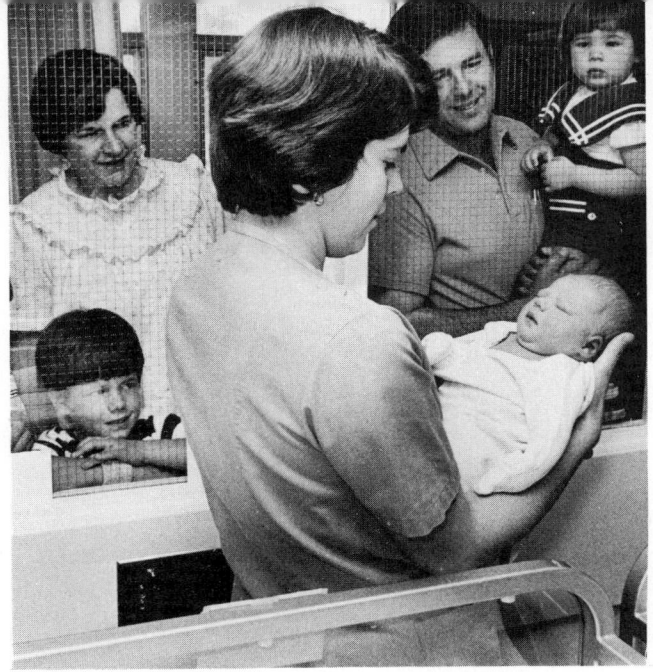

Consultant

Luigi Mastroianni, Jr
M.D., F.A.C.S., F.A.C.O.G.
William Goodell Professor and Chairman,
Department of Obstetrics and Gynecology,
University of Pennsylvania School of Medicine,
Philadelphia, Pennsylvania

Contributors

Ida Stanley Bird, R.N., M.N.
Assistant Clinical Professor, UCLA School of Nursing
UCLA Center for the Health Sciences
Childbirth Educator in private practice
Los Angeles, California

Chapter 20: Preparation for Parenthood; Appendix A: Exercises in Client Education

Roberta Gerds, R.N., M.N.
Associate Professor, Department of Nursing
California State College, Bakersfield
Bakersfield, California

Chapters 21, 28, 32, 33, 35, 38: Nutritional Care in Pregnancy; Immediate Care of the Newborn; Assessment of the Newborn; Nursing Care of the Normal Newborn; Nutritional Care of the Infant; Complications of Labor

Brett B. Gutsche, M.D.
Professor of Obstetrics and Gynecology
Professor of Anesthesia
University of Pennsylvania School of Medicine
Philadelphia, Pennsylvania

Chapter 27: Analgesia and Anesthesia During Childbirth

Deborah Koniak-Griffin, R.N., Ed.D.
Assistant Professor of Nursing
School of Nursing, UCLA
Los Angeles, California

Chapters 36 and 37: Complications of Pregnancy; Concurrent Diseases in Pregnancy

Mark Landon, M.D.
Assistant Professor, Department of Obstetrics and
  Gynecology
University of Pennsylvania School of Medicine
Philadelphia, Pennsylvania

Co-author, Chapters 42, 43: Fetal Diagnosis and Treatment; Intrapartum Fetal Monitoring and Care

Susan M. Ludington, R.N., C.N.M., Ph.D.
Assistant Professor of Nursing
School of Nursing, UCLA
Los Angeles, California

Chapter 34: Sensory Enrichment With the Newborn

Jane McAteer, R.N., M.N.
Assistant Professor
Dominican–St. Luke's School of Nursing
San Rapael, California

Chapters 44, 45, 46: The High-Risk Infant: Disorders of Gestational Age and Birth Weight; The High-Risk Infant: Developmental Disorders; The High-Risk Infant: Acquired Disorders

Margo McCaffery, R.N., M.S., F.A.A.N.
Consultant in the Nursing Care of People with Pain
Santa Monica, California

Chapter 26: The Nurse's Contribution to Pain Relief During Labor

Ann McDonnell, R.N.
Coordinator of Prenatal Genetic Diagnosis
Department of Obstetrics and Gynecology
University of Pennsylvania School of Medicine
Philadelphia, Pennsylvania

Co-author, Chapter 17: Genetic Counseling and Diagnosis During Pregnancy

Denise Main, M.D.
Assistant Professor
Department of Obstetrics and Gynecology
University of Pennsylvania School of Medicine
Philadelphia, Pennsylvania

Co-author, Chapters 42, 43: Fetal Diagnosis and Treatment; Intrapartum Fetal Monitoring and Care

Michael T. Menutti, M.D.
Professor
Department of Obstetrics and Gynecology
University of Pennsylvania School of Medicine
Philadelphia, Pennsylvania

Co-author, Chapter 17: Genetic Counseling and Diagnosis During Pregnancy

Philip Samuels, M.D.
Assistant Professor
Department of Obstetrics and Gynecology
University of Pennsylvania School of Medicine
Philadelphia, Pennsylvania

Co-author, Chapters 42, 43: Fetal Diagnosis and Treatment; Intrapartum Fetal Monitoring and Care

Mary E. Sheridan, R.N.C., M.N.
Clinical Nurse Specialist, Labor and Delivery
Perinatal Nursing Consultant, Perinatal Outreach
  Program
Memorial Medical Center, Long Beach
Long Beach, California

Chapter 25: Management of Normal Labor

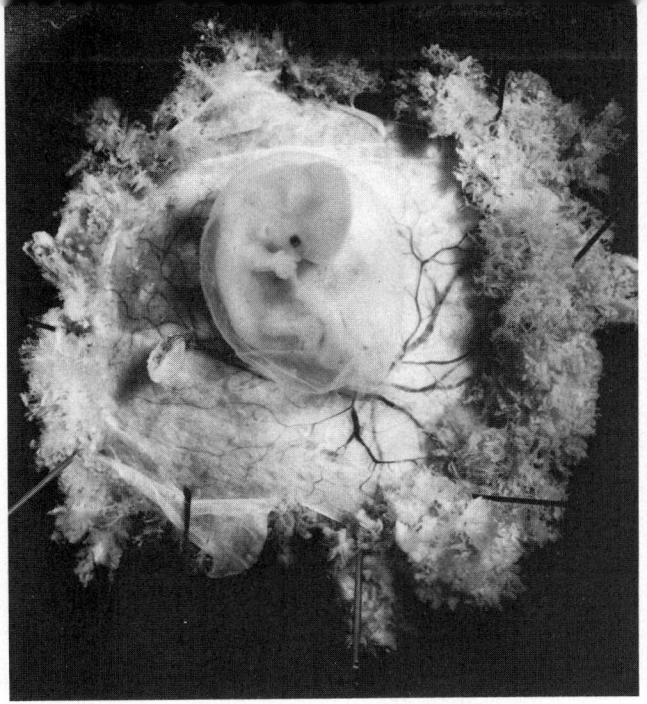

Preface

The 16th edition of *Maternity Nursing: Family, Newborn, and Women's Health Care* reflects extensive revision. The chapters have been reorganized and rewritten. Six new chapters, including a new unit, have been added. The nursing process has been delineated in detail and serves as a basis for nursing care throughout the book. All nursing care plans and clinical chapters reflect the nursing process.

Society continues to change at a phenomenal pace and the institutions in our society continue to reorganize, particularly the family and the educational and health systems. As society changes, clients change their orientations, values, and behavior and health providers must change in order to maintain a synchrony in their roles.

Family life-styles continue to evolve. With these various life-styles come a melange of attitudes and behaviors regarding reproduction, sexuality, and child-rearing. These factors broaden the scope of maternal care. Moreover, the continuing innovations that are occurring in the health care delivery system in response to health care economics are having a profound impact on the maternity specialty. These current issues are examined in depth to enable students to gain a better insight into their importance so that this knowledge can be incorporated into their care.

Unit I has been reorganized to provide a variety of fundamental concepts regarding the structure and function of the modern family and health systems, emerging multiple life-styles and various social factors relating to health. A new chapter on the nursing process serves as a basis for implementing nursing care throughout the book. Ethical and legal considerations in reproduction are introduced because of their profound impact on client care. These concepts are explored in depth in a new chapter as a basis for discussion of the current thinking regarding sexuality, changing role relationships in the family, nursing and parenting, reproductive behavior, and use of maternity services. This information provides a broad conceptual base that the student must comprehend in order to deliver high-quality nursing care to families.

In Unit II chapters dealing with the anatomy and the physiology of sexuality and reproduction have been combined. Affectional and relational aspects of sexuality have been retained because they are so inextricably bound to the cycle. This provides a further elaboration of the concepts introduced in Unit I and provides the student with a sound knowledge base in this fascinating area. Sections on the development and physiology of the embryo and fetus have been revised to reflect current data and thinking. This unit supplies the basic anatomy, physiology, and development necessary in the study of nursing care.

Unit III continues an in-depth examination of areas of sexuality and various facets of reproduction. Common concerns that individuals have regarding sexuality are addressed, and the chapters dealing with contraception, pregnancy termination, infertility, and genetic counseling provide additional necessary information for the delivery of quality maternity care.

Units IV through VI deal with the normal reproductive cycle from conception through the postpartum period. All of these chapters have been revised and updated. These chapters will enable the student to gain a knowledge of the total normal reproductive cycle and its management. Throughout these chapters and others in the book, dimensions of effective nursing care for each phase of the reproductive cycle have been expanded, based on recent research and conceptual developments in nursing practice and related disciplines. The nursing process is used throughout as a basis for care.

Units VII and VIII reflect current research and practice regarding the assessment and management of maternal and infant disorders and emergencies. The chapters on Complications in Pregnancy and Concurrent Diseases in Pregnancy have been extensively revised to update medical knowledge as well as expand and refine nursing care in these areas. Numerous nursing care plans based on the nursing process have been developed for these chapters to guide students in planning and implementing care. A full chapter has been devoted to fetal monitoring and its appropriate use. Nursing care in this area has been expanded. Fetal diagnosis and the management of the high-risk infant have been extensively updated to reflect current thinking and nursing management.

Three chapters are devoted to management of the infant with neonatal disorders. These chapters provide the student with a basic knowledge needed to observe who is at risk and to provide care for these newborns and their families. The information in these chapters is essential as the fields of perinatal medicine and nursing burgeon.

Unit IX examines several special considerations in maternity nursing. A chapter on the evolution of maternity nursing has been rewritten to reflect current trends. Health care is not carried out in a vacuum, nor did present-day maternity care spring from nothing. It was shaped and nurtured by a variety of economic and social factors. Thus, a thorough understanding of the history of the field will enable the student to appreciate current practice and predict future care patterns. The current issue of alternatives in maternity care is addressed and the topics of home deliveries, alternative birth centers, and nurse midwives are discussed to clarify the contribution of these providers in the total maternity spectrum.

A new unit—Assessment and Management in Women's Health Promotion—of three chapters has been added. It focuses on those areas of gynecology that a maternity/perinatal nurse is likely to see. It may very well be that the maternity nurse is the most important individual many women will ever consult on health matters. Therefore, one chapter deals with gynecological health promotion, while the other two chapters discuss menstrual and bleeding disorders and vaginal and pelvic infections.

This edition of *Maternity Nursing: Family, Newborn, and Women's Health Care* has been reformatted to provide greater readability. New photographs, drawings, illustrations, tables, and boxed highlights have been added to reinforce points made in the text and to provide the student with quick reference information. Again, at our readers' request, we have included study questions and conference material at the end of each of the units. In this edition we have placed answers to the questions at the back of the book, immediately preceding the Index. All of the suggested readings have been updated with references from current professional literature.

Sharon J. Reeder, R.N., Ph.D., F.A.A.N.
Leonide L. Martin, R.N., M.S., Dr. P.H.

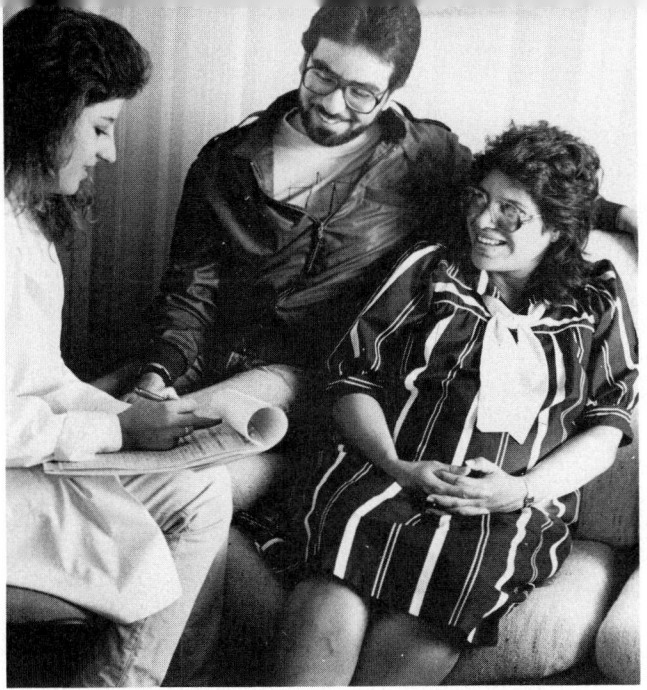

Acknowledgments

Once again, we wish to thank our contributors who have given a special dimension to the 16th edition of *Maternity Nursing: Family, Newborn, and Women's Health Care* with their varied expertise. We wish to express our gratitude for the help and encouragement of our many colleagues and friends in the revision of this edition. In particular, we would like to thank John Dodgson and Melody Butterfield for their scholarly and meticulous pursuit of the literature searches and revision of several of the care plans. We are also indebted to Carmen Methanges for her expert typing and editorial services.

We would like to extend our thanks to the Maternity Center Association of New York for permission to publish the exercises taught by the Center in its prepared childbirth program. We would also like to express our appreciation to colleagues, publishers, and organizations for the use of illustrations, assessment tools, and other tools that are found in the text. We are especially appreciative of the many parents, nursing students, and staff members who granted their permission for photographs appearing in *Maternity Nursing: Family, Newborn and Women's Health Care.*

Finally, we take this opportunity to thank the people of J. B. Lippincott Company for their suggestions and cooperation through the production of this edition. Most especially, we would like to thank Paul Hill, Editor, Eleanor Faven, Developmental Editor, and Shirley Kuhn, Manuscript Editor, whose steadfast assistance helped make this edition possible.

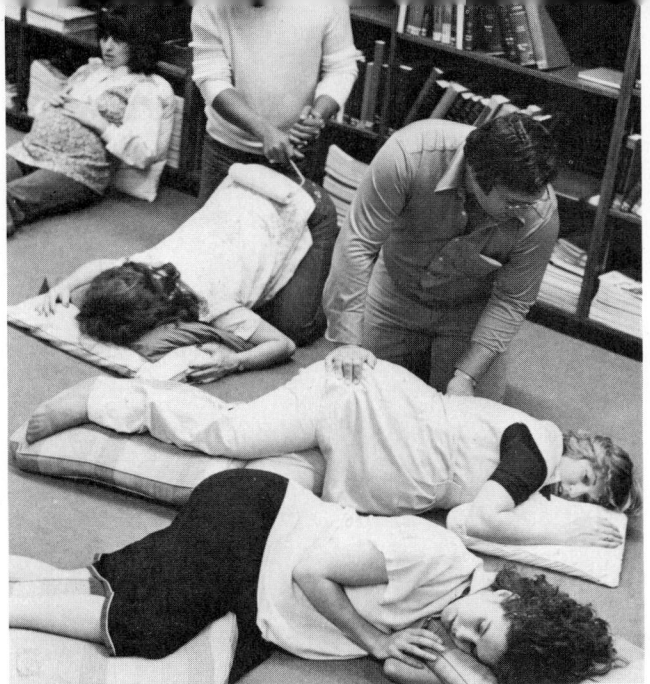

Contents

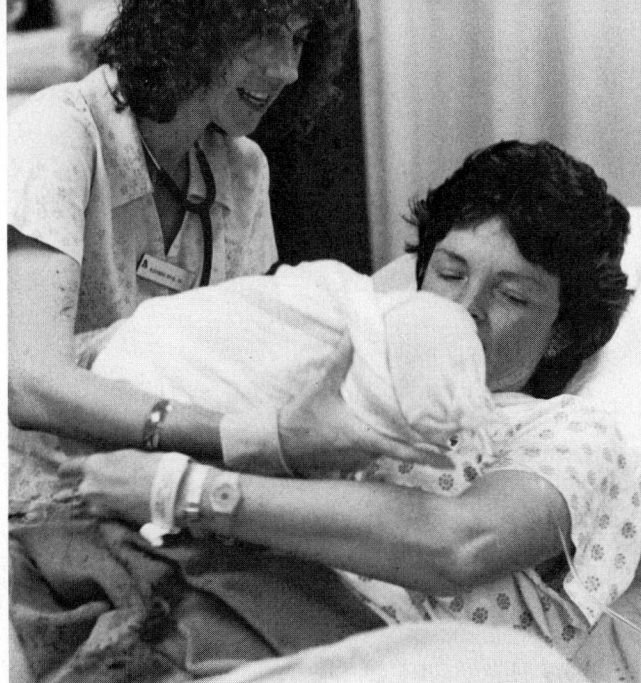

Expanded Contents

U N I T   I I

Biophysical Aspects of Human Reproduction 95

U N I T   I V

Assessment and Management in the Antepartum Period 281

C H A P T E R   1 8

Biophysical Aspects of Normal Pregnancy 283

C H A P T E R   1 9

Psychosocial Aspects of Normal Pregnancy 298

C H A P T E R   2 0

Preparation for Parenthood 312

U N I T   V

Assessment and Management in the Intrapartum Period 429

C H A P T E R   2 3
Assessment of the Passageway and Passenger 431

C H A P T E R   2 4
Phenomena of Labor 446

C H A P T E R   2 5
Management of Normal Labor 457

U N I T   I X

Special Considerations in Maternity Nursing   1073

C H A P T E R   4 7
Evolution of Maternity Nursing   1075

U N I T   X

Assessment and Management in Women's Health Promotion   1109

C H A P T E R   4 8
Promoting Gynecologic Health   1111

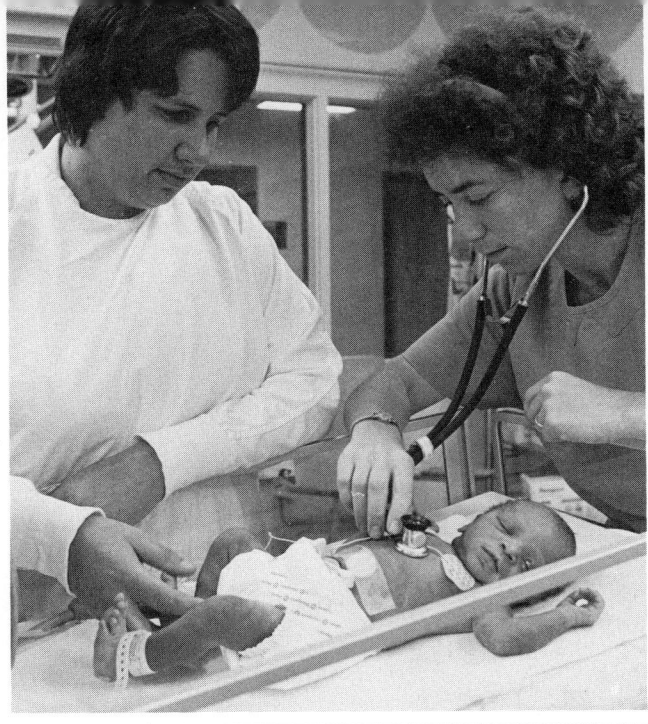

Nursing Care Plans

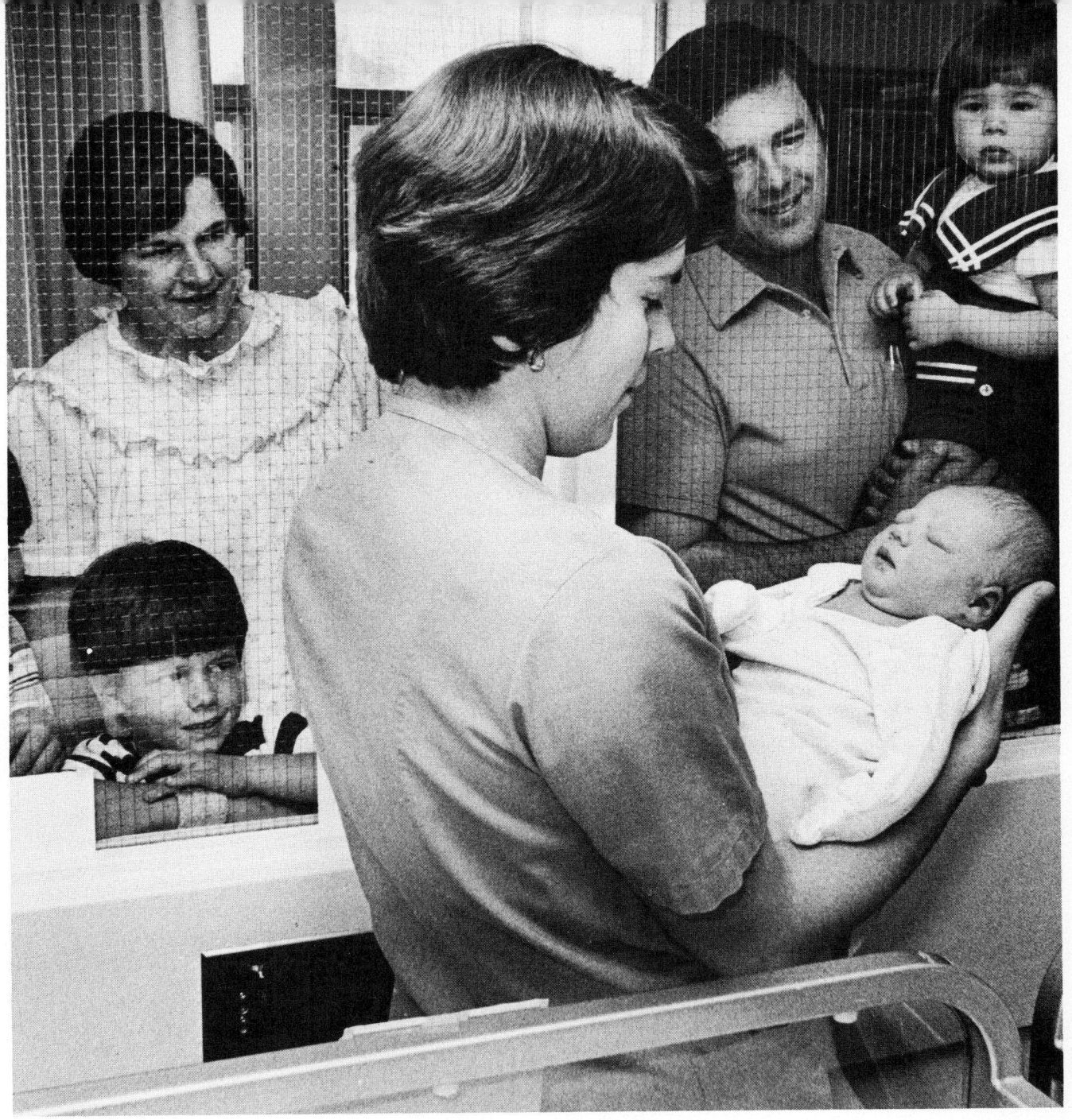

UNIT I

Nursing, Family Health, and Reproduction

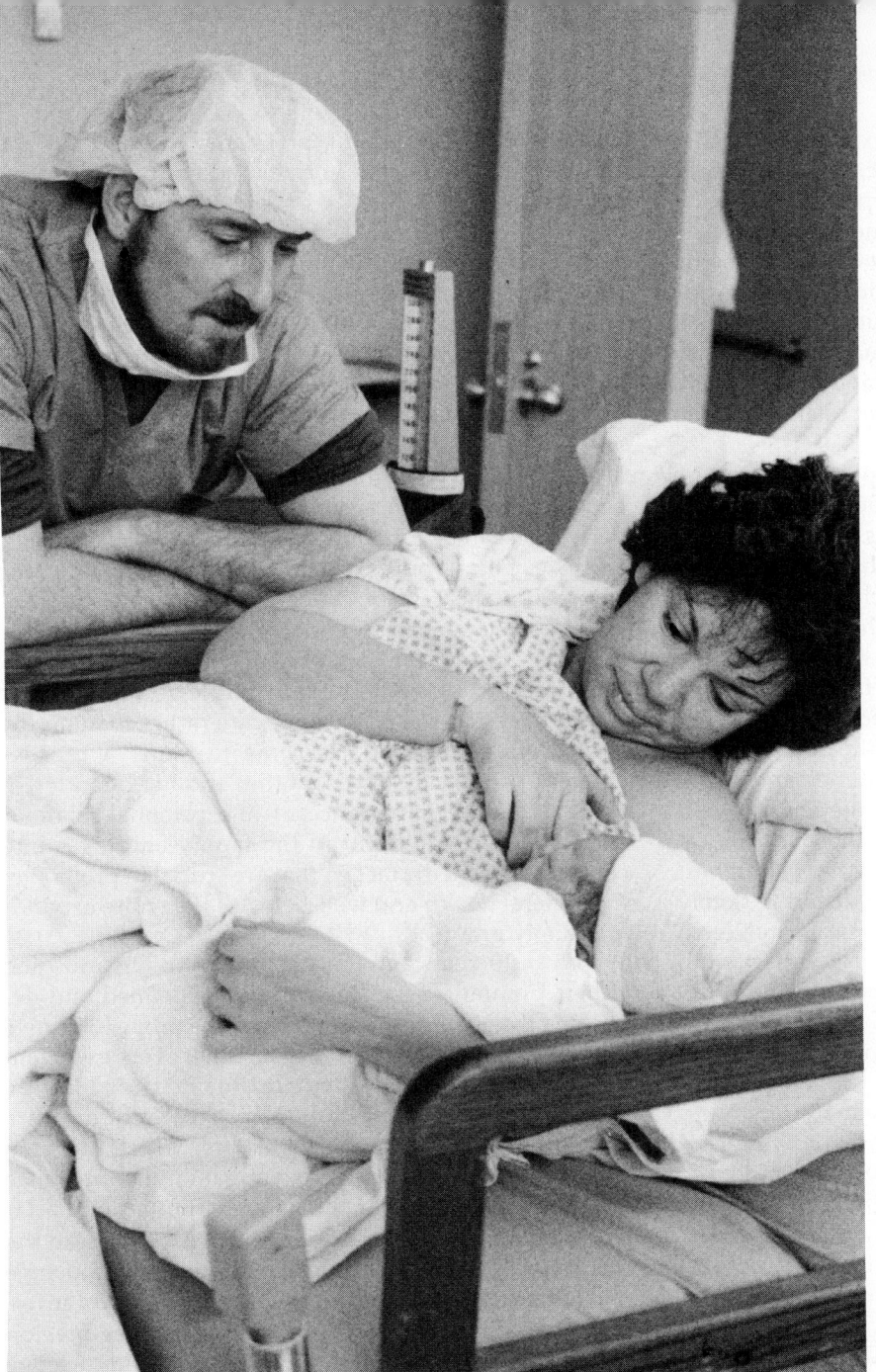

CHAPTER 1

Philosophy of Family-Centered Care

Of all the phenomena that humans experience, birth is perhaps the most emotional, dramatic, and awe-inspiring. Birth is a family affair, and the reproductive health of the total family is the cornerstone upon which a healthy society rests. Thus, the study of obstetrics and the nursing care of women and their families during childbearing includes not only the study of anatomical and physiological adaptations to human reproduction, but also the study of human growth and development and the many complex, interdependent relationships to the total society.

Knowledge of the anatomy and physiology of the reproductive organs and of the development of the unborn child from conception to birth is basic to the understanding required by everyone who participates in maternity care. The physiological mechanism by which conception takes place and the new human being develops is not only a fascinating story but also one that has far-reaching implications for the family. All that a person becomes depends on many factors—his or her heritage, the prenatal environment, the care at birth, and the care thereafter throughout infancy and childhood. Thus, it becomes apparent that the health, well-being, and safety of each mother, father, and infant must be protected, and simultaneously that the highest level of wellness possible for every childbearing family be achieved in the broadest sense of physical, emotional, and social well-being. Moreover, it is also important to understand the extent to which the structure and function of the family, as it relates to the larger society, influence the reproductive behavior and health of the childbearing family.

This chapter orients the student to maternity nursing. The philosophy and assumptions underlying care for the family during reproduction are given and basic concepts of care are examined. In the remainder of the unit, information and concepts relating to childbearing families and how they intermesh with society are explored.

Evolution of the Concept of Maternity Care

All definitions and modes of health care have a history. Maternity care is no exception. The student is referred to Chapter 48 for an in-depth presentation of the history of the field. For the moment, we will concern ourselves with a brief overview of some terms and the concepts of care that have become associated with them.

Obstetrics

Obstetrics is defined as that branch of medicine that deals with parturition, its antecedents, and its sequels. Thus, it is concerned principally with the phenomena and the management of pregnancy, labor, and the puerperium under both normal and abnormal circumstances.[1]

The word *obstetrics* is derived from the Latin *obstetricia* or *obstetrix*, meaning *midwife*. The verb form *obsto* (*ob*, before, plus *sto*, stand) means to stand by. Thus, in ancient Rome a person who cared for women at childbirth was known as an *obstetrix*, or a person who *stood by* the woman in labor. In both the United States and Great Britain, this branch of medicine was called *midwifery* until the latter part of the 19th century. The term *obstetrics* really came into use little more than a century ago, although reference to a variety of words of common derivation can be found occasionally in earlier writings.

The post-World War II era brought dramatic changes in the care of childbearing women and concomitant changes in terminology relating to them. In the then-current frame of reference, it seemed more appropriate to use the term *maternity* care because this term focuses on the *recipient* of care rather than on the *provider*. Moreover, it has come to imply a broader meaning of the care of the mother and her offspring; it emphasizes the importance of interpersonal relationships that are significant in the family and takes into consideration all the factors that are crucial in promoting the general health and well-being of the entire expanding family group.

Over 30 years ago the World Health Organization Expert Committee on Maternity Care defined and delineated the goals of maternity care. The proper objective of this care, they said, was to ensure that every expectant mother bore healthy children, maintained good health, and learned the art of child care. Not only did care consist of the mother's personal care, which included a safe delivery, a postnatal examination, maintenance of lactation, and care of the neonate, but also, in a far wider sense, it included care begun much earlier in the reproductive cycle. Health promotion of young people including personal health, family planning, and infertility counseling, together with helping couples develop appropriate approaches to family life and a knowledge of the family's place in society, were cornerstones in this concept.[2]

Thus, from the rather narrow definition that focused primarily on the provider of care, we expanded our concept of obstetrics to include not only the childbearing woman but all those significant persons in her social network.

Maternal–Child Health

The term *maternal–child health* has been used for more than 70 years. In 1912 the United States Children's Bureau was created by an act of Congress for the purpose of promoting maternal and child health "among all classes of people." Until its reorganization into The National Institutes of Health, the Children's Bureau continued to make significant contributions to the promotion of maternal–child health in this country.

Trends in Maternal–Child Care

There have been a number of strides, both technological and social, that have set the stage for influencing trends in the health-care delivery to families and their children.

High-Tech Advances in Information Exchange and in the Assessment, Management, and Delivery of Care. The development of sophisticated hardware and software information systems and the development of high-tech equipment and other testing measures used during the reproductive cycle have impacted not only on the health care needs of clients but also on the ability to respond to them. These advances have also influenced the ways in which efforts to meet these needs are viewed and received by clients. To the majority of providers and some consumers, these advances have been boons. To others, however, they are seen as evidence of an overpreoccupation with technology rather than with the client as a person. As a reaction to this high-tech trend, alternatives are emerging that again impact on the delivery of care (see Chap. 47).

Changes in Family Structure and Function. Owing to increased industrialization and urbanization, rapid transit, and mass communication, the family has become increasingly mobile. This has combined with the high divorce rate and the increasing trend to delay childbearing to fragment families. Contiguous, extended-family units often are nonexistent. Family supports previously available to members to help them manage childbearing and childrearing and cope with sexuality issues, health problems, and loss have become indirect, scattered, and, often, ineffective.[3] This is true at the societal level as well. In 1973 there was a drastic reorganization of federal child development and child health services under the Health Services Administration, which, while necessary in the opinions of some, resulted in the fragmentation of services and diminished the visibility of mothers' and children's health needs. Thus, there is no longer a clear single focus for the expression of concerns for those involved with the health of families.

Cost Containment. The seemingly limitless resources of the early 1950s, under pressure from escalating technology, have been reduced by stringent cost-containment measures and planning at the regional level. A prospective payment system was put into effect by the Social Security Amendments of 1983, and it has caused many ripples in the health-care system. As part of this prospective payment program, Diagnostic Related Groups (DRGs) were conceived to create a more competitive and cost-effective delivery system. This "front end" type of payment system is based on client diagnosis, irrespective of length of hospital stay or complexity of treatment. While certainly increasing incentives for cost efficiency, it is not ideal, since it does not take into consideration other health-care problems that may complicate or extend the client's recovery time.[4]

The Role of the Hospital. The role of the hospital has altered dramatically. Most care is institutionally based, but currently there is an upswing in ambulatory health care as hospitals attempt to cope with variable populations, increased technology, regulatory agencies, escalating costs, and families' increasing militancy in attempting to alleviate the stress accompanying hospitalization. Clients are no longer passive dependent; they are demanding active participation in their own care. Clients now wish explanations from all their health-care providers; they require informed consent, and they want to establish parameters for the type of care received.[3] This assertiveness has had implications for the nurses' role as well.

Similarly, modern perinatal management techniques have led to the recommendation of regional organization and coordination of services for the woman and her neonate. The intent of regionalization is to ensure pregnant women and their newborns prompt access to the level of care appropriate to the degree of obstetric or neonatal risk. Regionwide organization of these services would be expected to contribute to a reduction in poor outcomes through provision of risk assessment of pregnant women and infants and the development of mechanisms of facilitating the movement of patients within a graded care system. Delivery of the patients at highest risk would be centralized in those institutions offering the most complete and complex care available. Those patients at low risk would not need to be subjected to the cost and technology of these settings. Hence, regionalization is seen as cost-effective in avoiding duplication of costly technology and services, yet providing quality service at a needed level.[5]

Changes in Provider Role Relationships. Paralleling the changing client role are changes in the nurse's role. Nursing is redefining its role as a collaborative one within the team of health-care providers. Moreover, nurses are becoming increasingly aware that the definition and realization of their goals involve a true interactive process between the client and the health-care team. Hence, nurses, as well as society, are viewing themselves as increasingly accountable for their care and for safeguarding their clients' rights.

All of these changes can lead to confusion about practice standards for nursing. To clarify basic standards of practice, The Nurses' Association of the American College of Obstetrics and Gynecology (NAACOG) has developed Standards for Obstetric, Gynecological, and

---

Summary of Major Areas of Concern in Maternal–Child Health

- It is necessary to have integration of high-quality maternal–child health services within evolving comprehensive systems of prepaid (not necessarily prospective) group health-care plans. Services should include prevention, detection, and maintenance.
- Adequate funding of preventive and ambulatory services, especially during the newborn period, must be included in all the mechanisms for financing maternal–child health services.
- The present services and special projects must be extended to meet the needs of specific high-risk and disadvantaged groups.
- There is a need to resolve the dilemma of providing health services in settings that do not focus primarily on health, that is, schools.
- There must be a focus on concern for maternal and child health within the federal government and for mechanisms for child advocacy both within and without the federal government. The ongoing fragmentation has left the federal government without a clear point of entry for those interested in maternal–child health services.
- There is a need for continuing, critical evaluative research to explore innovations and alternative methods of delivery of care. For instance, it is necessary to have a much clearer idea about whether increased technology really results in higher quality of care.

Neonatal Nursing. According to NAACOG, these standards are not intended to limit innovations in nursing care. Rather, they should be viewed as part of an ongoing process with the knowledge that there needs to be constant revision.[3] The student is advised to familiarize herself with these important standards.

In view of all these trends, certain recommendations are made in major areas of concern (see Summary of Major Areas of Concern in Maternal–Child Health).

Philosophy About Maternity Care

Health providers' responses to their clients' needs in both health maintenance and illness management must take into consideration current attitudinal, social, and cultural changes. Health care is not delivered in a vacuum; it takes place in a larger social context and is greatly influenced by current thinking and change manifested by the host society. Philosophies of care evolve from this thinking and change.

We believe maternity care to be a philosophy of client care rather than a special area of medical services or nursing. We believe that begetting children is a family affair; thus, the medical and nursing care of maternity clients is properly a family-centered activity.

In almost no other normal physiological process does one find such individual extremes of reactions within a normal context. For both the woman and her partner, these reactions may be based on events going back to childhood or experienced as an adolescent and adult. Certainly, they are influenced by the immediate home environment from which the couple comes. Moreover, the expectant parents' level of satisfaction and the level of contentment of the newly delivered mother and infant are modified by the interpersonal relationships of those most significant to them in the health-care environment.

Assumptions About Maternity Care

Underlying the philosophy about maternity care are the following assumptions:

- All individuals have the right to be born healthy, and to ensure this right, every pregnant woman and every fetus has the right to quality health care.
- Individuals' sexuality is inextricably bound to reproduction but not subordinate to it; changing societal attitudes toward sexuality, role relationships, and childbearing, together with technological advances in fertility control, have combined to make parenthood increasingly a voluntary state.
- Reproduction is not experienced alone; whatever the circumstances, it involves one or more individuals.
- Reproduction is part of a normal psychophysiological process and can be physically and emotionally rewarding for the individuals involved.
- The childbearing experience is a developmental opportunity; it can also be a situational crisis during which family members benefit from the solidarity of the family unit.
- The profound physiological changes and adjustment that both the mother and her offspring experience during the childbearing process make them particularly vulnerable to changeable and noxious environments and situations that would ordinarily not prove hazardous.
- Each individual's attitudes, values, and health behavior are influenced by the culture and society from which he or she comes; thus, each individual's reproductive outcomes and childbearing experience will be influenced by his or her cultural heritage.

Maternity Nursing/ Family-Centered Care

Definition

Maternity nursing can be defined as the delivery of professional quality health care while recognizing, focusing on, and adapting to the physical and psychosocial needs of the childbearing woman, the family, and the newly born offspring.

Implicit in this definition is the notion of a family-centered approach. This approach assumes that the family is the basic unit of society and, as such, is to be viewed as a total unit within which each member is a distinct individual. It is further assumed that childbearing and the rearing and socialization of children are unique and important functions of the family. Therefore, the experience of childbearing is appropriate and beneficial to share as a unit.

When we speak of the "family," we do not necessarily mean the traditional nuclear family composed of a married pair and their children. In Chapters 4 and 5 we examine the various definitions and emerging family forms.

Maternity nursing involves direct, personal care to the childbearing woman and her infant, as well as the related activities of teaching, counseling, and supervising during the various phases of the childbearing experience. A cornerstone of care is client/consumer education with respect to health maintenance and reproductive health. It differs from the practice of nursing in other areas in that the clinical focus involves primarily the care of the childbearing unit (the mother, father, and infant) in contrast, for example, to the care of surgical or psychiatric patients. It is unique in that the nurse is called upon to attend, educate, and counsel all age-groups, from the fetus through childhood, adolescence, and adulthood, since the childbearing unit may span all those stages in the life cycle.

How the maternity nurse meets the needs of members of the childbearing unit cannot be spelled out in stereotyped activities. The nurse will intervene to relieve or reduce problems caused by physiological, psychological, or social stress. In addition, the nurse will make clients aware of the principles of health maintenance so that they may incorporate these into their preventive health behavior patterns.

A significant aspect of maternity nursing on the professional level is that the nursing care involves purposeful, sustained interaction during which the nurse makes an assessment of the client's problems and resources and then takes action to relieve the problem and support the strengths with appropriate nursing measures. If the condition requires additional services from the other members of the health team, referral or consultation is given.

Implementation

The successful implementation of family-centered nursing care includes recognition that the provision of high-caliber care requires a team effort by the woman and her family, the health-care providers, and the community. The composition of the team may vary from setting to setting and includes obstetricians, pediatricians, family physicians, certified nurse–midwives, nurse practitioners, and maternity clinical nurse specialists. While physicians are responsible for providing direction for medical management, other team members share appropriately in managing the health care of the family, and each team member must be individually accountable for the performance of his or her facet of care. The team concept includes the cooperative interrelationships of hospitals, providers, and the community in an organized care system so as to provide for the total spectrum of maternity/newborn care within a particular geographic region.[4]

Expanding Roles

Prior to the 19th century there was little interest by anyone in providing quality maternity care to mothers and families. Care was generally delivered by untrained women. In the mid-1900s physicians became more interested in obstetrics and in Britain nurse–midwifery educational programs were implemented. In 1925 Mary Breckinridge, who had trained in England as a midwife, spearheaded the organization of the Frontier Nursing Service in Kentucky. Also in 1925 the Frontier Graduate School of Midwifery opened its doors and for many years was the premier school of midwifery in the United States. Today there are numerous educational programs throughout the United States that are undertaking the preparation of nurses for various expanded roles in the field.

The main categories of nursing personnel are listed here. Several additional subspecialties are emerging; however, the following will provide a basis for later comparisons.

Nurse–Midwife

Certified nurse–midwives are registered nurses who have completed a specific program of study and clinical experience recognized by the American College of Nurse Midwives. They must also pass a certification test before beginning practice. They are qualified to take complete health histories and perform complete physical examinations for their clients. They can provide complete antepartal care, including teaching and counseling. They are qualified to give comprehensive care during the intrapartal period, including delivery of the infant. They are able to deliver care to the mother and infant in the postpartal period, including family-planning information and devices. Thus, they attend both the mother and the infant throughout the maternity cycle as long as the mother's progress is considered normal and uncomplicated. The student is directed to Chapter 47 for a more detailed examination of the role and functions of this practitioner.

Obstetric-Gynecological Nurse Practitioner

Obstetric-gynecological nurse practitioners are registered nurses who have completed an additional formal educational program that meets criteria specified for state licensure and certification. Such programs may be at the master's degree level. The practitioners work in collaboration with physicians and may have varying degrees of supervision from their physician colleagues. They function in somewhat the same way that nurse–midwives do; however, they do not deliver infants.

Obstetric-gynecological nurse practitioners provide immediate and continuing assessment of the newborn and its mother and aid the family in assuming the new parental role. Their focus of practice is on providing primary health care to normal pregnant and nonpregnant women with an emphasis on health maintenance. They can also diagnose and treat certain common abnormalities, such as uncomplicated cystitis or vaginitis, under the aegis of the collaborating physician's standing and contingency protocols.

Women's Health-Care Specialist

The women's health-care specialist may be a registered nurse or a licensed vocational nurse, or may have experience in another ancillary medical role. The length of training is variable, usually around 3 to 6 months, depending upon the entry level of professional education of the applicant. These programs do not have the in-depth preparation that the longer midwifery or master's degree programs do. Women's health-care specialists can screen for physical abnormalities in their patients; they then refer any person with suspected pathology to a physician. They can perform routine gynecologic examinations and provide family-planning counseling; they can also insert and remove intrauterine devices. Like the ob-gyn practitioner, they can, under physician's orders, treat simple gynecologic problems. Their focus of care is primarily on women, as their name implies, but many of these practitioners expand their focus to include a more family-centered approach in their patient teaching and counseling.

Maternity Clinical Specialist

The maternity clinical specialist is a registered nurse who has completed a university-based master's degree program of graduate courses designed to provide in-depth knowledge of the reproductive process and development of clinical expertise in the actual delivery of complex nursing care to the childbearing unit. Her functions include health education, counseling, dissemination of family-planning information, and assisting the family with their parenting role. These professionals may not have physical assessment (diagnostic) skills and hence would not do complete physical examinations or medically treat common disorders. Client and family education, counseling, and delivery of complex, expert nursing care is the focus of practice. They are also resource persons for staff education and client-care coordination.

New Directions/ Perinatal Nursing

During the past decade, as knowledge and technology have continued to burgeon, an effort has been made to provide a conceptual umbrella to encompass maternal–fetal health care as a unit. Consequently, the term *perinatal care* has evolved. By definition, the word *perinatal* means the 6-week period preceding or following birth; however, in actual use the connotation is much more encompassing. All of the definitions imply that both an obstetric and pediatric orientation is involved. Hence, perinatal care is a method of health-care delivery that would serve to decrease the segmentation and fragmentation of care for the mother and infant (Fig. 1-1).[6]

Perinatal care has also become associated with the high-risk mother and infant in those hospitals designated as tertiary care, or Level III. These hospitals have the resources and expertise to manage any complication of pregnancy or of the newborn. The personnel in Level III institutions provide care for normal patients and for all types of maternal–fetal and neonatal illnesses and abnormalities. By contrast, Level I hospitals provide for management of uncomplicated maternal and neonatal patients, and in these institutions there should be a strong component of preventive services and early detection of existing or potential problems, which then may be referred to the Level III institutions. Level II hospitals provide the same services as the Level I hospitals; however, they can provide for uncomplicated obstetric problems and certain types of neonatal illnesses that do not require the wide array of expertise and technology that are found in the Level III hospitals.[6]

Perinatal nursing is therefore emerging as a new subspecialty of professional maternity nursing. It has

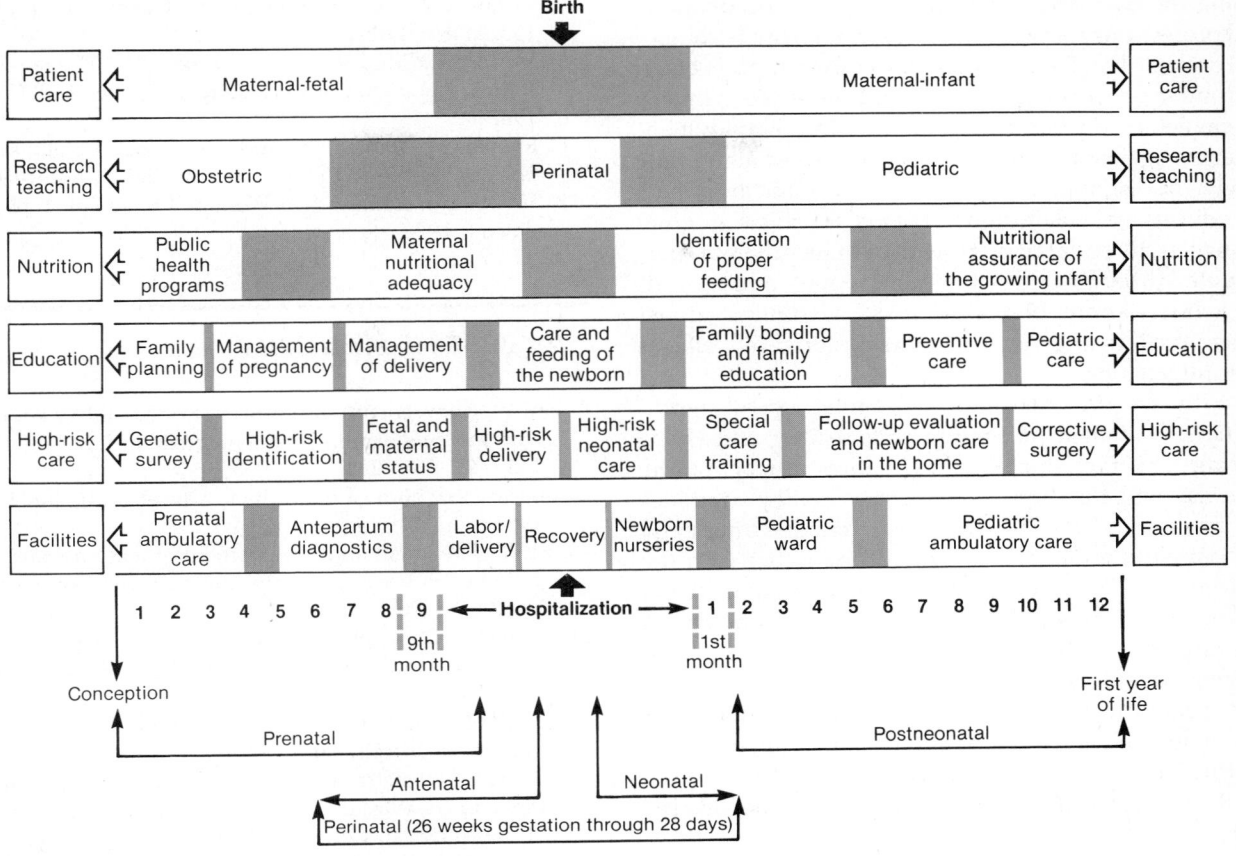

FIGURE 1-1

Paradigm of comprehensive perinatal services for the expectant family. (Hospital Planning Associates: Planning and design for perinatal and pediatric facilities, Columbus, Ross Laboratories, 1977)

evolved in response to a need that arose from past gaps, failures, and successes in the delivery of quality nursing care during the reproductive process. It encompasses many of the best features of the above roles, and the knowledge base is not significantly different from that of the midwife or master's-prepared maternity nurse practitioner.

Social Context of Maternity Care

Maternity care is practiced in the context of the total society and, as such, is influenced by the values, attitudes, and practices of that society. Of late, society is adopting a new stance, particularly with regard to women. At least half of the maternity nurse's clientele will be women, and attitudes and practices regarding them have great relevance for nursing practice. The maelstrom of social change this country has experienced,

particularly in the last 25 years, has greatly expanded the options of behavior.

Growing numbers of women and men no longer accept the traditional definitions of "feminine" and "masculine" identities and roles. They are seeking more individualized definitions of self that offer wider ranges of expression of their unique characteristics as *persons* rather than simply *woman* or *man*. Indeed, the common qualities shared by both women and men are felt to far outweigh their sex-related differences. Hence, social roles are developing that provide each sex with a much broader repertoire of behaviors.

Women, in particular, expect more choices of lifestyle. They may choose to marry or not, to have children or not, or to pursue any career or employment. They expect to have a voice in the determination of their lives and well-being. And, increasingly, they are demanding a large decision-making role regarding economic and social policies that affect their lives and the larger society in which they live.

At one time women had to make a choice between a family or a career; now women are increasingly combining the two. Moreover, many types of occupations and professions formerly closed to women are becoming more accessible. Federal legislation now supports equal treatment of working women, and more mechanisms to challenge discrimination and unfair employment practices against women are being developed at the state level. Antidiscrimination laws have also had an impact on educational institutions. This is forcing a gradual change in the social biases toward a male privilege, perpetuated through values taught in primary and secondary schools and culminating in the sex-linked admissions practices and career choices fostered by colleges and universities.[7]

Women who choose to rear families spend significantly less of their lifetime in childbearing and childrearing. This fact, of course, has a direct impact on the structure and function of the family. Today's families are smaller and for those who start childbearing early the last child is often born when the mother is in the mid- to late 20s or in the early 30s. The high degree of technology in the majority of American households has freed the woman from hours of household chores; thus, homemaking does not provide the full-time occupation that it once did. With her life span lengthened and her health improved, the 35- to 40-year-old woman can be healthy and vigorous and can look ahead to at least another 25 years of productivity in a sphere outside the home.[7]

It has been said that roles are differentiated in pairs; that is, every role has its complementary role. Thus, as women's roles change and broaden, so too must men's. Slowly more egalitarian relationships are developing between the two sexes. Increasingly, men are assuming more responsibility in childrearing and running the household as their partners are forging ahead with careers. When both parties are pursuing a career, there is a growing tendency for household management, chores, and child-related activities to be shared equally. Thus, social power is very slowly being equalized and sex-linked exploitation is very gradually being diminished. However, there is still a long way to go before true equality can be achieved.

References

1. Pritchard JA, McDonald P: Williams Obstetrics, 17th ed. New York, Appleton–Century–Crofts, 1983
2. World Health Organization Technical Report Series, No. 51. Geneva, Switzerland, World Health Organization, 1952
3. Standards for Obstetric, Gynecologic, and Neonatal Nursing, 2nd ed. Washington DC, The Nurses' Association of the American College of Obstetricians and Gynecologists, 1986
4. Lauver EB: Where will the money go? Economic fore-casting and nursing's future. Nurs Health Care 6:133–135, March 1985
5. McCormick MC, Shapiro S, Starfield BH: The regionalization of perinatal services. JAMA 253:799–804, Feb 8, 1985
6. Russell C (ed): Planning and design for perinatal and pediatric facilities. Columbus, Ross Laboratories, 1977
7. Martin L: Health Care of Women. Philadelphia, JB Lippincott, 1978

Suggested Reading

Callan VJ: Comparisons of mothers of one child by choice with mothers wanting a second birth. J Marr Fam 47:143–145, Feb 1985
Dunn PM: Newborn care in Britain. Lancet 1:156, Jan 17, 1981
Lesser AJ: The origin and development of maternal and child health programs in the United States. Am J Public Health 75:590–598, June 1985
McCormick MC, Shapiro S, Starfield BH: The regionalization of perinatal services. JAMA 253:799–804, Feb 8, 1985
Sonstegard L: Health care costs: Every nurse's problem. MCN 87ff, March/April 1985
Standards for Obstetric, Gynecologic, and Neonatal Nursing, 2nd ed. Washington DC, The Nurses' Association of the American College of Obstetricians and Gynecologists, 1986

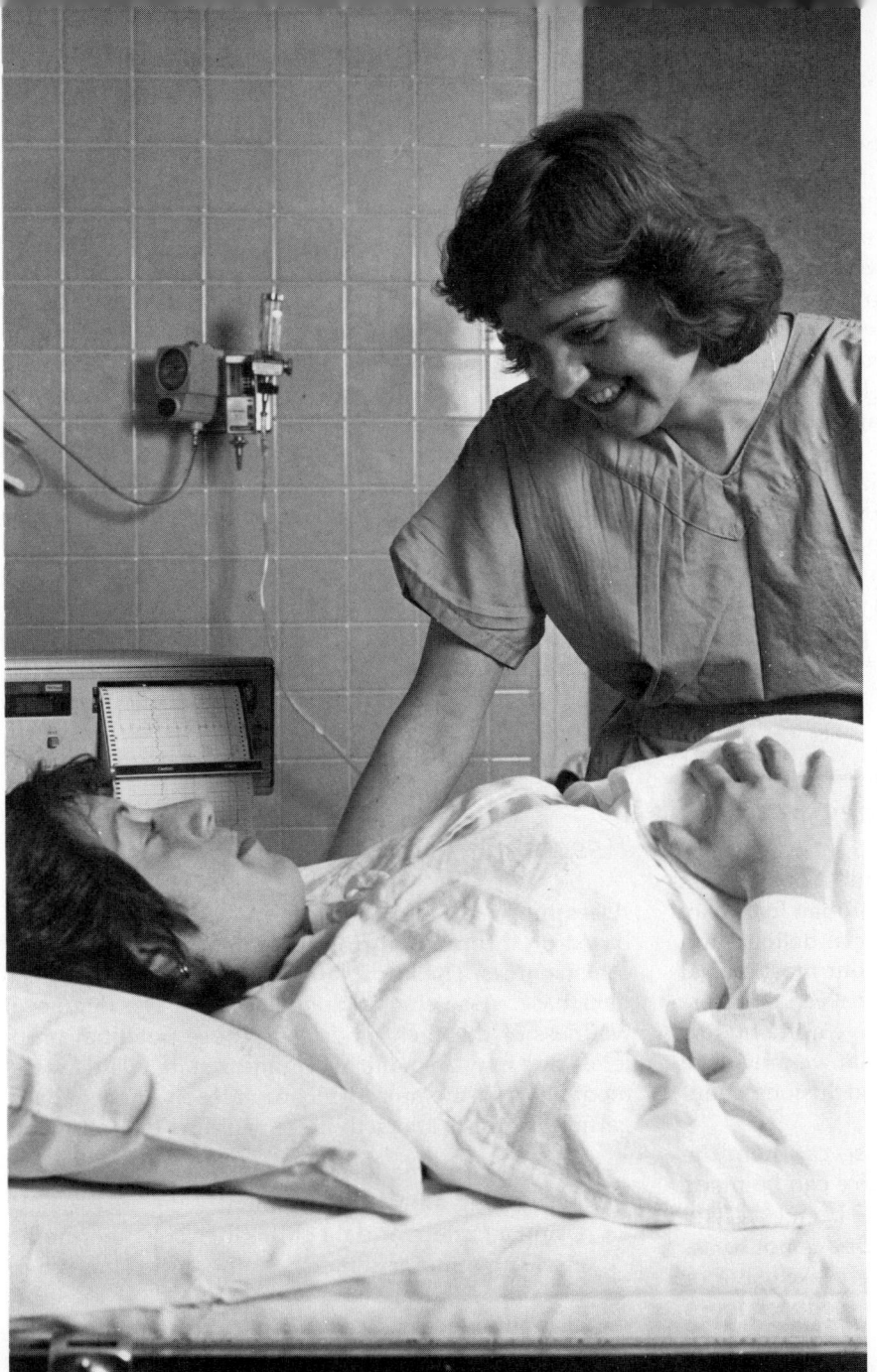

CHAPTER 2

The Nursing Process in Maternity Care

Implicit in the delivery of effective, professional nursing care is the ability to use a method that helps the nurse arrive at informed judgments about clients that have a sound data base. With the data base and these appropriate clinical judgments, nursing care can be planned and implemented so as to enable clients to maintain or return to a state of high-level wellness. This method has been conceptualized as *nursing process* by a variety of authors in an effort to describe a lucid, organized, scientifically based, problem-solving approach to professional nursing practice.[1-4]

Nursing process is the organizing conceptual framework used throughout this text to help the student learn to make nursing judgments appropriate to her nursing care. It supplies a mechanism that enables the nurse to arrive at a responsible valid judgment about clients from which to assess, diagnose, plan, implement, and evaluate nursing care that is responsive to the client's varied needs.

Components of the Process

It is important to point out that, in the midst of the press and crush of everyday practice, where human lives may be at stake, calm fact-finding and judicial deliberation become increasingly difficult. Some of our most crucial nursing problems arise from conflicts between principle and expediency. Hence, we need to have a method so internalized as to be second nature so that we can arrive quickly at appropriate decisions and conclusions about our patients.

The components of the process also can help the student understand how nursing practice can be made operational. The various operations have been classified under headings derived from Bloch.[2] One is not to assume that these categories are mutually exclusive or stand alone. Rather, there are constant feedback loops in the process.

The scientific method is used by other disciplines to provide a way of problem solving for their members and as a basis from which to formulate research that will expand the theoretical base of the discipline. Since nursing also has the concern of expanding its theoretical knowledge to provide a sound basis for its practice, it is very important that the nursing process be scientifically grounded (see the chart on Relationship of Scientific Method to Nursing Process).

The nursing process comprises assessment, planning, implementation or intervention, and evaluation.[5] Various authors have conceptualized the process as including assessment, problem identification, the diagnosis phase, validation, action, and evaluation.[6] Over the years new terminology has evolved, and as nursing science develops, other terminology will no doubt be employed. Thus, we have in the literature such terms as *nursing diagnosis, clinical judgment, assessment, nursing prescriptions, nursing orders,* and so on. While the components may be elaborated in slightly different ways by various authors, it is generally agreed that there are three basic components. In *assessment,* data are gathered on the state of the client's condition and nursing diagnoses are made from these data. Following the construction of the nursing diagnoses, *intervention* is planned and implemented. As the client's condition progresses, *evaluations* are made of the outcomes of the interventions. Additional assessments are made as indicated. Thus, a continuous feedback loop is in operation (Fig. 2-1).

Therefore, the use of the nursing process is twofold: to provide (1) a method that becomes second nature for quick but appropriate decisions and conclusions and (2) a scientific approach to problem solving, which is essential to a profession. For clarity, we use four steps in this book: assessment, nursing diagnosis, planning/intervention, and evaluation and reassessment.

Assessment

Assessing is the act of reviewing a human situation based on information from the client and a variety of other sources. The information gathered forms a crucial data base. Assessing is done to affirm the degree of wellness of the client and to diagnose potential problems; one may also affirm an illness state.[7] The assessment phase of the process incorporates a variety of data-gathering efforts and activities, including the following:

- Taking a nursing history
- Performing a health assessment
- Using a variety of data gathering tools: thermometer, sphygmomanometer, stethoscope, and other tools
- Using the techniques of physical examination: palpation, auscultation, percussion
- Using the five senses[7]

If these activities are used systematically, they will provide the information to make valid nursing judgments and diagnoses. Thus, it becomes clear that the purpose of the assessment phase is to identify and obtain data on the clients' needs that enable the nurse, client, and family to assess their degree of wellness, recognize actual and potential problems, and plan care that will ensure that the client and family will arrive at appropriate solutions.

In her assessments, the nurse will consider the interrelationships of such factors as the client's age, sex, education, stage of growth and development, and socioeconomic status. These factors are discussed more fully in Chapter 6.

Relationship of Scientific Method to Nursing Process

	Components of the Nursing Process	Scientific Method

Assessment	1. Collect data (subjective, objective).
	  a. Gather information on the physical, social, and psychological aspects of the health status of the individual and family.
	  b. Construct the data base by observation, interview, history taking, physical examination, and role taking.
	  c. Develop impressions.
		1. Recognize general problem area.
		  a. Survey pertinent information (literature, past experience, observation).
		  b. Construct data base (organize, select).
		  c. Develop "hunches."

Nursing diagnosis	2. Define the problem.
	  a. Make decisions regarding deficits or potential deficits in health status of the individual and family assigning resources.
	  b. Make nursing diagnoses based on clinical judgment and inference and review of related information, that is, theoretical formulations and research.
		2. Define specific problem.
		  a. Make decisions about relevance.
		  b. Review related information (research already done, theoretical formulations).

Planning/intervention	3. Plan the intervention.
	  a. Make decisions regarding the actions believed to be appropriate to effect a solution of defined problems.
	  b. Decisions include goal setting, priority setting, and nursing prescriptions.
	4. Implement the intervention.
	  a. Execute a nursing regimen by administering a prescribed medication or treatment, executing a medical regimen, providing comfort measures and physical care, providing counseling, providing referral services, coordinating services for the patient, and providing health education.
		3. Propose hypotheses.
		
		4. Test hypotheses.
		  a. Establish baseline data.
		  b. State criteria for acceptance or rejection.
		  c. Collect data.

Evaluation & reassessment	5. Evaluate the intervention. This in turn may lead to further reassessments.
	  a. Determine the degree of effectiveness of the actions taken in solving the defined problems by observation, interview of patient status and conditions, physical examination, and reading of current records.
	  b. Predict future nursing action and patient potential for change.
	6. Terminate or modify relationship.
		5. Analyze data and interpret results.
		
		6. Terminate or modify study.
		  a. Make recommendations and predictions for future research.

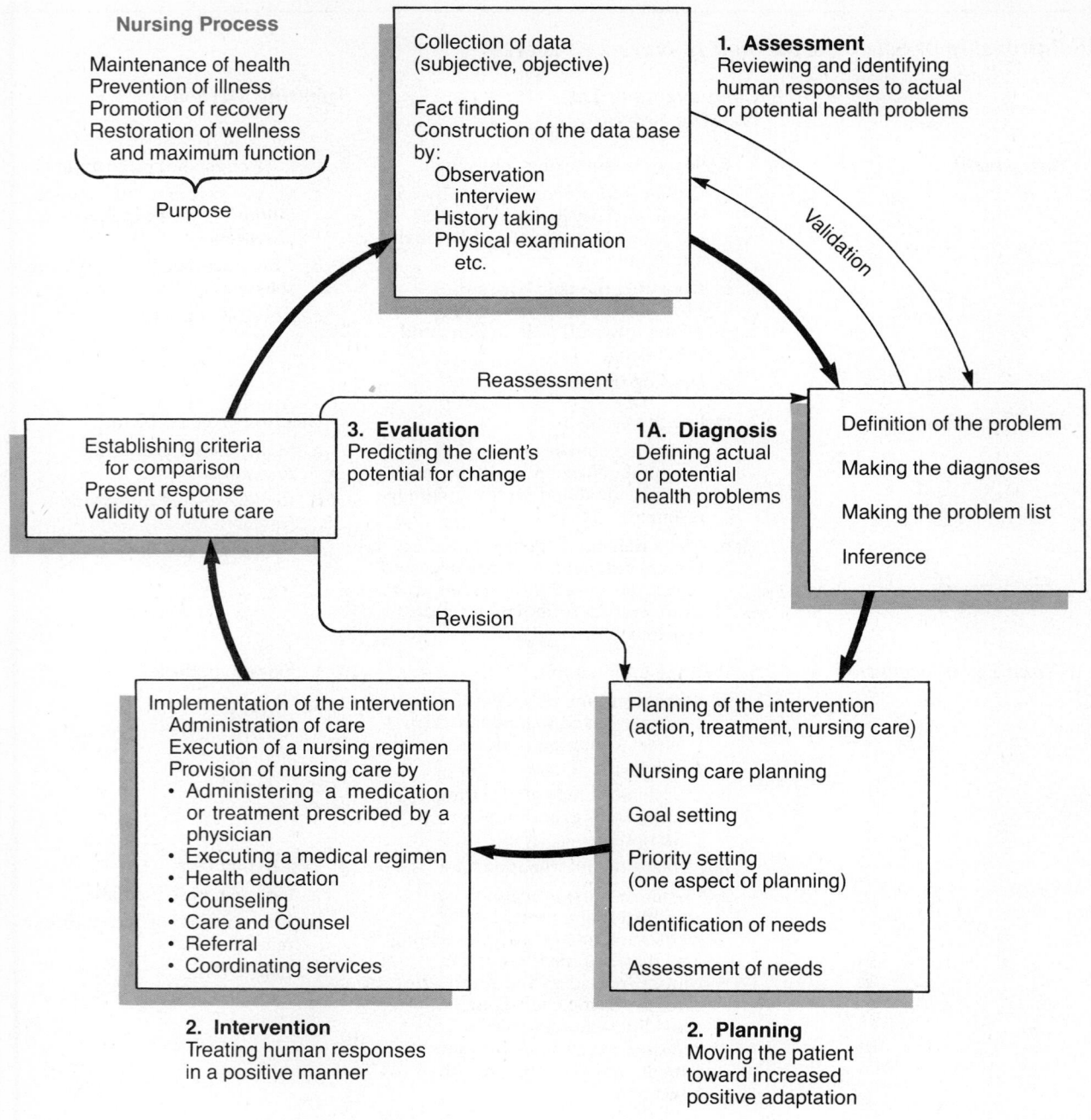

Nursing Process

Maintenance of health
Prevention of illness
Promotion of recovery
Restoration of wellness
and maximum function

Purpose

Collection of data
(subjective, objective)

Fact finding
Construction of the data base
by:
    Observation
    interview
    History taking
    Physical examination
        etc.

1. Assessment
Reviewing and identifying
human responses to actual
or potential health problems

Validation

Reassessment

3. Evaluation
Predicting the client's
potential for change

Establishing criteria
for comparison
Present response
Validity of future care

1A. Diagnosis
Defining actual
or potential
health problems

Definition of the problem

Making the diagnoses

Making the problem list

Inference

Revision

Implementation of the intervention
    Administration of care
    Execution of a nursing regimen
    Provision of nursing care by
    • Administering a medication
      or treatment prescribed by a
      physician
    • Executing a medical regimen
    • Health education
    • Counseling
    • Care and Counsel
    • Referral
    • Coordinating services

2. Intervention
Treating human responses
in a positive manner

Planning of the intervention
(action, treatment, nursing care)

Nursing care planning

Goal setting

Priority setting
(one aspect of planning)

Identification of needs

Assessment of needs

2. Planning
Moving the patient
toward increased
positive adaptation

FIGURE 2-1

Conceptualization of nursing care using the nursing process.

Specific data can be obtained by interviewing the client and performing a health examination. The interview and examination incorporate both physical and psychosocial dimensions, and a systematic format needs to be used. Previous records and charts should be considered to ensure completeness of information and avoid fragmentation of information with consequent impact on continuity of care.

While she collects data, the nurse validates inferences to ensure accuracy in interpretation. When she infers the existence of a problem, condition, or situation from the accumulated facts, she will confirm with the client. The mother then has the opportunity to confirm or deny the perceptions or diagnosis.[7]

Carpenito has pointed out that after the data are gathered and examined, alternative explanations need to be tested and ruled out.[5] At this point the nurse will have reached one of four conclusions:

- No problem is evident at the present time; hence, no health promotion/intervention is indicated.
- No problem is evident but health promotion activities are indicated to ensure and maintain the present level of wellness and to prevent health alterations.
- Actual or potential clinical problems are evident requiring medical referral or implementation of the medical regimen by the nurse.
- Actual or potential nursing problems are apparent that are within the legal and educational domain of the nurse and that require nursing orders.

Nursing Diagnosis

The assessment phase concludes with the nurse making one or more nursing diagnoses. In our text we will refer to "possible nursing diagnoses" in the care plans, since each client and each condition is different; without having an actual situation from which to extrapolate, it would be impossible to state what the diagnoses might actually be.

As we acquire our data, we become able to decide on the existence and extent of a problem. We can say in the most general terms that a problem does exist when there is a health goal to be obtained, but the client sees no well-defined, well-established means of attaining it. For instance, she may be too ill or too weak to help herself. Again, the goal may be so vaguely defined or unclear that the client cannot determine relevant means of achieving it. Thus, she may not understand or know how to accept conditions and instruction for achieving the goal of health.

As previously stated, a decision about the existence and extent of the problem or need initiates a diagnosis. The student will note that over the years, various definitions have been offered. See the chart listing some of these.

A review of the literature also reveals that the term *nursing diagnosis* has taken on two somewhat different meanings. In some situations the term is used to describe the process of problem solving; in other situations, it is used to mean an actual statement of the problem. This dual use has created a good deal of confusion. When the term is used to define the process of analyzing data and identifying a problem, the outcome of this process can be the delineation of both medical and nursing problems. The former must be referred to the physician, and the nurse may participate in the implementation of the medical regimen. Nursing problems, on the other hand, can be treated by the nurse, since they are within her legal and educational purview.[5]

For our purposes, we shall regard a nursing diag-

Definitions of Nursing Diagnosis

- An independent nursing function; an evaluation of a client's personal responses to his human experiences throughout the life cycle, be they developmental or accidental crises, illness, hardships, or other stresses[8]
- Actual or potential health problems that nurses by virtue of their education and experience are capable and licensed to treat[9]
- The judgment or conclusion that occurs as a result of nursing assessment[4]
- A statement that describes a health state or an actual or potential alteration in one's life processes (physiological, psychological, sociocultural, developmental, spiritual). The nurse uses the nursing process to identify and synthesize clinical data and to order nursing interventions to reduce, eliminate, or prevent health alterations that are in the legal and educational domain of nursing.[5]

---

nosis as a conclusion based on a systemic and scientific appraisal of an individual's health–illness condition, resulting from critical analysis of his or her behavior (alone and with others), the nature of the condition, and the numerous other factors (environmental, social, or psychological) that may affect the client's general state. This conclusion, in turn, serves as a guide for planning and implementing our nursing care.

The statement of the diagnosis may be several words and is more descriptive than etiologic. Carpenito suggests that the diagnosis be a two-part statement consisting of a diagnostic title linked to the etiologic and contributing factors.[5] She also cautions about the importance of not linking the statements with words that imply cause and effect, since such a relationship can result in legal and professional difficulty for the nurse. She suggests use of the words *related to* rather than *caused by* or *due to*. Thus, a diagnosis that the nurse might make while attending a maternity patient might be "anxiety about labor related to a knowledge deficit about the labor process," or "extreme discomfort during labor related to inefficient but painful contractions," or "elevated temperature related to inadequate hydration." Sometimes it is impossible to ascertain any etiologic factors despite a complete assessment. In this case, one might have a diagnosis: "fear of caring for the newborn related to unknown factors." Moreover, there may be several diagnoses relating to a constellation of interrelated problems the client has. The three diagnoses given above could conceivably apply to one client at any given time.

Finally, one can have the same nursing diagnosis but have different etiologic factors. In the case of a newly delivered infant, for instance, the diagnosis might be "inadequate oxygenation related to a possible congenital heart defect" or "inadequate oxygenation related to immature lungs associated with prematurity."

Planning / Intervention

Component 3 involves the planning and implementation of knowledgeable intervention in the form of nursing activities that encompass everything from the administration of comfort measures to counseling and health education. These activities are directed at moving the client toward increased positive adaptation to the environment and high-level wellness.

Nursing prescriptions or orders are given here. These are required to prevent, reduce, or eliminate the alteration in the client's health–illness continuum. Carnevali[1] states that nursing orders should be composed of the following: the date when written; a directive verb; what, when, how often, how long, and where the order is to be executed; and, finally, the signature of the nurse who wrote the order. The objective of the nursing prescription or order is to direct individualized care to the client. Orders differ from nursing actions in that the latter are broad interventions that can apply to any number of persons sharing a similar problem or health alteration.[5] For instance, we might have nursing orders and interventions for a mother who is recovering from dehydration and is having some difficulty establishing breast-feeding, as given in the Example of Nursing Orders and Interventions in a Given Situation.

Remember that the implementation phase is fluid

because it is based upon a diagnosis or diagnoses that may be reassessed at any point in the process. Moreover, as we administer care, the client's condition will be expected to change, which, upon evaluation, will necessitate possible new diagnoses and modification of care. Therefore, continuous feedback loops are built into the process.

In this phase, the nurse has the responsibility to disseminate her plan of care to her medical and nursing colleagues so that comprehensive care for the client can be attained. This can be done by means of the Kardex, verbal reporting, charting, and nursing-assessment care plans. Most hospitals have instituted these care-plan forms, and they provide a thorough but brief summary of pertinent patient data together with space to write and record nursing prescriptions, interventions, evaluations, and client response to care.

Evaluation and Reassessment

Component 4 includes both evaluation and prediction facets. A worthwhile evaluation includes an estimation of the results of our past nursing-care activities to help predict the validity of our future care. Carpenito suggests that appropriate evaluations consist of the following:[5]

- Establishing criteria to observe and measure
- Assessing the present response for evidence
- Comparing the present response to the established criteria

Any statement of the effectiveness and reliability of our actions is best made with qualifications indicating the

---

Example of Nursing Orders and Interventions in a Given Situation

Nursing Prescriptions / Orders	Nursing Planning / Intervention

Increase fluids to at least 2400 ml/24 hr.
    1000 ml 7–3
     700 ml 3–11
     100 ml 11–7
Likes all juices and carbonated beverages
Do not count coffee or tea in above amount.
	Increase fluid intake.

Nurse infant on each breast at each feeding. Time on each breast as tolerated	Ensure that breasts are emptied.
Nurse q2h or on demand; do not allow longer intervals than q4h between feedings. Can nurse sitting or lying down	Ensure that breasts are stimulated frequently.

TABLE 2-1

Primary Knowledge and Skills Needed to Implement the Nursing Process

Theoretical Knowledge	Communication Skills	Technical Skills	Therapeutic Use of Self
Basic science	Interviewing	Organization	Goal setting for self and others
General physiology	Mutual sharing	Use of equipment	Ability to use past experiences
General pathophysiology	Writing	Knowledge of general	and role take
Nursing research	Nonverbal	and specific:	Ability to appreciate others'
Social science	Listening	Techniques	value systems
Ethical/religious		Safety	Ability to recognize limitations
Family systems		Physics	in self and others
Reproductive:		Asepsis	
Physiology			
Pathophysiology			
Psychosocial			
Pharmacology			
Nutrition:			
Basic			
Relating to reproduction			

(Adapted from Carpenito LJ: Nursing Diagnosis: Application to Clinical Practice. Philadelphia, JB Lippincott, 1983)

degree or amount of effectiveness and the reliability claimed:

- What is the present state of the client?
- Were all symptoms relieved?
- What was the extent of the results?
- On what evidence (observation of self, others, verbal response, cessation of symptoms)?
- Who was involved (nurse, client, others)?
- In what contexts (what else was happening when the action was performed)?

When these points are established, we can begin to build categories of nursing action that are effective under certain circumstances for certain patients given certain conditions. As we ascertain the extent of our effective-

ness we are then in a better position to predict the client's potential for change toward stability or a wellness condition.

Knowledge and Skills in Implementing the Process

There are certain basic knowledge and skills that the nurse must have to implement the nursing process. Tables 2-1 and 2-2 give the student a handy referent for the knowledge and skills needed as the nursing process is used with the maternity client and her family. As the student increases in expertise in these areas and becomes

TABLE 2-2

Secondary Knowledge and Skills Needed to Implement the Nursing Process

Assessment	Nursing Diagnosis	Planning and Implementation	Evaluation
Ability to	Ability to	Ability to	Knowledge of
• Differentiate cues and inferences	• Differentiate nursing problems from medical clinical problems	• Identify goals	• Process criteria
• Observe systematically	• Identify and test alternatives	• Identify interventions	• Outcome criteria
• Perform a nursing health assessment	• Recognize patterns of problems	• Write nursing orders	
• Identify patterns of problems	• Correctly label patterns	Management skills	
• Validate impressions		Communication skills	
		Teaching skills	
		Ability to implement change theory	

(Adapted from Carpenito LJ: Nursing Diagnosis: Application to Clinical Practice. Philadelphia, JB Lippincott, 1983)

increasingly proficient in using the nursing process, she will find her relationship with her clients will develop more quickly and will be on a greater empathic level.

References

1. Carnevali DL: Nursing Care Planning: Diagnosis and Management, 3rd ed. Philadelphia, JB Lippincott, 1983
2. Bloch D: Some crucial terms in nursing: What do they really mean? Nurs Outlook 22:689–694, 1974
3. Kritek PB: The generation and the classification of nursing diagnosis: Toward a theory of nursing. Image 10(2):33–40, 1978
4. Gebbie K: Toward the theory development for nursing diagnoses classification. In Kim MJ, Maritz DA (eds): Classification of Nursing Diagnoses. New York, Mc-Graw-Hill, 1982
5. Carpenito LJ: Nursing Diagnosis: Application to Clinical Practice. Philadelphia, JB Lippincott, 1983
6. Little D, Carnevali DL: Nursing Care Planning, 2nd ed. Philadelphia, JB Lippincott, 1976
7. McCann/Flynn JB, Heffron PB: Nursing: From Concept to Practice. Bowie, Maryland, Robert J Brady, 1984
8. Bircher A: On the development and classification of nursing diagnoses. Nurs Forum 14:10–29, 1975
9. Gordon M: Nursing Diagnosis, Process and Application. New York, McGraw-Hill, 1982

Suggested Reading

Avant K: Nursing diagnosis: Maternal attachment. ANS 2(1):45–55, Oct 1979
Bockrath M: Your patient needs two diagnoses—medical and nursing. Nurs Life 2(2):29–32, 1982
Carnevali DL: Nursing Care Planning: Diagnosis and Management, 3rd ed. Philadelphia, JB Lippincott, 1983
Carpenito LJ: Nursing Diagnosis: Application to Clinical Practice. Philadelphia, JB Lippincott, 1983
Gordon M: Nursing Diagnosis, Process and Application. New York, McGraw–Hill, 1982
Harris RB: A strong vote for the nursing process. Am J Nurs 81:1999–2001, 1981
Urban DJ, Henkle CW, Rock JA: Nurse specialization in reproductive endocrinology. JOGN Nurs 11(3):167–170, 1982

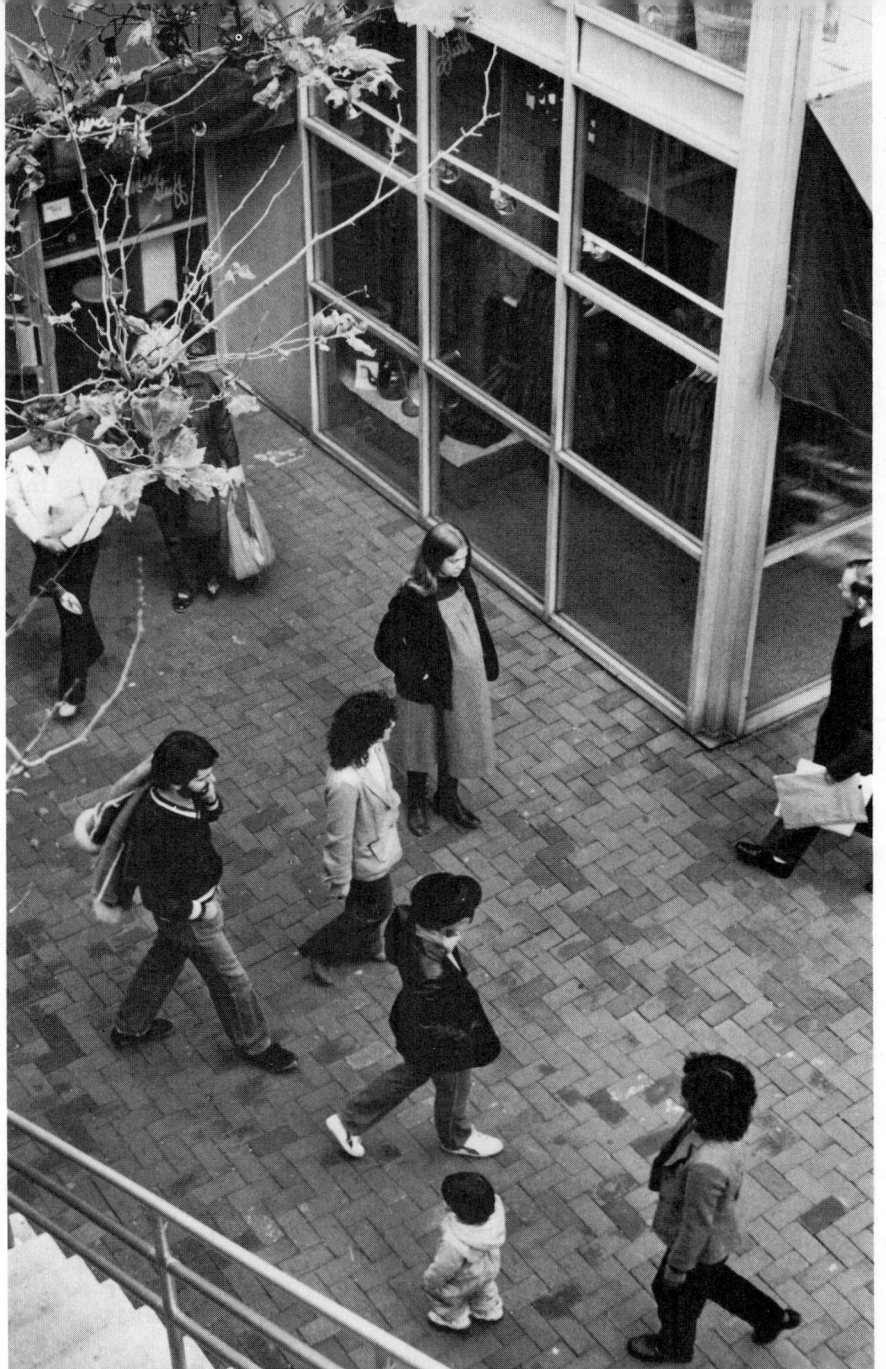

CHAPTER 3

Statistical Profiles

Statistical profiles are useful because they summarize a large amount of data about various populations and therefore supply health providers and policymakers with a valuable overview of needs and gaps in care.

Vital Statistics

In the United States vital statistics reports are published officially by the United States Public Health Service, National Center for Health Statistics, Vital Statistics Division. The terms listed in Definitions Pertaining to Vital Statistics have been defined by the National Center for Health Statistics. Mortality and morbidity terminology is classified according to the World Health Organization's Manual of International Classification of Diseases, Injuries and Causes of Death (ICD).

Natality

Overall, the number of registered births in the United States has decreased in the past 3 decades from over 4 million live births in 1957 to 3.5 million in 1968 and 3.15 million in 1975. However, there was a small 1% rise in the number of live births in 1976 as compared with the previous year. Similarly, in 1981 there was a 1% rise in the rate over 1980, and provisional data from the National Center for Health Statistics (NCHS) indicate a 2% increase in the birthrate in 1983 over 1981. NCHS has noted that while the latest increase is relatively small, it represents the highest birthrate level since 1971.[1]

Birthrates

The increase in the number of births is the result of the increase in the number of women in the childbearing ages (15–44). This number has risen rapidly owing to the high birthrates of the 1940s and the 1950s—the so-called baby boom of the post-World War II era. Although the fertility rate reached a record low in 1976 for the fifth consecutive year, the decline was not enough to offset the 2% increase in the number of women of childbearing age. Provisional data for 1982 indicate a rate of 16.0 per 1000, which is an increase from the 1980 rate of 15.8 per 100.[1]

Thus, an important consideration that influences the number of children being born annually is the size and the age composition of the female population of childbearing age. Although the fertility rate is computed on the basis of births per 1000 women between ages

---

Definitions Pertaining to Vital Statistics

Birthrate. The number of births per 1000 population. Also known as the crude birthrate

Marriage rate. The number of marriages per 1000 total population

Fertility rate. The number of births per 1000 women aged 15 through 44 years

Neonatal. The period from birth through the 28th day of life

Neonatal death rate. The number of neonatal deaths per 1000 live births

Stillbirth or fetal death. A death in which the infant of 20 weeks or more gestational age dies *in utero* prior to birth

Perinatal mortality. All stillborn infants whose gestational age is 28 weeks or more, plus all neonatal deaths under 7 days per 1000 births.* The 1979 revision of the ICD, however, uses birth weight rather than gestational age as a criterion. It also recommends two different categories of reporting. (For national data collection, the recommendation is that 500 g be used as the minimum weight of stillborn and live-born infants. For international compari-

* Current definition approved by WHO.

sons, however, the weight should be 1000 g or more. When weight is unknown, either gestational age [28 weeks] or body length corresponding to 1000 g may be used.) Obviously, these different criteria will make comparisons with previous data impossible and will also make national and international statistical comparisons difficult. There is current debate as to the efficacy of using the newly developed criteria.

Infant mortality rate. The number of deaths before the first birthday per 1000 live births

Maternal mortality rate. The number of maternal deaths resulting from the reproductive process per 100,000 live births

Race and color. Births in the United States are classified for vital statistics according to the race of the parents in the categories of white, black, American Indian, Chinese, Japanese, Aleut and Eskimo combined, Hawaiian and part-Hawaiian combined, and "other nonwhite." In most tables a less detailed classification of "white" and "nonwhite" is used. The white category includes births to parents classified as white, Mexican, Puerto Rican, or "not stated."

15 and 44, most of the childbearing continues to be concentrated among women in their 20s.[2]

There has been a slight rise in the rate of marriages since 1968.[2] However, more married couples are electing not to have children, and there are children being born more often now from social contract and other nonlegal unions.

Multiple Births

There has been a slight decline in the frequency of multiple births in the United States.[3] Changes in age and the racial composition of the population, as well as the use of certain ovulation-producing drugs for infertility, contribute to fluctuations in the rate over time. There are differences, for instance, in the occurrence of twins, depending on the number of births the mother has had before delivery of the multiple birth. There are differences between the rate of monozygotic, or identical, twins and dizygotic, or fraternal, twins, and the relative proportions of monozygotic and dizygotic twins are not the same for all races.

The Birth Certificate

All 50 states and the District of Columbia demand that a birth certificate be filled out on every birth and that it be submitted promptly to the local registrar. After the birth has been registered, the local registrar sends a notification to the parents of the child. Also, a complete report is forwarded from the local registrar to the state authorities and then to the National Office of Vital Statistics in Washington.

Complete and accurate registration of births is a legal responsibility (Fig. 3-1). The birth certificate gives evidence of age, citizenship, and family relationships and as such is often required for military service and passports and to collect benefits on retirement and insurance.

Population

The population of the United States more than doubled during the first half of this century and has continued to grow in tremendous proportions as was predicted.

Three vital factors determine the rate at which population grows: births, deaths, and migration. The decline in the death rate that was so apparent in the first half of this century has fluctuated near the same relatively low level. Recent modifications in immigration practices will undoubtedly exert an influence on this factor in our population growth.

The former decline in the annual number of births was partly related to the age and sex structure of the population. The majority of Americans are young. More than half are under 28 years of age, but the proportion is shifting because of the fluctuating birthrates. The young-adult group, composed of persons between ages 18 and 34, is now the fastest growing portion of the population, reflecting the high birthrates that followed World War II. This group increased to 28.5% of the total as of 1980. Moderately large increases are anticipated in the 65 years and over age-group.

According to population projections made by the Bureau of the Census, during the next 10 years the number of women of childbearing age will probably rise in this country. The uncertainty as to how much the population will grow rises from the unpredictable number of children who will be born to contemporary young couples. Though their fertility potential is huge, much will depend upon their choice in family size.

Mortality

Maternal Mortality

Maternal mortality refers to deaths that result from childbearing, that is, the underlying cause of the woman's death is the result of complications of pregnancy, childbirth, or the puerperium.

The maternal mortality rate in 1974 was about 15 per 100,000; in 1976, 12.3 per 100,000; and in 1978, 9.6 per 100,000. Provisional data for 1982 indicate a further decline to 7.9 per 100,000.[4]

The reduction in maternal mortality rates has been rather consistent since 1951. The dramatic decline in these rates began about the mid-1930s and continued until 1956. During the succeeding 5 years, the maternal mortality rate declined more slowly, reaching the all-time low in 1962. In 1963 the rate rose slightly but resumed its decline the following year and reached a record low in 1978.[5,6]

The risk of maternal death for all mothers is lowest at ages 20 to 24. It is slightly higher under age 20 and from age 25 on. Increasing age is associated with a steep rise in maternal mortality. At 40 to 44 years of age, the mortality rate is six times greater than at 20 to 24. At the oldest age in the reproductive age span, 45 years or older, the mortality is about 12 times greater than the low figure.

Causes of Maternal Mortality

The reduction in maternal mortality from the hemorrhage disorders of pregnancy and childbirth was the largest single factor responsible for the reduction in the

H105.142 Rev. 5-78

COMMONWEALTH OF PENNSYLVANIA
DEPARTMENT OF HEALTH
VITAL STATISTICS
CERTIFICATE OF LIVE BIRTH

TYPE OR PRINT IN PERMANENT INK

PRIMARY DIST. NO. _____

STATE FILE NO. _____

A. _____

B. _____

C. _____

D. _____

E. _____

F. _____

G. _____

H. _____

I. _____

CHILD—NAME FIRST MIDDLE LAST	SEX 2.	DATE OF BIRTH (Mo. Day Year) 3a.	HOUR 3b. _____ AM PM
1.			
HOSPITAL NAME (If not in Hospital, Give Street and Number) 4a.	City, Boro, or Twp. of Birth 4b.		COUNTY OF BIRTH 4c.
I CERTIFY THAT THE STATED INFORMATION CONCERNING THIS CHILD IS TRUE TO THE BEST OF MY KNOWLEDGE AND BELIEF 5a. (Signature) ▶	DATE SIGNED (Mo, Day, Year) 5b.	CERTIFIER—NAME AND TITLE (Type or Print) 5c.	
Name and Title of Attendant at Birth if other than Certifier (Type or Print) 5d.	CERTIFIER'S MAILING ADDRESS (Street or R.F.D. No., City or Town, State, Zip) 5e.		

MOTHER—MAIDEN NAME FIRST MIDDLE LAST	AGE (At time of this Birth) 6b.	STATE OF BIRTH (If not in U.S.A., Name Country) 6c.
6a.		
MAILING ADDRESS STREET AND NUMBER CITY AND STATE ZIP CODE 7.		
WHERE DOES MOTHER ACTUALLY LIVE? STATE COUNTY CITY, BORO, TWP. (Specify) 8.		

FATHER—NAME FIRST MIDDLE LAST	AGE (At time of this Birth) 9b.	STATE OF BIRTH (If not in U.S.A., Name Country) 9c.
9a.		

INFORMANT 10a.	Relation to Child 10b.	REGISTRAR'S SIGNATURE AND DATE RECEIVED 11. ▶

CONFIDENTIAL INFORMATION FOR MEDICAL AND HEALTH USE ONLY

Death Under One Year Of Age — Number of Death Certificate For This Child

Multiple Births Enter State File Number for Mate(s)

Live Birth(s)

Fetal Death(s)

RACE—MOTHER (e.g., White, Black, American Indian, etc. — Specify) 12.	RACE—FATHER (e.g., White, Black, American Indian, etc. — Specify) 13.	EDUCATION—MOTHER (Specify only highest grade completed)		EDUCATION—FATHER (Specify only highest grade completed)		IS MOTHER MARRIED TO FATHER?
		ELEMENTARY OR SECONDARY (0-12)	COLLEGE (1-4 or 5+)	ELEMENTARY OR SECONDARY (0-12)	COLLEGE (1-4 or 5+)	☐ Yes ☐ No
		14.		15.		16.

PREGNANCY HISTORY (Complete each section)		Date Last Normal Menses Began (Mo. Day, Year) 18.	Month of Pregnancy Pre-Natal Care Began (1st, 2nd, etc.) (Specify) 19a.	Pre-Natal Visits — Total (If none, so state) 19b.	Length of Pregnancy in weeks. 20.		
LIVE BIRTHS (Do not include this child)	OTHER TERMINATIONS (Spontaneous and Induced)						
17a. Now living / 17b. Now dead	17d. Before 16 wks. / 17e. After 16 wks.	BIRTH WEIGHT 21.	THIS BIRTH—Single, Twin, Triplet, etc. (Specify) 22a.	If NOT Single Birth — Born First, Second, Third etc. (Specify) 22b.	APGAR SCORE 1 Min. 23a. / 5 Min. 23b.		
Number ___ None ☐ / Number ___ None ☐	Number ___ None ☐ / Number ___ None ☐						
17c. Date of Last Live Birth (Mo. Year)	17f. Date of Last Other Termination (Mo. Year)	Method of Delivery 24.	COMPLICATIONS OF PREGNANCY (Describe or write "none") 25.				

CONCURRENT ILLNESSES OR CONDITIONS AFFECTING THE PREGNANCY (Describe or write "none") 26.	COMPLICATIONS OF LABOR AND/OR DELIVERY (Describe or write "none") 27.
BIRTH INJURIES OF CHILD (Describe or write "none") 28.	CONGENITAL MALFORMATIONS OR ANOMALIES OF CHILD (Describe or write "none") 29.

FIGURE 3-1

Certificate of live birth used by Pennsylvania Department of Health. Similar forms are used by other cities and states.

total maternal mortality rate (from 82.7 per 100,000 live births in 1949–1951 to 9.6 in 1978). The hypertensive disorders and sepsis (cases other than abortion) were next in importance as conditions affecting the mortality rate (Fig. 3-2). Subsequently, these three conditions will be discussed in detail, but it is important to stress the fact that deaths from these causes are for the most part preventable.[6]

It is also important to note that although *hemorrhage* is no longer the primary cause of maternal death as it once was, it still remains an important factor in the morbidity of mothers and in the underlying cause of death. For instance, according to the official classification, only the direct cause of death is considered, even though the predisposing cause may be an important factor. For example, in a case in which the mother has a massive hemorrhage and then (in her weakened condition) develops a puerperal infection that eventually causes her death, the death is classified as due to puerperal infection. Hemorrhage is often a predisposing factor, and in this manner its toll in maternal mortality cannot be underestimated.

Puerperal infection is a wound infection of the birth canal after childbirth, which sometimes extends to cause phlebitis or peritonitis. The nurse can play an important role in helping to prevent such infections by maintaining flawless technique in performing nursing procedures.

The *hypertensive disorders of pregnancy* are certain disturbances peculiar to gravid women, characterized mainly by hypertensive edema and albuminuria and in some severe cases by convulsions and coma. Antepartal care is an important part of prevention or early detection

Causes of Maternal Mortality

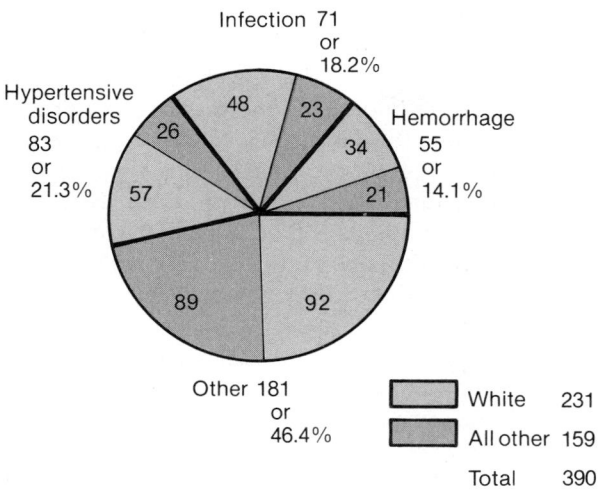

FIGURE 3-2

Percentage distribution for causes of maternal mortality. (Data from Vital Statistics of the United States, 1979, Vol II—Mortality, Part A, Table 1-15, U.S. Department of Health, Education, and Welfare, Public Health Service, 1979)

of symptoms, and with suitable treatment the disturbance often can be allayed.

Reduction in Maternal Mortality

Many factors are responsible for achieving the overall reduction in maternal mortality in this country during the past 25 years.

Medical management has improved. The widespread use of blood and plasma transfusions and antibiotics, together with careful maintenance of fluid and electrolyte balance and sophisticated anesthesia management, has changed obstetric practice substantially. Legalized abortion has also helped reduce the number of maternal deaths associated with abortion.

Perhaps more important is the development of widespread *training and educational programs* in obstetrics and maternity care, which have provided more and better qualified specialists, professional nurses, and other personnel to deliver care in this area. *Better hospital facilities* and the development of alternate hospital facilities to meet consumer demands for a more homelike setting for parturition may also prove to be a helpful factor.

The distinct *change in attitudes of physicians, nurses, and parents* has also contributed to this progressive saving of mothers. Childbirth is no longer an event to be awaited helplessly by the expectant mother with what fortitude she is able to muster; instead, it is the climax

of a period of preparation—a true state of preparedness attained through the cooperation of the physician, the nurse, and the expectant parents.

Antepartal care has been an important achievement in maternity care during the present century. This contribution to the mother's welfare was initiated by the nursing profession in 1901 when the Instructive Nursing Association in Boston began to pay antepartal visits to some of the expectant mothers who were to deliver at the Boston Lying-In Hospital. This work gradually spread until, in 1906, all of these women prior to confinement were paid at least one visit by a nurse from the association. By 1912 this association was making about three antepartal visits to each client. In 1907 another pioneer effort in prenatal work was instituted when George H. F. Schrader gave the Association for Improving the Condition of the Poor, New York City, funds to pay the salary of two nurses to do this work. In 1909 the Committee on Infant Social Service of the Women's Municipal League in Boston organized an experiment of antepartal work. Pregnant women were visited every 10 days, more often if necessary. This began the movement for antepartal care that has been extremely important in promoting the health and well-being of many pregnant women.

Another important factor in the reduction of maternal mortality has been the *development of maternal and child health programs* in state departments of public health, particularly the work of community-health nurses. These nurses visit a large number of the mothers who otherwise would receive little or no medical care, bringing them much-needed aid in pregnancy, labor, and the puerperium. This service fills a great need not only in rural areas, but also in metropolitan centers.

Perinatal Mortality

The two groups of problems in infant mortality that are of chief concern in maternity are those in which the fetus dies in the uterus prior to birth and those in which it dies within a short time after birth (neonatal death). The term *perinatal mortality* is used to designate the deaths in these two categories.

Fetal Death

In an effort to end confusion arising from the use of a variety of terms, such as *stillbirth, abortion, miscarriage,* and so on, the World Health Organization (WHO) recommended the adoption of the following definition of fetal death:

Fetal death is a death prior to complete expulsion or extraction from its mother of a product of conception, irrespective of duration of pregnancy; the

Infant Mortality
Per 1000 live births
1970-1982

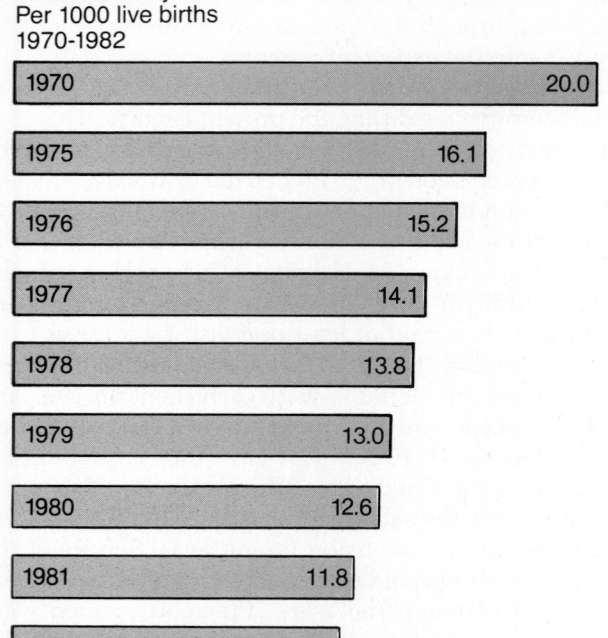

1970	20.0
1975	16.1
1976	15.2
1977	14.1
1978	13.8
1979	13.0
1980	12.6
1981	11.8
1982	11.2

FIGURE 3-3

Infant mortality rates per 1000 live births, 1970–1981. (National Center for Health Statistics, Annual Summary for the United States, 1982. Monthly Vital Statistics Reports 31: 13, October 5, 1983, DHHS Publication No. (PHS) 83–1120)

death is indicated by the fact that after such separation the fetus does not breathe or show any other evidence of life such as beating of the heart, pulsation of the umbilical cord, or definite movement of voluntary muscles.[7]

WHO further defined fetal death by indicating four subgroups, according to gestational age in weeks.

Infant Mortality

Two decades ago a total of 103,390 infant deaths before the first birthday was reported. Figure 3-3 indicates how the rate has dropped in the past 15 years. The leading causes of infant mortality are listed in Figure 3-4. A falling fertility rate, better contraceptive practices, and increasing availability of safe abortion, together with a higher standard of living in the general population, have been suggested as factors in this decline in infant mortality.

However, it has been pointed out that this national figure does not accurately reflect trends in the large urban areas and the southern states where the rate has declined less.

Many factors are responsible for infant mortality. The vast number of infant deaths is the result of several main causes: respiratory distress syndrome, preterm birth, asphyxia and atelectasis, congenital malformations, and birth injuries.

During the first 4 weeks of life, early gestational age and low birth weight are the chief causes of death. Birth injuries are another of the main causes of infant loss. Almost one third of these deaths are due to intracranial and spinal injury at birth. In the vast majority of these cases, death occurred within less than 7 days of life. These conditions will be discussed in detail later. It suffices to say that one of the first and most important of them, immaturity, is largely a nursing management problem.

The welfare of some 3,500,000 babies born annually in the United States is very much the concern of maternity nurses and obstetricians and one of the main objectives of the entire field of maternity care. To reduce the enormous loss of newborn lives, to protect the infant not only at birth but also in the prenatal period and during the early days of life, and to lay a solid foundation for his health throughout life are the problems and the challenge of maternity care.

Reproductive Wastage

The vast number of infants lost by spontaneous abortion is a matter of grave importance. About 10% of all pregnancies terminate in spontaneous abortion because of such factors as faulty germ plasm, unsatisfactory environmental conditions, and hormonal and many other unknown etiologic causes.[5]

Today the concerns for the United States stemming from the overall problem of maternal and fetal reproductive wastage reflect a symptom of far-reaching social change. The tremendous reduction in maternal and infant mortality rates presents concrete evidence of the progress that has been achieved in maternity care in this country. Nevertheless, the current major concern is that a large segment of our population is not receiving maternity care.

The needs resulting from problems of maternal and child health in rural areas continue today, but what is alarming is that now there is a parallel situation in the larger cities. The population still includes a large segment of disadvantaged, low-income families, as well as foreign immigrants, who recently have concentrated in the major cities. With the increased cost of health services in general and the cost of hospital care in particular, these low-income families are straining the local resources of the communities in which they reside. The most serious problem by far is that many of these women are receiving poor or, often, no antepartal care, owing in part to dissatisfaction with the kind of care provided. Inadequate care during pregnancy has been demonstrated to bear a direct relationship to the rate of immaturity.

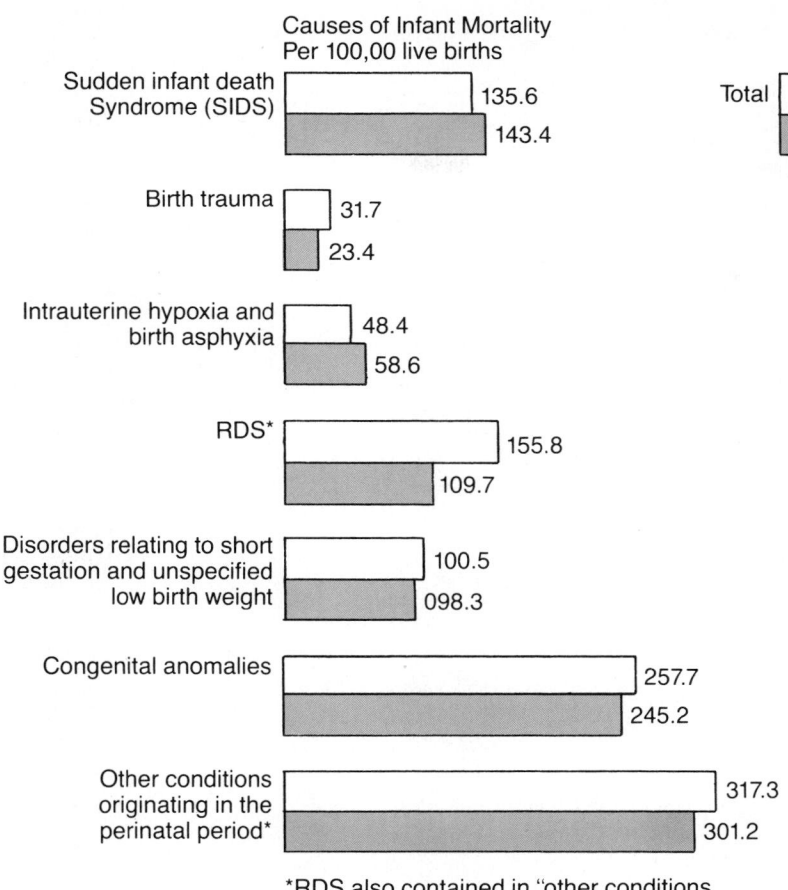

Causes of Infant Mortality
Per 100,00 live births

Sudden infant death Syndrome (SIDS) — 135.6 / 143.4

Birth trauma — 31.7 / 23.4

Intrauterine hypoxia and birth asphyxia — 48.4 / 58.6

RDS* — 155.8 / 109.7

Disorders relating to short gestation and unspecified low birth weight — 100.5 / 098.3

Congenital anomalies — 257.7 / 245.2

Other conditions originating in the perinatal period* — 317.3 / 301.2

Total | 1979 | 1047.0
| 1982 | 979.80

*RDS also contained in "other conditions originating in the perinatal period."

FIGURE 3-4

Causes of infant mortality per 100,000 live births in 1979 and 1982. (National Center for Health Statistics, Annual Summary for the United States, 1982. Monthly Vital Statistics Reports 33:9, December 8, 1982, DHHS Publication No. (PHS) 83-1120)

Moreover, with the recent economic fluctuations, it has been pointed out that middle-class couples are feeling the impact of not being able to afford adequate health care. They are not eligible for welfare coverage, yet not affluent enough to seek the kind of care that is appropriate.

Much of the difficulty in providing adequate care is due to a shortage of professional personnel in the maternity field. The rapid growth of the population has not been accompanied by a proportionate increase in physicians and nurses who are attracted to this area of specialization.

References

1. National Center for Health Statistics: Annual summary of births, deaths, marriages and divorces: United States, 1982. DHHS Publication No. (PHS) 83-1120. Monthly Vital Statistics Report 31:13, Oct 5, 1983
2. Statistical Abstracts of the United States, 1985. US Department of Commerce, Bureau of the Census, pp 57–83
3. United States Department of Health, Education and Welfare: Characteristics of births: United States, 1973–1975. DHEW Publication No. (PHS) 78-1908, Sept 1980
4. National Center for Health Statistics: DHHS Publication No. (PHS) 85-1120. Monthly Vital Statistics Report 34:2, May 28, 1985
5. National Center for Health Statistics: Annual summary of births, deaths, marriages and divorces: United States, 1979. DHHS Publication No. (PHS) 81-1120. Monthly Vital Statistics Report 30:12, March 18, 1982
6. Vital Statistics of the United States, 1976, Vol 11, Mortality, Part A, Table 1-15. US Department of Health, Education and Welfare (PHS)
7. National Summaries: Fetal Deaths, U.S., 1954. National Office of Vital Statistics 44:11, Aug 1956

Suggested Reading

Editorial: Not identifying the sources of the recent decline in perinatal mortality rates. Birth 10(1):33–37, Spring 1983
Elewood JM: The end of the drop in twinning rates? Lancet 1(8322):470–474, Feb 26, 1983

Elewood JM: Infant death gap widening. NAACOG Newsletter 10(8):1–11, Sept 1983

Ozorio P: Low birth weights throughout the world. Midwives Chronicle (Br) 98:66–69, Feb 1982

Rubin GW et al: The risk of childbearing re-evaluated. Am J Public Health 71:712–716, 1981

Savage JE: Obstetrics through the retrospectroscope. South Med J 73(11):1516–1520, 1980

Smith JC et al: An assessment of the incidence of maternal mortality in the United States. Am J Public Health 74: 780–783, Aug 1984

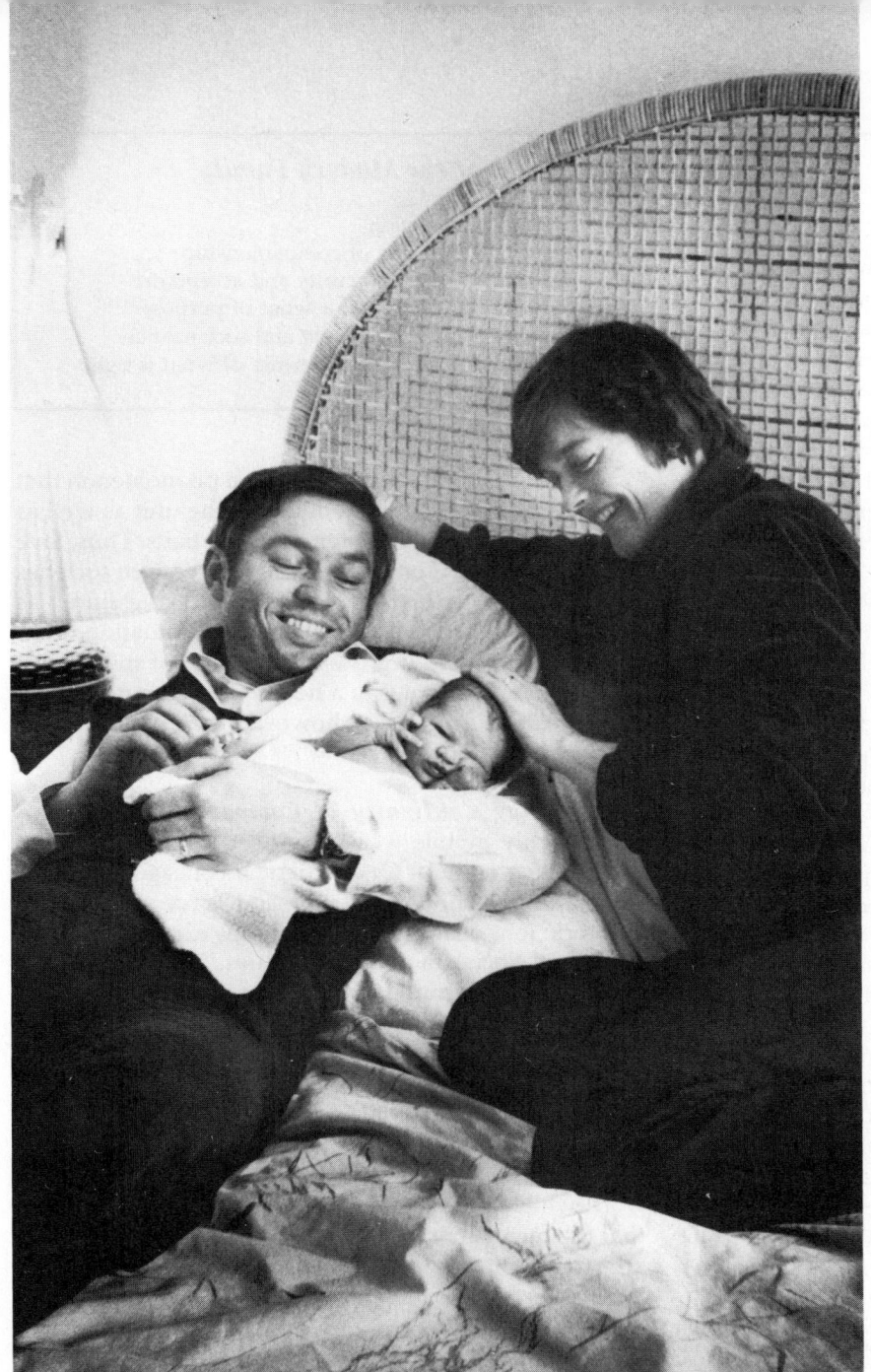

What is the Family?

Functions of the Modern Family

**Theoretical Approaches
to the Study of the Family**
Conceptual Frameworks in Family
Study and Practice
Symbolic Interaction Approach
Family Interaction and Stress

**Relationship of Family Theory
to Nursing Practice**
Family-Centered Care

**Roles, Role Theory, and
Implications for Nursing Practice**
Role and Status
Role vs Interaction
Complementary Roles
Socialization of Roles
and Role Models
Emotional Basis of Role Learning
Tension in Role Relations
Use of Social Power in the Family
Decision Making as an Indicator
of Power
Adjustment to the Role

Family Roles and the Nurse
Role of Mother
Attachment
Anxieties and Conflicts
in Motherhood
Role of Father
Attachment
Anxieties and Conflicts
in Fatherhood
Creative Fatherhood
Role of Child
Socialization of the Child
Role Induction Procedures
Role Modification
Role of Nurse
Aspects of the Nurse's Role

CHAPTER 4

The Family and Nursing Practice

What is the Family?

Most people know intuitively what they mean by "the family." They have known families throughout their lifetime, and intuitive definitions are sufficient for everyday conversation and action. However, when we begin to define what constitutes a family, or analyze the unit as a social institution, or attempt to deliver comprehensive care to its members, it becomes apparent that what we have considered as the family is inappropriate for systematic treatment. The characteristics of the families of our own personal experience often do not fit "families" of other segments of society or other cultures.

The family has been defined in a variety of ways. The US Census Bureau's definition, for instance, is simple and straightforward. According to this definition, a family is a group of two or more persons who are related by blood, marriage, or adoption and are residing together.[1] The concept of residing together is important for purposes of census enumeration, but, in fact, there are times and situations in which members do not share the same household. Other authors have defined the family as a system of roles or as a unit of interacting personalities who may not necessarily be sanctioned by law, but have some commitment to each other.[2,3] Generally, we can define the family as a group of kin united by blood, marriage, or adoption who share a common residence for some part of their lives, assume reciprocal rights and obligations with regard to one another, and are the principal source of socialization of its members.[4]

Common to all these definitions is the fact that the members relate to each other in some way, that is, they interact with specified patterns of behavior and in so doing differentiate and structure roles for themselves, thus providing valuable functions for the unit as well as society as a whole.

Functions of the Modern Family

It has been said that the modern family has been deprived of or has "lost" many of its former functions. Protective services are now provided by law enforcement, the fire department, child protective services, and the like. Education and religious training are now entrusted to schools and churches. Even the production, preservation, and preparation of food have become largely the domain of industry. Duvall and Miller state that there are still at least six basic functions left to the family and they are crucial for producing competent persons who must survive in a complex, ever-changing world:[5]

Functions of the Modern Family
• Generating affection
• Ensuring continuity of companionship
• Providing personal security and acceptance
• Giving satisfaction and a sense of purpose
• Providing social placement and socialization
• Inculcating controls and a sense of what is right

Generating Affection. This is a phenomenon that must go on between all members of the unit as well as among members of the different generations. Thus, love becomes a product of family living. In Western societies couples generally marry for love and have children as an expression of that love. In the ideal situation, both parents and children grow in a climate of mutual affection that contributes to a healthy development of all concerned. In actual fact, however, we know that the ideal is often not achieved.

Ensuring Continuity of Companionship. In today's highly mobile world, in most cases only family associations endure. One's friends, colleagues, neighbors, and acquaintances enter and leave one's social network; jobs change, neighborhoods expand and contract, and social mobility continues. The family unit provides a continuing presence of sympathetic companions who encourage family members to share both disappointments and successes.

Providing Personal Security and Acceptance. Most persons look to their family for the security and acceptance they need to make their lives dignified and worthwhile. It is within the family's protective security that the members can make mistakes, learn from them, and form complementary rather than competitive relationships. These relationships allow the members to develop naturally and at their own pace.

Giving Satisfaction and a Sense of Purpose. The family, at its best, can give its members a basic sense of satisfaction and worth that the other arenas in a person's life often do not fulfill. Family rituals, celebrations, gatherings, and the like serve to act as cohesive factors to dilute the frustrations and problems found in the larger society.

Providing Social Placement and Socialization. Every society demands that individuals learn what is expected of them and where they fit in the larger social hierarchy. At birth, the child automatically acquires a rich heritage by virtue of his family's attributes and position in society. These include such things as genetic, physical, national, ethnic, cultural, economic, political, religious, and educational attributes. Some of these the individual will change over time; some remain immutable. The family also acts as the transmitter of their personal as well as societal values, goals, and sentiments to the child. Thus, the child becomes socialized to the expectations of both the family and society.

Inculcating Controls and a Sense of What Is Right. Within the family unit, the child first learns the rules, obligations, responsibilities, rights, and privileges of the larger society to which he belongs. In the socialization process, family members criticize, correct, order, praise, blame, coerce, entice, reward, and punish in ways that would be unthinkable elsewhere. In this way, the family becomes the agent of the larger society, and its failure to perform its socialization tasks adequately means that the goals of the larger society may not be attained. No wonder those who are concerned with the "breakdown" of the family also are concerned with the loss of family functions.

The kinds of rewards and punishments that the child experiences influence his sense of right and wrong, and these carry into adulthood as moral values. Thus, the family becomes the primary source of transmitting human values that radiate into the society as a whole.[5]

Theoretical Approaches to the Study of the Family

In attempting to systematically study and delineate patterns of interaction in the family, scholars of the family, primarily sociologists, have developed several interpretive approaches to variations in family life, each one generating unique understanding about family organization while at the same time emphasizing a different aspect. These variations in emphasis result in slightly modified definitions of the family in each approach.

In 1960 Hill and Hanson wrote a seminal article describing the five major conceptual frameworks then extant for family study.[6] These included (1) symbolic interaction, (2) structural-functional, (3) situational, (4) institutional, and (5) developmental. Later literature surveys in the late 1960s and early 1970s found that the symbolic interaction, structural-functional, and developmental were those that were being used by the majority of family scholars.[7,8] In addition, Broderick found that the symbolic interaction framework had been used most frequently to produce research findings, while the structural-functional approach resulted in the generation of more theory papers.[9] In recent analyses of the use of frameworks in the field, symbolic interaction, structural-functional, systems and exchange theories

appear most highly used, although the developmental continues to attract the attention of some scholars.[10–14] These frameworks are summarized below to help the student understand the relationship between these important frameworks and her practice.[5,6,10,15]

Conceptual Frameworks in Family Study and Practice

The *symbolic interaction approach* views the family as a unit of interacting personalities. Each person has a position in the family in which he perceives the norms or role expectations held by the other individuals (or by the family as a whole) as the basis for his attitudes and behavior. The individual will define his role expectations primarily in light of their source and his own self-conception. The family is studied through analyzing the interactions and communication patterns of the role-playing members. The primary focus is on the internal structure of the family; this framework, however, neglects the family's relation to the community. The central theme is that actions, behaviors, and objects have a symbolic meaning and acquire shared meaning over time as a result of interaction between individuals, hence, socialization is a key concept, since it is the mechanism of transmitting values, goals, sentiments, and meaning to the family members.

The *structural-functional approach* views the family as a social system and one of the components of the complete social system, that is, society. Members have specific roles geared to maintaining internal and societal stability. In this formulation, traditional sex roles are conceptualized as universal and timeless and are not seen as dynamic, as in the interactional framework. This approach is useful in analyzing the relationship of the family to other societal institutions and the contribution of the family to society as a whole. It does not deal with change over time, and the emphasis has been on the statics of structure.

Systems approaches are used across various disciplines, including the natural and social sciences and engineering. The family is viewed as an open system comprised of interdependent subsystems that work toward common goals. Systems theory emphasizes sets of objects, their relationships, and their boundaries; the system as a whole experiences inputs and outputs from its own subsystems and from society as a whole and responds to feedback with control mechanisms. Family assessment depends on analysis of the interdependent parts, communication patterns, and the family's adaptation patterns.

The *exchange* approach has only recently been employed in family studies, but it is gaining in popularity. This perspective holds that all human interactions, including those in the family, can be viewed as social "exchanges." Individuals weigh rewards and costs in their interactions, and if the exchange is perceived as unequal, one person will be at a disadvantage and the other will control the relationship. The goal is to minimize costs and maximize rewards. Important concepts in this approach are rewards, costs, profits, and a normative context of reciprocity and equity. The ability to choose is also central to this formulation. While some authors say that this approach has relevance at both institutional and individual levels, to date, family assessment has been at the interpersonal level of analysis.

The *developmental* approach focuses on the family as it evolves over time. It holds that families have a predictable life cycle with changing developmental tasks and role expectations associated with each phase of the life cycle. Family assessment is based on analysis of task fulfillment at each stage, with consideration given to physical and emotional maturation, the development of personality and values, and the impact of social and cultural factors. It is an eclectic approach in that it borrows concepts from many disciplines. For instance, from sociology come the concepts of social class, social change, cultural influences, and the generational sweep of the life cycle; from psychology come learning theory concepts and interaction processes; and, finally, from home economics are taken the themes of home management, housing, and family practices.

Any of these frameworks can be used depending upon the problem under study. It is important to remember that these frameworks are helpful tools and are not to be considered "right" or "wrong." In choosing a framework, an individual must consider the assumptions he makes about human behavior, how he views people in relation to the environment, and the problem that he is trying to solve. Only one framework should be used for any one problem under study, since assumptions underlying the framework tend to become confused and conclusions then become spurious.

Symbolic Interaction Approach

One of the most useful of the above frameworks for those who must deal with the family as a unit is the interactional framework. This conceptual scheme provides a system for viewing the personal relationships between the man and woman and parents and children, as well as for viewing the impact of various health conditions on the family unit. The family is conceived of as a unit of interacting personalities and, as such, is a living, changing, growing thing. This conceptualization does not view the family in a legalistic way or in family contract sense, but rather as it exists by virtue of the interaction of its members. Thus, a single parent with a child is a family unit and a household with several monogamous couples with children can be a family unit, as is an unmarried couple with or without children.

Within the family, each member occupies a position or positions to which a number of roles are assigned or allocated. Through socialization and role differentiation (structuring a role) the individual perceives certain norms (rules) or role expectations that the other members of his family have set for his behavior in his role performance. The response of the others in the family reinforces or challenges this conception that he is developing. Thus, a person defines his role expectations in a given situation in terms of a reference group (others who are important to him) and also by means of his own self-concept.

Implicit in this formulation is the fact that human beings interpret or define one another's actions instead of merely reacting to them. For instance, a woman's response to her mate is not made merely on the basis of his actions; it also depends upon the meaning that both partners attach to such actions. Thus, the family members act and react by using symbols, and the key concept involved in the use of symbols is *communication*.

Interpersonal relations among family members based on communication is one of the major distinguishing aspects of the interactional approach. The emphasis in this framework is on the development of competence in interpersonal relations, and as such it describes a *process* rather than a *state*.[16]

Family Interaction and Stress

Several problems for investigation have grown out of these concerns and emphases on family unity, communication, and interpersonal competence. The one that is particularly important for health practitioners is that of the study of discontinuities in family life, particularly family crises or stress. This includes the impact of the reproductive process and parenthood on the family, stress created by acute or chronic illness of the various family members at any time during the life cycle, and the crisis brought about by death of a family member, particularly during the reproductive years.

Using this approach to the family, a practitioner can get inside the family group and analyze its coping as far as it involves interaction among members. Each family member, therefore, can be viewed as a developing member in a changing group. This approach can be particularly useful to the helping professions not only because it provides a practical way of inspecting the family, but also because it allows the professional to isolate and specify the potential sources of difficulty as family members relate to one another and to their society.[2]

Relationship of Family Theory to Nursing Practice

The structure and functioning of the family determines their use of health services. Hence, all members of the health team need to be aware of a variety of theories regarding human behavior and how families develop their various patterns of behavior. This awareness necessitates using knowledge from other specific disciplines when it is appropriate.

Family-Centered Care

The concept of family-centered care and its logical extension, family nursing, has always been a part of nursing. Some areas of practice, notably that of community health, have traditionally claimed more interest, expertise, and responsibility for total family care than others. Delivering care in the client's home has allowed the nurse more insights into the family and its workings and the implications its structure and function have for the health of its members. Moreover, it has allowed the nurse to assess the problems and progress of the family members as a whole.

However, other nursing specialists, notably those in maternal–child health, have also demonstrated interest in family care, focusing initially on the mother–child dyad and later on parenting. In addition, midwifery has used a family-centered approach to home delivery services by using family resources to prepare for care of the mother–infant couple in the home setting.[17] Parents' classes under the auspices of the Maternity Center Association and the Child Study Association in conjunction with the former Children's Bureau have also promoted the development of nursing care of the total family. The philosophy behind this approach has been to meet expressed needs and concerns of parents through the nurse's group leadership role, not necessarily through a course of preplanned instruction. Thus, as nursing has evolved to keep pace with today's health needs, it has become apparent that concepts from other disciplines are badly needed to supply a total picture of the family unit for which high-quality care is to be provided.

These multidisciplinary contributions have stimulated many teachers and students of nursing to seek advanced preparation and to conduct research about families that have implications for their practice. Perhaps most significant, nursing is now joining with other related disciplines whose basic interests and expertise in the family may someday ensure team approaches to research in clinical matters, multidisciplinary educational programs, and, most important, team effort in family care.[17] Society's demands, needs, and aspirations are causing rapid changes in all health fields, including nursing practice and educational programs. Tired of fragmentation in service, high costs, barriers to the entry into health services, and the inertia and unresponsiveness of the health-care system in general, consumers are taking action in what amounts to a social movement.[17,18]

As a result, health professionals find themselves in the center of a revolution in the health-care system.

Roles, Role Theory, and Implications for Nursing Practice

As background for understanding the family, we must deal with another concept that permeates both lay and professional language today. That concept is role, and it is an integral part of the structure and function of the family.

As with the concept of family, we have an intuitive sense of what a "role" is, but when attempts are made to systematically study the construct, we find a broad latitude in definitions and understandings of it. Psychological and sociological approaches to role are closely interrelated because an individual's personality develops within a social system, which in our culture is the family. Hence, roles may be viewed from a psychosocial viewpoint, which enables us to focus on the individual and how he integrates his role relationships, and also from a sociological viewpoint, which guides us in focusing on group or social relationships, primarily those within the family. We must also deal with culture, for the "self" can be viewed as the unit of personality, a person's "status" or position in a unit of society, or a role enacted in the culture.

Role and Status

Basic to any discussion of role are the definitions of role and status. *Status*, or position, generally refers to a person's location in a system of interaction. On the other hand, *role* applies to behavior that reflects the goals, values, and sentiments operating in a given situation. A further clarification of these definitions can be made by contrasting role as defined by two major theorists, Ralph Linton and George Herbert Mead. According to Linton, roles tend to be defined as constellations of rules or expectations for behavior associated with a given status or position.[19] In the Meadian, or interactionist, tradition, however, roles are defined, created, stabilized, or modified as a consequence of interaction between the self and others.[20]

Role vs Interaction

From an interactionist frame of reference, role is more than a series of dos and don'ts for the behavior expected of a person occupying a given position. Rather, it is a constellation of behaviors that emerges from interaction between the self and others that constitutes a meaningful unit and is an expression of the values, goals, or sentiments that provide direction for that interaction. It is true that these constellations of behaviors become patterned over time and that the actors proceed as if there were prescriptions for performance.

However, there is much more latitude in the Meadian or symbolic interaction conception of role because it allows for innovative, individualistic designing of a person's role performance on the basis of assignment of some sentiment or goal to the behavior of relevant others.

This conception of role is particularly salient for nursing practice as it allows for a broader interpretation of the behavior of all actors than do more traditional concepts. Moreover, it does not limit either the interpretation of the behavior or the nurse's response to the behavior to a prescribed set of dos and don'ts. Hence, it permits creativity and innovation in interaction with clients.

Complementary Roles

Another basic concept in role theory is that of the *complementarity* of roles, or the fact that all roles are learned in pairs. Thus, a role does not exist in isolation but is patterned to mesh with that of a role partner. For instance, the nurse's role meshes with the client's role, the husband's with the wife's, the child's with the parent's, and so on. Some of these roles that are basic in society, such as husband, wife, child, and so on, have become more patterned in the various cultures than others, and, thus, firmer expectations have come about. But we need only look at the innovative variation in recent family life-styles to appreciate how traditional role prescriptions and expectations can, and often must, be modified.

Whether there be firm or loose expectations, this pairing or complementarity of roles provides for reciprocal arrangements in interaction and therefore allows social interaction to proceed in an orderly fashion, since there emerges a predictability in interaction. The actors "know" what they are to do. Without this complementarity, it would be difficult to maintain stable interaction networks such as exist in the family system. Indeed, the family's equilibrium depends on this role pairing.

Socialization of Roles and Role Models

Roles are learned through the process of socialization. In socialization, individuals learn the ways of social groups so that they can function within these groups. Socialization takes place through both intentional and incidental instruction, that is, by providing specific instruction regarding a certain facet of behavior and by providing examples of desired behavior, in other words, role modeling. All of the various socialization agencies—the family in the beginning and later the church and schools—teach the child certain role behaviors through intentional programs of learning and study. Operating conjointly may be incidental learning in which the child adopts the ways of others in his environment through playacting, peer-group relations, and observations of adult and peer role models.

Thus, the significant others in the child's world teach him, both by defining the world for him and by serving as models for his attitudes and behavior. The child learns through a system of rewards and punishment, and if he behaves as the significant others desire, he receives positive attention and invitations to continue his participation and interaction. If, on the other hand, he behaves otherwise, he is refused attention, reprimanded, or physically punished.

It is important to remember that much of the role learning that takes place in the family is indirect. The child learns by observing and participating in the interpersonal relations patterns established by the family, the examples set by the other family members, and the role that he develops for himself within the family. Hence, he learns and adopts basic role skills from family members and concurrently adapts to the roles of the other family members.

Emotional Basis of Role Learning

Another important aspect of role learning is that it is not merely a cognitive process. It is associated with multiple emotional or affective ties that the individual makes with others. These attachments begin with the mother and gradually include increasing numbers of persons with whom the child interacts and comes to identify. As these attachments grow, the child develops a sense of self, in that he can take a position from the outside and view his own thoughts, feelings, and actions. In this way, he gradually internalizes the behavior that is expected of him as he figuratively stands back and looks at himself and guides, judges, and reflects on his own behavior according to his perceptions of others' expectations for his behavior.

It has been noted that, while individuals learn role behavior in much the same way, there are differences in respective role performances. This differential role performance may be due to differences in the ways persons respond in interpersonal situations, their knowledge of the role in general, their motivation to perform specific roles, their attitude toward themselves and, finally, their response to the behavior of other persons in the interaction.

Tension in Role Relations

Tension and discontinuities in role relations must also be considered when considering the concept of role. Many terms have been used to illustrate the idea of tension or interruptions in a smooth process of interaction. Terms such as role conflict, role strain, role change, and role transition have been used to convey the various aspects of tension that can occur in a role system.

We have made the point that role interaction is dynamic. As theories of the development of human nature change, so do socialization patterns. As these latter change, variant family life systems evolve, which in turn redefine reciprocal role relationships. Tensions and disruptions in smooth and rewarding role interaction may occur at any point.

Use of Social Power in the Family

As roles become differentiated (structured) and allocated (who gets what role), the element of social power comes into play. Various authors have defined this concept as the ability to influence a decision, to influence the emotions and behavior of others, or to achieve intended outcomes or goals.[15] It is a dynamic concept, and decision making is one indicator of power in the family. Moreover, several bases of power have been delineated:[21]

Legitimate power refers to the shared belief that one person in the family system has the right to make decisions for others in the system. The basis for such power is traditional. Thus, parents exert legitimate power over their children in much the way that elected officials enact laws for the society. In some families it is the father's traditional prerogative to make most of the decisions. Research indicates, however, that in families in which the woman works or in which role relationships are egalitarian, legitimate power is a more shared phenomenon.

Expert power is based on the perception that a family member or group has particular knowledge or skills. Thus, if the wife is a health provider, she may exert a good deal of power regarding health-related matters. Similarly, nurses are often seen by their clients as having requisite knowledge to effect a change in behavior.

Referent power refers to the influence of one person over another. This occurs through positive identification with the more powerful person, and there is the adoption of the behaviors, values, and attitudes of the powerful person. Role modeling is an example of this kind of power.

Reward power carries with it the expectation that the person has the resources to reward others. Parents certainly are invested with this type of power. The hierarchical structure of nursing also carries this power.

Coercive power is concerned with the expectation that punishment will occur if certain things are done or are not done, certain behavior is exhibited or is not exhibited, or certain expectations are met or are not met. Abuse among family members is an example of the use of this kind of power. In a less dramatic vein, a nurse must deny a child access to school if the parents have not had the child immunized.

Informational power is used to convey a message to convince the recipient of the message that change is necessary. The media is an example in this regard, although families use this when providing instruction to the members. In the family situation, this type of power is often used with expert power.[15]

Families do not use only one type of power. Indeed, each may be used at different times and several may be used simultaneously during the course of everyday family interaction. Some families do depend on one type predominantly, however.

Decision Making as an Indicator of Power

The decision-making process is a key indicator of power and dominance in the family.[15,22] To function in day-to-day living, family members must make a myriad of decisions. There are several areas that can be assessed:

- Who usually instigates a decision-making process?
- Who decides who will be involved in the decision?
- Who actually is involved and how did this come about?
- What processes are used in making decisions? For instance, are control, negotiation, persuasion, or authoritativeness modes employed and how frequently?
- Who seems to exert the most power during decision making?
- Who makes the final decision?
- How is it implemented?
- What is the significance of the decision for the family, and what are the effects on family interaction?

These are important questions, since decision making reflects how the family meets the needs of its members, which in turn has implications for family cohesion.

Adjustment to the Role

The major determinants of the degree of adjustment a person makes to a role can be summarized as follows: (1) the clarity with which a specific role and its complementarity is defined and demonstrated; (2) the clarity or definiteness of the transitional procedures in the acquisition of a new role; (3) how well the role is learned and enacted—this is partly dependent on 1 and 2 and the strength of the socialization process to the new role; (4) the consistency of the responses a role evokes; (5) a role's compatibility with the other roles in the person's set of roles; (6) a role's congruity with the emotional needs of the person; (7) the degree of complementarity that exists between reciprocal roles; and (8) the bases and use of social power in the family.

When there is a high degree of adjustment, the enactment of a person's set of roles can be rewarding in that they define for him his niche, his self-concept anchorage, a sense of belongingness and purpose. They give him social recognition and support, which in turn allow him to buy or earn desired conditions or things in the world and to view himself as a worthwhile, contributing member of society.[23]

Family Roles and the Nurse

Concepts from role theory encompass a body of knowledge that is vital for the nurse who works with families or individual family members. The application of these concepts can greatly increase the nurse's understanding of the role strains and changes inherent in the phenomenon of family stress that can be precipitated by childbearing, chronic or acute illness in the family, or death of any of the family members.

For example, consider the change in the interaction patterns that must be accomplished when a new infant is incorporated into the household—restructuring of all of the members' roles is necessitated, and this is doubly complicated when there are other children present. Sibling rivalry is only one aspect of the impact of a new infant on the family.

Also, consider the situational stress when parents bear a mentally retarded or otherwise defective child. Following the grief reaction and concomitant frustration, conflict, and high anxiety, the family equilibrium can be regained only when parents restructure their roles to either encompass or reject the afflicted member and learn to cope with the situation.

Finally, consider acute catastrophic illness in the father of a family with several children. When such an illness occurs, the man is thrust into the role of patient, which is, in essence, a dependent role. This necessitates a reorganization of the role behaviors of the other family members. The wife must become more dominant and the children generally must assume more responsibility; hence, their positions change vis-à-vis other family members. These few examples point out the necessity for the nurse to consider family role relations if she is to intervene in a holistic way.

Role of Mother

Each society provides many cues and signals that tell persons how it defines a role and identifies appropriate behavior for the role. These cues may be overt or covert and may be perceived in a subliminal way. In our culture, the ideal mother has been traditionally the nurturer, the one who gives sustenance and unconditional love (Fig. 4-1).

A woman's concept of the mother role is based on the norms of the culture, the social class and ethnic group to which she belongs, and the type of socialization she has received from her immediate family.

Attachment

There is a difference between the role of mother and feelings of attachment. In a sense, both are learned, but mothering, the enactment of the role of mother, involves skills and a certain understanding of the developmental process of the child. Thus, *attachment* can be thought of as an emotional feeling that develops over time as the mother has increasing contact with her infant. It is a feeling that the child is emotionally hers, and there is a need to identify the infant with the rewarding values and qualities that she considers part of herself and her life.

This development of attachment begins with the maternal claiming process and is evident in the initial and early mother–newborn contact when the mother touches (at first timidly) and later enfolds her infant and exclaims, "Oh, he is finally here! How did I ever produce that?"

Our hospital procedures often militate against this early claiming behavior, but fortunately we are now beginning to relax many of the restrictions that tend to disrupt the reality testing of this ownership process.

Anxieties and Conflicts in Motherhood

All mothers need reassurance that they are, indeed, mothers and adequate if not excellent ones. The disappointment the mother feels when the infant sleeps at the breast instead of nursing is very familiar to everyone. Mothers excoriate themselves with criticism when they are awkward in handling their firstborn. They try desperately to "pull themselves together," to assume care of the infant only hours after delivery. Al-

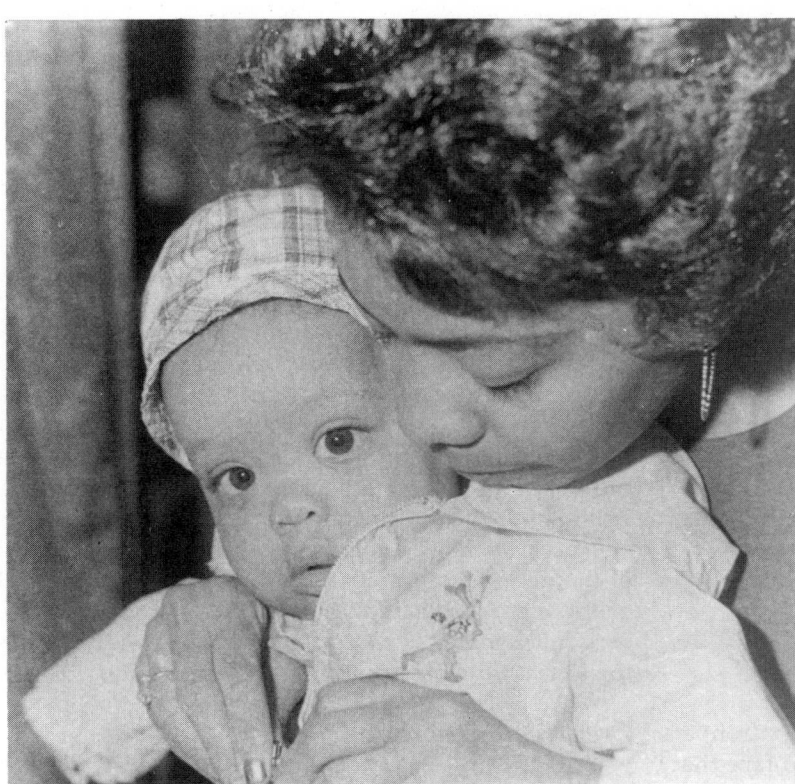

FIGURE 4-1

In our culture, the ideal mother has traditionally been the nurturer.

though seemingly small and unimportant, these initial anxieties are the basis of the future relationship between mother and child. Moreover, they are complicated by the many conflicts in modern society, where the role of mother has come into increasing competition with other social roles a woman may enact. Paramount among these conflicts are fantasies of idealized motherhood versus feelings of inadequacy in actual role performance; the need for dependency versus the adult goal of independence and responsibility; love versus resentment for the baby owing to fatigue and increased responsibility for such a dependent being; feelings for the baby versus feelings for the husband; and self-actualization versus the demands of motherhood.[23]

If the mother has had problematic relations with her own mother during the early socialization years, these may affect her role enactment. She may project many of these negative feelings onto her own child or, conversely, bend over backwards to avoid socialization techniques her mother used, thereby limiting or missing important features that she might have kept and used. Also, if the normal and increasing dependency needs of pregnancy and the early postpartum period are not met, she may not be able to easily care for and give love to her dependent child.

One final point deserves mention. For many, children of one age are more appealing than those of another. A mother may be able to respond to the needs of a dependent infant but not adapt readily to the 4-year-old's search for and insistence on autonomy.

Thus, the role of mother and its enactment is shaped by many interacting factors and therefore will have a wide range of behavioral manifestations.

Role of Father

Research on the dynamics of the father role and the development of attachment has received much less attention than that of motherhood. Recently, there has been impetus in research, but it will be some time before there is solid empirical evidence regarding this topic.

Attachment

As with the mother role and attachment, there is a difference between the father role or fatherhood and feelings of attachment. The role of father is learned, as is the role of mother, but feeling tones are not initiated physiologically as with the mother. This may be a very important difference. Moreover, the admission and enactment of a father's attachment in our culture is still wrought with conflicts stirred up by discontinuities in cultural conditioning. This is gradually changing with the more modern attitudes toward relaxed sex-role structuring. By and large, the image of the virile male is still not compatible with the demonstration of tender feelings that have usually been attributed to the female domain.

Traditionally, the father in our society was supposed to be a leader, a hero, a disciplinarian, a mentor, an authority figure, and the family bulwark against the outside, reality-oriented world. Yet attachment must involve feelings of tenderness and gentleness, empathic capacity, the ability to respond emotionally, the valuing of a love object more than the self, and, finally, the finding of a gratifying living experience in the experiences of others (Fig. 4-2). Obviously, these feelings are quite different from the simple pride of a man in his child as a symbol of his virility, or his feelings that the child represents a challenge to his own adequacy.[24]

It would seem that the coordination of the mother's and father's feelings of attachment in those who choose to be parents is essential to the mature, creative psychosexual development of both parents and eventually their children's development.

Anxieties and Conflicts in Fatherhood

It may be that the same basic problems that confront a woman in delineating her role as mother also face the man in defining his role as father. Interviews with young fathers indicate that they are immersed in many instrumental problems, such as rearranging work or study schedules, finding or preparing adequate housing, or taking on extra jobs to ease the finances. They also have basic questions and fears about their preparation for the parenting role, as well as changes in their wives during pregnancy and the postpartum periods. In some, the prospect of fatherhood also rekindles thoughts of the less happy aspects of their childhood and their relations with their parents. Their fears and concerns about their rest, quiet, and privacy, sexual relationships, and their wives' increasing demands for attention all become realities with the advent of childbirth.

We can speculate that these developments and problems may be due, at least partly, to our current lack of systematic obstetric care of the father. It is true that we invite him to childbirth classes (and this has been a big step) and that we are allowing him greater participation in the actual birthing process. However, there is still no systematic attempt (or even acknowledgment of the necessity) to prepare him for his father role. All of these problems are the common components of severe role conflict, and how they are resolved becomes the key to ultimate appropriate role transition.[23]

Creative Fatherhood

Several functions have been delineated that a father can creatively undertake to enrich and maintain a healthy family life.[25] First, a father can be a true com-

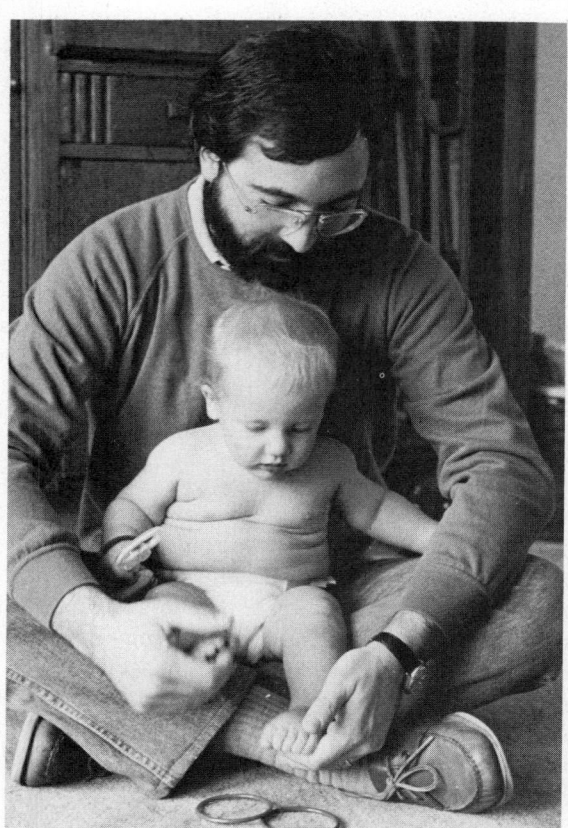

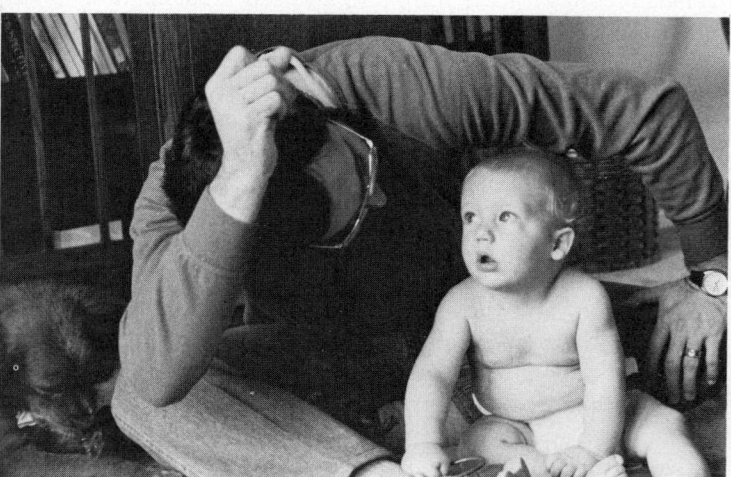

FIGURE 4-2

Although the father has traditionally been viewed as an authority figure and breadwinner, attachment to his infant must also involve feelings of tenderness and gentleness and a gratifying personal involvement with his children.

panion, help-mate, and inspiration for the mother. Second, he can be an awakener of emotional potential for his child, as well as a beloved friend and teacher. Third, he can present a role model for masculine love, ethics, and morality. Fourth, he can be a stabilizing influence as the child proceeds through his maturational stages. Fifth, he can be a model and mentor for social and occupational behavior. Sixth, he can provide a model as mentor and protector for children in general. Finally, he can be a counselor for and friend of the adolescent. While each of these activities will be modified to meet the needs of a rapidly changing society, it is apparent that they provide more of a basis for sound family interaction than does the traditional role of father as sire, disciplinarian, and breadwinner.

Role of Child

Of all the family roles, the child's role is perhaps the most dynamic because it is constantly evolving through techniques of socialization. These techniques are essentially future oriented, since they focus on and emphasize what the child is to become rather than what he or she is. Helping the child learn appropriate social roles requires that the parents be emotionally healthy and stable enough to keep the anxiety level at a point that will allow the child's self-esteem to be in relative equilibrium with the environmental demands that are made. This does not mean that there will be no demand or no anxiety; without these, no learning takes place. However, they must not be excessive or incompatible with reality.

Socialization of the Child

There are many techniques of socialization, and the evidence indicates that no one technique is better than another. Rather, each set of parents must choose and modify what is best for them, and this will depend on the many factors that we have previously alluded to. Spiegel has attempted to delineate the various steps in the maintenance of role complementarity so that the family can balance the demands society's expectations place on it, the family's attitudes, and the child's needs and eventually arrive at a progressively healthier family role equilibrium. He conceives of these steps along the torturous route of socialization as comprising two major groups of five steps, each linked by a sixth, or middle, step (Fig. 4-3).[26]

Role Induction Procedures

The first group consists of *role induction procedures* by which compliance of the child is elicited. These are primarily manipulative and ensure that the child gradually realizes that he must learn and that his parents are the chief source of learning.

The first and second steps are *coercion* and *coaxing*, in which punishment and rewards are used, respectively, to focus the child's attention on the fact that there are rules that must be observed and that the parents are the enactors of these rules.

The third step is *evaluation*, in which a value judgment of good or bad is placed on the behavior and implies or directly gives praise or blame to ensure appropriate behavior.

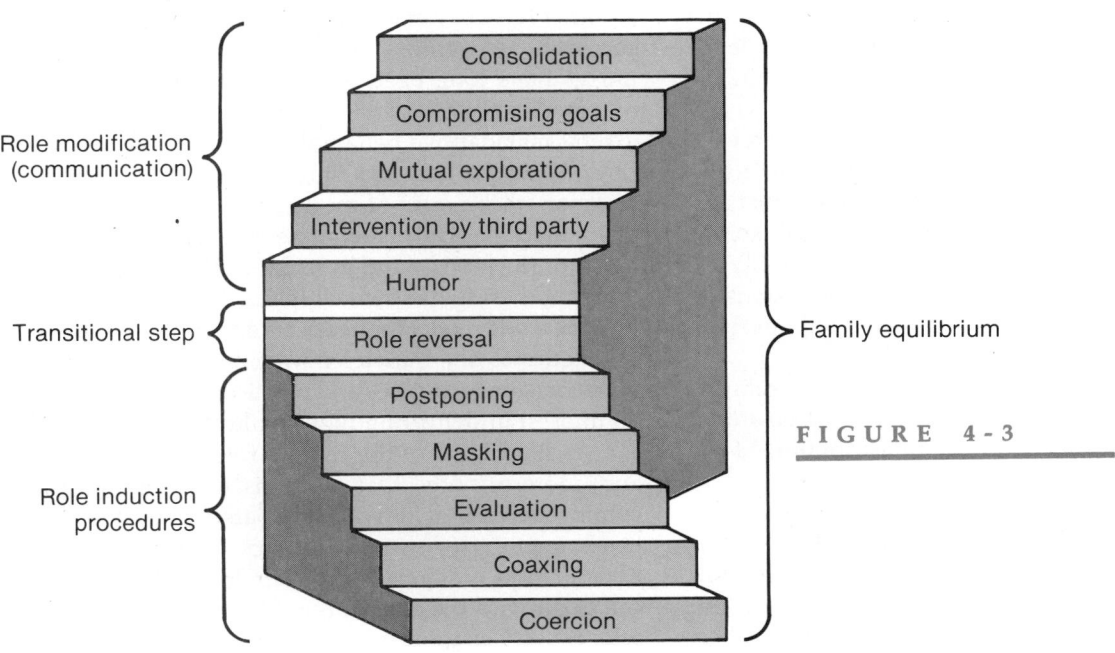

FIGURE 4-3

The fourth step is *masking*, or withholding correct information or giving wrong information for the sake of settling a conflict. This can be pernicious, and a crisis may occur if the child uncovers the truth; trust can be lost and reality is distorted.

Fifth is the technique of *postponing*, which can be useful because it puts off dealing with a conflict until a fresher look can be taken at the situation. Of course, if this maneuver is overused, it will intensify and prolong the difficulty.

The sixth step is the transitional step and has been called *role reversal* or *role taking*, that is, putting oneself in the role or position of the other and looking at the situation from the point of view of another. Some call this empathic ability. It is the first glimmer of adult thinking and requires a rather well-developed understanding of self and reality. The ability to perform this maneuver early and successfully depends on the degree of masking that goes on in the family. The less the extent of masking, the better the success of role taking.[26]

Role Modification

The second group of procedures has been called *role-modification* maneuvers. The basic characteristic here is *communication* and how persons learn to complement each other in role change.

Role modification begins with the seventh step of *joking*, or *humor*, in which persons develop the ability to laugh at themselves and each other (but affectionately). It is felt to be an outgrowth of role taking and the first of several tension-relieving mechanisms that families employ.

The eighth step employs the *intervention of a third party* (not necessarily a professional) who brings to the situation certain skills, a point of view, or knowledge that is not available to the parents or child within the family unit.

Mutual exploration is the ninth step, in which each person probes the capacity of the other to come to a solution regarding a conflict or problem. Here, trust and regard are expressed and invested in all members, including the children (to the extent of their capacity).

The tenth step, *compromising goals*, is an extension of mutual exploration. Here, goals are altered but to no single person's detriment.

Similarly, the last step, *consolidation*, is the refined, integrated effort of learning to compromise successfully. It is associated with adjustment, redistribution of rewards, and role clarification.

Needless to say, the evolution through these various steps does not necessarily proceed smoothly, nor at times are all accomplished, especially steps 8 through 10. However, the more frequently they can be used, the easier each subsequent role adaptation and transition will become.[26]

Role of Nurse

The understanding and application of role theory in nursing practice provides a conceptual base for understanding the populations that we serve and gives some anchorage to our therapeutic method. It increases our capacity to view the forces of personality, family interaction, social systems, the health condition, and nursing intervention as a unit. It provides a needed framework for studying motivations for childbearing, reproductive behavior, childrearing techniques, and cultural goals. In addition, it provides a basis for understanding ourselves and our colleagues who provide health care.

Nursing is an applied science. The broad implications of its scientific nature challenge its practitioners to document this aspect with intellectual experimentation, innovations in practice, and constant research. If we in maternity nursing define the family as the unit to be served, we must have a thorough knowledge of its dynamics, and that includes much more than the physiological and psychological stages the mother passes through during pregnancy, labor, delivery, and the postpartum period. The use of role theory provides a vehicle to tie all of these disparate aspects of childbearing into related units amenable for study and practice.

Aspects of the Nurse's Role

There are multiple facets or aspects of the nurse's role (Fig. 4-4). First, the nurse is a practitioner—she uses the nursing process to assess, prescribe, and implement nursing regimens for her clients and assists the physician in implementing his medical regimen for these clients. Another facet of her role is that of role model or mother surrogate. Maternity nurses and community-health nurses have long been experimenting with providing role models for mothers who are inexperienced or who exhibit maladaptive behavior in childrearing and child care. Again, in high-risk situations of child neglect or rejection, techniques of mothering the mother are implemented. Basically, the nurse meets the dependency needs of the mother and in so doing allows her to move on to mothering her own children. The nurse may also provide a role model for her peers and other professional colleagues as she initiates newcomers into the institutional or agency routines and practices and demonstrates an interest in delivering high-quality care.

Another facet of the nurse's role is that of teacher and, more recently, that of counselor. Nurses are becoming increasingly involved in parent education on all levels in order to socialize groups of parents expeditiously, thus avoiding the role strain and conflicts that can occur with the assumption of new roles. The counselor aspect has come into the fore with family-planning services and abortion and genetic counseling. Similarly,

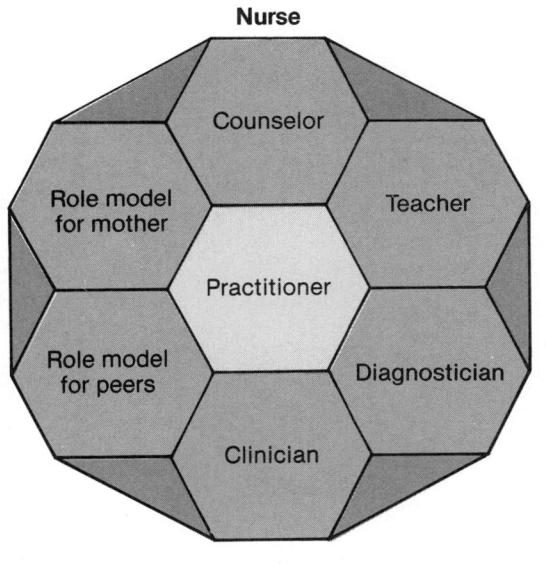

Nurse

Counselor

Role model for mother

Teacher

Practitioner

Role model for peers

Diagnostician

Clinician

FIGURE 4-4

Maternity nursing is a multifaceted role.

this aspect has become apparent in parental counseling with regard to health problems of the schoolchild, management of sibling rivalry, and childhood and maternal nutrition.

Finally, in her "expanded role" the nurse may bring new physical diagnosis-clinician skills to her basic role. She finds in many instances that her work in an ambulatory-care setting provides the bridge between the family in the community and the institution to which they must go from time to time for more severe conditions.

The potential for developing these multiple facets of the nursing role is unlimited and will be fully realized only when nursing recognizes its own unique and independent contribution to health.

When delivering care to individuals and families, nurses must observe and analyze the role behaviors of the persons involved, including their own. Cognizance must be taken of the various dimensions of the roles—the behaviors, values, expectations, and attitudes of the actors, as well as their underlying motivations and emotions. Role conflict and perceptions of inadequacy in role performance have the potential to undermine emotional and physical well-being. On the other hand, satisfactory role performance is a vital self-concept enhancing experience and can promote growth and emotional well-being.

References

1. US Bureau of the Census: Household and family characteristics: March 1980. Current Population Reports Series P20, No 286. Washington, DC, Department of Commerce, 1980

2. Schvaneveldt J: The interactional framework in the study of the family. In Reinhardt A, Quinn M (eds): Family Centered Community Nursing. St Louis, CV Mosby, 1973
3. Turner RH: Family Interaction. New York, John Wiley & Sons, 1966
4. Eshelman JR, Cashion BG: Sociology: An Introduction. Boston, Little, Brown & Co, 1985
5. Duvall EM, Miller BC: Marriage and Family Development. New York, Harper & Row, 1985
6. Hill R, Hanson DA: The identification of conceptual frameworks utilized in family study. Marr Fam Living 22:308–320, 1960
7. Klein JF, Calvert GP, Garland N et al: Pilgrims' progress: Recent developments in family theory. J Marr Fam 31:677–687, 1969
8. Cerny V, Dahl N, Kamiko T et al: International developments in family theory: A continuation of the initial "Pilgrims Progress." J Marr Fam 36:169–173, 1974
9. Broderick CB: Beyond the five conceptual frameworks: A decade of development in family theory. J Marr Fam 33:139–159, 1971
10. Burr WR, Hill R, Nye FI et al (eds): Contemporary Theories About the Family, Vols 1 and 2. New York, Free Press, 1979
11. Holman T, Burr WR: Beyond the beyond: The growth of family theories in the 1970's. J Marr Fam 42:729–741, 1980
12. Klein DM, Schvaneveldt JD, Miller BC: The attitudes and activities of contemporary family theorists. J Contemp Fam Studies 8:5–27, 1977
13. Hill R, Mattissich P: Family development theory and life span development. In Baltes PB, Brim OG (eds): Life Span Development and Behavior, Vol 2. New York, Academic Press, 1979
14. Nock SL: Family life cycle transitions: Longitudinal effects on family members. J Marr Fam 43:703–714, 1981
15. McCann/Flynn JB, Heffron PB: Nursing: From Concept to Practice. Bowie, Maryland, Robert J Brady, 1984
16. Foote N, Cottrell LS: Identity and Interpersonal Competence. Chicago, University of Chicago Press, 1955
17. Ford L: The development of family nursing. In Hymovich RD, Barnard M (eds): Family Health Care. New York, McGraw–Hill, 1973
18. Reeder LG: The patient-client as a consumer: Some observations on the changing professional-client relationship. J Health Soc Behav 13:400–412, 1972
19. Linton R: The Cultural Background of Personality. New York, Appleton–Century, 1945
20. Mead GH: Mind, Self and Society From the Standpoint of a Social Behaviorist. Chicago, University of Chicago Press, 1934
21. Blood RO, Wolfe DM: Husbands and wives. In Bell R (ed): Studies in Marriage and the Family. New York, Thomas & Crowell, 1973
22. Reeder SJ: The Impact of Disabling Health Conditions on Family Interaction. Unpublished doctoral dissertation, Department of Sociology, UCLA, 1974
23. Robischon P, Scott D: Role theory and its application in family nursing. Nurs Outlook 17:52–57, 1969
24. Hines JD: Father—the forgotten man. Nurs Forum 10:177–200, 1971

25. Josselyn I: Cultural forces, motherliness and fatherliness. Am J Orthopsychiatry 26:264–271, 1956
26. Spiegel JP: Resolution of role conflict within the family. Psychiatry 20:1–6, 1957

Suggested Reading

Getty C, Humphreys W: Power relationships in marriage: The fine print in oral tradition. In Understanding the Family: Stress and Change in the American Family. New York, Appleton–Century–Crofts, 1981
Roberts CS, Fleetham SL: Assessing family functioning across three areas of relationships. Nurs Res 31:231–235, July/Aug 1982
Schlesinger B: The ABCs of changing roles of family members. Fam Life Educator 3(4):18–19, Summer 1985

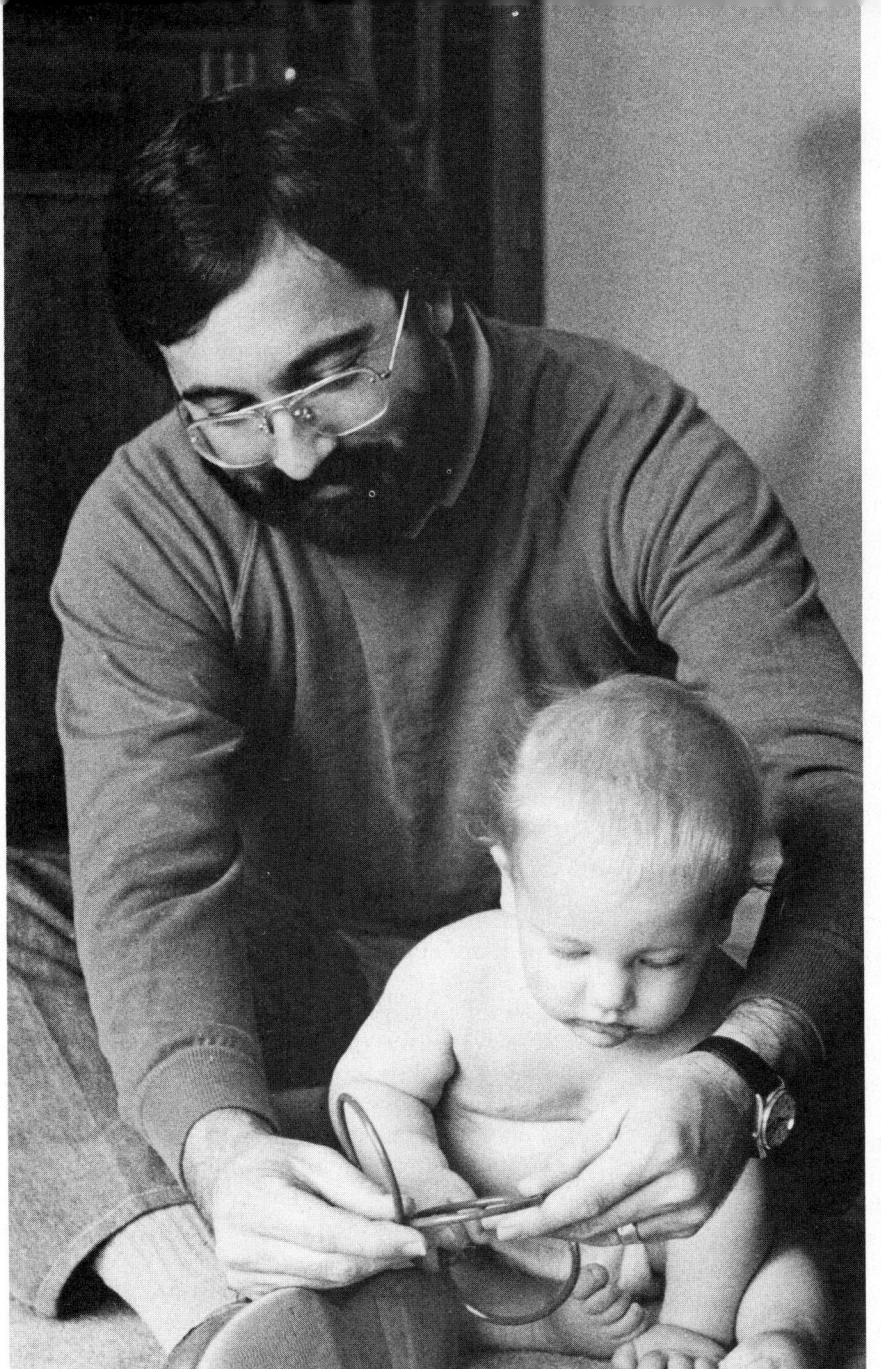

CHAPTER 5

Evolving Family Forms

Over the years there has been a good deal of discussion as to whether American society was a melting pot cooking an amalgam of ethnic and cultural distillates called "American," or a salad bowl with a variety of shapes, hues, and various ethnic, religious, and racial identities. The argument continues, but the salad bowl concept appears to be winning.

It appears that the family is a salad bowl also, and its varieties of character are slowly emerging. The family was thought of as having some "ideal" form, often religiously sanctioned and adhering to an ideal set of values. Thus, forms that vary from the traditional nuclear family of husband, wife, and children living together in their separate residence with the male as breadwinner and female as homemaker were viewed as deviant. Research in the 1950s and 1960s on single-parent families, working mothers, or dual-work families was, for the most part, concerned with the deleterious effects of the absence of spouses or the effect of gainful employment of mothers on the children. The implication was, of course, that the woman should be in the home and if a spouse was alone for any reason, he or she had the obligation to remarry (not just live with someone) as soon as possible.[1]

The Changing American Family

The structure and function of the American family has altered remarkably in the past quarter of a century. Among the most notable of the changes, documented through an analysis of census data, is the near tripling of one-parent and one-person households, together with the more than quadrupling of households comprised of unmarried couples. These shifts are the result of profound demographic and social changes in America.[2] A number of other social indicators suggest that the rapid changes in the roles of both men and women, begun in the 1960s and still continuing, are of primary importance in effecting change in the American family.

The changes in women's roles, particularly, have been caused primarily by three interrelated factors: changes in the economy affecting labor-force participation, changes in the age structure of our society due to the baby boom of the 1950s and the baby bust of the 1960s and 1970s, and, finally, changes in values.[3] The changes in roles and values have been intimately tied to what has been called the "contraceptive revolution" of the 1960s, and the continuing effective use of these products has allowed women to regulate their childbearing to a degree that was never possible before.[2] Now there are more younger women who may delay marriage or opt not to have children at all. More women are working outside the home (and more frequently in the professions) and choose to do so to realize themselves as individuals. There continues to be a restructuring of values and roles within the home toward a more egalitarian or democratic orientation, and the power base has shifted from a strong patriarchal orientation to one of egalitarianism or even to women oriented.[4,5] Pickett's research indicates that a new, "ideal type" of egalitarian family has emerged that he calls "romantic" monogamy. The partners are supposed to be dutiful parents, dual wage earners, fascinating lovers, and, finally, providers of unqualified emotional support for all concerned. Obviously the goals of this type of relationship are incredibly demanding, and a highly flexible divorce system has arisen as if in response. With divorce and remarriage, partners may shift, but the *monogamous ideal* remains.[4]

Some of the more startling changes in the family are highlighted here and in Figure 5-1:

- There have been approximately 30 million new households established since 1960. This constitutes a 58% increase.
- In 1960, 52% of the 53 million US households counted had no children under 18. By 1983, this proportion had grown to 63% of 84 million households. This has been due in part to the baby bust mentioned above and increasing rates of childlessness. Also, more older persons, especially women, are able to maintain their own households.
- More women are expecting to be childless. (In a 1982 survey, 16% of single childless women aged 18 to 24 said they would not have children.)
- Since 1960 the overall rate of married-couple households has increased slowly. In 1983 they accounted for six in ten households. Cohabitation, on the other hand, has skyrocketed, increasing by 331%! This increase has occurred primarily since 1970.
- There has been a swift rise also in the number of one-parent households. For instance, there has been a 175% increase in one-parent households compared with a 26% increase in married families. Again, the increase in one-parent households was most accelerated during the 1970s, when divorce rates greatly increased and the number of out-of-wedlock births also was greatest.[2]

As can be seen from this brief overview, not many persons remain in one type of family structure throughout their lifetime, although many will have some experience in the more traditional nuclear family.

Traditional Family Structures

There are a variety of forms in traditional family structures. The most prominent among these are the following:

The Changing American Family

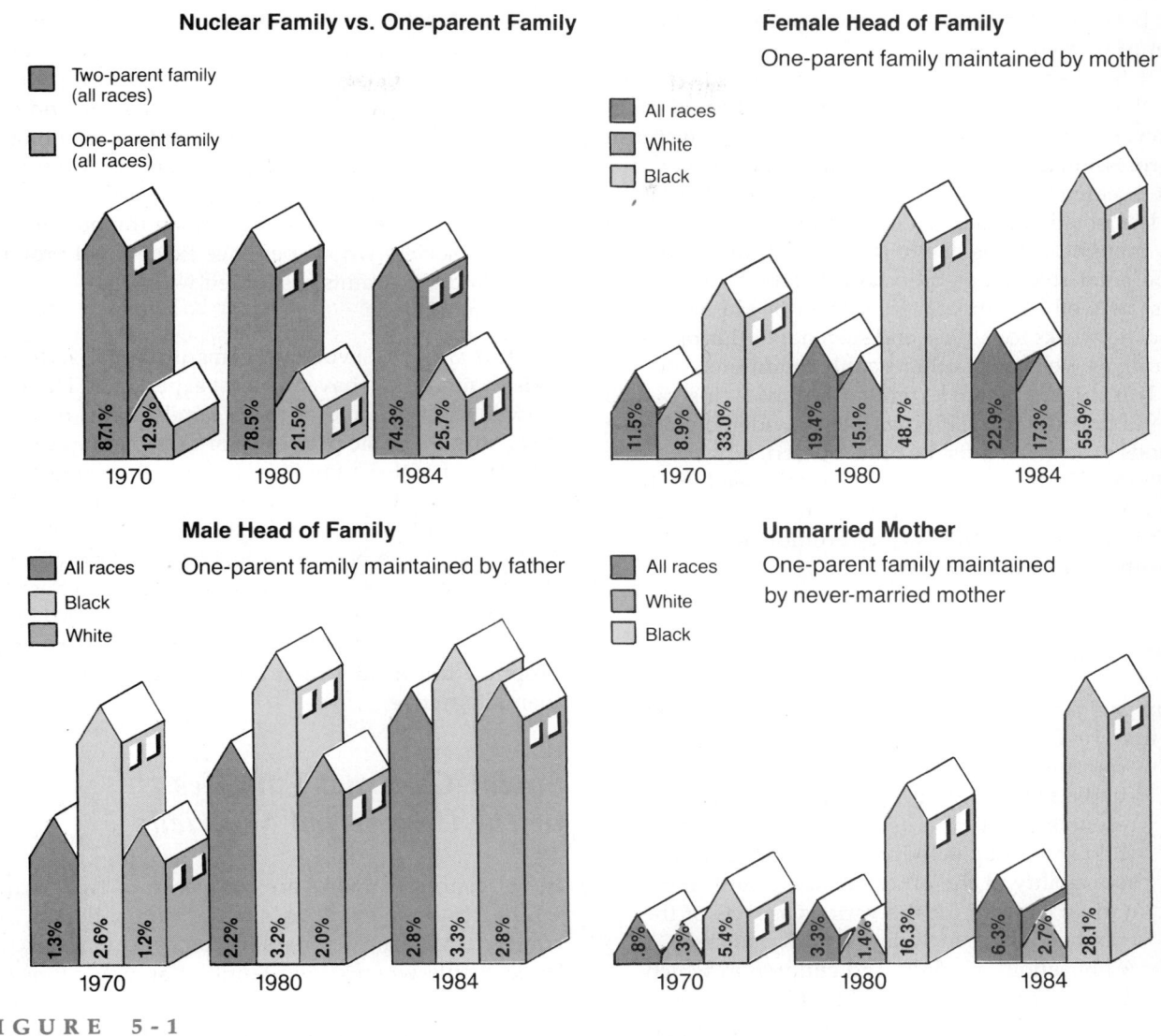

FIGURE 5-1

The changing American family.

- *Nuclear family* (husband, wife, and children live in a common household). A single or a dual career may be pursued, and in the case of the wife, her career may be continuous or interrupted as the children are born.
- *Nuclear dyad* (husband and wife live alone). They may be childless or not have children living at home. Again, there may be a single or dual career or a "second career," in which the wife enters the labor force after the children have left home.
- *Single-parent family* (one head as a consequence of death, divorce, abandonment, or separation). Here there are usually preschool or school-age children. There may or may not be a career;

when financial aid is not forthcoming from the absent spouse, there is usually some form of occupation pursued by the parenting spouse.
- *Single adult living alone*
- *Three-generation family or extended family.* These may be characterized by any variant of forms 1, 2, or 3.
- *Kin network* in which nuclear households or unmarried members live in close geographic proximity and operate within a reciprocal system of exchange of goods and services.[6]

Each of these will have its problems and resources with respect to health needs and utilization of services.

Generally, traditional households are looked upon more favorably by society because they are considered stable and provide a legitimating anchorage for the children born of these unions.

It has been said that nuclear families suffer from isolation and cannot cope with illness, repeated pregnancy, or reproductive wastage; hence, they must turn to professionals for sustenance and care. However, current research indicates that the nuclear family probably has less isolation and better coping ability than formerly was thought.[5] This is due to the fact that there appears to be great role adaptability and flexibility in time of stress as well as a greater utilization of kin and other social networks for advice and sustenance during childbearing as well as for other health conditions.

It is apparent that extended family forms can be helpful to counter isolation and to provide help during periods of stress. It must be remembered, however, that kin and friends can also deter family members from appropriately defining themselves in need of care and can prohibit or deter them from prompt and continued utilization of health services.

Evolving Family Structures

Communal family. This form can be further divided into the following:
- A household of more than one monogamous couple with children, sharing common facilities, resources, and experiences; socialization of the child is a group activity. Each member is a responsibility of the other members, and there is mutual concern for the various aspects of the members' lives, including health matters.
- A household of adults and children in which there is "group marriage," that is, all the persons are "married" to each other and all parent the children. A status system usually develops with the leaders believed to have charisma. These are very small in number and sometimes involve cultism.

Unmarried parent and child family. Often there is a mother for whom marriage is not desired or possible. Children can be natural offspring of the parent or adopted.

Unmarried couple and child family. Again, these may be of two varieties.
- A social contract marriage in which there is an ideologic commitment to a relationship not sanctioned by law, which usually is "worked at" to maintain its vitality and meaningfulness. Common value systems are shared that strongly emphasize humanism and personal relationships. A great deal of time is spent by the members, including the children, in sharing mutual

emotional experiences and ideas. The father plays a prominent role in the caretaking and socialization of the children, and both parents have intimate, continued, and sustained contact with their children.
- The second type of unmarried couple and child family is that usually referred to as common-law marriage with the children either born to the partners or informally adopted. These unions are often found among the poorer strata of society who experience exceptional problems and constraints associated with legal marriage.[6-8]

It is with the evolving forms of family styles that today's nurse may have the least experience. Therefore, we will discuss some of these family styles in greater detail and the basic principles of care that have special relevance for these families. It is worth noting that as recently as 10 years ago these families were known as "alternate" life-style families. However, their ethic and philosophy have become so much a part of the mainstream of society that they no longer can be so classified. Although we still use the term *alternate* or *alternative* from time to time in reference to them, it is more appropriate to consider their life-style as evolving rather than alternative.

Social-Contract Families or the Unmarried Marrieds

Social-contract families are composed of two partners whose structure exists as a social rather than a legal contract. Maternity nurses become acquainted with these clients when giving family-planning counseling and services during pregnancy and childbirth. The literature and current research suggests that in many ways this group shares the philosophy of the "turned-off," middle-class countercultures prominent in the 1960s. Living together in this form, however, has little similarity to the "shacking-up" of previous generations, or with the large number of common-law marriages found among some of the poor who experience constraints and problems associated with legal marriage, such as no finances to obtain a divorce or inability to manage the bureaucracy to facilitate legal severance. Rather, this form of marriage involves an ideologic commitment to a relationship instead of joint living by virtue of a legal status. Basic to this rejection of a legal marriage is the conviction that the bond of love and trust that binds the partners is more important and stronger than the legal bond authorized by church or state.[7,8]

In the family setting, parents spend long periods of time with one another and share emotional exchanges of closeness and rejection, desire and repulsion, and all of the certainties and uncertainties involved in living together and bearing and raising children. There is, for the most part, a great deal of frankness and openness about these statuses, which include the children. There is little secretiveness about their approach to life, and both names may be displayed on the mailboxes, in financial arrangements, and the like. There are no problems on their part regarding the legitimacy of the children.

Since the possible instability of the relationship can be critical to pregnancy outcomes and the children's development, researchers have explored these facets of alternate family forms.[7-9] Motivations for this life-style are very important. Some partners do not accept the civil contract *per se*. Others do not accept the relevance of the civil marriage contract to their relationship as it exists for them at the moment, wanting no civil constraints on their "splitting" if things change between them. Still others seek to avoid the obvious unhappiness in their own family life and upbringing. In general, from the participants' point of view, living together in this family structure is seen as representing true maturity and an acceptance of the faith placed in one another.

The women's liberation movement and the raising of women's consciousness have played a strong philosophical role in determining reproductive behavior and childrearing activities. The choice of having a child appears even more determined than in the traditional nuclear family. Contraception services appear to be used, and the option of termination of pregnancy is freely available and used without the apparent guilt associated with such termination in some of the traditional families. From this point of view, and because of the close interaction and caretaking when the children are born, this family style has been considered a very motivated form of parenting.[7]

Eiduson and her group have studied a variety of experimental family forms in their longitudinal *Family Styles Project*. These included social-contract families, communal groups, and single-parent families. A traditionally married group was also used for comparison. She states that the social-contract families are particularly interesting with respect to conflict and stress, since there is so much dependence on maintaining strong emotional involvement and positive interpersonal relationships.[10] Having a child apparently changed the parents' ideology somewhat. In these families were found the highest number of marriages in the first 3 years of the child's life and the highest number of divorces when the child was between the ages of 3 and 4. However, there was overall permanency in the relations: 68% of the social-contract partners were still together through the child's fourth year, and of these, half were married. These families are involved with the highest number of social-problem events (unemployment, short jail incarcerations, drug abuse), and in the

first 2 years of the child's life, they have the second highest total stress score, exceeded only by the single-mother families. Moreover, in the child's third year of life, the families' stress score is statistically significantly higher than in any other group; parental psychological stressors account for these scores. This is the same group of stressors that affect the single-parent families. The tension level between the mates, again, is higher than for any other type of family studied; however, it drops over the years, and by the time the child is 6, the tension level is the lowest in any family unit. This may well be due to the separation of the parents who truly did not get along. When the children were tested for the effect of this stress, they did appear to be adversely affected with respect to their social emotional competence and their cognitive intellectual development, at least at the early ages. Later testing will either confirm or deny these early findings.[10]

Single Parents

Single Mother

The single or unmarried mother is far from a new phenomenon in our society. In decades past, the unwed mother bearing the so-called illegitimate child was synonymous with single parent. However, with today's high divorce rate, the term has added a new dimension. Glick and Norton, in a review of national statistics, report that the proportion of children living with one parent has more than doubled from 1960 to 1978. A little more than 5.5 million American families (19% of the 30 million families with children) were headed by a single adult.[11] In fact, the popular notion of the intact, conventional family of mother, father, and children is a minority family form in the United States today. This form accounts for only 45% of Americans, whereas 55% are represented by single parents, couples without children, and reconstituted families (remarrieds with and without children).[2]

According to Census Bureau statistics for 1984, single parents headed 25.7% of the families with children under the age of 18. By 1990, it is estimated that one, and possibly two, of every three families will be headed by a lone parent. It is estimated that a quarter of the now-married mothers and fathers with children will be single parenting by the end of the decade. Moreover, it is predicted that approximately half of the children born in the 1980s will be living with only one parent.[12]

The quality of the single-parent experience will depend on the circumstances that result in this type of household. In the case of widows and widowers, for instance, when there is adequate insurance coverage and the remaining spouse has a high-paying occupation, there may not be the economic stringencies and social stigma that are often associated with households in which divorce has been the case of single parenting. However, it is important to remember that the one common characteristic shared by almost all female-headed, single-parent families is poverty or at best very reduced economic circumstances. Even with supplemental insurance or alimony and child support payments, the economic situation is often grim. And it is the mother who most often must be the ultimate financial support for her children. Even in today's so-called enlightened society, mothers are still awarded custody of the children in over 90% of all divorces.[13] Moreover, Ross and Sawhill state that child support and alimony supplements are less than is commonly believed and, in any event, inadequate to keep the divorced mother and her children from a poverty subsistence level.[14]

Unfortunately, our society is still dominated by the assumption that families headed by a single parent, particularly when that parent is a woman and in stringent economic circumstances, are deviant and pathological. Such families continue to be characterized as broken and disorganized rather than being recognized as a viable alternative family form. Instead of being seen as a solution to circumstances and assessed in terms of their strengths, they are often viewed negatively, particularly by health professionals, with an emphasis on their alleged weaknesses. This uncritical acceptance of the above assumption has led to biased governmental, employment, and social policies that have been very detrimental to these families. Moreover, many separated and divorced women have incorporated these negative images into their self-concepts, and this has become an obstacle to their readjustment to their new circumstances.[13]

Under such conditions, a variety of options need to be used because different supports are needed by these parents who are alone. Most importantly, the mother must enlarge her social support networks if she is to become economically independent and socially involved. The following paragraphs discuss several options and resources for the single parent that can be used to provide support and strategies.

Family Style Dwelling.   Among the family styles that have been encountered among single mothers (in addition to the single-family dwelling) are small group homes or boarding homes where a small number live together with their children, foster homes for mother and child, and apartment complexes where each family lives in its own unit.[15] The actual physical arrangements for the child differ among residences, but, in general, there are separate sleeping quarters for the parent and child, with common dining and living facilities. The opportunity for the children to eat and play together, share toys, and have a shared caretaker is considered one of the advantages for children in groups such as these.

Community and Organizational Support.   Many communities have developed programs that facilitate a mother's return to school or work so that she can gain skills that will enable her to be independent. These programs are still in the early stages and are largely experimental, but do indicate that society recognizes the complex needs of women who rear children alone. Child-care facilities, caretaking arrangements, and infant caretakers in the home reflect the kinds of assistance the community has developed, which means that children of single parents can be exposed to multiple caretaking as early as 6 weeks of life.

Societal recognition has also encouraged single parents to move toward developing organizations and social networks that provide them with tangible supportive contacts. The expansion of such organizations as Parents Without Partners, the Momma League, and the LaLeche League into activity programs, information and training centers, and consciousness-raising efforts suggests that middle-class parents have become more sensitive to their needs as persons as well as parents.

Single Male Parent

While voluntary single male parents are still much in the minority, they are becoming more numerous. Their living arrangements include group living as well as living alone with the child. Because the male's economic status is generally better than the female's, he has more options for child care and living quarters. Thus, caretakers in the home are found more frequently, although ample use is made of child-care centers and children's programs.[2,7]

In the case of divorce, while the number of male heads of households is still very small compared with female-headed households (2.8% male headed versus 22.9% female headed in 1984), the percentage has been growing. For instance, in 1970, 1.3% of divorced homes had a male head. In 1980 the number had risen to 2.2%, and in 1984 it was 2.8%. Thus, it is still unusual for the majority of fathers to assume custody of the children.[12] However, the beginnings of the breakdown in parental roles and postdivorce parental roles have begun to have some effect on custodial outcomes. Hence, a small but growing number of fathers are now requesting and getting both joint and sole custody of their children following divorce. In Gersick's study of fathers and custody, four interacting variables appear to be determinants of whether or not fathers consider assuming custody of their children. First, the father's own family relationships color his outlook toward his responsibility to his children. Many want to overcome, in their relationships with their children, the problems and the emotional detachment they experienced with their parents. Second, feelings toward the ex-wife affect the father's orientation. When he believes that the wife has betrayed him in some way, he is motivated to seek custody by a combination of a desire to punish his wife and a concern for the well-being of the children. The third variable is the fact that the wife gave pretrial consent, hence a court "battle" was not necessary and the father could assume custody with a minimum of conflict. The final factor has to do with the attorney's attitudes. If the attorney is reluctant to press for custody, the father tends to let the wife have the children.[13,16]

While Greif did not examine the determinants of seeking custody, he did find that those fathers in his study who wanted custody "very much" felt they shared in the marital breakup; were better prepared for assuming custody, having participated a great deal in rearing the children and doing household chores; and were generally more satisfied with their relationship with their children. Greif notes, however, that most of the custodial fathers "ended their marriages in an uncomfortable state." They did not want their marriages to end; they felt a good deal of stress when the marriage did end, and they blamed their spouses for the breakup.[17] Riley and Cochran found that approximately 27% of the fathers they studied did not use anyone in their networks for advice in childrearing. The networks were largely kin networks, and their former wives utilized networks less also. Interestingly, these fathers had large networks.[15]

As with the voluntary single male parent, divorced fathers generally have sufficient material wherewithal to provide at least an adequate life-style for their children. Research shows that many of the difficulties that the men experience are the same as those of the single-parent women. Economic circumstances become more stringent (but not as dire as for the women); arranging child care becomes a problem. Visits from the wife were anticipated with anxiety, and, in general, for many of the men, the strain of the divorce coupled with the new demands of total responsibility for the children made readjustment to the single life-style difficult. However, none of the fathers studied regretted their decision to assume custody of their children.[16]

Community and Organizational Support. As recently as 10 years ago, the idea of offering community and organizational support designed for fathers, whether single or married, would have been unthinkable. There was no "critical mass" of resources for and about fathers. In fact, there was barely any acknowledgment that the same social forces creating change in the needs, expectations, and opportunities for women might have implications for men.[18] However, there were researchers particularly interested in the changing roles of the American male, notably Levine and his group (who eventually designed and implemented The Fatherhood Project), Greif, Gersick, and others.[15-19] Data from The Fatherhood Project have resulted in a book that is invaluable as a ready reference for referrals for all fathers, married or single. It profiles a diverse collection of agencies, groups, and institutions that are making a broad commitment to fatherhood, particularly the single father. Levine points out that none of these organizations is self-contained; rather, each represents the combined efforts of both men and women who are committed to supporting one another and are reaching out to others in the community.[18] The student is referred to the publication *Fatherhood U.S.A.*, by Klinman and Kohl in the Suggested Reading for an excellent resource reference.

Communal Living Groups

The creation of a communal alternate to the isolated nuclear family is not new in this country. Generations have sought a new start and protested the status quo. Causes of their dissent and the ways in which they chose to organize their new communal existence varied in the past as they do with today's communards. Some were based upon religious conviction, some on economic idealism, and some on rebellion against authority. Some attempted to establish a model of government based upon an absence of central authority; others sought a strict line of hierarchical authority with the rejection of those members who did not adhere to the authority prescribed. Some had relatively long histories, while others dissolved rapidly.

Current Communal Life-style

Life-styles displayed by the current commune movement are perhaps even more varied than those of the historical models. This makes attempts to define this evolving life-style difficult. Communes vary today in type of membership, organizational structure, and general purpose. Some are involved in agricultural subsistence, seeking a closeness to the land characterized by the early close-knit communities reported to have existed in history, while others are composed of middle-class young professionals who do not wish to disengage from the urban scene and its various technological comforts. Size also varies from 12 or less to hundreds.

A significant number of present-day communes is based upon religious commitments of various persuasions. Eastern philosophy is often a guiding force in many of these religiously oriented communes. In others, the "Jesus movement" is central, with the members searching for a new way to live out the traditional Judeo–Christian convictions. There have been some tragic happenings in some of these communal groups. It remains to be seen what effect these events will have on the total commune movement.

Communes are often formed around common interests or crafts or some unifying goal. They start with people who like each other and share similar value systems, orientations, and convictions. This aspect is extremely important in these intentional communities, and some see their alternate family arrangement as the beginning of a social revolution that will bring about radical change in society.[9,20]

Family Structure Within Communal Living Groups

Some communes are reported to be group-marriage oriented, but they are in the minority. Children are shared with the group, and there is little concern about knowing or caring which persons have been biologically responsible for the conception of the child. The rearing of the child is considered more important than who the parents are.

Other groups are oriented as extended families, with couples remaining essentially monogamous in their own private quarters, although partners may change from time to time. Still others live together under a community concept rather than a family unit, sharing resources that are more effectively achieved in multiple-family cooperatives, such as expenses, household chores, and child-care responsibilities. The women's consciousness movement has given particular impetus to these groups.

The life span of the current communes varies. Such issues as organization of work and other aspects of living, interpersonal relationships, mutual values, economic feasibility, and ability to cope with outside community harassment have been suggested as important to the stability of communal arrangements.

Parent–Child Relationships. Living arrangements largely determine parent–child relationships. Great ingenuity is shown—tents, lean-tos, and cabins in the rural areas; apartment houses, motels, and sometimes single-family dwellings in the city.

The number of children varies from commune to commune. In general, the adults are conscious of the population explosion, and few parents with more than three biologic children are in evidence; however, there are some "families" who have eight to ten children. Birth, pregnancy, and children are esteemed and joyously regarded as an expression of a natural and ecologically appropriate experience.

Adult–child relations are often determined by proximity of living and sleeping quarters. Relations with biologic parents may be infrequent, with children being physically separated from them and assigned to caretakers, as is the case in some instances. In addition, the child's relationship with other adults is related to the extent of the existence of a hierarchical structure. In a family, multiple dwelling arrangements can permit a child to move among households, as when he is in conflict with other members or lonely for playmates or when his family is "splitting" for a time.[20] (See chart below.)

Childrearing Practices in Communal Groups

- Breast-feeding appears routine and there is usually close tactile contact between mother and child in the first year.
- There is often a clear break in the intense mother–infant relationship at around $2\frac{1}{2}$ years, when there is a push in the direction of independence and self-reliance.
- Good health, together with a desire for wholesomeness, is revered. Natural foods are stressed, and "junk" foods are restricted. Institutional medical and dental care may be limited to emergencies. The emphasis is on prevention through healthful, natural living.
- Nonviolence is generally espoused among the counterculture groups, although assertiveness among the children, especially the girls, is sanctioned.
- Humanistic and interpersonal relationships and the direct expression of affectional needs are valued. Artificial repression of sexuality and intimacy is eschewed; exposure to nudity and observation of adult sexual activity may be permitted.
- Children socialize each other.
- Early decision making is encouraged in the child.
- Parents experience some difficulty with serving as role models for their children. They appear to be quite reluctant to "lay their trip" on the child. The parents may not be willing to serve as sex role models because of their general acceptance of an antisexist philosophy. Yet many of the males are out and out sexists. There is also ambivalence about having the girls identify with the not completely emancipated women.
- Competency to handle daily life is stressed, while competition and achievement striving are played down; thus, individual potential and creativity are felt to be promoted. Sensory impressions, intuition, and the occult, as opposed to the rational, are data that are considered an enhancement of creativity.
- Materialistic values are seen as tied in with technological advances and nonhumanistic goals; thus, dependence on material possessions is minimized whenever possible. However, some of the children see the adults "ripping off" the outside society and ignoring the social contracts involved in personal ownership (*i.e.*, stealing).

Nursing Care Involving Families with Evolving Life-styles

There are several principles to remember when the nurse is assessing, diagnosing, planning, implementing, and evaluating care for those who may be involved in a variant life-style. A general rejection of so-called traditional values pervades our culture, with more and more emphasis placed on the right of each person to find values and a philosophy that are meaningful to him or her. Thus, couples involved in variant life-styles may assume a more questioning attitude, which may prove disconcerting to some health providers.

Evaluating Health Information

Health professionals often expect clients to accept their information as true because it is drawn from a scientific body of knowledge. However, some intelligent clients may regard modern science as attempting to bring forth more and more "laws" aimed at finding absolute truth in a relative world and, hence, having little to do with health and, more important, happiness.

On the other hand, information from other sources is also subjected to scrutiny and evaluation before acceptance. Thus, many practices that could be potentially harmful are often rejected.

The tendency to evaluate medical information given by the health professional on an experiential rather than a scientific basis does not preclude an interest in what the health professional has to say. In our experience, particularly in the free clinics, we find that the nurse is respected as a person who has knowledge in her field and who shares some of the client's concerns and feelings. Expectant parents will have many questions, and when the nurse responds to their inquiries, they may go on to relate information that they have gathered from other sources. It becomes important to discuss this information seriously and with respect because it is valuable to the parent. Health teaching documented with rational explanation and practical experiences is much more readily accepted. The advice and teaching must be practical also. To insist that a vegetarian eat meat, even if she may have anemia, is simply too impractical, especially if there are others in the family to consider.

Moreover, patients who follow evolving life-styles are, for the most part, well educated and, because of this and their value system, expect a fuller and more complete explanation than many other patients. If a mother prefers a vegetarian diet and wants to know the food values of the foods she wishes to include in her diet, she will not be satisfied with only a suggested menu. Exchanges and equivalents must be discussed. It is not sufficient to tell a mother in an antepartal clinic to return in so many weeks for another blood test without telling her the reason for returning and the purpose of the procedure. If clients reject some of the advice, this, too, is to be treated with respect.

Thus, the nurse will assess the mother's knowledge in the various pertinent areas and make a special effort to include her in the planning of her care.

Choosing Antepartal Services

The factors that affect the couple with an evolving family life-style include past experience with health personnel, geographic location, feelings about the pregnancy, the influence of significant others, and the parents' physical condition. These are all areas the nurse should assess.

Increasingly, there is a high priority placed on ambience and interpersonal relations during the pregnancy and at the time of delivery. Selection of services is made on the basis of consultation with friends, referrals from professionals, and past experience with health providers. In general, couples are taking a more militant stand regarding participation in the planning and execution of their care and tend to seek out health professionals who allow them this right. It becomes important then in planning care with the client to be sure that the couple is duly informed about the nature of their care, including their right to sign themselves out of the hospital. This information, together with a genuine indication of regard for the couple, is usually sufficient to lessen the apprehension about having a hospital delivery or seeking antenatal care from a "traditional" establishment provider.

Choosing the Place and Method of Delivery

Selecting a hospital for delivery or choosing between a hospital and home delivery involves many of the same factors as those considered in the selection of antepartal services. For most couples today, childbirth is regarded as a natural process; thus, prepared childbirth classes, an alternate birth center, and the Le Boyer method of delivery may be very popular. Modern up-to-date equipment and technological expertise may be much less important than an environment that simulates the home.

Today, parents come to their deliveries much more knowledgeable than previously. This is due, in part, to the large variety of books now available dealing with nutrition in pregnancy and the physiology of pregnancy, labor, and delivery; there are even "how to" books on home delivery. Parents therefore expect their requests to be considered. Hospitals that have the reputation for having a great deal of restrictions and "hassle" are avoided.

The need for control over one's own life may also be a strong motivating factor in the choice of a home delivery.[21] These types of deliveries still remain controversial. Safety of the mother and infant continues to be a grave concern for the health professionals, and there are data that indicate that this concern is well founded. However, birth carries a strong symbolic meaning and the home typifies this meaning. The traditional hospital setting is seen by many couples as a sterile place with little room for intimacy and family integration. Many hospitals have instituted birthing rooms (ABC rooms) or birth centers that simulate a homelike atmosphere free from many of the restrictions and rigidities imposed by the traditional delivery suite. It is hoped that this alternative will encompass both the symbolic atmosphere that is desired and adequate safety features for the mother and infant.

Ethnic, Social Class, and Cultural Variations

The recent emphasis on cultural pluralism and ethnic heritage in America seems to contradict the contention that ethnic groups tend to shed their distinctive family patterns as they become socially mobile. It can be seen, however, that the move toward the celebration of national origins represents an extolling of distinctive ethnic art, language, dress, and food patterns for the purpose of promoting a positive identity and ancestral pride in those who have had little of either.

If we examine the contemporary family roles of various ethnic groups, we see that the process of acculturation has been accelerated or delayed by several factors, including opportunity available in the new environment, the extent of discrimination, and the degree of cultural and physical similarity or difference between the acculturating group and the dominant society. There are many groups that comprise the "salad bowl" of America and, unfortunately, we cannot include all of them here. However, we will highlight some of the groups to give an indication of the current state of thought on contemporary family roles.

We would like to make clear at the outset that the variations among the different ethnic groups in family styles, health beliefs and practices, and utilization of health services are a function of the socioeconomic status of the individuals far more than their particular ethnicity. Since minority groups in general are often poorer than their white counterparts and because more individuals within each group tend to be poorer than the same proportion of whites, there has been an inability to gain access to education and other resources that money can buy. Thus, behavior and beliefs that differ from the mainstream white-middle-class–dominant society have come about or been retained, and misconceptions have arisen attributing these behaviors to ethnicity.

Native American Families

Of all the ethnic groups that abound in this country, the American Indian has perhaps the most remarkable history, one that reflects severe exploitation, astounding endurance, and incredible capability for adaptation. The Native American's history has been marred by disease, starvation, deliberate attempts at genocide, and blatantly inconsistent treatment by governmental agencies.[22]

Even today, there is no single accepted definition of American Indian or Native American. Governmental agencies and the Census Bureau rely on the individual to define himself as Indian; some require proof of at least one quarter Indian blood. Hence, even enumerating the number of tribes and individuals is difficult. In 1976 it was estimated that this population was increasing so that now there may be approximately 1 million Indians in the country, belonging to over 300 tribes.

Approximately one half of the Indian population lives on reservations whose development was a result of a racist governmental policy of exclusion. Reservation lands were much less acceptable than the lands originally inhabited by the various tribes. Life on the reservation, even today, is fraught with the twin plagues of poverty and substandard housing, which, in turn, give rise to myriad health problems.[23]

An urban resettlement program was attempted in 1952 that was supposed to aid the assimilation of the Indian into the mainstream American culture. Participants were given job training and limited aid in finding jobs and housing. The program is generally regarded as a failure. Because of bureaucratic red tape and disinterest, financial and other aid was so meager that it did not begin to achieve the goals originally outlined. Those who did leave the reservation often found themselves separated from their families because the housing allowance was inadequate to accommodate an entire family. Moreover, the traditional social supports found on the reservation disappeared in the city. Thus, the urban Indian became a true "marginal" man. He was distrusted by his own people and unable to participate in traditional tribal life. Moreover, he was stigmatized and ignored by those with whom he was supposed to assimilate. It is estimated that about half of those who attempted the urban move have returned to the reservation.[24]

An attempt is being made through the use of Urban Indian Centers to meet some of the needs of these urban migrants. These centers supply health services, educational services, and job counseling. It is still too early to comment on the success of this innovation, but it does seem as though these programs are achieving at least a modicum of success.[24]

The cultural background of the Native American varies according to tribal affiliation. Thus, generalizations about the American Indian family must be made with caution. In the main, family life is influenced by tribal beliefs, and there is a great deal of variation among the tribes with respect to holding to traditional values and customs. This variability occurs in both the reservation and urban Indian communities.

Family. For the most part, the family remains the basic unit of Native American society. The Indian idea of family is the extended family that includes grandparents, aunts, uncles, and even close friends. Children are valued and admired, and all members participate in the childrearing. Each has certain things that must be taught to the child, and the responsibility is taken seriously.

In many tribes, the lineage is matriarchal and the child automatically becomes a member of the mother's clan at birth (Fig. 5-2). Indian women have traditionally worked very hard, but they have also been very influential in tribal affairs. Indeed, they have been "the heart of the home," and several have also been leaders of their tribes.[23,25] Women are respected because they conceive and bear children and maintain the cohesiveness in the family. Children are considered assets, and the elderly are held in high regard.[26]

Beliefs and Health Providers. Health beliefs also vary according to tribal identity, and religion is a powerful force in giving direction to childbearing, childbirth, and childrearing. Again it is difficult to make generalizations, but a few principles will be attempted here. For the most part, pregnancy is thought of as a natural process in the normal cycle of life and death. In general, a harmonious prenatal period is stressed, with an attempt to help the mother be content, keep away from ill or evil persons and things, and think good thoughts. When facilities permit, prenatal care and hospital delivery is sought from obstetricians or other physicians. Tribal midwives are also used. The tribal medicine man is relied upon also to provide special foods and beverages that are believed to be helpful in increasing strength and preventing illness. He also supplies charms and amulets to aid in a healthy delivery.[27]

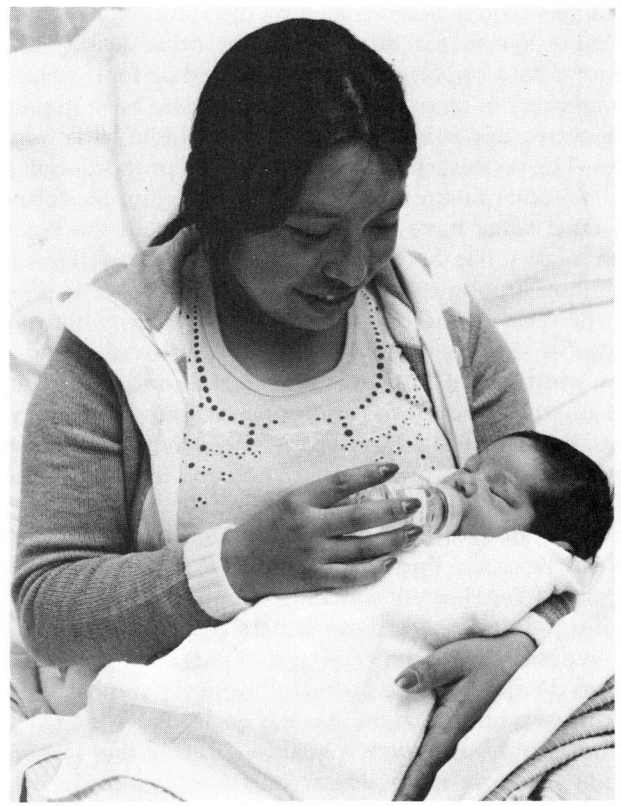

FIGURE 5-2

In many tribes, the lineage is matriarchal and the child automatically becomes a member of the mother's clan at birth.

In spite of the fact that the majority of Native American women deliver in hospitals, their maternal mortality rate is nearly 2% higher than the overall maternal mortality rate for the United States. It is becoming glaringly apparent that health providers who work with these clients must make more of an effort to become familiar with their customs and needs if they are to provide adequate services. A recent positive development has been a rapprochement between traditional western medicine and the native healers. Programs have been developed that permit sharing of each's beliefs and techniques. Thus, the best of each tradition can be incorporated into the care of clients, which results in an upgrading in the quality of care delivered.

Black Families

Family. One of the most significant factors affecting the family roles of the black population of the United States has been the concentration of a majority of these families at income levels that are grossly inadequate.

This has largely been caused by discrimination, which is more severe for blacks than for other less visible groups. New opportunities have opened up for the black community in recent years; however, these have mainly benefitted upper-working-class and middle-class families. The poorest strata have not gained proportionally.

Another factor that has been woven into the fabric of what some have called mythology about the black community has been the lack of a strong patriarchal tradition among the black family. The mother is seen as the head of the household and provider, while the father is seen as mostly absent, a nonprovider, and a powerless parent. However, research has indicated that, among the middle-class and upper-working-class families, there is no significant difference from whites with respect to family role differentiation and the acceptance of a middle-class value system.

In a thoughtful review and evaluation of the empirical research findings regarding lower-class black families, TenHouten concluded that the bulk of the findings do not show these fathers and husbands to be powerless in either their conjugal or parental roles. Black wives do appear to be powerful in their parental roles, but there is no indication that this emasculates the black father.[28] Indeed, there is a healthy effect in that fathers tend to be more expressive in their marital and parental roles and are helpful and willing to share in childrearing and homemaking chores. Moreover, this freedom from patriarchy has enabled the black woman to be more pragmatic, resourceful, and flexible than her counterparts from other cultures in which the tradition of authoritarianism and patriarchy is strong. Recent research indicates that black families are more likely to live in an extended-family household.[29]

Since they typically do not have authoritarian fathers, black children do not experience one of the psychological stresses of low-achievement motivations. The increased economic opportunities that will allow black fathers to become economic role models for their children, combined with an early emphasis on independence typical among black families and confident setting of standards by black mothers, should result in higher levels of achievement motivation among black children than among children whose fathers play a more repressive role. There is already evidence that middle-class black children have higher levels of motivation and aspiration than do their white counterparts.[28,30]

Blacks in the lower socioeconomic strata, especially when confined to the ghetto or rural areas and deprived of educational and other acculturating opportunities, tend to hold a traditional value system that includes a strong sense of family (or familism), superstition, religiosity, and fatalism. This is in contrast to the "middle-class" value system generally held by highly industrialized urban societies. These values—rationalism, pragmatism, individualism, egalitarianism, secularism, and achievement—have also become known as the dominant American values.

Beliefs and Health Providers.   Whether the person's value system is traditional or middle-class urban, it becomes part of his belief system and is incorporated into the roles of husband, wife, parent, and child. Thus, when dealing with these clients, health professionals often find their values competing with those of the clients. When the basic values are examined, it becomes clearer why certain health beliefs, differential use of health services, delay in seeking care, and often nonadherence to prescribed regimens are established.

Mexican–American Families

Mexican–Americans have been the forgotten minority in the United States, possibly because the Southwest has been somewhat neglected by both academicians and writers with the exception of John Steinbeck. There are more than 5 million Mexican–Americans, who are mainly second-generation offspring of peasant immigrants from Mexico. They are concentrated in the border states of Texas, Arizona, New Mexico, and California and constitute the second largest minority group in the United States.

Since World War II, the isolation of the Mexican–American has been declining, owing to the fact that many participated in the war, and gradually new perspectives and opportunities have come about that have had an impact on family roles and traditional value and belief systems (Fig. 5-3). Neighborhood enclaves (bar-

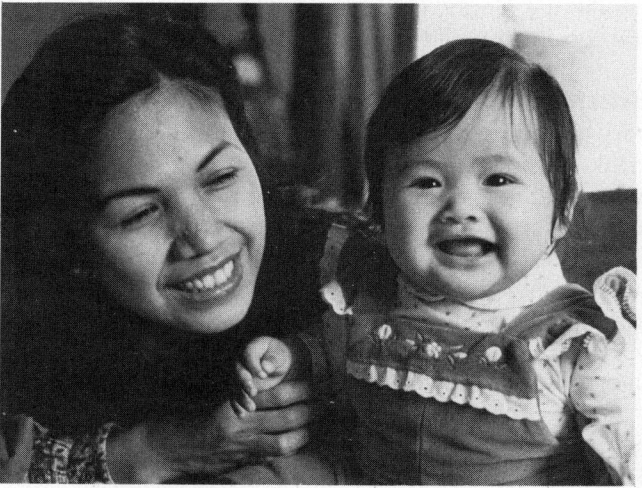

FIGURE   5 - 3

Since World War II many Mexican–American families have become less isolated as new perspectives and opportunities have had an impact on family life.

rios) still exist, of course, and in some small rural or isolated urban areas, even the middle-class Mexican–American tends to reside in them.

Family. Familism appears to be the strongest surviving traditional value within the older Mexican–American community, along with patriarchalism and machismo, the cultural ideal of masculinity that equates maleness with sexual prowess.[24] These traditional values and certain folk beliefs persist, particularly because of the isolation of the barrios, and the persistence of these values and beliefs makes the acceptance of modern health knowledge and practice difficult.

Beliefs and Health Providers. Mexican–Americans in the barrios who are educated and have had a positive experience with health services have accepted the ideas of scientific medicine and health care, allow their children to be immunized, attend clinics, and, in some cases, have accepted some kind of family planning. However, there are many others who have their own set of folk beliefs about illness and its treatment that they practice in conjunction with medical care or before seeking scientific health care. These beliefs about diseases and their cures are derived from experience and experimentation and are handed down from generation to generation. Two or more cures may be recognized for one disorder, and disorders generally fall into two categories, those of emotional origin and those of magical origin. Folk healers (primarily curanderas [women] or curanderos [men]) are often used, and some have an important and respected standing in the community. It is felt by the majority of the uneducated that physicians do not know how to treat folk disorders because they lack either faith, knowledge, or understanding of them.

Among those with little education, there is no distinction between the natural and supernatural, and many illnesses can be a result of evil forces, witches, spells cast by other persons, or punishment for some sin committed either knowingly or unknowingly. One common condition that health professionals should be aware of is the following: *mal aire,* or bad air, especially night air. It can enter through any of the body cavities under certain circumstances and results in illness of both mother and child. *Mal ojo,* or the evil eye, is a culturally defined disease, primarily of children. It is caused when someone looks admiringly or covetously on the child or adult. Its symptoms are restlessness, crying, and headache, as well as other nonspecific symptoms. *Susto,* or fright, can be caused by a frightening experience that can result in excessive nervousness, loss of appetite, and loss of sleep. *Mollera calda,* or fallen fontanelle, is a common disorder among infants. It is believed to be due to a fall or from taking the nipple out of the baby's mouth too suddenly, thus causing the fontanelle to be sucked in. Symptoms include irritability, crying, diar-

rhea, sunken eyes, and vomiting. There are other afflictions as well as their home remedies that it is wise for the nurse to know if she will be dealing with these clients.

Oriental Families

The Oriental family has been a part of the American scene for generations. As with the Native American families, one should not make sweeping generalizations about all types of Oriental families; however, there are some commonalities that exist. Especially among the older generations, roles tend to be clearly defined and differentiated.

Family. A woman marries to serve her husband and often his mother and others in the household as well. There is a good deal of extendedness in the Oriental family. While the modern family may not live in the paternal family home, they attempt to live as close as possible and keep in touch frequently with visits and calls. Grandparents and older members may reside with the younger couple. The elderly and children are both respected and valued. Grandparents are often the decision makers, advisors, and supervisors of the children's and grandchildren's upbringing. Filial respect is still expected. While more of the contemporary wives are employed, there is still the service orientation within the home despite career status. Harmony, patience, modesty, gentleness, and reserve remain important values. Confrontation is to be avoided even if unrealistic self-blame must be employed.[26,31,32]

Japanese–American Families

Of all the Oriental families the Japanese family system has received the closest scrutiny. We know, for instance, that in California, where the largest concentration of Japanese ancestry occurs, this segment of the population has the highest median levels of income and education of any minority group. Japanese–Americans also have very low rates of crime and delinquency, indicating at the same time the greater persistence of the traditional values of obedience and conformity to parental values and norms. The generational pattern of increasing acculturation is very clearly illustrated in the contemporary Japanese–American community, since other factors such as urban–rural residence do not vary significantly.

Issei. A majority of the Issei, or first-generation immigrants who were born in Japan, arrived here some time between the end of the 19th century and 1924, when immigration from the Orient and Eastern Europe was sharply restricted by the Johnson Act. While the Issei came largely from rural agricultural areas and occupations, they were unusual in that they were relatively literate, compared with peasant immigrants from Europe, and they valued education even before their arrival in this country.

Nisei. Second-generation Japanese–Americans, the Nisei, born largely before 1940, experienced an unusual push into modernity not only by the parents' preexisting emphasis on education, but by the West Coast evacuation of Japanese–Americans during World War II. Familistic values were weakened by the loss of confiscated family homes and businesses, which removed an important source of Issei control over their second-generation offspring. Thus, after the war, the Nisei, who were forced to seek out independent, nonfamily occupational opportunities, were thereby more speedily acculturated into the modern values of individualism and egalitarianism in family relationships, although a cultural lag in this respect is still quite pronounced among many Japanese–Americans.

Sansei. The third generation, the Sansei, born largely since World War II and now in the adult occupational world, were the first generation to become very acculturated. However, certain subcultural differences remain in family role conceptions, even within the third generation, which are traceable to the survival of traditional ethnic values in marital roles and in childrearing practices.

Frequent sources of role conflict in the Sansei generation are found in the greater prevalence of strict disciplinary measures in childrearing; the greater emphasis on conformity and unconditional obedience, on humility and emotional reserve (particularly the suppression of anger); the continued extensive use of shame and guilt as mechanisms of control; the greater submissiveness of women, even within the higher social strata; and the greater strength of extended-family pride and intergenerational emotional dependence. These are the residual of traditional values of the parents.

While recent studies of the Sansei generation have indicated a shift toward greater independence in this generation, both males and females remain, typically, less assertive, more deferent and conforming, and more emotionally reserved than their Anglo peers. The rigid conformity, status distinctions, and authority relations of traditional Japan that continue to affect family roles of Japanese–Americans in this country are likely to disappear with time, but more quickly in the occupational world than in the world of the family, where they appear less immediately dysfunctional.[26]

Yansei. The fourth generation, the Yansei, continue with acculturation patterns with the attendant role conflicts. While the continued emphasis within Japa-

nese–American homes on achievement and competitiveness has promoted educational and occupational success, the continuing stress of familism and authoritarian values has tended to retard the flexibility, independence, and self-reliance that are important attributes of individualistic achievement in highly industrialized society.

Beliefs and Health Providers. There are few folk beliefs, and, in general, scientific medicine is accepted especially by the second- and third-generation Japanese–Americans. Preventive medicine is solicited and, because of the high educational levels as well as high achievement aspirations, health and medical regimens are usually followed. There may be some reliance on herbal medicine and an interest in acupuncture among the older generation.

Southeast Asian Families

In 1975, almost 150,000 South Vietnamese refugees from all walks of life sought new homes and a new way of life in the United States. All of the states generously received these immigrants, but the highest concentration, approximately 27,000, is found in California.[24] The first wave of refugees in the early 1970s, prior to the collapse of the Vietnamese government, was, by American standards, middle class; these refugees had secondary-school educations and were largely multilingual in French, English, and their native tongue. About 23% held university degrees.[33] The second great wave, after the government's collapse, came in less fortunate circumstances. Many were penniless and poorly educated, with little or no command of English; in general, they were less likely to be exposed to Western culture. Moreover, the majority were in poor health, with such diseases and health conditions as malaria, tuberculosis, intestinal parasites, anemia, and malnutrition. These conditions, together with the cultural diversity and health belief systems, present a continuing challenge to the the American health-care system.[34,35]

Most of the available data about the homeland culture and mores and recent adjustment endeavors are experiential and anecdotal and derive from interviews with families as they make their varying adjustments.[24,36]

Beliefs and Health Providers. Vietnamese social concerns and problems including health needs are not significantly different from those of many Americans, especially those who live in reduced circumstances.[36] Economic opportunities may be limited for the unskilled and for the educated former urban dweller. Economic opportunities may not be commensurate with the Vietnamese's considerable skill and expertise. Culture shock and a language barrier may also prove troublesome. Moreover, the economic and emotional exigencies that the single parents, who are waiting for news or the arrival of their loved ones, face impact on their life-style just as severely as on an American family.[24]

The development of community agencies to assist these families to become acculturated has been helpful to some extent. Social support systems including friend and family networks have also eased the transition to the American culture.[24,36]

The Vietnamese family is not adverse to using the existing American health-care delivery system, including hospital care during parturition if the providers are sensitive to the family structure and try to use family members as resources for the care of the child in an extended-family manner. The use of a telephone outreach program based in the maternity ward and a well-monitored referral system to public health agencies have been found to be beneficial in the delivery of health services.[36]

There are several culture-based customs that have relevance for those providing maternity care to these clients.[37] As a sign of respect, the client may not look the provider in the eye when speaking and may often answer "yes" to a direct question when a "no" is more appropriate, again out of deference and fear of giving offense. Direct questions, loud conversation, getting on a first-name basis, touching, and other signs of easy conviviality, accepted to the Westerner, are considered with disdain and inappropriate by the Vietnamese. Thus, using questions that do not require a negative answer, making indirect rather than blunt requests, and maintaining a formal, respectful attitude will increase the family's comfort and therefore the effectiveness of the nurse's care.

References

1. Skolnick A: The Intimate Environment: Exploring Marriage and the Family. Boston, Little, Brown & Co, 1978
2. Glick PC: American household structure in transition. Fam Plann Perspect 16(5):204–211, Sept/Oct 1984
3. Lewis GL: Changes in women's role participation. In Frieze I et al (eds): Women and Sex Roles: A Social Psychological Perspective. New York, WW Norton & Co, 1978
4. Pickett RS: Monogamy on trial: II. The modern era. Alternate Lifestyles 1(3):281–301, 1978
5. Reeder SJ: The Impact of Disabling Health Conditions on Family Interaction. Unpublished PhD dissertation, UCLA, 1974
6. Sussman M: Family systems in the 1970's: Analysis, policies, programs. Ann Am Acad 396:5–10, 1970
7. Eiduson BJ et al: Alternatives in childrearing in the 1970's. Am J Orthopsychiatry 43:720–731, 1973
8. Alexander J, Kornfein M: Changes in family functioning amongst nonconventional families. Am J Orthopsychiatry 53(3):408–417, July 1983
9. Zimmerman IL, Bernstein M: Parental work patterns in alternative families: Influence on child development. Am J Orthopsychiatry 53(3):418–425, July 1983
10. Eiduson B: Conflict and stress in nontraditional families: Impact on children. Am J Orthopsychiatry 53(3):426–435, July 1983
11. Glick PC, Norton AJ: Marrying, divorcing and living together in the U.S. today. Population Bulletin 32(5). Washington, DC, Population Reference Bureau, 1982
12. Gelman D et al: The single parent's family albums. Newsweek, July 15, 1985
13. Hutter M: The Changing Family: Comparative Perspectives. New York, John Wiley & Sons, 1981
14. Ross HL, Sawhill IY: Line of Transition: The Growth of Families Headed by Women. Washington, DC, The Urban Institute, 1975
15. Riley D, Cochran MM: Naturally occurring childrearing advice for fathers: Utilization of the personal social network. J Marr Fam 47(2):275–286, May 1985
16. Gersick KE: Fathers by choice: Divorced men who received custody of their children. In Levinger G, Moles OC (eds): Divorce and Separation: Context, Causes and Consequences, pp 303–323. New York, Basic Books, 1979
17. Greif GL: Single fathers rearing children. J Marr Fam 47(1):185–191, Feb 1985
18. Klinman DG: Fatherhood U.S.A. New York, Garland Publishing, 1984
19. Greif GL: Custodial dads and their ex-wives. The Single Parent 27:17–20, Jan–Feb 1984
20. Eiduson B et al: Comparative socialization practices in alternative family settings. In Lamb M (ed): Nontraditional Families. New York, Plenum Press, 1981
21. Maralee J: Our Babies, Our Lives, Our Right to Decide. Chicago, Chicago Seed, 1972
22. Spradley JP, McCurdy DW: Conformity and Conflict, Readings in Cultural Anthropology, 4th ed. Boston, Little, Brown & Co, 1980
23. Billard JB (ed): The World of the American Indian, pp 311–382. Washington, DC, National Geographic Society, 1974
24. Clark AL: Culture, Childbearing and Health Professionals, pp 20–33. Philadelphia, FA Davis, 1978
25. Foreman CT: Indian Women Chiefs. Muskogee, OK, Hoffman Printing, 1954
26. Henderson G, Primeaux M: Transcultural Health Care. Menlo Park, CA, Addison–Wesley Publishing Co, 1981
27. Vogel G: American Indian Medicine. New York, Ballentine Books, 1973
28. TenHouten W: The black family: Myth and reality. Psychiatry 33:145–175, 1970
29. Hofferth SL: Kin networks, race, and family structure. J Marr Fam 46(4):791–806, Nov 1984
30. Martin EP, Martin JM: The Black Extended Family. Chicago, University of Chicago Press, 1978
31. Ho MK: Social work with Asian Americans. Soc Casework 57:195–202, March 1976

32. Benedict R: The Chrysanthemum and the Sword. Boston, Houghton–Mifflin, 1946
33. Benedict R: Making it in America: Story of the Vietnamese. U.S. News and World Report 85:45–49, Nov 27, 1978
34. Benedict R: The not so promised land. Time 83:24–26, Sept 10, 1979
35. Koval D, Brennan M, del Bueno D: Indochina moves to the mainstreet: Exotic diseases you're sure to see more of. RN 43:74–76, Sept 1980
36. Grosso C et al: The Vietnamese American family . . . and grandma makes three. MCH 6:177–180, 1981
37. Thomas RG, Tumminia PA: Maternity care for Vietnamese in America. Birth 9(3):187–190, Fall, 1982

Suggested Reading

Balik B, Foley MK: Developing a community-based parent education support group. JOGN Nurs 10(3):197–199, 1981
Blanton J: Communal child rearing: The Synanon experience. Alternative Lifestyles 3(1):87–116, 1980
Ellis J: Southeast Asian refugees and maternity care: The Oakland experience. Birth 9(3):191–194, Fall 1982
Glenn ND, Supancic M: The social and demographic correlates of divorce and separation in the United States: An update and reconsideration. J Marr Fam 46(3):563–575, Aug 1984
Greif GL: Single Fathers. Lexington, KY, DC Heath, 1985
Griffith S: Childbearing and the concept of culture. JOGN Nurs 11(3):181–184, May/June 1982
Grosso C et al: The Vietnamese American family and grandma makes three. MCN 6:177–180, 1981
Hanson FM: Single custodial fathers and the parent-child relationship. Nurs Res 30(2):202–204, 1981
Klinman DG, Kohl R: Fatherhood USA. New York, Garland Publishing, Inc, 1984

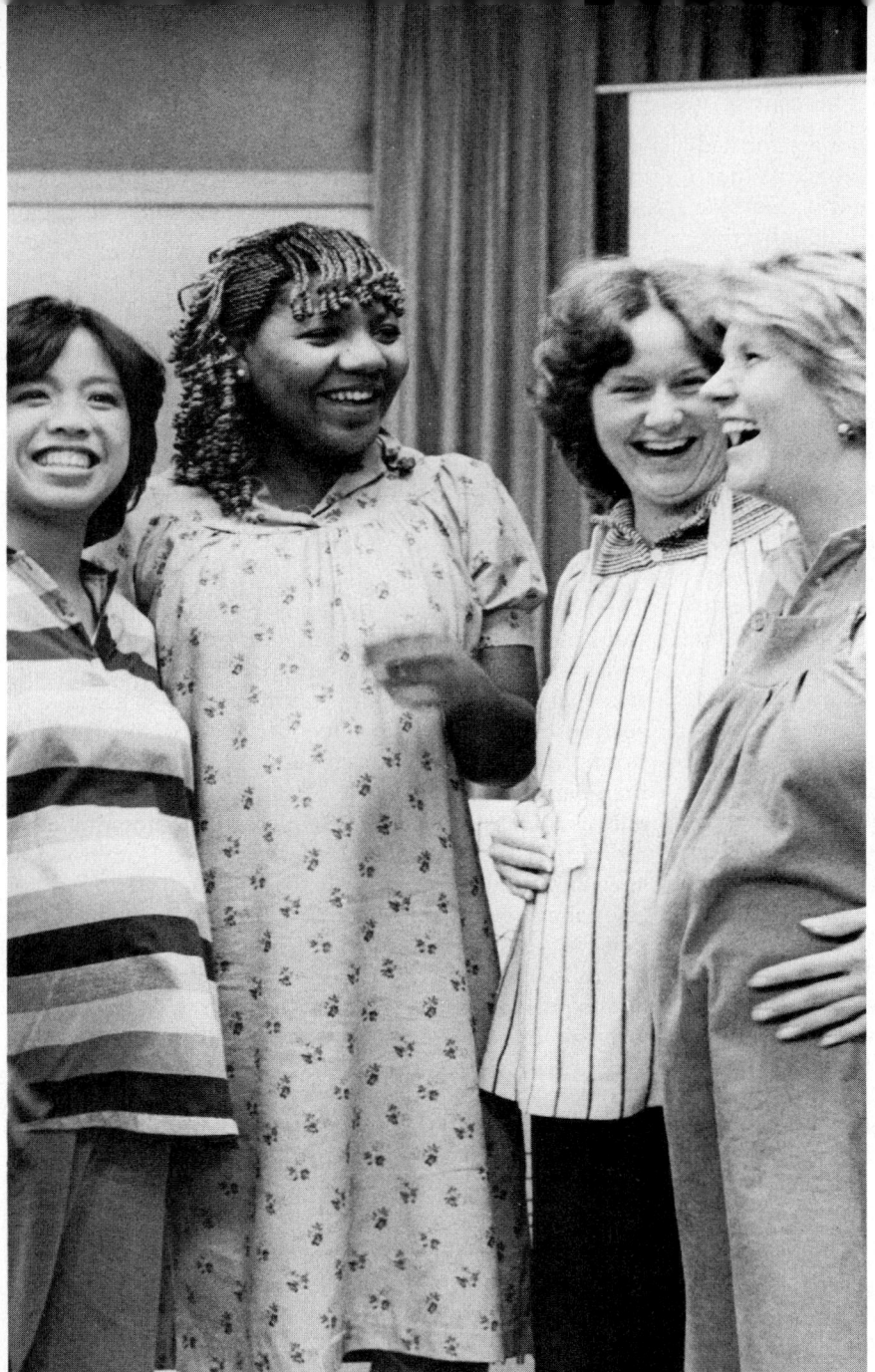

CHAPTER 6

Culture, Society, and Maternal Care

Values, attitudes, perspectives, and behavior are formed and conditioned by the social groups in which we participate from earliest childhood. Consequently, there are differing orientations to health and health care reflecting memberships in differing ethnic, racial, religious, and social-class groups. These varying health orientations become manifest both in the behavior of individuals and in the institutions that are organized to deliver health services.

In recent years, there has been a heightened awareness of the importance of social and cultural factors in health status, specifically maternal care. Although Americans are accustomed to thinking of their health status as being the best and highest in the world, their health care is still far short of its potential. Large segments of the population either do not have access to adequate medical care or are deprived of quality care in the services that they do receive. There has been a great stimulus to improve the prenatal care system, in particular, in order to improve the delivery of maternal-care services and thus reduce preterm, low birth weight, and infant deaths. Essentially, there has been an expansion and elaboration of the existing system of maternity services. Whether such an approach to maternity problems will have the desired effects depends on a variety of factors.

In this chapter the focus is upon those forces and features in society that influence the field of maternity services. First, it is important to examine the social and cultural meaning of pregnancy. What are the current social, cultural, and economic forces that influence motivations for childbearing? Second, we will discuss some of the critical issues in access and use of maternal services and finally present some aspects of the nurse's role in these matters.

Social and Cultural Meaning of Childbearing

For nurses to function appropriately, to use their talents more creatively than in the past, they must have an understanding of the social and cultural meaning of pregnancy. As discussed in Chapter 1, pregnancy itself needs to be considered in terms of the social context in which it occurs, namely, the family and the larger society. Moreover, pregnancy and childbearing in general have different meanings in various societies and even within any given society.

In Western society the expectations and the prescriptions for behavior surrounding pregnancy are relatively ill defined, and in some situations they do not exist. Consequently, women are often uncertain when and how often they ought to visit the physician and what is expected of them by significant others.

The Sick Role, Illness, and Pregnancy

How a society or groups within a society define pregnancy and cope with pregnancy tends to vary considerably. In some societies, pregnancy is regarded as a "normal" situation, a kind of status passage through which most women, at some time or other, will pass. In other societies, pregnancy may be regarded as an illness and is reacted to as other illnesses are. Moreover, there is considerable variation, even within societies, in the way health and illness are perceived by different social classes, ethnic groups, and age categories.

Concept of the Sick Role

The sick role has been developed as a concept by sociologists to study the role behavior of persons who are considered to be sick or to have an illness. In brief, the sick role concept refers to the process by which every society ensures that an adequate level of health and normative conformity exists among the majority of its members most of the time. Society has various mechanisms for accomplishing this purpose. It accommodates individuals or groups who are ill by placing them in a special position or status. The term *social role* refers to both the regular way of acting, which is expected of persons occupying a given position, and the social position itself. Typically there are certain rights, privileges, and expectations associated with given social positions. Parsons has presented an insightful and systematic analysis of the expectations associated with occupancy of the sick role.[1] There are two main rights in the sick role: (1) the sick person is allowed exemption from the performance of normal social-role obligations and (2) the sick person is allowed exemption from the responsibility for his own state. There are also two main obligations: (1) the sick person must be motivated to get well as soon as possible and (2) the sick person should seek technically competent help and cooperate with medical experts.

The sick role is generally thought of as only a theoretical model for the purposes of understanding the processes contributing to and the various conditions to be fulfilled in the legitimation of illness conditions. In reality, the concept is not universally applicable to all who claim to be ill; it varies depending on the unique background of the person, the particular illness involved, and the social context within which legitimation is sought.[2]

Behavioral scientists have made a number of criticisms concerning the sick role, including the fact that Parsons has left open the problem of the chronically ill, as well as some illness that is not considered serious enough to warrant more than a slight reduction in normal activities. Furthermore, much illness never reaches the stage of formal consultation with a qualified physician. Individuals who are ill may receive what they consider to be competent help from other than professional medical personnel. Finally, Parsons's formulation may not be relevant to all societies, and various studies have demonstrated that there are both intercultural and intracultural variations in the definitions of the conditions to which the sick role is thought to be applicable.

Pregnancy and the Sick Role

The state of pregnancy in its usual or normal situation, in which there are no resultant obstetric or delivery complications, must be considered in the discussion of the applicability of the sick-role concept. If a woman is experiencing complications of pregnancy, certainly this would make her eligible for the sick role as discussed above. The question that arises is whether pregnancy is in fact a "normal" state.

One may conceivably take the position that illness, or sickness, is statistically normal in most members of the population at some point in their lives; similarly, pregnancy can likewise be considered statistically normal in that most of the population of possible conceivers at some time are in this state. Pregnancy can also be considered normal in the sense that it is a necessary biologic function for the species. Indeed, it can even be considered a desirable state of affairs. In this latter sense, it is not similar to illness at all. McKinlay has noted that pregnancy differs from illness by "calling forth in both the woman and her significant others a set of responses which are in many ways different from those elicited with the onset of an illness."[3] Considering whether the sick-role expectations noted previously apply to pregnancy, McKinlay suggests that for a variety of reasons the state of pregnancy is in some ways different from illness and cannot be analyzed in terms of any of the expectations associated with the sick role.[3]

There is a tendency in the more advanced societies to consider some point during pregnancy as illness and to treat it in a manner similar to that of illness. For example, women are discouraged from home deliveries and are hospitalized for delivery. Blood pressure, height, weight, and other vital signs are usually checked at several points during the pregnancy. Treating women as if they are ill may perhaps encourage the adoption of certain behaviors because the women perceive this type of treatment as being similar to that for an illness. In sum, the state of pregnancy and the expectations covering it differ from routine illness behavior, and the situation is relatively unstructured. This relatively unstructured situation may produce a sense of role ambiguity in pregnant women. Women may take matters into their own hands and reduce the strain from ambiguity by structuring the situation in particular ways, including adopting the sick role.[4,5]

For women who are at greater risk and who react excessively or unfavorably under the strain of pregnancy, the sick role becomes meaningful and relevant.

Thus, both in the "normal" circumstances of pregnancy and in pathologic conditions, the sick role plays an important part in maternal care.

Childbearing Motivations

No biologic event has greater significance for society than reproduction and its outcome. Reproduction is important in family dynamics and population dynamics, which, in turn, have a heavy impact on individual and national welfare. Women begin their preparation for childbearing early in life. In a sense, they begin it at the time of their own conception.

As mentioned previously, society is primarily organized for families with children, and the argument for having children can be very persuasive. Even in this newer era of voluntary childbearing, couples without children are still generally made to feel "out of place," especially if they have been married very long. Research has indicated that the value of having children remains generally accepted by the vast majority of Americans.[6]

The availability of acceptable means for preventing conception should theoretically permit childbearing today to be a consequence of motivated human action rather than mere biologic happenstance. However, regardless of when pregnancies occur or if they are planned, the number of children a couple has and the time at which they have them are to a large extent a function of the couple's childbearing motivations, which, in turn, are influenced by cultural imperatives.

Childbearing Within a Cultural System

Griffith suggests that childbearing concepts can focus on four components of a cultural system:[7]

- Mores and value systems, involving notions of duty, obligation, and desirability
- Kinship system, prescribing reciprocal rights, duties, and obligations in relationships resulting from marriage and family descent
- Knowledge and belief system, defining conception, labor, and childbearing
- Ceremonial and ritual systems, providing reenactment of symbolic elements and allowing for their incorporation into daily lives

In attempting to understand the patterns of belief surrounding childbearing in other cultures, the nurse can keep in mind the Questions Involving Belief Systems Surrounding Childbearing, listed here, as she uses the nursing process in assessing, planning, implementing, and evaluating care for her clients.

Questions Involving Belief Systems Surrounding Childbearing

Antepartum

Who may have a child?

At what age?

By whom may one have a child?

How many children can one have?

Can one space pregnancies?

What should be the behavior during pregnancy?

Are there restrictions on the father?

Are there any restrictions on sexual activity?

Who may see and touch certain body parts?

How is a fetus formed?

What are the beliefs regarding conception?

Intrapartum

What causes labor?

How does one behave during labor?

How should one respond to pain?

Should one take medication?

Where should labor take place?

Postpartum

What general behavior is expected?

What behavior is expected of the father and others?

Are there restrictions on food or activity?

Care of the Newborn

When is he recognized?

What are the rules for his care?

Who cares for him?

(Adapted from Griffith S: Childbearing and the concept of culture. JOGN Nurs 11(3):181, May/June 1982)

Present Societal Trends Affecting Childbearing Motivation

Fertility Control. In Chapter 14, techniques of contraception and family planning are discussed. In this chapter we highlight certain implications of fertility control. A number of important trends have occurred in the United States and have resulted in lower fertility. The birthrate in 1974 reached an all-time low. Currently it is on the rise, but Americans are still restricting their families to approximately two children. This is particularly true of the middle class. Thus, in the opinion of many demographers, a revolution in the fertility regimen of American women that has profound implications for society, including maternity services, is taking place. At the core of the fertility changes is an apparent reassessment of the values associated with fertility control. Thus, the widespread use of the pill and the intrauterine devices (IUDs) has resulted not only in a more effective means of fertility control but also in an apparent change in the rules under which fertility decisions are made.[8]

First, it must be recognized that the extensive use of these more reliable contraceptives not only vastly improved contraceptive protection, but also separated contraception from sexual activity. Now childbearing can be voluntary in a radically different sense than ever before. Under the previous fertility regimen, women could not confidently plan a lifetime of childlessness or the prevention of unwanted pregnancy. Not surprisingly, under this regimen the role expectations of women were structured around motherhood. In fact, cultural values with respect to fertility can be thought of, in part, as rationalizations of the inevitable. For example, in the early 1960s about one half of all births were accidental and one fifth were reported by the mothers as unwanted.[8]

The widespread use of the pill has facilitated the adoption of other effective means of preventing unwanted births (the IUD, sterilization, and abortion) and has led to reductions in the number of children intended by women in the United States. Contraceptive sterilization had been a relatively infrequent occurrence in the population prior to the introduction of the pill. In recent years there has been a dramatic reversal of this pattern with majority approval and greater use of this procedure. Since 1970 sterilization has become the most prevalent contraceptive method among women older than 30.[8,9]

Competing Social Roles. These new fertility-control values have given more support to the equal opportunity concept by making nonfamilial roles a realistic and viable option for women. Thus, the potential for complete fertility control makes childbearing a matter of choice in a sense never before realized. Motherhood itself can now become a matter of rational evaluation. The costs as well as the virtues can now be weighed.[9] One of the consequences is to place motherhood more directly in competition with these alternative, socially desirable roles. As fertility becomes more a matter for decision, greater emphasis is placed on planning. Among the factors that must be taken into account in the decision are the direct social, psychological, and economic costs of children themselves, and also the loss of the wife's earnings and intrinsic satisfaction with her occupation (Fig. 6-1).

This is no small matter. Modern life-styles are significantly dependent on the wife's earnings. In a majority of the families in which both the husband and wife have incomes, the wife's income represents over one fifth of the total family income.[8]

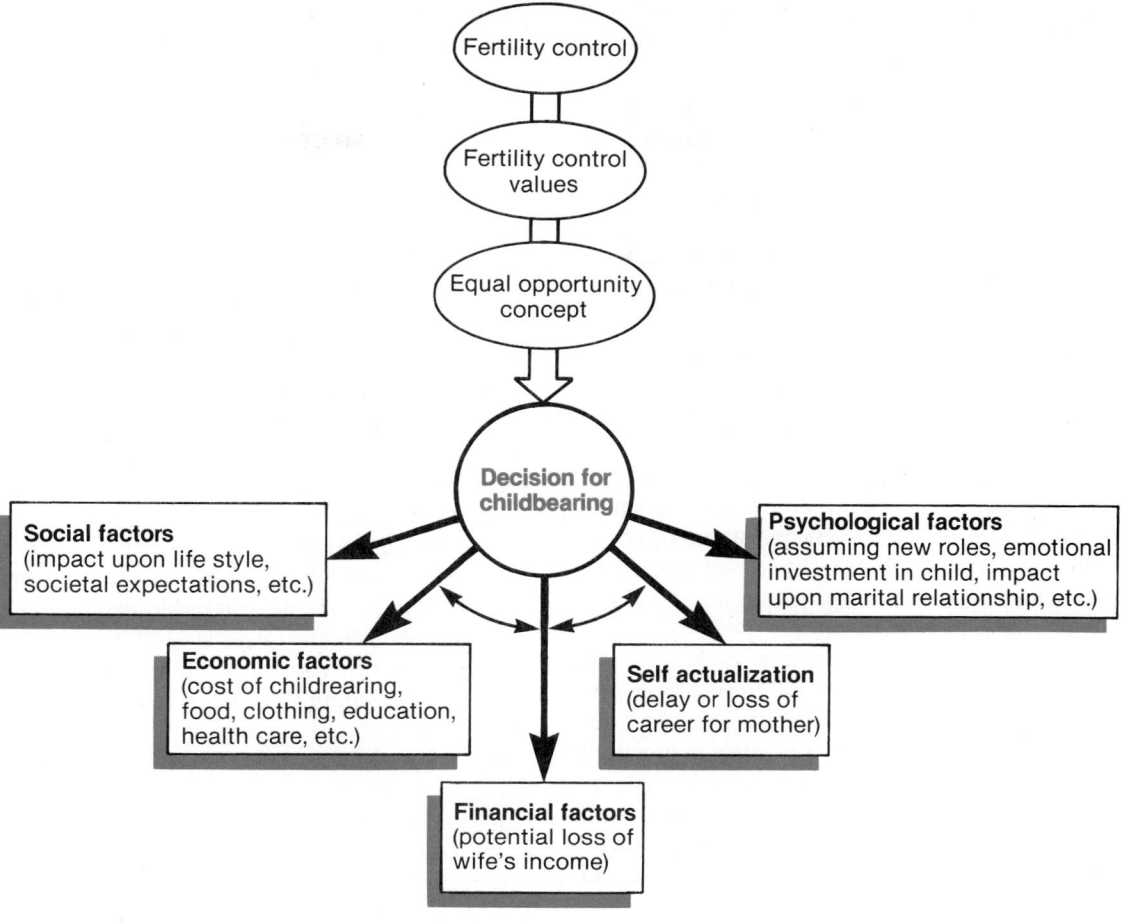

FIGURE 6-1

Fertility control has made childbearing a matter of choice. This illustration shows some of the factors that may be included in the decision for childbearing.

Impact on Maternity Services

The implications of all this are enormous, for fertility statistics influence almost every facet of our lives.

Two trends in particular are worth mentioning. First, not only are some hospitals closing their maternity units, but, perhaps more important, hospitals are merging their obstetric units and regionalization is an accomplished fact. It is hoped this will improve the quality of obstetric care for mothers and newborns, in addition to controlling costs and avoiding duplication of services. In addition, the experience of fertility control may make women more sensitive and aware of the need for better maternal care during pregnancy. Indeed, the increased availability of safe abortion after 1970 has been temporarily associated with a reduction in pregnancy-associated maternal mortality.[8] There is also good reason to connect the trends in fertility control to the recent rapid decline in infant mortality.

It should be recognized that no one knows for certain that the current pattern of fertility control will continue indefinitely. Nevertheless, it is important to note that the baby boom children of the 1950s are now forming their own families. Consequently, within the next few years there will be an increase of approximately 20% in the number of women in the childbearing age-groups of 15 to 44 years. Thus, the absolute number of births is rising even if the birthrate may not be.

Sociocultural Factors Affecting Childbearing

Sociodemographic Factors and the Use of Maternity Health Services

Social Class

Social class is an important determinant of maternal reproductive behavior and maternal use of services. Since socioeconomic status or social class has such a pervasive influence upon health and health care, it is important to briefly describe the central features of this concept.

Social class, or socioeconomic status, is a complex concept referring to a theoretical formulation of relationships between subgroups in our society. It is a term frequently used by sociologists and epidemiologists in medical research in an effort to subdivide populations into a few descriptive categories that differ in a variety of social and economic characteristics, background, and behavior.[4,10]

Typically, in determining socioeconomic status, the usual procedure is to select as indicators of social differences one or several characteristics, each of which is closely related to income, education, occupation, housing and place of residence, social values, and the general life-style of population subgroups. By far the most widely used indicator of socioeconomic status or social class is occupation. It is the best indicator of a person's income, education, standard of living, and social values, and of a variety of other attributes.

However, not all social differences stem from socioeconomic status. Dividing a population along one social dimension does not automatically provide categories that are socially meaningful in other respects. It can be demonstrated that such social variables as age, geographic region, height, parity, and ethnicity each contribute independently to the total picture of social variation in pregnancy outcome. The same may be said of other more complex social influences.

It is generally accepted that adequate medical care during pregnancy, particularly in the early stages of pregnancy, reduces the incidence of neonatal mortality, congenital malformations or other birth defects, maternal mortality, prematurity, and so on. The relationship between low socioeconomic status and failure to receive adequate antenatal care has been well documented. The data appear to be similar in the United States, Great Britain, and various other Western nations. Not only do the lower-class women typically comprise the highest proportion of those who have not received antenatal care, they are also the women, as a group, who contribute to the highest proportion of underusers of antenatal care.[11,12]

According to data for the United States, the average white mother had 60% more visits for medical care than the average nonwhite mother. This is undoubtedly related more to the influence of socioeconomic status than to the ethnicity of the mother. According to these data, as family income increased, the number of visits for medical care also increased. On the average, women living in families below the poverty level made 9.3 visits for medical care; women from middle-income families averaged 13.7 visits. Most of the women in the lowest-income group visited medical facilities (clinics, hospitals) for their care, as contrasted to the women in the highest-income group, the majority of whom visited physicians for medical care.[13,14]

Thus, income appears to be a major factor in the number of visits for prenatal care. There is a large jump in number of visits when the income goes over the poverty line.

Health-Care Organization and Social Class. Before discussing how the characteristics of lower-income persons influence their behavior in connection with the issues of health, illness, and the use of health services, it is appropriate to discuss briefly some aspects of health-care organization and care for the lower-income groups. In the 1970s there was a national commitment for equality of health care for all citizens, which led to a variety of important legislative acts. The emphasis was on extending and improving the system of health organization so that care could be offered more efficiently to the poor as well as to those more economically advantaged. For example, the federally subsidized maternal- and infant-care projects (MIC) were instituted to help reduce the incidence of mental retardation and other handicapping conditions caused by complications associated with childbearing and to help reduce infant and maternal mortality. These programs have been concentrated in the low-income areas of large and small cities and have emphasized early, comprehensive prenatal care for all clients in the geographic area served. The results, however, have been somewhat equivocal, although they have been considered to have had some success. With the current era of economic austerity in governmental subsidies, it remains to be seen whether or not these kinds of programs will continue to be viable and whether or not there will continue to be a national commitment to quality health services for all strata of society.[13,14] There is also a serious question as to whether the inequities in the medical care system can be overcome unless changes are made reflecting greater understanding of lower socioeconomic life-styles. It is well known that when health-care facilities are set up in convenient proximity to lower-income housing, they do not automatically draw clientele.

There are two factors that contribute to inequities of health care. The first of these relates to the way in which health organization facilities are structured, including the distribution of services and manpower concerns; the second is concerned with the characteristic life-styles of lower-income groups.

Health-Care Organization

What are the features of health-care organization that tend to blunt the effectiveness of medical care for lower-income clients?

Size

First, there is the massiveness of medical organization itself. Most lower-income women tend to visit medical facilities such as hospitals and clinics. These are often large and complex organizations, characterized by great specialization and a fair degree of impersonality. Lower-class clients are ill equipped by lack of education and experience to cope with complex bureaucratic organization.[13] Moreover, they often lack confidence in the community facilities for their care. They believe that adequate health care is a right of citizenship; however, when they seek it, they often find that two kinds of care exist, one for those who can pay and another for those who cannot. Since so many people now feel that proper health care is a right of citizenship, the provision of adequate health services for all requires a restructuring of present national priorities and an escalation of the public's social consciousness. Most health professionals agree that any worthwhile program should provide financial support and maintain the mother's dignity as well. The concept of comprehensive health planning by states and localities, including area health-education centers, community clinics, and innovative programs in hospital clinics, has been an attempt to provide a higher caliber of care for all segments of society.

Within the past 10 years, the focus of service in many outpatient departments and clinics of hospitals has changed from dispensing first aid to giving ambulatory care. As a result, the ambulatory-care department is now one of the most dynamic, change-oriented departments in many hospitals.[13,14]

As part of this change, nursing service in these ambulatory-care settings has replaced the managerial role with a care-centered, more independent role in which nurses are expanding their functions of educating clients, providing supportive guidance, and making observations. In this role, the professional nurse becomes the health professional who is primarily responsible for maintaining continuity of health care for a specific client population.[15,16]

Increasingly, expanded nursing roles such as the nurse practitioner and clinical specialist are used to provide routine prenatal care in outpatient, ambulatory settings.

Professionalization

A second feature of medical organization that tends to decrease the quality of care for lower-income clients is professionalization. Its perspectives toward work and clients result in a gap between the clients and the professionals. Lower-income people are less skilled in obtaining information from professionals. They tend to be less aggressive in demanding explanations. On the other hand, higher-income clients have greater aggressive and interactional skills and can cope more effectively with the professional's failure to communicate.

Lower-income clients also suffer from other, more subtle disadvantages stemming from professional stances. These have been discussed by a number of investigators in the field of mental disorders. That is, middle-class clients are preferred by most providers and are viewed as more treatable. In other words, there may be a distinct bias expressed against the lower-income client, based honestly on professional conceptions. Also, many regimens are impossible for low-income clients to carry out. The simple order that medication is to be taken "with each meal" may not recognize that many lower-income families eat irregularly and may not have three meals a day.[10]

Middle-Class Bias

Another characteristic of medical organization that influences the quality of medical care is the middle-class bias of most professional health workers. Typically, the staff members do not understand the perspectives, attitudes, customs, and life-styles of the lower-income clients. They often take for granted that the clients have the same attitudes about health as they do. Hence, they tend to issue orders that are not understood or cannot be easily followed by lower-income clients. Furthermore, there is a tendency to think of lower-income people in stereotyped terms: they cannot keep appointments, they have little sense of time or responsibility, and so on. Lower-income clients may perceive these class biases, and this may affect the underutilization of health-care services.

The many hours of waiting, the impersonal routines of institutional care in large hospitals or clinics, particularly in the municipal and county hospitals, and the real or imagined perceptions of racial and class bias all tend to maximize dissatisfactions of lower-income clients and reduce the possibility of use of health facilities. Furthermore, the distances that clients must travel to the facilities and the cost of transportation are realistic matters. Customarily, poor people organize their lives so as not to go far for the necessities of living. This is one of the factors in the relative success of the MIC program that reached into the lower-income communities and brought the clinic facilities into the neighborhood. Similarly, the neighborhood health centers have been relatively successful for this reason.[13,15,16]

Distribution and Manpower

The maldistribution of health personnel, which is characteristic of our urban specialty orientation in health care, contributes to the disparity in outcomes noted among various population groups. Rural and geographically isolated communities have traditionally experienced difficulties obtaining adequate health care because professional socialization and economic considerations promote practice in highly populated metropolitan areas. Inner-city areas also suffer a lack of health-care resources, largely due to economic factors and cultural differences between providers and clients.

It is felt that quality maternity care in the future will be provided by a closely integrated team of physicians, professional nurses, nurse–midwives or nurse practitioners, laboratory technicians, social workers, nutritionists, health educators, and homemakers. None of these is available in sufficient numbers at the present. However, the development of expanded roles for nurses and training programs for the education of paraprofessionals are proving to be viable efforts to ease this aspect of the present crisis. Research has indicated that when nurses use expanded roles and are integral members of the health-care team, there are considerably fewer broken antepartal appointments, better postpartal clinic attendance, better use of family-planning services and techniques, and reduction of infant mortality.[13,15,17]

Government programs have been developed to encourage health professionals to enter practice in medically underserved rural or inner-city urban areas. Efforts such as the National Health Service Corps, which supports team practices between physicians and nurse practitioners in rural communities; Medicare reimbursement of nurse practitioners and physicians' assistants in rural clinics; scholarships and educational subsidies for primary-care providers; and program grants for primary care to schools of nursing and medicine are steps toward ensuring greater availability and appropriate distribution of health personnel.

One of the most effective methods of providing care to underserved populations, whether they are geographically isolated or culturally unique, has been training of indigenous community members through decentralized educational programs. This often improves the quality of care. Their familiarity with the life-styles of childbearing families, their knowledge of the socioeconomic factors to be considered, and their willingness to provide whatever service is needed, be it transportation or referral for counseling, are salient factors in the improvement of reproductive outcomes. There is a very important message in the majority of the current research on the delivery of antepartal services to the various segments of society. Programs that are planned by outsiders and that do not consider the involvement of those whom they serve are doomed to failure and in no way deliver the quality of care that they ostensibly were designed to give.

Lack of coordination and overlap in agencies presents another dimension of maldistribution of health services. For example, there may be several community-health nursing services in one area, such as the health department, a voluntary nursing agency, and school nursing services. Many times they all serve one family, but they seldom communicate with one another regarding the total needs of the family. Similarly, some hospitals may be overcrowded, while others have empty beds.

The development of innovations such as community clinics and alternative birth centers are attempts by the health system to respond to consumer needs. Community clinics are initiated and organized by the indigenous population and are staffed largely by local people. Health professionals who share the ethnic and cultural background of the community are usually recruited. Supported largely by federal and state funds, community clinics can be very effective in responding to specific health-care needs of the population, served in a setting compatible with the values and style of the culture.

Alternative birth centers are special units associated with an acute hospital, which offer a more homelike atmosphere for labor and delivery. Low-risk mothers undergo labor in a comfortable room without the usual equipment and requirements of standard labor rooms and deliver in a natural position in the same bed (Fig. 6-2). Companions may be present in varying mix, and there is little intervention by the health provider beyond basic safety monitoring.

The National Health Planning and Resources Development Act of 1974.   Public Law 93-641, the National Health Planning and Resources Development Act of 1974, was intended to affect the distribution and quality of maternity services as well as other health-care services. This act established Health Systems Agencies, which are regional organizations within states that have primary responsibility for health planning and development of health services, manpower, and facilities to meet the needs of their service areas. These agencies are charged with four responsibilities, as listed in Responsibilities of Health Systems Agencies.

Guidelines for implementation of this law were issued by the Secretary of the former Department of

---

Responsibilities of Health Systems Agencies

1. Improving the health of residents of a health-service area
2. Increasing the accessibility (including overcoming geographic, architectural, and transportation barriers), acceptability, continuity, and quality of the health services provided them
3. Restraining increases in the cost of providing them health services
4. Preventing unnecessary duplication of health resources[18]

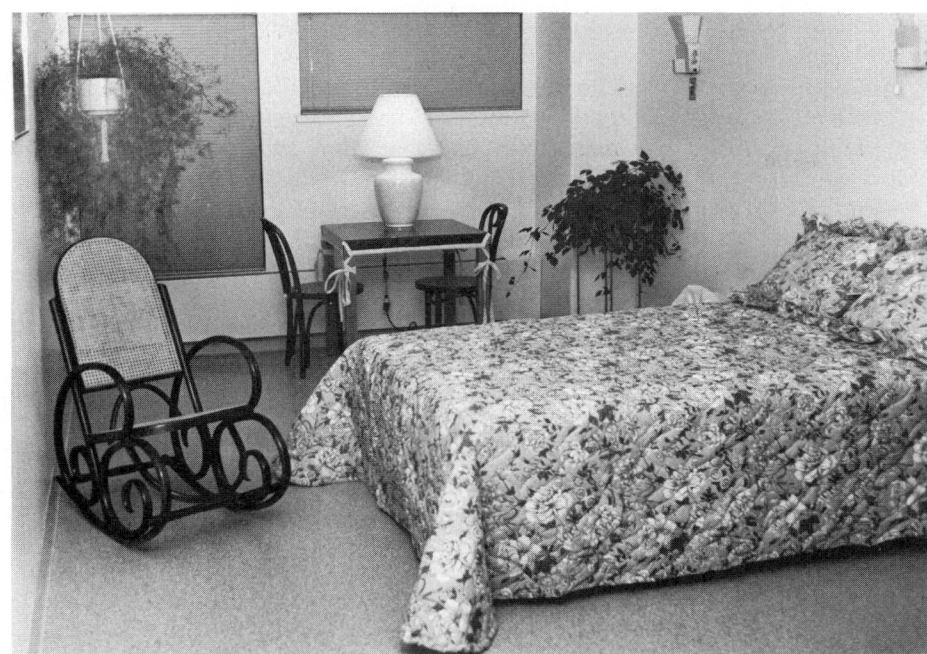

Health, Education, and Welfare. The general thrust is to set a minimum number of deliveries per year for a hospital to maintain an obstetric service, therefore promoting concentration of deliveries in larger regional centers to increase efficiency and cost-effectiveness. There are exception clauses for small, rural communities, isolated geographic areas, and transportation distances. The continued influence of Public Law 93-641 will depend upon the levels of support provided by Congress and the administration for operation of the Health Systems Agencies.

Life-styles and Social Class

It is important to take into account the characteristic life-styles of the poor. The lower-income person's experience of himself and his world is highly distinctive in our country. It is also distinctive for its problems and crisis-dominated character. Health concerns are minor to those who feel they confront much more pressing troubles. Health problems are just one crisis among many with which they must try to cope.

Indeed, the value orientations of the medical system reflect the values of the middle- and upper-middle classes. These have been characterized as activistic, rational mastery, future-time orientation to life. A large body of empirical research data suggests that the values of the middle class tend to result in a specific outlook on life that is reflected in health beliefs and behavior. Conversely, the lower classes, whose position in the social structure does not support a belief in the rational mastery of the world, tend to have quite a different orientation of the world. There is a feeling of lack of control over events; occurrences are viewed as luck or fate rather than as planned by rational design. Planning, education, and involvement in organized activity are less important in this framework; they seek help from those in their social network rather than from "experts" or professionals.[19]

Another problem is that many lower-income households are often much more understaffed than those of higher incomes. Understaffing of households means that each individual's health receives relatively little attention as far as preventive measures are concerned, and when someone is sick it is more difficult to care for him or her at home. When the main family member is sick, he or she will be in a disadvantaged position in caring properly for himself or herself. There is a necessity for poor people to learn to live with illness rather than to use their limited financial and psychological resources to do something about illness.

Lower-income people also do not conform to the expectations of how "good" and "considerate" clients should behave in medical settings. Their behavior is often frustrating and annoying to nursing and medical personnel for a variety of reasons.

Economic Concerns

Although the stated goals for health care on the national level include ensuring quality, access, and control of costs, methods of financing services continue to support disparities among population groups. The chief protection for the health needs of most of America's young parents in voluntary and commercial prepayment insurance. Unfortunately, the maternity benefits traditionally have been distressingly low. Young people with low incomes are frequently saddled with a large medical and hospital bill at a time when they can least afford to pay. Many professionals feel that maternity care should be entirely covered, but the actuarials believe that the rates for this kind of coverage would be prohibitive. However, it might be noted that insurance companies have had this opinion about other forms of coverage and under public pressure have increased benefits. Many community-health leaders feel that the resources of this country are so vast that full coverage is feasible if there is a public mandate to provide it.

Various bills for national health insurance have been introduced in the United States Congress, but conflicting goals and assumptions continue to make it very difficult for legislators to develop a comprehensive, widely acceptable plan. Many question the commitment of the majority to the concept that equitable health care is a right of all people. Certainly our values supporting individual rights and minimum government interference and our pluralistic governmental structure provide significant obstacles to a sense of national social purpose. The involvement of concerned health professionals in the governmental processes can help promote an equitable health-care system that is responsive to promotion of health and prevention of illness (Fig. 6-3).

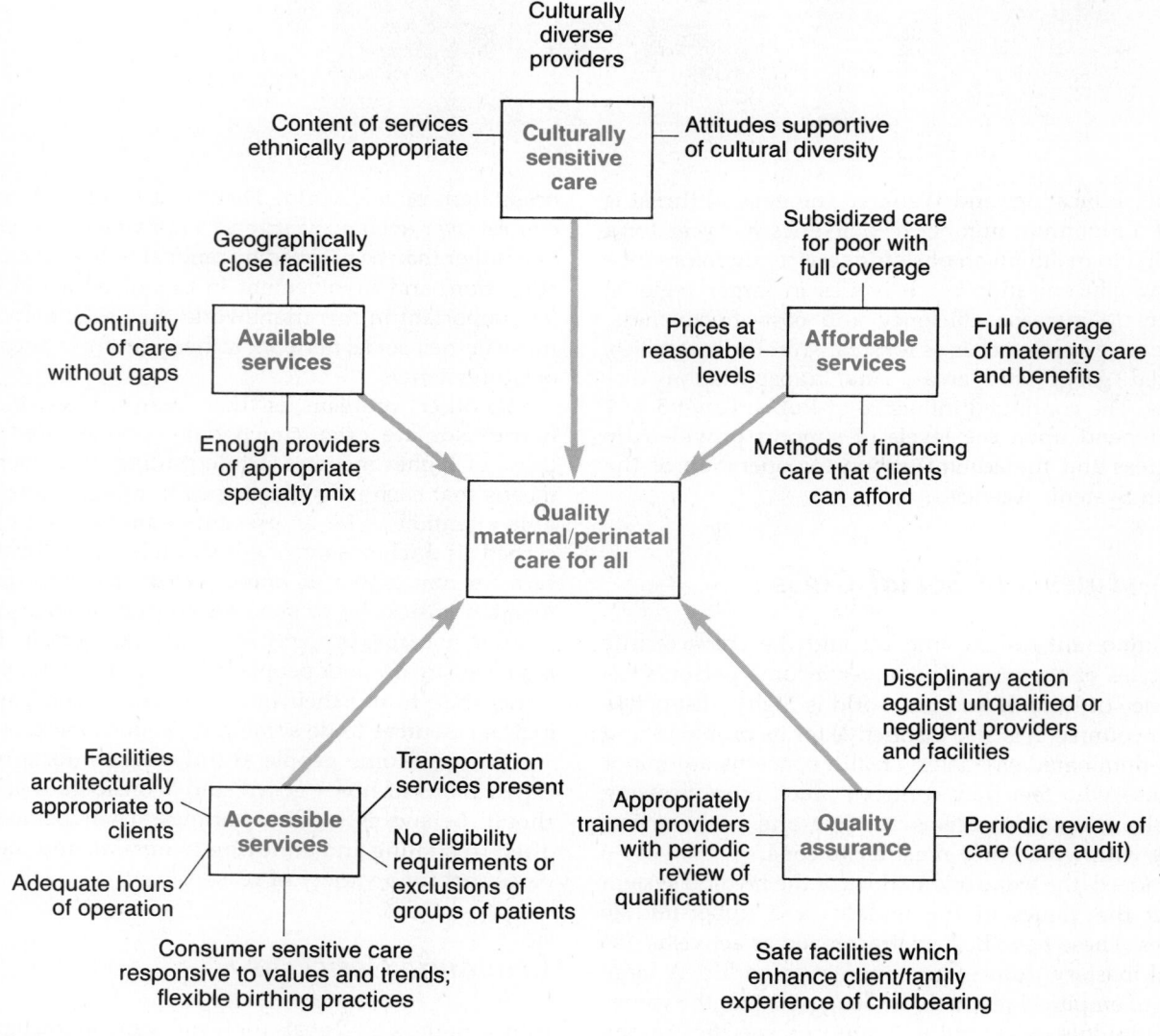

FIGURE   6 - 3

Health-care system requirements for providing quality maternity/perinatal care for all.

Ethnicity and Geographic Area

Evidence indicates that white mothers receive care earlier in pregnancy than nonwhite mothers. There is a consistent difference between white and nonwhite mothers in the receipt of medical care during each of the trimesters of pregnancy. There is evidence that women living in metropolitan areas receive care earlier than those outside metropolitan areas; this holds true for both white and nonwhite women. Furthermore, more nonwhite women in metropolitan areas are known to have received care than nonwhite women residing outside metropolitan areas. It is worth noting, though, that for any given income or educational group the differences between metropolitan and nonmetropolitan areas are insignificant with respect to the time when mothers first receive medical care.[20]

Age and Parity

Furthermore, there is a differential by age and parity; women in the younger age-group tend to come to prenatal care later than women in the other age-groups. This may be owing to the fact that the highest rates of unwed pregnancies are in the youngest age-groups. Both the young mother and the unwed mother tend to be latecomers to prenatal care. Multiparas who have had little trouble with previous pregnancies also tend to come later and be more lax in keeping appointments.

Additional Factors in the Use of Maternity Services

The issues discussed here are also related to the changing relationships between the client–patient and the providers of maternity services, physicians and nurses.

Consumers complain that it is becoming more and more difficult to find a primary-care physician who will give them the personal attention they want. Regardless of the social class level of the woman, it is very difficult for her to receive continuity of care from the personnel who provide maternity services. Regardless of its other merits, group practice sometimes disrupts the relationship between patient and physician; hospital structure requires nursing personnel to change with shift changes; clients have difficulty determining the status of the person in the medical office to whom they are speaking on the telephone. Patients feel that the obstetrician seems to relinquish his responsibility for the neonate during the postpartum period. Similarly, in this period, the pe-

diatrician (from the mother's perspective) does not appear to be centrally involved with the needs of the mother. All of these features of the medical-care system are reflected in the concept of "fragmented health care" and consumer dissatisfaction.[21]

Consumer Satisfaction

Consumer satisfaction, that is, the satisfaction of pregnant women, refers to the attitudes toward the health-care system of those who have experienced a contact with the system. It is different from the medical and health beliefs of the client in that it is concerned with the satisfaction of the client with the quantity or quality of care actually received. There are several dimensions to this concept, including (1) accessibility-convenience of services (convenience of care and emergency care); (2) availability (family physicians, hospitals, specialists, complete facilities); (3) continuity (regular family physician, same physician); (4) physician conduct (consideration of feelings, explanations, prudent risks, quality, regular checkup); and (5) financial aspects (cost of services, insurance coverage, payment mechanisms). However, little is known about the relationship of these features of client satisfaction to other social-psychological dimensions such as perceived health, values, psychological well-being, and general sentiments about life.

Communication

A crucial feature of this aspect of maternity care is the quality and quantity of client–provider communication. Here we refer not only to the physician, but also to the nurse in communicating with the client and her needs. One of the more important transactions that occurs in the provider–client relationship is effective communication from the provider to the client concerning the nature of her condition and the actions to be taken. The degree to which she has understood the physician and can verbalize the physician's advice and instructions depends on the quality of the relationship. Similarly, good health care results in communication from the client to the physician. In particular, the degree to which the woman's concerns, worries, and fears about her condition have been perceived by the physician are equally important.

Commentators on the physician–client relationship frequently have discussed the social-class and value differences between providers and clients as one barrier to communication and ultimately to utilization of health services. Numerous studies have demonstrated that working-class clients tend to be diffident in questioning physicians, especially about their health or illness condition. These studies indicate that middle-class clients tend to obtain most of their information about illness by asking their physicians and nurses direct questions. In contrast, working-class clients receive their information from a passive process in which they are given information without asking; they also tended to receive less information.[22]

Despite their reluctance to request information, working-class maternity clients are not much different from upper-class clients in their desire for information.[20] Although upper-class clients may desire more technical details regarding their health condition, there is no general social-class difference in clients' desires for as much information as possible presented in nontechnical language.

Part of the issue of better communication between provider and client results from a reflection of a general social-class difference in language use, which was alluded to previously. Working-class clients sense that physicians do not expect them to ask questions; they tend to hold the physicians in awe, and there is social distance. But even middle-class clients hesitate to freely communicate with their physician about troublesome problems or symptoms. A virtual legend has been created by the media about the hardworking, busy physician. It has become generally accepted throughout our society that all physicians are extremely busy professionals. Thus, although there may be some apparent social-class differences in the quantity and quality of communication with physicians, it is a matter of degree of communication.

Implications for the Nurse as Communicator

Given this situation, the maternity nurse has a crucial role to play. By and large the nurse is not perceived by the client in the same manner as the physician. Clients perceive the nurse as filling a substantially different role, with accompanying differences in expectations. Thus, the nurse has an opportunity to fill a much-needed role in the delivery of health care by seizing the initiative and closing the communication gap in the client–provider relationship. Such action would be congruent with client expectations; moreover, several studies have indicated that the nurse can perform roles involving the receiving and giving of information to clients far more effectively than can physicians.

These problems of communication have been emphasized here because, among other things, the client's perceived difficulties in communicating with medical providers has a direct influence upon the use of health services.

References

1. Parsons T: Definitions of health and illness in the light of American values and social structure. In Parsons T (ed): Social Structure and Personality, pp 257–291. Glencoe, IL, The Free Press, 1964
2. Segall A: The sick role concept: Understanding illness behavior. J Health Soc Behav 17(2):162–169, 1976
3. McKinlay JB: The new latecomers for antenatal care. Br J Prevent Soc Med 24:52–65, 1970
4. Bond J, Bond S: From the public point of view. Nurs Mirror 150(7):26–30, Feb 14, 1980
5. Bond J, Bond S: Changing images. Nurs Mirror 150(10):28–31, March 6, 1980
6. Hutter M: The Changing Family: Comparative Perspectives. New York, John Wiley & Sons, 1981
7. Griffith S: Childbearing and the concept of culture. JOGN Nurs 11(3):181–184, May/June 1982
8. Glick PC: American household structure in transition. Fam Plann Perspect 16(5):204–211, Sept/Oct 1984
9. Devore NE: Parenthood postponed. Am J Nurs 83(8):1161–1163, Aug 1983
10. Cox C: Where are we now? Midwives Chronicle 95(1128):3–6, Jan 1982
11. Flint C: Getting it right for mother and baby. Nurs Mirror 151(6):11–13, Aug 7, 1980
12. Hall MH, Chang PK, MacGillivray I: Is routine antenatal care worthwhile? Lancet 2(8185):78–82, July 12, 1980
13. Wilner S et al: A comparison of the quality of maternity care between a health maintenance organization and fee for service practices. N Engl J Med 304(13):784–789, March 26, 1981
14. Quick JD, Greenlick MR, Roghmann KL: Prenatal care and pregnancy outcome in an HMO and general population: A multivariate cohort analysis. Am J Public Health 71(4):381–389, April 1981
15. Lubic RW: Evidence that the childbearing center has influenced hospital maternity practice. Birth 10(3):179, Fall 1983
16. Baruffi G et al: A study of pregnancy outcomes in a maternity center and a tertiary care hospital. Am J Public Health 74(9):973–978, Sept 1984
17. Norton K: Beyond "choice" in childbirth. Birth 10(3):179–182, Fall 1983
18. Public Law 93-641, 88 Stat. 2236. 93rd Congress S 2994, 4 January 1975, pp 6–7
19. Hyman H: The value systems of different classes. In Bendix R, Lipset S (eds): Class Status and Power, pp 426–442. Glencoe, IL, The Free Press, 1953
20. Nelson MK: The effect of childbirth preparation on women of different social classes. J Health Soc Behav 23:339–352, Dec 1982
21. May KA, Ditolla K: In-hospital alternative birth centers: Where do we go from here? MCN 9:48–59, Jan/Feb 1984
22. Pratt L et al: Physicians' views on the level of medical information among patients. Am J Public Health 47:1277–1283, 1975

Suggested Reading

Bartley D: Preconceptual care. Nurs Mirror 157(16):ix–x, Oct 19, 1983

Bryant NB: Self help groups: An important strategy for perinatal health. J CA Perinatal Assoc IV(1):24–27, Winter 1984

Lubic RW: Childbirthing centers, delivering more for less. Am J Nurs 83(7):1053–1056, July 1983

Luegenbiehl DL: The birth system in Germany. JOGN Nurs 14(1):45–49, Jan/Feb 1985

Mercer RT, Hackley KC, Bostrom AG: Relationship of psychosocial and perinatal variables to perceptions of childbirth. Nurs Res 32(4):202–207, July/Aug 1983

Reinke C: Outcomes of the first 527 births at The Birthplace in Seattle. Birth 9(4):231–238, Winter 1982

Richards MPM: The trouble with "choice" in childbirth. Birth 93(4):253–260, Winter 1982

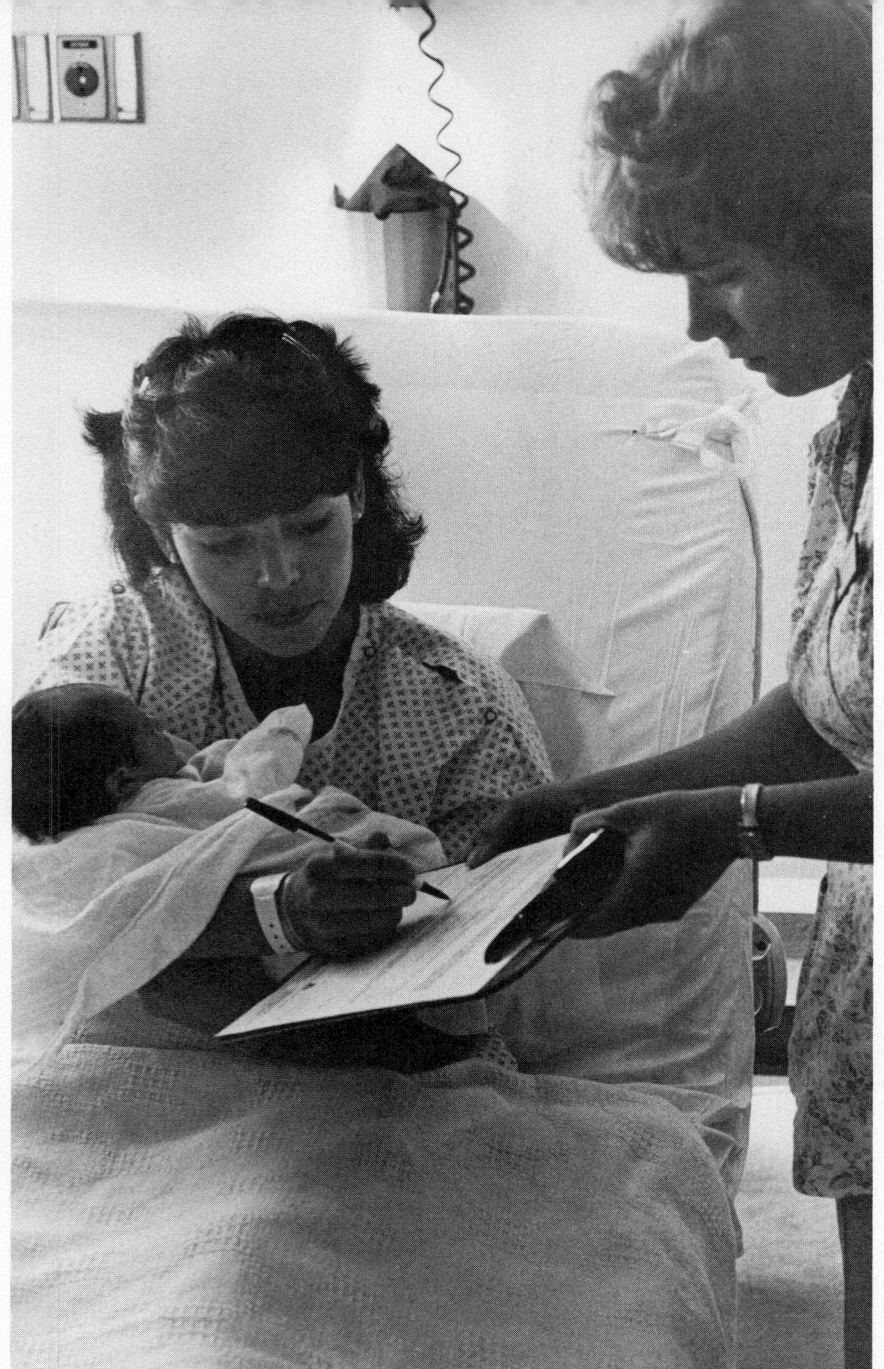

CHAPTER 7

Ethical/Legal Considerations in Reproduction

The direct personal encounters an individual has with himself and others constitute what he knows, that is, his experience, which over time becomes reality to him. As more encounters are experienced and data thought to be important are pursued and investigated, the individual's awareness and relationship to himself and others are expanded. Throughout this process, the person makes choices: what experiences to pursue, what data to discard, and so on. Rational choices are based on factual information, but they have a large subjective component that involves value judgments. The concept of choice necessarily involves freedom, that is, the ability to choose among alternatives, and the consequent responsibility for right or wrong action taken.[1] Thus, the unity of knowing and valuing that comprises an individual is put to the test when we make choices, particularly difficult ethical choices.

Curtin has made the point that not all choices or problems are ethical ones.[1] She outlines several characteristics that make ethical problems unique:

- *The problem cannot be resolved entirely from an appeal to empirical data.* For instance, should a healthy person be forced to donate an organ to someone who would otherwise die without the donor organ? Clearly any of the sciences cannot answer that question definitely; the various sciences and humanities can contribute information, but the answer lies beyond the competence of the scientific disciplines.

- *The problem is inherently perplexing.* There are a variety of conflicts of values and uncertainties about the amount or type of information needed to make a decision. If an infant is born with repairable multiple congenital anomalies, but has a chromosomal aberration that will eventually cause him to die at an early age, should aggressive efforts be made to keep him alive as long as possible, even if these efforts may cause pain and suffering for the parents as well as the neonate?

- *The answer to the ethical problem will have profound relevance for several areas of human concern.* It will have far-reaching effects on one's perception of his fellowmen, the relationships among human beings, the relationship of human beings to society, and the relationship of various societies to the world at large. If, for example, the decision is made to force a person to donate a body part to a family member, the decision is based on several premises and assumptions: a person's right to bodily integrity may be violated if someone else can benefit by it; one's right to life includes the right to require another to undergo painful surgery with the end result of permanent loss of a body part and damage to general body integrity; health professionals and others in authority can force or otherwise coerce a person to sacrifice body integrity for the well-being of another. The above choice involves the concepts of human rights, the limits of benevolence, and the power of those in authority. While the above example was dramatic and probably would not be put to a test, other issues are less clear-cut, such as a woman's right to choose an abortion or how long to prolong the life of an irreparably damaged neonate.

Curtin suggests that the above criteria be applied when the nurse is deciding whether a decision involves an ethical problem or not.[1]

Legal Aspects of Maternity/ Perinatal Care

Hankanson and others have pointed out that the maternity/perinatal field has become especially high risk for malpractice suits for several reasons.[2-4] Some hospitals are facing financial exigencies that cause them to implement staffing patterns that can be difficult and dangerous for the client and nurse alike. There has also developed an exceptionally high degree of technology for monitoring the mother and fetus preconceptually, conceptually, and postconceptually. A good deal of the techniques carry with them the risk of producing iatrogenic effects that can damage the mother or fetus and that may not be reversible. Moreover, and perhaps most importantly, there are potentially two claimants in any instance of mother–baby damage, and this doubles the risk to the nurse and other health providers. In the following paragraphs we discuss several basic legal issues that can provide a foundation for viewing and evaluating nursing practice.

Nursing Practice and Accountability

Nursing practice today is legislated by each state in the form of nurse practice acts. These practice acts define the boundaries of nursing practice by setting certain requirements regarding education, licensure, and standards of care. Since these vary among the states, it is the responsibility of the nurse to be familiar with the acts of the states in which she practices.[3,5]

Standards of care are developed by the nurse practice acts, by the hospitals or other institutions that employ the nurse, and by professional organizations such as the Nurses' Association of the American College of Obstetrics and Gynecology (NAACOG). It is important that the nurse know and implement the accepted standards of care in her community, since not to do so would result in a breach of duty or a charge of negligence. A breach of duty is considered to occur if the nurse performs an unauthorized act, fails to act, or carries out an authorized act improperly. If the nurse is found guilty of a breach of duty, she may lose her license or be a defendant in a malpractice lawsuit.[5,6] To be found guilty of negligence, the following facts must be established: (1) that the nurse had a responsibility to the client, (2) that the nurse failed to carry out that responsibility, (3) that injury was sustained by the client, and (4) that there was a causal relationship between the client's injury and the nurse's breach of duty (proximate cause). Thus, it can be seen that in nursing practice today the nurse is accountable for her care, not only morally and ethically but legally as well. In past decades, before health care became so complex and nurses expanded their roles, institutions and physicians were considered the primary responsible parties. However, with increasing independence in nursing came the responsibility to be accountable to the client for nursing care and hence to some degree for the client's well-being. Accountability also extends beyond the nurse's individual sphere of care. If the nurse knows that the quality of care given by other members of the health team is inappropriate or inferior, she also has the legal and ethical obligation to report such care to the appropriate authorities.[3,5]

One further point needs emphasis. Every nurse should carry professional liability insurance. This is in addition to any insurance provided by the institution that employs her. Institutional insurance generally covers the nurse only for the hours that she is on duty at the institution, not at other times when she might practice. The legal costs of a lawsuit can be truly horrendous; moreover, it is becoming more common for an institution to sue the nurse involved if the institution loses a malpractice suit.[5] Since adequate coverage can be purchased at a very reasonable price, it is well worth the investment for the nurse's personal protection.

Facts that Must Be Established to Prove Guilt of Negligence

1. The nurse had a responsibility to the client.
2. The nurse failed to carry out that responsibility.
3. Injury was sustained by the client.
4. There was a causal relationship between the client's injury and the nurse's breach of duty.

Breach of duty occurs if the nurse performs an unauthorized act, fails to act, or carries out an authorized act improperly.

Ethical and Legal Considerations Prior to Conception

Often a couple will have difficulty in conceiving. The reasons for infertility are many and varied (see Chap. 16).

Annas has noted that dependable birth control made sex without reproduction possible.[7] This separation of procreation from sex was viewed by some as an affirmation of love; however, it was also viewed by others as a sin against nature. One consequence, according to Annas, was the relaxation of inhibitions against sex with multiple partners, with sexually transmitted disease replacing pregnancy as the worst possible consequence. This, together with the infections associated with IUDs, the postponement of pregnancy until the late 30s, and other factors, has increased the incidence of infertility.

Now medical engineering is closing the circle of sex without reproduction by offering methods of reproduction without sex, including artificial insemination, husband (AIH); artificial insemination, donor (AID); *in vitro* fertilization (IVF); and surrogate embryo transfer (SET). As with contraception, artificial reproduction is defended by its proponents as life affirming and is denounced as unnatural by its detractors.[7]

In the following paragraphs we examine these techniques from an ethical–legal standpoint, since all have some element of controversy.

Artificial Insemination

As previously stated, artificial insemination employs two methods. In artificial insemination by the husband (AIH), the wife is inseminated within her reproductive tract with sperm from her husband. This is perhaps the least controversial of all of the "assisted parenthood" methods, since it is clear who the genetic and sociological parents are. Some religious denominations object to masturbation as a means of sperm collection, but in general this method is without grave ethical or legal questions.

The second method, artificial insemination, donor (AID), is more problematical. The woman is inseminated with the sperm of an anonymous donor. This method, of course, separates the sociological parent (the woman's husband) from taking part of his offspring's conception. This method has become the preferred treatment when the husband has an absence or marked decrease in the amount of sperm. AID is also used when the husband suffers from a genetic defect or is Rh sensitized. As long as the *husband* of the woman consents, the donor is not considered the *legal* father of the child. Thus, the husband replaces the genetic father as the legal father of the child. As can be seen, this therapeutic model places contracts among the parties ahead of genetic or "blood-line" considerations. This model has been suggested as a model for embryonic transfer, but there is a large question as to whether it fits or not.[7]

Legal obligations are satisfied by written informed consent by all parties—wife, husband, and donor. It is recommended that the donor and husband and wife all remain anonymous and that the physician be given the right to select the donor. This latter point raises questions as to the limits of authority for the professional. The consent usually includes a clause removing liability from the health professionals in the event the child is born with abnormalities. The question of the child's legitimacy can be resolved by adoption.[7]

In Vitro Fertilization

A variety of ethical and legal questions have been raised over time regarding *in vitro* fertilization (IVF). The first live birth using this technique occurred in 1978, and by January 1984 over 200 children had been born in the United States and abroad following IVF and embryo transfer. In this procedure, an egg or eggs are removed from a woman's ovary, fertilized by sperm in a laboratory dish, cultured, and then transferred back into the uterus. According to the American Fertility Society, at least 46 centers in the United States have or are planning to have IVF clinics.[8]

The demand keeps growing. The National Center for Health Statistics estimates that almost half of currently married women aged 15 to 44 suffer from some degree of infertility, and 10% of married couples fail to conceive after 1 year of no contraceptive use.[9] IVF is the only method of reproduction for women whose fallopian tubes are damaged or missing. It is also used for wives whose husbands have low sperm counts, women whose cervical mucus is nonreceptive to sperm, and women with infertility of unknown causes.[10]

While this procedure moves ahead clinically, there has been no *federally* funded research in humans since 1975 because of a *de facto* moratorium. Congress first imposed a temporary moratorium on fetal research on July 12, 1974 (Public Law 93-348). This was technically lifted on August 8, 1975 when regulations were issued by what was then the Department of Health, Education, and Welfare. These regulations required all proposals dealing with IVF and fetal research to be reviewed by a national Ethics Advisory Board (EAB) in addition to the usual Institutional Review Board (IRB) review and peer review for scientific merit. The EAB was duly but slowly constructed, and it examined the topic of IVF thoroughly and concluded in a report on May 4, 1979

Recommendations of the Ethics Advisory Board (EAB)

1. The department should consider support of carefully designed research involving *in vitro* fertilization and embryo transfer in animals, including non-human primates, to obtain a better understanding of the process of fertilization, implantation, and embryo development, to assess the risks to both mother and offspring associated with such procedures, and to improve the efficacy of the procedure.
2. Research involving human *in vitro* fertilization and embryo transfer is ethically acceptable provided that if the research involves human *in vitro* fertilization without embryo transfer, these conditions must be satisfied:
   - The research complies with regulations governing research with human subjects.
   - The research is designed to establish the safety and efficacy of embryo transfer and to obtain important scientific information not reasonably attainable by other means.
   - Informed consent is obtained.
   - No embryos will be sustained *in vitro* beyond the stage normally associated with the completion of implantation (14 days after fertilization).
   - The public is advised of possible risk.

   In addition, if the research involves embryo transfer following human *in vitro* fertilization, embryo transfer will be attempted only with gametes obtained from lawfully married couples.

(Adapted from Abramowitz S: The stalemate on (testtube) baby research: I. Test-tube. *Hastings Cent Rep*, 14:7, Feb 1984)

that, while controversy was legitimate, IVF with embryonic transfer was acceptable from an ethical standpoint.[8] The major conclusions of the EAB are listed in Recommendations of the Ethics Advisory Board. However, at subsequent public hearings and presentations to Congress the response was overwhelmingly negative and so a *de facto* moratorium set in.

The ethical–legal concerns have changed over the years. They can be summarized as follows:

1. *Concern over the moral status of the fetus.* The EAB concluded that the human embryo is entitled to profound respect, but this respect does not necessarily encompass the full array of legal and moral rights attributed to a person. Mainstream ethicists and theologians generally concur that IVF with embryonic transfer is not problematical as long as the EAB's guidelines are followed. The hierarchy of the Catholic church, conservative Protestants, and some Orthodox Jews, however, believe that

any tampering with the procreative process is unnatural and should not be attempted. Thus, while there is consensus among ethicists and theologians regarding the *clinical* application of the procedure, the *research* use of human embryos remains a problem.[8]

2. *Safety and efficacy.* During the 1970s there was only limited understanding about the risks involved in this procedure. As data have been collected over time, there is a good (but not conclusive) indication that there are no patterns of abnormality or short-term risks either in laboratory research with animals or in clinical experience with humans. Until further research is conducted, however, this concern will remain.[8]

3. *"The Slippery Slope."* This concern relates to the fear that research procedures performed on nonhuman mammalian species might be performed on human embryos and the results could lead to undesirable clinical applications. Other ethicists are concerned about extending the procedure to unmarried persons, including surrogate mothers, third-party donors, and the like. They see the basic relationship between husband and wife threatened and, indeed, the whole institution of marriage. These were the same concerns that artificial insemination sparked decades ago.[8]

4. *Funding and cost.* There is general acknowledgment that the procedure is costly. While some feel that it is ethical to federally fund research projects relating to IVF, it should have a low national priority, since there are many other national health problems that are far more pressing. Those who oppose the procedure strongly say that this approach to infertility is yet another high-tech, therapy-oriented, costly approach to disease and dysfunction and efforts would be better spent finding and preventing the causes of infertility and tubal obstruction.[11] Thus, the concerns persist, and it does not appear that they will be dispelled without definitive data from well-controlled research, which, as it looks now, has a very unlikely chance of strong federal support.

Surrogate Mothers and Surrogate Embryo Transfer

In surrogate embryo transfer (SET), a controversial procedure, a couple contracts with a woman to conceive and carry a child for them. At the time that the fetus is born, the surrogate mother relinquishes to the couple her rights to the infant as per the terms of a contract that has been drawn. Some have coined this only another instance of collaborative reproduction such as AID and IVF and state that we have already separated conception and gestation from childrearing through the use of adoption. However, ethical and legal issues remain.

First there is the issue of the "hiring" of the surrogate mother. The mother typically receives a fee for carrying the child. While this may seem only fair for the surrogate mother's efforts, for some the idea of the payment of money for producing a child is repugnant and morally offensive. Children are reduced to commodities to be bought and sold, and some have suggested that poor mothers may "sell" themselves as surrogates to keep their own families together.[7,12,13] Second, there is the stress of a complex relationship with a stranger in such an intimate context, which may be entangling and disturbing to the parties. For instance, the surrogate may experience depression upon giving up the child, or the couple may continue the relationship with the mother out of misplaced feelings of indebtedness. Third, the lineage of the children may become confused and the fabric of the marriage may be damaged. However, Robertson has argued that while these concerns are legitimate, they must be balanced against the deep desires of the infertile couple to have children.[14]

There are legal concerns surrounding the legality of the contractual arrangements. Gersz argues that a well-drawn contract may obviate some of the difficulties in the three-way relationship.[12] Furrow cites critics who are concerned about those cases in which no one wants the child born with impairments or in which the surrogate mother is reluctant to surrender the child.[13] The contract remains a knotty issue, since how binding it is has been disputed. The issue of the amount of control the couple can exert over the surrogate is also a difficult one. Certainly the couple wish to ensure the best possible "environment" for the fetus and may want to regulate the surrogate's nutrition and life-style. But what about the surrogate mother's right to privacy and freedom of choice?[7,12,13]

The world's first SET was born just 6 years after the birth of Louise Brown, the first baby born from IVF. The same legal and ethical considerations that surround IVF and surrogate mothers pertain here. Jones cautions that the use of a surrogate mother, even for so short a time, together with the inconvenience of synchronizing the menstrual cycles of the donor and recipient and the medical risks to the donor, will make this method less appealing to many.[15]

Amniocentesis

Amniocentesis has been available for over a decade and is discussed fully in Chapter 15. Legal issues relate to errors of omission or commission. For instance, if a woman is a candidate for the test because of age (over 35), has produced a child with a chromosomal anomaly, or has a history of genetic disease and is not made aware of the test, the physician may be culpable if she produces a defective infant. Risks and benefits of the test must also be given the patient in the form of a written consent. If the mother has the test and is told that her infant is normal and she subsequently produces a defective child, the physician and laboratory performing the test could be held accountable. If the physician has a personal belief about either the efficacy of the test or whether the woman should abort if the test shows a defective fetus, he nevertheless has the obligation to inform the patient about the test and refer her elsewhere if he feels he cannot do the test.[16]

Ethical and Legal Considerations in Abortion

The current controversy between the pro-choice and the pro-life groups has rekindled the fires that have raged around this topic. Thompson and Thompson have pointed out that nurses must understand their own ethical position on this matter if they are to render quality care to their clients.[17] Since the nurse is involved in counseling clients about abortions from a variety of standpoints, a brief review of the ethical and legal considerations is given in the following paragraphs.

Ethical Considerations

The ethics involved in this issue revolve around terminating the life of a fetus by removing it from the uterus, that is, from its life support system. It has been argued that if given a choice, humans would choose health and lack of suffering for themselves. Furthermore, the argument goes, humans do not have the right to inflict the tragic consequences of detectable diseases on a fetus. By aborting a defective fetus, "nothingness" is given rather than the pain of living with an abnormality, and the damaged fetus can be replaced with a normal one in a subsequent pregnancy.[18] While this line of reasoning supports aborting damaged fetuses, it does not address the ethics of aborting healthy (or undetermined) products of conception, and it raises the issue of who determines what is normal or healthy.

Pro-choice advocates take the position that the mother has the ultimate responsibility and freedom of choice regarding her body. It is important to remember that pro-choice is not pro-abortion. Pro-choice advocates stress using abortion only as a last resort. They uphold responsible use of contraception, amniocentesis to determine fetal defects, and adoption whenever possible. Pro-life advocates believe that the fetus is human from the time of conception and that to destroy human life is murder and, hence, indefensible morally.

Legal Considerations

Abortion Made Legal

In 1973, in the historical *Roe v. Wade* case, the US Supreme Court declared that abortion was legal anywhere in the United States. The basis of the decision was that existing state laws prohibiting abortion were unconstitutional because they invaded the mother's privacy. They also stipulated several other points: a state could not prevent a woman from obtaining an abortion from a licensed physician any time during the first trimester; during the second trimester the state could regulate the performance of an abortion to protect the woman's health; in the third trimester the state could regulate and even prohibit abortions except in cases in which the mother's life or health might be jeopardized. The state also had the right to impose safeguards for the fetus in that trimester. The decision did not provide for "abortion on demand." It was the intent that physicians

---

Legal Status of Abortion

In 1973 the United States Supreme Court ruled that abortion was legal; a summary of the decision follows:

1. The abortion decision and its implementation must be left to the judgment of the woman and her physician when pregnancy is in the first trimester.
2. After the first trimester and before the end of the second trimester, the state, in promoting its interest in the health of the pregnant woman, may choose to regulate abortions in ways that are reasonably related to health.
3. After pregnancy has reached the time of viability (defined as 24 to 26 weeks' gestation), the state, in promoting its interest in the potentiality of human life, may, if it chooses, regulate and even proscribe abortion except where it is necessary, in medical judgment, to preserve the life or health of the pregnant woman.

In 1976, the Supreme Court further ruled that the state cannot impose the requirement of consent by a third party on the woman's right to abortion; thus, abortion cannot be denied if a spouse or parent objects.

In 1983, the Supreme Court struck down state restrictions that imposed waiting periods for first-trimester abortions, that required specific informed consents, and that required hospitalization for second-trimester abortions.

Though states can implement requirements for parental notification of abortion services to pregnant minors, this can be waived by a state court or administrative agency if the minor is judged mature enough to give informed consent.

would still use their clinical judgment when clients requested abortion. The law also did not consider pregnant minors. Some states allow pregnant minors to have an abortion without parental consent. Somewhat of a precedent was set in 1981, however, when the Court upheld the constitutionality of a Utah law that required physicians to inform parents of a minor's request for abortion.[19,20]

One major problem with the ruling, which continues to be debated today, is that *there was no decision as to when life begins*. The Court felt that since no other scholars or scientists were able to come to a consensus on this matter, it would be presumptuous for the Court to do so. They did decide that the fetus was not a "person" for the purposes of the Fourteenth Amendment and that neither the father of the fetus nor the woman's husband had the right to interfere in or prevent the abortion.[21]

In many states there are laws with provisions for "conscience clauses," which allow institutions, health providers, and others to refuse to assist at abortions without risk of reprisal if participation is against their moral, ethical, or religious beliefs. However, public hospitals must allow the use of their facilities for abortion since they are supported by public funds.

Reaffirmation of Women's Rights.

Recent court decisions have upheld the original ruling on abortion and reaffirmed the conscience clause concept.[22] Opponents were frustrated in 1983 by the US Supreme Court's reaffirmation of a woman's constitutional right to terminate an unwanted pregnancy by striking down a variety of state restrictions. States were told they could not restrict first-trimester abortion services by requiring waiting periods or specific informed consents. Also, states could not require that second-trimester abortions be performed in hospitals. Though parental notification regarding abortion services for pregnant minors could be implemented by states, this could also be waived by a state court or administrative agency if the minor was judged mature enough to give informed consent.[23]

Senate activity in 1983 likewise gave abortion opponents little encouragement. The US Senate rejected a constitutional amendment to allow the states and federal government to prohibit abortion. The Senate also tabled a human life statute, which would allow a simple majority in Congress to outlaw abortion by declaring the fetus to be a human being from conception, therefore circumventing the bulky constitutional amendment process.[24]

With the current trend to conservatism, the issue of the legality of abortion continues to be debated and defended.

Hyde Amendment Restricting Federal Funds.

In 1978 the Hyde Amendment was passed restricting the use of federal funds for abortion. Three conditions were

---

> ### Stipulations for the Use of Medicaid Funds in Abortion According to the Hyde Amendment, 1978
>
> - The pregnancy is due to rape or incest and was reported promptly to a public-health agency or to the police.
> - The woman's life will be endangered by carrying the fetus to term (emotional well-being is not considered just cause).
> - Two or more physicians determine that the pregnancy will cause severe and long-term *physical* damage to the woman.

---

stipulated for the use of Medicaid funds for this procedure (see Stipulations for the Use of Medicaid Funds in Abortion According to the Hyde Amendment, 1978). Although a class action suit was filed in federal court against the Hyde Amendment, it was upheld as constitutional by the Supreme Court in 1980. The unfortunate result of this amendment is discrimination against poor women, since they tend to be dependent on general assistance for their health care.[22]

Abortion Opponents Continue to Seek Legislation

Abortion opponents continue to seek laws and regulations that discourage or restrict abortions. State laws that require physicians to take the same degree of care in aborting a possibly viable fetus as they would take in delivery of a live birth is one tactic. Another approach is to require physicians to use the abortion method most likely to result in fetal survival, unless this significantly increases risk to the woman. Such requirements have an impact on second-trimester abortions, many of which involve teenagers or cases of diagnosed fetal genetic abnormalities.

Increasing the burden of providers through reporting or information requirements is another tactic used by some states. One such requirement is that women be given a long list of statements including the gestational age of the fetus, descriptions of the fetus, possible unforeseeable physical or psychological sequelae, alternatives to abortion, and available services and benefits for continuing pregnancy. Reports filed with state health departments have also been used to discourage abortions. Data typically included are the woman's age, race, and marital status, the length and weight of the abortus, and many other facts.[25]

The constitutionality of such requirements is usually tested before the Supreme Court by such advocates of abortion as Planned Parenthood, the National Organization for Women, and the American Public Health Association. The Supreme Court has, in the past, upheld the principle that a woman's right to choose may not be burdened with excessive or discouraging regulations. However, the changing political composition of the Court leaves open the possibility of more conservative and restrictive interpretations.

Ethical and Legal Considerations for the Fetus and Sick Neonate

Perhaps there is no other area in perinatology/neonatology that is so fraught with dissention, discussion, and debate as the areas of neonatal intensive care and fetal research and treatment. Each of these is confronted with often profound and difficult ethical and legal dilemmas. Ironically many of the problems have been brought about by the extraordinary advances in the fields of neonatology and perinatology. Fetuses that would have aborted or been born dead 5 years ago now often can be treated *in utero* or brought to near term; infants who had no chance of survival a decade ago now may look forward to a relatively healthy, productive life. What then, is the cause for debate? As technology and expertise have increased, there are more attempts to salvage the heretofore "unsalvageable," with the consequent result of an infant with severe handicapping afflictions. Heroic efforts are made to prolong life when it is questionable if such efforts are warranted. Moreover, health providers and parents are often put in binds because of federal regulations and guidelines. In the following paragraphs we discuss the major ethical–legal problems encountered in these areas.

The Fetus

It is important to remember that the fetus has rights from the time of conception. He can be the beneficiary of a trust and inherit property. While not legally considered a person until he is born, the rights of the fetus have been upheld in the courts. Fletcher is cited in Patterson as describing the case of a woman who was ordered to have a cesarean section by the courts because of fetal distress. The woman had refused the procedure and wanted to leave the hospital and was adamant about doing so. After conferring with her, the legal staff of the hospital procured a court order. Fletcher notes that this was the first time a woman had legally been coerced into surgery. Similarly, the courts have ordered a mother who was a Jehovah's Witness to have a blood transfusion to save the life of her infant.[26]

Fetal Research

As previously stated, federal funding for fetal research is more or less at a standstill, although there are many advocates because of its alleged great potential for pre-

venting costly diseases. However, many states have made fetal research illegal, especially when the fetus is an abortus or is still *in utero*.[27] Several difficult questions have been raised regarding the mother's versus the fetus's rights: Does the mother have the right to determine what will be done with fetal remains? Does a mother who plans an abortion have the right to allow experimentation *in utero*? Can an aborted fetus be kept alive for experimental purposes?[7] Federal guidelines require that fetal research be designed to meet the needs of the fetus, be of minimal risk, and have the potential to develop important medical knowledge. These global guidelines allow for rather wide interpretation. Experts seem to agree that we are on the threshold of great discoveries. However, with this progress will come even more difficult decisions for expectant parents and those who care for them.[26]

Fetal Therapy

Elias and Annas note that we now have the capacity to drain spinal fluid from the brain of a fetus (cephalocentesis), catheterize the fetus *in utero*, remove its lower body from the uterus to repair a urinary tract obstruction, transfuse the fetus *in utero* for erythroblastosis, repair gastroschisis, and surgically repair skeletal defects.[27] While these are certainly milestones in the area of therapy, investigators generally advise caution and note the experimental nature of many of the treatments. Harrison and colleagues have stated that the only anatomical malformations that warrant consideration are those that interfere with fetal organ development and that, if alleviated, would allow *normal* fetal development to proceed.[28]

Fletcher and others have outlined some questions and possible conflicts as these treatments become more used.[26,27,29] What happens if a physician feels he can help a fetus, but the mother refuses consent or the surgical consent is ambiguous? If a court orders the mother to submit to fetal treatment, does this not invade her right to privacy and her own body integrity? Could she be charged with fetus abuse? Is the risk/benefit ratio favorable enough to cause this very costly therapy to be a national priority? Some would argue to the contrary, but Michejda and Hodgen state that if therapy on neural tube defects, for instance, could be perfected and applied to humans, it would provide an ethical alternative to abortion and a relatively inexpensive alternative to the average $60,000 per year spent caring for a child who suffers from this defect.[30]

The Neonate

How much should a child have to suffer for the sake of life? More importantly, which should be regarded more highly, the sanctity of life or the quality of life?

These and other dilemmas for face doctors, nurses, and parents increasingly as infant mortality rates continue to fall. Of the approximately 3.5 million babies delivered in the United States each year, some 250,000 come into the world with significant defects or victimized by birth injury.[31] Clearly, medicine is advancing in its effort to save lives, but the long-range outcomes may not be inevitably good.

Effects of Invasive Procedures and Supportive Care

Some of the procedures deemed necessary for a sick newborn can produce a disease or defect. This is known as an iatrogenic effect. Prolonged use of ventilators can scar respiratory passages. Oxygen therapy, if it is given at too high a concentration, can cause varying degrees of vision impairment (retrolental fibroplasia). Lyon notes that hospital staff stick needles in the neonate's heels, tubes down his throat, and catheters into his heart, bladder, and other orifices.[31] He cites Jameton, a medical ethicist, as observing that all too often in health care, medical suffering is seen as justifiable suffering. While Jameton concedes that it is natural for providers to uphold this point of view, because it enables them to practice with less guilt and, indeed, is often required by current legal regulations, it may be dismal from the infant's point of view. The Reverend James Bresnahan, a professor of ethics, makes the point that adults have the option of refusing treatment, but since the infant cannot consent or demur, deciding what is reasonable is more difficult.[31] Strong and others state that society must come to terms with several difficult questions in the next few years: Should we be saving the lives of certain infants only to have them lead lives of pain, disability, and deprivation? Or should we let those die who would not otherwise survive without major intervention? And if so, who makes the decision? What kind of care do you deny or give an infant to allow him to die with comfort and dignity? Some of these questions have received partial, albeit ambiguous, answers in the controversial "Baby Doe" regulations.[32-34]

Baby Doe Regulations

In March 1983 the first Baby Doe regulation was issued by the Secretary of the Department of Health and Human Services (DHHS). This was in response to a report that an infant with Down's syndrome had died in an Indiana hospital because her esophageal atresia was left uncorrected. The main thrust of the regulation was the threat to remove federal funding from hospitals that did not comply with a notice that was to be posted that stated that failure to feed or care for handicapped infants was against federal law. In addition, a Baby Doe hotline

was established by which suspected hospital failures to comply could be reported. Some alleged failures were reported, and "Baby Doe squads" were dispatched to the suspected hospitals. Needless to say there were major disruptions at all levels, including actual medical and nursing care, as charts were confiscated, providers interrogated, time taken from care, and the like. It was eventually proved that the hospitals in question were entirely blameless.

The American Academy of Pediatrics and others sought an injunction against the regulation. This was denied; however, a waiting period was granted in which public comment was to be solicited. Debate was heated, since health professionals felt the judiciary was interfering in a process of decision making that was in the purview of themselves and the parents and was insidiously labeling the parties "child abusers."[35]

In September 1983 the regulation was reissued with little change. One change was that hotline notices were to be posted only in nurses' stations, assumedly to encourage nurses to report "abuse," since they often were "afraid of reprisal" otherwise. Annas and others state that this was a demeaning rationalization of nurses, since it deprecates nurses as intelligent, participating members of the health team.[35,36]

On October 11, 1983, an infant was born in Port Jefferson, New York, with multiple neural tube defects, including spina bifida, microcephaly, and hydrocephaly. After consulting with physicians and their Roman Catholic priest, the parents chose conservative medical rather than surgical treatment to reduce the chance of infection rather than to correct the defects. A lawyer in Vermont, unrelated to any of the above participants, managed to get a court order to appoint a guardian *ad latem* for the child (depriving the parents of their parental authority) in order to have the surgery performed. The trial court's ruling was struck down eventually by New York's State Court of Appeals. The court commented upon the often "offensive activities of those who sought to displace parental responsibility for management of her medical care."[37] Nevertheless, fears were aroused once more as to the possibility of further interference in the provider–client relationship.[34]

In January 1984 what were thought to be the final regulations pertaining to handicapped infants were issued by the Secretary of DHHS. They were entitled "Nondiscrimination on the Basis of Handicap, 1984." Legal rights of handicapped infants were required to be posted, and state protective services were to develop procedures for protecting infants from medical neglect. The regulations did not require neonatal intensive care units (NICUs) to provide futile efforts to prolong the act of dying. Hospitals were encouraged (but not required) to set up infant-care review committees (ICRC) to review all cases of infants who might be deprived of care because of their health condition(s). The American

Further Regulations Resulting From the Child Abuse Amendments of 1985 to Public Law 98—The Child Abuse Prevention and Treatment Act

Medical neglect: withholding of medically indicated treatment from a disabled infant with a life-threatening condition

Definition of "withholding medically indicated treatment":

". . . the failure to respond to the infant's life-threatening conditions by providing treatment (including appropriate nutrition, hydration, and medication) which, in the treating physician's (or physicians') reasonable medical judgment, will be most likely to be effective in ameliorating or correcting all such conditions."

Withholding medical treatment is not "medical neglect" under three conditions:

i. The infant is chronically and irreversibly comatose;

ii. The provision of such treatment would merely prolong dying, not be effective in ameliorating or correcting all of the infant's life-threatening conditions, or otherwise be futile in terms of the survival of the infant; or

iii. The provision of such treatment would be virtually futile in terms of the survival of the infant and the treatment itself under such circumstances would be inhumane.

Definition of "reasonable medical judgment": "medical judgment that would be made by a reasonably prudent physician knowledgeable about the case and the treatment possibilities with respect to the medical condition involved."

(Adapted from Murray TH: The final anticlimactic rule on Baby Doe. Hastings Cent Rep 15(3):5–7, June 1985)

Academy of Pediatrics has developed guidelines for the composition and duties of such a committee and regards these committees as viable alternatives to hotlines and squads of investigators.[37]

On May 15, 1985 the latest Baby Doe regulation went into effect as the Child Abuse Amendments of 1985 to Public Law 98-457—the Child Abuse Prevention and Treatment Act.[38] The amendments authorized DHHS to draft a regulation explaining how to fulfill the intent of the legislation, and it provides for several more explicit definitions (see Further Regulations Resulting From the Child Abuse Amendments of 1985 to Public Law 98—The Child Abuse Prevention and Treatment Act). The rule also describes a brief set of requirements

that a state protective agency must fulfill to qualify for federal grants. Murray calls the final regulation anticlimactic and believes it will have minimal impact on medical and ethical decision making, since the trend is already to aggressive treatment of nonlethal conditions and the narrowing of parents' and physicians' discretion on treatment decisions (the "best interest of the infant" standard). Moreover, while "encouraging" hospitals to form ICRCs, DHHS is careful to maintain that these are guidelines only and does not offer sanctions or rewards for their establishment.[38] Thus, the future will continue to be fraught with these weighty ethical and legal issues. The student is referred to the article by Drane in the Suggested Reading for ethical guidelines in dealing with the dilemmas encountered in the NICU.

Ethical and Legal Considerations in Care of the Mother

The nurse has certain obligations to the mother. She must be familiar and skilled in the use of equipment that is necessary for the mother's care. Fetal monitors are increasingly used, and the nurse should become knowledgeable in their use. Guidelines for monitoring had been developed by the American College of Obstetrics and Gynecology (ACOG). The nurse is accountable for preparing herself (by a separate course of study, if necessary) to read the monitor accurately, make appropriate notations, and report complications promptly. She should also know that tapes need to be stored appropriately, since they are often used in malpractice suits. If she is not current in these matters, she can be held culpable in the event of a complication.

She must also observe the infant carefully after delivery and report and record signs of complications.

Dillon and his colleagues reported two cases of maternal complications that raised unusual ethical considerations.[39] They presented two cases of pregnant women with severe, and in one case total and irreversible, brain damage. The ethical question revolved around the appropriateness of using life support systems on the women for a short time to substantially improve fetal outcomes. Veach, an ethicist, notes in a commentary that the use of the mother's body to serve the interest of her infant would be permissible if her consent had been obtained or she had signed an anatomical donation card.[40] Without such consent, permission must be obtained from the next of kin, and there would be controversy if there were conflicting opinions among the kin and providers. However, Veach recommends that such cases are best reviewed by a multidisciplinary team of ethicists, lawyers, physicians, and clergy. Family should be consulted. That, of course, raises questions about the limits of benevolence and authority.

References

1. Curtin L, Flaherty MJ: Nursing Ethics, Theories and Pragmatics, Chap 4. Bowie, MD, Robert J. Brady, 1982
2. Hankanson EY: Reducing the risk involved in providing medical care for women, pp 24–32. Malpractice Digest, St. Paul, Fire and Marine, July–Aug 1980
3. Fiesta J: The Law and Liability: A Guide for Nurses. New York, John Wiley & Sons, 1983
4. Greenfield VR: Wrongful birth, what is the damage? JAMA 248:926–932, 1982
5. Tennenhouse DJ: Legal perils in nursing, pp 1–83. Symposium sponsored by Symposium Medicus, San Diego, California, March 19–21, 1982
6. Regan WA: Nursing malpractice: A giant leap on damages. RN 44(12):69–72, 1981
7. Annas GJ: Redefining parenthood and protecting embryos: Why we need new laws. Hastings Cent Rep 14(5):50–52, Oct 1984
8. Abramowitz S: A stalemate on test-tube baby research. Hastings Cent Rep 14(1):5–9, Feb 1984
9. Mosher WD, Pratt WF: Reproductive improvements among married couples: United States, pp 13, 32. Vital and Health Statistics, Series 23, No. 11, National Center for Health Statistics, Dec 1982
10. Marrs L et al: Clinical applications of techniques used in human *in vitro* fertilization research. Am J Obstet Gynecol 146(5):1146–1159, July 1, 1983
11. Kass L: Making babies revisited. Public Interest 54:54, Winter 1979
12. Gersz SR: The contract in surrogate motherhood: A review of the issues. Law Med Health Care 12(3):107–114, 1984
13. Furrow BR: Surrogate motherhood: A new option for parenting? Law Med Health Care 12(3):106, 1984
14. Robertson JA: Surrogate mothers: Not so novel after all. Hastings Cent Rep 13(5):28–30, Oct 1983
15. Jones HW: Editorial: Variations on a theme. JAMA 250:2182, Oct 28, 1983
16. Golbus MS et al: Prenatal genetic diagnosis in 3000 amniocenteses. N Engl J Med 300:157–162, 1979
17. Thompson JB, Thompson HO: Ethics in Nursing. New York, Macmillan, 1981
18. Camenisch PF: Abortion for the fetus' own sake. Hastings Cent Rep 6(2):38–40, June 1976
19. Fromer MJ: Abortion ethics. Nurs Outlook 30(4):234–236, 1982
20. Reizek SB: Ethical issues in childbirth technology. In Holmes HB, Haskins BB, Gross M (eds): Birth Controlling and Controlling Birth: Women Centered Perspectives. Clifton, New Jersey, The Humana Press, 1980
21. Baron CH: "If you prick us, do we not bleed?" of Shylock, fetuses and the concept of person in the law. Law Med Health Care 2(2):52–61, 1983
22. Annas GJ: Roe vs. Wade reaffirmed. Hastings Cent Rep 13(4):21–23, 1983
23. Hatcher RA, Guest F, Stewart F et al: Contraceptive Technology 1984–1985, pp 186–187. New York, Irvington Publishers, 1984
24. Donovan P: The holy war. Fam Plann Perspect 17(1):5–9, Jan/Feb 1985
25. APHA high court brief to oppose rules restricting abortions. Nation's Health 8:1; 8, Aug 1985
26. Patterson P: Fetal therapy, issues we face. AORN J 35(4):663–668, March 1982
27. Elias S, Annas GJ: Perspectives on fetal surgery. Am J Obstet Gynecol 145:807–815, 1983
28. Harrison MR, Golbus MS, Filly RA: Management of the fetus with a correctable congenital defect. JAMA 246:776–782, Aug 14, 1981
29. Ruddick W, Wilcox W: Operating on the fetus. Hastings Cent Rep 12(5):10–13, 1982
30. Michejda M, Hodgen GD: In utero diagnosis and treatment of nonhuman primate fetal skeletal anomalies. JAMA 246:1093–1097, Sept 4, 1981
31. Lyon J: New treatments, new choices. Nurs Life 4(2):48–52, 1984
32. Strong C: Defective infants and their impact on families: Ethical and legal considerations. Law Med Health Care 11(4):168–172; 181, 1983
33. Committee on the Legal and Ethical Aspects of Health Care for Children: Comments and recommendations on the "Infant Doe" proposed regulations. Law Med Health Care 11(5):203–209, 1983
34. Doudera AE: Section 504, handicapped newborns and ethics committees: An alternative to the hotline. Law Med Health Care 2(5):200–202, 1983
35. Annas GJ: Baby Doe redux: Doctors as child abusers. Hastings Cent Rep 13(5):25–32, 1983
36. Murphy CP: The changing role of nurses in making ethical decisions. Law Med Health Care 12(4):173–175; 184, Sept 1984
37. Fleischman AR, Murray TH: Ethics committees for Infant Doe? Hastings Cent Rep 13(6):5–9, Dec 1983
38. Murray TH: The final anticlimactic rule on Baby Doe. Hastings Cent Rep 15(3):5–7, June 1985
39. Dillon WP et al: Life support and maternal brain death during pregnancy. JAMA 248(9):1089–1091, Sept 3, 1982
40. Veach RM: Maternal brain death: An ethicist's thoughts. JAMA 248(9):1102–1103, Sept 3, 1982

Suggested Reading

Chervenak FA et al: When is termination of pregnancy during the third trimester morally justifiable? N Engl J Med 310(8):501–503, Feb 23, 1984
Drane JF: The defective child: Ethical guidelines for painful dilemmas. JOGN Nurs 13(1):42–48, Jan/Feb 1984
Frandel-Korenchuk DM: Informed consent, client participation in childbirth decisions. JOGN Nurs 11(6):379–381, Nov/Dec 1982
Infants' Bioethics Task Force and Consultants: Guidelines for infant bioethics committees. Pediatrics 72(2):306–310, Aug 1984
Murray TH: The final anticlimactic rule on Baby Doe. Hastings Cent Rep 15(3):5–7, June 1985
Zander LI: The place of confinement—a question of statistics or ethics? J Med Ethics 7:125–127, 1981

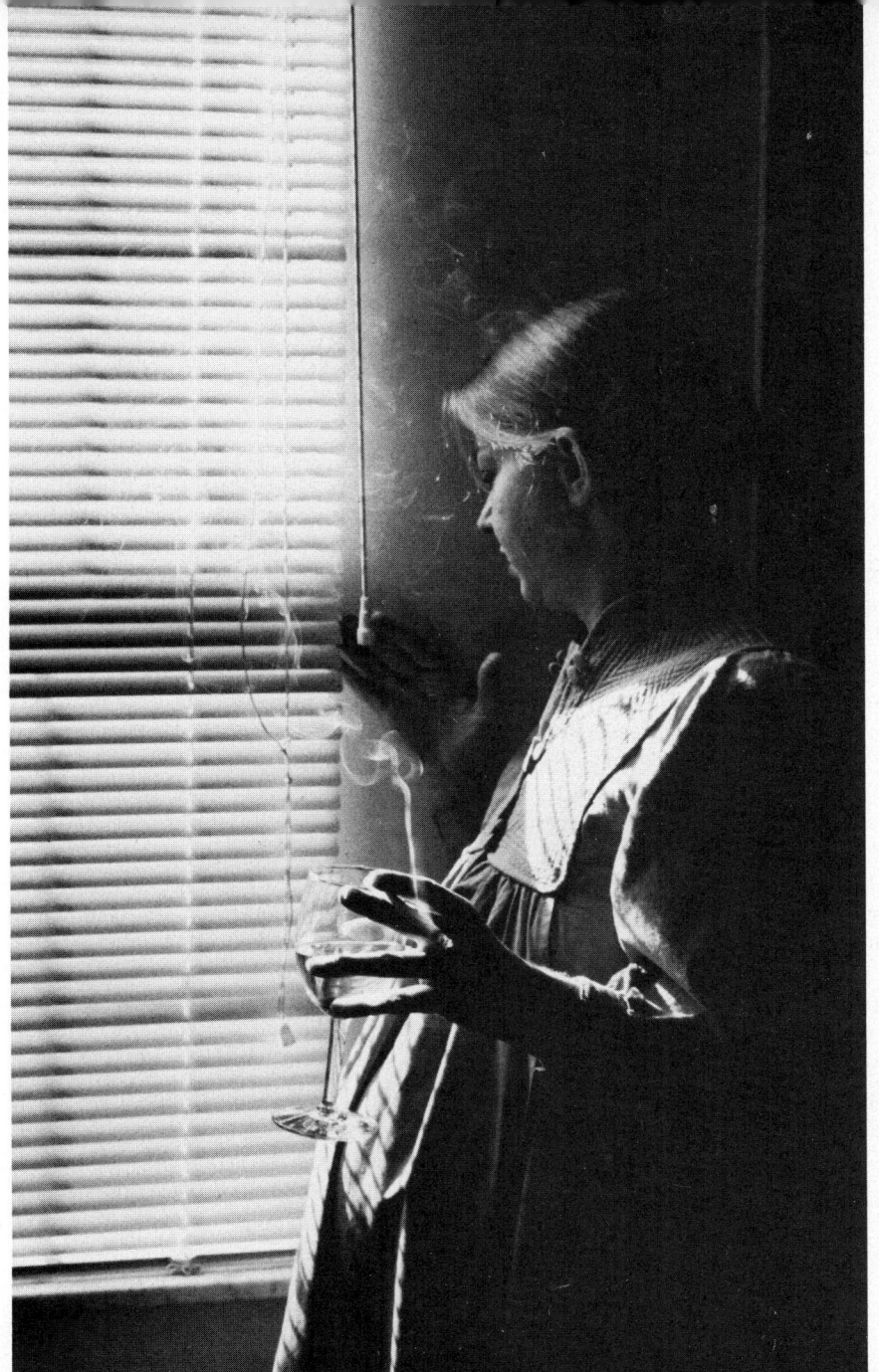

CHAPTER 8

Social Risk Factors and Reproductive Outcomes

In this chapter the focus is upon selected risk factors that are associated with such reproductive outcomes as infant and maternal mortality; low birth weight, and other complications of pregnancy.

Sociodemographic Risk Factors

Maternal Age

Findings indicate that mortality is higher among infants of the older primipara and multipara mother and among those of very young mothers.[1] Moreover, there is a strong correlation between socioeconomic status and age of the mother. In births to parents with more education or higher family income the mothers tend to be older. The lower the socioeconomic status, the greater the tendency for the mother to be younger.[2,3]

Late Pregnancy

Although women age 35 and older account for only about 5% of all births in the United States and statistics reveal that the number of births to women over 40 was 33,804 out of the total number of 3,136,965 live births, births to these women are viewed with interest and apprehension because they have come to be viewed as "high risk."[4,5] Heretofore attention has usually been focused on the maternal rather than the fetal results. More recently, because of the availability of sophisticated antenatal fetal assessment technology, the focus has gravitated to the fetal risk. Older women are considered high risk because they have more chance of neonatal mortality and morbidity, maternal mortality and morbidity, and spontaneous abortion.[6]

Thus, age and parity are two biologic categories that have specific social significance since they contribute to a general picture of poor reproductive outcomes for both mother and infant.

Nursing Implications. The role of the maternity nurse becomes particularly important here in terms of counseling women with respect to the problems they may encounter in such late pregnancies and the risks associated with some of the antenatal diagnostic techniques. Some popular articles give the impression that these diagnostic tests somehow cure fetal defects and can make pregnancy safer.[7,8] This is erroneous, and the mother and father need to be apprised of the limitations associated with these tests. They are not a panacea for a safe pregnancy outcome. They are useful because they can determine if some fetal defects do exist and, if so, the parents have the option of an abortion. They can also give a good indication of the age and well-being of the fetus, which helps if early delivery is indicated. Thus, these parents need meticulous antepartal care from all health providers as well as careful client education, particularly from the nurse.

Adolescent Pregnancy

Adolescent pregnancy is one of the problems associated with maternal age. Notable among the social and health costs of these pregnancies are the following: (1) about one half of school-age mothers will have a subsequent unwanted pregnancy within 2 years of the birth of the first child; (2) evidence indicates that approximately 60% of those who had their first baby at school age become welfare recipients; (3) young mothers have a disproportionate number of babies of low birth weight, which is associated with mental retardation and other handicapping conditions; (4) problems associated with pregnancy are particularly acute in mothers 15 years of age and younger.[9]

We cannot consider this issue systematically without placing it within a broader social context. The teenage sexual revolution is related to a number of concurrent trends. For example, there is an increased number and proportion of births to women under the age of 20. One third of all births are to girls 17 or younger, and about two fifths of these births are out of wedlock.[2,10] Thus, we shall consider out-of-wedlock births jointly with the problems of adolescent pregnancy.

Out-of-Wedlock Births. Out-of-wedlock birthrates have been increasing since 1940 among girls 19 years of age and younger. Among nonwhite individuals the

---

Factors Placing Mother or Fetus at Risk

Sociodemographic Risk Factors
  Maternal age
    Older woman
    Adolescent girl
      Out-of-wedlock birth
  Socioeconomic and ethnic factors
    Education of parent
    Ethnicity
    Family income
      Undernutrition

Behavioral Risk Factors
  Smoking
  Teratogenic foods and additives
  Substance abuse
    Drugs
    Alcohol

Life Events and Life Stress
  High life stress and low social support
  Attitudes and emotions

birthrates for girls aged 14 increased between 1940 and 1950 but have been rather stable since then. Similarly, there are variations for both whites and nonwhites in the period 1940 to 1976; the rate for nonwhites seems to be declining recently, but the rate for nonwhites is still higher than for whites.[10]

There are alternative explanations for the increasing out-of-wedlock birthrate in addition to the simple one of a "sexual revolution." Recent health status changes may explain a great deal of the increase. These changes concern the ability to conceive (fecundity rate) and the capacity to avoid spontaneous abortion. Specifically, research indicates that the mean age at menarche has decreased in the United States and western Europe as a result of improved nutrition and health during pre-adolescent years. Improved nutrition increases the rate of growth, which in turn decreases the age at menarche.[11-13] In addition, improved nutrition during pregnancy, particularly through participation in supplemental and therapeutic nutritional programs such as WIC and MDD (Montreal Diet Dispensary program), has impacted both on general health and consequently on spontaneous abortion in this high-risk group. When improved or adequate nutrition is coupled with adequate, monitored prenatal care, maternal and neonatal outcomes can be even better for these young mothers-to-be.[3,13,14] However, in reality these two crucial factors are often difficult to attain.[15]

Problems with Adolescent Pregnancies. Childbearing at any age is a momentous event. For the adolescent, however, it is often accompanied by a different set of problems from those experienced by older mothers. For the very young mother, under the age of 15, there is a greater probability that her infant will be stillborn or premature, will have a low birth weight (LBW), or will die soon after birth. In addition, the mother herself is at greater risk for pregnancy-induced hypertension (PIH) and its sequelae, cephalopelvic disproportion (CPD), iron deficiency anemia, and prolonged labor. Poor diets, inadequate prenatal care, and immaturity are all contributing factors.[3,16]

Health Problems. McCormick and co-workers found high levels of health problems among infants of two groups of mothers, primiparas who were 17 years old or younger and multiparas who were 18 to 19 years old and who began their childbearing under the age of 18.[3] They observed that despite decreases over the period of the study, neonatal mortality rates remained over one and a half times higher for infants of these mothers than for those of other mothers. This was due largely to the relatively high proportion of low-birth-weight infants born to these mothers. Postnatal mortality rates also remained high and showed a trend toward increasing. Morbidity was higher and was consistent with the socioeconomic disadvantagement of these mothers.

Moreover, these results could not be explained entirely by the difference in the proportion of low-birth-weight infants born to these mothers. The data further indicated the limited resources available to these adolescents to cope with their own and their infant's health needs. This group is particularly vulnerable to decreases in public programs supporting child health care.

Low Birth Weight. The increased risk of low birth weight may be the most important medical aspect of adolescent pregnancy. It has been observed that increased mortality is only one of the dangers facing infants of low birth weight. There are apparent linkages to additional sequelae: epilepsy, cerebral palsy, mental retardation, a variety of learning disabilities, and a higher risk of deafness and blindness.[2] The National Center for Health Statistics reports that, at all ages, and especially at the younger ages, infant mortality and morbidity are considerably higher for nonwhites than for whites.[17] Low birth weight is discussed further in Chapter 44.

Psychoemotional Problems. There can be some disturbing psychoemotional consequences of premature parenting. Sugar and others[18-20] observe that to the extent that becoming an adolescent parent constrains or prohibits freedom of choice in a variety of areas (*e.g.,* education, occupation, marriage), it inhibits the development of feelings of individual autonomy (*i.e.,* separation-individuation, feelings of independence from parents, and a sense of commitment to a heterosexual object). In short, adolescent motherhood can prematurely foreclose the process of identity formation, resulting in an ego structure characterized by the feeling that one's destiny is controlled by forces and events external to the self. This results in negative feelings of personal efficacy. McLaughlin and Micklin found that among equally educated women from equivalent socioeconomic backgrounds, the occurrence of a first birth by age 18 resulted in a decrease in perceived personal efficacy.[20] After age 18, neither the timing of the first birth nor the occurrence of that birth affected personal efficacy. Duncan and Morgan's research indicates that lower personal efficacy is a consequence of the occurrence of negative events and that those with low personal efficacy are more likely to experience negative events.[21] Thus, there appears to be a cyclical process in which every negative event lowers personal efficacy, which makes the individual vulnerable to repeated negative events. This is a finding that needs further research, especially as it relates to the very young teenager.

Implications for the Perinatal Team. What is the role of the health professional in preventing early childbearing? Any action must start with the assumption that these are not inevitable consequences. Many women wanted to become mothers, but the data indicate that a substantial proportion wish that their first child had come later.[21] What then might be the goals for dealing with adolescent pregnancy? Hayes and Crovitz have delineated two phases in goal setting for this population: (1) providing optimal services for adolescent unwed mothers and their families and (2) helping make real the option of "more mature" parenthood for adolescents in general.[22]

In the first phase of providing services, the researchers suggest that inexpensive pregnancy testing be made available by a nonjudgmental, well-trained staff who can inform the adolescent of the options available to her: termination of the pregnancy, adoption, or keeping the infant. Details of the advantages and disadvantages of each option, as well as how to go about each option, also need to be discussed. Each visit is to be personalized so that realistic short-term goals are set, preferably by the same health personnel.

Temporary foster-home care is another facet of services. For the youngster who wishes to keep her infant but cannot manage adequate baby-sitting to allow her to continue school or get a job, this service is a lifesaver.

A third service would be a comprehensive team approach to antepartal care, which includes the services of an array of personnel including a pediatrician who would be available for infant follow-up and to give anticipatory guidance as needed. Group educational and counseling services are recommended so that the adolescent takes responsibility for self-care and feels free to interact with professionals. Self-esteem is enhanced, and marketable skills are acquired. Thus, astute physical care as well as comprehensive counseling with referral to needed services lies within the purview of this perinatal team. It is also essential that the mother be encouraged to remain either in the public school system or in affiliated schools especially for pregnant adolescents.[22] Punitive efforts on the part of school systems to deprive the adolescent of schooling are anachronistic and have not worked in controlling the problem of unwed adolescent pregnancy.[21]

In the second phase, helping the younger generation realize "mature parenthood," the emphasis is on prophylaxis. Hayes and Crovitz suggest that there be early education in the area of life and health sciences. Ideally, there should be periodic parent–child discussions that begin as soon as the child expresses curiosity about sex and related matters and can comprehend accurate explanations. They recommend introduction of simple material as early as the third grade, with the content becoming more complex and detailed as the child grows. The overriding object is to ensure that by the time the child is a teenager, he or she has a clear understanding of how fertilization occurs and the events from fertilization through delivery and the postpartum periods, including both the biologic and the social consequences of pregnancy. In addition, the education should be handled by those knowledgeable and skilled in discussion groups. Parents need to be encouraged and given the chance to participate in these discussions.[22]

We cannot close this discussion without recognizing that knowledge, accessibility, and contraceptive technology are not the only variables in adolescent pregnancy. More than one study has documented that a large proportion of young mothers say that they had not used contraception because they did not care whether or not they became pregnant.[22] Thus, some do not appear to be motivated to take advantage of the opportunities to control their fertility, no matter how accessible these are. Altering their motivation appears to be a major undertaking for society.

Health-Care Goals for the Pregnant Adolescent

Optimal Health Services

1. Inexpensive pregnancy testing
2. Information regarding placement options
3. Information regarding operationalizing an option
4. Temporary foster-home care for the infant
5. Comprehensive perinatal team approach providing for continuity of care, which includes obstetrician, pediatrician, perinatal nurses, and nutritionists skilled with adolescents
6. Educational and personal group experiences that convey information and support for developmental and educational needs
7. Encouragement of parents to complete education
8. Supportive measures for enhancing self-esteem and developing marketable skills

Realization of Mature Parenthood

1. Emphasize anticipatory guidance before pregnancy occurs (prophylaxis)
   a. Early education in the life and health sciences
   b. Periodic parent–child discussion sessions regarding facts about sexuality
   c. Continued education during teen years to ensure accurate information regarding sexual facts and responsible sexuality
   d. Continual participation of parents

Socioeconomic and Ethnic Indicators of Risk

Certain indicators of socioeconomic status such as family income, education of mother and father, and ethnicity can be risk factors in pregnancy. Low-income individuals are considerably more predisposed to lowered health status and obstetric complications during pregnancy. Low birth weight is particularly prevalent in the lowest socioeconomic groups, especially the black population. The role of ethnicity becomes readily apparent when one analyzes data that have accrued since 1935 on racial background. Throughout this period marked differences have occurred on the basis of racial background, with nonwhites faring much worse than whites. Indeed, the relative differential has actually risen during this period. The racially related differentials in mortality have also been noted beyond the first year of life. It should be stressed that virtually all of the racially related differentials in mortality are socioeconomically related.[17,23]

Undernutrition

One of the most important sequelae of low socioeconomic status is undernutrition. Government studies have revealed that, compared with more affluent persons, the poor are twice as deficient in four essential diet ingredients. Most striking, poor persons had about four times as much clear-cut iron deficiency anemia and twice as many borderline cases as had the nonpoor. In three categories of essential diet ingredients—vitamin A, vitamin C, and riboflavin—the poor were found to have about twice as much of the clear-cut deficiency as the nonpoor. The survey also found a greater percentage of low height and weight measurements for children living below the poverty line than for those who were more affluent.[24]

Obviously, there is a complex interaction between undernutrition, poverty, and other environmental or genetic factors.

Effects on Fetal Brain Development. Studies have found that deficiencies in the diet of a pregnant woman can have profound effects on a number of pregnancy outcomes (Fig. 8-1). For example, it has been shown that nutritional and genetic factors may interact during prenatal development with consequent irreversible results on the development of the baby's brain. This is one of the most important recent discoveries in the field of mental retardation. It is estimated that one tenth of the children born today are seriously affected as a consequence of malnutrition. Recent work at the National Institutes of Health suggests that there is a correlation between the level of the amino acids in the blood of a pregnant woman and the subsequent intelligence of her baby.[14,15]

Low Birth Weight. Undernutrition has been identified as one of the causes of low-birth-weight infants born to poor urban mothers.[14] Extremely low birth weights have been reported among poorly fed groups in Asia and Africa. The relationship between low birth weight and malnourished populations may have a more complex explanation than simple nutrition. Rather than

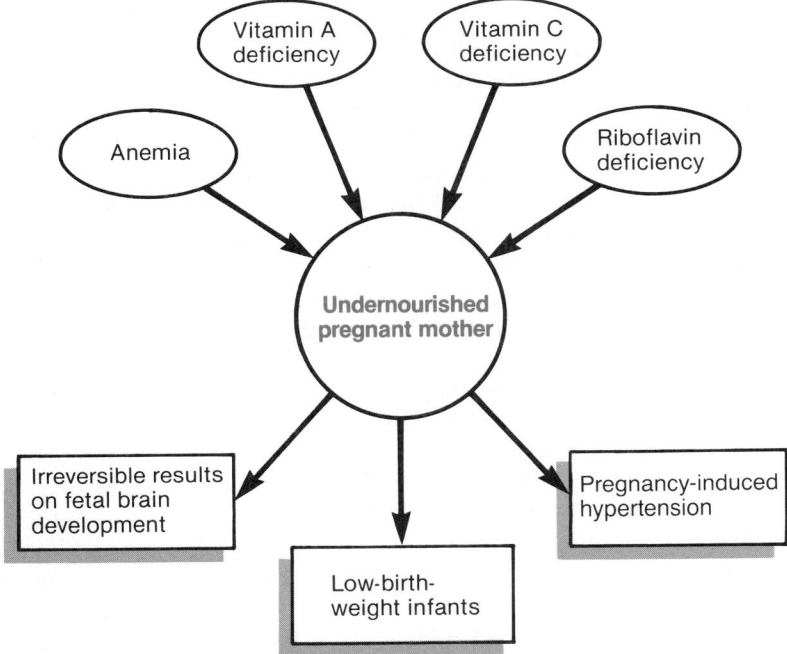

FIGURE 8-1

Some of the effects of undernutrition on pregnancy outcomes.

dietary deficiency in pregnancy, one specific factor, the small size of the baby, may reflect long-term maternal undernutrition dating back to the early childhood of the woman. Conceivably, malnutrition over many generations in underdeveloped societies may have favored the emergence of genetically different kinds of women with lower dietary requirements. This, however, is highly speculative and needs much carefully designed research to confirm such a possibility.

Hypertensive Disorders. The effect of socioenvironmental influences was most dramatically illustrated during World War II in Great Britain. During this period, the mortality from the pregnancy hypertensive disorders (toxemias) fell dramatically. The underlying reason for the drop in mortality resulting from this condition in England and Wales was that large numbers of women were evacuated from their homes in the cities into the country. The antenatal clinics were understaffed and improvisational. The major advantage brought about by this change of social environment was that the rationing system benefited expectant and nursing mothers and children. For the first time, women of the lower socioeconomic groups were fed as well as other population groups. Suffice to say that these disorders as a syndrome are most commonly seen in poor and badly nourished populations and that there is some evidence that the incidence has been modified by environmental changes, either situational or behavioral.[16,25,26]

Nursing Implications. The nurse can be a force both in the community and in the clinic setting to help improve preventive services to those at highest risk because of situational factors. Better ways can be devised to use the nurse and other health personnel to provide health education to the individuals at risk. This assumes that the nurse herself is equipped with the knowledge concerning nutrition and other precursors of problems of pregnancy to provide the appropriate knowledge to the client. Moreover, the nurse can be a positive force in the community to exert influence on other institutions, such as the schools, health departments, government agencies, and voluntary agencies, to provide preventive measures to the population at greatest risk.

In Chapter 22 specific care plans are given as the nurse uses the nursing process to render care to her clients.

Behavioral Risk Factors

Up to now, the discussion has been concerned primarily with factors that are not easily controlled by the nurse or other health personnel. A person's social position in society cannot be easily influenced by nursing intervention. As the following section will show, however,

the risk factors of smoking and substance abuse are mutable, and, hence, the nurse can have a greater degree of influence on the client.

Smoking

Literature reflects a heightened awareness of the important and substantial effects of smoking on pregnancy outcome. Studies demonstrate that mothers who smoke cigarettes have smaller babies than do nonsmoking mothers, and this finding has been attributed to the direct effect of smoking.

Unfortunately, cigarette smoking continues to be popular among women of childbearing age and some of these women are still not being advised by their physicians to stop. It is estimated that one half of pregnant women smoke.[27] Much of the research to date has focused on the relationship of maternal smoking to fetal and infant outcomes. Diebel has pointed out, however, that smoking has direct effects on the maternal organism, which in turn affects the fetus. The metabolism of several minerals including calcium, a variety of vitamins, hormones, glucose, fatty acids, and amino acids may be interfered with by smoking.[28,29]

Recent evidence, based on prospective studies and other well-designed research, has substantiated the fact that fetal size, growth, and mortality are related to smoking of cigarettes by the mother. According to the United States Public Health Service, some 4600 stillbirths each year in the United States probably can be attributed to women's smoking habits. Research indicates that women who smoke have a 30% higher rate of stillbirths than those who do not. These women also have a 26% higher rate of perinatal mortality.[30]

A positive association between maternal cigarette smoking and reduced infant birth weight in the range of 150 g to 200 g emerges from every study of these two characteristics. The hypothesis that the relationship between smoking and weight reduction in the infant is one of cause and effect is supported by several types of evidence. This relationship has been consistently observed in a wide variety of populations differing by geographic location, race, and social and economic circumstances. Furthermore, there is an inverse relationship between mean birth weights and the number of cigarettes smoked during pregnancy, an evident dose–response effect.[30–32]

However, there have been a few studies that have not confirmed these findings. Since smoking is a preventable behavior, the focus of concern is to determine whether babies who would otherwise be alive and healthy might die, before or after birth, because their mothers smoked.[31]

Meyer and her colleagues found that mothers who are young, reasonably healthy, having their first or second child, and smoking less than a pack of cigarettes a day have an increased risk of perinatal loss of less than 10%. "At the other extreme, heavy smokers who are high parity, public patients, those who have had previous premature births, or whose hemoglobin is under 11 g have an increased risk of perinatal loss of over 70%. Other groups are intermediate—perinatal mortality increased with maternal smoking, with the magnitude of increase ranging from 4% to 97%."[32] Thus, their data suggest that maternal smoking may interact with other factors in its influence on perinatal mortality.[31,32]

A relationship has also been shown between maternal smoking during pregnancy and the risk of spontaneous abortion.[33,34] This relationship has received much less study than that of smoking and intrauterine growth retardation, and the relationship of gestation to abortion is unclear. Nevertheless, subsequent studies indicate that these abortuses tend to be chromosomally normal.[34,35] There is no clear-cut evidence that there is a relationship between smoking and congenital malformations.[31,35] Stein and co-workers observe that not all the associations with smoking can be related solely to intrauterine exposure. They and others suggest that while the data are not definitive, there is some indication that the effect of smoking may be cumulative (*i.e.*, even though a woman does not smoke in a current pregnancy, but did at previous times in her life and in other pregnancies, the current fetus is still affected).[31,36] Thus, in conclusion, the consistent weight of evidence indicates that maternal smoking during pregnancy increases the infant's perinatal morbidity and mortality risk. Moreover, it interferes with maternal metabolism, which in turn impacts on the fetus. This risk increases directly with the number of cigarettes smoked, irrespective of the use of "reduced" tar and nicotine brands. In addition, the presence of other risk factors increases considerably the risks related to smoking.

Nursing Implications. The implications for prevention are clear. Counseling the client at the first visit, particularly in the case of mothers with other risk factors, can be done by the antepartal clinic nurse. Health education, although it needs to begin early in life, must be an essential part of prenatal care, and smoking is one behavior that is preventable. Moreover, the nurse can provide an appropriate role model for the mother and father through her own behavior. A detailed care plan is found in Chapter 22.

Teratogenic Foods and Additives

In the early years of the 20th century concern for the safety and quality of the food supply in the United States prompted the enactment of the Food and Drug Act, which prevented the addition of poisonous or other deleterious ingredients to foods. As technology has advanced and food production and processing, as well as advertising, have become increasingly sophisticated, there has been mounting concern as to the safety of foods and additives. It has been found that many heretofore unsuspected substances both naturally occurring and artificially added are, in fact, mutagens, teratogens, or embryotoxins. *Mutagens change the inherited chromosomal structure of cells, teratogens produce congenitally malformed infants, and embryotoxins kill or alter the embryo.*[37]

There are problems associated with the study of teratogens, particularly those relating to methodology; hence, there have not been the definitive data that we have for smoking and fetal morbidity. These problems revolve around the choice, dosage, and amount of the experimental substance, the choice of the subject animals (humans cannot be experimented upon), the difficulty in isolating variables and hence measuring results, the difficulty in determining preconditioning factors, and the need for multigenerational studies.[37] Some authors, in fact, maintain that there is little evidence that there has been an increase in rates of human malformations in the past few decades.[38,39] Nevertheless, consumer and health-provider concern has increased recently. Militant consumers feel that the Food and Drug Administration is too politically responsive to the demands of the food and drug industries and cite the use of rats and mice for testing instead of the use of a simian species that more closely approximates human responses. They also cite the hundreds of additives that have never been tested and that have been designated as "generally recognized as safe" (GRAS). Thus, it is particularly important that the prospective mother be made aware of the potential hazards, since ingesting large quantities of these substances may be harmful to her fetus. The groups of foods and additives are summarized in Potential Hazards of Foods and Additives.[37]

Substance Abuse

Drugs

There has been considerable interest in the potential genetic and teratogenic effects of drugs on the mother and fetus. Teenagers and young adults now make up the majority of the population for whom this interest applies. Many drug-abusing clients will admit to use or give some other evidence of use, such as inappropriate affect, general physical deterioration, and the like. Some even attempt to stop use during pregnancy, and some succeed if they are not "hard-core" abusers. Detection of maternal addiction is based on history or physical evidence, such as puncture marks and general debilitation.

The true prevalence of drug-abusing mothers is unknown. However, the indicators are that, in large urban

Potential Hazards of Foods and Additives

Nitrosamines (N-nitroso Compounds)

These compounds are potent carcinogens in all tested species, including amphibians, birds, fish, and mammals. While nitrosamines themselves are rarely found in foods, their precursors, nitrites (which combine with other nitrogen-containing compounds), are common. Sodium nitrite and sodium nitrate are added to most smoked and cured meat and fish to act as an antioxidant to ensure preserving the foodstuff. Nitrate, which may break down to nitrite, is found in soybean oil and naturally in leafy vegetables such as cauliflower, broccoli, lettuce, cabbage, and beets, especially when high levels of nitrate fertilizers are used. Drinking water in areas experiencing fertilizer runoff may also contain high levels. Ascorbic acid (vitamin C) can be used in place of nitrites as an antioxidant.

Aflatoxins

These substances are related to mycotoxins and are produced by fungal growths on a wide range of foodstuffs. Contamination is usually caused by excessive moisture before harvest or during storage. Aflatoxins are quite toxic to humans. For instance, the mycotoxin ergotism of rye can induce abortion in women as well as gangrene and other ills of the vascular system. Peanuts are particularly susceptible to infection, as are cereal grains, legumes, cocoa, cassava, sweet potatoes, improperly fermented foods and alcoholic beverages, and dairy products from animals fed contaminated feed. These toxins are not destroyed by home cooking or freezing, but milling is effective since the infected outer shells are removed. Regulation of harvest, storage, and marketing protects the consumer to a great extent.

US Certified Food Colorings

These are the "azo" dyes, which include red #2 (amaranth), red #4, yellow #6 (tartrazine), green (ferrous gluconate), and some others. Red #2 was found to be embryotoxic to rats and also to cause small litters in the same species; it has been banned since 1976. There is no clear-cut carcinogenic or teratogenic evidence regarding the other dyes; hence, Public Law 86-618 provides for setting "safe limits" for these and other food substances.

Artificial Sweeteners

Again there is no clear evidence of a carcinogenic or teratogenic effect with sodium cyclamate, saccharin, mannitol, and xylitol. Stone found that mothers who had taken cyclamates during pregnancy had children who suffered from hyperactivity and learning disabilities.[37] At present, research is continuing on these products, since the studies to date suffer from the methodological problems mentioned previously.

Caffeine

This substance is of concern because of its chemical structure, purine, one of the constituent groups of DNA. Moreover, it crosses the human placenta and is known to penetrate the preimplantation blastocyte in mammals. In addition, it has been found to cause chromosomal rearrangements in the sperm of mice. The data on human populations are not conclusive, and conflicting evidence is given. A recent large study in Finland, the country that leads the world in coffee consumption, did not produce any definitive data or recommendations.[40]

Thus, while there is reason for caution in using caffeine during pregnancy (and excessively in general), there is yet insufficient evidence to implicate it as a teratogen.

Trace Elements, Metallic and Chemical Contaminants

Such trace elements and metallic contaminants as lead, selenium, arsenic, cadmium, mercury, and methylmercury occur in the ground; in fish and crustaceans, especially when they come from contaminated waters; and in some fruits, cheeses, cereals, and other foodstuffs. When taken in large quantities they are known to be teratogenic, producing a variety of symptoms from congenital malformations to central nervous system problems.

Similarly, chemical contaminants, including pesticides, space sprays (DDVP, dichloros, vapona), herbicides, and fungicides, are embryotoxic, mutagenic, and teratogenic in mammals. The pesticide DVCP has been banned because of the occurrence of sterility in farm workers who used the substance in their work. Ingestion of these in pregnancy should be avoided.

centers, the ratio of drug-abusing mothers to total deliveries has increased greatly in the past 20 years, especially with the resurgence of adolescent use and the availability of such so-called recreational drugs as marijuana and cocaine. The abuse of the latter drug has been called an epidemic; it crosses all socioeconomic groups. Several studies are being done to ascertain the short-term and long-term effects of substance abuse on reproductive outcomes for both males and females.[41-44]

Woodward and colleagues observe that many mothers during their pregnancies take medications or use medicated products that have toxic or teratogenic potential because they have no information about these possible adverse effects.[45] These include Tylenol, Rolaids, aspirin, Bendectin, Maalox, Robitussin, ampicillin, Sudafed, Alka-Seltzer, and Massengill disposable douches. It is imperative that the nurse counsel the mother regarding all drug substances.

Use of Services. Most drug-abusing clients are latecomers for prenatal care. Indeed, most of these clients delay until they feel that they are ready for delivery in order to avoid a long labor without drugs and to satisfy their need for a last "fix" before submitting to the confinement of the hospital. As a result, there is evidence that a substantial proportion of deliveries to this population occurs at home, in the ambulance, or on the stretcher. This is especially true of the heroin addict. Also, addicts make considerable efforts to nourish their addiction during enforced periods of confinement in a hospital. Such clients will either hide the drug or obtain it from others in or outside the hospital. A portion of these clients supplement their supply with barbiturates, tranquilizers, or cocaine.

Effect on Mother and Infant. Very often the drug-abusing mother is also an alcohol abuser as well as a smoker. The combination of these three risk factors can have dire results for perinatal outcomes in both mother and infant.[44]

As far as heroin addicts are concerned, there is some difficulty in evaluating the data on total length of labor, but available evidence indicates that labor is not prolonged. Greatest difficulties tend to occur after delivery, when withdrawal in the infant and mother is a risk factor. Symptoms of withdrawal in the mother include nausea, tremors, sweats, abdominal pain, cramps, and yawning. (Chapter 46 discusses withdrawal symptoms in the infant.)

The attitude of the medical and nursing staff becomes a critical factor at this stage. The pregnancy outcomes of heroin-addicted mothers are typical of any nutritionally deprived groups of low socioeconomic status receiving inadequate prenatal care, with one important exception, congenital addiction of the baby.[46]

There is some suggestion in the literature that narcotic use by the mother may lead to intrauterine growth retardation. The long-term effects on growth and development are now being observed and evaluated in at least one prospective study. As yet, the effects of narcotic addiction on the reproductive process are not clearly reflected in our standard measures of maternal and perinatal mortality. Available evidence indicates that the addicted individual, even after withdrawal, detoxification, or rehabilitation, remains at risk, since subsequent intake, even years later, may result in the immediate urge for more drugs.

Thus, a pregnant woman who is a user of narcotic drugs of unknown potency and amount is carrying a potentially addicted fetus, and while detoxification of the newborn seems to be initially successful, a detoxified baby is still a problem infant. Even with use of methadone in the management of the pregnant addict, it is possible to magnify the effects on the fetus.[47]

The use of other drugs, such as marijuana, barbiturates, amphetamines, tranquilizers, and psychotropics (PCP, LSD), which are often taken in combination, impacts negatively on the mother's health and consequently on the health of the fetus. Since these drugs are often used with alcohol, the exact effects on the mother and fetus are confounded.[41] Congenital malformations, chromosomal damage, and intrauterine growth retardation have all been implicated with their use. This applies to marijuana use also.[41] Thus, it has been strongly recommended, even though results from the various studies vary, that the pregnant woman and her partner be strongly advised not to use any drugs during the pregnancy.[41,45-47] No over-the-counter medications should be used without first checking with the physician.

Alcohol

In 1968, a syndrome of prenatal and postnatal growth deficiency, mental retardation, developmental delay, cardiac defects, and a variety of skeletal–facial–limb problems was described, but these observations were neglected until 1973, when the term *fetal alcohol syndrome* was coined. Various studies document its existence.[48-50] A woman does not necessarily have to be an alcoholic to place her infant at risk for this condition. However, women who are chronic alcoholics run a much higher risk of having defective infants. Researchers have found that women who drink 2 to 4 ounces of hard liquor per day run a 10% risk of having an abnormal child. Women who drink 4 ounces or more per day have a 19% risk. If the average daily consumption is less than 2 ounces, the apparent risk is low but still present.[51]

Heavy alcohol consumption is most likely to affect fetal structure during the first trimester, when organogenesis is taking place. Frequently abortion will take place. During the second trimester, when there is mostly an increase in cell size rather than cell volume, the infant's weight is most likely to be affected.

However, Stein and Kline point out that the studies regarding the effect of alcohol on the fetus are less clear cut than those on smoking and that there are inconsistencies in the literature.[31] This is because of several methodological problems. Nevertheless, they maintain that the public health message is clear because every adverse outcome (and there are documented adverse outcomes, *e.g.*, spontaneous abortion, abruptio placentae, stillbirth, congenital malformations) calls for a separate evaluation. The relevant dose, time of drinking, type of beverage, and the like could be unique to each particular outcome.[31]

The infant born with fetal alcohol syndrome is discussed in Chapter 46.

Nursing Implications. The nurse has the obligation of making a careful assessment and evaluation with respect to the use of alcohol in the expectant mother's life-style. If the nurse suspects that her client has a drinking problem or even drinks moderately but consistently, it is important that she explore her reasons for drinking and refer the mother for counseling if necessary. Often clients' life-styles are such that "social drinking" is expected, and the mother may not realize the impact of her behavior on her fetus. The hazards of the syndrome can be clearly explained, and various counseling and assistance avenues can be used.

Life Events and Life Stress as Risks

Life events and life stress in the sense used here refer to such events as divorce, illness, death of a significant other, such as a family member, and job loss, rather than to the occurrence of the actual pregnancy itself, although this too may be a factor in pregnancy outcome. Appropriate intervention by nursing staff can be especially effective in meeting the needs and reducing the risks associated with such life stress. The interest in the relationship between the psychological and social world of the individual and human disorders and disease has a long history. Even the findings of carefully designed and conducted investigations have not always yielded clear-cut and unambiguous results concerning this relationship.[52] This is in sharp contrast to the dramatic results that have been obtained with animal experiments in which the various elements in the social environment have been correlated. Nevertheless, there is accumulating evidence of the intimate interaction between the social environment, physiological reactions, and pathologic outcome in the individual. This is particularly true of the chronic diseases, such as heart disease and cancer.[53,54]

Data on the relationship between disorders of pregnancy and life changes and experiences that may be stressful are relatively scanty.

High Life Stress and Low Social Support

Norbeck and Tilden have looked at the relationship of life stress, social support, and emotional disequilibrium to complications in pregnancy outcomes.[52,55] In a prospective study, they found that high life stress and low social support were significantly related to high emotional disequilibrium; social support and life stress were not significantly related to each other, however. They also found a relationship between high life stress, social support and gestational complications, as well as infant-condition complications. Social support appeared to play a mediating role. In a separate study, Tilden documented a significant relationship of life stress and social support to emotional disequilibrium during pregnancy.[55] However, she was not able to discern what contribution the pregnancy itself might have made to the overall relationship.

As these and other investigators point out,[54,56] additional research is needed, but their data help to explain some of the discrepant results in the literature. In short, the research and the approach cast serious doubt on the utility of specificity (as far as current clinical syndromes are concerned) in research concerned with psychosocial factors in disease etiology. Similar psychosocial factors may be related to different disease syndromes. At the present, this research approach is very promising, and additional work needs to be done using this approach.[54,56]

Attitudes and Emotions

Much has been written in recent years on the role of emotional and attitudinal factors and psychological stress during pregnancy, as these may be related to pregnancy outcomes. The evidence is inconclusive, but more important, much of it is based on poorly designed research and inadequate samples of the population at risk. Despite this poor state of affairs, there is a general consensus in medical science that psychological factors are in some way associated with various aspects of the maternity cycle. Indeed, some investigators have asserted that early psychological assessment of pregnant women holds promise of being predictive of the course and outcome of pregnancy. Most of the literature makes an attempt to measure the attitudes of the woman toward her pregnancy and to measure other psychosocial factors as these may influence the outcome.[57]

Surely there are attitudinal differences among women toward their individual pregnancies. There is also an intimate interaction between the psychological stress experienced by the person and psychological reactions, as the Colmans have noted.[58] Complications of pregnancy, labor, and delivery are obscured by this interaction. Thus, physiological changes and discomfort may trigger psychologically negative attitudes toward the pregnancy and, conversely, life stress may precipitate somatic problems.[59]

Nursing Implications. There is no doubt that many women, perhaps a majority, experience some psychological stress and anxiety during pregnancy. However, the literature in medical and nursing journals alike tends to assume that some of these conditions are psychosomatic or emotional in origin. In a paper critical of the cloudy thinking that has characterized such conditions as menstrual pain, nausea of pregnancy, and pain in labor as caused or aggravated by psychogenic factors, Lennane and Lennane suggest sexual prejudice as the basis for such thinking. Such scientific evidence as exists clearly suggests organic causes for these conditions.[60]

The point here is that nurses must not unwittingly and uncritically accept long-established attitudes that are rooted in prejudice rather than in scientific evidence. Stereotypic thinking is not only poor in scientific terms, but, equally important, it tends to influence the course and quality of treatment of women clients. Nursing staff has an important role to play in assisting the pregnant woman to use her psychosocial assets to the fullest in coping with the fears, anxieties, somatic complaints, and other problems associated with the pregnancy in the prenatal and intrapartal periods. Emotional and social support during and following the pregnancy cannot only be a comfort to the client but may also assist in reducing problematic outcomes.

A S S E S S M E N T   T O O L

High-Risk Pregnancy Factors

Prenatal Factors

1. Maternal disease
   a. Diabetes mellitus
   b. Preeclampsia and eclampsia
   c. Hypertension
   d. Cardiopulmonary disease
   e. Renal disease
   f. Infection: syphilis, rubella, tuberculosis
   g. Drug addiction
   h. Chronic alcoholism
   i. Endocrinopathy
   j. Severe anemia and blood dyscrasias
   k. Malnutrition
   l. Malignancy during pregnancy
2. Maternal practices
   a. Taking of medications associated with adverse fetal effects
   b. Smoking more than one cigarette a day
   c. Excessive exposure to radiation
   d. Less than three prenatal visits
3. Age: <16 years and >35 years
4. Short maternal stature
5. Severe isoimmunization (Rh or other)
6. Multiple gestation (particularly second of twins, third of triplets, etc)
7. Premature rupture of the membranes: <37–38 weeks (not considered here as a high-risk factor since all preterm infants are PROM)
8. Prolonged rupture of membranes: >18–24 hours (predisposes to neonatal sepsis, intrauterine pneumonia, and infections)
9. Polyhydramnios, oligohydramnios
10. Evidence of intrauterine growth retardation
11. Previous perinatal and neonatal deaths, preterm or low-birth-weight deliveries
12. Lower socioeconomic status

Previous Labor and Delivery Factors

1. Placental accident/hemorrhage
   a. Abruptio placentae
   b. Placenta previa
2. Cesarean section
3. Mechanical factors
   a. Abnormal presentation (*i.e.*, breech, transverse)
   b. Anatomy of the birth canal: cephalopelvic disproportion (CPD)
4. Fetal distress
5. Prolonged or obstructed labor that leads to fetal asphyxia (>24 hr for primigravidas; >18 hours for multigravidas)
6. Prolonged second stage of labor
7. Prolapsed, knotted, or entangled umbilical cord leading to fetal asphyxia
8. Maternal fever
9. Depressant drugs given to mother near delivery (*e.g.*, meperidine [Demerol])

(Adapted from Trotter CW, Chang P-N, Thompson T: Appendix: High-risk pregnancy factors. JOGN 11:90, March/April 1982)

Assessment and Nursing Care

The Assessment Tool provides a guide for assessing the variety of high-risk factors, both social and obstetric, discussed in this chapter. Specific care plans can be found in those chapters dealing with complications of pregnancy and the high-risk infant.

References

1. National Center for Health Statistics: Annual Summary for the United States, 1979. DHHS Publication No. (PHS) 81-1120, Monthly Vital Statistics Reports 28:13, November 13, 1980

2. Phipps-Yonas S: Teenage pregnancy and motherhood. Am J Orthopsychiatry 50(3):403–431, 1980

3. McCormick L, Shapiro S, Starfield G: High-risk young mothers: Infant mortality and morbidity in four areas in the United States, 1973–1978. Am J Public Health 74(1):18–23, January 1984

4. Hogan LR: Pregnant again—at 41. MCN 4:174–176, 1979

5. National Center for Health Statistics: Vital Statistics of the United States, 1973, Vol 1, Natality (HRA) 77-113, pp 1–12, 1977

6. Trotter CW, Chang P, Thompson T: Prenatal factors and the developmental outcome of preterm infants. JOGN Nurs 11(2):83–90, March/April 1982

7. Siegal M: A first baby after 40—It's safer now. Parade: Sunday Supplement, pp 6–7, Detroit Free Press, August 1976

8. Calton L: Prenatal tests help cure defects and save babies. Parade: Sunday Supplement, pp 10–12, Detroit Free Press, April 1976

9. Card JJ, Wise LL: Teenage mothers and fathers: The impact of early childbearing on the parents' personal and professional lives. Fam Plann Perspect 10(4):199–205, 1978

10. National Center for Health Statistics: Monthly Vital Statistics Report 1980, No. 8. DHHS Publication No. (PHS) 83-1120, November 1982

11. Tietze C: Teenage pregnancies: Looking ahead to 1984. Fam Plann Perspect 10(4):205–207, 1978

12. Lawrence RA, Merritt TA: Infants of adolescent mothers: Perinatal, neonatal and infancy outcomes. Semin Perinatol 5:19–32, 1981

13. Teenage Pregnancy: The Problem That Hasn't Gone Away. New York, Alan Guttmacher Institute, 1981

14. Jacobson HN: Diet therapy and the improvement of pregnancy outcomes. Birth 10(1):29–31, Spring 1983

15. Committee on Nutrition of the Mother and the Preschool Child, Food and Nutrition Board, National Research Council: Nutrition Services in Perinatal Care. Washington, DC, National Academy Press, 1981

16. Carey WB et al: Adolescent age and obstetric risk. Semin Perinatol 5:9–15, 1981

17. Infant mortality rates: Socioeconomic factors, United States. Washington, DC, Vital Health Statistics, Series 24, No. 14, 1980

18. Sugar M: Developmental issues in adolescent motherhood. In Sugar M (ed): Female Adolescent Development, pp 330–343. New York, Brunner/Mazel, 1979

19. Lasselson R: Ego development in adolescence. In Adelson J (ed): Handbook of Adolescent Psychology, pp 188–210. New York, John Wiley & Sons, 1980

20. McLaughlin SD, Micklin M: The timing of the first birth and changes in personal efficacy. J Marr Fam 45(1):47–55, February 1983

21. Duncan GJ, Morgan JN: The incidence and some consequences of major life events. In Duncan GL, Morgan JN (eds): Five Thousand American Families: Patterns of Economic Progress, Vol 8. Ann Arbor, ISR, 1980

22. Hayes L, Crovitz E: Adolescent pregnancy. South Med J 72(7):869–874, 1979

23. Cranley MS: Perinatal risk. JOGN Nurs 12(6):13s–18s, May/June 1983

24. Kotelchuck M et al: WIC participation and pregnancy outcomes: Massachusetts Statewide Evaluation Project. Am J Public Health 74(10):1086–1092, 1984

25. Parapakkam SA: An epidemiologic study of eclampsia. Obstet Gynecol 4:26–36, 1979

26. Lechtig A: Studies of nutrition intervention in pregnancy. Birth 9:115–121, 1982

27. Kretzehmar RM: Smoking and health: The role of the obstetrician gynecologist. Obstet Gynecol 55:403–418, 1980

28. Deibel P: Effects of cigarette smoking on maternal nutrition and the fetus. JOGN Nurs 9(6):333–336, 1980

29. Taper LJ et al: Influence of maternal weight, smoking and socioeconomic status on infant triceps, skinfold thickness and growth during the first year of life. Birth 11:97–101, Summer 1984

30. A Report of the Surgeon General. DHEW Publication No. (PHS) 79-50056, 1979

31. Stein Z, Kline J: Smoking, alcohol and reproduction. Am J Public Health 73:1154–1156, October 1983

32. Abel EL: Smoking during pregnancy: A review of effects on growth and development of offspring. Hum Biol 52:593–625, 1980

33. Kline J et al: Smoking, a risk factor for spontaneous abortion. N Engl J Med 297:793–796, 1977

34. Harlap S, Shiono PH: Alcohol, smoking and incidence of spontaneous abortions in the first and second trimester. Lancet ii:173–176, 1980

35. Stein Z, Kline J, Kharazzi M: What is a teratogen? Epidemiologic criteria. In Kalter H (ed): Issues and Reviews in Teratology. New York, Plenum Press, 1984

36. Wainwright RL: Change in observed birth weight associated with change in maternal cigarette smoking. Am J Epidemiol 117:665–675, 1983

37. Streitfeld PP: Congenital malformation: Teratogenic foods and additives. Birth Fam J 5:7–19, Spring 1978

38. Wilson T (ed): Handbook of Teratology. New York, Plenum Press, 1977

39. Wilson T: Teratogenic effects of environmental chemicals. Fed Proc 36:1698–1703, 1977

40. Kurppa K et al: Coffee consumption during pregnancy

and selected congenital malformations: A nationwide case-control study. Am J Public Health 73:1397–1400, December 1983

41. Linn S et al: The association of marijuana use with outcome of pregnancy. Am J Public Health 73:1161–1164, October 1983
42. Bogdanoff B et al: Brain and eye abnormalities: Possible sequelae to prenatal use of multiple drugs including LSD. Am J Dis Child 123:145–148, 1972
43. Fried PA: Marijuana use by pregnant women: Neurobehavioral effects in neonates. Drug Alcohol Depend 6: 415–424, 1980
44. Hingson R et al: Effects of maternal drinking and marijuana use on fetal growth and development. Pediatrics 70:539–546, 1982
45. Woodward L et al: Exposure to drugs with possible adverse effects during pregnancy and birth. Birth 9(3): 165–171, Fall 1982
46. Connaughton JF et al: Perinatal addiction: Outcome and management. Am J Obstet Gynecol 129:679–686, 1977
47. Chasnoff IJ, Hatcher R, Burnes WJ: Early growth patterns of methadone addicted infants. Am J Dis Child 134:1049–1056, 1980
48. Lindor E, McCarthy AM, McRae MG: Fetal alcohol syndrome: A review and case presentation. JOGN Nurs 9(4):222–228, 1980
49. Herrmann J et al: Teratoectodactyles and other skeletal manifestations in the fetal alcohol syndrome. Eur J Pediatr 133:221–226, 1980
50. Clarren SK, Smith DW: The fetal alcohol syndrome. N Engl J Med 298:1063–1067, 1978
51. Tennes K, Blackard C: Maternal alcohol consumption, birth weight and minor physical anomalies. Am J Obstet Gynecol 138:774–780, 1980
52. Norbeck JS, Tilden VP: Life stress, social support, and emotional disequilibrium in complications of pregnancy: A prospective, multivariate study. J Health Soc Behav 24:30–46, March 1983
53. Gore S: The effect of social support in moderating health consequences of unemployment. J Health Soc Behav 19:157–165, 1978
54. LaRocco JM, House JS, French JR Jr: Social support, occupational stress and health. J Health Soc Behav 21: 202–218, 1980
55. Tilden VP: The relation of life stress and social support to emotional disequilibrium during pregnancy. Res Nurs Health 6:167–173, 1983
56. Thoits PA: Conceptual, methodological and theoretical problems in studying social support as a buffer against life stress. J Health Soc Behav 23:145–159, 1982
57. Beck NC et al: The prediction of pregnancy outcomes: Maternal preparation, anxiety and attitudinal sets. J Psychosom Res 24:343–351, 1980
58. Colman A, Colman L: Pregnancy as an altered state of consciousness. Birth Fam J 1(1):7–11, 1973
59. Glazer G: Anxiety levels and concerns among pregnant women. Res Nurs Health 3:107–113, 1980
60. Lennane KJ, Lennane RJ: Alleged psychogenic disorders in women—a possible manifestation of sexual prejudice. N Engl J Med 6:288–292, 1973

Suggested Reading

Conger RD, Yang RK, Burgess RL: Mother's age as a predictor of observed maternal behavior in three independent samples of families. J Marr Fam 46:411–424, May 1984

Council on Scientific Affairs: Effects of toxic chemicals on the reproductive system. JAMA 253:3431–3437, June 21, 1985

Emkin MW: Smoking and pregnancy: A new look. Birth 11(4):217–224, Winter 1984

Howley C: The older primipara: Implications for nursing. JOGN Nurs 10(3):182–185, 1981

LaRocco JM, House JS, French JR Jr: Social support, occupational stress and health. J Health Soc Behav 21:202–218, 1980

Makinson C: The health consequences of teenage fertility. Fam Plann Perspect 17:132–139, May/June 1985

Norris FD, Williams RL: Perinatal outcomes of Medicaid recipients in California. Am J Public Health 74:1112–1117, October 1974

Norwicki P et al: Effective smoking intervention during pregnancy. Birth 11(4):217–224, Winter 1984

Silverstein B et al: The availability of low-nicotine cigarettes as a cause of cigarette smoking among teenage females. J Health Soc Behav 21:383–388, 1980

Verny T, Kelly J: The Secret Life of the Unborn Child. New York, Dell Publishing, 1981

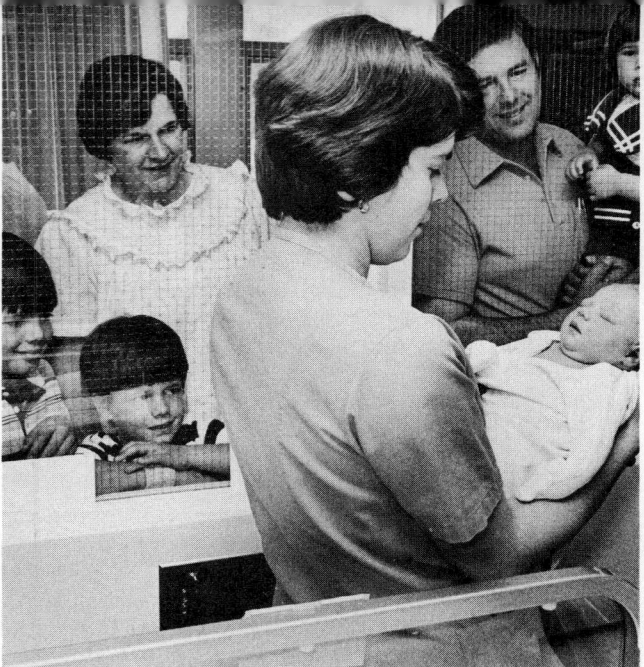

2. Which of the above is true until the time of fetal viability (defined as 24 to 26 weeks' gestation)? ____

3. The 1976 Hyde Amendment (upheld by the U.S. Supreme Court, 1980) made which provision relative to use of federal funds for abortions?
A. No federal funds could be used for abortions.
B. Federal funds could be used only for abortions when continuation of the pregnancy threatens the woman's life.
C. Federal funds could be used only for abortions in the first trimester. ____

S T U D Y   A I D S

Unit I:
Nursing, Family Health and Reproduction

Conference Material

1. Discuss the expanding roles of the maternity/perinatal nurse. Is there a difference between these roles? If so, how do they differ? Include a discussion of the rationale of why/why not the roles differ.

2. How would you go about refining the nursing diagnoses related to maternity care? Include a discussion of the present categories of nursing diagnoses. How do they relate to maternity/perinatal care?

3. What are the evolving family forms in your geographic area? Discuss how these may have an impact on nursing care.

4. Discuss the behavioral risk factors that you see threatening the clientele you serve.

Multiple Choice

1. The 1973 U.S. Supreme Court decision on abortions held that, in the first trimester of pregnancy
A. The abortion decision must be left to the woman and her physician
B. The state may regulate abortions in ways reasonably related to health
C. The state may proscribe abortions except where necessary to preserve the life or health of the pregnant woman ____

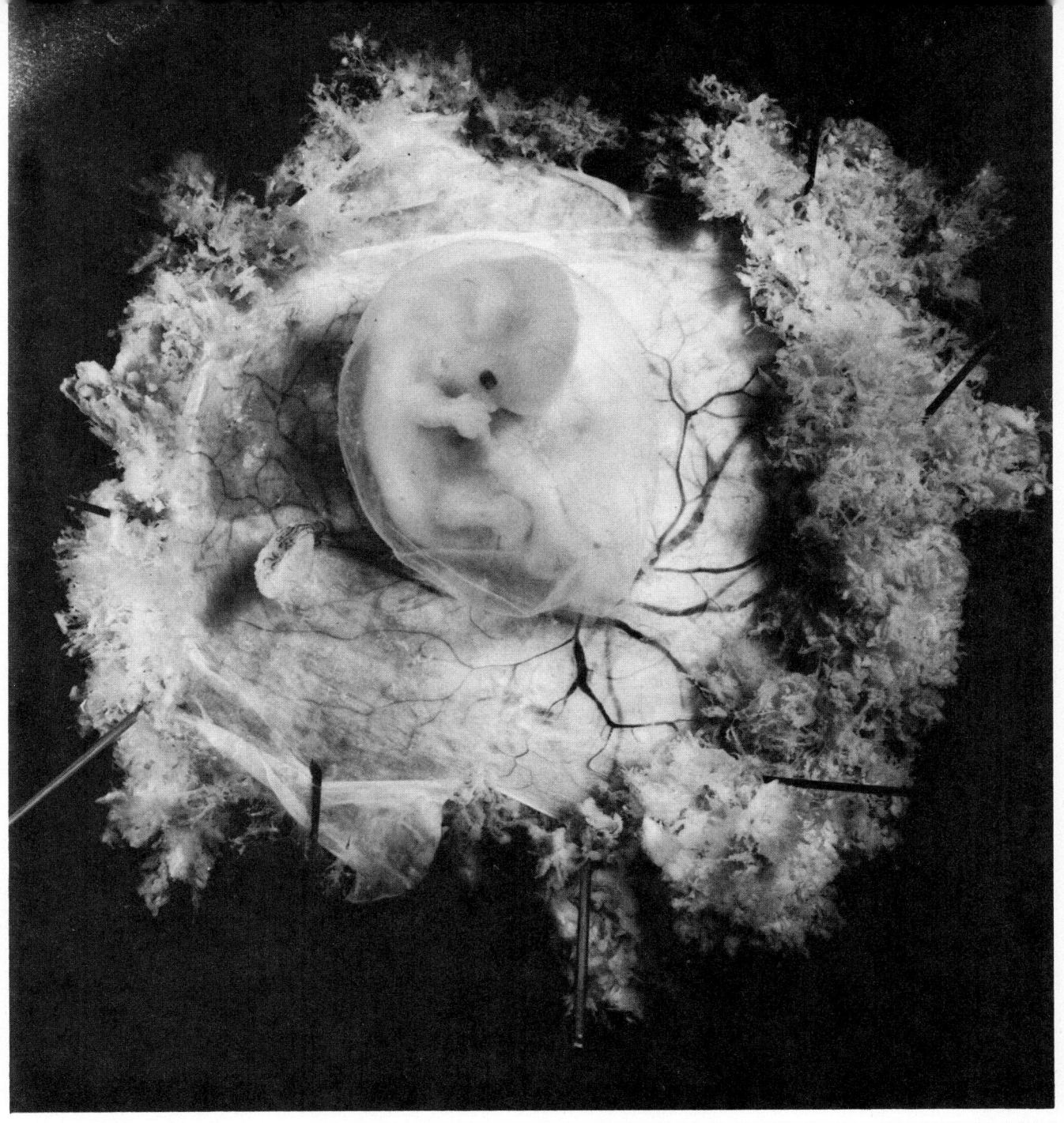

UNIT II

Biophysical Aspects
of Human Reproduction

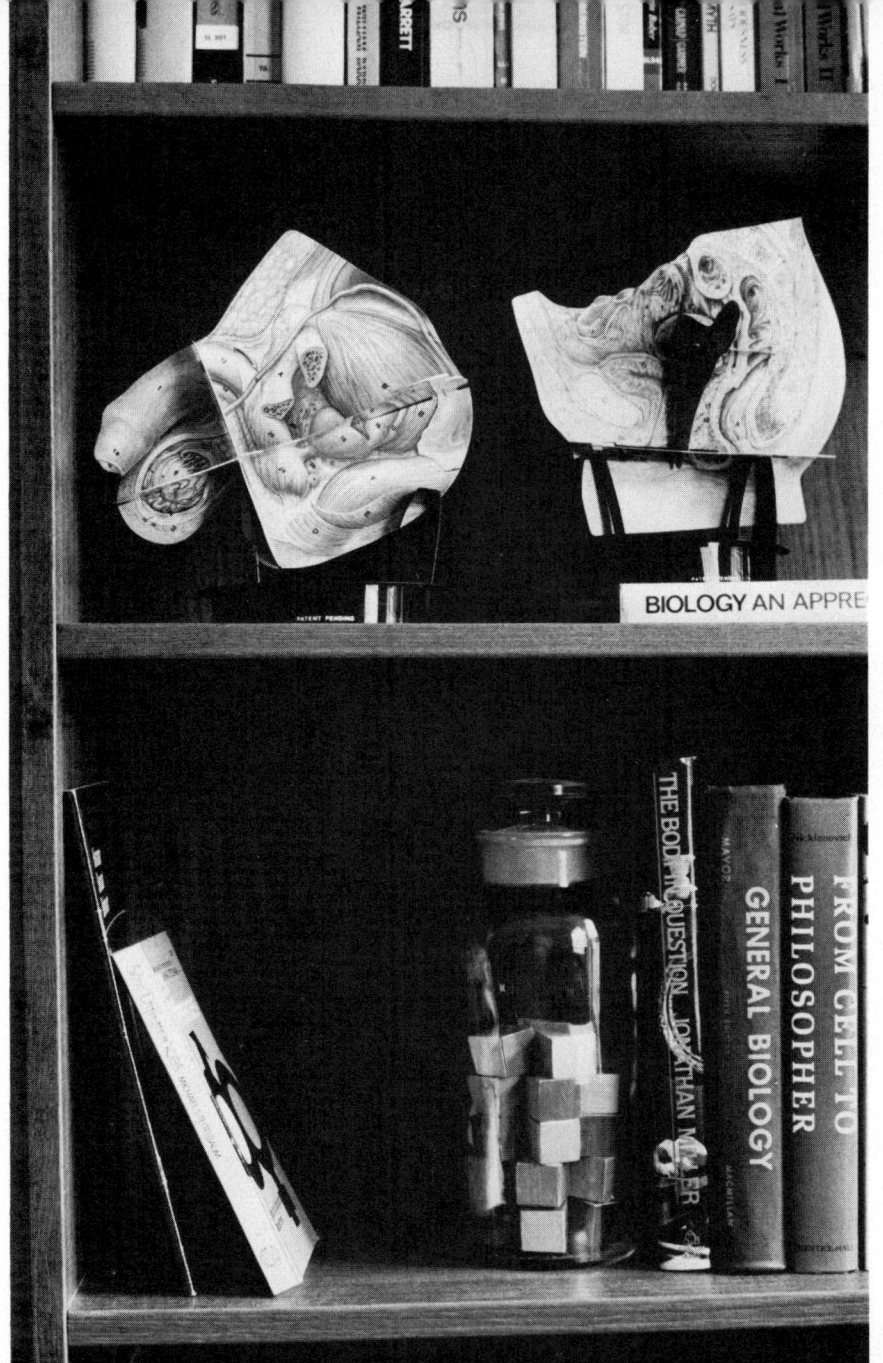

CHAPTER 9

Sexual and Reproductive Anatomy and Physiology

Women have a limited reproductive life span, beginning soon after the first menstrual period, declining somewhat in the late reproductive years, and finally terminating at the menopause. No more than 500 eggs or ova may be released during the course of reproductive life. In the male, sperm production is initiated at the time of puberty and continues well into senescence. The number of mature spermatozoa produced by the testes during this very long interval are in the billions, and the reproductive capacity of a given fertile male is nothing short of phenomenal.

Another important difference is that in the male the capacity to reproduce is necessarily associated with sexual excitement, erection of the penis, and ejaculation. However, the capacity of the female to reproduce may be disassociated from sexual excitement and receptivity. Consider that conception can occur by mechanical placement of the ejaculate through artificial insemination. The capacity of the woman for sexual pleasure, however, is extremely important. There is no doubt that the physical aspects of a relationship play a critical role in the communication process that brings a couple closer together.

Anatomy and physiology of the reproductive organs are discussed in this chapter, while orgasm is discussed in Chapter 10 and ovum and sperm development and fertilization are discussed in Chapter 11.

Male Organs of Reproduction

The male reproductive system consists of the penis, the testes, and an excretory duct system with their accessory structures (Fig. 9-1). Embryological development and genital differentiation of the male reproductive system are discussed in Chapter 10.

Penis

The penis, the male organ of copulation, consists of two lateral, cavernous bodies (two corpora cavernosa) and a central core of erectile tissue (corpus spongiosum) that encloses the urethra. The enlarged conic structure at the free end of the penis, an extension of the corpus spongiosum, is called the glans penis. The glans contains the external orifice of the urethra and is covered by a fold of retractable skin called the foreskin, or prepuce. Sometimes the foreskin is removed by circumcision.

The two corpora cavernosa are surrounded by a thick but elastic fibrous envelope. They are intimately connected along their course but are separated at their base into two *crura*, strong tapering fibrous processes that are firmly attached to the pubic bone. The corpora cavernosa receive their blood supply from branches of the dorsal artery of the penis. These divide further and terminate in a capillary network, the branches of which open directly into the cavernous spaces. These are usually quite empty, and the organ is flaccid. When these spaces fill with blood, the organ becomes turgid. This is called an erection. The flow of blood is controlled by the autonomic nervous system (vasodilator fibers) and varies with sexual arousal. When the erect penis is stimulated further, impulses from the autonomic nervous system trigger pulsatile release of semen along the urethra.

Testes

The functional capacity of the male reproductive tract is governed principally by the testes. Like their coun-

terpart in the female, the testes are dependent upon an interplay between the brain, the hypothalamus, and the pituitary gland. Like the ovary, the testes have two functions, in this case, secretion of the male hormone (testosterone) and spermatogenesis (the production and release of spermatozoa). Both are initiated at about the time of puberty and, under normal circumstances, continue well into senescence. Testosterone production can occur independently of spermatogenesis, but spermatogenesis cannot occur independently of testosterone production.

The testes are approximately 5 cm long and are contained in a fibrous protective covering, the tunica albuginea, which subdivides the testes into lobules (Fig. 9-2). Each lobule contains seminiferous tubules, coiled ducts in the walls of which spermatogenesis occurs. The

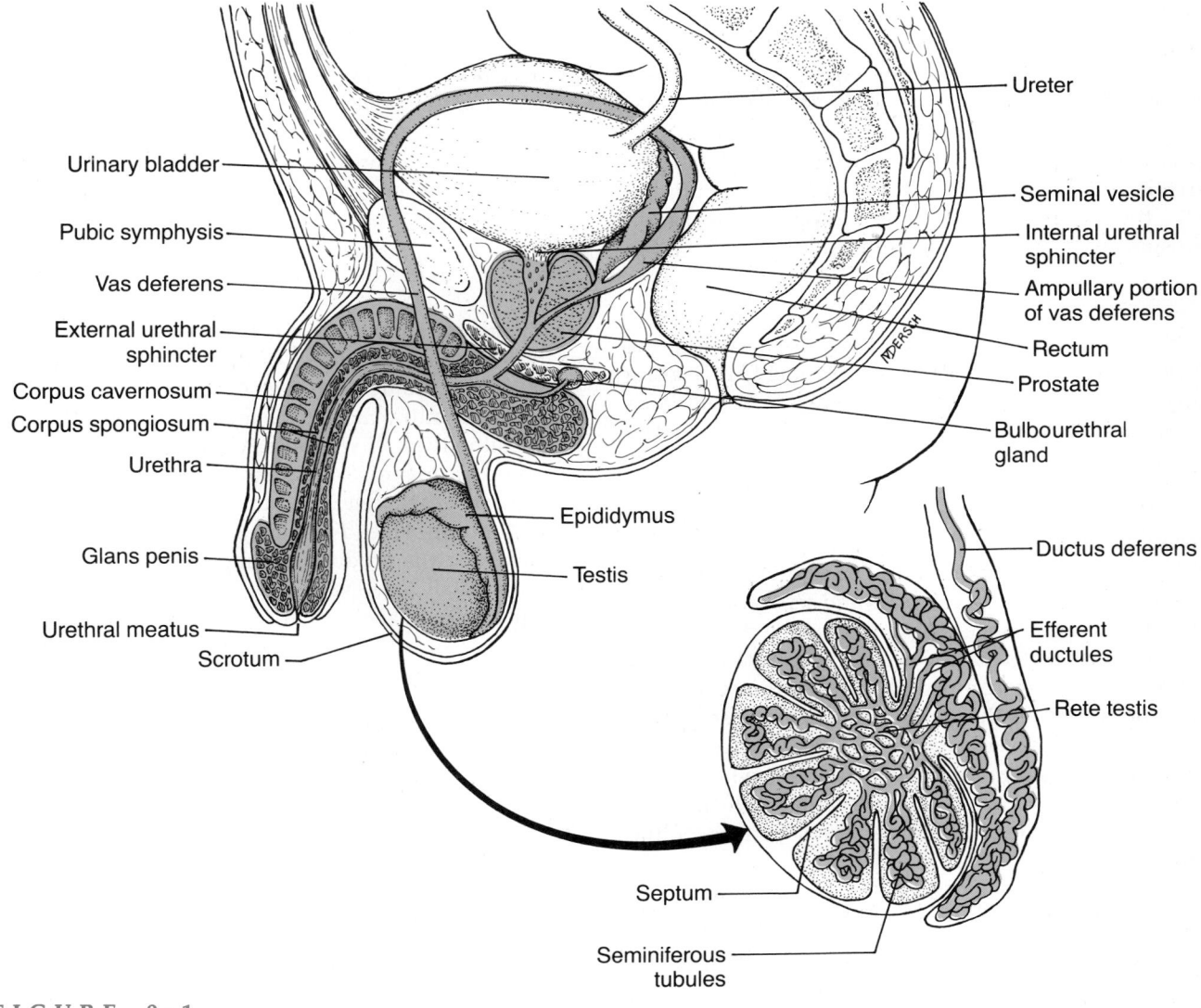

Urinary bladder

Pubic symphysis

Vas deferens

External urethral sphincter

Corpus cavernosum

Corpus spongiosum

Urethra

Glans penis

Urethral meatus

Scrotum

Epididymus

Testis

Ureter

Seminal vesicle

Internal urethral sphincter

Ampullary portion of vas deferens

Rectum

Prostate

Bulbourethral gland

Ductus deferens

Efferent ductules

Rete testis

Septum

Seminiferous tubules

FIGURE   9 - 1

Organs of the male reproductive system.

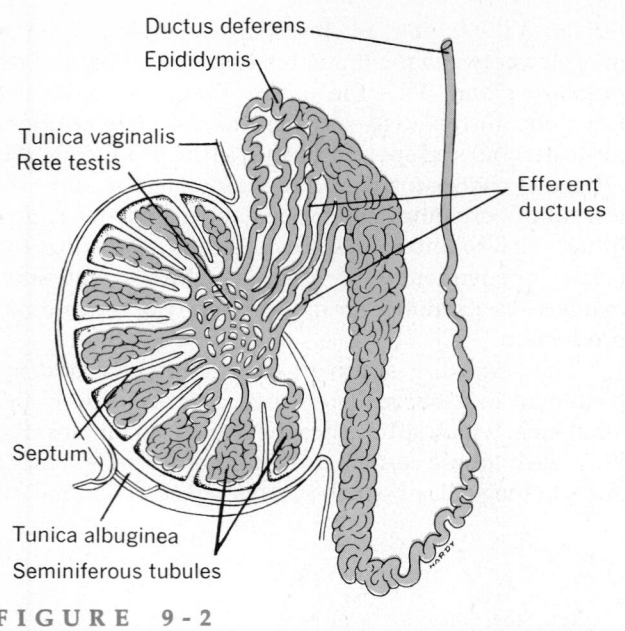

FIGURE 9-2

Diagram of structural features of the testis and epididymis.

testes also contain testosterone-producing cells, the interstitial cells of Leydig, as well as larger supporting cells, the Sertoli cells, which are important for sperm transport within the seminiferous tubules.

Scrotum

Unlike the ovaries, the testes are located outside the abdominal cavity in the scrotum (meaning bag). During early fetal life, the testes are abdominal. As the fetus develops, the testes move downward and enter the scrotum through the inguinal canal shortly before birth. The scrotum is located between the penis and the anus. It is a saclike structure composed of fascial connective tissue containing smooth-muscle fibers (dartos fascia) with overlying corrugated skin. The skin of the scrotum is pigmented with scattered hairs and sebaceous glands. Its wrinkled appearance is produced by the dartos fascia that underlies it. The muscle contained in dartos fascia responds to cold by contracting, accentuating the wrinkled appearance as the scrotum is drawn closer to the body wall. The two testes are separated from each other by a medial septum within the scrotum, which is an extension of the dartos fascia. Its location in the midline is marked by a ridge on the external surface of the scrotum.

Testicular Hormone Production

The adult testes produce a continuous supply of the male hormone, testosterone. Testosterone is synthesized and released by the interstitial cells, also referred to as Leydig cells. The interstitial cells are located in the interstitial connective tissue that surrounds and supports the seminiferous tubules. The interstitial cells are stimulated to produce testosterone by luteinizing hormone (LH), which is released from the anterior pituitary gland. This is identical to the LH that is released in large amounts at midcycle to trigger the onset of ovulation in the female. In the male, LH is sometimes referred to by another name, interstitial cell stimulating hormone (ICHS). ICHS does not display the marked cyclic variation in concentration seen during the menstrual cycle, although, as in the female, its release from the pituitary gland is controlled by releasing hormones from the brain and hypothalamus. There is a reciprocal relationship between LH release and testosterone production by the interstitial cells.

Testosterone establishes and maintains the secondary sex characteristics of the male, such as development and maturation of the external genitalia, prostate, and seminal vesicles; growth of body and facial hair; and maturation of the larynx. It also contributes to body growth and general development.

The principal role of testosterone in terms of reproduction is maintenance of spermatogenesis. Unless this hormone is present in normal amounts, fertility is impaired.

Spermatogenesis

Production of spermatozoa is initiated and maintained in the seminiferous tubules of the testes (Fig. 9-3). The seminiferous tubules are long coiled structures containing a lumen into which spermatozoa are released from their epithelial wall where they are produced. During this process, meiosis occurs, and the number of chromosomes in each cell is reduced to half, which is the haploid number (see Fig. 10-2). A structurally mature spermatozoon is produced, complete with head, midpiece, and tail (see Fig. 11-5). The maturation of the human spermatozoon occupies an interval of 60 days.

Spermatogenesis is a heat-sensitive process. The 2° to 3° difference between scrotal and abdominal temperatures allows spermatogenesis to proceed normally in the cooler environment. Testosterone production is not affected by temperature. When there has been failure of the testes to descend, spermatogenesis is severely impaired, but testosterone production remains unaffected.

Testicular Release of Sperm. The wall of the seminiferous tubules is separated into two physiologically distinct compartments by specialized supporting cells, the Sertoli cells. These cells are large, easily identifiable structures that are joined to each other by firm cell-to-

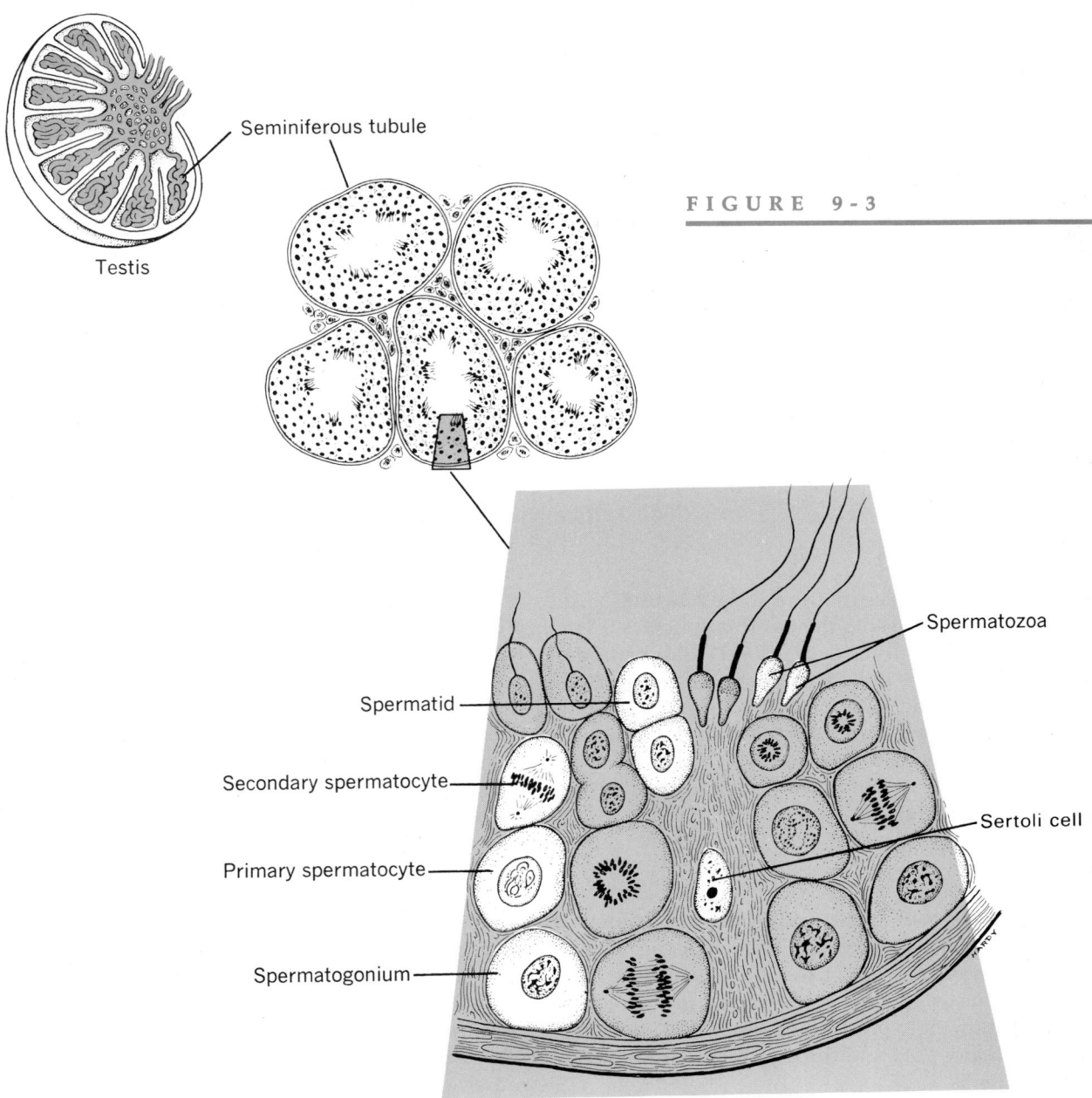

Testis

Seminiferous tubule

FIGURE 9-3

Spermatozoa

Spermatid

Secondary spermatocyte

Sertoli cell

Primary spermatocyte

Spermatogonium

cell connections. They separate the epithelium into a basal and a luminal compartment. This arrangement produces an effective separation of the basal compartment from the circulation and provides a blood–testes permeability barrier. In this way the early-developing sperm-forming elements are protected from harmful substances that may be circulating in the bloodstream.

The Sertoli cell plays an active role in the release of spermatozoa into the lumen of the seminiferous tubules. The tight junctions between the Sertoli cells break down transiently to permit upward movement of sper-

matocytes into the compartment adjacent to the lumen. They are then drawn into the cytoplasm of the Sertoli cell, moved upward toward the surface of the cell, and finally extruded by contractions of the cytoplasm of the apex of the Sertoli cells (Fig. 9-4).

Duct System

Leading from the testes are the transporting and storage ducts of the male reproductive tract.

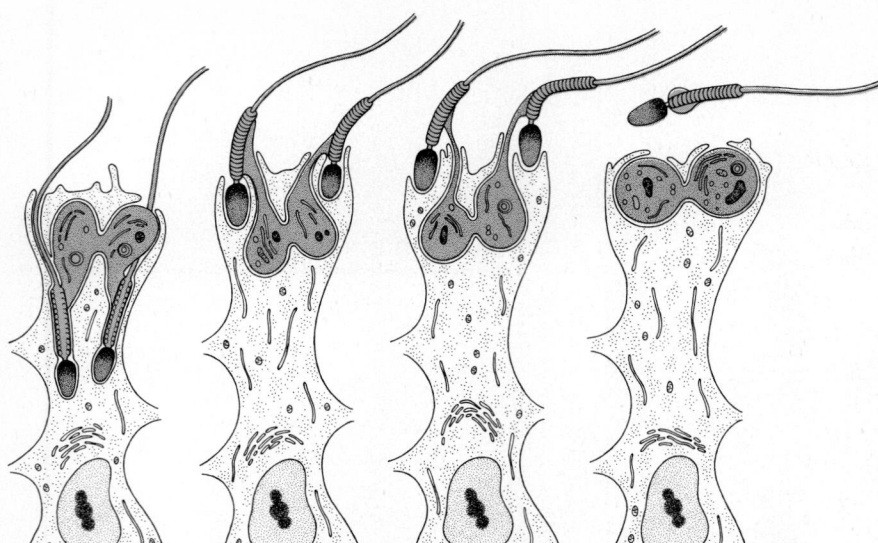

FIGURE 9-4

Diagram of the stages of sperm release. The conjoined cell bodies of the advanced spermatids are retained in the epithelium while the nucleus, neck region, and tail are gradually extruded into the lumen. The narrow stalk connecting the neck region with the cell body becomes increasingly attenuated and finally gives way. Individual spermatozoa are thus separated from the syncytial cell bodies. (Redrawn from Greep RO, Koblinsky MA (eds): Frontiers in Reproduction and Fertility Control. Cambridge, MIT Press, 1977)

Epididymis

The seminiferous tubules coalesce at the rete testis (see Fig. 9-2) and enter the epididymis. This structure is located adjacent to the testis (see Fig. 9-1) and serves as a reservoir for sperm. It is divided into a head portion (caput) and a tail (cauda).

When spermatozoa are released into the seminiferous tubules, although endowed with tails, they are not yet capable of motility. They acquire motility as they pass along the epididymis.

Vas Deferens

The ducts of the epididymis lead to the vas deferens, which provides the transporting passage along which spermatozoa traverse to the base of the penis (see Fig. 9-1). The ductus deferens or vas deferens has contractile power that allows it to propel the spermatozoa upward to the ejaculatory duct and through the urethra to the base of the penis.

Accessory Structures

The accessory structures consist of the seminal vesicles, the prostate gland, and the bulbourethral glands (see Fig. 9-1). The seminal vesicles are sacculated structures located behind the bladder and in front of the rectum; the prostate gland surrounds the base of the urethra and the ejaculatory duct; and the bulbourethral glands, or Cowper's glands, lie at the base of the prostate and on either side of the membranous urethra. The function of the accessory sex organs is maintained by testosterone. The bulbourethral glands produce a mucinous substance that lubricates the urethra and coats its surface.

The prostate rests upon the rectum, through which it can be felt. In shape and size it resembles a chestnut. It consists of two lateral lobes of equal size and a much smaller middle lobe. The ejaculatory ducts pass through the gland between the middle and lateral lobes, and the urethra traverses it. It sometimes becomes enlarged in men past middle age (benign prostatic hypertrophy) and causes urinary obstruction that requires surgical treatment.

Semen and Ejaculation

During ejaculation, the semen receives contributions from the seminal vesicles and the prostate gland. The seminal vesicles deliver the secretions to the urethra through the ejaculatory ducts, discharging a fructose-rich product. The seminal vesicles are a major source of prostaglandins, substances that stimulate smooth-muscle contractions. The prostate transmits its contents into the urethra during ejaculation through a number of small ducts. It secretes a clear fluid with a slightly acid *p*H that is rich in acid phosphatase, citric acid, zinc, and a number of proteolytic enzymes.

Two additional accessory glands, the bulbourethral, or Cowper's, glands, empty into the bulbous urethra. They produce a lubricating fluid that maintains moisture within the urethra. At the height of sexual excitement and full erection, their contents may be released, sometimes carrying with them a few spermatozoa. The functions of the secretions of the accessory glands are to facilitate transportation of spermatozoa along the urethra during the ejaculatory process and to provide a temporary milieu where spermatozoa can survive. Thus, the ejaculate or semen is made up of spermatozoa contained in seminal vesicular and prostatic secretions with a small contribution from Cowper's glands. On intravaginal ejaculation some spermatozoa leave the ejaculate almost immediately and begin to traverse the cervical mucus. Within a matter of minutes some spermatozoa are on their way to the site of fertilization.

Male Sexual Maturity

On the average, changes associated with puberty in the male occur somewhat later than in the female and span an interval of approximately 4 years. These include development of axillary, pubic, and body hair and maturation and growth of the testes and penis over a 2- to 3-year period, accompanied by a growth spurt and general muscular development.

Development of internal glands (prostate, bulbourethral, seminal vesicles) occurs syncronously with penile and testicular growth. Ejaculation of fluid with penile erection may occur as soon as a year after the beginning of growth of the penis, even before it is of mature size. Generally, the ability to grow a full beard signifies the completion of male sexual maturity.

Female Structures and Organs of Reproduction

Female Pelvis

The pelvis, so named because of its resemblance to a basin, is a bony ring interposed between the trunk and the thighs. The vertebral column, or backbone, passes into the pelvis from above and transmits the weight of the upper part of the body to it. Then the pelvis in turn

---

Female Organs of Reproduction

External	Internal
Vulva	Ovaries
Mons veneris	Fallopian tubes
Labia majora	Uterus
Labia minora	Corpus (body)
Clitoris	Cervix (neck)
Vestibule	
Perineum	

---

transmits weight to the lower limbs. From an obstetric point of view, however, it is the cavity that contains the generative organs and is the canal through which the fetus must pass during birth.

Bony Structure

The pelvis is made up of four united bones: the two hipbones (*os coxae,* or innominate), situated laterally and in front, and the sacrum and the coccyx, situated behind (Fig. 9-5).

Anatomically, the hipbones are divided into three parts: the ilium, the ischium, and the pubis. These bones become firmly joined into one by the time the growth of the body is completed (between the ages of 20 and 25) so that when the pelvis is examined, no trace of the original edges or divisions of these three bones can be discovered. Each of these bones may be briefly described as follows.

The *ilium,* the largest portion of the bones, forms the upper and back parts of the pelvis. Its upper flaring border forms the prominence of the hip, or crest of the ilium (hipbone).

The *ischium* is the lower part below the hip joint, and from it projects the tuberosity of the ischium, on which the body rests when in a sitting position.

The *pubis* is the front part of the hipbone; it extends from the hip joint to the joint in front between the two hipbones, the symphysis pubis, and then turns down toward the ischial tuberosity, thus forming, with the bone of the opposite side, the arch below the symphysis, the pubic or subpubic arch. This articulation of the two pubic bones encloses the pelvic cavity anteriorly.

The *sacrum* and the *coccyx* form the lowest portions of the spinal column. The sacrum is a triangular wedge-shaped bone that consists of five vertebrae fused together. It serves as the back part of the pelvis. The coccyx forms a tail end to the spine. In the child, the coccyx consists of four or five very small, separate vertebrae; in the adult, these bones are fused into one. The coccyx is usually movable at the point of attachment to the sacrum, the sacrococcygeal joint, and may become pressed back during labor to allow more room for the passage of the fetal head.

The marked projection formed by the junction of the last lumbar vertebra with the sacrum is of special importance. This is the *sacral promontory,* one of the most important landmarks in obstetric anatomy.

Articulation and Surfaces

There are four *articulations,* or joints of the pelvis, that have obstetric importance. Two are behind, between the sacrum and the ilia on either side, and are termed the *sacroiliac articulations;* one is in front, between the

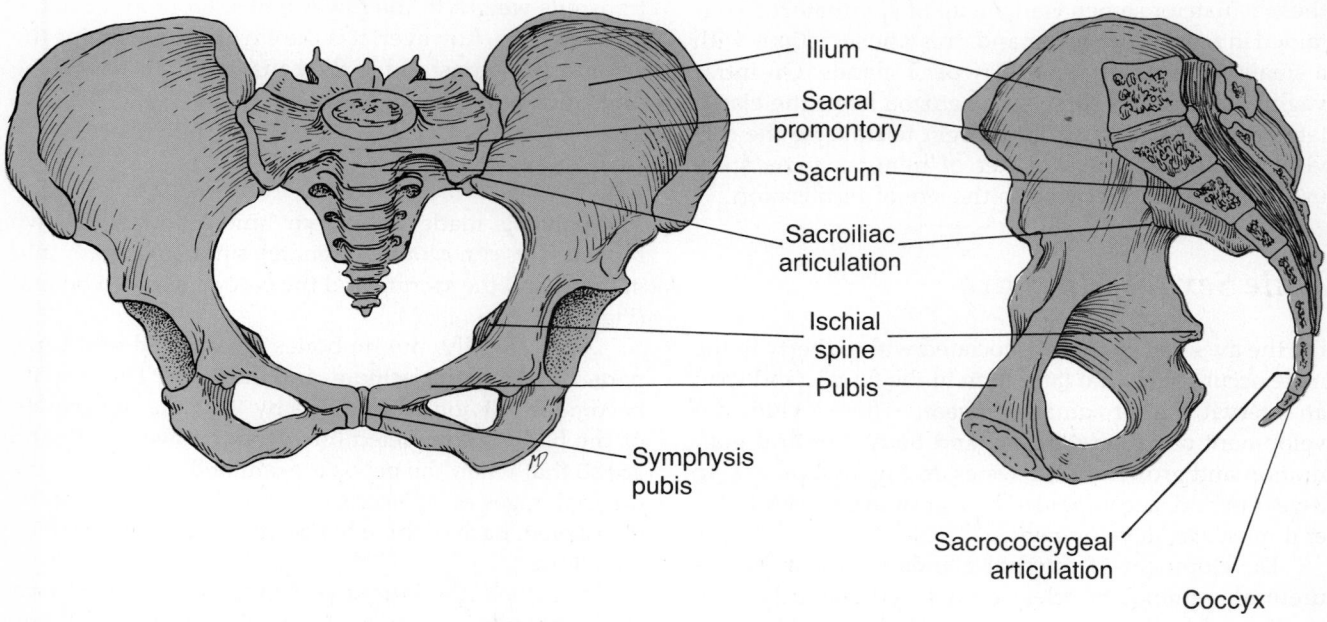

Ilium
Sacral promontory
Sacrum
Sacroiliac articulation
Ischial spine
Pubis
Symphysis pubis
Sacrococcygeal articulation
Coccyx

FIGURE 9-5

Front and lateral views of the pelvis showing major bones and articulations.

two pubic bones, and is called the *symphysis pubis;* and the fourth is the *sacrococcygeal articulation,* located between the sacrum and the coccyx.

All of these articular surfaces are lined with fibrocartilage, which becomes thickened and softened during pregnancy; likewise, the ligaments that bind the pelvic joints together become softened, and as a result greater mobility of the pelvic bones develops. A certain definite, though very limited, motion in the joints is desirable for a normal labor; however, there is no change in the actual size of the pelvis. From a practical standpoint, the increased mobility that these joints develop in pregnancy produces a slight "wobbliness" in the pelvis and throws greater strain on the surrounding muscles and ligaments. This accounts for much of the backache and leg ache in the later months of pregnancy.

The pelvis is lined with muscular tissue that provides a smooth, somewhat cushioned surface for the fetus to pass over during labor. These muscles also help to support the abdominal contents.

True and False Pelves

Regarded as a whole, the pelvis may be described as a two-story, bony basin that is divided into two parts by a natural line of division, the *inlet* or *brim.* The upper part is the false pelvis, and the lower part is the true pelvis (see Fig. 23-1).

The *false pelvis,* or upper flaring part, is much less concerned with the problems of labor than is the true

pelvis. It supports the uterus during late pregnancy and directs the fetus into the true pelvis at the proper time.

The *true pelvis,* or lower part, forms the bony canal through which the fetus must pass during parturition. For descriptive purposes it is divided into three parts: an inlet or brim, a cavity, and an outlet. The importance of these three parts and the various ways of assessing them during pregnancy and labor are discussed in Chapter 23 under material concerning the passageway of birth.

External Organs

The external female reproductive organs are called the *vulva,* from the Latin word meaning *covering.* This includes everything that is visible externally from the lower margin of the pubis to the perineum, namely, the mons veneris, the labia majora and minora, the clitoris, the vestibule, the hymen, the urethral opening, and various glandular and vascular structures (Fig. 9-6). The term *vulva* has often been used to refer simply to the labia majora and minora.

The *mons veneris* is a firm, cushionlike formation over the symphysis pubis that is covered with crinkly hair.

The *labia majora* are two prominent longitudinal folds of adipose tissue that are covered with skin and extend downward and backward from the mons veneris and disappear in forming the anterior border of the per-

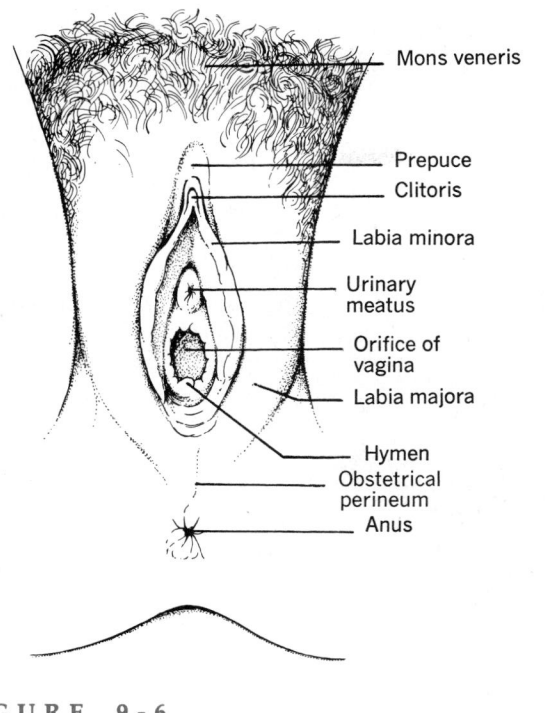

Mons veneris

Prepuce

Clitoris

Labia minora

Urinary meatus

Orifice of vagina

Labia majora

Hymen

Obstetrical perineum

Anus

FIGURE 9-6

External genitalia of the female.

ineal body. These two thick folds of skin are covered with hair on their outer surfaces after the age of puberty but are smooth and moist on their inner surfaces. At the bottom they fade away into the perineum posteriorly, joining together to form a transverse fold, the posterior commissure, which is situated directly in front of the fourchette. This fatty tissue is supplied with an abundant plexus of veins that may rupture as the result of injury sustained during labor and give rise to an extravasation of blood, or hematoma.

The *labia minora* are two thin folds entirely covered with thin membrane that are situated between the labia majora. The outer surfaces join with the inner surfaces of the labia majora. The labia minora extend from the clitoris downward and backward on either side of the orifice of the vagina. In the upper extremity, each labium minus separates into two branches, which, when united with those of the opposite side, enclose the clitoris. The upper fold forms the prepuce, and the lower fold forms the frenum of the clitoris. At the bottom, the labia minora pass almost imperceptibly into the labia majora or blend together as a thin fold of skin, the fourchette, which forms the anterior edge of the perineum or perineal body.

The *clitoris* is a small, highly sensitive projection that is composed of erectile tissue, nerves, and blood vessels and is covered with a thin epidermis. It is analogous to the penis in the male and is regarded as the chief area of voluptuous sensation. The clitoris is par-

tially hidden between the anterior ends of the labia minora.

The *vestibule* is the almond-shaped area that is enclosed by the labia minora and extends from the clitoris to the fourchette. It is perforated by four openings: the urethra, the vaginal opening, the ducts of Bartholin's glands, and the ducts of Skene's glands. *Bartholin's glands* are two small glands situated beneath the vestibule on either side of the vaginal opening. *Skene's glands* open on the vestibule on either side of the urethra.

The *hymen* marks the division between the internal and the external organs. It is a thin sheath of mucous membrane situated at the orifice of the vagina. It may be entirely absent, or it may form a complete septum across the lower end of the vagina.

The hymen changes in shape and consistency throughout the life cycle. In the newborn it projects beyond the surrounding parts. In adult virgins it is a membrane of varying thickness that presents an aperture that varies in size from a small opening to one that readily admits one or even two fingers. The opening is circular or crescent shaped. In rare instances, the hymen may be imperforate and cause retention of menstrual discharge if it occludes the vaginal orifice completely.

The *perineum* consists of muscles and fascia of the urogential diaphragm and lies across the pubic arch and the pelvic diaphragm (Fig. 9-7). The pelvic diaphragm itself consists of the coccygeus and the levator ani muscles, together with the fascia covering their internal and external surfaces. It is the most inferior portion of the body wall and stretches across the pelvic cavity like a hammock. The levator ani forms a slinglike support for the pelvis. It can generally be separated into two parts, the pubococcygeus and the iliococcygeus. The pubococcygeus, as its name implies, arises from the dorsal surface of the pubis. It is separated from its counterpart on the opposite side by the urethra, vagina, and rectum. Behind the rectum the two pubococcygeus muscles join, forming a loop or sling. The more superficial fibers of these muscles are attached to the perineal body. The iliococcygeus is the most lateral portion of the levator ani, arising from the ischial spine and inserting in the last two segments of the coccyx as well as in the perineal body. Between the anus and the vagina the levator ani is reinforced by a central tendon of the perineum, where three pairs of muscles converge: the bulbocavernous, the superficial transverse muscles of the perineum, and the external sphincter ani. These structures, which constitute the perineal body, are also joined by fibers of the levator ani and together form the main support of the pelvic floor. They are often lacerated during delivery.

The pubococcygeus muscle then is the muscle located immediately adjacent to the urethra, vagina, and rectum. By virtue of the fact that it forms a sling around the structure, it is one of the most important muscles

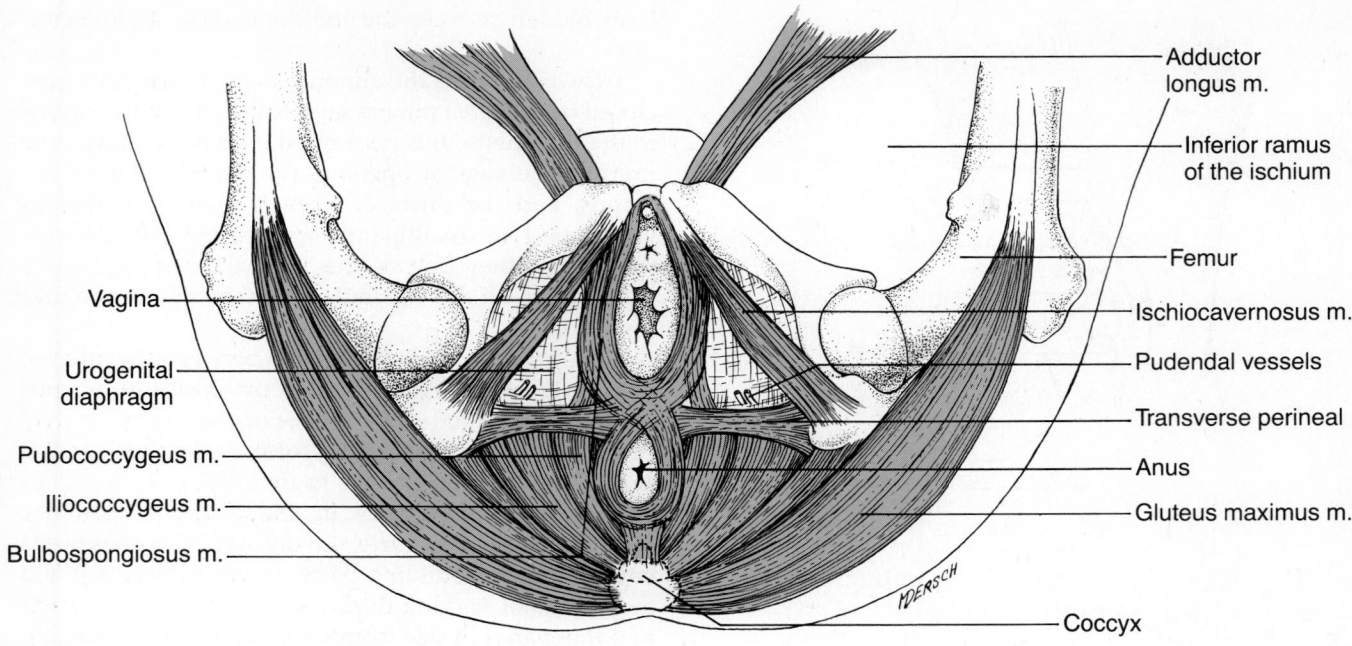

Vagina

Urogenital
diaphragm

Pubococcygeus m.

Iliococcygeus m.

Bulbospongiosus m.

Adductor
longus m.

Inferior ramus
of the ischium

Femur

Ischiocavernosus m.

Pudendal vessels

Transverse perineal

Anus

Gluteus maximus m.

Coccyx

FIGURE 9-7

Muscles of the pelvic floor (female perineum).

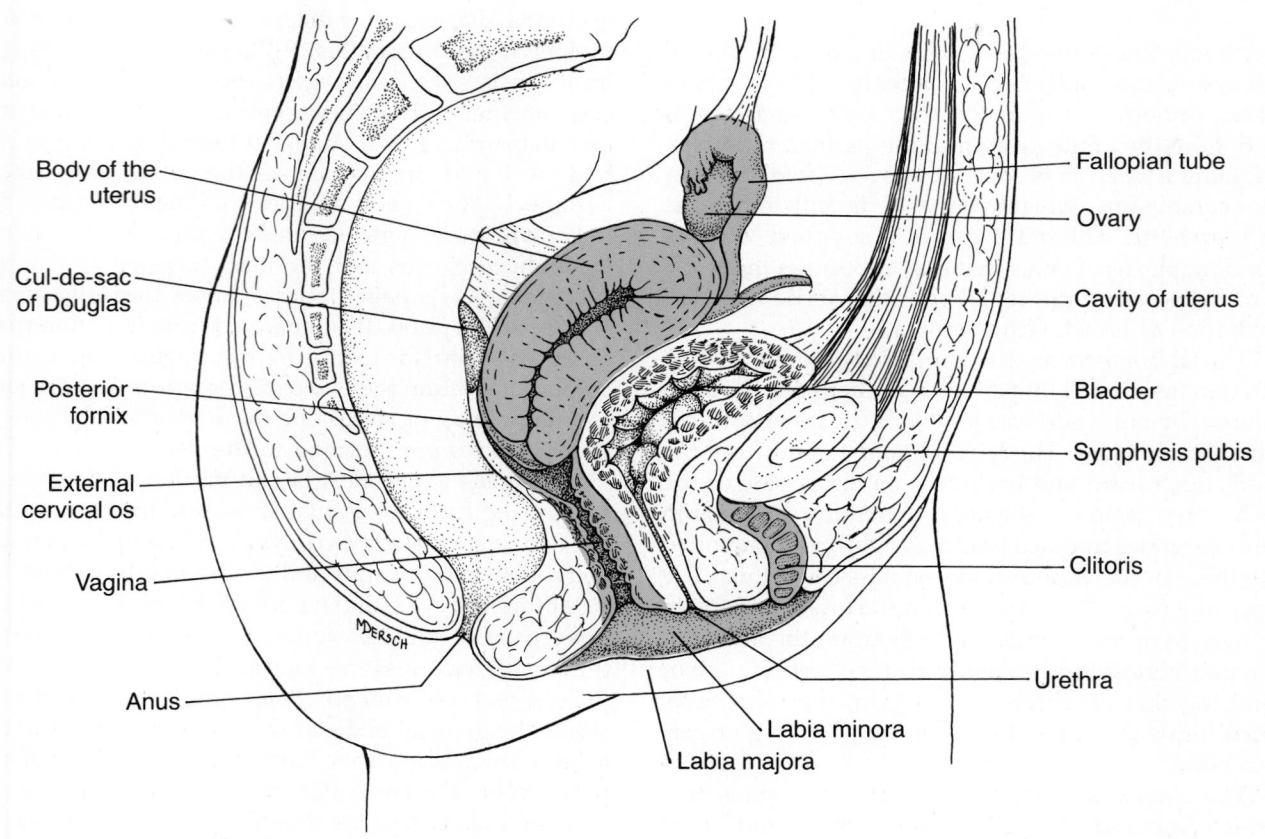

Body of the
uterus

Cul-de-sac
of Douglas

Posterior
fornix

External
cervical os

Vagina

Anus

Fallopian tube

Ovary

Cavity of uterus

Bladder

Symphysis pubis

Clitoris

Urethra

Labia minora

Labia majora

FIGURE 9-8

Female reproductive organs as seen in sagittal section.

in terms of pelvic support. When this muscle has become attenuated as a result of childbirth, the support of these structures is altered, with herniation of the bladder (cystocele) and rectum (rectocele) as well as descent into the vagina of the cervix and uterus. Associated symptoms of this condition include urinary stress incontinence (inability to retain urine with coughing or sudden movement). Correction of these conditions can sometimes be accomplished with the use of exercises designed to strengthen the pubococcygeus muscles. Patients can be instructed to contract these muscles, and successful use of such exercises can sometimes obviate the necessity for corrective surgical procedures.

Internal Organs

The internal organs of reproduction are the vagina, the uterus, the fallopian or uterine tubes, and the ovaries (Figs. 9-8 and 9-9).

Ovaries

The *ovaries* are two almond-shaped organs that are situated in the upper part of the pelvic cavity on either side of the uterus. Their chief functions are the devel-

opment and the expulsion of ova and the provision of certain internal secretions, or hormones. These organs correspond to the testes in the male. They are embedded in the posterior fold of the broad ligament of the uterus and are supported by the suspensory, the ovarian, and the mesovarium ligaments (see Fig. 9-9).

Each ovary contains a large number of germ cells, or primordial ova, in its substance at birth. This huge storage of primordial follicles present at birth more than suffices the woman for life. It is believed that no more are formed and that this large initial store is gradually exhausted during the period of sexual maturity. Beginning at puberty, one of the follicles that contain the ova enlarges each month and ruptures. The ovum and the fluid content of the follicle are released from the ovary; then they are swept into the tube. The development and the maturation of follicles containing the ova continue from puberty to menopause.

The arteries that supply the ovaries are four or five branches that arise from the anastomosis of the ovarian artery with the ovarian branch of the uterine artery (Fig. 9-10). The veins that drain the ovary become tributaries to both the uterine and the ovarian plexus. Superiorly, the ovarian vein drains into the inferior vena cava on the right and into the renal vein on the left.

The nerves supplying the ovaries are derived from

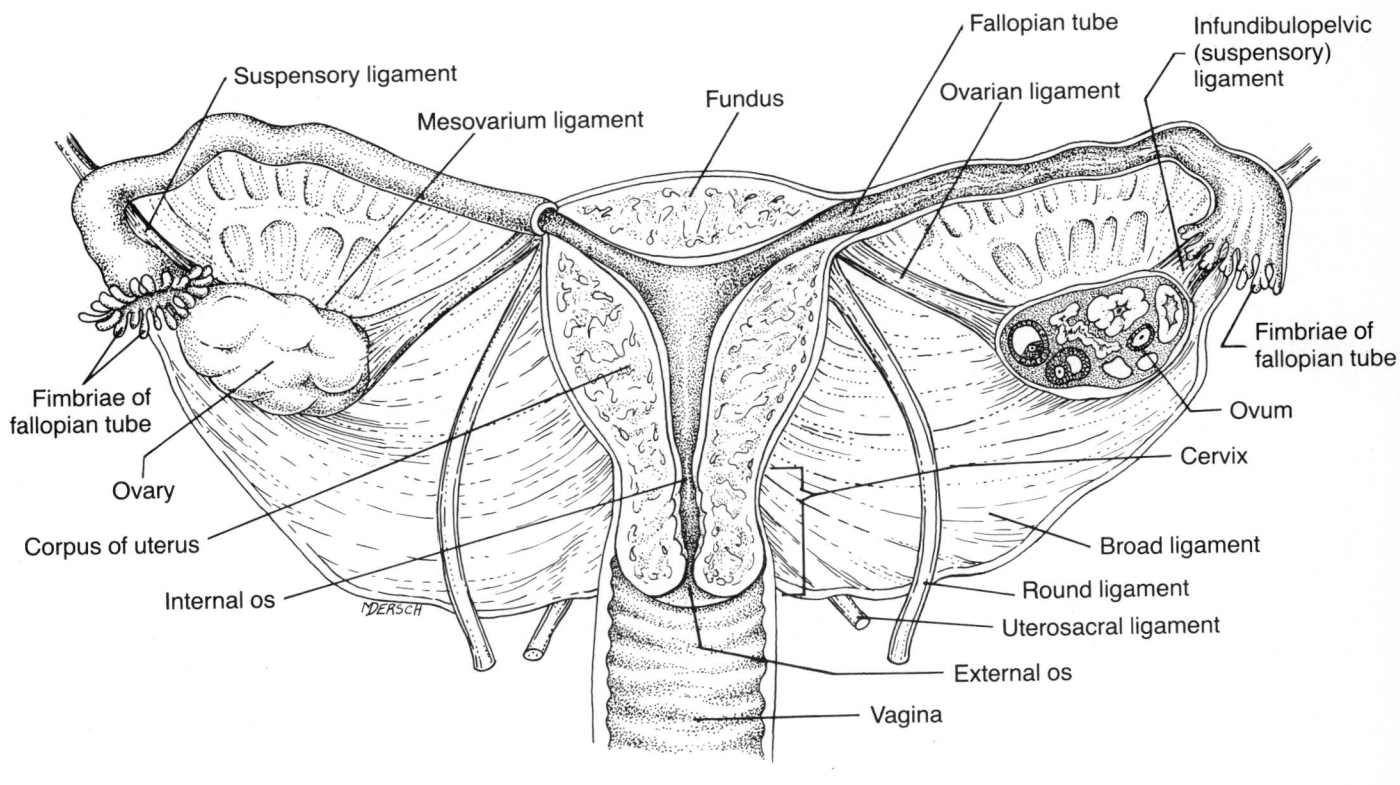

FIGURE 9-9

Anterior view of the uterus and related structures.

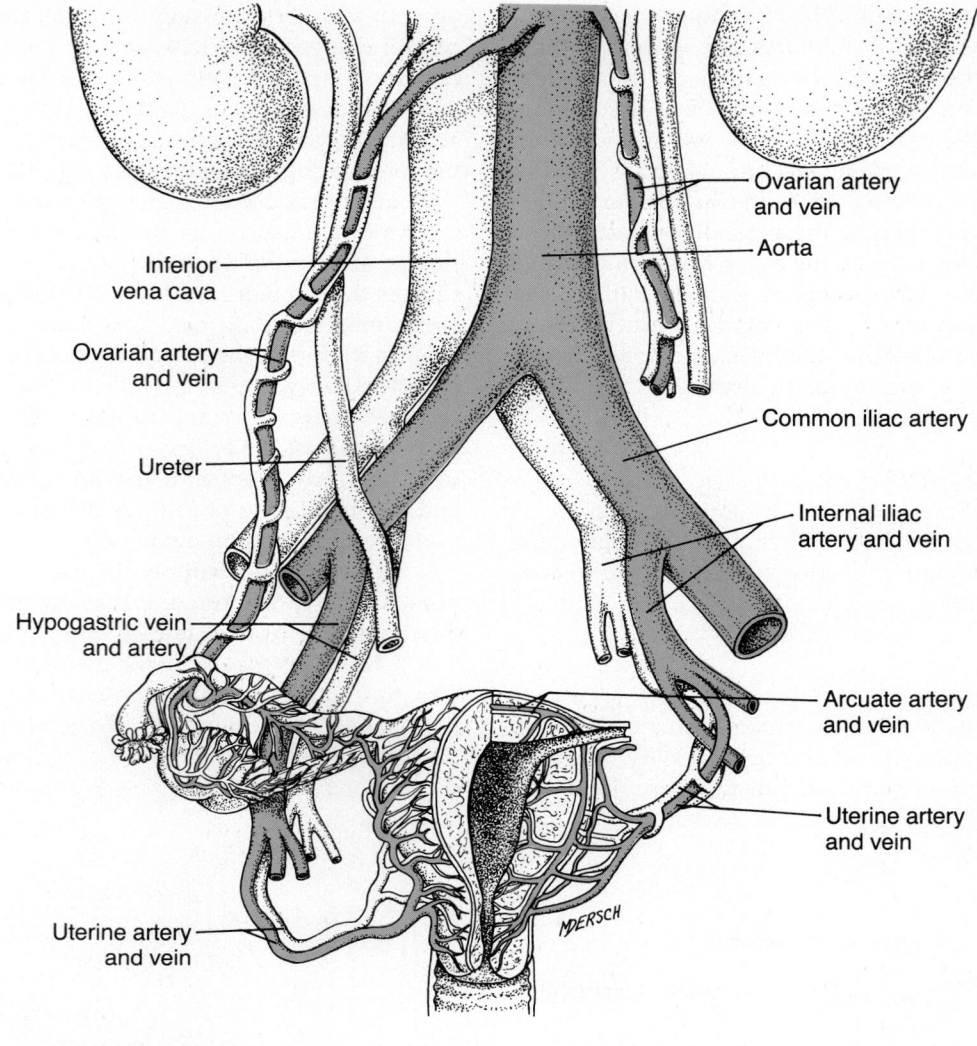

FIGURE 9-10

Blood supply of the uterus and the adnexa.

the craniosacral and the thoracolumbar sympathetic systems. The postganglionic and visceral afferent fibers form a plexus that surrounds the ovarian artery, which is formed by contributions from the renal and the aortic plexuses and corresponds to the spermatic plexus in the male.

Fallopian Tubes

The fallopian tubes are two trumpet-shaped, thin, flexible, muscular tubes that are about 12 cm long. They extend from the uterine cornua along the upper margin of the broad ligaments to the ovaries. They have two openings, one into the uterine cavity and the other into the abdominal cavity.

The opening into the uterine cavity is minute and will admit only a fine bristle. The abdominal opening is larger and is surrounded by a large number of fine fringes or fimbriae. The fimbriated extremity lies near the ovary, but it is not necessarily in direct contact with it. It is generally believed that the cilia on the fimbriated end of the tube create a current in the layer of fluid that surrounds the various pelvic organs.

The tubes convey the ovum by ciliary action and peristalsis to the cavity of the uterus. The fimbriated ends of the tube convey the escaped ovum into the tube, where fertilization occurs.

The tubes are lined with mucous membrane that contains ciliated and secretory epithelium. The muscular layer is made up of longitudinal and circular fibers that provide peristaltic action. The serous membrane covering the tubes is a continuation of the peritoneum, which lines the whole abdominal cavity.

The fallopian tubes receive their blood supply from

the ovarian and the uterine arteries (see Fig. 9-10). The veins of the tubes follow the course of these arteries and empty into the uterine and the ovarian trunks. The nerves that supply the uterus also innervate the tubes.

Uterus

The uterus is a hollow, thick-walled, muscular organ (see Fig. 9-9). It serves two important functions: (1) it is the organ of menstruation and (2) during pregnancy it receives the fertilized ovum and retains and nourishes it until it expels the fetus during labor.

The uterus varies in size and shape according to the age of the woman and whether or not she has borne children. The uterus of the adult nullipara weighs approximately 60 g and measures 5.5 cm to 8 cm in length.

It resembles a flattened pear in appearance and has two divisions, the upper triangular portion, the *corpus,* and the lower constricted cylindrical portion, the *cervix,* which projects into the vagina. The fallopian tubes extend from the *cornu* (the Latin word meaning *horn*) of the uterus at the upper outer margin on either side. The upper rounded portion of the uterus between the points of insertion of the tubes is the fundus (see Fig. 9-9).

The nonpregnant uterus is situated in the pelvic cavity between the bladder and the rectum. Almost the entire posterior wall and the upper portion of the anterior wall is covered by peritoneum. The lower portion of the anterior wall is united with the bladder wall by a layer of loose connective tissue. The lower posterior wall of the uterus and the upper portion of the vagina are separated from the rectum by the Douglas cul-de-sac, or pouch of Douglas.

Because of its muscular composition, the uterus is capable of enlarging to accommodate a growing fetus; at the termination of pregnancy it weighs about 1 kg or 2 lb. It is made up of involuntary muscle fibers that are arranged in all directions, making expansion possible in every direction to accommodate the products of conception. The arrangement of the uterus enables the fetus to be expelled at the end of a normal labor. Arranged between these muscular layers are many blood vessels, lymphatics, and nerves.

The cavity of the uterus is somewhat triangular. It is widest at the fundus, between the small openings into the fallopian tubes, and narrowest at the opening into the cervix. The anterior and posterior walls lie almost in contact, so that if a cross section of the uterus could be examined, the cavity between them would appear as a mere slit. The body of the uterus is lined with endometrium.

Cervix. The *cervix* is less movable than the body of the uterus. Its muscular wall is not as thick, and its lining is different in that it is much folded and contains crypts that produce mucus and are the chief source of

the mucous secretion during the menstrual cycle and in pregnancy. The cervix has an upper opening, the *internal os,* leading from the cavity of the uterine body into the cervical canal, and a lower opening, the *external os,* opening into the vagina. The cervical canal is small in the nonpregnant woman, barely admitting a probe, but at the time of labor it dilates to a size sufficient to permit the passage of the fetus.

Ligaments. The uterus is supported by ligaments extending from either side of the uterus and by the muscles of the pelvic floor. The ligaments that support the uterus in the pelvic cavity are the broad ligaments, the round ligaments, and the uterosacral ligaments (see Fig. 9-9).

The *broad ligaments* are two winglike structures that extend from the lateral margins of the uterus to the pelvic walls and divide the pelvic cavity into an anterior and a posterior compartment. Each consists of folds of peritoneum that envelop the fallopian tubes, the ovaries, and the round and ovarian ligaments. Its lower portion, the *cardinal ligament,* is composed of dense connective tissue that is firmly joined to the supravaginal portion of the cervix. The median margin is connected with the lateral margin of the uterus and encloses the uterine vessels.

The *round ligaments* are two fibrous cords that are attached on either side of the fundus, just below the fallopian tubes. They extend forward through the inguinal canal and terminate in the upper portion of the labia majora. These ligaments aid in holding the fundus forward.

The *uterosacral ligaments* are two cordlike structures that extend from the posterior cervical portion of the uterus to the sacrum. They help to support the cervix. The uterovesical ligament is merely a fold of the peritoneum that passes over the fundus and extends over the bladder. The rectovaginal ligament is a fold of the peritoneum that passes over the posterior surface of the uterus and is reflected upon the rectum.

Uterine Blood Supply. The uterus receives its blood supply from the ovarian and the uterine arteries (see Fig. 9-10). The uterine artery, the principal source, is the main branch of the hypogastric artery, which enters the base of the broad ligament and makes its way to the side of the uterus. The ovarian artery is a branch of the aorta. It enters the broad ligament and as it reaches the ovary it breaks up into smaller branches that enter that organ, while its main stem makes its way to the upper margin of the uterus, where it anastomoses with the ovarian branch of the uterine artery.

The uterovaginal plexus returns the blood from the uterus and the vagina to the venous circulation. These veins form a plexus of thin-walled vessels that are embedded in the layers of the uterine muscle. Emerging from this plexus, the trunks join the uterine vein, which is a double vein. These veins follow on either side of the uterine artery and eventually form one trunk that empties into the hypogastric vein, which makes its way into the internal iliac.

Uterine Nerve Supply.
The uterus possesses an abundant nerve supply that is principally derived from the sympathetic nervous system and partly from the cerebrospinal and parasympathetic system. Both the sympathetic and the parasympathetic nerve supplies contain motor and a few sensory fibers. The functions of the nerve supplies of the two systems are in great part antagonistic. The sympathetic system causes muscular contraction and vasoconstriction, and the parasympathetic system inhibits contraction and leads to vasodilatation.

Position of Uterus.
Since the uterus is a freely movable organ that is suspended in the pelvic cavity between the bladder and the rectum, the position of the uterus may be influenced by a full bladder or full rectum. The uterus can be pushed backward or forward. The uterus also changes its position when the patient stands, lies flat, or turns on her side. Also, there are variations in position, such as anteflexion, in which the fundus is tipped far forward; retroversion, in which the fundus is tipped far backward; and prolapse, which occurs when the muscles of the pelvic floor and the uterine ligaments are attenuated (Fig. 9-11).

Lymphatic Vessels.
The lymphatic vessels drain into the lumbar lymph nodes.

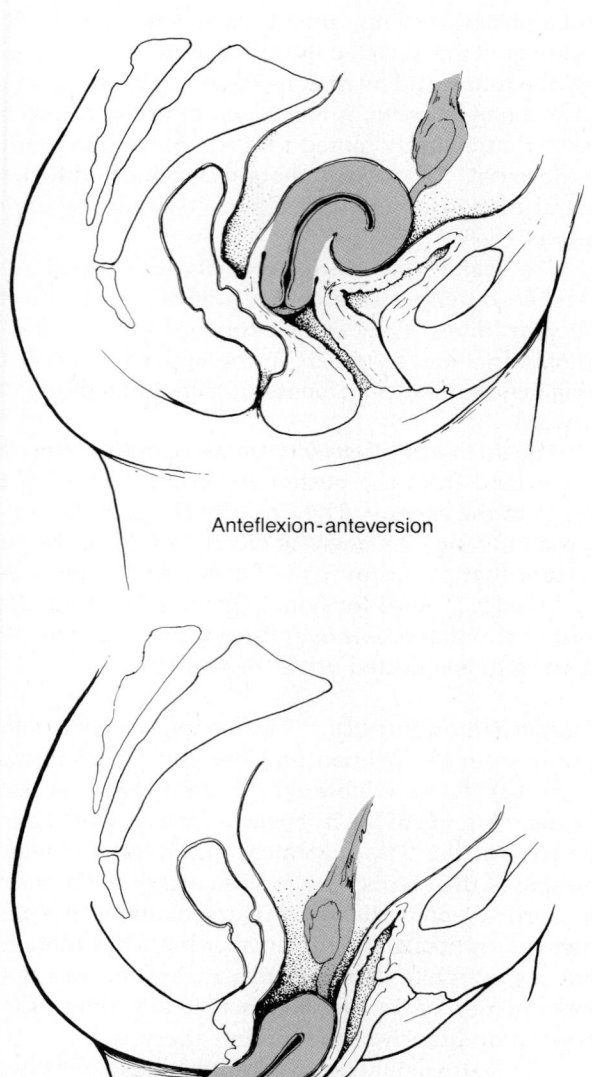

Anteflexion-anteversion

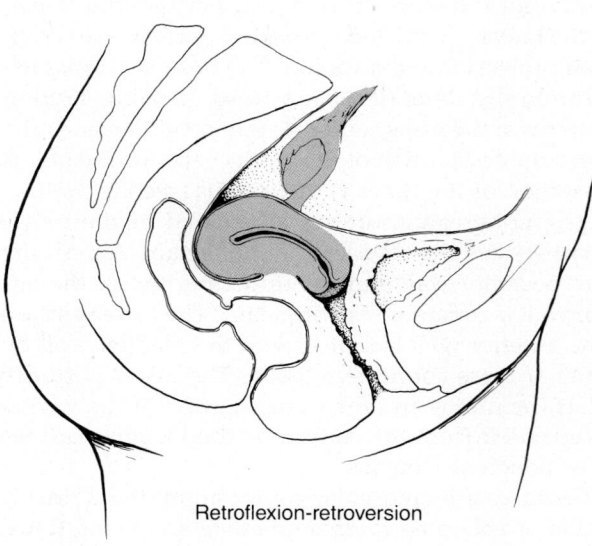

Retroflexion-retroversion

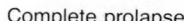

Complete prolapse

FIGURE 9-11

Positions of the uterus, showing anteflexion-anteversion, retroflexion-retroversion, and complete prolapse.

Vagina

The *vagina* is a dilatable, mucous membrane–lined passage between the bladder and the rectum (see Fig. 9-8). The vaginal opening occupies the lower portion of the vestibule. The vagina is from 8 cm to 12 cm long, and at the upper end is a blind vault, commonly called the *fornix,* into which the lower portion of the cervix projects.

The fornix is divided into four parts for descriptive purposes. The lateral fornices are the spaces between the vaginal wall on either side and the cervix; the anterior fornix is between the anterior vaginal wall and the cervix; and the posterior fornix is between the posterior vaginal wall and the cervix. The posterior fornix is considerably deeper than the anterior fornix because the vagina is attached higher up on the posterior than the anterior wall of the cervix. The fornices are important because the examiner is usually able to palpate the internal pelvic organs through their thin walls.

The vagina serves three important functions: it represents the excretory duct of the uterus through which secretion and the menstrual flow escape, it is the female organ of copulation, and it forms part of the birth canal during labor. Its walls are arranged into thick folds, the columns of the vagina, and, in women who have not borne children, numerous ridges, or *rugae,* which extend outward and almost at right angles to the vaginal columns and give the surface a corrugated appearance. Normally, the anterior and the posterior walls of the vagina lie in contact, but they are capable of stretching to allow marked distention of the passage, as in the process of childbirth.

The vagina receives an abundant blood supply from branches of the uterine, the inferior vesical, the median hemorrhoidal, and the internal pudendal arteries. The passage is surrounded by a venous plexus; the vessels follow the course of the arteries and eventually empty into the hypogastric veins. The lymphatics empty into the inguinal, the hypogastric, and the iliac glands.

Related Pelvic Organs

Bladder

The *bladder* is a muscular sac that serves as a reservoir for urine. It is situated in front of the uterus and behind the symphysis pubis (see Fig. 9-8). When empty or moderately distended, it remains entirely in the pelvis, but if it becomes greatly distended, it rises into the abdomen. Urine is conducted into the bladder by the ureters, two tubes that extend down from the basin of the kidneys and over the brim of the pelvis beneath the uterine vessels to open into the bladder at about the level of the cervix. The bladder is emptied through the urethra, a short tube that terminates in the urethral meatus. Lying on either side of the urethra and almost parallel with it are two small glands, less than 2.5 cm long, known as Skene's glands. Their ducts empty into the urethra just above the meatus. Often in cases of gonorrhea, Skene's glands and ducts are involved.

Anus

The *anus* is the entrance to the rectal canal. The rectal canal is surrounded at the opening or anus by its sphincter muscle, which binds it to the coccyx behind and to the perineum in front. It is supported by the muscles passing into it; these are the muscles that help to support the pelvic floor (see Fig. 9-8). The rectum is considered here because of the proximity to the field of delivery.

Mammary Glands

Although the mammary glands are not actual organs of reproduction, they are discussed in this section because of their importance as accessory glands, especially in the female body, and because they are directly affected by the female hormones.

The *breasts,* or mammary glands, are two highly specialized cutaneous glands located on either side of the anterior wall of the chest between the third and the seventh ribs (Fig. 9-12). They are abundantly supplied with nerves. The breasts contain tissue that responds to hormones. Thus, breast development at puberty and lactation during pregnancy occur as a result of endocrine influences.

The internal mammary and the intercostal arteries supply the breast glands, and the mammary veins follow these arteries. Also, there are many cutaneous veins that become dilated during lactation. The lymphatics are abundant, especially toward the axilla. These breast glands are present in the male, but exist only in the rudimentary state.

Internal Structure

The breasts of a woman who never has borne a child are conic or hemispheric in form, but they vary in size and shape at different ages and in different persons. In women who have nursed one or more babies, the breasts tend to become pendulous. At the termination of lactation, certain exercises aid in restoring the tone of the breast tissue.

The breasts are made up of glandular tissue and fat. Each organ is divided into 15 or 20 lobes, which are separated from each other by fibrous and fatty walls. Each lobe is subdivided into many lobules, which contain numerous acini cells. The *acini* are composed of a

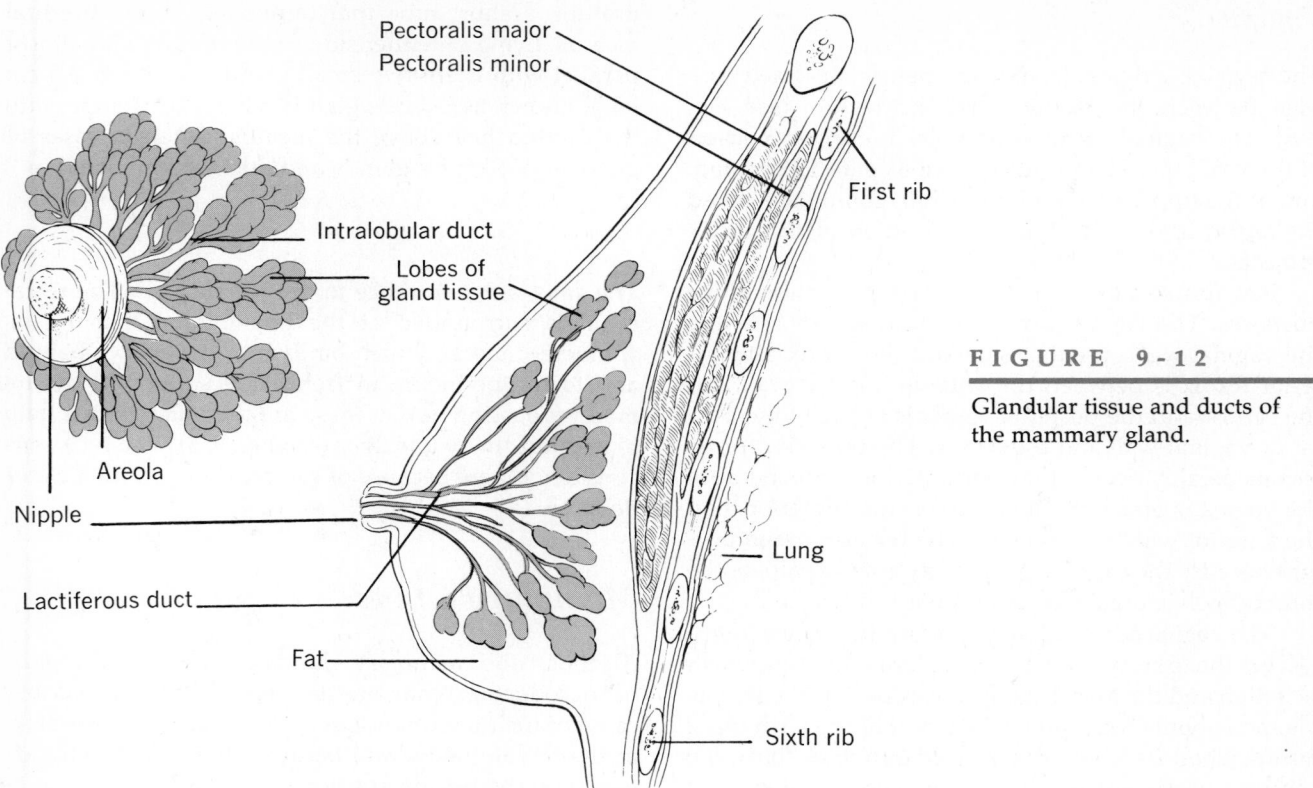

Pectoralis major
Pectoralis minor
First rib
Intralobular duct
Lobes of
gland tissue
Areola
Nipple
Lung
Lactiferous duct
Fat
Sixth rib

FIGURE 9-12

Glandular tissue and ducts of
the mammary gland.

single layer of epithelium, beneath which is a small
amount of connective tissue richly supplied with capillaries. The products necessary for the milk are filtered
from the blood by the process of osmosis, but the secretion of the milk really begins in the acini cells. As
the ducts leading from the lobules to the lobes approach
the nipple, they are dilated to form little reservoirs in
which the milk is stored; they narrow again as they pass
into the nipple. The size of the breast depends on the
amount of fatty tissue present and in no way denotes
the amount of lactation possible.

External Structure

The external surface of the breast is divided into three
portions. The first is the smooth and soft area of skin
extending from the circumference of the gland to the
areola.

The second is the *areola,* which surrounds the nipple
and is of a delicate pinkish hue in blondes and a darker
rose color in brunettes. The surface of the areola is
roughed by small fine lumps of papillae, known as
Montgomery's glands. These enlarged sebaceous glands,
which are white and are scattered over the areola, become more marked during pregnancy. Under the influence of gestation, the areola becomes darker, and, in
many cases, this pigmentation constitutes a helpful sign
of pregnancy in the primigravida.

The *nipple* is largely composed of sensitive, erectile

tissue; it forms a large conic papilla projecting from the
center of the areola, and its summit is at the openings
of the milk ducts. There are 3 to 20 milk duct openings.

Breast care (see Chaps. 22 and 31) constitutes one
of the important phases of the nursing care of the
maternity patient throughout pregnancy and the
puerperium.

Female Sexual Maturity

Sexual maturity in the female begins at the time of puberty, with the onset of dramatic bodily changes. Early
in the course of puberty, axillary and pubic hair appear.
Shortly thereafter, there is a gradual change in the contour of the labia. The breasts also begin to mature at
this time, and there is a sudden increase in bodily
growth.

These changes usually precede the onset of the first
menstruation, the *menarche.* Establishment of the menstrual cycle is the most clearly identifiable sign of puberty and serves as an indication that the internal sex
organs are approaching maturity. These physical
changes are accompanied by emotional changes. The
whole process of puberty spans about 3 years and is
completed with the menarche.

The time sequence of changes that culminates in
the attainment of reproductive potential varies considerably from person to person (Fig. 9-13). Bodily mani-

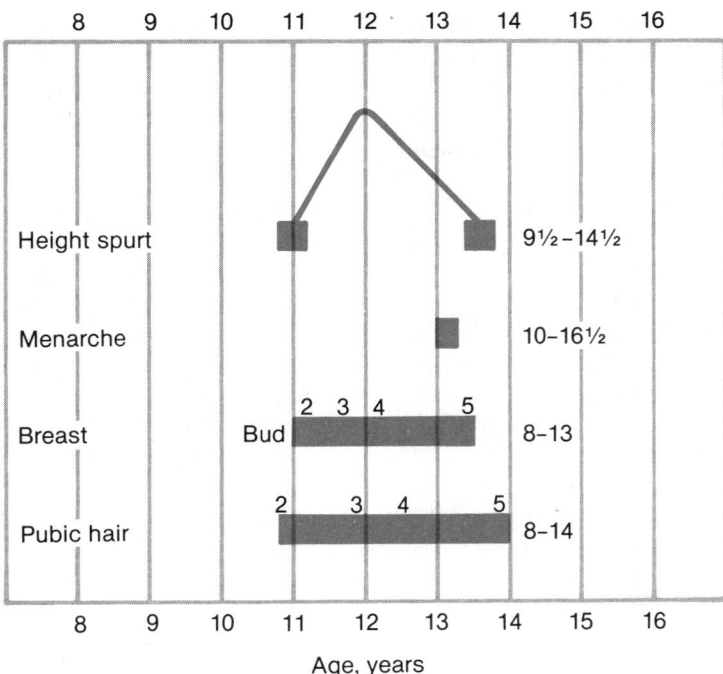

Age, years

F I G U R E   9 - 1 3

Sequence of events at adolescence in girls. An average girl is represented; the range of ages within which some of the events may occur is noted. Breast development progresses from the development of the breast bud (2) through full development (5). There is progression from downy pubic hair (2) through complete development of hair over the mons (5). (After Tanner JM: Growth at Adolescence, 2nd ed. Oxford, England, Blackwell Scientific Publications, 1969. Pierson EC, D'Antonio WV: Female and Male: Dimensions of Human Sexuality. Philadelphia, JB Lippincott, 1974)

festations of puberty, such as the beginning of breast development, the appearance of pubic hair, and a spurt of growth, precede the actual onset of menstruation by a variable amount of time.

Throughout puberty there is an interplay of physiological and sociocultural forces, and often the nurse is called upon to explain the bodily and psychological changes in puberty to mothers who have daughters approaching their teens. There is often anxiety about the onset of pubertal changes that are thought to be occurring too early or too late. Therefore, it is important to recognize the wide variability from one young woman to the next.

Menstruation and Ovulation

Menstruation is the periodic discharge of blood, mucus, and epithelial cells from the uterus. It usually occurs at monthly intervals throughout the reproductive period, except during pregnancy and lactation, when it is usually suppressed.

The monthly flow of blood is only one phase of a marvelous cyclic process that not only makes childbearing possible, but also profoundly influences both body and mind. For this reason, the time of the onset of menstruation is a critical period in the life of a young woman.

The span of years during which childbearing is possible, that is, from about ages 12 to 45, corresponds to the period during which ovulation and menstruation

occur. In general, a woman who menstruates is able to conceive, whereas one who does not is probably infertile. Ovulation and menstruation are closely interlinked, and because no process of nature is purposeless, menstruation must play some vital and indispensable role in childbearing.

Menarche

Puberty is the age at which reproductive organs become functionally active. *Menarche* marks the beginning of menstruation and usually occurs between the ages of 9 and 16, although heredity, race, state of nutrition, climate, and environment may influence its initial appearance. For example, maturity tends to occur earlier in warm climates and later in cold regions. The reproductive period spans about 35 years, from some point after the beginning of menstruation until its cessation during menopause, between ages 45 and 50.

Throughout childhood the *gonadotropins*, hormones produced by the pituitary gland to stimulate the ovaries, appear in very low concentrations. Estrogen, produced by the ovaries in the adult, remains undetectable. Puberty begins when there is a rise in the release of gonadotropins from the pituitary gland. These stimulate the ovary to secrete increasing amounts of *estrogen*, the hormone responsible for many of the bodily changes of puberty.

An orderly sequence of endocrinological events resulting in ovulation may not occur initially. The first few menstrual cycles following the menarche may not be associated with ovulation. However, once menstruation has occurred, it must be assumed that there is ovulation and, therefore, fertility and the potential for pregnancy.

Ovulation and the Ovarian Cycle

Each month, with considerable regularity, a blisterlike structure about 1 cm in diameter develops on the surface of one of the ovaries. Within this bubble, almost lost in the fluid and cells around it, lies a tiny speck, scarcely visible to the naked eye (a thimble would hold 3 million of these specks). This speck is the human ovum, a truly amazing structure. It not only has the potential to develop into a human being, but it also embodies the mental as well as physical traits of the woman and her forebears (*e.g.,* her own brown eyes, her father's tall stature, her mother's genius at mathematics, or her grandfather's love of music). These and a million other potentials are contained in the ovum, which is so small that it is about one fourth the size of the period at the end of this sentence.

In the process of ovulation, one blister on one ovary ruptures at a given time each month and discharges an ovum. The precise day on which ovulation occurs is a matter of no small significance. For instance, because the ovum can only be fertilized (impregnated by the spermatozoon, or male germ cell) within hours after its escape from the ovary, the day after ovulation a woman is no longer fertile. However, a woman is potentially fertile for a number of days preceding the actual time of ovulation because spermatozoa survive in the female reproductive tract for hours, even days, awaiting the arrival of the ovum.

In a given cycle, the time of ovulation is unpredictable. Even the woman who consistently has regular menstrual periods could experience a delayed or early ovulation in any one cycle. This possibility of irregularity, combined with the potential for fertility any time prior to ovulation due to the fact that spermatozoa retain their ability for fertilization, makes it difficult to identify accurately the fertile phase of a given cycle.

It should be remembered that the only really infertile interval is after ovulation has occurred. The time between ovulation and menstruation is relatively constant (14 ± 2 days); the time between menstruation and ovulation is variable enough that ovulation cannot be accurately predicted from one cycle to the next.

Graafian Follicle

In delving further into the process of ovulation, we find that at birth each ovary contains a huge number of undeveloped ova, probably more than 400,000. These are rather large, round cells with clear cytoplasm and a good-sized nucleus occupying the center. Each ovum is surrounded by a layer of a few small, flattened or spindle-shaped cells. The whole structure, ovum and surrounding cells, is a *follicle,* but in its underdeveloped state at birth it is a *primordial follicle.*

The formation of primordial follicles ceases at birth or shortly after, and the large number contained in the ovaries of the newborn represents a lifetime supply. The majority have disappeared before puberty, so that there are then perhaps 30,000 left. This disintegration of follicles continues throughout reproductive life until menopause when, usually, none are found.

Meanwhile, from birth to the menopause a few of these primordial follicles show signs of development. The surrounding granular layers of cells begin to multiply rapidly until they are several layers deep; at the same time, they become cuboid in shape. As this proliferation of cells continues, a very important fluid develops between them, the *follicular fluid.*

After puberty, the cells within the developing follicles produce estrogenic hormones, which in turn act on the reproductive organs and bring about cyclic bodily changes. During each menstrual cycle, several follicles develop further. One of these is finally selected, by a process not as yet completely understood, for complete maturation and ovulation.

Follicular fluid accumulates in such quantities that the multiplying follicle cells are pushed toward the margin; the ovum itself is almost surrounded by fluid and is suspended from the periphery of the follicle by only a small neck of cells. The structure is now known as the *graafian follicle,* named after Von Graaf, a Dutch physician who first described it in 1672.

As it increases enormously in size, the graafian follicle naturally pushes aside other follicles that form each month and a very noticeable, blisterlike projection appears on the surface of the ovary. At one point the follicular capsule becomes thin, and as the ovum reaches full maturity, it breaks free from the few cells attaching it to the periphery and floats in the follicular fluid. The thinned area of the capsule now ruptures, and the ovum is expelled from the ovary in the process of ovulation (Fig. 9-14).

Changes in the Corpus Luteum

After the discharge of the ovum, the ruptured follicle undergoes a change. It becomes filled with large cells containing a special yellow matter. The follicle then is known as the *corpus luteum,* or yellow body. If pregnancy does not occur, the corpus luteum reaches full development in about 8 days, then retrogresses and is gradually replaced by fibrous tissue, the *corpus albicans.*

If pregnancy occurs, the corpus luteum enlarges

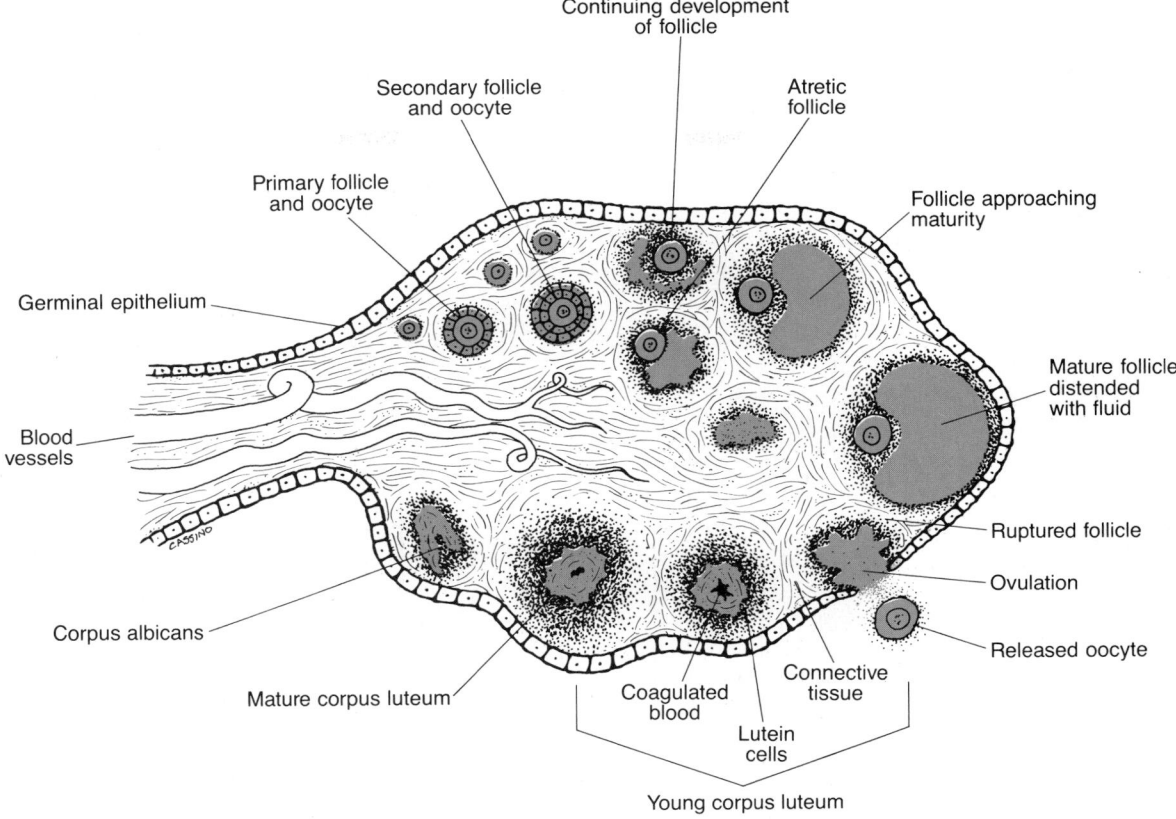

FIGURE 9-14

Schematic design of an ovary, showing the sequence of events in the origin, growth, and rupture of an ovarian follicle. (Modified from Patten BM: Human Embryology, 3rd ed. New York, McGraw-Hill, 1968)

somewhat and persists throughout the period of gestation, reaching its maximum size about the fourth or fifth month and retrogressing slowly thereafter. The corpus luteum secretes an extremely important substance, progesterone, which will be discussed later in this chapter.

In the absence of pregnancy, the corpus luteum remains active for about 2 weeks. The corpus luteum produces progesterone for the standard duration of the postovulatory phase of the menstrual cycle, 14 ± 2 days.

The Menstrual Cycle

If day by day we were privileged to watch the *endometrium*, the lining membrane of the uterus, we would observe some remarkable alterations (Fig. 9-15). These changes have only one purpose, to provide a suitable bed for the fertilized ovum to secure nourishment and to grow. If an ovum is not fertilized, these alterations serve no useful function.

The menstrual cycle may be broken into three phases: proliferative, secretory, and menstrual. The menstrual cycle is related directly to the ovarian cycle, and both are under hormonal influences. Hormones are discussed after this section.

Proliferative Phase

Immediately following menstruation the endometrium is very thin. During the subsequent week or so it proliferates markedly. The cells on the surface become taller, while the glands that dip into the endometrium become longer and wider. As the result of these changes, the thickness of the endometrium increases sixfold or eightfold. Its glands become more and more active and secrete a rich, nutritive substance.

Each month during this phase of the menstrual cycle (from approximately the fifth to the 14th days), a graafian follicle is approaching its greatest development and is manufacturing increasing amounts of follicular fluid. This fluid contains the estrogenic hormone *estrogen*. Be-

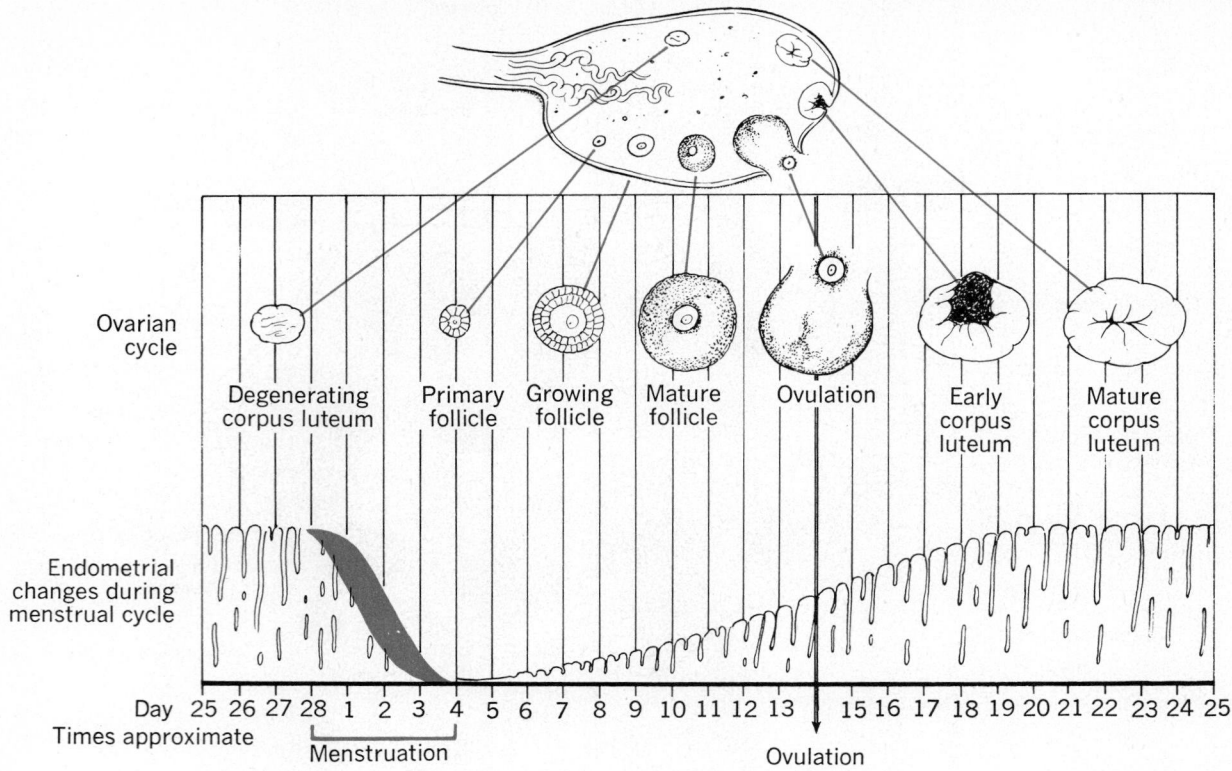

Ovarian cycle

Degenerating corpus luteum | Primary follicle | Growing follicle | Mature follicle | Ovulation | Early corpus luteum | Mature corpus luteum

Endometrial changes during menstrual cycle

Day 25 26 27 28 1 2 3 4 5 6 7 8 9 10 11 12 13   15 16 17 18 19 20 21 22 23 24 25
Times approximate

Menstruation

Ovulation

F I G U R E   9 - 1 5

Schematic representation of one ovarian cycle and the corresponding changes in thickness of the endometrium. It is thickest just before the onset of menstruation and thinnest just as it ceases.

cause estrogen causes the endometrium to grow or proliferate, this phase of the menstrual cycle is commonly called the *proliferative phase.* Sometimes it is referred to as the *follicular,* or *estrogenic, phase.*

Secretory Phase

Following the release of the ovum from the graafian follicle (ovulation), the cells that form the corpus luteum begin to secrete another important hormone, *progesterone,* in addition to estrogen. This supplements the action of estrogen on the endometrium in such a way that the glands become very tortuous or corkscrew in appearance and are greatly dilated. This change occurs because the glands are swollen with a secretion.

Meanwhile, the blood supply of the endometrium is increased, and it becomes vascular and succulent. The process reaches its height; the endometrium is now of the thickness of heavy, downy velvet and has become soft and succulent with blood and glandular secretions. At this time the ovum, if it has been fertilized, is embedded into this luxuriant lining.

Since these effects are directed at providing a bed

for the fertilized ovum, it is easy to understand why the hormone that brings them about is called progesterone, meaning *for gestation.* It is also clear why this phase of the cycle, occupying the last 14 ± 2 days, is commonly called the *secretory phase* and why occasionally it is referred to as the *progestational, luteal,* or *premenstrual phase.*

Menstrual Phase

Unless the ovum is fertilized, the corpus luteum is short lived. Since corpus luteum cells secrete both progesterone and estrogen, cessation of corpus luteum activity means a withdrawal of both of these hormones. As a result, the endometrium degenerates. This is associated with rupture of countless small blood vessels in the endometrium with innumerable minute hemorrhages. The disintegrated endometrium and blood and glandular secretions escape into the uterine cavity, pass through the cervix, and flow out through the vagina, carrying the tiny unfertilized ovum with them. In other words, menstruation represents the abrupt termination of a process designed to prepare lodging for a fertilized ovum. It forecasts the breakdown of a bed that is not needed because fertilization did not occur. Thus, its purpose is to clear away the old bed so that a new and fresh one may be created the next month. This phase of the cycle (from approximately the first to the fifth days) is called the *menstrual phase.*

Hormonal Control of the Cycles

The menstrual cycle is regulated primarily through the highly coordinated function of the brain, the hypothalamus, the pituitary, the ovaries, and the uterus. If it were possible to inspect the ovaries from day to day during the menstrual cycle, it would be noted that the uterine alterations are directly related to certain changes that take place in the ovary. If it were possible to look further, it might be seen that the alterations that occur regularly in the ovarian cycle are directly related to certain phenomena that take place in the anterior pituitary gland and the hypothalamus, a portion of the brain that lies above the pituitary. Thus, the whole sequence represents the harmonious, integrated reactions of several processes within the human organism, all of which are necessary to maintain proper relationships in the menstrual cycle.

Role of the Pituitary Gland

The pituitary gland is essential in the function of the reproductive system.* The anterior lobe of the pituitary, the "master clock," releases the gonadotropins, to stimulate the ovary, as well as other hormones. These hormones produce the ovarian alterations associated with ovulation. There are two principal gonadotropins. One is *follicle-stimulating hormone (FSH);* as its name implies, FSH stimulates the development of the follicle. The other is *LH,* which is principally active during ovulation and the luteal phase of the cycle.

The release of the gonadotropic hormones by the pituitary is regulated by the *hypothalamus,* a specialized structure within the brain located just above the pituitary. The hypothalamus has a vascular connection to the pituitary gland, as well as nerve connections to the central nervous system. Indeed, its function can be modified by influences within the central nervous system. Thus, the function of the pituitary gland may be affected by the brain. The cyclic release of gonadotropin by the pituitary gland is controlled by a hormonal agent released by the hypothalamus. This is called gonadotropin-releasing hormone or LH/FSH-releasing hormone (GnRH or LH/FSH-RH), since it triggers the release of both FSH and LH from the pituitary gland.

* The posterior lobe of the pituitary gland produces oxytocin, a hormone that has an important role in obstetrics but one that differs altogether from the purpose of the present discussion.

Cyclic Pattern

Sensitive laboratory methods now allow accurate measurement of day-to-day changes in circulating pituitary and ovarian hormones (Fig. 9-16). The interplay between the pituitary and the ovary, influenced in turn by the central nervous system through the hypothalamus, brings about orderly development of the follicle and ovulation.

At the end of a given cycle and at the beginning of the subsequent cycle (see Fig. 9-16), the pituitary gland releases increased amounts of FSH. With the help of small amounts of LH, FSH stimulates maturation of several ovarian follicles. Together, LH and FSH produce modest amounts of the estrogen estradiol. The levels of estradiol in the bloodstream begin to rise, and estradiol in turn acts negatively on the central nervous system at the hypothalamic–pituitary level by inhibiting the release of additional amounts of FSH. Consequently, the level of FSH in the circulating blood begins to fall. FSH also acts on the follicle to make it more sensitive to LH.

About 2 days before ovulation, all but the one follicle that is destined to ovulate begin to regress in a process called atresia. That one follicle undergoes rapid growth, and estrogen production rises sharply. The increased amount of estrogen produced at this point then acts positively at the central nervous system–hypothalamic level, stimulating a rapid increase in GnRH levels. In turn, GnRH causes large amounts of LH, as well as additional FSH, to be released from the pituitary gland. This dramatic rise in LH stimulates the completion of maturation of the follicle and, within 24 hours after the LH surge, ovulation takes place.

The increased levels of preovulatory estrogen prepare the genital tract for sperm migration. The secretions of the cervix, scanty and viscous early in the cycle, become thin and watery and more receptive to spermatozoa. The vaginal wall also reflects the effects of estrogen. A vaginal smear taken at this time reveals a large percentage of mature, or "cornified," cells. The endometrium displays maximal proliferation (see Fig. 9-15).

Following ovulation, the cyclic pattern continues. The ruptured follicle is transformed into a corpus luteum. The second function of LH is to maintain the corpus luteum. These endocrine events are associated with further modifications in the cervical mucus, vagina, and endometrium. The mucus becomes thick, "tacky," and viscous and is no longer as receptive to spermatozoa. The vaginal smear reflects the influence of progesterone with a decreasing "maturation index." The endometrium takes on secretory changes preparatory to implantation.

Progesterone secretion by the corpus luteum reaches its maximum about 5 to 7 days after ovulation (see Fig. 9-16). This is the time when the fertilized egg, now a *blastocyst,* is ready to implant. If pregnancy has occurred,

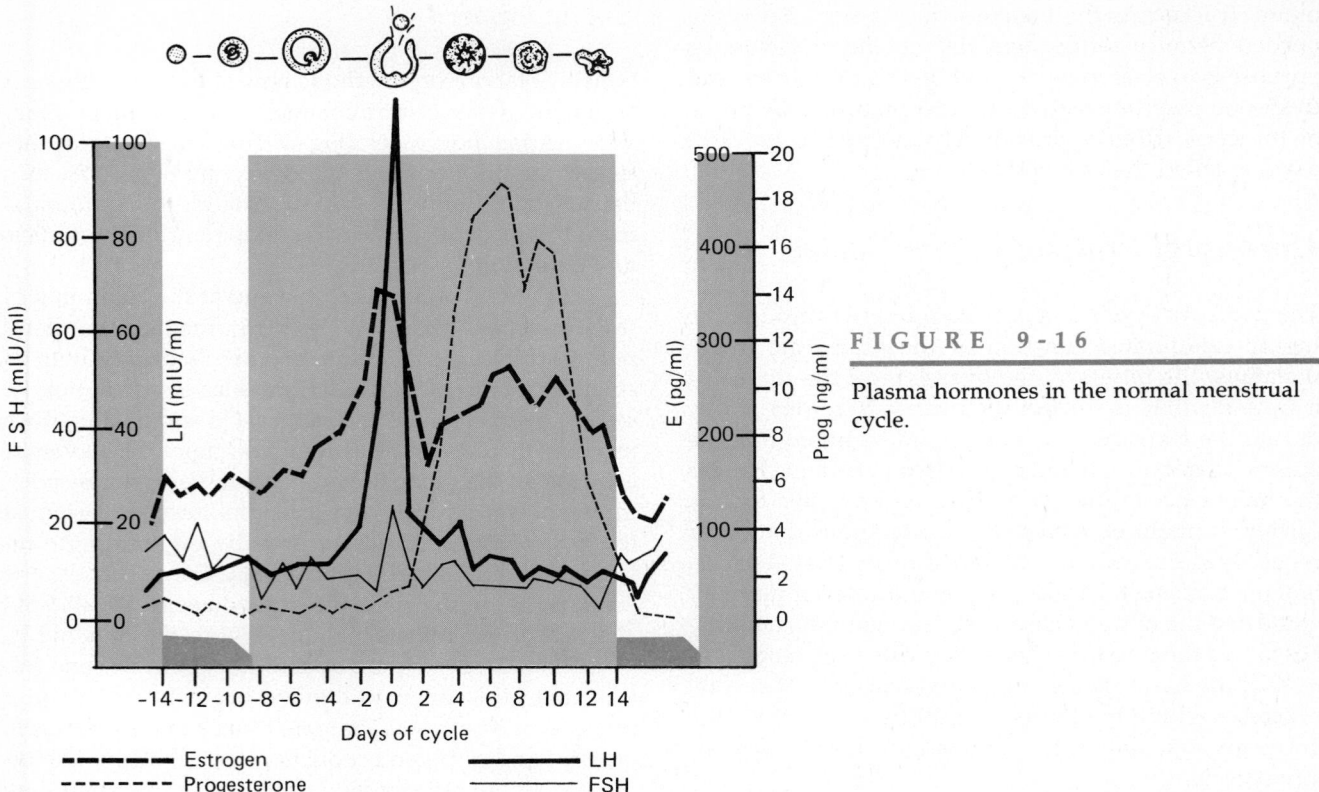

FIGURE 9-16

Plasma hormones in the normal menstrual cycle.

another hormone, *human chorionic gonadotropin (hCG)*, appears within 2 to 3 days of implantation. This hormone, which is produced by the conceptus, acts on the corpus luteum, maintaining its progesterone-providing function, and transforms it into a corpus luteum of pregnancy. If pregnancy has not intervened, the corpus luteum begins its demise at this time. Approximately 10 to 11 days after ovulation, progesterone levels decline precipitously, and on about the 14th postovulatory day, no longer receiving hormones, the endometrium begins to shed in the process of menstruation.

Other Functions of Estrogen and Progesterone

In addition to their role in controlling menstruation, estrogen and progesterone serve other important functions. Estrogen is responsible for the development of the secondary sex characteristics, that is, all those distinctive sex manifestations that are not directly concerned with the process of reproduction. Thus, the growth of the breasts at puberty, the distribution of body fat, the size of the larynx and its resulting influence on the quality of the voice, as well as mating instincts, are all the results of estrogenic action. Thus, it may almost be said that a woman is a woman because of estrogen.

Aside from its action on the endometrium, progesterone also helps to relax the uterine muscle. Thus, it plays an important role in preserving the life of the embryo in early pregnancy, by preventing its expulsion from the uterus and by preparing the endometrium to receive and nourish it.

Variations in Cycles

Although the interval of the menstrual cycle, counting from the beginning of one period to the onset of the next, averages 28 days, there are wide variations even in the same woman. Indeed, a woman rarely menstruates exactly every 28 or 30 days each month. This has been the subject of several studies on normal young women. These investigations show that the majority of woman (almost 60%) experience variations of at least 5 days in the length of their menstrual cycles; differences in the same woman of even 10 days are not uncommon and may occur without explanation or apparent detriment to health.

The degree and intensity of the outward manifestations of the ovulatory cycle vary from one woman to the next. Some women consistently experience pelvic discomfort during ovulation, or *mittelschmerz*, so named because it typically appears in the middle of a 28-day menstrual cycle. Slight staining or occasional bleeding may occur in association with ovulation. In the post-ovulatory interval there may be breast tenderness and fullness, which typically reaches a peak just before menstruation.

Premenstrual Syndrome. Clinically, it has become evident that many women suffer not only tension but other affective and somatic symptoms premenstrually. Consequently, the term *premenstrual syndrome,* or *PMS,* has largely replaced *premenstrual tension.* While the term *PMS* sounds definitive, it really does not describe a definite diagnostic entity. It is, nevertheless, an important entity in the lives of those women whom it affects. In discussing PMS with clients it is important to differentiate it from normal premenstrual awareness, which most ovulatory women experience to some degree. PMS involves symptoms that occur in repetitive fashion prior to menses, which seriously affect a woman's life, and subside with the onset of menses or a few days into the period. Severity of symptoms is the critical factor. PMS should also be separated from other menstrual complaints, such as dysmenorrhea. Although the search continues for a clear-cut physiological basis for PMS, it is recognized that this syndrome is certainly real and, in fact, can be documented. It is a bona fide psycho-neuro-endocrine disorder. Characteristically, it involves three symptom clusters: hostility, depression, and somatic complaints. In a self-selected series of clients reviewed at the University of Pennsylvania, women complained of irritability, tension, frequent outbursts of temper, shouting, and throwing things. Depression may or may not accompany this hostility, but when it does, it is characterized typically by low energy level, blaming one's self for things that happen, feeling blocked in getting things done, and forgetfulness. The somatic symptoms include the classic ones associated with the premenstrual state: breast tenderness and swelling, abdominal tenderness, bloating, and joint pains. Interestingly, clients who have the somatic symptoms may not always have the psychiatric symptoms. Those with psychiatric symptoms often find their somatic symptoms to be relatively minor. One of the problems in establishing PMS as an entity has been that most studies are retrospective, based on a woman's recollection of what has happened in the past. It is therefore important to document the symptoms in relation to the menstrual cycle. A useful assessment instrument is the menstrual calendar (see Daily Symptom Checklist). Treatment of this poorly understood entity is not always successful. About 40% of the clients seem to respond to dietary therapy alone, a diet low in simple sugars, caffeine, and salt, with adequate protein and complex carbohydrates. Since a substantial number of clients with PMS respond to placebo, it is difficult to establish the efficacy of any one treatment. Vitamin B$_6$ seems to offer some advantage, and encouraging a regular exercise program seems to be useful. PMS is an evolving clinical entity in which there is substantial current interest, and until it is better understood, treatment by and large will be unsatisfactory.

Dysmenorrhea. Normal menstruation should not be accompanied by incapacitating pain. There may, however, be some cramp and general malaise, together with a feeling of weight and discomfort in the pelvis. Painful menstruation is known as *dysmenorrhea.* The menstrual discharge contains substances referred to as prostaglandins. These cause smooth-muscle contractions and a cramping sensation. Ovulatory women produce more endometrial prostaglandins than do anovulatory women; hence, dysmenorrhea is rarey observed in the absence of ovulation. Recently developed prostaglandin inhibitors that can be taken orally are very effective in the treatment of dysmenorrhea.

Amenorrhea. If there is great irregularity, extremely profuse flow, or marked pain, a pathologic condition may be present. Absence of menses is known as amenorrhea. The most common cause of amenorrhea is pregnancy, but sometimes it is brought about by emotional disturbances (*e.g.,* fear, worry, fatigue), which work through the central nervous system and hypothalamus, or by debilitating diseases (*e.g.,* anemia, tuberculosis), and sometimes by prolonged strenuous exertion (*e.g.,* marathon running).

Determinants of Phases of Cycles

Not all menstrual cycles are of 28-day length, and ovulation cannot be determined by counting 14 days from the last menstrual period. Therefore, other means of establishing phases of ovulation have been determined. Two useful means of determining ovulation are the following. Both are used in infertility clinics and natural methods of contraception (see Chaps. 14 and 16).

Variations in Cervical Mucus

Under the influence of rapidly rising preovulatory levels of estrogen (see Fig. 9-16) the cervical mucus, scant and tacky early in the cycle, becomes copious and clear. It is most abundant on the day preceding ovulation and, not surprisingly, is most receptive to spermatozoa at that time. Following ovulation, under the influence of progesterone, the mucus becomes scanty, thick, and sticky once again.

These cyclic changes in the quality of the cervical mucus are often easily detected by the normally men-

Menstrual Calendar

Daily Symptom Checklist

DATE (Mo/Da/Yr)																																	
Check, if Menstruating																																	
Medication																																	

*Symptoms (Grade 0 to 4)***

** Rate Symptoms Using This Scale:
0 = Not at all   1 = A little bit   2 = Moderate   3 = Quite a bit   4 = Very much

Nervous Tension																																	
Mood Swings																																	
Irritability																																	
Swelling																																	
Breast Tenderness																																	
Headache																																	
Craving Foods																																	
Fatigue																																	
Depression																																	
Insomnia																																	
Confusion																																	
Aches																																	
Sexual Desire																																	
Cramps																																	
Crying																																	
Out of Control																																	
Avoid Social Activities																																	
Poor Coordination																																	
Other:																																	

(Courtesy of Hospital of University of Pennsylvania, Philadelphia, PA, PMS Program).

struating woman once she is made aware of them. In some cases, a clear translucent mucus appears at the labia or may be wiped from the cervix to provide suggestive evidence of impending ovulation. In the postovulatory phase of the cycle, the sticky and less abundant mucus is not as easily detected. Daily observations of cervical mucus changes have been suggested as a useful parameter in using the rhythm method of contraception, also referred to as the symtothermal approach.

Basal Body Temperature

Beginning about the first year of life, slight daily variations in body temperature normally occur in all human beings. These temperature variations are relative to the time of the day and the nature of the circumstances surrounding the person. For example, the body temperature is lowest in the morning before breakfast, after a good night's rest, and before activity. After a day of normal activity, the body temperature is usually highest toward afternoon and early evening. The fact that physiological variations in basal body temperature also occur in relation to the menstrual cycle is important here because it can be useful in estimating the time of ovulation. Such an index becomes extremely important in studies of fertility and sterility.

In the woman who is ovulating, there is normally a rhythmic variation in the basal body temperature curve during the course of the menstrual cycle (see Basal Body Temperature Graph and Directions for Using). The basal temperature is lower during the first part of the menstrual cycle, the proliferative phase. It rises in association with ovulation and remains relatively higher during the luteal phase of the cycle. The rise in the basal temperature occurs as a result of the influence of progesterone, produced by the corpus luteum following ovulation. Progesterone causes this thermogenic effect through its influence on the central nervous system. The basal temperature rises as much as 0.5 of a degree, and a relatively higher temperature is sustained until just before the onset of the menstrual period. This interval occupies the 14 ± 2 terminal days in the cycle.

If pregnancy occurs, the progesterone level is maintained, and under its influence the basal temperature remains high past the expected time of the period. In the absence of pregnancy, the basal temperature usually drops a day or so before the menstrual period.

The Use of the Basal Temperature Graph. The basal body temperature is one of the most practical means of diagnosing ovulation. It is the relative difference in basal body temperature during the course of the cycle that is the important diagnostic criterion for ovulation. It is only useful in the timing of ovulation retrospectively. Thus, when there is infertility, efforts

to time intercourse to coincide with changes in the temperature chart have not proved worthwhile. In fact, such regulation of coital habits is not recommended. However, for the diagnosis of ovulation, the temperature chart has proved valuable. The temperature chart is also useful as an adjunct to the rhythm method of family planning (see Chap. 14).

Menopause

Menopause means the cessation of menstruation. In about 50% of women this usually occurs between the ages of 45 and 50. About 25% will reach menopause before the age of 45, and 25% after the age of 50. In common use, menopause generally means cessation of *regular* menstruation. Ovulation may occur sporadically or may cease abruptly. Hence, periods may end suddenly, may become scanty or irregular, or may be intermittently heavy before ceasing altogether. Markedly diminished ovarian activity, that is, significantly decreased estrogen production and cessation of ovulation, causes menopause. Often the terms *menopause* and *climacteric* are used synonymously, but the use is not accurate. Climacteric encompasses the total syndrome of endocrine, somatic, and psychic changes occurring at the termination of the reproductive period in the female. It is derived from the Greek word meaning *rung of the ladder*, or critical point in human life. The termination of cyclic estrogen production associated with greatly decreased ovarian function causes the ovary, the uterus, and the breasts to decrease in size. The external genitals become flattened, and the vaginal walls lose their folds, elasticity, and lubrication, becoming shiny and smooth. The decrease in estrogen levels may also produce intermittent "hot flashes" and some emotional instability, for example, irritability and sudden outbursts of tears much like the emotional lability associated with PMS.

Each woman reacts somewhat differently to this withdrawal of estrogen. These reactions are unpredictable, vary from woman to woman, and depend to some extent on her previous emotional history and her present support systems within the family and to a very real extent on the fact that the menopausal reproductive-endocrine system may be quite labile during this interval, which may last as long as 8 or 9 years.

Hot flashes are not an old wives' tale; they are real and a result of vasomotor instability. This instability also results in sweating and brief sensations of being cold "all over." There may be redness and perspiration that are visible, or the sensations may be equally intense but with no visible signs. Their daily frequency may vary, and there can be long intervals, sometimes weeks, with no symptoms at all.

BASAL BODY TEMPERATURE RECORD

NAME:_____

AGE:_____

↓ COITUS

■ MENSES

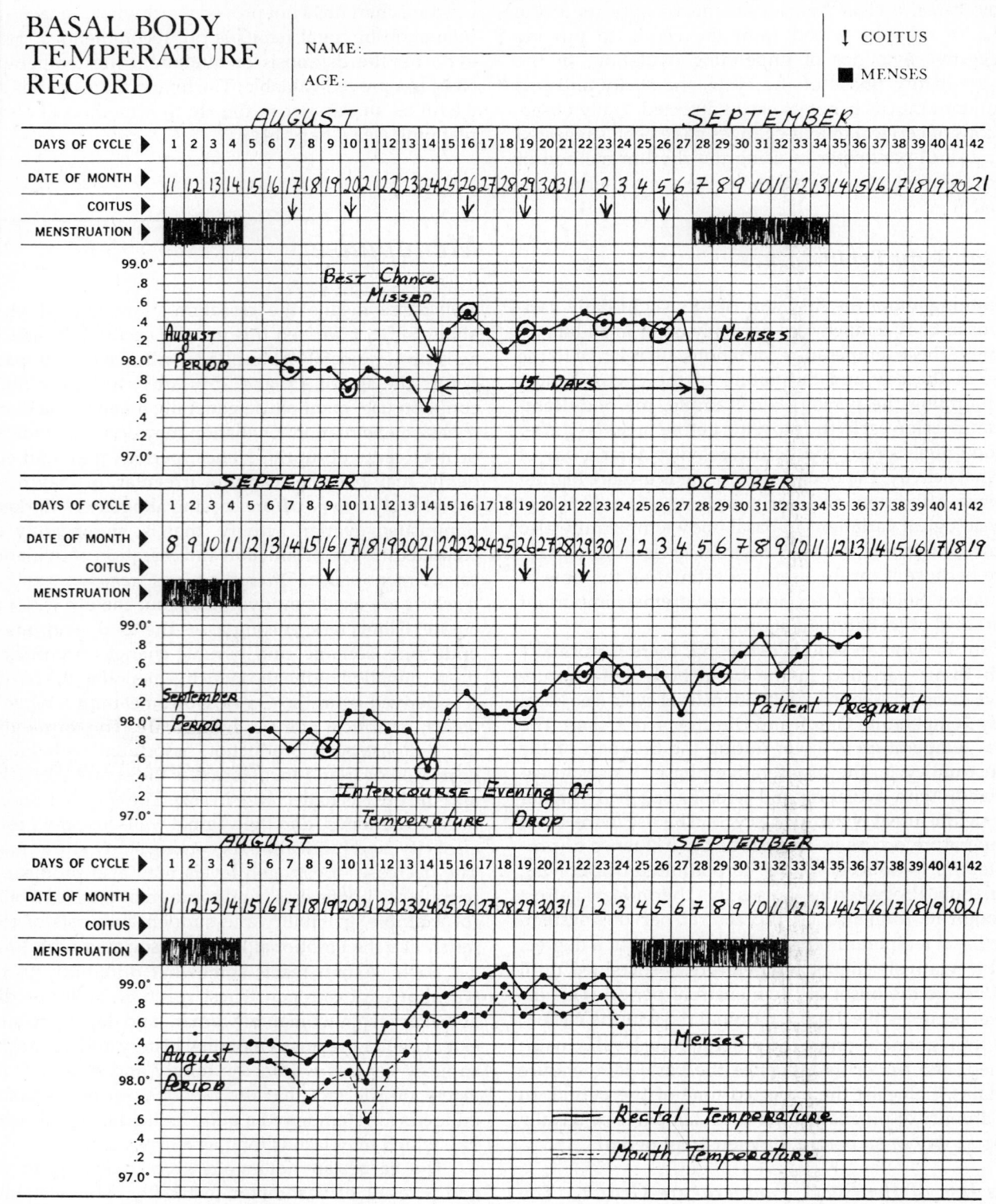

Samples of basal temperature charts indicating menstrual cycles and daily temperature readings. Temperature drops are clearly indicated on all charts, with optimal time for fertilization. Phases of the cycles are determined by these charts. Charts may be used in family planning or in management of infertility. The bottom chart contrasts oral and rectal temperatures. Directions for using this chart are given on the facing page.

(Published by Merrill-National Laboratories, Div. of Richardson-Merrill Inc., Cincinnati, Ohio 45215.)

ASSESSMENT TOOL

Directions for Using the Basal Temperature Graph

1. The first day of menses is considered to be the first day of the menstrual cycle. The duration of menstrual flow is recorded, beginning on cycle day 1 (see graph). The date of onset of flow is recorded, and each subsequent date is recorded in the spaces provided. Following cessation of flow, the morning temperature is taken. Oral temperatures are as satisfactory as rectal recordings and are certainly more convenient. The temperature should be taken immediately after waking and before getting out of bed, talking, eating, drinking, or smoking. Ideally, it should be taken at about the same time every morning.
2. The thermometer is read to within 0.1 of a degree, and the reading is recorded on the chart.
3. Any known cause for temperature variation should be noted on the chart, for example, interrupted or shortened sleep, a cold, indigestion, or emotional disturbance. If intercourse has occurred, that fact should be recorded with a circle around the recording the following morning.
4. Some women can recognize ovulation by mittelschmerz; others have vaginal bleeding or clear preovulatory vaginal discharge. Such manifestations should also be recorded on the chart.

Artificial Menopause. Menopause may result from other than the natural physiological alterations of the climacteric. The term *artificial menopause* describes the cessation of menstruation produced by some artificial means, such as an irradiation of the ovaries or surgical operation for the removal of the ovaries (oophorectomy) or the uterus (hysterectomy). As a result of either surgery, the woman will no longer menstruate, but beyond this the manifestations in the client are not identical.

Certain misunderstandings based on incorrect interpretation of terminology are rather widespread and should be clarified. The fact that a woman has had a hysterectomy and ceases to menstruate does not mean that her healthy ovaries will not function. Hysterectomy involves only the removal of the uterus. On the other hand, if the ovaries are also removed surgically or are treated by irradiation, the source of estrogen is withdrawn abruptly and thus the symptoms caused by the sudden withdrawal of this hormone will occur. Because there is much misinformation among the public on this point, sometimes intensive preoperative and postoperative counseling is required. Abrupt interruption of ovarian function in a woman who is still having regular periods may create more withdrawal symptoms than in a woman who is in her menopausal years. The younger woman may need estrogen replacement to alleviate signs and symptoms of estrogen withdrawal. The need for estrogen replacement in the older woman after surgical removal of ovaries will vary from client to client.

Physiology of the Menopause

When one considers that menopause is experienced by all middle-aged women, it may seem surprising that the endocrine and metabolic changes associated with it are still not completely understood. This lack of information is due, in part, to difficulties associated with long-term, longitudinal studies spanning many years. In addition, the sensitive endocrine assays that would allow study of the endocrinological events associated with menopause have only recently become available. Because of this, estrogen replacement therapy with its possible short-term or long-term effects has created much controversy in both lay and scientific literature.

It is now known that several years before menopause there is an increase in circulating levels of both FSH and LH. The actual levels of estrogen and progesterone produced by the ovaries are decreased. These are only slight changes, and in spite of them, ovulation and menstruation continue to occur. The decreasing production of estradiol and progesterone undoubtedly allows release of increased amounts of gonadotropins from the pituitary, resulting in higher circulating levels of FSH and LH.

In normal postmenopausal women, FSH and LH levels are consistently high. The ratio of FSH to LH is always greater than one. Both of the gonadotropins are released in a pulsating fashion, similar to that seen in younger women but much more pronounced, with bursts occurring every 10 to 20 minutes. There is also periodic fluctuation in gonadotropin levels that occurs about every 2 hours. After removal of the ovaries in regularly menstruating women, gonadotropin levels begin to rise within 2 days. The rise in the FSH is more dramatic than that of LH.

Estrogen production by the postmenopausal ovary is minuscule. Surgical removal of the ovaries after menopause does not affect circulating estrogens in any significant way. However, the postmenopausal ovary does continue to produce androgens, and in increased amounts. The appearance of dark hair on the upper lip and chin is seen in some women. Since varying amounts of circulating estrogen are found in postmenopausal women, it has been suggested that estrogen may be produced elsewhere in the body and also that other tissues are able to convert the circulating androgens to estrogen. Fat, the liver, and some areas of the hypothalamus are capable of this conversion. Such estrogen production varies from one postmenopausal woman to the next, and this variability may account for some of the variations in menopausal symptoms.

The mechanism responsible for *vasomotor symptoms* is only partially understood. Obviously, neuroendocrinological factors are at work. It has been suggested that catecholamines that act as neurotransmitters in the brain—they transfer information from one neuron to another—may respond to fluctuating gonadotropin or ovarian hormone levels. Catecholamines are responsible for modulating behavior and motor activity as well as the function of the hypothalamus and pituitary. Disturbance in catecholamine activity produces vasodilatation in the brain that could bring about hot flashes. Many other environmental influences operate in the life of a postmenopausal woman, and it is difficult to separate these from the physiological events associated with decreased ovarian function. Although it is clear that emotional and physical stress can be related to increased frequency of vasomotor symptoms and signs, this relationship does not always occur in a predictable fashion. Hot flashes are the result of vasomotor instability and are clearly related to the estrogen deficiency associated with the cessation of ovarian function.

Changes in the vaginal mucosa also vary among menopausal women. Even minimal changes may result in painful intercourse (*dyspareunia*). Thinning of the vaginal lining and the decrease in lubrication can be corrected with estrogen administered orally or locally with vaginal suppositories or cream. Dyspareunia is a common symptom that should not be overlooked in the management of the postmenopausal woman.

Suggested Reading

Chaffee EE, Lytle IM: Basic Physiology and Anatomy, 4th ed. Philadelphia, JB Lippincott, 1980

Cutler W, Garcia CR: Medical Management of the Menopause and the Premenopause. Philadelphia, JB Lippincott, 1985

Goss CM (ed): Gray's Anatomy of the Human Body, 30th ed. Philadelphia, Lea & Febiger, 1984

Greep RO, Koblinsky MA: Frontiers in Reproduction and Fertility Control. Cambridge, MIT Press, 1977

Greep RO, Koblinsky MA, Jaffe FS: Reproduction and Human Welfare: A Challenge to Research. Cambridge, MIT Press, 1977

Mastroianni L, Paulsen CA (eds): Reproduction, Aging and the Climacteric. New York, Plenum Press, 1986

Speroff L, Glass RH, Kase NG: Clinical Gynecologic Endocrinology and Infertility, 3rd ed. Baltimore, Williams & Wilkins, 1984

Yen SS, Jaffe RB: Reproductive Endocrinology: Physiology, Pathophysiology and Clinical Management, 2nd ed. Philadelphia, WB Saunders, 1985

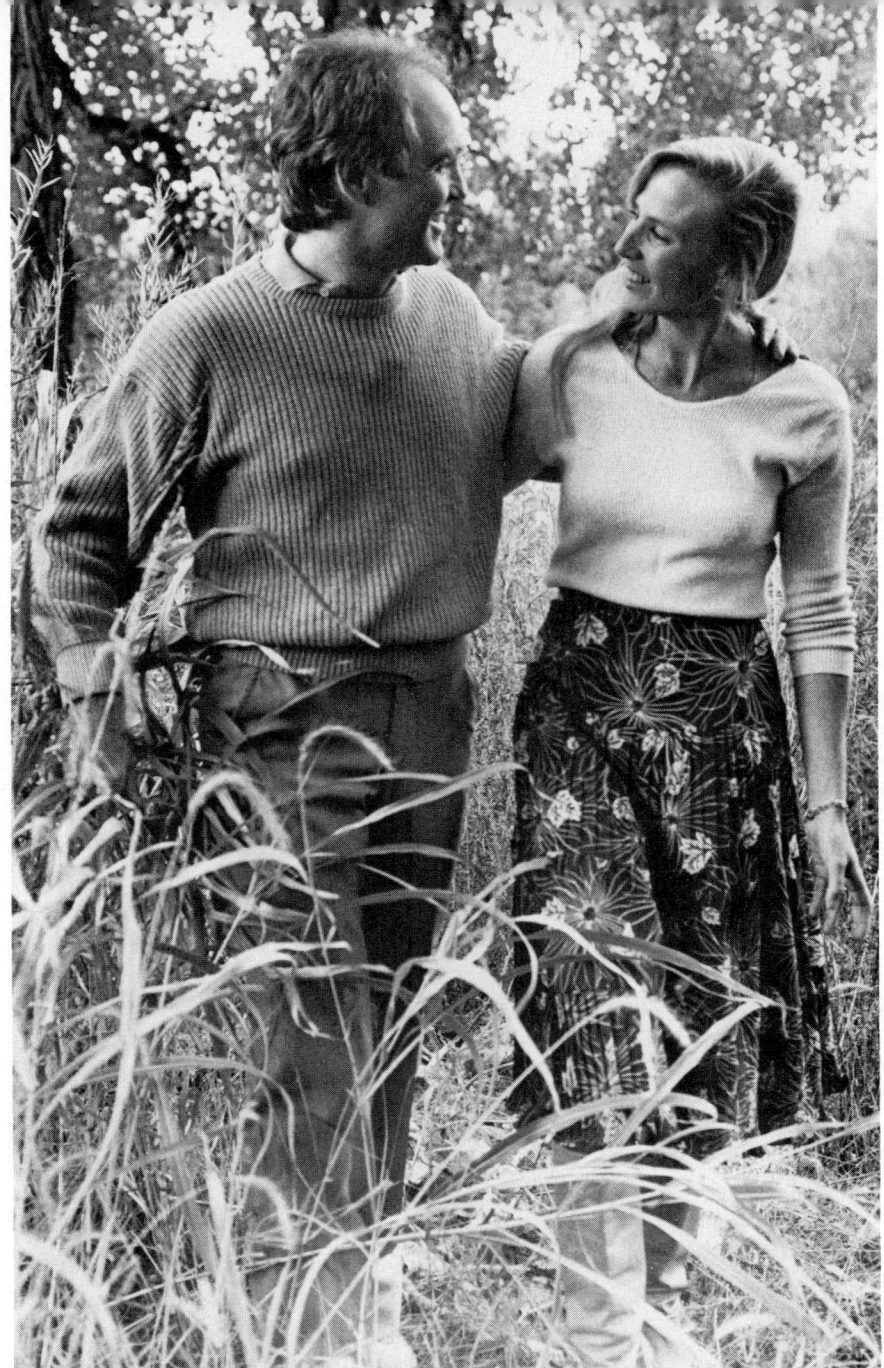

CHAPTER 10

Human Sexual Response

Sexual response in men and women is a complex process with both psychological and physiological components. Sex can be considered one of the basic human drives, but is much more malleable in expression than food and sleep, for example. Although a nearly universal behavior among humans, sex can be postponed for long periods or, in some instances, never activated, without adverse effects. Although cultural expression leads to a wide variety of sex-related behaviors, the biologic roots of sexual interaction lead to more underlying similarities than differences among peoples.

The apparent sexual differences between men and women have received much emphasis and have been viewed as both a source of delight and pleasure and a cause of conflict and strain. However, since the advent of sex research, it has been found that male and female sexual responses are more alike than different. The woman's sex drive, in an era of greater social support and openness, is assumed to be as powerful as the man's, although an adequate measurement is lacking. The common stereotype that women need affection and intimacy to respond sexually, while men respond regardless of the relationship has been found to have numerous exceptions. Sexual responses of both men and women are direct and simple at times, and mysterious and complex at others.

The basic similarities of physiological sexual responses between both sexes have been stressed by such researchers as Kinsey and Masters and Johnson. Aside from the obvious anatomical differences, men and women are homogeneous in their physiological responses to sexual stimuli. There are direct parallels in male and female anatomical responses to effective sexual stimulation, and the same underlying physiological mechanisms are involved: vasocongestion and myotonia. For example, vaginal lubrication in the woman is parallel to penile erection in the man, and both responses occur as a result of vasocongestion. Increases in muscle tension (*myotonia*) and changes in heart rate, blood pressure, and respiration are common to both men and women during sexual excitement. The reflexive contractions of orgasm are virtually identical in both sexes, although there are variations in the results that these contractions produce. And, there is a considerable overlap in the subjective experience of orgasm.

The psychological and physiological components of human sexual response cannot really be separated because these are intricately interrelated and create numerous feedback loops that can enhance or inhibit sexual response. The changes in bodily function and the perceptions and emotions that precede or accompany these are closely related to physiological processes.

Nursing and Sexuality

Historically, nurses' sexuality has been repressed. Nightingale's rules prohibited jewelry, ribbons, or ornaments, and homely women were chosen for students. Well into the mid-1900s, student nurses were required to live in dormitories under close supervision by a matron, with strict curfews and rules requiring that nurses go out in pairs. Students were expelled for pregnancy or overt sexual activity. Along with the norms of cleanliness and neatness, such practices represent the value of personal purity and asexuality felt necessary for women who touched bodies of others intimately in giving nursing care.

From the 1930s to the late 1960s, nursing literature reflected little information about sexuality. With a more holistic approach in the 1970s, awareness grew that sexuality was a proper concern for nurses. Journal articles and nursing curricula began to include various aspects of human sexuality, and professional conferences were devoted to this subject. In the past 2 decades, nurses have acted as leaders in such sexually oriented organizations as the American Association of Sex Educators, Counselors and Therapists; the Society for the Scientific Study of Sex; and the Society for Sex Therapy and Research.[1]

Nurses who are knowledgeable about sexuality and comfortable with their own sexuality have many opportunities to promote sexual health. Although about 90% of nursing programs include content in this area, it is usually integrated into other courses or offered in elective courses. In a 1980 survey, 83% of schools responding agreed that graduates and the public are not well served by programs that omit study of sexual behavior.[2] Many nurses are only prepared to deal with a narrow range of sexual behavior, however, and feel ill equipped to handle sexual problems.

Sexuality is a sensitive area in which personal values exert strong influences. Conflicts about the nursing role frequently exist. Nurses with strong religious beliefs about the immorality of certain sexual practices often have difficulty providing care to clients whose practices contradict these beliefs. Nurses may also find some sexual behavior shocking, embarrassing, or repulsive if it differs dramatically from their norms or experiences. Not every nurse will agree that sexuality is a valid area for nursing practice. Some are convinced it is a personal matter and not part of nursing; others see sexuality as part of being human and a valid area for a profession that cares for the whole person.

Sexism and Stereotyping

The nursing profession has been subject to negative influences of sexism and sexual stereotyping. Sex discrimination has resulted in decreased financial opportunities, uneven power relationships, communication barriers, job insecurity, and sexual harassment. Sexual harassment is now prohibited by law, including such behaviors as sexist remarks, demeaning and offensive jokes, promise of reward for sexual favors, and threat of punishment unless cooperation is given. Strides are being made to redress financial and power inequities, though progress is slow. Changing roles and relationships between the sexes (and nurses and physicians) are leading to increasing autonomy, independence, and assertion of goals by women.[3]

Traditional sex stereotyping leads to anxiety, low self-esteem, and low acceptance of self. It restricts behavior and decreases flexibility to respond to new situations. The relatively late development of nursing theory in the profession's history and the lack of research emphasis in nursing curricula have been related to nurses' stereotyping of their (female) sex. Nurses tend to see themselves as nonintellectual and nontheoretical and to focus on practice for its own sake. Most nurses' needs to combine many roles (wife, mother, professional) are also seen as contributing to this by preventing leisure time necessary for thinking and theory building.[4]

Sexism affects both female and male nurses and creates disharmony between these groups. Overemphasis of tenderness and compassion (affective role) to the exclusion of the theoretical and analytical domains (cognitive role) produces an unbalanced practitioner. A complex postindustrial society needs nurses of both sexes with greater theoretical interests who are also comfortable and competent in affective behaviors. Indeed, autonomy and independence are necessary to promote values of caring, gentleness, and responsibility.[5] The former will not be attained without using cognitive tools accepted by a scientifically oriented society. Eventually, a balance can be attained that promotes healthy behavior and growth for both women and men.

The nursing process and nursing roles in providing care for sexual needs or problems are discussed in Chapter 13.

Components of Sexuality

A person's sexuality may be thought of as a complex of emotions, attitudes, preferences, and behaviors that are related to erotic expression. Among the many components of sexuality are a person's genetic (chromo-

somal) sex, gonadal sex, hormonal sex, morphological sex, gender identity, behavioral sex (sex role), and sexual partner preference. Usually there is congruence among these components, but this is not necessarily true. *Homosexuality* is an example of genetic, gonadal, and hormonal sex being incongruent with behavioral sex and sexual partner preference, at least by the dominant social definitions. *Transsexualism* (desiring to have the body, sexual organs, and sex role of the opposite sex) is an example of conflict between gender identity and genetic, gonadal, hormonal, and morphological sex.

In the more common case, in which there is congruence among the components of sexuality, it appears that the person's biologic equipment provides a frame through which sociocultural definitions of sexuality can be expressed. There is considerable evidence that the expression of sexuality is largely learned, although the significance of relations among gonadal hormones, anatomical structures, and sexual behavior is only in the beginning stages of exploration.[6,7] Among humans, there are very few imperative, or unalterable, sexual behaviors, including ejaculation in the male and menstruation, pregnancy, and childbirth in the female. These are necessary to carry out reproductive functions. All other sexual behaviors are, in a sense, optional. They are subject to environmental influences and comprise a very large sociocultural expression of sexual behavior. The following are key components of sexual expression that are largely shaped by culture rather than biology.

Gender Identity

Gender identity is the personal and private sense of being male or female, the personal experience of one's sex role. The sense of being male or female begins by the time a child is 3½ years of age. This is also the age at which a child develops conceptual language, which is involved in establishing a gender-differentiated self-concept. Information about the development of gender identity was gained from studies of children born with ambiguous genitalia, in whom it was impossible to clearly distinguish the baby as male or female. Sometimes a child is initially assigned the wrong sex according to its chromosomal sex. If during the first 12 months to 18 months of life an error is discovered through chromosomal analysis, the child's identity may be changed to the opposite sex. With each subsequent month, however, changing gender identity becomes increasingly difficult.[8] Although the range of behavioral expression is extremely wide, this basic sense of maleness or femaleness persists throughout life (Fig. 10-1).

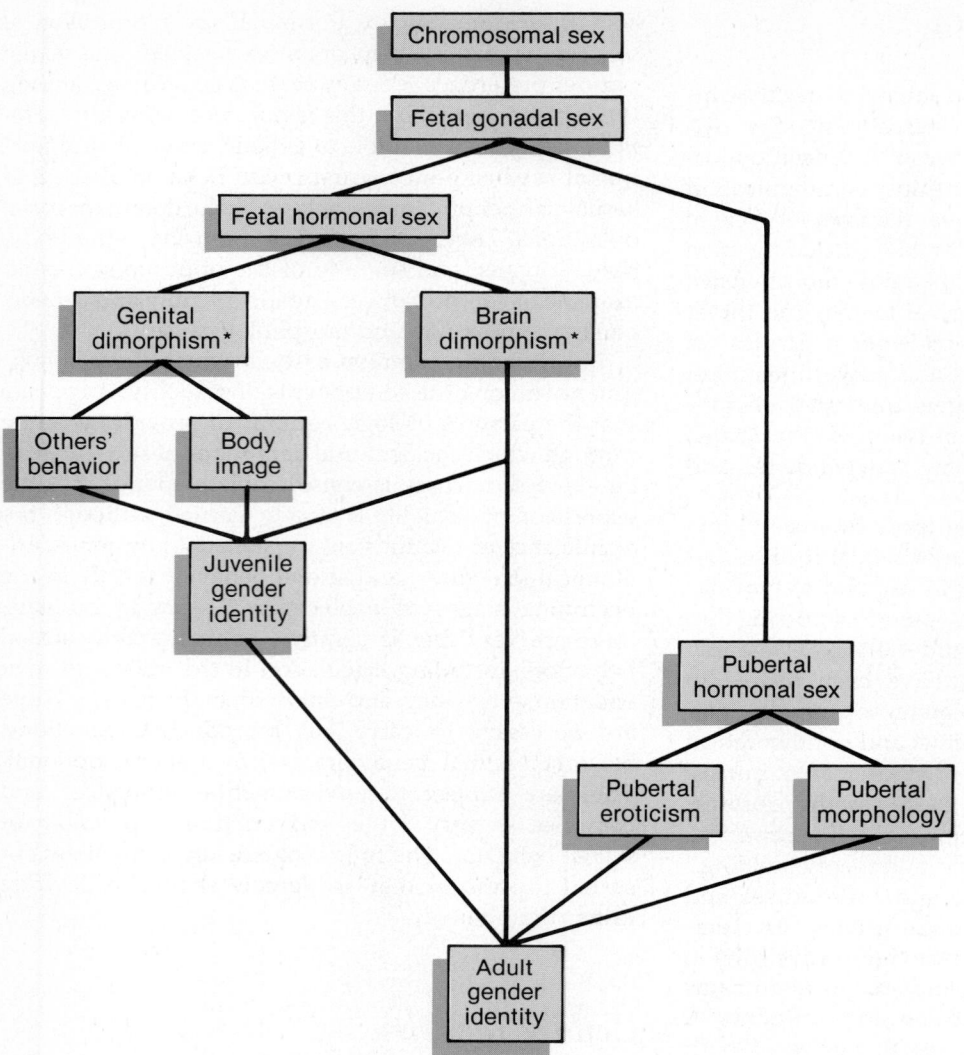

FIGURE   10-1

The sequence and interaction of components involved in development of gender identity are diagramed, showing the interaction of genetics and the environment. *Dimorphism is the manifestation in the same species of two forms, such as male and female; it refers to both bodily form and appearance and to sex differences in behavior and language. (After Money J, Ehrhardt AA: Man & Woman, Boy & Girl. Baltimore, The Johns Hopkins University Press, 1972)

Sex Role

Sex role is the public expression of gender identity. A person's sense of what are appropriate behaviors, attitudes, beliefs, and emotions for a female or male constitutes sex-role identification. In most Western societies, masculine (male sex role) behavior has been considered to be more aggressive, independent, and logical, while feminine (female sex role) behavior is seen as more submissive, dependent, and emotional. However, expressions of masculinity and femininity vary widely among cultures, and there are some societies in which what is considered male and female is exactly opposite of the Western stereotype.

Although most cultures place the women in the role of caretaker to children, and men in the role of breadwinner, there is no necessity that roles be assigned in this manner. Sex roles and definitions of masculinity and femininity are based on arbitrary criteria, rather than anatomical and physiological differences. Femininity and masculinity are not absolute conditions, and they can have overlapping behaviors. All humans are a mixture of maleness and femaleness and have the same types of impulses, wishes, attitudes, and basic emotional and physiological equipment (except those imperative parts of sexual function and behavior, and the obvious anatomical differences). The different expressions of sex role observed in various cultures is a result of society's selective development of behavioral potentials. Sex roles are developed through family interactions, the effects of peers, social codes of dress and manners, all forms of media communication, and numerous social structures that encourage certain behaviors and inhibit others for males and females.

Sexual Partner Preference

Preference for a sexual partner may be heterosexual, homosexual, or bisexual, and this preference may change during one's lifetime. Despite considerable research, it is far from clear how preferences for a sexual partner develop, even among heterosexuals. Sexual partner preference also appears to be on a continuum, rather than an all-or-none situation, and it probably varies with the circumstances for some people. There is a difference between actual sexual experiences and sexual responsiveness in regard to partner preference. For example, a person may be exclusively heterosexual in actual experience, but feel somewhat sexually attracted to people of the same sex.

There is enormous variety in sexual partner preference and associated sex-role behavior. A homosexual man may appear very masculine, carry out the role of a typical man, and have a strong gender identity as male, yet prefer a person of the same sex as an erotic partner. An effeminate-appearing male working at an occupation dominated by women may have a clear sense of male gender identity and opposite-sex erotic preference. A woman who appears and acts very masculine may have male gender identity and prefer women as sexual partners.

Many studies have examined social, psychological, and biologic factors as possible causes of homosexuality, but none are conclusive. It is well established that many people have sexual experiences with persons of the same sex, usually during childhood and adolescence. Homosexual preferences often develop before any actual sexual experience, however. Most people who have same-sex encounters do not develop homosexual partner preferences. Recent biologic research suggests that there may be a "sex center" in the fetal brain that is influenced by prenatal hormones and affects later sex-role behavior and choice of sexual partners. The mothers of some homosexuals were found to have atypical hormonal events during the critical period of sex center development during pregnancy, and it has been found that emotional stress during pregnancy causes reduced maternal androgen output, which might have contributed to feminization of male infants.[8]

The biologic linkage of sex-role and sexual partner preference in humans is far from established. "Tomboy" girls and "sissy" boys do not necessarily, or even usually, become homosexuals. The development of sexual partner preference is probably shaped by such diverse and complex factors as the prenatal hormonal environment, early mother–infant interactions, imitation by the child of the most valued parent, family dynamics and interstructure that selectively fosters and inhibits behaviors, the privileges and drawbacks of social sex roles

affecting value formation, and society's tolerance of variation in sexual expression.

Sexual Psychophysiology

Psychophysiology is a term that describes the interaction between psychological and physiological processes, between higher mental processes and the responses of muscles, glands, and organs. Two important fundamental psychophysiological principles are that a physiological response to a stimulus is influenced by past experiences and that current experiences and emotions are influenced by the body's responses. For example, a woman whose past experiences include frequent, intense orgasm may respond rapidly to sexual stimulation, while a woman who has learned not to expect to reach orgasm may have little response to the same type of stimuli. Also, awareness of the body's responses, such as vaginal congestion and lubrication in women and erection in men, can heighten pleasure and sexual feelings.

Human sexual response is determined by a delicate interaction between psychology and physiology. The nervous system has a central role in mediating sexual response by processing sexual signals of both cognitive and somatic origin. The causes of sexual arousal may be sought in the interplay between the brain and the sexual organs, to gain an understanding of the characteristics of sexual stimuli and the wide individual variation found.

Reflexogenic and Psychogenic Stimuli

Direct stimulation of erogenous areas, usually genitals and breasts, causes sexual arousal in a reflexive, or automatic, manner. When the penis or clitoris is stroked, the peripheral nerves send a signal to a relay center in the lower part of the spinal cord, which in turn sends a signal back to the penis for erection and to the clitoris and vagina for congestion and lubrication. The cerebral cortex and higher brain centers are not involved in this transmission of signals; it is a reflexogenic response that is mediated in the same way as the knee-jerk response. This is the mechanism through which some men with spinal cord injuries are able to have erections even though they have no sensation in the pelvic area.

Psychogenic stimuli are processed through the higher brain centers and can include sensory input such as sights, sounds, tastes, smells, and touches, as well as cognitive events such as thoughts, fantasies, memories, and images. Without direct stimulation of the genitals, it is possible to become sexually aroused through any one of these types of psychogenic stimuli. Watching an erotic movie, having the earlobe stroked, listening to a song with provocative lyrics, fantasizing a favorite sexual drama, or remembering a sexual encounter can all produce sexual arousal.

Most often, a combination of reflexogenic and psychogenic stimuli is used to produce sexual arousal, and they work in a synergistic way to enhance the level of excitement. Many men have found women more rapidly responsive sexually after an evening of candlelight, soft music, and romantic interaction. After seeing an erotic picture or movie, a man will often need considerably less (maybe no) direct stimulation to have an erection. On the other hand, feelings such as anger, guilt, or anxiety inhibit sexual response when direct stimulation is being used.

Neurologic Pathways

The neurologic pathways of reflexogenic stimuli are easier to trace than those of psychogenic stimuli, which involve complex mental processes and functions such as learning, emotions, and memory. The past experiences of a person are very important in determining which types of psychogenic stimuli are perceived as arousing. Early childhood experiences of pleasurable genital touching occurring in an environment with certain smells, sights, or sounds may lead to later association of these sensations with sexual arousal. The pro-

cess continues during adolescence and adulthood as sexual experience widens and different stimuli are associated with negative or positive sexual consequences. Being interrupted during sex by parents can lead to associations of anxiety or guilt with future sexual encounters. Circumstances in which a man has difficulty with erection can result in future erection problems under similar conditions. Situations in which intense sexual pleasure was felt tend to be sought again.

The central nervous system plays a key role in processing psychogenic stimuli and mediating the interplay between these and the activity of the peripheral nervous system. Central nervous system output travels through either the somatic or autonomic branch of the peripheral nervous system (Fig. 10-2). Generally speaking, the somatic nerves connect the central nervous system with the striated muscles. The muscle tension (myotonia) during sexual arousal is caused by stimulation of the somatic nerves. The autonomic nervous system, however, is responsible for most of the physiological changes during sexual arousal. In general, the autonomic nervous system controls the smooth muscles of the heart, internal organs, and glands whose functions are largely involuntary, or not under conscious control. Thus, sexual response has a large involuntary component, with conscious inhibition generally more effective than conscious activation.

The sympathetic and parasympathetic branches of the autonomic nervous system, with their different anatomical pathways and chemical activators of the smooth muscles and glands, are the immediate media-

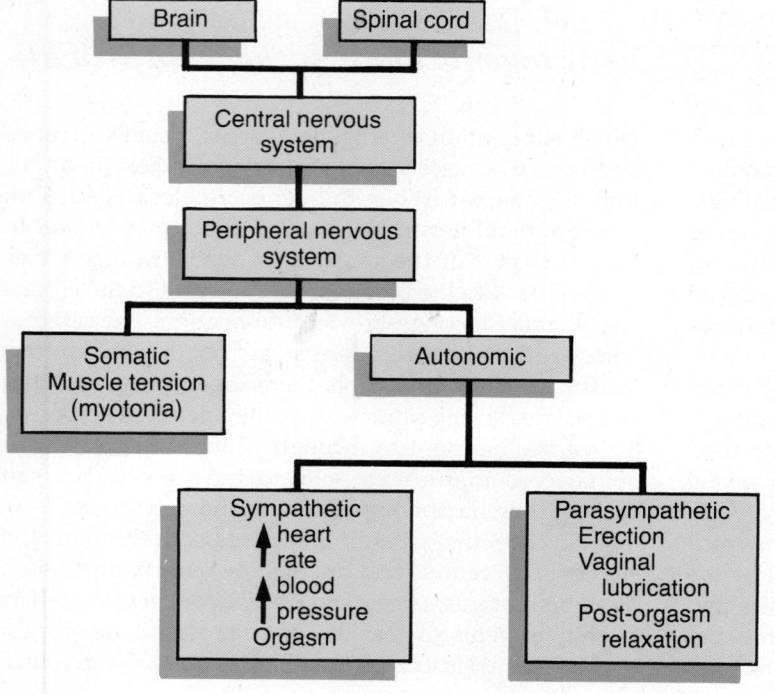

FIGURE 10-2

Neurologic pathways of sexual response.

tors of sexual response. The parasympathetic branch is also called cholinergic because its nerve endings release acetylcholine to transmit their messages, and the sympathetic branch is called adrenergic because it releases adrenaline and noradrenaline. These two branches serve different functions, with the sympathetic nervous system usually responding during times of stress, when there is a need for vigorous activity (thus the release of adrenaline), and the parasympathetic system dominating during periods of relaxation.

The sexual organs receive messages from both the sympathetic and parasympathetic systems, as do most other body organs. Penile erection and vaginal lubrication are caused by the effects of the parasympathetic system, which produce vasodilatation. As arousal progresses, the sympathetic system plays a larger role, causing increases in heart rate and blood pressure. The sympathetic system may take over completely at orgasm, with ejaculation and vaginal spasms set off by a sudden discharge of adrenaline. The autonomic imbalance produced by this sudden release of adrenaline is quickly compensated for by a release of acetylcholine that comes from the parasympathetic system. This parasympathetic rebound phenomenon, with its vasodilatation, contributes to the subjective feelings of warmth and relaxation that many people feel after orgasm.

Psychological Mediators of Sexual Response

The psychogenic stimuli that affect sexual response work largely through the relatively simple process of conditioning by association, or conditioned response. However, sexual meanings can be attached to stimuli through more complex psychological processes. The mental state in which people are likely to initiate or respond to sexual advances is created by a complex interplay of many factors. Sometimes a person can identify why he or she is "in the mood" for sex or why he or she is not, but at other times the sources of a reaction to sexual stimuli are elusive. Sexual feelings can be spontaneous and uncomplicated at times, but in other instances there may be conflicts, uncertainty, resistance, or hesitation. Human emotions and thoughts are very complex, so it is not surprising that sexual responsiveness varies greatly among different people, and in the same person at different times.

Major psychological mediators of responses to sexual stimulation have been identified as informational responses, emotional reactions, imaginative capacity, attention, and love. These factors interact with each other and exert a direct influence upon experiences in one area or another or create conflicts in responses to stimuli when there is disagreement among them. There is also a feedback loop between physiological response and the erotic stimulus; upon becoming aware of physical arousal, the stimulus causing arousal will be perceived as increasingly arousing (Fig. 10-3).

Informational Responses

The informational component that acts as a psychological mediator of sexual response consists of beliefs, knowledge, and labels concerning various aspects of sexuality. If a certain sexual practice is considered a perversion, such as oral-genital stimulation, then a person is unlikely to engage in this behavior and the idea of doing it would be repulsive, acting as a sexual "turn-off." If a sexual partner suggests or initiates oral-genital sex, this would effectively decrease sexual arousal and probably generate a number of negative feelings or expressions.

A person without this belief, however, who sees oral-genital sex as healthy and desirable, and who has had pleasurable past experiences, would respond with increased arousal to the idea, suggestion, or initiation of this activity. The expectations that are built upon beliefs, experiences (experiential knowledge), and the labeling–categorizing process exert powerful influences upon sexual responsiveness. These can either effectively shut down the physiological response or greatly enhance it.

Emotional Reactions

The emotional components in psychological mediation consist of subjective feelings and perceptions about a sexual stimulus. These follow beliefs and expectations very closely; emotions are the affective expression of values and beliefs. Feelings about sexual stimuli can range from the very positive, such as joy, happiness, and excitement, to the very negative, such as guilt, anxiety, repulsion, anger, and fear. A man exhibiting very "macho" behavior with the flavor of male superiority would probably evoke anger and repulsion in a feminist woman; therefore, he would be an ineffective visual and auditory sexual stimulus.

Many people report heightened arousal and increased intensity and rapidity of sexual response when there are deep, powerful feelings of love and commitment between partners. The boredom and diminished intensity of sexual experiences that are common among long-time married couples probably derive, at least in part, from a flattening of emotional response to each other. The sense of knowing someone too completely

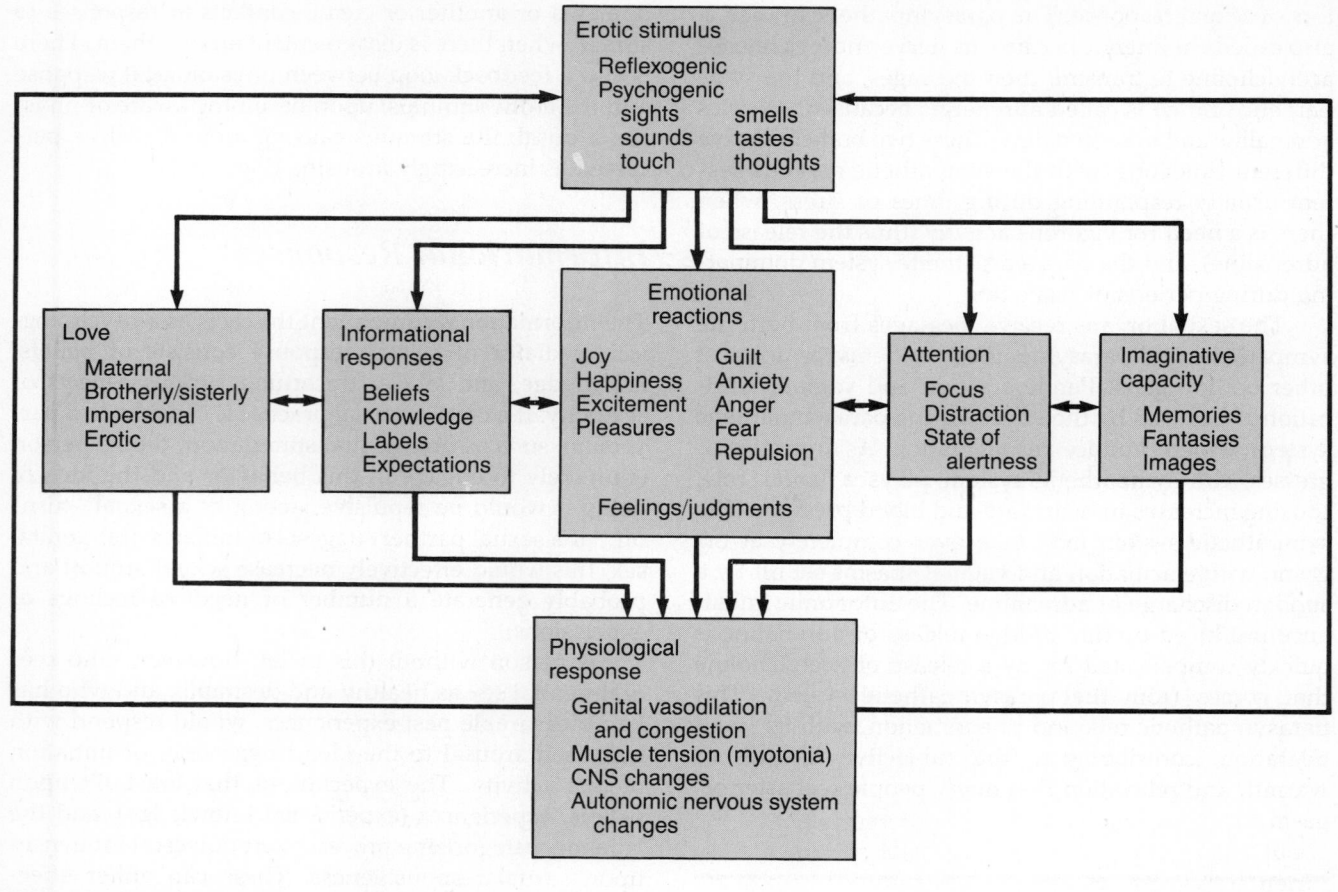

FIGURE 10-3

Psychological mediators of sexual response and the processing of erotic stimuli. (After Rosen R, Rosen LR: Human Sexuality. New York, Alfred A Knopf, Inc., 1981)

so there is no excitement of the unknown and unpredictable, and the little resentments that build up over years of unexpressed or unresolved conflicts so there is a smoldering anger just under the surface constitute emotions that detract from sexual response. The directness, honesty, and humility necessary to grow out of such traps require conscious cultivation by both partners.

As previously mentioned, guilt is one of the most effective inhibitors of sexual response. Many men and women with sexual problems find early inculcation of guilty feelings about themselves as sexual beings and sex-related activities at the base of their difficulties. Making judgments about oneself or one's partner, whether related to appearance or behaviors, sets up an acceptable or not acceptable dichotomy that may screen out many sexual stimuli. Judging something as "good" or "bad" is a way of expressing values and beliefs and lays the foundation for associated feelings.

Imaginative Capacity

The imaginative component in psychological mediation of sexual response includes the memories, images, and fantasies that are invoked by sexual stimuli. Almost everyone has sexual fantasies. Some people can create or enhance arousal by just thinking about them. Because some fantasies are bizarre, there is often guilt associated with them, producing a conflict in psychological input. Sexologists state that any fantasy that increases arousal is acceptable as long as it is not acted out in a way that will harm others, physically or emotionally.

Mental images have been found by sex researchers to be very important in determining sexual response. Arousal tends to be greatest with evocation of memories of the person's own past sexual acts, when what was personally experienced produced significant pleasure in sexual encounters. Imagery is so powerful that people can quickly learn to arouse themselves sexually or turn off sexual response, just by using appropriate fantasies and images.

Attention

The importance of attention in mediating sexual response is so direct and obvious that it is often overlooked. If a person is not paying attention to a sexual stimulus, then it will have very little effect, if any. Sexual response will be limited, or may not occur at all, if a person is unattentive or distracted. This was well demonstrated in a laboratory experiment in which subjects listened to an erotic tape recording through one side of an earphone headset, while simple mental arithmetic problems were played through the other earphone. Using instruments to measure the subjects' penile erections, it was found that the distraction of the math problems definitely reduced the amount of erection produced in response to the erotic tape.

The effects of distraction have been felt by most people at some time. People do not respond as readily to sexual stimuli when also aware of the noises of their children in a nearby room, when thoughts of housework or office work to be done arise, when hungry and smelling food cooking, or when dissatisfied with something about their appearance or the circumstances of sex. When no environmental distractions are present, the ability to focus on the sexual encounter becomes an important part of attention processes. For no apparent reason, a person may find his or her mind wandering to totally unrelated subjects. Although the body is physically going through the motions, the level of arousal may be quite low, delaying or inhibiting orgasm when a person is not focused upon the sexual experience. The state of alertness is also important; if a person is drowsy and drifting off into sleep, sexual responses will also be sluggish. This applies to the effects of certain drugs such as alcohol, which decreases mental alertness as well as depressing physiological responses.

Sex and Love

Another important psychological mediator in sexual response is love. Similar to sexuality, love is a complex phenomenon and is variously defined and understood. There appear to be many types of love that can affect sexual development and expression. Maternal love is uncritical caring for the weak and helpless, or specifically for one's own child. It provides a crucial foundation for developing security and self-esteem. Brotherly (sisterly) love is affection between friends or relatives, usually one's peers and close companions. It supports the sense of identity and belonging. Love of humanity is caring for all people. This love is selfless and nonsexual; it is impersonal love (because it encompasses all people and not individuals). Such love is the basis for altruism and self-transcendence.

Erotic love is most clearly expressed in sexual relationships. The feelings of affection, caring, and intimacy shared between sexual partners are often inseparable from their sexual behaviors. Some believe that sexual "freedom" means separating sex from love, something that men have long been accused of, but which now seems frequent among women also. Subordination of sex needs to love needs and expressing sexuality only in a loving (or socially approved) relationship were traditionally expected of women. Pursuit of sexual liberation through separating sex and love may prove to be unsatisfying or anxiety producing, however. More sexual activity and less emotional involvement creates an emptiness for many people. The fusion of sex with feelings of love and intimacy creates one of life's most intense experiences.

Love has developmental aspects with sexual components. Generally, a person's ability to love progresses throughout life. Some elements of sexual pleasure or sex-role expression occur in almost all types of love. When love relationships are inadequate or interrupted, sexual problems can develop. Love is essential for growth, human development, and being. In its impersonal form, it is the path to self-transcendence.

The Sexual Response Cycle

The systems of sexual anatomy and physiology that are organized around the clitoris in women and the penis in men are exact homologues of each other. Each part in one sex has its counterpart in the other. These counterparts may be structurally the same in both women and men, may be modified to perform the same function in a different way, or may perform a different function. The sexual response cycle, with its two basic physiological mechanisms of vasocongestion and myotonia, progresses through identical phases with corresponding changes in genital and other body organs in both women and men. There are certain differences in timing and patterns characteristic of each of the sexes within this common physiological process.

Prenatal Sexual Differentiation

The physical similarities in sexual anatomy stem from the first few months of embryonic life. The XX (female) configuration or XY (male) configuration of the chro-

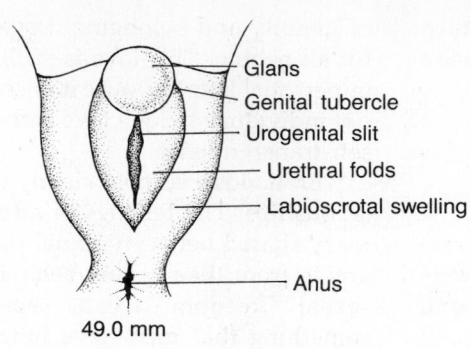

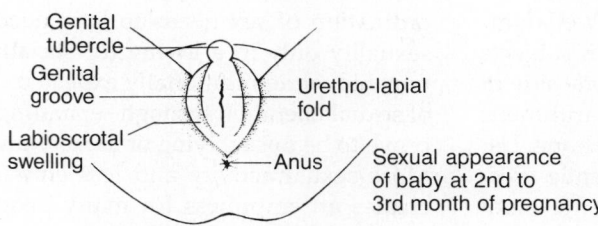

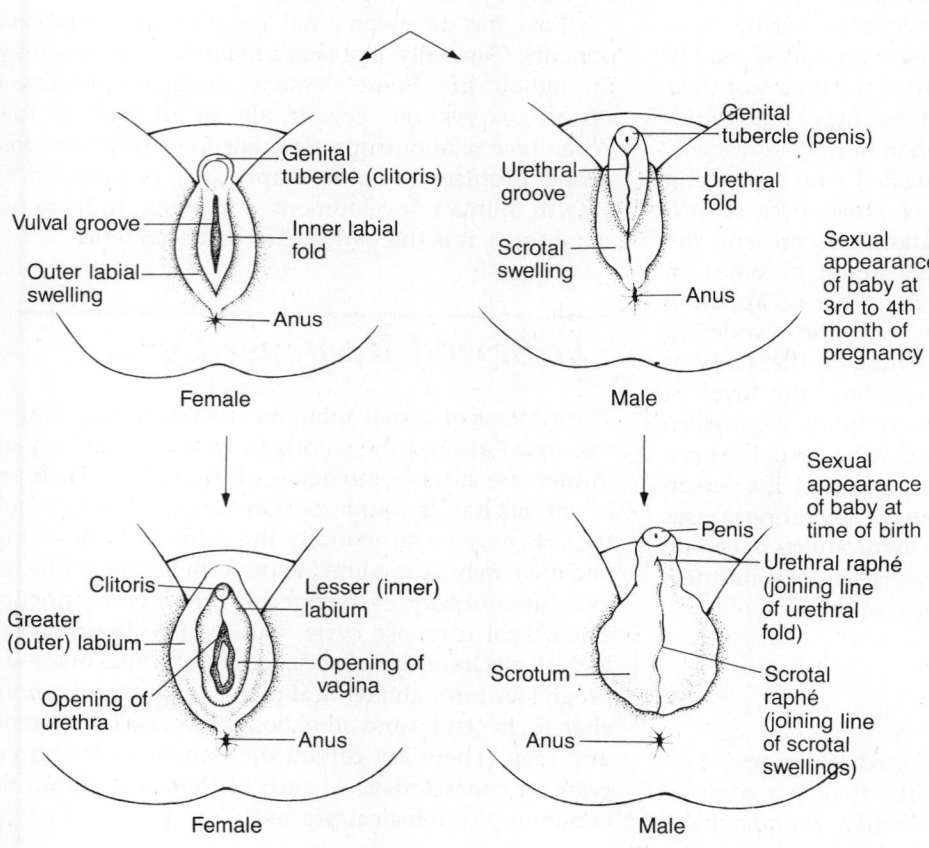

F I G U R E   1 0 - 4

Fetal genital differentiation. (*A*) Undifferentiated external genitalia of 7-week embryo. Male and female appear the same; sex can be determined only by the Barr body chromosome test. (*B*) Differentiation of external genitalia into male and female in the fetus. (*C*) Differentiation of internal sex organs into male and female in the fetus.

mosomes after conception passes the sexual program to the primordial gonad. The primitive genital ducts of the embryo are identical until about 6 weeks' gestation. At that time, under chromosomal influence, the gonads of the embryo become ovaries with the XX pattern or testes with the XY pattern. In the male embryo, androgenic hormones secreted by the testes stimulate development of the wolffian ducts, which give rise to most of the male reproductive system. The müllerian ducts produce the female reproductive system and are probably suppressed in the male embryo. Even though the female embryo's ovaries secrete estrogen, this is not necessary

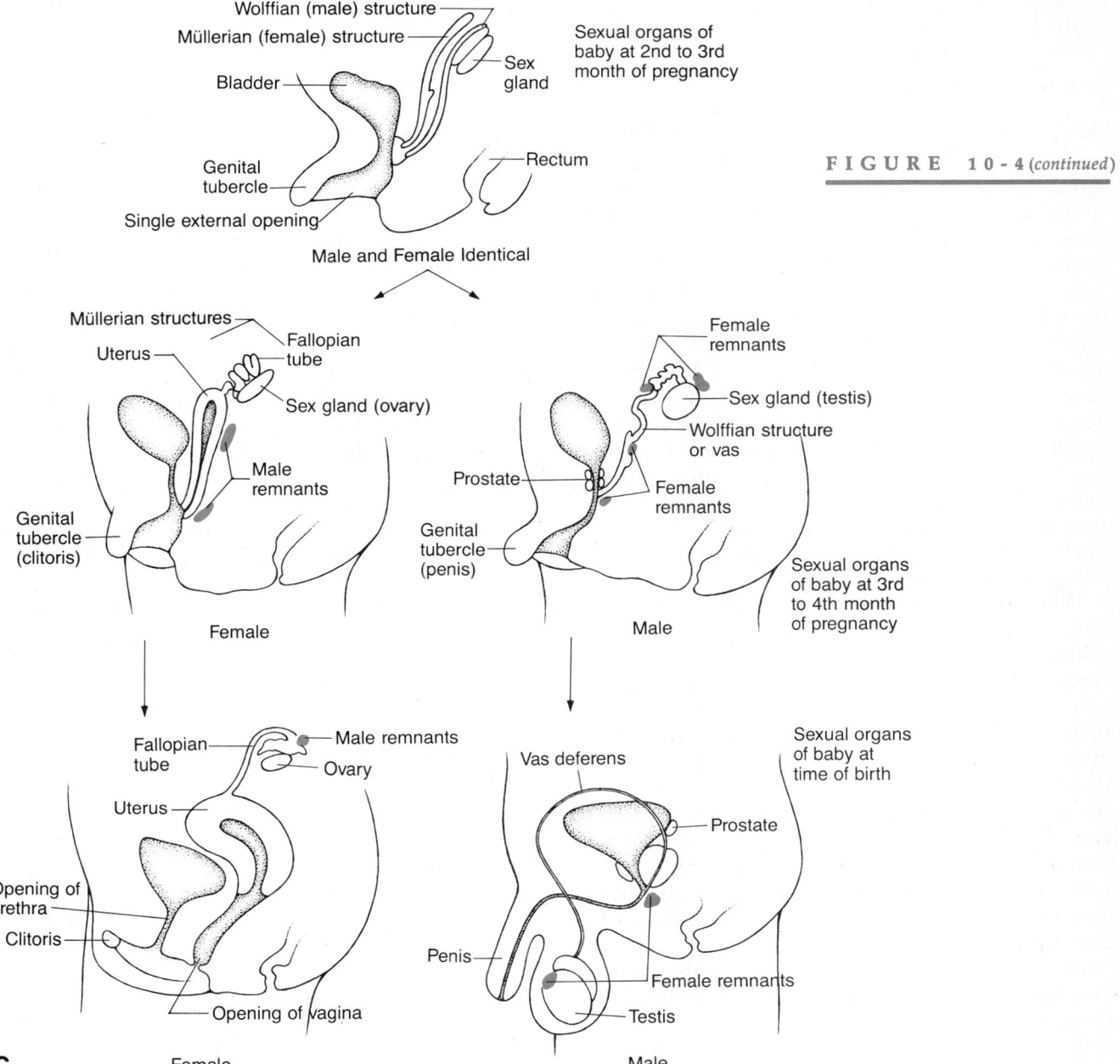

Wolffian (male) structure
Müllerian (female) structure
Sex gland
Bladder
Sexual organs of baby at 2nd to 3rd month of pregnancy
Genital tubercle
Rectum
Single external opening

Male and Female Identical

FIGURE 10-4 *(continued)*

Müllerian structures
Fallopian tube
Uterus
Sex gland (ovary)
Male remnants
Genital tubercle (clitoris)

Female remnants
Sex gland (testis)
Wolffian structure or vas
Prostate
Female remnants
Genital tubercle (penis)
Sexual organs of baby at 3rd to 4th month of pregnancy

Female   Male

Fallopian tube
Male remnants
Ovary
Uterus
Vas deferens
Opening of urethra
Clitoris
Prostate
Penis
Opening of vagina
Female remnants
Testis
Sexual organs of baby at time of birth

C   Female   Male

for female sexual differentiation. If fetal gonads do not secrete hormones, and even if embryonic reproductive tracts (without gonads) are removed in experiments and kept alive, the genital structures continue to develop in the female pattern. Androgens must be added to produce male sexual differentiation, while their absence leads to female differentiation. This implies that nature's basic propensity, at least in mammals, is to produce a female.[10]

The embryonic glans and genital tubercle develops into the clitoral system in the female and the penis in the male. The labioscrotal swelling becomes the female labia or male scrotum, and the urogenital slit and ure-

thral folds form the different urethral systems in males and females. Internally, the müllerian structures become the female fallopian tubes, uterus, and vagina, and the wolffian structures become the male vas deferens, prostate, and seminal vesicles (Fig. 10-4).

Anatomy and Physiology of Sexual Response

Male and female sexual and reproductive anatomy and physiology have been presented in Chapter 9. A brief review of the most pertinent structures is included in this section, with a more detailed discussion of sexual physiology.

Female Sexual Response

The *labia majora,* which are well endowed with fat, hair, sweat glands, blood vessels, lymphatic vessels, and nerves, respond to vasocongestion with sexual excitation by spreading apart, becoming more flattened and elongating anteroposteriorly. The *labia minora,* which are continuous with the prepuce (clitoral hood), are well supplied with blood vessels, nerves, and lymphatics. The labial skin has a pink pigmentation that deepens in color with arousal, becoming bright red or purplish red with high levels of sexual excitement. The labia minora increase in size and extend outward with vasocongestion, protruding past the labia majora and functionally elongating the vagina. Often called the "sex skin," the labia minora are highly sensitive to touch and play a major role in arousal and orgasm through their draping over the clitoris, providing continual clitoral stimulation as tension is increased and decreased with penile thrusting (see Fig. 10-6).

The *clitoris* is a complex anatomical structure with both external and cryptic, or hidden, parts. Its role in arousal and orgasm is central, and it appears that the sole purpose of the clitoral structure is to enhance female sexual pleasure. There are four parts to the clitoris: the glans, shaft, crus, and vestibular bulbs. The glans and shaft are the most external and smallest portions and are largely hidden under the prepuce. Comprising only one tenth of the volume of the clitoris in its resting state, the glans and shaft represent even a smaller proportion during sexual arousal when the cryptic structures may increase in size up to three times. The clitoral shaft contains two small erectile cavernous bodies enclosed in a dense fibrous membrane, similar to the male penis. The length of the shaft is about ¼ inch to ¾ inch, although there are marked variations. The glans is on average 4 mm to 5 mm in diameter, though normal range encompasses 2 mm to 1 cm.

The clitoral glans is the most sensitive female erogenous area, with its mucous membrane so densely packed with nerve endings that there is little room for blood vessels. The entire female sexual cycle can be initiated and maintained to orgasm by stimulation of only the glans. At rest, the shaft is sharply retroflexed posteriorly. With sexual stimulation, it becomes congested, leading to erection, moving the tip through an 180° arc in a forward elliptical curve. As arousal proceeds, it is retracted under the prepuce and appears shorter because of the actions of muscles and the cryptic structures pulling it inward.

The cryptic structures of the clitoris include the crus and vestibular bulbs. At the end of the shaft, the clitoris bifurcates and branches into two crura, which extend inward bilaterally following the inferior rami of the symphysis pubis downward. The crura lie below the ischiocavernous muscles and bodies, with a tough, tendinous lower portion that anchors the clitoris to the inner surface of the ischium. The clitoral crus is homologous to the corpus cavernosum in the male, which becomes the crus of the penis. The crura play a lesser role in distention during arousal in the female than the vestibular bulbs because of their tendinous nature (Fig. 10-5).

The vestibular bulbs also divide and descend into the pelvis from the clitoral shaft. Extending outward bilaterally, they wrap fully three quarters of the way around the lower portion of the vagina. Each bulb presses closely against the lower third of the vagina, just above the vaginal opening. The vestibular bulbs are erectile and highly distensible and are covered with a mass of coiled blood vessels (*commissure of the bulbs*). These blood vessels also become distended during arousal and convey blood between the bulbs and the clitoral shaft. The greater vestibular glands (Bartholin's glands) are located at the bottom of the bulbs. The vestibular bulbs become greatly distended during arousal, contributing to the buildup of the orgasmic platform in the lower third of the vagina. The homologous structure

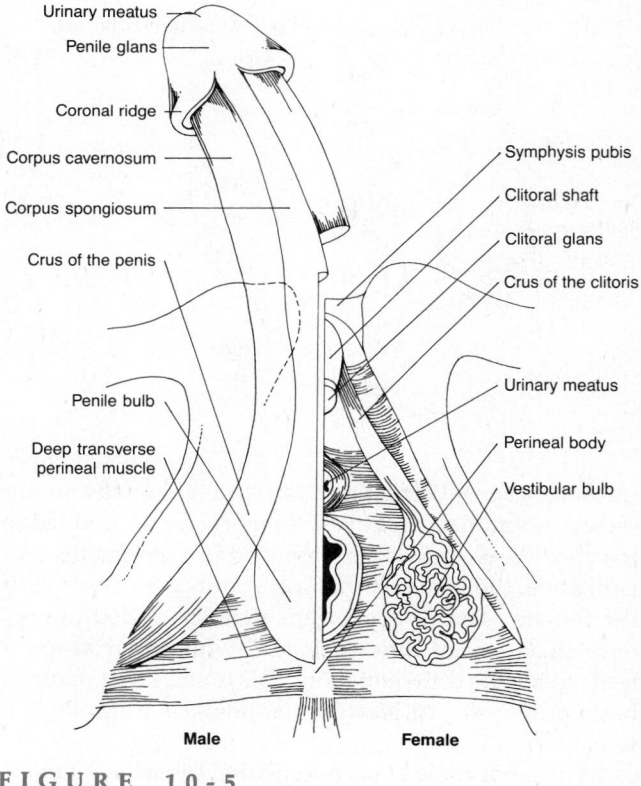

Urinary meatus
Penile glans
Coronal ridge
Corpus cavernosum
Corpus spongiosum
Crus of the penis
Penile bulb
Deep transverse perineal muscle

Symphysis pubis
Clitoral shaft
Clitoral glans
Crus of the clitoris
Urinary meatus
Perineal body
Vestibular bulb

Male   **Female**

FIGURE   10-5

Comparison of female and male cryptic structures.

in the male is the corpus spongiosum, which becomes the bulb of the penis.

The female *pelvic muscles* participate in engorgement during sexual arousal and have an important function in orgasm. The *ischiocavernous muscles* envelop the clitoral crura, and the *bulbocavernous muscles* surround the vestibular bulbs and the lower third of the vagina. Ascending from the vagina, the bulbocavernous muscles terminate in fibrous tissue dorsal of the clitoris and overlie the crura, and join the ischiocavernous to form the striated sphincter of the urethra. The *transverse perineal muscles* and *levator ani muscles* converge on the lateral walls of the lower third of the vagina and unite behind the vaginal opening to form the perineal body. These pelvic muscles become congested during arousal, and many women are aware that voluntary contractions of perineal muscles can heighten arousal. The muscles press on distended clitoral and vaginal structures, and when a critical point is reached in this distention, a reflex stretch mechanism is set off in the muscles and the contractions pressing on the distended clitoral crura, vestibular bulbs, and lower vaginal area cause orgasm.

The *vagina* is a muscular tube that is lined with mucous membranes and is richly supplied with blood vessels, glands, and lymphatics. The lower third of the vagina has many nerve endings, but the upper portion is not as well endowed and may be distended considerably laterally and posteriorly without discomfort. The circumvaginal venous plexus is a dense grouping of blood vessels surrounding the lower third of the vagina, and these vessels provide the blood supply for the massive congestion that produces vaginal lubrication during sexual arousal. They also contribute to building the orgasmic platform in later stages of excitement.

With effective sexual stimulation, pelvic venous dilatation and congestion occur quickly, and fluid from these venous networks passes into tissue spaces and causes edema. Within 10 to 30 seconds, droplets of clear fluid called transudate appear on the vaginal walls, coalesce, and produce vaginal lubrication. Concurrently, the upper two thirds of the vagina begins to lengthen and distend. As excitement progresses, the upper vagina balloons outward as the uterus and cervix are pulled upward into the false pelvis. In the lower pelvis, a broad platform of distended tissues forms as pelvic congestion and edema reach a peak. The vestibular bulbs and labia minora are also highly distended and congested at peak excitement. The thickened area of congested tissue surrounding the lower vagina and vaginal opening is called the *orgasmic platform* (Fig. 10-6).

When this vasocongestive distention reaches a critical point, orgasm is triggered in a mechanism involving the clitoral shaft and glans, clitoral cryptic structures, vaginal platform, and pelvic muscles. The muscles contract vigorously at intervals of 0.8 second, expelling the blood and fluid trapped in the tissues and venous plexi, and create the sensations of orgasm. Orgasm usually consists of 8 to 15 contractions; the first five or six are the most intense. Mild orgasms may only have three to five contractions. Because of the extent of pelvic congestion and the capacity for distention of pelvic structures, much of the blood and edema cannot be removed and may flow back into the distended structures. As a result of this, many women are capable of restimulation seconds after orgasm and may have repeated orgasms.

The *cervix* and *uterus* have less dramatic roles in female sexual response. The uterus enlarges owing to vascular engorgement and rises gradually with increasing excitement until it is out of the true pelvis. It also pulls the upper vagina upward. Uterine contractions occur during orgasm; they are usually pleasurable, but sometimes they are not consciously perceived. For some women, however, these contractions may be painful owing to prolonged spasm; most often this occurs during menopause or pregnancy, with dysmenorrhea, or when an intrauterine device is used.[11] The cervix may undergo some congestion, but there is no significant response until the cervical os opens slightly after orgasm. During the final, resolution phase of the sexual cycle, the uterus drops back down into its usual position. The cervical os opens more widely during this time and is positioned in the seminal pool in the upper vagina; this is believed to be an aid to sperm entry into the cervix and ultimately to conception (see Fig. 10-6).

The breasts and other nongenital areas are also involved in sexual response. During sexual excitement, the *breasts* become enlarged and the nipple becomes erect owing to congestion. Both of these are erotic areas for women. Some women are able to reach orgasm by breast stimulation alone. The *skin* in some women may show the "sex flush," a mottled pinkish discoloration that is most prominent on the chest and trunk. Spasms of the abdomen, buttocks, and thighs may also occur with high levels of excitement.

Recently, interest has surfaced in a phenomenon called *female ejaculation*, the emission of fluid during orgasm by women. It has been thought that orgasmic muscle contractions squeezed out some vaginal lubrication to cause this sensation. It is now postulated that a homologous female structure to the male prostate secretes the jet of fluid from the vulval area during orgasm. The paraurethral ducts (Skene's ducts) develop from the same primitive tissue as the male prostate and consist of two small glands and their ducts, which are located on either side of the urethra. It is possible that the Skene's ducts emit fluid during orgasm like the male prostate. There is a great deal of variability in the amount and location of this tissue among women. One descriptive study of both heterosexual and homosexual

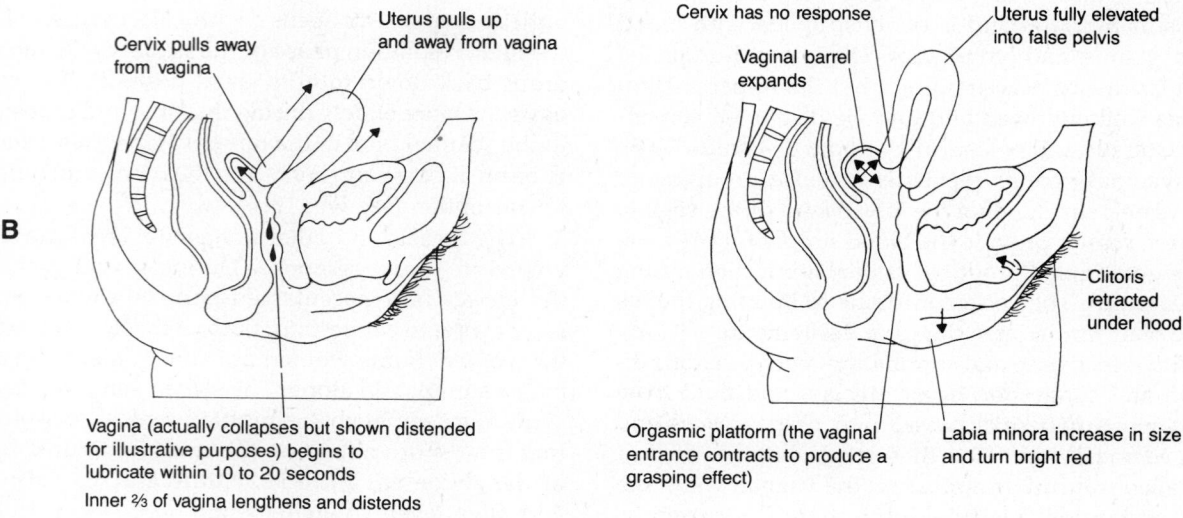

Excitement Stage

Clitoris increases in length
two to three times

A

Labia majora
spread flat and
anteroposteriorly

Labia minora
increase in size
and extend outward

Cervix pulls away
from vagina

Uterus pulls up
and away from vagina

B

Vagina (actually collapses but shown distended
for illustrative purposes) begins to
lubricate within 10 to 20 seconds

Inner ⅔ of vagina lengthens and distends

Plateau Stage

Clitoris retracts under hood
(it is difficult to locate and
so tender that efforts to touch it
directly may cause discomfort)

Bartholin glands
secrete 1 to 3
drops

Labia majora
(no further response)

Labia minora turn bright red and increase
in size (if stimulation continues, orgasm
occurs 1 minute or 1½ minutes after
the bright red color appears)

Cervix has no response

Vaginal barrel
expands

Uterus fully elevated
into false pelvis

Clitoris
retracted
under hood

Orgasmic platform (the vaginal
entrance contracts to produce a
grasping effect)

Labia minora increase in size
and turn bright red

FIGURE 10-6

Female sexual response cycle. (*A*) Changes in external genitalia. (*B*) Changes in
internal genitalia.

women found that 54% in the sample reported ejaculation, which was defined as orgasmic expulsion of
fluid.[12]

Male Sexual Response

The *penis* consists of three long cylinders of erectile tissue that are surrounded by an elastic sheath. Each cylinder contains blood vessels and spaces that fill up with
blood during sexual arousal. The two upper cylinders,

the corpora cavernosa, are responsible for the rigidity
and the increase in length and width of the penis with
erection (Fig. 10-7). At the base of the penile shaft,
where it joins the body, the corpora cavernosa diverge
into the crura, which become tough tendinous fibers
that attach to the pelvic bones. These are homologous
to the clitoral crura in the female. On the underside of
the penis is the third cylinder, the corpus spongiosum.
On the external end it terminates in the glans, and on
the internal end it terminates in the bulb. The urethra

Orgasm Stage

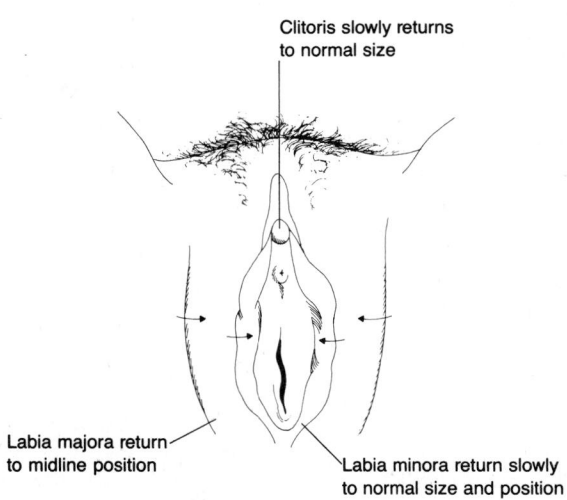

Clitoris retracted under hood

Urinary meatus dilates in some women

Labia majora (no specific response)

Labia minora (no specific response)

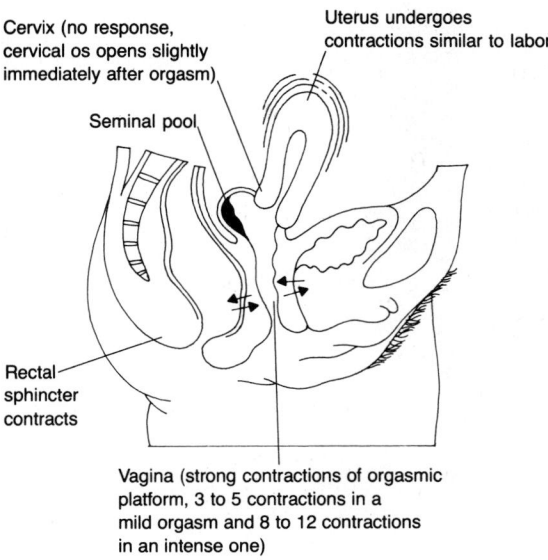

Cervix (no response, cervical os opens slightly immediately after orgasm)

Uterus undergoes contractions similar to labor

Seminal pool

Rectal sphincter contracts

Vagina (strong contractions of orgasmic platform, 3 to 5 contractions in a mild orgasm and 8 to 12 contractions in an intense one)

Resolution Stage

Clitoris slowly returns to normal size

Labia majora return to midline position

Labia minora return slowly to normal size and position

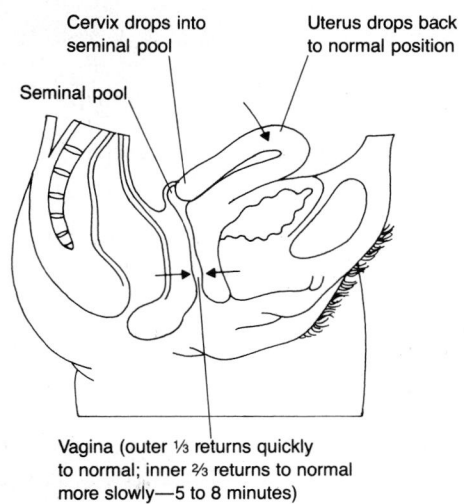

Cervix drops into seminal pool

Uterus drops back to normal position

Seminal pool

Vagina (outer ⅓ returns quickly to normal; inner ⅔ returns to normal more slowly—5 to 8 minutes)

FIGURE 10-6 (*continued*)

runs through the corpus spongiosum. During erection, the spongy body remains softer than the corpora cavernosa. The glans enlarges when it is excited to almost twice its quiescent size and provides a soft protective cushion for the rigid corpora cavernosa (Fig. 10-8). The glans is highly endowed with nerve endings, and it is the male's area of maximum erotic sensation.

The penile bulb becomes very rigid and distended during sexual arousal, lengthens, and increases markedly in diameter. It nearly fills the space between the pubic rami and presses downward on the testicles. The bulb of the penis is homologous to the female vestibular

bulbs, but is not as large. The penile structures continue to distend and enlarge until the peak of excitement is reached. Clear mucoid fluid is secreted from the urethra, probably from Cowper's glands or the prostate. At the critical point of vasocongestive distention, the reflex stretch mechanism is set off in the muscles and orgasm occurs. The same muscles are involved in the male as in the female, primarily the bulbocavernous, the ischiocavernous, the levator ani, and the transverse perineum.

As muscle contractions beginning around the seminal vesicles and prostate cause emission of the semen

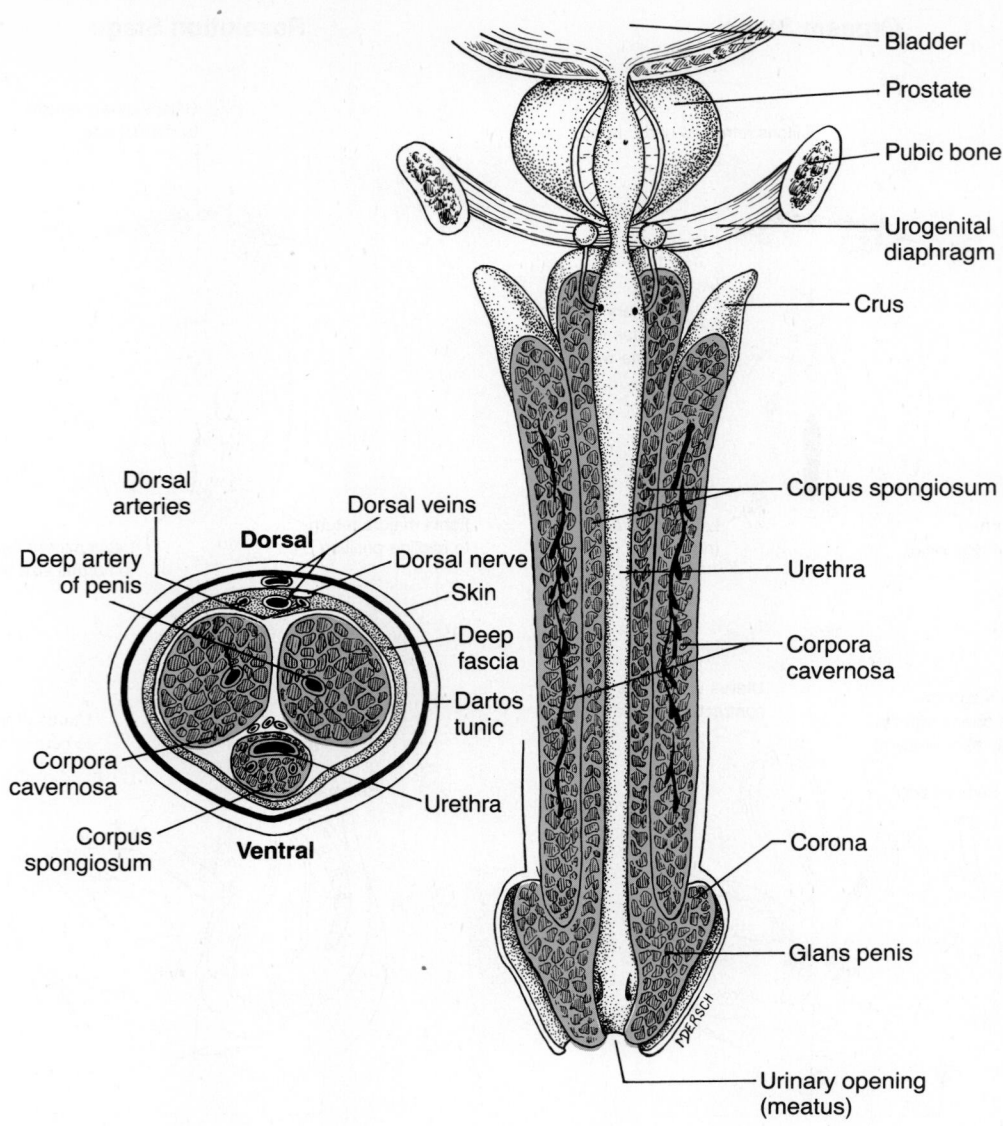

Bladder

Prostate

Pubic bone

Urogenital diaphragm

Crus

Corpus spongiosum

Urethra

Corpora cavernosa

Corona

Glans penis

Urinary opening (meatus)

Dorsal arteries

Dorsal

Dorsal veins

Deep artery of penis

Dorsal nerve

Skin

Deep fascia

Dartos tunic

Corpora cavernosa

Corpus spongiosum

Ventral

Urethra

FIGURE 10-7

Internal structures of erect penis.

into the upper urethra, the man feels the sensation of "ejaculatory inevitability," immediately followed by the propulsive orgasmic contractions. Semen spurts out of the urethra at 0.8-second intervals in three to seven ejaculatory spurts. Contractions of the penis and urethra are felt with each spurt of semen.

The skin of the *scrotum* begins to thicken and wrinkle with sexual excitement, and the *testes* begin to elevate closer to the perineum. The cremaster muscle elevates the testes and also helps to heat and to cool the testes by bringing them closer to or farther away from the body, maintaining an even temperature for effective sperm production. As excitement progresses, the scrotum thickens more and the testes increase up to 50%

in size and rotate anteriorly. Vasocongestion causes increase in testicular size. At the time of orgasm, the testes are elevated closely against the perineum and are maximally engorged. Following orgasm, the testes descend and decrease in size, and the scrotal skin thins and returns to its former texture (see Fig. 10-8).

The *prostate* is located just below the bladder and surrounds the urethra, and it contains an intricate series of ducts that secrete prostatic fluid. This fluid contains prostaglandins, hormonal substances that cause contractions of the uterus and are thought to aid fertilization, and other biochemical substances, including fibrinogenase, which causes temporary coagulation of semen in the vagina to prevent its dripping out. Prostatic

Excitement Stage

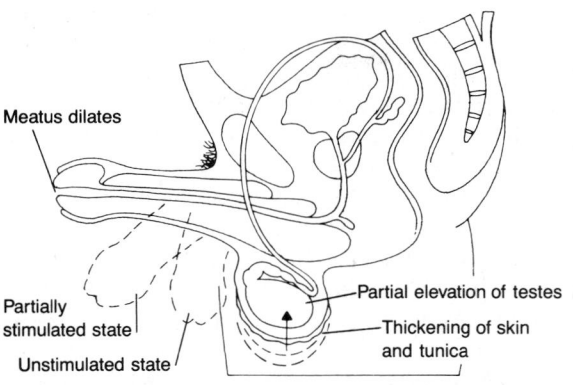

Meatus dilates

Partially stimulated state

Unstimulated state

Partial elevation of testes

Thickening of skin and tunica

The smaller flaccid penis tends to enlarge proportionately more in erection, thus decreasing the difference between the larger and the smaller flaccid penis.

Plateau Stage

As seminal fluid collects in prostatic urethra, there is a feeling of ejaculatory inevitability. Larger fluid volume is experienced as more pleasurable.

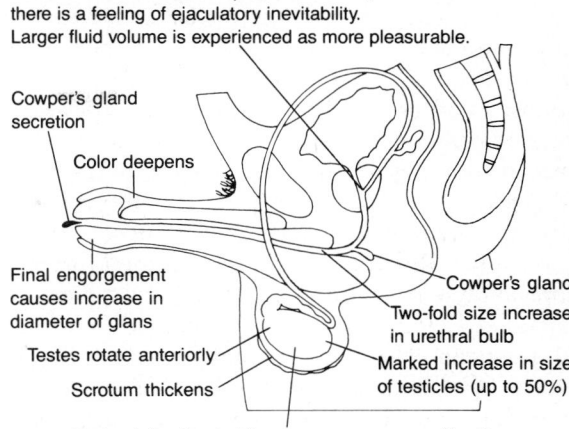

Cowper's gland secretion

Color deepens

Final engorgement causes increase in diameter of glans

Testes rotate anteriorly

Scrotum thickens

Cowper's gland

Two-fold size increase in urethral bulb

Marked increase in size of testicles (up to 50%)

Testes fully elevated (orgasm never occurs without elevated testes, though they may be less elevated in men over 50 years of age.)

Orgasmic Stage

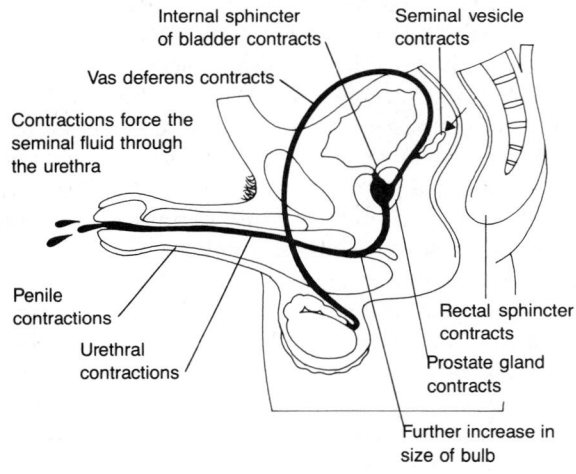

Internal sphincter of bladder contracts

Vas deferens contracts

Contractions force the seminal fluid through the urethra

Penile contractions

Urethral contractions

Seminal vesicle contracts

Rectal sphincter contracts

Prostate gland contracts

Further increase in size of bulb

Resolution Stage

Duration of this stage varies proportionately with length of excitement and plateau stages

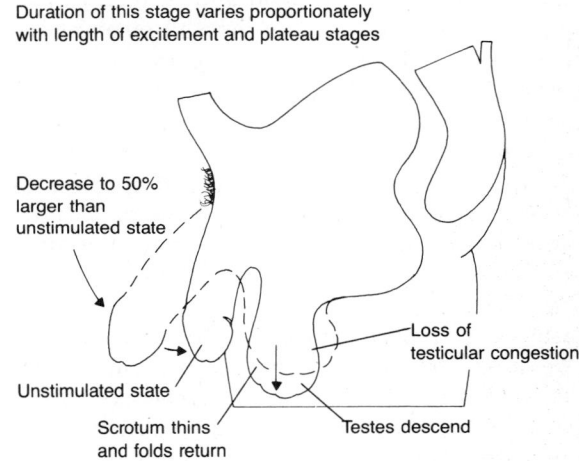

Decrease to 50% larger than unstimulated state

Unstimulated state

Scrotum thins and folds return

Loss of testicular congestion

Testes descend

FIGURE 10-8

Male sexual response cycle.

fluid is alkaline and buffers the acidity of the vagina, allowing sperm to survive longer. It provides a vehicle for sperm transportation through the urethra and is secreted during orgasm to make up the largest part of the semen.

The *seminal vesicles* are coiled tubal structures that join the vas deferens with the ejaculatory ducts that enter the prostate. Sperm from the vas deferens mix with secretions, which are triggered by orgasm, from the seminal vesicles and pass through the prostate by way of the ejaculatory ducts. These secretions are high in fructose, a natural sugar that aids sperm motility.

The two *Cowper's glands* are the size of a pea and are located between the prostate and urethra. They produce an alkaline secretion that neutralizes the acidity

of the urethra, which is caused by transporting urine. It is important to neutralize this acidity before sperm are transported through the urethra because the acidity can damage sperm. The Cowper's glands usually secret a drop or two of fluid, but the amount varies considerably. This fluid appears as preejaculate, and it is possible that sperm secreted into the urethra from the ejaculatory ducts might be carried along in the Cowper's gland fluid prior to orgasm. This accounts for the risk in using withdrawal for contraception, as sperm may be present in the fluid secreted before orgasm. The secretions from Cowper's glands usually appear during the plateau phase of sexual arousal, just before orgasm.

Men also experience nipple erection during sexual arousal, and they may have the sex flush, as well as spasm of the buttocks and thighs. Although no muscles play an important role in initial erection of the penile shaft, pelvic muscles are the key to the final surge to orgasm in the male. The penile bulb and corpora cavernosa are enclosed in a muscular coat, which, along with almost all other muscles in the area, is responsible for complete erection and ejaculation. Contracting in a coordinated, downward rhythm, these muscles compress the prostate, seminal vesicles, and the internal structures (penile bulb and corpora cavernosa), which in turn compress the urethra and force semen forward with considerable pressure. Blood also is forced out of the distended cavernous spaces, leading to detumescence of the penis. The penis gradually becomes flaccid and returns to its original size after orgasm; the length of time varies for different occasions in the same man.

Patterns of Sexual Response

The sexual response cycle in men and women can be divided into several stages. The most popular model was introduced by Masters and Johnson in *Human Sexual Response*.[13] An orderly sequence of psychophysiologic events takes place and brings about marked changes in the shape and function of the genital organs, as described in the preceding section. Regardless of whether sexual stimulation is reflexogenic or psychogenic, reactions in the neurologic, vascular, muscular, and hormonal systems occur that affect many parts of the body.

Masters and Johnson developed a four-stage model, which progresses from excitement to plateau, to orgasm, and finally to resolution. The *excitement stage* begins with the onset of erotic feelings and sensations. This produces an immediate and intense vasocongestion and increased myotonia if stimulation is effective. Excitement in the man is signaled by erection, with scrotal thickening and elevation of the testes. In the woman, vaginal lubrication occurs rapidly, the clitoris enlarges and becomes erect, the uterus enlarges and begins to rise, and the vagina begins to enlarge and balloon in the upper portion.

As excitement progresses, the *plateau stage* is reached; this is the stage immediately preceding orgasm. In men, the penis is fully distended and erect at its maximum size; the testes are enlarged and elevated closely against the perineum; and drops of fluid from the Cowper's glands appear at the urethral meatus. In women, pelvic congestion and edema are at a peak with maximum distention of the vestibular bulbs, labia minora, lower third of the vagina, and uterus. The orgasmic platform builds up in the lower vagina, and the uterus ascends from the true pelvis while the upper vagina widely balloons. The clitoris is completely retracted under the prepuce, is enlarged, and has completed its upward arc.

The *stage of orgasm* is reached when vasocongestion passes a critical point and a reflex stretch mechanism is set off in the pelvic muscles of both sexes. The muscles contract vigorously, pressing on distended structures and expelling blood that is trapped in tissues and vessels, which then creates the sensation of orgasm. Ejaculation occurs in the man, with spurts of semen from the urethral meatus and contractions of the penis and urethra. In the woman, contractions occur at the same time interval (0.8 second) as blood and fluid moves out of distended pelvic tissues and veins. The main sites of orgasmic sensation involve the clitoris and lower part of the vagina.

Resolution is the final stage of the sexual response cycle. The changes in genitals and other organs and structures are reversed. The testes decrease in size and descend immediately and the scrotum relaxes and returns to its usual position. The penis becomes flaccid, usually in two stages. It reduces to half the erect size soon after orgasm and completes detumescence in 30 minutes or less. In the woman, the clitoris returns to its original position rapidly and the orgasmic platform undergoes detumescence. The vagina returns to a relaxed state in about 15 minutes, the uterus descends, and the cervical os gaps for about 30 minutes. The labia minora lose their deep coloration rapidly, but the edema takes longer to resolve. Genital swelling persists in most women for variable periods of time.

Some men and women perspire heavily and have a thin film of sweat over much of the body. There is often a feeling of calm and relaxation as muscle tension ceases; laughing or crying also happen frequently. Some people feel exhausted after orgasm and rapidly fall asleep, while others feel invigorated and refreshed. Some may feel mildly depressed or have a sense of letdown; others feel elated or euphoric. There do not seem to be any consistent differences in postorgasmic responses between men and women.

If orgasm does not occur, resolution follows the same physiological processes but takes considerably longer. Muscle tension and vasocongestion recede more gradually, and the pelvic area may remain congested for several hours. Responses to sexual experiences without orgasm vary by occasion and individual. In some instances, it may be desirable to avoid orgasmic release, and even if not sought, occasional occurrences will probably not be problematic. Consistent absence of orgasm, however, often leads to frustration, resentment, feelings of inadequacy, and unhappiness. There are cultural differences between the male and female responses to nonorgasm; a man generally is not satisfied with sex unless he has ejaculated, while women do not find it unusual to have some percentage of nonorgasmic sexual encounters. However, a long-term, high proportion of encounters without orgasm in women gradually can lead to less interest in sex.[14]

A biphasic model of sexual response has been proposed by Kaplan.[14] The two phases consist of (1) vasocongestion of genital and pelvic structures, causing erection in the male and vaginal congestion and lubrication in the female, and (2) reflex, clonic muscular contractions of the striated and nonstriated muscles in both men and women during orgasm. This model is not as widely used as that of Masters and Johnson.

Male Sexual Pattern

There appears to be less variability in the man's pattern of sexual response than the woman's. Generally, excitement progresses continuously in the man unless prolonged by deliberate use of delaying tactics, until

the plateau stage is reached. Plateau lasts for a relatively short period of time, then peaks in one definitive, usually strong orgasm. Resolution occurs rather rapidly, with a supposed refractory period during which restimulation of the penis is not possible. This refractory period is much shorter in younger men, who may have another erection in a few minutes, and is longer in older men. Some have questioned the concept of a time during which the man cannot respond to sexual stimuli (Fig. 10-9). Men report experiencing orgasms of different intensity.

Female Sexual Patterns

There are three basic types of sexual response patterns in women. One pattern resembles the male pattern, in that excitement builds rapidly to plateau, with some peaks and dips along the way, leading to one intense

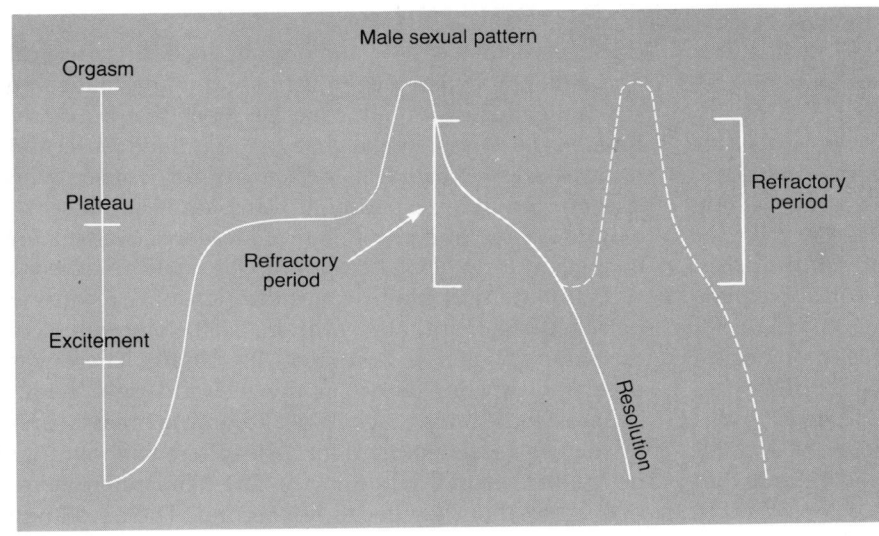

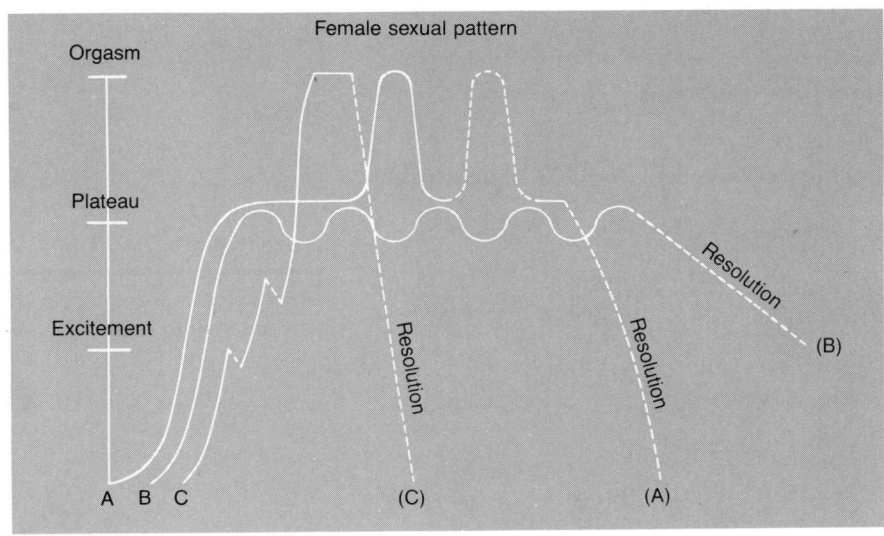

FIGURE 10-9

Male and female sexual response patterns. Female Sexual Patterns—(*A*) Steady progression to plateau stage is followed by intense orgasm; subsequent orgasms may occur; resolution is slower. (*B*) Slower progression to plateau stage is followed by minor surges toward orgasm causing prolonged pleasurable feelings without definitive orgasm; resolution is slowest. (*C*) Rapid progression to plateau stage with some peaks and dips; one intense orgasm follows with rapid resolution. This most closely resembles male pattern.

orgasm and a rapid resolution stage (see Pattern C, Fig. 10-9). A second pattern among women involves a slower progression of excitement and a longer plateau stage. An intense and definite orgasm is then experienced, followed by a slower resolution stage. Or, after orgasm the woman may return to plateau for a while, then have another orgasm that may be either more or less intense. Some women can have multiple orgasms while rising and falling into plateau levels of arousal, followed by slower resolution (see Pattern A, Fig. 10-9). In the third pattern, excitement progresses more slowly until plateau is reached, then there are minor surges toward orgasm causing repeated and prolonged pleasurable and tingly sensations without a definite orgasm. Resolution tends to be longest with this pattern (see Pattern B, Fig. 10-9).[13]

Although this model is widely used, there is both subjectively and physiologically little difference between excitement and plateau. These tend to be continuous as most of the physiological changes that occur during excitement continue into the plateau stage. However, it is still a useful abstraction for studying human sexual response.

There are a few other differences between the male and female sexual response that warrant discussion. Erection is attained within 3 to 5 seconds, while vaginal lubrication takes about 30 seconds. It takes longer for the woman to fill the much larger structures in her pelvic area, and greater amounts of vasocongestion and edema are required. The man has three erectile bodies to fill (two corpora cavernosa and one corpus spongiosum with its bulb), while the woman has five bodies to fill (two corpora cavernosa, two vestibular bulbs, and a large circumvaginal plexus). With all the bulbs and venous plexi maximally distended, the blood volume that a woman has to remove during orgasm is considerably greater than that of a man. Women need longer pelvic muscles to do this because the female pelvic outlet is greater in diameter. In the man, the greatest strength of muscle contractions occurs in the first three to four orgasmic contractions. This strong, concentrated muscular activity assures deposition of semen deep within the vaginal barrel. This results in a short, intense orgasm that enhances conception. The woman's orgasmic contractions generally last twice as long as the man's, and their strength is not as markedly concentrated in the first few contractions. These types of contractions remove a greater amount of the woman's more widespread pelvic congestion. However, as discussed previously, there is wide variation in a woman's orgasmic response with a generally greater range in intensity and duration than a man's.

Orgasm and Changes in Brain Waves

Because sexual response and orgasm are both a physical and a mental experience, it is not surprising that some striking changes in brain function have been found to parallel the physiological changes. A unique pattern in brain waves occurred in both men and women who participated in an experiment using an electroencephalogram (EEG) and physiological measures to check for changes during sexual response. The data revealed a typical pattern of brain waves through EEG recording before, during, and after orgasm. These patterns were the same for men and women (Fig. 10-10). There was a clear distinction between the left and right hemispheres of the brain just before and during orgasm. Frequency decreased in the right hemisphere to about four cycles per second, while in the left hemisphere it remained at about ten cycles per second. The amplitude

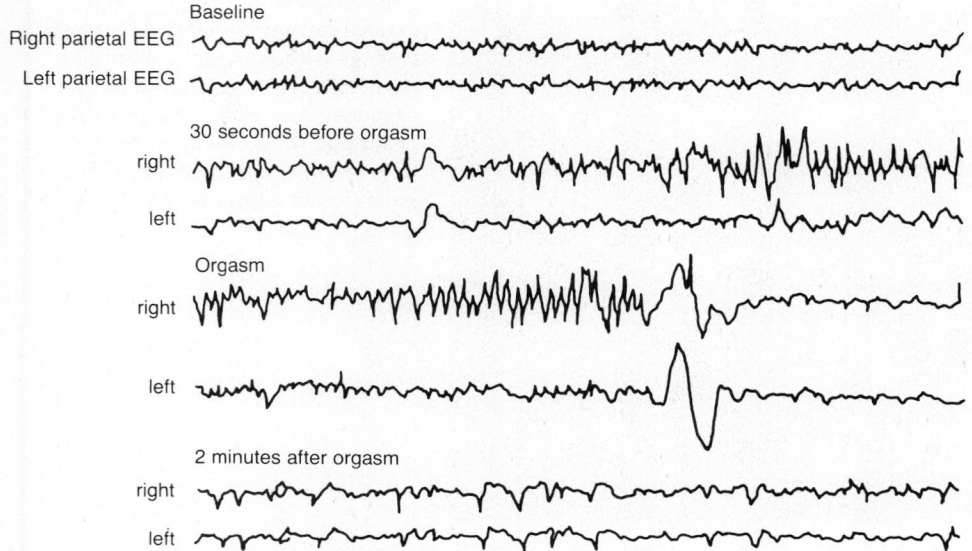

FIGURE 10-10

Brain wave changes associated with orgasm.

response was also found much greater in the right hemisphere than in the left hemisphere.

The two hemispheres have been connected with different types of mental functions and cognitive activities. The left hemisphere is associated with verbal, logical, and rational thought processes. The right hemisphere has a larger role in spatial, intuitive, and emotional thought processes; it is considered the source of artistic and creative abilities. The slowing of brain wave cycles and increases in amplitude that occur in the right hemisphere with orgasm indicate its emotional-intuitive character. These brain wave patterns are unique to orgasm and do not occur with other types of activities studied in laboratories. It seems likely that the experience of orgasm is a unique state of consciousness. This may be one reason why people find the orgasmic experience difficult to describe.[15]

References

1. Hott JR, Ryan-Merritt M: A national study of nursing research in human sexuality. Nurs Clin North Am 17: 429–447, Sept 1982
2. Whipple B, Gick R: A holistic view of sexuality: Education for the health professional. Top Clin Nurs 1:34, 1980
3. Hogan RM: Human Sexuality: A Nursing Perspective, pp 15–16. Norwalk, CT, Appleton-Century-Crofts, 1985
4. Keller MC: The effect of sexual stereotyping on the development of nursing theory. Am J Nurs 79:1584–1586, Sept 1979
5. Pinch WJ: Feminine attributes in a masculine world. Nurs Outlook 29:596–599, Oct 1982
6. Green R: Sexual Identity Conflict in Children and Adults. New York, Basic Books, 1974
7. Money J, Ehrhardt AA: Man & Woman, Boy & Girl. Baltimore, The Johns Hopkins University Press, 1972
8. Nass GD, Libby RW, Fisher MP: Sexual Choices. Monterey, CA, Wadsworth Health Sciences Division, 1981
9. Rosen R, Rosen LR: Human Sexuality. New York, Alfred A. Knopf, 1981
10. Sherfey MJ: The Nature & Evolution of Female Sexuality. New York, Random House, 1972
11. Bragonier JR: Uterine spasms elicited by orgasm. Medical Aspects of Human Sexuality 14(11):99–103, 1980
12. Bullough B, David M, Whipple B et al: Subjective reports of female orgasmic expulsion of fluid. Nurse Pract 9(3):55–59, March 1984
13. Masters W, Johnson VE: Human Sexual Response. Boston, Little, Brown & Co, 1966
14. Kaplan HS: The New Sex Therapy. New York, Brunner/Mazel, 1974
15. Cohen H, Rosen RC, Goldstein L: Electroencephalographic laterality changes during human sexual orgasm. Arch Sex Behav 5:189–199, 1976

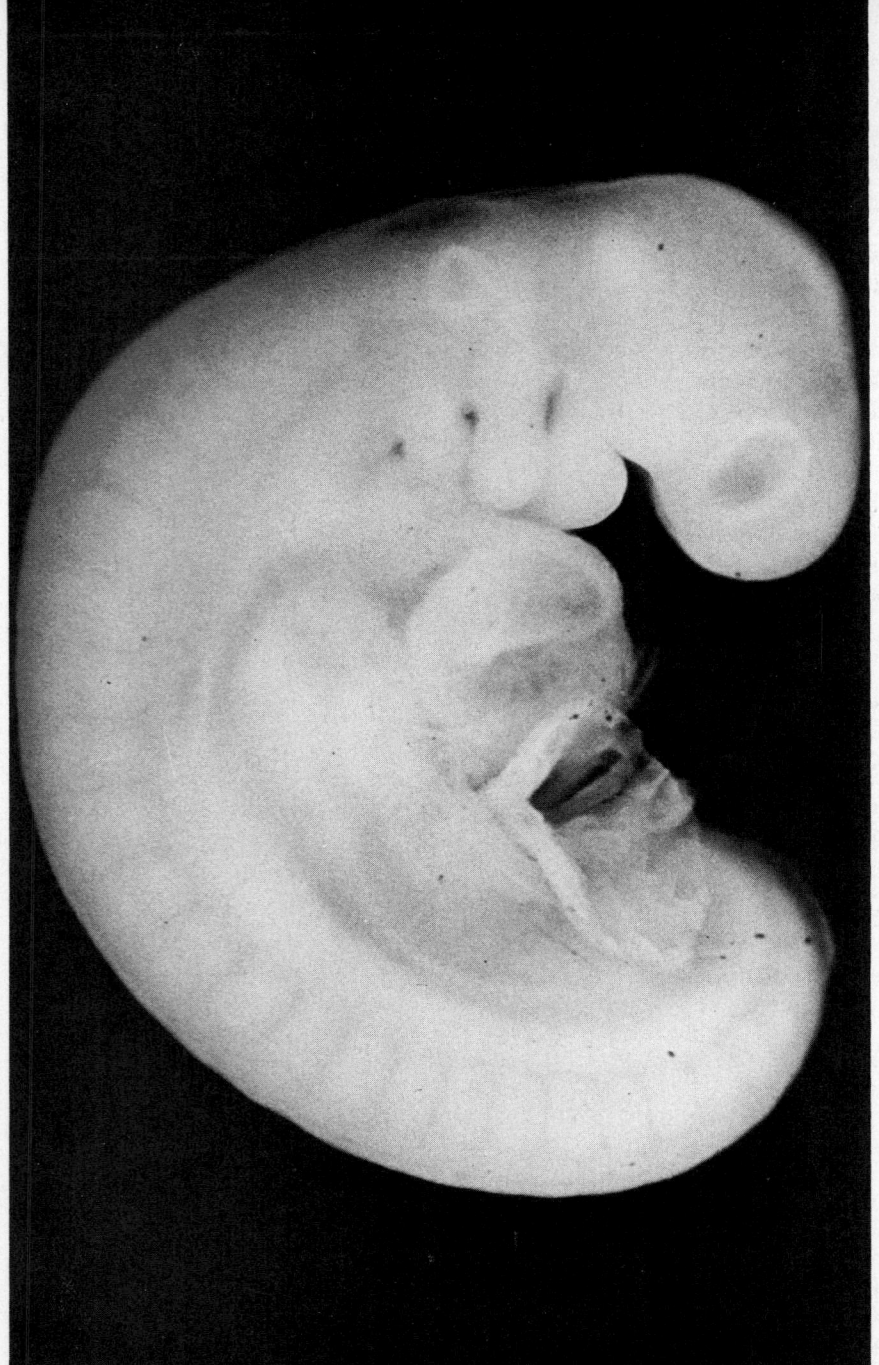

CHAPTER 11

Conception and Ovum Development

In all of nature's wide universe, there is no process more wondrous and no mechanism more fantastic than the one by which a tiny speck of tissue, the human egg, develops into a 7-pound baby. Primitive peoples considered this phenomenon so miraculous that they frequently ascribed it to superhuman intervention and overlooked the fact that sexual intercourse was a necessary precursor. Throughout unremembered ages, our own primitive ancestors doubtlessly held similar beliefs, but now we know that pregnancy comes about in only one way: from the union of a female germ cell, the egg, or ovum, with a male germ cell, the spermatozoon. These two germ cells, or *gametes*, become fused into one cell, or *zygote*, which contains the characteristics of both the female and the male.

Maturation of Ovum and Sperm Cells

The ovum remains in a resting stage of development until about 2 days before ovulation. Its nucleus is large and round and has been described as vesicular because it resembles a bleb or vesicle. The ovum undergoes the process of *meiosis*, the special method for cell division, while still in the follicle. Through meiosis the ovum matures and its genetic material (chromosomes) prepares for fertilization.

The spermatozoon is fully matured when it is discharged in the ejaculate. It has undergone a meiotic process in preparation for fertilization before it leaves the testis.

In all human cells, with the exception of the mature sex cells, there are normally 46 chromosomes (chroma, color; soma, body). Normally, the chromosomes within each somatic cell are paired. Thus, each cell contains 22 pairs of autosomes (auto, self) and one pair of sex chromosomes. Female cells normally contain two X chromosomes, and male cells normally contain one X and one Y chromosome. The sex chromosome of the mature ovum is always of the X type. The mature spermatozoon may have either an X chromosome or a Y chromosome (Fig. 11-1). When fertilization occurs with a spermatozoon containing the X chromosome, a female is produced. When an ovum is fertilized by a spermatozoon containing a Y chromosome, a male is produced.

Thus, in the human being, age, state of health, and physical strength have nothing to do with the determination of the sex of the offspring. The sex is determined at the time of fertilization by the spermatozoon, not by the ovum. At the completion of the fertilization process, the fertilized ovum contains 46 chromosomes, the number normally present in all somatic cells.

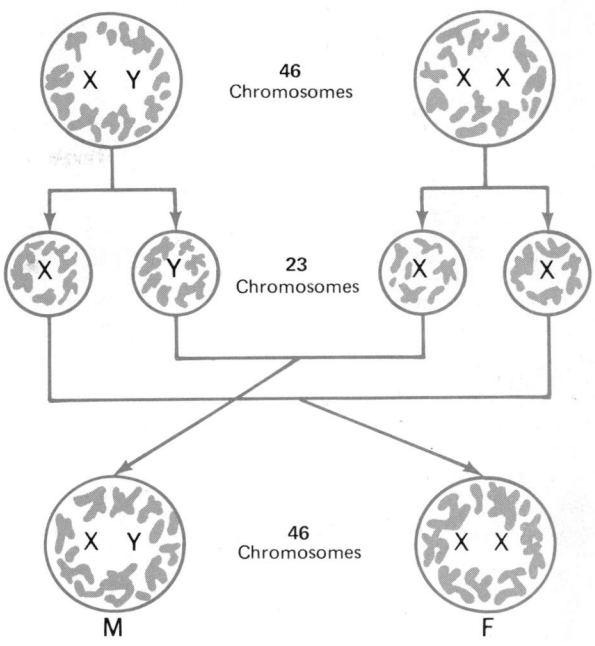

FIGURE 11-1

The sex of the offspring is determined at the time of fertilization by the combination of the sex chromosomes of the spermatozoon (either X or Y) and the ovum (X). The ovum fertilized by a sperm cell containing the X chromosome produces a female (44 regular chromosomes + 2X chromosomes). If it is fertilized by a spermatozoon containing the Y chromosome, the union produces a male (44 regular chromosomes + X + Y). Note that the structures depicted as chromosomes are diagrammatic only. In this illustration it was not possible to include the total correct number.

Prior to fertilization, each gamete undergoes a reduction in its total number of chromosomes to one half of the usual number, the *haploid number*. This reduction occurs through the process of meiosis (see Fig. 11-2). In the meiotic process, each gamete normally receives only one chromosome of each pair. Thus, each mature spermatozoon has 23 chromosomes in its nucleus, and each mature ovum also contains 23 chromosomes, the haploid number.

The cells that will eventually produce mature spermatozoa within the seminiferous tubules are called spermatogonia. These are located at the periphery of the seminiferous tubules (see Fig. 9-3). They divide by mitosis, forming a new generation of germ cells, the primary spermatocytes. In time these cells undergo a reduction division through the process of meiosis (see Fig. 11-2). Although their cytoplasm divides, the chromosomes do not split; instead, they are divided between each of two new cells, each now containing 23 chro-

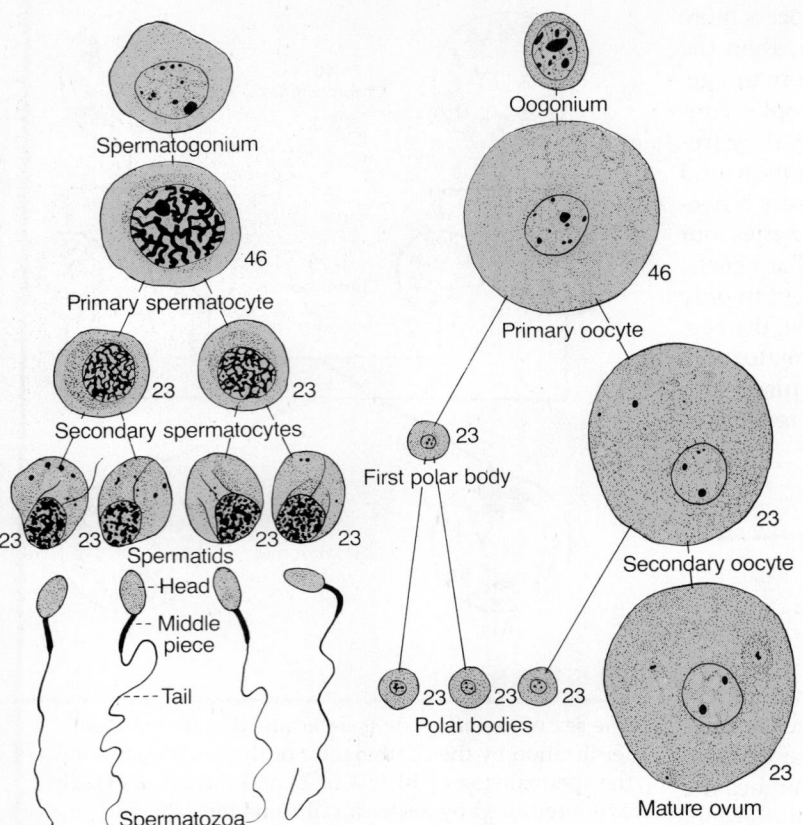

FIGURE   11-2

Diagram of gametogenesis. The various stages of spermatogenesis are indicated on the left; one spermatogonium gives rise to four spermatozoa. On the right, oogenesis is indicated; from each oogonium, one mature ovum and three abortive cells are produced. The chromosomes are reduced to one half the number characteristic for the general body cells of the species. In man, the number in the body cells is 46, and that in the mature spermatozoon and secondary oocyte is 23.

mosomes, the haploid number. These new haploid cells are called *secondary spermatocytes*. One contains 22 regular chromosomes (*autosomes*) and an X chromosome. In the other, there are 22 autosomal chromosomes and a Y chromosome. These cells divide again and form four spermatids, each with 22 autosomal chromosomes, two with X and two with Y sex chromosomes. Each spermatid develops a tail and eventually becomes a mature spermatozoon.

The reduction division of the oocyte begins as the follicle is being prepared for ovulation (see Fig. 11-2). While the primary oocyte is still within the follicle, it divides through meiosis into two cells, a secondary oocyte and a first polar body, so called because it is observed at one pole of the developing ovum. A second polar body is released upon penetration by the spermatozoon, and as a result of its release, the number of chromosomes is halved. The final product, the fertilized ovum, once again contains a set of 46 chromosomes, 23 from the ovum and 23 from the spermatozoon.

The individual chromosomes differ in form and size, ranging from small, spherical masses to long rods. By the use of cell culture techniques, it is possible to photograph the individual chromosomes in a given cell. (Techniques for chromosome analysis are discussed in Chapter 17.)

Ovum

As described in Chapter 9, one ovum per month is normally discharged from the human ovary. Under the influence of the gonadotropins, the graafian follicle, which is destined to release an ovum, has matured. The ovum itself has been pushed to one side of the fluid-filled cavity of the follicle. It is surrounded by a translucent coat, the *zona pellucida*. Immediately adjacent to and connected to the zona pellucida is a layer of follicular cells, the *corona radiata*, which are arranged in a radial pattern. The *cumulus oophorus* is a more loosely structured layer of cells peripheral to the corona radiata. The ovum, surrounded by this entourage of cells, having matured through release of its first polar body, is released through the process of ovulation. The ovum, within its sticky cumulus mass, rapidly and efficiently is transported into the fallopian tube, the site of fertilization. The ovum is now about 0.2 mm ($^1/_{25}$ of an inch) in diameter and is barely visible to the naked eye.

Transport Through the Fallopian Tube

The fallopian tube is an important structure that serves a number of functions in reproduction (Fig. 11-3). It is responsible for transferring the ovum into its lumen

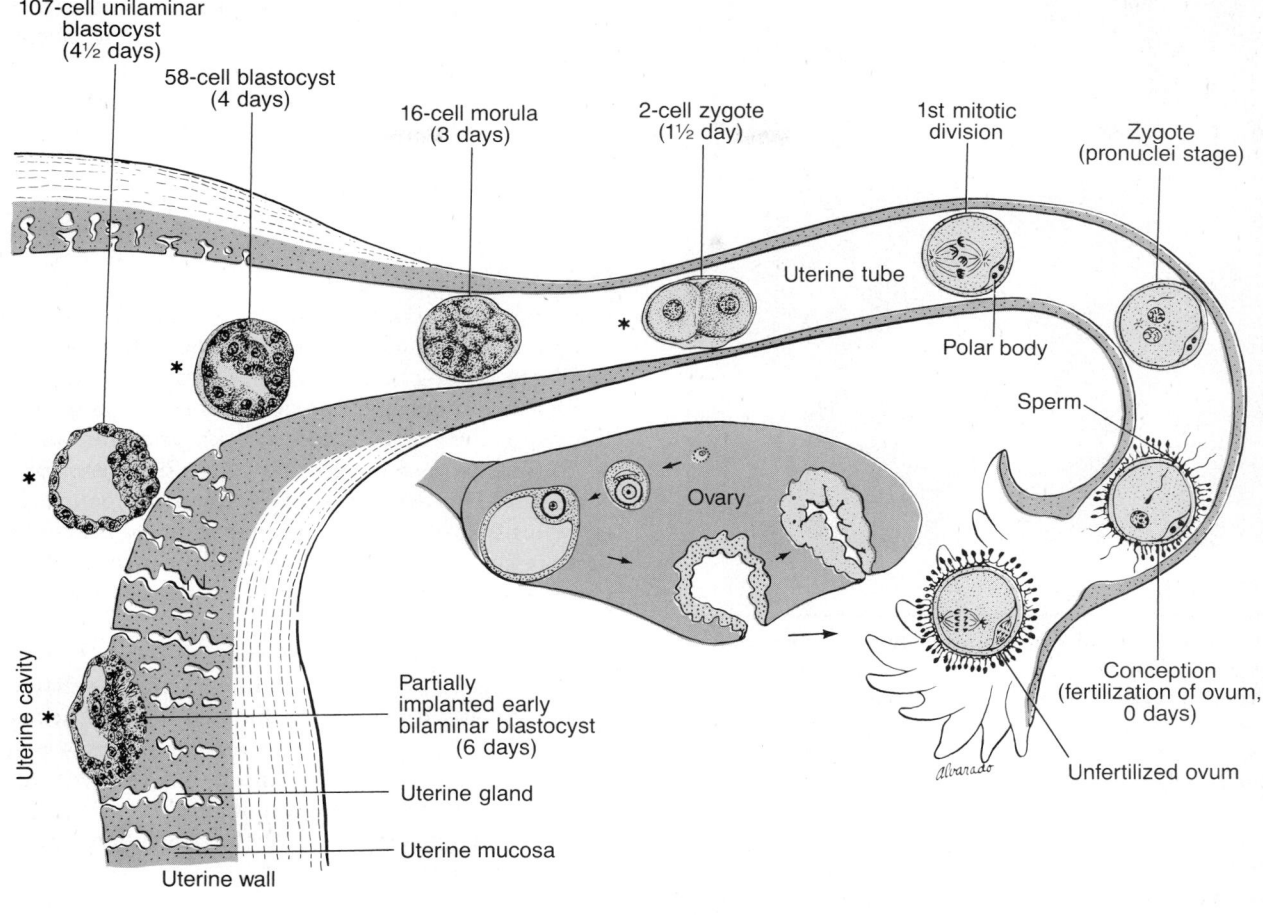

FIGURE 11-3

Transport of the ovum into the fallopian tube, and fertilization within the tube followed by cleavage (cell division) to the 8- to 16-cell stage. The product, now referred to as a morula, is delivered into the uterus where it develops into a blastocyst and implants in the endometrium on the sixth to seventh postfertilization day. (Modified from Gasser RF: Atlas of Human Embryos. Hagerstown, Harper & Row, 1975)

from the rupturing follicle and for providing a temporary environment for the ovum and the spermatozoon. It is also where fertilization occurs and where the ovum passes through several cell divisions during the early stages of human life. Finally, this tube is responsible for transporting the fertilized, cleaving ovum into the uterus after a 3-day interval.

The tube is uniquely designed anatomically for its various functions. The ovarian end is endowed with *fimbriae.* These are arranged in fronds and are lined with hairlike projections called *cilia,* which beat to direct any overlying fluid, as well as any particles contained therein, in the direction of the uterine cavity. The rest of the fallopian tube is also lined with cilia, which are important in transporting the newly released ovum along the tube (Fig. 11-4). The cilia create a current that

courses along the tube. They are partially responsible for transporting particles through the tube.

The anatomical arrangement at the fimbriated end of the tube is important in ovum pickup mechanisms. A separate strand of fimbriae, the *fimbria ovarica,* extends from the tube to the ovary to which it is attached. This contains a separate bundle of smooth muscle. During ovulation this muscle contracts and pulls the ovary in the direction of the tubal opening. The remainder of the fimbriae are thought to embrace the ovary near or over the point of ovulation. They exercise muscular movement that moves them to and fro over the rupturing follicle. Thus, the cilia lining the fimbriae soon come into contact with the cumulus oophorus surrounding the ovum, and as they beat in the direction of the tubal lumen, they carry the sticky cumulus mass

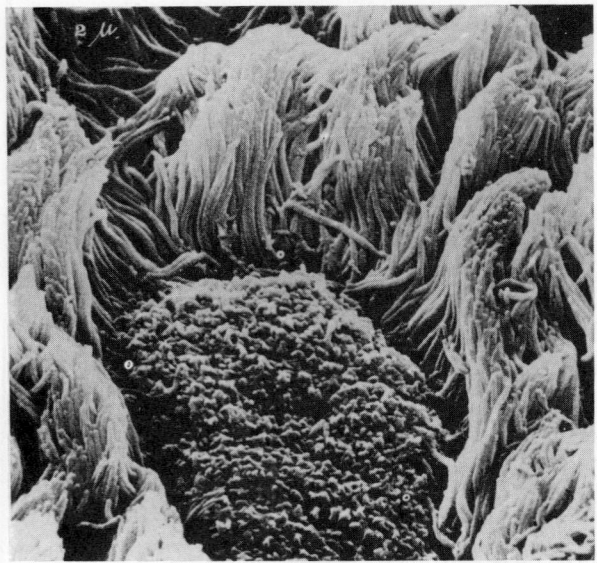

FIGURE   11-4

Scanning electron micrograph of the human fallopian tube showing ciliated cells surrounding a nonciliated cell in the midproliferative phase of the menstrual cycle. (Patek E, Nilsson L, Johannisson E: Scanning electron microscopic study of the human fallopian tube: The proliferative and secretory stages. Fertil Steril 23:459, 1972)

past the tubal ostium to a point well within the fallopian tube. An efficient process of ovum transfer is arranged through these mechanisms, and ovum pickup is practically assured, despite the fact that the ovum is minuscule in size.

Once the ovum is safely past the tubal ostium, it is rapidly transported to a point well within the fallopian tube. Fertilization occurs there. The fertilizing spermatozoon has been previously conditioned in the female reproductive tract so that it has acquired the ability to fertilize an ovum.

After fertilization, the ovum passes through several cell divisions, during which it is retained in the fallopian tube for approximately 3 days. Eventually it develops into a solid mass of cells, a *morula*. It is finally transferred into the uterus at the 8- to 16-cell stage.

In the human, the mechanism by which the ovum is retained in the tube is not as yet clear. However, the importance of the 3-day residence within the tube can be extrapolated from experiments in other mammals. In the rabbit, for example, if the fertilized ovum is removed from the tube and placed in the uterus prematurely, it degenerates and fails to implant. Although for obvious reasons this experiment has not been carried out on humans, it is generally accepted that the 3-day residence within the human tube is important. Premature expulsion of the ovum from the tube could result in failure of implantation. Prolonged retention could

result in ectopic pregnancy, causing tubal rupture and hemorrhage. The latter condition is a serious obstetric emergency. The importance of the fallopian tube, a once-neglected organ that bridges the space between the ovary and the uterus, is now quite evident.

Spermatozoa

The minute, wriggling *spermatozoa* are in some respects even more remarkable than the ova that they fertilize. They resemble microscopic tadpoles, with oval heads and long, lashing tails about ten times the length of the head. The human spermatozoon consists of three parts: the head, the middle piece (neck), and the tail (Fig. 11-5). The head of the spermatozoon is covered by the acrosome. This acrosomal cap is an envelope in which enzymes that play an important role in sperm penetration are contained. The nucleus, and consequently the chromatin material, is in the head; the tail serves as a propeller.

Spermatozoa are much smaller than ova; their overall length measures about one quarter the diameter of the egg, and it has been estimated that the heads of 2 billion of them—enough to regenerate most of the population of the world—could be placed, with room to spare, in the hull of a grain of rice.

The wriggling motions of the tails allow spermatozoa to swim with a quick vibratory motion, as fast as

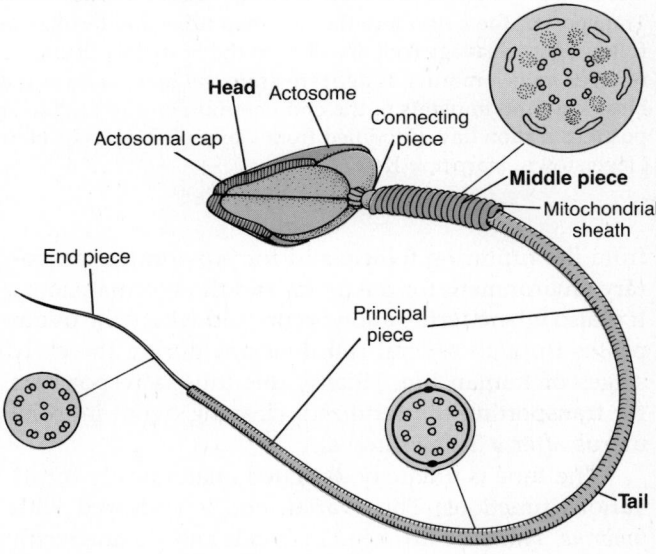

FIGURE   11-5

Drawing of a mammalian spermatozoon with the cell membrane removed to show the arrangement of the underlying structural components. The appearance of cross sections as seen in electron micrographs at various levels is also depicted.

3 mm a minute. To ascend the uterus and the fallopian tube they must swim against the same currents that waft the ovum downward; they are assisted by the muscular action of the uterus, which propels them upward in the direction of the tube. Spermatozoa have been observed in the fallopian tube within minutes of insemination.

The most amazing feature of spermatozoa is the huge number of them. At each ejaculation during intercourse, approximately 300 million are discharged into the vagina. If each of these could be united with an ovum, the babies that would be created would exceed the total number born in the United States during the past 100 years.

Of the millions of spermatozoa deposited in the vagina during coitus, many are expelled immediately and some remain in the vagina for an interval and are later extruded. Those retained in the vagina lose their motility in about an hour because of the acidic environment provided by the vagina.

Some spermatozoa reach the cervix almost immediately after ejaculation. Those transferred into the secretions of the cervix find a more favorable environment and may remain motile for as long as several days, especially in the preovulatory phase of the cycle.

Thousands of spermatozoa find their way into the cavity of the uterus; fewer still reach the lumen of the fallopian tube. Only one is afforded the privilege of continued biologic life through fertilization and, at that, only occasionally. The remainder are disposed of in the reproductive tract or in the peritoneal cavity, and as they degenerate they are phagocytized by white blood cells. However, once the spermatozoon is in the female reproductive tract it may retain its motility, and therefore its potential ability to fertilize, for hours or days.

Spermatozoa are conditioned to fertilize an ovum after they are exposed to the female reproductive tract, a process called *capacitation,* that is, they attain the capacity to penetrate the ovum. This mechanism involves the removal of a protein layer that coats the head of the spermatozoon as it traverses the male reproductive tract. The removal of this protein is accomplished in the fluids of the female reproductive tract and is an essential requisite to fertilization.

Fertilization and Changes Following Fertilization

After the ovum is well within the fallopian tube, the cumulus oophorus disperses. These cells begin to separate, partly as a result of the influence of the enzyme hyaluronidase that is contained in the acrosome surrounding the head of the spermatozoon. The spermatozoon makes its way through this peripheral layer of

cells; meanwhile the densely packed corona radiata has undergone certain changes. These cells become looser under the influence of tubal fluid, and the spermatozoon then finds its way through this layer to the zona pellucida. It is now thought that the zona pellucida is penetrated by the spermatozoon because of a trypsinlike enzyme that is present in the sperm acrosome. Prior to penetration, openings are created in the outer membrane of the acrosome through which the enzyme-rich contents of the acrosome escape. This process, called the *acrosome reaction,* leads to a loss of the membrane over the anterior half of the sperm head. The spermatozoon makes a channel through the zona pellucida as the trypsinlike enzyme, referred to as acrosin, dissolves the protein containing zona with which it comes into contact. After the spermatozoon traverses the zona pellucida, it is in a position to penetrate the membrane of the ovum. As the spermatozoon penetrates the ovum, it brings its tail with it.

Once penetration is complete, a physiological barrier occurs and penetration of the ovum by other spermatozoa is prevented. Soon after penetration, the nucleus of the spermatozoon and the nucleus of the ovum undergo characteristic changes. They become pronuclei, distinct, clearly identifiable bodies of chromatin, each contained in a membrane. The male pronucleus and the female pronucleus then fuse. The new cell presents the full complement, or *diploid number,* of chromosomes, one half from the spermatozoon and one half from the ovum. Soon thereafter the first cell division occurs. In this process, the male and female chromosomes and their genes are mingled and finally split, forming two sets of 46 chromosomes, one set of 46 going to each of the two new cells. This process is repeated again and again until masses containing 8, 16, 32, and 64 cells are produced successively. These early cell divisions produce a morula. At the 8- to 16-cell stage, the dividing ovum is delivered into the uterus.

The ovum remains in the fallopian tube for about 3 days. The fertilized ovum then spends about 4 days in the uterine cavity before actual embedding takes place. Thus, a total interval of some 7 days elapses between ovulation and implantation.

Meanwhile, important changes are taking place in the internal structure of the fertilized ovum. Fluid appears in the center of the mulberry mass that pushes cells to the periphery of the sphere. At the same time it becomes apparent that this external envelope of cells is actually made up of two different layers, an inner and an outer. After some 260 days a specialized portion of the inner layer will have developed into the long-awaited baby. The outer layer is a sort of foraging unit called the *trophoblast,* which means ''feeding'' layer, it is the principal function of these cells to secure food for the embryo (Fig. 11-6).

While the ovum is undergoing these changes, the

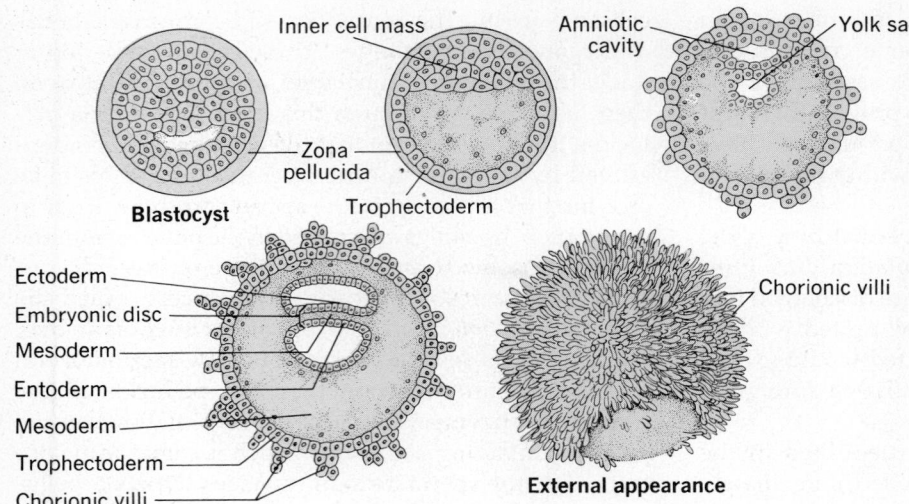

FIGURE   11-6

Early stages of development. (*Top, left* and *center*) The cells are separated into a peripheral layer and an inner cell mass. The peripheral layer is called the trophoblast, or trophectoderm; the entire structure is called a blastodermic vesicle. (*Top, right*) The formation of the amniotic cavity and yolk sac is indicated. The former is lined with ectoderm, the latter with entoderm. (*Bottom, left*) The location of the embryonic disc and the three germ layers is shown, together with the beginning of the chorionic villi. (*Bottom, right*) The external appearance of the developing mass is shown; the chorionic villi are abundant.

lining of the uterus is preparing for its reception. Considering that ovulation took place on the 14th day of the menstrual cycle and that the tubal journey and the uterine sojourn required 7 days, 21 days of the cycle will have passed before the ovum has developed its trophoblastic layer of cells. This is the period when the lining of the uterus reaches its greatest thickness and succulence.

Implantation of the Ovum

The *trophoblast* is responsible for embedding the ovum. This process is carried out by means of enzymes. In this manner these cells not only burrow into the endometrium and eat out a nest for the ovum, but they can also digest the walls of the many small blood vessels that they encounter beneath the surface. The mother's bloodstream is thus tapped and the ovum finds itself deeply sunk in the lining epithelium of the uterus, with tiny pools of blood around it. Fingerlike projections, or chorionic villi, now develop out of the trophoblastic layer and extend greedily into the blood-filled spaces. Another name for the trophoblast, and one more commonly used as pregnancy progresses, is the *chorion*. These chorionic villi contain blood vessels that are connected to the fetus and are extremely important because they are the sole means by which oxygen and nourishment are received from the mother. The entire ovum becomes covered with villi, which grow out radially and convert the chorion into a shaggy sac.

The cells of the chorionic villi begin to produce hCG. This hormone maintains progesterone production by the corpus luteum. In turn, progesterone stimulates and supports endometrial growth by providing a suitable environment for continued development of the conceptus.

Suggested Reading

England MA: Color Atlas of Life Before Birth. Chicago, Year Book Medical Publishers, 1983

Hafez ESE, Evans TN (eds): Human Reproduction: Conception and Contraception, 2nd ed. Philadelphia, Harper & Row, 1980

Mastroianni L, Biggers J, Sadler W: Fertilization and Embryonic Development in Vitro. New York, Plenum Press, 1981

Moore K: The Developing Human, 3rd ed. Philadelphia, WB Saunders, 1982

Yen SS, Jaffe RB: Reproductive Endocrinology: Physiology, Pathophysiology and Clinical Management, 2nd ed. Philadelphia, WB Saunders, 1985

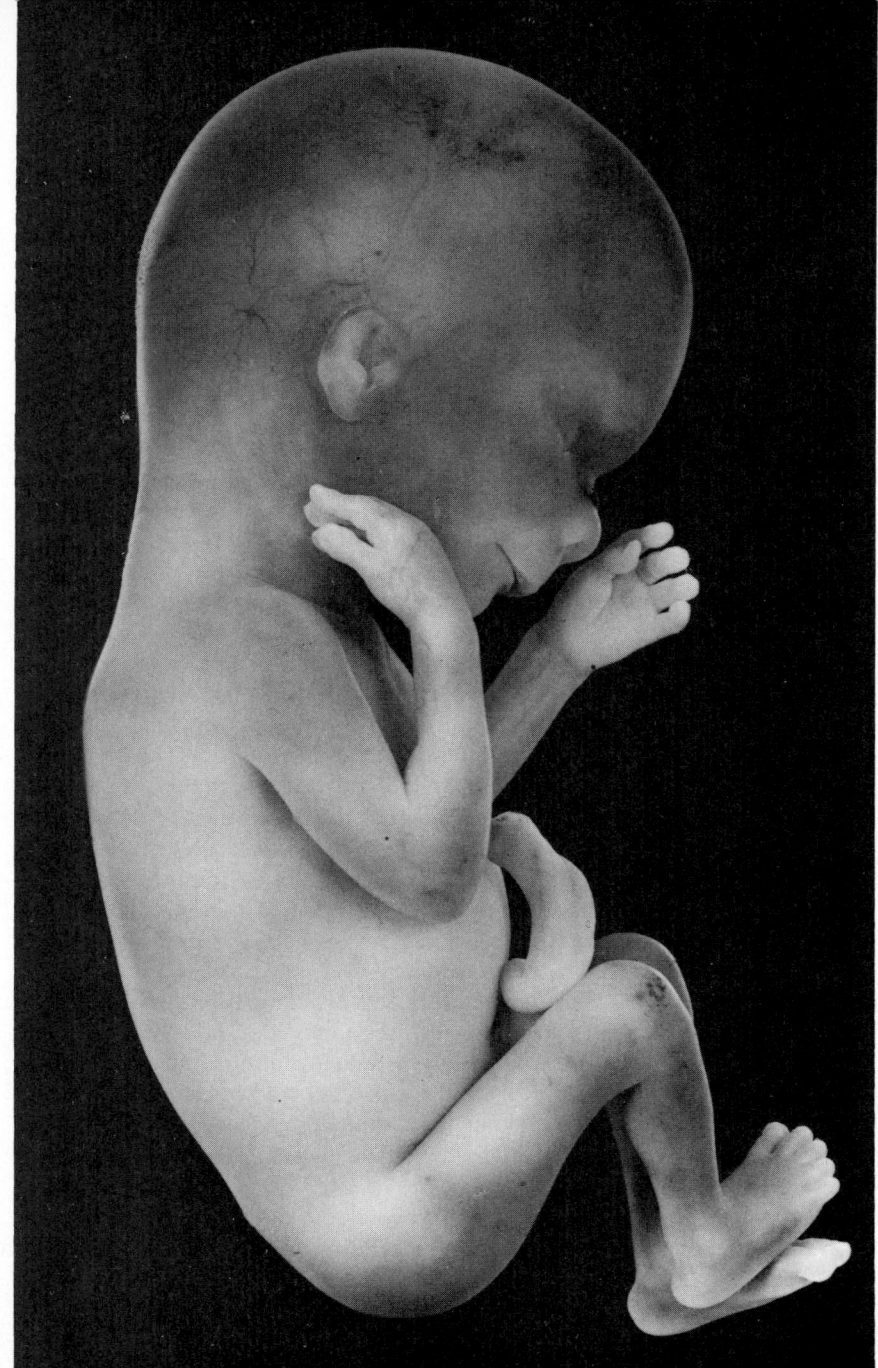

CHAPTER 12

Development and Physiology of the Embryo and Fetus

By the time of implantation, the fertilized ovum has survived a series of delicately programmed events. It has been released from its ovarian follicle after resumption of the meiotic process. Following ovulation the ovum has been transported successfully into the lumen of the fallopian tube. There a single, properly conditioned spermatozoon has traversed the barriers surrounding the ovum to initiate the fertilization process. Ovum meiosis is completed and there is fusion of the male and female genetic components, followed by a series of mitotic divisions. Three days later the multicellular ovum is ushered out of the fallopian tube into the uterus. It lingers freely in the uterine cavity and bathes in uterine fluid while it develops further into a blastocyst. Implantation occurs on about the seventh postfertilization day, and the conceptus begins to derive its nourishment from the blood and tissue juices of the endometrium.

As development continues, the conceptus begins to produce human chorionic gonadotropin (hCG), which maintains production of progesterone by the corpus luteum. Thus, the newly formed pregnancy is now essentially self-sufficient and is in control of its own environment. Support of the corpus luteum by hCG results in continued maintenance of the endometrium by progesterone, and the next expected menstrual period is missed. At this point the conceptus is traditionally referred to as an *embryo*.

Throughout this 2-week interval, there is a substantial incidence of pregnancy loss. It is estimated that 35% of fertilized ova develop abnormally and fail to progress beyond 2 weeks. Such a pregnancy loss is not surprising when one considers the complicated series of events that culminate in a successfully implanted pregnancy.

From the second week on, development occurs relatively rapidly. The mechanisms that support pregnancy as the now nearly self-sufficient embryo develops are considered in this chapter.

Physiology of the Embryo

Decidua

The thickening of endometrium, which occurs during the premenstrual phase of menstruation, was described in Chapter 9. If pregnancy ensues, this endometrium becomes even more thickened, the cells enlarge, and the structure becomes known as the *decidua*. It is a direct continuation, in exaggerated form, of the already modified premenstrual endometrium.

For descriptive purposes, the decidua is divided into three portions. The part that lies directly under the embedded ovum is the *decidua basalis* (Fig. 12-1). The portion that is pushed out by the embedded and growing ovum is the *decidua capsularis*. The remaining portion, which is not in immediate contact with the ovum, is the *decidua vera*. As pregnancy advances, the decidua capsularis expands rapidly over the growing embryo and at about the fourth month lies in intimate contact with the decidua vera.

Amnion, Chorion, and Placenta

Amnion

Even before the previously noted structures become evident, a fluid-filled space develops around the embryo. This space, the amniotic cavity, is lined with a smooth, slippery, glistening membrane, the *amnion* (see Fig. 12-1). Because it is filled with fluid, it is often called the bag of waters; the fetus floats and moves in the amniotic cavity. At full term this cavity normally contains from 500 ml to 1000 ml of liquor amnii, or the "waters."

The amniotic fluid has a number of important functions. It keeps the fetus at an even temperature, cushions the fetus against possible injury, and provides a medium in which the fetus can easily move; furthermore, the fetus drinks this fluid.

At the end of the fourth month of pregnancy, the amniotic cavity has enlarged to the size of a large orange and, with the fetus, occupies the entire interior of the uterus. At this point, the amniotic fluid, which contains viable cells that are cast off by the fetus, can be sampled by amniocentesis and the chromosomal makeup of the

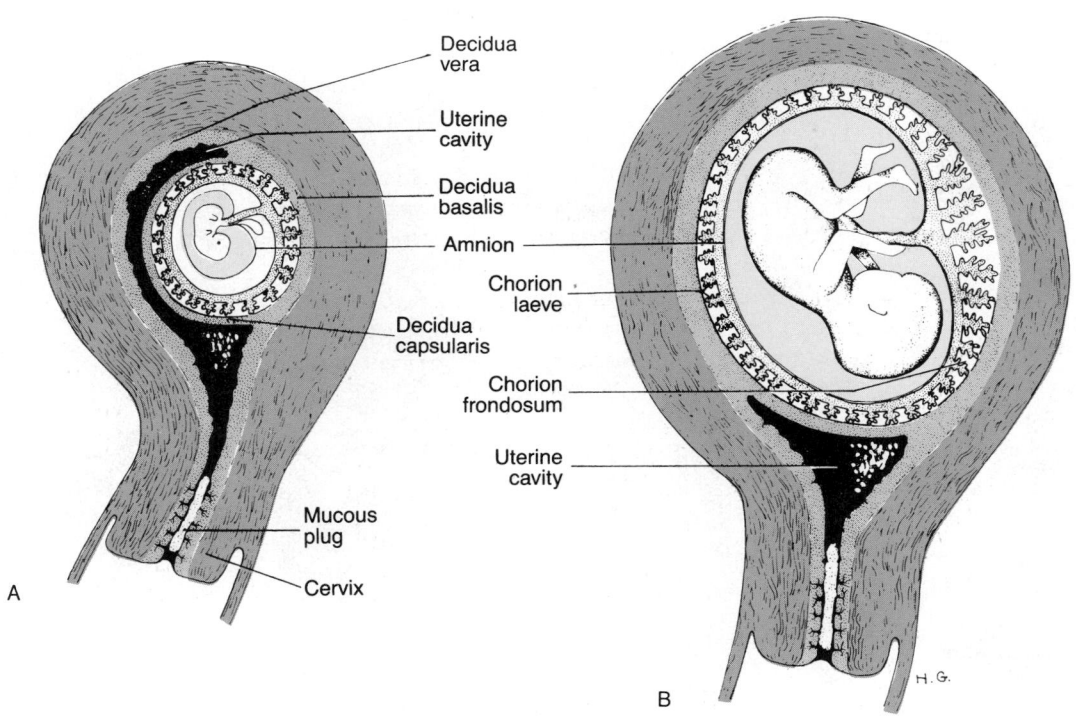

Decidua vera
Uterine cavity
Decidua basalis
Amnion
Chorion laeve
Chorion frondosum
Uterine cavity
Decidua capsularis
Mucous plug
Cervix
A
B

FIGURE 12-1

Diagrams illustrating enlargement of the chorionic vesicle and progressive obliteration of the uterine cavity. (*A*) At 6 weeks after fertilization. (*B*) At 16 weeks after fertilization. (Modified from Fitzgerald MJT: Human Embryology: A Regional Approach. Hagerstown, MD, Harper & Row, 1978)

fetal cells evaluated in culture for prenatal diagnosis of genetic abnormalities (see Chap. 17).

Chorion

As explained in Chapter 11, the early ovum is covered on all sides by shaggy chorionic villi, but in a short period of time the villi that invade the decidua basalis enlarge and multiply rapidly. This portion of the trophoblast is the *chorion frondosum* (leafy chorion). Conversely, the chorionic villi covering the remainder of the fetal envelope degenerate and almost disappear, leaving only a slightly roughened membrane, the *chorion laeve* (bald chorion). The chorion laeve lies outside the amnion and has contact with its outer surface. The outer surface of the chorion laeve lies against the decidua vera. The fetus is thus surrounded by two membranes, the amnion and the chorion.

At about the eighth week a sample of chorionic villus can be obtained by aspiration needle biopsy (see Chap. 17). Since villi are fetal tissue, their chromosomal makeup, which can be analyzed, is the same as that of the embryo; hence, this approach is useful for prenatal diagnosis of genetic abnormalities and can be used as an alternative to amniocentesis.

Placenta

By the third month the placenta (Latin meaning *flat cake*) has formed. This is a fleshy, disklike organ that measures about 20 cm in diameter and 2 cm in thickness late in pregnancy.

The placenta is formed by the union of the chorionic villi and the decidua basalis (see Fig. 12-1). A thin layer of the uterine bed clings to the branching projections of chorionic villi, and together they make up the organ that supplies food to the fetus, like the roots and the earth provide nourishment for a plant.

At term the placenta weighs about 500 g. The fetal surface is smooth and glistening and is covered by amnion. Beneath this membrane a number of large blood vessels may be seen. The maternal surface is red and fleshlike and is divided into a number of segments, or *cotyledons*, about 2.5 cm in diameter (Fig. 12-2).

The placenta is connected to the fetus by the *umbilical cord*, which is usually about 45 cm in length and about 1.5 cm in diameter. The cord usually leaves the placenta near the center and enters the abdominal wall of the fetus at the umbilicus, just below the middle of the median line in front. It contains two arteries and one large vein, which are twisted upon each other and

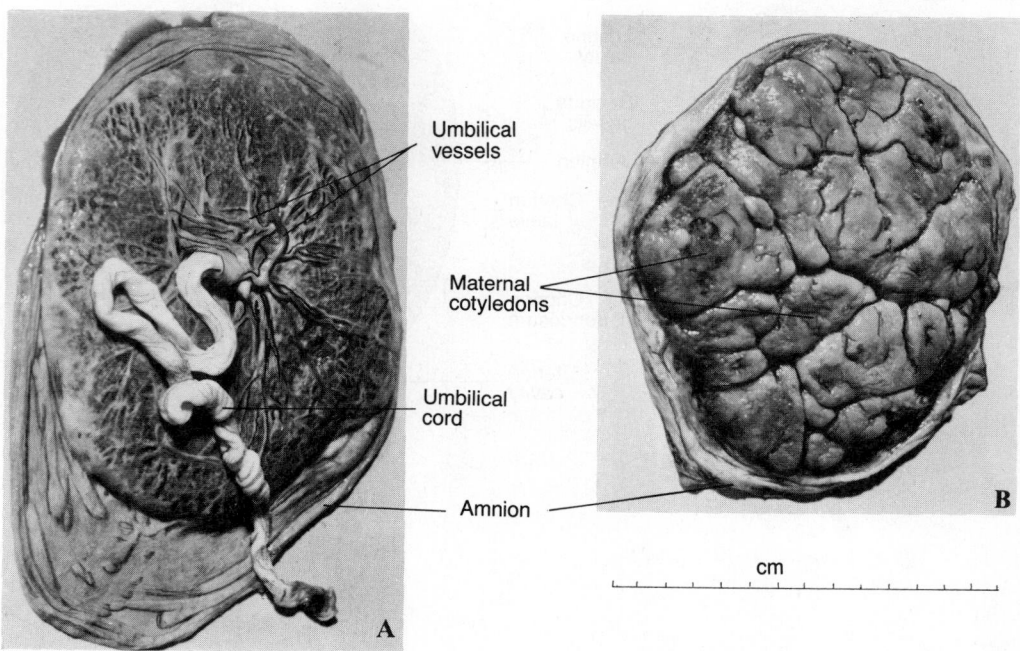

Umbilical vessels

Maternal cotyledons

Umbilical cord

Amnion

cm

FIGURE 12-2

Full-term placenta. (*A*) Fetal surface. (*B*) Maternal surface. (Fitzgerald MJT: Human Embryology: A Regional Approach. Hagerstown, MD, Harper & Row, 1978)

are protected from pressure by a transparent, bluish white, gelatinous substance called *Wharton's jelly.*

Three Germ Layers

The cells that are destined to form the baby grow rapidly with nutritional facilities provided. At first they all look alike, but soon after embedding, certain groups of cells assume distinctive characteristics and differentiate into three main groups: an outer covering layer (ectoderm), a middle layer (mesoderm), and an internal layer (entoderm).

The epithelium of the skin, hair, nails, sebaceous glands, sweat glands, and nasal and oral passages; the salivary glands and mucous membranes of the mouth and nose; the enamel of the teeth; and the nervous system are all derived from the *ectoderm.*

Muscles, bone, cartilage, the dentin of the teeth, ligaments, tendons, areolar tissue, kidneys, ureters, ovaries, testes, the heart, blood, lymph and blood vessels, and the lining of the pericardial, pleural, and peritoneal cavities are formed from the *mesoderm.*

The *entoderm* structures the epithelium of the digestive tract and the glands that pour secretion into this tract, the epithelium of the respiratory tract (except for the nose) and the bladder, the urethra, the thyroid, and the thymus.

Size and Development of the Fetus

Size of Fetus at Various Months

The nurse is sometimes called upon to estimate the intrauterine age of a fetus that has been expelled prematurely.

In general, length is a more accurate criterion of the age of the fetus than weight. Hasse's rule suggests that for clinical purposes, the length of the embryo in centimeters may be approximated during the first 5 months by squaring the number of the month of pregnancy; in the second half of pregnancy, the month may be multiplied by five to estimate the length of the fetus. Conversely, the approximate age of the fetus may be obtained by taking the square root of its length in centimeters during the first 5 months and thereafter by dividing its length in centimeters by five. For instance, a fetus that is 16 cm long is about 4 months old; a fetus that is 35 cm long is about 7 months old.

Development of Fetus from Month to Month

Conception does not take place until ovulation, 14 days after the onset of menstruation in a 28-day cycle, and an embryo does not attain the age of 1 month until about a fortnight after the first missed period (assuming a 28-day cycle). Its "birthday" by months regularly falls 2 weeks or so after any numerically specified missed period (Fig. 12-3). If the cycle is longer than 28 days, or if ovulation was delayed in the conceptive cycle, the duration of actual pregnancy, relative to the last menstrual period, will be shorter. This should be remembered in evaluating the month-by-month development of the fetus.

Physicians refer to the age of a pregnancy as *lunar months,* that is, periods of 4 weeks. Since a lunar month corresponds to the usual length of the menstrual cycle, it's easier to calculate this way (see Fig. 12-3).

End of First Lunar Month

The embryo is about 7 mm long if measured in a straight line from head to tail and recognizable traces of all organs are differentiated. The backbone is apparent but is so bent upon itself that the head almost touches the tip of the tail. The head is extremely prominent, representing almost one third of the entire embryo. The head is very large in proportion to the body throughout intrauterine life. This is still true at birth, but to a lesser degree.

The rudiments of the eyes, the ears, and the nose now make their appearance (Fig. 12-4). The tube that will eventually form the heart has been formed, producing a large, rounded bulge on the body wall; even at this early age, this structure is pulsating regularly and propelling blood through microscopic arteries. The rudiments of the future digestive tract are also discernible. A long, slender tube leading from the mouth to an expansion becomes the stomach; connected with the latter, the beginnings of the intestines may be seen. The incipient arms and legs resemble buds.

End of Second Lunar Month

The fetus, the term used for the product of conception after the fifth week of gestation, now begins to assume human form (Fig. 12-5). As the brain develops, the head becomes disproportionately large so that the nose, the mouth, and the ears become relatively less prominent. It has an unmistakably human face, as well as arms and legs, with fingers, toes, elbows, and knees (Fig. 12-6). During the past 4 weeks it has quadrupled in length and measures about 2.2 cm from head to buttocks. It is

(text continued on page 160)

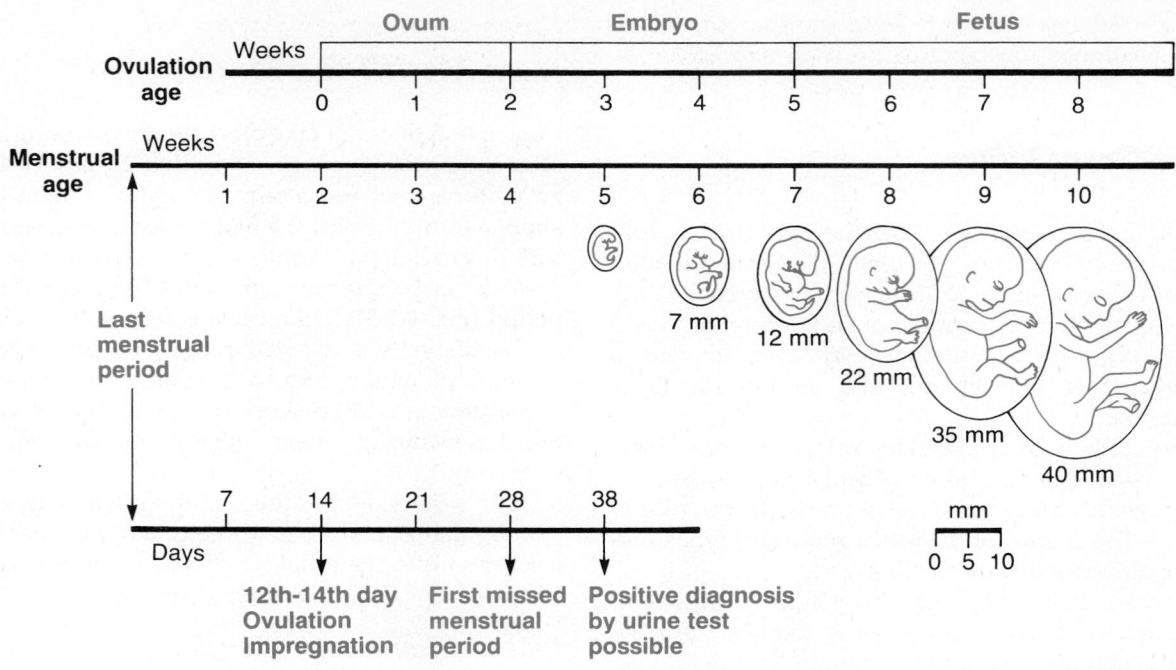

FIGURE 12-3

Growth of the ovum, embryo, and fetus during the early weeks of pregnancy.

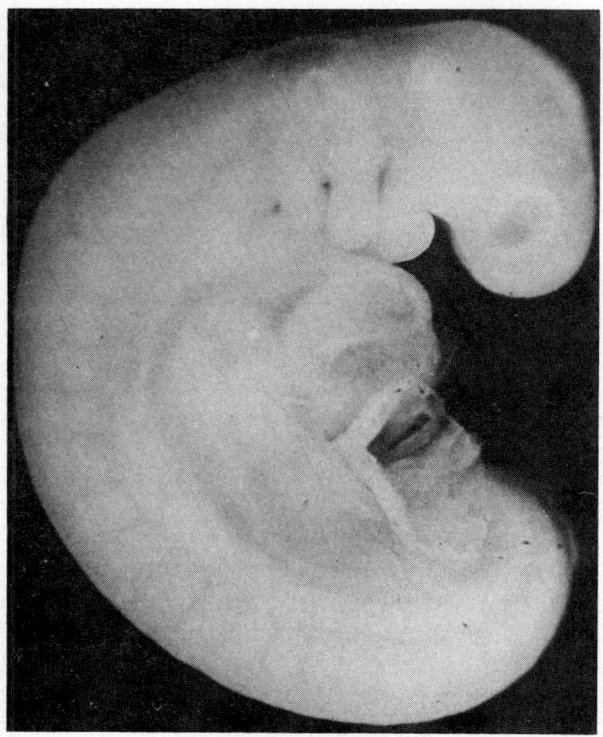

FIGURE 12-4

Human embryo in the first lunar month of development. (Carnegie Institution, Washington, DC)

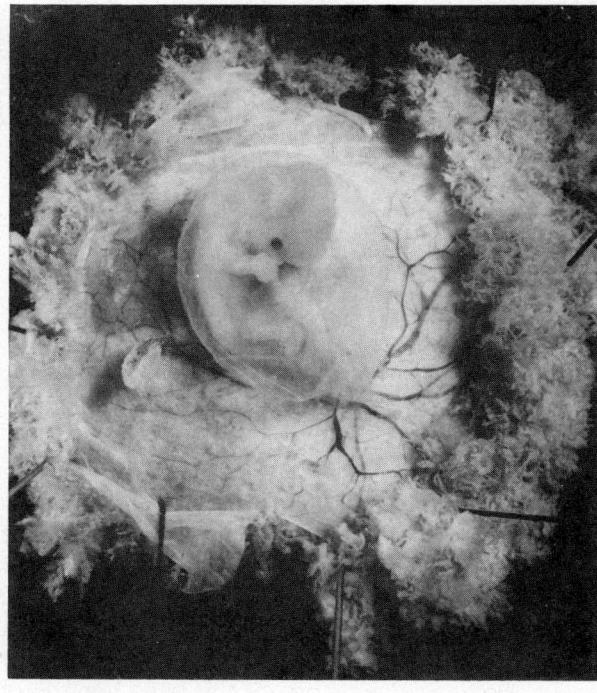

FIGURE 12-5

Human embryo photographed by Chester F. Reather. This specimen represents about 40 days of development and is shown in the opened chorion. Original magnification ×1.7. (Carnegie Institution, Washington, DC)

Fetal Development

1st Lunar Month

The fetus is 0.75 cm to 1 cm in length.

Trophoblasts embed in decidua.

Chorionic villi form.

Foundations for nervous system, genitourinary system, skin, bones, and lungs are formed.

Buds of arms and legs begin to form.

Rudiments of eyes, ears, and nose appear.

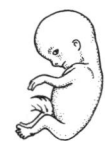

4 weeks

2nd Lunar Month

The fetus is 2.5 cm in length and weighs 4 g.

Fetus is markedly bent.

Head is disproportionately large, owing to brain development.

Sex differentiation begins.

Centers of bone begin to ossify.

8 weeks

3rd Lunar Month

The fetus is 7 cm to 9 cm in length and weighs 28 g.

Fingers and toes are distinct.

Placenta is complete

Fetal circulation is complete.

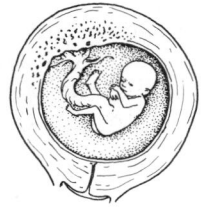

3 months

4th Lunar Month

The fetus is 10 cm to 17 cm in length and weighs 55 g to 120 g.

Sex is differentiated.

Rudimentary kidneys secrete urine.

Heartbeat is present.

Nasal septum and palate close.

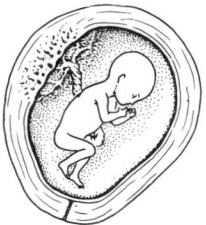

4 months

5th Lunar Month

The fetus is 25 cm in length and weighs 223 g.

Lanugo covers entire body.

Fetal movements are felt by mother.

Heart sounds are perceptible by auscultation.

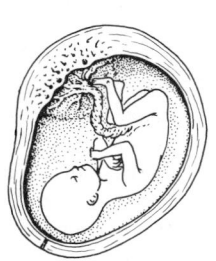

5 months

6th Lunar Month

The fetus is 28 cm to 36 cm in length and weighs 680 g.

Skin appears wrinkled.

Vernix caseosa appears.

Eyebrows and fingernails develop.

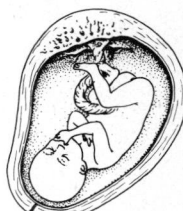

6 months

7th Lunar Month

The fetus is 35 cm to 38 cm in length and weighs 1200 g.

Skin is red.

Pupillary membrane disappears from eyes.

The fetus has an excellent chance of survival.

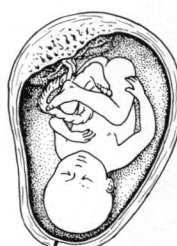

7 months

8th Lunar Month

The fetus is 38 cm to 43 cm in length and weighs 2.7 kg.

Fetus is viable.

Eyelids open.

Fingerprints are set.

Vigorous fetal movement occurs.

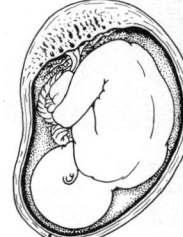

8 months

9th Lunar Month

The fetus is 42 cm to 49 cm in length and weighs 1900 g to 2700 g.

Face and body have a loose wrinkled appearance because of subcutaneous fat deposit.

Lanugo disappears

Amniotic fluid decreases.

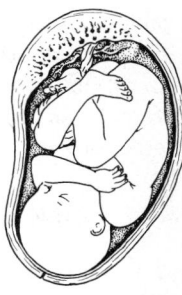

9 months

10th Lunar Month

The fetus is 48 cm to 52 cm in length and weighs 3000 g.

Skin is smooth.

Eyes are uniformly slate colored.

Bones of skull are ossified and nearly together at sutures.

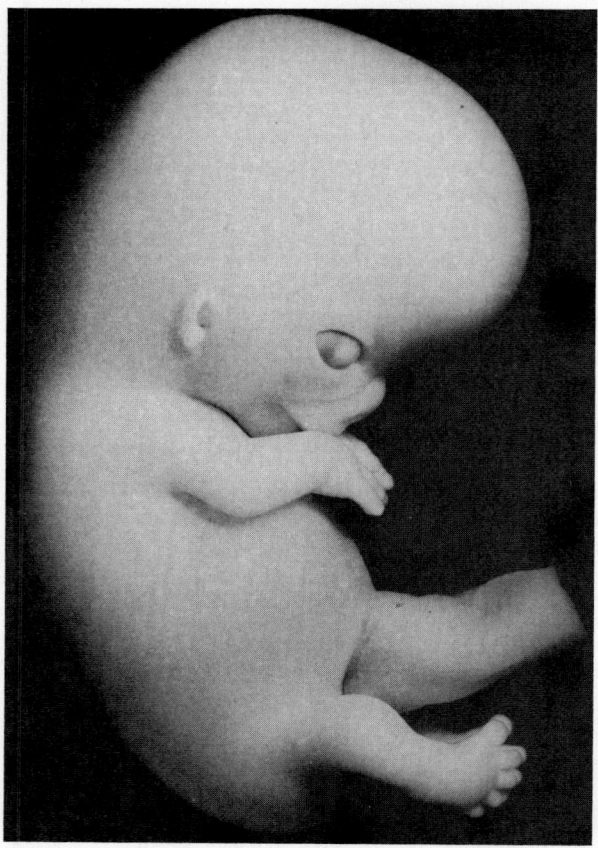

FIGURE 12-6

Human fetus at about 8 weeks of development. Note the prominence of the head and the continuing development of the extremities. (Carnegie Institution, Washington, DC)

(text continued from 157)

during this period that the external genitalia become apparent, but it is difficult to distinguish between male and female. In the seventh week a fetal heartbeat can be detected with real-time sonography.

End of Third Lunar Month

The fetus is over 7.5 cm long and weighs almost 28 g. The sex can now be distinguished because the external genitalia are beginning to show definite signs of sex. Centers of ossification have appeared in most bones; the fingers and the toes have become differentiated, and the fingernails and the toenails appear as fine membranes. Early in this month, buds for all the temporary "baby" teeth are present, and sockets for these develop in the jawbone. Rudimentary kidneys have developed and secrete small amounts of urine into the bladder, which probably escape later into the amniotic fluid. Movements of the fetus are known to occur at this time, but they are too weak to be felt by the mother.

End of Fourth Lunar Month

The fetus is now 16 cm long from head to toe and weighs about 110 g (Fig. 12-7). The sex, as evidenced by the external genital organs, is now quite obvious.

End of Fifth Lunar Month

The length of the fetus now approximates 25 cm, and it weighs about 223 g. A fine, downy growth of hair, *lanugo*, appears on the skin over the entire body. Usually, the mother now becomes conscious of slight fluttering movements in her abdomen, as a result of fetal movement. Their first appearance is called *quickening*, or the perception of life. Fetal heart tones can easily be detected by auscultation at the end of the fifth lunar month. If a fetus is born now, it may make a few efforts to breathe, but its lungs are insufficiently developed to cope with conditions outside the uterus, and it invariably dies within a few hours at most.

End of Sixth Lunar Month

The length of the fetus is 36 cm and its weight is 680 g. It now resembles a miniature baby, with the exception of the skin, which is wrinkled and red with practically no fat beneath it. At this time, however, the skin begins to develop a protective covering, *vernix caseosa*, which means cheesy varnish. This fatty, cheesy substance adheres to the skin of the fetus and at term may be 0.3 cm thick. Increasing numbers of fetuses of this size now survive in intensive-care nurseries.

In Utero *Fetal Behavior*

Sonographic techniques have contributed greatly to our understanding of *in utero* behavior. As pregnancy progresses the fetus becomes capable of carrying out increasingly complex movements. By the eighth week, movements of the trunk can be observed; the limbs begin to move a week later. By the 11th week there is movement of the fetal chest and soon thereafter the fetus becomes capable of moving amniotic fluid in and out of the respiratory tract—intrauterine fetal "breathing." The fetus also actually swallows amniotic fluid and, since the taste buds are already developed, can actually react to substances injected into the amniotic fluid, which are swallowed by the seventh month. The internal and middle ear are well developed by mid-pregnancy, and the fetus is capable of reacting to sudden noise with active movement at about the 24th week.

End of Seventh Lunar Month

The fetus measures about 37 cm in length and weighs approximately 1 kg. If it is born at this time, it has an excellent chance of survival.

End of Eighth Lunar Month

The fetus measures about 40 cm and weighs approximately 1.8 kg. Its skin is still red and wrinkled and vernix caseosa and lanugo are still present. The fetus resembles a little old man. With proper incubator and good nursing care, infants born at the end of the eighth month have a better than 90% chance of survival in many nurseries in the United States.

End of Ninth Lunar Month

For all practical purposes the fetus is now a mature infant. It measures some 47 cm and weighs approximately 2.7 kg. Because of the deposition of subcutaneous fat, the body has become more rotund and the skin less wrinkled and red. The fetus devotes the last 2 months in the uterus to putting on weight; during this period it gains 220 g a week. Its chances of survival are now as good as though it were born at full term.

Middle of Tenth Lunar Month

Full term has now been reached and the fetus weighs on an average 3 kg if it's a girl and 3.4 kg if it's a boy, and it is about 50 cm long. Its skin is now white or pink and thickly coated with the cheesy vernix. The fine, downy hair that previously covered its body has largely disappeared. The fingernails are firm and protrude beyond the end of the fingers.

Duration of Pregnancy

The length of pregnancy varies greatly; it may range between 240 days and 300 days and yet be entirely normal in every respect. The average duration from the time of conception is 9½ lunar months, that is, 38 weeks or 266 days. From the first day of the last menstrual period its average length is 10 lunar months, that is, 40 weeks or 280 days. However, scarcely one pregnancy in ten terminates exactly 280 days after the beginning of the last period. Less than one half terminate within 1 week of day 280. In 10% of all pregnancies, birth occurs a week or more before the theoretical end of pregnancy, and in another 10%, it takes place more than 2 weeks later than expected. Indeed, it does appear

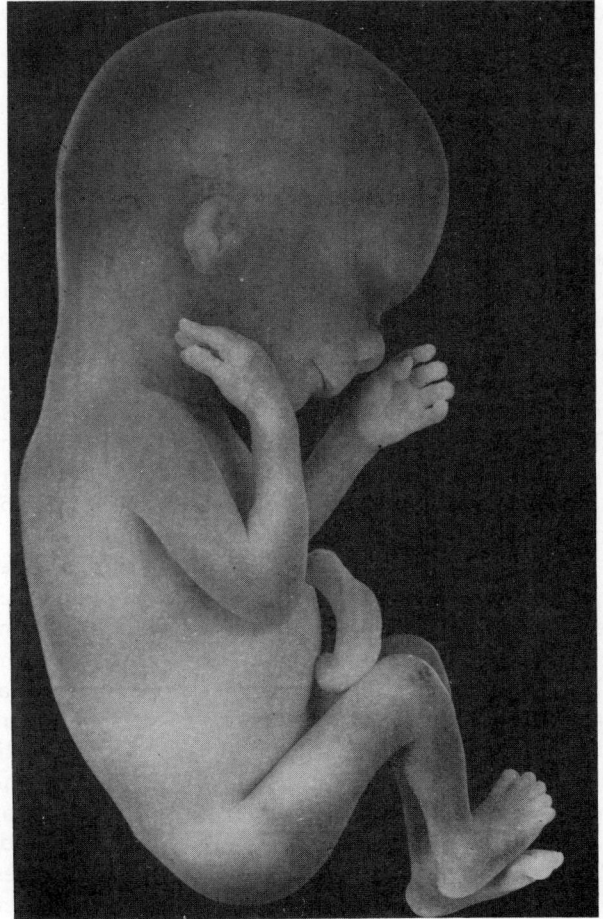

FIGURE 12-7

At about 4 months external features are easily identified. Most organ systems have been formed and will continue to grow and mature. (Carnegie Institution, Washington, DC)

that some fetuses require a longer time and others a shorter time in the uterus for full development.

Physiology of the Fetus and Placenta

During the period when the ovum lies unattached in the uterine cavity, its nutriment is provided by an endometrial secretion that is rich in glycogen. The ovum lies in a lake of fluid that represents the broken-down product of endometrial cells and obtains nourishment from this source.

Very early in pregnancy, by the third or the fourth week, the chorionic villi develop blood vessels within them (connected with the fetal bloodstream). Since these villi have already opened up the maternal blood vessels, nourishment is available from the maternal blood through the placenta.

Placental Function

The human placenta is a truly versatile organ. It functions as a lung in the transfer of gases, as a gastrointestinal tract in the transport of nutrients, as a kidney in the excretion of wastes, as skin in the transfer of heat, much like a liver in its conjugation of drugs and hormones, and as an endocrine gland through production of various protein and steroid hormones. The normal weight of a full-term human placenta is approximately 500 g, and it covers about one quarter of the uterine wall. During the course of pregnancy its weight and mass increase in proportion with that of the fetus. The normal fetal/placental weight ratio at term is 6:1.

The structure and function of the placenta differ among mammalian species. *Homo sapiens* has a villous hemochorial placenta because the fetal vessels are contained within fingerlike villi that extend into an intervillous space (Fig. 12-8). There they are bathed by maternal blood (hemo), which transfers nutrients from across the chorionic membrane (chorial), which constitutes the outer surface of the villi. Nutrient-rich and well-oxygenated blood enters the intervillous space by way of the maternal spiral arteries. This blood surrounds the villi that contain fetal blood that has been delivered to them by the umbilical arteries and therefore has been depleted of both nutrients and oxygen. Oxygen and nutrients from the blood in the intervillous space are delivered into the blood that is contained in the villous capillaries. The newly restored blood is then returned

Functions of Placenta
Transfer of gases
Transport of nutrients
Excretion of wastes
Transfer of heat
Hormone production

to the fetus along the veins contained within the villi, which converge into the umbilical vein.

Fetoplacental Oxygen Exchange

The partial pressure of oxygen (PO_2) in the intervillous space is approximately 40 mm Hg. This is the highest oxygen tension that the fetal circulation is exposed to. At any given time, the oxygen that is contained in the intervillous space is capable of satisfying fetal oxygen consumption for approximately 1½ minutes. On their way to the intervillous space, the spiral arteries traverse the muscular wall of the myometrium. The spiral arteries are compressed by the myometrium, and blood flow through these vessels is interrupted with each uterine contraction. Thus, delivery of oxygen to the intervillous space is interrupted. The normal fetus can tolerate this brief period of oxygen deprivation without damage. In certain cases of abnormal labor, when the contractions are unusually prolonged, the resulting anoxia could cause fetal damage.

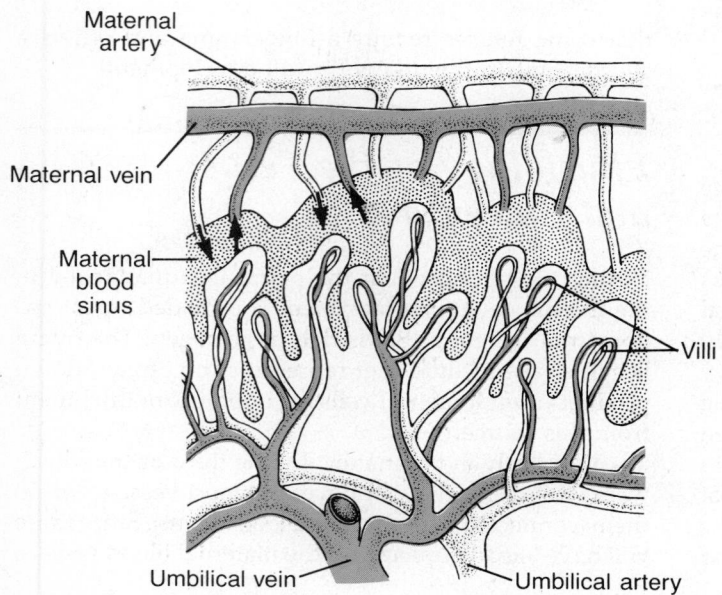

FIGURE 12-8

Diagram of placental circulation. Note that maternal and fetal circulations are completely separate.

The umbilical cord is the other vulnerable link in the system for maternal–fetal exchange of oxygen. Under certain conditions of labor the umbilical cord can be compressed, for example, between the fetal head and the pelvis, or entangled above the fetus. Prolonged interference with cord circulation can seriously affect fetal oxygenation.

On gross examination of the maternal side of the placenta, one can usually see approximately 20 cotyledons or lobes. These are further divided into approximately 200 lobules, each of which is a circulatory unit containing a single spiral artery. When a spiral artery becomes obstructed, as when there has been a thrombosis or development of a clot within its lumen, the blood supply to that circulatory unit is interfered with, resulting in tissue destruction or infarction of the area. Many term placentas contain an area of infarction. Fortunately, the placenta is endowed with a substantial reserve. It has been estimated that only half of the placental surface is required for maintaining a normal maternal–fetal exchange.

At the microscopic level, three layers of tissue separate the fetal circulation from the maternal blood. A molecule passing from the fetus to the mother must traverse these tissues. The outermost layer is the fetal trophoblast, which contains an outer syncytiotrophoblast and inner cytotrophoblast. Immediately beneath the trophoblast is a connective tissue layer. The innermost layer is the endothelial layer of the fetal capillary. As pregnancy progresses, the fetal capillaries are brought closer and closer to the surface of the villi and exchange is facilitated. At term, the diffusion distance for a molecule is approximately 3.5 μ, as compared with 0.5 μ in the adult lung.

Placental Transmission of Nutrition

There are six well-documented mechanisms for the transport of nutrients from the mother to the fetus: diffusion, facilitated diffusion, active transport, bulk flow, pinocytosis, and defects in placental membrane.

1. *Diffusion* is the passage of a substance from one area to another on the basis of its concentration gradient. Materials that are transported by diffusion include the respiratory gases, oxygen and carbon dioxide, the electrolytes sodium and chloride, and some lipid-soluble vitamins. The transport of gases depends on their partial pressures. The mechanism of diffusion is important because it is clinically evident that placental failure is generally the result of a limitation in substances exchanged by diffusion.
2. *Facilitated diffusion* involves passage along a concentration gradient that occurs when the concen-

Placental Transport

Mechanism	Key Substances Exchanged
Simple diffusion	O_2, CO_2, sodium, chloride, lipid-soluble vitamins
Facilitated diffusion	Glucose
Active transport	Amino acids, iron, calcium, iodine, water-soluble vitamins.
Bulk flow	Water
Pinocytosis	Immunoglobulins
Membrane breaks	Red blood cells

tration of material on the maternal side is greater than that on the fetal side. This kind of transfer occurs without the use of energy, but at a faster rate than can be explained on the basis of the concentration gradient alone. This mechanism is carrier mediated, that is, it is transferred by cellular elements that carry it into and through the membrane. Glucose, a most important fetal fuel, is transported by facilitated diffusion.

3. *Active transport* requires the passage of substances from one area to another against a concentration gradient, and it is energy dependent. This mechanism requires the expenditure of energy by the cells. Amino acids are transported against a 2:1 concentration gradient from mother to fetus. Iron, calcium, iodine, and water-soluble vitamins are transported by the mechanism of active transport.
4. *Bulk flow* involves the transfer of substances by hydrostatic or osmotic gradients through micropores in the membrane. This mechanism is important in maintaining maternal–fetal exchange of water.
5. *Pinocytosis* involves the transfer across a cell of materials contained in small vessels located at or near the cell membrane. Microdrops of plasma are taken up by the trophoblasts, which transport immunoglobulins to the fetus.
6. *Breaks in the placental membrane* is the final mechanism by which substances are transported from mother to fetus. Defects in the placental membrane can allow the transfer of very large materials, such as red blood cells. This process is responsible for sensitization of the Rh-negative woman carrying an Rh-positive fetus. Rh-positive fetal red blood cells are carried into the maternal circulation and produce antibodies. This most frequently occurs at delivery, when the incidence of breaks in the placental membrane is greatest.

Placental Permeability

Diffusion is the most important mechanism regulating the transfer of substances between mother and fetus. Thus, impaired diffusion is often the cause of clinically evident placental dysfunction. Diffusion depends upon the characteristics of the placental membrane. It is purely a physical process and requires no energy. The process is governed by certain principles, which, in combination, are described in Fick's law. Fick's law states that the rate of transfer of materials is directly proportional to the permeability of the membrane and to the actual area of the membrane, but inversely proportional to the thickness of the membrane. This means that the more permeable the membrane and the greater the area presented by the membrane, the greater the rate of transfer. Conversely, the thicker the membrane, the slower the rate of transfer.

Other determinants of permeability for any molecule include the size of the molecule, as well as its molecular charge and lipid-solubility properties. In general, molecules with a molecular weight greater than 1000 do not cross the placental membrane. For example, the anticoagulant heparin is a large molecule that, because of its size, will not traverse the placental membrane; hence, heparin treatment can be used safely in pregnancy. In contrast, the anticoagulant dicumarol is a much smaller molecule that readily crosses the placenta and, when used in pregnancy, may affect the fetus.

Lipid solubility is an extremely important characteristic in the transport of drugs from mother to fetus, as is the electrostatic charge on the molecules themselves. Many of the narcotic agents and analgesics used in labor and delivery are designed to reach the maternal brain quickly to provide rapid pain relief. The characteristics that allow this rapid transport to the brain also allow them to rapidly cross the placental membrane, and thus they can equally quickly affect the fetal central nervous system.

Factors Influencing Placental Exchange

Blood Flow to Uteroplacental Circulation

In general, impaired exchange of carbon dioxide and oxygen is not usually related to problems of diffusion. There is little, if any, resistance to the diffusion of these molecules. Their transfer is most often affected by interference with blood flow into the intervillous space and back to the fetus. Oxygen is brought to the intervillous space by the maternal uterine circulation. Uterine blood flow is approximately 600 ml/minute to 700 ml/minute, representing 10% of the total maternal car-

diac output at term. Almost 90% of the total uterine blood flow goes into the intervillous space, while 10% supplies the myometrium. The amount of blood that flows into the intervillous space is directly affected by the perfusion pressure within the uterine arteries. Uteroplacental circulation is widely dilated at rest and therefore has little capacity to expand further. This circulation is, however, capable of marked vasoconstriction, which occurs through hormonal or neural mechanisms. Hence, uterine blood flow during pregnancy can be increased significantly by only one mechanism, maternal bed rest. At rest, blood flow to other organs and tissues, such as muscle and fat, is diminished and the supply of blood to the placenta and fetus is enhanced.

Many mechanisms exist by which blood flow to the uteroplacental circulation may be diminished. Each uterine contraction interrupts the supply of blood into the intervillous space. A contraction that lasts 45 seconds stops the blood flow for approximately 30 seconds. During this interval, the fetus must exist on stored nutrients or on those present in the stagnant blood of the intervillous space. This stress is well tolerated by the normal fetus. Abnormally prolonged uterine contractions or a decrease in maternal blood pressure can diminish blood flow to the uteroplacental circulation. For example, the large term uterus may compress the inferior vena cava, interfering with the return of blood to the right heart. Cardiac output and, therefore, delivery of blood to the uteroplacental unit are decreased. Diminished uterine blood flow can also result from chronic hypertension and pregnancy-induced hypertension owing to vasoconstriction. Various pharmacologic agents, such as vasopressors, may also cause constriction of these vessels. Finally, vigorous maternal exercise will increase blood flow to the muscles and may divert blood from the uteroplacental circulation.

Fetal Blood, Fetal Hemoglobin, Bohr Effect

Several other important determinants of oxygen transfer from mother to fetus should be considered. These include the actual affinity of fetal blood for oxygen, the concentration of fetal hemoglobin within the fetal blood, and the Bohr effect (to be discussed). *Fetal hemoglobin,* because of its special characteristics, has a greater affinity for oxygen than does maternal blood. By virtue of certain biochemical constituents, maternal hemoglobin has a greater capacity to unload oxygen, while fetal hemoglobin is endowed with a greater ability to accept oxygen. The actual concentration of hemoglobin in fetal blood is also greater than in maternal blood. Fetal blood contains 15 g of hemoglobin per deciliter and adult blood contains approximately 12 g/dl. Since hemoglobin is the agent that actually carries the oxygen, and since the fetus has more hemoglobin, a given unit of fetal blood can carry much more oxygen than can maternal blood.

The *Bohr effect* is the effect of *p*H on the ability of hemoglobin to accept or unload oxygen. A more acidic *p*H is associated with an increased ability of hemoglobin to unload oxygen, while a more alkaline *p*H will increase the ability to accept oxygen. Blood returning from the fetal circulation in the umbilical artery is more acidic and therefore has a greater capacity to unload oxygen. It reaches the intervillous space, where it gives up its hydrogen ions and carbon dioxide, and its *p*H rises. Concomitantly, these hydrogen ions and carbon dioxide are accepted by the maternal circulation, and the *p*H of the maternal blood decreases. The increased fetal *p*H results in a greater capacity to accept oxygen, and the decreased maternal blood *p*H results in a greater capacity to deliver oxygen.

Adjustments in Fetal Blood Flow

Fetal blood flow is redistributed during periods of oxygen deprivation. Increased amounts of blood are supplied to the fetal brain and heart, while blood flow to the fetal gastrointestinal tract is diminished. This helps to ensure survival of the most vital fetal organs during a time of temporary oxygen lack. Nature has endowed the fetoplacental unit with a unique system of checks and balances whose purpose is to preserve the fetal well-being throughout pregnancy.

The Placenta as an Endocrine Organ

From very early pregnancy the cells that eventually form the placenta are hormonally active. Even before the skipped menstrual period the trophoblastic cells that have been responsible for allowing the embryo to invade into the endometrium have begun to secrete hCG.

Human Chorionic Gonadotropin

Human chorionic gonadotropin is produced by the syncytial cells of the trophoblast. It is a glycoprotein with a very large molecular weight of 36,000 to 40,000. It is similar to pituitary luteinizing hormone in both structure and activity, but it differs physiologically in that its levels are maintained in the circulation for longer periods of time. It is composed of two subunits, an alpha subunit, which is similar to the alpha subunit of pituitary glycoprotein hormones, and a beta subunit, which is specific and unique to hCG. The beta subunit has recently been used to make antibodies for a pregnancy test, which is specific for hCG levels.

Human chorionic gonadotropin appears in maternal blood by the eighth day after ovulation in the fertile cycle. Its levels increase steadily in early pregnancy,

reaching a maximum in 60 to 90 days, and then the levels in the blood begin to fall. Very little hCG is secreted into the fetal compartment in comparison to the large quantities that are released in the maternal circulation. It is the circulating hCG that has served as the basis for all of the commonly used pregnancy tests.

Human Placental Lactogen or Human Chorionic Somatomammotropin

The placenta produces a second protein hormone, human placental lactogen (hPL), also called human chorionic somatomammotropin (hCS). This hormone is also formed in syncytial cells within the trophoblast of the placenta. Its production increases progressively during pregnancy, with a very marked increase after the 20th week. Very little hPL reaches fetal circulation. There is a distinct correlation between hPL levels and placental weight. For example, maternal hPL levels are higher in multiple gestations. This hormone has an action similar to human growth hormone, and its purpose is to regulate maternal metabolism to maintain a supply of nutrients for the fetus. Specifically, hPL facilitates transport of glucose across the placenta by the process of facilitated diffusion. As its name implies, hPL also has a mammotropic effect.

Progesterone and Estrogen

The placenta also produces the steroid hormones progesterone and estrogen. Throughout pregnancy there is a steady increase in *progesterone* levels, which reach maximum just prior to delivery. This progesterone maintains the endometrium and endometrial blood supply, brings about uterine growth, inhibits the activity of the uterine muscle, and stimulates alveolar development in the maternal breast. It also has significant effects on the mother's metabolism.

The *estrogens*, estriol, 17β-estradiol, and estrone, are products of the placenta. Estriol is biologically the weakest of the three major estrogens, but it is produced in greatest quantity. Its production by the placenta involves a unique interplay between the fetal adrenals, fetal liver, and placenta. Estriol is produced by a weak androgen, dehydroepiandrosterone (DHA) sulfate, which comes from the fetal adrenal gland. Ninety percent of all the estriol that is seen in pregnancy is derived from fetal adrenal DHA-sulfate. The fetal liver further modifies DHA-sulfate and converts it to a hormone, which the placenta can then use in estriol production. Thus, the requisites for the placenta to produce significant quantities of estriol are an intact fetal adrenal gland and a normally functioning fetal liver.

The placenta itself converts the modified DHA-sulfate into estriol. The estriol levels in the blood rise steadily during pregnancy. There is a positive correlation between urinary estriol excretion and fetal weight. The levels of the other two hormones, estradiol and estrone, parallel the estriol levels in maternal blood.

The physiological functions of the estrogens during pregnancy are multifold. They stimulate the growth of the uterus and uterine placental blood flow, and they stimulate contractile activity of the myometrium and growth of mammary tissue. The estrogens also have significant effects on maternal metabolism.

Clinically, it is important to understand the mechanism behind estrogen production by the placenta because estrogen levels can be used to detect certain deficiencies in the fetoplacental unit. If, for example, the placenta is not functioning properly (as in diabetes), the estrogens are not produced in normal amounts. Periodic determination of estrogen levels, either in the urine or in the blood, can be clinically useful in assessing the progress of such affected pregnancies.

Effects on the Newborn. Maternal estrogen is transmitted to the fetus and produces very striking effects in the newborn. First, as the result of the action of this hormone, the breasts of both boy and girl babies may become markedly enlarged during the first few days of life and even secrete milk—the so-called witch's milk (see Chap. 32). Second, estrogen causes hypertrophy of the endometrium of the female fetus as it does in an adult woman. When this hormone is suddenly withdrawn after birth, the endometrium breaks down and bleeding sometimes occurs. For this reason, perhaps one girl baby in every 15 manifests a little spotting on the diaper during the first week of life. This is entirely normal and clears up by itself within a few days.

Fetal Circulation

As the placenta acts as the intermediary organ of transfer between mother and fetus, the fetal circulation differs from that required for extrauterine existence. The fetus receives oxygen through the placenta because the lungs do not function as organs of respiration in the uterus. To meet this situation, the fetal circulation contains certain special vessels ("bypasses" or "detours") that shunt the blood around the lungs, with only a small amount circulating through them for nutrition.

The oxygenated blood flows up the cord through the umbilical vein and passes into the inferior vena cava; on the way to the inferior vena cava, part of the oxygenated blood goes through the liver, but most of it passes through a special fetal structure, the *ductus venosus*, which connects the umbilical vein and the inferior vena cava. The liver is proportionately large in a newborn because it receives a considerable supply of freshly vitalized blood directly from the umbilical vein.

From the inferior vena cava, the current flows into the right auricle and goes directly on to the left auricle through a special fetal structure, the *foramen ovale*. It then flows into the left ventricle and out through the aorta. The blood that circulates up the arms and the head returns through the superior vena cava to the right auricle again, but instead of passing through the foramen ovale as before, the current is deflected downward into the right ventricle and out through the pulmonary arteries. Part of it goes to the lungs (for purposes of nutrition only), but most of it goes into the aorta through the *ductus arteriosus*.

The blood in the aorta, with the exception of that which goes to the head and the upper extremities (this blood has been accounted for), passes downward to supply the trunk and the lower extremities (Fig. 12-9). Most of this blood finds its way through the internal iliac, or hypogastric, arteries and back through the cord to the placenta, where it is again oxygenated, but a small amount passes back into the ascending vena cava to mingle with fresh blood from the umbilical vein and again makes the circuit of the entire body.

Circulation Change at Birth

The fetal circulation is so arranged that the passage of blood to the placenta through the umbilical arteries and back through the umbilical vein is possible up to the time of birth, but it ceases entirely the moment the baby breathes and begins to take oxygen directly from its own lungs. During intrauterine life the circulation of blood through the lungs is for the nourishment of the lungs and not for the purpose of securing oxygen.

To understand, even in a general way, the course of the blood current and how it differs from the circulation after birth, it must be remembered that in infants after birth, as in the adult, the venous blood passes from the two venae cavae into the right auricle of the heart, then to the right ventricle and through the pulmonary arteries to the lungs, where it gives up its waste products and takes up a fresh supply of oxygen. After oxygenation, the arterial blood flows from the lungs, through the pulmonary veins to the left auricle, then to the left ventricle and out through the aorta, to be distributed through the capillaries to all parts of the body and eventually collected, as venous blood, in the venae cavae and discharged again into the right auricle.

Circulation Path After Birth

As soon as the baby is born and breathes, the lungs begin to function and the placental circulation ceases. This change not only alters the character of the blood

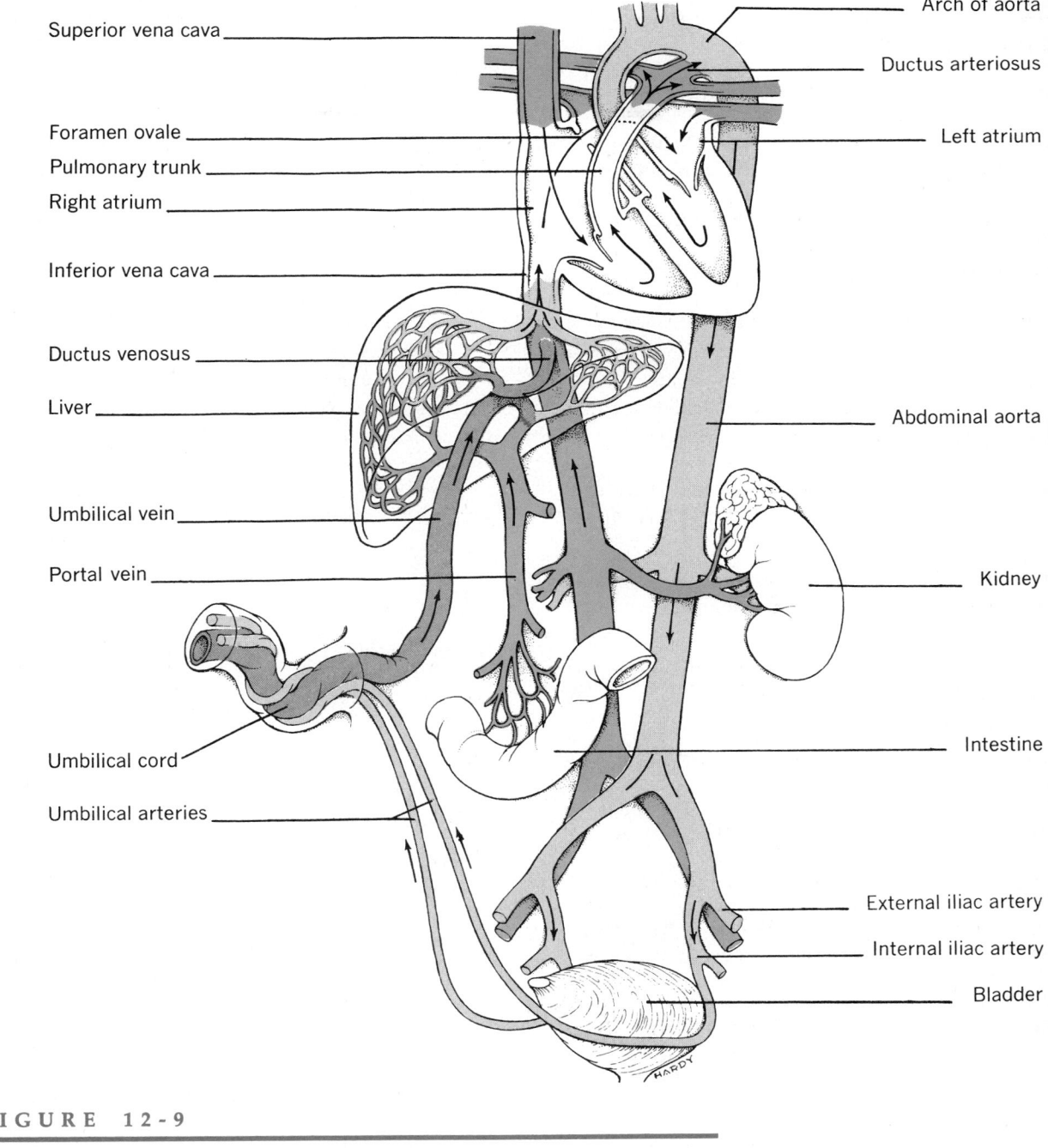

Superior vena cava

Foramen ovale

Pulmonary trunk

Right atrium

Inferior vena cava

Ductus venosus

Liver

Umbilical vein

Portal vein

Umbilical cord

Umbilical arteries

Arch of aorta

Ductus arteriosus

Left atrium

Abdominal aorta

Kidney

Intestine

External iliac artery

Internal iliac artery

Bladder

FIGURE 12-9

Diagram of the fetal circulation shortly before birth. The course of blood is indicated by arrows.

in many vessels, but it also makes many of these vessels useless. The umbilical arteries within the baby's body become filled with clotted blood and are ultimately converted into fibrous cords, and after occlusion of the vessel, the umbilical vein within the body becomes the round ligament of the liver. After the umbilical cord is tied and separated, the large amount of blood returned to the heart and the lungs, which are now functioning, causes equal pressure in both of the auricles. This pressure causes the foramen ovale to close. The foramen ovale remains closed and eventually disappears, and the ductus arteriosus and the ductus venosus finally shrivel up and are converted into fibrous cords or ligaments in the course of 2 or 3 months. The instantaneous closure of the foramen ovale changes the entire course of the blood current and converts the fetal cir-

T A B L E 1 2 - 1

Changes in Fetal Circulation After Birth

Structure	Before Birth	After Birth
Umbilical vein	Brings arterial blood to liver and heart	Obliterated; becomes round ligament of liver
Umbilical arteries	Brings arteriovenous blood to placenta	Obliterated; become vesical ligaments on anterior abdominal wall
Ductus venosus	Shunts arterial blood into inferior vena cava	Obliterated; becomes ligamentum venosum
Ductus arteriosus	Shunts arterial and some venous blood from pulmonary artery to aorta	Obliterated; becomes ligamentum arteriosum
Foramen ovale	Connects right and left auricles (atria)	Obliterated usually; at times open
Lungs	Contain no air and very little blood	Filled with air and well supplied with blood
Pulmonary arteries	Bring little blood to lungs	Bring much blood to lungs
Aorta	Receives blood from both ventricles	Receives blood only from left ventricle
Inferior vena cava	Brings venous blood from body and arterial blood from placenta	Brings venous blood only to right auricle

Guyton AC: Medical Physiology, 7th ed. Philadelphia, WB Saunders, 1986.

culation into the adult type. The changes in the fetal circulation after birth are shown in Table 12-1.

Suggested Reading

England MA: Color Atlas of Life Before Birth. Chicago, Year Book Medical Publishers, 1983

Klopper A, Genazzani A, Grosignari PG (eds): The Human Placenta: Serono Symposium No. 35. New York, Academic Press, 1980

Moore KL: The Developing Human, 3rd ed. Philadelphia, WB Saunders, 1982

Shawker TH, Schueth WH, Whitehouse W et al: Early fetal movement: A real-time ultrasound study. Obstet Gynecol 55:195, 1980

Simpson ER, McDonnald PC: Endocrine physiology of the placenta. Ann Rev Physiol 43:163, 1981

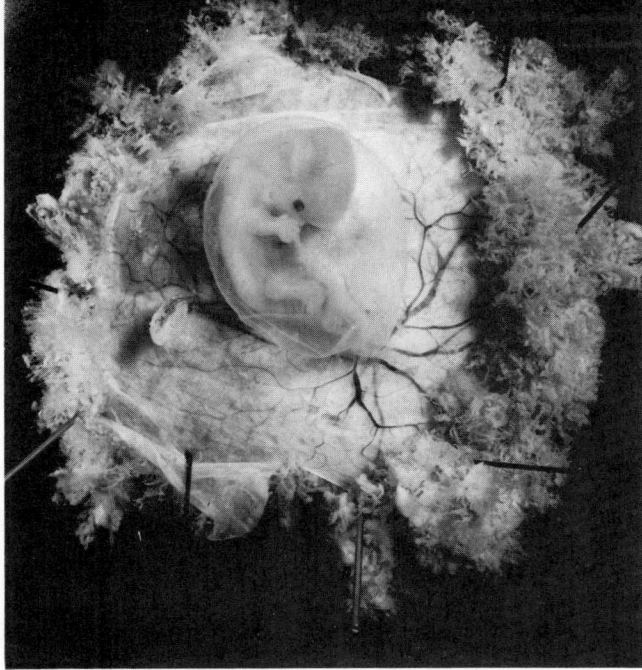

S T U D Y   A I D S

Unit II:
Biophysical Aspects of Human Reproduction

Conference Material

1. Discuss the internal and external parts of the clitoral system in women and the penile system in men, and their significance in the sexual response cycle. In the discussion include their role in initiating sexual arousal, in developing vasocongestion, and in producing orgasm. Describe how the male and female systems are homologues of each other, and their homologous origins in embryonic development. Include a discussion of the critical factors for male and female embryologic sexual differentiation.

2. Describe the various patterns of male and female sexual response cycles according to the four-stage model of Masters and Johnson. What are the main differences between the male and female patterns? What are the main similarities? What anatomic and physiologic explanation can you find for the differences in male and female patterns?

Multiple Choice

Read through the entire question and place your answer on the line to the right.

1. A patient who was in the later part of her pregnancy reported to the nurse that she was suffering from backache and wanted to know the cause. What is the most likely reason that the nurse could give her?
   A. The larger size of the fetus tires her more easily.
   B. Increased mobility of joints throws greater weight on surrounding muscles.
   C. She must have some abnormality in pelvic structures.
   D. The descent of the presenting part into the pelvic cavity prior to labor increases pressure against the sacrum.   _____

2. A patient's chart shows pelvic measurements of 10.5 cm for the diagonal conjugate and 9 cm for the true conjugate; therefore, the nursing care for the patient in the labor room should anticipate that the patient might have which of the following?
   A. An easy, rapid delivery
   B. A labor and delivery of reasonable duration
   C. A protracted labor with difficult delivery   _____

3. To give adequate care to the patient during and after delivery, the nurse should fully understand the structure of the uterus. Which of the following are true of the uterus?
   A. Its muscular tissue is
      1. Chiefly striated
      2. Chiefly nonstriated
      3. Entirely striated
      4. Entirely nonstriated   _____

   B. Its muscle fibers are arranged to run
      1. Circularly
      2. Longitudinally
      3. In all directions
      4. In three layers, the inner and the outer circularly, the other longitudinally   _____

   C. Its blood is supplied directly from
      1. Ovarian and uterine arteries
      2. Abdominal aorta and uterine arteries
      3. Internal iliac and ovarian arteries
      4. Internal iliac and uterine arteries   _____

   D. Normally, the uterus is
      1. Attached anteriorly to the bladder wall
      2. Suspended and freely movable in the pelvic cavity
      3. Suspended between the bladder and the rectum
      4. Attached posteriorly to the anterior wall of the sacrum   _____

4. The perineum lies between the vagina and the rectum. This structure has
   A. A single, strong elastic muscle
   B. A strong elastic tendon
   C. A tendon to which muscles are attached
   D. Two strong muscles, the anal and the transverse perineal   _____

5. A patient with small breasts in her first pregnancy is worried about her ability to feed her baby.
   A. The nurse could respond correctly to the patient by telling her that
      1. She probably would be unable to feed her baby

2. The size of the breasts do not influence the amount of lactation possible

3. Mothers with small breasts usually have less difficulty feeding their babies

4. Her baby would be fed better by means of a formula ____

B. The structure most directly involved in milk production is
1. Papillae
2. Glands of Montgomery
3. Acini cells
4. Areola
5. Lactiferous ducts ____

6. The structures in the testes that are responsible for spermatogenesis are
A. The Sertoli cells
B. The seminiferous tubules
C. The interstitial cells of Leydig
D. The tunica albuginea ____

7. Seminal plasma is made up of secretions derived from
A. The seminal vesicles
B. The prostate gland
C. The bulbourethral glands
D. All of the above ____

8. The time sequence of changes that occur at puberty in the female is
A. Appearance of axillary and pubic hair, breast development, and menarche
B. Menarche, breast development, and appearance of axillary and pubic hair
C. Breast development, menarche, and appearance of axillary and pubic hair
D. Breast development, appearance of axillary and pubic hair, and menarche ____

9. The interval between ovulation and menstruation is normally
A. Extremely variable
B. 14 ± 2 days
C. 28 ± 2 days
D. 10 ± 2 days ____

10. What are the ovarian hormones produced by the graafian follicle and the cells of the corpus luteum?
A. Progesterone and gonadotropin
B. Estrogen and progesterone
C. Gonadotropin and FSH
D. FSH and estrogen ____

11. The release of gonadotropins from the pituitary gland is directly regulated by
A. GNRH
B. HGH
C. Insulin
D. Androgens ____

12. The post ovulatory increase in basal body temperature is brought about by
A. Gonadotropins
B. Estrogen
C. Progesterone
D. GNRH ____

13. Spermatozoa are delivered into the lumen of the seminiferous tubules by
A. Action of the Sertoli cells
B. Their own motility
C. Contraction of Leydig cells
D. Effect of testosterone ____

14. A young mother-to-be told a nurse that she was sure that she would have a boy because her husband was such a strong, physically well-developed man. The nurse could respond correctly by saying
A. "It is the female cell that determines the sex of the child."
B. "It is unlikely because there are more girls born than boys."
C. "Physical strength does not influence the sex of the child."
D. "You are probably right." ____

15. Fertilization normally occurs in
A. The uterus
B. The ovarian follicle
C. The fallopian tube
D. The cervix ____

16. Following fertilization the ovum is
A. Transported into the uterus immediately
B. Retained in the tube for three days and then transferred to the uterus
C. Retained at the uterotubal junction for six days
D. Transferred to the abdominal cavity ____

17. Human chorionic gonadotropin (hCG) is produced by
A. The uterus
B. The ovarian follicle
C. The trophoblastic cells of the embryo
D. The uterine decidua ____

18. A patient expelled a 16-cm fetus prematurely. What would be the approximate age of the fetus?
A. 2 months
B. 3 months
C. 4 months
D. 5 months ____

19. Although the exact date of delivery cannot be predetermined, if a pregnant woman's last menstrual period began on September 10, the estimated due date would be nearest
A. May 6
B. May 10
C. June 10
D. June 17 ____

20. The only direct connection between the fetus and any other structure is through the umbilical cord. The umbilical cord contains which of these important structures?
    A. Umbilical artery
    B. Umbilical arteries
    C. Umbilical vein
    D. Umbilical veins
    E. Umbilical nerves
    F. Umbilical lymphatic duct
    G. Wharton's jelly
    Select the number corresponding to the correct letters.
    1. A, D, and F
    2. B, C, and G
    3. C, E, and G
    4. All of the above   ——

21. The placenta is formed by the union of
    A. The chorion frondosum and the decidua basalis
    B. The chorion laeve and the decidua capsularis
    C. The amnion and the chorionic cavity
    D. The decidua basalis and the chorion laeve   ——

22. During a uterine contraction the blood flow to the uteroplacental circulation is
    A. Unchanged
    B. Increased
    C. Decreased   ——

23. When genetic, gonadal, and hormonal components of sexuality are incongruent with behavioral sex and sexual partner preference, yet the person has appropriate gender identity, the condition is
    A. Transvestism
    B. Homosexuality
    C. Transsexualism   ——

24. Core gender identity has been established by age
    A. 1½ years
    B. 2½ years
    C. 3½ years
    D. 4½ years   ——

25. Sexual partner preference is believed to be influenced by all but which of the following?
    A. Early sexual experiences
    B. Prenatal hormonal environment
    C. Early mother–infant interactions
    D. Values assigned to social sex roles   ——

26. Stimuli leading to sexual arousal that include thoughts, fantasies, sights, or sounds are classified as
    A. Reflexogenic stimuli
    B. Psychogenic stimuli   ——

27. Which branch of the nervous system is most immediately responsible for the sexual responses of erection in the man and vaginal lubrication in the woman?
    A. Parasympathetic nervous system
    B. Sympathetic nervous system   ——

28. Which biochemical substance triggers orgasm?
    A. Noradrenaline
    B. Acetylcholine
    C. Androgen
    D. Adrenaline   ——

29. Which psychological mediator of sexual response invokes erotic images and fantasies?
    A. Informational responses
    B. Emotional reactions
    C. Imaginative capacity
    D. Attention   ——

30. In order for an embryo to differentiate as male, what hormonal event must occur?
    A. Decrease in maternal estrogen secretion
    B. Secretion of androgen by the fetal gonad
    C. Secretion of estrogen by the fetal gonad
    D. Increase in maternal androgen secretion   ——

31. The process by which proteins in the uterine wall are broken down during involution is called
    A. Hemostasis
    B. Catabolysis
    C. Autolysis
    D. Regeneration   ——

32. Involution is complete by 8 weeks after birth at all sites except
    A. Fallopian tubes
    B. Placental site
    C. Cervix
    D. Vagina   ——

33. Lochia serosa usually begins on which postpartum day?
    A. Third
    B. Fourth
    C. Fifth
    D. Tenth   ——

34. The shape of the cervical os in nulliparas is
    A. Round
    B. Transverse
    C. Oblong
    D. Truncated   ——

35. Muscular-fascial relaxation of the vagina after birth may cause
    A. Cystocele
    B. Rectocele
    C. Gaping introitus
    D. Cervical erosion
    E. Increased vaginal infections
    Select the number corresponding to the correct letters.
    1. A, B, and C
    2. A, B, C, and D
    3. A, B, C, and E
    4. All of the above   ——

36. Hemodynamic changes in the postpartal period include
   A. Up to 30% increase in blood volume the first 2 to 3 days
   B. Hemodilution leading to a fall in the hematocrit
   C. Up to 35% increase in cardiac output
   D. Transient bradycardia in the first 24 to 48 hours
   E. Leukocytosis for several days
   Select the number corresponding to the correct letters.
   1. A, B, and C
   2. B, C, and D
   3. A, B, C, and D
   4. All of the above   ____

37. The average time for first menstruation after delivery in nonlactating women is
   A. 6–7 weeks
   B. 7–9 weeks
   C. 9–12 weeks
   D. 12–14 weeks   ____

38. The average weight loss after delivery is
   A. 5–10 lb
   B. 10–15 lb
   C. 15–25 lb
   D. 25–30 lb   ____

39. What is the cause of postpartal afterpains?
   A. Tonic uterine contraction
   B. Intermittent uterine contractions
   C. Irritation at the placental site
   D. Inflammation of the uterine cavity   ____

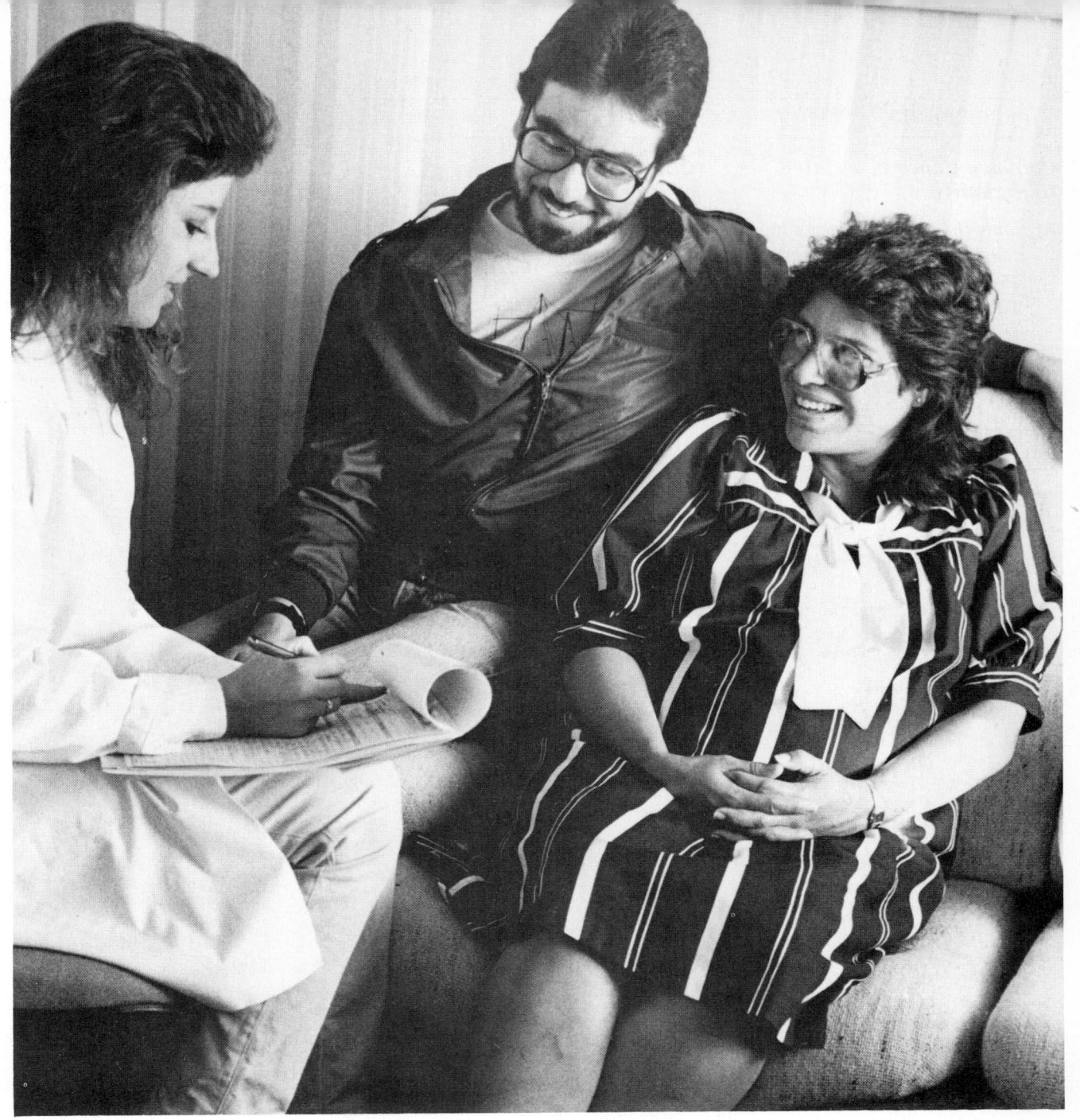

UNIT III

Assessment and Management of Sexuality and Reproduction

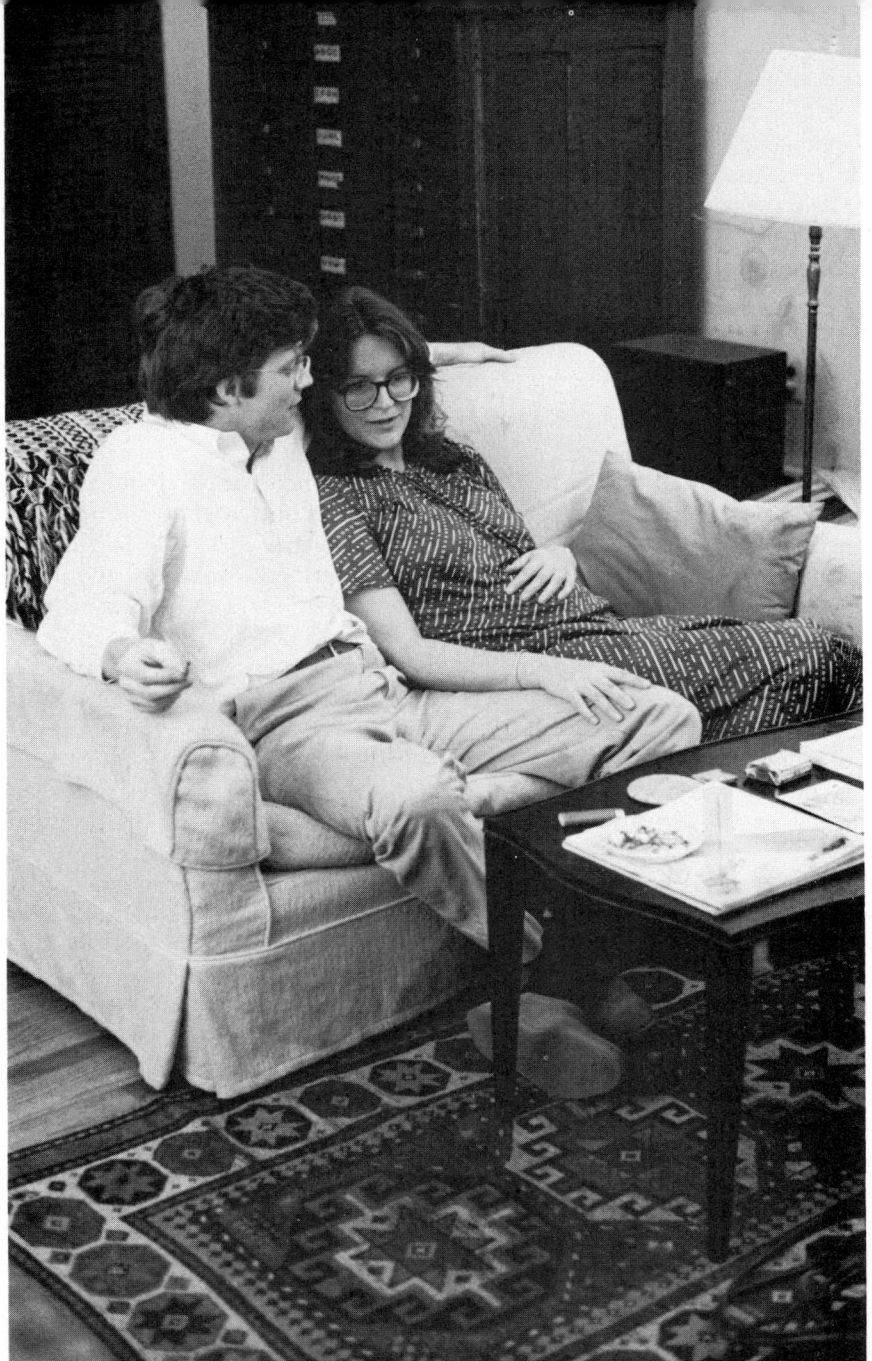

CHAPTER 13

Common Concerns Related to Sexuality

Maternity nurses have an important responsibility in promoting sexual health. The integration of sexuality into the practice of nursing, assessment of sexual health and concerns of clients, and nursing intervention to promote health or alleviate problems are all part of this nursing responsibility. Assembling a data base by taking a sexual history and planning interventions have become integrated into the nursing role.

The area of human sexuality has become a specialty within the health-care field. Professionals from various disciplines have undergone preparation with all degrees of formality to become equipped to handle sexual problems. As more professionals participate in sex therapy, more research and empirical data are generated to expand the knowledge of sexuality. Across the country "institutes of human sexuality" are being formed by groups interested in this new branch of health care. They offer services ranging from sex education to intensive therapy. Groups and individuals in private practice or associated with health-care institutions are providing many other opportunities for diagnosis and treatment of sexual problems. Many resources are available with prepared specialists, although their therapeutic approaches often vary significantly.

Although the field of sexual therapy has become a sophisticated and complex specialty in certain ways, there are actually different levels of practice within the field related to the nature of sexual problems. Because of changing public attitudes toward sex and a great increase in openness about sexuality in many channels of public communication and media, there is a greater expectation on the part of clients that health professionals will respond to sexual problems and concerns.

The nurse is an ideal member of the health-care team to assume responsibility for counseling clients about sexuality because of a background in the social, behavioral, and physical sciences as well as knowledge of counseling techniques. A comprehensive view of nursing care requires nurses to understand the relationship of sexuality to the particular client's health needs or illness and the context of current living situations and sexual-affectional relationships in order to access and use support systems. Clients need adequate sex information whether they are coping with an illness or striving to attain a higher level of health. The importance of a positive integration of one's sexuality has been repeatedly demonstrated.

Few authorities in human behavior would deny that sexual adjustment is prerequisite to an individual's maturation and successful adaptation to his environment. Indeed, history has demonstrated that the mental health of whole nations has been markedly influenced by the sexual attitudes and behavior of their citizenry—young and old, male and female alike. Scientific investiga-

tions and clinical observations have confirmed the premise that sexual adjustment is positively correlated with well-timed, ongoing, accurate sex education presented in a wholesome, guilt-free manner.[1]

Applying the Nursing Process to Sexual Health Care

Sexual health care is readily incorporated in the nursing process. The same principles and approaches apply to this area of nursing care as apply to others. The assessment phase concerns gathering information about the client's past and current experiences with sex, how sexual knowledge was obtained, key attitudes toward sexuality, and difficulties. The person's sexual self-concept, relationship with sexual partner(s), and the health status of both partners are also explored in the history. From the assessment phase the nurse is able to form conclusions about the nature of sexual concerns or problems and to diagnose the problem. Identifying the problem is the basis for planning care or intervention.

Nursing planning and intervention are directed at assisting the client or couple to find methods of alleviating their sexual difficulties. Many approaches may be used in this process, including the nurse providing facts about the sexual response cycle and the ranges of normal sexual experiences, teaching techniques to heighten sexual arousal or delay orgasm, facilitating better communication between partners, and assisting the couple to find sources of in-depth sexual therapy or marital counseling through referral. When illness or physical problems are involved, consultation with a physician is often necessary. A wide range of resources can be used to deal with problems from economic relief to child care, as any of these may adversely affect sexual functioning.

Evaluation of the effectiveness of care is an essential component of the nursing process. This is accomplished through return visits in which progress is assessed.

Assessment

Sexual History

A sexual history can be incorporated into the usual health history, such as the menstrual and contraceptive history, pregnancy history, and gynecologic history. It flows nicely when included in assessment of the reproductive system; in fact, it should be a standard part of data gathering regardless of setting or area of practice. In clinics dealing specifically with sexual problems, the sexual history will, of course, be more detailed and the center of focus. But, even in the absence of indications of sexual problems, the information gathered serves a number of purposes that enhance the nurse–client relationship and provide a broader base for nursing care.

Taking a sexual history provides a base for identifying present or potential sexual problems, from which nursing intervention can be planned, either therapeutic or preventive. Additionally, gathering information about the couple's sexual experiences and attitudes demonstrates that the nurse is comfortable talking about sex. By taking the initiative in bringing up the subject, the nurse implicitly gives them permission to discuss sexual concerns. This legitimizes sexuality as an important component of health and an integral part of care for reproductive families and indicates that sexual counseling is an appropriate part of care they can expect to receive from health providers.[2]

Varying degrees of formality may be used in taking a sexual history, although it is generally best to have a flexible structure so the discussion can go in the direction the client wants it to go. If forms are used, they should be relatively short and simple to keep writing at a minimum and allow the nurse to focus attention on the interaction. A sexual history should proceed from more general to specific areas, from common to unusual, from simple to complex. Conditional statements which assume a range of behavior should be used.

The sexual history generally begins with a conditional or universal statement about why sexual health is included in the health history. The nurse might use a statement such as the following:

> "Sexual health is an important part of people's lives. A person's physical health sometimes affects sexual experiences, and sexual health can have effects on physical well-being. As part of your health history, I'd like to ask some questions about your sexual health that will help me to better understand your health status."

It is important to have a quiet, private place to talk and enough time for discussion and client education to conduct a history. Confidentiality must be stressed. The client should be assured that all questions are optional, and the nurse must continually assess the client's readiness as the history taking progresses. The acceptability of declining to answer must be clearly communicated. A short form for a sexual history of an adult is shown below.

The advanced sexual history is taken in conjunction with beginning of sex therapy. The guidelines for taking a sexual history prior to brief sex therapy for a specific sexual problem include the following:

1. Description of current problem
2. Onset and course of problem
   a. Onset (age, gradual or sudden, precipitating events, contingencies)

ASSESSMENT TOOL

Taking an Adult Sexual History

As part of the general health history, these questions about sexual experiences and concerns can be included.

1. When you were a child, how were your questions about sex answered (where did your sexual information come from)?
2. When you were a teenager, how were your questions about sex answered?
3. How did you first find out about sexual intercourse (how babies are made)?
4. How would you describe your current sexual activity?
5. What, if anything, would you change about your current sexual activity?
6. At this time in your life, how important is a sexual relationship to you?
7. Do you have any concerns about birth control?
8. Do you have any health problems that, in your opinion, affect your sexual health or happiness?
9. Are you taking any medicines that, in your opinion, affect your sexual health or happiness?
10. Is there anything about these questions that you would like clarified or explained?

(Mims FH, Swenson M: Sexuality: A Nursing Perspective. New York, McGraw–Hill, 1980)

---

   b. Course (change over time—increase, decrease, or fluctuation in severity, frequency, or intensity; any functional relationships)
3. Client's concept of cause and maintenance of problem
4. Past treatment and outcome
   a. Medical evaluation (specialty, date, form of treatment, results, medication taken)
   b. Professional help (type and results)
   c. Self-treatment (type and results)
5. Current expectancies and goals of treatment (concrete or ideal)[3]

Sexual History During Pregnancy

Sexual expression during pregnancy is influenced by the physical and emotional changes that happen at this time, as well as attitudes and beliefs about sex during pregnancy. Difficulties can arise as a result of myths, misconceptions, and a lack of understanding of the physiology and emotional dynamics of couples during pregnancy. Questions related to the sexual self-concept, relationship, physical status, and attitudes are included in the sexual history as shown below.

Even if there are no significant sexual problems associated with the pregnancy, most couples have many

Sexual History During Pregnancy

As part of the prenatal health history, these questions about sexual experiences and concerns can be included. Most questions are appropriate for both partners, and a joint history-taking session is recommended.

1. How does the pregnancy make you feel? (asked of both)
2. How do you feel about changes in appearance and emotions?
3. How do you feel about each other's experience of the pregnancy?
4. What are your feelings about sex during pregnancy?
5. Has the pregnancy made many changes in your life and sexual relationship?
6. How do you think having a baby will change your life? How do you plan to manage these changes?
7. What have you heard about what you should or should not do sexually during pregnancy?
8. How do you feel physically? What medications do you take? Have you had any recent changes in your health?
9. Are there any concerns or worries about your sexual relationship during pregnancy or afterward?

questions about sexual activities and their sexual responses during this time and appreciate the opportunity to discuss them. Openly discussing the many changes during pregnancy with implications for sexuality can prepare the couple for potential reactions and prevent the development of conflicts and tensions in their relationship stemming from misunderstandings of physiological changes and psychodynamics.

Nursing Diagnosis

Analysis of data obtained from the sexual history and from physiological and psychosocial factors may lead to the identification of problems related to sexuality. Sexual dysfunction is a nursing diagnosis accepted by the Fifth National Conference on the Classification of Nursing Diagnoses. It is defined as:

> *Sexual Dysfunction:* The state in which an individual experiences, or is at risk of experiencing, a change in sexual health or sexual function that is viewed as unrewarding or inadequate.[4]

Problematic alterations in sexual patterns can result from pathophysiologic problems, such as endocrine, genitourinary, cardiovascular, and neuromuscular diseases. Psychological factors such as anxiety, guilt, depression, fear of failure, and fear of pregnancy can also contribute to sexual difficulties. Many situational factors can be involved in sexual dysfunctions. The sexual partner may be unavailable (divorce, separation), abusive, uninformed, or unwilling to participate in satisfactory sexual relations. The environment may be unconducive, such as being in the hospital or having no privacy. Financial worries, work problems, religious proscriptions, or value conflicts may be stressors that affect sexual expression. Alcoholism, medications, chronic pain, obesity, and fatigue are other factors that affect sexuality. Lack of knowledge is a common cause of minor sexual dysfunctions.

Maturational factors can contribute to sexual problems. Absent or negative sexual teaching often leads to problems related to lack of knowledge, as well as anxiety and guilt. Ineffective role models, such as parents with sexual dysfunctions or negative attitudes toward sexuality, can lead to problems. The aging process may be a factor through loss of sexual partner, separation (through hospitalization, for example), or declining physiological functioning.

During pregnancy and the postpartum period, sexual dysfunctions are often related to lack of knowledge, fatigue, anxiety (*e.g.*, over possibly harming the fetus), discomfort, and pathophysiological genitourinary problems. Alterations in the self-concept of both the mother and the father can contribute to ineffective sexual expression. In addition, couples during pregnancy are subject to many of the other causes of sexual dysfunction mentioned above.

Nursing Planning/Intervention

The care of the reproductive family is concerned with events intimately associated with sexual functioning and expression. This special area of nursing practice embraces a wide spectrum within the sexual-affectional system, although older concepts of "maternity care" viewed the processes largely in asexual terms. Pregnancy is a time of unusual sensuousness, with increased feelings of masculine and feminine potency, voluptuous sexual expression in fantasy and behavior, and profound primitive satisfactions in bearing, nursing, and nurturing children. Nurses have often sensed that the essence of the childbearing experience involves the mystery of life, as it springs forth in a sexual expression of creativity. Sexuality is undeniably an integral part of maternity nursing, and the nurse's view must expand to recognize that sexuality is more than reproduction; self-concept, roles, and interpersonal relations are modes of expressing sexuality in all phases of childbearing and parenting.

Maternity nurses can easily provide sexual teaching and counseling as they work in prenatal, postnatal, and family-planning clinics; physician's offices; hospital maternity units; and public-health agencies. Nurses frequently conduct classes for expectant parents and classes in parenting and contraception. In any of these areas, concerns related to sexuality are likely to surface if the atmosphere is comfortable and accepting. The nurse who is prepared to deal with both information and feelings about sex has much opportunity to assist clients in a wide variety of settings.

The Nurse's Comfort with Sexuality

Although it is always important for the nurse to be aware of his or her own feelings and attitudes toward a particular area of practice, human sexuality requires a level of self-understanding beyond that of most other areas. Nurses bring their personal experiences, values, and attitudes to the professional relationship, which may either facilitate or obstruct the process of caring for clients with sexual concerns and problems. A nurse who plans to provide sexual teaching and counseling must become comfortable with sexuality both generally and personally.

The first step in becoming comfortable with sexuality involves gathering information through reading books and articles, viewing films, and attending workshops and symposia. It is a good idea to read popular as well as professional books, because this is where the public gets its information. Knowing the facts about sex enables the nurse to provide accurate information, teach with authority, and refute commonly held myths and misconceptions. Resources and organizations are listed in Appendix E.

Examination and reexamination of personal attitudes is an ongoing part of becoming comfortable with sexuality. The nurse must identify prejudices and blind spots as well as positive and healthy feelings about different sexual practices. Personal definitions of normal and acceptable sexual expression must be carefully identified, and the extent to which these may affect the ability to assist clients in these areas must be assessed.[5]

The nurse–client encounter is a constant feedback loop, and how the nurse is perceived by the client when sexual matters come up is an important part of the nurse's effectiveness. Attitudes are communicated in verbal and nonverbal ways, and people are always reading each other's subtle behavioral cues and responding accordingly. The nurse who is aware of her or his own attitudes and feelings and is comfortable with sexuality will be less likely to react with shock, ambivalence, or discomfort when clients reveal unusual or unexpected sexual information. The ability to be accepting and understanding and to avoid passing judgment on others' sexual behaviors or concerns enables the nurse to provide more effective care.

Framework for Sexual Counseling

Sexual counseling is basically talking to people about their sex-related problems and concerns. This can occur at various levels of depth and complexity and may involve problems of differing severity and character. The role of the maternity nurse in providing sexual counseling is determined by the individual nurse's background and expertise, as well as the origin and severity of the sexual problem of the client. Sexual problems range from those involving gender identity, such as hermaphroditism and transsexualism, to those resulting from misinformation, confusion about the normal sexual response cycle, and minor sexual dysfunctions. The dif-

---

Developing Comfort With Sexuality

The nurse must be personally comfortable with the topic of sexuality to counsel effectively. Some approaches to developing this comfort include the following:

Information and Knowledge

Read books and articles.

View educational films.

Attend workshops.

Enroll in classes.

Join discussion groups.

Read popular books (source of the public's information).

Attitudes and Values

Join discussion groups (as part of classes, workshops, community activities) that cover topics such as human sexuality or values clarification.

Take self-administered questionnaires, inventories, or tests related to sexual values and attitudes found in textbooks and journals.*

* Examples of these are found in each issue of the journal Medical Aspects of Human Sexuality, and in appendices of textbooks, such as "Inventory for Self-Evaluation," Appendix A, in Nass GD, Libby RW, Fisher MP: Sexual Choices: An Introduction to Human Sexuality. Monterey, CA, Wadsworth Health Sciences Division, 1981

Framework for Sexual Counseling

	Knowledge Problems	Relationship Problems	Attitudinal Problems
Occurrence	Most common Most simple	Quite common Intermediate complexity	Quite common Most complex
Origins	Misinformation Ignorance	Communication patterns Goals or intent in relation-ships and interactions	Internalized beliefs and values Psychological conflicts
Typical Problems	Concern over normalcy of sexual practices Labeling activities as ab-normal or dangerous Worry over changes in sexual response patterns (*i.e.*, during pregnancy) Avoidance of certain prac-tices or sexual activity under different circum-stances (*i.e.*, in late preg-nancy) Fears about effects of birth control Ineffective arousal due to lack of proper stimula-tion Unsatisfying sex due to mistiming of arousal or orgasm	Painful intercourse Lack of interest in sex Early ejaculation Nonorgasm in women Ineffective arousal Unsatisfying sex	Male erectile dysfunction Premature ejaculation Nonorgasm in women Vaginismus Lack of arousal
Type of Counseling	Information, clarification Reassurance of normalcy Discussion of feelings	Encourage discussion be-tween partners Information, clarification Family or marital counsel-ing Sex therapy	Sex therapy Psychotherapy
Level of Nurse's Involvement	Major responsibility Provide entire counseling	Initial identification and discussion; marital or family therapy if nurse is a trained therapist	Initial identification Must be trained sex thera-pist or psychologist to undertake therapy

ferent levels of sexual problems can be approached by dividing them into three (often overlapping) categories: problems of knowledge, relationship, and attitudes.

Problems of Knowledge. Problems of knowledge are the most common and simple types of sexual prob-lems and usually arise out of misinformation or igno-rance. A couple may fail to appreciate the erotic signif-icance of the clitoris, be unaware of differing tempos of sexual arousal, have the idea that sex during pregnancy might injure or mark the baby, think that oral sex in-dicates latent homosexuality, expect the woman's sex

drive to be decreased during pregnancy and be worried when it increases, and so forth. Lack of knowledge about changes in sexual drive and eroticism during pregnancy, which often happen to both partners, can be a cause of misunderstanding and conflict.

Fears created by minor unpleasant symptoms may lead to avoidance of sex when there is no understanding of the physiology or of what can be done about them. For the woman, the common symptom of painful in-tercourse during pregnancy can be related to a number of factors: vaginitis causing perineal or vulval irrita-tion, insufficient vaginal lubrication due to inadequate foreplay, normal uterine contractions during orgasm setting off Braxton Hicks contractions, or increased pelvic pressure due to the presenting part deep in the pelvis. These can be alleviated with proper medical treatment, explanation of physiological causes of the pain, and teaching of techniques to heighten arousal or increase comfort. In this way, a potential stressor to the relationship and the couple's adaptation to pregnancy can be removed.

Couples need specific information about practical matters regarding sex and pregnancy. For instance, there is no reason in the absence of complications to avoid sex during late pregnancy or in the postpartum period once lochia has ceased. The couple's own comfort and desires are their best guide when there is no physical pathology. However, understanding the vagaries of sexual drive during this time could prevent development of conflicts that might set up negative patterns as the couple tries to cope with the many demands of impending or new parenthood.

Nurses working with adolescents and young adults, as in family-planning clinics, will find innumerable problems of knowledge related to sexuality. This is a setting in which provision of information can have an enormous impact on developing sexual practices and adjustments and can prevent many potential future problems involving unwanted pregnancy and sexual dysfunctions. Problems of knowledge related to sexuality are clearly within the scope of maternity nursing practice, and with the addition of specific factual content and a sense of comfort with sexuality to the nurse's repertory, this kind of sexual counseling can be readily carried out.

Problems of Relationship. A second level of sexual problems involves relationships between partners, and these may or may not fall within the scope of maternity nursing practice. This would depend largely on the nature of the given problem and the individual nurse's counseling skills. Communication problems between the partners are the most common types of relationship problems. The sending and receiving of messages between people is a highly complex symbolic process, with many variations of style and receptivity. Both sender and recipient must be attuned and ready for clear communication to take place; consequently, there are often garbled messages and lack of communication.

Good communication regarding sexual needs and preferences is even more difficult than in most interpersonal situations. Some people find it hard to talk about their own sexual feelings or to accept criticism or suggestions regarding sexual performance. Communication concerning sexual practices that one partner may dislike but is embarrassed to discuss or may desire but is unable to ask for is often faulty. Open and candid discussion of sexual preferences between partners can

often dramatically improve satisfaction, but many fears about propriety, hurting the other's feelings, not knowing how to say it, or being embarrassed prevent this communication from occurring.

A first step, and one that the maternity nurse could take in dealing with common sexual problems such as painful intercourse, lack of interest in sex, early ejaculation, and nonorgasm, is to encourage the couple to talk with each other about what they like and do not like in sex. If they can settle on practices that are comfortable and enjoyable to both of them, often the problem will be resolved.

However, many other factors complicate communication. The bedroom as a battlefield and sex with a hidden agenda are familiar syndromes to those involved in marital counseling. Perceptions of male and female roles may hamper communication (*e.g.,* the notion that the woman is there to serve the man sexually and that her enjoyment of sex is secondary and her sexual needs do not deserve much attention.) Some couples may be in a struggle for power, attempting to frustrate the other sexually or doling out sex as a reward for compliance. Anger over real or imagined wrongs may interfere with giving oneself freely to the sexual experience or may be expressed in a desire to hurt the other partner, either mentally or physically.

Such situations create barriers to clear communication about sexual needs and preferences. They represent problems in the couple's relationship that must be worked out before the sexual problem itself can be resolved. If the maternity nurse is skilled in family or marital counseling, then she is able to deal with these relationship problems. Because sexual difficulties are part of the symptomatology, it is frequently necessary for the counselor to have an understanding of sexual physiology and to be familiar with basic sex therapy techniques to provide effective care.

Problems of Attitudes. Attitudes toward sexuality and the sexual self are established through internalized beliefs and values, originating from earliest childhood and often rooted in the unconscious levels of the psyche. This represents the third and most complex level of sexual problems. Arising from the individual's psychological conflicts, the more common of these sexual problems include male and female orgasmic dysfunction, premature ejaculation, male erectile dysfunction, vaginismus, and lack of arousal. The underlying mechanism in the great majority of these sexual dysfunctions is fear. Whether this fear has its origins in sociocultural values, religious inhibitions and guilt, negative early experiences, familial patterns of dominance and discipline, or temporary functional failures of performance, it is the catalyst that sets into motion the psychodynamics that produce the sexual problem. This fear of inadequacy in sexual performance is the most significant deterrent to effective sexual functioning because it completely distracts the person from natural responsiveness by blocking reception of sexual stimuli. Both partners eventually become self-conscious, worrying about their own and each other's sexual performance. Crippling tensions can develop in the relationship as frustrations and dissatisfactions mount. Obviously, problems of attitudes and relationship often overlap. It is unlikely that the partner can remain uninvolved when a sexual problem occurs.

Numerous therapeutic approaches have been developed to help people with such sexual problems. These range from intensive residential sexual therapy to short-term behavior modification. Frequently a process of reeducation is used to modify negative attitudes and counteract inhibitive beliefs. These approaches combined with teaching effective techniques for sexual stimulation have a reasonably good success rate.

When deep anxieties, unresolved guilt or conflict, or other psychopathology are present, the person usually receives some kind of psychotherapy aimed at the specific problem. Many sex therapists prefer not to delve into old conflicts, but focus on changing the problematic behavior with a variety of sexual techniques. Whatever the cause, they reason, removal of the symptom will bring immediate relief and perhaps result in satisfactory long-term functioning without the need for extensive insight therapy.

Nurses have become involved in this type of sex therapy after undergoing additional education in human sexuality and training in specific techniques for treating sexual problems. This level of sexual counseling is specialty practice and is often provided by a team, using the cotherapist approach (one therapist of each sex) in an extensive program involving education, attitude change, setting a permissive environment for sexual experiencing, marital counseling or psychotherapy, and application of appropriate techniques of sex therapy. The scope of maternity nursing practice usually does not include this kind of sexual therapy, unless the nurse has been specially trained and works in a setting that provides these services.

Evaluation

Progress is assessed during return visits. It is often necessary to alter approaches, try new approaches, or examine what factors are interfering with satisfactory resolution of the problem, which in itself is frequently therapeutic. Simple sexual problems may resolve surprisingly rapidly through the reassurance of accurate information and by altering the context in which sexual activity occurs. However, there may be many layers of difficulty, and dealing with an apparently simple problem may reveal more deep-seated conflicts that require specialty referral.

Common Sexual Problems During Pregnancy and the Postpartum Period

There is a wide range of sexual problems that couples may encounter during pregnancy. Sexual problems of a dysfunctional nature include dyspareunia (painful intercourse), changing and conflicting sexual drives, and male erectile dysfunction.[2] These problems may be specifically related to the pregnancy and a function of the couple's psychobiologic responses, or they may represent deeper-seated difficulties brought to the surface by the psychological effects of pregnancy. Other common problems include the avoidance of intercourse, breastfeeding and erotic response, and lack of arousal or dyspareunia during the postpartal period.

Changes in Sex Drive

Alterations in the woman's level of sensuousness and sexual responsiveness are undoubtedly very widespread during pregnancy. These may be a problem for some couples and rather insignificant for others. In early pregnancy, some women experience a heightened sexuality, enjoy sex more, and seek it frequently. Their general level of sensuousness may increase, with heightened awareness and responsiveness to stimuli. Other women have decreased sex drive during the first 2 to 3 months of gestation, often because of nausea, bloating, breast soreness, fatigue, and the many other physical changes women experience at this time. As pregnancy reaches its midpoint, heightened sexuality becomes more common. Many women report an increase in erotic feelings, more interest in sex, actively seeking sexual encounters with partners, and, not uncommonly, occurrence of first orgasms. The physiological changes of pregnancy, including increased pelvic vascularity and vasocongestion, contribute to this phenomenon.[6]

During the first trimester, the pregnant woman is very aware of her pelvis. The feeling of fullness, the sharpened sensations, and the round ligament twinges that may occur deep in the groin with sudden movement all give rise to some anxiety. Even though she may have had previous successful pregnancies and enjoyed sexual relations, she still tends to view these symptoms as possible threats to the pregnancy. If there is occasional (common) spotting, there is all the more reason for her to believe (however mistakenly) that the pregnancy is in danger. Very different sensations from those usually experienced occur with deep penile penetration when the woman has an enlarging soft uterus, although the uterus is still entirely in the pelvis. This does not imply that intercourse should not take place or that thrusting or movement need be curtailed. However, it does have implications for the woman's immersing herself in the pleasures of sexual stimulation, as she may be preoccupied with these other thoughts and sensations. Hence, she may not be orgasmic on all occasions or as often as is usual for her. This preoccupation may also give rise to unpredictableness in her general sexual desire. If there appear to be large changes from what is usual, concern may be generated in both partners. It is important for them to understand that the time of pregnancy can be one of the most anxiety-free, spontaneous sexual interludes of a couple's life. They can be counseled that intercourse poses no threat to pregnancy under normal circumstances. If they have been reasonably comfortable with their sexuality before the pregnancy, and there are no unusual problems, there is no reason to anticipate that their sexual activity need be curtailed.

If there are times when intercourse is not the desired sexual mode, there need be no limitation of any of the other variations of sexual stimulation and orgasmic release for either the man or the woman. Sexual techniques may need modification because of increased sensitivity of the breasts and genitals. As the secretions increase and change in character, there may be an accompanying odor, which is not unpleasant if standards of hygiene are maintained daily. Candidal vaginal infections, which are common to pregnancy, can cause irritation and odor. The physician will prescribe treatment as needed, and the nurse can be helpful in eliciting the needed information about the existence of such problems.

In the second trimester, early in the fourth month, the uterus enlarges rather rapidly and becomes an abdominal organ rather than a pelvic organ. The expectant mother has usually adapted to increased pelvic awareness and is comfortable with intercourse. However, with the rapidly enlarging abdomen, new concerns are engendered regarding crushing the fetus. While there is no danger that this will happen, such concern is very real to both partners. The fetus is very well protected by the uterus and the abdominal wall, but the enlarging uterus can get in the way about the fifth month if the partners assume face-to-face, prone, and supine positions for intercourse. Hence, modifications in positioning may be needed. Since the uterus is not pressing down in the vagina, there is not the feeling of hitting an immovable object with penetration.

Vaginal bleeding during the second trimester is very unusual. Even abortions and premature deliveries during this period are not generally preceded by bleeding, but by cramping and a gush of amniotic fluid. Stress incontinence of urine (losing urine with coughing, sneezing, or orgasm) may occur because the uterus is pressing on the bladder even though it is out of the pelvis. This incontinence is sometimes confused with loss of amniotic fluid and can be frightening during intercourse.

Intercourse using the side position may be preferred as the uterus enlarges. From a purely mechanical point of view, it is necessarily gentle. As the uterus grows larger, the expectant mother is usually much more comfortable lying on her side, with her uterus supported by a pillow. If she is on her back for any length of time, with the enlarged uterus pressing on the abdominal aorta and the vena cava, there may be problems with hypotension and lightheadedness. Using a pillow under the hips during intercourse can be helpful in avoiding hypotension.

It is well to remember that sexual activity does not have to include intercourse *per se,* and often the female genitalia are so sensitive that the woman is not interested in intercourse and many prefer alternate practices or caressing.

As the woman's abdomen increases in size, giving evidence of the pregnancy, the couple may respond with feelings of shame or pride. For some women, the change in body image is an unwelcome development, making them feel unattractive; others take pleasure in this evidence of the growing fetus and feel a sense of heightened potency. These feelings also affect sexual response. Men react to the woman's changing shape too: some feel that their partner is more beautiful and sexy; others are turned off by the perceived distortion of the woman's body. Such feelings have a significant impact upon the man's sexual responsiveness, and naturally upon the woman's response to him. The woman's emotional lability and fluctuating sexual drives are often confusing for both the expectant father and mother. Fathers undergo psychological processes in pregnancy resembling those of the mother and may have symptoms and alternating periods of emotional stability and well-being and times of anxiety, unexplained fears, and compulsions.[7]

Communication between the expectant parents is very important if they are to understand their own and each other's responses to this time of emotional change and uncertainty. There is a tendency for women to withdraw as they become preoccupied with their physical and emotional changes and the psychological tasks related to incorporating and differentiating the baby, as well as preparations for motherhood. The father may at times feel excluded and seek other sources of understanding, support, and companionship.

Dyspareunia During Pregnancy

Painful intercourse during pregnancy can be caused by a number of things. Pressure on the pregnant abdomen may cause a generalized discomfort. Deep penile thrusting may be painful when there is pelvic congestion, when the presenting part is deep in the pelvis, or when certain positions are assumed that exaggerate pressure. Although vaginal secretions are increased during pregnancy, in some instances there may be a relative lack of lubrication owing to inadequate stimulation, which leads to discomfort with intercourse. Irritation of the perineum or introitus, secondary to vaginitis, causes burning or pain on penetration and during intercourse. Cramps and backache may occur following coitus due to increased vasocongestion of sexual arousal combined with that of pregnancy. Orgasm may initiate Braxton Hicks contractions, which may continue and cause considerable pain. Aching postcoital pain may result from lack of orgasm to assist removal of the pelvic congestion associated with plateau levels of sexual arousal. If the woman experiences conflicts about having intercourse while pregnant, there may be a psychological overlay with the dyspareunia.

Avoidance of Sex

Misinformation and fears about the effects of intercourse during pregnancy on the mother and the fetus can prompt couples to avoid or abstain from intercourse. Common fears are that the baby will be injured or marked in some way or be aware of the parents having sex. If a previous baby was born with some kind of physical or mental impairment, this fear may be strong though rarely expressed. Some couples also fear injury to the mother, particularly if she experiences painful intercourse. The widespread practice of advising sexual abstinence during the last part of pregnancy may reinforce these fears of injury. For couples accustomed to frequent, regular intercourse, prolonged abstinence can be a real hardship and may encourage extramarital relations. It is now generally accepted that intercourse poses no problems in late pregnancy if there are no complications. Once membranes have ruptured or labor has begun, or if there is vaginal bleeding, intercourse should be avoided. When premature labor threatens and intercourse is proscribed because orgasm can initiate uterine contractions, the couple must also be advised against oral or manual stimulation that can produce orgasm.

Male Erectile Dysfunction During Pregnancy

Occasionally men find themselves unable to attain or maintain an erection during their partner's pregnancy. This is a type of secondary erectile dysfunction; it may be a situational phenomenon with no long-term reper-

cussions, or it may indicate a more significant psychological problem with sexual dysfunction. Almost all men, at one time or another, will fail to have an erection during a sexual encounter for a vast complex of reasons. This does not indicate significant dysfunction and is usually connected with being upset, tired, or preoccupied or having too much alcohol. As men experience emotional upheavals during pregnancy, they may at certain times be disinterested in sex because of other psychological processes. For some men, a reawakening of maternal relationships and the projection of this relationship onto their pregnant wife create conflicts interfering with erotic response. If the woman's body is perceived as unattractive, sexual arousal may be blocked. This may also occur when the man fears injuring the mother or fetus, or if he is feeling a close identification with his partner in vicariously experiencing the pregnancy.

Inability to attain erection on occasion during pregnancy, as at other times, does not indicate a true sexual problem unless the couple perceives it as such. Expectations of male performance create enormous pressures on men and often exaggerate fears of inadequacy, which further interfere with sexual arousal, perpetuating the difficulty in having or maintaining erections. A man is considered to have significant erectile dysfunction when he cannot achieve penile erection in 25% of his sexual attempts.[8]

Breast-Feeding and Erotic Response

The physiology of sexual responses includes changes in the breasts, which have characteristic variations during lactation. The contractile tissues surrounding the milk ducts contract during orgasm and may result in milk spurting out during sexual arousal and orgasm. Sexual stimulation may produce a "let down" reflex, causing milk to leak or spurt. If this is a concern to the couple, the woman can wear a bra with absorbent pads and avoid pressure on the breasts. Breast tenderness can also present a problem during the postpartal period, but this is a temporary condition and the couple can avoid breast stimulation until the soreness subsides.

Another relatively common occurrence is sexual arousal in response to the baby's suckling. This may range from pleasant, mild excitation to orgasm. If women are aware that this is a normal response and does not indicate that they are somehow perverted, they may become comfortable with this experience. Some women discontinue breast-feeding, however, because they cannot accept these responses. Women who breast-feed also tend to resume intercourse sooner postpartally than those who do not, presumably because of increased eroticism associated with breast-feeding.

Nursing Care: The Couple with Sexual Problems in Pregnancy and Post Partum

Nursing Objectives

1. Provide the pregnant couple with accurate information about sexuality during pregnancy and post partum.
2. Identify problems and concerns pertaining to sexual needs and functions related to the effects of pregnancy and the puerperium.
3. Assist the couple to resolve sexual problems and concerns during pregnancy and in the postpartum period by creating an accepting environment, encouraging expression of concerns, and providing appropriate nursing care.
4. Provide referrals for sexual, family, or psychological counseling for couples with problems beyond the scope of nursing care.

Assessment	Potential Nursing Diagnosis	Intervention	Evaluation
Changes in Sex Drive			
Stage of pregnancy and associated physical and emotional symptoms Level of couple's understanding of psychophysiology of pregnancy Attitudes toward sex in pregnancy Communication patterns	Sexual dysfunction related to physical and emotional changes of pregnancy, lack of knowledge, anxiety or guilt, conflicting values	Reinforce accurate knowledge Teach correct information, clear misconceptions Reassure about normality of fluctuating sex drives Support clear communication	Couple feels comfortable with changing sex drives
Dyspareunia in Pregnancy			
When this occurs, associated factors and symptoms Techniques of intercourse Adequacy of stimulation Perineal irritation due to vaginitis	Sexual dysfunction related to physical changes of pregnancy, lack of knowledge, pain	Instruct on alternate techniques and positions Discuss arousal patterns Refer for treatment of vaginitis Teach normal variations of pregnancy (Braxton Hicks contractions with orgasm, backache)	Couple attains comfortable intercourse or finds acceptable alternative
Avoidance of Sex			
Reasons why sex is avoided (fears, misconceptions, told by physician) Difficulties this poses for the couple Attitudes toward sex in pregnancy	Sexual dysfunction related to lack of knowledge, anxiety, value conflicts, fatigue	Correct misinformation and teach normal fetal–maternal development Inform when sex should be avoided and reasons why Discuss alternatives to intercourse	Couple clarifies that fears and misinformation have been cleared Couple no longer avoids sex when not medically necessary Couple uses acceptable alternatives if indicated
Male Erectile Dysfunction			
Extent of the problem, how often this occurs Level of couple's concern Level of understanding of the man's psychophysiology in pregnancy	Sexual dysfunction related to stressors, fears, anxiety or guilt, lack of knowledge, conflicting values	Teach about normal male reactions and psychological processes Reassure normality of occasional inability to maintain or attain erection Refer to specialist if problem is extensive	Concern decreased Able to have intercourse often enough to satisfy both partners

(continued)

185

Assessment	Potential Nursing Diagnosis	Intervention	Evaluation
Breast-Feeding and Erotic Response			
Loss of milk with arousal or orgasm	Sexual dysfunction related to physical changes of postpartum period, lack of knowledge, anxiety, guilt	Advise regarding normality of milk loss	Comfortable with methods to prevent milk loss from interfering with sex
Extent to which this poses problem to the couple		Suggest wearing bra with absorbent pads if a problem	Able to accept erotic feelings and continue nursing
Arousal or orgasm with nursing, level of concern about this		Avoid pressure or stimulation of breasts	
		Advise of normality of arousal during nursing	
		Discuss discomfort and concern, and meaning of this to woman	
Postpartum Dyspareunia and Lack of Arousal			
When symptoms occur, how often, associated with what factors	Sexual dysfunction related to physical changes of postpartum period, lack of knowledge, fatigue, value conflicts, altered self-concept, pain, lack of privacy, depression	Teach normal postpartal physiology and hormonal effects	Concern decreased
Weeks or months post partum and stage of involution		Reinforce that arousal levels are often lower at this time	Comfortable with level of sexual arousal
Contraceptive use		Discuss techniques of arousal, advise lubricants if needed	Comfortable intercourse attained or acceptable alternative found
Techniques of arousal and intercourse		Refer for treatment of vaginitis	
Level of understanding of postpartal physiology		Discuss approaches to managing home and family demands to provide the couple with private time	
Perineal irritation due to vaginitis			

Postpartal Dyspareunia or Lack of Arousal

During the first 6 months following delivery, the vagina does not lubricate well because of relatively low levels of steroid hormones, which inhibit the vasocongestive response to sexual stimulation. There is also a time period of 3 to 6 weeks needed for healing to occur after childbirth, including the episiotomy; cervical, vaginal, or perineal lacerations; and the site of placental attachment. Couples are usually advised to resume intercourse by the third or fourth postpartal week, if the bleeding has stopped and if the episiotomy is not painful. Their own comfort and sexual desires are used as the guide for resumption of intercourse if there are no contraindications.

However, women are at times concerned with their lack of sexual response in the months following childbirth. Taking their mothering responsibilities into consideration, with the lack of sleep, fatigue, and juggling of activities this usually requires, it is not surprising that their sexual interest might be low even without the additional factor contributed by their sexual physiology after delivery. Understanding this may alleviate fears and enable women to await full restoration of their hormonal and physical status. Residual tenderness of the perineum or vagina can also contribute to painful intercourse as well as to a lack of interest in sex. Vaginitis can result from low estrogen levels, further creating problems with dyspareunia. Fears that intercourse may be permanently affected by pregnancy, labor, and delivery grow out of the belief that these cause damage to the woman's genitalia. Painful intercourse and lack of arousal during the postpartal period can be taken as evidence that these fears have been realized unless the couple can be assisted in understanding the physiological processes of childbirth and of the postpartal period and their true effects on sexual functioning.

Educating Children About Sex

Parents are often concerned about sex education for their children, and a wide range of values are connected with where sex education occurs and who is responsible for this. Developing positive attitudes toward sexuality is very important, but so is conducting sexual activities responsibly. Guilt or conflicts arising from inadequate sex knowledge interfere with learning and schoolwork, happy relationships, and future adjustments with sexual partners. Anxiety due to lack of understanding and confusion about sexual feelings inhibits the freedom of the sexual response, which can lead to various types of sexual dysfunctions. The greater the amount of accurate sex information, the less the anxiety; therefore, sex education is an important method of preventing sexual problems.

Opponents of sex education argue on the basis of invasion of privacy, danger to society, and threat to moral behavior. They believe parents should provide instruction in sexuality to their children. Those arguing for formal sex education point out that no studies have demonstrated greater sexual activity among students who have taken sex education courses. Considerable evidence supports the central influence of parents and family on sexual attitudes and behaviors.[9]

Objectives of Sex Education

Given that there are differences in religious traditions, philosophies, and personal–familial values related to sexual information and expression, the objectives for sex education set forth by the Sex Information and Education Council of the United States (SIECUS) provide an excellent framework for approaching this sensitive area. (See Objectives of Sex Education chart.)

Sex Education in the Schools

Public schools are assuming increasing responsibility for sex education, and about 71% of parents do favor this as part of school curricula.[1] However, parents are often concerned about the quality of sex education in the schools. Some feel that the information is presented in a dry, dehumanized way that does not assist children in understanding the emotional components of sexuality. Others fear that too much will be presented too

rapidly and that the children will not be well assisted to process this information or that the ethical issues will not be addressed. Valid concerns over the qualifications of those teaching sex education are voiced because few schools specifically train teachers for this sensitive subject. Teachers who are embarrassed, uncomfortable, and ill informed or who conduct their classes in a strained, mechanical manner will not enhance the development of healthy, positive attitudes toward sexuality.

Parental Responsibility

Parents need to assume a major responsibility in teaching their children about sex, recognizing that inevitably much information will come from other sources, such as peers, older children, pornography, and mass media. One of the best ways of teaching is by the example of a caring, committed relationship between parents and the parents' comfort in answering sexual questions as they arise. Touching and physical expression of love among family members helps create a climate of acceptance of one's sexuality and body. Flexibility in habit training and weaning also prevents conflicts from developing over these primitive levels of sexuality and allows the young child's emotional and physical needs to unfold naturally.

Genital Exploration

Infants and small children touch their genitals as part of necessary exploration of the body, and parents need not discourage this activity. When the child is about 3 years old, parents can advise him or her that handling genitals in public is not polite. Children usually will not spend an inordinate amount of time with this self-stimulation if they are comfortable in their family environment. Any compulsive behavior that preoccupies a child can signify an emotional conflict, however, whether the behavior is masturbation, scratching, eating, talking, or something else. Giving the child the message that any part of his or her body or normal functions is bad or dirty can create guilt and conflicts later.

"Playing doctor" and other games involving genital exploration among children are very common. Parents occasionally find children at such games. Most feel the need to intervene in some way to assist children in learning the socially acceptable modes of sexual expression, but want to avoid causing a negative conditioning toward sexuality. Letting the children know this is not the time or place for such activities, without making them feel they are doing something terrible, can accomplish this goal.

Nudity in the home may be one way to dignify sexuality and body comfort. However, parents should be comfortable with nudity if they want to use this

Objectives of Sex Education

To provide the individual with an adequate knowledge of his or her own physical, mental, and emotional maturational functions as they relate to sex

To eliminate fears and anxieties regarding the individual's sexual development and adjustments

To develop objective and understanding attitudes in the individual toward the self and toward others, regarding sex in all of its various manifestations

To give the individual insight concerning relationships with members of both sexes, and to help him or her understand obligations and responsibilities to others

To provide an appreciation of the positive good that wholesome human relations can bring to both the individual and the family group

To build an understanding of the fact that ethical and moral values form the only rational basis for making decisions regarding one's behavior

To provide enough knowledge about sexual abuse and aberration so that the individual can protect himself or herself against exploitation and damage to physical and mental health

To provide an incentive to work for a society in which prostitution, illegitimacy, archaic sex laws, irrational sex-related fears, and sexual exploitation are nonexistent

To provide the insight and the climate conducive to the individual's eventually using his or her sexuality effectively and creatively in the roles of spouse, parent, community member, and citizen.

(Sex Information and Education Council of the U.S.)

method, or else a negative or strained attitude might be communicated, which can confuse the child. Also, parents need to be ready to deal with the child touching breasts or genitals, which is a natural way children explore and learn. If parents act shocked or slap the child's hand, another double message is communicated; parents can limit touching with gentle expression of personal preferences and privacy needs.

Basic Explanations

When children encounter objects they do not recognize, their natural curiosity leads them to ask what these are for, as with sanitary napkins, tampons, or contraceptives. Simple explanations about normal body functions in a matter-of-fact tone are readily accepted by children. Usually short answers are enough, but if parents discuss more than they think the child can absorb, the child will not be dismayed as long as there is no sense of

fear, embarrassment, or discomfort. Children will ask additional questions later to clarify what they have not fully understood.

Accurate explanations of the processes of menstruation, childbirth, erection and nocturnal ejaculations, development of secondary sex characteristics, and sexual intercourse will enable children to attain comfortable sexual feelings. These explanations usually occur over many years, may be repeated several times at various levels of sophistication, and can occur spontaneously following the child's questions or be deliberately planned by parents. Actually, the process involves a combination of both, with reinforcements and clarifications as the child processes the information. The basic sex education should probably be completed by about age 9, as girls may menstruate around 10 to 11 and boys begin having wet dreams at this age also. More discussion of intercourse, sexual expression, and contraception is needed during the early adolescent years.

Sexual Terminology

Using correct anatomical and physiological terms when discussing genitals or sexual matters aids understanding and prevents problems in communicating. It is no more difficult for a child to learn to say penis or vagina than such slang terms as pee-pee and ding-dong, and it gives more dignity and acceptability to the sexual parts of the body.

Children pick up sexual words from many sources and usually sense when such terms or expressions are provocative or inappropriate. They may test parents' responses by suddenly saying the word with a straight face. Again, a calm reply with a straightforward explanation of the meaning of the obscene or sexual term is best. Then the child can be advised as to how the family feels about the use of the word or expression. By repeating the word, parents demonstrate that they are not upset or hurt by its use or by other expressions, such as swear words or obscenities, and that it is useless to use them as a weapon or an attention-getting device. Children also learn that parents are willing to respond to sensitive areas of sexuality in a comfortable manner.

Sexual Abuse of Children

Adult sexual molestation of children has been recognized as a widespread problem. Most sexual activity with children involves relatives, neighbors, or friends of the family. Considerably more girls are molested than boys, and the most common age for adult–child sexual activities is when the child is between 11 and 17 years. However, even infants have been subjected to sexual abuse. Sexual activity between close relatives (incest) typically involves fathers and daughters, although both parents are involved psychologically. It usually takes place over a long time period, in unbroken homes, and when the mother is indifferent and easily intimidated.

Children need to learn that their sexual parts are private and they need not allow any person, adult or child, to touch these parts. They can learn to avoid situations in which they are asked to undress at an unusual time and place or to go to a secluded place without clear purposes. Children also need encouragement to tell parents or trusted adults about sexual experiences. The burden of secrecy, with its guilt and fear of repercussion, may well be more harmful than the sexual activity itself. However, family dysfunction underlies much childhood sexual abuse, making it difficult for children to recognize their exploitation and find adult confidants.

Some signs of sexual victimization in children include excessive bathing, sudden bedwetting, school absenteeism, change in sleep patterns, truancy, delinquent behavior, running away, fearfulness, and crying. Physical problems such as urinary tract infections, stomachaches, and frequent upper respiratory tract infections may be more indirect reactions to the stress of sexual abuse.

Teenage Sex

Parents find teenage sex a thorny issue and one they are often uncomfortable with. For many good reasons, they desire children to postpone intensive sexual involvements until they are emotionally mature enough to handle the powerful feelings associated with these kinds of relationships. Helping teenagers to recognize that there are many types of sexual expression not involving intercourse may be one approach, as is teaching sexual ethics about respecting the other person and relating with concern and caring. Teenagers can find a wide range of expression through masturbation, close physical contact without intercourse, dating and doing activities together, kissing, daydreaming, and having caring friendships with each other. Postponing intercourse until they feel ready can do much to prevent conflicts and tensions or the establishment of dysfunctional sexual patterns that can later plague the individual's expression of sexuality. Parents need to communicate the idea of responsible sex to adolescents in terms of avoidance of pregnancy, venereal disease, and emotional exploitation or injury to others.

The intercourse decision among teenagers is affected by such factors as fear of pregnancy, cultural and peer-group influence, religious and moral values, suitability of partner, access to an appropriate place, and respect and concern for oneself and others. Individual sexual needs and psychological pressures toward developing a comfortable sexual identity are also important. Nurses can help adolescents clarify values and make the best long-range decisions. In high school education programs or in contacts in health-care settings, nurses can emphasize that no one need enter a sexual relationship if it causes emotional discomfort.

A teenager has the right to be a virgin without harassment and may need to be reminded that abstinence is normal and healthy. A Gallup survey reported that 62% of teenagers thought premarital sex was acceptable, but paradoxically 51% also felt that virginity was important in a marriage partner.[10] Since sexual activity among adolescents has increased during the past decade,[9] contraceptive information and accessibility are important. Adolescents need to know that no method of contraception is perfect, that there are always some risks, but that birth control is essential to prevent pregnancy if their decision is to have sexual intercourse. Assisting adolescents in this decision-making process and guiding them toward acceptable and effective contraception during sexual activity is a primary responsibility of the nurse.

References

1. McCary JL: Human Sexuality. New York, D Van Nostrand, 1973
2. Zalar MK: Sexual counseling for pregnant couples. MCN 1(3):176–181, May/June 1976
3. Mims FH, Swenson M: Sexuality: A Nursing Perspective. New York, McGraw–Hill, 1980
4. Carpenito JL: Handbook of Nursing Diagnosis, p 64. Philadelphia, JB Lippincott, 1984
5. Tanner LM: The maternity nurse as counselor in human sexuality. In Anderson EH (ed): Current Concepts in Clinical Nursing, Vol IV, pp 169–178. St Louis, CV Mosby, 1973
6. Martin LL: Health Care of Women. Philadelphia, JB Lippincott, 1978
7. Coleman AD, Coleman LL: Pregnancy: The Psychological Experience. New York, Herder and Herder, 1971
8. Masters WH, Johnson VE: Human Sexual Inadequacy. Boston, Little, Brown & Co, 1970
9. Hogan RM: Human Sexuality: A Nursing Perspective, pp 108, 109; p 175; pp 236–238; p 249. Norwalk, CT, Appleton-Century-Crofts, 1985
10. Gallup G: Sexual attitudes reveal conflict, Sect c, p 7. The Plain Dealer, December 20, 1981

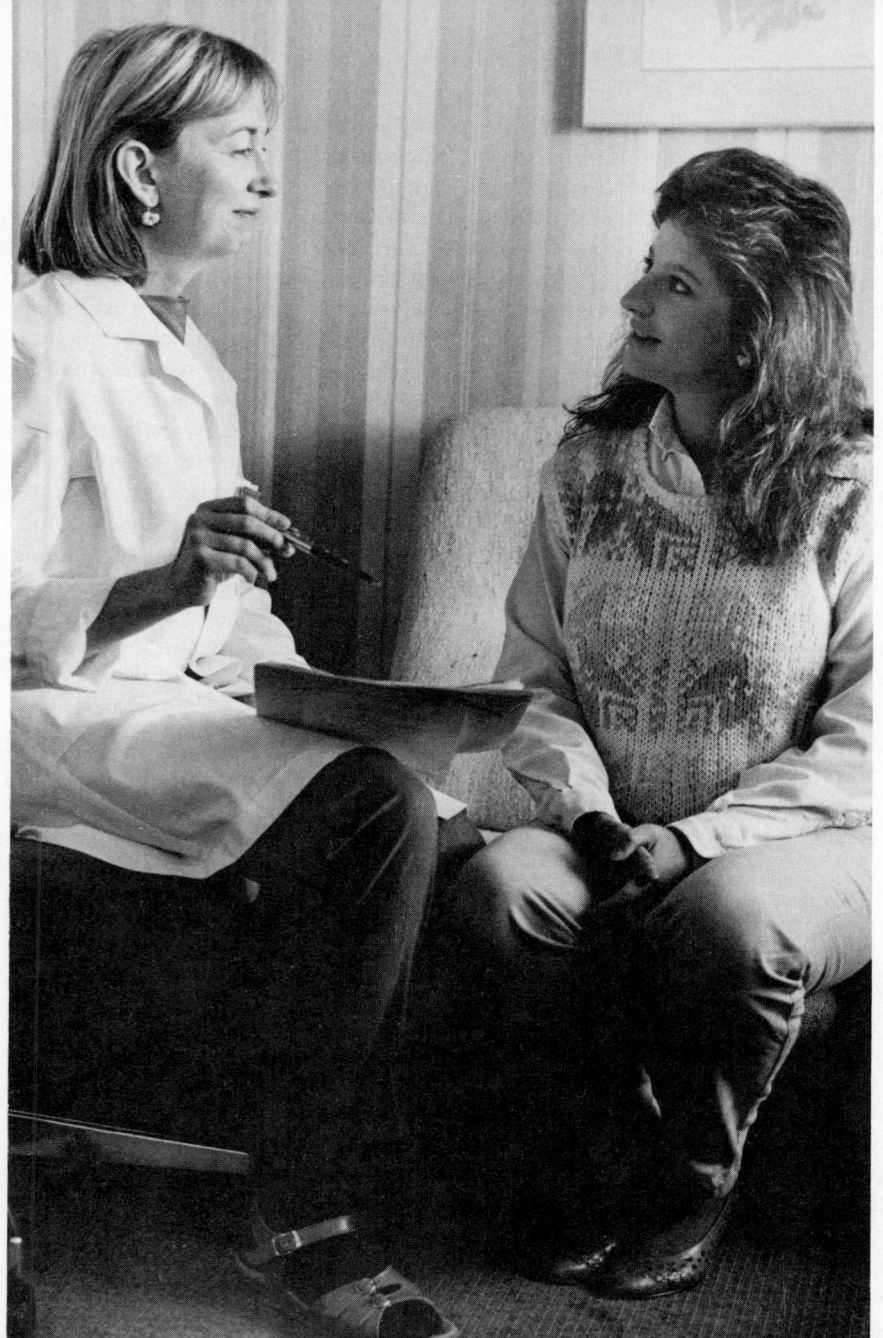

CHAPTER 14

Management of Family Planning

The ability to regulate fertility effectively, introduced in the 1960s with oral contraceptives and the intrauterine device (IUD), has profoundly affected the character of the American family. Extensive demographic and social changes have occurred, producing different household patterns and shifting economic relationships among women, men, and children. Changes in the patterns of family structure are associated with transformations in the roles and expectations of women. The contraceptive revolution helped shape the reproductive and work aspirations of women, freed them from reproductive determinism, and opened a wide range of life choices.

The trend toward smaller families continues in the United States. The fertility rate (number of children per woman) has dropped below replacement level to about 1.8, in contrast to a high of 3.8 in 1957.[1] Approximately 30 million new nontraditional households have been established since 1960. This includes a 175% increase in one-parent households and a 331% increase in households composed of unmarried couples. Women have been postponing marriage and childbearing to later ages, and divorce rates have been rising.[2]

Women have increasingly acquired the education, employment experience, and economic independence to be able to maintain their own households. This depends upon well-regulated fertility. Exposure to sexual activity and the risk of pregnancy is clearly no longer confined primarily to married women. The need for effective and dependable contraception is critical, therefore, to very large numbers of women. A deepening feminization of poverty has been occurring, with the rising divorce rates and increasing births to unwed mothers. Half of the children in households maintained by women live in poverty.[3]

While highly effective contraceptive methods are available, their effectiveness is often lowered by inappropriate use. In addition, their safety has not yet reached levels at which risk is truly minimal. The ideal contraceptive would be a method that is 100% safe and 100% effective, inexpensive, simple to use and understand, not directly connected to intercourse, totally reversible at any time, and readily available. No currently available contraceptive method meets all these criteria, nor does it seem probable that research will find such a method in the near future. Despite the risks involved, people desire the benefits of reproductive choice and must therefore make decisions about methods based on personal values and a full understanding of the risks and benefits involved.

The majority of American women, regardless of religious affiliation, approve of and use contraception. For the poor, having fewer children puts less strain on the family's resources and enhances the family's opportunities for economic and personal advancement. A better informed public, supported by changing social values that encourage individual choice and smaller family sizes, has demanded access to professional advice and contraceptive techniques as an integral part of health-care services.

Motives for contraceptive use are unique, and the choice of method and its meaning are highly individual. Therefore, differences must be respected by the nurse, without presumption based on external characteristics, and the full range of contraceptive possibilities needs to be discussed with each individual or couple so a fully informed and satisfactory choice can be made.

Applying the Nursing Process to Contraceptive Care

Both the maternity and the community-health nurse play an important role in the care of the client seeking contraceptive advice. While not advocating any particular method of contraception, the professional nurse has a responsibility to see that help, understanding, and guidance in family planning are made available.

The nurse who gives contraceptive advice needs to be aware of all the available methods of birth control and should be conversant with the advantages and disadvantages of each method, both at the functional and at the psychological level.

The nurse also should be acquainted with the increasing availability and acceptability of vasectomy and tubal ligation. Studies report dramatic increases in sterilization; 61% of all couples look to this permanent method of contraception when their families are completed.[4] Currently available methods of contraception are listed in Table 14-1.

Pregnancy prevention ideally involves the participation of both male and female partners. Family-planning programs generally encourage participation of the male and provide an opportunity for him to share responsibility for fertility control. A discussion of some of the methods of male contraception, such as withdrawal, the use of condoms, vasectomy, or even rhythm when it is the method of choice, should be included in the program.

The steps of the nursing process are followed in providing care to clients seeking family planning.

Assessment

Since family planning deals with people's sexuality, a private setting should be arranged whenever possible. Feelings about contraception must be explored in a nonjudgmental way and the variety of choices summarized to allow selection of a method that fits the unique circumstance of the individual or couple. There is no "best method" of contraception, but there is always

T A B L E   1 4 - 1

*Current Contraceptive Methods**

Female	Male	Both
Barrier methods	Withdrawal	Abstinence
Jellies, creams, foams	Condoms	Total
Diaphragm	Vasectomy	Periodic
Vaginal sponge		Calendar
Cervical cap		BBT
Hormonal methods		Cervical mucus
Combination pills		Masturbation
Progestin-only pills		Oral-genital
Injections		Anal intercourse
Subdermal implants		Mutual pleasuring
Morning-after pill		
Intrauterine devices		
IUDs (plastic, copper, hormone-impregnated)†		
Tubal ligation		

* Douching, breast-feeding, and abortion are not considered contraceptive methods.
† The Copper 7 and Copper T were withdrawn by Searle, and the Lippes Loop was withdrawn by Ortho in 1985–1986.

a method that can work best in the circumstances at hand.

The nurse should recognize that some clients appearing in a family-planning clinic may be there because of an infertility problem or because they wish to have a Pap smear, a breast examination, or an evaluation for venereal disease. Family-planning clinics often serve as a client's initial introduction to the health-care system and offer opportunities for general health maintenance.

The postpartal period is an optimal time for exploring methods of family planning. Choices can conveniently be reviewed with the client at that time so that knowledgeable selection of a method can be made. The availability of contraceptive advice has resulted in a marked increase in the number of clients returning for postpartal care.

The choice of a suitable contraceptive depends on factors that can vary even from year to year in any couple's contraceptive life span. These factors include expense, bathroom facilities, frequency of intercourse, number of children, the risk of pregnancy the couple wishes to accept, illness, and physical problems.

Assessment covers the client's knowledge, understanding, and experience using various birth-control methods. Historical data include general health, menstrual and reproductive histories, sexual patterns, family structures and relationships, and other significant demographic or socioeconomic information. Certain minimal laboratory work is indicated when the method of choice is the IUD or an oral contraceptive. More historical and physical data are needed for these two methods and when tubal ligation and the diaphragm are under consideration.

History

It is important to know whether there is a history in the immediate family of diabetes, bleeding, or clotting problems, heart problems or high blood pressure, migraine headaches or seizure disorders, kidney or liver disease, anemia, tuberculosis, stroke, cancer, or mental problems. This information provides a baseline on diseases for which the client may be at risk and helps identify contraindications, especially when oral contraceptives are being considered. The woman's own past medical history is elicited, covering the above problems in addition to previous hospitalizations, operations, and other major illness. Menstrual and obstetric histories are of particular importance, with any complications or abnormalities carefully noted. Previous use of and experience with contraceptives also are included. Allergies and the current use of medications alert the practitioner to potential problems.* Key points in the history include the following:

- *When did menarche occur, and have menses been irregular or skipped?* Late menarche and irregular menses indicate a possible endocrine abnormality, and the woman may be having anovulatory cycles. In this case, oral contraceptives should not be used until her endocrine status has been investigated. Otherwise, permanent anovulation with subsequent infertility could result.
- *Are menstrual periods heavy with clotting and cramping?* The IUD will cause these problems to become worse, and often oral contraceptives will improve them. However, extremely heavy flow, particularly in the woman over 30, needs investigation before the pill is prescribed. The diaphragm may be a better choice in this situation.
- *Is there a history of pelvic inflammatory disease?* This is a contraindication for the IUD.
- *Is there a history of severe migraine, cerebral arterial insufficiency, cardiovascular disease, liver disease, severe diabetes, genital or breast cancer, thrombotic problems, high blood pressure, or a family history of stroke?* These are contraindications for oral contraceptives.
- *What type of contraceptive was used before? Was it effective or did a pregnancy occur?* Information is gained here about the probability of the successful use of certain contraceptive methods, and

some idea is provided about the client's level of knowledge and understanding of these methods.
- *What are the most important reasons for contraceptive use?* This question helps the health provider assess the presence of realistic or unrealistic expectations on the part of the client. Misconceptions should be cleared up in discussion, and the client should be helped to understand the practical benefits of contraception. Goals and priorities can also be identified; if the woman feels strongly that pregnancy must be prevented, a highly effective method is indicated. If delay or spacing of pregnancy is actually the goal and if the woman is quite concerned about any alterations in her body physiology and functions, a method with somewhat greater pregnancy risk but no systemic or local alterations would be more appropriate.

Any positive responses in the history must be fully explored and considered in making decisions about the appropriateness of any particular method.

Physical Examination

The extent of the physical performed will depend upon policies and practices in the particular setting, positive responses from the history, and the type of contraceptive method desired. A breast check, pelvic examination, and Pap smear constitute a minimum; at least some health screening should be done when the woman presents this opportunity. A preferred screening physical examination, mainly with the IUD and oral contraceptives in mind, would include those items listed in the Nursing Guidelines.

Laboratory Tests

A Pap smear should be performed during the pelvic examination, and it is also wise to obtain a culture for gonorrhea in sexually active women. Urinalysis is simple and inexpensive and provides some screening for diabetes, urinary tract infections, and kidney function. A complete blood count rules out anemia or systemic infection in most cases and gives an indication of the condition of the platelets. If there is any question about liver function, liver enzymes should be obtained because impaired liver function is an absolute contraindication to oral contraceptives. A VDRL or other serological test for syphilis would also be a good screening measure.

Nursing Diagnosis

The nursing diagnosis is made based on historical and physical examination data and nursing assessments. The nursing diagnosis focuses nursing care upon problems

---

* Parts of the History, Physical Examination, and Laboratory Tests sections are adapted from Martin LL: Health Care of Women. Philadelphia, JB Lippincott, 1978.

Nursing Guidelines: Abnormalities Found Upon Physical Examination That Contraindicate Use of Particular Types of Contraceptives

- *Eyes.* Check for signs of glaucoma such as narrow anterior chamber and cupping of discs or increased cup/disc ratio; conditions of veins and arteries, particularly arteriolar narrowing or venous nicking; and condition of retina.

- *Thyroid.* Examine for nodules and diffuse enlargement. Oral contraceptives alter thyroid function tests, although there is no evidence at present that they cause either hypothyroidism or hyperthyroidism.

- *Chest.* Examine lung fields, heart, and great vessels. Any heart murmurs, bruits, or adventitious lung sounds indicate the need for consultation.

- *Breasts.* Any masses, nodules, or discharge from the nipples contraindicates oral contraceptives, at least initially, and calls for consultation. There is some evidence that the pill may be helpful in certain types of benign breast disease, but it is recommended that the pill not be used in cases of suspected or proved breast cancer.

- *Abdomen.* Examine for bruits, masses, and hepatosplenomegaly.

- *Skin.* Signs of chloasma (mask of pregnancy) or history of this is a relative contraindication for oral contraceptives. Acne may be improved.

- *Extremities.* Varicose veins are a relative contraindication for oral contraceptives. Peripheral pulses that are weak or absent indicate circulatory or arteriosclerotic problems, and further investigation is necessary with avoidance of oral contraceptives until the safety of their use is determined.

- *Pelvic examination.* Significant pelvic relaxation with prolapse, cystocele, or rectocele makes effective use of the diaphragm impossible. Anatomical anomalies such as a small cervix or short anterior vaginal wall also dictate against this method. An infantile cervix and uterus suggests endocrine problems, and oral contraceptives or an IUD should not be used until this possibility has been ruled out. Pelvic inflammatory disease and extensive cervicitis contraindicate the use of IUDs. Suspicious cervical lesions should be biopsied before any contraceptive method is instituted. Uterine myomas make IUD placement difficult and may be stimulated to increase with the use of oral contraceptives; therefore, foam, a condom, or a diaphragm would be the method of choice. Ovarian or tubal masses should be referred at once for consultation, and no contraceptive should be given until their nature has been ascertained and the problem treated. Vaginitis is not a contraindication to either the IUD or an oral contraceptive, although it may influence the type of pill used and should, of course, be treated. Severe retroversion or anteversion of the uterus contraindicates use of the IUD.

- *Weight.* Obesity must be viewed as a serious problem when oral contraceptives are desired. Some consider it a contraindication owing to the pill's effects on carbohydrate and lipid metabolism. It definitely puts the client at increased risk for several complications. The obese woman also presents difficulties in fitting a diaphragm and inserting an IUD. It is difficult to find anatomical landmarks and determine the size and position of the uterus. Foam or condoms seem to be the contraceptives of choice until weight is lost.

- *Age.* Oral contraceptives carry a greater risk for the very young woman, whose endocrine system is immature, and for the woman over 35, who is increasingly susceptible to thromboembolic problems and hypertension.

- *Blood pressure.* Even marginal elevation of the blood pressure contraindicates the use of oral contraceptives. There is a direct relation between the estrogen in the pill and hypertension, and even a certain percentage of normotensive women will develop high blood pressure under the influence of these drugs. When there is already marginal or established hypertension, the risk of serious complication and of a higher blood pressure is increased. Another method of contraception is indicated.

Positive findings and abnormalities indicate further consultation or referral.

---

or needs to which nurses, by virtue of their particular expertise, are able to respond effectively. In family-planning care, these often include needs for further education and information about risks and benefits of various contraceptive methods. Other diagnoses commonly made include home or family problems adversely affecting contraceptive use and the need for specific teaching on the use of a given contraceptive method.

Planning/Intervention

The nursing plan is based on the diagnoses. Interventions are designed and carried out that will improve or affect the problem/need identified. The nurse may carry out interventions directly or may facilitate or arrange for others to provide the necessary services.

Potential Nursing Diagnoses

Knowledge deficit related to
- Lack of information or exposure to specific contraceptive method
- Information misinterpretation (*e.g.*, about side-effects of specific method)
- Cognitive limitations (intellectual)
- Lack of motivation to learn

Noncompliance related to
- Health beliefs and value systems
- Prior unsuccessful experience with contraceptive method
- Increase in symptoms with method
- Disturbed self-esteem (not taking responsibility for self-care)

Intervention focuses upon assisting the client or couple through the decision-making process in selecting an appropriate contraceptive method. Knowledge deficits are remedied through teaching about various contraceptives, correcting misinformation as needed. Decision making is fostered by thorough discussion of the risks and benefits of each potential contraceptive choice. Fears need to be expressed, uncertainties clarified, and personal preferences identified.

When the client has experienced prior difficulties with certain methods, intervention focuses upon the meanings attached and perceived reasons for problems. The nurse can assist in values clarification, so the client may better understand the psychodynamics of unsuccessful contraceptive use. The client's health beliefs, values, fears related to physical or psychoemotional harm, and personal reactions to contraceptive experiences are explored. This process assists the client in clarifying values, understanding behaviors, and making personal choices that work better in achieving goals.

Evaluation

Evaluation of the plan involves observing for desired changes in knowledge, understanding, or behavior in the client. Often evaluation leads to another round of assessment, diagnosis, and planning as problems are refined and better understood (see Nursing Care: Couples Seeking Contraceptive Methods).

The most basic level of evaluation is whether or not the client uses the selected method of contraception effectively. Prevention of pregnancy is the basic outcome criterion. Other levels of evaluation consider the client's satisfaction with the method, ease in use, compatibility with life-style, acceptability in relation to values and cost, response of sexual partner, and concern with side-effects. If difficulties are experienced in any of these areas, the nurse reassesses the situation in partnership with the client or couple. A new diagnosis is made, and appropriate intervention is planned and evaluated.

Effectiveness, Risk, and Informed Consent

Contraceptive Effectiveness

The effectiveness of a contraceptive method is of primary concern to both clients and professionals. When counseling clients on effectiveness, professionals must be familiar with the two types of effectiveness rates, maximal (theoretical) effectiveness and typical (use) effectiveness. *Maximal effectiveness* is the method's effectiveness in preventing pregnancy under ideal conditions, that is, when it is completely understood and used perfectly. This is the method's lowest observed failure rate; if a pregnancy occurs it is due to a failure of the method itself, not how it is being used. *Typical effectiveness* takes into consideration the method's effectiveness under actual use, in which some people use the method correctly and others use it carelessly or incorrectly. Typical effectiveness rates are lower, naturally, because the human error factor is included.

In answering questions about effectiveness, the counselor may allow his or her bias to show by quoting maximal effectiveness figures for preferred contraceptive methods and typical effectiveness figures for those methods not favored. This provides misleading data to the client and is an attempt to influence choice according to the counselor's preference. Ethical counseling requires consistency in presenting effectiveness data. Some counselors present both sets of figures, so the potential for error in use can be clearly assessed. Figures for maximal (theoretical) and typical (use) effectiveness of common contraceptive methods are shown in Table 14-2. When assisting clients to select a contraceptive method, it is good to keep in mind that the "best method" of contraception is one that a couple will use most consistently and correctly, and this is often the one that feels most natural and comfortable. The assessment questions for use effectiveness provide a guide to factors that might lower effectiveness in contraceptive use. Any "yes" response indicates potential problems, and most people will have several "yes" answers for any contraceptive method. The one with the fewest "yes" responses would be best for that couple.

(text continued on page 198)

Couples Seeking Contraceptive Methods

Nursing Objectives

1. Provide accurate information about modes of action, methods for use, risks, and benefits of all contraceptives.
2. Clarify misunderstandings and alleviate knowledge deficits regarding particular contraceptive methods.
3. Assist in selection of appropriate contraceptive method, considering indications, client characteristics, and acceptability.
4. Instruct in use of selected contraceptive method, with opportunity for questions and method for assessing client understanding and ability to use effectively.
5. Educate about potential side-effects and complications and the need for immediate evaluation of problems.

Assessment	Potential Nursing Diagnosis	Intervention	Evaluation
All types			
Understanding of sexuality, characteristics of sexual activity (*i.e.*, regular or occasional intercourse, one or several partners)	Knowledge deficit related to sexual and reproductive functions, contraceptive methods (use, effectiveness, risks, mechanisms of action)	Reinforce accurate knowledge	Affirms understanding, no further questions
Knowledge of contraceptives and understanding of their use		Teach correct information, clear misconceptions	Able to select method and feel comfortable with it
Satisfaction and dissatisfaction with previous contraceptive practices	Noncompliance related to health beliefs/values, prior unsuccessful experience with method, increased symptoms with method, or disturbed self-concept (not taking responsibility for self-care)	Provide information about methods not well understood	Effective contraceptive use (*i.e.*, no unwanted pregnancies)
Menstrual and pregnancy history		Provide feedback about effectiveness rates, reasons why method not effective	
General health history		Provide feedback about risks and contraindications of various methods	
Expectations of benefits from contraceptive method		Reinforce accurate expectations, clear misconceptions	
Concerns about various methods related to religious affiliation, life-style, and values such as naturalism		Discuss various methods, mechanisms of action, and implications	
Oral contraceptives			
Determine if contraindications are present from history and physical examination	Knowledge deficit related to contraindications, monitoring needs, use, side-effects and complications, risks and benefits of oral contraceptives	Advise if contraindicated	Finds method suitable and uses effectively
Explore understanding of requirements for this method to be effective (*i.e.*, regularity of pill taking)		Discuss regular use of medication, need for periodic checkup, blood pressure, and Pap smears	Comfortable with decision not to use
	Knowledge deficit related to learning ability that impairs ability to follow regimen	Explain how to begin and discontinue pills	
	Health beliefs/values inconsistent with oral contraceptive use	Discuss side-effects, serious complications, when to seek medical care, what to do if one or more pills are forgotten	
		Discuss advantages and disadvantages	

(continued)

Assessment	Potential Nursing Diagnosis	Intervention	Evaluation
IUD			
Determine if contraindications are present from history and physical examination Explore understanding of requirements for this method to be effective (*i.e.*, checking IUD strings)	Knowledge deficit related to contraindications, insertion/removal techniques, monitoring needs, side-effects and complications, risks and benefits of IUDs Health beliefs/values inconsistent with IUD use Disturbance in self-concept with inability to touch body part (genital)	Advise if contraindicated Discuss techniques and experience of IUD insertion and removal, need for periodic checkup and Pap smears Explain method, discuss side-effects, serious complications, and when to seek medical care Note when IUD must be replaced if it contains copper or hormone Discuss advantages and disadvantages	Finds method suitable and uses effectively Comfortable with decision not to use
Diaphragm/sponge			
Determine if contraindications are present from history and physical examination Explore understanding of requirements for this method to be effective (*i.e.*, insertion/removal techniques, checking for tears, using with every act of intercourse)	Knowledge deficit related to contraindications, requirements for effective use, risks and benefits of sponge or diaphragm Disturbance in self-concept with inability to touch body part (genital) Inappropriate environment/life-style for use requirements Deficit in psychomotor skills that impairs ability to follow regimen	Advise if contraindicated Discuss insertion/removal techniques, instruct and have client practice until correctly done Explain method and necessity for constant use, applying more spermicide with additional acts of intercourse, and for leaving in 6–8 hours (diaphragm); wet sponge before insertion, remove within 30 hours Advise that diaphragm must be refitted after each delivery and if substantial amount of weight is lost or gained Discuss advantages and disadvantages	Finds method suitable and uses effectively Comfortable with decision not to use
Fertility Awareness			
Explore understanding of requirements for this method to be effective (*i.e.*, long periods of abstinence, regular menstrual periods, ancillary techniques to increase effectiveness)	Knowledge deficit related to requirements for effective use, risks and benefits of fertility awareness Knowledge deficit related to learning ability that impairs ability to follow regimen Alteration in family processes related to goal conflicts with sexual partner.	Discuss methods to establish baseline menstrual patterns and identify ovulation Instruct on calculating fertile period Discuss advantages and disadvantages	Finds method suitable and uses effectively Comfortable with decision not to use

(continued)

Assessment	Potential Nursing Diagnosis	Intervention	Evaluation
Spermicides and condom			
Explore understanding of requirements for this method to be effective (*i.e.*, timing of application, regular use, precautions to avoid leakage or decreasing spermicide effectiveness)	Knowledge deficit related to requirements for effective use, risks and benefits of spermicides and condom Inappropriate environment/life-style for use requirements Lack of motivation for regular and consistent use	Instruct on proper insertion of spermicides and application of condom Advise on repeated acts of intercourse and reapplications, care in condom removal, no douching for 6–8 hours when spermicides are used Discuss advantages and disadvantages	Finds method suitable and uses effectively Comfortable with decision not to use
Sterilization			
Determine understanding of procedure as ending fertility and irreversible Obtain childbearing history, ages and health of children, marital situation, and values assigned to reproductive role	Knowledge deficit related to indications for sterilization, types of procedures, permanence of procedures, risks and benefits Health beliefs/values inconsistent with sterilization Disturbance in self-concept due to loss of body function	Discuss permanence of sterilization Explore meanings to couple Explain various procedures and required follow-up	Affirms understanding of permanence, desire to end childbearing; accepts requirements of procedure; satisfied with outcome

(text continued from page 195)

Informed Consent and Contraceptive Risk

There is a certain amount of risk in every contraceptive method, either the method itself or the risk of pregnancy due to contraceptive failure or misuse. It should be noted that the mortality associated with pregnancy is greater than that of any commonly used contraceptive method. Often the risk a given method poses for the individual cannot be completely determined in advance, although in many instances contraindications can be identified for known health problems or personal characteristics. Still, an apparently healthy woman with no major contraindications to a given method can develop serious complications, some of which are life threatening. Although the incidence of such complications is low, it is the client's right to be well informed about the risks, benefits, and effectiveness of all contraceptive methods (see Table 14-2).

The issue of informed consent is particularly critical in the field of contraception, because the services are not "therapeutic" in the traditional medical sense.

Healthy clients request family-planning methods, which are initiated without health indications in most instances. In evaluating possible malpractice considerations, the legal approach uses the "reasonable person" standard. Did the client receive all the information a reasonable person would need to make a sound decision and give a truly informed consent to care? The professional counselor has the responsibility of ascertaining that the client has sufficient information about the proposed method (treatment) and that the client is competent to consent on his or her own behalf.

The key factors to sufficient information include discussion of the benefits and risks (all major and all minor) of the method, discussion of alternatives (including abstinence and no method), that the client has a right and responsibility to ask questions about the method, that the client may decide to withdraw or not use the method at any time without penalty, and an explanation of the use and results of the method. All the above information must be documented; a written consent form and signature alone are not enough. Legally, the professional must enter a record of the information covered in the client's chart and make some notation to document client understanding. Often,

TABLE 14-2

Effectiveness and Risks of Contraceptives and Pregnancies per 100 Women per Year

Method	Maximal (Theoretical) Effectiveness	Typical (Use) Effectiveness	Continuing Pregnancies	Deaths due to Pregnancy	Deaths due to Contraception	Major Morbidity (%)	Minor Morbidity (%)
No contraception			90	0.016	0		
Oral contraceptives (combined)	0.5	2–4	0.5	0	0.003	1	40
Low-dose oral progestin	1–1.5	5–10					
IUD	2	5	3	0.001	0.001	1	40
Diaphragm	2–3	13–19	12	0.002	0		
Rhythm (calendar)	14	21	25	0.005	0		
BBT only	7	21					
Cervical mucus only	2	25					
Early abortion*	0	0	0	0	0.003	1	8
Laparoscopic tubal ligation	0	0.04	0.04	0	0.03	0.6	1
Vasectomy	0	0.15	0.15	0	0	1	5
Condom†	3	10–15					
Spermicides†	3	13–22					
Condom + spermicide	<1	5					
Coitus interruptus†	3–16	15–25					
Cervical cap†‡	8	16					
Vaginal sponge†‡	3	16–20					

* Abortion is not a method of contraception, but is included here for comparison.
† Data on continuing pregnancies and deaths due to pregnancy are not available, but typical effectiveness figures indicate these would be in the range found for the diaphragm.
‡ Data are inadequate for accurate comparisons.
(After Hatcher RA, Stewart GK, Stewart F et al: Contraceptive Technology 1984–1985, p 3. New York, Irvington Publishers, 1984, and Romney SL et al: Gynecology and Obstetrics: The Health Care of Women, pp 551, 552. New York, McGraw–Hill, Blakiston, 1975)

clients are asked to sign a statement at the end of the record of information, such as, "I have read and discussed the above information about contraception (or the specific method) and I fully understand these points." The importance of a voluntary decision by the client, without coercion or professional bias, is clearly evident.

The basic criteria for competence to consent are that the client is capable of understanding the proposed treatment (method) and its alternatives and risks and is capable of rational decision making. Competence to consent may be difficult to evaluate in some instances, such as the very young teenager or the mentally ill or mentally retarded person. Legal consultation is recommended when there is doubt about a client's ability to give consent to care. Documentation of such consultation is critical.

Informed consent is both a safeguard for the client and a way of increasing proper contraceptive use. When the woman or couple fully understand the technique, have weighed the possible adverse effects against the convenience and acceptability of the method for them, and have made a choice based on which method best meets their needs, the likelihood of discontinuation and

misuse is reduced. Guidelines for informed consent suggested by the United States Department of Health and Human Services are included in Nursing Guidelines: Contraceptive Teaching.

Adolescent Family Planning and the Law

The legal rights of adolescents to obtain contraceptive services without parental consent constitute an area of concern to many professionals involved in family planning. The laws related to minors' rights to contraceptive services, sterilization, and nonprescription contraceptives vary from state to state. In all 50 states, minors can consent to treatment for venereal disease, and in many they can consent to contraception and pregnancy-related care. In 1977 the United States Supreme Court ruled that minors have a constitutional right to contraceptives. Although there are no rulings on the rights of minors to prescription contraceptives, Planned Parenthood Federation of America reports no record of a suit being won against a physician or health service for providing contraceptive services to minors without parental consent. However, the rights of family-planning counselors to provide confidential services and the rights of women, teens, and indigents to obtain services are being challenged. Nurses need to clarify personal values on these issues, remain informed of new developments, and participate in the legislative or regulatory processes by which decisions about family-planning rights are made.

Contraceptive Methods

Oral Contraception

Oral contraceptives ("the pill") are hormonal agents consisting of a combination of estrogen and a synthetic progestational agent or only progestin. They act principally at the central nervous system level to inhibit ovulation through suppression of follicle-stimulating hormone (FSH) and luteinizing hormone (LH). There are secondary effects on endometrial development, tubal motility, and cervical mucus. Under the influence of the progestational agent, the cervical mucus becomes thick, viscous, and unreceptive to spermatozoa. However, the most important effect of standard-dose combination pills is the inhibition of ovulation, which means that there is no ovum to be fertilized.

Oral contraceptives are available in 21- and 28-day packages; in the 21-day packs a pill is taken each day for 3 weeks, followed by a week without any pills. In the 28-day pack, a pill is taken every day for 4 weeks, but only those taken during the first 3 weeks will have active hormonal ingredients; those pills taken during the last week consist of lactose or ferrous sulfate, but no hormones. The purpose of a week of nonhormonal pills is to keep the woman in the habit of taking a pill a day, and in some instances to provide an iron supplement for prevention of anemia. When the 21-day approach is used, the pill is taken daily beginning on the fifth day of the menstrual cycle through day 25. Two or 3 days after the last pill is taken there is usually a "withdrawal" menstrual flow.

There is a large number of oral contraceptives available, with differing combinations of estrogen or progestin doses (Table 14-3). Basically there are two types, the combination pills, which contain estrogen and progestin and are available at the standard or low (micro) dosage levels, and the progestin-only type (minipills). Because the majority of serious side-effects are due to estrogen, the trend has been toward reducing this hormonal agent from the original dosage of 80 mcg to 100 mcg to doses ranging from 50 mcg to 20 mcg. However, use of 20- or 30-mcg pills is associated with higher rates of breakthrough bleeding and unpredictable menses, making them less acceptable to some women. Similar problems are encountered with progestin-only pills, with increased incidence of amenorrhea, spotting, and irregularity of menses.

Biphasic Oral Contraception. Biphasic oral contraception was introduced in 1982 to simulate a woman's normal hormonal pattern. The low-dose estrogen (35 mcg) is kept constant throughout the cycle, while the progestin is increased (0.5 mg–1.0 mg) from day 11 through day 21. The biphasic pill is intended to reduce total steroid exposure while alleviating problems with breakthrough bleeding and spotting common with lower-dose pills.[5] The benefits of decreasing progestins might be reduction in the following: hypertension, high-density lipoprotein levels, pelvic congestion, acne and oily skin, depression, fatigue, and headaches. However,

9 tablets containing 1.0 mg norethindrone and 0.035
   mg ethinyl estradiol, then
5 tablets containing 0.5 mg norethindrone and 0.035
   mg ethinyl estradiol, then
7 inert tablets

Triphasic oral contraceptives are available in 28-day regimens, as shown above, and in 21-day regimens in which the seven inert pills are omitted. The woman waits 7 days, then begins the next pack of pills.[7]

The maximal (theoretical) effectiveness of the combined-formulation pill approaches 100%. In fact, the method failure rate—failure when properly used—is negligible. When client error is included (client failures to take the pill for one or more days during the cycle), effectiveness falls to approximately 90% to 95%. The discontinuation rate has been reported to be from 20% to as high as 50%. The appearance of side-effects and untoward symptoms, as well as variations in motivational factors in the populations studied, often are reasons for discontinuation of oral contraceptives.

Contraindications and Side-Effects

Generally accepted absolute contraindications to oral contraception include a history of thrombophlebitis, thromboembolic disorders, cerebrovascular accident, hepatic adenoma, or malignancy of the breast or of the reproductive tract, the presence of marked impairment of liver function, and, of course, pregnancy. Strong relative contraindications include migraine, hypertension, diabetes, gallbladder disease, sickle cell disease, undiagnosed vaginal bleeding, age over 35, abortion within the past 10 to 14 days, fibrocystic breast disease, and less than 4 weeks postpartum.

Common side-effects of the pill include accentuation of such premenstrual symptoms as mastalgia, irritability, edema, nausea, headaches, spotting, weight gain, missed periods, and increased yeast vaginal infections. The major life-threatening side-effects include blood clots in the legs, pelvis, lungs, heart, or brain. The risk of heart attack is increased in women over 40, especially if they smoke. Liver tumors (adenomas), gallbladder disease, and hypertension also are serious complications.

The side-effects of oral contraceptives, according to the excess or deficiency of hormone responsible for the symptom or condition, are shown in Table 14-4.

Systemic Effects of Synthetic Hormones

Initially oral contraceptives were believed to affect only the reproductive system through suppression of ovulation and alteration of menstrual flow. However, there is increasing recognition that these powerful synthetic hormones affect many systems of the body, causing metabolic and endocrine changes with far-reaching im-

Informed consent is the voluntary, knowing assent from the individual on whom any procedure is to be performed after she or he has been given the following:
- A fair explanation of the procedures or method
- A description of attendant discomforts and risks, including all major (life-threatening) and all common minor risks
- A description of the benefits to be expected
- An explanation of alternative methods and effectiveness rates with indication that nothing is 100% and that sterilization is permanent
- An offer to answer any questions about procedures or method
- An instruction that the individual is free to withdraw consent to the procedure or method at any time prior to the procedure, or to discontinue the method, without affecting future care or loss of benefits
- A written consent document detailing the basic elements of informed consent and the information provided; this should be signed by the client, an auditor–witness of the client's choice, and the person obtaining the consent

some noncontraceptive benefits of progestins also might be lost, such as protection against pelvic inflammatory disease, less dysmenorrhea and menstrual blood loss, and protection against endometrial cancer and fibrocystic breast disease.[6]

Triphasic Oral Contraception. Triphasic oral contraceptives appeared in 1985, intended to even more closely approximate the hormonal fluctuations of the menstrual cycle. Both low-dose estrogen and progestin change in a "low-higher-low" pattern, or estrogen is constant while progestin rises at midcycle and falls prior to the onset of bleeding. The triphasic pill reduces total steroid exposure, provides greater protection at midcycle, and reduces problems with breakthrough bleeding. Two examples of the hormonal patterns in triphasic pills follow:

Example 1
6 tablets containing 0.05 mg levonorgestrel and 0.03
   mg ethinyl estradiol, then
5 tablets containing 0.075 mg levonorgestrel and 0.04
   mg ethinyl estradiol, then
10 tablets containing 0.125 mg levonorgestrel and
   0.03 mg ethinyl estradiol, then
7 inert tablets

Example 2
7 tablets containing 0.5 mg norethindrone and 0.035
   mg ethinyl estradiol, then

T A B L E 1 4 - 3

Most Currently Available Combination, Microdose, and Progestin Oral Contraceptives

Product/Manufacturer	Type	Estrogen	Progestin
Envoid-E/Searle	Combination	100 mcg mestranol	2.5 mg norethynodrel
Ortho-Novum/Ortho	Combination	100 mcg mestranol	2 mg norethindrone
Norinyl/Syntex	Combination	100 mcg mestranol	2 mg norethindrone
Ovulen/Searle	Combination	100 mcg mestranol	1 mg ethynodiol diacetate
Ortho-Novum 1 + 80	Combination	80 mcg mestranol	1 mg norethindrone
Norinyl 1 + 80/Syntex	Combination	80 mcg mestranol	1 mg norethindrone
Norlestrin/Parke–Davis	Combination	50 mcg ethinyl estradiol	2.5 mg norethindrone acetate
Norinyl 1 + 50/Syntex	Combination	50 mcg mestranol	1 mg norethindrone
Ortho-Novum 1 + 50/Ortho	Combination	50 mcg mestranol	1 mg norethindrone
Norlestrin/Parke–Davis	Combination	50 mcg ethinyl estradiol	1 mg norethindrone acetate
Ovral/Wyeth	Combination	50 mcg ethinyl estradiol	0.5 mg norgestrel
Demulen/Searle	Combination	50 mcg ethinyl estradiol	1 mg ethynodiol diacetate
Ovcon-50/Mead Johnson	Combination	50 mcg ethinyl estradiol	1 mg norethindrone
Brevicon/Syntex	Combination	35 mcg ethinyl estradiol	0.5 mg norethindrone
Ovcon-35/Mead Johnson	Combination	35 mcg ethinyl estradiol	0.4 mg norethindrone
Modicon/Ortho	Combination	35 mcg ethinyl estradiol	0.5 mg norethindrone
Norinyl 1 + 35/Ortho	Combination	35 mcg ethinyl estradiol	1 mg norethindrone
Demulen 35/Searle	Combination	35 mcg ethinyl estradiol	1 mg ethynodiol diacetate
Ortho-Novum 10/11/Ortho	Combination-Biphasic	35 mcg ethinyl estradiol	0.5 mg norethindrone (days 1–10) 1 mg norethindrone (days 11–21)
Nordette/Wyeth	Combination	30 mcg ethinyl estradiol	0.15 mg levonorgestrel
Loestrin 1.5 + 30/Parke–Davis	Combination	30 mcg ethinyl estradiol	1.5 mg norethindrone acetate
Lo/Ovral/Wyeth	Combination	30 mcg ethinyl estradiol	0.3 mg norgestrel
Loestrin 1 + 20/Parke–Davis	Combination	20 mcg ethinyl estradiol	1 mg norethindrone acetate
Micronor/Ortho	Progestin		0.35 mg norethindrone
Nor-QD/Syntex	Progestin		0.35 mg norethindrone
Ovrette/Wyeth	Progestin		0.075 mg norgestrel

pact. The possible long-term consequences and risks of taking the pill are creating a climate of concern among women and health professionals and have led to a call for a more conservative and cautious approach involving careful selection and frequent monitoring.

Thrombotic Effects.   Several factors seem to be involved in the increased risk of death or disability due to clotting disorders (*e.g.,* stroke, pulmonary embolism,

retinal vein thrombosis, myocardial infarction, thrombophlebitis) in women taking the pill. There is more rapid fibrin formation with increased clot firmness among pill users than among nonusers, as well as an increase in certain blood factors associated with coagulation, an increase in platelet count with changes in electrophoretic mobility of platelets, and an increase in vascular lesions and venous stasis.[8,9] Women who use the pill have a seven to eight times greater risk of death

TABLE 14-4

Hormonal Basis of Side-Effects of Oral Contraceptives

Estrogen		Progestin		Androgen
Excess	Deficiency	Excess	Deficiency	Excess
Nausea, vomiting	Amenorrhea	Acne, oily scalp	Hypermenorrhea with clotting	Acne
Fluid retention (premenstrual tension, irritability, breast tenderness, corneal swelling, cramping, edema)	Oligomenorrhea	Increased appetite	Late-cycle spotting	Oily skin
	Early-cycle or midcycle spotting	Weight gain	Delayed onset of menses	Rashes
		Fatigue	Dysmenorrhea	Increased hair growth in male pattern
	Loss of pelvic tone	Depression	Weight loss	Increased interest in sex
Increased vaginal discharge	Hot flashes	Hair loss		Cholestatic jaundice
Chloasma	Nervousness, irritability	Headaches when not taking pills		Increased appetite
Headaches	Decreased interest in sex	Increased breast size		Pruritus
Increased breast size		Increased muscle mass		
Weight gain		Increased monilial vaginitis (*Candida*)		
Increased cervical ectropion		Breast tenderness not related to fluid retention		
Increased size of fibroids		Short menses		
Telangiectasia		Relative endometrial atrophy		
Thromboembolic disorders		Decreased interest in sex		
Reduction of lactation		Cholestatic jaundice		
Possible hypertension		Decreased carbohydrate tolerance		
Hepatic adenoma		Dilated leg veins		

from thromboembolic disease than nonusers. The incidence of complications is dosage related. There is a significant difference between women taking pills with less than 50 mcg of estrogen per day and those taking dosages above 50 mcg of estrogen per day. The risk of death from clotting disorders secondary to oral contraceptives is age related, the risk increasing after age 35.

Effects of Cigarette Smoking. Evidence indicates that there is an increased death rate from cardiovascular complications among women over 35 who use oral contraceptives and smoke. Studies have shown that women over age 30 who both smoke and use oral contraceptives have a greater risk of fatal heart attack than younger women who use the pill and women over 30 who do not smoke. While other risk factors such as hypertension and high cholesterol are also associated with higher incidence of myocardial infarction, cigarette smoking was considered the most important factor. Women who smoke heavily and use the pill have 39 times the risk of cardiovascular disease, including heart attack, stroke, and thromboembolism, compared with

women who neither smoke nor use the pill. Half of all the deaths associated with oral contraceptive use would be avoided if women who take birth control pills would not smoke.[10] Apparently women without these risk factors can continue taking oral contraceptives with relative safety between the ages of 30 and 44.[11] The Food and Drug Administration (FDA) has required the following antismoking warning be added to package inserts accompanying oral contraceptives:

Cigarette smoking increases the risk of serious cardiovascular side-effects from oral contraceptive use. The risk increases with age and with heavy smoking (15 or more cigarettes per day) and is quite marked in women over 35 years of age. Women who use oral contraceptives should be strongly advised not to smoke.[10]

Hypertensive Effects. Blood pressure increases in some women who take oral contraceptives. Usually this is rapidly reversible once the pill is discontinued, but it can lead to permanent complications if the blood pressure elevation is high enough or persists for some time. In normotensive women, it is difficult to predict who will develop hypertension, so blood pressure monitoring is essential for all pill users. One study based on a sample of 2700 black women found that black women are less prone to develop clinical hypertension than are white women. However, all the women in the study were under the age of 35, most had higher baseline blood pressures than white women of similar ages, and almost all were taking pills with 50 mcg of estrogen. Those women in both study and control groups who did have significant blood pressure elevations (20 mm or more increase in diastolic pressure) were those who had gained the most weight in the 2-year study period.[12]

Liver and Gallbladder Effects.
Changes in liver function due to oral contraceptives are related to estrogen dosage levels and apparently are reversible. An increased risk of liver adenomas develops after 5 years of pill use; it is predominantly associated with mestranol (an estrogen).[13] The incidence of these benign tumors is about 3 to 4 per 100,000 long-term pill users; death, which is rare, is caused by internal bleeding.[14] An increase in gallbladder disease among pill users was reported in the early 1970s, but the Walnut Creek Contraceptive Drug Study, a prospective study by the federal government, has not yet confirmed this association.[10]

Carbohydrate Metabolism.
About 20% to 25% of women taking oral contraceptives have elevated fasting blood sugar, and an additional 20% show abnormal glucose tolerance test curves. Human growth hormone is significantly increased with a compensatory increase in insulin, which usually allows women to maintain a normal glucose tolerance test even though blood sugar levels are increased. A history of diabetes or the presence of obesity places women at a greater risk for abnormalities of carbohydrate metabolism with pill use. Although short-term studies show reversal of these changes after discontinuation of oral contraceptives, the long-term effects have not been established.

Lipids.
Increases in plasma triglycerides and phospholipids among women taking the pill are related to dosage levels of estrogen. Increased hepatic production of lipids may possibly be involved, and although the long-term effects are not yet known, it is speculated that these changes may be associated with cardiovascular disease and acute vascular accidents.[15]

Fetal Abnormalities.
Although there appears to be no increase in fetal abnormalities among women who have used oral contraceptives prior to conception, studies have indicated an association between use of progestins in the first 4 months of pregnancy and congenital heart and limb reduction defects. There was a 4.7-fold increase in the risk of limb reduction defects in infants exposed to sex hormones *in utero*, including oral contraceptives, hormone withdrawal tests for pregnancy, and treatment for threatened abortion.[16] Cardiovascular malformations occurred at an increased rate of 8.6 per 1000 among infants of women receiving progestins only during pregnancy.[17] These concerns are reflected in physician labeling and client warnings that are now required by the FDA when progestational drugs are used during pregnancy.

A long-term, prospective British study found that pill users have no higher risk than other women of bearing a low-birth-weight or malformed infant or of having a stillbirth, miscarriage, or ectopic pregnancy.[18]

Cancer.
Considerable evidence suggests that oral contraceptives protect users against both ovarian and endometrial cancer. The study by the Centers for Disease Control (CDC) in Atlanta found pill users to be 40% less likely to develop ovarian cancer and 50% less likely to develop endometrial cancer than those who had never used the pill. The protective effect persisted for 10 or more years after discontinuing oral contraceptives.[19,20] The CDC study also found that pill use does not seem to increase the risk of breast cancer. Women with a family history of breast cancer and women with fibrocystic breast disease are not at increased risk for breast cancer if they use oral contraceptives.[21]

Other studies either have supported the protective effect of oral contraceptives against ovarian, breast, and endometrial cancer or have not found evidence of an increased incidence with pill use.[22–24]

Evaluation and Reassessment

Clients on the pill should undergo regular checkups every 6 months. The initial visit should include assessment of the client for contraindications to the pill, a blood pressure determination, Pap smear, hematocrit or hemoglobin, and urinalysis, and, when circumstances dictate, a culture for gonorrhea and a serologic test for syphilis. An alternate method of birth control should be reviewed thoroughly, in case the client discontinues the pill without consulting the physician.

In many family-planning centers, an early follow-up visit after 6 to 12 weeks is suggested. At that time, evidence of side-effects and the client's general attitude are reviewed, with specific questions about headaches, blurred vision, chest pain, and leg pain, as well as a blood pressure check and an evaluation to be sure the pills are being taken correctly.

Teaching clients the "ACHES" system of remembering early danger signs is an effective method. Some women may experience these symptoms for weeks or months before seeking help. Women should call the clinic or physician right away if any of these danger signals develop (see Client Education: "ACHES" System: Pill danger signs).

When the pill is discontinued, ovulation and menstruation will usually return by the next monthly cycle. Some women, however, may experience a delay in ovulation and, therefore, menstruation for several months. There is no evidence that future pregnancies are affected by the prior use of oral contraceptives.

Intrauterine Device

Use of the IUD (actually an ancient practice but only recently validated scientifically) involves inserting a small, usually flexible appliance into the uterine cavity (Figs. 14-1 and 14-2) that remains in the uterus for as long as contraception is desired. Devices have been made in various shapes (spirals, loops, rings) and of various materials (plastic tubing, nylon thread, stainless steel). The only IUD presently used is Progestasert. Although the mechanism by which these appliances pre-vent conception is not completely understood, there appears to be a local inflammatory effect on the endometrium making it unfavorable to implantation or causing cytolysis. An immunologic antifertility mechanism may also be operating, or a dislodging effect may occur mechanically.

IUDs have about 97% maximum effectiveness and 93% typical effectiveness. They rank second only to the oral contraceptives in the protection they afford. The advantages of IUDs are that they are inexpensive and, once inserted, require no further attention, provided they remain in place. The main drawback of the appliances is that they are frequently expelled and at times cause bleeding and cramps, requiring that they be removed. Spontaneous expulsion or necessary removal occurs in 15% to 20% of clients.

Many commonly used IUDs have a nylon string attached. This serves two purposes: it aids in removal, and it allows the client to check for its presence by palpating the strings at the cervix. The nurse should emphasize to the client that it is important to check for the presence of the IUD before each sexual exposure during the first several months of use. Beyond this time the chance of spontaneous expulsion without the client's knowledge is reduced, and it is at this time that the quoted 97% rate of effectiveness is valid.

The metallic copper in some IUDs appears to be associated with a lower expulsion rate and an increased effectiveness. The copper is slowly delivered from the device into the uterine fluid. For this reason, it was recommended that the copper device be replaced every 2 to 4 years. IUDs that contain progesterone slowly release the hormone from the device to provide a local effect on the endometrium; this is also reported to increase effectiveness. However, these types have to be replaced at intervals because the progesterone gradually disperses.

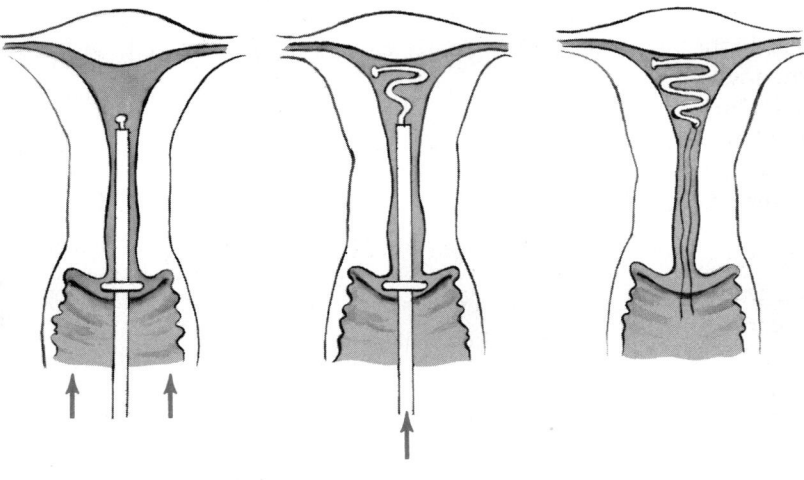

A   **B**   **C**

FIGURE 14-1

The Lippes loop is inserted by a health-care provider. (*A*) The inserter is placed in position with the stopcock at the external cervical os. (*B*) The plunger is advanced and the IUD is released into the uterine cavity. (*C*) The inserter is removed when the IUD is in place in the uterine cavity with strings protruding from the external cervical os. (Whitley N: A Manual of Clinical Obstetrics. Philadelphia, JB Lippincott, 1985)

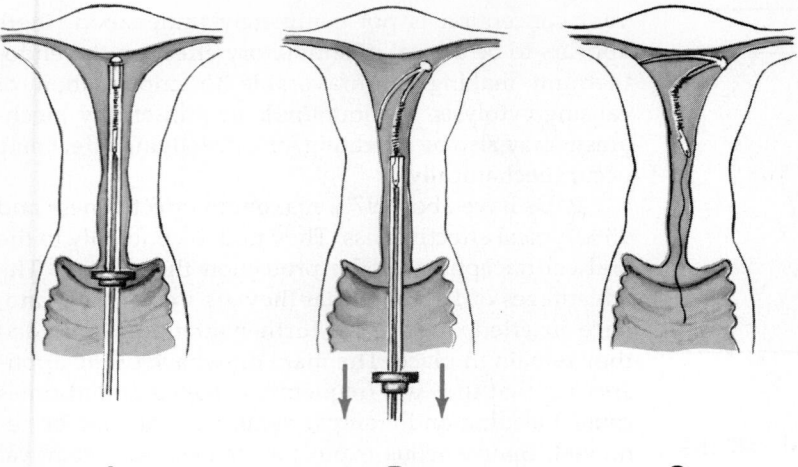

A   **B**   **C**

FIGURE 14-2

The Cu-7 is inserted by a health-care provider. (*A*) The inserter is in position with the stopcock at the external cervical os. (*B*) The plunger is held steady while the inserter is withdrawn, thus releasing the IUD into the uterine cavity. (*C*) With the inserter removed, the IUD fully expands in place in the uterine cavity with string protruding from the external cervical os. (Whitley N: A Manual of Clinical Obstetrics. Philadelphia, JB Lippincott, 1985)

Contraindications and Side-Effects

The major contraindications to IUDs include active pelvic infection, recent or chronic pelvic infection, postpartum endometritis or septic abortion, pregnancy, endometrial hyperplasia or carcinoma, and abnormalities of the uterus, such as myomatosis, polyps, or bicornate uterus, making insertion problematic. In women with a small uterus (sounding to less than 6 cm) or with marked anteflexion or retroflexion, insertion is more difficult but may be accomplished with the smaller devices.

Commonly reported side-effects of the IUD include increased menstrual flow, dysmenorrhea, and intermenstrual spotting. Since flow is sometimes excessive, clients should be checked routinely for anemia. They should be instructed to report any fever, pelvic pain or tenderness, or unusual vaginal bleeding because these may be signs of pelvic infection. If pregnancy occurs when the IUD is in place, removal is recommended. An increased danger of intrapartum infection and deaths from sepsis has been reported among clients whose IUD was allowed to remain in place during pregnancy. The risk of spontaneous abortion is somewhat higher when the IUD remains in place (about 50%) than when it is removed at the time pregnancy is discovered (25%).

Uterine infections pose a special problem when an IUD is present. As many as 95% of IUD users who abort show signs of infection. Pelvic inflammatory diseases account for the majority of IUD-related deaths and hospitalizations. Women with a Dalkon Shield are at significantly increased risk of infection (the Dalkon Shield was removed from the market several years ago, but a number of women still have these in place). The IUD is usually removed when infection occurs, to prevent persistent smoldering infection and reduce the risk of serious complications.[6,25]

Another major complication is uterine perforation, which usually occurs at the time the IUD is inserted.

When perforation occurs through the uterine wall into the abdomen, it is generally recommended that the IUD be removed. This can be done with the use of a laparoscope, avoiding an exploratory laparotomy.

Occasionally on insertion, the IUD may produce enough pain and stimulation to result in syncope. The nurse should be aware of this complication and should be ready to place the client in a recumbent position if there are any signs of lightheadedness, sweating, or nausea.

Ectopic pregnancy also may be related to the use of an IUD. The incidence of ectopic pregnancy is considerably higher with the Progesterone T (Progestasert) IUD than with unmedicated or copper-containing IUDs. About 3% to 4% of women with unmedicated or copper IUDs who become pregnant have ectopic pregnancies, as compared with about 16% ectopic pregnancies with the progesterone IUD or no contraception. The FDA has alerted health professionals to carefully evaluate clients who become pregnant with progesterone IUDs in place to determine if the pregnancies are ectopic.[26]

Nurses should teach clients the "PAINS" system of recognizing early danger signs of the IUD. A late or

---

CLIENT EDUCATION

"PAINS" System: IUD Danger Signs

P   Period late, or skipped period

A   Abdominal pain (severe)

I   Increased temperature (fever), chills

N   Noticeable vaginal discharge, foul-smelling discharge

S   Spotting, bleeding, heavy periods, clots (unusual)

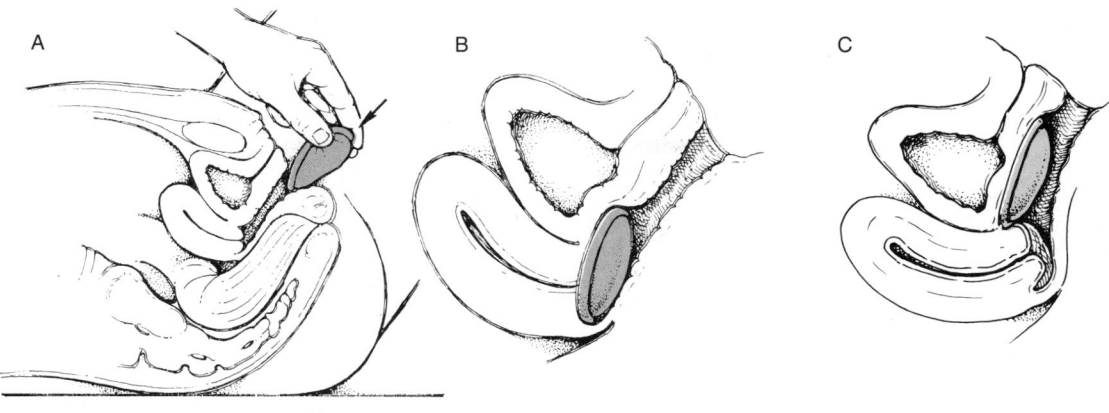

FIGURE 14-3

User method of manual insertion of diaphragm. (*A*) Prior to insertion, contraceptive cream or jelly is placed over the dome around the edges of the diaphragm. Plastic inserters are also available for ease of insertion of the diaphragm. (*B*) Diaphragm proper position. (*C*) Diaphragm positioned improperly.

absent menstrual period, abdominal pain, fever, a foul vaginal discharge, and spotting or bleeding that is unusual or very heavy may signal complications. The physician or clinic should be contacted if any of these danger signs develop (see Client Education: "PAINS" System: IUD danger signs).

Diaphragm

The diaphragm, a dome-shaped rubber cap ranging in diameter from 7 cm to 10 cm, is inserted into the vagina and over the anterior vaginal wall and cervix prior to intercourse (Fig. 14-3). The diaphragm, by itself, is not a contraceptive device; it must be used with a spermi-

cidal jelly or cream that is placed in the diaphragm between it and the cervix. The use of the diaphragm ensures the placement of spermicidal jelly over the cervix (Fig. 14-4).

When the diaphragm is properly used—each time intercourse occurs, without exception—it is associated with a failure rate of two to three pregnancies during the first year per 100 women, which is a very acceptable rate. In practice, however, the overall failure rate varies from 13 to 19 pregnancies during the first year per 100 women. This may be a result of inconsistent use. A diaphragm requires motivation and premeditation, but despite these drawbacks it has again gained favor as some of the disadvantages of the pill and IUD are weighed.

Advantages of the diaphragm include safety, few

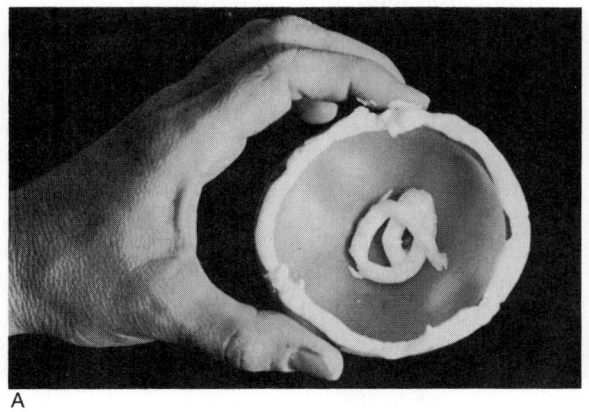
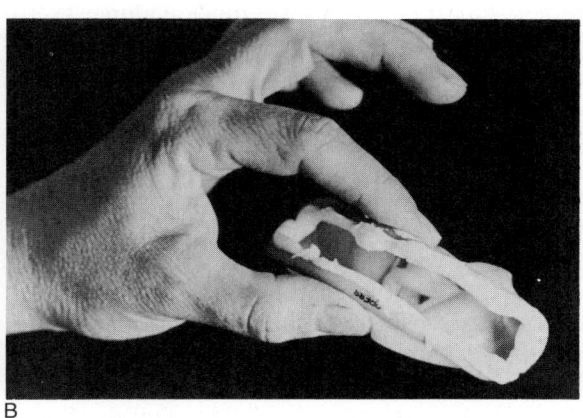

FIGURE 14-4

(*A*) Diaphragm with spermicidal cream applied. (*B*) Compressed diaphragm that is ready for manual insertion.

CLIENT EDUCATION

Instructions for Inserting and Removing Diaphragm

1. When being fitted for a diaphragm, practice insertion and removal several times before leaving the physician's office or clinic and have the provider check your placement of the diaphragm after practice. If the diaphragm feels uncomfortable, or if you think it may be too small or too large, return to the office with it in place for a reexamination.
2. Apply contraceptive jelly or cream by holding the diaphragm with the dome down, like a cup. Place about one tablespoon of cream or jelly into the dome and spread a thin layer around the rim also. The cream or jelly remains an active spermicide for up to 6 hours, so the diaphragm can be inserted well before intercourse.
3. With the dome down, insert the diaphragm by squeezing the opposite sides of the rim together. Spread the lips of the labia with one hand and insert the folded diaphragm with the other. The best positions for insertion are standing with one foot propped up, squatting, or lying down. Push the diaphragm downward into the vagina as far back as it will go, then tuck the front rim up behind the pubic bone inside the vagina. Check for proper placement by feeling for the cervix, which should be covered by the rubber dome of the diaphragm.
4. If you have intercourse more than once, you must apply more spermicidal cream or jelly with an applicator before each act of intercourse. Do not remove the diaphragm, but place the cream or jelly in front of it. You may use condoms for subsequent intercourse instead of more applications of spermicide.
5. After intercourse, the diaphragm must be left in place for 6 to 8 hours. Do not douche during this time.
6. Remove the diaphragm by placing your index finger behind the front rim and pulling down and out. If the suction is tight, insert a finger between the diaphragm and the pubic bone to break suction. If the rim is hard to reach, bear down to bring it forward. Be careful not to puncture the diaphragm with long fingernails.
7. After use, clean the diaphragm with soap and water, rinse thoroughly, and dry with a towel. You may dust it with cornstarch, but do not use talcum or perfumed powder, as these damage the diaphragm and may irritate the vagina and cervix. Store the diaphragm in its plastic container in a cool, dry place.
8. Inspect the diaphragm each time you use it for tears or holes. Do not use petroleum jelly, as it can cause deterioration of the rubber of the diaphragm. Use K–Y Jelly or spermicidal jelly for additional lubrication. The diaphragm will become darker, mottled brown over time, but will last several years if properly cared for.
9. Have your diaphragm fitting checked if you gain or lose more than 10 to 20 pounds, have a pregnancy or abortion, have pelvic surgery, if the diaphragm causes discomfort or pain, or if you think it is too large or too small.

side-effects, and flexibility according to frequency of intercourse. Since it can be inserted up to 2 hours before sex, it is relatively separated from coitus. Once in place it is unobtrusive, as its presence cannot be felt by either partner if it is properly fitted, and less cream or jelly is left in the vagina than with a spermicide alone. Well-motivated women have used the diaphragm effectively to limit pregnancies since the end of the 19th century.

A common objection to the diaphragm is the vaginal manipulation necessary for insertion, a procedure which is repugnant to some women. This problem is easily solved if the client is fitted with a flat or coil-spring diaphragm (in contrast to the arc flex diaphragm). These diaphragms may be used with an "inserter," which allows the client to insert it like a tampon, without touching the genital area (Fig. 14-5). The arc flex diaphragm cannot be used with an inserter. It was designed for ease of manual insertion and may, in some cases, give a better fit in the presence of a mild cystocele. Some women after one or more pregnancies cannot be fitted with a diaphragm.

One of the stated disadvantages of prescribing a diaphragm is the office time consumed during fitting and instruction on its use. Increasingly, the nurse is called upon to play an active role in both. Sample diaphragms or rings of known size are inserted until a size is found that will cover the cervix and fit snugly behind the symphysis pubis (Fig. 14-6). The client is asked to remove the diaphragm by hooking a finger over it just beneath the symphysis and then to reinsert it (Fig. 14-7). Before the client leaves the office, she should be able to insert and remove the diaphragm with ease. She should be instructed to always use a spermicidal cream or jelly around the rim and in the dome of the diaphragm. If intercourse occurs a second or third time, additional spermicidal agent should be inserted for added protection. The diaphragm should be left in place for at least 6 hours following intercourse. A douche is recommended after removal to cleanse the remaining jelly or cream.

The diaphragm may be an excellent contraceptive for younger, nulliparous women who do not have intercourse with great regularity. In a study at the Sanger Bureau in New York, involving 2175 women over 2 years, an actual failure rate of two pregnancies per 100 users per year was documented. Significantly, most of the women in the study were under 30 (80%) and were unmarried (70%).[27] Proper fitting (a flat or coil-spring

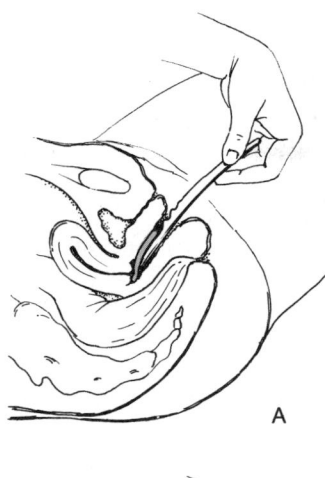

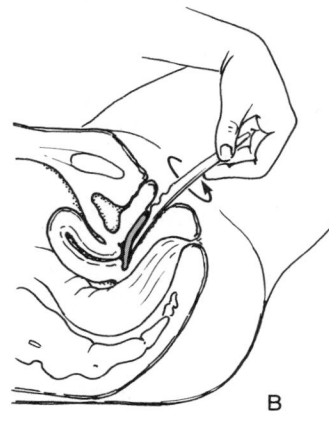

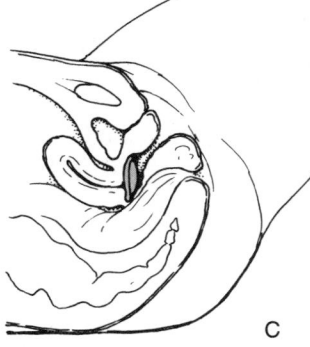

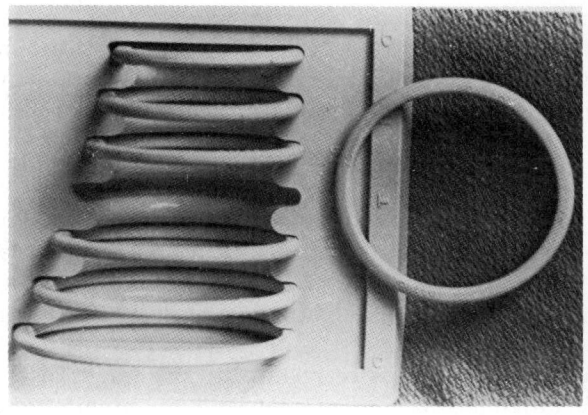

FIGURE 14-6

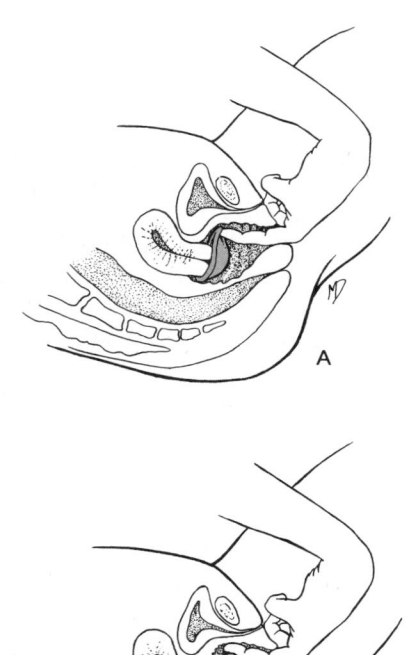

FIGURE 14-5

Personal use of an inserter to position the diaphragm minimizes genital touching and may be easier for some women. (*A*) The inserter with diaphragm in place is positioned deep in the posterior fornix. (*B*) The inserter is twisted to release the diaphragm. (*C*) The diaphragm is pushed behind the symphysis pubis with a finger; here it is correctly positioned over the cervix. (Whitley N: A Manual of Clinical Obstetrics. Philadelphia, JB Lippincott, 1985)

FIGURE 14-7

Removal of diaphragm. (*A*) A finger is hooked around the diaphragm rim just below the symphysis pubis; diaphragm is pulled forward. (*B*) Alternate method in which a finger is slipped between the diaphragm rim and the symphysis pubis; diaphragm is pulled forward. (Whitley N: A Manual of Clinical Obstetrics. Philadelphia, JB Lippincott, 1985)

diaphragm is generally better for women with firm vaginal tone), thorough contraceptive counseling, and unhurried positive education and practice in insertion and removal are the key factors in the success of this method.

Side-Effects and Complications

Although there are few serious complications with use of the diaphragm, studies have reported several cases of toxic shock syndrome (TSS) occurring immediately after diaphragm use.[6] Recurrent cystitis can occur owing to upward pressure of the diaphragm rim against the urethra, and cramps or rectal pressure might also be felt. Often the diaphragm is too large or too small when these occur. Some women or their partners have allergic reactions to rubber or spermicides. Vaginitis or foul vaginal discharge may be caused by spermicide or leaving the diaphragm in the vagina too long.

Cervical Cap

The cervical cap resembles a diaphragm that is small and has a tall dome (Fig. 14-8). It fits snugly over the cervix and is held in place by suction between its firm but flexible rim and the cervix. Although not marketed for contraceptive use in the United States, caps can be obtained through some women's health centers, college health services, and public and private clinics or offices that are participating in a research study (using protocols approved by the FDA). Caps are widely available in Europe and were developed about the same time as the diaphragm.

Cervical caps are made of impermeable plastic or soft rubber. The plastic ones can be left in place as long as 3 to 4 weeks, but the rubber ones cause a strong vaginal odor after 36 to 48 hours. Rubber caps are most commonly used, and approximately one third of the

inside of the cap is filled with spermicide. Time rules for insertion and removal are virtually the same as for diaphragms. When properly positioned, the cap is a barrier to sperm entering the cervix, producing the same contraceptive effect as the diaphragm. Insertion and removal of the cervical cap are somewhat more difficult than with the diaphragm.

Research data on effectiveness are contradictory and limited. Failure rates from 8.0 to 16 per 100 women during the first 6 to 12 months of use have been reported.[28,29] Most studies have been small and differed in criteria for acceptable cap fit, use of spermicide, and research design. Contraindications to cervical cap use include allergy to rubber or spermicide, anatomical abnormalities or variations (extremely shallow or long cervix, severe lacerations), inability to learn insertion/removal technique, lack of privacy or facilities for washing and cleaning cap, acute cervicitis, pelvic or vaginal infections, abnormal Pap smear, recent delivery or cervical surgery, and history of TSS.

Side-Effects and Complications

Although there is little published information on safety and side-effects of the cervical cap, problems may arise owing to prolonged cervical exposure to secretions, spermicide, and bacteria trapped within the cap. Trauma could result to the cervix or vagina from insertion/removal or prolonged retention of the cap. There may be interference with the normal flow of cervical mucus or menstrual blood. Clinicians providing cervical caps have observed acute pelvic infection, acute cervicitis, and development of abnormal Pap smears associated with cap use.[6] However, whether or not the cap caused these problems has not been determined. Vaginal lacerations or abrasions and chronic irritation of the vaginal mucosa have also been reported.[30]

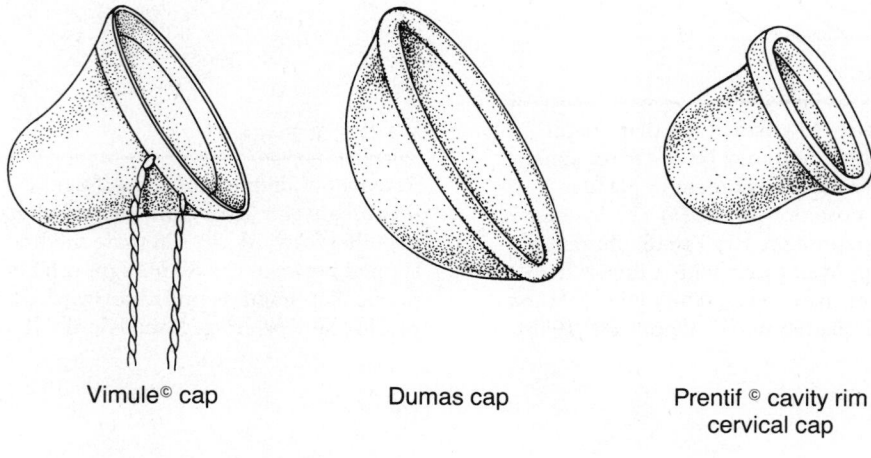

Vimule© cap   Dumas cap   Prentif © cavity rim
                                        cervical cap

FIGURE 14-8

The cervical cap fits snugly over the cervix and is held in place by suction.

Vaginal Sponge

Since ancient times, natural sea sponges have been used for contraception. In the 1970s natural collagen and synthetic sponges were developed incorporating spermicide, with eventual FDA approval in 1983 of vaginal contraceptive sponges made of polyurethane containing 1 g of nonoxynol-9 spermicide. The sponge is 2.5 cm thick and 5.5 cm in diameter, with a central dimple that fits over the cervix and reduces chances of dislodgment during intercourse. A braided cord is attached to the other side and is used to remove the sponge. Sponges must be soaked in water before inserting and may be left in place for 24 to 30 hours (Fig. 14-9).

The sponge exerts its contraceptive effect by providing a barrier between sperm and the cervix, by trapping sperm within the sponge, and by releasing spermicide at a steady rate while in place. After use, it is discarded. No additional spermicide is needed for repeated intercourse. Sponges are available without prescription as an over-the-counter item.

Studies on effectiveness indicate wide ranges: between 3 and 16 pregnancies per 100 women over 6 to 12 months.[31,32] After 6 months of use, effectiveness improves. The main problems reported with sponge use are difficulty removing it from the vagina, unintended pregnancy, and allergic reactions. TSS is the most serious potential complication, but rates are lower with use of the sponge than with use of the diaphragm.[33] To prevent TSS, users are advised to remove sponges within 30 hours and not to use them during menstruation. Women with a history of TSS or evidence of vaginal colonization with *Staphylococcus aureus* should not use sponges.

Vaginal sponges offer some advantages common to barrier contraceptives, such as protection from sexually transmitted diseases and possibly protection against cervical neoplasia. Certain complaints about diaphragms and vaginal spermicides, such as their messiness and distastefulness, are avoided with use of sponges. Some women find sponges make the vagina dry, however, by absorbing vaginal lubrication.

Condom

Condoms ("rubbers") are thin sheaths of rubber or processed collagenous tissue that are placed over the penis to act as a mechanical barrier to prevent sperm from entering the vagina. Also effective in preventing venereal infections, condoms are a male method of contraception that has been used since ancient times. The condom is applied over the shaft of the penis after erection. Before withdrawal of the penis from the vagina, the condom should be held in place on the penis so that it does not slip off into the vagina. Some condoms are packaged with a lubricant and some have a small pouch at the tip to collect the ejaculate, which reduces the danger of tearing. In some cases, lubricants cause an irritation at the introitus and an unpleasant "stinging" sensation. In general, a lubricant should not be necessary if there is sufficient foreplay to produce the natural lubrication associated with female sexual arousal.

If it is used properly, the condom is an effective contraceptive. However, it must be applied before any penile–vaginal contact. Condoms are advantageous because they are available without a medical prescription, are easy to use, do not present any serious side-effects, are low in cost, and prevent transmission of sexual infections.

The major criticism of condoms is that they decrease sensation for both partners or, more commonly, for the man. In addition, the sex act must be interrupted to apply the condom; this may be distracting for some

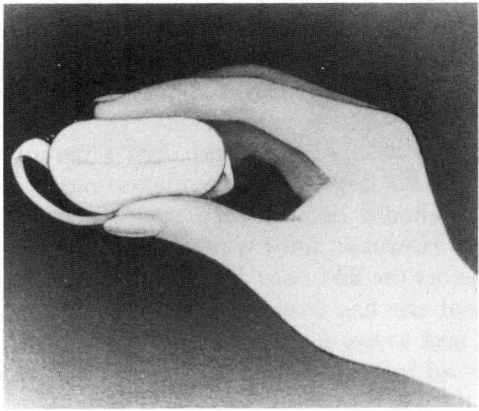
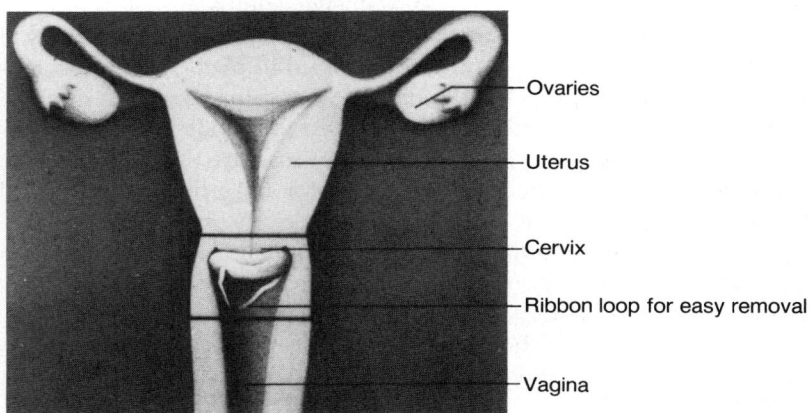

Ovaries

Uterus

Cervix

Ribbon loop for easy removal

Vagina

FIGURE 14-9

The contraceptive sponge is inserted manually by the user into the deepest part of the vagina just below the cervix. (Courtesy of *Today*)

couples. There is also frequent worry that the condom might break.

The nurse might point out that no method of contraception is perfect (all have some disadvantages for one or both partners and have some anxiety-producing aspects). If they are used before any penetration, condoms are safe and rarely break. This information will help those couples who have anxiety over other forms of contraception.

Natural Methods and Fertility Awareness

The rationale underlying natural methods of birth control based on fertility awareness is that when there are regular periods, ovulation occurs at approximately the same time in each cycle, that is, 14 days prior to the beginning of the next cycle. The ovum is capable of being fertilized only for a period of 48 hours at the most after ovulation. Theoretically, therefore, abstinence from sexual intercourse on that day and for the 2 days before and after (a total of 5 days) should forestall conception.

In actual experience, however, even normal, regular cycles can be off by 1 or 2 days in either direction (*e.g.*, 28 ± 2 days). This puts the day of ovulation in the same 4-day range ± 2 days, and the period of abstinence must then be at least 8 days. Because of the normal variability of menstrual cycles, however, the interval of fertility will often be as long as 15 or more days, or about half of the cycle.

There are three basic variations of natural methods of birth control. One is based on calendar calculations of ovulation, another on use of a record of the basal body temperature (BBT) to determine ovulation, and the last on noting changes in the condition of cervical mucus for this purpose. Advantages of these methods are that they are devoid of any side-effects that may be caused by introduction of drugs or substances into or on the body, they are relatively inexpensive, they are acceptable to religious groups that oppose other contraceptive methods, and they are very helpful in planning pregnancy owing to the familiarity with signs of fertility that results. Disadvantages of these methods include the need to keep records for several menstrual cycles before they can be used, the need for diligent record keeping to ensure accuracy, the necessity for considerable initial and ongoing counseling in their use, a restriction of sexual spontaneity, and the need for abstinence or use of another contraceptive method for a considerable portion of the cycle. The inability of some women to recognize cervical mucus changes, and the problem of irregular cycles make cervical mucus, calendar, and BBT methods difficult and unreliable.

Another consideration is the failure rates of these methods, which in actual use are in the range of 21 to 25 pregnancies per 100 women per year. Should pregnancy occur, there is increased risk that an "old" egg will be fertilized. When the ovum and sperm are at their outer limits of functioning, some deterioration has occurred and there are associated increases in fetal abnormalities from such fertilizations.[34] The longevity of sperm adds to this problem; sperm have been found in cervical mucus as long as 7 days after ejaculation.

Calendar Method

A menstrual calendar in which the woman records the length of each menstrual cycle over an 8-month span must be kept. With the first day of bleeding counted as day 1, the earliest fertile day is computed by subtracting 18 days from the length of the shortest cycle. Subtract 11 days from the length of the longest cycle to determine the latest day of fertility. These two numbers represent the beginning and end of the fertile period. During these days, intercourse must be avoided or another method of birth control used (Table 14-5).

This method is more effective if the woman has regular cycles and if intercourse is avoided (or other forms of contraception are used) through the entire first part of the menstrual cycle until the last fertile day. Women who are younger and postpartum, postabortion, and premenopausal women often have irregular menstrual cycles, so this method may be contraindicated unless it is the only acceptable method. In this case, it should be supplemented by the BBT or cervical mucus method to increase effectiveness.

Basal Body Temperature Method

The resting temperature or BBT of a fertile woman normally rises each cycle just after ovulation. It will then remain higher until the next menstrual period begins. Most women can observe this temperature change if they take and record their temperature every day with a special thermometer before they get out of bed or begin any kind of activity, including smoking. The thermometer can be used orally or rectally and should be left in place a full 5 minutes. It is recorded on a special BBT chart (see Chap. 9, Assessment Tools).

There is usually a slight drop and then a rise of about 0.4 degree to 0.8 degree when ovulation has occurred. This rise should be sustained until the next menstrual period. However, some women have no preliminary drop before the BBT rises. Because the woman cannot know that she has ovulated until after it has happened, it is best to use another method of contraception or to avoid intercourse the entire first part of the cycle until the sustained rise in BBT is seen. The fertile period can be assumed to end after the BBT has remained elevated for 3 full days.

Many factors such as illness, nightmares, and

TABLE 14-5

Calculating the Interval of Fertility

No. of Days Shortest Cycle	First Fertile Day	No. of Days Longest Cycle	Last Fertile Day
21	3rd day	21	10th day
22	4th day	22	11th day
23	5th day	23	12th day
24	6th day	24	13th day
25	7th day	25	14th day
26	8th day	26	15th day
27	9th day	27	16th day
28	10th day	28	17th day
29	11th day	29	18th day
30	12th day	30	19th day
31	13th day	31	20th day
32	14th day	32	21st day
33	15th day	33	22nd day
34	16th day	34	23rd day
35	17th day	35	24th day

changes in daily schedule can influence the BBT. When the pattern of rise is not clear or sustained, it is advisable to assume it is not safe to have intercourse. This method is more effective when combined with the calendar or mucus methods, which give earlier signs that ovulation is near.

Cervical Mucus Method

Many women can observe physiological changes relating to ovulation that help determine when their fertile period begins. Changes in the character and appearance of cervical mucus occur just before ovulation in some women. In addition, ovulatory pain may be experienced. Characteristically, in the ovulatory cycle there is a rapid increase in the quantity of cervical mucus just prior to ovulation. At that time, the mucus becomes clear and stringy. The woman may observe the presence of such mucus at the introitus or may wipe the cervix to obtain a sample for observation. Subsequent to ovulation, mucus becomes more viscous. When this change is associated with a rise in temperature, it is assumed that ovulation has occurred.

The woman must be careful not to confuse other substances in the vagina, such as semen, lubricants, spermicides, and discharges due to infections, with cervical mucus at midcycle. Women who douche cannot observe changes because they wash the mucus away. This method is more effective when intercourse is restricted to the postovulatory phase of the cycle and

when it is used in combination with the calendar or the BBT method.

Women need to observe their mucus changes for several cycles before relying upon this method. They need to check vaginal secretions several times a day and record the most fertile observation for that day. The peak of fertility occurs when the vagina feels very wet and mucus is abundant, clear, slippery, and very stretchable (can be stretched 3–4 inches between the thumb and forefinger). When this type of mucus has decreased and is no longer detectable, there may be thick, cloudy, sticky mucus or no mucus. When this change is observed, the women is no longer fertile.

Jellies, Creams, Suppositories, and Foams

Spermicidal agents are inexpensive and available without consulting a physician. However, they are relatively ineffective, because the woman cannot be sure of their placement or retention (Fig. 14-10). For proper use, the spermicidal agent should be inserted vaginally no more than one half hour before intercourse; a separate application must be made for each act of intercourse. In addition, the woman should not douche for at least 8 hours after intercourse. The aerosol foams expand rapidly when inserted, covering the vaginal folds and seeming to disappear. They also leave less vaginal residual than jellies or creams, which take longer to spread over the vaginal surface.

The major disadvantage of spermicides is their low effectiveness when used alone. Many couples find them aesthetically unpleasant, and there is limited usefulness for repeated acts of intercourse. However, these preparations are particularly useful as short-term contraceptives. During the postpartum period, spermicides are useful until the 6-weeks checkup, when a more effective method can be instituted. They are frequently recommended for 2 weeks to 1 month after insertion of an IUD or initiation of an oral contraceptive regimen, as a precaution before these methods should be relied on alone. When the pill or IUD is discontinued, spermicides can be used for a few cycles until another method is begun or pregnancy is attempted.

Withdrawal

Withdrawal, or *coitus interruptus,* is an extensively used method of contraception and appears to be satisfactory for some couples. However, withdrawal as a method of contraception is a compromise at best. It requires concentration and willpower on the part of the male and trust on the part of the female. This trust is not always well founded and creates anxiety. Neither of these factors is conducive to relaxation and pleasure

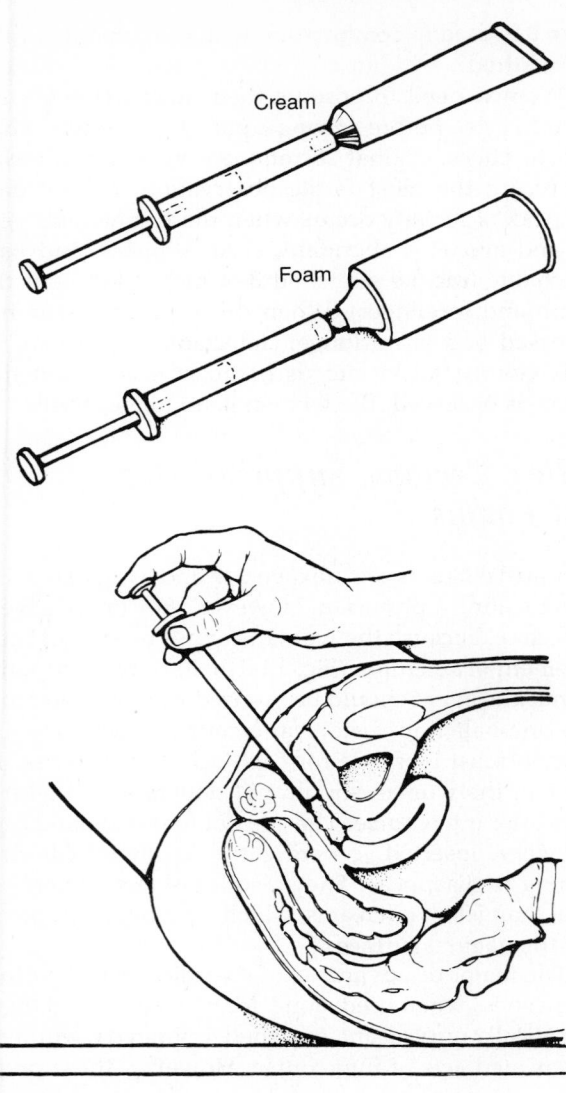

Cream

Foam

FIGURE 14-10

The user inserts foam or cream near the cervix.

and may leave the couple with a distorted idea of what sexual pleasure is or can be. Also, preejaculatory secretion may contain motile spermatozoa, especially when there has been prolonged erection.

Withdrawal is one of the more ineffective contraceptive methods, with a failure rate of about 16 to 25 pregnancies per 100 women per year. However, it is always available and costs nothing. This method, often used by young people just beginning their sexual activities, can contribute to later sexual difficulties through a conditioning process. When intercourse occurs in circumstances associated with haste, fear, and guilt, and withdrawal is used in a way that interferes with communication and fulfillment, patterns of premature ejaculation in the male and orgasmic dysfunction in the female may be established.

Unreliable Approaches

Douching after intercourse is actually not a contraceptive method. Sperm enter the cervix within 20 seconds of ejaculation, and it is highly unlikely that douching could occur before this time. The douche must simply be considered a method of cleansing the vagina or a means of inserting a medicated solution to treat vaginal infections.

Lactation has been considered a method of postponing pregnancy by delaying ovulation. It is widely used in developing countries with some effectiveness for varying periods of months, which is probably related to the nutritional status of the mother. However, in the United States, women generally have good nutrition, and the lactation period is shorter because infants are given formula supplements and solid foods at an earlier age. These factors contribute to an earlier and unpredictable return of fertility, making breast-feeding an unreliable approach to contraception.

Postpartal Contraception

In the absence of complications, intercourse is commonly resumed 2 weeks to 3 weeks following delivery. The practice of advising couples to abstain from intercourse for 6 weeks has generally been discarded because there is no reason to avoid sex once lochia has ceased and the episiotomy is adequately healed. Although the incidence of ovulation within the first 6 weeks post partum is small, fertility does occasionally return and women are well advised to use a contraceptive method during this time. The condom is probably the most practical method to use during this period because it does not involve introducing chemicals into the vagina. However, spermicidal foams and creams are frequently advised, either in combination with the condom or alone, if the condom is unacceptable. If foams and creams are not used too early in the postpartum period, there does not appear to be a problem with infection.

Insertion of an IUD within the first 6 weeks post partum is generally not recommended, since the expulsion and infection rates are higher during this time. Estrogen-containing oral contraceptives are contraindicated because of the increased incidence of thromboembolic complications associated with their use in the postpartum period. Nursing mothers are usually advised to use progestin-only oral contraceptives because lactation may be suppressed with estrogen, particularly higher-dose pills. Synthetic hormones are excreted in breast milk, but the amount that actually passes through the milk is very small (approximately one fifth to one tenth of the mother's dose). Although not known for certain, it is presumed that hormonal contraceptives pose no hazard to infants if these contain 2.5 mg or less of progestogen and 50 mcg or less of estradiol or 100 mcg or less of mestranol.[6]

Generally the progestin-only pill (minipill) is the best hormonal contraceptive during the postpartal and breast-feeding phases. Minipills may be given immediately post partum or at the 6-weeks checkup. These pills have little effect on lactation and do not pose thromboembolic risks. The American Academy of Pediatrics has approved use of combined pills in breast-feeding women, however, once lactation is well established.[35]

Sterilization

Vasectomy in the male and tubal ligation in the female are being used with increasing frequency as a means of limiting family size. Approximately 61% of contraceptive users in the United States intending no additional births depended on sterilization in 1982, compared with 36% in 1973.[4] For married couples over 30, sterilization is the most common means of birth control. Since both tubal ligation and vasectomy are permanent methods of contraception, the decision to undergo these procedures must be very carefully considered. In many settings, the role of the nurse in the decision-making process is pivotal. The counselor is responsible for making sure that both husband and wife are aware that these methods are considered irreversible. Total family circumstances that could influence the decision should be reviewed in depth, and such factors as the number of children, stability of the marriage, age of marital partners, and ability to use nonpermanent methods should be considered. The following laws and regulations are important in counseling couples about sterilization:

- Strict adherence to informed consent procedures and voluntary choice are absolutely essential, both legally and practically.
- There is no legal requirement for partner consent.
- When federal funds are used, clients must be 21 years old and mentally competent.
- Federal and some state regulations relating to use of Medicaid funds for sterilization require prescribed waiting periods of various lengths after counseling and before the procedure can be performed.[6]

Vasectomy

The *vas deferens* is a tube that leads from the testis to the urethra in the male and carries spermatozoa from the testis to the urethra. It is a firm structure somewhat less than 0.5 cm in diameter that can be felt bilaterally in the scrotum, lateral to the base of the penis. *Vasectomy*

involves surgical interruption and ligation of the vas and is a relatively minor operation. It can be carried out under local anesthesia and is associated with minimal risk and only slight morbidity. It is a simple procedure that takes about 15 minutes and can be done on an outpatient basis (Fig. 14-11).

The major disadvantage is that it is permanent. Although surgical methods have been developed to re-anastomose the ligated vas, the success rate is variable. Anatomical success ranges between 40% and 90%, but clinical success (pregnancy, normal active sperm in ejaculate) is only 18% to 60%.[6] Successful reanastomosis of the vas depends upon the type of initial procedure and the training and skill of the surgeon. The length of vas removed, use of coagulation, type of ligature, and amount of time between vasectomy and the reversal procedure all affect outcome.

Over half of the men with vasectomies develop sperm antibodies, but there is no physiological evidence of pathologic complications from this. Limited animal studies found that monkeys developed atherosclerotic plaques after vasectomy, and these were attributed to sperm antibodies. The reliability of these studies and their applicability to humans are questionable. Human studies have found no connection between vasectomy and plaques.[36]

Vasectomy failure is the result of recannalization of the ends of the ligated vas and occurs in 0.15 per 100 cases. Additional pregnancies occur following vasectomy when unprotected intercourse takes place before the male reproductive tract is cleared of spermatozoa. Couples must be advised that the first few post-vasectomy ejaculates contain active spermatozoa. Except for the absence of spermatozoa, vas ligation does not affect the ejaculate itself, nor does it affect the ejaculatory process.

The fear of a reduction of potency or masculinity prevents many men from accepting vasectomy. However, the vast majority of men who have had vasectomies are satisfied with their decision and report that sexual performance is unchanged. Less than 2% report decreased sexual pleasure or other dissatisfaction with vasectomy.

Tubal Ligation

Tubal ligation is designed to eliminate the tubal conduit that spermatozoa and ova pass through. A number of approaches have been used to interrupt the continuity of the fallopian tubes (Fig. 14-12). The procedure may be carried out by way of an abdominal incision and is commonly done along with cesarean section or in the first few postpartal hours. Many workers in family planning feel that women should be encouraged not to accept a permanent form of contraception during emo-

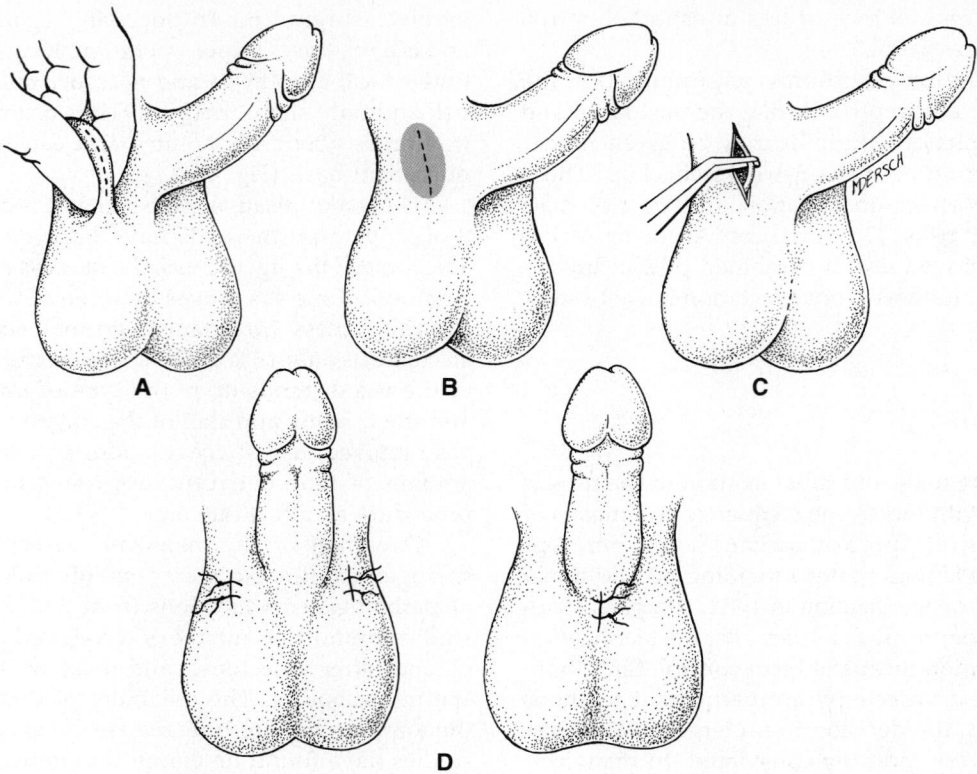

FIGURE 14-11

Vasectomy procedure. (*A*) The vas deferens is identified. (*B*) A small area of the skin and subcutaneous tissue is anesthetized. (*C*) The vas deferens is isolated from surrounding tissue and lifted through the incision. (*D*) Skin sutures showing one- and two-incision approaches.

tionally charged intervals in their lives. An "on the spot" decision to have a tubal sterilization following an abortion or delivery should be explored with great care.

Coagulation and interruption of the fallopian tubes can be carried out using a *laparoscopic approach* (Fig. 14-13). In some centers this procedure is carried out under local anesthesia, but often a general anesthetic is used. After the abdomen is distended with carbon dioxide, the laparoscopic trocar is introduced through a small incision in the umbilicus. The laparoscope is then passed into the peritoneal cavity. Visualization of the adnexa is usually complete. Forceps are used to grasp the fallopian tubes and the tubes are occluded using a clip, ring, or band, coagulated, or cut and tied (resection).

Because the procedure is relatively simple, it can be carried out on an outpatient basis. Although it is associated with a relatively low morbidity, the morbidity is considerably higher than for vas ligation.

The *interval minilaparotomy* is a sterilization technique in which a small suprapubic incision is usually made below the pubic hair line in order to enter the abdominal cavity. The fallopian tubes are isolated with grasping instruments and may be crushed, ligated,

embedded, clipped, or plugged as in other tubal ligation methods.

The procedure may be done under local, spinal, or general anesthesia. It is suitable for outpatient surgery (*e.g.*, in surgicenters). Women are instructed to rest for 2 days postoperatively, avoid intercourse for a week, and avoid lifting for a week. Tubal ligations may also be done vaginally, but higher complication rates (infection, hemorrhage) have discouraged widespread use in this country.

Complication rates of tubal ligation range from 0.4% to 1% and include wound infection, hematoma, uterine perforation, bladder injury, and sterilization failure. Most deaths associated with these procedures are a result of general anesthesia. Other mortality risk results from sepsis, hemorrhage, and cardiovascular events. The overall case fatality rate is reported at 3.6 per 100,000. Put in perspective, the risk of a one-time sterilization procedure is far less for a healthy woman over 35 to 40 years than that posed by use of oral contraceptives or a term pregnancy.[6]

Most women who undergo tubal ligation are satisfied with their decision, but about 10% to 15% regret

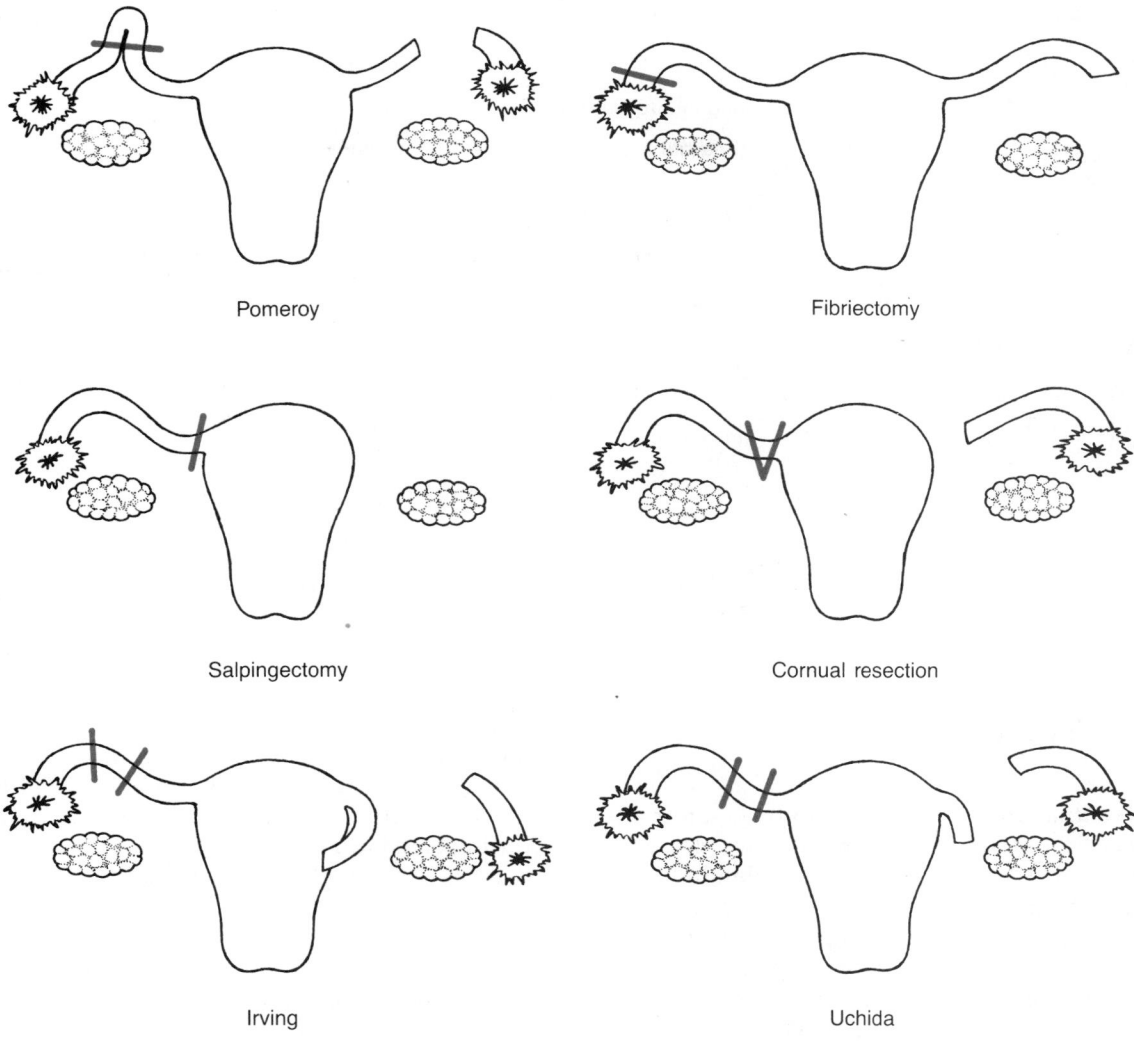

Pomeroy

Fibriectomy

Salpingectomy

Cornual resection

Irving

Uchida

FIGURE 14-12

Tubal ligation techniques interrupt the continuity of the fallopian tubes. The various techniques may be carried out through an abdominal incision. (Redrawn from Shain RN, Pauerstein CJ: Fertility Control. Hagerstown, MD, Harper & Row, 1980)

the termination of fertility or express other dissatisfactions, including diminished sexual enjoyment, dysmenorrhea, menorrhagia-metrorrhagia, and premenstrual tension. Although tubal interruption theoretically has no effects on hormone cycles, it is possible that interference with lymphatic and vascular drainage secondary to scar tissue formation could contribute to increased pelvic congestion.

Although tubal ligation must be considered a permanent method, surgical techniques have been developed to reunite the fallopian tubes. These are difficult procedures at best. The success rate is variable, depending upon the experience of the surgeon and the extent of the segment of tube that was damaged or removed. Success rates of 50% to 70% are reported by experts using careful microsurgical techniques.[6] A decision to attempt reanastomosis is usually based on social circumstances, such as the death of a child, divorce and remarriage, or an agonizing reappraisal of an earlier decision that was made in haste.

Contraceptive Research

Improvements in contraception are constantly being sought through research. The most significant trends are toward multiple options, long-term effects, simplicity and self-administration, lower doses, and additional noncontraceptive benefits.

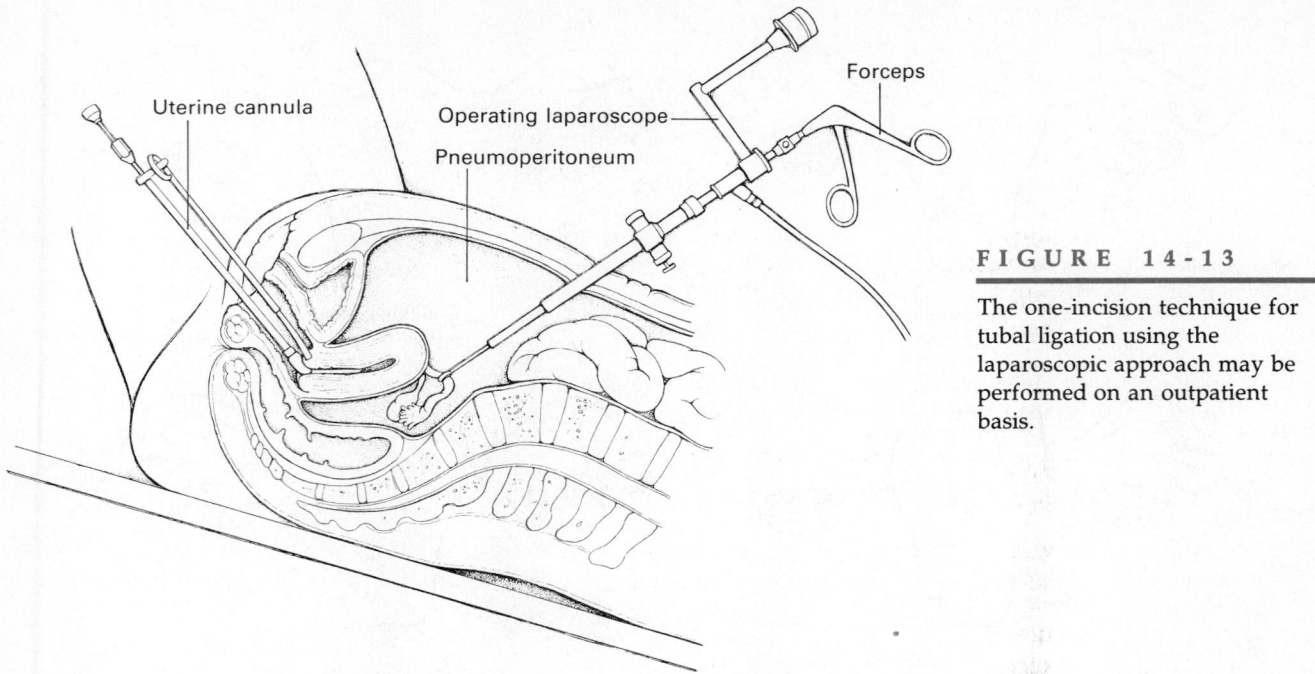

Forceps

Uterine cannula

Operating laparoscope

Pneumoperitoneum

FIGURE 14-13

The one-incision technique for tubal ligation using the laparoscopic approach may be performed on an outpatient basis.

Female Methods

Hormonal contraceptives may have improved safety and reduced cardiovascular risks through slow-release estrogen and synthesis of new analogues to diminish effect on high-density lipoprotein. Once-a-month pills, which use luteinizing hormone releasing hormone (LHRH) analogues to produce luteolysis or suppress ovulation, are under investigation. Time-release dermal implants using steroidal hormones are in advanced stages of clinical testing, but there are problems with bleeding disorders and the need for removal. More promising are steroid-releasing vaginal rings, designed to be worn intravaginally for from 3 weeks each month to 3 months continuously. These act by inhibiting ovulation and have side-effects of irregular menses and expulsion.

Prostaglandins are now used to interrupt pregnancy, and research is in progress on using analogues for menses induction, either once a month or when menses are delayed by a few days. In early first-trimester pregnancy, prostaglandins can be self-administered on an outpatient basis.

Medroxyprogesterone acetate still stirs considerable interest and research and is particularly in demand in developing countries. It is injected every 3 months and is about as effective as oral contraceptives. However, there are many side-effects, including irregular bleeding, amenorrhea, and, possibly, delayed fertility after discontinuation. Interest persists in a long-acting injectable hormonal contraceptive, but progress is slow.

IUDs of copper and silver are being clinically tested and appear to be superior to plastic ones in preventing pregnancy, avoiding expulsion, and extending continuation rates. These may have action lasting as long as 16 years.[37] New forms of IUDs might be impregnated with compounds such as diamidine instead of steroids, reducing blood loss while protecting against pregnancy.

Immunization against pregnancy is under investigation, and a vaccine has been developed for clinical testing. Antibodies produced at the onset of pregnancy are being used for a vaccine against chorionic gonadotropin (hCG), which would interfere with implantation. As subunits of hCG are characterized, more selective immunization may be possible, and vaccines against LH as well as hCG may be developed. The goal is to produce a vaccine that would be effective for at least 1 year.[37]

Immunizations against antigens of the ovum are being studied in animals. Extracts of ova antigens have been found to interfere with fertilization and hatching of the blastocyst. Antibodies against the trophoblast have produced chronic rejection of implanted embryos in animals. Human placental antigens are being tested on monkeys for similar effects.

Ovarian follicular fluid shows inhibinlike activity and might possibly interfere with FSH production (thus inhibiting ovulation) or affect ovum transport. Investigation of these effects is not expected to produce clinically useful results until between the years 1990 and 2000.

Ovulation prediction would be ideal, rather than detecting ovulation after the fact (as current fertility awareness methods do). If accurate prediction were possible, the period of abstinence would be greatly reduced. However, present technological sophistication is not adequate for such investigations.

Reversible sterilization in several forms is being pursued. Plastic or Silastic devices, tissue adhesives, and methods to cause inflammatory occlusion (quinacrine, silver nitrate, zinc chloride, phenol, heat cauterization) have been used inside the uterine cavity to occlude the cornual insertions of the fallopian tubes. The promise of easily performed, effective, low-cost, and reversible occlusion contraception is exciting. This is being further investigated, but there are problems of reversibility, failure to prevent pregnancy, and risk of ectopic pregnancy.

Male Methods

Gossypol is a derivative of cottonseed oil and is used effectively in China for male contraception. The drug suppresses sperm production and affects the structure and motility of sperm in the epididymis. It is excreted slowly, and Chinese trials show that fertility returns in about 3 months. Side-effects of weakness, gastric discomfort, nausea, and decreased sex drive have limited its acceptability in this country. Animal studies are underway in the United States, and analogues of gossypol are being synthesized in hopes of avoiding side-effects.

Hormonal contraceptives under investigation include analogues of LHRH, which appear to depress spermatogenesis, but which also produce loss of libido and other signs of androgen deficiency. Androgen supplementation might be used to counteract these effects, but it is not known if using LHRH and androgens together will produce effective contraception. Testosterone is also being studied as a method to suppress spermatogenesis.

Sperm vaccines are being studied, since a number of potential antigens against sperm have been identified. Sperm enzymes and peptides derived from FSH appear to depress spermatogenesis. An anti-FSH vaccine would be particularly attractive, because its specific action would inhibit sperm production while not affecting secretion of testosterone, thus avoiding androgen-deficiency effects. If inhibin could be isolated and purified, it might possibly interfere with FSH production when administered orally.

References

1. Editorial: The changing American family. Fam Plann Perspect 16(5):204, September/October 1984
2. Glick PC: American household structure in transition. Fam Plann Perspect 16(5):205–211, September/October 1984
3. US Bureau of Census: Families maintained by female householders 1970–1979. Current Population Reports, Series P-23, No. 107, 1980
4. Bachrach CA: Contraceptive practice among American women, 1973–1982. Fam Plann Perspect 16(6):253–259, November/December 1984
5. Sasso SC: Biphasic oral contraceptives. Matern Child Nurs J 9:101, March/April 1984
6. Hatcher RA, Guest F, Stewart F et al (eds): Contraceptive Technology 1984–1985, 12th ed, pp 48, 100, 101, 123, 168, 212, 214, 216. New York, Irvington Publishers, 1984
7. Syntex Laboratories, Palo Alto, CA, product information. Nurse Pract 10:11, November 1985
8. Romney SL, Gray MJ, Little AB et al: Gynecology and Obstetrics: The Health Care of Women. New York, McGraw–Hill, Blakiston, 1975
9. Ory HW, Rosenfield A, Landman LC: The pill at 20: An assessment. Fam Plann Perspect 12(6):278–283, November/December 1980
10. Digest: Cigarettes plus pill: Deadly for women 30 and over. Fam Plann Perspect 9(1):36, January/February 1977
11. Drug data up-date. Am J Nurs 79(1):137, January 1979
12. Digest: Black women, unlike white women, not prone to hypertension while using orals, study finds. Fam Plann Perspect 13(1):40–42, January/February 1981
13. Edmondson HA, Henderson B, Benton B: Liver-cell adenomas associated with use of oral contraceptives. N Engl J Med 294(9):470–472, February 26, 1976
14. Rooks JB, Ory HW, Ishak KG et al: Epidemiology of hepatocellular adenoma: The role of oral contraceptive use. JAMA 242:644, 1979
15. Stern MP, Brown BW, Haskell WL et al: Cardiovascular risk and use of estrogens or estrogen-progestogen combinations. JAMA 235(8):811–815, February 23, 1976
16. Janerich DT, Piper JM, Glebatis DM: Oral contraceptives and congenital limb-reduction defects. N Engl J Med 291:697, 1974
17. Heinonen OP, Slone D, Monson RR et al: Cardiovascular birth defects and antenatal exposure to female sex hormones. N Engl J Med 296:67, 1977
18. Vessey M, Meisler L, Flavel R et al: Outcome of pregnancy in women using different methods of contraception. Br J Obstet Gynaecol 86:584, 1979
19. Division of Reproductive Health, Centers for Disease Control: Oral contraceptive use and the risk of endometrial cancer. JAMA 249:1600–1604, 1983
20. Division of Reproductive Health, Centers for Disease Control: Oral contraceptive use and the risk of ovarian cancer. JAMA 249:1596–1599, 1983
21. Division of Reproductive Health, Centers for Disease Control: Long-term oral contraceptive use and the risk of breast cancer. JAMA 249:1591–1595, 1983
22. Kowal D: OCs do not raise breast, endometrium, ovary cancer risks. Contraceptive Tech Update 3:69, 1982
23. Ory HW: The noncontraceptive health benefits from oral contraceptive use. Fam Plann Perspect 14:182–184, 1982
24. Rosenberg L, Shapiro S, Slone D et al: Epithelial ovarian cancer and combination contraceptives. JAMA 147:3210, 1982
25. Lee NC, Rubin DL, Ory HW et al: Type of intrauterine device and the risk of pelvic inflammatory disease. Obstet Gynecol 62:1, 1983

26. Progestasert IUD and ectopic pregnancy. FDA Bulletin, DHEW-PHS No. 8, 6:37, December 1978/January 1979
27. Lane M, Arleo R, Sobrero AJ: Successful use of the diaphragm and jelly in a young population: Report of a clinical study. Fam Plann Perspect 8(2):81–86, March/April 1976
28. Denniston GC, Putney D: The cavity rim cervical cap. Adv Plann Parent 3:77–80, 1981
29. King L: The Cervical Cap Handbook for Users and Fitters. Monograph published by Emma Goldman Clinic for Women, Iowa City, 1981
30. Bernstein GS, Kilzer LH, Coulson AH et al: Studies of cervical caps: I. Vaginal lesions associated with use of the Vimule cap. Contraception 5:443–446, 1982
31. Edelman DA: Barrier contraception: An update. Adv Plann Parent 4:144–148, 1980
32. Edelman DA, McIntyre S, Harper J: Comparative trial of the contraceptive sponge and diaphragm. Am J Obstet Gynecol 140:869–876, 1984
33. Darney PD: New developments in barrier methods of contraception. Sexual Med Today 3:5–9, March 1985
34. Jongbloet PH, quoted by Ross MA, Pietrow PT: Birth control without contraceptives. Popul Rep (I), No. 1, June 1974
35. American Academy of Pediatrics: Breast-feeding and contraception. Pediatrics 68(1):138–140, 1981
36. Association for Voluntary Sterilization: Immunologic aspects of vasectomy and atherosclerosis. Biomed Bull 1:2, 1980
37. Standley CC, Kessler A: Contraception tomorrow. Int Nurs Rev 31(3):73–75, 1984

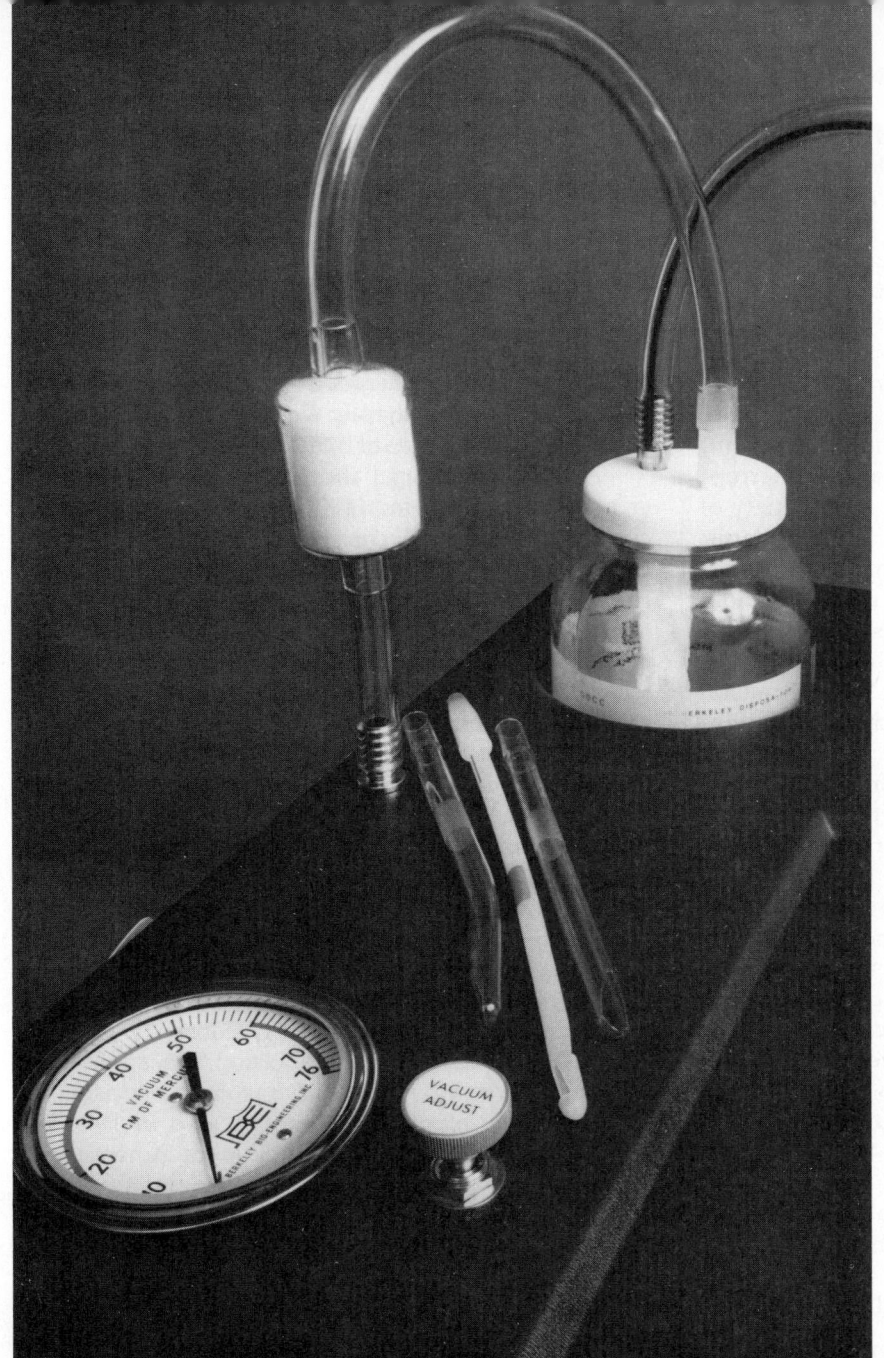

CHAPTER 15

Clinical Interruption of Pregnancy

In general, attitudes toward abortion and the availability of abortion procedures are strongly influenced by prevailing societal values. Whether the society's approach is permissive or restrictive depends on several factors: culture, economy, and ecology. For example, the existence of a predominant religion in a country can affect abortion laws and practices, as can the country's economic or sociopolitical system and its population trends, level of technology, and standard of living.

Women have long sought abortion as a solution to unwanted pregnancy, regardless of whether their culture approved or disapproved of this practice. Interruption of pregnancy is sought by women for a variety of reasons, including health, economics, marital status, family stability, the circumstances of conception, personal goals, age, and many other social and psychological factors. Although accurate abortion statistics are difficult to obtain, especially in countries where the procedure is illegal, it is estimated that from 30 to 55 million pregnancies are purposefully ended each year throughout the world.[1]

The number of abortions in the United States increased steadily from 1963 to 1981, then decreased slightly in 1982. Just over 1 million abortions were performed in 1975, rising to a high of 1.58 million in 1981 and dipping to 1.57 million in 1982. In 1982, approximately 3% of American women of reproductive age obtained an abortion, and about 26% of all pregnancies were terminated by abortion.[2] Abortion services are highly concentrated in metropolitan areas, and 87% of nonmetropolitan counties do not have any abortion providers. Only about 2% of abortions are performed in nonmetropolitan counties, although over one quarter of women of reproductive age live in these counties. Over 80% of abortions are performed in nonhospital facilities, half of these in specialized abortion clinics. The average cost of a first-trimester abortion in 1983 was $200.[2] Statistics on the number of reported abortions in the United States are presented in Table 15-1.

Factors Affecting Abortion Decisions

Legal Factors

Ethical and legal considerations in abortion are discussed in Chapter 7. In this chapter we discuss how these legal factors become important in making abortion decisions.

Availability of legal abortion has dramatically decreased the maternal mortality and morbidity previously associated with illegal, criminal abortion (see Chap. 36). Death from illegal abortion in the United States declined from 39.3 per year in the five-year period (1972–1976) to zero in 1979 and one in 1980, the lowest rates ever reported. Infant mortality rates also have declined in recent years, with fewer premature births. While causes are complex, some of this decline can be attributed to effects of legal abortion availability. One other effect has been a reduction in the number of babies available for adoption.[3]

The courts and legislatures have been a battleground for the opponents and proponents of abortion. Since liberalization of abortion laws in 1973, opponents have tried many strategies to restrict or prevent legal abortions. In 1976, the Supreme Court ruled in the case of *Planned Parenthood of Missouri v. Danforth* that a state cannot impose the requirement of consent by a third party on a woman's right to abortion.[4] This foiled the attempt to give veto power over a woman's decision for an abortion to a spouse or parent. Also in 1976 the United States Congress passed the Hyde Amendment, which forbids the expenditure of federal funds for abortion services except in cases in which continuation of the pregnancy threatens the woman's life. The Supreme Court declared the Hyde Amendment constitutional in 1980. The result has been a virtual withdrawal

TABLE 15-1

Abortion Rates and Ratios in the United States: 1973–1982

	1973	1975	1977	1979	1981	1982
No. of abortions (000s)	744.6	1034.2	1316.7	1497.7	1577.3	1573.9
Abortion rates						
(Abortions per 1000 women between 15 and 44 years of age)	16.6	22.1	26.9	30.2	29.3	28.8
Abortion ratio						
(Abortions per 1000 live births 6 months later)	193	249	286	303	300	299

(Henshaw SK, Forrest JD, Blaine E: Abortion Services in the United States, 1981 and 1982. Fam Plann Perspect 16(3):119–127, May/June 1984)

of federal funds since 1981 to subsidize abortions for indigent women. This is discussed as a social factor in the next section.

The antiabortion movement was disappointed with Senate activity in 1983 and, as a result, has taken a more radical form with the overall goal of shutting down the abortion industry through continuous harassment of clinics and clients. In 1984, at least 161 acts of violence were recorded against abortion and family-planning clinics. Damage from bombings and fires, as well as vandalism, costs millions of dollars, and some abortion clinics have been forced to close. Although there have not yet been any serious injuries or deaths, physicians have been accosted at gunpoint and kidnapped.[5]

Although abortion is legal, it is still viewed with misgivings by many because of religious and personal attitudes. Most, if not all, agree that abortion is not a happy substitute for pregnancy prevention and that the procedures necessary for bringing about termination, though generally safe, are associated with a higher morbidity than are most contraceptive methods.

Psychological Factors

The highest value placed on women in most societies is their role as mothers, and powerful systems of reinforcement operate to make motherhood central to women's lives. A decision to interrupt a pregnancy is rarely taken without some conflict because of the complex meanings and values associated with reproduction and motherhood. Even if the outcome of pregnancy (a child) is consciously unwanted, the woman may on some level desire to be pregnant as a symbol of potency, vitality, or reconnection with primal inner forces. While pregnancy can be completely accidental, it is often used to affect relations with important people in the woman's life, such as parents, husband, or lover.

A teenage girl may become pregnant to demonstrate her maturity, prove her sexuality, or bolster her self-concept as a woman. She may become pregnant because her romantic ideals of motherhood and man–woman relations preclude the use of contraceptives, which imply premeditated sexual activity. Or pregnancy may result from sexual experimentation when neither partner takes responsibility for avoiding unwanted consequences. A woman at any age may use pregnancy as a means of alleviating feelings of inadequacy or doubts about her femininity. A woman entering menopause may conceive to reinforce her sexual self-image or to avoid facing the loss of reproductive capacity. Although pregnancy *per se* may be desired in these instances, the woman may find she cannot face the responsibilities of caring for and raising a child and so elects abortion as the most reasonable solution.

Marital status can also affect the decision to continue or interrupt a pregnancy. Many unmarried women feel

---

Psychological Factors in Pregnancy and Abortion

Purpose for Becoming Pregnant (complex meanings and values associated with reproduction and motherhood)
- Symbol of potency, vitality, or reconnection with primary inner forces
- Symbol of man's virility, potency
- Manipulation of relationships with particular people
- Maturity, sexuality, self-concept
- Elimination of feelings of inadequacy or doubts about femininity
- Avoidance of facing loss of reproduction capacity in the older woman

Purpose for Interrupting Pregnancy
- Marital status
- Quality of man–woman relationship
- Realization that motives for pregnancy were not appropriate
- Poor physical health (risk to life)
- Poor mental health (drain on energies; unable to cope)
- Educational or professional goals
- Conception too early in marriage
- Conception too soon after birth of previous child
- Emotionally unable to handle parenthood
- Financially unable to handle parenthood
- Hereditary genetic defects
- Possible fetal anomalies
- Possible reactions of peers, family, community

---

incapable of raising a child outside of marriage, although there are increasing numbers of single parents and more social acceptance of this situation. A critical factor is the quality of the man–woman relation and its meaning for the woman in terms of commitment and dependability. Pregnancy has historically been used to force a man into marriage, but has proven to be a poor basis on which to build a lifetime relationship. In marriages that are in trouble and facing dissolution, pregnancy may be used as an attempt to prevent a breakup. A woman may also become pregnant, even though she does not truly desire a child, in order to meet her partner's expectation, for example, if the man's sense of masculinity or potency requires that "his woman" become pregnant. In many of these cases, however, the pregnancy does not produce the desired result, and the woman may seek abortion when she realizes that motives for pregnancy were not appropriate for her.

Poor physical or mental health can lead a woman to interrupt her pregnancy if pregnancy poses a risk to her life or a drain on her already depleted energies. A life crisis or emotional upheaval may lead a woman to feel incapable of coping with pregnancy and motherhood until her life becomes less chaotic.

Abortion may also be chosen when a pregnancy is untimely. Education or professional goals may have higher priority at the time, or pregnancy may occur too early in a marriage or too soon after the birth of a child. Or the couple may feel emotionally or economically unable to manage parenthood. Couples frequently seek abortion for economic reasons. They prefer to strive for a higher standard of living and greater social opportunity for themselves and their children and are unwilling to be subjected to increased material hardship.

Abortion may be sought for eugenic reasons, even if pregnancy and the child are desired. Clients are becoming better informed about the hereditary genetic defects that may be of risk to their offspring. They are taking advantage of screening programs to detect such conditions as Tay-Sachs disease, hemophilia, Down's syndrome, sickle cell disease, and other genetic abnormalities. Awareness of fetal anomalies caused by rubella, exposure to radiation, and teratogenic drugs may cause some women to elect abortion if they have been exposed during the first trimester.

Sociocultural factors play an important role in a decision to seek abortion. If abortion is illegal, the woman risks criminal prosecution, and if social values condemn abortion she faces disapproval by peers, family, and community. When abortion is legal and there are generally accepting social values, deciding to have an abortion does not present such a traumatic experience and is usually emotionally well accepted. Studies have demonstrated that there are few negative psychological reactions to abortion when positive attitudes on the part of professional staff encourage acceptance. It also has been shown that psychological sequelae are usually of short duration and reflect the circumstances surrounding abortion and attitudes conveyed by peer groups, family, and health providers.[6]

Results of Unwanted Pregnancies

The rates of admission to psychiatric hospitals were found to be higher among postpartum and postabortion women who were separated, divorced, and widowed than among those currently or never married. Among this latter group, the admissions following abortion were considerably higher than those following delivery. The interaction of stress, lack of social support, and reversal of original intention for a previously desired pregnancy was felt to account for the higher rates among postabortion women.[7]

In a longitudinal study of children born to women who had been denied an abortion for that pregnancy, persistent and significant differences were found between children in the study group and those in control groups. When the children were 9 years of age, the study group children had a higher incidence of illness despite the same biologic start in life, had poorer grades in school despite the same levels of intelligence, and

had worse integration in the peer group. At ages 14 to 16, more children in the study group did not continue into secondary education but began jobs without vocational training and found their mothers inconsistent in emotional behavior toward them. In the latest report, when these children were 16 to 18 years of age, the boys in the study group more often reported that they felt neglected or rejected by their mothers than did the controls; however, no difference could be found among the girls. These boys also felt that their parents' marriages were less happy, that they were insufficiently informed about sexual matters (especially contraception), and that they held more conservative views on such social issues as resolution of unplanned pregnancies, divorce, and coping with alcohol and drugs. The study concluded that "unwantedness" during early pregnancy is a significant risk factor for the subsequent life of the child.[8]

Social Factors

Although the United States law places no restrictions on early abortions, and very few requirements for later abortions, this does not mean that every woman who desires to interrupt a pregnancy can do so. The ability to obtain an abortion is greatly influenced by such factors as availability and accessibility of abortion facilities, methods of financing health-care services, and personal and economic resources.

Facilities

For women with health insurance or adequate means to pay for an abortion, the main problem may be a lack of facilities. Eight of every ten counties in the United States have no facility where legal abortions are performed. It is estimated that about one fourth of the women in need of abortion services reside in these counties, which have no physician, clinic, or hospital that would perform abortions. Over 1 million women would need to travel to other counties to seek abortions, and it is likely that a large proportion of these women could not obtain abortion services at all (Table 15-2).

Abortion rates vary widely among the states, from highs of 170 abortions per 1000 women between the ages of 15 and 44 in the District of Columbia and 45 abortions per 1000 women in California and New York, to lows of seven to nine abortions per 1000 women in West Virginia, Mississippi, and Wyoming.[2] Those states with the lowest abortion rates also tend to have the highest proportion of residents obtaining abortions in out-of-state facilities.

Although many women are able to travel to obtain abortions, this still creates a hardship. There is a high correlation between the proportion of women living in counties with abortion services and the number of state

Percentage of Women Traveling Out of State to Obtain Abortions

Year	Percent
1973	21
1974	12
1975	10
1976	10
1977	9
1978	8
1981	6

residents who obtain abortions.[9] The need to travel to obtain an abortion increases costs, reduces privacy owing to prolonged absence from home and work, may delay abortion until later in gestation (which increases the risk of morbidity and mortality), and decreases effective treatment for postabortion complications.

Financing Health-Care Services

The situation for poor women is made more difficult by the enactment of the Hyde Amendment, which restricts the use of public funds to provide abortions for indigent women. As a result of this amendment, federal funding of Medicaid abortions fell by 99%. Many states adopted the Hyde restrictions, or narrower ones, instead of picking up the costs of abortions for poor women. Some of the more populous states, namely, New York, California, Pennsylvania, Michigan, and Illinois, maintained more liberal standards for Medicaid abortions, however, and paid almost the entire cost from state monies. In fiscal year (FY) 1978, 99% of abortions were funded with state funds only, and 1% involved federal funding. The District of Columbia and 18 states spent over 51 million dollars in FY 1978 to provide 191,700 abortions for which federal funding was unavailable. Those states with liberal policies accounted for 98% of all public funds expended for abortion services during FY 1978. Ten states had no publically funded abortions, and another 11 had ten or less publically funded abortions.[10]

There was a 34% decrease in the number of publically funded abortions from 1977 to 1978. This aggregate United States figure does not adequately represent the plight of poor women in those states that severely restricted payment from public funds, because it is raised by the efforts of those few states that continued to pay for abortions largely out of state monies. The Alan Guttmacher Institute estimated that nearly one third of the Medicaid-eligible women in need of publically funded abortion services in 1977 were unable to obtain them. After the Hyde Amendment went into effect in 1978, this figure increased to over 54%.[10]

Although the restrictions on publically funded abortions did not completely eliminate use of federal funds, they have had a major impact. The number of subsidized abortions decreased by more than one third, and in states with restrictive policies regarding use of state funds, abortions for poor women with public support were virtually eliminated. A large estimated unmet need for publically funded abortions existed before these funding restrictions, and it has increased substantially following the institution of these restrictions.

The impact of this decrease in publically funded abortions is felt in several ways. Indigent women who are able to raise the money to pay for their own abortions often do so at the expense of their rent or utility bills, by pawning household goods, by diverting food or clothing money, or possibly by fraudulent use of a relative's insurance policy. Some women have been driven to theft. It was found that the price Medicaid-eligible women were paying for abortions was almost the same as that paid by those not eligible; they paid the full price themselves. The distress and hardship involved in obtaining or foregoing an abortion are hardly reflected in the statistics; cases have been reported of indigent women attempting self-induced abortion or suicide after being denied publically funded abortions.[11]

Medicaid-eligible women can obtain medically necessary abortions in those states in which public funds are approved for abortions. However, many states do not receive Medicaid funds or approve their use for abortions. In 1983, 14 states and the District of Columbia covered abortions through state Medicaid mechanisms. Even in these states, more than one fourth of all providers did not accept public reimbursement.[2] The proportions of hospitals, clinics, and physicians' offices that accepted state Medicaid payment for abortions are shown in Table 15-3.

Applying the Nursing Process to Abortion Care

The nurse is often a key professional in providing counseling to clients considering abortion. The need to weigh alternatives and make responsible decisions about an unwanted pregnancy may become apparent in the prenatal or family-planning clinic or other health-care setting. As part of client education and the supportive role, the nurse may offer initial discussion and assistance in problem solving to women or couples facing the problem of an undesired conception.

The nurse must recognize that attitudes toward abortion are varied and personal and that there are strong religious and moral influences in these attitudes. One is entitled to one's own conclusions on this matter, but the opinions of others should be respected. Personal convictions of health professionals in this area are generally respected, and those who do not feel that abortion is ethically acceptable should make their views known so that arrangements can be made well in advance for substitute medical personnel.

An outline of the nursing process is used in Nursing Care: The Woman/Family Who Is Interrupting a Pregnancy.

Assessment

Nursing assessment includes physiological data such as last menstrual period, use of contraceptives, signs and symptoms of pregnancy, and other past health history. Psychosocial data include circumstances surrounding unwanted conception, reaction to pregnancy, involvement of partner and others, life situation related to choices about pregnancy, level of ambivalence, and consideration of all options. The nurse also assesses whether the client is in crisis and needs further counseling.

Nursing Diagnosis

The nursing diagnosis is based largely on psychosocial data that were obtained during assessment. Although several diagnoses may be made, much of nursing intervention will provide care for the client/family with a knowledge deficit. Initially this deficit will be related to options available and procedures to be used. Later knowledge deficit is related to self-care, expected bleeding or cramping, signs and symptoms of complications, sexual activity, contraception, and community resources. Ineffective coping and alteration in family processes are two other potential diagnoses for this situation.

Planning/Intervention

Nursing intervention usually covers such areas as assisting the client to fully consider all choices, to understand requirements for various abortion procedures, to examine supports and resources, to understand her reactions and find expression for emotional needs, to locate or take advantage of facilities or financing methods, and to provide education about the processes of abortion and contraception.

Exploring Alternatives

Many women need help to think beyond their first reaction to the unwanted pregnancy. They need to be encouraged to consider other options available to them. Many women feel ambivalent and confused and are

TABLE 15-3

Proportions of Hospitals, Clinics, and Physicians' Offices Accepting State Medicaid Payment for Abortions, 1983

State	Total	Hospitals	Clinics	MDs' Offices
Total	72	87	74	53
Alaska	73	60	100	67
California	80	85	90	70
Colorado	60	90	47	42
Connecticut	43	58	67	17
D.C.	82	100	86	0
Hawaii	87	100	100	82
Maryland	65	90	46	0
Massachusetts	70	94	70	22
Michigan	96	100	91	100
New Jersey	41	76	28	9
New York	67	91	60	38
Oregon	87	100	100	63
Pennsylvania	51	73	63	4
Washington	88	81	96	88
West Virginia	100	100	100	100

Percentages are based on the 70% of providers whose policies regarding acceptance of public reimbursement are known. Respondents were asked whether they accept "Medicaid payment for abortions"; North Carolina funds abortions for low-income women, but is omitted from this table because reimbursement is not provided through the Medicaid system.
(Adapted from Henshaw SK, Forrest JD, Blain E: Abortion Services in the United States, 1981 and 1982. Fam Plann Perspect 16(3):119–127, May/June 1984)

under pressure from family or their own social values. It is important that the nurse encourages the woman to make the decision for herself, because there is less regret and emotional sequelae when the choice is not perceived as being forced by other people. Exploring alternatives realistically helps clarify the situation and places manageable boundaries within which the decision can be made. Thinking through what each choice means not only for present feelings and relations but also for future circumstances, goals, and needs, both from a practical and from an emotional-values standpoint, encourages a carefully weighed choice. While the counseling is in progress, tests are carried out to confirm the pregnancy and determine the length of gestation, and the type of abortion procedure indicated is discussed. These factors alone in and of themselves may influence the decision. Simply knowing that the pregnancy has progressed beyond the time when simple curettage can be used and that the abortion may actually involve labor and expulsion of the fetus may cause a woman to decline abortion. In any event, understanding the nature of the procedure required is essential to informed decision making (Fig. 15-1).

The Woman/Family Who Is Interrupting a Pregnancy

Nursing Objectives

1. Assist woman/family in reaching acceptable decision regarding continuing or interrupting pregnancy.
2. Provide early confirmation of pregnancy and implement first-trimester abortion to minimize risk and trauma, or provide early prenatal care if pregnancy is to be continued.
3. Provide information about various procedures as indicated by gestational age; clarify misunderstandings.
4. Provide or refer for psychological counseling if indicated.
5. Educate about effective contraception to avoid future unwanted pregnancy.

Assessment	Potential Nursing Diagnosis	Intervention	Evaluation
Menstrual history and last menstrual period, use of contraceptives	Knowledge deficit related to options available, procedures, normalcy of emotions, self-care, postprocedure care, expected bleeding or cramping, signs and symptoms of complications, resumption of sexual activity, contraception, sexuality, community resources, follow-up care	Advise of length of gestation and what type of procedure this indicates; discuss various types of abortion procedures, time in hospital or if outpatient, techniques and what the experience entails, risks, and complications	Able to reach decision about pregnancy termination with which client feels comfortable
Assist in physical examination, collection of specimens, pregnancy tests to determine length of gestation			Accepts requirements of various procedures as indicated by gestational age
Understanding of physiology of conception and contraceptive methods		Explore alternate choices (*i.e.*, have abortion or continue pregnancy and either keep baby or give baby for adoption) and meanings these have for woman, partner, and family	Affirms understanding of process of conception and effective use of contraception
Consideration of alternatives to abortion			Returns for follow-up visit and institutes contraceptive method
Pregnancy and health history to identify special needs and risks		Assist during procedures, provide support and clarification, and keep client informed of process	Feels accepting of abortion if undertaken; no serious emotional problems
		Advise of postabortion complications, when to seek medical care, preventive measures, and when to resume activities and sex	Seeks prenatal care if abortion decided against
		Discuss contraception, follow-up visits, and emotional reactions	Avoids future unwanted pregnancies
		For midtrimester abortion, monitor during labor, provide pain relief and supportive care, and facilitate presence of companion if desired	
Circumstances surrounding unwanted conception	Ineffective individual coping leading to depression related to unresolved emotional responses (guilt, regret)	Initiate referral to psychological counseling if indicated	Initiates psychological counseling if emotionally distressed
Level of ambivalence or certainty about abortion decision		Provide opportunity to express emotional responses, conflicts, problems	Expresses emotional responses openly, seeks resolution to conflicts and problems

(continued)

227

Assessment	Potential Nursing Diagnosis	Intervention	Evaluation
Involvement of partner, family, parents, and sources of support	Alteration in family processes related to the effects of abortion on relationships (disagreements, marital and personal conflicts, adolescent identity problems)	Initiate referral to psychological counseling if indicated	Initiates psychological counseling if emotionally distressed
Presence of crisis, need for further psychological counseling		Provide opportunity to express emotional responses, conflicts, problems	Expresses emotional responses openly, seeks resolution to conflicts and problems

Abortion Procedures

The approach to pregnancy termination varies according to gestational age. Prior to the 12th week, abortion is generally a relatively uncomplicated vaginal procedure, employing dilatation and evacuation (D&E, suction curettage) or standard dilatation and curettage (D&C). In the early stages of pregnancy, prostaglandins may be used in the form of vaginal suppositories, intramuscular injections, or transcervical instillation to induce abortion. Or a suctioning method for menstrual extraction or regulation may be carried out by means of a very small cannula (Fig. 15-2). This procedure is occasionally used during the first 2 weeks after a missed menstrual period, frequently before pregnancy is confirmed.

Beyond the 11th to 12th week, interruption requires more complex procedures, often involving amniocentesis, for which 1 to 3 days of hospitalization are often necessary and the complication rate is considerably higher. Suction curettage is the most frequently used method and the safest in the 13- to 16-week interval, but has an increased rate of morbidity and mortality over first-trimester procedures. Serial intramuscular injections of prostaglandins (15-methyl analogues) have been successful during this time, but with significant effects on temperature regulation and gastrointestinal symptoms. Intra-amniotic instillations of saline, urea, or prostaglandins are most effective after 16 weeks' gestation, but with substantially increased complication rates.

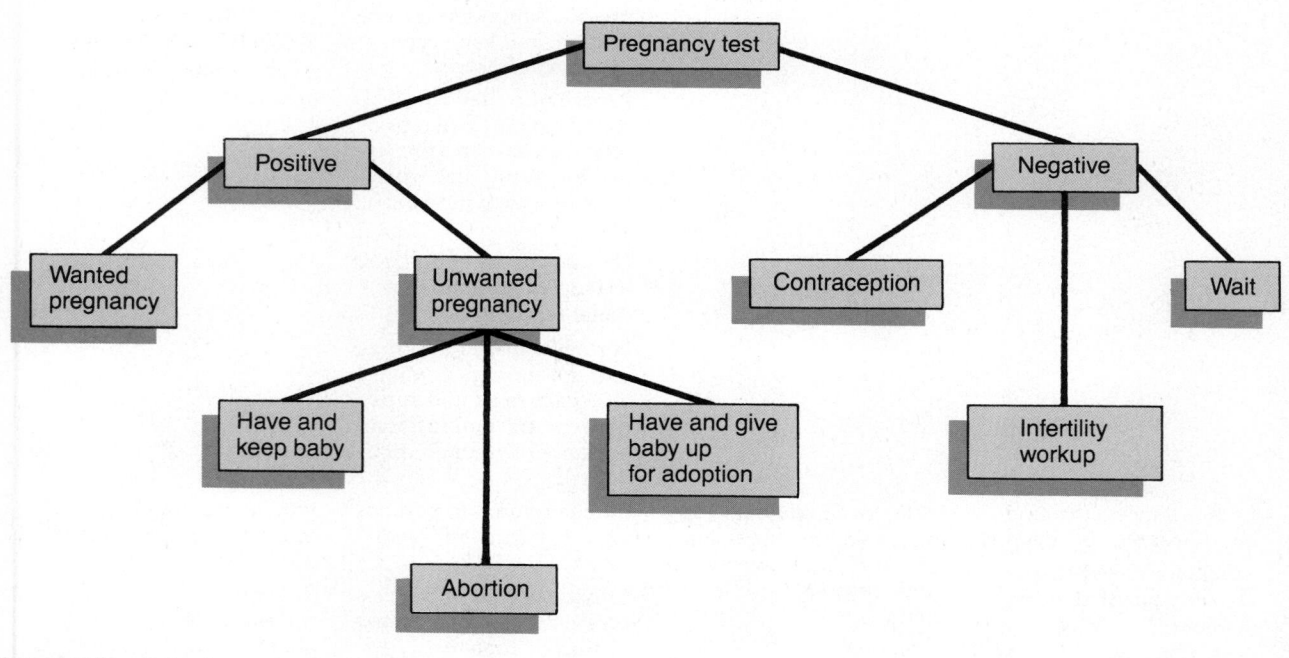

FIGURE 15-1

Decision tree for pregnancy alternatives.

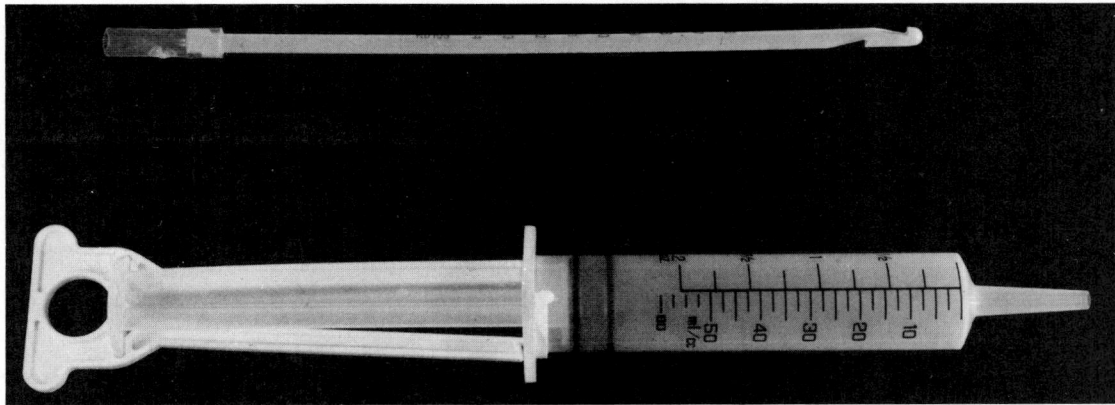

FIGURE 15-2

A flexible plastic Karman cannula and a self-locking syringe for menstrual extraction. (Rocket of London)

Techniques Used Prior to 12 Weeks' Gestation.

First-trimester abortions may be carried out as outpatient procedures. Nonhospital facilities have been established, and many hospitals have designed facilities for outpatient procedures. Over 80% of abortions now take place in nonhospital facilities. Many physicians or hospitals will not perform abortions beyond the 20th to 24th week of gestation.

Suction (Vacuum) Curettage. Increasingly, the procedure of choice for the termination of early pregnancy is *suction curettage* (Figs. 15-3 and 15-4). A local anesthetic (paracervical block) or a spinal anesthetic may be used. The cervix is dilated with graduated dilators, and a suction curet is placed into the endometrial cavity to the fundus. Suction is applied, usually by an electric pump, and the products of conception are evacuated into a container. These are usually sent to the pathology laboratory for confirmation of the pregnancy and to rule out unusual conditions such as hydatidiform mole. Generally, recovery takes from 2 to 3 hours, during which time the client is observed for excessive bleeding.

In some circumstances, the cervix is prepared for the abortion by the use of *laminaria.* These are lengths of sterile hydroscopic material derived from seaweed, which absorb moisture at a rapid rate. When placed in the cervical canal, they expand in 3 to 6 hours and cause cervical dilatation. Insertion of laminaria several hours prior to a first-trimester abortion can reduce the need for mechanical cervical dilatation. Some feel that using them decreases the incidence of cervical lacerations. The most common complications of suction curettage are infection, hemorrhage, and retained products or blood clots in the uterus, and cervical or uterine trauma.

Surgical (Sharp) Curettage. Standard D&C, which is used for first-trimester abortions, often requires

a general anesthetic and the usual preoperative precautions. The cervix must be dilated more than for suction curettage, and there is more danger of cervical laceration

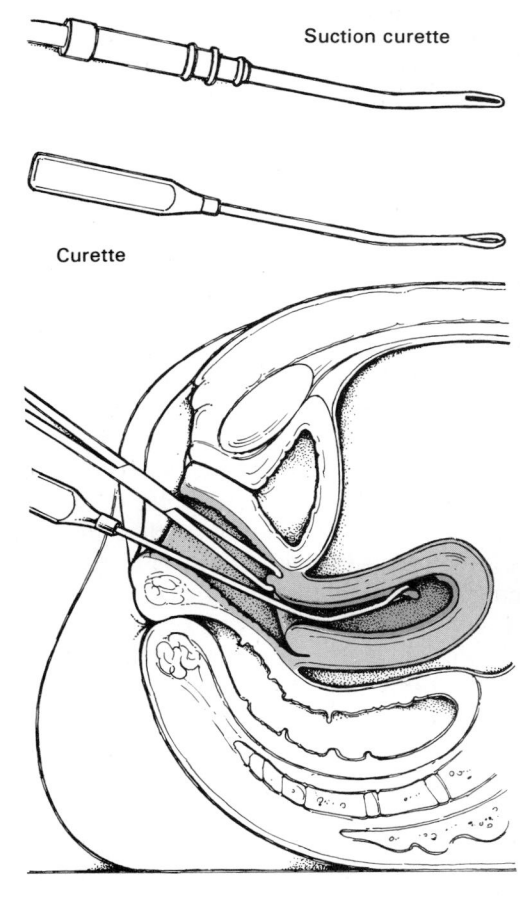

FIGURE 15-3

Curettage or vacuum aspiration for first-trimester abortion.

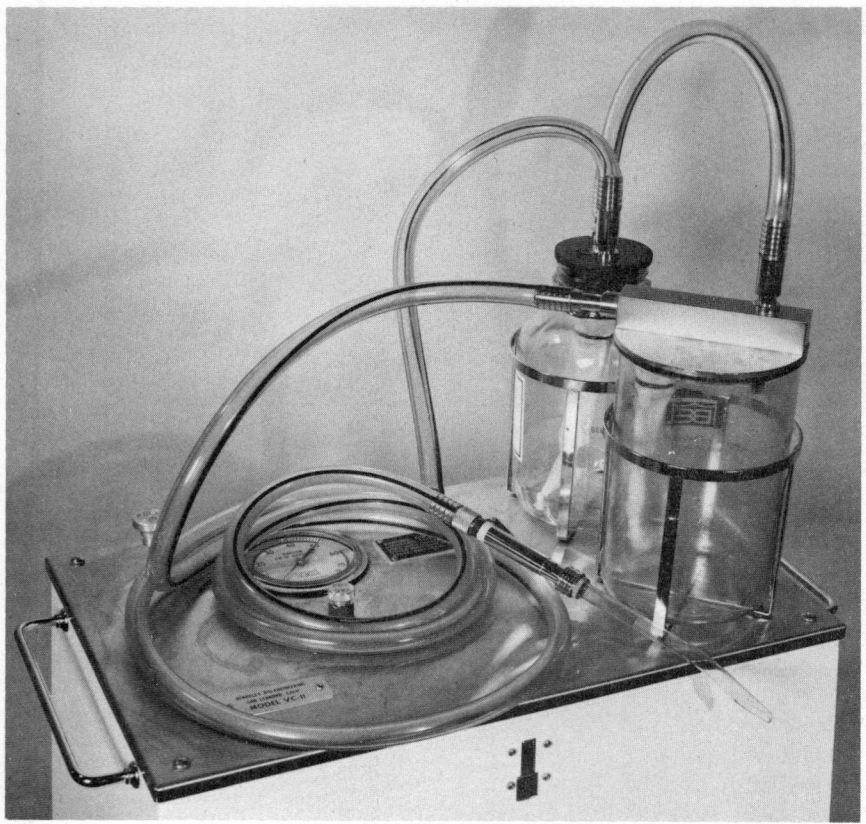

FIGURE 15-4

An electric suction apparatus with a swivel handle and a curet. (Model V C II by Berkeley Bio-Engineering, Inc.)

and blood loss. The advantage of this technique is that it is widely used and known by family physicians, general practitioners, and obstetrician–gynecologists.

Menstrual Extraction.   Aspiration of the endometrium on an outpatient basis performed from 5 to 7 weeks after the last menstrual period is called menstrual extraction, menstrual regulation, menstrual induction, minisuction, miniabortion, and interception. The procedure is simple and relatively atraumatic; little or no cervical dilatation is required, and usually no anesthetic is given. A 4-mm to 6-mm flexible plastic cannula and a syringe or other low-pressure suction are used. The uterus does not need to be clinically enlarged, and often a pregnancy test is not required, since one of the advantages of the procedure is that the woman need not know for certain if she is pregnant. Although this procedure has been taught and used among women's groups as a self-administered technique, it is not safe to use it this way because of the dangers of hemorrhage, retained products, and infection.

Prostaglandins.   Prostaglandins, a group of fatty acids found in the semen, are very effective abortifacients at any stage of pregnancy. The exact mechanisms by which they work are not clearly understood. Oral administration is impractical because of the high incidence of side-effects, the most common being vomiting, diarrhea, fever, and shaking. Vaginal, intramuscular,

and transcervical administration produce fewer side-effects, and serious complications are rare. Prostaglandins may be used more frequently as preparations are refined and side-effects are minimized.[12]

Techniques Used After 12 Weeks' Gestation

Dilatation and Evacuation.   Over two thirds of all second-trimester abortions are done by D&E.[13] It is particularly used in the 13- to 15-week interval, when intra-amniotic procedures are often ineffective. The procedure is an extension of vacuum curettage and traditional D&C. The cervix requires greater dilation, since the products of conception are larger. Usually a laminaria is inserted for gradual cervical dilation prior to the procedure. Following administration of a paracervical block or general anesthesia, graduated metal dilators are introduced until the cervix is adequately dilated. A large suction cannula (14 mm–16 mm) is used to remove pregnancy tissue. Forceps or crushing instruments may be needed to completely remove fetal tissue.

After the uterus has been emptied, a sharp curet is often used to explore the cavity for any remaining tissue. All fetal parts must be accounted for before administration of oxytocins. Some providers use prophylactic antibiotics (usually tetracyclines) to reduce the risk of infection. The most common complications are infections, retained products, hemorrhage, and cervical injury. Dilatation and evacuation has about half the mortality associated with instillation methods. Data on late complications are incomplete; however, there is some evidence that the greater cervical dilation required for D&E in the second trimester is associated with a higher risk of delivering a subsequent low-birth-weight infant.[14]

Dilatation and evacuation abortions are less stressful for women than instillation abortions, which involve labor and fetal expulsion. Because D&E often requires a destructive procedure, the psychological impact of second-trimester abortion may be transferred from the woman to the physician.

Hypertonic Saline. When pregnancy has progressed beyond the 16th week, termination is often carried out by instilling *hypertonic saline* into the amniotic cavity. This procedure is most easily carried out when there is sufficient fluid in the amniotic cavity to be identified and aspirated. The bladder is emptied, and the client is placed in the supine position. The skin is prepped and draped with sterile towels and infiltrated with a local anesthetic over the injection site. An 18-gauge spinal needle is then inserted through the uterus into the amniotic cavity. When properly placed, clear amniotic fluid flows into the syringe attached to the needle. After a small amount of fluid is removed to verify proper placement of the needle, hypertonic saline is injected into the amniotic cavity. Initially, a small amount is placed, and if there is no reaction, the remainder is delivered over approximately 15 minutes.

Following a latent period of several hours, labor usually ensues and the fetus with part or all of the placenta is delivered within 24 to 72 hours. If the placenta cannot be extracted completely after delivery, a curettage must be carried out to complete the abortion. During the course of labor, the contractions can cause considerable discomfort. As the cervix dilates, the client should be medicated at intervals; generally a substantial amount of emotional support is needed during this process. The previable fetus is usually dead at the time of delivery, but at this late stage of gestation it has human form.

Oxytocin infusion is often used as an adjunct to saline abortion to decrease the time needed for completion of the process. Oxytocin is used in a manner similar to that employed for induction of labor (see Chap. 38), except that a more concentrated solution is used. The oxytocin drip is begun 6 to 12 hours after amino infusion of saline. Maximum time of oxytocin use should be limited to 24 hours. If it is used longer, there is an increased incidence of water retention, which could lead to water intoxication.

In cases in which the hypertonic saline fails to induce contractions, a repeat dose must be administered. In some circumstances, as in severe hypertension, infusion of hypertonic saline is contraindicated. Complications most often include hemorrhage, infection, and retained placenta. Occasionally more serious compli-

cations occur as a result of the intravenous injection of saline, including hypernatremia, amniotic fluid embolism, disseminated intravascular coagulation, and necrosis of the myometrium from saline entering the uterine musculature.

Intra-amniotic Prostaglandins. Instillation of prostaglandins into the amniotic cavity by a similar amniocentesis technique is another method of inducing midtrimester abortions; it has a lower complication rate than saline instillation in the 16- to 20-week interval and a more rapid onset of labor with subsequent expulsion. Medication can be used to control the gastrointestinal side-effects. Women with asthma or pulmonary disease are at increased risk because the drug can cause marked bronchospasm. Other rare serious complications are arrhythmias, cardiovascular changes, and grand mal seizures. These complications are more frequent when the prostaglandins enter systemic circulation; therefore, careful placement in the uterine cavity reduces the incidence of such complications.

Over half of the women given intra-amniotic prostaglandins abort within 24 hours, and 93% abort within 48 hours.[15] Although these drugs are more expensive than sodium chloride, this may be offset by shorter hospitalization and fewer complications. The increased potential for expulsion of a live fetus is often reduced by the concomitant instillation of urea.

Intramuscular Prostaglandins. Serial intramuscular injections of the 15-methyl analogues of prostaglandins are effective in interrupting pregnancies of between 10 weeks' and 17 weeks' gestation. Contractions begin rapidly and are intense within 40 minutes. Abortion is completed within 12 hours in 76% of the clients and within 24 hours in 96%. One type of prostaglandin causes greater gastrointestinal symptoms, and the other type causes more temperature elevation, shaking, and chills. This method is managed as an inpatient procedure because repeated injections are necessary and labor must be carefully monitored.

Hysterotomy. When other methods of midtrimester abortion fail, or if D&E, saline, or prostaglandins are contraindicated for various reasons, a hysterotomy or minicesarean section may be performed. The operation is major surgery and may be done abdominally or vaginally. This procedure requires the standard preoperative preparations and general or spinal anesthesia. The morbidity and mortality from this procedure are greater than for other techniques, and a live fetus may be delivered. Advantages of this method include the opportunity for concomitant sterilization by tubal ligation or hysterectomy, and treatment of pelvic disease. Mortality rates for the commonly used methods of pregnancy interruption are summarized in Table 15-4.

TABLE 15-4

Mortality Rates (Death-to-Case) for Legal Abortions by Type of Procedure and Length of Gestation, 1972–1981†*

Type of Procedure	Total‡	≤8	9–10	11–12	13–15	16–20	≥21
				Length of Gestation (in weeks)			
Total†	**1.8**	**0.5**	**1.2**	**2.0**	**4.8**	**12.5**	**15.1**
Curettage	0.9	0.5	1.1	1.9	0.0	0.0	0.0
D&E	4.9	0.0	0.0	0.0	3.2	9.2	12.0
Instillation	9.6	0.0	0.0	0.0	5.5	12.0	13.3
Saline	11.6	0.0	0.0	0.0	1.7	15.2	12.9
Prostaglandin and others§	6.4	0.0	0.0	0.0	12.1	6.0	14.2
Hysterectomy/hysterotomy	47.8	0.0	50.4	34.7	64.9	84.5	123.0

* Deaths per 100,000 abortions.
† Based on distributions of abortions for which the type of procedure and the weeks of gestation are known.
‡ Total includes four deaths for which the type of procedure was classified as "other" and two for which it was unknown.
§ Denominators for these rates include abortions reported as "other" types of procedures (1% of all abortions for which the procedure was known).
(Grimes DA: Second-trimester abortions in the United States. Fam Plann Perspect 16(6):260–266, November/December 1984)

Nursing Care

If a support person from the family or a friend cannot be present, it is the nurse's responsibility to be a support person before, during, and after the procedure. Support may involve holding a hand, listening, or just being present as a friend. Some of the procedures involve physical discomfort, and the nurse should prepare the woman for this in addition to providing comfort as discomforts arise. The nurse monitors vital signs and intake and output and assists during procedures.

The nurse keeps the client informed of the progress of the procedure and clarifies directions and terminology. Self-care pertaining to the procedure is taught to the client, and other self-care needs of the client may be addressed (see Instructions for Clients Following an Abortion). The nurse advises of complications that may occur after the procedure and suggests preventive measures. Sexual matters are discussed, including such topics as when intercourse may be resumed and contraceptive use.

The nurse needs to be a good listener and to know when to give advice and when to let the woman talk. The nurse should always be further assessing for psy-

CLIENT EDUCATION

Instructions for Clients Following an Abortion

- Bleeding and cramps are not unusual for the first 2 weeks following an abortion. Some spotting may occur for as long as 4 weeks after the procedure.
- Medical attention should be sought if bleeding is severe or if bleeding is heavier than the heaviest day of her normal menstrual period for 2 consecutive days.
- The next normal menstrual period may begin in about 4 to 6 weeks, except when birth control pills have been prescribed. If birth control pills are used, the normal period should resume at the end of the first month on the pill. If the menstrual period does not resume within 8 weeks, medical attention should be sought.
- Sanitary pads, instead of tampons, should be used for the first week after an abortion to help reduce the chance of infection.
- Douching is prohibited during the first week following the abortion to help prevent infection.
- Sexual intercourse is avoided for at least the first week following the abortion to help prevent infection.
- Temperature should be taken twice each day during the first week, preferably at noon and at bedtime. If temperature reaches 100°F or more, the client should seek medical attention. If she is taking aspirin or other pain medications, her temperature should be taken before she takes the medication.
- If the client experiences severe pain or breaks out in a rash or hives, or if the symptoms of pregnancy such as breast tenderness or nausea persist for over a week after the abortion, medical attention should be sought.
- A follow-up examination 2 weeks after the procedure should be scheduled.

chological complications involving the abortion. When the nurse is aware of psychological problems, the client should be referred to counseling or psychiatric care for follow-up.

Specifics in nursing care are outlined in the nursing-care plan given earlier in the chapter.

Follow-Up Care

After a first-trimester abortion, the woman is instructed about signs and symptoms of complications and how to contact the clinic or physician if these occur. Fever and chills, foul-smelling discharge, heavy bleeding, severe abdominal pain, and nausea and vomiting can indicate complications. Abstinence from intercourse and avoidance of tampons and douching for 2 weeks are advised. Normal activity may be resumed in 1 or 2 days in most instances. Contraception is discussed, and occasionally an IUD is inserted at the time of abortion, but perforation and expulsion rates are high. Oral contraceptives may be given with instructions that they be started 1 week after the abortion.

It is standard to have a follow-up office visit in 2 weeks, at which time contraceptives are prescribed if not already begun. The client's adjustment to termination of pregnancy, as well as her partner's or family's reactions, can be discussed and referral made if needed for psychological, social, or economic reasons.

Following midtrimester abortion, RhoGAM is administered to unsensitized Rh-negative women. Instructions about signs and symptoms of infection and hemorrhage are given, and clients are advised to avoid sex, tampons, and douches for 2 weeks. Women need to be prepared for frequently occurring depression, which is probably related to drastic hormonal changes. A return visit is scheduled for 2 weeks after the abortion, at which time uterine size should be normal and bleeding ceased. Contraception is usually initiated and reactions to the abortion discussed with referral as needed.

Evaluation

The client's care has been successful when the client has been able to make a decision (whether to interrupt the pregnancy or to continue the pregnancy), feels comfortable with her decision, and follows through in an acceptable manner. The latter involves choosing an acceptable method for abortion or seeking prenatal care for herself and her baby. She has adjusted well if she expresses emotional responses openly and seeks resolution to her conflicts and problems.

Effective care also results in her returning for a follow-up visit and using a suitable contraceptive method to prevent further unwanted pregnancies.

References

1. Tietze C: Incidence of legal abortion. In Omran AR (ed): Liberalization of Abortion Laws: Implications, pp 1–4. Chapel Hill, University of North Carolina, Carolina Population Center, 1976
2. Henshaw SK, Forrest JD, Blaine E: Abortion services in the United States, 1981 and 1982. Fam Plann Perspect 16(3):119–127, May/June 1984
3. Hatcher RA, Guest F, Stewart F et al: Contraceptive Technology 1984–1985, pp 186–187. New York, Irvington Publishers, 1984
4. United States Supreme Court: Planned Parenthood of Central Missouri v. Danforth, Opinion Nos. 75–73 and 75–109, July 1, 1976
5. Donovan P: The holy war. Fam Plann Perspect 17(1): 5–9, January/February 1985
6. Osofsky JD, Osofky JH: The psychological reaction of patients to legalized abortion. Am J Orthopsychiatry 42(1):48–60, 1972
7. David HP, Rasmussen NK, Holst E: Postpartum and postabortion psychotic reactions. Fam Plann Perspect 13(2):88–91, March/April 1981
8. David HP, Matéjćek Z: Children born to women denied abortion: An update. Fam Plann Perspect 13(1):32–34, January/February 1981
9. Henshaw SK, Forrest JD, Sullivan E et al: Abortion services in the United States, 1979 and 1980. Fam Plann Perspect 14(5):5–8, 10–15, 1982
10. Gold RB: After the Hyde Amendment: Public funding for abortion in FY 1978. Fam Plann Perspect 12(3): 131–134, May/June 1980
11. Trussel J, Menken J, Lindheim BL et al: The impact of restricting Medicaid financing for abortion. Fam Plann Perspect 12(3):120–130, May/June 1980
12. Bygdeman M, Martin JN, Eneroth P et al: Outpatient postconceptional fertility control with vaginally administered 15 (S) 15-methyl-PGF, a-methyl ester. Am J Obstet Gynecol 124(5):495–498, March 1, 1976
13. Grimes DA: Second-trimester abortions in the United States. Fam Plann Perspect 16(6):260–266, November/December 1984
14. Grimes DA, Schulz KF: Morbidity and mortality from second-trimester abortions. J Reprod Med 30(7):505–514, 1985
15. Brenner WE: The current status of prostaglandins as abortifacients. Am J Obstet Gynecol 123(3):306–328, October 1, 1975

Suggested Readings

Atrash HK, Peterson HB, Cates W et al: The risk of death from combined abortion-sterilization procedures: Can hysterotomy or hysterectomy be justified? Am J Obstet Gynecol 142:269, 1982

Berger C, Gold D, Andrew D et al: Repeat abortion: Is it a problem? Fam Plann Perspect 16(2):70–74, 1984

Callahan S, Callahan D: Abortion: Understanding differences. Fam Plann Perspect 16(5):219–221, September/October 1984

Cates W: The Hyde Amendment in action. JAMA 246:1109, 1981

Chervenak FA, Farley MA, Walters L et al: When is termination of pregnancy during the third trimester morally justifiable? N Engl J Med 310:501, 1984

Corsaro M, Korzeniowsky C: A Woman's Guide to Safe Abortion. New York, Holt, Rinehart & Winston, 1983

Frohock FM: Abortion: A Case Study in Law and Morals. Westport, CT, Greenwood Press, 1983

Grimes DA, Cates WC, Selik RM: Abortion facilities and the risk of death. Fam Plann Perspect 13(1):30–32, January/February 1981

Henshaw SK, Binkin NJ, Blaine E et al: A portrait of American women who obtain abortions. Fam Plann Perspect 17(1):90–96, 1985

Henshaw SK, Wallisch LS: The Medicaid cutoff and abortion services for the poor. Fam Plann Perspect 16(4): 170–180, July/August 1984

Hogan R: Human Sexuality: A Nursing Perspective, Chap 20, pp 307–325. Norwalk, CT, Appleton–Century–Crofts, 1985

Hogue CJR, Cates W, Tietze C: The effects of induced abortion on subsequent reproduction. Epidemiologic Rev 4: 66, 1982

Merton AH: Enemies of Choice: The Right-to-Life Movement and Its Threat to Abortion. Boston, Beacon Press, 1982

Sarvis B, Rodman H: Social and cultural aspects of abortion: Class and race. In Ostheimer N, Ostheimer JM (eds): Life or Death—Who Controls? pp 104–118. New York, Springer–Verlag, 1976

Tanis JL: Recognizing the reasons for contraceptive non-use and abuse. Am J Maternal Child Nurs 2(3):364–369, May/June 1977

Tietze C: The public health effects of legal abortion in the United States. Fam Plann Perspect 16(1):26–28, January/February 1984

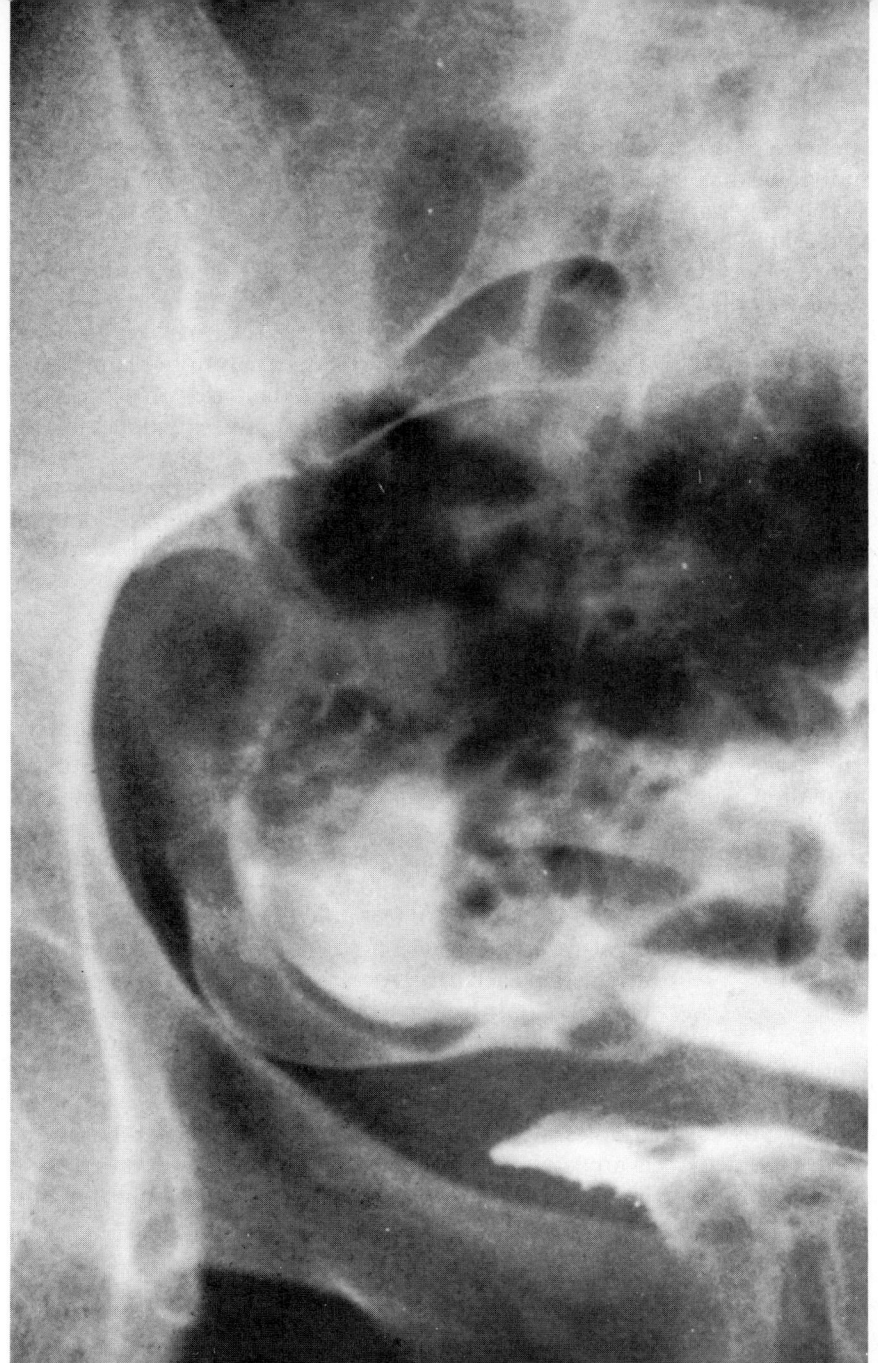

CHAPTER 16

Management of Infertility

Technology has introduced an element of choice in reproduction. The right of choice of the individual has been emphasized by international bodies. The General Assembly of the United Nations has declared that, "The size of the family should be the free choice of each individual family." The concept was later expanded to include the right to the means to space and limit births. Fertility is not always a matter of choice. The generally accepted estimate is that about 10% of couples are infertile.

One can realistically project a rise in the incidence of infertility due to social causes. The increase in the prevalence of gonorrheal and chlamydial salpingitis, and recent changes in women's social orientation—with the concomitant trend toward postponement of childbearing until the late reproductive years—have materially influenced reproductive potential. A shortage of children for adoption has created additional pressures.

Basic reproductive mechanisms were discussed and events beginning with spermatogenesis and oogenesis and ending in the development of the term fetus were explored in preceding chapters. This information will now serve as a basis for understanding the clinical approach to problems of human reproduction.

Assessment

Since infertility is usually caused by abnormalities in the anatomy and physiology of the male or female reproductive tract, management of the problem involves both marital partners. Emotional support is provided most effectively when the couple is approached as a unit, without singling out one of the partners for exclusive attention.

Before selecting a method of treatment, efforts should be made to identify the underlying cause of infertility. Appropriate therapy can be selected only after the cause for infertility is determined. Shotgun measures involving use of so-called fertility drugs are useless. There is no quick substitute for a carefully planned investigative program. Minimal standards that are suggested for a complete infertility investigation include evaluation of seminal, cervical, ovarian, tubal, peritoneal, and uterine factors. In addition, the frequency and technique of intercourse should be explored. Some of the outpatient procedures used in a standard infertility investigation are outlined in Table 16-1.

Initiating Investigation

When one considers the complexity of reproductive processes, it is not surprising that unprotected coitus at about the time of ovulation does not always result in a pregnancy. In fact, under normal circumstances an average of six cycles of exposure is required. It is generally felt that infertility should be explored after a year's exposure without contraception. However, it is unwise to insist on an interval of 1 year before investigation is initiated in each case. A reassuring consultation is often helpful, if only to dispel doubts concerning the existence of major abnormalities. Because fertility declines with age, it would seem justifiable for couples in their 30s to seek advice somewhat earlier. Even among younger couples, when the nurse or physician senses that there is anxiety over failure to conceive or when on cursory exploration there is an obvious reason for infertility, for

T A B L E   1 6 - 1

Standard Outpatient Procedures for Infertility

Test	Timing	Interpretation
Semen analysis ♂	Suggested as initial procedure Repeated if questionable 2–3 days of abstinence prior to collection	Volume 2–5 ml Count >20 million/ml Motility >60% with good quality Morphology >60% normal
Postcoital test ♀♂	1–2 days prior to ovulation (days 12–14 in a 28-day cycle)	10–20 sperm/high-power field in favorable mucus is considered normal
Plasma progesterone ♀	Presumed postovulatory phase (last 10 days of cycle)	>4 ng/ml strongly suggests ovulation
Endometrial biopsy ♀	Luteal (postovulatory) phase of cycle (days 21–24 of a 28-day cycle)	Secretory changes as interpreted in relation to onset of next menses Absence or presence of chronic endometritis
Hysterosalpingogram ♀	Preovulatory (before day 12 in the 28-day cycle)	Contour of uterus and patency of tubes as seen on fluoroscopy and roentgenograms

example, amenorrhea or a history of acute salpingitis or postabortal infection, early evaluation is in order.

Initial Interview

In the initial interview, sexual habits should be reviewed with both husband and wife. Although the frequency of coitus varies greatly from one couple to the next, patterns of intercourse do influence fertility. Only about 16% of couples who are having intercourse less than once a week will conceive in less than 6 months. Over 80% conceive in the same interval when exposure occurs four or more times weekly. When intercourse occurs infrequently the sexual adjustment in the marriage should be explored. There is no evidence to suggest a relationship between female orgasm and conception. Nevertheless, the frequency of coitus is influenced by sexual satisfaction; intercourse may be infrequent because it is associated with discomfort (dyspareunia) or because it is simply not a pleasurable experience for the wife.

The uninitiated health professional is often uncomfortable when matters of sexuality are reviewed. The role of the nurse is especially important because often the nurse may be called upon to elicit the initial history. When emotionally charged matters of reproductive failure are at issue, a sympathetic, nonjudgmental approach, coupled with the competence that comes only from knowledge and experience, contributes greatly to client management. Nurses who are most effective in this regard are those who are most comfortable with their own sexuality and those who have had the opportunity to share the care of infertility clients with seasoned practitioners.

Some centers have found self-assessment forms such as those included here to be useful. Both the husband and the wife are asked to complete them prior to their initial interview. Emphasis is placed on those aspects of the history that could have impact on infertility. The forms include details of the menstrual history, past medical–surgical history, fertility and sexual history, details of personal habits such as alcohol consumption, smoking, and drug use, and past contraceptive programs. This approach allows clients to review the various factors that could influence fertility, but also provides easy entrance into the sexual area, since each is asked for an appraisal of frequency of coitus and sexual satisfaction.

Male Factors

Male abnormalities are responsible in at least 35% of infertility in couples, and evaluation of the husband early in the course of the investigation is mandatory. Because evaluation of the male is much less complicated

than the series of tests required to explore female infertility, his reproductive potential should always be assessed first. The postcoital test—examination of cervical mucus for the presence of spermatozoa—is useful in this regard. This test is discussed later in the chapter.

Physical Examination

Physical examination of the genitalia may immediately reveal abnormalities that would explain the infertility. The testes may be undescended or hypoplastic. Postpubescent mumps orchitis may have resulted in testicular atrophy. Herniorrhaphy may have impaired the blood supply to the testes. Varicocele, varicose veins around the testes, is sometimes associated with decreased spermatogenesis and may also affect the quality of sperm motility. The extra heat delivered to the testicular area by the dilated veins is thought to influence sperm production adversely. It is important to examine the client for the presence of a varicocele in the standing position to allow the veins to fill with blood. Surgical correction of the varicocele by high ligation of the veins is followed by significant improvement in semen quality in over 50% of cases.

Semen Evaluation

Unless adequate numbers of spermatozoa are seen in the cervical mucus following coitus, the semen should be evaluated. This involves assessment of the fresh ejaculate obtained by masturbation after at least 3 days of abstinence. The ejaculate is collected in a clean, dry container and brought to the laboratory as soon after collection as practical. The client should be cautioned not to lose the first few drops of the ejaculate because the majority of active spermatozoa are located in the first portion of the specimen. Normally, seminal fluid becomes coagulated immediately upon ejaculation. Liquefaction of the coagulum occurs within 20 minutes. Examination should be deferred until liquefaction is complete because the coagulum interferes with the distribution of spermatozoa in the counting chamber.

The interval from the time of last coitus should be recorded. Although frequent coitus is of little consequence when the ejaculation is normal, the relatively infertile male undergoes a marked reduction in sperm count when ejaculation occurs too frequently. It is recommended that the first specimen for analysis be collected after a period of abstinence that is roughly equivalent to the customary interval between intercourse for that couple. If the specimen reveals differences, the semen analysis can be repeated after a longer interval of abstinence.

The volume of the specimen, sperm density, percentage of motile forms, quality of the motility, and percentage of abnormal spermatozoa are determined. The volume of the normal ejaculate ranges from 2 ml

(text continued on page 242)

ASSESSMENT TOOL

Husband's Medical History Form, Infertility Clinic

Name: Date:
Address: Tel.:
Occupation: Age: Religion:
Employer: Ins.:
Bus. Tel.:   Cert. No.:
Referred by: Gr. No.:
Birth Place: Name Rel./Friend:
Birth Date: Address:

All previous occupations:	List all states or countries in which you have lived:

Education:	Please encircle the last grade you completed	Grade	5	High School	1 2 3 4	Post Grad. _____ yrs.
		6 7 8		College	1 2 3 4	Degrees

CHIEF COMPLAINTS   P. I. Please do not write in this space.
Please list all symptoms you have NOW.
1. _____
2. _____
3. _____
Routine checkup—no symptoms [ ]

FAMILY HISTORY	Age	If Living Health	Age at death	If Deceased Cause	Has any blood relative had (Please Encircle)		Who
Father					Cancer	no yes	
Mother					Tuberculosis	no yes	
Brother or sister 1.					Diabetes	no yes	
2.					Heart trouble	no yes	
3.					High blood pressure	no yes	
4.					Stroke	no yes	
5.					Epilepsy	no yes	
Husband or wife					Mental illness	no yes	
Son or daughter 1.					Suicide	no yes	
2.					Congenital deformities	no yes	
3.					NOTE:		
4.					This is a confidential record of your medical history and		
5.					will be kept in this office. Information contained here		
6.					will not be released to any person except when you		
7.					have authorized us to do so.		

PERSONAL HISTORY
ILLNESS: Have you had
(Please Encircle all Answers no or yes)

Measles or German measles	no yes	Gonorrhea or syphilis	no yes	Mycins or other antibiotics	no yes
Chickenpox or mumps	no yes	Anemia or jaundice	no yes	Merthiolate or mercurochrome	no yes
Whooping cough	no yes	Epilepsy	no yes	Any other drug	no yes
Scarlet fever or scarlatina	no yes	Migraine headaches	no yes	Any foods	no yes
Pneumonia or pleurisy	no yes	Tuberculosis	no yes	Adhesive tape	no yes
Diphtheria or smallpox	no yes	Diabetes or cancer	no yes	Nail polish or other cosmetics	no yes
Influenza	no yes	High or low blood pressure	no yes	Tetanus antitoxin or serums	no yes
Rheumatic fever or heart disease	no yes	Nervous breakdown	no yes	INJURIES: Have you had any	
Arthritis or rheumatism	no yes	Food, chemical or drug poisoning	no yes	Broken bones	no yes
Any bone or joint disease	no yes	Hay fever or asthma	no yes	Sprains or dislocations	no yes
Neuritis or neuralgia	no yes	Hives or eczema	no yes	Lacerations (extensive)	no yes
Bursitis, sciatica or lumbago	no yes	Frequent colds or sore throat	no yes	Concussion or head injury	no yes
Polio or meningitis	no yes	Frequent infections or boils	no yes	Ever been knocked out	no yes
Bright's disease or kidney infection	no yes	Any other disease	no yes	TRANSFUSIONS: Have you ever had	
		ALLERGIES: Are you allergic to		Blood or plasma transfusion	no yes
		Penicillin or sulfa	no yes	Weight: now _____ one year ago _____	
		Aspirin, codeine or morphine	no yes	Max _____ when _____ Height _____	

Please review the section you have just completed and wherever you answered "yes" fill in the year (guess if necessary) and also where there is more than one illness to a line encircle the ones you have had. Example: Chickenpox or mumps ....1961 ....no (yes)

(continued)

ASSESSMENT TOOL (continued)

SURGERY: Have you had

Tonsillectomy .... no   yes
Appendectomy .... no   yes
Any other operation (give details)   no   yes

Give DETAILS below of all hospitalizations for surgery or illness including name and address of Doctor and Hospital . . . .

Have you ever been advised to have any surgical operation which has not been done? [1] no   [2] yes   what ....

Systems: Please check those you have had.

Eye disease [ ], Eye injury [ ], Impaired sight [ ], Ear disease [ ], Ear injury [ ], Impaired hearing [ ],
Trouble with: Nose [ ], Sinuses [ ], Mouth [ ], Throat [ ], Have you checked any in this group? .... no   yes
Fainting spells [ ], Loss of consciousness [ ], Convulsions [ ], Paralysis [ ], Frequent or severe headaches [ ], Dizziness [ ], Depression or anxiety [ ], Hallucinations [ ], Have you checked any in this group? .... no   yes
Enlarged glands [ ], Goiter or enlarged thyroid [ ], Skin disease [ ], Have you checked any in this group? .... no   yes
Chronic or frequent cough [ ], Chest pain or angina pectoris [ ], Spitting up of blood [ ], Night sweats [ ], Shortness of breath [ ], Palpitation or fluttering heart [ ], Swelling of hands, feet, or ankles [ ], Varicose veins [ ], Extreme tiredness or weakness [ ], Have you checked any in this group? .... no   yes
Kidney disease or stones [ ], Bladder disease [ ], Albumin, sugar, pus, etc. in urine [ ], Difficulty in urinating [ ], Awake to urinate nightly [ ], Have you checked any in this group? .... no   yes
Stomach trouble or ulcers [ ], Indigestion [ ], Liver or gallbladder disease [ ], Colitis or other bowel disease [ ] Appendicitis [ ], Hemorrhoids or rectal bleeding [ ], Constipation or diarrhea [ ], Recent change in bowel action or stools [ ], Recent change in appetite or eating habits [ ], Have you checked any in this group? .... no   yes

HABITS: Do you

Sleep well? .... no   yes
Use alcoholic beverages .... no   yes
  Every day? .... no   yes
Smoke? .... no   yes
  How much? ....
Exercise enough .... no   yes
Is your diet well balanced? .... no   yes

List any drugs or medications you take regularly or frequently:

MARITAL HISTORY

Prior marriage? ....
Was pregnancy achieved? ....

Is sex entirely satisfactory? ....
Reaction of wife: ....

When? (Dates) ....
Any other proof of fertility? ....

Estimated frequency of coitus (intercourse) per month: ....
Remarks: ....

INFERTILITY STUDIES

	Result	Date	Where Done
Semen analysis			
Thyroid tests:			
Hormone tests:			
Medicines given:			
Other tests:			

(Courtesy of Division of Human Reproduction, Hospital of the University of Pennsylvania, Philadelphia, PA)

A S S E S S M E N T   T O O L

Wife's Medical History Form, Infertility Clinic

Name:	Date:	Unit No.:
(Nee):	Tel.:	Husb.:
Address: Age:	Ins.:	Occupation: Age:
Occupation:	Cert. No.:	Employer
Employer:	Gr. No.:	Bus. Address:
Bus. Tel.:	Name Rel./Friend:	Bus. Tel.:
Referred by:	Address:	Religion: Husb. Wife:
Birth Place:		[ ] Single [ ] Divorced
Birth Date:		[ ] Married [ ] Widow (er)

All previous occupations:	List all states or countries in which you have lived:

Education:	Please encircle the last grade you completed	Grade 5 6 7 8	High School 1 2 3 4 College 1 2 3 4	Post Grad. _____ yrs. Degrees

Date of last physical exam.

Chief Complaints: Please list all symptoms you have NOW.

1. _____
2. _____
3. _____

Routine checkup—no symptoms [ ]

P. I. Please do not write in this space.

FAMILY HISTORY	Age	If Living Health	Age at death	If Deceased Cause	Please Encircle Has any blood relative had		Who
Father					Cancer	no yes	
Mother					Tuberculosis	no yes	
Brother or sister 1.					Diabetes	no yes	
2.					Heart trouble	no yes	
3.					High blood pressure	no yes	
4.					Stroke	no yes	
5.					Epilepsy	no yes	
Husband or wife					Mental illness	no yes	
Son or daughter 1.					Suicide	no yes	
2.					Congenital deformities	no yes	
3.					NOTE: This is a confidential record of your medical		
4.					history and will be kept in this office. Information contained		
5.					here will not be released to any person except when		
6.					you have authorized us to do so.		

PERSONAL HISTORY

ILLNESS: Have you had
(Please Encircle all Answers no or yes)

Measles or German measles	no yes
Chickenpox or mumps	no yes
Whooping cough	no yes
Scarlet fever or scarlatina	no yes
Pneumonia or pleurisy	no yes
Diphtheria or smallpox	no yes
Influenza	no yes
Rheumatic fever or heart disease	no yes
Arthritis or rheumatism	no yes
Any bone or joint disease	no yes
Neuritis or neuralgia	no yes
Bursitis, sciatica or lumbago	no yes
Polio or meningitis	no yes
Bright's disease or kidney infection	no yes

Gonorrhea or syphilis	no yes
Anemia or jaundice	no yes
Epilepsy	no yes
Migraine headaches	no yes
Tuberculosis	no yes
Diabetes or cancer	no yes
High or low blood pressure	no yes
Nervous breakdown	no yes
Food, chemical or drug poisoning	no yes
Hay fever or asthma	no yes
Hives or eczema	no yes
Frequent colds or sore throat	no yes
Frequent infections or boils	no yes
Any other disease	no yes

ALLERGIES: Are you allergic to

Penicillin or sulfa	no yes
Aspirin, codeine or morphine	no yes

Mycins or other antibiotics	no yes
Merthiolate or mercurochrome	no yes
Any other drug	no yes
Any foods	no yes
Adhesive tape	no yes
Nail polish or other cosmetics	no yes
Tetanus antitoxin or serums	no yes

INJURIES: Have you had any

Broken bones	no yes
Sprains or dislocations	no yes
Lacerations (extensive)	no yes
Concussion or head injury	no yes
Ever been knocked out	no yes

TRANSFUSIONS: Have you ever had

Blood or plasma transfusion   no   yes

Weight: now _____ one year ago _____

Max _____ when _____ Height _____

Please review the section you have just completed and wherever you answered "yes" fill in the year (guess if necessary) and also where there is more than one illness to a line encircle the ones you have had. Example: Chickenpox or mumps ....1961 .... no (yes)

(continued)

A S S E S S M E N T   T O O L   *(continued)*

SURGERY: Have you had   no   yes   Give DETAILS below of all hospitalizations for surgery or illness including name and address of
Tonsillectomy ....   Doctor and Hospital . . . .
Appendectomy ....   no   yes
Any other operation (give details)   no   yes

Have you ever been advised to have any surgical operation which has not been done? [1] no   [2] yes   what ....

Systems: Please check those you have had.
Eye disease [ ], Eye injury [ ], Impaired sight [ ], Ear disease [ ], Ear injury [ ], Impaired hearing [ ],
Trouble with: Nose [ ], Sinuses [ ], Mouth [ ], Throat [ ], Have you checked any in this group? .... no   yes
Fainting spells [ ], Loss of consciousness [ ], Convulsions [ ], Paralysis [ ], Frequent or severe headaches [ ], Dizziness [ ], Depression
or anxiety [ ], Hallucinations [ ], Have you checked any in this group? .... no   yes
Enlarged glands [ ], Goiter or enlarged thyroid [ ], Skin disease [ ], Have you checked any in this group? .... no   yes
Chronic or frequent cough [ ], Chest pain or angina pectoris [ ], Spitting up of blood [ ], Night sweats [ ], Shortness of breath [ ],
Palpitation or fluttering heart [ ], Swelling of hands, feet, or ankles [ ], Varicose veins [ ], Extreme tiredness or weakness [ ], Have you
checked any in this group? .... no   yes
Kidney disease or stones [ ], Bladder disease [ ], Albumin, sugar, pus, etc. in urine [ ], Difficulty in urinating [ ], Awake to urinate
nightly [ ], Have you checked any in this group? .... no   yes
Stomach trouble or ulcers [ ], Indigestion [ ], Liver or gallbladder disease [ ], Colitis or other bowel disease [ ], Appendicitis [ ],
Hemorrhoids or rectal bleeding [ ], Constipation or diarrhea [ ], Recent change in bowel action or stools [ ], Recent change in appetite
or eating habits [ ], Have you checked any in this group? .... no   yes

---

HABITS: Do you

Sleep well? .... no   yes
Use alcoholic beverages ...... no   yes
    Every day? .... no   yes
Smoke? .... no   yes
    How much? ....
Exercise enough .... no   yes
Is your diet well balanced?   no   yes

List any drugs or medications you
take regularly or frequently:

_____
_____
_____
_____
_____
_____

OBSTETRICAL-GYNECOLOGICAL REVIEW

Age at first menstruation _____ Age at first coital
experience ____ Number of living children (at present) _____
Number of pregnancies _____
Number of live births _____ Number of multiple
pregnancies _____
Number of stillbirths (more than 20 weeks) _____
Number of abortions, miscarriages (20 weeks or less) _____
Number of children dead _____ Age of oldest child _____
Number of births with deformities _____

GYNECOLOGICAL HISTORY

Are menstrual cycles regular? .... Are your periods similar? ....
Interval between periods ....
Length of flow .... Date of last menstrual cycle ....
Amount of flow ....[1] Light   [2] Moderate   [3] Heavy
Was the quality, quantity, and duration of flow for this last cycle similar in
comparison with previous cycles? ....
   [1] No (specify how it differed) ....
   .... [2] Yes
Has there been any bleeding in between periods? ....
   [1] No   [2] Yes (specify) ....
Were any medications taken during cycle? ....
   [1] No   [2] Yes (specify)
Dysmenorrhea (menstrual discomfort) ....
   [1] None   [2] Intermittent   [3] Constant
Type of menstrual discomfort experienced
   [1] None   [3] Dull   [5] Cramp
   [2] Sharp   [4] Ache   [6] Backache

PREMENSTRUAL SYMPTOMS

Bloating .... no   yes
Breast tenderness .... no   yes
Pelvic pain .... no   yes
Backache .... no   yes
Headache .... no   yes
Irritability .... no   yes
Edema .... no   yes
Acne .... no   yes

INTERMENSTRUAL DISCHARGE

Type [1] None   [3] Yellow [5] White
       [2] Tan   [4] Bloody [6] Other (specify)
Amount .... Scant Heavy
Itching .... no   yes
Odorless .... no   yes
Frequent .... no   yes
Regular pattern .... no   yes

MARITAL HISTORY

Prior marriage? .... when? (Dates) ....   Was pregnancy achieved? ....
Is sex entirely satisfactory? ....   Dyspareunia (discomfort during coitus): no .... yes ....
Estimate frequency of coitus (sexual   Does coitus occur during menses?   Yes .... No ....
intercourse) per month: ....
Reaction of husband: ....   On which days of flow? ....
Remarks: ....   Is this consistent? ....
....
....

(continued)

ASSESSMENT TOOL   *(continued)*

INDICATE THE INFORMATION FOR ANY OF THE FOLLOWING STUDIES WHICH YOU HAVE HAD.

	Date	Result	Doctor
Basal body temperature record:			
Biopsy test:			
Thyroid test:			
Gas (Rubin) test:			
X-ray of uterus and tubes:			
Postcoital test: (survival of seed in your secretions)			
Cautery of cervix:			
Hormone test:			
Inseminations:			
Medicines given:			
Other:			

(Courtesy of Division of Human Reproduction, Hospital of the University of Pennsylvania, Philadelphia, PA)

(text continued from page 237)

to 5 ml. A volume greater than 5 ml is often associated with a lower than normal concentration of spermatozoa and, if such is the case, is considered abnormal. A volume of less than 1 ml is also abnormal and may result in infertility probably because it is less likely that the ejaculate will reach the cervix during intercourse. A sperm count of more than 20 million/ml is considered normal, provided the quality and percentage of motility in the specimen are also normal. The single most useful criterion is the actual quality of motility, the ability of spermatozoa to progress. Pregnancies do occasionally occur when the counts are much lower than 20 million/ml.

Because there is usually some variation in the quality of semen ejaculated at various times, assessment of the husband's fertility potential should never be based on a single analysis. Since maturation of spermatozoa within the testis occurs over a 60-day interval, the quality of semen could be influenced by an event, such as a viral infection, that took place many days before the spermatozoa appeared in the ejaculate.

If the postcoital test is abnormal, but the semen analysis is within normal limits, the possibility that semen is not being ejaculated deep in the vagina during intercourse should be considered. In such cases, further investigations of coital techniques and examination of the male genitalia are often helpful. Hypospadias, a condition in which the opening of the urethra is located along the shaft of the penis and not at the glans, may result in semen not being ejaculated deep in the vagina. Discussion may uncover unsuspected sexual difficulties such as premature ejaculation or even impotence.

When the semen analysis or postcoital test is abnormal, the male partner should be evaluated further for anatomical, genetic, or endocrine abnormalities. These evaluations are usually carried out by urologists who specialize in infertility.

When there is azoospermia (absence of spermatozoa in the ejaculate) the client should be evaluated for genetic abnormalities. If the testes are grossly normal to palpation and there is azoospermia, obstruction of the duct system should be considered. Such obstruction may be congenital or may be the result of a postinflammatory process such as tuberculosis or gonorrhea. Testicular function can be assessed further by microscopic examination of the specimen removed by testicular biopsy. When there is ductal occlusion and the testicular biopsy reveals evidence of normal spermatogenesis, patency can sometimes be reestablished by microsurgery. The most common cause of duct obstruction is, of course, vasectomy, carried out for purposes of sterilization. This can also be reversed surgically with moderate to good success.

Postcoital Test—Evaluation of Insemination

The postcoital test is sometimes referred to as the Sims–Huhner test, named for the two physicians who introduced and popularized it initially. A couple is instructed to have intercourse during the 12 hours preceding the examination. The test is timed for within a day or two before expected ovulation, that is, the 12th or 13th day in the 28-day menstrual cycle. At that time, the cervical mucus, under the influence of estrogen, is normally clear and abundant and is most receptive to spermatozoa. At other times in the cycle, the mucus is scanty, thick, turbid, and generally unreceptive.

A sample of cervical mucus is obtained in the following manner. The cervix is exposed with a vaginal speculum, and after secretions and debris are gently wiped from the exocervix, mucus is removed from well within the endocervical canal with fenestrated intestinal forceps or nasal polyp forceps, or the mucus may be aspirated from the cervix into a polyethylene tube. Its gross characteristics, quantity, and clarity are evaluated, and its ability to form a thin continuous thread (a quality referred to as *spinnbarkeit*) is assessed. Spinnbarkeit is determined by stretching the mucus between the tips of the forceps until the thread breaks. Normal preovulatory mucus can be stretched for a distance of up to 10 cm. The sample is then placed on a clean, dry slide and a coverslip is applied. The specimen is then examined microscopically for spermatozoa. The test is normal when there are more than 20 motile spermatozoa per high-power field in areas of clear, abundant cervical mucus. In addition to assessing the placement of spermatozoa during coitus, the postcoital test permits evaluation of the quality of cervical secretions and their ability to support the life of the spermatozoon—the cervical factor.

Female Factors

Physical Examination

A complete general physical examination is an integral part of an infertility study. Obviously, one would want assurance that there are no medical conditions that could adversely affect the health of the mother during pregnancy or conditions that might affect a pregnancy adversely, such as diabetes or chronic hypertensive vascular disease.

At the time of pelvic examination, abnormalities are sought that could influence fertility, such as ovarian cysts, stigmas of past pelvic inflammatory disease (such as thickening of the adnexa), subacute pelvic inflammatory disease as evidenced by tenderness in the adnexa, and physical signs of endometriosis, such as nodularity along the uterosacral ligaments or a fixed retroverted uterus. Some centers make it a practice to culture the cervix for organisms that are associated with venereal disease, such as *Chlamydia trachomatis* or even gonococci, at the time of the initial examination. If there is a history of intrauterine diethylstilbestrol exposure, one should pay particular attention to the status of the cervix for evidence of abnormalities.

Cervical Factor

To assess the quality of the cervical secretions and to diagnose abnormalities at that level, the timing of the recovery of the mucus in the cycle is critical. The healthcare professional should be aware of the normal variations in mucus quality in the menstrual cycle. If the mucus never demonstrates the characteristics of normal ovulatory mucus after serial evaluation on alternate days during the presumed ovulatory period, the possibility that mucus production is deficient should be seriously considered. Inability of spermatozoa to penetrate and survive in such mucus may reasonably be inferred to be a cause of infertility.

Ovarian Factor

Clearly, conception cannot occur when there is failure of ovulation, and fertility is impaired when ovulation is infrequent. Thus, ovulation detection is an integral part of the infertility investigation. Clues as to the occurrence of ovulation are derived from menstrual history, evaluation of characteristic changes in cervical mucus, and the basal body temperature chart. The use of the temperature chart is discussed in detail in Chapter 9. Additional parameters used to assess ovulation include histologic evaluation of a sample of endometrium obtained by biopsy, a plasma progesterone determination obtained late in the cycle, and determination of the preovulatory luteinizing hormone (LH) peak by evaluating urinary LH levels.

Endometrial biopsy is a simple office procedure that offers the additional advantage of ruling out a chronic inflammatory condition in the endometrium (Fig. 16-1). It is usually scheduled 5 days to 7 days before the expected onset of the next menses or on days 21 to 24 of a 28-day cycle. Any one of the available specially designed biopsy curets may be used.

After the position of the uterus is determined, a curet is gently introduced through the cervical canal to the level of the fundus and one or two samples of tissue are removed. The endometrial sample is then sent to the pathologist's laboratory for evaluation.

Following ovulation the glands of the endometrium exhibit secretory changes under the influence of progesterone. These changes are progressive and predictable and are characteristic enough from day to day to allow retrospective timing of ovulation.

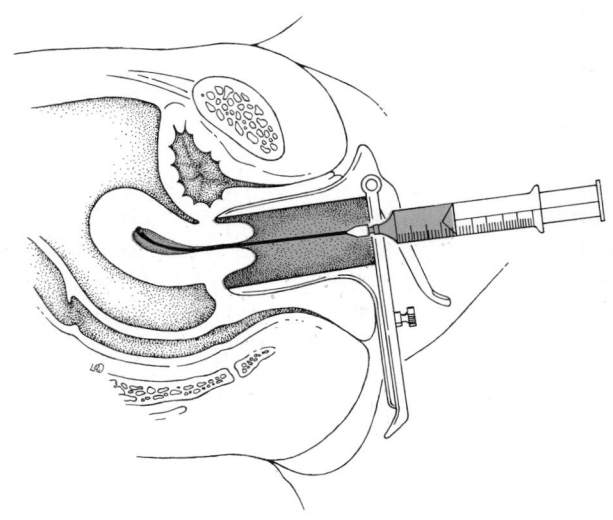

FIGURE 16-1

A simple office procedure of endometrial biopsy helps to rule out a chronic inflammatory condition of the endometrium.

Hormonal Determinations. Plasma progesterone levels increase significantly after ovulation following the formation of the corpus luteum. Evidence of corpus luteum function, and therefore indirect evidence of ovulation, is provided when plasma progesterone levels are greater than 4 ng/ml.

Monoclonal antibody technology has resulted in the development of a simple home kit for evaluating urinary LH levels. An enzymatic reaction causes a color change when LH is present in urine, and the intensity of the color can be correlated with the concentration of LH. Thus, when daily observations are carried out, the peak in LH level that precedes ovulation can be determined and, therefore, ovulation can be reasonably accurately timed in the course of a given cycle. The assay is carried out by the client at home beginning several days before expected ovulation. This approach has proved useful in evaluation of the ovulatory pattern and has particular application in the timing of artificial insemination.

Tubal Factors

The clinical approach to tubal disease involves assessment of tubal and peritubal anatomy. Because the human tube is a conduit that provides a passage between the ovary and the uterus, tubal obstruction, of course, results in infertility. In addition, since the fimbriated end of the tube is important in transferring the ovum from the rupturing follicle to the tubal lumen, when the relationship between it and the ovum is distorted by pelvic adhesions, fertility is also diminished.

Anatomical defects in and about the fallopian tubes are generally a result of a past infection or pelvic irritation. Acute gonorrheal salpingitis is a common offender. A ruptured appendix associated with pelvic peritonitis may also cause peritubal and periovarian adhesions.

Endometriosis, a condition in which the endometrium has been displaced into the peritoneal cavity around the tube and ovaries, may also result in pelvic adhesions and distortion of pelvic architecture.[1,2] Anatomical tubal disease is treated surgically with lysis and excision of the adhesions and special techniques to reestablish the patency of the fallopian tubes.

The commonly used tests for evaluation of tubal function include uterotubal insufflation (the Rubin test), hysterosalpingography, and endoscopy.

Uterotubal insufflation involves the introduction of carbon dioxide into the uterus through a cannula. If one or both of the tubes are patent, the carbon dioxide flows along the uterus and tubes into the peritoneal cavity. When the client sits up, the carbon dioxide rises to the diaphragm, causing pain in the shoulder referred there by way of the phrenic nerve. This test was used extensively in the past, but, increasingly, physicians have substituted other methods for it.

Hysterosalpingography involves introduction of radiopaque material into the uterus and fallopian tubes (Fig. 16-2). This is usually done under fluoroscopic visualization, and x-ray films are taken at intervals to provide a permanent record. When the tubes are patent, the radiopaque material enters the peritoneal cavity and is evenly distributed there. When the tubes are closed, the peritoneal egress is prevented by the obstruction, and a diagnosis of tubal occlusion can be made without further delay.

Peritoneoscopy involves direct visualization of the tubes and ovaries with an endoscope. This may be carried out through the cul-de-sac (*culdoscopy*) or through the umbilicus (*laparoscopy*). The former is carried out under local anesthesia with the client in the knee–chest position. In expert hands, visualization is usually satisfactory. It is a more difficult procedure, however, than laparoscopy, which has become the procedure of choice.

Diagnostic laparoscopy is generally carried out under general anesthesia (Fig. 16-3). This is the same procedure that is used for tubal sterilization. A needle is introduced through the umbilicus, and carbon dioxide is passed under controlled pressure into the abdominal cavity. This intra-abdominal gas causes the abdominal wall to balloon, pushing it away from the abdominal contents. The needle is removed and a trocar is introduced through an incision at the umbilicus through which a fiberoptic telescope can then be passed. This system usually allows complete visualization of the abdominal contents. The anatomy of the uterus, ovaries, and fallopian tubes is assessed visually. To manipulate these structures so as to allow the most complete evaluation, a second puncture is usually made just above the symphysis pubis through which a calibrated wand can be introduced. This allows the operator to move the ovaries and tubes about, to explore the fimbriated ends of the fallopian tubes and to view the undersurface of the broad ligaments and ovaries to detect endometriosis or pelvic adhesions. Prior to the initiation of the procedure a cannula is placed at the cervix for manipulation of the uterus for more complete visualization. The cannula is also used for introduction of a dilute solution of dye while the ends of the tubes are under visualization. Dye can be seen spilling from the ends of patent tubes. In addition, the area in and about the fallopian tubes can be evaluated directly for the presence of adhesions or endometriosis.

Uterine Factors

Pathologic conditions of the uterus associated with decreased fertility include uterine fibroids, congenital malformations, and intrauterine adhesions. Inflammatory lesions of the endometrium also occur.

Congenital defects of the uterus, as well as uterine fibroids, are more often related to habitual abortion than

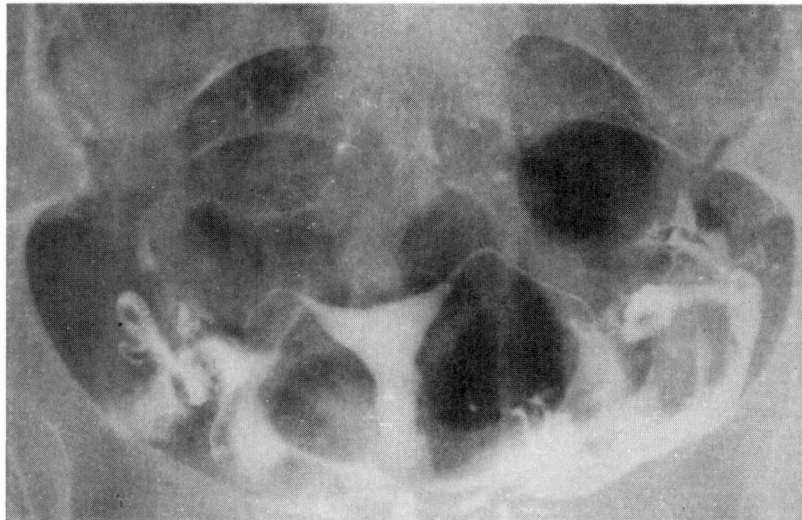

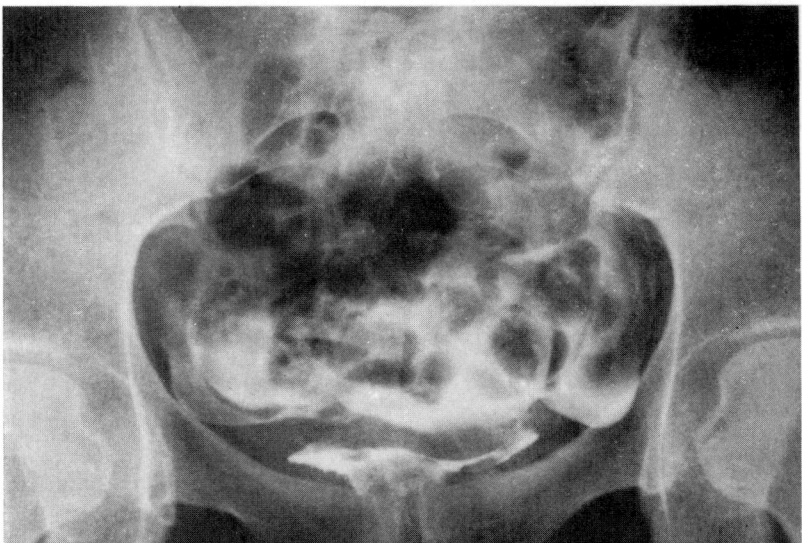

FIGURE 16-2

A normal hysterosalpingogram revealing bilateral tubal patency with spill of radiopaque material into the peritoneal cavity. (Mastroianni L Jr: Variations of Fertility. In Romney SL, Gray MJ, Little AB (eds): Gynecology and Obstetrics: The Health Care of Women. New York, McGraw-Hill, 1975)

to infertility. Fibroids may distort the endometrial cavity, and if they are strategically located and large enough, they presumably could interfere with implantation. If located adjacent to the tube, they may cause tubal obstruction. When a causal relationship is thought to exist, *myomectomies* (removal of the fibroids), with preservation of the uterus, are usually technically possible. Treatment of congenital abnormalities, more commonly associated with habitual abortion than infertility, is also surgical.

Asherman's syndrome, or adhesions within the uterine cavity, is usually the result of a postpartal or postabortal infection or pelvic tuberculosis. There is often a history of a previous dilatation and curettage followed by a stormy postoperative course. Increasing use of abortion as a backup for contraceptive failure may be associated with an increased incidence of this uncommon but potential fertility-impairing lesion.

Nursing Diagnoses

Infertility invariably represents a life crisis situation. It involves many feelings that must be recognized and dealt with. The infertile couple is often sensitive and extremely vulnerable. It is important to acknowledge the pressures associated with infertility and to allow opportunities to review the sense of isolation, guilt, depression, and even anger that often accompanies infertility.

The following are potential nursing diagnoses that may be seen at this time: anxiety related to the unknown or the outcome, fear related to the outcome or unknown, alterations in comfort (pain) related to tests or treatment, ineffective individual or family coping, knowledge deficit related to sexual anatomy or physiology, power-

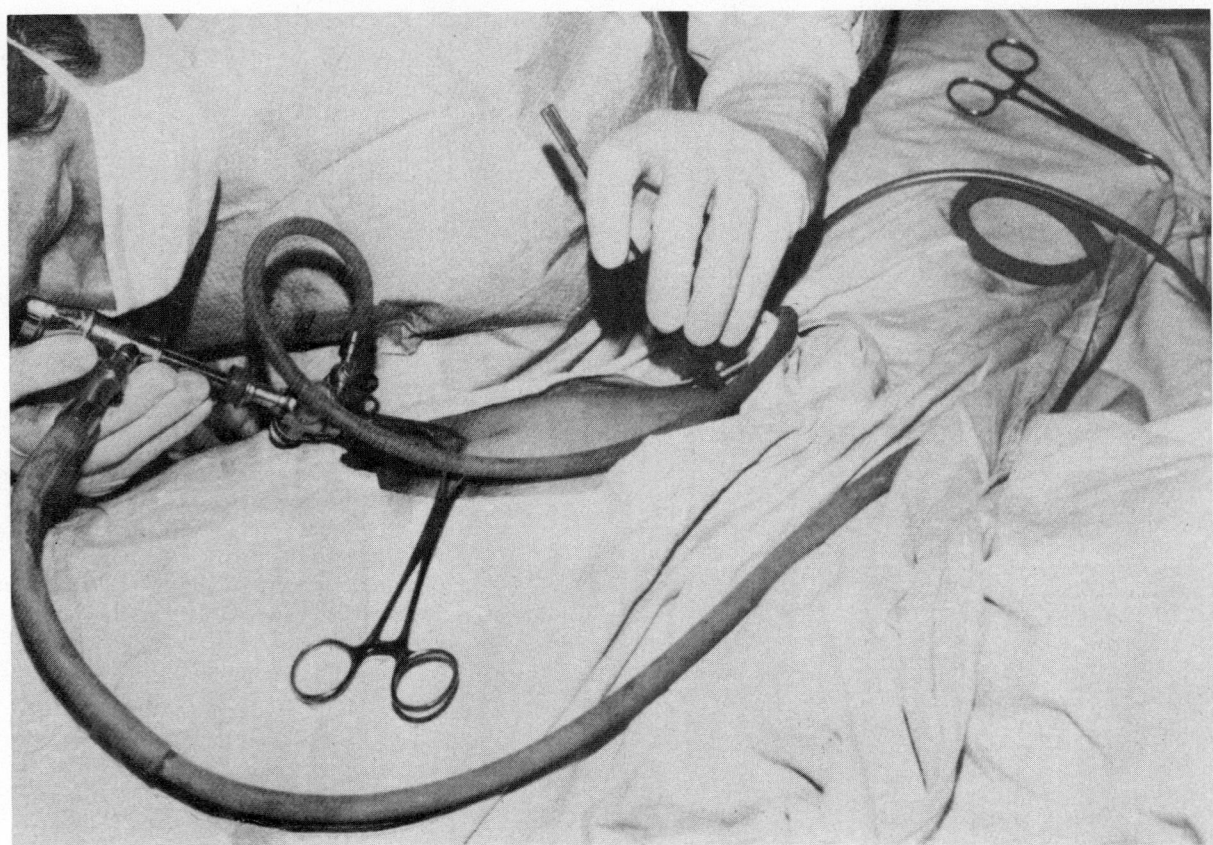

FIGURE   16-3

The double-puncture laparoscopic technique using the probe to position the pelvic structures for optimum visualization. (Seitz HM Jr, Rosenfeld RL: Endoscopy in the management of infertility. Clin Obstet Gynecol 17:86, 1974)

lessness over reproductive processes, disturbance in self-concept, and sexual dysfunction.

The ultimate goal of infertility investigation is not solely that of a successful pregnancy. It is equally important to establish a prognosis and to help couples who, after careful evaluation, are finally adjudged hopelessly sterile plan their lives realistically.

Treatment

General Treatment of Infertile Couples

Clients who make it a habit to arise from bed immediately after intercourse, spilling much of the ejaculate shortly after it is placed in the vagina, should be advised to remain in bed for at least 30 minutes following coitus. Occasionally, couples admit to using lubricants during intercourse or to douching postcoitally, which may in-

terfere with sperm migration. Petroleum jelly and some of the water-soluble lubricants have been shown to be spermicidal. These factors may not cause infertility when the husband's fertility potential is normal, but may play a role when sperm production is marginal. In some clients, there is even anatomical evidence that normal intercourse is not occurring (*e.g.*, an intact hymenal ring or a rigid perineal body). Other sexual problems such as premature ejaculation may result in failure of proper placement of sperm. Sympathetic and knowledgeable advice in these areas is often useful not only in the treatment of infertility but also in bringing about a better sexual relationship.

Some clients, for reasons that are not understood, conceive during the course of the diagnostic evaluation for infertility. Occasionally, conception occurs after not more than a preliminary examination and discussion of the diagnostic approach to follow. It is tempting to conjecture that, in some cases, the decision to seek aid for infertility is associated with a release of emotional tension followed, somehow, by improved reproductive performance. With the exceptions of ovulatory failure, which may have a psychological basis, and decreased frequency of intercourse, which sometimes has a psychological basis, there is as yet no proved somatic basis for psychologically induced infertility. The general impression that adoption is often followed by conception has not been substantiated. Nevertheless, throughout the infertility investigation, the emotional support provided by those involved in client management is especially important.

Artificial Insemination

In selected cases, artificial placement of semen is an effective therapeutic modality. The technique involves insertion of a freshly ejaculated specimen at the cervical os with a cannula and syringe within a day or two of the estimated time of ovulation (Fig. 16-4). Alternatively, the specimen can be injected into a plastic cervical cap that is placed around the cervix. The cap retains the specimen at the cervix and is removed several hours later. To be sure that ovulation has been covered, insemination is repeated on alternate days until it has been determined by the temperature chart that ovulation has occurred.

AIH

Artificial insemination with the husband's specimen (AIH) is especially useful in cases in which the postcoital test consistently reveals few or absent spermatozoa in cervical mucus of good quality. In selected cases, the use of a "split ejaculate" is recommended. Here, the specimen is collected into two containers. By and large,

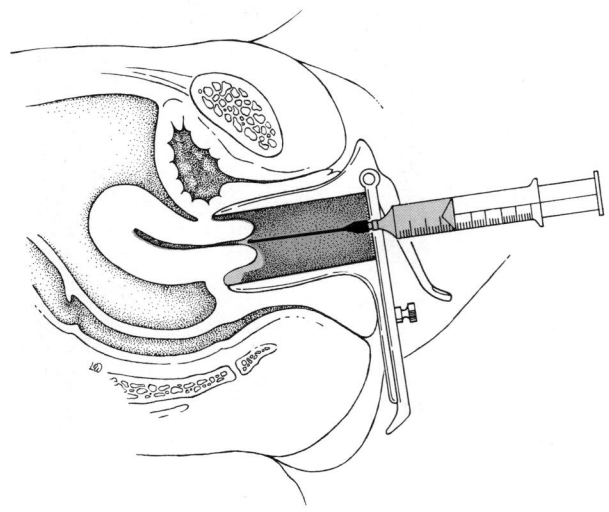

FIGURE 16-4

One technique for artificial insemination involves placing fresh semen at the cervical os with a cannula and syringe. The timing is based on the ovulatory phase of the female.

the first portion of the ejaculate contains a significantly higher portion of normal motile spermatozoa and it is this first portion that is used for the insemination.

AID

In cases of azoospermia (absence of spermatozoa in the ejaculate) or severe oligospermia (markedly decreased numbers of spermatozoa in the ejaculate) that has failed to respond to treatment, insemination of a specimen from a donor (AID) may be employed. AID is sometimes called semiadoption and has gained increasing popularity and acceptability in recent years. Willingness of a couple to consider AID has been influenced to a large degree in recent years by the lack of availability of children for adoption. AID is also used in cases in which the husband suffers from a genetic defect or in cases of Rh sensitization. In the latter instance, an Rh-negative donor is used.

The physician who wishes to use AID should settle on an organized approach and must be willing to give this procedure the necessary time and attention it demands. Selection of the donor must be carried out with great care, with attention to general state of health, genetic background, Rh type, and physical characteristics that at least to some degree resemble those of the husband. Those advising clients on this matter should be aware of the social and ethical implications of the procedure and should allow adequate time to explore matters with the couple in depth before proceeding. On the positive side, when AID is accepted by informed consenting partners, the end result is usually satisfactory. There is a remarkable marriage stability among properly selected couples who have been treated with AID.

The fresh ejaculate can be frozen and stored for future use. The use of frozen semen for AID offers several distinct advantages. The specimen is readily available, and the client's visits need not be timed to coincide with the delivery of a fresh ejaculate. A wider selection of donor specimens is possible, and it is easier to plan repeated inseminations in a given cycle. For a subsequent pregnancy, the same donor can conveniently be used if several of the specimens have been stored. More than 600 pregnancies have been reported following the use of frozen semen. There is no evidence of an increase in genetic abnormalities, and the spontaneous abortion rate is below that expected in the general population. There is evidence of a somewhat decreased pregnancy rate with frozen semen, but the difference is slight. Many physicians, nevertheless, are still uneasy.

Treatment of the Cervical Factor

Because little is known about the physiology of cervical mucus production, treatment of the cervical factor has not been uniformly successful. Local treatment of the cervix when there is a cervicitis and the use of small doses of estrogen prior to ovulation to have been suggested to produce a mucus more favorable to sperm migration, but success with such treatment has been limited.

Treatment of Ovulatory Failure

When failure of ovulation is suspected, a thorough endocrine evaluation is in order. The defect may occur at the level of the hypothalamus, the pituitary, or the ovaries themselves. Ovulation is also influenced by the client's general state of health and thyroid and adrenal abnormalities.

Ovulatory failure can be caused by a pituitary adenoma, a space-occupying tumor within the pituitary gland. Such tumors produce the breast-stimulating hormone prolactin and thus are often associated with secretions from the breasts (galactorrhea). Clients with ovulatory failure should be screened for this condition by careful examination of the breasts.

Recent availability of effective agents for the induction of ovulation has made careful evaluation of clients suspected of anovulatory infertility all the more important. In properly selected cases, mainly clients with clinical evidence of continued estrogen production, the use of an estrogen antagonist, *clomiphene citrate*, is associated with more than a 50% success rate. Clients with hyperprolactinemia may be candidates for treatment with *bromocriptine*, an agent capable of inducing ovulation by reducing prolactin levels. In clients whose ovulatory failure is the result of a defect at the hypothalamic–pituitary level, the use of *human menopausal gonadotropin* (hMG), which is derived from the urine of postmenopausal women, is associated with some success. Multiple pregnancies, which have received considerable attention from the press, are usually the result of hMG treatment. Even in expert hands, it is difficult to avoid overstimulation of the ovary with hMG and induction of more than one ovulation in a given cycle. The incidence of multiple pregnancy can be reduced significantly by careful monitoring with plasma estrogen levels and sonography. The final step in the treatment regimen is the administration of a second hormone, hCG, which has an action similar to that of LH. It triggers the final maturation of the follicle and ovum release. If multiple follicles are observed in sonography, the ovulation triggering injection of hCG can be withheld and the treatment resumed in a subsequent cycle.

Surgical Treatment of Pelvic Disease

Surgical techniques have been developed for the treatment of pelvic adhesions and tubal occlusion. The postoperative prognosis depends on the extent of the previous damage to adnexal structures. It is also greatly influenced by the skill of the surgeon and has been enhanced in recent years by using the principles of

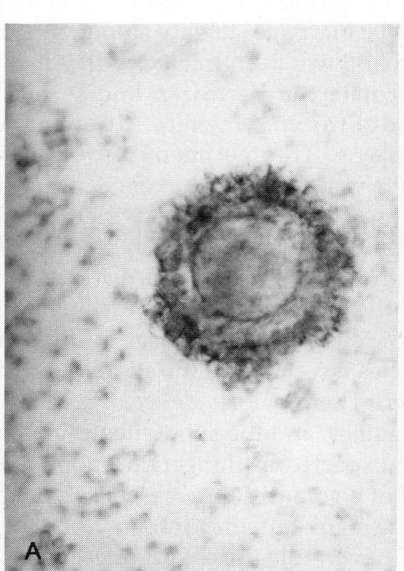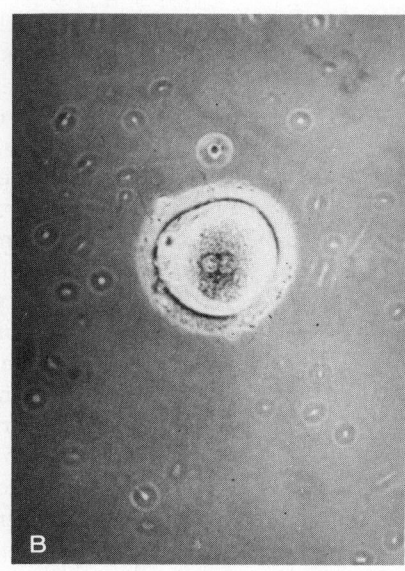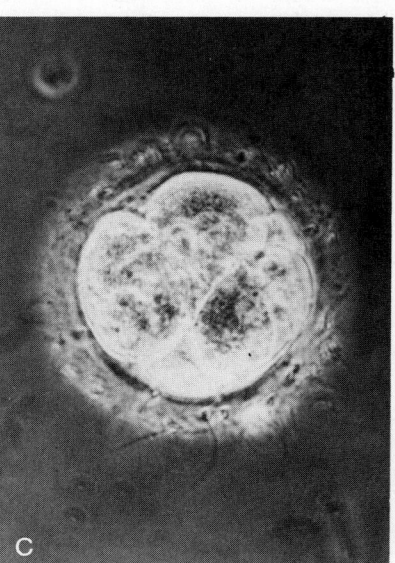

FIGURE 16-5

In vitro fertilization involves obtaining an oocyte, fertilizing it, and then transferring it to the uterus. (*A*) Mature egg just aspirated. (*B*) Fertilized egg (two pronuclei seen) 16 hours after insemination. (*C*) Four-cell embryo shortly before embryo transfer. (Pace-Owens S: In vitro fertilization and embryo transfer. JOGN Nurs Supplement 14:44s–48s, Nov/Dec, 1985)

plastic surgery. Microsurgery with the operating loupe or an operating microscope has also been particularly helpful.

Laparotomy should not be considered until all of the other causes of reproductive failure have been conscientiously investigated. For example, an operation is not generally justifiable if the husband is severely oligospermic or if the wife suffers from ovulatory failure that is refractory to treatment. In some cases, the tubes have been so extensively damaged and the ovaries so severely compromised by periovarian adhesions that pelvic reconstruction is ill advised. Prior to surgery for infertility, the couple should be given a realistic appraisal of the prognosis.

In large measure, this is based on the appearance of the adnexa at the time of laparoscopy. Risks of this procedure should be thoroughly reviewed, and the mistaken impression that failure to accept treatment will affect general health later on should be dispelled. The decision to accept an operative procedure solely to enhance fertility is a serious matter deserving the most careful review.

The role of pelvic adhesions in infertility depends on their location in relation to the tubes and ovaries. When the tubes are patent, pelvic adhesions present the best prognosis, with postoperative pregnancy rates in the 40% to 50% range.

Tubal obstruction usually occurs in the proximal (uterine) or distal (fimbrial) segments. A diagnosis of nonpatency at the uterotubal junction should be made with extreme caution. Obstruction in this area may be caused by tubal spasm, and actual anatomical obstruction must be corroborated by both hysterosalpingogram and laparoscopy. With the use of the operating microscope, the point of obstruction near the uterus can be accurately identified, and a tubal anastomosis is carried out. When the intrauterine portion of the tube is completely occluded, reimplantation of the patent segment into the uterus can be carried out. The prognosis following these procedures is relatively poor, in the 10% to 30% range.

When the tube is occluded at its fimbriated extremity, efforts are made to salvage any remaining fimbriae and the distal end of the tube is reconstructed microsurgically. The prognosis depends on the extent of prior tubal damage, but in the hands of a skilled surgeon it is in the 20% to 30% range. Subsequent to tubal surgery, the possibility of a tubal ectopic pregnancy must be seriously considered when conception occurs. The incidence of ectopic pregnancy is 5% to 10%.

Treatment of Uterine Problems

When a causal relationship is thought to exist, *myomectomies* (removal of the fibroids), with preservation of the uterus, are usually technically possible. Treatment of congenital abnormalities, more commonly associated with habitual abortion than infertility, is also surgical. Intrauterine adhesions are treated with surgery plus steroid and estrogen therapy to decrease the incidence of repeat formation of adhesions. Surgery for intrauterine adhesions can be carried out vaginally with the use of the hysteroscope. This is a fiberoptic instrument similar to a laparoscope that is introduced past the cervix into the uterine cavity. This system allows visualization of the interior of the uterine cavity and the introduction of microscissors, which are used to incise any adhesions that may be present.

In Vitro *Fertilization and Embryo Transfer*

One of the most dramatic events in the treatment of infertility was the birth of baby Louise in England in 1978, following successful *in vitro* fertilization and embryo transfer (IVF-ET). This first recorded success was in a client whose fallopian tubes had been previously surgically removed. This breakthrough offers hope for clients with extensive tubal disease or whose tubes are absent.

A number of principles have been applied in the successful application of this approach to infertility. The development of multiple follicles is stimulated with ovulation-inducing agents. At a precisely timed interval, a laparoscopy is carried out. The ovarian follicles, matured under the influence of ovarian stimulation, are aspirated (Fig. 16-5A). Oocytes can also be retrieved by ultrasonographically directed needle aspiration. The needle is inserted into the peritoneal cavity transvesically or transvaginally and is directed into the follicles under sonographic visualization. The oocytes retrieved are then cultured *in vitro* with the husband's treated spermatozoa under carefully controlled laboratory conditions. If fertilization is successful, the oocyte divides and is transferred into the uterus at the four- to eight-cell stage (Fig. 16-5B and C). As techniques have been refined, there has been a gradual improvement in the success rate.

These procedures have engendered a great deal of controversy among those who feel, for moral and ethical reasons, that the creation of new life *in vitro* is inappropriate (ethical considerations of *in vitro* fertilization are discussed in Chap. 7). In 1982, the American Fertility Society drafted the following position on IVF-ET, "In view of the current rate of success in programs of *in vitro* fertilization, it is the sense of the Board of Directors of the American Fertility Society that in appropriately staffed and equipped institutions that have demonstrated proficiency and success, *in vitro* fertilization must now be recognized as the acceptable treatment for achieving pregnancy for couples whose wives have absent or irreparably damaged fallopian tubes."

It is clear that this technology represents a significant advance in our ability to treat otherwise hopeless cases of infertility, and knowledge gained from this work has done much to improve our understanding of human reproductive processes.

While the potential benefit of IVF-ET treatment is obvious, the psychological costs of involvement in such a program are enormous. Among 200 consecutive couples seen in the IVF-ET program at the University of Pennsylvania, 50% of the women and 15% of the men reported that infertility was the most upsetting experience of their lives.[3] One fifth of both males and females displayed test results suggesting dysfunctional emotional distress or personality difficulties, although one half displayed test scores indicating effective functioning and ability to withstand stress. Couples who seek IVF-ET treatment do so in spite of the likelihood of negative outcome. It is important to provide them with emotional support and to develop better understanding of the psychological components of IVF. A coordinated approach that should include psychological counseling enables infertile couples to make informed choices about treatment options and certainly increases understanding of IVF-ET treatment outcomes. Of equal importance is sharing with the clients a realistic appraisal of the success rate in the setting in which the IVF-ET is to be carried out.[4]

Surrogate Embryo Transfer

The world's first surrogate embryo transfer (SET) was born in 1984, so the procedure is still young. It was developed by a research team at Harbor-UCLA Medical Center with funding from Fertility and Genetics Research, a for-profit company. SET involves five steps[5]:

1. Synchronization of the ovulation times between the recipient and donor women
2. Insemination of the donor woman with sperm from the husband of the infertile recipient
3. Washing out of the donor's uterus about 5 days following fertilization
4. Recovery of the embryo from the lavage fluid
5. Transfer of the embryo to the recipient's uterus

At any step problems can arise. The reported success rate is less than 7% despite enthusiastic claims from the procedure's proponents[6] (ethical and legal considerations of this method are discussed in Chap. 7).

Nursing Intervention

Infertility is a threatening condition, and both husband and wife inevitably display anxiety. The role of the nurse in such situations is to understand the purpose of the various diagnostic procedures for infertility and to provide the couple with information so that both partners can cope with the problem knowledgeably.

The nurse is often called upon to schedule tests. In that role the nurse must be thoroughly familiar with the physiological basis for the diagnostic tests and for any treatment that is planned after the testing is completed.

The nurse's role is particularly important in the interpretation of changes in the temperature chart and, more recently, in the interpretation of changes observed in the urine when the kit for urinary LH determinations is used. The timing of tests and even the timing of intercourse is a subject that engenders a great deal of anxiety and, in some cases, resentment. This combination results in frequent client contact, often by phone. In some settings the nurse may actually be called upon to carry out some of the diagnostic tests and treatment. Increasingly, the nurse practitioner with special training in the management of infertility has become part of the team, sometimes acting as coordinator for special programs such as artificial insemination or IVF-ET. It goes without saying that this role requires special counseling skills and is especially appropriate for nurses, given the emphasis placed on this area in modern nursing education.

An Emotionally Charged Situation

Often the nurse is called upon to act as counselor in what is an emotionally charged situation: as a couple faces the prospect of a barren marriage. Infertility involves many feelings that must be recognized and dealt with; the infertile couple is often sensitive and extremely vulnerable. It is important to acknowledge the pressures associated with infertility and to allow opportunities to review the sense of isolation, guilt, depression, and even anger that often accompanies infertility.

The need for addressing the emotional aspects of human infertility has prompted organization of a national support group, Resolve, Inc., which now has chapters in many cities in the United States. Barbara Eck Menning, former Executive Director of Resolve, outlines the feelings of infertile couples that most frequently surface during support group meetings. The first reaction is commonly one of shock. Most couples have not considered the possibility that they will be infertile and are unaware of how common infertility is. The next reaction is usually denial—"this can't happen to me." Denial is a useful mechanism that allows time for adjustment to a threatening situation.

Help is not sought until after the couple comes to grips with the problem. Anger may occur in response to the discomfort and inconvenience of infertility testing or perhaps as a result of social pressure from well-intended friends and family members. Infertile people

NURSING CARE PLAN

The Infertile Couple

Nursing Objectives:
1. Obtain a complete assessment through history taking, records, and behavioral observation.
2. Provide thorough explanation as necessary of infertility conditions and options for remedial help.
3. Allay anxiety through information and emotional support.

Assessment	Potential Nursing Diagnosis	Intervention	Evaluation
Couple's knowledge about the reproductive process	Knowledge deficit related to sexual anatomy and/or physiology	Take complete history regarding this area Provide accurate information as needed Allow time for feedback and questions	Couple demonstrates that they have accurate information
Couple's knowledge and technique regarding sexual behavior	Knowledge deficit related to foreplay and/or coital techniques	Same as above	Same as above
Couple's family coping styles (e.g., cohesiveness, blaming, sharing responsibility)	Ineffective coping styles	Take complete history in this area Observe family interaction Clarify observations Feedback behavior when appropriate	Couple demonstrate realistic appraisal of the situation
Couple's general life-style including substance use, nutrition, etc.	Knowledge deficit related to impact of life-style on fertility Negative impact of life-style on fertility	Take complete history (use self-assessment form as necessary) Clarify misinformation Feedback negative aspects of life-style if appropriate	Couple can verbalize accurate information and make positive changes as indicated
Feelings of self-esteem	Lowered self-esteem related to inability to conceive	Clarify misinformation Support positive feelings	Couple demonstrates more positive attitude
Degree of anxiety and/or fear regarding conditions and treatment options	Anxiety/fear related to the unknown and treatment procedures and outcomes	Provide adequate time for questions Provide accurate information and clarification of treatment procedures as indicated Provide opportunity to verbalize concerns Provide referrals as necessary Schedule tests and procedures carefully, with the clients' interest in mind	Couple indicates that their fear and anxiety have lessened Couple follows through with regimen

may direct their anger at the nurse or physician, who is perceived as exercising an element of control over them. Allowing an opportunity to express rage is the most effective way to dissipate it. When faced with irrational anger the health-care professional should strive to avoid becoming defensive. Nonjudgmental acceptance of the client's feelings and sincere empathy are essential in these circumstances.

People facing infertility commonly experience a sense of isolation. The infertile couple may find it difficult to share their problem with others, even with those close to them.

Infertility is often associated with a sense of guilt. This may be engendered by a completely unrelated past event such as an induced abortion, an extramarital affair, venereal disease, premarital sex, or homosexual acts or thoughts. When guilt feelings are intense, they are associated with a sense of worthlessness. For the above reasons, clients should be encouraged to discuss their feelings at every visit during the course of investigation and treatment. It is especially important to provide an opportunity to consider marital and sexual conflicts that may have arisen out of the infertility.

References

1. Garcia C-R, David SS: Pelvic endometriosis: Infertility and pelvic pain. Am J Obstet Gynecol 129:740–747, 1977
2. Schenken RS, Malinak LR: Conservative surgery versus expectant management for the infertile patient with mild endometriosis. Fertil Steril 37:183–186, 1982
3. Freeman E, Boxer A, Rickels K et al: Psychological evaluation and support in a program of *in vitro* fertilization and embryo transfer. Fertil Steril 43:48–53, 1985
4. Soules MP: The *in vitro* fertilization pregnancy rate: Let's be honest with one another. Fertil Steril 43:511, 1985
5. Annas GJ: Surrogate embryo transfer: The perils of parenting. Hastings Cent Rep 14(3):25–26, June 1984
6. Bustillo M et al: Nonsurgical ovum transfer as a treatment in infertile women: Preliminary experience. JAMA 251:1171–1179, March 2, 1984

Suggested Reading

Bernstein J, Potts N, Mattox JH: Assessment of psychological dysfunction associated with infertility. JOGN Nurs Supplement, pp 63s–66s, November/December 1985
Clapp D: Emotional responses to infertility: Nursing interventions. JOGN Nurs Supplement, pp 32s–35s, November/December 1985
Garcia CR, Mastroianni L, Amelar R et al (eds): Current Therapy of Infertility, Vols 1 and 2. St Louis, CV Mosby, 1982 and 1985
Mastroianni L Jr, Biggers JD: Fertilization and Embryonic Development *In Vitro*. New York, Plenum Press, 1981
Menning BE: The emotional needs of infertile couples. Fertil Steril 34:313, 1980
Pace-Owens S: *In vitro* fertilization and embryo transfer. JOGN Nurs Supplement, pp 44s–48s. November/December 1985
Smith PM: Ovulation induction. JOGN Nurs Supplement, pp 37s–43s. November/December 1985
Sperott L, Glass RH, Kase HG: Clinical Gynecologic Endocrinology and Infertility, 3rd ed. Baltimore, Williams & Wilkins, 1985
Wallach E, Kempers RD (eds): Modern Trends in Infertility and Conception Control, Vols 1, 2, and 3. Baltimore, Williams & Wilkins, 1979, 1982, and 1985

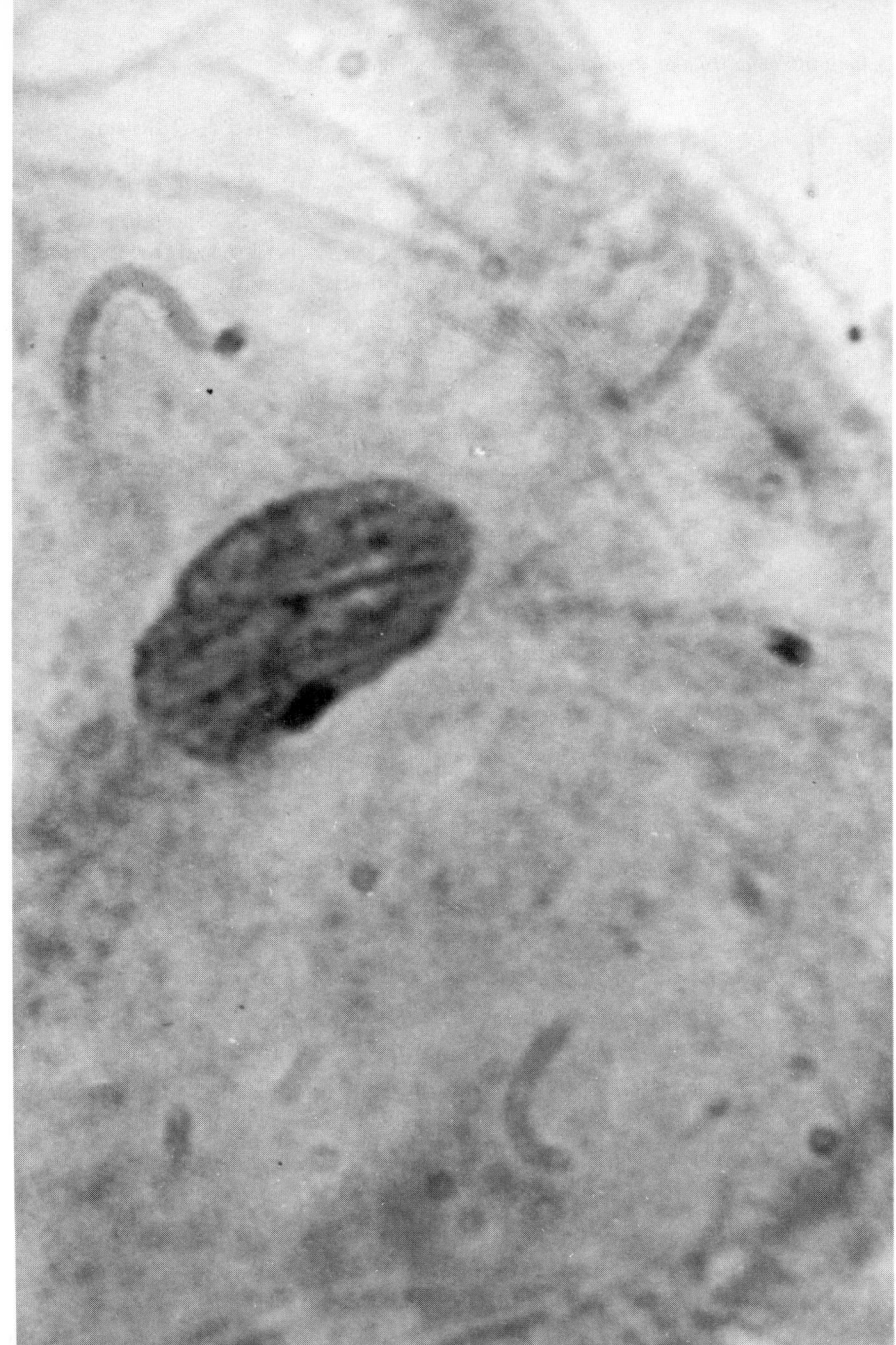

CHAPTER 17

Genetic Counseling and Diagnosis During Pregnancy

Procedure for Amniocentesis

NURSING CARE PLAN:
Families Involved in Genetic Counseling

Counseling After Amniocentesis

Since 1956, when it was determined that human cells contain 46 chromosomes, the knowledge gained from research in human genetics has expanded rapidly.[1,2] During that time, clinical genetics has developed as a medical discipline, which uses and integrates expertise from all other medical fields. Genetic information has been disseminated beyond the academic community and research laboratory to the practicing physician. The amount of genetic information available to the lay public has also increased markedly in the past few years. Magazine and newspaper articles and television programs frequently discuss genetic disease, often focusing on dramatic new advances in diagnostic methods or therapy. As a result, clients, as health-care consumers, expect providers to respond to their increasing sophistication and needs in this area. Many more clients are requesting genetic counseling and are willing to make decisions about their health care. These changes in information and attitudes facilitate the counseling process.

Accordingly, the field of prenatal genetic diagnosis has developed rapidly. The number of genetic disorders and birth defects that can be diagnosed continues to increase dramatically. Public education has resulted in a large number of clients who consider having these studies performed.

Genetic Counseling

Genetic counseling is a communication process that deals with the human problems associated with the occurrence, or risk, of a genetic disorder in a family.[3] This information may deal with a genetic disease in the individual, a family member, or future offspring. While the basic approach and principles are the same as those used at other times, certain situations, such as critical time limitations for decision making, occur more frequently in pregnancy. The aspects discussed during the counseling process include medical considerations, genetic mechanisms, and the options available. Medical considerations include a description of the disease or defect, the clinical manifestations, therapy, and prognosis. The burden of the disease for the affected person, as well as the family, should be presented during the counseling process. For example, in the case of maternal age, it is important that the client understands not only the risks of having a child with Down's syndrome, but also the burden associated with it. Only with this understanding can the couple make a fully informed decision regarding prenatal diagnosis.

The genetic mechanism by which the disorder occurs and the risk of occurrence or recurrence should be explained to the client in terms that can be readily understood. It may be necessary to review and summarize the information several times. Having the client relate the information back to the counselor is a useful way of assessing the effectiveness of the counseling.

During counseling any alternatives that may reduce the risk for or alter the course of the genetic disease are discussed. It may also be important to discuss new or anticipated developments in therapy when they are relevant.

Counseling should enable the client to make decisions regarding a genetic disease in the present family or in future generations. These decisions may involve selecting reproductive options (*e.g.*, childless marriage, selective abortion of affected fetus, donor insemination, or sterilization). The impact of how genetic counseling and testing may alter a client's view of herself and family members in terms of health and disease is significant.

Referral for Genetic Counseling

Although any client who requests genetic information should be referred for counseling, initiation of the referral by the health-care provider is most appropriate for clients with more than one course of action available to them. Many clients who suspect that their child might have an increased risk for a birth defect use denial effectively until a pregnancy occurs. The reality of the pregnancy and concern for the fetus motivate them to seek information for the first time during early pregnancy. It is also important to recognize that clients may presume that a risk is not significant if it is not specifically mentioned by the nurse or physician. Occasionally, clients with the greatest anxiety are identified among those seeking pregnancy terminations. Their concerns for having a malformed child may be based on misinformation. Genetic counseling in these circumstances should allow the clients to make an informed and appropriate decision. Moreover, counseling may provide reassuring information by clarifying the actual risk. The gestational age of the pregnancy, the availability of pregnancy interruption, and the client's attitude regarding this option should be assessed very early in the course of genetic referral for counseling.

Multidisciplinary Approach

As a necessity, comprehensive genetic service programs employ a multidisciplinary approach to the care of clients and their families. A team composed of physicians (geneticists with specialty backgrounds in obstetrics, pediatrics, and internal medicine), nurses, genetics associates, laboratory personnel, and other support services is required.

Methods Used in the Prenatal Detection of Birth Defects

Several techniques may be employed in the prenatal diagnosis of genetic disorders or birth defects. Ideally, these methods should define the genotype (genetic constitution) of the fetus; however, in some instances only techniques to delineate the phenotype (observable characteristics) of the fetus are available. The latter include fetal visualization by roentgenogram, ultrasound, and fetoscopy.

Roentgenograms

Roentgenograms performed as early as 20 weeks of pregnancy have been used to examine the fetus for skeletal manifestations of certain genetic disorders or birth defects.[4,5] Because the fetal skeleton is rather poorly visualized at this gestational age, *amniography* is often employed. In this procedure, a water-soluble contrast material is injected into the amniotic fluid to provide a more distinctive outline of the fetus and improve the identification of skeletal structures. The usefulness of radiographic procedures is limited to the diagnosis of severe disorders with major skeletal manifestations

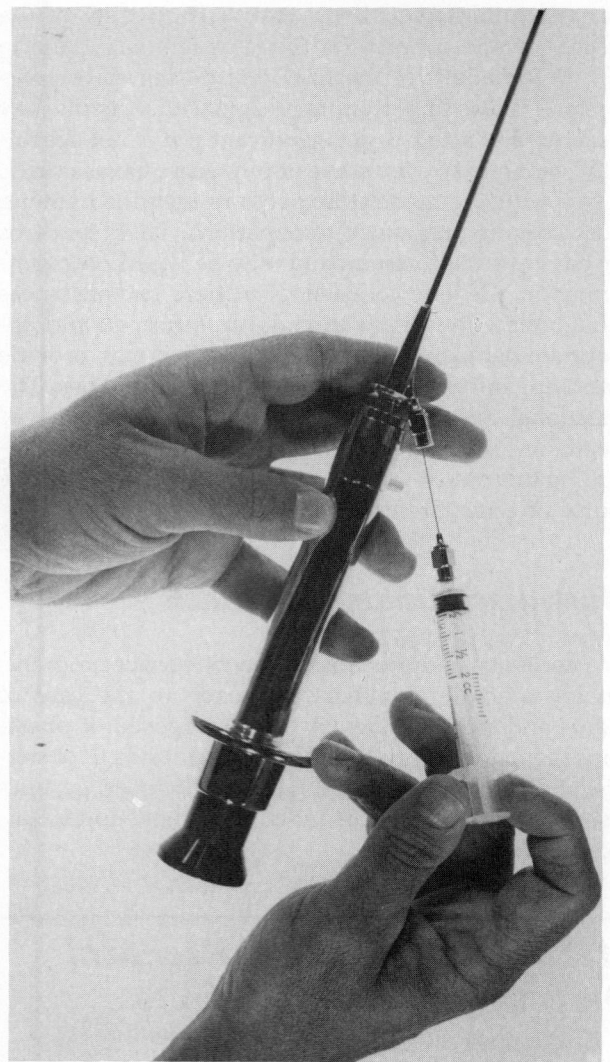

FIGURE   17-1

Amnioscope. Endoscope for transabdominal amnioscopy with needle for aspiration.

early in development or, occasionally, large soft-tissue defects, such as a bulging myelomeningocele.[6,7] Unfortunately, many skeletal disorders can only be diagnosed so late in pregnancy that the option of termination is not feasible.

Ultrasound

Rapid advances in *ultrasound* have enabled the definition of fetal anatomy to a remarkable degree. Fetal organs may be evaluated and single organ defects can be detected with this technique.[8,9] Additionally, the examination of one organ may permit the diagnosis or define the risk of certain multiple malformation syndromes. Examination of the cerebral ventricles for dilation due to hydrocephalus, renal evaluation for the

diagnosis of renal agenesis (Potter's syndrome) or polycystic kidneys, and evaluation for short-limbed dwarfism are only a few examples.[10,11]

Fetoscopy

Delineation of other defects will require more direct examination of the fetus by *fetoscopy*. Under local anesthesia, a fine-caliber endoscope, about the thickness of a 14-gauge needle, is inserted percutaneously into the amniotic cavity to visualize the fetus (Fig. 17-1). Although it is easy to imagine the great potential of this instrument, wide-scale use for direct visualization awaits improvement in the optics of the system and further experience for evaluation of its safety. Small amounts of fetal blood obtained from the placental vessels during fetoscopy have been used for fetal diagnosis of a number of diseases, particularly those with abnormality of blood elements, such as hemophilia A, hemoglobinopathies, and platelet or white blood cell disorders.[12,13]

Amniocentesis

Prenatal genetic diagnosis is most often performed when the fetus is at risk of having a disorder that may be diagnosed by studying cells obtained by *amniocentesis*. This relatively simple and safe outpatient procedure may

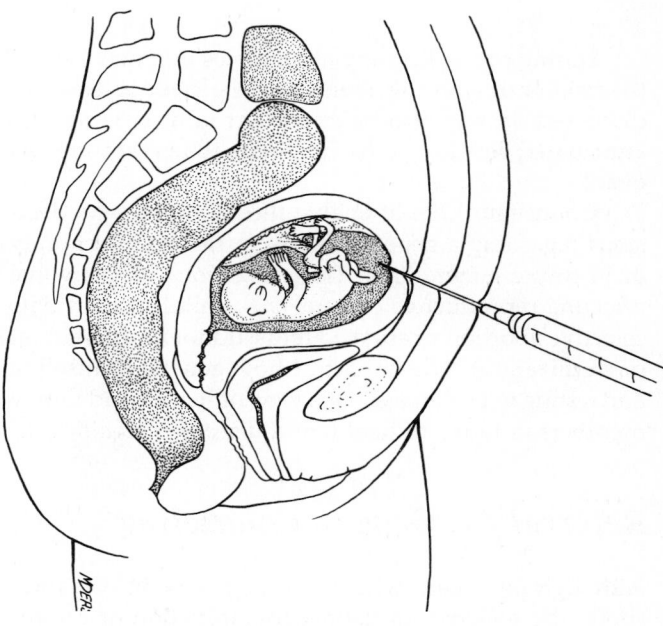

FIGURE   17-2

Amniocentesis. Amniotic fluid is withdrawn for analysis by transabdominal needle aspiration.

be performed as early as 14 weeks of pregnancy to 16 weeks of pregnancy (Fig. 17-2).[14] Amniotic fluid contains desquamated fetal cells that are separated from the fluid by centrifugation. The supernatant fluid contains a number of hormones, proteins, and other elements that are useful for diagnosis, for example, α-fetoprotein (AFP) measurement for the prenatal diagnosis of neural tube defects. Although the cells present in amniotic fluid come from a variety of sites (amnion, skin, and the gastrointestinal and the genitourinary tract), all are of fetal origin. Of these desquamated cells, a large proportion are dead or dying. Generally, enough viable cells are collected to permit cell culture. The cells are placed in plastic flasks or dishes containing a nutrient medium. The temperature, pH, and atmospheric conditions of the culture are adjusted and controlled in specially designed incubators. After a period of time, viable cells will attach to the flask and begin to multiply by cellular division. Chromosome analysis, detection of enzyme defects, and, more recently, DNA isolation procedures can be performed following adequate cell growth.[15-17] With the latter methods, the absence of a gene or a mutant gene may be detected by sophisticated molecular genetic techniques. Amniocentesis is discussed in greater detail at the end of the chapter.

Chorionic Villous Sampling

Chorionic villous sampling (CVS) is the newest method of prenatal diagnosis. It is performed during the first trimester of pregnancy, usually between the ninth and twelfth weeks of gestation. Small fragments of the developing placenta are obtained for study. CVS has the potential for diagnosis of the same disorders detected by amniocentesis, with the exception of neural tube defects. Several techniques have been used to obtain the tissue samples. The use of a polyethylene catheter to obtain a transcervical aspiration biopsy at the placental site under direct ultrasound guidance is the most commonly applied technique. Old and colleagues reported the diagnosis of β-thalassemia major by CVS in 1982.[18] In 1983 Brambati and Simoni used this technique for the diagnosis of Down's syndrome with their newly developed laboratory methods for direct (same-day) chromosome analysis.[19] The potential benefits of early biopsy and rapid chromosome analysis met with immediate enthusiasm for the procedure, and within a few months CVS was clinically applied in the United States.

The potential advantages of CVS when compared with amniocentesis are obvious. The testing is performed during the first trimester of pregnancy. Diagnosis is available much more quickly, from one to several days for cytogenetic studies and a few days to two weeks for diagnosis by metabolic tests or DNA analysis. Additionally, if a positive diagnosis is made, the option of late first-trimester D&E for pregnancy termination is available.

The potential risks of CVS have not, as yet, been accurately established. In a December 1984 report from the World Health Organization, the rate of pregnancy loss was 3.7%.[20] Although the rate of spontaneous abortion is low, the background rate (corrected for maternal age, gestational age, normality of ultrasound findings, and normal chromosome results) has not been established. Thus, the absolute risk of pregnancy loss due to this procedure has not been defined. The issue of safety of this procedure has prompted the National Institutes of Health to initiate a randomized collaborative study in the United States to compare the risks of CVS using a plastic catheter under ultrasound guidance during the first trimester with the risks of amniocentesis during the second trimester. In addition to the risks of pregnancy loss, rupture of membranes, and infection, a number of other *potential* risks have been considered. The latter include fetal injury, fetal hypoxia, fetal malformations, focal placenta accreta, placental insufficiency, placenta previa, and Rh sensitization. Administration of Rh immunoglobulin at the time of CVS should effectively prevent this last complication. Though theoretical, the other potential risks are important.

The accuracy of diagnosis by CVS must be confirmed by follow-up studies of abortuses and live-born children. Thus far, the accuracy of chromosome analysis, biochemical testing, and DNA studies using direct methods applied to CVS samples appears comparable to amniocentesis. The use of cultured CVS samples can provide additional material for study but results in more potential for maternal cell contamination of tissue cultures than do amniocentesis samples. This has been reported to be a problem particularly during the early learning phase in some laboratories.[21] Other potential pitfalls of CVS diagnosis, such as chromosome mosaicism or equivocal biochemical results, may require follow-up by amniocentesis or other standard methods of diagnosis until considerably more experience is obtained.

Disorders Amenable to Prenatal Diagnosis

Chromosomal Abnormalities

The nucleus of a normal human cell contains 46 chromosomes (diploid number of 2N), which includes 22 pairs of autosomes and one pair of sex chromosomes (XX in females and XY in males). Each chromosome is composed of DNA strands containing thousands of genes and a supporting protein structure. The mature gamete contains only 23 chromosomes (haploid number

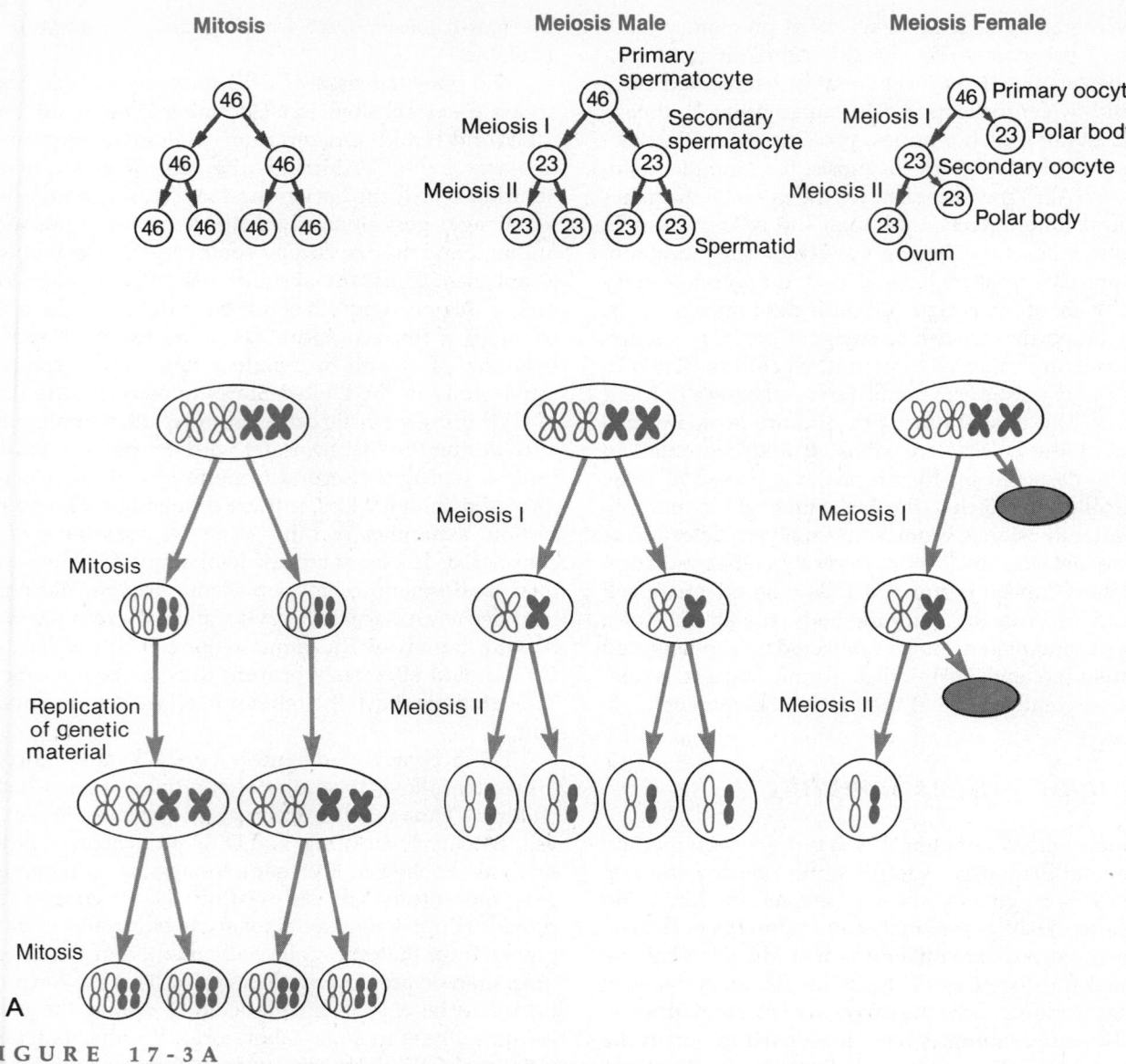

FIGURE 17-3A

Normal mitosis and meiosis. Upper portion demonstrates the segregation of chromosomes numerically, and lower portion depicts the segregation of two of the 23 chromosome pairs. (*Left*) Two normal mitotic divisions. (*Center*) Normal meiosis in the male. (*Right*) Normal meiosis in the female.

of N), one member of each chromosome pair and one sex chromosome (an X in the ova and either an X or a Y in the sperm) as a result of meiosis (Fig. 17-3A). At the time of fertilization, the diploid number is restored, and one member of each chromosome pair is inherited from each parent.

Studies Performed. The chromosomes of an individual may be examined by arresting the metaphase of dividing cells with colchicine or related agents. This can be done with lymphocytes, cultured skin fibroblasts, or amniotic fluid cells. After appropriate preparation,

the chromosome content of the cell is analyzed microscopically, photographed, and karyotyped (Fig. 17-4). Pretreatment of the chromosomes with a number of different chemical agents will cause distinctive staining patterns (banding), which allows the identification of each chromosome pair and definition of small subsegments of the chromosomes. The successful culture and cytogenetic study of human amniotic fluid cells was first reported in 1966.[22] Since that time, cytogenetic analysis of cultured amniotic fluid cells has been the most frequently used method for prenatal diagnosis of genetic disorders.

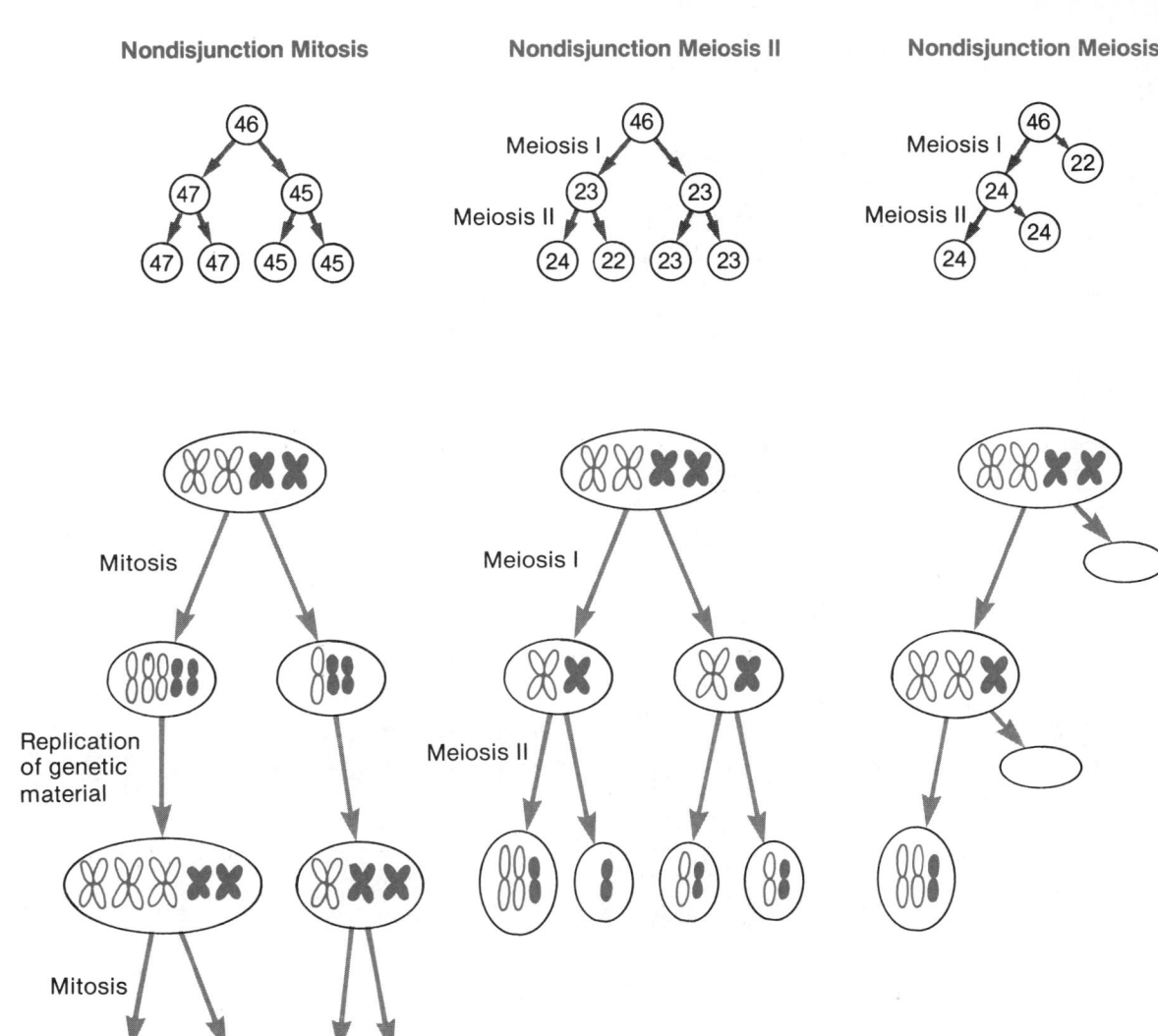

Nondisjunction Mitosis   **Nondisjunction Meiosis II**   **Nondisjunction Meiosis I**

B

FIGURE 17-3B

Nondisjunction in mitosis and meiosis. Upper portion demonstrates the segregation of chromosomes numerically, and lower portion depicts the segregation of two of the 23 chromosome pairs. (*Left*) Mitosis, two mitotic divisions with nondisjunction occurring in the first and the error passed through the subsequent division. (*Center*) Meiosis in the male, with nondisjunction occurring in the second division of meiosis resulting in normal and abnormal spermatids. (*Right*) Meiosis in the female, with nondisjunction occurring in the first division of meiosis resulting in an abnormal ovum.

Numerical Chromosome Errors

An abnormal number of chromosomes (*aneuploidy*) in conception results in major developmental defects. When there is an extra chromosome in each cell, the disorder is termed a *trisomy* and when there is a missing chromosome in each cell, the disorder is termed a *monosomy*. These disorders may originate at conception because the egg or sperm had an abnormal chromosome content, or after fertilization as a result of misdivision of the chromosomes to daughter cells during mitosis.[23] *Nondisjunction*, meaning that there is unequal distribution of chromosomes to daughter cells during either meiotic or mitotic division, accounts for the majority of numerical chromosome abnormalities (Fig. 17-3B). Trisomic conceptions are most often lost during the first trimester of pregnancy. Nevertheless, conceptions with certain abnormalities may be live-born.

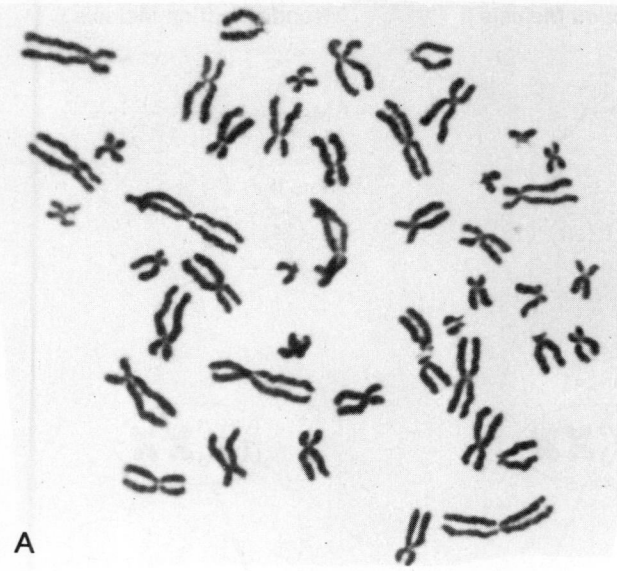

A

FIGURE 17-4

(*A*) Chromosomes of normal human female. (*B*) Karyotype of normal human male.

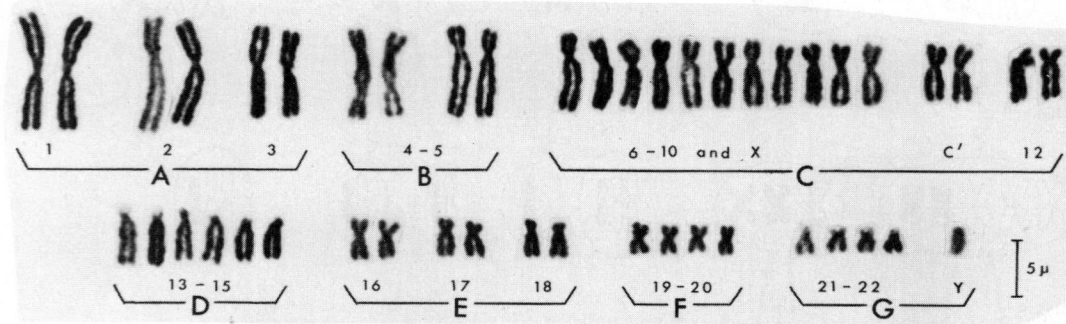

B

The cells of a conception may contain 69 (3N or triploid) or even 92 (4N or tetraploid) chromosomes. These conditions, known as *polyploidy*, can be caused by an error in fertilization, for example, two sperm (*dispermy*) penetrating an egg, resulting in a triploid (3N) conception. Polyploid conceptions usually abort, although occasional cases of the prenatal diagnosis or live birth of triploid fetuses are reported.

Anaphase Lag. Anaphase lag occurs when homologous chromosomes fail to attach or separate correctly on the spindle during cell division, resulting in the loss of one member of the pair. This results in monosomy and is believed to be the mechanism responsible for the majority of X chromosome monosomy (45,X) in human conceptions.

Frequency of Occurrence

The frequency of numerical chromosome errors in human conceptions is much higher than previously suspected, but the vast majority of these pregnancies are lost by spontaneous abortion. It is estimated that in 50% of early spontaneous abortions there is an abnormal number of chromosomes. Autosomal trisomies, 45,X (Turner's syndrome), and polyploidy are the most common abnormalities detected in early abortuses. Surveys of late pregnancy loss, including stillbirth and neonatal deaths, have shown chromosome abnormality in 5% to 10% of these infants.[24] An abnormal chromosome constitution occurs in approximately 1 of every 200 live births (Table 17-1). The most common numerical abnormalities encountered in newborn surveys are autosomal trisomies (trisomy 21, 18, 13) and sex chromosome aneuploidy (45,X; 47,XXY; 47,XYY; 47,XXX).[25]

Age Factor. The frequency of meiotic nondisjunction resulting in trisomic conceptions increases with maternal age. This is exemplified by the well-defined association between the age of the mother and the birth of children with Down's syndrome (trisomy 21). The increased frequency of Down's syndrome births is most dramatic in pregnancies of women over the age of 35 (Table 17-2). For this reason, it has become generally accepted that pregnant women in the later reproductive years should have the opportunity to consider amniocentesis. Analysis of the frequency of chromosome abnormality by maternal age in women having prenatal diagnosis has

TABLE 17-1

Incidence of Chromosome Abnormalities in Newborns

Type	Incidence
Sex Chromosome	
Males	1:400
47,XYY	1:1100
47,XXY	1:1100
Other	1:1300
Females	1:700
45,X	1:9500
47,XXX	1:950
Other	1:2700
Autosome	
Trisomies	1:700
Trisomy 13	1:19,000
Trisomy 18	1:8000
Trisomy 21	1:800
Other	1:5500
Autosomal Structural Abnormalities	
Unbalanced	1:1700
Balanced	1:500

TABLE 17-2

Incidence of Down's Syndrome Births Related to Maternal Age

Age	Ratio	Age	Ratio
<20	1:2300	34	1:527
20–25	1:1600	35	1:413
25–30	1:1200	36	1:333
		37	1:266
30–35	1:880	38	1:183
35–40	1:290	39	1:135
		40	1:106
40–45	1:100	41	1:83
>45	1:46		

(Retrospective data for maternal age–related risk of Down's syndrome taken from Collman RD, Stoller A: A survey of mongoloid births in Victoria, Australia 1942–1957. Am J Public Health 52:813, 1962; Hook EB: Estimates of maternal age—specific risks of a Down's-syndrome birth in women aged 34–41. Lancet 2:33, 1976)

uniformly indicated a higher incidence of Down's syndrome than that observed in newborn studies. Mothers between 35 years of age and 40 years of age had approximately a 1.5% rate of positive diagnosis; mothers over 40 years of age had a rate of approximately 5%.[26] The marked discrepancy between newborn and amniocentesis data is probably largely due to the natural loss of chromosomally abnormal fetuses after 16 weeks' gestation.[27]

It had been believed that nondisjunction in female meiosis accounted for the majority of trisomic conceptions. Recently, banding techniques have enabled identification of the parental origin of the extra chromosome in some cases. The paternal contribution to Down's syndrome births is more substantial than previously estimated. Currently, there is controversy surrounding a paternal age effect and the clinical counseling that should be given for this.

Although the likelihood of bearing children having different autosomal trisomies (*i.e.,* trisomy 13 or trisomy 18) increases with age, these are much less common abnormalities, and the numerical risk is not as well defined as that for trisomy 21. Children with trisomy 18 and trisomy 13 most often do not survive the first year of life. Thus, the burden of these disorders differs from that of Down's syndrome, which is compatible with prolonged survival. In younger women who have had a child with trisomy 21, there is a recurrence risk of 1% to 2%, irrespective of their age.[28] These clients, as well as those who have had children with other trisomies, often request amniocentesis.

Structural Chromosome Abnormalities

Structural chromosome abnormalities occur as a result of breakage and reunion of chromosomes. Exchange of material between chromosomes of different pairs is known as a *translocation* (Fig. 17-5). If all the genetic material is conserved, the individual is unaffected by this and is designated a balanced carrier of the rearrangement. There are no phenotypic consequences for the balanced carrier except the reproductive problems associated with the conceptions of pregnancies with an unbalanced chromosome constitution. The gametes that are produced by a balanced translocation carrier may

I   II   III   IV

FIGURE 17-5

Mechanism of reciprocal translocation. I. Two normal chromosome pairs. II. Breakage of one member of each pair. III. Exchange of broken segments. IV. Reunion to form balanced rearrangement (translocation).

Chromosomes of translocation carrier parent	Possible gametes	Chromosome constitution of resulting conception	Normal gametes	Normal parental chromosomes

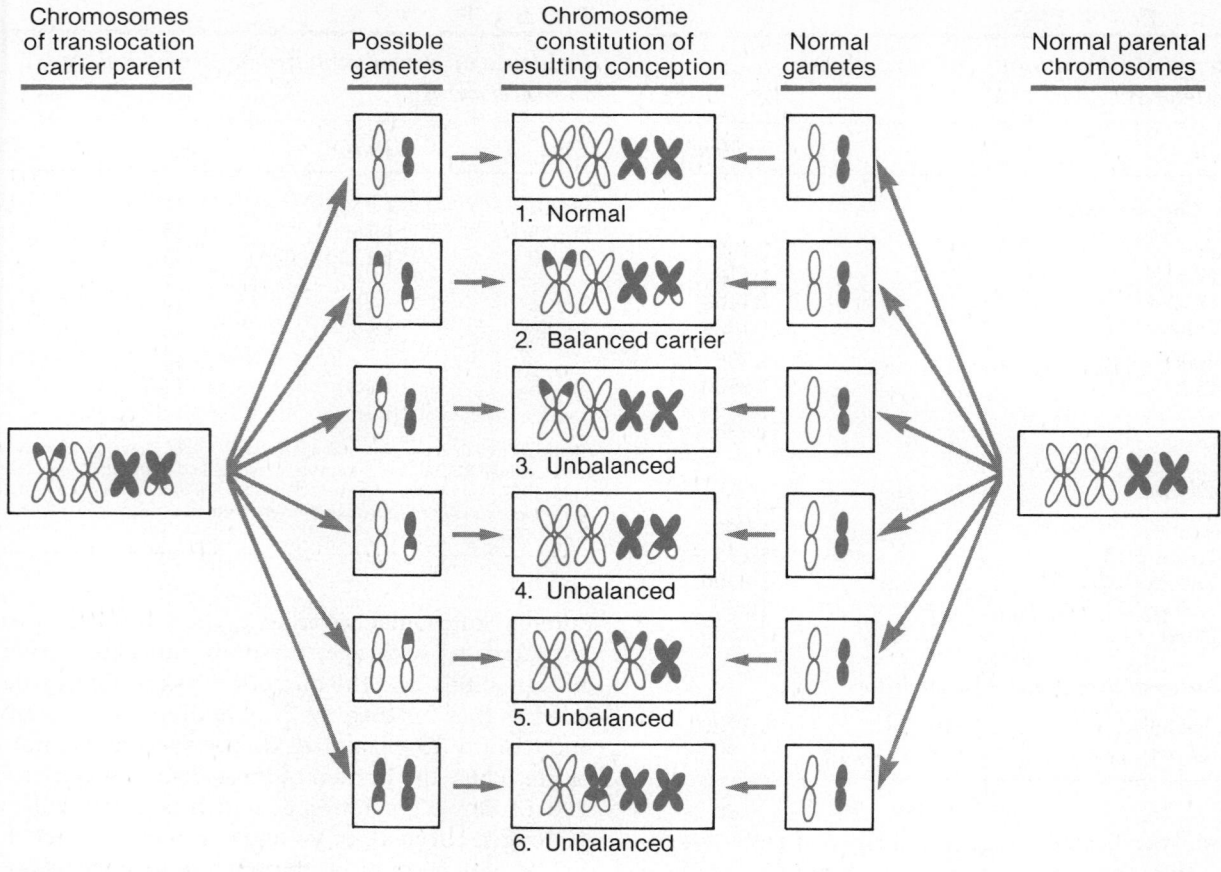

F I G U R E   1 7 - 6

Gametes formed by parent with translocation shown in Figure 17-5 and resulting conceptions after fertilization with normal gametes. 1. Normal. 2. Balanced translocation carrier. 3 through 6. Conceptions with unbalanced chromosomal segments.

contain a normal chromosome constitution, the balanced rearranged chromosomes, or a combination of the two chromosome pairs, which would result in deleted or duplicated chromosome segments (Fig. 17-6). In the latter case, spontaneous abortion may occur; however, if there are live-born infants with missing or extra chromosome segments they are likely to have serious physical and mental defects.

Since the development of banding, which helps to identify chromosome regions, many more children are being diagnosed as having structural chromosome abnormalities. This may occur *de novo* (as a new event) or may be secondary to a balanced translocation or other structural rearrangement in one parent. Persons with translocations are usually detected by a history of habitual abortion or the birth of a child with an abnormal chromosome constitution. The majority of balanced structural rearrangements detected in humans are familial.

Translocations involving chromosome 21 may result in children born with Down's syndrome due to additional chromosome material. Because a balanced trans-

location may be passed from one generation to another, a family history of Down's syndrome should be investigated. Chromosome analysis of the affected child will indicate whether the abnormality is due to nondisjunction (sporadic) or is secondary to a familial translocation. If an unbalanced translocation is found, chromosome studies to identify relatives who are translocation carriers are indicated. The reproductive risk when a parent carries a translocation varies with the sex of the carrier and the particular rearrangement. In these cases the parents may elect amniocentesis to determine if the fetus has an unbalanced chromosome constitution. If the family member with Down's syndrome is unavailable for study, chromosome analysis performed on the client's blood will readily determine if he or she is a carrier of a translocation involving chromosome 21.

On occasion, clients without the usual indications request cytogenetic testing of a pregnancy by amniocentesis. In many instances, the motivation for this request is previous experience with Down's syndrome. Often this contact is with a family member who has the disorder or is the result of occupation, as with nurses, physicians, or educators. Counseling is given based on the client's particular age-related risk. The risks and accuracy of the testing are presented. It is explained to the client that she and her partner are the only ones who can decide whether the benefit of the reassurance gained by testing justifies the risk involved.

Mendelian Disorders

A large number of genetic disorders that follow the inheritance patterns described by Mendel (*i.e.,* dominant gene, recessive gene, X-linked gene) have been delineated. For some of these diseases, the expression of the gene in cultured cells can be studied, permitting fetal diagnosis by amniotic cell culture (Table 17-3).

Dominant Disorders

Dominant disorders are those in which the presence of a single abnormal gene results in important phenotypic changes or disease, even though the other member of the gene pair is normal. Dominant disorders may occur as a result of a new mutation of a gene or by transmission of an abnormal gene from one of the parents. When one parent has a dominant disorder, the chance that he or she will contribute the abnormal member of the gene pair to a fetus is 1 in 2, or 50%. Because the penetrance and expression of some dominant genes vary greatly, the diagnosis of the disorder in a parent may be made only after the birth of an affected child. It is important that the counselor be familiar with the frequency of penetrance and the variability of expression of the gene for a disease when discussing the concepts of risk and burden with the family (see Principal Characteristics of Autosomal Dominant Traits).

Studies Performed. The biochemical expression of the gene for many dominant disorders is not known at the cellular level, and they are not detectable by amniocentesis. In some instances, anatomical defects associated with the disorder may be diagnosed by methods that define fetal anatomy. Prenatal diagnosis may be possible when the gene for a dominant disorder is linked (*i.e.,* in close proximity) on the chromosome to other traits that can be studied. The risk of the disease in this instance is defined by studying the linked gene rather than the gene for the disease. The applicability of this approach is limited at present, but it may become considerably more useful in the future. Several requirements must be met before a linkage study may be used for prenatal diagnosis: close linkage of the genes for the disease and marker (*i.e.,* the linked trait being studied), assignment of the gene and marker in the family by studying affected and unaffected family members, and an information mating (*i.e.,* transmission of the abnormal gene can be determined or excluded with a high level of confidence by studying the linked markers in the fetus).

Recessive Disorders

Recessive disorders are those in which both members of the gene pair are abnormal or deficient. When only one member of the pair is abnormal, the individual is unaffected but is heterozygous for, or a carrier of, the gene (see Principal Characteristics of Autosomal Re-

TABLE 17-3

Prenatal Diagnosis of Metabolic Diseases

Disease	Diagnostic Test
Lipid Metabolism	
Tay–Sachs	Hexosaminidase A
Sandhoff	Hexosaminidase A and B
Gaucher	β-Glucosidase
GM$_1$ gangliosidosis	β-Galactosidase
Niemann–Pick	Sphingomyelinase
Fabry	α-Galactosidase
Metachromatic leukodystrophy	Arylsulfatase A
Krabbe	Galactosylceramide-galactosidase
Wolman	Acid esterase
Familial hypercholesterolemia	Low-density lipoprotein cell-surface receptor
Mucopolysaccharidoses and Related Disorders	
Hurler (MPS I-H)	α-Iduronidase
Scheie (MPS I-S)	α-Iduronidase

(continued)

TABLE 17-3 (continued)

Prenatal Diagnosis of Metabolic Diseases

Disease	Diagnostic Test
Mucopolysaccharidoses and Related Disorders	
Hunter (MPS II)	Sulfoiduronate sulfatase
Sanfilippo A (MPS III-A)	Heparan sulfate sulfamidase
Sanfilippo B (MPS III-B)	α-N-acetylglucosaminidase
Maroteaux-Lamy (MPS IV)	Arylsulfatase B
Mucolipidosis II (I-cell disease)	Lysosomal hydrolases
Mucolipidosis III	Lysosomal hydrolases
Mucolipidosis IV	Electron microscopic ultrastructure
Fucosidosis	α-Fucosidase
Mannosidosis	α-Mannosidase
Sialidosis (variant)	Neuraminidase $+ \beta$-galactosidase
Amino Acid Metabolism	
Argininosuccinicaciduria	Argininosuccinate
Cystinosis	^{35}S-cystine uptake
Citrullinemia	Argininosuccinate synthetase
Homocystinuria	Cystathionine synthetase
Maple syrup urine	α-Keto acid decarboxylase
Methylmalonic acidemia	
$\quad$B$_{12}$-responsive	Deoxyadenosyl-B$_{12}$ synthesis
$\quad$B$_{12}$-nonresponsive	Methylmalonyl-CoA mutase
Propionic acidemia	Propionyl-CoA decarboxylase
Carbohydrate Metabolism	
Glycogen storage type II	α-Glucosidase
Glycogen storage type IV	Amylo-(1,4 $\rightarrow$ 1,6) transglucosidase
Galactosemia	Gal-1-P uridylyl transferase
Pyruvate decarboxylase deficiency	Pyruvate decarboxylase
Blood	
Hemophilia A	Factor VIII/Factor VIII antigen
Sickle cell anemia	β-Chain synthesis/restriction enzyme analysis
Homozygous β-thalassemia	β-Chain synthesis/restriction enzyme analysis
Homozygous α-thalassemia	c-DNA hybridization
$\beta°\delta°$-Thalassemia	c-DNA hybridization
Chronic granulomatous disease	NBT/superoxide formation
Miscellaneous	
Combined immunodeficiency	Adenosine deaminase
Lesch–Nyhan syndrome	HGPRT
Menke's disease	Copper uptake
Xeroderma pigmentosum	DNA repair
Hypophosphatasia	Alkaline phosphatase isoenzymes
Acute intermittent porphyria	Uroporphyrinogen I synthesis
Congenital adrenal hyperplasia (21-hydroxylase)	HLA-B linkage
Lysosomal acid phosphatase deficiency	Acid phosphatase
Congenital nephrosis	α-Fetoprotein

Principal Characteristics of Autosomal Dominant Traits

- Every affected child has at least one affected parent (except mutations).
- An affected person need only be heterozygous for the given allele.
- Male and female offspring are equally affected.
- There are affected individuals in several generations.
- There is a 50% risk of involvement of each sibling of an affected individual if the parent is affected.
- Examples of dominantly inherited diseases
  Apert's syndrome
  Crouzon's disease
  Achondroplasia
  Hereditary spherocytosis
  Huntington's chorea
  Marfan's syndrome
  Osteogenesis imperfecta
  Treacher Collins syndrome

(Waechter EW, Phillips J, Holaday B: Nursing Care of Children, 10th ed. Philadelphia, JB Lippincott, 1985)

Principal Characteristics of Autosomal Recessive Traits

- Each parent of an affected individual must carry at least one mutant allele (normal parents are carriers).
- Every affected individual is homozygous for the given allele.
- Individuals possessing a single mutant allele do not show the trait.
- Either sex may be affected.
- There is a 25% risk of involvement of the siblings of an affected individual.
- The disease tends to be rare and more severe than dominantly inherited conditions.
- Examples of recessively inherited diseases
  Albinism
  Cystic fibrosis
  Galactosemia
  Microcephaly
  Sickle cell anemia
  Tay–Sachs disease
  Thalassemia

(Waechter EW, Phillips J, Holaday B: Nursing Care of Children, 10th ed. Philadelphia, JB Lippincott, 1985)

cessive Traits). Production of a child with recessive disorders can only occur when both parents are carriers of the same abnormal gene. In this instance there is a 50% chance (1:2) that the child will inherit the abnormal gene from either parent. The likelihood that the child will inherit the abnormal gene from both parents and, thus, have the disease (homozygous) is 25% ($1/2 \times 1/2 = 1/4$). For prenatal diagnosis of a recessive disorder it is essential that the test be able to discriminate between the heterozygous (carrier) and the homozygous (affected) because two thirds of normal offspring will be carriers. (Fig. 17-7).

Everyone carries recessive genes for several rare disorders. Although these may be passed from generation to generation, the likelihood that a carrier will reproduce with another carrier of the same rare gene is quite low. In some instances, a couple are carriers of the same abnormal gene because they are closely related (consanguinity). The genes for some disorders that are otherwise quite rare have a relatively higher frequency in certain geographic areas or ethnic groups. Common examples of this were previously cited. Most often, couples in which both members are carriers of the gene for a rare recessive disorder are not identified until birth of an affected child. If laboratory testing can detect carriers for a recessive disorder, counseling and monitoring of pregnancies can be offered prior to the birth of an affected child. Screening programs for *Tay–Sachs disease* (hexosaminidase A deficiency) are examples of this approach. The carrier frequency for this disorder in United States population is about 1 in 300. Thus, the chance

that both members of any couple are carriers of the gene is $1/300 \times 1/300 = 1/90,000$. Because the risk to a "carrier couple" of having a child is 1 in 4, the frequency of the disease is $1/90,000 \times 1/4 = 1/360,000$. The likelihood that a person of Eastern European Jewish origin carries this gene is 1 in 30. Thus, the frequency of a carrier couple is $1/30 \times 1/30 = 1/900$ and the frequency of the disease is $1/900 \times 1/4 = 1/3600$. Because reliable prenatal diagnosis is available for this

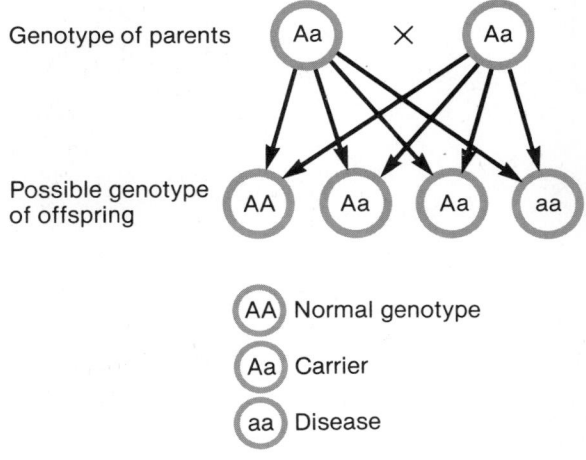

FIGURE 17-7

Recessive inheritance (A, normal gene; a, abnormal gene; AA, normal genotype; Aa, carrier; aa, disease). Note that the frequency of aa children when both parents are Aa carriers is 1:4, or 25%.

lethal disease, many Jewish communities support voluntary screening programs for carrier detection.

Studies Performed. More than 50 recessive disorders may be diagnosed by amniocentesis. For many of the disorders, the availability of diagnosis is limited to a few research laboratories.

X-Linked Recessive Disorders

The genes of X-linked recessive disorders are present on the X chromosome. In women, one X chromosome is inactivated in each cell. This inactivated X chromosome may be visualized as a chromatin mass in the periphery of the cell nucleus and is called a *Barr body* (Fig. 17-8). In women with Turner's syndrome (45,X), the single X chromosome is active in each cell and Barr bodies are absent. Individuals with more than two X chromosomes (47,XXX) maintain only one active X in each cell.

Inactivation of the X chromosome in normal women occurs randomly (*i.e.*, in some cells the maternally inherited X chromosome is active and in the other cells the paternally inherited X chromosome is active). Thus, when a woman has a gene for an X-linked recessive disorder on one of her two X chromosomes, it will be genetically active in only a portion of her cells. The woman is a carrier of the gene for the disorder, and in some instances the X chromosome with the abnormal gene will be active in enough cells to allow laboratory identification of the carrier state. Unless the normal X chromosome happens to be inactivated in the vast majority of cells, the disease will not be manifested.

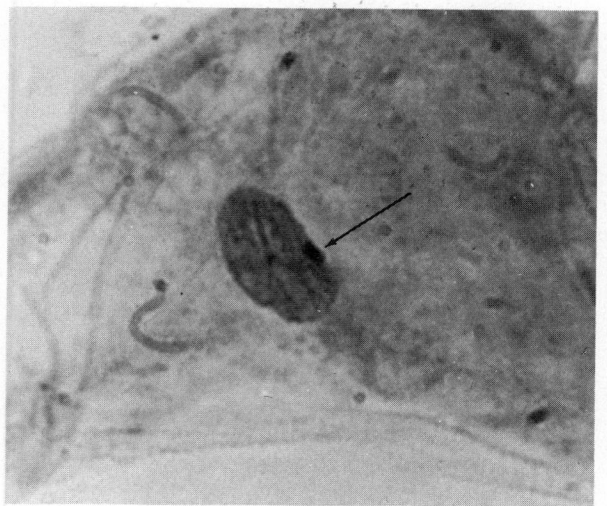

FIGURE 17-8

Cell from buccal mucosa. Arrow points to Barr body.

The single X chromosome that is present in the male is active in each cell. When a gene for an X-linked recessive disorder is present on that chromosome, the male will manifest the disease. Commonly cited examples of X-linked recessive disorders are hemophilia (Factor VIII deficiency) and Duchenne type muscular dystrophy. In some instances, a male child will have the disorder by new mutation. When the gene is inherited in the family, there may be a history of the disease in the mother's brothers or her uncles. Half of the daughters born to a carrier mother will also be carriers of the gene. Likewise, half of the sons born to a carrier mother will inherit her X chromosome with the mutant gene and will have the disease (see Principal Characteristics of X-Linked Recessive Traits).

Studies Performed. Amniotic fluid studies can detect affected males for a few X-linked recessive disorders such as Lesch–Nyhan and Hunter's syndromes. Hemophilia A may be diagnosed by using fetal blood obtained by fetoscopy in male fetuses at risk. In the majority of cases when a woman is a carrier of an X-linked recessive disorder, the risk can be refined only by identifying the sex of the fetus. Sex identification of the fetus is most reliably performed by chromosome analysis.

Nonspecific Mental Retardation. A proportion of nonspecific mental retardation in males is due to X-linked recessive genes. Recently the expression of a fragile site on the X chromosome of some of these males using specific cell culture conditions has enabled diagnoses of one form of X-linked mental retardation. A fragile site on a chromosome is a specific segment or band of the chromosome that demonstrates breakage with a higher frequency than expected as a random phenomenon.

Studies Performed. Methods for carrier identification and prenatal diagnosis of the fragile X chromosome associated with mental retardation are being actively investigated and will probably be clinically applied in the very near future.

When the fetus of a mother who is a carrier for an X-linked recessive disorder is male, there is a 50% risk that the child will have the disease. If the disorder cannot be specifically diagnosed by other methods, the client and her husband face the dilemma of selective termination based on the sex of the fetus.

Multifactorial Defects

Multifactorial defects occur when several genes predispose the fetus to or lower the threshold for an abnormality in development. In addition to the genetic constitution, environmental factors are thought to play a part in the development of these defects. Many of the most common birth defects are multifactorial in origin.[29,30] Most often, these are single defects such as cleft palate, pyloric stenosis, congenital heart disease, or neural tube defects (*e.g.,* anencephaly and myelomeningocele).

The occurrence risks in close relatives are based on empirical studies of families in which the defect has occurred. The risk for siblings is frequently in the range of 2% to 7% and increases with each affected child. The risk to other close relatives (*e.g.,* nieces, nephews, and first cousins), although low, is often higher than that of the general population.[31] More distantly related persons (*e.g.,* second cousins) are usually not at a substantially increased risk compared with the population.

Studies Performed. Advances in the methods used to detect structural abnormalities in the fetus, especially ultrasound and fetoscopy, may be useful for the diagnosis of some of these defects.

Neural Tube Defects

The only group of the more common multifactorial disorders that can be reliably diagnosed by amniocentesis at present are neural tube defects (NTDs). These defects arise during early fetal development owing to a failure of fusion or disruption of the neural tube, which will form the central nervous system. Although they may be associated with chromosome abnormalities or certain recessive disorders, the majority of NTDs are multifactorial in origin. The frequency of NTDs in the United States population is 1 to 2 per 1000 live births. Neural tube defects rank second only to cardiac abnormalities

as a cause of major congenital malformations in the United States.[11] The risk of recurrence when there has been an affected child is 3% to 5%.[32] Following two affected pregnancies, this risk increases to 10% to 12%.[33]

NTDs are described according to their location and anatomical structure. *Anencephaly,* a failure of development of the brain and skull, is the most severe NTD and is incompatible with survival. *Myelomeningocele* (spina bifida), in which there is a defect in formation of the spinal cord, surrounding tissues, and spinal column, is the other most common NTD. NTDs are also seen in children with other malformations. In some situations these may be sporadic or chromosomal. In other cases, the defect is caused by a single mutant gene (*e.g.,* Meckel's syndrome, which is autosomal recessive and may be confused with trisomy 13). Because of the heterogeneity of these defects, accurate diagnosis before counseling is essential to present accurate information.

Advances in neurosurgical techniques and aggressive medical management have improved the survival and quality of life for children with NTDs. Nevertheless, the likelihood of serious handicaps remains quite high for most of these children.

Studies Performed. The prenatal diagnosis of NTDs by amniotic fluid analysis is based primarily on measure of the AFP concentration in the amniotic fluid. AFP is produced in large quantities by the fetal yolk sac and liver during early fetal life, resulting in high concentrations in the fetal blood.[34,35] A substantially lower concentration of AFP is normally present in amniotic fluid. When a highly vascularized, non-skin-covered defect such as a meningomyelocele is present, the leakage of AFP from the fetal circulation into the amniotic fluid will elevate the levels of AFP in the amniotic fluid. Other abnormalities in which there are skin defects, such as omphalocele, may also be associated with elevated AFP levels in the amniotic fluid. To enhance the accuracy of this testing, confirmatory amniotic fluid tests and definition of the anatomical defect by ultrasound or amniography have been developed.

Very low concentrations of AFP are measurable in maternal blood by sensitive radioimmunoassay techniques. Maternal serum AFP concentration increases during the second trimester and peaks at approximately 34 weeks' gestation to 36 weeks' gestation. Studies have shown that maternal serum testing is a reasonably reliable method of identifying a large percentage of fetuses with an open NTD.[36,37] Because of the changing levels of maternal serum AFP as pregnancy advances, cut-off values for normal results must be established on a week-by-week basis and interpretation of results requires accurate gestational dating.

Voluntary, large-scale maternal serum AFP testing (MS-AFP) has been studied and utilized effectively in the United Kingdom for a number of years. Many similar programs have now been established in the United States.

In order to help patients make an informed decision about this testing, counseling and/or written information should be provided. In addition to neural tube defects, MS-AFP levels can be elevated due to errors in gestational dating, multiple gestation, or other fetal abnormalities (*e.g.*, renal agenesis, omphalocele). In the event of an elevated MS-AFP level, it is critically important to make an accurate diagnosis. Many women who have a single elevated MS-AFP level are found, on further evaluation, to have normal pregnancies. Further evaluations and testing may include a second MS-AFP measurement, ultrasound examination, and amniocentesis. MS-AFP screening should not be implemented unless a clinical geneticist, skilled ultrasonographer, and the diagnostic laboratory support for amniotic fluid studies are available.[38]

Other than ultrasound evaluation, MS-AFP screening might be considered the earliest form of evaluation of fetal well-being. Both elevated as well as lower than normal MS-AFP levels have been associated with impending spontaneous abortion. Approximately 5% of patients with serially elevated MS-AFP have subsequently aborted, while 38% of women with very low MS-AFP (<0.25 multiple of median) have had spontaneous abortions.[39–41] In addition, low MS-AFP has recently been associated with an increased risk of chromosome abnormality.[42,43] Combining low MS-AFP results with maternal-age–related risk may establish a level of risk for Down's syndrome at which it is appropriate to offer amniocentesis.

Nursing Process in Prenatal Genetic Counseling and Diagnosis

The nurse's role in genetic counseling often parallels that of the genetics associate with a master's degree in human genetics and counseling. Both are involved in the initial client contact, assessing clients for referral, and taking family histories. They perform preliminary counseling and coordinate appointments with physicians for evaluation and extended counseling. Throughout the counseling, the rapport that has been established permits them to serve as a client advocate. Through continued contact after counseling, they are able to evaluate the client's understanding of the information presented to her and her response to it. The nurse works with the client during the decision-making process and identifies resources for implementation of decisions.

A nurse–counselor or nurse–coordinator is especially suited to the prenatal genetic diagnostic team. In addition to having a basic knowledge of human genetics, the educational preparation of the nurse in reproduction and in obstetric procedures makes her invaluable for both client education and emotional support during prenatal diagnosis. The nurse's role is easily adapted to these services because nursing has traditionally espoused the philosophy of treating the whole client, including family members in client care, rather than focusing on the disease process or therapeutic regimen in itself. Additionally, in other areas of health-care delivery, nurses often assume the role of coordinating total client care.

Nurses in Maternity Care

Nurses involved with the health care of women should be aware of genetic counseling services and be able to identify clients who might benefit from them. (See the list in Reasons for Seeking Genetic Counseling.) In an extended role of the maternal–child health nurse, the nurse–counselor is ideally suited to coordinate and deliver essential elements of this care.

Identification of Those at Risk

An important aspect of primary maternity care is identifying families who have an increased risk of having a child with a genetic disorder or birth defect. Ideally, these factors should be recognized prior to pregnancy; however, it cannot be assumed that couples are aware of a specific risk, no matter how obvious it may seem.

Reasons for Seeking Genetic Counseling

- A medical problem has affected more than one individual in the family.
- A child with a previously diagnosed congenital defect or a group of malformations has been born.
- A medical condition that is suspected to be genetic has been diagnosed within a family.
- A family has one or more children who are mentally retarded.
- A child has delayed physical or mental developmental milestones.
- An individual has a birth defect that has been previously undiagnosed.
- The individual or family is concerned that some environmental agent (*e.g.*, x-ray, LSD, pesticides) with which they have come in contact might cause abnormalities in the offspring.
- Closely related couples want to know their risk of having a child with a birth defect.

(Waechter EW, Phillips J, Holaday B: Nursing Care of Children, 10th ed. Philadelphia, JB Lippincott, 1985)

The nurse's interview during the first obstetric visit can identify clients who might benefit from genetic counseling. A brief screening questionnaire may be used effectively to identify the majority of clients who might wish to consider prenatal diagnosis (see sample questionnaire). The following aspects should be reviewed with the client:

- Maternal age. The risk of having a child with Down's syndrome increases significantly when the mother is over 35.
- Ethnic background. A number of rare genetic disorders occur with higher frequency in certain ethnic groups. For example, Eastern European Jews have a ten times greater chance of carrying the Tay–Sachs gene than the general population in the United States; descendants of Mediterranean forebears have a greater chance of carrying the gene for thalassemia; and blacks have a much greater chance of carrying the sickle cell trait.
- Family history. Specific diseases (*e.g.,* Huntington's chorea and hemophilia), birth defects (*e.g.,* NTDs), or mental retardation may be hereditary.
- Reproductive history. Spontaneous abortions, stillborns, and previous live-born children with

birth defects, slow development, or mental retardation may indicate an increased risk.
- Maternal disease. Several maternal disorders are associated with higher frequency of birth defects (*e.g.,* diabetes mellitus and seizure disorder) or with mental retardation (*e.g.,* maternal phenylketonuria).

Assessment

While the majority of clients referred for genetic counseling and prenatal diagnosis are aware of the reason for referral, most are unsure of what to expect. Contact with the client should be made as soon as possible after referral. Any delay can serve only to intensify the client's anxiety, while the advancing gestational age may limit the options available to her.

Sensitivity. Clients invariably feel anxious as they approach genetic counseling. Many have only a limited understanding of the inheritance of diseases and what the counseling process will involve. Often these clients are in the process of grieving over the birth of a mal-

ASSESSMENT TOOL

Screening Questionnaire to Identify Candidates for Prenatal Diagnosis

1. Will you be age 35 or older when the baby is due? ___ YES ___ NO
   Age when due? _____
2. Have you or the baby's father or anyone in either of your families ever had:
   a. Down's syndrome or mongolism? ___ YES ___ NO
   b. Spina bifida or meningomyelocele (open spine)? ___ YES ___ NO
   c. Hemophilia? ___ YES ___ NO
   d. Muscular dystrophy? ___ YES ___ NO
3. Have you or the baby's father had a child born dead or alive with a birth defect not listed in question 2? ___ YES ___ NO
   If yes, describe: _____
4. Do you or the baby's father have any close relatives who are mentally retarded? ___ YES ___ NO
   If yes, list cause if known: _____
5. Do you or the baby's father or close relatives in either of your families have any inherited genetic or chromosomal disease or birth defect not listed above? ___ YES ___ NO
   If yes, describe: _____
6. Have you, or the spouse of this baby's father in a previous marriage, had 3 or more spontaneous pregnancy losses? ___ YES ___ NO
7. Do you or the baby's father have any close relatives descended from Jewish people who lived in Eastern Europe (Ashkenazic Jews)? ___ YES ___ NO
   If yes, have either you or the baby's father been screened for Tay–Sachs disease? ___ YES ___ NO
   If yes, indicate results and who was screened: _____
8. If client or her spouse is black:
   Have you or the baby's father or any close relative ever been screened for sickle-cell trait and found to be positive? ___ YES ___ NO
9. If client or her spouse is of Mediterranean ancestry:
   Have you or the baby's father or any close relative ever been screened for or found to have a trait for thalassemia or Cooley's anemia? ___ YES ___ NO

formed child or a serious illness of a family member. Guilt frequently compounds this anxiety. One or both parents may feel that there is something inherently wrong with themselves because a "defective" child has been born. On the other hand, they may blame the child's problems on the other partner or his or her "side of the family." The anxiety associated with counseling is easily exaggerated during pregnancy; therefore, it is important that genetic counselors be particularly sensitive to the pregnant client's concerns and family dynamics, so that disruption of the marriage or other family relationships may be avoided.

The nurse–counselor must assume an attitude of calm reassurance from the beginning to ensure good rapport. At the outset, the nurse–counselor should make it clear that the decision to have a study performed will rest with the couple, and a nondirective approach should be maintained throughout the counseling.

History

During the initial interview, it is useful to assess any factors that may alter the approach to counseling. First, determine how the referral was made and by whom (physician, nurse, advice of a friend or family member, or self-referred because of publicly available knowledge). The client's response to the referral and her perception of prenatal diagnosis are then discussed.

Factors Surrounding Current Pregnancy. The gestational age of the pregnancy is determined, and the couple's feelings concerning the pregnancy are explored. The counselor should determine if the pregnancy was planned or if there is ambivalence about continuing the pregnancy. It is extremely important to allow the client to express her ideas and anxieties prior to counseling. If the opportunity for this is not given, the focus during counseling may be diverted from the information presented and may be clouded by prior misinformation or denial.

Pedigree. To ensure comprehensive counseling, the nurse–coordinator obtains a detailed family history (pedigree) (Fig. 17-9). The outcome of all previous pregnancies and the health and development of live-born children are reviewed. The health and reproductive histories of the couple's parents, their siblings, and both sets of grandparents are taken. In addition, the ethnic origin of the families and any possibility of consanguinity of families are noted.

Cause of Death of Family Members. If a family member is deceased, it is important to know the cause of death and approximate age at which death occurred. When there is a history of a birth defect or mental retardation, there may be a need to review medical records including autopsy reports, x-ray films, photographs, and pathologic slides. This permits the most precise definition of identifiable genetic risks for the couple.[44] If a hereditary disorder in the family is ascertained, this may have great impact on the counseling. For example, if a woman is referred for prenatal cytogenetic diagnosis at age 35 with a 1 in 400 chance of having a child with Down's syndrome and it is learned from the pedigree that her father recently died from Huntington's chorea (a dominant disorder with late onset of neurologic deterioration), the entire focus of the counseling changes. In that instance, although the chance for a child with Down's syndrome is quite low, the chance that the child will develop Huntington's chorea is 25% (a 50% chance that the client herself has the gene and will develop the disease and a 50% chance if she has the gene that the fetus will inherit it from her). Although prenatal diagnosis of Down's syndrome is available through amniocentesis, there is no predictive study for Huntington's chorea. Thus, this new information may become the most important factor for this couple in selecting options.

Medical Records. When review of family medical records becomes important because of the medical history, it is essential that they are requested in a nonthreatening manner. Many families with malformed or retarded children are very protective of these individuals. Often, their diagnosis is not discussed outside the immediate family and a long-standing silence about their problem has prevailed. Since medical records are confidential, permission is required to obtain them. To obtain cooperation, the client must understand the reason for and value of these records. The release forms are sent to the client and forwarded to the relatives by her. While family members should not be contacted independently by the counselor, it is vital that the client be assured that relatives should feel free to contact the counselor for any explanation or clarification. Through this approach, the counselor may create opportunities to offer services to the extended family, while maintaining the privacy of the individual.

A review of medical records may enable the nurse or the physician to determine that the health problems of other family members do not indicate an increased risk for the fetus. If there have been unspoken or denied anxieties about the medical problems of close relatives, the reassurance provided by the counselor is of great value to the couple and, frequently, to other family members.

Intervention

Once the background information has been gathered and the scope of the counseling has been established, the counseling process begins. In most cases, prenatal counseling can be done by the nurse–counselor. In the

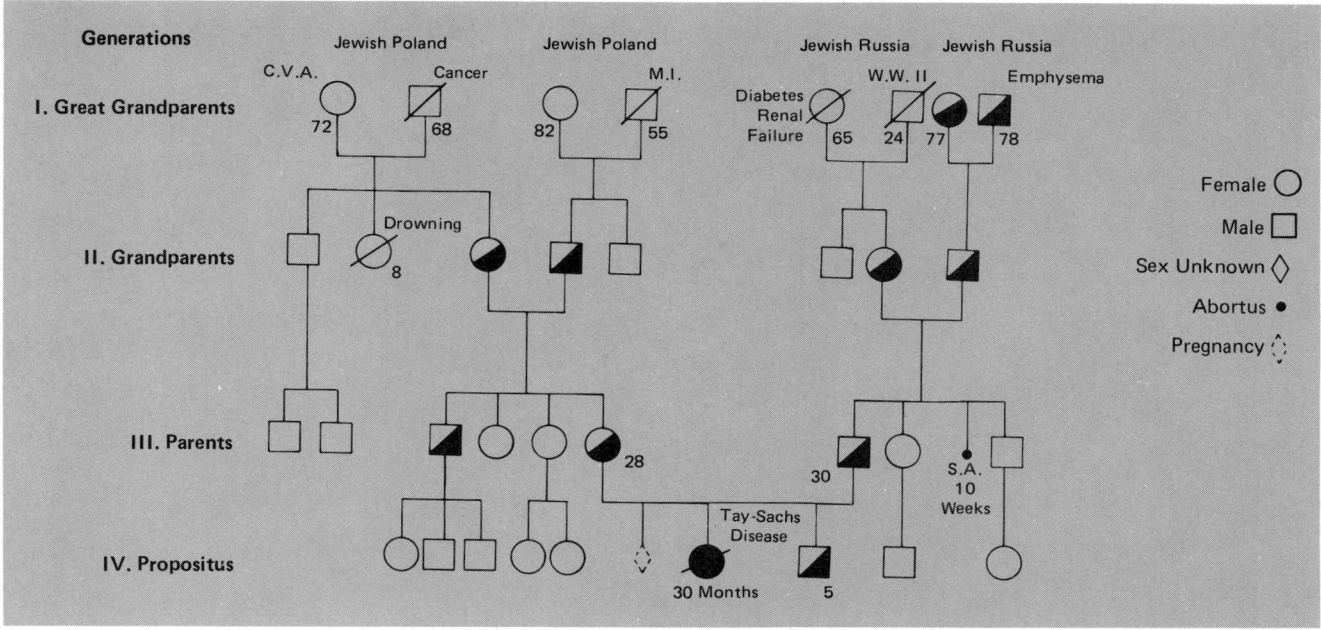

FIGURE 17-9

Sample pedigree demonstrating recessive inheritance of Tay–Sachs disease and the carrier state. Slanted line (/) through symbol represents deceased individual. Carriers are depicted by partially blackened symbol. Affected individual is depicted by totally blackened symbol.

usual situation (advanced maternal age without significant family history), an explanation of chromosomes, genes, and their functions is given. The mechanism for, and the numerical risk of, having a child with Down's syndrome at the client's age are explained and contrasted to the risk at other ages. The couple's knowledge of Down's syndrome is assessed and their information is clarified and supplemented. Studies in genetics clinics have found that, in addition to numerical risk, the perception of burden is of paramount importance in the decision-making process. The presentation of burden must not be biased by the opinion or experience of the counselor, but must be well founded in fact.

The medical procedures involved in prenatal diagnosis and the rationale for them are explained. It is vitally important to conduct the discussion in terms that the client can readily understand. The vocabulary must be individualized for each client. The risks and diagnostic limitations of the procedure are discussed in detail. For example, when ultrasonography is to be performed prior to amniocentesis, it is often necessary to distinguish this procedure from x-ray films. The reasons for performing this test are explained. Ultrasonography allows localization of the placenta. Placental puncture or injury during amniocentesis may be avoided when the implantation site is defined (Fig. 17-10). Measurement of the biparietal diameter of the fetal skull by ultrasound confirms the gestational age. The detection of multiple gestation is also a benefit of the procedure.

It is also explained that ultrasound is not painful and requires no special preparation by the client (*i.e.*, fasting); however, the bladder must be full during the study. The anatomical relationship of the bladder to the anterior lower segment provides a landmark for the evaluation of the uterus and its contents.

Counseling for Amniocentesis. Following a description of the technical aspects of the test, the client must consider the limitations, safety, and diagnostic accuracy of the procedure.

Limitations. The nurse–counselor should explain to the client that amniocentesis is not invariably successful. If ultrasound or clinical examination indicates that the pregnancy is earlier than 14 to 16 weeks' gestation, the procedure is postponed. If amniotic fluid is not obtained by the initial needle insertion, the physician may suggest another attempt or postponing the procedure for 7 to 10 days until a slightly more advanced gestational age. Once an adequate fluid sample is obtained, successful completion of the study depends upon the growth of cells in tissue culture. The client is told that if culture failure occurs (less than 1% of cases) a repeat amniocentesis must be considered. Most important, the couple must understand that the study is not a general test for birth defects or mental retardation, but is designed to detect the specific disorder that has been discussed in the counseling. It should be explained

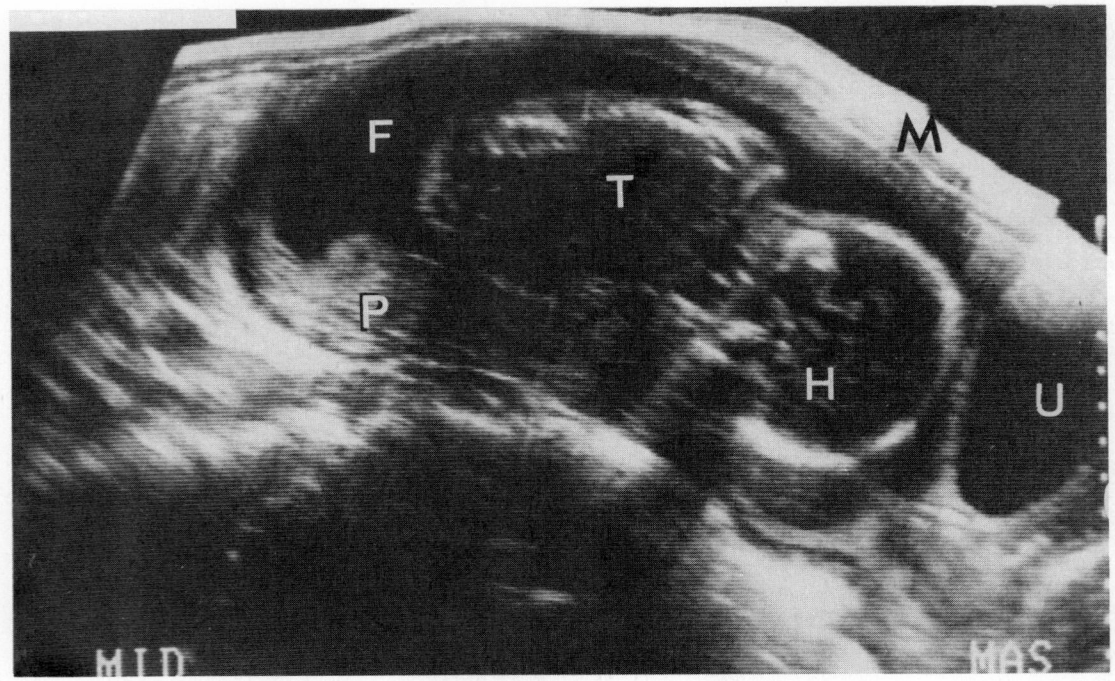

A

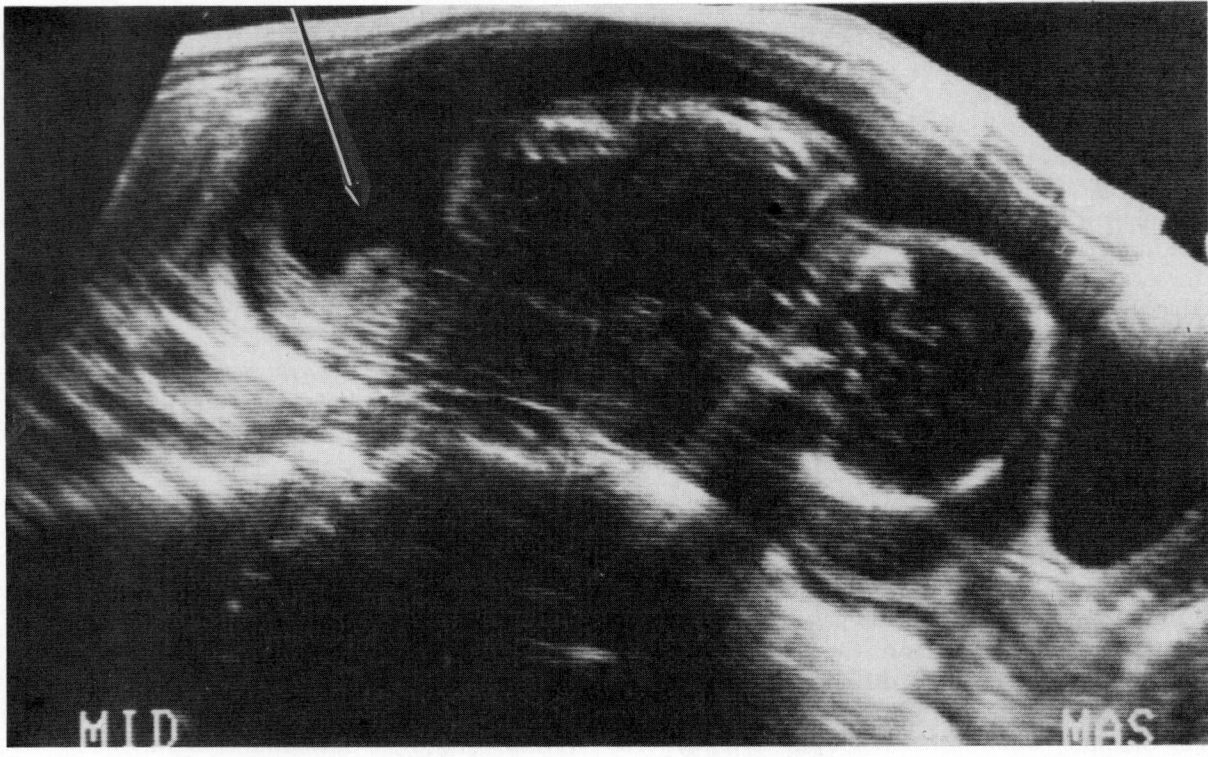

B

FIGURE 17-10

(*A*) B-mode gray-scale ultrasound of intrauterine pregnancy. (*M,* maternal abdominal wall; *H,* fetal head; *T,* fetal trunk; *P,* posterior placenta; *F,* amniotic fluid; *U,* maternal urinary bladder). (*B*) Same ultrasound. Arrow shows site selected for amniocentesis.

that any pregnancy has a 2% to 3% chance of resulting in a child born with a birth defect or congenital malformation and that the vast majority of these defects will not be detected by amniocentesis.[45] Chromosome analysis and AFP determination are usually offered even when these are not the primary studies being performed. The parents are told that if they wish to know the sex of the child when the chromosome studies are completed, the information will be available to them.

Risks. The risks of amniocentesis must be explained in detail. Concerns regarding spontaneous abortion related to the procedure prompted a collaborative controlled study by a number of centers in the United States.[14] The frequency of pregnancy loss in approximately 1000 clients undergoing midtrimester amniocentesis and in the controls was not significantly different; the incidence of pregnancy loss in both groups was approximately 3.5%. The results were confirmed by a similar study performed in Canada.[46] These studies indicate that the risk of pregnancy loss related to midtrimester amniocentesis is probably considerably less than 1%. More important, if pregnancy loss occurs following amniocentesis, it is most likely unrelated to the procedure. Instances of septic abortion due to chorioamnionitis following midtrimester amniocentesis have been reported. Most often, parents express a fear of fetal injury by the needle. Minor skin scars, secondary to midtrimester amniocentesis injury, occur infrequently,[47] and more significant injuries have rarely been reported.[48] Because of the large number of studies being performed, it is reasonable to assume that the likelihood of serious fetal injury is exceedingly low.

Entry of fetal blood cells into the maternal circulation as a result of amniocentesis occurs in approximately 10% of cases.[49,50] When the woman is Rh negative and the fetus is Rh positive, Rh sensitization may occur. Many centers administer Rh immunoglobulin prophylaxis to Rh-negative women in conjunction with amniocentesis.[51] When the potential for Rh sensitization is present, the rationale for this approach is explained.

Other complications following amniocentesis are spotting of blood or leakage of a small amount of fluid from the vagina. These occur in about 1% of cases and are generally limited to an isolated episode. Many clients will experience mild discomfort at the needle site for 1 to 2 days and a few may have ecchymosis or, more rarely, abdominal wall hematoma.

Accuracy. It is of paramount importance that prenatal genetic diagnosis be highly accurate. Nevertheless, every laboratory test has limitations. Every effort is taken to avoid human error, including independent duplicate analysis. When cultured amniotic fluid cells are used for testing, error owing to maternal cell contamination may be unavoidable. In less than 1% of cases, maternal cells are "picked up" by the needle as it penetrates the abdominal wall, and these cells grow in the tissue culture. When this occurs, the study may reflect the genotype of the mother rather than of the fetus.

During counseling, it is not unusual for the client to ask for the nurse–counselor's opinion or advice regarding the testing. The counselor must emphasize that the decision to have prenatal diagnosis is one that belongs only to the couple. The same information is interpreted differently by each couple based on personal factors. For example, a 40-year-old primigravida with a long-standing infertility problem may view any risk of spontaneous abortion associated with a procedure as unacceptable and her risk for having a child with Down's syndrome as low (99% chance that it will not occur). When clients ask for advice it should be explained that the opinion of the counselor may not be appropriate to their particular situation.

Evaluation: Postcounsel Follow-Up

After counseling, the couple needs time to discuss all of the information presented with each other and to explore their feelings about the diagnostic procedure. Ideally, the evaluation is given at a time when they have several weeks to make a decision regarding the testing. Even when the initial contact is made late in gestation (16–18 weeks), the couple should have at least several days to consider the procedure. It should be emphasized that both the husband and the wife must feel comfortable with the decision, and the nurse must evaluate their response to her counseling.

Several days after the counseling the nurse contacts the client. Any questions that have arisen are answered. If there is a great deal of ambivalence, difficulty, or disagreement about the decision, additional counseling is offered. The decision-making process is influenced by many factors outside the realm of genetics: the marital relationship, the presence and needs of other children, religious beliefs, attitudes of other family members, career aspirations, financial considerations, self-images, and concepts of parenthood to name just a few.[52]

Procedure for Amniocentesis

Shortly prior to amniocentesis, the obstetrician reviews the counseling and answers any additional questions from the couple. The client is asked to sign a consent form, which includes statements regarding the risks and limitations of the procedure. Because of the rapport that has been established, the presence of the nurse–counselor during the procedure is invaluable in minimizing anxiety. The steps in the procedure and possible sen-

NURSING CARE PLAN

Families Involved in Genetic Counseling

Nursing Objectives

1. Assist client(s) to obtain appropriate information regarding options for anticipated or present pregnancies.
2. Assist client(s) with feeling comfortable regarding their choices.

Assessment	Potential Nursing Diagnosis	Planning/Intervention	Evaluation
Past history of pregnancy and so forth	Anxiety related to actual or perceived threat to biologic integrity	Take general health and obstetric history Obtain attitudes toward pregnancy, nuclear-family composition, initiation of referral, general knowledge and attitude toward prenatal diagnosis	Couple indicates feeling of rapport with nurse Couple discusses health problems Couple indicates readiness for referral and counseling
Genetic history of extended family Psychological status of pregnancy	Alteration in family processes related to birth history of previous pregnancy or of other family members	Obtain multigeneration family pedigree (when necessary, request medical records, arrange appropriate consultations, and perform laboratory studies)	Couple understands implications of high risk factors Couple understands vocabulary used by nurse/counselor Couple freely discusses genetic history of family Couple weighs advantages and risks for their situation

(continued)

sations that the client will feel are anticipated by the nurse and explained.

After emptying the bladder, the client is instructed to rest on the examining table in a supine position with her legs extended. The site selected for needle insertion is determined by abdominal examination and the ultrasonic findings. The skin is prepared with antiseptic solution, and a sterile field is established. Local anesthesia is injected into the skin and through the abdominal wall to the peritoneum. A stinging or burning sensation upon injection of the local anesthetic is usually the most uncomfortable aspect of amniocentesis. An 18-gauge or a 20-gauge spinal needle is inserted through the anesthetized area and uterine wall into the amniotic cavity. The client may have a sensation of deep pelvic pressure during the procedure.

Amniotic fluid will often spill spontaneously after the amniotic sac is entered with a needle. One milliliter to 2 ml of fluid is discarded to help avoid contamination of the sample with cells from the maternal abdominal wall. If blood is obtained at first, the fluid may become clear again before the specimen is collected. The amount of fluid withdrawn varies with the studies performed, but generally it ranges from 5 ml to 30 ml. The fluid specimen is collected in two or more separate, sterile syringes, which are capped and labeled immediately. The samples are transported to the laboratory in the same syringes to avoid the possibility of bacterial contamination during transfer to another container. The volume of fluid withdrawn rapidly reaccumulates.

Following the procedure, the needle puncture site is dressed with a bandage and the client is asked to rest on the examining table for several minutes. There are usually no symptoms after the procedure. Although apprehension and anxiety levels are quite high prior to amniocentesis, most clients state that the experience involves less discomfort than a dental appointment.

At the conclusion of the procedure, the client is often shown the labeled sample before it is transported to the laboratory. This helps to alleviate concerns regarding mislabeling of samples, especially if a positive diagnosis occurs. Signs or symptoms of complication, such as bleeding, leakage of amniotic fluid, and fever, are reviewed and instructions for contacting the nurse or physician are given. The length of time required for completion of the studies, usually 2 to 4 weeks, is discussed again, and the mechanism for notifying the client of the results is decided.

Assessment	Potential Nursing Diagnosis	Planning/Intervention	Evaluation
Need for counseling related to prenatal diagnosis and amniocentesis	Knowledge deficit related to purpose of tests and procedures of examinations	Provide precise, detailed information (e.g., ultrasonography and its purposes, length of time for procedures and results) in objective, nonjudgmental manner	Couple asks additional questions to clarify details
Knowledge related to ultrasound and amniocentesis			Mother is comfortable and at ease. Father feels included in procedure
		Brief overview of initial counseling (by nurse–counselor and physician)	Parents continue to develop rapport with nurse–counselor
		Assist client to examination table; position and drape client; direct father to best position to observe ultrasound	
Understanding of outcome of tests	Knowledge deficit related to outcome of tests	Review possible aftereffects and complications; provide couple with phone number for answering service (24-hour availability)	Couple expresses reduced anxiety
			Couple exercises control in receiving information
		Arrange per couple's preference (call directly, referring physician call with results, or arrange return visit to review results with nurse–counselor or physician)	Couple indicates that they feel diagnosis is accurate
			Couple evaluates options and makes decisions
		Arrange appointment with couple to return for detailed objective discussion of findings; be prepared to answer any questions regarding diagnosis, prognosis, and pregnancy termination	

Counseling After Amniocentesis

Prior to amniocentesis, much of the client's anxiety is focused on the procedure. Following amniocentesis, her concerns shift to possible complications and the test results. Several days later, the nurse may contact the client to determine if there are any unusual symptoms related to the procedure. Most often there are none. If necessary, an examination may be arranged. The client is aware that the successful completion of the study depends on the adequate growth of fetal cells in culture and that delays or, rarely, failure of culture can occur. The success of the cell culture can usually be determined by the examination of the sample after 7 to 10 days, and the client is notified immediately. If repeat amnio-

centesis is required, this should be discussed with the client as soon as possible. The client is reassured that failure or delays in establishing cell culture are not indicative of a problem with the pregnancy. If this occurs or, more commonly, if fluid is not obtained after the initial amniocentesis is attempted, the decision regarding a repeat amniocentesis must be made by the couple.

The interval between successful amniocentesis and final results is also accentuated by physiological changes and social pressures. Amniocentesis involves considerably more than a simple medical procedure; major psychosocial concomitants that may have important consequences for the couple and the family are involved as well.[53] In some cases, the couple have not announced the pregnancy to relatives and friends and wish to wait until the diagnostic results are known. During the 16th week of gestation to the 20th week of gestation, the uterus grows and the pregnancy begins to "show" or be more apparent. The mother may feel fetal movement for the first time while awaiting the results of the studies. This will intensify her fears of an abnormal result and her ambivalence about termination. It is interesting that many clients ignore or deny fetal movement until after the studies are completed. A most important aspect of the nurse–counselor's role is giving emotional support to the couple during this waiting period. There should be ample telephone communication with the couple and they should feel free to call as frequently as necessary for reassurance.

Normal Results. Giving the couple the normal results following amniocentesis does not end the nurse–counselor's contact; follow-up is also important. The accuracy of prenatal diagnosis is not confirmed until the baby is born. After delivery, the nurse may also wish to discuss the client's reactions to amniocentesis once again.

Positive Diagnosis. When a positive diagnosis occurs, the nurse–counselor and physician notify the couple, preferably in person. Prior to informing couples of positive results, all studies should be completed and verified; most clients will ask about the certainty of the results. After counseling, these clients often desire termination of the pregnancy as rapidly as possible. The method of termination is selected with maternal safety as the greatest priority. Confirmation of the diagnosis for scientific purposes and parental information are important but should be secondary. Because detailed information regarding pregnancy termination during the second trimester is not offered prior to the test results, this information must be presented to the client at this time. The nurse–counselor maintains contact with the client throughout the termination procedure and recovery.

Following selective abortion of an affected fetus, the couple experiences grief. Observation of these clients has documented a high frequency of depression and marital discord. Because of the emotional stress following selective abortion of a wanted pregnancy, the couple is dissuaded from making permanent decisions about their future reproduction. Sterilization is not advisable at this time. Several weeks to months later, one or more visits are arranged for the couple to assess their resolution of grief and, if they wish, to discuss future reproduction. In the interval between these visits, the nurse–counselor maintains close contact with the client. Often she may be the only person with whom the couple can freely discuss their feelings about the pregnancy and termination. Communication between the husband and wife is fostered, and psychiatric care or marriage counseling is offered when appropriate.

References

1. Ford CE, Hamerton JL: The chromosomes of man. Acta Genetica 6:264–266, 1956
2. Tijo JH, Levan A: The chromosome number of man. Jereditas 42:1–6, 1956
3. Fraser FC: Genetic counseling. Am J Med Genet 26:636–659, 1974
4. Omenn GS, Figley MM, Graham CB et al: Prospects for radiographic intrauterine diagnosis: The syndrome of thrombocytopenia with absent radii. N Engl J Med 288:777, 1973
5. Grisom NT: Radiographic fetal diagnosis. In Milunsky A (ed): Genetic Disorders and the Fetus. New York, Plenum, 1980
6. Queenan JT, Gadow EC: Amniography for detection of congenital malformations. Obstet Gynecol 35:648, 1970
7. Mennuti MT, Moranz JC, Schwarz RH et al: Amniography for the early detection of neural tube defects. Obstet Gynecol 49:25, 1977
8. Robinson HP, Hood VD, Adam AH et al: Diagnostic ultrasound: Early detection of fetal neural tube defects. Obstet Gynecol 56:705, 1980
9. Hobbins JC, Grannum P, Berkowitz RL et al: Ultrasound in the diagnosis of congenital anomalies. Am J Obstet Gynecol 135:331, 1979
10. Grannum P, Bracker M, Silverman R et al: Assessment of fetal kidney size in normal gestation by ratio of kidney circumference to abdominal circumference. Am J Obstet Gynecol 136:249, 1980
11. Hobbins JC, Mahoney MJ: The diagnosis of skeletal dysplasia with ultrasound. In Sanders R, James AE (eds): Ultrasonography in Obstetrics and Gynecology. New York, Appleton-Century-Crofts, 1980
12. Alter BP, Friedman S, Hobbins JC et al: Prenatal diagnosis of sickle cell anemia and alpha G Phila. N Engl J Med 294:1040, 1976
13. Mibashan RS, Peake IR, Rodeck CH et al: Dual diagnosis of prenatal haemophilia A by measurement of fetal factor VIIIC and VIIIC antigen (VIII CAg). Lancet 2:994, 1980
14. The NICHD Amniocentesis Registry: The Safety and Accuracy of Mid-Trimester Amniocentesis. DHEW Publication No. (NIH) 78-190, 1975
15. Mennuti MT, Cormbleholme WR, Zackai EH et al: Amniocentesis for prenatal diagnosis: A seven year experience in a University based service. ACM Meeting, American Association of Obstetricians and Gynecologists, Hot Springs, Virginia, September 1979
16. Crandall BF, Howard T, Lebherz TB et al: Follow-up of 2000 second trimester amniocenteses. Obstet Gynecol 56:625, 1980
17. Golbus MS, Loughman WD, Epstein CJ et al: Prenatal genetic diagnosis in 3000 amniocenteses. N Engl J Med 300:157, 1979
18. Old J: First trimester fetal diagnosis for haemoglobinopathies: Three cases. Lancet 2:1413–1416, 1982
19. Brambati B, Simoni G: Diagnosis of fetal trisomy 21 in first trimester. Lancet 1:586, 1983
20. Jackson L: Chorionic villi sampling. Registry Newsletter, December 10, 1984

21. Cheung SW, Burgess AC, Crane JP: Reliability of cytogenetic studies using chorionic villus biopsy (CVB) for first trimester diagnosis. Society for Gynecologic Investigation 31st Annual Meeting, San Francisco, March 21–24, 1984

22. Steele MW, Breg WR Jr: Chromosome analysis of human amniotic fluid cells. Lancet 1:383, 1966

23. Warburton D, Kline J, Stein Z et al: Monosomy X: A chromosomal anomaly associated with young maternal age. Lancet 1:167, 1980

24. Dhadial RK, Machin AM, Tait SM: Chromosome anomalies in spontaneously aborted human fetuses. Lancet 2:20, 1970

25. Hook EB, Hamerton JL: The frequency of chromosome abnormalities detected in consecutive newborn studies. In Hook EB, Porter IH (eds): Population Cytogenetics Studies in Humans. New York, Academic Press, 1977

26. Magenis RE, Overton KM, Chamberlin J et al: Parental origin of the extra chromosome in Down's Syndrome. Hum Genet 37:7–16, 1977

27. NICHD National Registry for Amniocentesis Study Group: Midtrimester amniocentesis for prenatal diagnosis: Safety and accuracy. JAMA 236:7, 1976

28. Holmes LB: Current concepts in genetics: Congenital malformations. N Engl J Med 295:204, 1976

29. Warkany J: Spina bifida. In Congenital Malformations: Notes and Comments. Chicago, Year Book Medical Publishers, 1971

30. Yen S, MacMahon B: Genetics of anencephaly and spina bifida. Lancet 2:623, 1968

31. Carter CO, David PA, Lawrence KM: A family study of major central nervous system malformations in South Wales. J Med Genet 5:81, 1968

32. Carter CO, Roberts JAD: The risk of recurrence after two children with central nervous system malformations. Lancet 1:306, 1967

33. Brock DJH: The prenatal diagnosis of neural tube defects. Obstet Gynecol 31:32, 1976

34. Weiss RR, Macri JN, Elligers KW: Origin of amniotic fluid alpha-fetoprotein in normal and defective pregnancies. Obstet Gynecol 47:697, 1976

35. Brock DJH, Sutcliffe RG: Alpha fetoprotein in the antenatal diagnosis of anencephaly and spina bifida. Lancet 2:197, 1972

36. Brock DJH, Bolton AE, Monaghan JM: Prenatal diagnosis of anencephaly through maternal serum alpha fetoprotein measurement. Lancet 2:923, 1973

37. Report of U.K. collaborative study on alpha-fetoprotein in relation to neural tube defects, maternal serum alpha fetoprotein measurement in antenatal screening for anencephaly and spina bifida in early pregnancy. Lancet 1:1323, 1977

38. Main D, Mennuti M: Neural tube defects: Issues in prental diagnosis and counseling. Am J Obstet Gynecol 67:1–16, 1986

39. Macri JN, Weiss RP: Prenatal serum alpha-fetoprotein screening for neural tube defects. Obstet Gynecol 59:633, 1982

40. Burton BK, Sowers SG, Nelson LH: Maternal serum alpha-fetoprotein screening in North Carolina: Experience with more than twelve thousand pregnancies. Am J Obstet Gynecol 146:439, 1983

41. Davenport DM, Macri JN: The clinical significance of low maternal serum alpha-fetoprotein. Am J Obstet Gynecol 146:657, 1983

42. Merkatz IK, Nitowsky HM, Macri JN, Johnson WE: An association between low maternal serum alpha-fetoprotein and fetal chromosome abnormalities. Am J Obstet Gynecol 148:866, 1984

43. Cuckle HS, Wald NJ: Maternal serum alpha-fetoprotein measurement: A screening tool for Down's Syndrome. Lancet 1:926, 1984

44. World Health Organization Expert Committee: Genetic counseling. WHO Tech Rep Ser 416:1, 1969

45. Leonard CD, Chase GA, Childs B: Genetic counseling: A consumer's view. N Engl J Med 287:433, 1972

46. Simpson NE et al: Prenatal diagnosis of genetic disease in Canada: Report of a collaborative study. Can Med Assoc J 75:115, 1976

47. Broome DL, Wilson MG, Weiss B et al: Needle puncture of fetus: A complication of second trimester amniocentesis. Am J Obstet Gynecol 126:247, 1976

48. Epley SL, Hanson JW, Cruikshank DP: Fetal injury with midtrimester diagnostic amniocentesis. Obstet Gynecol 53:77–80, 1979

49. Mennuti MT, Brummond W, Crombleholme WR et al: Fetal-maternal bleeding associated with genetic amniocentesis. Obstet Gynecol 55:48–54, 1980

50. Blajchman MA, Maudsley RF, Uchida I et al: Diagnostic amniocentesis and fetal maternal bleeding. Lancet 1:993, 1974

51. Hill LM, Platt LD, Kellogg B: Rh sensitization after genetic amniocentesis. Obstet Gynecol 56:459, 1980

52. Levine C: Genetic counseling: The client's viewpoint. In Capron A, Lappe M, et al (eds): Genetic Counseling: Facts, Values and Norms. New York, Alan R Liss, 1979

53. Grobstein R: Amniocentesis counseling. In Kessler S (ed): Genetic Counseling Psychological Dimensions. New York, Academic Press, 1979

Suggested Reading

Cohen EJ, Cohen C: A birth defects prevention curriculum for inner city junior high school students. J Sch Health 51:97–100, 1981

Fibison WJ: The nursing role in the delivery of genetic services. Issues Health Care Women 4(1):1–15, 1983

Fletcher JC: Ethical issues in genetic screening and antenatal diagnosis. Clin Obstet Gynecol 24(4):1151–1168, 1981

Kasper AS: Maternal serum alpha fetoprotein testing: Some public policy considerations. Women's Health 6:147–153, 1981

LaRochelle D: Prenatal genetic counseling: Ethical and legal interfaces with the nurse's role. Issues Health Care Women 4(1):77–92, 1983

Thompson J, Thompson M: Genetics in Medicine, 4th ed. Philadelphia, WB Saunders, 1986

Tishler C: The psychological aspects of genetic counseling. Am J Nurs 81:732, 1981

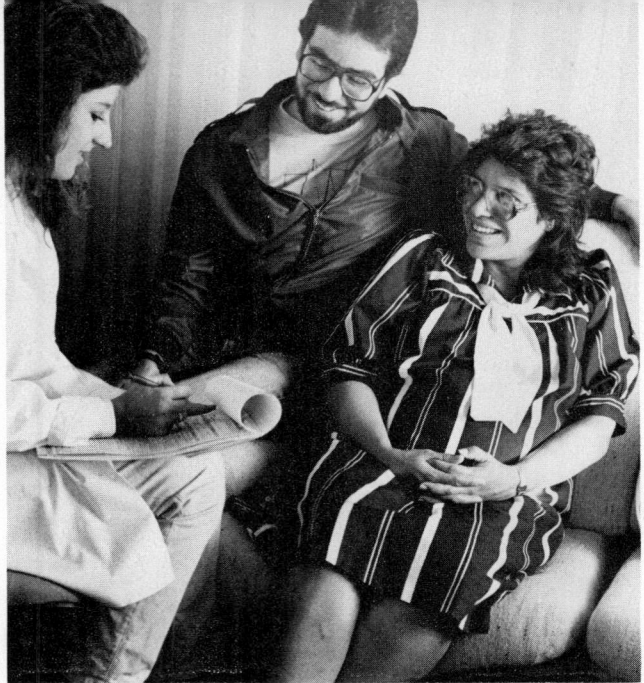

Unit III:
Assessment and Management of Sexuality and Reproduction

Conference Material

1. Ruth W. is 24 years old, pregnant for the first time, and in the eighth month of pregnancy. She and her husband Tom report a generally satisfying sexual relationship during pregnancy. For the last week, however, intercourse has been quite painful on deep thrusting, and she notices continued uncomfortable contractions for one half hour after sex. Because of this, Ruth has been avoiding sex, which is creating tension in their relationship. What additional information would you need, and how would you assist this couple in understanding what is happening and finding approaches to alleviate this problem?

2. Sally and Bill S. are having their second child, and in early pregnancy they seek counseling about the changes in sex drive and responsiveness during pregnancy. They were worried and confused about these changes during the first pregnancy, and did not enjoy their childbearing experience as much as they wanted. Both usually have an intense, enjoyable sexual experience, and this is an important part of their lives. To counsel this couple effectively, what information do you need, and what specific knowledge about sexuality in pregnancy can you draw from?

3. Louise H. is a 34-year-old mother of three who has used oral contraceptives successfully for a total of seven years. Her weight and blood pressure are normal, and there is no history of thromboembolic disease in her family. She smokes a half pack of cigarettes per day and has smoked for 15 years. She is currently taking a combination pill with 50 mcg estrogen. Louise has a stable marriage, her husband is 38 years old, and they feel their family is complete. On this visit for her biannual examination, how would you counsel Louise concerning continuation of oral contraceptives and alternative methods of birth control?

4. Aurora and Saadi are in their early 20s, unmarried and have been living together for 2 years. She had an IUD in place, but became concerned about complications and had the IUD removed last week. They are now interested in a natural method of birth control, which would be more compatible with their life-style and philosophy (includes avoiding the introduction of unnatural substances into the body). In discussing their options, what information do you need to know about Aurora's menstrual cycles, the pattern of their sexual relations, and their feelings about an accidental conception? Outline the benefits and risks of using one or a combination of natural contraceptive methods.

5. Vikki is 16, a high school sophomore who is active in student government and has a part-time job. She and her boyfriend Chris have been going steady for 3 months. Vikki has come to the family planning clinic requesting birth control pills, because she and Chris want to begin having sex but strongly want to avoid pregnancy. In counseling Vikki about contraception, what information about teenage sexuality will you draw upon? How would you present their options regarding intercourse and contraception to her? What would be the main considerations in their using the following contraceptive methods: the pill, the IUD, condom, spermicidal cream or foam, diaphragm, and withdrawal?

6. A 44-year-old woman has just been evaluated for a first trimester abortion. She has four children, ages 6 to 17, and had two miscarriages. Presently she is divorced and receiving both state welfare assistance and Aid to Dependent Children, and she has no job. The pregnancy is 10 weeks' gestation, and she is definite about wanting an abortion. She desires no further children, and had been using foam and condom as contraception. Although receiving Medicaid, she lives in a state that does not provide funds for abortions. What factors will you take into consideration in discussing the patient's options with her? Since she feels strongly about wanting to have the abortion, what types of assistance can you provide her in carrying out this decision? (Her state of health is good.)

7. Marianne is 17, unmarried, and 12 weeks pregnant. No one but her boyfriend knows that she has come to the clinic for pregnancy evaluation. She is from a middle-class family, her parents have been divorced for 5 years, and she is the oldest of three children. A junior in high school, she is not very interested in her studies and has no clear career plans. Marianne and her boyfriend Jeff have talked about getting married, but he is reluctant because he wants to go to college. She is unhappy with her home situation because she feels she has too much responsibility for her younger siblings since her mother works. She has mixed feelings about the pregnancy, is confused about what she wants to

do, and has little understanding about what her choices entail. How would you counsel Marianne and Jeff about their decision making and implementing their choice?

Multiple Choice

Read through the entire question and place your answer on the line to the right.

1. Cervical mucus is not receptive to spermatozoa when it is
   A. Clear, abundant, and acellular
   B. Turbid and thick
   C. Under the influence of progesterone
   D. Under the influence of estrogen
   Select the number corresponding to the correct letters.
   1. A and C
   2. A and D
   3. B and C
   4. B and D   ____

2. A pituitary tumor should be suspected and ruled out in the patient with amenorrhea who exhibits
   A. Elevated levels of FSH and LH
   B. Elevated prolactin levels
   C. Low estrogen levels
   D. Pregnanediol in the urine   ____

3. A 35-year-old nulligravida has had unprotected intercourse for 10 months. She and her husband both want a pregnancy. She should be told
   A. Not to worry; it will happen in time
   B. To consider having a fertility investigation if pregnancy does not ensue soon
   C. Patients over 35 years of age have a higher incidence of children affected by Down's syndrome, and therefore, pregnancy is unwise   ____

4. The maternity nurse without training in sex therapy can most effectively intervene in which type of sexual problem?
   A. Knowledge problems
   B. Relationship problems
   C. Attitudinal problems   ____

5. Sexual responsiveness might decrease during early to mid pregnancy because of
   A. Physiological changes (*e.g.*, nausea, fatigue)
   B. Increased pelvic vascularity and vasocongestion
   C. Heightened sensual responsiveness   ____

6. Intercourse should be avoided during pregnancy
   A. After the seventh month
   B. When the uterus is large enough to press on the vena cava
   C. If vaginal bleeding or loss of amniotic fluid occurs
   D. If cramping occurs   ____

7. Intercourse should be resumed after delivery
   A. Following the six-week check-up
   B. When bleeding has ceased and intercourse is comfortable
   C. When the physician permits it   ____

8. Couples who fear harming the fetus by pressure or crushing during intercourse in later pregnancy can be advised
   A. To avoid intercourse after 6 to 7 months' gestation
   B. To use the side position for intercourse
   C. To use noncoital methods   ____

9. Physiologic causes of postpartal dyspareunia or lack of arousal include all but which of the following?
   A. Low levels of steroid hormones
   B. Perineal tenderness due to episiotomy or lacerations
   C. Fatigue and lack of sleep
   D. Postpartal diuresis   ____

10. In discussing contraceptive effectiveness, the method's lowest observed failure rate, when used perfectly and understood completely, is called
    A. Maximal (theoretical) effectiveness
    B. Typical (use) effectiveness   ____

11. Ethical contraceptive counseling requires the nurse to
    A. Quote effectiveness data for all methods using only one type of failure rate
    B. Quote maximal rates for the more effective methods and typical rates for the less effective methods
    C. Avoid quoting any type of failure rates and letting the client follow her/his own inclinations   ____

12. Which of these statements is not a component of informed consent?
    A. Discussing benefits and risks of the methods being considered
    B. Discussing alternative methods
    C. Encouraging the client to ask questions
    D. Assuring that the client may stop using a method at any time without penalty
    E. Explaining how to use the method
    F. Discussing results expected by using the method
    G. Written documentation in the chart
    H. Written, signed client consent form
    I. All of these are components of informed consent   ____

13. Which of these statements is accurate regarding contraceptives for minors?
    A. It is illegal to provide contraceptives to minors.
    B. Minors may receive contraceptives only after pregnancy or abortion.
    C. Minors have a constitutional right to contraception.   ____

14. Absolute contraindications to use of oral contraceptives include all but which of the following?
    A. Thromboembolic disorders
    B. Migraine headaches
    C. Pregnancy
    D. Malignancy of breast or reproductive tract ____

15. Life-threatening side-effects of oral contraceptives include
    A. Edema, headaches, weight gain
    B. Vaginal spotting and amenorrhea
    C. Thrombosis or embolus
    D. Liver adenomas ____

16. The risk of cardiovascular complications, particularly fatal heart attacks and strokes, is substantially increased in women using oral contraceptives who
    A. Use alcohol moderately (2 drinks per day)
    B. Are over age 30 to 35
    C. Smoke heavily (15 or more cigarettes daily)
    D. Do not exercise regularly
    E. Are hypertensive
    Select the number corresponding to the correct letters.
    1. A, B, and C
    2. B, C, and D
    3. B, C, and E
    4. B, C, D, and E
    5. All of the above ____

17. Major contraindications to IUD insertion include all but which of the following?
    A. Small uterus (sounds less than 6 cm)
    B. Acute or chronic pelvic infection
    C. Pregnancy
    D. Uterine myomas ____

18. The most common life-threatening complication of IUDs is
    A. Increased bleeding
    B. Pelvic infection
    C. Uterine perforation
    D. Thrombosis ____

19. The contraceptive of choice for short-term use during the first six weeks postpartum or for 2 to 4 weeks after IUD insertion or beginning oral contraceptives is
    A. Abstinence
    B. Withdrawal
    C. Jellies, creams, or foams
    D. Fertility awareness methods ____

20. The rationale underlying natural methods of birth control based on fertility awareness includes which of the following?
    A. With regular menses, ovulation occurs at approximately the same time in each cycle.
    B. The ovum remains fertile for about 48 hours and sperm are viable for about 3 to 5 days.
    C. Abstinence can occur during a calculated fertile period to prevent pregnancy.

    D. Intercourse is safe during the pre- and postfertile phases.
    E. Intercourse is safe only during the postfertile phase.
    Select the number corresponding to the correct letters.
    1. A, B, C, and D
    2. A, B, C, and E ____

Discussion

21. What preparation is necessary for the maternity nurse to provide basic sexual counseling to pregnant families?

22. What areas should be covered in taking a sexual history? What areas should be covered in taking a sexual history during pregnancy?

23. What are the common dysfunctional sexual problems during pregnancy?

24. What general principles would you discuss with parents who are concerned about how to respond to their children's questions about sex?

25. Discuss four reasons why a woman might want to terminate her pregnancy.

26. What have been three findings of studies on the psychological sequela of abortions?

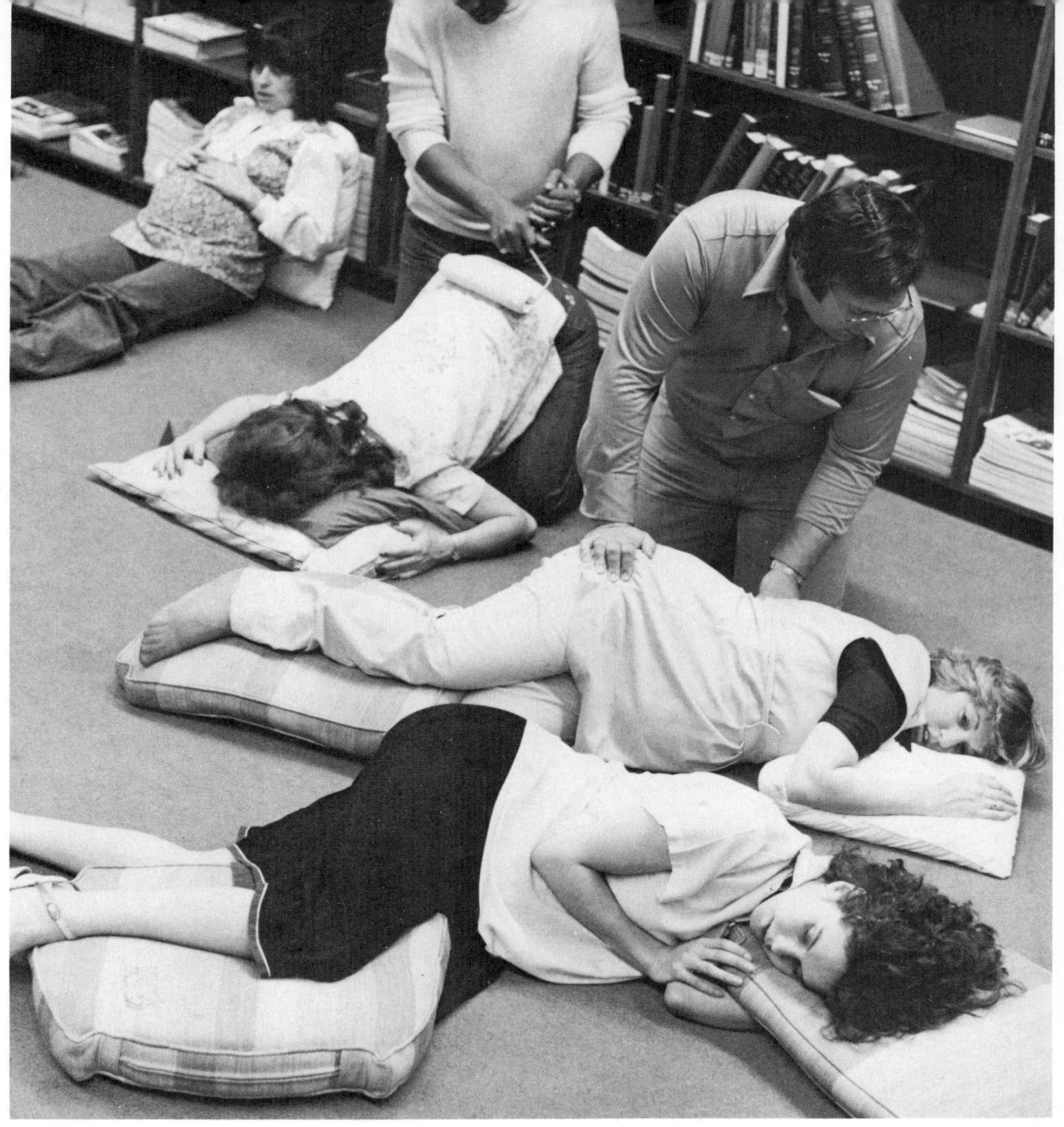

UNIT IV

Assessment and Management in the Antepartum Period

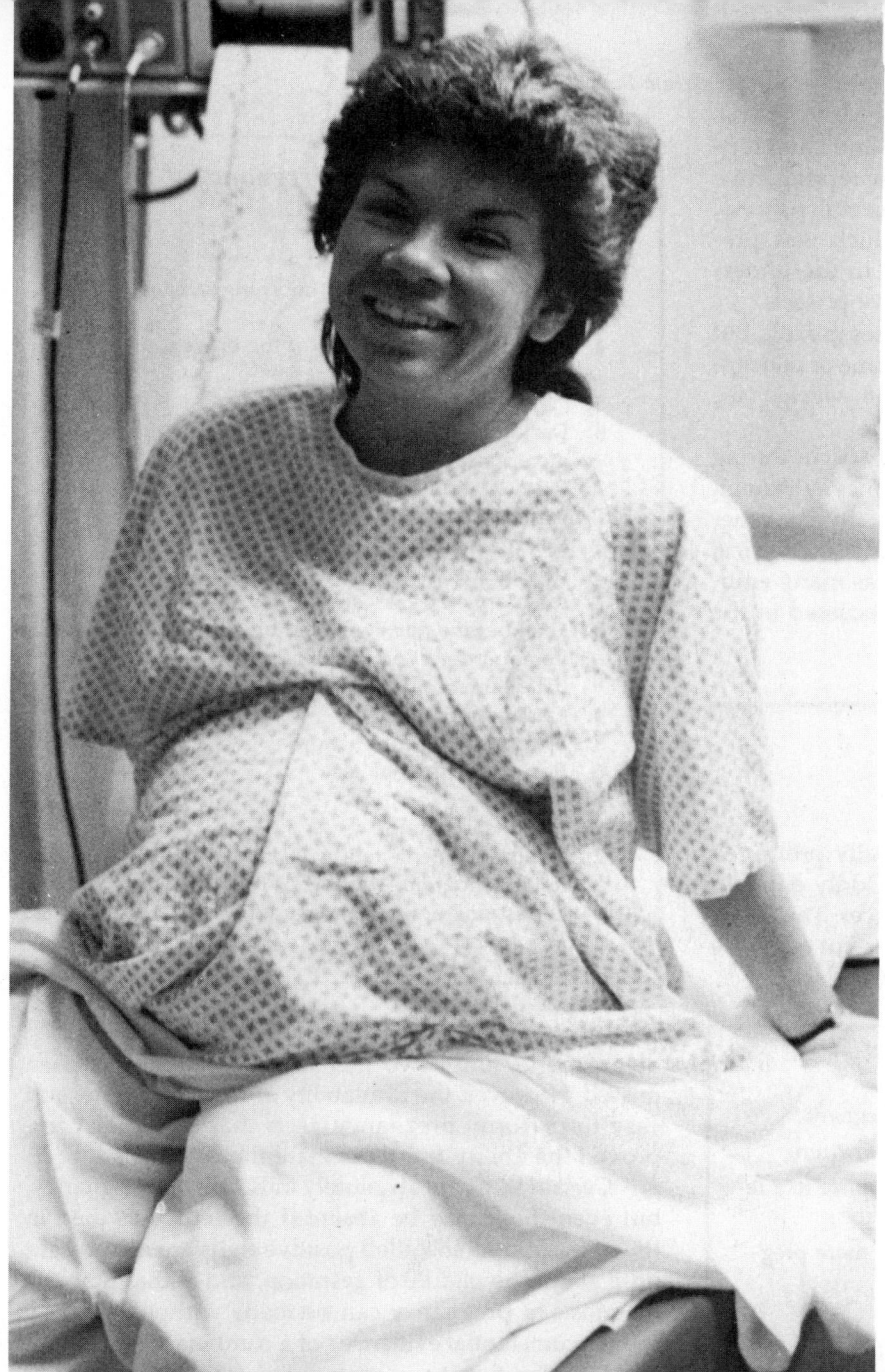

CHAPTER 18

Biophysical Aspects of Normal Pregnancy

From a biologic point of view, pregnancy and labor represent the primary function of the female reproductive system and should be considered a normal process. Knowledge of human reproduction, which was presented in the previous unit, is essential to the understanding of this phase of the reproductive process.

The length of human pregnancy varies greatly, but the average duration, counted from the time of conception, is approximately 267 days or 38 weeks (see Chap. 11).

Many changes in maternal physiology occur during pregnancy. These adaptations to pregnancy, although most apparent in the reproductive organs, involve other body systems as well. In addition to these physical changes, the expectant mother usually has many emotional adjustments to make; these are discussed in the next chapter.

Signs and Symptoms of Pregnancy

The expectant mother's first visit is usually prompted by the query, "Am I really pregnant?" Oddly enough, this is one question that is difficult to answer. The initial pelvic examination will rarely reveal clear-cut evidence

---

Signs and Symptoms in Pregnancy

A. Presumptive signs
 1. Menstrual suppression
 2. Nausea, vomiting, and "morning sickness"
 3. Frequency of micturition
 4. Tenderness and fullness of the breasts, breast pigmentation, and discharge
 5. "Quickening"
 6. Dark blue discoloration of the vaginal mucous membrane (Chadwick's sign)
 7. Pigmentation of the skin and abdominal striae
B. Probable signs
 1. Enlargement of the abdomen
 2. Changes in the size, shape, and consistency of the uterus (Hegar's sign)
 3. Fetal outline, distinguished by abdominal palpation and detection of a fetal part vaginally by ballottement
 4. Changes in the cervix
 5. Braxton Hicks contractions
 6. Positive pregnancy test
C. Positive signs
 1. Fetal heart sounds
 2. Fetal movements felt by examiner
 3. Roentgenogram—outline of fetal skeleton
 4. Ultrasonographic demonstration of the presence of a conceptus

---

Important Definitions

Gravida. A woman who is or has been pregnant

Primigravida. A woman pregnant for the first time

Primipara. A woman who has given birth once to a fetus that has reached the stage of viability

Multipara. A woman who has had two or more pregnancies to the stage of viability

Para I. A primipara

Para II. A woman who has had two children of viable age (and so on up numerically: para III, para IV, and so forth)

The term *gravida* refers to a pregnant woman, regardless of the duration of pregnancy. In reference it includes the present pregnancy. The term *para* refers to past pregnancies that have produced an infant of viable age, whether or not the infant is dead or alive at birth. The terms *gravida* and *para* refer to pregnancies, not to fetuses.

In many centers it is customary to describe the past obstetric history with a series of digits connected by dashes. The first digit refers to the number of term infants delivered, the second to the number of premature infants delivered, the third to the number of abortions, and the fourth to the number of children currently alive.

---

of pregnancy until two menstrual periods have been missed. However, the availability of rapid, accurate, and easy-to-perform pregnancy tests has markedly improved the ability to substantiate the diagnosis.

Certain signs are absolutely indicative of pregnancy, but even these may be absent if the fetus has died in the uterus. Some so-called positive signs are not present until about the middle of gestation, and at that time the diagnosis of pregnancy can be made without them by the "circumstantial evidence" of a combination of earlier and less significant symptoms. The signs of pregnancy are usually divided into three groups: presumptive, probable, and positive.

Presumptive Signs

Menstrual Suppression

In a healthy woman who has previously menstruated regularly, cessation of menstruation strongly suggests pregnancy. However, not until the date of the expected period has been passed by 10 days or more can any reliance be put on this symptom. When the second period is also missed, the probability naturally becomes stronger.

Although cessation of menstruation is the earliest and one of the most important symptoms of pregnancy, it should be noted that pregnancy may occur without prior menstruation and that occasionally menstrual periods may continue after conception. An example of the former circumstance is noted in certain cultures in which girls marry at a very early age; here pregnancy may occur before the menstrual periods are established. Nursing mothers, who usually do not menstruate during the period of lactation, may conceive at this time from the first postpartal ovulation. More rarely, women who think they have passed the menopause are startled to find themselves pregnant.

Conversely, it is not uncommon for a woman to have one or two periods after conception, but almost without exception these are brief and scant. In such cases the first period ordinarily lasts 2 days instead of the usual 5, and the next lasts only a few hours.

Although some women claim that they menstruated every month throughout pregnancy, these claims are of questionable authenticity and can probably be ascribed to some abnormality of the reproductive organs. Indeed, vaginal bleeding at any time during pregnancy should be regarded as abnormal and reported at once.

Absence of menstruation may result from a number of conditions other than pregnancy. Any condition that affects the function of the CNS–hypothalamic-pituitary-ovarian-endocrine axis may cause amenorrhea. Probably one of the most common causes of delay in the onset of the period is psychic influence. In addition, certain chronic systemic diseases, such as tuberculosis, advanced thyroid disease, chronic malnutrition, and the like, may be associated with amenorrhea. Amenorrhea may also occur as a result of sustained strenuous exertion and is often seen among marathon runners.

Nausea and Vomiting

Approximately half of pregnant women suffer no nausea whatsoever during the early part of pregnancy; the other half do experience waves of nausea. Of these, perhaps one third experience some vomiting. *Morning sickness* usually occurs in the early part of the day and subsides in a few hours, although it may persist longer or may occur at other times. When morning sickness occurs, it usually begins about 2 weeks after the first missed menstrual period and subsides spontaneously 6 or 8 weeks later.

Since this symptom is present in many other conditions, such as ordinary indigestion, it is of no diagnostic value unless it is associated with other evidence of pregnancy. When the vomiting is excessive, lasts beyond the fourth month, begins in the later months, or affects the general health, it must be regarded as pathologic. Such conditions are termed *hyperemesis gravida-*

rum, or pernicious vomiting, and are discussed with complications of pregnancy in Chapter 36.

Frequent Micturition

Irritability of the bladder with resultant frequency of urination may be one of the earliest symptoms of pregnancy. It is attributed to the fact that the growing uterus stretches the base of the bladder, so that a sensation results identical with that felt when the bladder wall is stretched with urine. As pregnancy progresses, the uterus rises out of the pelvis and the frequent desire to urinate subsides. Later on, however, the symptom is likely to return, because during the last weeks of pregnancy the head of the fetus may press against the bladder and give rise to a similar condition.

Although frequency of urination may be somewhat bothersome, it should never be a reason for reducing the quantity of fluid consumed.

Breast Changes

Slight temporary enlargement of the breasts, causing sensations of weight and fullness, is noted by most women prior to their menstrual periods. The earliest breast changes of pregnancy are merely exaggerations of these changes. After the second month, the breasts begin to become larger, firmer, and more tender (Fig. 18-1). A sensation of stretching fullness, accompanied by tingling in the breasts and in the nipples, often develops, and in many instances a feeling of throbbing is experienced also. As time goes on, the nipple and the elevated, pigmented area immediately around it, the *areola,* become darker. The areola tends to become puffy, and its diameter, which in the nulligravida rarely exceeds 3 cm (1½ inches), gradually widens to reach 5 or 6 cm (2–3 inches). Tiny sebaceous glands, which take on new growth with the advent of pregnancy and appear as little protuberances or follicles, are embedded in the areola.

In a few cases, patches of brownish discoloration appear on the normal skin immediately surrounding the areola. This discoloration is known as the secondary areola and is a sign of pregnancy, provided the woman has never nursed an infant previously.

With the increasing growth and activity of the breasts, it is not surprising that a richer blood supply is needed; consequently, the blood vessels supplying the area enlarge. As a result, the veins beneath the skin of the breasts, which previously may have been scarcely visible, now become more prominent and occasionally exhibit intertwining patterns over the whole chest wall.

The alterations in the breasts during pregnancy are directed ultimately to the preparation for breast-feeding

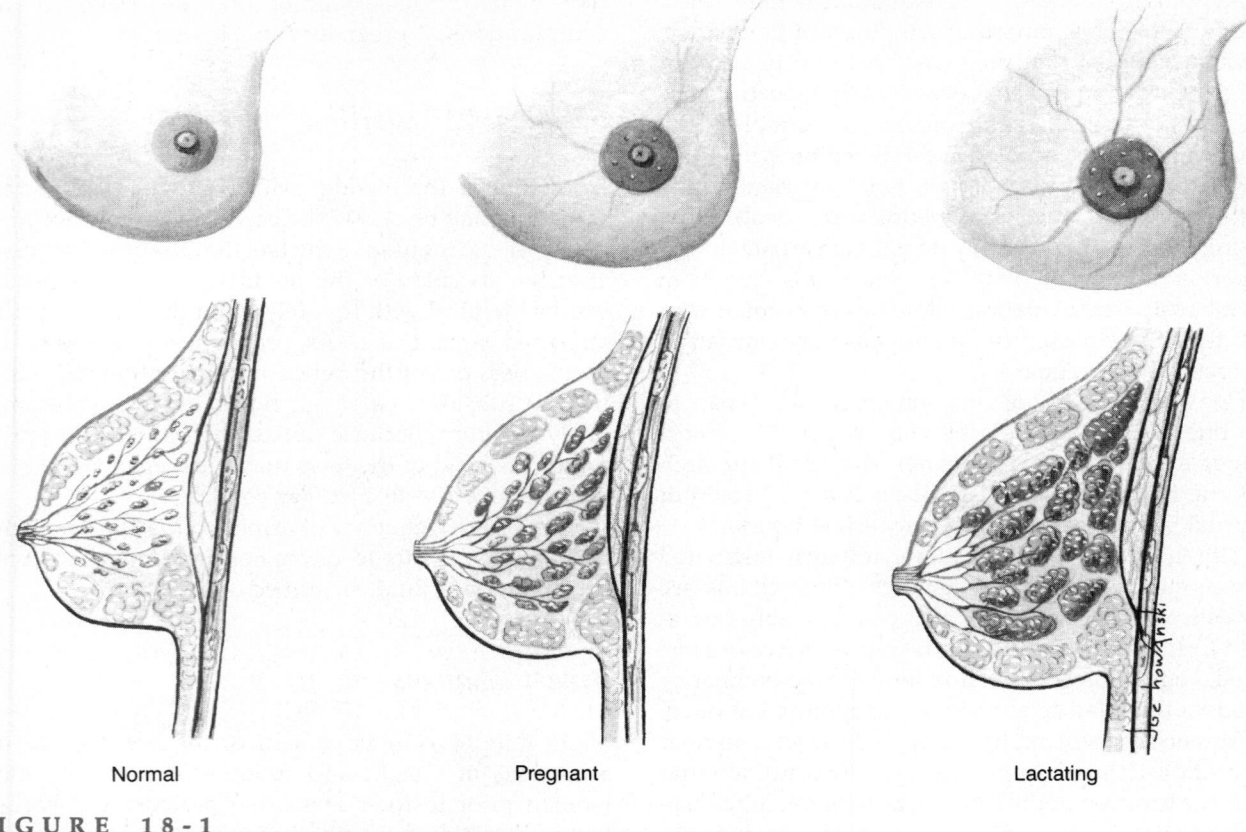

Normal   Pregnant   Lactating

FIGURE 18-1

Breast changes during pregnancy. (Whitley N: A Manual of Clinical Obstetrics.
Philadelphia, JB Lippincott, 1985)

the baby. After the first few months, a thin, viscous, yellowish fluid may be expressed by gentle massage or may appear spontaneously from the nipples. This is a watery precursor of breast milk, *colostrum.*

In primigravidae breast changes are helpful adjuncts in the diagnosis of pregnancy, but in women who have already borne children, particularly if they have nursed an infant within the past year, these changes are much less significant.

"Quickening"

Quickening is an old term derived from an idea prevalent many years ago that at some particular moment of pregnancy, life is suddenly infused into the infant. At the time this notion was in vogue, the first tangible evidence of intrauterine life lay in the mother's feeling the baby move, and the conclusion was only natural that the infant "became alive" at the moment these movements were first felt. The term is still used in obstetric terminology, whereas the common synonym among the laity is "feeling life." As used today, quick-

ening refers only to the active movements of the fetus as first perceived by the mother.

Quickening is usually felt as a tremulous fluttering low in the abdomen toward the end of the fifth month. The first impulses caused by the stirring of the fetus may be quite faint; later on, however, they grow stronger and become clearly perceptible.

Many fetuses, although alive and healthy, seem to move about very little in the uterus, and, not infrequently, a day or so may pass without a movement being felt. Inability to feel the baby move for brief periods of time does not mean that it is dead or in any way a weakling, but, in all probability, that it has assumed a position in which its movements are not felt so readily by the mother. If 3 or 4 days pass without movements, the nurse or physician should listen for the fetal heart sounds. If fetal heart sounds are heard, it means that beyond doubt the fetus is alive and presumably in good condition.

It might seem that the sensations produced by the baby's movements would be so characteristic as to make this a positive sign of pregnancy, but, oddly enough, women occasionally misinterpret movements of gas in the intestines as motions of a baby and, on this basis, imagine themselves to be pregnant. Therefore, the woman's statement that she feels the baby move cannot be regarded as absolute proof of pregnancy.

Vaginal Changes

On inspection of the vagina, one is able to observe discoloration of the vaginal mucous membrane owing to the influence of pregnancy. The mucosa about the vaginal opening and the lower portion of the anterior wall frequently becomes thickened and of a dark bluish or purplish congested appearance because vascularity is greatly increased. This increase in the blood supply of the genital canal gives a dark violet hue to the tissues (Chadwick's sign), in contrast with the ordinary pink color of the parts, and is often described as a valuable sign of pregnancy. As a result of the succulence of the parts, the vaginal secretions may be considerably increased toward the end of gestation. The increased vascularity extends to the various structures in the vicinity (*i.e.*, tissues in the perineal region, skin, and muscle) and effects changes in preparation for labor.

Chadwick's sign is of no special value in women who have borne children, and, since it may be due to any condition leading to the congestion of the pelvic organs, it can be considered only a presumptive sign of pregnancy.

Skin Changes

Striae Gravidarum. The abdomen naturally enlarges to accommodate the increase in size of the uterus. The distention of the abdominal wall causes (in the later months of pregnancy) certain pink or slightly reddish streaks, or *striations,* to form in the skin covering the sides of the abdomen and the anterior and the outer aspects of the thighs. These streaks, or *striae gravidarum,* are caused by the stretching, rupture, and atrophy of the deep connective tissue of the skin. They grow lighter after labor has taken place and finally take on the silvery whiteness of scar or cicatricial tissue. In subsequent pregnancies new pink or reddish lines may be found mingled with old silvery-white striae. The number, size, and distribution of striae gravidarum vary, and some clients have no such markings whatever, even after repeated pregnancies.

Striae are not peculiar to pregnancy but may be found in other conditions that cause great abdominal distention, such as the accumulation of fat in the abdominal wall or the development of large tumors of rapid growth.

Striae gravidarum often develop in the breasts, the buttocks, and the thighs, presumably as the result of deposition of fat in those areas with consequent stretching of the skin.

Pigment Changes. Certain pigmentary changes are also common, particularly the development of a black line running from the umbilicus to the mons veneris, the so-called *linea nigra.*

The external genitalia and pigmented nevi also darken. In certain cases, irregular spots or blotches of a muddy brown color appear on the face. This condition is *chloasma,* or the "mask of pregnancy." Oral contraceptives may also cause chloasma in some women. These facial deposits of pigment often cause the woman considerable mental distress, but her mind may be relieved by the assurance that they will often disappear after delivery. However, the increased pigmentation of the breasts and the abdomen never disappears entirely, although it usually becomes much less pronounced.

All these pigmentary deposits vary exceedingly in size, shape, and distribution and usually are more marked in brunettes than in blonds.

Vascular Markings. Vascular spiders are minute, fiery-red blemishes on the skin with branching legs coming out from a central body. They develop more often in white women; however, they are of no clinical significance and will disappear.

Variations in Skin Changes. The changes in the skin that may accompany pregnancy (*i.e.*, striae gravidarum, linea nigra, chloasma, and pigmentation of the breasts) vary exceedingly in different women; often they are entirely absent. The pigmentation changes are frequently absent in blonds and exceptionally well marked in pronounced brunettes. As already mentioned, this pigmentation may remain from former pregnancies and cannot be depended on as a diagnostic sign in women who have borne children previously.

Sweat Glands. In addition to the aforementioned skin changes, there is a great increase in the activity of the sebaceous glands, the sweat glands, and the hair follicles. The augmented activity of the sweat glands produces an increase in perspiration, an alteration that is helpful in the elimination of waste material.

Probable Signs

Abdominal Changes

The size of the abdomen during pregnancy corresponds to the gradual increase in the size of the uterus, which at the end of the third month is at the level of the symphysis pubis. At the end of the fifth month it is at the level of the umbilicus, and toward the end of the ninth month it is at the ensiform cartilage. Mere abdominal enlargement may be due to a number of causes, such as accumulation of fat in the abdominal wall, edema, or uterine or ovarian tumors. However, if the uterus can be distinctly felt to have enlarged progressively in the proportions stated above, pregnancy may properly be suspected.

Changes in the Uterus

Changes in shape, size, and consistency of the uterus that take place during the first 3 months of pregnancy are very important indications. These are noted in the bimanual examination, which shows the uterus to be more anteflexed than normal, enlarged, and of a soft, spongy consistency. About the sixth week, the so-called Hegar's sign is perceptible (Fig. 18-2). At this time, the lower uterine segment, or lower part of the body of the uterus, becomes much softer than the cervix. It is so soft that in its empty state (for it has not yet become encroached upon by the growing embryo) it can be compressed almost to the thinness of paper. This is one of the most valuable signs in early pregnancy.

The uterus increases in size to make room for the growing fetus. It increases from approximately 6.5 cm long, 4 cm wide, and 2.5 cm deep to about 32 cm long,

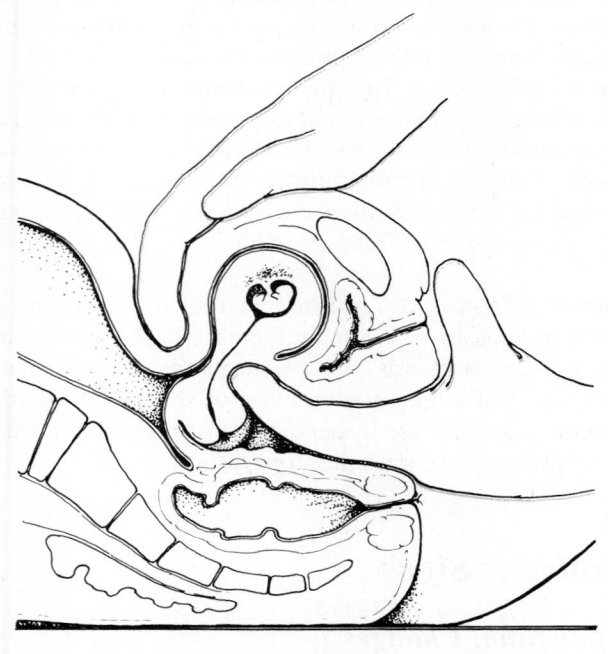

F I G U R E   1 8 - 2

Hegar's sign.

24 cm wide, and 22 cm deep. The uterine wall thickens during the first few months of pregnancy from about 1 cm to almost 2 cm, but thereafter it thins to about 0.5 cm or less. By the end of pregnancy, the uterus becomes a soft-walled muscular sac that yields to the movements of the fetal extremities and permits the examiner to palpate the fetus easily. Its weight increases from 50 g to 1000 g. The small, almost solid organ that has a capacity of about 2 ml increases to become a thin-walled muscular sac capable of containing the fetus, the placenta, and over 1000 ml of amniotic fluid.

The tremendous growth is due partly to the formation of new muscle fibers during the early months of pregnancy but principally to the enlargement of preexistent muscle fibers that are seven to 11 times longer and two to seven times wider than those observed in the nonpregnant uterus. Simultaneously, fibroelastic tissue develops between the muscle bands and forms a network around the various muscle bundles. This is of great importance in pregnancy and labor because it strengthens the uterine walls. During early pregnancy, the hypertrophy of the uterus is probably due to the stimulating action of estrogen on muscle fibers.

The muscle fibers are arranged in three layers: the external hoodlike layer, which arches over the fundus; the internal layer of circular fibers around the orifices of the fallopian tubes and the internal os; and the figure-eight fibers in the middle layer, which make an interlacing network through which the blood vessels pass. This last group plays an important role in childbearing and will be referred to particularly in the care of the mother during labor and after delivery. When these muscle fibers contract, they constrict the blood vessels.

Fetal Outline

After the sixth month, the outline of the fetus (head, back, knees, elbows, and so on) can usually be identified sufficiently well by abdominal palpation to justify a diagnosis of pregnancy. As pregnancy progresses, the outline of the fetus becomes more and more clearly defined. The ability to outline the fetus makes pregnancy extremely probable. In rare instances, however, tumors of the uterus may so mimic the fetal outline as to make this sign fallible.

Ballottement.   Another valuable sign suggesting the presence of a fetus is ballottement (from the French *balloter*, to toss up like a ball). During the fourth and the fifth months of pregnancy, the fetus is small in relation to the amount of amniotic fluid present; during vaginal examination, a sudden tap on the presenting part makes it rise in the amniotic fluid and then rebound to its original position and, in turn, tap the examining finger. When elicited by an experienced examiner, this response is the most certain of the probable signs.

Cervical Changes

Softening of the cervix usually occurs about the time of the second missed menstrual period. In comparison with the usual firmness of the nonpregnant cervix (which has a consistency approximate to that of the cartilaginous tip of the nose), the pregnant cervix becomes softened, and on digital examination the external os feels like the lips or like the lobe of the ear (Goodell's sign).

Softening of the cervix may be apparent as early as a month after conception. The softening of the cervix in pregnancy is due to increased vascularity, edema, and hyperplasia of the cervical glands.

As shown in Figure 18-3, the glands of the cervical mucosa undergo marked proliferation and distend with mucus. As a result they form a structure resembling a honeycomb and make up about one half of the entire structure of the cervix. This is the so-called mucous plug and is of practical importance for a number of reasons. First, it seals the uterus from contamination by bacteria in the vagina. Second, it is expelled at the onset of labor and along with it a small amount of blood; this gives rise to the discharge of a small amount of blood-stained mucus, or *show*. Frequently, the onset of labor is heralded by the appearance of show.

Braxton Hicks Contractions

Uterine contractions begin during the early weeks of pregnancy and occur at intervals of from 5 to 10 minutes throughout pregnancy. These contractions are painless, and the client may or may not be conscious of them. They may be observed during the later months by placing the hand on the abdomen and during the bimanual examination. By means of these contractions, the uterine muscles contract and relax, thereby enlarging to accommodate the growing fetus. These contractions are called the Braxton Hicks sign, after a famous London obstetrician of the last century who first described them. They often account for false labor.

Pregnancy Tests

Since the dawn of civilization efforts have been made to devise a satisfactory test for pregnancy. In the earliest writings handed down to us the priest–physicians of ancient Egypt tell of a test that was based on the seeming ability of pregnancy urine to stimulate the growth of wheat and barley seeds. The itinerant physicians of classical Greece employed similar tests, and during the Middle Ages the omniscient physician merely gazed at

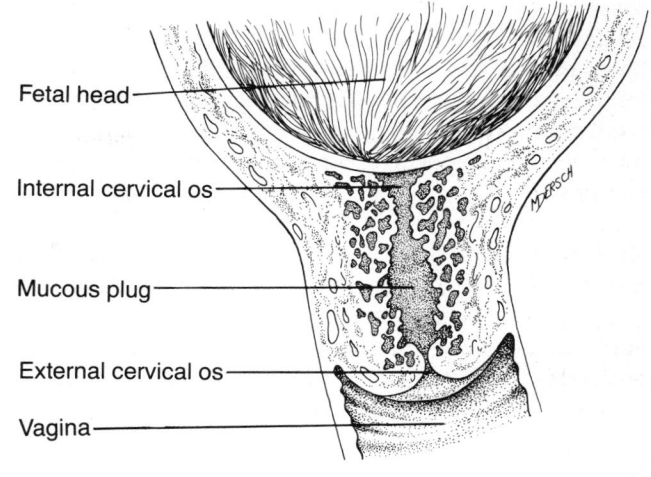

Fetal head

Internal cervical os

Mucous plug

External cervical os

Vagina

FIGURE 18-3

Cervix with mucous plug.

the urine and claimed to be able to diagnose not only pregnancy but also many other conditions.

Today, interestingly enough, as in the tests of old, urine is used in a large number of tests for pregnancy. The tests are based on the fact that the early chorionic villi of the implanted ovum secrete human chorionic gonadotropin (hCG), which appears in the maternal blood and is excreted in the urine. This hormone may be detected in maternal serum or urine by biologic or immunologic methods. Some of the biologic tests that were used extensively in the past include the Aschheim–Zondek test (immature female mouse), the Friedman test (female rabbit), the Hogben test (southern African toad), and the American male frog test.

Immunologic Pregnancy Tests. Numerous systems for immunologic pregnancy testing have been devised. Since hCG is an antigen capable of producing specific antibodies when injected into an animal such as the rabbit, the serum of the animal so injected will contain an antibody specific for hCG. This serum then can be used by reliable immunologic methods to establish the presence or absence of hCG in maternal serum or pregnancy urine.

Kits for immunologic pregnancy testing are available and have been simplified so that with a little practice the test can be carried out within minutes. Immunologic tests have two main advantages over the older biologic ones: they provide an answer within a few minutes rather than many hours, and they eliminate the need for maintaining an animal colony. These tests are more accurate than the older biologic methods.

The great value of the endocrine tests is that they become positive very early in pregnancy. The standard office pregnancy tests are usually positive approximately 10 days after the first missed menstrual period, sometimes even a few days earlier than this. If any of the tests have been carried out properly, the results are accurate in more than 95% of cases. They are not, therefore, absolutely positive signs of pregnancy, but very nearly so.

Radioimmunoassay Test.

Recently, very accurate tests to detect hCG in maternal serum by radioimmunoassay have been developed. These methods are capable of detecting pregnancy from about the eighth postfertilization day on, and thus pregnancy can be diagnosed even before the skipped menstrual period. Human chorionic gonadotropin is made up of an alpha and a beta subunit. The alpha subunit is common to the pituitary gonadotropic hormones. The beta subunit has molecular characteristics that are specific for hCG. Antibodies specific for this subunit have been produced. These antibodies are used in a radioimmunoassay for hCG. This assay system has the advantage of being specific for hCG, and it is capable of detecting minute amounts of hCG in blood. It is a much more elaborate assay than those used in the office to detect urinary hCG, and it must be carried out in the laboratory with radioisotope techniques (radioimmunoassay).

The radioreceptor assay is another radioimmunoassay test for hCG, which is based on a slightly different principle. In this system, antibodies against the combination of hCG and the intracellular receptor for hCG (the constituent in the cell to which hCG attaches when it exerts its effects) are used. This method is also highly sensitive, but is not quite as specific as the beta subunit assay. As there is some cross-reaction with pituitary (LH), LH levels are also detected by this method. These tests have found increasing use for the early diagnosis of pregnancy and are especially useful clinically to diagnose abnormalities, such as ectopic pregnancy, as well as to follow the course of early pregnancy when abnormalities of embryonic development are suspected.

Radioimmunoassay for beta subunit hCG is extremely reliable and accurate. Serum levels of hCG can be used to follow the course of a pregnancy. A rising beta hCG titer most assuredly denotes pregnancy.

Positive Signs

Although some of the signs mentioned above, particularly the hormone tests, ballottement, and palpating the fetal outline, are nearly positive evidences of pregnancy, they are not 100% certain; errors in technique occasionally invalidate the hormone tests, and on rare occasions the other signs may be simulated by nonpregnant pathologic states. If the term *positive* is used in the strict sense, there are only four positive means of detecting pregnancy, namely, the presence of fetal heart sounds, fetal movements felt by the examiner, the roentgenogram outline of the fetal skeleton, and delineation of a pregnancy by ultrasonography.

Fetal Heart Sounds

When fetal heart sounds are heard distinctly by an experienced examiner, there is no longer any doubt about the existence of pregnancy. Ordinarily, they become audible at about the middle of pregnancy, or at approximately the 20th week. If the abdominal wall is thin and conditions are favorable, they may become audible as early as the 18th week, but obesity or an excessive quantity of amniotic fluid may render them inaudible until a much later date.

Although the usual rate of the fetal heart is approximately 140 beats per minute, it may vary under normal conditions between 120 beats per minute and 160 beats per minute. The use of the ordinary bell stethoscope, steadied by rubber bands, is entirely satisfactory, but in doubtful cases the head stethoscope is superior because the listener receives bone conduction of sound through the headpiece in addition to that transmitted to the eardrum (Fig. 18-4). Contractions of the fetal heart can also be detected by use of the Doppler principle with ultrasound. Using this approach fetal heartbeats can almost always be detected by the 10th to 12th week.

Office electronic fetal heart monitors that detect fetal heartbeat by ultrasound are now available (see Fig. 18-4). The heartbeat is transmitted to a monitor and amplified so that it can be heard by both the examiner and the client. The use of this instrument provides an exciting experience and can be appreciated by all, including the client's mate who is present at the time.

Learning Technique.

It is advantageous to determine the fetal position by abdominal palpation before attempting to listen to the fetal heart tones, since ordinarily the heart sounds are best heard through the fetus's back (see Chap. 23). One method to use while learning the characteristics of the fetal heart sounds is to place one hand on the maternal pulse and feel its rate at the same time that the fetal heart tones are heard through the stethoscope. Occasionally, the inexperienced attendant, particularly when listening high in the abdomen, may mistake the mother's heart sounds for those of the fetus. Since the two are not synchronous (fetal, 140 beats per minute; maternal, 80 beats per minute), the method suggested above will obviate this mistake; in other words, if the rate that comes to the ear through the stethoscope is the same as that of the maternal pulse, it is probably the mother's heartbeat. On the other hand, if the rates are different, it is undoubtedly the sound of the fetal heart.

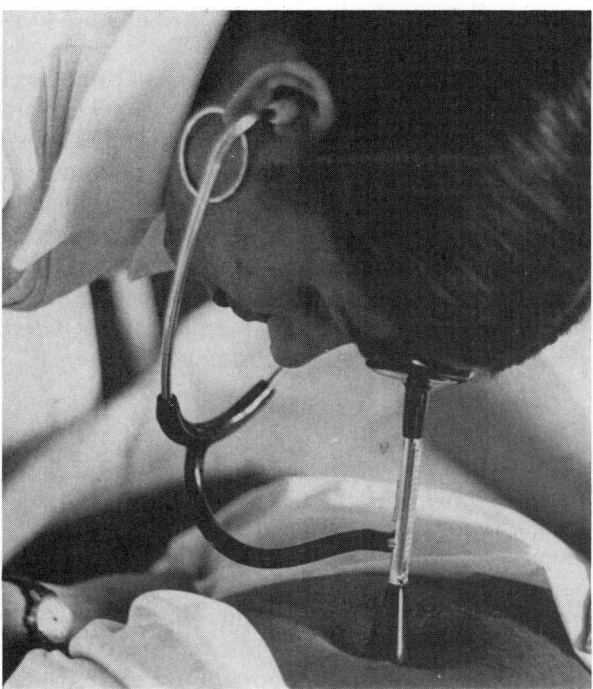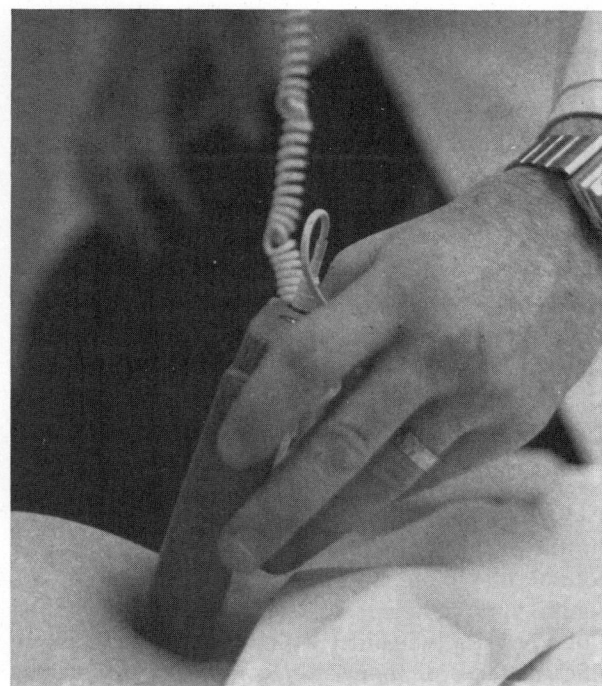

FIGURE 18-4

Auscultation of fetal heartbeat by means of a head stethoscope (*left*) and by ultrasound (*right*).

Funic and Uterine Souffles.   Two additional sounds may be heard in listening over the pregnant uterus: the funic souffle and the uterine souffle. Since the word *souffle* means a blowing murmur, or whizzing sound, the nature of these two sounds is similar, but their timing and causation are quite different.

The word *funis* is Latin for umbilical cord; accordingly, the term *funic souffle* refers to a soft blowing murmur caused by blood rushing through the umbilical cord. Since this blood is propelled by the fetal heart, the rate of funic souffle is synchronous to that of the fetal heart. It is heard only occasionally, perhaps in one case of every six.

The funic souffle is a positive sign of pregnancy, but it is not usually so listed, because it is almost always heard in close association with the fetal heart sounds.

The *uterine souffle* is produced by blood rushing through the large vessels of the uterus. Since this is maternal blood, propelled by the maternal heart, it is synchronous to the rate of her heartbeat. In other words, the rate of the funic souffle is ordinarily approximately 140 beats per minute (or the same as that of the fetal heart rate); the rate of the uterine souffle is near 80 beats per minute (that of the maternal heart rate). The fetal heart may also be detected electronically or with ultrasound techniques described in detail in Chapter 42.

Fetal Movements Felt by Examiner

As already noted, fetal movements supposedly felt by the client may be very misleading in the diagnosis of pregnancy. However, when an experienced examiner feels the characteristic thrust or kick of the fetus against the hand, this is positive evidence of pregnancy. Often this can be felt after the end of the fifth month.

Roentgenogram

A roentgenogram showing the outline of the fetal skeleton is, of course, undeniable proof of pregnancy. How early the fetal skeleton will show in the roentgenogram depends on the thickness of the abdominal wall, the x-ray equipment, and other factors. It has been demonstrated as early as the 14th week and is quite easily demonstrated as a rule after the 20th week. Because of the potential hazards of ionizing radiation and because the fetus can now be outlined sonographically, this approach is rarely used today.

Sonography

The presence of an early embryo can be detected by the use of ultrasound techniques. This test is most useful clinically when the diagnosis of intrauterine pregnancy is in question. A fetal sac within the uterus usually provides an unmistakable pattern on the ultrasonogram. Sonography is of great clinical use when tubal ectopic pregnancy is suspected. The test is increasingly accurate as pregnancy advances, and ultrasonographic outline of a fetus within the fetal sac is a positive sign of pregnancy. This technique is described in greater detail in Chapter 42.

Physiological Changes of Pregnancy

The physiological changes of pregnancy are both local and general alterations that affect the maternal organism as a result of pregnancy but subside at or before the end of the puerperium. Such changes are to be regarded as normal, inevitable, and purely temporary. They are present in varying degrees in every instance, and in the case of a physically healthy woman there should be no significant traces of them after convalescence is complete. It must be remembered, however, that after pregnancy the uterus does not return to its normal nulliparous size, though it does return to a normal nonpregnant state. The adult parous uterus is slightly larger than that of a woman who has never borne a child.

Bodily Changes Associated with Uterine Growth

Between the third month and the fourth month of pregnancy, the growing uterus rises out of the pelvis and can be palpated above the symphysis pubis. It rises progressively to reach the umbilicus at approximately the sixth month and almost impinges on the xiphoid process at the ninth month (Fig. 18-5).

In the majority of pregnancies the uterus is rotated to the right as it rises out of the pelvis. This dextrorotation is probably caused by the presence of the rectosigmoid on the left.

As the uterus becomes larger, it comes in contact with the anterior abdominal wall and displaces the intestines to the sides of the abdomen.

Coincident with the uterine and abdominal enlargement, the umbilicus is pushed outward until about the seventh month, when its depression is completely obliterated and it forms merely a darkened area in the smooth and tense abdominal wall. Later, it is raised above the surrounding integument and may project, becoming about the size of a hickory nut.

When the abdominal wall is unable to withstand the tension created by the enlarging uterus, the recti muscles become separated in the median line, so-called *diastasis recti.*

About 2 weeks before term, in most primigravidae, the fetal head descends into the pelvic cavity. As a result, the uterus sinks to a lower level and at the same time falls forward. Since this relieves the upward pressure on the diaphragm and makes breathing easier, this phenomenon of the descent of the head has been called *lightening.* These changes usually do not occur in multiparas until the onset of labor. By palpating the height of the fundus, experienced examiners can determine the approximate length of gestation.

Effects on Posture

Since the full-term pregnant uterus and its contents weigh about 6000 g (12 lb), a gravid woman may be likened to a person carrying a heavy basket pressed against the abdomen. Such a person will instinctively lean backward to maintain equilibrium. This backward tilt of the torso is characteristic of pregnancy. From a practical viewpoint it is important to note that this posture imposes increased strain on the muscles and the ligaments of the back and the thighs and in this way is responsible for many of the skeletomuscular aches and cramps so often experienced in late pregnancy.

An additional contributing factor is a relaxation of the ligaments that support the joints of the spinal column and pelvis. This feature is increasingly prominent as pregnancy progresses. Relaxation of the sacroiliac joints and the pubic symphysis creates a certain amount of pelvic instability, producing additional strain on the back muscles and thighs. These changes account for the waddling gait observed in late pregnancy and in the early postpartal period.

Changes in the Body Systems

Metabolic Changes

The presence of a rapidly growing fetus and placenta and the demands of these structures bring about a number of significant metabolic changes. Although there is a notable alteration in weight, only a small portion of this increase occurs as a result of metabolic alteration; most weight gain is associated with the presence of the growing fetus, placenta, fetal membranes, and amniotic fluid.

Pregnancy has a decided influence on carbohydrate metabolism. In general, levels of fasting blood sugar are lower, and it has been suggested, but not proved, that secretion of insulin by the pancreas is increased. The stress of pregnancy may actually bring to light subclin-

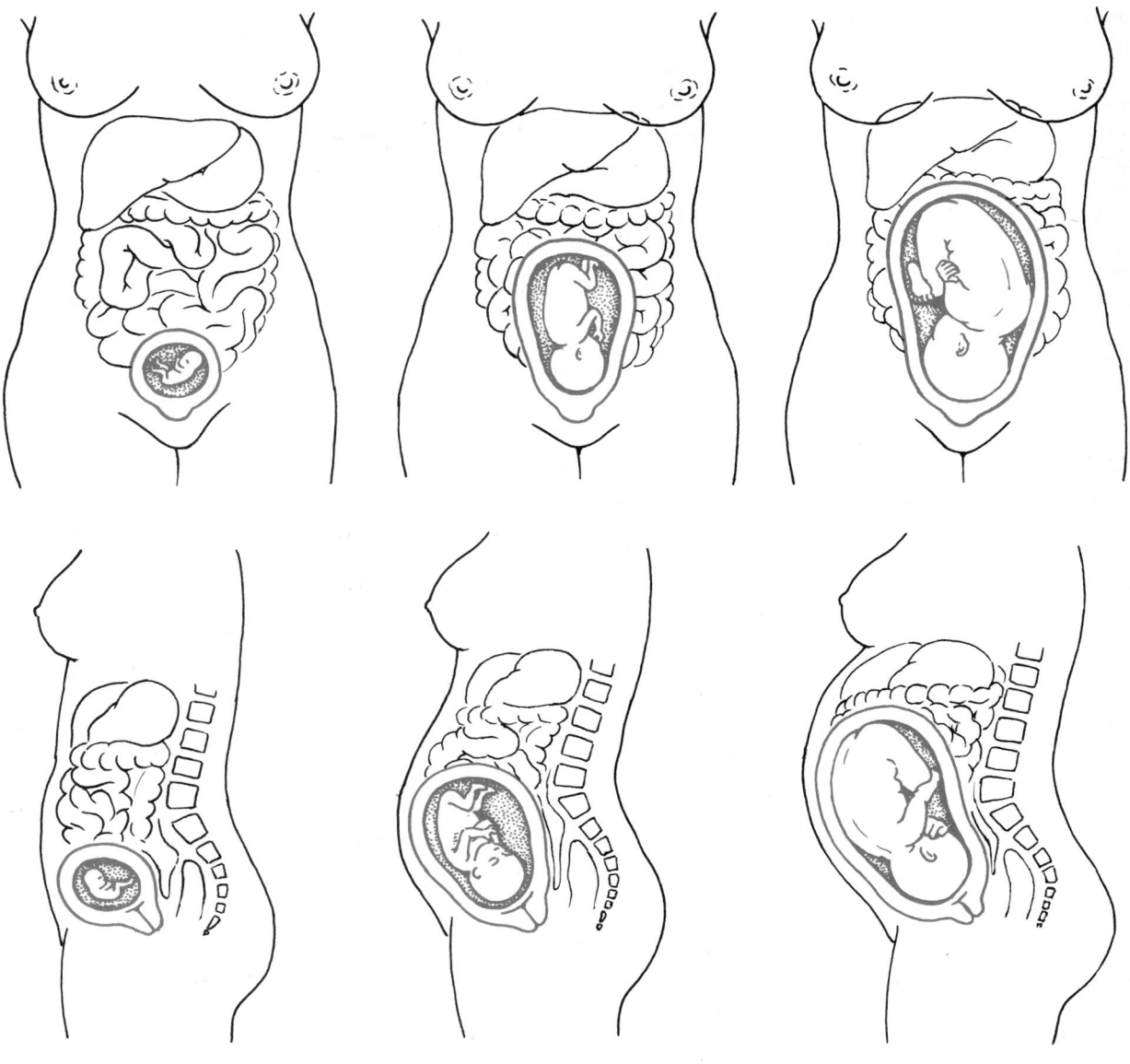

FIGURE 18-5

Front (*top*) and lateral (*bottom*) views of the relative size of the growing uterus, showing the fetus at 4, 6, and 9 months of gestation. The fundus reaches a height between the symphysis pubis and the umbilicus by the fourth month, is about the level of the umbilicus at the sixth month, and almost impinges on the xiphoid process at about the ninth month of gestation.

ical diabetes, which may be detected for the first time during the course of prenatal care (see Chap. 37).

The uterus, maternal blood, and products of conception contain more protein than fat or carbohydrate. There are significant alterations in several plasma proteins. During pregnancy, albumin concentration decreases and fibrinogen levels increase while immunoglobulin levels fall somewhat. In the latter half of pregnancy there is an appreciable increase in plasma lipid,

including total lipids, cholesterol, phospholipids, free fatty acids, and lipoproteins.

Circulatory Changes

Blood. The total volume of blood in the body increases approximately 30% during pregnancy. The minimal hematologic values for both nonpregnant women and pregnant women is 12 g of hemoglobin,

3.75 million erythrocytes, and 35% hematocrit. If there are adequate iron reserves in the body, or if sufficient iron is supplied from the diet, the hemoglobin, the erythrocyte count, and the hematocrit values remain within normal limits during pregnancy.

During pregnancy, there is an increased production of red blood cells by the bone marrow. At the same time, the maternal blood volume, the total amount of fluid circulating in the vessels, increases. Thus, the actual concentration of red blood cells is more or less the same as under normal conditions.

Iron Needs.   The marked increase in production of red blood cells places an inordinate demand on bodily iron stores. Iron stores in the female are often marginal anyway because of the normal loss at menstruation. Iron deficiency anemia is often present prior to pregnancy, especially when there has been inadequate dietary intake of iron, frequently the case among clients in poor socioeconomic circumstances. Iron deficiency is markedly aggravated by pregnancy because of the heavy demand for iron by the growing fetus, especially late in gestation. The increased demand for iron as a result of the changes associated with pregnancy should be kept in mind during the course of prenatal care, and the use of supplementary iron should be seriously considered.

Heart.   An important aspect of this increase in blood volume relates to its effect on the heart. During pregnancy, the heart has about 50% more blood to pump through the aorta per minute. This augmented cardiac output attains a peak at the end of the second trimester, then declines to the nonpregnant level during the last weeks of gestation. Immediately following delivery there is a sharp rise again. In women with normal hearts this is of no particular concern. However, in women with heart disease this increase in the work that the heart has to do may add to the seriousness of the complication (see Chap. 37).

Palpitation of the heart is not uncommon. In the early months of pregnancy this is due to sympathetic nervous disturbance; toward the end of gestation it is due to the intra-abdominal pressure of the enlarged uterus.

Blood Pressure.   The arterial blood pressure of the pregnant woman is affected by her posture. Pressure in the brachial artery is highest when she is sitting and lowest when she is in the lateral recumbent position. Ordinarily, arterial blood pressure falls during the second or early third trimester of pregnancy and rises slowly thereafter.

In the supine position, femoral venous pressure rises during the course of pregnancy, increasing from about 8 cm of water in early pregnancy to 24 cm at or near term. There is a retarded blood flow in the legs except when the gravida is in the lateral recumbent position. This stagnation in late pregnancy is the result of occlusion of the inferior vena cava and pelvic veins by pressure of the enlarged uterus. When the gravida lies on her side, relieving pressure on these veins, the venous pressure in the lower extremities returns to normal. These alterations are in large measure responsible for the dependent edema of the lower extremities often seen as term approaches, and also for the tendency toward development of hemorrhoids and varicose veins of the legs and vulva. The pressure of the uterus on the vena cava and the venous system that drains the lower half of the body may actually reduce cardiac filling and cardiac output. Occasionally, the net result is arterial hypotension, which results in light-headedness in the supine position.

Respiratory Changes

In the later months of pregnancy the lungs are subjected to pressure from the underlying uterus, and the diaphragm may be displaced upward. As a consequence, shortness of breath at that period is common. It might seem that this upward displacement of the diaphragm would decrease the capacity of the lungs, but a concomitant widening of the thoracic cage occurs that more than compensates for the other change. Actually, the pregnant woman breathes in much more air than the nonpregnant woman. This is necessary because the mother must oxygenate not only her own blood, but, by osmosis, that of the fetus too.

The increased respiratory level occurs largely from the influence of progesterone and estrogen acting directly on the respiratory center of the brain.

Gastrointestinal Changes

The intestines and stomach are displaced upward by the enlarging uterus. These positional changes may alter the physical findings in certain diseases such as appendicitis. The appendix itself is usually displaced somewhat laterally and upward and at times may be located as high as the right flank. The motility in the gastrointestinal tract is decreased during the course of pregnancy. These changes result in a prolonged gastric emptying time and a longer intestinal transit time. A generalized relaxation of the smooth musculature of the gastrointestinal tract occurs under the influence of the progesterone that is produced by the placenta. Gastric emptying time is especially prolonged during the course of active labor. Gastric contents are retained when a general anesthetic is administered for delivery. There is danger of regurgitation of the highly acid stomach contents and lung aspiration, and special precautions must be taken to avoid this complication (see Chap. 27). The altered position of the stomach contributes to the increased frequency of heartburn in pregnancy, most likely caused by reflux of acidic secretions into the lower esophagus. Muscular tone about the stomach and esophagus is altered, resulting in lower intraesophageal pressures and higher intragastric pressures, and slower esophageal peristalsis. All of these changes contribute to gastroesophageal reflux.

There is often a vascular swelling of the gums, referred to as epulis of pregnancy. The gums become hyperemic and softened, with an increased tendency toward bleeding after brushing the teeth. These changes *per se* do not lead to an increased incidence of tooth decay and regress spontaneously after delivery.

Digestion. The function of the digestive organs may be somewhat altered during pregnancy. During the early months the appetite may be diminished, particularly if nausea exists. Since the nutritional requirements to meet the needs of the mother's body and the growing fetus demand quality of the diet rather than an appreciable increase in the quantity of food ingested, this temporary manifestation should not produce injurious effects. As pregnancy advances and the digestive apparatus seems to become accustomed to its new conditions, the appetite is increased and may be voracious. Heartburn and flatulence may occur at this time. Also, the pressure from the diaphragm and the diminished tone may delay the emptying time of the stomach.

Constipation is exceedingly common in pregnancy; at least one half of all gravid women suffer from this disorder. This suggests that the entire gastrointestinal tract is limited by diminished tone and pressure of the growing uterus during gestation.

Liver and Gallbladder. Although no characteristic changes in liver morphology occur during the course of normal pregnancy, there are alterations in some of the laboratory tests for hepatic function. Such changes could erroneously suggest hepatic disease. The total alkaline phosphatase activity in serum doubles, reaching levels that would be abnormal in the nonpregnant state. This is caused not by intrinsic changes in the liver, but rather by the effect of alkaline phosphatase isoenzymes produced by the placenta. Serum cholinesterase activity normally falls during pregnancy, a change seen in certain liver diseases, and lucine aminopeptidase activity as measured in serum is markedly elevated. Palmar erythema and spider nevi, lesions in the skin that are characteristically seen in clients with liver disease, are commonly found in normal pregnant women. These are thought to be caused by the dramatic increase in circulating estrogens; they disappear shortly after delivery. Gallbladder function is also altered, with a tendency toward decreased tone and distention. Gallbladder contents are thickened, and these changes could account for the increased predisposition to gallstones during pregnancy.

Urinary and Renal Changes

The urine in pregnancy usually is increased in amount and has a lower specific gravity. Pregnant women show a tendency to excrete dextrose in the urine. Although a reduction in the renal threshold for sugar is often associated with pregnancy, the presence of any sugar in the urine should always be reported to the physician. Lactosuria may be observed at times, especially during the latter part of pregnancy and the puerperium. Lactosuria is associated with the presence of milk sugar, which is from the mammary glands and is not of any significance.

Some of the commonly used tests for renal function may be altered during gestation. Plasma creatinine and urea concentrations decrease. Urine concentration tests may be altered, and in the normal pregnant woman there may be failure to concentrate urine after withholding fluids. The kidney simply mobilizes extracellular fluid.

The *ureters* become markedly dilated in pregnancy, particularly the right ureter. This change apparently is due in part to the pressure of the gravid uterus on the ureters as they cross the pelvic brim and in part to a certain softening that the ureteral walls undergo as the result of endocrine influences. These dilated ureters, the walls of which have now lost much of their muscular tone, are unable to propel the urine as satisfactorily as previously; consequently, stasis of urine is common. Following delivery, the ureters return to normal within 4 to 6 weeks. The stretching and the dilatation do not continue long enough to impair the ureter permanently unless infection has developed or pregnancies are repeated so rapidly that a subsequent pregnancy begins before the ureters can return to normal.

The dilatation of the collection system may result in retention of urine there, altering some of the commonly used dye excretion tests for kidney function.

The *bladder* functions efficiently during pregnancy. The urinary frequency experienced in the first few months of pregnancy is caused by pressure exerted on the bladder by the enlarging uterus. This is observed again when lightening occurs prior to the onset of labor.

Endocrine Changes

Placenta. In Chapter 12 the placenta was considered as an organ designed to transmit nutritive substances from mother to fetus and waste products in the reverse direction. The role of the placenta as an important organ of internal secretion was also reviewed. As discussed previously, the early chorionic villi of the implanted ovum secrete hCG, which prolongs the life of the corpus luteum. The result is the continued production of estrogen and progesterone, which are so necessary for the maintenance of the endometrium. During pregnancy this hormone appears in maternal blood and is excreted in the mother's urine, which makes the standard urine tests for pregnancy possible.

The chorionic cells of the placenta produce yet another unique protein hormone, human chorionic somatomammotropin (hCS), which is also known as human placental lactogen (hPL). This hormone is detectable in placental cells as early as the third week after ovulation and is found in maternal serum by the sixth week. Its name suggests its actions. It influences somatic cell growth of the fetus and facilitates preparation of the breasts for lactation.

In addition to its function in the formation of hCG and hCS, the placenta takes over the production of estrogen and progesterone from the ovaries and, after the first 2 months of gestation, becomes the major source of these two hormones. The increase in these hormones in the maternal organism is thought to be responsible for many important changes that take place during pregnancy, such as the growth of the uterus and the development of the breasts. In the breasts, the development of the duct system is promoted by estrogen and the development of the lobule-alveolar system, by progesterone.

Pituitary Body.
The pituitary gland enlarges somewhat during pregnancy, but, as such, is not essential for the maintenance of pregnancy.

Anterior Lobe.
The *anterior lobe* of this small gland, located at the base of the brain, has already been referred to as the "master clock," which, under the influence of the hypothalamus, controls the menstrual cycle (see Chap. 9). In addition to gonadotropins, the anterior lobe secretes hormones that act on the thyroid and adrenal glands and yet another hormone that influences the growth process. Production of these hormones continues during the course of pregnancy. Gonadotropins, on the other hand, are no longer released cyclically. The estrogen and progesterone produced by the placenta inhibit their release from the pituitary gland.

Posterior Lobe.
The *posterior lobe* of the pituitary secretes an oxytocic hormone, *oxytocin*, which has a very strong stimulating effect on the uterine muscle. The portion of the pituitary gland that contains oxytocin is widely used in obstetrics to cause the uterus to contract after delivery, thereby diminishing postpartal hemorrhage. It is sometimes used to initiate labor and to stimulate contractions during labor when they are of poor quality. Oxytocin also has an influence on the breasts. It causes *milk let-down*, or ejection of milk from the nipples. This effect is of clinical use in the care of the nursing mother. Oxytocin is marketed under the names Pitocin and Syntocinon, the latter a synthetic product, and is administered either parenterally or, for milk let-down, by a nasal spray.

Other Endocrine Glands.
It is quite clear that the placenta is the major endocrine gland in pregnancy. Other endocrine glands display alterations during normal pregnancy.

Thyroid.
During the course of pregnancy, there is slight to moderate enlargement of the thyroid. It is now known that this hypertrophy of thyroid tissue is not associated with increased thyroid activity, although there is an elevation in the basal metabolic rate that increases throughout the course of pregnancy. This is merely a reflection of the increased oxygen consumption as a result of the metabolic activity of the products of conception.

Other parameters for the measurement of thyroid function also display changes. The serum protein-bound iodine (PBI), butyl extractable iodine (BEI), and thyroxine (T_4) levels increase, and the elevated levels are maintained until shortly after delivery. The increase is due not to increased thyroid activity as such, but rather to an elevation in the level of thyroid-binding protein normally present in the blood. Thus, although there is an increase in the amount of circulating thyroid hormones and, therefore, the total concentration of hormone is elevated, the actual amount of unbound or available hormone remains within normal limits.

The triiodothyronine (T_3) uptake test displays decreased values in pregnancy, which indicates an increase in the binding of circulating triiodothyronine. A similar increase in the level of thyroid-binding proteins is seen in the nonpregnant client following the administration of estrogen, and it is likely that in pregnancy the increase is a reflection of the high level of circulating estrogen.

Adrenals.
The *adrenal cortex* hypertrophies during pregnancy, and it is believed that its activity increases. The actual secretion of cortisol by the adrenals is unchanged, although there are alterations in the metabolism of cortisol as a result of the influence of estrogen. There is clearly an increase in the production by the adrenal glands of aldosterone, the hormone responsible for the retention of sodium by the kidneys. This increase begins early in pregnancy and continues throughout. The net result of the increase is a decreased ability of the kidneys to handle salt during pregnancy. In the absence of proper dietary control of salt intake, there is often fluid retention and either occult or overt edema.

Ovary.
The *ovary*, except for the activity of the corpus luteum of pregnancy, remains relatively quies-

cent. Gonadotropin levels are low, inasmuch as their release is inhibited by the estrogen and progesterone produced by the placenta. Thus, follicular activity in the ovary remains in abeyance, and there is no further ovulation until after delivery.

Suggested Reading

Pritchard JA, MacDonald PC, Gant NF: Williams' Obstetrics, 17th ed. New York, Appleton–Century–Crofts, 1985

Quilligan EJ: Prenatal care. In Romney SL, Gray M, Little AB (eds): Gynecology and Obstetrics: The Health Care of Women, pp 579–594. New York, McGraw–Hill, 1980

Simpson ER, MacDonald PC: Endocrine physiology of the placenta. Ann Rev Physiol 43:163, 1981

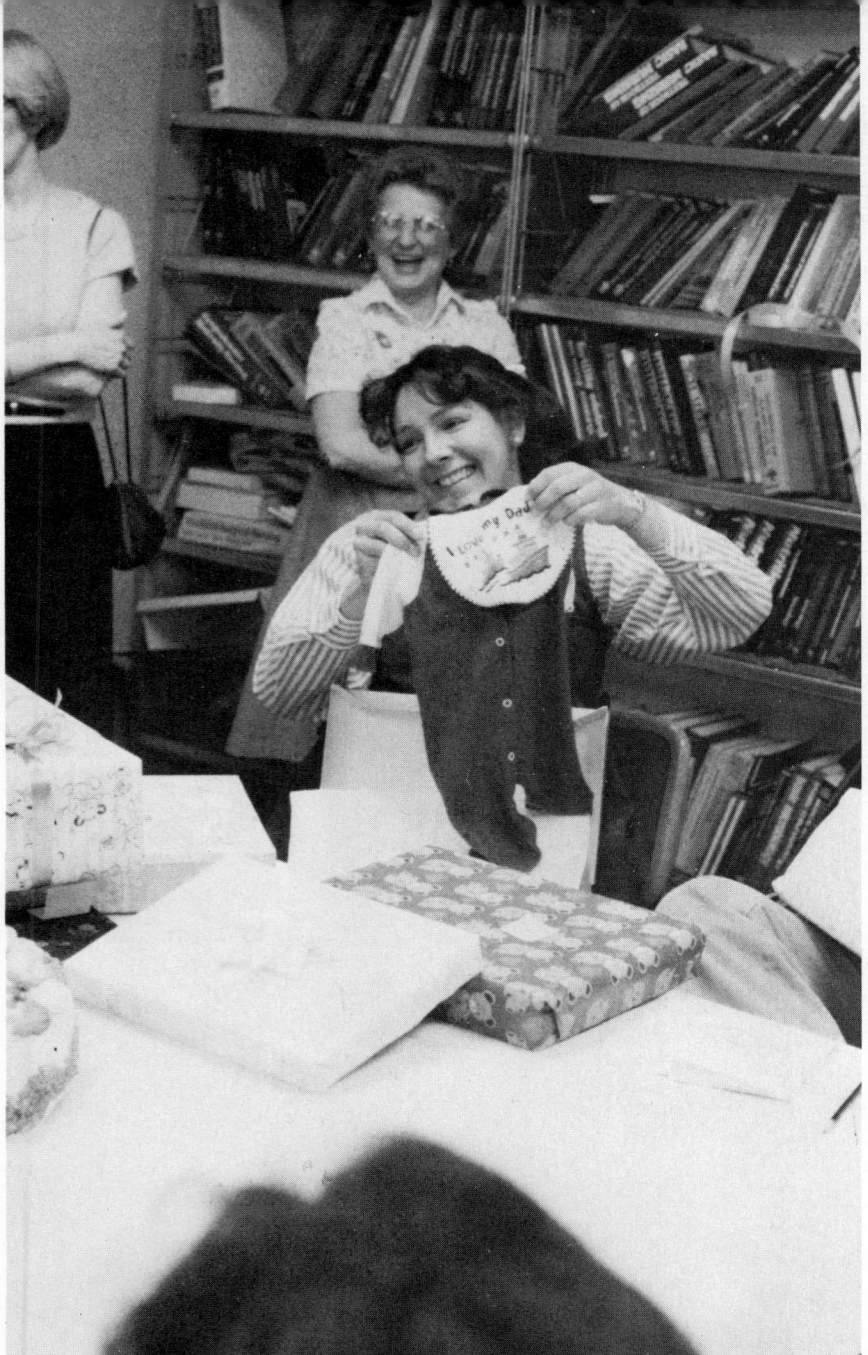

CHAPTER 19

Psychosocial Aspects of Normal Pregnancy

Cultural Influences on Perceptions of Pregnancy

As indicated previously, the family is society's most basic unit, surviving through the centuries as it has because it serves vital human needs. We have seen that there may be very different styles of family living and different ways of relating the family to the larger society. However, whatever the form, the family will no doubt continue to exist as long as humans continue to populate this planet.

In the family, as previously noted, each member assumes roles for which the culture dictates overt and covert behavioral expectations. Each member's perceptions of these roles also vary according to the manner of socialization and the kind of interaction he or she has had with others. As the society evolves and changes, so do the various role expectations. Each successive generation may hold different expectations as they adapt to changing times and needs, although there are always socially imposed limitations.

So it has been with childbearing. Pregnancy and birth are very important events in most cultures. However, attitudes toward these processes vary considerably among different cultures and even within one society. In some cultures, birth is a social event, with open attendance by all friends and family; in other cultures it is conducted in secrecy.[1] Similarly, pregnancy may be seen as a normal uneventful preparatory phase to a desired change in status connoting achievement; conversely, it may be viewed as mysterious, crisis ridden, and the harbinger of possible disaster. Again, it may be looked upon as atonement for simply being a lowly female.[2]

Pregnancy in the American Culture

There have been two competing views of pregnancy in our culture. One conceptualizes pregnancy and childbirth as a "crisis" situation, and the other regards them as more of a role transition experience. Each of these attitudes has quite different assumptions that if carried to their logical conclusions have very different implications for the delivery of health care. Unfortunately, assumptions and terminology have not always been clearly articulated and when the rhetoric has been uncritically accepted and applied to the health-care scene, some peculiar innovations and traditions have been incorporated into the delivery of care. In this chapter we discuss these two orientations to pregnancy so that the implications of these attitudes for actual maternity care can be seen.

Pregnancy as Crisis vs Stress

A couple's first pregnancy, in particular, is a critical period in the evolution of a family. During the past 3 decades, there have been a variety of disciplines interested in this critical event. Psychologists and psychiatrists, notably Bibring, Hass, Larsen, Menninger, Caplan, and Coleman and Coleman, have all written about the critical nature of this event and have at least alluded to the assumed crisis implications.[3-8] Shainess, in fact, refers to this period as a "crucible tempering the self" and recognizes the possibility that the tempering process may go wrong, resulting in damage to the person and to the person's relationships with others.[9] Chertok speaks of pregnancy as a progressively developing crisis with the labor and delivery as the peak of the crisis since parturition results in separation of the mother and child and isolation from significant others.[10]

It is important to note that these writings are based largely on experiential or clinical impressions of individuals who have experienced difficulty. There have been no comparison studies with control groups. Moreover, samples have been small and skewed to the pathological end of a normal–abnormal continuum. There have been problems in analysis also, since small skewed samples do not lend themselves to multivariate analysis, which is more appropriate when dealing with the multiple variables involved in family research.[11,12]

Another tradition of research in the crisis vein has led to the formulation of the "normal" crisis of parenthood, a contradiction in terms to say the least. While the focus of this crisis research was originally on parenthood, the time of pregnancy was often uncritically included, rather by default, and has become intermingled with the general research in this area with little basis in empirical fact. The early work of Le Masters, Dyer, and Hobbs laid the foundation for this unfortunate extrapolation.[13-15]

In many of the conceptual formulations, both psychological and sociological, a crisis appears to be considered a critical event but not necessarily one that is totally psychologically or interpersonally disruptive. However, the authors' true meaning was often subverted because they did not precisely define their terms.

In the original stress research on the family as exemplified by Hill and Hansen and Hill,[16,17] the term *crisis* connoted a sharp change. Specifically, crisis was a sharp, decisive change for which old patterns of behavior were inadequate.[17] Thus, there was an interruption in the family's routine and new patterns of interaction had to be developed. There was also the implication that resolution and reintegration were not only possible (*i.e.*, "normal" crisis) but quite expected and well within the family's capabilities. McCubbin and others, in more recent work, have done much to clarify and refine concepts, definitions, and measurement of family stress, crisis, and role transition.[11,18,19] This topic is addressed more fully in Chapter 30.

In summary, then, there has been some confusion, both semantically and conceptually, over the way the term *crisis* has been applied to the events of pregnancy, childbirth, and parenthood. At times this has led to the uncritical acceptance of pregnancy as always being disruptive and potentially damaging emotionally or psychologically.

Pregnancy as a Role Transition

Rossi suggested that the term *normal crisis* was a misnomer as applied to parenthood because the concepts of "normal" and "crisis" are basically incongruous since one implies natural successful resolution and the other plainly indicates the possibility of nonresolution.[20] She suggested that parenthood be viewed as a role transition and be based on a stage–task conceptual framework such as is found in the work of Erickson, Benedek, and Hill.[17,21,22] This type of orientation puts parenthood and other phases of the reproductive cycle, including pregnancy, into a developmental task formulation and allows these phenomena to be seen as essentially normal or usual, but also respects the fact that deviation, stress, or disruption can occur, depending on a variety of circumstances. It is also the orientation that more recent researchers of parenthood have adopted.[11,18,19] In Chapter 30 we discuss this concept as applied to the postpartum period, when parenthood becomes very tangible. In this chapter we limit the discussion to pregnancy.

If one views the total life span in terms of a developmental task interaction, then we can view individuals' life spans as having cycles composed of stages or phases, each with its unique tasks. As the various cycles occur, social roles develop out of interaction with others in our social network. By analogy, social roles may be said to have cycles and each stage in the cycle has its set of tasks and adjustments. Rossi has outlined four broad stages in the role cycle that have implications for pregnancy as well as parenthood.[20]

1. *Anticipatory stage.* Almost all social roles have some kind of formal or informal training, either through formal schooling, role modeling, or watching others. This stage serves to socialize or train the potential actor for the role he or she is to assume. As its name implies, this stage precedes the assumption of the role and may take place years ahead of the actual role assumption.
2. *Honeymoon stage.* This is the time period immediately following the full assumption of the role. Here intimacy and exploration occur as the person tries to adjust the "fit" of his or her personality to

the role demands. Reality testing takes place rather than the fantasizing that often accompanies the anticipatory phase.
3. *Plateau stage.* This is the protracted middle period of a role cycle during which the role is fully exercised. In this phase, the individuals validate themselves as adequate or inadequate depending on how well they and others see themselves performing in the role.
4. *Disengagement–termination stage.* This period immediately precedes and includes the actual termination of the role. For some roles, this stage is quite tangible. The marital role, for instance, ends abruptly with death or divorce. For other roles, such as parenthood or pregnancy, the distinction is much less clear because there is little cultural prescription about when the authority and obligations end.[20]

The Meaning and Effect of Pregnancy on the Couple

As we discuss the impact of pregnancy on the potential father and mother, we will relate some of the psychosocial aspects to the stages of the role cycle. We can see that pregnancy is a unique experience in which a sexual union between a male and female leads to the creation of a new life. This new life in turn will result in the creation of many new and unprecedented relationships.

One example of the profound influence that pregnancy has on the couple lies in the realm of body image. Body image refers to the way one pictures his or her own body. It is a composite of attitudes, feelings, and perceptions that each individual has regarding how his body appears.[23] Research indicates that it is not only the mother that experiences a change in body image perception as she literally grows during pregnancy, but her mate as well.[24] Fawcett found that both husbands and wives demonstrate statistically similar patterns of change in perceived body space from the eighth month of pregnancy through the 12th postpartal month. The data also show that the couple's ability to identify with one another plays a mediating role in the process. Interestingly, marital adjustment did not.[24]

Other studies have found that husbands have a variety of signs and symptoms that mimic or imitate the pregnancy signs and symptoms that their wives are experiencing.[25,26] The British researchers Trethowen and Conlon, for instance, found that the men in their study experienced symptoms of physical illness during their wives' pregnancies. These include increased and decreased appetite, gastrointestinal disorders, toothache, and backache. It was noted that these men did not ordinarily experience these conditions at other times.[27]

Similarly, studies of American men found that they expressed concerns about body intactness and tended to demonstrate "sympathetic" pregnancy symptoms. These included nausea and vomiting, dizziness, fainting, weight gain, backache, and leg cramps.[25,28] Coleman and Coleman have made the observation that was documented in Fawcett's study that the father's close proximity to the mother influences his response to the pregnancy. They also postulate that the more closely the men identifies with his mate, the more intensely he will experience changes in his own body during pregnancy.[29] Thus, we can see what a momentous physiological, psychological, and emotional milestone pregnancy can be.

Mother

Although the normal female may love her partner greatly and desire a child very much, there still are major developmental changes that she must make to become a mother. In the process of childbearing, she is creating from the union of herself and her mate another individual *inside* herself that must ultimately grow to become a separate person *outside* herself. Hence, the coming child represents the synthesis of three distinct entities: the mother's relationship to her partner, the relationship of the mother to the child as a representative of herself, and the relationship to the unique individual, which is the unborn child itself (Fig. 19-1). As with puberty, when the individual can never again be a child, or with menopause, when the individual can never again reproduce, with pregnancy the individual can never become a completely single unit again. As long as the child lives, it will never cease to exist as a representative of the woman, her mate, and itself.[30]

Psychological Tasks of Pregnancy

Several psychological tasks that the pregnant woman must accomplish have been delineated. First, she must believe she is pregnant and incorporate the fetus into her body image.[31] Rubin has spoken of the two questions that the pregnant woman continues to ask during the course of her pregnancy: "Now?" and "Who, me?" The woman questions if this is the right time to have the infant and acknowledges the ever-present surprise she feels being in the pregnant state.[32] As the mother feels the fetus move and her body change in both subtle and very apparent ways, she begins to realize that the fetus inside her is a real and separate being complete with its own boundaries and identity.[30] With this comes a lessening of the surprise and gradual integration. This is not to say there is no turmoil; there is a great range of behavioral displays: mood swings, introspection, physical and psychological weariness. Hence, we have

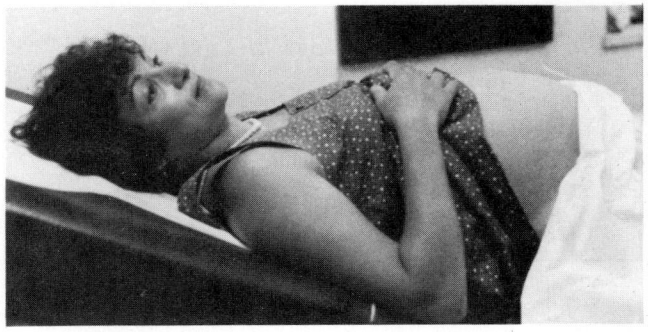

FIGURE 19-1

The mother can never again be a single unit. Her baby represents her relationship to her partner, her relationship to her baby as a representative of herself, and her relationship to the unique individual who will soon become a separate person outside herself. (Courtesy of Booth Maternity Center)

many descriptions of the emotional lability of pregnancy. We must note, however, that there is ample evidence that the physiological and hormonal changes play an additional role in this lability.

The mother's second task is to prepare for the physical separation, the birth of the infant. As with all aspects of pregnancy, there are various responses. Many women are eager to have the baby; they are "tired" of being pregnant. Some even state they are frightened to have this intrusive "invader" within them. However, others do not want to let the fetus go; they anticipate delivery as a loss of a loved object, and this anticipation may actually cause depression. Nevertheless, the task must ultimately be resolved, for every fetus lost is, in a moment, a baby gained.[31]

A third task is to resolve the identity confusions that accompany role transition and thus prepare for the smooth functioning of the family after birth. Coleman and Coleman suggest that as the woman progresses in pregnancy, she becomes one with "mother," the primitive memory of the omnipotent being who nurtured her. Moreover, she becomes increasingly prone to evaluate her partner with respect to his appropriateness as a father. She may criticize his current behavior patterns to bring them more into line with her idea of what constitutes and ideal father.[31] Fishbein found that concordance between the partners about the expectations of the father role was important in reducing the father's anxiety during pregnancy.[33] Similarly, the pregnant father watches his partner become transformed into "mother" as her body changes, her behavior becomes more nesting, and so on. He is simultaneously confronting his own feelings and aspirations as he metamorphoses into father. Pregnancy may be the first occasion in the relationship when the partners realize the extent to which they are interdependent psychologically,

---

**The Mother's Psychological Tasks
of Pregnancy**

1. Incorporation of the fetus into her own body image
2. Perception of the fetus as a separate object
3. Readiness to assume the caretaking relationship
   with the baby

---

socially, and economically. On the one hand, this represents a physiological union that can be mystical; on the other hand, however, the merger may be experienced as a trap.[31] No wonder this resolution of identity confusions requires energy, commitment, and work.

Emotional Reactions to Pregnancy

Although physiological changes are overt manifestations of pregnancy, psychological changes are more subtle but just as important.

At various times throughout pregnancy, a woman's emotional reactions have been described as ambivalence/uncertainty, introversion/narcissism, passiveness/dependency, and fear/anxiety. These feelings predominate at different periods of pregnancy; others fade in and out as pregnancy progresses. There are certainly happier, more positive feelings also. The more ambivalent reactions are discussed here, since these are the ones that the nurse will assist the mother to resolve.

First Trimester

Ambivalence. At the outset, many women experience ambivalent feelings about being pregnant. Even those who have planned their pregnancy are plagued by doubts as to whether it is the "right time" to have a child. A woman who is pregnant for the first time may wonder if she is really ready for a child. A frequently heard question, asked by both parents, is "What kind of parent will I be?" "How will I be able to cope with the total responsibility of a child—24 hours a day, 7 days a week?" Assuming that these women will carry to term, there is no going back for them. Whatever their life-style, a drastic change is in the making; some of the ambivalence they feel may be the result of a reluctance to let go of old and familiar ways. For a woman who has other children and has already made the transition to parenthood, doubts may exist as to whether the spacing between that last child and the expected child is suitable. These basic uncertainties may be compounded by other concerns related to the timing of the pregnancy, the impact on the other children (if there are other children), the economic considerations of providing for another family member, the possibility of giving up a job and losing a second income—all of these

doubts and concerns can contribute to the unsettling prospects of pregnancy. Added physical discomforts such as nausea and vomiting that may accompany early pregnancy only serve to underscore the sense of ambivalence felt by so many women.

This is not to say that a woman does not feel positive about her pregnancy. At the same time that she is struggling with her doubts she may also be experiencing joy and excitement as well as happiness and anticipation. The point is that in all likelihood her feelings will fluctuate between doubts and joys, and she may need to be reassured that what she is feeling is not unnatural and that she need not feel guilty about her ambivalence.

Fears and Fantasies. The first trimester is a time of speculation and anticipation on the part of the mother as she works her way toward accepting the fact that she is pregnant and deals with the physical changes and possible discomforts that she is experiencing. Much time is spent fantasizing about her pregnancy and the impact it will have on her life and the lives of other family members. Mixed with the sense of anticipation is a sense of concern over whether the baby will be normal and healthy, especially if the mother has been recently exposed to a questionable infection.[32]

Shereshefsky and Yarrow noted that mothers who visualized themselves with confidence and clarity during the first trimester tended to make satisfactory adaptations during the entire pregnancy.[34]

If the fantasies become moribund or are characterized by fear and despair, professional intervention may be necessary. If concrete evidence for concern exists (*e.g.,* the presence of genetic defects in the mother's or father's family, the exposure to infection, or the use of drugs or alcohol), the mother should be encouraged to discuss these conditions with the nurse or physician. In some cases, counseling may be necessary if the nurse is not able to allay the mother's fear by simply listening and clarifying misconceptions.

In general, it is important for the nurse to be aware that pregnancy has been recognized as a source of anxiety, particularly for the mother, for the reasons discussed previously. Research has indicated for some time that emotions, although perceived and interpreted by the cerebral cortex, have physiological effects on the body. When the emotion is anxiety, there is motor tension, restlessness, tachycardia, sweating, and flushing. These symptoms are mediated by the sympathetic nervous system through the release of catecholamines and through changes in circulating levels of adrenocortical hormone and other hormones. Animal studies indicate that when catecholamines are released in pregnant animals, there is an increase in maternal blood pressure, a decrease in placental blood flow, and more infant stress than is produced by the administration of oxytocin. Studies with humans indicate that anxiety, as measured by a variety of psychological tests, has been correlated with fetal/neonatal abnormalities, decreased infant birth weight, maternal obstetric complications, and parity.[35-39] It is important to note that these data are not definitive and conclusive as yet. However, there is enough evidence to warrant a very careful family assessment, particularly in terms of the mother experiencing undue anxiety during her pregnancy.

Sometimes, old wives' tales underlie the mother's concern. For example, some mothers believe that eating certain foods (*e.g.,* strawberries or watermelon) will cause the baby to have birthmarks. Other mothers believe that if they are frightened during the pregnancy, their babies will be adversely affected. Assessing the mother's fears, beliefs, or notions provides the nurse with a framework from which to work. Adequate data collection allows the nurse to know what factors are likely to influence the mother. This information allows the nurse to plan a more appropriate, individualized strategy for working with the expectant mother.

Second Trimester.
The second trimester is often marked by a feeling of well-being as the body adjusts to the hormonal changes and some of the early discomforts of pregnancy (nausea and vomiting) subside. Usually, the woman has adjusted to the reality of the pregnancy and reconciled herself to whatever inconvenience it carries. Many of the fears regarding the health and well-being of the infant are forgotten temporarily. Feeling the baby move and hearing the heartbeat are immensely reinforcing and rewarding events for both the expectant mother and father. Allowing the father and the children to share in the experience of feeling fetal movement and hearing the fetal heart tone is a tangible way of incorporating the entire family into the pregnancy.

In the second trimester, mothers become particularly engrossed in fetal growth and development. Both parents become fascinated with pregnancy and the birth process and extremely conscious of the behavior of infants and children with whom they come in contact. At this time parents begin to plan for the actual birth of the baby. They may arrange to attend childbirth classes, read books on infant care, and prepare to face the issues of parenthood.

It is during the second trimester that the mother has been described as becoming narcissistic, passive, and introverted as she concentrates on her own needs and the needs of the fetus growing inside her. As she prepares for her transition to parenthood she may reflect upon her own childhood and her relationship with her mother, from whom she may draw her sense of maternal identity.

Because of her preoccupation with her own thoughts and feelings, the mother may seem to be self-centered and egocentric to those around her. Her moods may change drastically from happy to sad for no apparent reason. At times she may seem romantic and preoccupied with daydreams.

Because her preoccupations may be somewhat troublesome to both her and those around her, people close to the mother should be alerted to her passiveness and dependency needs. In this way they can provide the extra love and attention she needs. This, in turn, will enable her to give more of herself to others. Family members should also be reassured that the mother's behavior and emotional lability are not abnormal but are part of the reaction to pregnancy.[40]

Third Trimester.
The third trimester adds further psychosocial dimensions. As the woman's body changes, so does her self-image, reflected at times in a feeling of awkwardness and clumsiness. She may feel more unfeminine than at any point in pregnancy and may worry about how her husband or mate perceives her.

The third trimester is a time of heightened introversion marked by periods of thinking back on her own childhood and projecting forward in thoughts of her yet-to-be-born child (Fig. 19-2). New fears arise at this time concerning the health and well-being of the baby, as well as her own health and well-being as she contemplates the approach of labor. Mothers frequently distress family members by talking about the possibility of dying during labor. This may reinforce fears that the father is likely to have concerning the outcome of labor.

Furthermore, the mother is likely to wonder how she will "perform" during labor and will be interested in hearing about labor and what she can expect. She may wish to discuss the labor experience with other mothers or to read about it in books and pamphlets.

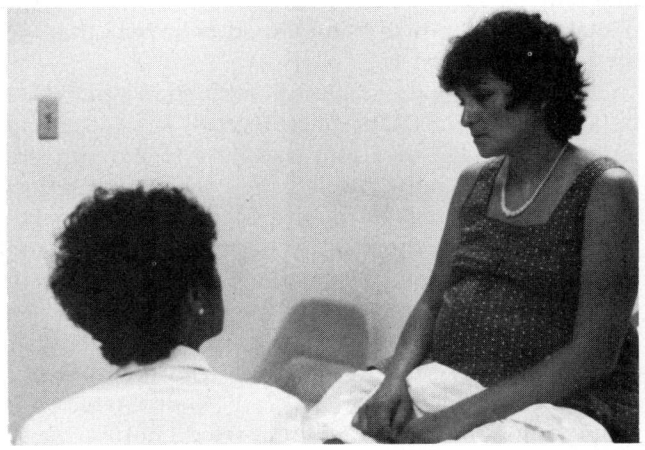

FIGURE 19-2

The third trimester is marked by heightened introversion as the woman looks back to her own childhood and forward to her child's future. (Courtesy of Booth Maternity Center)

Regardless of the apprehension she may feel about labor, as the mother approaches the end of pregnancy, she wonders if "her time" will ever arrive. Many mothers cannot seem to wait for pregnancy to be over as they approach full-term. The obsession with delivery frequently finds expression in dreams about labor and the birth of the child. In conscious fantasies, the mother's thoughts center on the appearance of her infant. Toward the end of pregnancy, many expectant parents can clearly conceptualize what the baby will look like and imagine what characteristics he or she will have.[41]

As she contemplates her own labor, the mother may again wonder what kind of parent she will be. Because both father and mother may share the same feelings, some form of role playing may take place with the parents presenting each other with hypothetical situations in an effort to think out what their responses should be. Such "fantasies" seem to be useful to parents during the transition to parenthood. For the couple expecting their first child, the birth of the baby will signal the crossing of a one-way bridge, that of parenthood. No matter what happens, the new parents cannot go back developmentally to a time prior to the conception.

Pregnancy as a Social Role

Although there have been positive attempts to describe the various stages of pregnancy, emotional reactions together with the developmental tasks that need to be accomplished, we still do not have definite boundaries, expectations, and prescriptions for the pregnant role. How are the imcumbents supposed to act? What kinds of behaviors are really expected? Does one act "ill," or is pregnancy essentially a well state? Is it "business as usual," or are there special restrictions or exemptions that may be claimed? There are several interesting explanations of the many and varied behaviors that we see in parents to be.

If we examine the stages we outlined in a role cycle transition, we find that being pregnant is, in itself, an anticipatory stage in a role transition to parenthood. This can cause confusion at the outset. As she enters the *anticipatory* stage of the pregnant role, the woman attempts to learn the role by observing others, both family and friends, and she recalls how other significant people in her life acted when they were pregnant. She also takes cues from her physician, who may overtly or covertly influence her thinking, even to the extent of regarding pregnancy as a "sick" or "well" state.[42,43] It is interesting that, in our culture, we do not have any socialization or role modeling for the pregnant role—little girls play at being mothers, but not at being pregnant. Thus, although there are certain behaviors that directly relate to women and their fetuses during pregnancy and are essential for the collective well-being of the entire family (to say nothing of the happiness), the prescriptions for these activities are very amorphous and vary considerably in different social classes. These include such behaviors as assuming positive personal health habits, cutting down on activities (or, conversely, exercising to maintain fitness), prompt and consistent attendance to prenatal care, and adequate nutrition practices.

The *honeymoon* and *plateau* stages of the role cycle come quickly upon the anticipatory stage. The showers, coffee klatches, and conversations with mother and pregnant friends or new mothers help the woman adjust the "fit" of the pregnant state to her personality. Some women find that they adore being pregnant. They feel at one with the earth and sky and see themselves at the center of the universe. They find that they seem to bloom physically and emotionally. Others find the condition almost unbearable. They feel unwell, ugly, and put upon and cannot wait to be "unpregnant." By far the more usual are those women who come to accept this condition and tolerate the discomforts and inconveniences. They see it as a necessary stepping stone to another larger role change.

With the infant's birth comes a relatively sudden *disengagement* stage. As we stated previously, there are few cultural norms concerning when the duties and privileges of pregnancy end and parenting begins. It is this role ambiguity that makes this condition difficult. The student is referred to the Suggested Reading for articles that examine this issue in depth.

Father

Men undergo far less social preparation than women do for parenthood and there is little to prepare them for pregnancy *per se*. Experience with fathers who have actively involved themselves in pregnancy indicates that men, like women, go through various phases during the pregnancy.

The introduction comes with the confirmation of the diagnosis of pregnancy. This places fathers almost immediately into a honeymoon stage. As we know, the reactions are as many and varied as with the women. There may be very unclear feelings because the intellectual focus is on the impending fatherhood, rather than the immediate state of pregnancy.[1] Like his partner, he must assimilate the fact that the baby is his. He may not have the physiological changes to help him in this as the woman does, although we have seen some men who do experience many of the same physical symptoms of early pregnancy. How men accomplish this psychological task is still unclear and should be the topic of some fascinating research. We do know that there

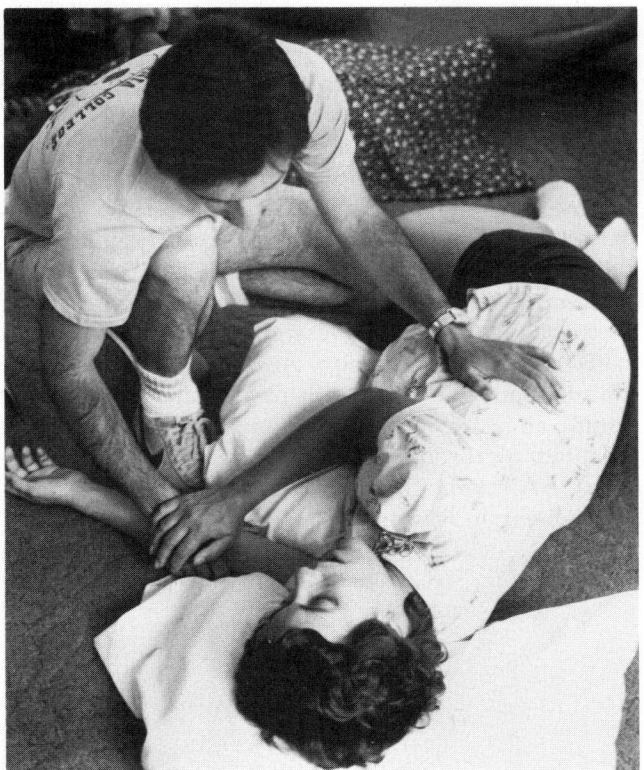

FIGURE 19-3

It is believed that men who take an active part in the pregnancy are more likely to have positive psychological outcomes to the birth, thus strengthening the parental bond. (Courtesy of Booth Maternity Center)

may be guilt reactions about getting the partner pregnant or causing her to be sick and uncomfortable. On a more positive note, there may be feelings of pride at his virility or mutual pride that "We did it!" There may also be feelings of distance between him and his partner as she continues through her introverted first trimester. Jealousy, worry about the change in sexual relationships, and concern about his own competence as a man and provider may occur.[44]

The first perceptible movement of the fetus generally creates a profound feeling that the fetus is real; most men, when questioned, recall the time when "I first felt the baby move" or he viewed the fetus through ultrasound. In the second trimester, more thought is given to what it means to be a father and the plateau stage is entered. Men observe children and pregnant women more intently and become more acutely aware of their partners' growing uterus. A myriad of thoughts and concerns may sweep over the father just as with the mother. Often these center on his ability to provide for the expanding family. However, there is also concern

and thought about how well he will be able to "father" the new progeny and meet the newly evolving expectations of the mother.[1]

As with pregnancy for the woman, there is a good deal of literature that describes this period as a crisis time for fathers. Yet there is evidence to indicate that psychologically healthy men cope without major problems.[1] What is clear, however, is that pregnancy requires as much adjustment for the father as it does for the mother.

As is true for the mother, labor and delivery mark the disengagement–termination stage of the role transition of pregnancy for the father. How these proceed can have a profound effect on the father. Most health providers who have had experience with pregnant couples believe that men who take an active part in the pregnancy by attending childbirth and parent education classes, participating in preparations for the infant, and so on are more likely to participate in the birthing with positive psychological outcomes and this, in turn, strengthens the building of the parental bond (Fig. 19-3).

Applying the Nursing Process to Psychosocial Aspects of Normal Pregnancy

The nurse can function in collaboration with other members of the health team by providing emotional support together with counseling and teaching for the pregnant couple. Regarding pregnancy as a role transition rather than a crisis helps emphasize the normality of the condition. Care then is structured to support the resources of the couple rather than looking for problems that may not exist. The key to appropriate intervention in this instance is *family* assessment.

Family Assessment

There are certain extrafamilial stressors, both developmental and situational, that must be taken into account. Pregnancy, parenthood, and other family life-cycle changes are examples of developmental or normative stressors.[11] Major illness, loss of a job, destruction of property through natural catastrophes, divorce, and separation of families because of war are examples of situational stressors (Fig. 19-4). These extrafamilial stressors work in conjunction with the intrafamilial stressors (e.g., inadequate communication, personal disorganization, inadequate role relationships) to affect the role relationships within the family by producing varying amounts of difficulty in role transition. The amount of difficulty produced is related to how well the family roles are organized, how good their resources are, and how flexible they can be in defining positively the discomfort produced by the stressor.[11]

The way the family is organized (their role structure) depends on each member's values, goals, and ability to perceive and put meaning on events (definitions of the situation). On the basis of these goals and definitions, roles are given to the members and certain behaviors become associated with each role (role allocation and differentiation). Strength is gathered from the family resources, which can be material (e.g., finances, material support from relatives) or interpersonal (integration,

cohesiveness, good communications). Appropriately structured roles and a reservoir of family resources serve to buffer the family from the impact of the various stressors and make role transition easier.

McCubbin has pointed out that, in reality, it is infrequent that the family copes with only one stressor at a time.[11] There can be preexisting stressors or new stressors that accrue, often because of the immediate stressor, causing what McCubbin calls a "pile up" of stressors. This calls for the garnering of new resources to consolidate with the old and the redefinition of the current emerging situation. According to McCubbin's formulation, this will result in the adaptation of the family along a continuum of "good" adaptation (bonadaptation) through "poor" adaptation (maladaptation).[11] A schematic rendering of McCubbin's model can be seen in Figure 19-5.

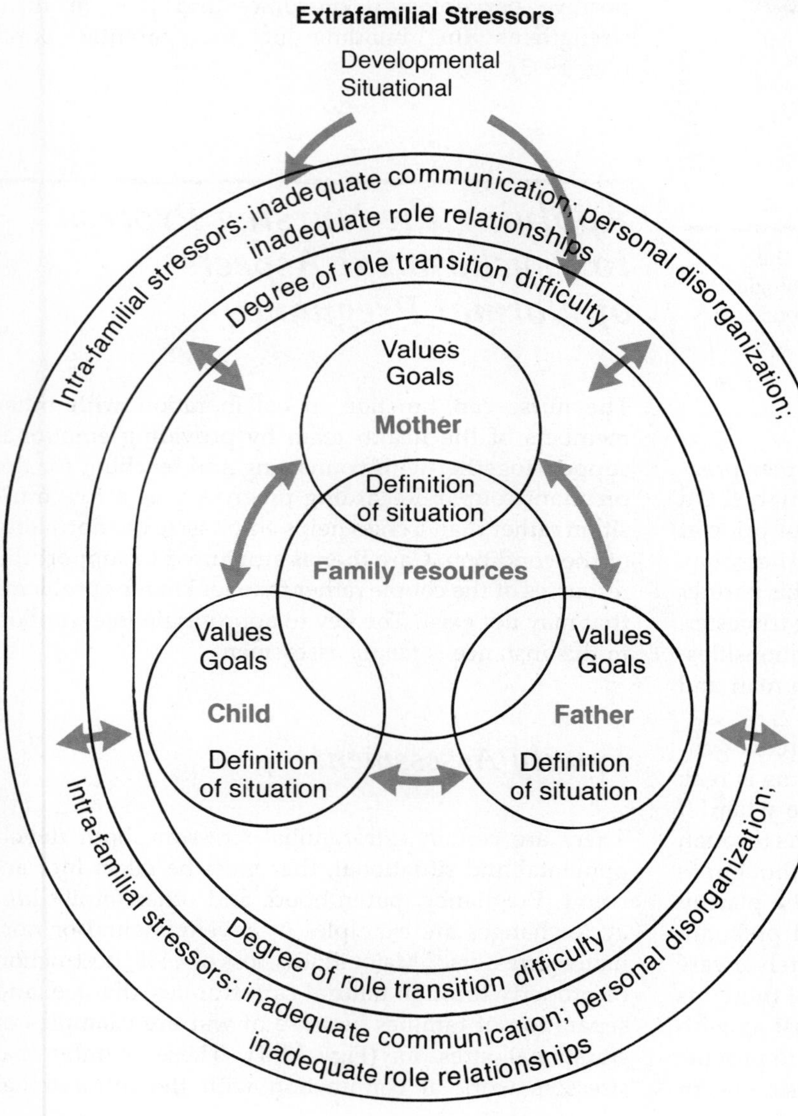

FIGURE   1 9 - 4

Model of family interaction during role transition and components of assessment.

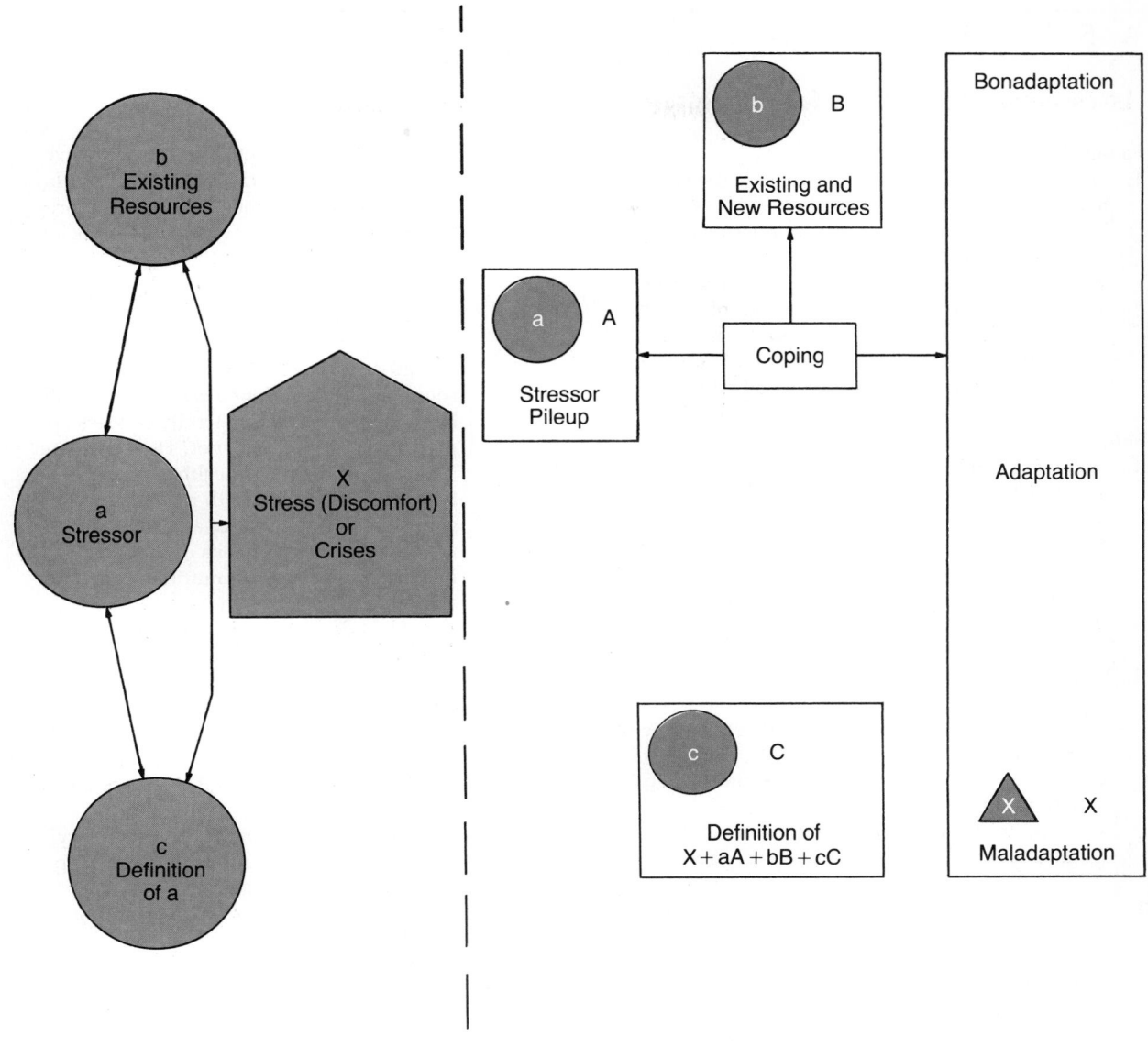

FIGURE 19-5

Modification of the McCubbin model for the family stress process (double ABCX). (McCubbin HI, Sussman JM, Patterson M (eds): Social Stress and the Family, p 12. New York, Haworth Press, 1983)

The following is a tool for the development of a family-care plan. These questions are the type of questions the nurse would include during an assessment.

Nursing Diagnosis

Assessment will help the nurse determine if members of the family are fulfilling role behaviors. If they are at this time, what are potential problems for the remainder of pregnancy or post partum? If they are not fulfilling roles, what are the interfamilial and extrafamilial stressors determined by the assessment? Diagnoses, in this case, deal with psychosocial problems: alteration in family processes, alteration in personal/social integration, inefficient individual coping, and knowledge deficit. Both the client and the family should be considered in making diagnoses.

Intervention

Intervention is aimed at helping the parents define possible stressors and resources within their family unit and developing strategies for coping with manifest or

A S S E S S M E N T   T O O L

Assessment of Psychosocial Aspects of Pregnancy

Family Composition
1. Who are the family members? (Include the extended family.)
   a. What are their ages? What are their relationships to one another?
   b. Where do they live? Do they interact frequently?
   c. Are they "close" emotionally if not physically?
   d. What is the family's relationship to the larger educational community? Is the family involved in community affairs and religious activities? What is its community support structure?

Family Functioning
1. How are the roles allocated and differentiated?
   a. Who does what in the house? Is this mutually satisfactory?
   b. Who makes decisions? How are they made? Is there mutual discussion?
   c. What are the changes that members would like?
   d. How do the parents see their roles being changed with the new infant?
2. How do members usually define situations that happen?
   a. Does the family generally consolidate in time of trouble?
   b. Do they tend to be optimistic, pessimistic, or do attitudes vary with situations?
   c. What are the communication patterns? Who talks to whom? Do problems usually get solved with discussion?
3. What are the family's material and emotional resources?
   a. Is the general and health status of the family and the environment safe and healthful?
      Is housing safe and adequate? Is the house in good repair and is there appropriate room

for the expected infant? If not, what plans are being made to remedy the situation? Is the housing environment structured to prevent accidents? If not, what plans are being made to remedy this?

What is the general health status of the family? Have there been or are there now illnesses? If so, has appropriate medical (or dental) care been sought? Is there a regular source of medical/dental care for the family? Does the mother use maternity services appropriately? If not, why not? How does the family usually pay for health services? Is health insurance or health maintenance organization (HMO) service available? What are the usual health habits of the family members (exercise, rest, nutrition, smoking, substance abuse)?
   b. Are finances adequate? Who contributes? Will the pregnancy make a difference?
   c. Who turns to whom for emotional support? Who is the mother's main support at this time? Who is the father's main support at this time?
4. Are there interpersonal or intrapersonal difficulties?
   a. Are there long-term problems? What are the attempts to resolve them?
   b. Are there problems specific to this pregnancy?
   c. What alternatives for solution for the existing problems do the parents see?
5. What are the specific plans for the baby and for themselves during pregnancy?
   a. What are their plans for themselves as parents?
   b. What are their plans for the infant?
   c. Are siblings anticipated (if this is the first child)?
   d. What are plans for siblings?

possible disruptive elements. By helping parents become aware of their resources and supporting them in their decision making, the nurse can minimize a great deal of stress associated with this role transition. Parents need to validate their impressions of what is happening to them, both physically and emotionally, with an outside person. Family, friends, and health professionals all can be useful in this way. The nurse will want to encourage the parents to use their network of family and friends if it is determined that this network can supply material and emotional support.

Evaluation

Intervention can be evaluated as effective if the family unit is perceived as drawing together (by the family as well as the nurse), if there is open discussion of problems and experiences, and if concrete plans are made for the infant's arrival and the parents have a realistic perception that the infant will change their lives and that adjustment is possible for this momentous new role.

A care plan for the psychosocial aspects of the pregnant family follows.

The Family with Psychosocial Needs

Nursing Objectives:

1. Identify possible needs during the pregnancy arising out of the family composition.
2. Identify possible needs during the pregnancy arising out of family functioning.

Assessment	Potential Nursing Diagnosis	Intervention	Evaluation
Family Composition Ages; relationships to one another Where they live; frequency of interaction Emotional closeness Family's relationship to larger community; family's involvement in community affairs and religious activities; community support structure Additional members in its social network; other relatives or friends available for support	Alteration in personal/social integration related to lack of support in the family/social network	Identify potential stressors and sources of support within family and between family and community Support family in their decision making Allow family to validate their impressions of what is happening to them Encourage family to use identified support systems	Family verbalizes understanding of stressors or potential stressors Family uses support systems appropriately

Family Functioning
Role allocation and differentiation
  Who does what; mutually satisfactory?
  Decision maker; how made
  Any changes members would like
  Parents' views of role changes with new infant
Member definitions of situations that happen
  Family consolidation in times of trouble
  Tone of attitudes: optimistic, pessimistic, or varying
  Communication patterns; who talks to whom; problem solving with discussions
	Alteration in family processes related to pregnancy
	Alteration in family processes related to disturbance in communication patterns
		Identify potential stressors and sources of support within familial roles or in decision making
		Encourage family to use identified support systems
		Identify family's realistic views of role changes
		Identify potential stressors and sources of support within family communication patterns
		Share with the family any nurses' perceptions of healthy communication patterns
			Family verbalizes understanding of stressors or potential stressors
			Family uses support systems appropriately
			Family has realistic perception that infant will change their lives and adjustment is possible
			Family verbalizes understanding of stressors or potential stressors
			Family uses support systems appropriately
			Family is perceived as drawing together by family and nurse

Family's material and emotional resources Is the general/health status of the family/environment safe and healthful?	Ineffective individual coping related to inadequate resources Alteration in health maintenance related to inadequate resources	Identify stressors in systems: environmental, emotional, and financial Identify alternative support systems Refer family to financial services as necessary	Family shows adequate emotional and financial support systems Family uses support systems appropriately

(continued)

Assessment	Potential Nursing Diagnosis	Intervention	Evaluation
Is housing safe/adequate with appropriate room for expected infant?			
What is the health status of the family? Recent illness? Appropriate medical/dental care sought? Regular source of medical/dental care? Clinic, insurance, HMO available?			
Maternity services appropriately used? General health habits of family healthful?			
Adequate finances; who contributes; differences with pregnancy			
Who turns to whom for emotional support; mother's support; father's support			
Interpersonal or intrapersonal difficulties	Social isolation related to demands of pregnancy	Identify any long-term problems or problems specific to this pregnancy	Family's long-term problems are resolved
Long-term problems; resolution attempts		Determine support systems and solutions best for this family	Family's problems specific to this pregnancy are resolved
Problems specific to this pregnancy			
Alternative solutions for existing problems			
Specific plans for baby and selves during pregnancy	Knowledge deficit related to pregnancy and inadequate resources	Identify whether plans are realistic or not	Family has realistic plans for the pregnancy
Plans for themselves as parents		Identify potential sibling rivalry situations	Parents have realistic expectations of selves as parents
Plans for infants		Offer individualized family solutions	Minimal sibling rivalry experienced
Siblings anticipated			
Plans for siblings			

References

1. Phillips CR, Anzalone SJ: Fathering, Participating in Labor and Birth. St Louis, CV Mosby, 1978
2. Brown ML: A cross-cultural look at pregnancy, labor and delivery. JOGN Nurs 5(5):35–38, September/October 1976
3. Bibring GL et al: A study of the psychological processes in pregnancy and of the earliest mother-child relationship. In Psychoanalytic Study of the Child, vol 16, pp 9–72. New York, International Universities Press, 1955
4. Hass S: Psychiatric implications in gynecology and obstetrics. In Ballak (ed): Psychology of Physical Illness. New York, Grune & Stratton, 1952
5. Larsen VL: Stresses of the childbearing years. Am J Public Health 56:32–36, 1966
6. Menninger WC: The emotional factors in pregnancy. Bull Menninger Clin 7:15–24, 1943
7. Caplan G: Patterns of parental response to the crisis of premature birth: A preliminary approach to modifying the mental health outcome. Psychiatry 23:365–374, 1960
8. Coleman AP, Coleman L: Pregnancy: The Psychological Experience. New York, Herder and Herder, 1971

9. Shainess N: The structure of the mothering encounter. J Nerv Ment Dis 136:146–161, 1963
10. Chertok L: Motherhood and Personality. London, Tavistock, 1969
11. McCubbin HI, Sussman MB, Patterson JM (eds): Social Stress and the Family: Advances and Developments in Family Stress Theory and Research. New York, Haworth Press, 1983
12. Kitson GC et al: Sampling issues in family research. Marr Fam 44:965–981, November 1982
13. Le Masters EE: Parenthood as crisis. Marr Fam Living 19:352–355, 1957
14. Dyer ED: Parenthood as crisis: A restudy. Marr Fam Living 25:196–201, 1963
15. Hobbs DJ Jr: Parenthood as crisis, a third study. J Marr Fam 27:367–372, 1963
16. Hill R, Hansen DA: The identification of a conceptual framework utilized in family study. Marr Fam Living 22:299–311, 1960
17. Hill R: Generic features of families under stress. Soc Casework 39(2–3):32–54, 1958
18. Belsky J, Rovine M: Social network contact, family support, and the transition to parenthood. J Marr Fam 46:455–462, May 1984
19. Steffenmeier RH: A role model of the transition to parenthood. J Marr Fam 44:319–347, May 1982
20. Rossi AS: Transition to parenthood. J Marr Fam 30:26–39, February 1968
21. Erickson E: Identity and the life cycle: Selected papers. Psychol Issues 1:1–171, 1959
22. Benedek T: Parenthood as a developmental phase. J Am Psychoanal Assoc 7(8):389–417, 1959
23. Schilder P: The Image and Appearance of the Body. New York, International Universities Press, 1950
24. Fawcett J: Body image and the pregnant couple. MCN 3:227–233, July/August 1978
25. Lamb GS, Lipkin M Jr: Somatic symptoms of expectant fathers. MCN 7:110–115, March/April 1982
26. May KA: Active involvement of expectant fathers in pregnancy: Some further considerations. JOGN Nurs 7:7–12, March/April 1978
27. Trethowen WH, Conlon MF: The Couvade syndrome. Br J Psychiatry 111:57–66, January 1965
28. Munroe RL, Munroe RH: Male pregnancy symptoms and cross-sex identity in three societies. J Soc Psychol 89:147–158, February 1973
29. Coleman AD, Coleman LL: Pregnancy: The Psychological Experience. New York, Herder and Herder, 1971
30. Osofsky HJ: Psychological and sociological aspects of normal pregnancy. Med Services J (Can) 23(4):512–521, 1967
31. Coleman AD, Coleman L: Pregnancy as an altered state of consciousness. Birth Fam J 1(1):7–11, 1974
32. Rubin R: Cognitive style in pregnancy. Am J Nurs 3:502–508, 1970
33. Fishbein EG: Expectant fathers' stress—due to the mothers' expectations. JOGN Nurs 13:325–328, September/October 1984
34. Shereshefsky P, Yarrow L (eds): Psychological Aspects of a First Pregnancy and Early Postnatal Adaptation. New York, Raven Press, 1973
35. Ascher BH: Maternal anxiety in pregnancy and fetal homeostasis. JOGN Nurs 7(3):18–21, May/June 1978
36. Greiss FG, Gabble FL: Effect of sympathetic nerve stimulation on the uterine vascular bed. Am J Obstet Gynecol 21:295, 1967
37. Shabanah EH, Tricorni EV, Suarez J: Fetal environment and its influences on fetal development. Surg Gynecol Obstet 129:556, 1969
38. Adamson KE, Mueller-Heubach KE, Myers R: Production on fetal asphyxia in the rhesus monkey by administration of catecholamines to the mother. Am J Obstet Gynecol 190:248, 1971
39. Shaw JA, Wheeler JP, Morgan W: Mother-infant relationship and weight gain in the first month of life. J Am Acad Child Psychiatry 9:428, 1970
40. Stichler J, Bowden JM, Reimer E: Pregnancy, a shared emotional experience. MCN 4:153–157, May/June 1978
41. Pharis ME, Manosevitz M: Parental models: A means for evaluating different prenatal contexts. In Sawin DB, Hawkins RC II, Walker LO et al (eds): Exceptional Infant: IV. Psychosocial Risks in Infant-Environment Transactions. New York, Brunner/Mazel, 1980
42. Rosengren W: The sick role during pregnancy: A note on research in progress. J Health Hum Behav 3(3):213–218, Fall 1962
43. Rosengren W: Social instability and attitudes toward pregnancy as a social role. Social Problems 9(4):371–378, Spring 1962
44. May KA: Active involvement of expectant fathers in pregnancy: Some further considerations. JOGN Nurs 7:7–12, March/April 1978

Suggested Reading

Antle K: Psychologic involvement in pregnancy by expectant fathers. JOGN Nurs 4(4):40–42, July/August 1975

Hern WM: The illness parameters of pregnancy. Soc Sci Med 9:365–372, 1975

May KA: Active involvement of expectant fathers in pregnancy: Some further considerations. JOGN Nurs 7(2):7–12, March/April 1978

Pridham KF, Schutz ME: Parental goals and the birthing experience. JOGN Nurs 12:50–55, January/February 1983

Rosengren WR: Social instability and attitudes toward pregnancy as a social role. Social Problems 9(4):371–378, 1962

Rossi AS: Transition to parenthood. J Marr Fam 30:26–39, February 1968

Steinberg MC: The relationship between anticipated life change and nausea and vomiting of the first trimester of pregnancy of primiparas. J Perinatol IV:24–31, Summer 1984

Tilden VP: The relation of selected psychosocial variables to single status of adult women during pregnancy. Nurs Res 33:102–106, 1984

Wollery L, Barkley N: Enhancing couple relationships during prenatal and postnatal classes. MCH 6:184–188, May/June 1981

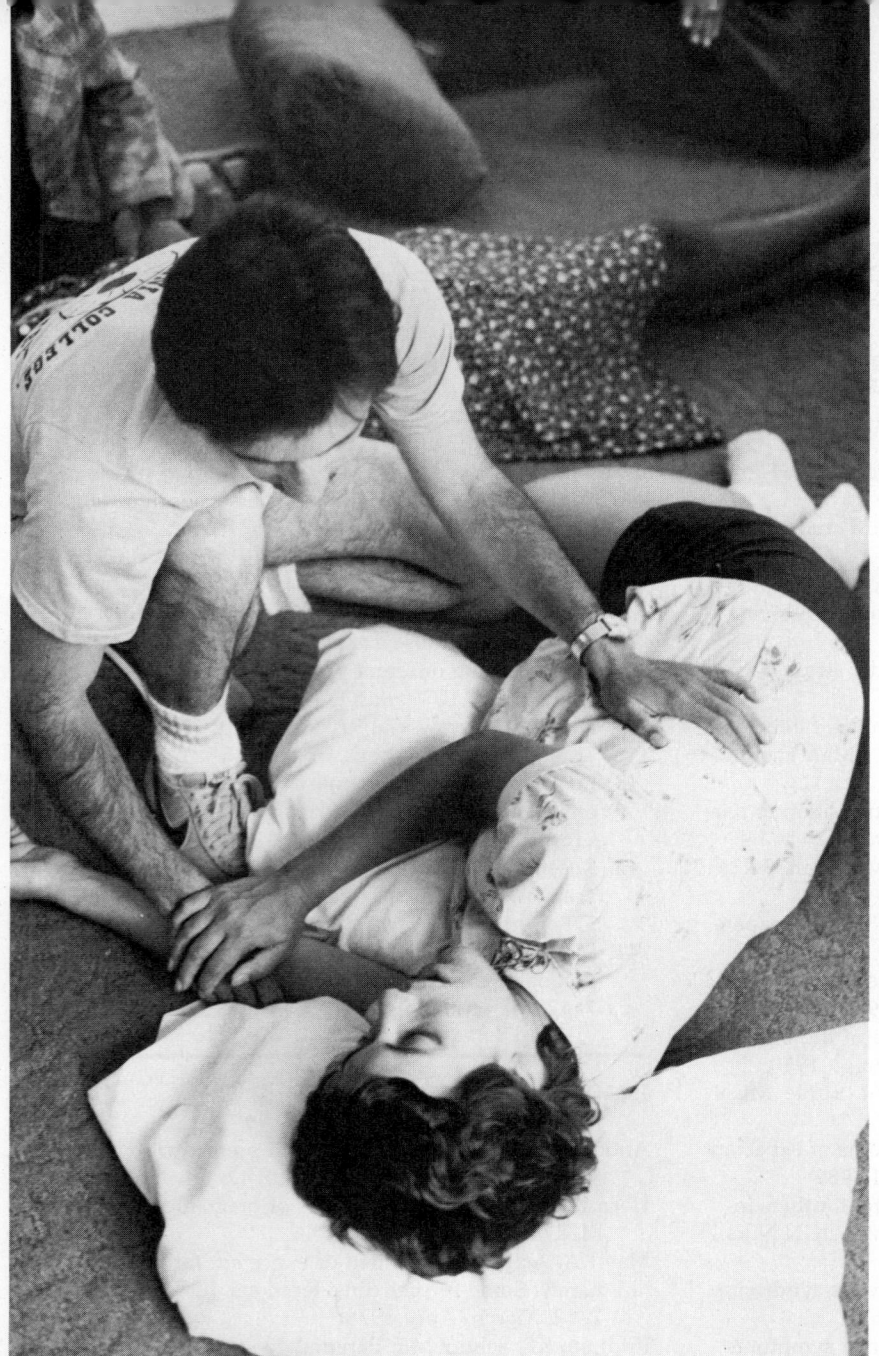

CHAPTER 20

Preparation for Parenthood

Pregnant women and their families not only are interested in learning about maternity care but also have come to view such knowledge as their right. They expect the nurse to be both willing and prepared to assist them in acquiring knowledge and to take their individual wants and needs into consideration.

The increased involvement of childbearing couples in all phases of the reproductive cycle benefits not only the parents, as receivers of care, but also nurses, as givers of care. A concerned and knowledgeable woman will follow a more healthful regimen during pregnancy, including nutrition, exercise and rest, physical care, and psychological processes. A prepared woman and an involved partner can cope positively with the stresses of labor, enriching their relationship and promoting psychological maturation. Parents who are informed and who actively seek understanding of their child's numerous needs for comfort, security, and stimulation during the early formative years can attain a happier, more satisfying parent–child relationship and foster optimal growth and development of the child.

The cornerstone of client education is recognition and respect of the learning needs of clients. The nurse may design content, but if it does not meet the family's learning needs, it is pointless and ineffective. The nurse is responsible for developing the skill to assess these learning needs accurately. Therefore, the teaching–learning process is a complex entity composed of various interrelated parts:

- Identifying the need or needs of the learner
- Determining the motivation of the learner
- Establishing the objectives of learning
- Evaluating the results in terms of desired learning

Many factors affect the teaching–learning process, and the nurse must be aware of those that might either enhance or interfere with learning. The concepts treated in Factors Affecting the Teaching–Learning Process illustrate some of these influences.

Factors in Parent Preparation

Psychological Tasks of Pregnancy and Women's Interests

Nurses have long observed that pregnant women ask different kinds of questions and express different concerns in early pregnancy than in later periods of gestation.

Professional interest in the many behavior changes characteristic of pregnant women led to identification of the specific and unique psychological tasks that apto information about fetal growth and development and about maintaining her own health and the baby's health. As pregnancy draws to an end, the woman becomes concerned about preparing for the baby's arrival and becomes interested in preparation for childbirth, infant behavior, and caretaking activities including feeding, handling, bathing, and so on. By tailoring the information presented to the different interests of each group and providing women with the opportunity to express their own learning needs, nurses can conduct meaningful antepartal educational programs.

Importance of Labor and Postpartum Processes

Although the experience of labor is undoubtedly significant for the woman's self-concept, maternal–infant bonding, and possibly the couple's relationship, few data are available to substantiate what impact nursing intervention during labor might have on these perceptions. Advocates of prepared childbirth believe that women move more rapidly into the caretaking role when they are awake and actively participating in their labor. There is some empirical evidence that fathers who act as labor coaches develop stronger and more recognizable paternal feelings toward the babies of these labors than toward their other children.

Effective client teaching must take into account what is known about the processes occurring during labor and the puerperium, as well as individual variation and specific need. If the labor experience is as important as we suspect, health professionals have an obligation to assist parents in preparing for it and supporting them during this stressful time. When labor has started, a certain amount of teaching is possible, and sensitive care can be helpful, but this is not as effective as antenatal preparation.

Other physiological and psychological changes occur during the puerperium that are part of the process of regeneration undergone by the mother. There is a *taking-in* period, which lasts for the first day or two, possibly three. During this restorative period the mother has a great need for sleep. Among other normal reactions associated with this taking-in phase is the mother's passive and dependent behavior. However, when the *taking-hold* phase follows, the mother is physically and psychologically ready to assume active care of her infant and seeks information and support to facilitate her mothering behaviors. Once her dependency needs have been met in the taking-in phase, she needs to move toward greater independence. For further details of nursing care during the puerperium, refer to Chapters 29 and 30.

pear to be a universal phenomenon of pregnancy. Viewing pregnancy as a developmental process, involving profound endocrine and general somatic as well as psychological changes, it can be understood as a period of disequilibrium and a significant turning point in the woman's (and probably her partner's) life. Certain specific psychological tasks are necessary to cope with the numerous changes, and these seem to occur at specific times during gestation (see Chap. 19).

During early pregnancy, when the woman is working through the idea of being pregnant, informational needs center on validating the pregnancy, understanding physical changes, and recognizing normal emotions and feelings. In midpregnancy, a woman begins to identify the baby as a unique individual and is receptive

Socioeconomic Factors

The learning process will vary according to culture and the socioeconomic situation. Mothering practices in lower-income groups are influenced by economic circumstances that limit equipment, supplies, and mobility; by the organization of the family group and the authority structure; and by the accumulated folk knowledge that establishes specific practices for many common activities and problems of childrearing. Standard educational programs about breast-feeding or formula preparation, clothing and supplies for the baby, integration of the baby into the family, and the mother's nutritional and rest needs are often meaningless to low-income mothers because of a lack of resources and a different value system. Family and friends are generally viewed as more reliable consultants for health concerns than professionals, whose assistance is sought only when community knowledge cannot solve the problem. Sometimes the use of language itself precludes useful exchange of information, as differences in terms used, accent, and speed of delivery vary substantially between middle-class nurses and low-income mothers. In lower socioeconomic levels, the grandmother's word about baby care is often law, and she may be the major caretaker of the baby. Teaching given solely to the mother may thus be of little consequence to the actual care given to the baby. Different cultural groups also have their unique approaches to childrearing and patterns of assistance to new mothers. Values, language, style, and knowledge will exert influences within other cultural groups in a manner similar to that discussed previously.

The nurse must come to understand different cultural and low-income life-styles if effective antepartal and postpartal teaching is to occur. The approach to teaching used with these groups will probably need to shift from the giving of information to assessing present practices, supplementing these practices when necessary with information presented in a form that can be understood and accepted.

Types of Preparation for Childbearing

Preparation for parenthood is influenced by an accumulation of experiences through infancy, childhood, adolescence, and maturity. Schools are increasingly incorporating information about childbearing and parenthood into "health education" and "family life" courses. Classes about pregnancy, sexuality, and parenthood are becoming more common in college and university curricula, as well as more widely available in continuing education and private adult educational

---

Types of Education for Childbearing

Individual teaching and counseling
Groups and classes
    Informational groups
    Discussion or counseling groups
    Prepared childbirth and related classes
        Dick-Read
        Lamaze or psychoprophylaxis
        Bradley
        Wright
        Kitzinger or psychosexual
        Yoga
        Hypnosis

---

programs. Couples thus bring a wealth of previous learning to their experience of childbearing, some of it useful and positive and some frightening and inaccurate. With the advent of pregnancy, preparation for parenthood begins in earnest.

Individual Teaching and Counseling

One-to-one teaching is widely used in all nursing settings and is frequently effective in assisting clients to understand and adapt to a variety of health problems. In most nurse–client contacts, some individual teaching occurs. Numerous opportunities are present during pregnancy for nurses to enhance the effectiveness of medical care through explanations of treatments and procedures, interpretations of what the physician tells parents, and specific instructions for carrying out the regimen of care. When the client asks questions about symptoms or feelings or seeks general information, an on-the-spot response by the nurse meets that particular learning need.

Some clinics and offices have pamphlets or audio-visual material intended to provide individualized instruction to parents during the antepartal period. The amount of structure necessary to ensure that these materials are actually used varies widely. The effectiveness of written or media information without reinforcement through discussion is questionable.

Counseling, an interchange of opinions or giving of advice to help direct the judgment or conduct of others, is often hard to separate from teaching. While counseling is more personal and feeling oriented, its use in combination with presentation of facts usually results in enhanced learning. Appropriate use of counseling takes into consideration the client's viewpoint and works within an acceptable framework to bring about increased understanding, which leads to a change in behavior in the desired direction through the client's internalization of the new goals.

Individualized nursing care in which the woman is assisted to recognize her feelings and fears, reassured that such feelings are normal, and given certain facts to dispel myths or anticipate and prepare for coming events is a common example of how teaching and counseling are combined in antepartal care.

Groups and Classes

Although individual teaching and counseling will continue to be a major mode of nursing intervention, concerns for more efficient use of the health professional's time have led to increased use of groups for antepartal education. Groups are also beneficial because the exchange of experiences among parents with common concerns provides support and encouragement, and expertise and knowledge of the group members combined often exceeds that of the professional alone.

Most institutions providing maternity care also offer some type of antepartal group instruction, but the goals and purposes of these groups vary widely. Many private organizations also offer programs in antepartal education, prenatal exercise and yoga, and preparation for childbirth and parenthood. Classes may be affiliated with continuing education programs in colleges and universities, adult education programs in local communities and high schools, health professionals in private practice, or national health-care organizations such as the Red Cross. The teachers in these groups or classes usually have some type of preparation or certification. They may represent one or, less commonly, several disciplines.

These educational programs can enhance, strengthen, and broaden the care and services provided by the physician and maternity nurse. Programs in parent education should be related segments in the total constellation of services provided to families. To make these sessions truly a preparation for parenthood and family-centered nursing, special attention has to be given to timing and availability of these courses. Sometimes hospitals and institutions arrange classes at times that are not feasible for the parents attending, especially for the father and often for the mother (*e.g.*, in the middle of a busy day). Therefore, attendance is sparse and limited and many valuable aims of the programs may be thwarted.

Informational Groups

The informational group is the most widely used type of program in this country. These groups are planned to serve everyone in the community and place emphasis on a general type of "education for childbirth." Courses usually include the physiology of childbearing, general hygiene, including nutrition during pregnancy and lactation, preparations for the baby, and the care of the mother and baby after birth. In this type of program a multidisciplinary approach may be used in the teaching, or the nurse may be responsible for teaching all of the content.

In general, the material is usually covered in a lecture format with time allowed for questions and discussion. At times a semistructured approach may be used, with certain topics being suggested by the participants and additional relevant information introduced by the nurse–discussion leader as it seems appropriate. Audiovisual materials such as films and slides are often used, with a film depicting actual childbirth a standard component. Tours of the hospital labor unit, postpartum floor, and nursery are usually included.

Some of these classes are given for expectant mothers or fathers separately; in other classes the parents attend together. In the latter group the classes aid the parents in their mutual appreciation of the value of antepartal preparation and tend to promote the idea of sharing parenthood. The goals set for the parents in any of these classes are similar, namely, to gain increased knowledge about childbearing and increased understanding of ways to promote and to maintain optimum health through the practice of good health habits in daily living.

These classes are included as a part of the programs of private "public-health" agencies such as the Visiting Nurse Association, official community-health agencies such as the local and state departments of health, private organizations such as the Maternity Center Association in New York City, and many hospitals throughout the states.

Breast-feeding classes for antepartum clients are becoming extremely popular. These classes usually consist of 10 to 15 women in their last trimester. Husbands, grandmothers, or other support persons are welcome in some classes. Emphasis is placed on knowledge of the lactation process, nutrition, how to prevent and overcome the common minor problems of breast-feeding, myths and misconceptions, and information about the working mother and breast-feeding. Often a mother and infant from a previous class return to demonstrate proper positioning, manual expression, and how to use breast pumps. These classes are often taught by certified lactation educators or certified lactation consultants, who are either hired by a hospital to teach or are in private practice.

Discussion or Counseling Groups

In discussion or counseling groups no structured curriculum is set in advance. Group discussion is developed from the contributions of the group members. The leader is responsible for guiding the discussion and for opening essential areas not probed by the group members. The various areas described in informational programs (physiology of childbearing and general hygiene) are covered as the nurse–leader introduces these topics when they fit with the areas brought up by the participants.

The group situation demands that the nurse develop a new concept of self as a leader and acquire new skills. Knowledge and understanding of what material is relevant are essential so that it can be drawn upon as the group needs it. Hence, the nurse must be totally prepared each time that the group meets because the discussion may range from nutrition in the first trimester of pregnancy to the physiology of labor. In addition, she must be skilled in listening, probing, and reflecting so that she can help the group elaborate on germane comments and statements.

The nurse must recognize the importance and the implication of "iceberg questions," sometimes spoken of as "the question behind the question," knowing that such questions may indicate an underlying concern of the questioner. For example, an expectant mother in the last trimester of pregnancy asks, "How common is going crazy after having a baby?" In such instances the professional nurse should be able to explore and to sift alternatives until the real question can be asked and appropriate action may be taken. In this instance the client really was not concerned with how often people became psychotic after childbirth but rather whether she is likely to experience this malady. Because of a history of mental illness in her family and her own extreme emotional lability during this pregnancy she was afraid that she might become psychotic after delivery.

Because training group leaders is a costly and time-consuming business (and it is essential that those who manage parents in this way be trained in the techniques), group education is not a commitment to be undertaken lightly by either the participating nurses or the sponsoring agencies. Unfortunately, many of these agencies rate the success of the program by the numbers attending, and in the group situation, by definition, only *small groups* can be served at any time.

Group discussion programs are usually well received by those who become involved on a continuing basis, with high levels of professional and client satisfaction. Small groups are also quite effective in bringing about behavior change. Moreover, group education has the advantage of not limiting the discussion to certain topics usually discussed by particular class groups, and it can focus upon any of the aspects of pregnancy or childbearing that are of interest to the group.

Whatever the approach, the nurse who participates in parent classes is in a favorable position to help the clients and families develop a better understanding of their immediate situations, together with a balanced view of the sociology of pregnancy and parturition, growth and development, and the psychological and emotional aspects of family life.

Prepared Childbirth Methods

The late Grantly Dick-Read, a British obstetrician, emphasized certain psychological aspects of labor—that "fear is in some way the chief pain-producing agent in otherwise normal labor." The woman builds up a state of tensions because she is frightened, and these tensions create an antagonistic effect on the muscular activity of normal labor and result in more pain. The pain causes more fear, which further increases the tensions, and so on, creating a vicious circle.

Dick-Read's approach included an educational component to help women comprehend the physiological processes of labor, exercises to improve muscle tone, and techniques to assist in relaxation and prevent the fear-tension-pain mechanism. These three components are included in most childbirth preparation programs that developed after Dick-Read's work became well known.

The educational component during pregnancy is designed to eliminate fear. Facts that concern the anatomy and the physiology of childbearing and the appropriate care of the woman are taught. The woman not only learns how labor progresses but also is helped to gain an understanding of the sensations likely to accompany labor and methods of working cooperatively with them. The exercises that are included are designed for the muscles that will be used in labor, as well as those that will promote the general well-being of the body. The performance of any skill is more efficient if the muscles involved are in the best condition. The exercises are not strenuous and, for the most part, are ones that will contribute to improved posture, body balance, agility, and increased flexibility, strength, and endurance. The woman and her partner learn breathing techniques that will aid her ability to relax in the first stage of labor and techniques that will help her to work effectively with muscles used in the birth.

Components Included in Most Childbirth Preparation Programs

- Education to help women comprehend the physiological processes of labor
- Exercises to improve posture, muscle tone, and flexibility and techniques to assist in relaxation
- Breathing and pushing techniques

An important consideration throughout such programs is "to help the woman help herself," so that her pregnancy will be a healthy, happy experience and at the time of labor she will be better able to participate actively in having her baby.

Early Resistance. Early in the movement in the United States, prepared childbirth earned a bad name through publicity about its more overzealous advocates. "Painless childbirth" was held up as a goal by some extremist groups, and the woman who did experience pain and resorted to pain medication during labor was made to feel a failure. This can be extremely destructive to the woman's self-concept at a time when she needs positive reinforcement in her abilities to achieve and perform competently. Fortunately, current thinking recognizes the variability in individual responses to stress and the differing character of individual labors and teaches that pain medication used judiciously may enhance the woman's ability to use relaxation techniques, thus helping her to cope better with labor and to achieve a satisfying outcome.

For some years many obstetricians and labor room nurses resisted prepared childbirth. Couples who had been trained in a particular method often had to buck staff pressures in their attempt to use the relaxation and breathing techniques they had learned. Medication was at times forced upon the laboring woman because the physician felt it would be best for her, even when she protested that it was not necessary. Such practices as laboring in a semiupright position instead of lying flat, having ice chips or sips of water, eliminating the perineal shave, holding and putting the baby to breast immediately after birth, and constant presence of the father throughout labor and birth caused much staff consternation and were often vetoed.

Although prepared childbirth advocates had long been reporting the increased satisfaction the couple experienced and the reduction of depressed babies when these methods were used, it took economic consumer pressure to bring about widespread acceptance of prepared childbirth. When childbearing couples began avoiding physicians and hospitals because they were not allowed to practice their method, the recalcitrants began to see the benefits of involvement and participation of the parents.

Father Involvement. Currently most prepared childbirth programs include the father as an active participant in helping the woman cope with labor. In this way the father is made to feel involved and useful, and through learning the physiological and emotional processes of pregnancy, he may gain an appreciation of the woman's experience. He is also able to explore his feelings and role as a parent and to prepare psychologically for fatherhood.

Fathers also play another important role in labor. A study by Sosa, Kennel, and Klaus suggests that there may be major perinatal benefits of constant human support during labor.[2] The control group (no labor companion) showed a higher rate ($P < 0.001$) of subsequent perinatal problems (*e.g.*, cesarean section and meconium staining). It was necessary to admit 103 mothers to the control group and 33 to the experimental group (supportive companions in labor) to obtain 20 in each group with uncomplicated deliveries. Also, in the final sample, the length of time from admission to delivery (primigravidas) was shorter in the experimental group (8.8 versus 19.3 hr $P < 0.001$). In another study, by Gaziano and colleagues, the women rated medication during labor of less importance than the presence of a labor companion.[3]

Selecting a Class. Because prepared childbirth classes differ, it is important that couples are aware of how to shop around for a teacher and class that suits their particular needs (see Variables to Consider in Selecting a Childbirth Class).

Lamaze or Psychoprophylactic Method

The psychoprophylactic method (PPM), or Lamaze method, is the most widely used prepared childbirth method in the United States today. It was first propounded by two Russian doctors, Nicolaiev and Vel-

---

Variables to Consider in Selecting a Childbirth Class

1. Professional credentials of instructor and type of training as a childbirth educator
2. Class size
   a. Eight couples or less—ideal for group interaction and supervised practice
   b. More than 12 couples—limited group interaction, limited supervised practice, and decreased relaxation skills mastered by couple
3. Location of class
   a. Home—usually limits class size and provides informal, relaxed atmosphere
   b. Office, school, church, or hospital—class size may escalate and atmosphere may be less than ideal
4. Total hours of class time for the fee
5. Amount of supervised practice time per session
6. Fee payment by couple
   a. Directly to instructor—instructor accountable to consumer
   b. To group or sponsoring health facility—instructor accountable to agency

vovsky. The rationale of the program was based on Pavlov's concept of pain perception and his theory of conditioned reflexes (*i.e.,* the substitution of favorable conditioned reflexes for unfavorable ones).

The theory intrigued a Paris obstetrician, Ferdinand Lamaze, who studied Russian-trained mothers-to-be in a Leningrad clinic. Lamaze returned to France and began to prepare his clients in *psychoprophylaxis,* or *mental prevention* of pain in childbirth. He gradually introduced certain adaptations, the most important of which was the rapid shallow breathing that came to characterize the Lamaze method.

As the technique spread throughout Europe and Latin America, the *Lamaze method* and *psychoprophylaxis* became synonymous. The late Marjorie Karmel was perhaps the most responsible for introducing this technique to America. There are now programs in psychoprophylaxis throughout this country. Many are under the auspices of the American Society for Psychoprophylaxis in Obstetrics, Inc. (ASPO), which was founded through joint efforts of Mrs. Karmel and a physical therapist, Elizabeth Bing, and others.

In general, the teaching in the program consists in combating the fears associated with pregnancy and childbirth by instructing the pregnant woman and her labor partner in the anatomy and the neuromuscular activity of the reproductive system and the mechanism of labor. The underlying theory of these programs remains firmly based on the neurophysiology of cortical excitation and conditioned response. That is, the woman is taught to replace responses of restlessness and loss of control with more useful activity. Its usefulness lies in the fact that a high level of activity can excite the cerebral cortex sufficiently to inhibit other stimuli, in this case, the pain usually associated with labor. The responses also allow the woman to see herself as someone who is able to cope, which reinforces the probability of continued coping behavior (Fig. 20-1).

In some programs nutrition and general hygiene are included. Exercises that strengthen the abdominal muscles and relax the perineum are taught, and breathing techniques to help the process of labor are practiced (Fig. 20-2). Thus, the mother is conditioned to respond with respiratory activity and dissociation (or relaxation) of the uninvolved muscles. She then controls her perception of the stimuli associated with labor.

Techniques. Several changes have occurred in the Lamaze method as a result of experiences gained over many years of use. Class content, flexible breathing techniques, theories of learning and motivation, and emphasis on the childbirth team constitute the major changes. Class content originally dealt mostly with exercises, relaxation, breathing techniques, and the normal labor and birth experience. Childbirth educators have added information on such subjects as prenatal nutrition, infant feeding, cesarean birth, and other variations from usual labor, as well as discussions concerning sexuality, early parenting, and coping skills for the postpartum period.

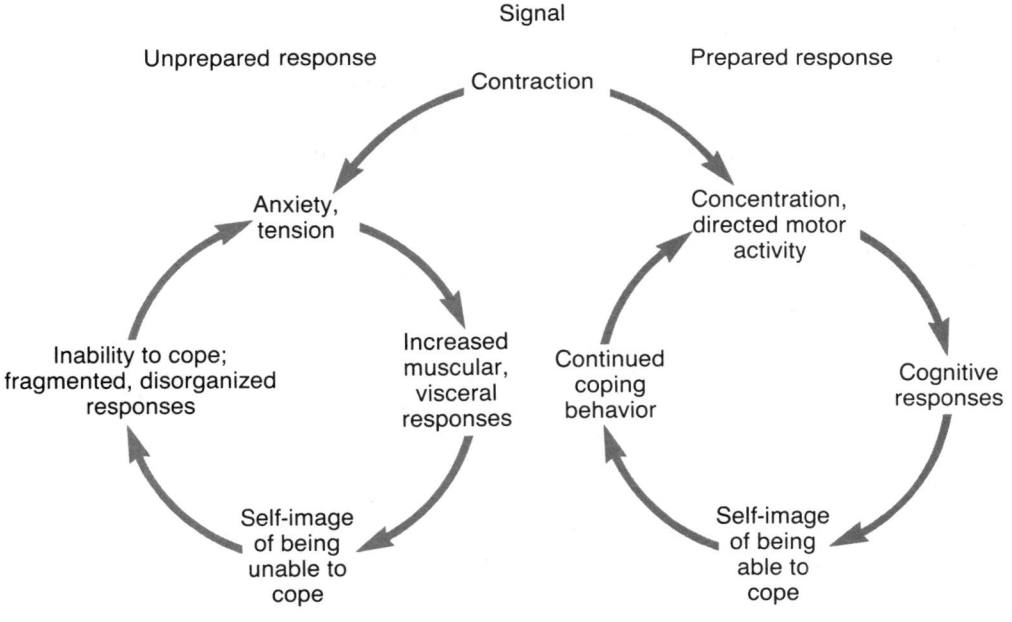

FIGURE 20-1

The continuum of responses in the prepared and unprepared woman. (Redrawn from Hassid P: Textbook for Childbirth Educators, 2nd ed. Philadelphia, JB Lippincott, 1984)

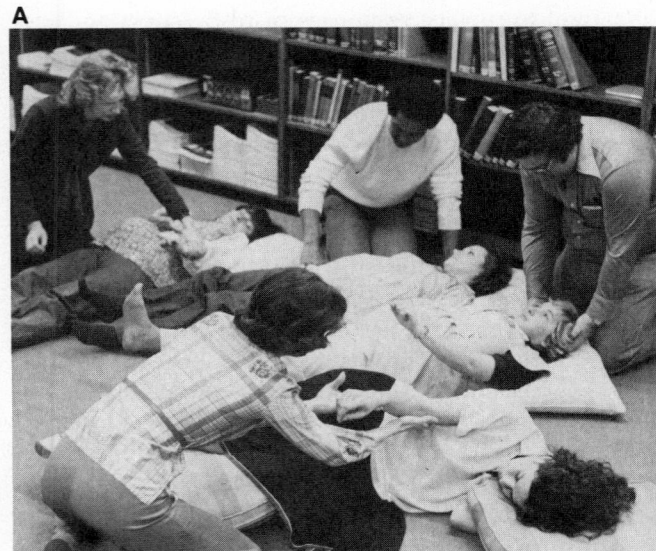

FIGURE 20-2

(A) Couples practicing muscle relaxation for labor. (B) Couples practicing different positions and breathing for labor. (C) Couples practicing various positions for pushing: leg holding, squatting, relaxing legs, and lying on side.

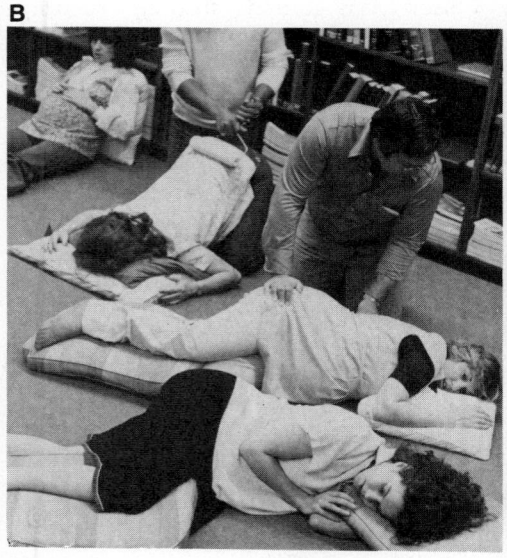

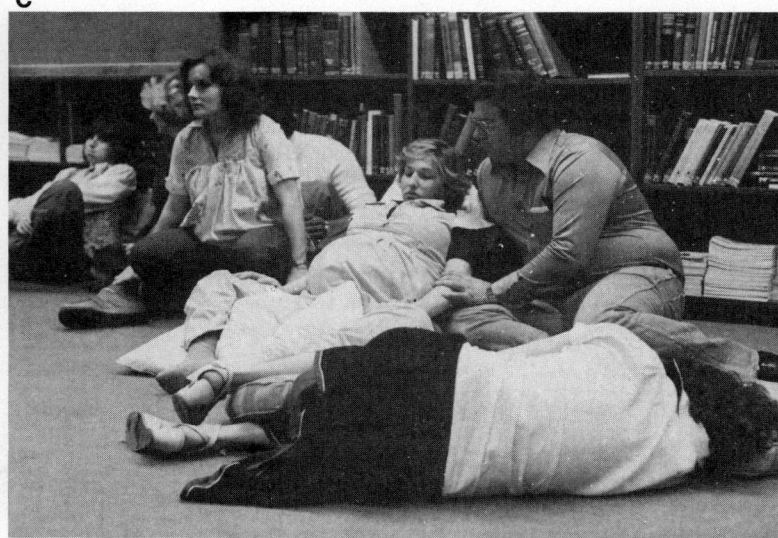

The breathing techniques have been modified in recent years. The first breathing for labor is slow-paced breathing and is done at a maximum rate of half the individual woman's resting respiration rate. As labor progresses some women will want to move into modified paced breathing, which is a maximum rate of twice the individual woman's resting rate of respiration. For the last part of the first stage some women find moving into a patterned breathing more calming. The rhythmical breathing is patterned with soft blows that do not change the rate or the volume of air exchange. This breathing continues at a maximum rate of twice the woman's individual resting respiration rate. All breathing techniques may be inhale/exhale nose, inhale/exhale mouth, or inhale nose/and exhale mouth.

In the second stage of labor, the woman may assume any comfortable physiological position, a semi-sitting position, squatting, or sidelying (as in Fig. 20-2C). Pushing then may take one of two forms. The woman will take two deep breaths, hold her breath, relax the perineum (slightly bulge), and push out through the vagina. Grunting noises may accompany this effort and indicate the woman is responding to the physiological need to release air. Using the other method, the woman will take two deep breaths, relax the perineum and push out through the vagina while exhaling slowly through her mouth.[4]

This pushing effort is repeated throughout the contraction, timed, and coached by the partner. (For more specific techniques see the Second Stage of Labor in Chap. 26.) Caldeyro–Barcia[5] found that when women *hold their breath* for pushing, bearing-down efforts that last more than 5 seconds resulted in late decelerations of the fetal heart rate and marked falls in the maternal systolic and diastolic blood pressures. He suggests that if the woman is not urged to bear down long and hard, which often occurs with the "cheering section" approach to pushing, her *spontaneous* efforts are usually within physiological limits—5 to 6 seconds long—and fetal acidosis is avoided.

Goal Setting. Lamaze has progressed to a more individualized approach to learning and motivation. The original psychoprophylactic training was rather rigid, with goals set by the teacher. Now, the couple sets their own goals for labor and birth and the teacher assists the couple in learning ways in which these goals can be realized. This approach removes any set criterion for the success of the labor experience, avoiding the disappointment of externally imposed goals that may be unrealistic for the particular couple.

Greater emphasis is also given to the childbirth team, in which the couple, obstetrician, nurse, and Lamaze teacher work together toward a satisfying birth experience. Rather than anticipating a thwarting of their goals, the couple is encouraged to discuss their goals with their physician so he or she can understand what they hope to do. They also gain appreciation of some of the physician's responsibilities and alternate plans, should labor not progress normally.

Other Childbirth Methods

Several other approaches to prepared childbirth are used, some of which are popular in specific geographic regions or even specific areas of a particular city.

Although these programs may derive from different theories and vary in specific techniques, they have many points in common, including the following basic beliefs:

- Fear enhances the perception of pain but may diminish or disappear when the parturient knows about the physiology of labor.
- Psychic tension enhances the perception of pain, but the parturient may relax more easily if childbirth takes place in a calm and agreeable atmosphere and if good human contacts have been established between her and the personnel attending her.
- Muscular relaxation and a specific type of breathing diminish the pain of labor.

Another reason for teaching correct breathing techniques is to avoid hyperventilation during labor. Nurses are often concerned about hyperventilation during labor when prepared childbirth breathing techniques are used. Undue fatigue, hyperventilation, and subsequent carpopedal spasm have been observed when breathing techniques are improperly used. Maternal respiratory alkalosis and a paradoxical acidosis in the fetus are also possibilities if hyperventilation is prolonged.

Hyperventilation can occur in any labor when the woman breathes improperly. Correct use of prepared childbirth breathing techniques can help prevent hyperventilation from occurring, which is another benefit of these programs.

The *Bradley method*, also called husband-coached childbirth, emphasizes slow, deep breathing along with complete deep relaxation. The Academy of Husband-Coached Childbirth is the organization that trains teachers to conduct classes in the Bradley method.

The *Wright method* is based on psychoprophylaxis but uses less active breathing than is taught in the Lamaze method. The breathing "levels" become more complex as labor progresses. This method is also referred to as the *new childbirth*.

The *psychosexual method* of Shelia Kitzinger is not based on psychoprophylaxis but on a method using sensory memory as an aid to understanding and working with the body in preparation for birth. Included also is the Stanislavsky method of acting as a basis for teaching relaxation. Kitzinger advocates chest breathing but teaches release of the abdomen at the same time. Her method is called the psychosexual method because she saw sexuality as part of the larger whole encompassing family relationships, birth, cuddling, and feeding.[6]

Yoga, although not a method of prepared childbirth, has been used by numerous women in labor, sometimes in combination with other specific methods of childbirth preparation. Yoga teachings include relaxation, concentration, and a combination of abdominal and chest breathing called "complete breathing." It is not unusual to see childbirth educators teaching different techniques from several methods in an eclectic or "holistic" preparation for childbirth.

Hypnosis is a technique that induces a state of extreme suggestibility in which the client is insensible to outside impressions, except the suggestion of her attendant. There is no particular "program" associated with the use of this technique; rather, training in achieving a hypnotic state or autohypnosis is usually given by a person who is specially trained in this area. Although there is no general regimen for learning this technique, the conditioning required is usually presented in several individual sessions, usually in the latter half of pregnancy.

The *modus operandi* of hypnotically induced relaxation has been explained by suggesting that whenever all the voluntary muscles are completely relaxed during labor, the uterus has a monopoly on available energy and hence can work more efficiently. In addition, it is likely that when fears are abolished or diminished, efficient uterine action is promoted. The use of comfort measures, such as low back massage, has also been suggested as enhancing the hypnotic state. The major drawback to this technique lies in the difficulty of securing adequately prepared therapists in some areas of the country. However, much of what is taught in childbirth education classes can be called self-hypnosis.

Comfort During Pregnancy

The majority of women can maintain their usual work and play activities during pregnancy. However, since changes do occur in weight and weight distribution, comfort in pregnancy can be significantly improved by good posture and body mechanics in everyday activities. It is often possible to reduce or overcome discomfort by correct positions, body movements, and exercises (Table 20-1). Since the major postural changes begin in the second trimester of pregnancy, this is the logical time for learning. Correct posture for standing, sitting, and stair climbing and good body mechanics for carrying packages or lifting objects must be reinforced. The spinal muscles and joints should be protected from undue strain; thus, the woman needs to know how her feet can be used efficiently for balance and for movement (see Principles for Activities of Daily Living (ADL) During Pregnancy).

CLIENT EDUCATION

Principles for ADL During Pregnancy

- Activities need to be varied (walking, standing, sitting).
- Time period should be of short duration.
- Walking back and forth is preferable to standing still.
- Standing posture should be with one leg forward so that weight can be shifted easily and efficiently from foot to foot and the body turned comfortably.
- Walking posture should be head erect, back upright, and chin up and pelvis tilted.
- Use a footstool when sitting.
- When climbing stairs, the entire foot should be placed on stair and leg muscles used to lift self up each step without leaning forward.
- Stooping and lifting should be avoided; if stooping is necessary, it is best to squat down and reach and lift, with feet wide apart and back straight. The alternate squatting position, with one foot placed forward, may also be used. The body is lowered slowly to the other knee. The front foot, which should be flat on the floor, will be used for lifting. The rear foot, flexed at the toes, will serve for pushing and will act as a balance.
- When carrying bulky packages (groceries) the load should be divided and carried in two hands. A cart that rolls easily should be used for heavy loads.

TABLE 20-1

Exercises and Positions to Relieve Common Discomforts of Pregnancy

Discomfort	Exercise or Position
Swelling of feet, ankles	Leg elevating
Leaking urine when coughing, laughing	Pelvic floor contraction
Heaviness in pelvis	Pelvic floor contraction
Hemorrhoids and swelling around vagina	Pelvic floor contraction
Low back pain	Rotating legs
Cramps in legs	Leg elevating; calf stretching
Tired legs	Leg elevating; calf stretching
Varicose veins in legs	Leg elevating; calf stretching
Shortness of breath	Good posture; good body mechanics; rib cage lifting; shoulder circling
Low backache	Pelvic rocking; good posture; pushing position; squatting
Middle backache	Pushing position
Upper backache	Shoulder circling; good posture
Numbness in arms and fingers	Shoulder circling; lying on side
Abdominal muscle spasm (stitch)	Pelvic rocking; deep abdominal breathing

For rest and comfort during pregnancy, the woman can learn the positions for lying on her side and on her back, the side relaxation position, and, equally important, how to get up and out of bed without strain.

Backache is one of the most common complaints, and the *pelvic tilt* performed daily will help to relieve abdominal pressure and low back pain during pregnancy and early labor. This exercise is also used to firm the abdominal muscles following the birth of the baby.

Other exercises to promote comfort and give relief from some of the common discomforts of pregnancy include *rib cage lifting, shoulder circling, leg elevating,* and *calf stretching* (see Appendix A, Prenatal Exercises).

Posture and Body Mechanics

Maintaining correct posture and practicing good body mechanics are important in avoiding some of the more common discomforts of pregnancy. For example, a frequent cause of backache during pregnancy is poor posture. As pregnancy progresses, body proportion and weight distribution are altered. As the body's center of gravity is gradually shifted forward, the abdominal muscles often relax and the natural curvature of the spine becomes exaggerated, shortening the muscles of

CLIENT EDUCATION

Posture Checklist

Incorrect posture

Head

Neck sags, chin pokes forward, and whole body slumps

Shoulders and chest

Slouching cramps the rib cage and makes breathing difficult

Arms turn in

Abdomen and buttocks

Slack muscles cause a hollow back

Pelvis tilts forward

Knees

Pressed back strains joints and pushes pelvis forward

Feet

Weight on inner borders strains arches

To correct posture

Head

Straighten neck and tuck chin in so body lines up

Shoulders and chest

Lift up through rib cage and pull shoulder girdle back

Roll arms out

Abdomen and buttocks

Contract abdominals to flatten back

Tuck buttocks under and tilt pelvis back

Knees

Bend to ease body weight over feet

Feet

Distribute body weight through center of each foot

(Essential Exercises for the Childbearing Year, 1982 Elizabeth Noble, Houghton Mifflin Company)

the lower back. The woman often compensates for this by leaning backward slightly at the waist, which shifts her weight to her heels when walking. This results in an awkward, waddling gait and frequently contributes to backaches, particularly of the lower back.

It is important to encourage the woman to be constantly mindful of her posture and to provide her with information on correcting her body alignment (see Posture Checklist). Some exercises, such as the pelvic tilt, which strengthens the muscles of the abdomen and lower back, are also helpful in correcting poor posture and relieving backaches (see Appendix A, Prenatal Exercises).

The importance of practicing good body mechanics should also be taught to the pregnant woman. Body mechanics involve the efficient use of the body to evenly distribute weight and stress among several muscle groups rather than overtaxing a particular muscle group with undue strain. For example, pregnant women

should be instructed to avoid stooping when lifting or reaching for low objects. Bending forward or stooping may put the woman off balance and will require the muscles of the back to assume the burden of returning the trunk (and any weight that is lifted) to an erect posture. A squatting posture is much preferred when reaching for low objects (Fig. 20-3). The woman should be instructed to squat with the back straight and the body properly aligned. Any weight to be lifted should be pulled close to the body and the muscles of the thighs and legs should be used to raise the body to an erect posture.

Good body mechanics relate directly to good posture. Throughout daily activities, such as household chores, walking, and climbing stairs, the woman should be encouraged to keep the back straight (but not rigid) and the body in proper alignment. Learning to maintain a correct posture and practicing good body mechanics often require a considerable amount of conscious

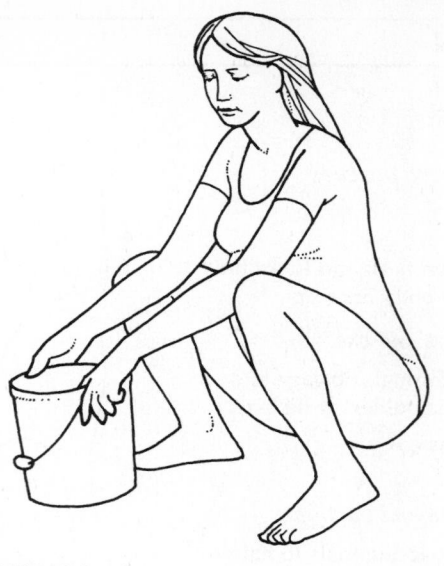

The squatting posture is the preferred method of lifting or reaching for low objects during pregnancy.

thought and practice at first. It is not unusual for a person who has previously had a poor posture to feel strange or even uncomfortable when her body is in proper alignment. However, it should be emphasized that good posture and body mechanics are beneficial throughout life, and it is hoped that the lessons learned during pregnancy will carry over to a more healthful future.

Comfort Positions

Pregnant women often comment that they find it difficult to relax because they are unable to find a comfortable position or that heartburn, backaches, or other common discomforts interfere with their ability to relax. A variety of positions have been found effective in providing comfort and in relieving some of the discomforts of pregnancy. A comfort method for sleeping is illustrated in Figure 20-4.

It should be noted that a position that works effective for one woman may not necessarily work equally

as well for another. For example, some women find the squatting position (see Fig. 20-3) relaxing and effective in relieving backaches and others find a pushing posture or some other position or exercise more effective. Women should be encouraged to try a variety of positions until they find what works best for them.

Tailor Sitting

The tailor sitting position is helpful in stretching the muscles of the thighs, hips, and lower back. If is often helpful in relieving lower backache, and many women find it relaxing. The woman should sit on the floor with her knees spread as far apart as comfortable, with one leg resting on the floor or chair in front of the other and the back straight. Many women find it more comfortable to assume this position with the back against a wall or some other support. The beginner should remain in this position for about 5 minutes at a time, gradually increasing to intervals of 15 to 30 minutes. Since this position significantly decreases circulation to the legs and feet, the woman should "shake out" her legs every few minutes and then return to the position. Many women find this a very comfortable position and assume it several times each day for relaxation. They may also find the tailor sitting exercise beneficial in strengthening thigh, hip, and lower back muscles and in providing additional relief from backache. (The tailor sitting position is illustrated in Appendix A, Prenatal Exercises.)

It should be noted that the tailor sitting position is not exactly the same as the "Indian sitting" position that many people learn as children. In the Indian sitting position the legs are often crossed with one leg resting on the other. Generally, the comfort positions in pregnancy place the body in good alignment, with no body part resting on any other body part to interfere with circulation.

Leg Elevation

Among the more common discomforts of pregnancy are fatigue, swelling, cramps, and varicosities of the legs. One method of relieving these discomforts and increasing circulation to the legs is to have the woman elevate her legs for 2 to 5 minutes several times each day. It is often convenient to have the woman lie supine on her

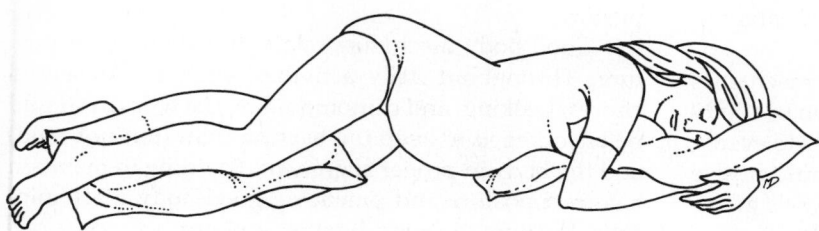

FIGURE 20-4

Comfort positions. The comfort positions for pregnancy are positions in which the body is in alignment, with no body part resting on any other body part to interfere with circulation.

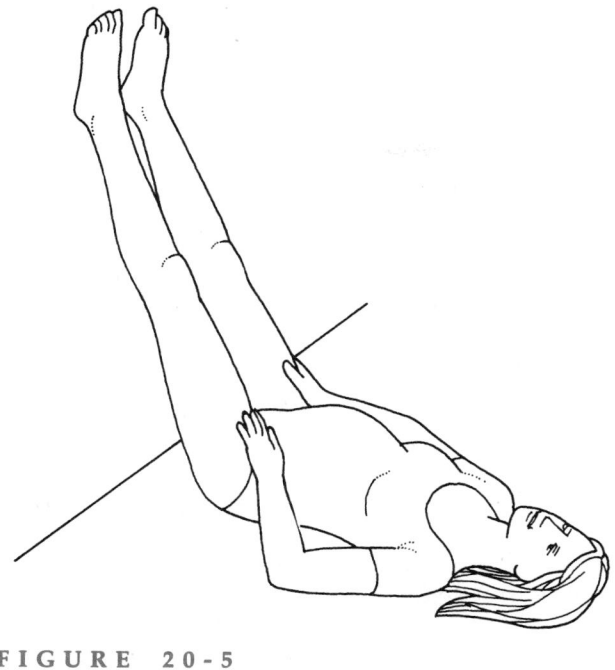

FIGURE 20-5

Elevating the legs is helpful in relieving fatigue, swelling, cramps, and varicosities in the legs.

bed or on the floor with her heels resting against a wall (Fig. 20-5). Early in pregnancy, the body and legs can be nearly at a right angle with the buttocks either against the wall or very close to it. However, as pregnancy progresses, the right-angle position may become uncomfortable because of pressure on the diaphragm, and the woman may find it more comfortable to move her body slightly away from the wall to reduce the angle. Eventually, she may find it more comfortable to lie with her legs supported by a footstool or chair. Women who experience swelling and varicosities of the vulva should be instructed to elevate both the legs and hips. When rising from the supine position, the woman should be instructed to relax for a few moments after lowering her legs and to rise slowly to avoid dizziness.

Exercises*

Exercises done during pregnancy increase circulation, improve muscle tone, aid in prevention of fatigue, promote physical comfort, and encourage good posture. Exercises should be done smoothly, avoiding exaggerated or jerky movements. The woman should not do any exercise that causes pain or discomfort. Breathing should be coordinated with exercises, generally exhaling while doing the effort part of the exercise.

* Prenatal exercises are illustrated in Appendix A.

Many communities offer special exercise classes for pregnant and postpartum women. A group setting is often helpful because motivation is enhanced.

The following exercises are provided as a general guide for the pregnant woman.

Pelvic Floor Contractions

Pelvic floor exercises are useful in relieving the discomforts of heaviness in the pelvis and the leaking of urine during activity or when coughing or laughing. These exercises strengthen and increase the flexibility of the pelvic floor muscles. They also help the woman develop an awareness of tension and relaxation in the perineal area, which is important during childbirth. Pelvic floor contractions may also be helpful after childbirth to promote healing, provide comfort, and to help regain muscle tone after birth.

Pelvic floor contractions can be performed in a standing, sitting, squatting, or lying position. Instruct the woman to draw up the muscles of the pelvic floor as she would if she were attempting to avoid urinating. She should feel the squeeze as the muscles surrounding the vagina and urethra are tightened. She should hold this tightness for 2 or 3 seconds and then relax for a couple of minutes. Next, she should perform the same exercise, tightening the muscles around the rectum and, eventually, tightening all of the muscles of the perineum at the same time. She should progress to doing 50 or more pelvic floor contractions each day in a series of five contractions, holding each contraction for 5 seconds.

Pelvic Tilt

The pelvic tilt is useful in strengthening the muscles of the abdomen and lower back and is also helpful in relieving backache. The pelvic tilt exercise may also be used during labor to relieve backache and to help in rotating the fetal head when the presentation is posterior.

To perform this exercise the woman should be on her hands and knees, with her hands directly under the shoulders and the knees under the hips. Her back should be in a neutral position with the small of the back flattened, *not hollowed*. Her head and neck should be aligned with a straight back, and her elbows and knees should remain stationary throughout the exercise. Instruct the woman to pull in the abdominal muscles and buttocks and to press up with her lower back. She should hold this position for a few seconds and then relax to a neutral position. Initially, many women will need assistance in assuming the neutral position and avoiding a sagging or hollow back posture. She should repeat the exercise about five times, maintaining a slow rhythmic motion. The pelvic tilt exercise may also be performed in a standing or supine position.

Rib Cage Lifting

Rib cage lifting is a useful exercise for increasing the flexibility of the intercostal muscles and for improving general muscle tone. This exercise may also be used to help relieve shortness of breath.

This exercise can be performed in either a standing, sitting, or tailor sitting position. The tailor sitting position is often recommended because performing the exercise in this position also helps to tone the muscles of the hips, thighs, and lower back. Instruct the woman to inhale while extending the right arm with the elbow slightly flexed above her head. With the arm extended, she should then exhale, extending the arm further as she feels the muscles of her right side stretch. She should inhale again, return to the starting position, and repeat the exercise with the left arm. Initially, the exercise can be repeated five times with each arm and gradually increased to ten times.

Shoulder Circling

The shoulder circling exercise is useful in strengthening the muscles of the upper back and may be used to relieve upper backache and numbness in the arms and fingers.

This exercise can be performed in either a standing or a supine position. The woman should be instructed to keep her back, neck, and head straight throughout the exercise and to allow her arms to hang loosely at her sides. She should slowly rotate her shoulders up and back as far as they can comfortably go in a circular motion. She should inhale as the shoulders are rotated and exhale as the circle is completed and the shoulders have returned to the starting position. The exercise can be repeated ten times, relaxing momentarily between each rotation.

Calf Stretching

The calf stretching exercise is a particularly effective means of relieving leg cramps. If performed regularly, calf stretching is also helpful in preventing the cramps.

Instruct the woman to stand with her feet slightly apart and her hands on the back of a chair or some other object that will provide secure support. She should slide the heel of her right leg back as far as possible without letting her heel leave the floor. She should then bend the knee of her left leg, lowering herself slightly as she feels the stretching of the calf muscles in her right leg. She should return to her original standing position, relax for a few minutes, and repeat the exercise with the opposite leg. The exercise can be repeated several times, using the alternate leg each time. If the woman is performing the exercise to relieve a leg cramp, she may repeat the exercise several times with the affected leg until the cramp is relieved.

Preparation for Labor and Birth

Whether or not the maternity nurse is involved in offering classes for parents, it is important that education for childbirth be part of the professional repertoire. This information can be used for individual teaching or for reinforcing what has been learned from other sources. Including the father in this instruction will assist him to understand his partner's needs during the childbearing process and offer support.

Choices in Childbirth

Today, in most areas of this country, women and their partners have choices surrounding their birth experience. While in some geographic areas choices may be few, in other areas the choices are many and varied. Some parents-to-be decide to choose their birth attendant and then allow the birth attendant to make all the other choices, either because they don't want to decide or don't know about their options. Other expectant parents decide what they want in a birth experience and then go out and find a birth attendant and facility they are comfortable with who can help them achieve the experience they want. Choices in Childbirth gives some specific labor and birth options expectant parents may want to consider. (To obtain a detailed pamphlet entitled "Planning Your Baby's Birth," see the Suggested Reading at the end of this chapter.)

Relaxation

The use of relaxation as a coping skill during labor is the foundation of all the childbirth education techniques.

Many authorities regard the ability to release tension under stress as *the* most important skill being taught or learned in childbirth education classes. It is the core of all other skills, including breathing and expulsion techniques.[7] Humenick found that prenatal relaxation skill achievement was significantly related to medication used in childbirth.[8] She also found that larger childbirth class size correlated negatively with achievement of relaxation skill for expectant mothers.[9]

Tensing during labor is a natural response to the contracting uterus. Tension, however, causes exhaustion and oxygen depletion, lowers the pain threshold, and prolongs labor. Adrenaline, the hormone that accompanies the fear-tension-pain syndrome, inhibits the effects of oxytocin, which causes the uterus to contract. This interference with oxytocin actually makes the contractions of the uterus less effective and prolongs labor.[10] There has been research documenting significantly shorter labors with increased relaxation skill.[11]

(text continued on page 330)

CLIENT EDUCATION

Choices in Childbirth

The two lists below do not represent an "either–or" situation. Most parents choose their options from both pathways. Very few doctors or midwives practice completely in accordance with either pathway. Consider and discuss each option and then decide which you prefer. Flexibility is necessary to ensure that the Birth Plan will apply in difficult or complicated labors as well as normal and typical labors.

Medical Pathway

Physiological Pathway

(Which of these are routines and which are options in your hospital or birth center? Most parents choose some options from each list.)

Labor

Medical Pathway	Physiological Pathway
• Mother in wheelchair upon arrival at hospital	• Mother walks to labor and delivery
• Shave, minishave, or clipping of long hairs on perineum	• No shave or clipping of hair
• Enema	• Bowels emptied spontaneously, or enema self-administered at home
• Partner asked to leave during prep and exams	• Partner present throughout labor and delivery
• Limit to one support person during labor and birth	• Presence of other friends, relatives, and siblings
• Confinement to bed or one position	• Freedom to walk and change positions as desired
• Induction of labor Methods: stripping membranes, amniotomy, oxytocin	• Spontaneous labor Alternatives: making love, breast stimulation
• IV fluids for hydration and energy	• Drinking fluid or eating as desired
• Frequent vaginal exams	• Vaginal exams when requested by mother or for medical reasons
• Electronic fetal heart monitor	• Listening to fetal heart with fetal stethoscope
• Pain relief through medication: analgesics or anesthetics	• Relaxation, emotional support, massage, breathing

Birth

Medical Pathway	Physiological Pathway
• Lithotomy position or semisitting in labor bed for pushing	• Choice of position and freedom to move
• Prolonged breath holding and bearing down for expulsion	• Mother follows her urge to push
• Limit of 2 hours on 2nd stage, then forceps or cesarean birth	• Allow for longer 2nd stage and position variations to help progress
• Delivery table for birth	• Birth in labor bed, birth chair, or bean bag
• Lithotomy position with stirrups for birth	• Side lying, all fours, squatting, standing with leg up, semireclining with back support, no stirrups
• Mother not allowed to touch sterile field	• Mother allowed to touch baby's head as it crowns
• Catheterization in 2nd stage	• No catheterization and frequent voiding in first stage
• Episiotomy	• No episiotomy: massage, warm compresses, slower delivery, coaching to pant out baby, support to perineum Late episiotomy with no anesthetic
• Forceps or vacuum extraction	• Spontaneous delivery

After Birth

Medical Pathway	Physiological Pathway
• Intubation/suctioning	• Waiting to see if baby can handle own mucus
• Immediate care of baby done out of sight of mother (e.g., identification, Apgar, heat lamp, replace hemostat with cord clamp	• Care done on mother's abdomen. Baby skin to skin with mother with heat lamp or blanket over them Delay in nonessential routines

(continued)

CLIENT EDUCATION (continued)

Medical Pathway

- Limit of 15–20 minutes on 3rd stage followed by manual extraction of the placenta
- Pitocin drip or injection for contraction of uterus after placenta is delivered

Baby
- Baby to isolette or nursery for 4–24 hours. Mother to recovery room for observation
- Eye drops—silver nitrate applied shortly after birth
- Baby's first feeding—glucose water by nurse
- Baby in nursery except for scheduled 4-hour feedings
- Circumcision
- Home in 3 or more days after delivery

Physiological Pathway

- Allow for longer time for placenta. Allow mother to move around, nurse baby. Let cord drain
- Evaluation of uterus before using uterine stimulant routinely
  Breast-feeding

- Baby held by mother or father on delivery table or in recovery
- Omit eye drops or delay administration up to 2 hours
- Colostrum by mother who plans to breast-feed or plain water given by mother
- Demand feeding, baby to mother when crying Twenty-four hour rooming in
- No circumcision
  Parents present to comfort baby after operation
- Early discharge from hospital

The Unexpected

Common Medical Procedures

Cesarean Birth

- Scheduled surgery
- Mother without her support person in surgery
- General anesthesia
- Screen to prevent viewing surgery
- Mother not allowed to wear contacts or glasses
- Baby sent to intensive care nursery

Possible Options

- Surgery after labor begins
- Father present to support mother
- Spinal or epidural
- Screen lowered at time of birth or baby held up for mother and father to see
- Mother to wear contacts or glasses
- Father to hold baby and mother to see baby, if baby is not in distress
  Mother allowed to breast-feed in recovery if her and her baby's condition permits

Premature/Sick Infant

- Baby cared for by professionals
- Baby rushed to intensive care
- Baby sent to another hospital or another part of hospital
- Baby transported to hospital with intensive care unit
- Limited visits to baby from mother only
- IV and bottle feeding

- Parents involved in care of baby, diapering, touching, talking to baby in incubator, feeding baby
  Mother allowed to hold and see baby, if not distressed
- Baby close to mother in same part of hospital
- Father goes with the transport team, mother goes if she is able
- Father or extended family allowed to see baby
- Mother allowed to express her colostrum for the baby and encouraged and helped to get started at breast-feeding

(Simpkin P, Reinke C: Planning Your Baby's Birth. Seattle, The Pennypress, 1980)

TABLE 20-2

Approaches to Teaching Relaxation

Name and Type	Description	Feedback
Progressive relaxation (modifies muscular responses)	Consists in systematically tensing and releasing muscles. Developed by Edmond Jacobson, modified by J. Wolpe into a 6-week approach with home practice.	Primary feedback initially described as the awareness of participant who focuses on the sensation of tensing and relaxing each muscle. Either a coach or electromyograph can provide feedback.
Neuromuscular dissociation (modifies muscular responses)	Follows progressive relaxation by asking the participant to tense some muscles and relax others simultaneously. Introduced in this country by Elisabeth Bing.	Feedback by having the coach check relaxation and tension was introduced by Karmel and Bing—not mentioned in books by either Fernand Lamaze or Irwin Chabon
Autogenic training (mental control modifying muscular and autonomic systems responses)	Training through suggestions including "my right arm is heavy" or "my left arm is warm." Includes slowing of the heart and respiration as well as cooling of forehead. Developed by J. Schultz and W. Luther.	Feedback initially described as the awareness of the participant with no outside feedback. Has been used with biofeedback equipment, thermometers, etc.
Meditation (modifies vascular and neurotransmitter responses)	Defined by Herbert Benson as dwelling on an object (repeating a sound or gazing at an object) while emptying all thoughts and distractions in a quiet atmosphere in a comfortable position. Used in transcendental meditation and yoga.	Concentration on a focal point and on breathing patterns would be forms of meditation by Benson's definition. Participant can monitor self but also receives coach's feedback on both activities.
Visual imagery	Includes techniques such as visualizing oneself on a warm beach or as a bag of cement or going down a staircase. Often precedes introduction of other kinds of relaxation. May also be used to visualize and potentially affect specific body parts as in cancer therapy. May be used in desensitization in which one relaxes while visualizing a potentially threatening situation. Used in labor rehearsals.	
Touching/massaging	Touch has always been a way for one person to calm another. There is evidence of actual transfer of energy taking place in some forms of touching. In childbirth preparation, touching is associated with muscular relaxation (Sheila Kissinger).	Feedback from coach includes informing when muscle tension is felt, necessitating advanced coaching. Coaches may need first to discern relaxation by moving a limb.
Biofeedback	Electromyograph measures neuromuscular tension.	
	Thermometer measures skin temperature at extremities.	
	Galvonic skin reflex records conductivity changes because of the action of sweat glands at the surface of the skin.	
	Electroencephalograph distinguishes alpha, beta, and theta waves in the brain.	Feedback from all of these machines is in one or more of these forms: visualization of a meter, listening to a sound, or watching a set of flashing lights.

(Humenick S: Teaching relaxation. Childbirth Educator, Summer 1984)

(text continued from page 326)

Learning to relax involves an active building of awareness of the state of the muscles, either tensed or relaxed, and a conscious control by the mind of that state. It is a learned activity, a process of isolating muscle groups, differentiating between tenseness and relaxation, and a conscious letting go of or total release of muscle groups. Relaxation is an active involvement of mind over body, which requires awareness, concentration, and practice.

Constant practice or repetition of a relaxation technique is necessary to maintain a conditioned response of this nature. Continued practice establishes patterns that can be depended on if thought processes become cloudy in active labor. The response will be well ingrained and the body will respond as automatically as possible during labor and birth with this conditioning.

The woman and her labor partner should practice relaxation exercises during the last weeks of pregnancy. During labor, the exercise is not practiced as such, but the skill the woman has learned by consciously relaxing her body while other body parts have been tensed will be used. During labor and birth all muscles that can be voluntarily controlled with the brain should be as relaxed as possible so the muscles of the uterus can work undisturbed, at maximum efficiency, and with the least amount of pain.

The skill of relaxation is not only helpful for birth but is a lifelong skill that can be called upon during the daily stresses of life.

There are many ways of teaching relaxation, including progressive relaxation, focusing, meditation, and touching.[12] Some of the methods are listed in Table 20-2.

To begin teaching relaxation it is important to start first with the simple techniques and after they are mastered to move to the more complex. A simple general-body relaxation technique is presented to begin with (see Conditioned Relaxation), followed by a progressive relaxation (see Preparatory Exercises for Controlled Relaxation) and finally a neuromuscular dissociation technique (see Practice Drill for Controlled Relaxation). All of these Client Education charts are in Appendix A.

Many people find an audiocassette recording of a relaxation technique helpful to supplement their practice with their partner. Several are listed in the Suggested Listening/Viewing at the end of this chapter. It is also possible for an individual to record her own relaxation tape by reading the Conditioned Relaxation exercise slowly into a tape recorder, with pauses for 3 seconds for . . . and about 6 seconds between paragraphs.

Guided Imagery

Coupled with relaxation, guided imagery can be a powerful coping mechanism for labor. Also called visual-

ization, imagery is a form of daydreaming with direction and purpose. It is a conscious experience in which an individual maintains a focus on one object of concentration. The physiological basis of how imagery decreases pain is not understood. However, several theories are currently proposed. It is known that when a person is in a highly relaxed state her electroencephalographic (EEG) recordings show brain waves in the alpha state and sometimes in the theta state[13] (Table 20-3). The alpha state is most easily created in a relaxed person. This state allows an individual to more efficiently use the functions of the right brain.

Some researchers have explored the theory that there is anatomical division of the brain into two hemispheres with separate functions (Table 20-4). The suggestion has been made that the different hemispheres allow the brain to access the central nervous system

TABLE 20-3

Brain Wave States

Beta	Alpha	Theta
Focus attention	Pleasant feelings	Drowsiness
Visual scanning	Well-being	Daydreaming
Anxiety, worry	Tranquility	Creative processes
Concentration	Relaxation	Problem solving
Fear	Relief from attention	Uncertainty
Frustration		Future planning
Excitement	Concentration	
Hunger	Wordless images	
Surprise	Blank nothingness	

(Bressler D: Free Yourself From Pain. New York, Simon and Schuster, 1979)

TABLE 20-4

Functions of Brain Hemispheres

Left hemisphere	Right hemisphere
Speech	Images
Words	Symbols
Analytic	Impulsive
Rational	Creative
Logical	Receptive
Sequential	Intuitive
Active	Emotional
Cognitive	Spiritual
Somatic control	Autonomic control

(Bressler D: Free Yourself From Pain. New York, Simon and Schuster, 1979)

Couples Participating in Training for Relaxation for Pregnancy/Labor and Birth/Life Stress

Nursing Objectives

1. The client will be able to state two sensations of relaxation that she felt while doing Conditioned Relaxation. (Appendix A)
2. The client will be able to correctly demonstrate tension and release during Preparatory Exercises for Relaxation. (Appendix A)
3. The client will tense stated muscle groups while releasing all others during Practice Drill for Controlled Relaxation. (Appendix A)
4. The client will be able to imagine a calm, serene environment and demonstrate this by increased relaxation during the Imagery Exercises. (Appendix A)
5. The client will demonstrate integration of relaxation, breathing and imagery by maintaining proper pacing of breathing and relaxation during a practice contraction.

Assessment	Potential Nursing Diagnosis	Intervention	Evaluation
1. Knowledge of benefits of relaxation in pregnancy, labor and birth, and life stress management	Knowledge deficit related to relaxation skills	After finding out what woman and partner know explain other benefits of relaxation. Include benefits for right now, labor and birth, and later life.	Verbalizes understanding May contribute some benefits No further questions
a. ↑ O_2 to baby/uterus		Give other examples in everyday life that may be familiar, for example, "tension headache" (tension causes ↑ pain).	
b. ↓ Fatigue			
c. ↓ Pain perception			
d. ↑ Feeling of competency and mastery			
3. Aids breathing for labor and expulsion of baby			
f. Facilitate labor process			
g. ↓ Blood pressure and stress disease			
h. Enhances feeling of well-being			
2. Past use of relaxation or hypnotic techniques, meditation, or yoga in any life situation and its effectiveness		Build on what she already knows. May be able to omit more basic techniques if she is currently skilled in a technique. Encourage her to use what she knows best or what has worked in the past.	
3. Partner's or friends' willingness to help her learn and practice new skill	Noncompliance related to: a. Partner's knowledge deficit about importance of relaxation skills	Include partner in teaching when possible. Discuss health benefit for partner also. Have partner participate by doing relaxation with woman as you teach. Teach partner how to assess woman's level of relaxation and how to give positive nonjudgmental feedback to her.	Partner assists with woman's learning, practice, and evaluation; gives appropriate feedback during practice
4. Motivation to practice consistently, 15–20 min/day	b. Powerlessness		
	c. Learning deficit: ineffective teaching		

(continued)

Assessment	*Potential Nursing* Diagnosis	*Intervention*	*Evaluation*
		Explain it will take time and daily practice (15–20 min) to be effective in labor/stress.	
5. Determine whether client(s) learn best with cognitive or effective modes.		Motivate by making sure couple understands benefits and physiological consequences resulting from unnecessary tension. Help couple plan specific home practice schedule with self-reward system to help motivate.	Couple practices, evidenced by verbal reports and by woman's increasing ability to relax as observed by nurse during practice sessions:
6. Determine whether the staff at client's chosen birth place are knowledgeable and willing to assist her with specific labor skills.		Tailor teaching to individual or with class provide multimodal approach. (See Table 20-2)	a. Relaxed jaw
			b. Slow, regular breathing
		1. Week 1: Start with basic whole body relaxation. (See Conditioned Relaxation—Appendix A)	c. Smoothed out facial muscles
			d. Legs rolled out and feet at 45° angle to each other
		2. Week 2: Progress to tense-release exercise. (See Preparatory Exercises for Controlled Relaxation—Appendix A)	Couple acts as team during observed practice session.
		3. Week 3: Progress to neuromuscular disasssociation exercise. (See Practice for Controlled Relaxation—Appendix A)	
		4. Week 4: Add Imagery Exercises (Appendix A)	
		5. Week 5: Have client integrate relaxation, breathing, and imagery during practice contractions.	

with two different and separate methods of communication. Access to the somatic nervous system is thought to be verbal, and access to the autonomic nervous system is thought to be the language of imagery, dreams, and intuition. The autonomic nervous system prepares the body for action through the sympathetic nervous system (SNS) and prepares the body for rest through the parasympathetic nervous system (PNS). When the PNS is activated, a feeling of tranquility occurs as the breathing and heart rate slows. The person who can learn to influence those activities of the body that previously were thought to be out of one's ability to control can benefit by stress reduction and pain control.[14]

To start a learning session on imagery the nurse must first create an atmosphere in which relaxation can occur. It should be as quiet as possible, lights lowered, and everyone should be in a sitting or comfortable reclining position. Selected music often helps (see Suggested Listening at the end of this chapter for suggestions). The teacher's position in the room should be where self-consciousness or embarrassment by the individual or group will be minimized. Once the physical setting has been established, the next task is to orient those present to the activity. This should include explaining what sensations to expect and emphasizing the need to just "let things happen." Occasionally, as individuals relax, they experience new or unusual feelings, which may include a feeling of losing control. The group, however, needs to be reassured that they will always remain in control and that to gain control, they first must learn to let go. It is important to set a low achievement level and allow anyone who does not want to participate to refrain from doing so. It is important also to mention that their minds may wander and closing the eyes may help by avoiding visual distraction. If someone prefers, keeping the eyes open is fine. Once the group is oriented, first the relaxation process is begun. Generally, any relaxation technique or breathing exercise can be used either in part or whole (see Conditioned Relaxation, Appendix A). When the group is relaxed, the next step is to begin the exercise in imagery (see Imagery Exercises, Appendix A).[15]

Because the experience of imagery may supercede time and space, upon completion of the exercise each person needs to be directed to slowly return to the physical realities of the room and their surroundings.[13] Afterward, the group needs to process the experience. Some people want to talk about what it was like, some find drawing or writing helpful, and others desire to be alone with their thoughts. The nurse needs to assess which may be most useful for the individual, and with a group it is not unusual to need to use all three types of activities.[11]

Breathing and Pushing Techniques

There are similarities between the breathing techniques used by the Maternity Center, in New York City, and those used in other prepared childbirth methods; therefore, we present the Maternity Center's breathing techniques (see Appendix A) as a general guide. The nurse must be aware, however, that these may vary in different parts of the country.

Postpartum Teaching

Parenthood often constitutes a stress in the developmental processes of both mothers and fathers. The postpartum period is particularly stressful because of the numerous physical changes the mother undergoes, the incomplete integration of her pregnancy and labor experiences, the changing roles that must occur within the family complex, and the uncertainty of the nature of the early mother–child relationship. Fatigue, confusion, feelings of helplessness and inadequacy, and depression often complicate this period. Isolation from the extended family, lack of community resources, economic strains, and pressures upon the woman to resume her full previous role within the family as rapidly as possible create additional stresses. Factors that may influence teaching and learning in the postpartum period are outlined in Table 20-5.

The nurse working on the postpartum unit has a unique opportunity to intervene early in the developing mother–child relationship and to assist the parents to anticipate and plan for the first few critical weeks at home. If the mother can attain a level of confidence in her ability to perform caretaking tasks and begin to recognize her baby's behavioral messages, a good foundation can be laid and later difficulties minimized.

Priorities for postpartum teaching focus on information concerning bodily changes and methods for relieving physical discomforts. Exercises and diet are important, and specific instruction is helpful.

The needs of the hospitalized postpartum woman may conflict with the nursing staff's needs to maintain the routine or provide the teaching they believe necessary. Mothers will progress at different speeds in assuming the caretaking role and will have individualized concerns. Finding a way to respond to individual needs yet conduct an efficient postpartum educational program is a major challenge to postpartum nurses.

Sources for continuing care and counseling need to be available to parents during the baby's first few months at home, and the postpartum nurse can direct them to such sources in the particular community.

Individual Teaching

Part of the postpartum nurse's daily responsibility is to provide individual instruction and support to mothers who are under her care. This can range from information about infant sleep and activity patterns, growth and development, and how to dress the baby for different types of weather to sibling rivalry, contraception, and organizing the household to get the necessary tasks done. Mothers' concerns may be small and particular, such as getting the baby to stay awake and suck well, or they may be larger and more general, such as the changes in her own and the father's life-style after the advent of the baby. The nurse needs to be informed about a wide variety of topics, including contraception,

T A B L E   2 0 - 5

Factors Influencing Teaching and Learning

Factor	Implications
Infant's condition	Preparation of the parents of a preterm infant or an infant with significant neonatal problems differs considerably from that of parents of the healthy, full-term infant.
Parental age	Parental age reflects development status. For example, the adolescent may need more concrete examples and be less able to assimilate written material.
Marital status	Marital status may influence the paternal role. Whether married or not, there is need to determine desired paternal involvement. Father should be included in caretaking activities when interested. Marital instability usually increases the anxiety level and makes teaching more difficult.
Parity	When there are other siblings, the family usually needs more of a review of child care than actual teaching. Some teaching should be directed at interaction with the other children and meeting their needs as well as the infant's.
Socioeconomic status	Socioeconomic status influences the parent's ability to provide material things for the infant, and it usually influences childrearing practices.
Educational level of the parents	Appropriate vocabulary should be used for verbal instruction and written material.
Experimental readiness	Previous learning transfers to the new situation. Insight enables the learner to apply older learning to a new situation.
Health beliefs and behaviors of the family	When health beliefs deviate from the usual, teaching may be difficult and more time required to convince the family of the need to change.
Emotional state of the learner	Some anxiety may enhance the learning process, but high anxiety militates against learning. Efforts should be made to lower high anxiety levels before proceeding with instruction. Attempts should be made to help parents work through feelings about their child's illness before attempting to teach.
Physical state of the learner	Physical discomfort may preclude or reduce learning.
Parental questions	The type of questions asked indicates learning needs.
Parental motivation	Motivated parents are usually easier to teach. The nurse needs to find ways of stimulating the apparently unmotivated.
Interest in the infant	Lack of interest in the infant makes teaching very difficult. When interest appears slight, there should be exploration of apparent disinterest.

(Oechler JM: Family Centered Neonatal Nursing Care. Philadelphia, JB Lippincott, 1961)

sexuality, and family dynamics, as well as infant care and involutional physiology.

Individual teaching allows the nurse to respond to the personal questions and concerns of mothers and to relate information to that particular situation. Reinforcement of mothering skills is particularly effective on an individual basis, as is counseling regarding family problems or emotions. However, the nurse may not have the time to give each mother the amount of individual teaching and counseling needed. Certain types of teaching can be effectively done in groups, and the use of postpartum groups has increased on hospital postpartum units. Baby-care classes seem well suited to group methods because the more experienced mothers can add their wisdom and practices to the pooled knowledge available.

Postpartum Classes

The organization of classes for postpartum mothers and fathers differs considerably from one institution to another. Each unit must work out the most convenient time for both staff and parents and a method of communication to ensure maximum attendance. Sometimes a conference room on the unit is used, or a large patient room can be adapted and extra chairs brought in. The teachers may be postpartum nurses only, or they may be nursery nurses, physicians, social workers, nutritionists, and public health nurses. A variety of media aids can be used, ranging from films to flip charts, books, or other printed material. Closed-channel television, which can be viewed by each mother in her room, has also been explored as a method of postpartum group instruction.

The content of postpartum teaching varies, but generally it includes content about the mother and her needs and information about the care of a newborn. Content about the mother should include getting enough rest, postpartum blues, family adjustment to a new baby, involutional physiology, pericare, breast care, sexuality, contraception, nutrition, and postpartum exercises. Mothers should be instructed in bathing and dressing the baby, breast-feeding or bottle feeding, holding and handling, cord care and care of the circumcision, routine tests (*e.g.*, the PKU test), and the normal range of newborn behaviors, including sleeping and crying. Some classes may include time for the mother to practice what she has just been taught while the nurse is available for assistance.

Special Classes

Some postpartum units organize special classes for mothers with particular needs, for example, there may be breast-feeding classes. The mothers are instructed in techniques of nursing, and possible problems and their prevention are discussed. Mothers whose babies are in the neonatal intensive care nursery, but who plan to nurse, may also be invited to these classes, or, better yet, special breast-feeding classes for a group of mothers of neonatal intensive care unit babies can be held. More experienced mothers can be encouraged to attend, as they are most helpful to new mothers who have never breast-fed before.

Common situations that breast-feeding mothers might encounter are discussed, and group solutions are developed. Questions such as what foods should be avoided, does breast-feeding ruin the breasts, and what to do when the mother plans to be away for several hours are elicited from the mothers. Answers to these questions can be provided by the nurse or other mothers in the group. Having the telephone number of the nurse for consultation if problems arise after discharge is very helpful to mothers and promotes continued success with breast-feeding. Hospitals are now beginning to hire certified lactation educators and consultants to provide specialized service and expertise to this growing population of clients.

If the hospital is large enough to have a regular census of diabetic, adolescent, or low-income mothers, postpartum classes to address their particular needs and concerns are helpful. Perhaps women who had a cesarean birth could make up another group, as their physiological problems often affect accomplishment of mothering tasks. If, however, the maternity service is relatively small and cannot support many different postpartum groups, the common concerns of baby care can be taught to a group of varied composition, with needs for particular information handled on an individual basis.

Outpatient Classes

Nurses and other health professionals are increasingly aware of the need to extend services to parents after discharge from the hospital. This care may be provided through the public-health department, hospital-affiliated clinics, private physicians' offices, a community liaison nurse from the postpartum unit, or health professionals in private practice.

Parenting Groups

The importance of the first year of life in the child's development, both behaviorally and physically, has led to establishment of "parenting groups" in a variety of settings. Because most couples are unprepared for the realities of parenthood, there is a need to educate parents with respect to basic processes of parenting in order to foster more realistic expectations.

Such groups often meet prenatally and continue into the postpartum period. The goal is generally to promote healthy parent–child relationships by educating parents about the physical and psychological aspects of pregnancy, childbirth, infant care, parenting, and child development. The group also promotes problem-solving skills, enhances parenting skills, and facilitates growth.

Post partum, the groups serve four primary functions: a source for socioemotional support, a forum to address a mother's specific problem, a setting in which the leader serves as a role model, and an arena in which to address common problems of all new mothers.[16]

These groups are often under the auspices of community adult education groups, large teaching hospitals (department of psychiatry), and sometimes professionals in private practice.

Mothers' Groups

Mothers' groups provided by local facilities can also be helpful to new mothers. If mothers receive little or no instruction in the hospital before discharge, these groups can offer answers to many common concerns about care of the baby and support in mothering abilities. Cultural differences must be respected, and the structure must be informal and friendly if such groups are to be effective.

The content of each class varies, but information about infant nutritional needs and feeding methods is important and should be covered in detail, as inadequate nutrition and protein deprivation are common problems among this group, which may create serious implications for the baby. General care of the infant, particularly bathing, diaper care, and causes of simple skin rashes, is another standard topic.

Sharing among the mothers can also enhance learning. If the atmosphere is comfortable, these mothers can be encouraged to examine practices that might be contributing to the baby's health problems, and possibly to modify these practices.

The nurse has the opportunity to observe the infants for signs of illness and refer them to the pediatrician if needed. She is also able to identify serious emotional problems and make appropriate referrals.

The LaLeche League provides a mothers' group in support of breast-feeding. Distribution of information and group sharing of solutions to breast-feeding and other common questions of new mothers make this a valuable source of support for new and expectant mothers.

Cluster Visits

Cluster visits constitute one approach to pediatric care that uses the group method. A small number of mothers and their babies, usually four pairs, are scheduled for a joint visit with the pediatric nurse practitioner or pediatrician. Each baby is examined with the mother standing by, findings are explained, and instructions are given for minor illness or problems. Subjects of general interest are postponed until discussion time, which follows the examinations. While one mother and baby are involved in the examination, the others are getting acquainted and comparing notes.

During the discussion period, the nurse and mothers talk about childrearing, feelings related to motherhood and baby care, changes in the family structure, or other topics relevant to the baby's age or the mother's needs. The groups are formed to include mothers with babies of about the same age. The mothers generally take the lead in the discussion and often provide specific information and teaching for one another. During the last 10 minutes, the next cluster visit is planned and immunizations are given to the babies as needed.

These cluster visits are usually alternated with individual visits. They permit more care to be provided to mothers and babies using less professional time. The mothers involved tend to respond very positively, as they enjoy the camaraderie, the sharing of problems and anxieties, the chance to observe other babies, and the knowledge and support gained through the discussion. This group experience increases parental confidence and shows how babies are individuals whose weight and development vary. There appears to be no increased cross-contamination. Cluster visits are one way of providing improved health care at a lower cost to parents.

Parent Effectiveness Training

Other outpatient groups for parents are those that train parents how to prevent behavior problems in their children. Parent Effectiveness Training (PET) was started in the early 1960s by Dr. Thomas Gordon, a clinical psychologist from Pasadena, California. Parents attend class one night a week for 8 weeks and learn active listening and other communication skills, behavior modification, and methods of resolving parent–child conflicts. Content also includes dealing with infants and toddlers. PET classes are available in many communities in all 50 states and are sometimes sponsored by schools, social agencies, or organizations serving parents, as well as health professionals in private practice.

Postpartum Exercises

During the puerperium, the 6 weeks following childbirth, the body undergoes major changes. In effect, a bodily transformation that took 9 months to complete is being reversed in the course of a few weeks.

Good nutrition and adequate rest are essential during this period. A new mother needs at least one rest period each day. Lying on the abdomen may help the uterus to return to good position (Fig. 20-6). A pillow under the hips and ankles when she is lying in this position prevents back strain.

Postpartum exercises are important in restoring muscle tone and the woman's figure. Many of the ex-

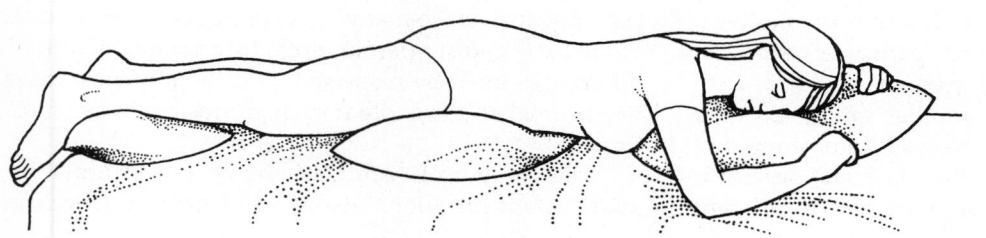

FIGURE 20-6

Prone position for rest and relaxation post partum.

ercises that are used during the prepartum period are also useful in the postpartum exercise program. In an uncomplicated delivery, simple exercises may be started during the first postpartum day. If the woman had an abnormal delivery or extensive perineal repair, exercises may need to be delayed.

A postpartum exercise program should progress in phases, beginning with simple exercises and progressing to more strenuous ones. When the mother is able to comfortably accomplish the repetitions of one phase, she is ready to progress to the next. Women progress at different rates, and the same woman does not progress through all phases at the same rate. For example, the chart Postpartum Exercises (Appendix A) suggests two series of progressive exercises, and it is not uncommon for a woman to easily progress through all of the phases of one series, but experience difficulty with one of the exercises in the other series. This should not be a matter of concern. The woman should progress through all exercises at her own pace. As with prepartum exercises, emphasis should be placed on avoiding fatigue, and the mother should not do any exercise that causes pain. If the exercises are practiced properly, they should not be tiring. They should be done slowly and rhythmically, only a few times at first, and gradually increased.

The postural reflex needs to be reestablished post partum so that the woman doesn't continue the stance she had during pregnancy. This means she must consciously contract the abdominal and pelvic floor muscles to balance the pelvis again after the sudden loss of its load. Because of the hormones of pregnancy, the joints are still at risk for a few weeks and good body mechanics are essential to protect the joints and ligaments. The abdominal muscles are obviously in need of exercise.

The goal is to achieve a flat abdomen and good posture, with the pelvis tilted back to realign correctly with the spine.[4]

Diastasis Recti. It is not uncommon for the longitudinal muscles (recti) of the abdomen to separate (diastasis) during pregnancy, labor, or delivery (Fig. 20-7). The gaping can be slight or severe. If these muscles are not corrected, the abdominal wall will remain weakened and will not be supportive for a subsequent pregnancy. Because the recti muscles are important in controlling the tilt of the pelvis, their weakness can give rise to poor posture and pain in the lower back. A postpartum check of the recti muscles is done about the third day after delivery. Until this time the entire abdominal area feels so slack that the test is not reliable.

The following exercise may be done to see if diastasis has occurred. Lie on back with knees bent. Press the fingers of one hand firmly into the area around the navel. Slowly raise head and shoulders until neck is about 8 inches from the bed. The bands of muscles on each side will pull toward the midline, pushing the fingers out of the way. A slight gap, one or two fingers, is just tissue slackness and will tighten by itself. A gap of three, four, or more fingers between the muscles requires a special exercise to restore the integrity of this area.

There is an exercise to correct it. If diastasis has occurred, the exercise is done by lying on the back with knees bent. Cross hands over the abdominal area to pull the muscles toward the midline as head is raised. Take a deep breath. Raise the head (and later the shoulders to a 45° angle) off the bed while exhaling, and at the same time pull the muscles together. Return slowly to original position. Repeat exercise often and gradually work up to at least 50 times a day. Until the diastasis

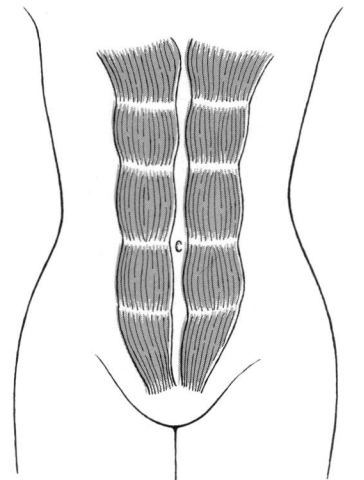
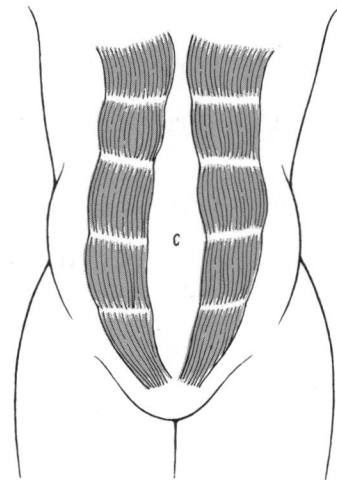

Abnormal   Normal

FIGURE 20-7

Diastasis recti.

has closed, the woman should avoid exercises that rotate the trunk, twist the hips, or bend the trunk to one side.[4]

The purpose of the pelvic floor exercise after delivery is to enable the muscles to resume their role in supporting pelvic contents and to reestablish sphincter control. It is an excellent exercise to maintain lifelong pelvic floor tone and to enhance sexual enjoyment. It is also widely used for women with sexual dysfunction to increase their capacity for orgasm, and it is helpful for minor degrees of cystocele.

Applying the Nursing Process to Parenthood Preparation

Assessment

The nursing process is especially important in the area of client education. One of the important aspects of any educational program is to begin where the learner is. This is accomplished by careful assessment of a specific client's or group's knowledge base. In assessing this knowledge base, the maternity nurse must take into consideration a whole range of knowledge the client should have from the cause and alleviation of the normal discomforts of pregnancy to knowledge necessary to understand and comply with the dietary changes necessary for the gestational diabetic. This process should be carried out by means of a systematic written assessment to ensure a thorough assessment that is available to all the staff.

Nursing Diagnosis

Potential nursing diagnoses common to maternity client education include specific knowledge deficits (unaware of what dietary changes are necessary during pregnancy), powerlessness (not learning how to cope with labor because it won't help anyway), noncompliance (not taking a full course of antibiotics because she felt better and was not told why it is important to do so), and fear and anxiety that interfere with learning (not "hearing" how to rotate injection sites for newly diagnosed Class B diabetic because fear of giving her own injection was not dealt with first).

Planning/Intervention

Nursing intervention is based on the diagnoses. The nursing care plan displayed earlier in this chapter gives examples of interventions for a client (couple) who has a knowledge deficit about relaxation for labor.

Evaluation and Reassessment

The nurse's evaluation of the success of instruction is both observable and measurable. Has there been a change in the client's eating habits? What changes? Is the couple practicing labor-coping strategies at home? Did the client take all the antibiotics as prescribed? Is the client feeling more comfortable about giving her own injections? Did the nurse observe a change in her performance? Can she state why site rotation is necessary? With evaluation the feedback loop of reassessment occurs and the nursing process begins anew.

References

1. Gorman AH: Teachers and Learners in the Interactive Process of Education. Boston, Allyn and Bacon, 1969
2. Sosa R, Kennell J, Klaus M: The effect of a supportive companion on perinatal problems, length of labor, and mother–infant interaction. N Engl J Med 303:597–600, 1980
3. Gaziano E, Garvis M, Levine E: An evaluation of childbirth education for the clinic patient. Birth Fam J 6:89, Summer 1979
4. Noble E: Essential Exercises for the Childbearing Year. Boston, Houghton-Mifflin, 1982
5. Caldeyro–Barcia R: The influence of maternal bearing-down efforts during second stage on fetal well-being. Birth Fam J 6:17, Spring 1979
6. Bean CA: Methods of Childbirth. New York, Doubleday & Co, 1972
7. Shrock P: Relaxation Skills: Update on Problems and Solutions. Genesis (ASPO) Vol 6, No. 5, October/November 1984
8. Humenick S: Assessing the quality of childbirth education: Can teachers change? Birth Fam J 7:82–90, Summer 1980
9. Humenick S, Marchbanks P: Validation of a scale to measure relaxation in childbirth education classes. Birth Fam J 8:141, Fall 1981
10. Ewy D, Ewy R: Preparation for Childbirth. New York, New American Library, 1976
11. Gregg, R: Biofeedback and biophysical monitoring during pregnancy and labor. In Busmajian JV (ed): Biofeedback Principles and Practice for Clinicians. Baltimore, Williams & Wilkins, 1979
12. Humenick S: Teaching relaxation. Childbirth Educator, Summer 1984
13. Blattner B: Holistic Nursing. Englewood Cliffs, NJ, Prentice-Hall, 1981
14. Bressler D: Free Yourself From Pain. New York, Simon and Schuster, 1979
15. Steffes S: Relaxation plus: The use of guided imagery or visualization. In Humenick S (ed): Expanding Horizons In Childbirth Education. Arlington, VA, ASPO/Lamaze, 1983
16. Heinicke C, Carlin E, Given K: Parent and mother–infant groups. Young Children, March 1984

Suggested Reading

Artal R: Exercise during pregnancy and the postnatal period. ACOG, May 1985

* Bing E: Six Practical Lessons for an Easier Childbirth. New York, Bantam Books, 1977

Hilbers S: Paced breathing: Terminology changes and teaching techniques. Genesis (ASPO) Vol 5, No 6, January 1984

Humenick S: Relaxation tapes for childbirth preparation: A review. Birth, Vol 9, No 4, Winter 1982

* Karmel M: Thank You, Dr. Lamaze. Philadelphia, JB Lippincott, 1959

McKay S, Roberts J: Second stage labor: What is normal? JOGN Nurs, Vol 14, No 2, pp 101–106. March/April 1985

* Noble E: Essential Exercises for the Childbearing Year. Boston, Houghton-Mifflin, 1982

* Rozdilsky ML, Banet B: What Now? A Handbook for New Parents. New York, Charles Scribner's Sons, 1975

* Salk L: Preparing for Parenthood. New York, Bantam Books, 1975

Shrock P: Relaxation skills: Update on problems and solutions. Genesis (ASPO) Vol 6, No 5, October/November 1984

Simkin P, Reinke C: Planning Your Baby's Birth. The Pennypress, 1100 23rd Avenue East, Seattle WA 98112 (50¢)

Snyder M: Progressive relaxation as a nursing intervention: An analysis. Adv Nurs Sci, pp 47–58. April 1984

Suggested Listening/Viewing

Relaxation Tapes for Childbirth Preparation—Audiocassettes

"Labor-eze" by Kenneth and Gloria Price, 2 sides 20 minutes each, $12.95 plus tax and handling, 12800 Hillcrest Rd., Suite 116, Dallas, TX 75230

"Preparing for Easier Childbirth: Home Practice Exercises" by Elizabeth Bing, 2 sides 29 minutes each, $9.95, 200 Park Ave. South, New York, NY 10003

"Relaxation Tapes for Childbirth . . . and After" by Rae Grad, 6 sides 12 to 15 minutes each, $18.00 plus $1.00 shipping, Box 6358, Alexandria, VA 22306

Music For Relaxation/ Labor—Audiocassettes

"Celtic Harp" by Patrick Ball, Fortuna Records, 1982

"Fairy Ring" by Mike Rowland, Sona Gaia Productions, 1982

* If not available locally write to International Childbirth Education Association Book Center, PO Box 20048, Minneapolis, MN 55420 USA.

* $8.50 plus $1.50 shipping for each audiocassette, ASPO of LA, 7761 Airport Blvd., Los Angeles, CA 90045; $42.00 plus $2.50 shipping for each VHS videocassette

"Pachabel Canon and Other Baroque Favorites" by Paillard Chamber Orchestra, RCA Corp., 1983

"Pachabel's Greatest Hit, Canon in D" by Pachabel, RCA Corp., 1984

"Seascapes" by Michael Jones, Narada Productions, 1984

*Videotapes

"The Lamaze Method: Techniques for Childbirth Preparation," narrated by Patty Duke Astin, ASPO/Lamaze, Embassy Home Entertainment, 1983 (45 minutes, color, VHS)

"Postnatal Exercise Program," American College of Obstetricians and Gynecologists, Feeling Fine Programs, Inc., 1985 (55 minutes, color, VHS)

"Pregnancy Exercise Program," American College of Obstetricians and Gynecologists, Feeling Fine Programs, Inc., 1985 (51 minutes, color, VHS)

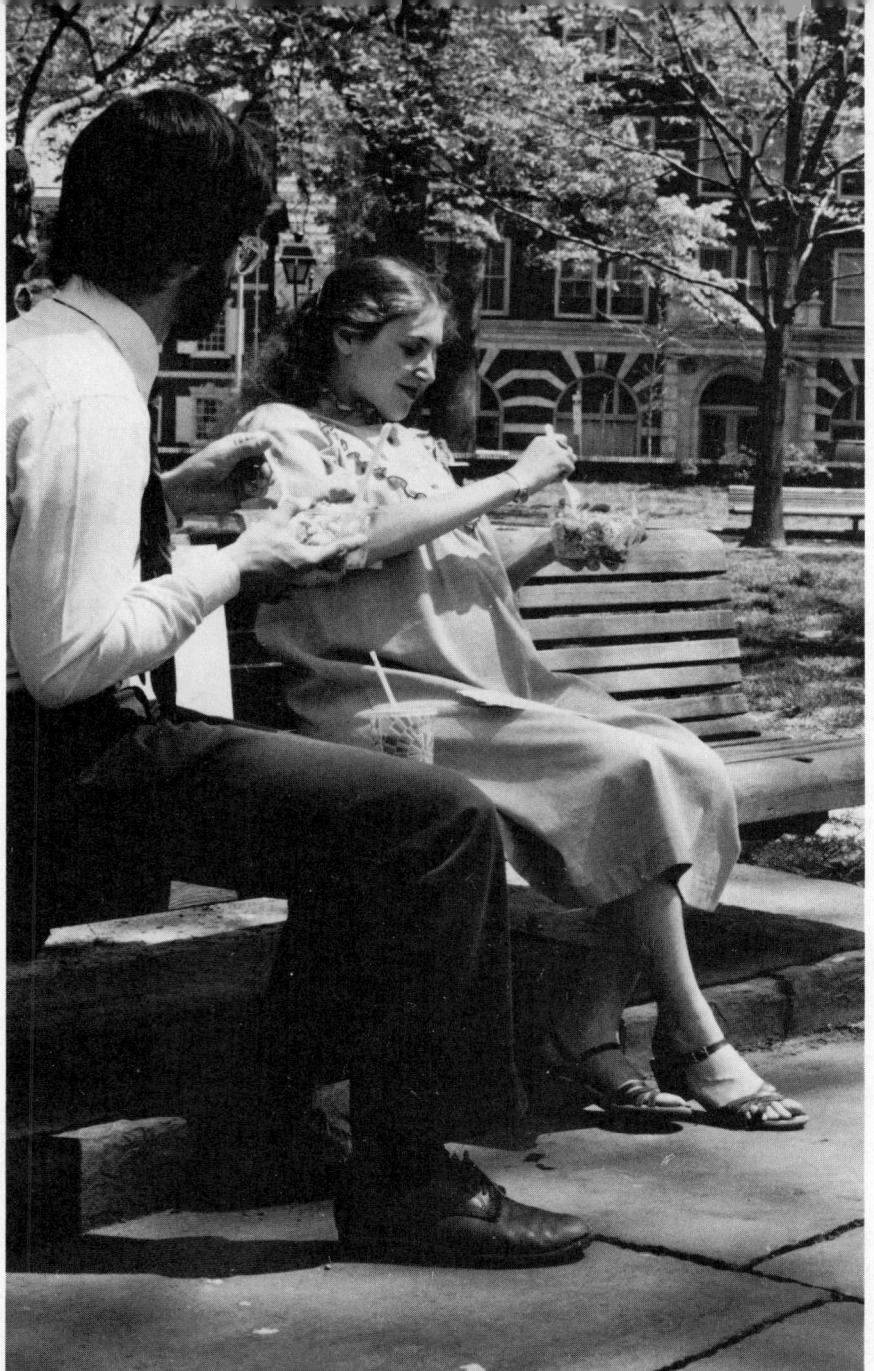

CHAPTER 21

Nutritional Care in Pregnancy

Nutrition plays a key role in the outcome of pregnancy. A woman's nutritional status at conception and the quality of the diet she consumes during the following months help to determine her health and well-being and that of her child. Ensuring optimum nutrition for all childbearing women might not eliminate all the problems of pregnancy, but it is a giant step in the right direction.

If counseling is to be effective and the results lasting, the nurse should strive to elicit wholehearted cooperation from the client. This may be facilitated by involving her in the planning; considering her needs, background, preferences, and attitudes and those of her family; providing information; encouraging and reinforcing appropriate choices and preparation; providing gentle but firm limit setting when indicated; and giving careful, thorough explanation regarding the rationale behind the advice.

If the pregnant woman is helped to understand the importance of good nutrition for herself and her fetus, she may be more motivated than at other times in her life to improve her dietary habits. She should be encouraged to continue her new interest in nutrition after the baby arrives. These improvements can have long-lasting effects on her family. Not only does improved nutrition promote better health for the present family, but it can have a positive effect on future pregnancies of the mother and her children.

Importance of Nutrition During Pregnancy

The importance of maternal nutrition during pregnancy has long been recognized. Evidence of its importance was provided in 1970 when the National Academy of Sciences issued a report that reviewed studies of reproductive experiences and concluded that adequate prenatal nutrition is one of the most important environmental factors affecting the health of pregnant women and their babies.[1]

Over the years a wide variety of dietary advice has been given to the pregnant woman. This includes instructions that ranged from severe restriction of intake to admonitions to eat large quantities, and from limitation of protein to high-protein diets.[2] The final words on the effects of nutrition during pregnancy have not been written, but at present, stress is being placed on the importance of adequate nutrition before, during, and after pregnancy.

Effects of Poor Nutrition

Controlled studies on animals have shown a direct relationship between maternal diet and pregnancy out-

*Possible Adverse Effects of Poor Nutrition on the Reproductive Cycle**

Infertility

Reproductive casualty
  Abortion
  Stillbirth
  Neonatal death

Pregnancy problems
  Preeclampsia and eclampsia
  Placental abnormalities
  Gestational diabetes

Difficult labors and deliveries

Low-birth-weight infants

Slow postpartum recovery of mother

Difficulties with lactation

Delayed mental and physical development of infant

* Obviously there are many other factors that influence the occurrence of these problems, but prepregnant nutritional status and nutrient intake during pregnancy play a significant role.

come. Although it is not possible to show a direct cause-and-effect relationship between specific nutrients and specific problems in human studies, general correlations have been found. Chronic malnutrition in developing countries and in low-income populations of developed countries has been shown to be related to reproductive problems, including difficulties during pregnancy, labor, and delivery; increased perinatal mortality; and low birth weight and other problems of the newborn.

Some historical occurrences have provided study populations that demonstrate the effects of nutritional deprivation under conditions that would not have been purposely set up. During World War II, a 7-month food embargo of western Holland decreased the population's average daily food ration to fewer than 750 calories. In a retrospective study, women who were pregnant or who conceived during the famine were shown to have a higher incidence of stillbirth and neonatal mortality and decreased infant birth weight.[3] Similar effects on pregnancy were found during the siege of Leningrad in 1941 and 1942.

Effects of Supplementation

There have been a number of studies in the past few decades that are designed to demonstrate the effects of improved nutrition on the pregnancies of women with deficient nutrition. In some of these studies supple-

mentation is by means of additional food and in others it is by provision of a prepared supplement of either protein and calories or just calories. One such study, in which supplemental food was used, was carried out at the Montreal Diet Dispensary. In this study, women who were determined to be at risk nutritionally and who were given supplemental foods showed a lower incidence of preeclampsia and other diseases of pregnancy, had easier deliveries with fewer cesarean sections, and had infants with a greater mean birth weight and considerably lower neonatal morbidity and mortality rates.[4]

Other studies, especially those using prepared protein and calorie supplements, have sometimes shown less promising results. Generally they have substantiated the belief that adequate nutrition during pregnancy is important for optimal maternal and fetal outcome, but they have also shown that supplementation is not always the answer to improving perinatal outcome.[5]

Effects on Mental Development

When discussing the effects of nutrition on mental development, it is difficult to differentiate between prenatal and postnatal nutritional effects. The critical period for brain cell development begins during pregnancy and continues during the first year of life. The nutritionally deprived fetus may have decreased development of brain cells, but if optimum nutrition is provided after birth, the effects may be reversible.[6]

Inductees into the Dutch armed forces whose conception, gestation, or birth occurred during the 1944 to 1945 famine were compared with other Dutch inductees who were born in the same time period, but not living in the famine area. Although birth weights in the famine area were significantly lower than in other areas, intelligence tests failed to show significant differences between famine and nonfamine subjects.[6] A possible explanation for the good mental outcomes of the survivors of the famine in spite of their prenatal nutritional deprivation is that the Dutch were generally well nourished before and after the famine, in contrast to many other study populations who suffer from chronic malnutrition and other deprivations.[7]

On the other hand, when malnutrition during and following pregnancy is associated with other forms of environmental deprivation, mental retardation and severe, long-lasting behavioral effects, such as learning disabilities, are more frequent. The Montreal Diet Dispensary study indicates that improved nutrition during pregnancy and lactation improved the mental development of the children in the study, compared with siblings who were born before the mother received supplements.[8]

Assessment

Each pregnant woman has a unique nutritional background. Many factors influence her nutritional status and her daily food intake. To be able to help these women choose the best possible diets during their pregnancy, the nurse needs to be aware of the factors, their effect on each individual, and ways of obtaining information about them.

Assessing Dietary Intake

To gather information about the client's food habits and actual food intake, an atmosphere and opportunity must be provided for the woman to discuss her concerns about food and diet and to give information about her current dietary patterns. Nutritional evaluation requires information on what is eaten, as well as the quantities and the method of preparation. Information regarding purchasing practices is also needed. Certain foods may not be purchased because of cost and more economical substitutions may be needed.

The *Nutrition Questionnaire* that was developed by the California Department of Health Services is a useful tool in assessing the client's food habits. It should be completed by the client on her first prenatal visit and used as a basis for a nutritional counseling interview. Some questions may not be applicable to all client populations, and other questions may need to be added in some areas.

To provide appropriate guidance for the woman and to better assess her level of understanding and knowledge about her diet, a *diet history* can be taken to determine actual eating patterns. The nurse may ask the woman to describe or write down her food intake for the past 24 hours or for a typical day. This should include the time, place, and the type and amount of food eaten. These are a variety of forms available that may be useful in obtaining a diet history (see Diet History and Evaluation Form).

Another method of obtaining the information is to have the woman keep a *diary* of everything she eats for 2 or 3 days. She should be advised to avoid holidays or days with atypical diet patterns, to record everything as soon after eating as possible, to write down amounts of each food as accurately as she can, and to describe sauces and condiments, such as cheese sauce or soy sauce. Some women have difficulty remembering to write things down, but even if the diary is incomplete, it can still provide useful information.

The *Guide to Food Frequency* can provide useful information for identifying food preferences and dislikes that might lead to diet inadequacies. However, it should be used only with a diet history or food intake diary because it does not show daily food patterns and amounts.

Assessing Nutritional Status

Gathering information about a variety of maternal characteristics can help in assessing a woman's nutritional status.

Anthropometric evaluation includes various measurements of the body. Height and weight are the most common measurements taken. Comparing height to pregravid weight gives an estimate of body build, which is useful in determining standard weight and identifying the underweight person. Recording weight at intervals throughout the pregnancy also allows comparisons of the individual's weight gain pattern with the recommended pattern (see Prenatal Weight Gain Grid). Measurement can also include the use of tape measures and calipers for skin fold width, but these are not usually done and are not necessary for most women.

Laboratory tests are used to determine the presence of adequate amounts of certain nutrients. Hemoglobin and hematocrit are done routinely to evaluate the woman's iron status and need for supplements. The serum folacin level may be used as an indicator of nutritional intake.[9] Determination might also be made of serum albumin, total serum protein, and serum vitamin B_{12}. Additional hematologic values may be obtained in assessing specific nutrient-related problems.[10]

General physical assessment of the pregnant woman can provide useful information in assessing nutritional status. Alone, the signs may not be reliable indicators, but considered together, and with laboratory tests and dietary history, they can provide useful clues for further investigation (Table 21-1).

Assessing Individual Dietary Factors Involved in Food Choices

The *psychological aspects of nutrition* are important determinants of food choice, but do not lend themselves to clear-cut analysis. Food is a basic need for survival, and hunger is one of the most fundamental of all sensations.

Related to hunger, but of a very different origin, is appetite. Appetite is Nature's primary defense for the prevention of hunger. Based on the anticipation of eating, the impulse is determined by the person's previous experience. Only by coincidence and training does appetite become associated with health-giving foods. Factors affecting food-seeking behavior are the main de-
(text continued on page 351)

T A B L E   2 1 - 1

Physical Indicators of Nutritional Status

Body Area	Normal Appearance	Signs Associated With Malnutrition
Hair	Shiny, firm, not easily plucked	Lack of natural shine; hair dull and dry; thin and sparse; fine, silky, and straight; color changes (flag sign); can be easily plucked
Face	Skin color uniform; smooth, pink, healthy appearance; not swollen	Skin color loss (depigmentation); skin dark over cheeks and under eyes (malar and supraorbital pigmentation); lumpiness or flakiness of skin of nose and mouth; swollen face; enlarged parotid glands; scaling of skin around nostrils (nasolabial seborrhea)
Eyes	Bright, clear, shiny; no scores at corners of eyelids; membranes a healthy pink and are moist; no prominent blood vessels or mound of tissue on sclera	Eye membranes are pale (pale conjunctivae); redness of membranes (conjunctival injection); Bitot's spots; redness and fissuring of eyelid corners (angular palpebritis); dryness of eye membranes (conjunctival xerosis); cornea has dull appearance (corneal xerosis); cornea is soft (keratomalacia); scar on cornea; ring of fine blood vessels around cornea (circumcorneal injection)
Lips	Smooth, not chapped or swollen	Redness and swelling of mouth or lips (cheilosis); especially at corners of mouth (angular fissures and scars)
Tongue	Deep red in appearance; not swollen or smooth	Swelling; scarlet and raw tongue; magenta (purplish color) of tongue; smooth tongue; swollen sores; hyperemic and hypertrophic, and atrophic papillae
Teeth	No cavities; no pain; bright	May be missing or erupting abnormally; gray or black spots (fluorosis); cavities (caries)
Gums	Healthy; red; do not bleed; not swollen	"Spongy" and bleed easily; recession of gums
Glands	Face not swollen	Thyroid enlargement (front of neck); parotid enlargement (cheeks become swollen)
Skin	No signs of rashes, swellings, dark or light spots	Dryness of skin (xerosis), sandpaper feel of skin (follicular hyperkeratosis); flakiness of skin; skin swollen and dark; red, swollen pigmentation of exposed areas (pellagrous dermatosis); excessive lightness or darkness of skin (dyspigmentation); black and blue marks due to skin bleeding (petechiae); lack of fat under skin
Nails	Firm, pink	Nails are spoon shaped (koilonychia); brittle, ridged nails
Muscular and skeletal systems	Good muscle tone; some fat under skin; can walk or run without pain	Muscles have "wasted" appearance; baby's skull bones are thin and soft (craniotabes); round swelling of front and side of head (frontal and parietal bossing); swelling of ends of bones (epiphyseal enlargement); small bumps on both sides of chest wall (on ribs)—beading of ribs; baby's soft spot on head does not harden at proper time (persistently open anterior fontanel); knock-knee or bowlegs; bleeding into muscle (musculoskeletal hemorrhages); person cannot get up or walk properly
Internal systems		
Cardiovascular	Normal heart rate and rhythm; no murmurs or abnormal rhythms; normal blood pressure for age	Rapid heart (above 100 tachycardia); enlarged heart; abnormal rhythm; elevated blood pressure
Gastrointestinal	No palpable organs or masses (in children, liver edge may be palpable)	Liver enlargement; enlargement of spleen (usually indicates other associated diseases)
Nervous	Psychological stability; normal reflexes	Mental irritability and confusion; burning and tingling of hands and feet (paresthesia); loss of position and vibratory sense; weakness and tenderness of muscles (may result in inability to walk); decrease and loss of ankle and knee reflexes

(Reprinted with permission from Nutritional Assessment in Health Programs, American Journal of Public Health, 63: November, 1973 Supplement)

A S S E S S M E N T   T O O L

Nutrition Questionnaire

A nutritional questionnaire such as this one developed by the California Department of Health Services can be an invaluable tool in helping to assess a client's nutritional intake.

Name: _____ Date: _____

Please answer the following by checking the appropriate box or filling in the blank. Answer only those questions that apply to you. All information is confidential.

I. a) Before this pregnancy, what was your usual weight?
  _____ lbs. ( ) Don't Know
  b) During your last pregnancy, how much weight did you gain?
  _____ lbs. ( ) Don't Know
  c) How much weight do you expect to gain during this pregnancy?
  _____ lbs. ( ) Don't Know
  d) Have you ever had any problems with your weight?
  ( ) Yes ( ) No
  If yes, what? ( ) Underweight
  ( ) Overweight
  ( ) Other _____

II. a) How would you describe your appetite?
  ( ) Hearty ( ) Moderate ( ) Poor
  b) With this pregnancy, have you experienced either of the following?
  ( ) Nausea ( ) Vomiting

III. a) How would you describe your eating habits?
  ( ) Regular ( ) Irregular

IV. a) Indicate the person who does the following in your household:
  Plans the meals _____
  Buys the food _____
  Prepares the food _____
  b) How much is spent on food each week for your household:
  $ _____ ( ) Don't Know
  How many people does this feed? _____
  c) Indicate the types of kitchen equipment you have in your home:
  ( ) Refrigerator ( ) Stove
  ( ) Hot plate

V. a) Are you *now* taking any vitamin or mineral supplement?
  ( ) Yes ( ) No
  b) Do you take any pills to control your weight?
  ( )Yes ( ) No

c) Do you take diuretic (water) pills?
  ( ) Yes ( ) No

VI. a) Are you now on a diet to lose weight?
  ( ) Yes ( ) No
  b) Are you *now* on a special diet (low salt, diabetic, gallbladder)?
  ( ) Yes ( ) No
  If yes, what kind of diet? _____
  c) If you have been on a special diet in the past, indicate what kind and when.
  _____
  _____

VII. a) Is there any food you *can't* eat?
  ( ) Yes ( ) No
  If yes, what foods? _____
  _____
  What happens when you eat this food? _____
  _____
  b) Do you have any cravings for things such as the following:
  ( ) cornstarch
  ( ) plaster
  ( ) dirt or clay
  ( ) other _____

VIII. Do you have any of the following problems?
  ( ) constipation
  ( ) diarrhea

IX. a) Do you smoke? ( ) Yes ( ) No
  b) Do you drink any alcoholic beverages (liquor, wine, beer)? ( ) Yes ( ) No

X. Are you receiving either of the following?
  ( ) food stamps
  ( ) WIC vouchers

XI. How do you want to feed your baby?
  ( ) breast feed
  ( ) evaporated milk formula
  ( ) commercial formula
  ( ) undecided

(Nutrition During Pregnancy and Lactation. Maternal and Child Health Unit, California Department of Health, 1975)

A S S E S S M E N T   T O O L

A Diet History

A "diet history" or "food diary" could use a simple form such as the one below.

Daily Food Intake

Patient's name: _____

Date: _____ Food intake recorded by: _____

Instructions

1. Include everything eaten from the time she gets up until she goes to bed.
2. Food should be described in terms of how it was prepared and served (*e.g.*, mashed potatoes and gravy; salad of raw carrots with raisins and mayonnaise).
3. Approximate amounts should be listed for each individual food (*e.g.*, 1 small carrot, ¼ cup raisins; 1 tablespoon mayonnaise).

Time	Place	Food Eaten (description)	Amount

(Nutrition During Pregnancy and Lactation. Maternal and Child Health Unit, California Department of Health, 1975)

ASSESSMENT TOOL

Diet History and Evaluation Form

It is desirable to obtain a dietary history as early as possible in pregnancy and before recommending a specific diet for an individual mother. This history should include information concerning the expectant mother's usual food practices, meals often omitted, typical menu patterns, food likes and dislikes, cultural factors, methods of food preparation, financial situation, and so on. Nutritional gaps will be obvious from an evaluation of this information. During the process of taking a diet history, useful information is obtained concerning the patient's level of nutrition knowledge and clues to methods of counseling. Explaining any recommended changes will help the expectant mother understand her present needs. If history is kept in patient's chart and information is recorded elsewhere, interviewer may prefer to omit some questions. Sample form may be changed to fit situation.

Name _____ Date _____
_____ Due Date _____
Patient's childhood home _____ Height _____
  (State or country) _____ Present weight _____
Patient's occupation _____ Pregravid weight _____
Last year school completed _____
Husband's occupation _____ Birth date _____
Money available for food weekly _____ Number in household _____
Food currently bought by _____
Meals currently prepared by _____
Foods liked especially, including cravings _____

Foods never eaten and why (storage problems, equipment, and so on) _____

Nutritional supplements currently used during pregnancy (kind and amount used) _____

Diet modified previously or currently (type of diet and date) _____

Meals and snacks often eaten at the following times:
Morning: _____

Midmorning: _____

Midday: _____

Afternoon: _____

Evening: _____

Before bedtime: _____

(continued)

A S S E S S M E N T   T O O L   *(continued)*

Prenatal diet prescribed and date ————————————————————————————
Instruction received on prenatal diet including materials given ————————————————

——

Additional information ——————————————————————————————————

Follow-up remarks ———————————————————————————————————

Prenatal dietary history recorded by: ———————————————————————

——

——

——

(Cross AT, Walsh HE: Prenatal diet counseling. Reprod Med 7:269–270, 1971. From Nutrition—During Pregnancy and Lactation. Berkeley, CA, California State Dept. of Public Health, 1971)

A S S E S S M E N T   T O O L

Guide to Food Frequency

This guide to food frequency can be a helpful tool in a nutritional assessment. However, it should only be used with a diet history or food intake diary.

Name: ————————————————————————— Date: ————————————————

Instructions

Indicate whether or not you eat the following foods by checking the columns "Don't eat" or "Do eat" for each item. For each food you have checked "Do eat" write the approximate number of times you eat it in a week. If you eat any particular food less than once a week, do not write anything in the column "Times eaten per week."

In some cases more than one food has been listed on a line. If you do not eat all of these foods, underline the specific foods you eat. A space has been provided at the end for you to write in foods not listed which you regularly eat.

Food	Don't Eat	Do Eat	Times Eaten Per Week	For Office Use Only
I. Chicken				
Beef, hamburger, veal				
Liver, kidney, tongue				
Lamb				
Cold cuts, hot dogs				
Pork, ham, sausage				
Bacon				
Fish				

(continued)

A S S E S S M E N T   T O O L   (continued)

Food	Don't Eat	Do Eat	Times Eaten Per Week	For Office Use Only
Kidney beans, pinto beans, lentils (all legumes)				
Soybeans				
Eggs				
Nuts or seeds				
Peanut butter				
Tofu				
II. Milk (fluid, dry, evaporated)				
Cottage cheese				
Cheese (all kinds other than cottage)				
Condensed milk				
Ice cream				
Yogurt				
Pudding and custard				
Milkshake				
Sherbert				
Ice milk				
III. Whole grain bread				
White bread				
Rolls, biscuits, muffins				
Bagel				
Crackers, pretzels				
Pancakes, Waffles				
Cereals				
White rice				
Brown rice				
Noodles, macaroni, grits				
Tortillas (flour)				
Tortillas (corn)				
IV. Tomato, tomato sauce, or tomato juice				
Orange or orange juice				

(continued)

A S S E S S M E N T   T O O L   (continued)

Food	Don't Eat	Do Eat	Times Eaten Per Week	For Office Use Only
Tangerine				
Grapefruit or grapefruit juice				
Papaya, mango				
Lemonade				
White potato				
Turnip				
Peppers (green, red, chili)				
Strawberries, cantaloupe				
V. Dark green or red lettuce				
Asparagus				
Swiss chard				
Bok choy				
Cabbage				
Broccoli				
Brussels sprouts				
Scallions				
Spinach				
Greens (beet, collard, kale, turnip, mustard)				
VI. Carrots				
Artichoke				
Corn				
Sweet potato or yam				
Zucchini				
Summer squash				
Winter squash				
Green peas				
Green and yellow beans				
Hominy				
Beets				
Cucumbers or celery				

(continued)

A S S E S S M E N T   T O O L   *(continued)*

Food	Don't Eat	Do Eat	Times Eaten Per Week	For Office Use Only
Peach				
Apricot				
Apple				
Banana				
Pineapple				
Cherries				
VII. Cakes, pies, cookies				
Sweet roll, doughnuts				
Candy				
Sugar or honey				
Carbonated beverages (sodas)				
Coffee or tea				
Cocoa				
Wine, beer, cocktails				
Fruit drink				
VIII. Other foods not listed which you regularly eat				

(Nutrition During Pregnancy and Lactation. Maternal and Child Health Unit, California Department of Health, 1975)

(text continued from page 343)

terminants of eating (*i.e.,* hunger, appetite, and custom). The great deterrents to normal appetite are worry, fear, and preoccupation with troublesome or difficult problems. These may be reflected in either an increase or a decrease in appetite. Some of the positive emotional stimulants include situations that encourage feelings of calm contentedness, mild elation, or ego-stimulation.

Present-day food choices are a combination of heritage, superstition, custom, knowledge, and opportunity. Subtle cravings are passed along from one generation to the next by the process of training and imitation. Unique methods of food preparation as well as food selection, combinations, and prejudices are embodied in this training. Congeniality and hospitality are en-

hanced by the serving of good food, and it has become the custom to serve food at practically all functions, business as well as social.

From infancy onward, food and closeness are associated with love and security. Food and eating are looked upon as symbolizing interpersonal acceptance, warmth, and sociability. Throughout all societies this symbolic undertone is unmistakable; from the "breaking of bread" in antiquity to the modern banquet, the serving of food is a vehicle for expressing honor, joy, or mutual bonds. It is easy to see why food has become associated with the symbolism of motherliness. Feeding is not only kindly and warm in its emotional meaning to those who receive food, but it is also essential to growth and well-being; hence, it has become bound up

ASSESSMENT TOOL

Prenatal Weight Gain Grid

Guide to prenatal weight gain grid.

Recommended weight gain during pregnancy is 2 to 4 pounds (1 kg–2 kg) during first trimester and 0.9 pound (0.5 kg) per week for second and third trimesters. For optimum care, the prenatal weight gain grid should be used with all pregnant women. This tool provides a visual representation of the patient's weight gain during pregnancy by plotting the patient's weight gain at every visit.

Patient's Name: _____

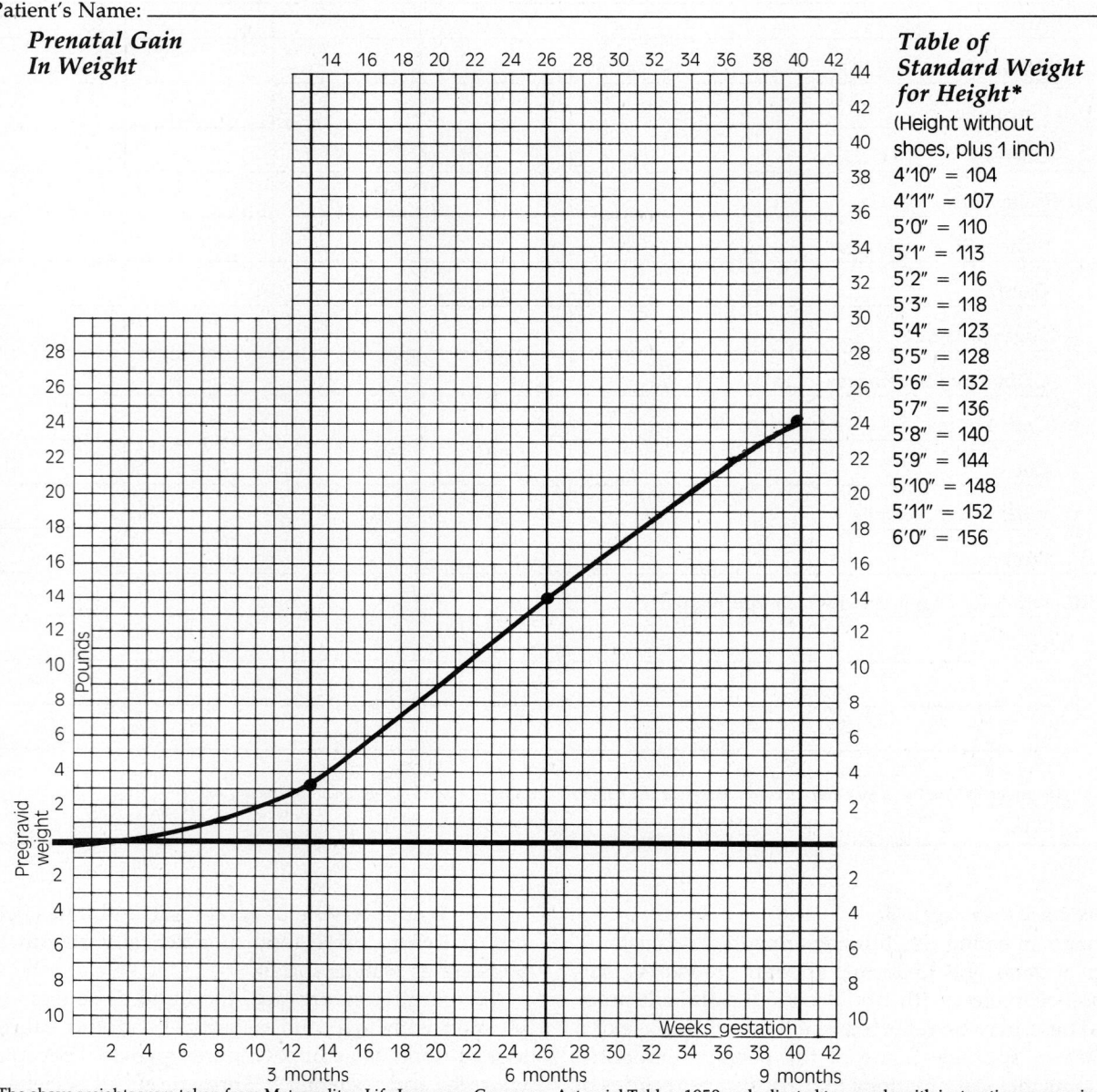

Prenatal Gain In Weight

Pounds

Pregravid weight

Weeks gestation

3 months   6 months   9 months

Table of Standard Weight for Height*
(Height without shoes, plus 1 inch)

Height	Weight
4'10"	= 104
4'11"	= 107
5'0"	= 110
5'1"	= 113
5'2"	= 116
5'3"	= 118
5'4"	= 123
5'5"	= 128
5'6"	= 132
5'7"	= 136
5'8"	= 140
5'9"	= 144
5'10"	= 148
5'11"	= 152
6'0"	= 156

* The above weights were taken from Metropolitan Life Insurance Company, Actuarial Tables, 1959 and adjusted to comply with instructions appearing on the Prenatal Weight Gain Grid, namely, height in inches without shoes plus 1 inch to establish a standard for heels. Patients should be weighed with shoes as normally worn. The table above is for medium body build and except for extreme body build deviations, these figures should be used. For example, a patient whose height, measured without shoes, is 5 feet 4 inches would have one inch added; therefore, her standard weight for height would be 128 pounds.

Ranges are not acceptable in estimating standard weight since this is an objective observation and represents the midpoint. This midpoint must be used for recording purposes.

For patients under age 25 one pound should be deducted for each year.

(Nutrition During Pregnancy and Lactation. Maternal and Child Health Unit, California Department of Health, 1975)

with the idea of the mother, the one who originally nurtured, loved, and supported.

The pregnant woman makes a close identification with the concept of the mother, and selections and choices may be influenced profoundly by these symbolic meanings of food. She may crave certain foods and reject others, and not because of physiological factors. For instance, she may feel that certain foods will "mark" her baby or will give him strength. It is crucial that the meaning food has for the client be explored and that her feelings and attitudes be respected.

The *stage of growth and development* of the client may also influence her food choices. For instance, foods enjoyed by adolescents are often different from those enjoyed by older people.

When people marry younger and become parents at an earlier age, they carry these eating patterns into marriage with them. In addition, adolescence is a time for developing independence, and this is healthy. However, many foods may be rejected (*e.g.*, milk, vegetables, cereal, and the like) because they are associated with "home" and a dependency period. The desire to be free and to select the "forbidden" foods is very strong.

The *religious, racial,* and *ethnic background* of the client and her family is also an important consideration. Certain foods may be highly valued and others excluded from the diet. Methods of preparation may also be different. Many families are fond of their regional or national diet and prefer it to the American "meat and potatoes" regimen.

Knowing the client's ethnic background can be helpful in understanding her dietary habits (Table 21-2), but there is much variation within ethnic groups. These differences may be related to climate, growing conditions, geographic relocation, intermarriage, and individual differences. Therefore, assumptions should not be made about a client's food habits based only on surname or language spoken.

An *individual dietary pattern, vegetarianism,* has become the dietary choice of an increasing number of people in recent years. Some abstain from eating meat

TABLE 21-2

Ethnic Dietary Characteristics

Ethnic Group	Protein Foods	Milk and Milk Products	Grain Products	Vegetables and Fruits	Counseling Suggestions
Mexican–American	Variety of meats; poultry, legumes, eggs	Not usual part of adult diet as beverage; small quantities of cheese in cooking	Tortillas and rice are staples	Tomatoes, chili peppers, fried potatoes, other raw or boiled vegetables, oranges, apples, bananas	Increase cheese and milk in cooking, and milk as beverage. Encourage variety of vegetables eaten raw or cooked for short time in small amount of water Decrease consumption of carbonated beverages and other empty-calorie foods Encourage use of enriched flour for tortillas
Puerto Rican	Beans, chicken, pork, beef, eggs; ham butts and sausage used for flavoring, not	Limited use— "cafe con leche" may contain 2 oz to 5 oz milk	Rice; French bread, rolls, crackers, increasing use of cereals	Pumpkins, carrots, green pepper, tomatoes, sweet potatoes, special boiled	Encourage milk and cheese Suggest meat source with bean meal

(continued)

TABLE 21-2 *(continued)*

Ethnic Group	Protein Foods	Milk and Milk Products	Grain Products	Vegetables and Fruits	Counseling Suggestions
	as a protein source			root vegetables, canned fruits and nectars	Urge more leafy green vegetables Increase use of citrus and other fresh fruits and use of whole grain or enriched breads, cereal, and rice
Black/Southern	Beef, pork, chicken; legumes as accompaniment	Some milk, buttermilk, cheese, ice cream	Rice, biscuits, white and corn bread	Greens, sweet potatoes, okra, cabbage, corn, green beans, usually boiled; seasonal fruits, limited citrus	Increase milk and decrease carbonated beverages Encourage whole grain cereals and bread Decrease water and time for cooking greens and other vegetables Eat some raw vegetables Increase vitamin C sources
Chinese	Fish, chicken, pork, legumes, eggs, nuts	Ice cream, flavored milk, some milk in cooking	Rice, millet, noodles	Variety of vegetables, often stir-fried with minimal nutrient loss; many fruits, usually fresh	Increase serving sizes of protein foods, or use as snacks Increase calories Encourage dairy products in cooking and use of tofu (soybean curd) Discourage washing rice because of nutrient loss
Japanese	Variety of meat and fish, eggs, nuts, legumes, tofu (soybean curd)	Milk and milk products limited	Polished rice, some wheat products	Variety of fruits and vegetables	Encourage use of dairy products to overcome major dietary problem Use calcium and vitamin D supplements if necessary Avoid par-cooking of vegetables and washing of rice to avoid nutrient loss

for religious or health reasons, while others choose the vegetarian way to make more efficient use of the world's resources or to economize on their food bills. Vegetarian diets vary in the extent to which they exclude animal sources of protein. Lacto-ovovegetarians exclude meat, but include eggs and dairy products and sometimes fish, poultry, and liver. Lactovegetarians exclude all animal protein sources except dairy products. A small minority of vegetarians in the United States are "pure" vegetarians, or *vegans*, who exclude *all* animal sources of protein. Besides the obvious need to make sure the pregnant vegetarian obtains enough high-quality protein, it is also important for the nurse to be aware that some vegetarians, especially the vegans, may have diets lacking in other nutrients. Their caloric intake may be low, leading to low prepregnancy weight and low pregnancy weight gain. Owing to avoidance of dairy products, they may not get enough calcium in their diets. They also run the

risk of developing a vitamin B_{12} deficiency, since this vitamin is found only in foods of animal origin.[11]

Food allergies or *intolerances* can develop to a number of different foods. Adjustments in the diet may be required to avoid these foods and still obtain adequate amounts of the essential nutrients. Intolerance to the milk sugar lactose is a particular problem during pregnancy because it is difficult to meet the pregnant woman's need for calcium, protein, and certain vitamins and minerals without using milk.

Assessing Nutritional Risk Factors

There are certain factors that place women "at risk" for nutritional problems related to pregnancy and require special attention to nutritional needs. These factors can be grouped into categories (Table 21-3).

TABLE 21-3

Nutritional Risk Factors

Category	Factor	Significance
Age	Adolescence	Increased nutritional needs; possible poor food habits
	Older gravidas	Possible increased incidence of other risk factors
Obstetric history	High parity or frequent conceptions	Depletion of maternal nutrient stores
	Previous obstetric complications	Possible nutritional relationship may recur
Medical history	Preexisting medical problems	May affect ingestion, utilization, or absorption of nutrients
Complications of current pregnancy	Development of complications, such as anemia, preeclampsia, or gestational diabetes	Development of nutritional deficiencies due to increased nutritional needs
Maternal weight	Low prepregnancy weight	Increased incidence of pregnancy and neonatal complications
	Insufficient weight gain	Indication of poor maternal and fetal nutrition; increased number of low-birth-weight infants
	Obesity	Possible poor nutritional habits; increased incidence of pregnancy complications
	Excessive weight gain	If sudden, may indicate preeclampsia; lack of agreement on other possible risks
Dysfunctional dietary patterns	Dietary faddism	Diets often inadequate to meet fetal or maternal nutritional needs
	Pica	Displacement of nutritious foods, often related to iron deficiency anemia
	Excessive use of alcohol, drugs, or tobacco	Interference with appetite and with utilization of some nutrients
Socioeconomic status	Low income	Limited ability to buy sufficient food; possible chronic malnutrition
Cultural or ethnic group	Ethnic or language differences	Interference with ability to find usual foods; misinterpretation of dietary instructions
Psychological conditions	Depression, anorexia nervosa	Possible reduced caloric and nutrient intake

Age

A woman's age can affect her nutritional needs during pregnancy as well as her dietary habits. *Women under the age of 17* who become pregnant have their own growth needs to satisfy in addition to their pregnancy needs and those of the fetus. This increases their nutritional requirements at a time when they may be reluctant to follow dietary instructions or to gain weight. Adolescent pregnancies have been associated with low birth weight, prematurity, and increased perinatal mortality (see the section Counseling the Pregnant Adolescent for further discussion of nutrition and the adolescent who is pregnant).

Older gravidas may also be at increased nutritional risk, mostly because they have a greater chance of being in one of the other risk categories.

Obstetric History

High parity or *frequent conceptions* can cause depletion of maternal nutrient stores, leading to pregnancy complications, unless the diet is of very high quality.

Previous obstetric complications, such as inadequate weight gain, preeclampsia/eclampsia, anemia, gestational diabetes, antepartum hemorrhage, premature or small-for-gestational-age infants, and fetal or neonatal death, have nutritionally related factors and may recur in the present pregnancy. These women need very good nutritional guidance.

Pregnancy Complications

Complications that develop during the current pregnancy, such as anemia, gestational diabetes, or preeclampsia, may indicate the development of nutritional deficiencies due to increased nutritional needs. Continuing emphasis on a well-balanced diet is important, as well as specific help, possibly from a dietitian, to meet the individual needs related to the condition.

Medical History

Preexisting medical problems, including anemia, cardiac disease, diabetes, hypertension, and infections, may affect the ingestion, absorption, or utilization of nutrients. These clients will need nutritional guidance to meet their pregnancy needs and to incorporate any diet therapy for the particular condition.

Maternal Weight

Low prepregnancy weight is defined as 10% or more under the standard weight for height. Underweight women have been shown to have more pregnancy complications, and their infants a higher incidence of

prematurity and low birth weight, lower Apgar scores, and increased neonatal morbidity. Improved nutrition with adequate weight gain during the pregnancy has been shown to improve the outcome.

Insufficient weight gain during pregnancy has been shown to be correlated with low-birth-weight infants and may indicate poor maternal and fetal nutrition. Pitkin defines it as a gain of 1 kg or less per month during the second or third trimester.[12] Jacobson suggests failure to gain 10 pounds by the 20th week of pregnancy as a means of identifying the woman at risk.[13]

Obesity is defined as a weight 20% above the standard weight for height (see Prenatal Weight Gain Grid on p. 352 for standards). The obese maternity client is at risk for developing such problems as hypertension, gestational diabetes, and thrombophlebitis. The obesity also indicates, in most cases, that her nutritional habits are not optimal. It is sometimes tempting for the obese client to try to lose weight during pregnancy, but this can be dangerous to the fetus. When caloric intake is low enough to cause weight loss, maternal fat stores are catabolized for energy, resulting in ketonemia. Evidence suggests that ketosis is poorly tolerated by the fetus, and maternal acetonuria during pregnancy has been associated with significant lowering of the IQ scores of the offspring.[14]

Kitay advised that "education in the proper foods to eat, rather than weight reduction, should be paramount during pregnancy" for the obese patient.[9] Improved dietary habits learned during pregnancy may lead to easier weight reduction after pregnancy.

Excessive weight gain during pregnancy has not been well defined, nor is there agreement on whether or not it should be considered a risk factor.

Pitkin defines excess weight gain as a gain of 3 kg or more per month.[14] Some studies have shown that pregnancy outcome continues to improve as maternal weight gain increases, but others indicate that there can be problems above a certain optimal gain.[15] Those favoring unrestricted weight gain cite concern that any limitation will possibly limit needed nutrients.

Dysfunctional Dietary Patterns

Dietary faddism refers to diets that are very restrictive or food habits that concentrate on certain foods or food groups to the exclusion of others. Food regimens such as the macrobiotic diet, the Atkins diet, or the Stillman diet are insufficient for even a nonpregnant woman if pursued for a prolonged period of time. For the pregnant woman, with her increased nutritional needs, they should not be used at all. Besides endangering the fetus, they sometimes induce harmful metabolic changes in the mother.

Pica is usually defined as the craving for and ingestion of nonnutritive substances such as clay, laundry starch, raw flour, or ice. In some cases there are regional preferences for certain substances. The cause is unknown, but in many instances it appears to be related to iron deficiency anemia as either a cause or an effect. Some studies indicate that the ingested substances could lead to anemia by displacing iron-containing foods, but others have demonstrated that iron therapy can stop the cravings.[16] When large quantities are ingested there is usually some displacement of nutritious foods to the detriment of the woman's nutritional status.

Excessive use of alcohol, drugs, or *tobacco* can interfere with appetite and with the utilization of some nutrients, sometimes resulting in congenital anomalies, low birth weight, and, in the case of alcohol and drugs, withdrawal symptoms in the infant after delivery. See Chapter 8 for further discussion.

Socioeconomic Status

Low income limits the amount of money available for food and may be related to an inadequate nutrient intake. Low maternal nutrient stores may also be a problem owing to chronic malnutrition. There is an increased likelihood of low-birth-weight babies and other reproductive problems in low socioeconomic groups.

Ethnic or Language Differences

Ethnic or language differences may contribute to nutritional problems in the pregnant woman. She may not be able to find the foods she is used to cooking, and substitutions may not furnish the same nutrients. Also, if English is not spoken, she may misunderstand or misinterpret dietary instructions or recipes.

Psychological Conditions

Mental illness such as depression, and eating disorders such as anorexia nervosa or bulimia, may lead to a reduced caloric and nutrient intake. The result may be poor maternal weight gain with the possibility of low-birth-weight infants and increased perinatal mortality. See "Eating Disorders" in the section on Counseling the Pregnant Adolescent, for further discussion of this topic.

Nursing Diagnosis

Nutritional assessment of the pregnant woman can lead the nurse to a variety of nursing diagnoses that can then be used in planning and implementing care. Most of these nursing diagnoses would involve the diagnostic category Alteration in Nutrition and then be related to different factors that might put the expectant mother

or fetus at increased risk for problems. Some possible diagnostic statements would be:

Alteration in nutrition: less than body requirements, related to inadequate caloric intake
Alteration in nutrition: less calcium than required for pregnancy, related to decreased intake of dairy products secondary to lactose intolerance
Alteration in nutrition: inadequate weight gain, related to self-imposed limitation of calories

Knowledge deficit is another diagnostic category that might be appropriate for nutritional problems of the pregnant woman. A possible diagnostic statement would be: knowledge deficit regarding nutritional needs during pregnancy, related to lack of informational resources.

Planning/Intervention: Dietary Counseling

In her contacts with women during the reproductive cycle the nurse has many opportunities to use the nursing process in assisting each individual woman to improve her nutritional status. Drawing from the information in the previous section on assessment, the nurse can work with individuals or groups of clients to plan and implement nutritious food choices.

The responsibility for initial and ongoing dietary evaluation and counseling varies from one prenatal setting to another. If a dietician or nutritionist is available, she may see all clients at least one time, or her services may be limited to seeing high-risk clients and consulting with staff concerning other clients. In the absence of a nutritionist or dietician, the primary responsibility for nutrition counseling may rest with the nurse. Whether it is her primary responsibility or a shared responsibility with other members of the health-care team, the nurse plays an important role because she usually sees the client at each visit and often is the one available to answer questions. If more than one person is involved in the counseling, it is important that there be consistency in the nutritional information taught and the advice given. Nutrition counseling ideally begins at the first prenatal visit, starting during the assessment of dietary intake.

As the nurse and the woman plan together, the client's likes and dislikes are recognized, and those foods that provide the essential nutrients are encouraged. Suggestions may be given for the addition of certain foods or the modification of existing methods of selecting or preparing it. Incorporating the woman into the planning and allowing her choices whenever possible, helping her to increase her knowledge of nutrients, encouraging and reinforcing correct choices or willing adaptations, and giving firm guidance when indicated, all help the client and the nurse to achieve their respective goals.

Many women are already eating an adequate diet. They may only need reinforcement of their dietary habits and encouragement to continue what they are doing. For those women whose dietary intake is not adequate or whose history indicates one or more risk factors, consistent counseling toward optimum nutritional intake is vitally important.

The nurse must have a tolerant and nonjudgmental attitude and should respect the client's right to reject dietary information if she chooses. This attitude may be difficult for the nurse to achieve, since health-care providers traditionally expect their advice to be followed. However, more may be gained in the long run by accepting the "client's right to choose." A client is more likely to seek care from those she feels respect her views, even when these views differ from those of the provider.

Dietary counseling should be an ongoing aspect of prenatal care. It is not enough to talk about it at the first visit and hand out a suggested diet plan or food guide. There should be some discussion of nutrition at each follow-up visit, with reinforcement or additional suggestions as needed. Periodic use of diet recall or a food diary can be helpful in assessing the extent to which the suggestions are being followed. The following sections include information on specific areas that may be helpful in counseling.

Calorie Intake and Weight Gain

Calories provide the energy requirements for the body and are needed to maintain bodily processes, thermal balance, and physical activity. Caloric allowances are established to provide for adequate energy requirements and to support growth and body weight levels for the fetus and mother that are commensurate with health and well-being.

In the past, it was generally recommended that weight gain be limited by caloric restriction, with the purpose of preventing and controlling preeclampsia and eclampsia. However, in recent years, controlled studies have not supported the contention that caloric intake as reflected by weight gain causes preeclampsia. To the contrary, there is evidence that limiting weight gain decreases essential nutrient intake, which is thought to be one of the contributing factors in the development of preeclampsia.

In pregnancy there is an increased need for calories to meet the energy requirements for building fetal and placental tissue and for maintaining the woman's tissue requirements. The recommended dietary allowance (RDA) is 300 kcal/day above the woman's usual RDA.

For the individual woman actual needs could vary according to many factors, including her size and activity. Vermeersch suggests calculating individual needs by allowing approximately 40 kcal/kg of pregnant body weight or about 18 kcal/lb.[17] In a study group at the Montreal Diet Dispensary, additional calories are recommended for specific conditions such as protein deficiency, underweight, and special conditions of stress.[8]

One of the main risks to the newborn is low birth weight and the problems that accompany it. The outcome for the infant has been shown to improve as the birth weight increases. Many studies have shown the relationship between maternal weight gain and birth weight. It is these findings, coupled with concern over the relatively high United States perinatal mortality rate, that have led to the recommendation of more liberal weight gain for the mother during pregnancy. The weight gain recommended varies from one source to another. Some suggest that unlimited weight gain might be best to ensure an adequate intake of nutrients. Others advocate a minimum gain of 24 or 25 lb, with a range of 24 lb to 30 lb.

In a study conducted by Naeye, optimum pregnancy weight gain was shown to be related to prepregnancy weight.[15] According to his findings mothers who began pregnancy very overweight had the lowest perinatal mortality when they gained 15 lb to 16 lb. For the very thin mothers, the most favorable gain was about 30 lb, and for the average-weight mothers, about 20 lb. Ademowore and colleagues demonstrated that maternal weight gain alone is less important as an indicator of birth weight than the quality of nutrition.[18]

Components of Weight Gain

For some time, it was taught that maternal weight gain was adequate if it consisted only of the amount necessary for the products of conception and that anything over that would just be stored by the mother as "unwanted fat." Although the exact components of weight gain and the proportions of each are not known, and probably vary from one pregnancy to another, a possible distribution of average weight gain is shown in Figure 21-1. Table 21-4 indicates weight gain as shown in Figure 21-1. These figures are rough estimates only, and if actual weights could be measured, they might differ. The fat component is sometimes quoted as being closer to 2 kg, and in some analyses, part of the maternal gain is credited to lean muscle mass.

It is apparent from Figure 21-1 that most of the gain during the second trimester is related to maternal tissues, while the fetus gains the most during the third trimester. The pattern of total weight gain is also illustrated in this figure. This pattern is believed to be much more important than the actual amount of weight gained. The usual pattern consists of a 1-kg to 2-kg (2 lb–4 lb)

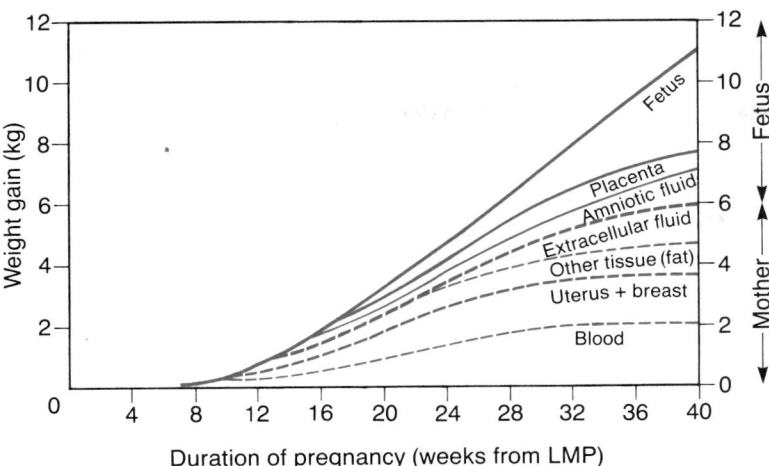

FIGURE 21-1

Pattern and components of cumulative gain in weight during pregnancy, assuming total gain of 11 kg. (Pitkin RM: Nutritional support in obstetrics and gynecology. Clin Obstet Gynecol 19(3):491, September 1976)

weight gain during the first trimester, followed by an average, fairly steady, gain of about 0.4 kg (0.9 lb) per week during the last two trimesters.[12]

The Prenatal Weight Gain Grid on page 352 shows the recommended pattern. It can be used to plot the pattern of each individual's weight gain and to detect any deviation. For example, a sudden, sharp increase in weight after the 20th week may indicate excessive water retention and the onset of preeclampsia. Inadequate weight gain or weight loss can also be noted.

Promoting Adequate Weight Gain

Counseling in regard to weight gain varies from one client to another. Some women have been counseled to restrict weight with previous pregnancies or have heard about this practice from friends and believe it is the best way. They may need reassurance that gaining over 20 lb is beneficial for both themselves and the baby. Other women may think that they can limit the size of the baby and have an easier delivery if they eat less. They can be helped to understand that if the mother's nutritional status is poor, the labor and delivery might be difficult regardless of the size of the baby.

Some women are very weight conscious and may resist gaining adequate weight because of fears that they will not be able to lose it after the baby is born. Careful explanation of the distribution of the additional weight and the importance of good nutrition to the outcome of pregnancy may help them accept the weight gain. Holey states, "Knowing from her first prenatal visit that her 'temporary pounds' will influence her unborn child and prepare her for the work of motherhood is not only fascinating to the mother, but makes sense of the puzzle—'Why should I gain so much weight?' "[19]

Women who gain weight rapidly during the first two trimesters may reach what they consider to be maximum gain by the seventh month. They then attempt to cut down on what they eat to try to avoid gaining any more weight. This deprives them of adequate nutrients at the time when fetal brain cells are growing the fastest and when the fetus is depositing a protective layer of fat.[20] These women need encouragement to continue eating adequately.

Making Calories Count

"Making calories count" is not the same as saying that pregnant women should count their calories; it is to emphasize the importance of eating only foods that contribute necessary nutrients to the diet. "Empty calories" are to be avoided, especially if the woman's appetite is poor or her food dollar is limited. The obese woman also benefits from this kind of instruction, not only during pregnancy, but also in planning a weight reduction program after pregnancy. "Eat to appetite" may be a good slogan to promote adequate weight gain during pregnancy, but it is only valid when the woman is taught which foods to eat to obtain the most nutrients.

The woman whose diet consists mainly of foods such as doughnuts, candy bars, and soda pop may satisfy her appetite, but her nutritional status suffers

TABLE 21-4

Components of Weight Gain During Pregnancy

	kg	lb
Fetal components		
Fetus	3.4	7½
Placenta	0.6	1½
Amniotic fluid	1.0	2¼
Maternal components		
Uterus and breasts	1.6	3½
Blood	2.0	4½
Extracellular fluid	1.6	3½
Other tissue (fat)	0.8	1¾

and she gets a very poor return for her food dollar. This does not mean that desserts must be eliminated from the diet. Custard, made from eggs and milk, is an example of a nutritious dessert. The nutritive value of other desserts such as baked goods can be improved by the use of whole grain flour and the addition of wheat germ or extra eggs and milk.

Nutrient Needs

A brief review of basic nutrition may be helpful to the nurse in teaching her clients about good nutrition during pregnancy. All foods are made up of a combination of classes of nutrients: carbohydrates, proteins, fats, vitamins, minerals, and water. Carbohydrates, proteins, and fats constitute the group referred to as "energy nutrients" because they contribute energy or "calories" to the diet. Vitamins, minerals, and water do not contribute to the caloric content of food.

Recommended Dietary Allowances

The Food and Nutrition Board of the National Research Council sets standards for the daily intake of calories and nutrients by people in the United States (Table 21-5). The RDA is set for 18 of the 40 or so nutrients known to be needed to promote growth and maintain health. The allowances are based on available scientific data and are updated periodically. In the near future some of the RDAs will probably be lowered, and others, such as the recommendation of calcium for women, are expected to be increased. The allowances for the adult woman are based on the needs of a well-nourished, semisedentary reference woman between 23 years of age and 50 years of age, who weighs 120 pounds and is 64 inches tall. Allowances vary for the older or younger woman and are increased for pregnant or lactating women. They are meant to be used as a basic reference and changed according to individual needs.

Carbohydrate

The main function of a carbohydrate is to produce energy. It is necessary in adequate amounts to spare protein for growth needs. The main sources of carbohydrate in the diet are fruits, vegetables, and grain products. The unrefined sources contribute valuable fiber. Sugars and sweets are also sources of carbohydrates, but are often called empty calories because they do not contribute many nutrients to the diet.

Fat

Fat is a concentrated source of energy, yielding over twice as many calories per gram as carbohydrates. Besides supplying energy, fat in the diet provides essential fatty acids and supplies and carries the fat-soluble vitamins, A, D, E, and K. Also, fats, such as butter, margarine, and salad oil, add to the palatability of food.

Protein

The main function of protein is to build and repair all body cells. An increased amount is needed during pregnancy for growth and maintenance of maternal and fetal tissues. Proteins are made up of different combinations of the more than 20 amino acids. Eight of these cannot be synthesized by the body and are referred to as *essential amino acids,* which must be supplied by the diet. All eight must be present in the correct proportion at the same meal in order to be used by the body.

Proteins that contain adequate amounts of all eight essential amino acids are called *complete proteins.* Most animal sources fall into this category. Most vegetable protein sources are deficient in one or more of the essential amino acids. Those amino acids that are in short supply in any given protein are called *limiting amino acids.* The body can only use the protein to the level of the limiting amino acid, and what is left over is used for energy. Two or more "incomplete" protein sources with different limiting amino acids can be combined in the same meal and are then used by the body as a complete protein.[21]

Vitamins

Vitamins are organic substances that are essential to life and must be supplied by the diet in minute amounts daily. They are directly involved in regulating the metabolism of carbohydrate, protein, and fat, and they assist in regulating reactions by which body tissues are maintained. Many reactions in the body require more than one vitamin, and the lack of any one can interfere with the function of another. Most vitamins cannot be synthesized by the body.

Fat-Soluble Vitamins. Fat-soluble vitamins are stored by the body, so large doses, especially of vitamins A and D, can be toxic. Excesses usually come from excessive supplementation, not from food sources.

Vitamin A assists in maintaining the integrity of the mucous membrane, which increases the body's resistance to infection. It is also essential for normal skeletal and tooth development and plays a role in night vision. Carotene, which is synthesized by plants and is the usual form of the vitamin in foods, is the precursor of vitamin A. Dark green and deep yellow vegetables and fruits are the best sources of vitamin A. Some foods, such as milk, are fortified with vitamin A.

Vitamin D is important for its role in the absorption and utilization of calcium and phosphorus in skeletal and tooth bud formation. Egg yolk, liver, and some fish contain small amounts of vitamin D. Cod liver oil was

TABLE 21-5

Recommended Daily Dietary Allowances for Pregnancy

	Age				Differences for Lactation
	11–14	15–18	19–22	23–50	
Body size					
Weight					
kg	46	55	55	55	
lb	101	120	120	120	
Height					
cm	157	163	163	163	
in	62	64	64	64	
Nutrients					
Energy, kcal	2500	2400	2400	2300	+200
Protein, g	76	76	74	74	−10
Vitamin A, RE*	1000	1000	1000	1000	+200
IU*	5000	5000	5000	5000	+1000
Vitamin D,† μg	15	15	12.5	10	same
Vitamin E,‡ α-TE	10	10	10	10	+1
Ascorbic Acid, mg	70	80	80	80	+20
Niacin, mg NE§	17	16	16	15	+3
Riboflavin, mg	1.6	1.6	1.6	1.5	+0.2
Thiamin, mg	1.5	1.5	1.5	1.4	+0.1
Vitamin B$_6$, mg	2.4	2.6	2.6	2.6	−0.1
Folacin, μg[11]	800	800	800	800	−300
Vitamin B$_{12}$, μg	4.0	4.0	4.0	4.0	same
Calcium, mg	1600	1600	1200	1200	same
Phosphorus, mg	1600	1600	1200	1200	same
Iodine, μg	175	175	175	175	+25
Iron, mg#	18+	18+	18+	18+	#
Magnesium, mg	450	450	450	450	same
Zinc, mg	20	20	20	20	+5

The allowances are intended to provide for individual variations among most normal persons as they live in the United States under usual environmental stresses. Diets should be based on a variety of common foods in order to provide other nutrients for which human requirements have been less well defined.
* RE, retinol equivalent; 1 retinol equivalent = 1 μg retinol or 6 μg β-carotene. 1 RE = 10 International Units.
† As cholecalciferol. 10 μg cholecalciferol = 400 IU of vitamin D.
‡ α-Tocopherol equivalents. 1 mg d-α-tocopherol = 1 α-TE.
§ 1 NE (niacin equivalent) is equal to 1 mg of niacin or 60 mg of dietary tryptophan.
[11] The folacin allowances refer to dietary sources as determined by *Lactobacillus casei* assay after treatment with enzymes (conjugases) to make polyglutamyl forms of the vitamin available to the test organism.
The increased requirement during pregnancy cannot be met by the iron content of habitual American diets or by the existing iron stores of many women; therefore, the use of 30 mg–60 mg of supplemental iron is recommended. Iron needs during lactation are not substantially different from those of nonpregnant women, but continued supplementation of the mother for 2 to 3 months after parturition is advisable to replenish stores depleted by pregnancy.
(After Food and Nutrition Board, National Research Council, National Academy of Sciences, Recommended Dietary Allowances, 9th ed, Washington, DC 1980)

used as a supplement for years to prevent rickets in children. Currently, most milk is fortified with 400 IU of vitamin D per quart. Although some vitamin D can be produced by the body from sunlight on the skin, this is not a reliable source because of the variability of exposure to the sun and interferences with the rays, such as smog or dust.

Vitamin E is primarily an antioxidant. It reduces oxidation of the polyunsaturated fatty acids, helping to maintain the integrity of the cell membranes. It is also involved in certain enzymatic and metabolic reactions. The main sources of vitamin E in the diet are vegetable fats and oils, leafy green vegetables, grains, nuts, and egg yolks.

Vitamin K is an essential factor in the formation of prothrombin and is therefore necessary for normal blood clotting. Leafy green vegetables and pork liver are excellent dietary sources of this vitamin. Vitamin K is also synthesized by bacteria of the lower intestinal tract. Dietary deficiency is not usually a problem.

Water-Soluble Vitamins. Water-soluble vitamins are not stored in any significant amount, so deficiencies develop more easily than with the fat-soluble vitamins. The *B complex* actually consists of a number of different vitamins that are essential to good nutrition. The Food and Nutrition Board lists allowances for thiamin (vitamin B_1), riboflavin (vitamin B_2), niacin (vitamin B_6), folacin (folic acid), and vitamin B_{12}. They serve as components of enzymes and coenzymes in many reactions in the body, such as cell respiration, glucose oxidation, and energy metabolism. Requirements are increased to meet the increased metabolic and growth needs of pregnancy. The B vitamins are not all found together in the same foods; however, if the diet includes milk, organ and other meats, eggs, whole grain or enriched cereals and breads, legumes, and dark green vegetables, most of them will probably be present. Vitamin B_{12} is only found in foods of animal origin.

Folic acid is one of the B vitamins that has received increasing attention in recent years. It is involved in deoxyribonucleic acid (DNA) and ribonucleic acid (RNA) synthesis. If there is a lack of folic acid, cell division cannot proceed normally. Needs are increased during pregnancy for growth of the fetus and expansion of maternal blood volume. Maternal serum folate levels are often low during pregnancy, but megaloblastic anemia, a sign of folic acid deficiency, is seldom seen. Leafy green vegetables, other green vegetables, liver, yeast, legumes, nuts, and whole grains are sources of folic acid, but as much as 80% of the vitamin may be destroyed in cooking or storage, so supplementation is often advised.[22]

Vitamin C (ascorbic acid) is essential for the formation of *collagen*, which is sometimes called the "cement" that holds the body's cells and tissues together. This helps explain the importance of vitamin C in building strong bones and teeth, healing wounds, and aiding the ability of the body to withstand the stresses of injury and infection. Vitamin C is found in fresh vegetables and fruits, especially citrus fruits. Fresh strawberries, cantaloupe, pineapple, guavas, tomatoes, and the green vegetables are also good sources. Other fruits and vegetables can be important dietary sources if eaten in sufficient quantity. Vitamin C is easily destroyed by exposure to air, overcooking, or cooking in too much water. The exact amount of vitamin C needed in the diet to promote optimum health is not known, but it probably varies from person to person. Infections and stress may increase requirements. The current RDA is 60 mg for adults, with an additional 20 mg for pregnant women.

Minerals

There are 14 or more mineral elements that are essential for good nutrition. Some of these are found in fairly large amounts in the body, and others, called *trace elements* or *micronutrients,* are found in minute amounts. The minerals are constituents of vital body materials, and some act as regulators and activators of body functions.

Calcium is an important constituent of bone and teeth. It is also used by the body for other functions, such as normal blood clotting, promoting muscle tone, and regulating the heart beat.

Although two thirds of the calcium in the fetus is deposited during the last month of pregnancy, the mother's daily requirement of calcium is increased during the entire course of pregnancy to prepare adequate storage for this demand. The principal foods from which calcium is obtained are cheese, eggs, oatmeal, vegetables, and milk. A quart of milk alone supplies 1.2 g of calcium.

Phosphorus is an essential constituent of all the cells and the tissues of the body. Milk provides an abundant source of phosphorus. Actually, because phosphorus is an almost invariable constituent of protein, a diet that includes sufficient protein-rich foods, such as eggs, meat, cheese, oatmeal, and green vegetables, will provide also an adequate amount of phosphorus.

Iron is one of the chief components of hemoglobin, the substance in the blood responsible for carrying oxygen to the cells. During pregnancy iron is needed to manufacture hemoglobin for fetal red blood cells as well as maternal red blood cells. During the first two trimesters of pregnancy, iron is transferred to the fetus in moderate amounts, but during the last trimester, when the fetus builds up its reserve, the amount transferred is accelerated about ten times. The diet should be rich in iron-containing foods (*e.g.,* liver, wheat germ, egg yolks), but dietary sources of iron and limited maternal stores often cannot supply the amounts needed for pregnancy. Therefore, supplementation of 30 mg to 60 mg of elemental iron daily is recommended. A glass of citrus juice taken with the iron can enhance absorption.[22]

Iodine is only needed in very small amounts for the health of the woman and the fetus. This mineral is obtained very readily from seafoods and cod liver oil. In certain localities around the Great Lakes and in parts of the Northwest the water supply and the vegetables grown are poor in iodine. Hence, daily use of iodized salt ensures an adequate intake of iodine and prevents deficiency.

Zinc has recently been shown to be important during pregnancy. Deficiency has been linked to congenital malformations and labor and delivery complications, including prolonged labor.[23] Lack of sufficient zinc in the diet is also thought to predispose to bacterial infections of the amniotic fluid, which may lead to preterm labor and delivery.[24] Meats, fish, egg yolks, and most other protein foods have a relatively high zinc content, so a diet meeting the RDA for protein should also furnish sufficient amounts of zinc.[23]

Sodium is present in foods of animal origin and in

some vegetables, but the major dietary source is salt. There is increasing recognition of the importance of adequate sodium intake during pregnancy. In the past, like calorie restriction, restriction of salt was thought to be an important factor in the prevention of toxemia. Clinical and laboratory data now indicate that the sodium requirement is increased during pregnancy. Restriction, therefore, can be harmful when imposed indiscriminately. Flowers has noted that there is a mechanism present in pregnancy that increases sodium reabsorption and retention when there is a reduction in sodium intake.[25] An adequate renal and placental blood flow demands an adequate circulating blood volume. When there is a stringent reduction in sodium intake, there is a reduction in circulating blood volume, which is intolerable during pregnancy and causes damage to both mother and fetus. Thus, the routine restriction of salt is no longer practiced. The use of diuretics for reduction of edema that was previously thought to be associated with sodium retention caused by excessive salt in the diet has also been discontinued.

Many physicians now advise clients early in the pregnancy to simply salt their food to taste. However, this does not mean that salt intake needs to be increased, because the usual diet of most women in the United States easily meets even the increased pregnancy needs.[26]

Vitamin and Mineral Supplements

The use of vitamin and mineral supplements during pregnancy is not universally agreed upon. Ideally, the diet should supply all the nutrients needed so that supplements are not necssary. Iron and folacin are the most frequently recommended supplements, since they are difficult to obtain by diet alone. Some physicians prescribe a multivitamin and mineral supplement to be "on the safe side." Calcium supplements might be advised for women who drink little or no milk and vitamin B_{12} for the vegan vegetarian, who eats no animal protein. If any vitamin or mineral supplements are used, it is important for the woman to understand that these are in addition to, not instead of, her recommended dietary intake.

Megadoses of Vitamins and Minerals.
The idea that if a little is good, a lot will be even better is applied by some individuals to vitamin supplementation. As more is learned about vitamins and their uses in the body, it is becoming more apparent that doses far in excess of body requirements may cause chemical imbalances that can lead to adverse effects. Toxic effects have been seen in individuals consuming large amounts of certain vitamins. Evidence of detrimental effects during pregnancy is limited at present, but the embryo/fetus is thought to be particularly vulnerable to toxic effects of vitamin and mineral megadoses.[27] One reason

for this is that the placental transport system concentrates some nutrients in fetal blood in an effort to make sure that the fetus has a sufficient amount, and thus excessive maternal intake exposes the fetus to unusually high levels. Another reason is that the excretory capacity of the fetus is limited. Susceptibility to damage is greatest during early pregnancy, when organ systems are developing.[28]

The fat-soluble vitamins, especially *vitamin A* and *vitamin D*, have been linked to birth defects by both human case reports and animal studies. Some infants whose mothers took large doses of vitamin A during pregnancy have been born with urinary tract malformations, and others have developed behavioral problems and learning disabilities.[27] Vitamin D has the smallest margin of safety of any of the vitamins. Among the adverse conditions associated with an excessive intake during pregnancy is infantile hypercalcemia, which is characterized by damage to the cardiovascular and renal systems and the brain.

Although water-soluble vitamins are not stored in the body in the same way fat-soluble vitamins are, some of them have been shown to have adverse effects in excessive amounts. There is some evidence that the fetus may become accustomed to the high levels during pregnancy and show withdrawal symptoms after birth. Some infants of women who took large amounts of *vitamin C* during pregnancy have shown scurvylike symptoms when their high prenatal intake was cut off at birth.[28]

To help avoid potential dangers of vitamin overdosage, questions about vitamin supplementation should be included in the initial dietary assessment of the pregnant woman. As with other aspects of dietary counseling, the nurse can assist the expectant mother in planning a diet that includes appropriate amounts of nutrients and avoids excesses.

Water and Other Fluids

Water is often omitted when nutrients are listed, but it is, in fact, a very essential nutrient. It is an important solvent that is necessary for digestion, nutrient transport to the cells, and removal of body wastes. It is also a lubricant and helps regulate body temperature.

Fluids should be taken freely. The woman should drink an average of six to eight glasses daily. Water and juices are good choices. Some beverages contain ingredients that should be used sparingly in the prenatal diet. For example, regular soft drinks contain many empty calories, dietetic soft drinks contain artificial sweeteners, and cola, tea, and coffee contain caffeine (see Food Additives, p. 371). Women who drink large quantities of any of these beverages should be counseled to decrease their intake.

Although there is no definite evidence at present that tea and coffee should be eliminated from the prenatal diet, women are usually advised to at least cut down. Using decaffeinated coffee or tea and removing the teabag promptly when brewing regular tea help to decrease the amount of caffeine per cup.

Planning the Diet

The following discussion and tables provide guidelines to assist the nurse in helping the pregnant woman plan her diet. Planning a menu to include all the essential nutrients would seem impossible if each nutrient had to be considered individually. Fortunately, they are found in foods in certain combinations, so division of foods into groups according to the nutrients they supply can simplify the planning. The four basic food groups are protein foods, milk and milk products, breads and cereal, and fruits and vegetables. The Daily Food Guide further differentiates between vitamin C–rich fruits and vegetables, dark green vegetables, and other fruits and vegetables (Table 21-6).

The Daily Food Guide is meant to be used to plan nutritionally adequate diets with clients. The woman should eat the number of servings recommended from each food group every day. The Nutritional Teaching Guides are helpful in selecting the foods. The Sample Meal Plan illustrates how the guide can be used. Note that the guide serves as a framework for the menu, but does not limit the foods that can be included. The nurse can assist the woman in deciding where ethnic foods fit into the plan. Intake varies depending on the foods selected, but using the guide leads to an average intake of adequate amounts of most of the essential nutrients. The woman should be counseled to include additional nutritious food to meet her caloric needs.

Protein Foods

Four or more servings of beef, pork, lamb, veal, or organ meats are recommended daily. Legumes (*e.g.*, dried beans, peas, and lentils) or nuts may be used as alternates. In addition to their main value of providing amino acids, these foods are also good sources of many vitamins and minerals.

Often the family's budget restricts the quantity and the variety of these proteins, especially meat. The substitution of cheese, peanut butter, poultry, fish, or legumes may then be suggested. The mother may also need advice regarding the preparation and the use of the organ meats that are so rich in protein, vitamins, and minerals. Because some of these are relatively inexpensive, many women do not realize their nutritional worth and further avoid them because of the aesthetics that may be involved in the preparation, such as skinning and soaking. Taste also is sometimes a factor. Nevertheless, with a little ingenuity and suggestions from a good nutrition book or cookbook, the nurse can do

TABLE 21-6

Daily Food Guide*

Food Group	Nonpregnant	Daily Servings Pregnant	Breast-Feeding
Protein foods	4	4	4
Milk and milk products	2	4	5
Breads and cereals	4	4	4
Vitamin C–rich fruits and vegetables	1	1	1
Dark green vegetables	1	1	1
Other fruits and vegetables	1	1	1

* Additions: (a) 2 tablespoons (30 ml) fats and oils each day (*e.g.*, vegetable oil, margarine, mayonnaise, salad dressing); fats and oils provide essential nutrients such as fatty acids and vitamin E; (b) Plenty of liquids—at least six 8-ounce (240 ml) glasses each day during pregnancy, plus eight 8-ounce glasses a day during breast-feeding (*e.g.*, water, milk, cocoa, fruit juice, soups, coffee, tea). (Eating Right for Your Baby. Sacramento, CA, California Department of Health Services, 1978)

much to help the family use this valuable and inexpensive source of protein. Liver, for instance, can be lightly broiled, ground, and incorporated into a meatloaf or ground meat patties. The taste and looks are disguised, the nutritional value is retained, and the meat goes further.

Another group of women who may need assistance in meeting their protein needs are those who follow a vegetarian diet, especially the vegans (see p. 355). Vegetarian diets can be adequate in protein if the individual is knowledgeable about the complementarity of protein foods with different limiting amino acids to ensure the presence of complete proteins (Table 21-7). However, some of the people who adopt vegetarian diets do not have the knowledge or the resources to select or obtain the appropriate foods. They will need help in finding sources of information and in planning menus.

Milk and Milk Products

A quart of milk or its equivalent daily is the recommendation for the expectant mother. Milk is nature's most nearly perfect food and is invaluable as a nutrient. It contains all the different kinds of mineral elements that are needed for fetal development. The high content of calcium and phosphorus in milk makes it almost indispensable for good growth of bone and teeth; it provides these minerals in the correct proportions and in a digestible form that permits optimum utilization by both mother and fetus. It is not only an excellent source of protein, but it is also the most readily digested and easily absorbed of all food proteins.

(text continued on page 368)

CLIENT EDUCATION

Nutritional Teaching Guides

Protein Foods

Protein builds muscle and tissue for the mother and the fetus. Besides protein, protein foods provide B vitamins and iron. B vitamins help you obtain energy from food. Iron is needed to form red blood cells.

Protein comes from both animal and vegetable sources. Each day eat a total of four servings. Try to include two servings from animal protein foods and two servings from vegetable protein foods.

Animal Protein

A serving is two oz (60 g) unless otherwise noted.

Beef (ground, cube, roast, or chop)	
Clams	4 large or 9 small
Eggs	2 medium
Fish (fillet or steak)	
Fish sticks	3 sticks
Frankfurters	2
Lamb (ground, cube, roast, or chop)	
Luncheon meat	3 slices
Organ meats: heart, kidney, liver, tongue	
Oysters	8–12 medium
Pork, ham (ground, roast, or chop)	
Poultry (chicken, duck, turkey)	
Rabbit	
Sausage links	4 links
Shellfish (crab, lobster, scallops, shrimp)	
Spareribs	6 medium ribs
Tuna fish	
Veal (ground, cube, roast or chop)	

Vegetable Protein

Beans are the best choice from vegetable protein foods. A serving of beans contains more vitamins and minerals than a serving of nuts or seeds. A serving is any of the following:

Canned beans (garbanzo, kidney, lima, pork and beans)	1 cup (240 ml)
Dried beans and peas	1 cup (240 ml)
Nut butters (cashew butter, peanut butter, *etc*)	¼ cup (60 ml)
Nuts	½ cup (120 ml)
Sunflower seeds	½ cup (120 ml)
Tofu (soybean curd)	1 cup (240 ml)

One can get the protein needed by eating only vegetable protein foods. However, these foods should be combined with eggs and milk. Ask the physician, dietitian, or nutritionist for further information.

Milk and Milk Products

Milk and milk products are the best food sources of calcium. Calcium builds strong bones and teeth in your baby. It also keeps nerves and muscles healthy.

Milk and milk products also contain protein, several B vitamins, and vitamins A and D. Vitamin D helps the body use calcium. Vitamin A is needed for growth and vision. It also protects you from infection.

Choose four servings of milk and milk products each day if you are pregnant. Choose five servings if you are breast-feeding. A serving is 1 cup (8 oz or 240 ml) unless otherwise noted.

Cheese (except Camembert and cream)	1 slice (1½ oz or 45 g)
Cheese spread	4 tablespoons (60 ml)
Cocoa made with milk	1¼ cups (10 oz or 300 ml)
Cottage cheese	1⅓ cups (320 ml)
Custard (flan)	
Ice cream	1½ cups (360 ml)
Ice milk	
Milk	
buttermilk	
chocolate (not drink)	1¼ cups (10 oz or 300 ml)
evaporated	½ cup (4 oz or 120 ml)
goat	
low-fat	
nonfat	
nonfat (made from dry milk powder)	
nonfat dry milk powder	⅓ cup (80 ml)
whole	
Milkshake	
Pudding	

(continued)

C L I E N T   E D U C A T I O N   (continued)

Soups made with milk   1½ cups (12 oz or 360 ml)

Yogurt (plain)

Not all milk and milk products contain vitamins A and D. Check the label.

Breads and Cereals

Breads and cereals have several nutrients important for you and your baby, including B vitamins and iron. These foods may be either whole grain or enriched. It's best to eat whole grains because they contain more vitamins and minerals. Whole grains also provide fiber that helps prevent constipation.

Choose four servings of breads and cereals each day. A serving is any of the following:

Whole Grain Items

Bread (cracked, whole wheat, or rye)	1 slice
Cereal, hot (oatmeal, rolled oats, rolled wheat, cracked wheat, wheat and malted barley)	½ cup cooked (120 ml)
Cereal, ready-to-eat (puffed oats, shredded wheat, wheat flakes, granola)	¾ cup (180 ml)
Rice (brown)	½ cooked (120 ml)
Wheat germ	1 tablespoon (15 ml)

In some communities you can also buy whole wheat macaroni, noodles, and spaghetti.

Enriched Items

Bagel	1 small
Bread (all except those listed above)	1 slice
Cereal, hot (cream of wheat, cream of rice, farina, cornmeal, grits)	½ cup cooked (120 ml)
Cereal, ready-to-eat (all except those listed above)	¾ cup (180 ml)
Crackers	4
Macaroni, noodles, spaghetti	½ cup cooked (120 ml)
Pancake, waffle	1 medium (5-in or 13-cm diameter)
Rice (white)	½ cup cooked
Roll, biscuit, muffin, dumpling	1
Tortilla	1 (6-in or 15-cm diameter)

Doughnut, cakes, pies, and cookies are not included in the breads and cereals group. These foods contain mostly calories and very few nutrients.

Vitamin C–rich Fruits and Vegetables

Vitamin C–rich fruits and vegetables contain ascorbic acid (vitamin C). This vitamin is needed to hold body cells together and to strengthen blood vessel walls. Ascorbic acid also aids in healing wounds.

Choose one serving of Vitamin C–rich fruits and vegetables each day. A serving is ¾ cup (180 ml) unless otherwise noted.

Vegetables

Bok choy	
Broccoli	1 stalk
Brussels sprouts	3–4
Cabbage	
Cauliflower	
Chili peppers (green or red)	¼ cup
Greens (collard, kale, mustard, turnip)	
Peppers (green or red)	½ medium
Tomatoes	2 medium
Watercress	

Fruits

Cantaloupe	½ medium
Grapefruit	½ large
Guava	½ small
Mango	1 medium
Orange	1 medium
Papaya	½ small
Strawberries	
Tangerine	2 large

Juices

Fruit juices and drinks with vitamin C added

Grapefruit	½ cup (4 oz or 120 ml)
Orange	½ cup (4 oz or 120 ml)
Pineapple	1½ cups (12 oz or 360 ml)
Tomato	1½ cups (12 oz or 360 ml)

Dark Green Vegetables

Dark green vegetables are an excellent source of vitamin A and folacin. A fetus needs vitamin A for bone

(continued)

CLIENT EDUCATION *(continued)*

growth and tooth formation. Vitamin A is also important for vision and resisting infections.

Folacin, a B vitamin, is needed to form red blood cells and other body cells. Cooking temperatures destroy folacin, so eat dark green vegetables raw whenever possible.

Choose one serving of dark green vegetables each day. A serving is 1 cup (240 ml) raw or ¾ cup (180 ml) cooked.

Asparagus
Bok choy
Broccoli
Brussels sprouts
Cabbage
Chicory
Endive
Escarole
Greens (beet, collard, kale, mustard, turnip)
Lettuce (dark leafy, red leaf, romaine)
Scallions
Spinach
Swiss chard
Watercress

Other Fruits and Vegetables

Other fruits and vegetables add vitamins and minerals to your diet. Those dark yellow in color contain vitamin A. Fruits and vegetables also provide fiber, which is important for normal bowel movements.

Choose one serving of other fruits and vegetables each day. A serving is ½ cup (102 ml) unless otherwise noted.

Vegetables

Artichoke	1 medium
Bamboo shoots	
Beans (green, wax)	
Bean sprouts	
Beet	
Burdock root	
Carrot	
Cauliflower	
Celery	
Corn	
Cucumber	
Eggplant	
Hominy	
Lettuce (head, boston, bibb)	
Mushrooms	
Nori seaweed	
Onion	
Parsnip	
Peas	
Pea pods	
Potato	1 medium
Radishes	
Summer squash	
Sweet potato	1 medium
Winter squash	
Yam	1 medium
Zucchini	

Fruits

Apple	1 medium
Apricot	2 medium
Banana	1 small
Berries	
Cherries	
Dates	5
Figs	2 large
Fruit cocktail	
Grapes	
Kumquats	3
Nectarine	2 medium
Peach	1 medium
Pear	1 medium
Persimmon	1 small
Pineapple	
Plums	2 medium
Prunes	4 medium
Pumpkin	¼ cup (60 ml)
Raisins	
Watermelon	

Dark yellow fruits and vegetables, such as carrots, sweet potatoes, yams, winter squash, apricots, and persimmons are an excellent source of vitamin A.

(After Eating Right for your Baby. Sacramento, CA. California Department of Health Services, 1978)

C L I E N T   E D U C A T I O N

Sample Meal Plan

	Pregnant Woman		**Lactating Woman**	
Breakfast	1 svg Vitamin C–rich fruits and vegetables 1 svg grain products 1 svg milk and milk products	4 oz orange juice ½ c oatmeal with brown sugar* 8 oz milk coffee or tea*	1 svg vitamin C–rich fruits and vegetables 1 svg grain products 1 svg milk and milk products	4 oz orange juice ½ c oatmeal with brown sugar* 8 oz milk coffee or tea*
Morning Snack	Optional	*	Optional	*
Lunch	2 svgs grain products 1 svg protein foods 1 svg other fruits and vegetables 1 svg milk and milk products	1 tuna fish sandwich made with 2 slices whole wheat bread, ½ c tuna fish, diced celery and onion to taste*, mayonnaise*, lettuce* 1 small banana 8 oz milk	2 svgs grain products 1 svg protein foods 1 svg other fruits and vegetables 1 svg milk and milk products	1 tuna fish sandwich made with 2 slices whole wheat bread, ½ c tuna fish, diced celery and onion to taste*, mayonnaise*, lettuce* 1 small banana 8 oz milk
Afternoon Snack	1 svg protein foods ½ svg milk and milk products	½ c salted peanuts 4 oz milk	1 svg protein foods 1 svg milk and milk products	½ c salted peanuts 8 oz milk
Dinner	2 svgs protein foods 2 svgs leafy green vegetables 1 svg milk and milk products	6 oz roast beef ½ c egg noodles* with sauteed poppy seeds* ¾ c cut asparagus salad made with 1 c torn spinach, sliced mushrooms, and radishes to taste*, and oil and vinegar* 8 oz milk coffee or tea*	2 svgs protein foods 2 svgs leafy green vegetables 1 svg milk and milk products	6 oz roast beef ½ c egg noodles* with sauteed poppy seeds* ¾ c cut asparagus salad made with 1 c torn spinach, sliced mushrooms and radishes to taste*, oil and vinegar 8 oz milk coffee or tea*
Evening Snack	½ svg milk and milk products	2 oatmeal raisin cookies* 4 oz milk	1 svg milk and milk products	2 oatmeal raisin cookies* 8 oz milk

* This food is optional and is added to the basic diet.

(After Nutrition During Pregnancy, Sacramento, CA, California Department of Health Services, pp 35–36)

(text continued from page 364)

Finally, milk contains some of the most important vitamins, particularly vitamin A, which increases resistance to infection and safeguards the development of the fetus.

When a woman indicates that she does not drink milk or drinks very little, it is important to pursue the subject and find out the basis for the avoidance. She may not like milk or be able to tolerate it well. After the cause is established, a plan can be developed with

Basic Guidelines for Good Nutrition During Pregnancy

1. Use the Daily Food Guide to plan each day's meals.
2. Include a wide variety of foods.
3. Gain weight gradually and steadily.
4. Salt food to taste with iodized salt.
5. Do not diet to lose weight.
6. Use supplements as prescribed.

her to make milk more palatable or to include adequate substitutes.

The instant nonfat and whole dry milks may be used in a quantity that provides an adequate intake. Approximately 5 tablespoons of dried skim milk equals 1 pint of fluid milk. The milk may be used dry and worked into meatloaf, mashed potatoes, cereals, sandwich spreads, baked articles, and so on. Reconstituted with less than the usual amount of water, it has a richer taste than the regular liquid skim milk. Certain condiments and flavorings (*e.g.,* vanilla, nutmeg, cinnamon) enhance the flavor of milk. Some clients may prefer evaporated milk, buttermilk, nonfat, or low-fat milk instead of whole milk. Milk can also be taken in some other form, such as soups or custards.

Other dairy products, such as cottage cheese, ricotta cheese, farmer's cheese, hoop cheese, yogurt, and the hard cheeses, are also adequate substitutions. One ounce of cheese contains approximately the same amount of minerals and vitamins as a large glass of whole milk. However, the total protein and fat content varies and must be considered when making substitutions. Cream cheese has a high percentage of fat and a low calcium content so it is not a good substitute for the other cheeses. Also, products such as "cheese foods" and "cheese spreads" are diluted and therefore contain fewer nutrients per serving.

TABLE 21-7

Complementary Plant Protein Sources

Food	Amino Acids Deficient	Complementary Protein
Grains	Isoleucine Lysine	Rice + legumes Corn + legumes Wheat + legumes Wheat + peanuts + milk Wheat + sesame + soybean Rice + sesame Rice + brewer's yeast
Legumes	Tryptophan Methionine	Legumes + rice Beans + wheat Beans + corn Soybeans + rice + wheat Soybeans + corn + milk Soybeans + wheat + sesame Soybeans + peanuts + sesame Soybeans + peanuts + wheat + rice Soybeans + sesame + wheat
Nuts and seeds	Isoleucine Lysine	Peanuts + sesame + soybeans Sesame + beans Sesame + soybeans + wheat Peanuts + sunflower seeds
Vegetables	Isoleucine Methionine	Lima beans Green peas Brussels sprouts } + sesame seeds or Brazil nuts or mushrooms Cauliflower Broccoli Greens + millet or converted rice

(After Lappé FM: Diet For a Small Planet. Ballantine, NY, 1975. By Frances Moore Lappé, Friends of the Earth/Ballantine, New York, 1975)

Lactose Intolerance.   Many adults, especially those from certain geographic areas, have difficulty digesting milk because of an insufficient amount of the enzyme lactase in the small intestine. Lactase is responsible for breaking down lactose (milk sugar) into glucose and galactose. If the available lactase is not sufficient to hydrolyze the amount of lactose ingested, fermentation occurs in the large intestine and causes abdominal cramps, diarrhea, bloating, and flatulence.

Groups of people most likely to be lactose intolerant include those whose traditional cultural food habits did not include much milk in the adult diet. These include Eskimos, aborigines of Australia, natives of New Guinea, Chinese, Thais, Filipinos, and most African blacks.[29] Lactose intolerance is not, of course, limited to these groups. On the other hand, not every woman who says "I don't like milk" or "Milk doesn't agree with me," is lactose intolerant.

In counseling these women, special attention should be directed to meeting calcium, protein, vitamin, and mineral requirements. Some dairy products are lower in lactose than others and can be used in place of milk (Table 21-8). Encouraging the lactose intolerant individual to "drink more milk" can be counterproductive if it causes symptoms. Besides the discomfort from the symptoms, the increased stool frequency and mass can lead to the increased loss of nutrients, including calcium, in the feces. This, in turn, can cause a negative calcium balance.

Bread and Cereal

Four or more servings should be included from this group daily. Women should be encouraged to substitute whole grain products for white bread and cereals. Whole grains contain vitamins and minerals not found in re-

T A B L E   2 1 - 8

Composition and Comparison of Dairy Products

Products and Amount	Calories	Protein (g)	Lactose (g)	Lactose Ratio to Milk	Calcium (mg)	Calcium Ratio to Milk
Sandwich cheese (2 oz)						
American	210	12.6	0.96	0.09:1	364	1.4:1
Cheddar	230	14.2	1.18	0.11:1	386	1.5:1
Cream cheese	196	4.8	1.14	0.11:1	40	0.15:1
Swiss	210	15.6	0.96	0.09:1	522	2.0:1
Cottage cheese (4 oz)						
Plain, creamed	108	14.0	2.4	0.23:1	68	0.3:1
Low fat (2%)	96	15.6	3.7	0.36:1	100	0.4:1
Uncreamed	92	21.2	0.8	0.08:1	28	0.1:1
Ice Cream (4 oz)						
Vanilla (12% fat)	254	4.4	8.0	0.77:1	164	0.6:1
Ice Milk (4 oz)						
Vanilla	166	4.4	8.4	0.8:1	156	0.6:1
Milk (8 oz)						
Whole milk (3.5% fat)	141	7.3	10.4	1:1	260	1:1
Chocolate drink	136	7.3	9.6	0.9:1	247	0.95:1
Egg nog (6% fat)	304	10.4	12.8	1.2:1	343	1.3:1
Skimmed	73	7.3	10.4	1.1	266	1:1
Yogurt (8 oz)						
Blueberry	257	9.6	10.4	1:1	282	1:1
Plain	134	12.0	13.6	1.3:1	362	1.4:1
Strawberry	232	10.4	12.0	1.2:1	314	1.2:1
Vanilla	195	11.2	12.8	1.2:1	336	1.3:1
Milk (reconstituted; 8 oz)						
Nonfat dry	80	8.0	12.4	1.2:1	300	1.2:1
Evaporated whole	174	8.8	12.5	1.2:1	325	1.3:1
Evaporated skim	96	9.6	13.9	1.3:1	350	1.4:1
Liquid breakfast mix (1-serving envelope)						
Vanilla	130	7.0	12.2	1.2:1	50	0.2:1

Figures are calculated from nutritional analysis information provided by the Kraftco Corporation and the Carnation Company on their own products.
(Luke B: Lactose intolerance during pregnancy: Significance and solutions. MCN 2(2)95, March/April 1977)

fined flour and not replaced by the enriching process. When cereals are supplemented by milk, they become adequate for growth, as well as for maintaining life. The *germ* of the grain, removed in the refining process, also contains protein of value comparable to that from animal sources. Wheat germ can be purchased separately and eaten as a cereal or added to foods, such as baked goods or meatloaf, to increase the nutritional value.

Cereal products are a primary source of energy in the diet, and they make an important contribution to every nutrient need except calcium, ascorbic acid, and vitamin A. When bread is buttered, it even contributes to the vitamin A intake. Whole grain cereal and breads also add fiber to the diet to help counteract constipation.

Vegetables and Fruits

Three or more servings should be included from this group. At least one serving of dark green vegetables and one serving of citrus fruits or tomatoes should be included. Some fruits and vegetables each day should be served raw.

Vegetables. Vegetables are particularly rich sources of iron, calcium, and several vitamins. The dark green vegetables are good sources of vitamin A, folacin, and iron. The deep yellow fruits and vegetables are also good sources of vitamin A. Fresh or frozen vegetables can be used interchangeably. Canned vegetables may be used if necessary, but some nutrients are lost in the cooking and canning process.

Careful preparation and cooking of vegetables helps to retain the maximum vitamin and mineral content. Presoaking should be avoided. Steaming and stir-frying are preferred methods of cooking. Steamer baskets to fit standard size pans are widely available. Some vegetables contain incomplete proteins that add to the total protein intake.

In addition to their value as nutrient agents, these vegetables deserve an important place in the diet as laxative agents because their fibrous framework increases the bulk of the intestinal content and thereby stimulates elimination.

Fruits. Citrus fruits such as oranges, lemons, and grapefruit are the best sources of vitamin C. Most of these fruits also supply vitamins A and B. Tomatoes are also an excellent source of vitamin C; the amount eaten, however, must be twice that of the citrus fruits to supply the same amount of vitamin. Other fruits, raw and cooked, such as prunes, raisins, and apricots, contain important minerals (*e.g.*, iron and copper) as well as vitamins. Fruits may stimulate a lagging appetite and counteract constipation. They may be used as juices, combined in salads, as additions to cereals or plain yogurt, as in-between-meal refreshments, and in desserts, such as gelatins and puddings. Fruits contain some incomplete proteins but only supplement the other proteins.

Food Quality

Women may need to be reminded to select foods that are fresh and of good quality, as they are more appealing and safer as well. Foods that have been on the shelf a long time are more likely to begin to deteriorate or become rancid, interfering with their nutritive value. Aflatoxins and other mycotoxins are produced by fungal growths on a wide variety of foodstuffs. They can be toxic to humans and are suspected of being teratogenic and carcinogenic. Therefore, pregnant women should be warned against eating any foods that are fermented, moldy, rotten, discolored, or malodorous because they are potentially contaminated.[30]

Food Additives

Food additives are substances, added either directly or indirectly to a food, that become a component of the food or affect its functional characteristics.[31] Some additives are necessary to our food supply to prevent spoilage and ensure that certain products are safe to eat. Other additives are used to improve the flavor, odor, texture, color, or the nutritional quality of foods.

The FDA monitors additives and bans those that cause cancer or other problems in animals. There is often controversy over the safety of additives. Nitrates and nitrites, for example, can be converted by the body to nitrosamines, which have been shown to be teratogenic and carcinogenic in rats, but they are still used to preserve processed meats and other foods until adequate substitutes can be found. The safety of artificial sweeteners has been questioned in recent years. The use of saccharin as an additive in commercial products has decreased markedly since it was linked with the development of bladder cancer in animal studies. There is no real evidence that other artificial sweeteners such as aspartame (Nutra-Sweet) are harmful, but most dieticians recommend that they be used with caution during pregnancy. BHA and BHT, which are used in many foods, including cereals, oils, and snack foods, are other additives whose safety has been questioned.

Although caffeine is not really an additive, it is a substance of potential concern to the pregnant woman. There have been conflicting results, but it has been shown to be teratogenic and mutagenic in some experiments on rats and mice. There is insufficient evidence to label it as a teratogen in humans, but it should be used with caution (see Chap. 22 for further information).

Teratogenicity is usually considered to be dose related, so that, although it may be impossible to eliminate

NURSING CARE PLAN

The Pregnant Woman and Her Nutritional Needs

Nursing Objectives

1. Identify nutritional deficiencies in the pregnant woman.
2. Provide information and counseling to promote an adequate prenatal diet.
3. Promote fetal/neonatal well-being and weight gain by assisting the mother to obtain optimal dietary intake to provide adequate intrauterine nutrients.

Assessment	Potential Nursing Diagnosis	Planning/Intervention	Evaluation
Nutritional status	Alteration in nutrition: less than body requirements, related to: inadequate caloric intake or inadequate financial resources or dysfunctional dietary patterns	Use assessment tools to determine individual client needs	Absence of nutritionally related problems such as preeclampsia and anemia
Physical indicators		Provide dietary counseling as needed:	Repeat dietary recall or food diary indicates use of Daily Food Guide and implementation of suggested changes
Prepregnant weight		Involve client in planning	
Pregnancy weight gain	Alteration in nutrition: less calcium than pregnancy requirements, related to: lactose intolerance	Consider individual needs, preferences, attitudes, family needs, and cultural or ethnic background	Weight gain is adequate and follows recommended pattern
Laboratory values (hemoglobin, hematocrit)			
Current dietary habits		Provide information about nutrient needs	
Daily food intake	Knowledge deficit regarding nutritional needs during pregnancy, related to lack of information	Encourage and reinforce appropriate food choices and preparation	
Individual factors in food selection			
Nutritional risk factors		Plan menus with client, including foods she likes, can afford, and is able to prepare	
Client understanding of nutrition	Alteration in nutrition: inadequate weight gain, related to self-imposed limitation of calories		
Importance of good nutrition during pregnancy		Give careful, thorough explanation of rationale for any suggested changes	
Important nutrients		Teach importance of weight gain; use and discuss weight gain grid at each visit	
Importance of weight gain		Refer to dietitian when appropriate	

additives from the diet, reducing the amount during pregnancy would lower the risks.[31] Until more is known, it is wise for the pregnant woman to read labels carefully and choose products with as few additives as possible.

Resources

The nurse should be aware of available resources for nutritional counseling, education, and support. This will assist her in keeping her own nutritional education up

to date and also enable her to make appropriate referrals.

When consultation with a nutritionist is advisable and one is not available on the clinic or hospital staff, it may be possible to locate one in the area through the local community-health department or a home economist's office. Publications, visual aids, charts, and so on may be secured from city, county, and state health departments. The March of Dimes Birth Defects Foundation also provides many teaching aids and reminders about nutrition during pregnancy.

The United States Government Printing Office is

another invaluable source of publications. The Food and Nutrition Board, National Research Council, Council on Foods and Nutrition, American Medical Association, American Home Economics Association, and American Public Health Association are all professional organizations that offer additional resources. The above associations are only a few of the resources that the nurse and the physician have to assist their clients in planning for adequate nutrition.

WIC

A source of nutritional help for some pregnant women is the *Special Supplementary Food Program for Women, Infants and Children,* better known as *WIC.* This program was initiated in 1974 to provide food for low-income families at critical times of growth and development. Funds for the program come from the United States Department of Agriculture and are administered at the state and local levels by state health departments.[32]

At the local level specific foods are provided for pregnant and lactating women, infants, and children up to 5 years of age who are determined to be at risk nutritionally and who otherwise would be unable to afford an adequate diet. Food vouchers or supplemental foods are distributed at designated health clinics. The WIC program seeks to do more than just provide food for needy families. Nutrition education is mandated to be an integral part of the program. The educational component of the program uses a variety of teaching modalities, including lectures, films, group or individual discussions, and written material. It is planned to take into account socioeconomic, educational, and cultural factors and the level of understanding of the recipients.

Counseling the Pregnant Adolescent

Special nutritional concerns arise when the pregnant client is in her teenage years. She not only has the same added nutritional needs of other pregnant women, but these may be superimposed on age-related growth needs and possible dysfunctional dietary patterns. Other factors leading to inadequate nutrition for the pregnant adolescent include the desire to be slim, peer food practices, and resistance to adult advice. Eating nutritionally may also be of low priority to the pregnant adolescent, who may be much more concerned with meeting her social and emotional needs.

Food Selection. The teenager's food choices may include many "fast foods" and snacks. This leads to a low intake of fresh fruits and vegetables, which in turn limits the intake of vitamins and minerals, especially vitamins A and C. If milk and milk products are also

avoided, there may be a lack of vitamin D, B vitamins, calcium, and protein.

Weight Gain. Theoretically, the ideal weight gain would include the usual pregnancy recommendation plus the amount the girl would have gained in the process of maturation during the 9-month period if she hadn't become pregnant. Younger adolescents (13–15 years) would therefore be expected to gain more than older adolescents (16 and over), whose growth rate would have slowed down.[32] Weight-conscious teenagers may resist continuous weight gain, especially if they gained a lot in early pregnancy. They need extra help in understanding the dangers of dieting during pregnancy.

Eating Disorders. Weight consciousness and equating thinness with attractiveness have led to an increased incidence of eating disorders. Anorexia nervosa and bulimia are found most frequently in the adolescent and young-adult age-groups. Fertility is usually reduced in the anorexic female, who is rarely able to conceive or carry a pregnancy. Bulimia, however, which is becoming more common among teenagers, is less likely than anorexia to affect fertility. The bulimic, through her binging and purging, is in far from an optimum nutritional state in spite of near-normal body weight. Since recognition of bulimia is relatively recent, little research is available on how best to manage the pregnant bulimic female.[33]

Some possible effects from the practices of bulimia, besides the nutritional deficits, are tooth decay and possible esophageal damage caused by the repeated vomiting, rectal bleeding and electrolyte imbalance caused by the continual use of laxatives, and possible diabetes or hypoglycemia resulting from the stimulus of food without its nutritional effects.[34] Theoretically, the primary problem during pregnancy is the effect on the fetus of the potentially detrimental changes in its biochemical environment resulting from the maternal binging, vomiting, and purging.[33]

To provide sufficient nourishment to support the pregnancy and attempt to avoid detrimental effects on the fetus, the bulimic woman needs psychological intervention. The nurse's primary role with these individuals is detection of the problem and referral to an appropriate source for psychological help.

Counseling. The pregnant adolescent will benefit most from counseling designed to meet her individual needs. Many teenagers do eat nutritionally sound diets and just need reinforcement of their good eating habits and information about additional pregnancy needs. Others will need more specific assistance. Although some may respond to the appeal to eat well for a healthy baby, to many the unborn child does not seem very real until late in the pregnancy or after the birth.

The nurse working with these girls may find it more helpful to stress the girl's own growth and development needs.[32] When pregnant teenagers are well nourished throughout their pregnancy they are much less likely to develop complications and much more likely to produce a healthy infant.

References

1. Committee on Maternal Nutrition, Food and Nutrition Board, National Research Council: Maternal Nutrition and the Course of Pregnancy. Washington, DC, National Academy of Sciences, 1970
2. Luke B: Maternal Nutrition. Boston, Little, Brown & Co, 1979
3. Rosso P, Cramoy C: Nutrition and pregnancy. In Winick M (ed): Nutrition—Pre and Postnatal Development, p 176. New York, Plenum Press, 1979
4. Primrose T, Higgins A: A study in human antepartum nutrition. J Reprod Med 7(6):257–264, December 1971
5. Lechtig A: Studies of Nutrition Intervention in Pregnancy. Birth 9(2):115–119, Summer 1982
6. Winick M: Malnutrition and mental development. In Winick M (ed): Nutrition—Pre and Postnatal Development, p 52. New York, Plenum Press, 1979
7. Stein Z (ed): Famine and Human Development: The Dutch Hunger Winter of 1944–1945. New York, Oxford University Press, 1975
8. Higgins A: Montreal diet dispensary study. In Nutritional Supplementation and the Outcome of Pregnancy, pp 93–110. Washington, DC, National Academy of Sciences, 1973
9. Kitay DZ: Dysfunctional antepartum nutrition. J Reprod Med 7(6):251–256, December 1971
10. Nutrition During Pregnancy and Lactation, Maternal and Child Health Unit, California Department of Health, 1975
11. Dwyer J: Vegetarian diets in pregnancy (Proceedings of a Workshop). In Committee on Nutrition of the Mother and Preschool Child, Food and Nutrition Board, Commission on Life Sciences, National Research Council: Alternative Dietary Practices and Nutritional Abuses in Pregnancy, pp 61–83. Washington, DC, National Academy Press, 1982
12. Pitkin RM: Nutritional support in obstetrics and gynecology. Clin Obstet Gynecol 19(3):489–513, September 1976
13. Jacobson HN: Diet therapy and the improvement of pregnancy outcomes. Birth 10(1):29–31, Spring 1983
14. Pitkin RM: Nutritional influences during pregnancy. Med Clin North Am 61(1):3–14, January 1977
15. Naeye RL: Weight gain and the outcome of pregnancy. Am J Obstet Gynecol 135(1):3–9, September 1979
16. Luke B: Understanding pica in pregnant women. MCN 2(2):97–100, March/April 1977
17. Vermeersch J: Physiological basis of nutritional needs. In Worthington B (ed): Nutrition in Pregnancy and Lactation, 3rd ed. St Louis, CV Mosby, 1985
18. Ademowore AS, Courey NG, Kime JS: Relationships of maternal wieght gain to newborn birthweight. Obstet Gynecol 39:460, 1972
19. Holey ES: Promoting adequate weight gain in pregnant women. MCN 2(2):86–89, March/April 1977
20. Shearer M: Malnutrition in middle-class pregnant women. Birth Fam J 7(1):27–35, Spring 1980
21. Lappe FM: Diet for a Small Planet. New York, Ballantine Books, 1975
22. Robinson CH: Basic Nutrition and Diet Therapy, 4th ed. New York, Macmillan, 1980
23. Lemasters GK: Zinc insufficiency during pregnancy. JOGN Nurs 10(2):124–125, March/April 1981
24. Naeye RL: Effects of maternal nutrition on fetal and neonatal survival. Birth 10(2):109–113, Summer 1983
25. Flowers CE: Editorial: Nutrition in pregnancy. J Reprod Med 7:264–274, November 1971
26. Food and Nutrition Board: Recommended Dietary Allowances, 9th rev ed. Washington DC, National Research Council, Committee on Dietary Allowances, 1980
27. Luke B: Megavitamins and pregnancy: A dangerous combination. MCN 10(1):18–23, January/February 1985
28. Pitkin RM: Megadose nutrients during pregnancy. (Proceedings of a Workshop). In Committee on Nutrition of the Mother and Preschool Child, Food and Nutrition Board, Commission on Life Sciences, National Research Council: Alternative Dietary Practices and Nutritional Abuses in Pregnancy, pp 203–211. Washington, DC, National Academy Press, 1982
29. Luke B: Lactose intolerance during pregnancy: Significance and solutions. MCN 2(2):92–96, March/April 1977
30. Streitfeld PP: Congenital malformation: Teratogenic foods and additives. Birth Fam J 5:1, Spring 1978
31. Green ML, Harry J: Nutrition in Contemporary Nursing Practice, p 228. New York, John Wiley & Sons, 1981
32. Ritchey SJ, Taper LJ: Maternal and Child Nutrition. New York, Harper & Row, 1983
33. Worthington-Roberts BS, Rees JM: Nutritional needs of the pregnant adolescent. In Worthington-Roberts BS, Vermeersch J, Williams SR (eds): Nutrition in Pregnancy and Lactation, 3rd ed, pp 207–235. St Louis, Times Mirror/Mosby, 1985
34. Williams SR: Nutrition and Diet Therapy, 5th ed, pp 809–813. St Louis, Times Mirror/Mosby, 1985

Suggested Reading

California Department of Health Services: Eating Right for Your Baby, Using Vitamin/Mineral Pills and Salt, Your Weight and Weight Gain, Relief from Common Problems: Nausea, Constipation, Heartburn. In Nutrition for Pregnancy and Breastfeeding Series. Sacramento, California, 1978*

* Available without charge by writing to Department of Health, 714 P. Street, Sacramento, California 95814.

Hinton SM, Kerwin DR: Maternal Infant & Child Nutrition: A Resource Book for Health Professionals. Chapel Hill, Health Sciences Consortium, 1981

Lappe FM: Diet for a Small Planet. New York, Ballantine Books, 1975

Luke B: Maternal Nutrition. Boston, Little, Brown & Co, 1979

Nutrition During Pregnancy and Lactation. Sacramento, California, Maternal and Child Health Unit, California Department of Health, 1975*

Rang ML: Bibliography for nutrition in pregnancy. JOGN Nurs 9(1):55–58, January/February 1980

Ritchey SJ, Taper LJ: Maternal and Child Nutrition. New York, Harper & Row, 1983

Rush D, Stein Z, Susser M et al: Diet in Pregnancy: A Randomized Controlled Trial of Nutritional Supplements. New York, AR Liss, 1980

Worthington–Roberts BS, Vermeersch J, Williams SR et al: Nutrition in Pregnancy and Lactation, 3rd ed. St Louis, CV Mosby, 1985

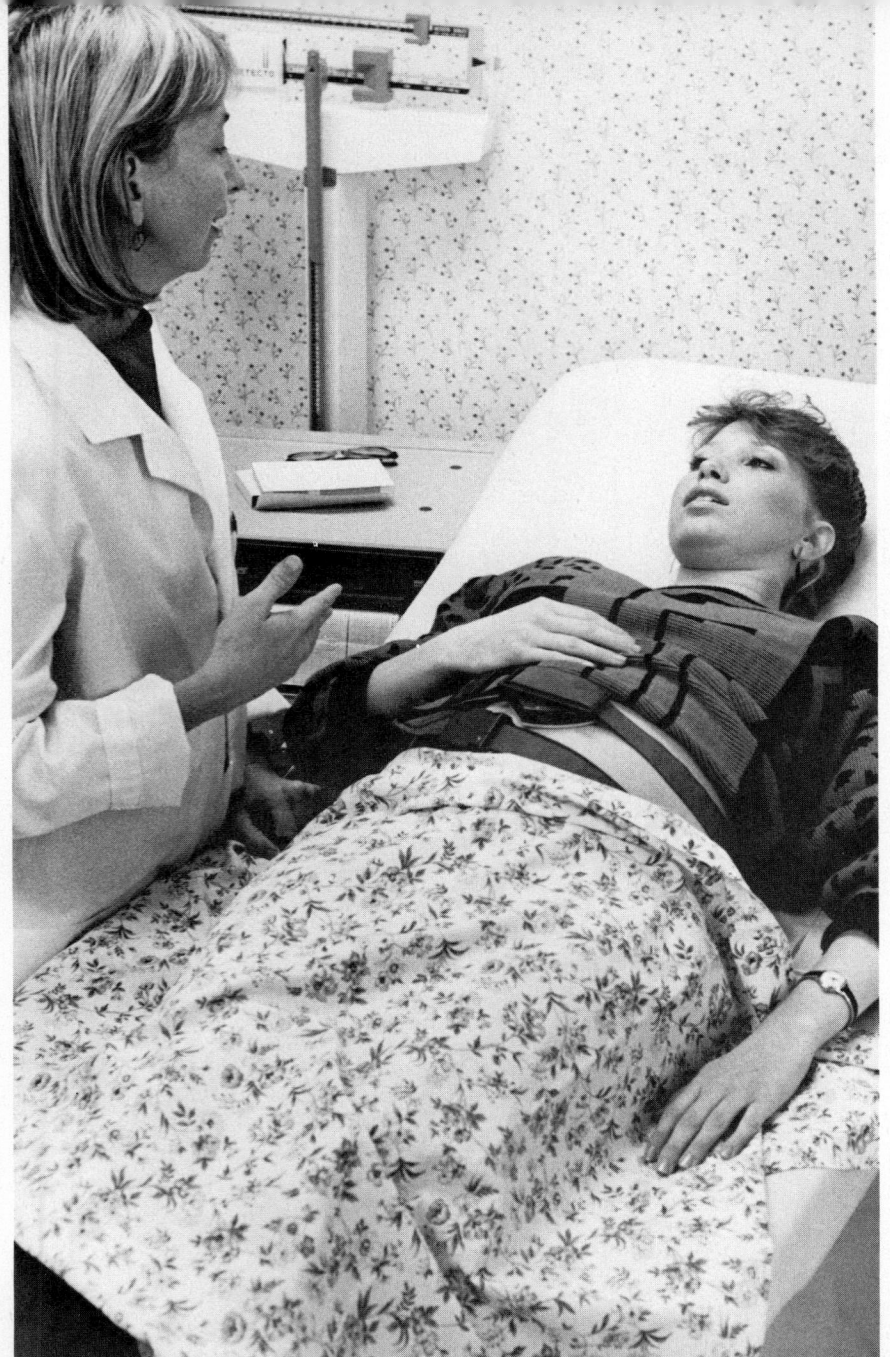

CHAPTER 22

Nursing Care in the Antepartal Period

Pregnancy is a normal physiological process. The vast majority of births do not require active management by health professionals, since the natural reproductive process unfolds according to biologic patterns. Normal pregnancy does, however, significantly alter the woman's physiological systems, and there is always the potential for reduction of general health status and the development of hazards for mother and fetus.

Modern prenatal care is a relatively recent development, in which the organized health-care system assumes primary responsibility for the supervision of pregnancy and the conduct of labor and delivery.

Antepartal care refers to the medical and nursing supervision and care given to the pregnant woman during the period between conception and the onset of labor. Adequate antepartal care generally considers the physical, emotional, and social needs of the woman and her unborn baby, her partner, and their other children, if any. It attempts to provide the best of medical and nursing science to protect the life and health of the mother and fetus. In addition, it takes into consideration the social conditions under which the family lives (*i.e.*, its economic status, educational level, housing, nutrition, support systems, and so on; see Chap. 6) so that the mother and fetus may progress through pregnancy, labor, and the puerperium with a maximum of mental and physical fitness.

The goals of antepartal care are accomplished through the combined efforts of the expectant parents, the physician, the nurse, and the various other members of the health team. These goals include increasing the knowledge of the mother-to-be and her family, so that all members may experience pregnancy in a positive way, the health of mother and infant are promoted, and the family transition to include its new member proceeds smoothly.

Antepartal care may be considered the foundation for the normal development, adequate growth, and good health of the baby. During this formative period, the teeth, bones, and various systems of the body have their beginnings, and the foundations for the infant's future health are laid. Adequate antepartal care also aids in stabilizing the daily health of the mother. As pregnancy advances, the demands of the fetus increase. Since individuals react differently to pregnancy, the careful monitoring of regular care is of the utmost importance in detecting these reactions.

Nurses provide essential care to prenatal women and their families. An ongoing relationship can be established, with regular contact and much opportunity to assess and appreciate client and family needs. Nursing responsibilities for prenatal care include physiological and psychosocial assessment, education and counseling for pregnant women and their families, and identification of needs for other types of services with appropriate community and specialty referrals.

Initial Prenatal Visit

When the woman thinks she may be pregnant, she makes an appointment with the physician or clinic. The visit for confirmation of pregnancy may be combined with the prenatal work-up, or two visits may be required, depending upon office or clinic routines. The prenatal work-up consists of a thorough history, a physical examination, and laboratory tests. Prenatal forms are used by most facilities to summarize data and to serve as a flow sheet for continuing visits throughout pregnancy. Frequently the nurse is responsible for obtaining the history, collecting specimens, participating in or conducting the physical examination, and providing client education and orientation to the services that are offered.

Initial contact is particularly important. By greeting the client in a pleasant and professional manner the nurse can initiate a productive relationship that conveys interest and concern.

Assessment

The woman's name and address, her age and parity, and the date of the latest menstrual period (LMP) are recorded, and the date of delivery is estimated.

Calculation of the Expected Date of Confinement

Nägele's Rule. It is impossible to predict the expected day of confinement (EDC) with accuracy. However, the time-honored method, based on the average duration of pregnancy, is simple. Count back 3 calendar months from the first day of the LMP and add 7 days (Nägele's rule). For instance, if the LMP began on June 10, we would count back 3 months to March and, adding 7 days, arrive at the date of March 17. An easier way to calculate this is to substitute numbers for months. Then, this example becomes as follows: $6/10 - 3$ months $= 3/10 + 7$ days $= 3/17$. Although it may be satisfying to the curiosity to have this date in mind, it must be understood that only approximately 5% of all pregnant women go into labor on the EDC. Most women deliver within a 2-week period surrounding the EDC, from 7 days before to 7 days after the EDC.

Actually, women seldom go beyond term; in most of these cases it is the system of calculation and not nature that has erred. For example, ovulation and, therefore, conception may have occurred days later than calculated; this error would make the beginning and the end of pregnancy that many days later. If, in addition to this circumstance, the fetus required a slightly longer stay in the uterus for complete development, it

---

Estimated Date of Confinement (EDC)

Nägele's Rule

Count back 3 months from the first day of the LMP and add 7 days. Correct for year if necessary.

$$EDC = LMP - (3\ months) + 7\ days$$

Considerations for using Nägele's rule: Assumes a 28-day menstrual cycle with conception occurring on the 14th day. Adjustments must be made for shorter or longer cycles.

McDonald's Rule for Fundal Height

Height of fundus (cm) $\times 2/7$
   = gestation in lunar months
Height of fundus (cm) $\times 8/7$
   = gestation of pregnancy in weeks

Considerations in using fundal height measurements: Such factors as hydramnios, multiple gestation, very large fetus, and obesity affect the accuracy of measurement. For women weighing over 200 lb, subtract 1 cm from the measurement obtained. Technique can vary measurements; providers need to standardize approaches when more than one person takes serial measurements.

Ultrasonography

Four methods for estimating fetal age are the following:
- Determination of gestational sac dimensions (used as early as 6–10 weeks; fetus appears in sac about 7–8 weeks after the LMP, fetal heart activity appears by 9–10 weeks, and fetal movement is seen by 11 weeks)
- Measurement of crown–rump length (between 7 and 14 weeks)
- Measurement of femur length (after 12 weeks)
- Measurement of biparietal diameter (BPD) of fetal head (after 12 weeks. BPD is frequently used for diagnosis of term pregnancy. Fetal weight and BPD are well correlated, and at 36 weeks BPD should be about 8.7 cm. At term the BPD is usually greater than 9.8 cm.)

---

would be clear that the apparent delay was quite normal and for the best.

Fundal Height. Measurement of fundal height helps in determining the age of the fetus and, thus, the EDC. Directions for measurement of fundal height are given later in this chapter.

Ultrasonography. Indications for ultrasonographic estimation of fetal age include uncertain dates for the LMP, recent discontinuation of oral contraceptives, first-trimester bleeding, discrepancy between uterine size and estimated gestation by dates, previous cesearean delivery, and other high-risk conditions. Ultrasonography is discussed in Chapter 42.

History

Inquiries are made into the family history, with special reference to any condition likely to affect childbearing, such as hereditary diseases, tuberculosis, or multiple pregnancy. Then the personal history of the client is reviewed, not only with regard to previous diseases and operations, but particularly in relation to any difficulties experienced in previous pregnancies and labors, such as miscarriages, prolonged labor, death of infant, hemorrhage, and other complications.

Inquiry is made into the history of the present pregnancy, especially in relation to nausea, edema of the feet or the face, headache, visual disturbance, vaginal bleeding, constipation, breathlessness, sleeplessness, cramps, heartburn, lower abdominal pain, vaginal discharge, and varicose veins. A sample prenatal history form is given below.

As time permits, the nurse can use the initial visit to expand upon historical information for assessment purposes, both nursing and medical. The following areas are generally included:

1. Social and personal characteristics of the client: age, marital status, occupation, ethnicity, religion, height, weight, number of children in the home
2. Information summary of spouse (father of baby): name, address, age, height, weight, ethnicity
3. Characteristics influencing the course of pregnancy: EDC, LMP, blood type and Rh, pertinent

medical conditions or hospitalizations, current medications and medication habits, usual bowel patterns, usual sleep patterns, resumé of dietary habits
4. Attitudes toward the pregnancy:
Was this child planned?
What are the client's goals and values regarding this pregnancy and other relevant areas?
Does she view this pregnancy positively or as an interference in her life?
What is her knowledge about health in general and pregnancy and childrearing in particular?
Does she have any previous experience with pregnancy or childrearing?
What are her expectations and concerns about this pregnancy, birth, and care of the infant?
What is her apparent willingness or disinclination to prepare herself in the areas that need attention?
5. Resources:
What appears to be her general level of intelligence or education?
What is the level of economic stability?
Is the family intact?
Is there extended family available to her?
Does she have sufficient friends from whom she can get tangible help and emotional support if necessary?
6. Resumé of antenatal classes and instruction: antenatal classes and films attended, individual and group instruction and counseling

(text continued on page 382)

ASSESSMENT TOOL

Prenatal History

Name _____ Date _____
Address _____ Phone number _____
_____ Date of birth _____
Physician _____

I. HEALTH HISTORY
Family History
Health status of parents, siblings (if deceased, note cause of death):
_____
_____
_____
_____

Occurrence or history of the following diseases in parents, siblings, and close relatives:
diabetes mellitus ____   hypertension ____   renal disease ____   vascular disease ____
tuberculosis ____   cardiopulmonary ____   neuromuscular disease ____
complications of pregnancy or congenital anomalies (specify) _____
psychiatric disorders (specify) _____
cancer (specify) _____

(continued)

A S S E S S M E N T   T O O L   *(continued)*

Personal and Health History

Personal characteristics:

age _____

racial/ethnic background _____

relationships (husband, partner, children,

support networks) _____

_____

_____

habits:

smoke _____

alcohol ____   drugs ____

exercise _____

relaxation _____

misc. _____

Past medical history:

childhood diseases: _____

_____

immunizations (including rubella): _____

_____

hospitalizations (reasons, years): _____

_____

surgery (type, year): _____

_____

blood transfusions: _____

drug sensitivities: _____

allergies (foods, allergens): _____

_____

diseases:

diabetes mellitus ____   vascular disease ____   endocrinopathy ____

rheumatic fever ____   sexually transmitted disease ____   severe anemia ____

cardiopulmonary ____   asthma ____   blood dyscrasias ____

hypertension ____   psychiatric disorders ____   malnutrition ____

tuberculosis ____   cancer ____   malignancy ____

renal/urinary tract disease __

injuries (especially to pelvic organs or structures): _____

_____

Menstrual history:

age at menarche ____

describe present cycle (interval between menses _____, amount of flow _____, pain _____, clots _____,

intermenstrual bleeding): _____

problems and procedures (*e.g.*, D&C _____, conization, _____, irregular bleeding _____, amenorrhea _____):

Sexual history:

sexual learning and understandings of sexual functions: _____

_____

sexual self-concept and identity: _____

_____

attitudes toward sexuality, particularly as affected by pregnancy: _____

_____

current sexual practices and satisfaction with these: _____

_____

contraceptive history and practice: _____

method _____ effective/satisfied with use _____ problems _____

method _____ effective/satisfied with use _____ problems _____

method _____ effective/satisfied with use _____ problems _____

(continued)

ASSESSMENT TOOL *(continued)*

sexually transmitted diseases and treatment: _____
    type of STD _____ date _____ Rx _____
    type of STD _____ date _____ Rx _____
    type of STD _____ date _____ Rx _____

II. PREGNANCY HISTORY
Past Obstetric History

Year	Length Gest.	Probs During Preg	Onset Labor	Length Labor	Complications Labor

Current Pregnancy
Last menstrual period (LMP): _____ Prior menstrual period (PMP): _____
Date fetal movement first felt: _____
Symptoms: nausea _____ urinary frequency _____ headache _____ leukorrhea _____
edema _____ constipation _____ bleeding _____ abdominal pain _____
others _____

Drugs or medications taken since pregnancy began:
_____

Exposure to communicable disease (especially rubella if not immune): _____

Illnesses since beginning of pregnancy (colds, flu, etc): _____

Occupation: _____ Possible workplace exposure to toxins: _____

Reactions and adaptation to pregnancy (Was pregnancy planned? Is woman pleased or concerned?): _____

Reactions of partner and family: _____

Data about father:
    age _____ height _____ weight _____
    racial/ethnic origins _____
    health status _____
    medical history: _____

    response to pregnancy: _____

    relationship with client and family: _____

    occupation: _____ potential health hazards: _____

Interviewed by: _____ Date: _____

Comments:

A S S E S S M E N T   T O O L

Components of the Prenatal Physical Examination

Part Examined Examination Technique	Normal Findings	Abnormal Findings
Head and neck		
Palpation, inspection with otoophthalmoscope, and visual inspection of mouth	Hyperemia of nasal and buccal mucous membranes, slight diffuse enlargement of thyroid	Enlarged lymph nodes, thyroid nodules or irregular enlargement, lesions of eyes or mouth, caries and abscesses of teeth, ear infections
Chest and heart		
Auscultation with stethoscope, percussion and visual inspection	Lungs clear, heart in regular rhythm (occasionally a soft, short functional murmur due to hemodynamic changes of pregnancy)	Adventitious lung sounds (rates, wheezes, ronchi), irregular cardiac rhythm, nonphysiological murmurs
Breasts		
Palpation and visual inspection	Enlargement of breasts with increased vascular patterns, darkened areola with prominent tubercles, clear fluid from nipples in later pregnancy	Masses or nodules, bloody or serosanguinous nipple discharge, nipple lesions, erythema
Skin		
Visual inspection	Pigmentation changes (linea nigra, mask of pregnancy), enlargement of nevi, appearance of spider angiomas, mottled erythema of hands	Pallor, jaundice, rash, skin lesions
Extremities		
Visual inspection and palpation, percussion with reflex hammer	Mild pretibial and ankle edema in third trimester, slight edema of hands in hot weather	Limitations of motion, varicosities, more than slight pretibial, hand, or ankle edema, edema of face or sacrum, hyperreflexia and clonus

(continued)

(text continued from page 379)

Physical Examination

A thorough physical examination is usually performed to establish a baseline for the woman's general state of health and to evaluate the pregnancy. Vital signs including temperature, blood pressure, pulse, respiration, height, and weight are taken. Components of the Prenatal Physical Examination summarizes the techniques for examination and normal and abnormal findings, which are generally included in the prenatal physical examination.

The nurse who is alert to the clues and the events that transpire during the physical examination may use this information to interpret instructions or answer questions that the client may ask afterward. Often a client hesitates to discuss some matter with a physician because she considers it too trivial, but she may feel comfortable talking about it with the nurse. In turn, the nurse may consider this a problem of some importance and on reporting it to the physician may find that it has a bearing on the course of treatment that is prescribed.

Since the initial examination is thorough, it is desirable that the client disrobe completely and wear a gown that opens easily. In addition, the expectant mother should be covered with a small sheet to prevent unnecessary exposure and chilling. The nurse should

ASSESSMENT TOOL *(continued)*

Part Examined Examination Technique	Normal Findings	Abnormal Findings
Abdomen		
Palpation, visual inspection, auscultation, percussion	Enlarged uterus, palpation of fetal outline in later pregnancy, fetal heart sounds, contractions in last trimester	Uterus too large or too small for dates, absence of fetal heart sounds beyond 10 weeks (using Doppler), transverse lie of fetus, fetal head in fundus, tonic uterine contractions, enlarged liver or spleen
Pelvis		
Speculum exam, bimanual exam with inspection and palpation, collection of specimens	Speculum exam: Bluish discoloration of mucosa of vagina and cervix, congested cervix, ectropion in multigravidas, increased leukorrhea Bimanual exam: Cervix soft, admits a finger or two (depending upon gravida and length of pregnancy), uterus soft and enlarged, fetal head or parts may be felt in lower uterine segment, gynecoid pelvic configuration Pap smear: Squamous metaplasia, negative or normal, adequate or increased estrogen, endocervical cells present, hyperplasia is considered borderline	Speculum exam: Yellow, purulent, frothy, cheesy white or homogeneous gray, foul-smelling discharge, friable, bleeding lesions of cervix; vaginal lesions; bleeding from cervical os, amniotic fluid Bimanual exam: Cervix dilated and effaced (unless labor has begun); cervical or vaginal masses; excessive amniotic fluid (uterus unusually enlarged); adnexal masses or fullness; rectal masses; hemorrhoids; contractions of the pelvic inlet, midpelvis, or outlet Pap smear: Inflammation, presence of *Trichomonas* or fungi, diminished or absent estrogen, atypical or suspicious cells, atypical hyperplasia, dysplasia, neoplasia, or carcinoma

instruct the woman to empty her bladder, because a full bladder is uncomfortable and may interfere with the manipulations carried out during the examination. A good footstool is imperative if the woman is to mount the table in safety and comfort.

During the physical examination particular attention is paid to the teeth and throat, thyroid gland and lymph nodes, lungs, heart, breasts, skin, extremities, and abdomen (Fig. 22-1). Characteristic changes of pregnancy are noted (see Chap. 18), and signs of infection or systemic disease are identified if present.

Physical indicators of high-risk pregnancy can often be determined in initial examination, such as obesity, hypertension, severe varicosities, preeclampsia, or inappropriate uterine size for dates.

Pelvic Examination. Pelvic examination provides data relevant to confirming the pregnancy and deter-

mining the length of gestation, pelvic characteristics, and any abnormalities that might produce complications of pregnancy. At the same time, specimens are obtained to screen for potential problems. The pelvic examination includes both speculum and bimanual examinations. On speculum examination, the characteristics of the vaginal and the cervical mucosa are examined, and vaginal discharge is evaluated. Unusual lesions are identified and biopsies are taken, as well as smears for vaginitis and cultures for gonorrhea. Pap smears to screen for cervical cancer are done routinely.

The bimanual examination provides information about the consistency of the cervix; the size, shape, and consistency of the uterus; the condition of the fallopian tubes and ovaries; and the configuration of the bony pelvis. Uterine size is useful in determining length of gestation, and pelvic measurements enable a clinical appraisal of potential pelvic contractions which might

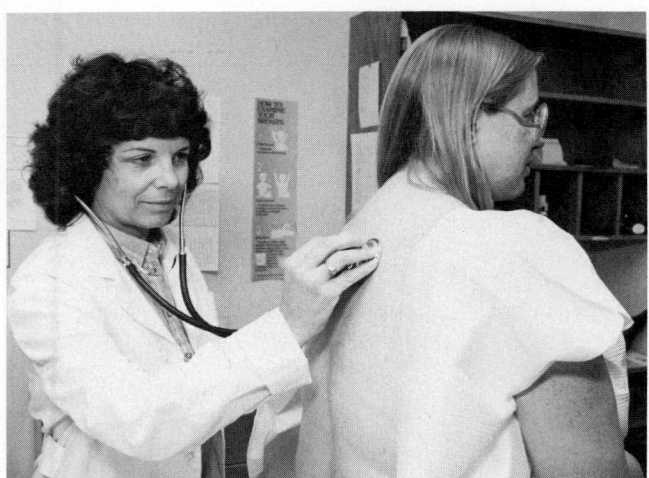

FIGURE 22-1

A thorough physical examination is done early in pregnancy to assess the mother's health and the status of the pregnancy. (Courtesy of Media Services, Sonoma State University)

lead to cephalopelvic disproportion in labor. Other abnormalities of the birth canal, such as soft-tissue masses, can also be identified.

The vaginal or pelvic examination deserves special consideration because often it is the most stressful part of the experience for the client. This examination is carried out with the woman in the dorsal recumbent position. In this position she lies on her back with the lower extremities flexed and rotated outward. Her heels are supported in stirrups, which are level with the table, perhaps a foot in front of her buttocks. In this position the anxious woman, already under stress during the physical examination, is likely to tense her abdominal, pelvic, and thigh muscles, attempting to adduct her thighs. Moreover, if she arches her back as her tension increases, her pelvis will be tilted downward, a position that makes the pelvic examination almost impossible to achieve.

The nurse can be most effective in assisting the client to relax if she encourages her to keep breathing naturally, reminds her to breathe if she holds her breath, and reminds her to press the small of her back down on the table. Merely telling the anxious woman to relax is of no avail; thus, the nurse needs to give the client direct guidance, often step by step. For example, if the client is clenching her fists, the nurse may say, "See, your wrists and hands are tense. Try to let them go limp—very limp—like a rag doll's. That's it—very limp." And a moment later, "Keep breathing naturally." Such short, explicit requests and instruction give the mother a simple task that she can do with guidance. This diverts her attention from the anticipated discomfort and promotes relaxation.

Steps in the Pelvic Examination. To see the cervix clearly, the examiner sits on a stool and focuses a good light into the vagina. Any equipment that is needed, such as vaginal speculum, swabs, cotton balls, slides, and lubricating jelly, should be within reach.

The pelvic examination begins with an examination of the external genitalia, including the urethra and Skene's and Bartholin's glands. If any unusual discharge is present, a specimen may be obtained for culture or microscopic examination.

Usually, the next step is to insert a speculum into the vagina to distend the folds so as to provide a clearer view of the cervix (Fig. 22-2). If a Pap smear is to be taken, no lubricating jelly is used; instead, the speculum may be rinsed under *tepid* running water to facilitate the ease of insertion. Occasionally, the dilatation of the vagina by the speculum may cause an unpleasant sensation of stretching (Fig. 22-3).

As the examination proceeds, the cervix is visualized, and the examiner notes its color and character. Normally, the cervix of the primigravida is pink or bluish and smooth, with a dimple for the os. The cervix of a multigravida may have an irregular os owing to lacerations from previous deliveries (Fig. 22-4). Ectropion is often present around the os in multigravidas; this is a darker pinkish-red, bumpy tissue composed of columnar epithelium, which lines the endocervical canal. Unless infection is present, this tissue is considered a normal variant during the years of active estrogen secretion. Any discharge that is purulent, greenish, or frothy is considered to be abnormal, and a specimen may be secured for microscopic examination or culture.

After the cervix has been examined, the examiner withdraws the speculum and proceeds with the bimanual examination to evaluate the uterus and the adnexa (Fig. 22-5). The size, consistency, and contour of these organs, as well as the relationship of the uterus to the pelvis, are determined. Pelvic measurements are taken

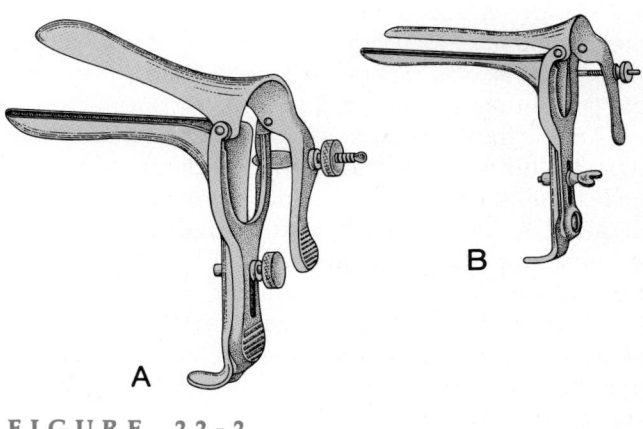

A   B

FIGURE 22-2

Instruments of the gynecological examination. (*A*) Graves speculum. (*B*) Pederson speculum.

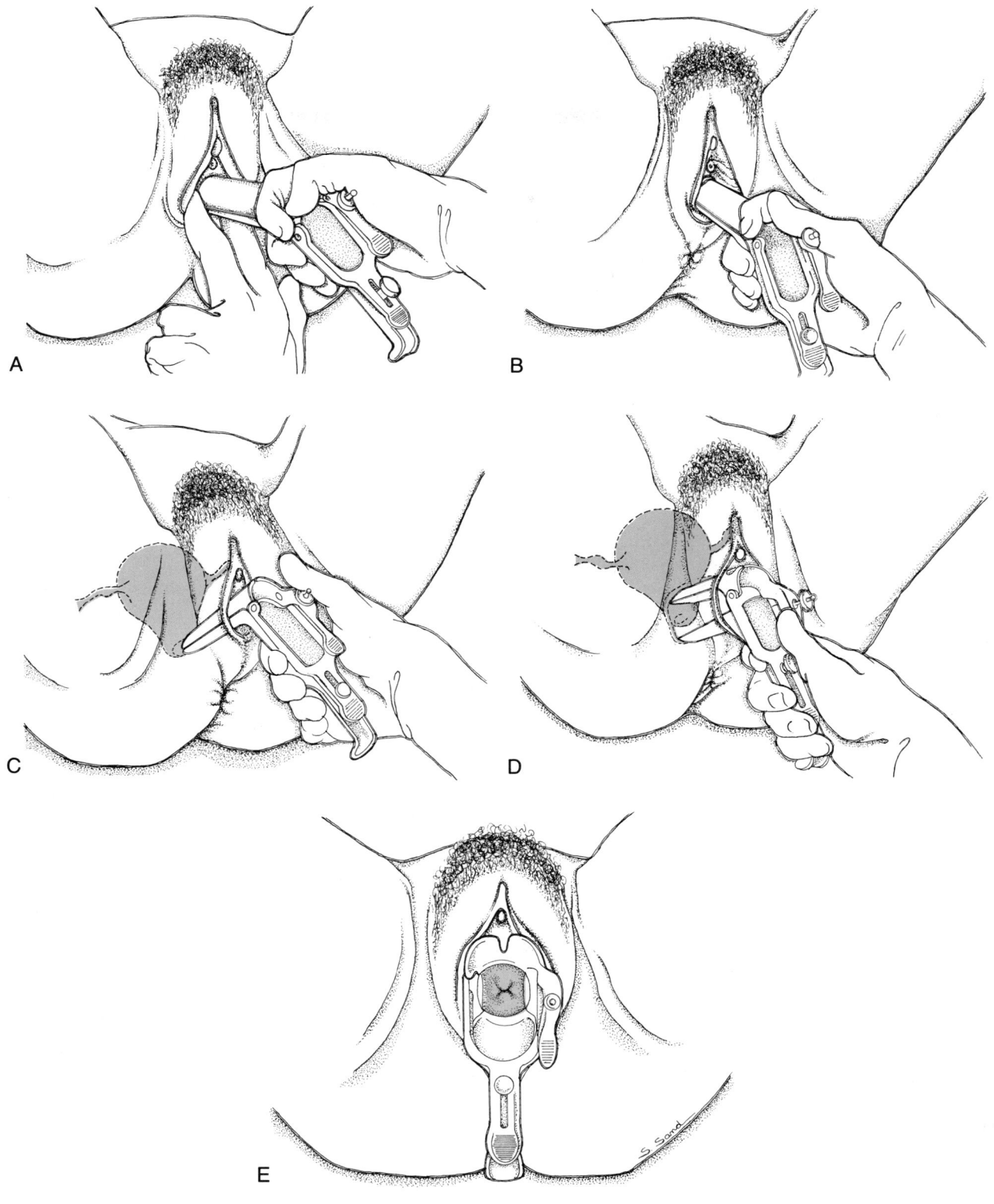

FIGURE 22-3

Insertion of the speculum. (*A*) Opening the introitus. (*B*) Oblique insertion of the speculum. (*C*) Final insertion of the speculum. (*D*) Opening the blades of the speculum. (*E*) View of the cervix through the speculum.

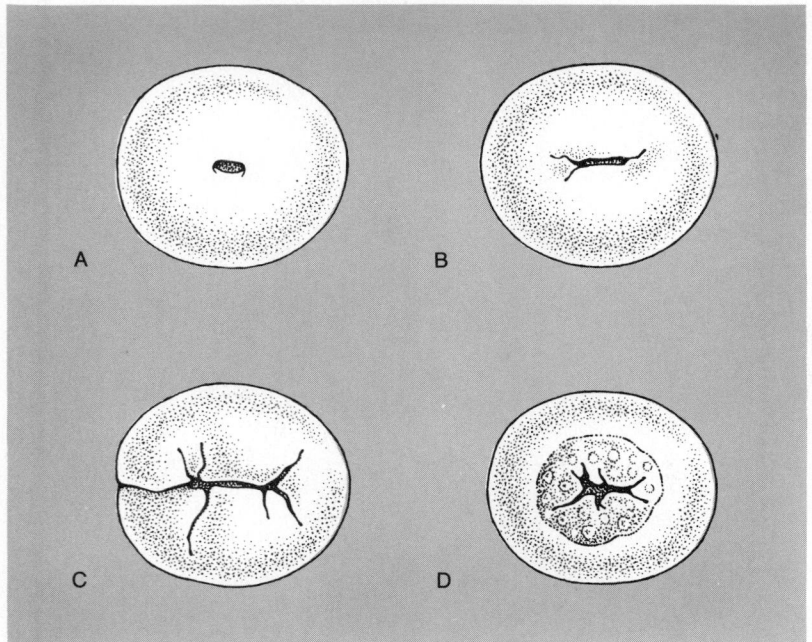

F I G U R E   2 2 - 4

Common appearance of the cervix. (*A*) The nulliparous cervical os is small and either round or oval. (*B*) After childbirth the os presents a slitlike appearance. (*C*) Difficult deliveries may tear the cervix, producing permanent lacerations. (*D*) Ectopion, often present in multigravidas, is a pinkish-red, bumpy tissue composed of columnar epithelium. (Redrawn from Bates B: A Guide to Physical Examination, 2nd ed. Philadelphia, JB Lippincott, 1979)

at the same time. The examination is usually completed with an examination of the rectum to ascertain the presence of hemorrhoids, polyps, or other abnormalities. When the examination is completed, disposable tissues should be offered the client to wipe the perineum adequately.

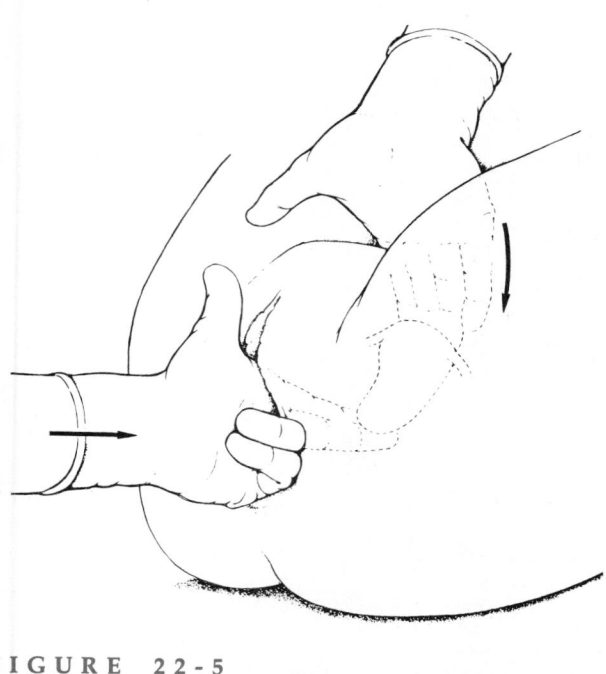

F I G U R E   2 2 - 5

Bimanual palpation of the uterus.

Pap Smear. The Pap smear is obtained during speculum examination. The cervix is cleansed with a dry cotton ball to remove excess mucus, and a saline-moistened cotton-tipped applicator is introduced into the endocervical canal. It is rotated several times, withdrawn, and rolled on a glass slide. The smear is fixed immediately with commercial fixatives or immersed in 95% ethyl alcohol to prevent the specimen from drying, which distorts the cells. Next, a wooden or plastic spatula is used to obtain the ectocervical sample. The shaped end is introduced slightly into the cervical os and turned firmly several times to scrape the tissue of the squamocolumnar junction (where the endocervical epithelium meets that of the ectocervix) (Fig. 22-6). This is the area where most malignancies arise and can be seen as a color change of cervical epithelium. This specimen is smeared on a glass slide and fixed as above. Some providers place both endocervical and ectocervical specimens on one slide. A vaginal pool sample may also be taken by introducing the rounded end of the spatula into the posterior vaginal fornix or by aspirating fluid with a vaginal pipette. The smears should be accompanied by data about the woman's age, LMP, pregnancy or postpartum status, gynecologic surgery, and use of hormones.

Laboratory Tests

The laboratory tests carried out in antepartal care are the urine examination, the blood test for syphilis, complete blood count or hemoglobin, tests for the Rh factor and blood type, and often rubella titer (tests for the

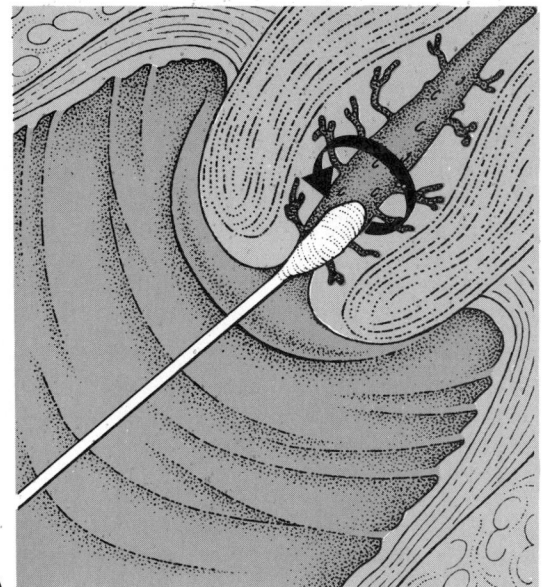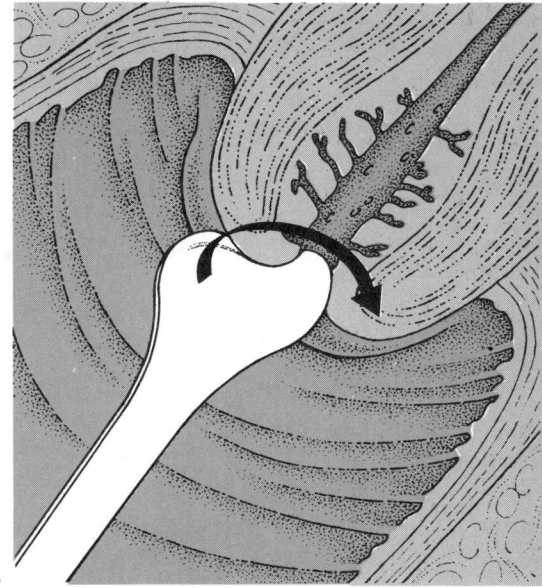

FIGURE 22-6

The Pap smear. (*A*) Obtaining the endocervical sample. (*B*) Obtaining the ectocervical sample.

mother's status to rubella immunity), gonorrhea culture, and antibody screening (Table 22-1).

Urine Test. At the first and subsequent examinations, the urine is tested for albumin and sugar. If indicated, the client is instructed to collect part of the first urine voided in the morning before breakfast. Glucose may spill into the urine of a normal pregnant woman owing to a decreased kidney threshold for glucose. Hence, it is more likely to appear in the urine after a meal. The test for sugar is the same as that used to test a diabetic's urine; several simple dipstick tests are available today and may be completed quickly and accurately in a matter of minutes.

Any positive reaction to sugar is reported so that the possibility of diabetes or a prediabetic condition can be ruled out.

The test for albumin is simple, also using a dipstick. *The presence of albumin in the urine is another symptom of possible preeclampsia and should be reported immediately.*

At least once a full urinalysis is performed, including chemistry and microscopic examination. This allows identification of clients with unsuspected diabetes, renal disease, hypertensive disease, and bacteriuria. The examination reports specific gravity, color, character, *p*H, glucose, protein, ketones, blood, and the presence of microorganisms, cellular components (RBCs, WBCs, epithelials, casts), and crystals.

Blood Tests. Blood for the Venereal Disease Research Laboratories (VDRL) or other serologic tests for syphilis is usually obtained by venipuncture. A sufficient quantity of blood is drawn at this time so that a portion may be used for the Rh factor and complete blood count (CBC) or hemoglobin estimation. Since many pregnant women develop anemia, the latter examination is highly important.

If the test for the *Rh factor* shows that the client is Rh negative, it may be necessary to check the father and do serial antibody titers throughout pregnancy. It is also a wise precaution to obtain the father's blood type (see Chap. 36).

In some states, a blood test for presence of rubella antibodies is required. Since maternal rubella during the first trimester has such devastating effects upon the fetus, it is important to know the mother's immune status so she may be counseled about possible rubella exposure during pregnancy. If the mother's titer is negative, she has no immunity and is strongly advised to stay away from small children, particularly with any symptoms of upper respiratory tract infections (rubella prodromal symptoms). Immunization is not done during pregnancy but should be done in nonimmune women after delivery.

Gonorrhea Culture. It is often routine to perform gonorrhea cultures as part of the prenatal work-up, without ascertaining a history of exposure. This is done

Laboratory Tests During Pregnancy

Test	Source of Specimen	Purpose

Urinalysis
  Sugar
  Albumin
  Microscopic
	Clean voided urine	Sugar (glycosuria)—screen for diabetes
		Albumin (proteinuria)—screen for preeclampsia, kidney stress, or renal problems
		RBCs, WBCs, epithelial cells, casts, microorganisms—screen for renal disease, urinary tract infection

CBC
  Hematocrit and hemoglobin
  White blood cell count and differential
  Platelets
	Venous blood	Hematocrit and hemoglobin—screen for anemia
		White blood cell count and differential—identify infectious processes; screen for blood dyscrasias, folic acid deficiency
		Platelets—assess blood-clotting mechanisms

Urine culture	Clean voided urine	Diagnose urinary tract infections; often done routinely on all pregnant women; done when urinary symptoms are present to identify organism
Serologic test for syphilis	Serum	Screen for syphilis (if positive must confirm with FTA-ABS)
Rh factor and blood type	Venous blood	Determine the blood type and Rh factor (positive or negative): blood type is important in case of hemorrhage; Rh factor alerts providers to possible incompatibility disease in fetus
Rh titers	Venous blood	Done when mother is Rh negative and father is Rh positive to assay danger to fetus (signified by rising titer)
Rubella antibodies	Venous blood	Determine if mother has been exposed previously to rubella and has built up antibodies (*i.e.*, is immune or not)
Gonorrhea culture	Cervical discharge	Diagnose gonorrhea; often done routinely because gonorrhea is frequently asymptomatic in women
Pap smear	Cervix	Screen for cervical intraepithelial neoplasia; herpes simplex type 2
Tuberculin skin test	Applied to skin	Screen high-risk women for tuberculosis
BUN, creatinine, total protein, electrolytes	Serum	Evaluate renal function and diagnose renal disease
ECG, chest x-ray	Heart, lungs	Evaluate cardiac and pulmonary function
Hemoglobin electrophoresis	Blood	Diagnose hemoglobinopathies (*e.g.*, sickle cell anemia, thalassemias)

because gonorrhea is frequently asymptomatic in women and is a widespread infectious disease. If the culture is positive, treatment during pregnancy can prevent possible maternal and fetal complications. Any regular sexual partner and known contacts also must be treated.

Nursing Diagnosis

The purpose of the first prenatal visit usually is to confirm the pregnancy. The woman and her family may be excited or upset about her pregnancy. Their reactions and the woman's health status and physiological re-

sponse to pregnancy will largely determine nursing diagnoses and interventions. Potential diagnoses, unless high-risk factors are found, may include anxiety, knowledge deficits, ineffective individual or family coping, or alteration in comfort as a result of physiological changes. Further diagnoses are discussed in the section concerning return visits.

Planning/Intervention

At the initial visit, counseling and education should be brief and focused on immediate and short-term needs. The mother's initial questions should be answered and an overview given of prenatal care. It is better to postpone further health teaching and counseling until a subsequent visit, when the mother is not so overloaded with new stimuli.

Return Visits

Regular return visits are scheduled throughout pregnancy to provide continuing monitoring of maternal and fetal status, to institute treatment and further diagnostic tests as necessary, and to offer ongoing opportunity for support and education. The usual schedule of visits is once a month until the seventh month, every 2 weeks during the seventh and eighth months, and weekly during the ninth month until delivery. Visits are scheduled more frequently if problems arise. Routine return visits consist of follow-up history, physical examination, and client education (see Schedule of Return Prenatal Visits).

Assessment

Nursing assessment includes physiological data on maternal adaptations to changes of pregnancy, measures of fetal well-being, identification of signs or symptoms of complications, maternal and family psychological adaptation to pregnancy, compliance with medical regimens, and preparations for parenthood. There is also great opportunity to identify other health problems within the pregnant family, but not directly related to pregnancy. Such problems may need immediate attention or may be appropriately dealt with in the future.

General inquiry is made about how the client and family are feeling and the presence of any concerns or symptoms. New signs or physical findings, such as excessive weight gain or glycosuria, are explored through a series of questions. The woman is queried about any untoward signs and symptoms, including edema of the fingers or face, bleeding, constipation, and headaches. During these visits the woman is encouraged and giv-

---

Schedule of Return Prenatal Visits

First through sixth month—visits once per month
Seventh and eighth months—visits every 2 weeks
Ninth month until delivery—visits once per week

Included in Visit	When Done
Weight	Each visit
Blood pressure	Each visit
Fundal height (McDonald's)	Each visit
Fetal heart rate	Each visit
Check for edema	Each visit
Pelvic examination	Middle of ninth month, then weekly as indicated
Other examination	As indicated by symptoms
Inquiry about symptoms, signs, or problems	Each visit
Prenatal education*	Each visit
Nutrition and appetite	Each visit
Family and personal adjustment	Each visit
Urinalysis for glucose and albumin	Each visit
Hematocrit and hemoglobin	At 32 to 34 weeks (more often if anemic)
Urine culture	As indicated by symptoms or signs
Rh titers	If initially negative, twice more during pregnancy; if positive, more often as indicated by titer levels
Other tests	As indicated by symptoms or signs

* See Prenatal Education Checklist later in the chapter.

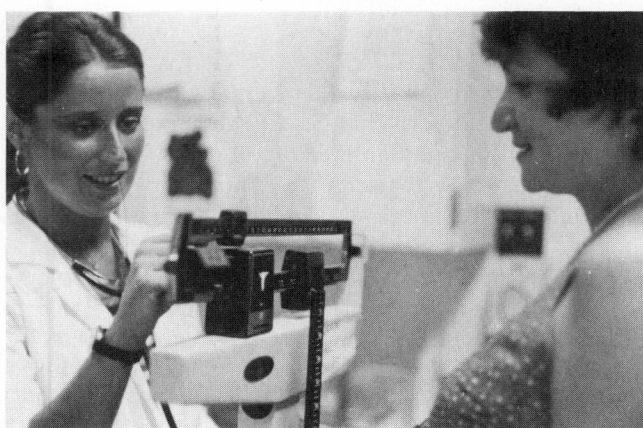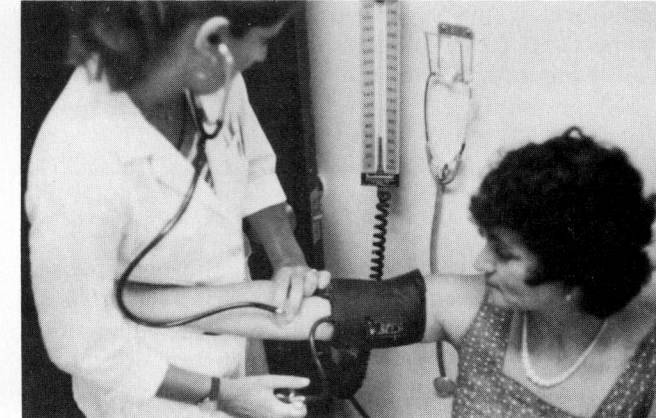

FIGURE 22-7

Weight gain is measured and blood pressure is taken at each return visit.
(Courtesy of Booth Maternity Center, Philadelphia)

en ample opportunity to ask any questions of concern to her.

Weight, blood pressure, fundal height, and fetal heart tones are taken during each return visit (Fig. 22-7). Weight is plotted on a graph or flow sheet, and deviations from expected progression are noted and explored.

Legs and feet are examined for edema and development of varicosities. Other aspects of the physical examination are performed if indicated by signs or symptoms.

Vaginal examinations are usually not done on return visits until the client nears term. Frequently vaginal examinations begin about 2 or 3 weeks from EDC to assess the status of the cervix, fetal presentation, and the degree of engagement. The urine is tested on each return visit for sugar and protein (albumin), and hematocrit is repeated at 32 to 34 weeks as a precaution against anemia.

Abdominal Examination

Abdominal examination is useful in providing information about the position of the fetus after the 13th week of gestation (Fig. 22-8). Leopold's maneuvers help determine position and presentation of the fetus, and auscultation of the fetal heart tones can provide an indication of fetal conditions. (Leopold's maneuvers are discussed in Chap. 23. Monitoring of fetal heart tones is discussed in Chap. 42.)

Fetal activity can be assessed, and the height of the fundus can be used to approximate the length of gestation by means of McDonald's technique. A flexible tape measure is used to measure the distance from the upper border of the symphysis pubis to the top of the uterine fundus. Frequently the tape measure is curved over the mother's abdomen, although some providers

hold it straight between the fingers with the hand at a right angle to the top of the fundus (Fig. 22-9). The distance measured in centimeters, multiplied by two and divided by seven gives the duration of pregnancy in lunar months. During the first 24 to 26 weeks the fundal height in centimeters is roughly equal to the weeks of gestation (*e.g.*, 20 cm fundal height equals 20 weeks' gestation). Using *McDonald's rule* increases accuracy during the second and third trimesters (see rule given earlier in this chapter).

Other Tests

Additional diagnostic tests are done as indicated during pregnancy. Tuberculin skin testing is advisable in high-risk and symptomatic clients. Renal function tests such

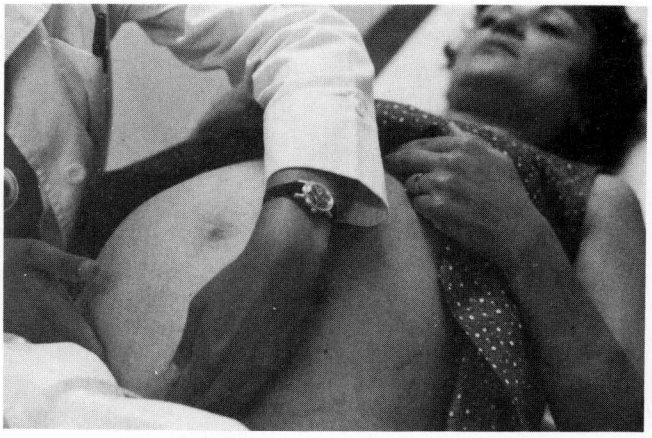

FIGURE 22-8

Leopold's maneuvers are used to determine fetal presentation and position. (Courtesy of Booth Maternity Center, Philadelphia)

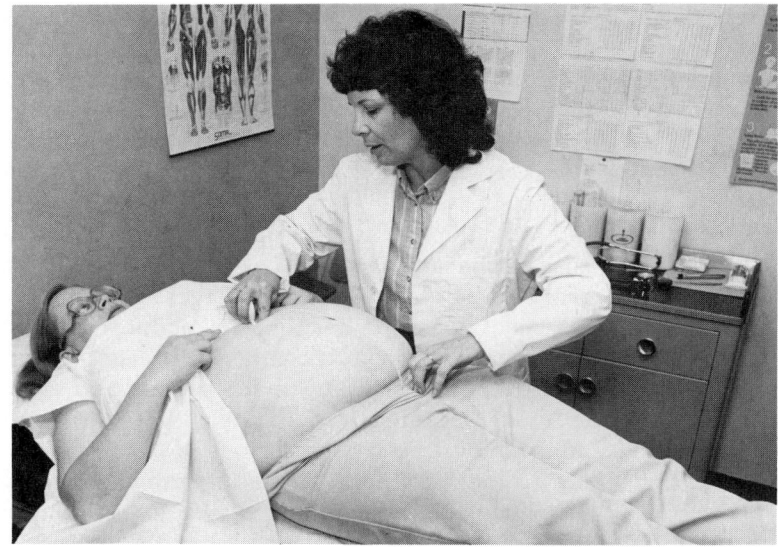

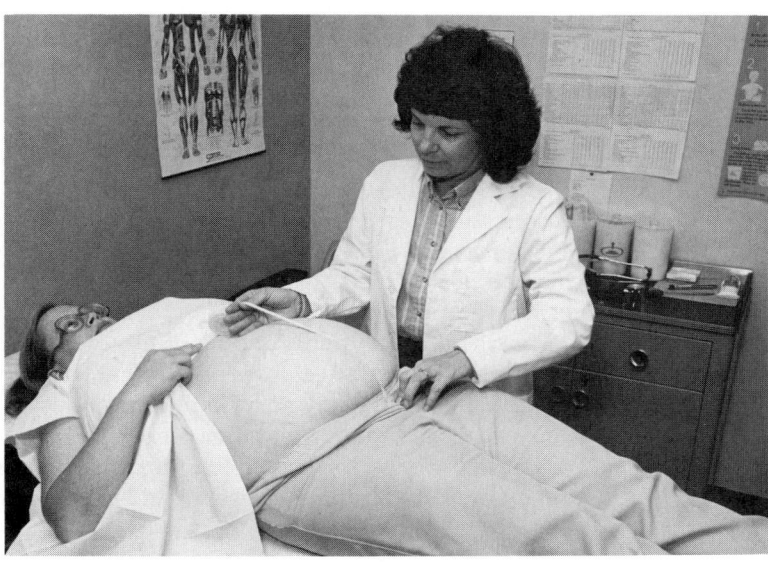

as blood urea nitrogen (BUN), creatinine, electrolytes, and total protein excretion are obtained when renal complications or conditions are suspected. Some clinics or offices obtain routine screening urine cultures because of the prevalence of asymptomatic bacteriuria. Urine cultures are definitely indicated with urinary tract symptoms or the presence of bacteria or WBCs on microscopic urinalysis. Specific problems such as cardiac disease are evaluated with electrocardiogram (ECG) and echocardiogram, pulmonary problems with chest x-ray and pulmonary function studies, and hemoglobinopathies with hemoglobin or protein electrophoresis (see Table 22-1).

Nursing Diagnosis

A variety of nursing diagnoses may be made during the antepartum period because pregnancy causes numerous physiological and psychosocial changes to which the woman and her family must adapt (see Chaps. 18 and 19). Diagnoses may involve all the functional patterns identified by Gordon: health perception–health management, nutritional-metabolic, activity-exercise, sleep-rest, cognitive-perceptual, self-perception, role relationship, sexuality-reproductive, coping-stress tolerance, and value-belief.[1] Diagnoses are discussed not only in the nursing-care plan in this chapter but also throughout the book using the North American Nursing Diagnosis Association (NANDA) categorization.

Planning/Intervention

Nursing intervention uses techniques of teaching, support, advice, self-care preparation, direct physical care, and referral or coordination of services. The scope of nursing care includes helping client and family understand and adapt to physiological and emotional changes of pregnancy, deal with minor discomforts effectively, recognize and if possible avoid potentially serious complications, plan for parenthood and integrating the new baby into the family, understand and comply with the medical regimen, and attain optimal health status.

Weight Gain

The routine estimation of weight at regular intervals during pregnancy is an important detail of antepartal care. At first the average gain in weight of the fetus is 1 g daily; nine tenths of the weight is gained after the fifth month, and one half of the weight of the fetus is acquired during the last 8 weeks. Most specialists agree that a weight gain of about 25 to 30 pounds is desirable for a woman who is average or "normal" in her prepregnant weight. However, there is increasing evidence among investigators that the weight gain for pregnancy needs to be individualized for every client, particularly those under and over average prepregnant weights. In the former case, a gain of 30 pounds or more has had no deleterious effects on the mother and has resulted in a healthy infant of normal weight. For all clients the emphasis is becoming less on gain *per se* than on a balanced nutritional status related to the woman's general physical condition.

Certainly no woman should try to lose weight during pregnancy, and even those who begin pregnancy significantly overweight must expect to gain additional weight. Explaining to the client how pregnancy weight is distributed (see Chap. 21) helps her understand why it is necessary for normal progression of fetal development.

Instructions and Anticipatory Guidance

During prenatal visits the client may be instructed regarding diet, rest and sleep, daily intestinal elimination, proper exercise, fresh air and sunshine, bathing, clothing, recreation, and dental care. Therefore, it is necessary for the nurse to have broad knowledge and understanding about the physiology of pregnancy and childbearing, general hygiene, nutrition, the emotional, psychological, and socioeconomic aspects of family living, and the part played by a family in the larger community.

Danger Signals to Be Reported Immediately

Vaginal bleeding, no matter how slight
Swelling of the face or the fingers
Severe continuous headache
Dimness or blurring of vision
Flashes of light or dots before the eyes
Pain in the abdomen
Persistent vomiting
Chills and fever
Sudden escape of fluid from the vagina

It is always desirable to assure the woman when the findings on examination are normal. Barring complications, such clients may anticipate an uneventful pregnancy followed by an uncomplicated delivery. However, all prenatal clients must be tactfully instructed about certain danger signals that must be reported immediately.

In addition, the client needs an explanation of the changes that are taking place within her body. This point cannot be stressed enough. Intelligent exploration with the client regarding her concerns about these changes and appropriate instruction give her greater reassurance and self-confidence. An understanding and empathic attitude does much to buoy the client's morale and to diminish unnecessary anxiety.

As the client approaches full term, she can also be instructed about the signs and symptoms of oncoming labor, so that she may know when the process is beginning and when to notify the physician. At this time she needs to report the frequency of contractions and any other pertinent symptoms. See the accompanying Prenatal Education Checklist for items to be discussed.

Teaching sessions are individualized for each client and should include instruction in ways of maintaining good health habits in daily living, interpretation of the reasons that these practices are important, and suggestions of ways in which undesirable habits may be changed or modified.

The first step toward this goal is to identify the level of knowledge and understanding of the client through exploration of what she knows and feels about the topic in question. Second, any misinformation or misconceptions must be clarified. The final step is to add to the base of knowledge and understanding through reinterpretation, clarification, reemphasis, and reinforcement.

Visual Aids and Teaching Groups

In hospitals and offices where the appointment system is used, the waiting time for the client is minimized. In others the client may have to wait longer periods. Waiting time in any setting may be used advantageously by providing reading material that contributes to the client's knowledge of her condition. Visual aids such as posters and charts may be both instructive and diverting. Some simple computerized programmed instruction or interactive computer educational programs are being used more frequently.

Offices and, increasingly, clinics are using a group approach for discussion, teaching, and guidance. These groups are usually under the leadership of the nurse and provide a maximum amount of instruction for a large number of clients in a short period of time. In addition, in the large, busy clinic, this group discussion technique provides clients with a feeling of continuity of care, since the nurse leader remains a stable figure (see Chap. 20, Preparation for Parenthood).

Hospital Tour

Most hospitals conduct routine tours of the maternity division for the expectant parents. It is advisable to encourage parents to take advantage of this opportunity sometime during the pregnancy. Becoming familiar ahead of time with the surroundings where the mother-to-be will deliver the baby reduces the anxiety that may be experienced in going to a strange hospital for the first time after labor begins (Fig. 22-10). The details of

---

A S S E S S M E N T   T O O L

Prenatal Education Checklist

Pregnancy and Health Status

Date   Initials

_____ _____ Prenatal history and physical examination results discussed
_____ _____ Prenatal laboratory panel results discussed
_____ _____ Medications and teratology discussed
_____ _____ Nutritional counseling
_____ _____ Preferred weight gain _____
_____ _____ Emotions of pregnancy
                The following minor problems discussed:
_____ _____   Constipation or hemorrhoids
_____ _____   Backache
_____ _____   Leg cramps
_____ _____   Stretch marks
_____ _____   Difficulty sleeping
_____ _____   Ankle edema
_____ _____   Nausea and vomiting
_____ _____   Heartburn
_____ _____   Varicosities
_____ _____   Headache
_____ _____   Stuffy nose and allergies

                The following danger signs discussed:
_____ _____   Vaginal bleeding
_____ _____   Swelling of face and fingers
_____ _____   Severe continuous headaches
_____ _____   Dimness or blurring of vision
_____ _____   Flashes of light before eyes
_____ _____   Severe abdominal pain
_____ _____   Persistent vomiting
_____ _____   Chills and fever
_____ _____   Sudden escape of fluid from vagina

Preventive Health Care

_____ _____ Smoking discussed
_____ _____ Activity, exercise, travel, working discussed
_____ _____ Sexual activity discussed
_____ _____ Accident prevention
_____ _____ Dental care
_____ _____ Alcohol discussed
_____ _____ Community-health resources
_____ _____ Contraception discussed. Plans: ____ birth control pills, ____ IUD, ____ diaphragm, ____ foam and condom, ____ tubal ligation, ____ vasectomy, ____ rhythm or ovulation, ____ none

(continued)

ASSESSMENT TOOL (continued)

Preparation for Labor, Delivery, and Parenthood

_____	_____	Prenatal classes discussed
_____	_____	Enrolled in class: date _____ type _____
_____	_____	Hospital arrangements discussed (visit and register)
_____	_____	Breast-feeding versus bottle feeding discussed
		Type selected _____. Breast care taught _____.
_____	_____	Management of labor and delivery discussed
		Anesthesia/analgesia _____
		Prepared childbirth _____
_____	_____	Partner in delivery room discussed. Yes ____ No ____
_____	_____	Signs of labor discussed (when to go to hospital)
		Instructed on what to do about the following:
_____	_____	Ruptured membranes
_____	_____	Bleeding
_____	_____	Fever
_____	_____	Fetal monitoring equipment discussed
_____	_____	Circumcision discussed
_____	_____	Special requests related to birth _____
_____	_____	Infant care
_____	_____	Rooming-in
_____	_____	Pediatrician
_____	_____	Layette

the hospital admission routine are explained, so that the parents are familiar with this procedure before admission for delivery.

Referrals

The problems that come to light are not always of a physical nature; emotional and social problems also may interfere with the client's ability to derive full benefit from health services. It is the responsibility of the nurse to find out in what ways the client needs help and to make appropriate referrals when they are indicated (*e.g.*, to the nurse in the community, to community services, or to other members of the extended health team). Through the use of such referrals, lines of communciation can be kept open between the particular health agency, the community, and the members of the health team. This is one of the nurse's most important functions. Thus, comprehensive care for the client is assured.

Community Resources

The nurse in the office or clinic who is alert to actual or potential health problems that affect both the woman and her family recognizes that a home visit by a community-health nurse (CHN) often is very helpful. If such a situation arises, the woman can be informed about available community-health services and what the CHN might do while making a home visit and how such a visit can be beneficial. A referral can be made through

the proper channels. Each institution or agency has its own procedure.

Community-Health Nurse. The nurse in the community may work in either an official or a voluntary agency. The official health agency may have an antepartal clinic offering complete antepartal services for families with financial need.

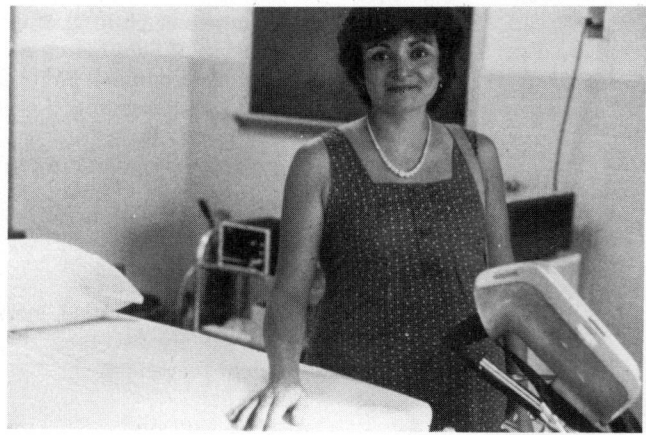

FIGURE 22-10

When the expectant mother visits the maternity center during pregnancy she can see the labor and delivery rooms and the monitoring systems used. This gives her more confidence when she enters to have her baby. (Courtesy of Booth Maternity Center, Philadelphia)

Home Visits. Real value may be derived from a visit in which the nurse is able to see the woman in her usual surroundings. For instance, if the woman has the problem of excessive weight gain and is not responding to clinic therapy, the CHN can visit the home and gain some insight into the basis of the problem. In her report to the clinic or the office staff, she relates information that contributes to both the medical and the nursing management of this pregnancy.

In situations in which the clinic program is limited in educational opportunities, such as parents' classes or individual guidance, the CHN's visit to the home may be necessary to supplement the health-care teaching and anticipatory guidance done in the clinic.

The CHN orients the home visit to what the woman wants and needs to know. Repeated visits based on the *nurse's* needs (to impart certain information, instruction, and so on) may result in a firmly closed door and a consequent severing of the nurse–client relationship.

Astute assessment of the situation at each visit includes, first of all, finding out what the woman needs to know. Communication and observation skills are of paramount importance. It is the wise nurse who takes her cues from the mother and handles each need as it arises without feeling compelled to "teach" a certain amount of material each visit. If the visits are managed in this way, topics may include basic information about pregnancy, hygiene, and nutrition; specific preparations for the baby; how to handle sibling rivalry; and so on. These subjects may come up naturally in the course of the visits, or the nurse can guide conversation around to them as she explores with the mother certain areas of need. By the end of the antepartal supervision period, all necessary counseling usually can be accomplished.

Opportunities for Family-Health Supervision. During the course of antepartal care, the nurse has many opportunities for family-health supervision. In her observation of other children in the home, she may be the first person to notice a neglected orthopedic condition, to suspect a need for a chest roentgenogram, or to observe a possible vision or hearing difficulty. In addition, observation of the mother's interaction with her children may give valuable clues to the woman's mothering patterns. This aids the nurse in planning more effective anticipatory guidance and health teaching.

Medical Social Worker. The medical social worker, a member of the health team, works closely with the nurse in the care of the pregnant woman. Most hospitals and community-health agencies have a social service department.

The function of social service workers is to help people meet and cope with problems that interfere with social functioning. These problems may include unmarried parenthood, divorce, desertion, placing older children during the mother's hospital stay, arranging for a working housekeeper, planning convalescent care for the mother, or arranging financial or material assistance.

In their professional role, social workers are called on to evaluate these problems. Then, with the client's cooperation, they help her to mobilize her resources and assist her, when necessary, through referral and counseling to alleviate the condition. They may make home visits and interview the client, and perhaps other family members, to aid them in diagnosing the extent of the problems.

Social problems may seem overwhelming if the client's physical condition is affected, and these concerns, in turn, may interfere with the benefit that the client may derive from medical services. The social worker may act as an understanding counselor between the family and the client during her hospital stay. In many hospitals the need for a social service referral is apparent when the client is registered early in pregnancy. In that event, the client is interviewed after the initial medical examination, and from both the physical and the social findings plans are made with the client to mobilize her resources.

By observation, counseling, and liaison work, the social worker combines efforts with the other members of the health team to see the client not only as an individual maternity client, but also as an important member of the family, and the family as an integral part of the community.

Summary. Comprehensive antepartal care is concerned with the total health and the well-being of the pregnant woman and her family. With this as the central objective, the combined efforts of several disciplines, in addition to those of medicine and nursing, may be required in the cooperative plan.

A positive effort on the part of the health team becomes possible if each member has a clear understanding of his or her own role, appreciates and understands the contribution of the other professions represented on the team, knows something of the processes involved in the differing approaches, recognizes commonality of interest and skill, and has the intellectual and the emotional capacity to enter into a team relationship.

General Health Maintenance in Pregnancy

Pregnancy ought to be a normal, happy, healthy experience for a woman. If a woman has a good general state of health, there is no reason why pregnancy should produce physical or emotional symptoms that would significantly interfere with her ability to function and participate in her usual activities. Women are encouraged to continue their usual habits with very little

NURSING CARE PLAN

The Pregnant Woman

Nursing Objectives

1. Assure early diagnosis of pregnancy and regular prenatal care.
2. Assess accurately and monitor carefully the progress of pregnancy.
3. Provide pertinent and timely education for mother and family to promote maximum health and well-being during pregnancy.
4. Assist to alleviate minor discomforts of pregnancy.
5. Identify potential or actual complications and make early referral.

Assessment	Potential Nursing Diagnosis	Intervention	Evaluation
Physiological status of pregnancy (vital signs, weight, urine, fundal height, fetal heart rate and activity, symptoms, test results)	Knowledge deficit of effects of pregnancy on body systems Knowledge deficit of fetal growth and development Concomitant medical conditions	Take general health history and obstetric history, physical examination, and laboratory tests as part of antepartal work-up; continue surveillance at return visits	Client repeats EDC Client understands implications of minor health problems and complications
Psychosocial status of pregnancy (responses to pregnancy, family adaptations, knowledge of psychosocial effects)	Knowledge deficit related to effects of pregnancy on psychosocial domain Knowledge deficit of effects of pregnancy on sexuality Disturbance in self-concept related to effects of pregnancy on biopsychosocial patterns	Discuss client profile, identifying data, family composition, attitudes toward pregnancy, knowledge levels, expectations related to pregnancy, family and personal resources, coping mechanisms, and economic situation	Client discusses expectations of pregnancy Client realizes who support persons are Client clarifies her understanding of (or lack of) information
Health maintenance needs (self-care, diet, rest and exercise, substance use, medications, sexuality)	Knowledge deficit of nutritional requirements Knowledge deficit of hazards of smoking, alcohol, drugs Alterations in health maintenance related to increased psychophysical needs	Provide information about ways to promote health and well-being during pregnancy (*i.e.,* rest, exercise, work, recreation, travel, medications and immunizations, skin care, breast care, clothes, teeth, bowel habits, douching, smoking, sexual relations, drug and alcohol use) Refer to appropriate health professional or agency when significant problems are identified	Client acknowledges areas needing improvement Client seeks information on changing behavior Client follows through on referrals, recommendations, and treatment plans
Minor discomforts (symptoms in specific systems: genitourinary, gastrointestinal, urinary, musculoskeletal, neurologic)	Alteration in comfort: nausea or vomiting, heartburn, constipation, headaches, hemorrhoids, flatulence, backache, dyspnea, leg cramps, vaginal discharge Activity intolerance related to fatigue and dyspnea	Provide information and instruction about occurrence and alleviation of such discomforts as urinary frequency, nausea and vomiting, heartburn, constipation, flatulence, hemorrhoids, backache, dyspnea, varicosities, leg cramps, and vaginal discharge	Client identifies discomforts Client understands remedies for symptoms Client receives comfort from remedies

(continued)

Assessment	Potential Nursing Diagnosis	Intervention	Evaluation
	Potential for vaginal infection due to hormonal changes	Refer to physician or other health professional if difficulties persist or if there is present significant interference with daily activities	Client follows through on referral
Prenatal educational needs (knowledge of effects of pregnancy, fetal development, prenatal routines, preparing for delivery and child care)	Knowledge deficit of fetal growth and development Knowledge deficit of effects of pregnancy on body systems Knowledge deficit related to effects of pregnancy on psychosocial domain Knowledge deficit of childbirth preparation resources	Provide specific information and instruction related to growth and development of the fetus, progression of pregnancy, physical and emotional changes, prenatal management routines, and preparation for childbirth, or refer to sources providing these educational services (*i.e.,* childbirth classes, nutritionist)	Couple attends childbirth classes Couple indicates understanding of fetal development, effects of pregnancy, and prenatal routines Couple makes plans for labor and delivery Couple makes plans for infant care at home
Indicators of complications of pregnancy (*i.e.,* rising blood pressure, facial edema, bleeding, excessive weight, inappropriate fundal measurements for dates)	Potential for pregnancy complication (related to specific symptoms) Anxiety/fear related to potential complication	Notify physician, obtain additional physical data and laboratory tests as indicated, explain to client the meaning of symptoms and signs and the plan of care	Client affirms understanding of complications Client cooperates with treatment Client controls signs and symptoms of complications
Indicators of stress and psychosocial problems (*i.e.,* missed appointments, noncompliance, affect, direct expression of concerns, acting out behavior of children, complaints)	Potential disturbance in self-concept related to pregnancy or other life situations Potential alteration in parenting or family processes related to psychosocial problems Potential for pregnancy complication (related to specific behaviors)	Determine sources of problems, whether economic, interpersonal, or due to emotional illness, cultural discrepancies, or conflicts with the system of health care; provide counseling according to level of skills, refer as needed for more intensive therapy; use community resources for socioeconomic, cultural disparity problems; work with agency and health team to improve client relations if this is a problem	Client keeps appointments Client follows through on referrals Client implements suggestions and recommendations Client reports recommendations have been helpful Client affirms improvement of problems

change, unless they have previously been living in ways not conducive to health and well-being. Although pregnancy creates numerous physiological and psychoemotional changes, women with basically positive attitudes and good health are able to adapt without undue stress. Many find these changes intriguing and enjoyable—part of the mystery of the phenomenon of childbearing. During the months of antepartal care, the nurse has many opportunities to assist clients to attain healthier patterns of living and to reinforce health-promoting behaviors.

Rest, Relaxation, and Sleep

Because rest and sleep are so essential to health, it is important to emphasize this detail in parent teaching. Pregnant women become tired more readily. Nature has made provision for some reduction in normal energy without injury to health. Beyond this limit the symptoms of fatigue are evidenced in irritability, apprehension, a tendency to worry, and restlessness. These symptoms are sometimes very subtle and misleading. The pregnant woman should rest to prevent this fatigue.

The expectant mother ought to get as much sleep as she feels she needs. Some people need more than others. In addition to a good night's sleep, it is advisable that the mother take a nap or at least rest for a half hour every morning and afternoon. If this is not possible, shorter rest periods, preferably taken lying down (several times a day), are beneficial.

Not all mothers are able to follow the recommended rest periods. Both the woman who works throughout her pregnancy and the mother of preschool children need special attention in planning for adequate rest. Rigid recommendations are to be avoided, and the nurse can search with the mother for minutes in her busy day that can be used for rest. Counseling the family may be necessary to maximize the mother's free moments. It can be explained that rest means not only to lie down and to sleep, but also to lie down or to sit comfortably— to rest the body, mind, abdominal muscles, legs and back, and to stretch out whenever possible, so it is easier for the heart to pump the blood to the extremities.

During the last months of pregnancy, a small pillow used for support of the abdomen while the pregnant woman lies on her side does much to relieve the discomfort common at this time and adds to the degree of rest that the client gets in a given time.

It can be suggested that the client sit whenever possible, even while doing her housework. Sitting to rest for brief periods during the course of the day can be beneficial if the feet and legs are elevated.

Conscious relaxation can be used to advantage by the pregnant woman. Various techniques are available, including such approaches as progressive relaxation, breathing exercises, attention focusing, imagery, and forms of meditation. Practiced regularly, relaxation is refreshing, energizing, and effective in counteracting stress. If the mother does not already practice relaxation, the nurse can teach her a simple technique. Relaxation and techniques are discussed in Chapter 20; exercises are given in Appendix A.

Benefits from conscious relaxation can include relief of minor discomforts of pregnancy, increased ability to cope with everyday stress, heightened self-awareness, building of trust in the personal capacity to establish control over responses, reduction of stress, and decreased pain and discomfort during childbearing.

Exercise

Outdoor exercise during pregnancy is usually beneficial. However, the degree of exercise recommended depends on the individual woman, her general condition, and the stage of pregnancy.

There are differences in the amount of exercise for the early and late periods of pregnancy. When pregnancy is advanced, exercise may be limited in comparison with the amount advised previously. Exercise provides a welcome diversion, reduces anxiety and tension, quiets the mind, promotes sleep, helps decrease constipation, and stimulates the appetite, all of which are valuable aids to the pregnant mother.

Walking is generally a preferred form of exercise during pregnancy because it stimulates the muscular activity of the entire body and is available to all women. Exercise of any kind should not be fatiguing; to secure the most beneficial results, it should be combined with periods of rest.

Interest in active exercise has been increasing among pregnant women, as in the general population. More women are exercising strenuously during pregnancy than in previous years. It is not unusual to see pregnant women regularly engaged in physically demanding work or sports and doing aerobic exercises such as running, bicycling, climbing stairs, and swimming. The research to date indicates that most fetuses can tolerate strenuous maternal exercise when women are accustomed to this level of activity and continue exercise programs into their pregnancies. New strenuous exercise should not begin during pregnancy, and women need their physician's approval before undertaking any strenuous exercise program. In physically fit women, the ventilatory reserve and cardiovascular changes of pregnancy contribute to increased fetal tolerance of the circulatory and respiratory challenges of strenuous maternal exercise.[2]

Prenatal exercises have been standard components of childbirth education, but approaches vary widely and there is question about effectiveness. Exercises to strengthen abdominal muscles, relax muscles of the pelvic floor, teach the pelvic tilt, stretch and adduct the thighs, and limber specific body parts have been used. Data supporting these effects are controversial. For women who are not accustomed to exercising regularly, data indicate that even well-motivated clients do not remember to practice more than three exercises daily.[3] (Prenatal Exercises are given in Appendix A.)

Standing or sitting for long periods of time should be avoided. Adequate exercise generally promotes a sense of well-being and can also aid in preventing several minor discomforts of pregnancy. Lifting heavy objects, moving furniture, reaching to hang curtains, any activity that might involve sudden jolts, and sudden changes in balance that might result in a fall or the likelihood of physical trauma should be avoided.

Employment

Women frequently continue work during pregnancy. The type of work, level of physical activity, environmental risks or occupational hazards, and obstetric or medical problems of the woman affect whether she should work and the length of time she should continue working during pregnancy. Avoidance of work environments that expose the pregnant woman to fetotoxic substances is a major consideration.

In general, jobs requiring moderate manual labor should be avoided if they must be continued over long hours or if they require delicate balance, constant standing, or constant working on night shifts. Actually, the woman who has a "desk job" in an office often does less strenuous work than the average homemaker who does not go out to work. Nevertheless, positions that require the worker to sit constantly can be extremely tiring. Adequate rest periods should be provided for all pregnant women employed in such positions.

Many women are employed in industry, and the problem of pregnancy for the working mother in this type of employment is a most important one. To safeguard the interests of expectant mothers so engaged, the Standards for Maternity Care and Employment of Mothers in Industry have been recommended by the United States Children's Bureau (see accompanying list).

The environmental risks to pregnant women and occupational hazards to those employed in certain industries have received considerable attention in recent years. Ten percent of all birth defects are known to be caused by environmental agents, and another 65% to 70% are of unknown origin. Environmental and workplace exposure to toxins may be responsible for most of these developmental defects. With women composing nearly half of the work force, the problem of intrauterine exposure to toxic substances is one of major proportions. Many industrial chemicals have been found hazardous to reproduction. Vinyl chloride, used in the plastic industry; the agricultural pesticide dibromochloropropane; chloroprene, used in rubber industries; and hydrocarbons, used in numerous industries, are capable of causing reproductive failure in both men and women. Among wives of male operating room personnel exposed to anesthetic gases, a 25% increase over expected incidence of birth defects was found. Hexachlorophene and radiation exposures among health workers are associated with congenital malformations and diseases. Hair dyes used by beauticians are capable of causing mutations in laboratory experiments. Textile workers exposed to cotton dust are at risk for byssinosis (brown lung), which reduces fetal oxygenation as a result of maternal bronchial disorders. Benzene, used in textile industries, can cause chromosomal aberrations. Exposures to lead, mercury, lithium, and the solvents toluene and xylene occur among workers in the arts and crafts industry. Chronic poisoning by such compounds has implications for fetal development and well-being.[4]

Environmental contamination poses a risk to any pregnant woman exposed to toxic substances. The use of pesticides in agriculture, forestry, and lawn care is of growing concern. Dioxin, a degradation product of the pesticide 2,4,5T (Agent Orange, used as defoliant in Vietnam), is known to cause mutations and birth defects and miscarriages in laboratory animals. When this agent was sprayed in Alsea, Oregon, in 1979, the incidence of miscarriage among women living in the area increased significantly. Two other widely used pesticides, heptachlor and chlordane, are carcinogenic in animals and possibly linked to causing neuroblastomas and leukemia in prenatally and postnatally exposed children.[4] Pregnant women are advised to avoid using such agents at home (on lawn and gardens) and to prevent exposure at work (*i.e.,* nurseries).

The prenatal history should include assessment of possible work, home, or environmental exposure to toxins. Appropriate teaching and counseling by the nurse helps the client to make a more informed decision about the risks and benefits of working in a potentially hazardous environment. Steps to avoid or minimize exposure can be identified. Occupations commonly held by women, potential occupational hazards, and known or suspected effects on reproduction are summarized in Table 22-2.

Recreation

Recreation is as necessary during pregnancy as it is at any other time in life. The woman is preparing for one of the most important role changes that she will undergo during her lifetime, and some anxiety naturally accompanies such change. A certain amount of concern about the impending labor no doubt will be present; the additional responsibility of having a new baby in the household, caring for and integrating him into the family unit, is also anxiety provoking. The parents may wonder whether they are equal to the enormous responsibility of rearing children and whether or not they will be "good" parents. Therefore, activities that are diverting, healthful, and relaxing help the client and the family to keep things in proper perspective. The nurse can discuss with the mother some types of recreation that are most relaxing and pleasing for her and her family. Family group activities can still be enjoyed, even though the mother's energy and dexterity may be somewhat curtailed.

Consideration and understanding on the part of the father, the family, the physician, and the nurse can do much to relieve any uncertainties or concerns that the mother may have. When the father, in particular, understands more about the processes involved in the pregnancy (see Suggested Reading), his helpfulness can be increased. The nurse can discuss with the family ways in which they might help to diminish strain and tension. This may call for changes in attitudes, understanding, and habits. Certainly, it means increased tolerance and forbearance on the part of those involved; yet, this is

400 UNIT IV: Assessment and Management in the Antepartum Period

Standards for Maternity Care and Employment (United States Children's Bureau)

1. Facilities for adequate prenatal medical care should be readily available for all employed pregnant women, and arrangements should be made by those responsible for providing prenatal care, so that every woman has access to such care. Local health departments should make the services of prenatal clinics available to industrial plants, and the personnel management or physicians and nurses within the plant should make available to employees information about the importance of such services and where they can be obtained.

2. Pregnant women should not be employed on a shift including the hours between 12 midnight and 6 AM. Pregnant women should not be employed more than 8 hours a day or more than 48 hours per week, and it is desirable that their hours of work be limited to not more than 40 hours per week.

3. Every woman, especially a pregnant woman, should have at least two 10-minute rest periods during her work shift, for which adequate facilities for resting and an opportunity for securing nourishing food should be provided.

4. It is not considered desirable for pregnant women to be employed in the following types of occupations, and they should, if possible, be transferred to lighter and more sedentary work:
   a. Occupations that involve heavy lifting or other heavy work
   b. Occupations that involve continuous standing and moving about

5. Pregnant women should not be employed in the following types of work during any period of pregnancy:
   a. Occupations that require a good sense of bodily balance, such as work performed on scaffolds or stepladders and occupations in which the accident risk is characterized by accidents causing severe injury, such as operation of punch presses, power-driven woodworking machines, or other machines having a point-of-operation hazard
   b. Occupations involving exposure to toxic substances considered to be extra hazardous during pregnancy, including the following:
      Aniline
      Benzene and toluene
      Carbon disulfide
      Carbon monoxide
      Chlorinated hydrocarbons
      Lead and its compounds
      Mercury and its compounds
      Nitrobenzol and other nitro compounds of benzol and its homologues
      Phosphorus
      Radioactive substances and x-rays
      Turpentine
      Other toxic substances that exert an injurious effect upon the blood-forming organs, the liver, or the kidneys.

   Because these substances may exert a harmful influence upon the course of pregnancy, may lead to premature termination, or may injure the fetus, the maintenance of air concentrations within the so-called maximum permissible limits of state codes is not, in itself, sufficient assurance of a safe working condition for the pregnant woman. Pregnant women should be transferred from workrooms in which any of these substances are used or produced in any significant quantity.

6. A minimum of 6 weeks' leave *before* delivery should be granted with the presentation of a medical certificate of the expected date of confinement.

7. At any time during pregnancy, a woman should be granted a reasonable amount of additional leave with the presentation of a certificate from the attending physician to the effect that complications of pregnancy have made continuing employment prejudicial to her health or to the health of the child.

   To safeguard the mother's health she should be granted sufficient time off after delivery to return to normal and to regain her strength. The infant needs her care, especially during the first year of life. If it is essential that she return to work, the following recommendations are made:
   a. All women should be granted an extension of at least 2 months leave of absence after delivery.
   b. Should complications of delivery or of the postpartum period develop, a woman should be granted a reasonable amount of additional leave beyond 2 months following delivery with presentation of a certificate to this effect from the attending physician.

one of the ways that others can make their contribution to a successful pregnancy. The father's gentleness and tenderness are especially appreciated and therapeutic at this time; the mother can help him maintain his supportive attitude and behavior by letting him know when his actions are helpful. This type of feedback conveys her appreciation to the father and leads to reinforcement of his positive behavior. He is perhaps the key person in helping the mother to secure the kind of social relaxation that she enjoys most.

The mother should avoid situations that are likely to cause discomfort. Amusements, exercise, rest, and

T A B L E   2 2 - 2

Occupations Commonly Held by Women Working in Industry and Potential Occupational Hazards

Occupation	Potential Hazard	Known or Suspected Effects on Reproduction
Hospital workers Nurses Anesthetists Lab technicians Physicians Dentists Dental assistants	Radiation	Chromosomal aberrations, sterility, birth defects, leukemia, miscarriages, retarded fetal development, carcinogen
	Benzene	Chromosomal aberrations, aplastic anemia and leukemia, prolonged menstrual periods
	BIS (chloromethyl ether)	Known human carcinogen, possible fetal effects (BIS ether formed by combination of formaldehyde and HCl in warm, moist air)
	Toluene	Chromosomal aberrations (derivative of benzene, less toxic)
	Anesthetic gases	Birth defects, miscarriages, infertility, low-birth-weight infants
	Hexachlorophene	Congenital malformations
	Mercury	CNS damage in humans, cerebral palsy symptoms in exposed infants, behavioral alterations in animal offspring
	Estrogens	Birth defects (teratogenic), carcinogenic in offspring (DES), heavier and more frequent menses, enlarged breasts and impotence in male workers
Clerical workers	Asbestos	Chronic lung disease (asbestosis) with reduced fetal oxygenation
	Trichloroethylene	Liver and kidney damage, suspected carcinogen
	Benzene	See above
	Toluene	See above
Laundering and dry cleaning	Perchlorethylene	Liver damage, suspected carcinogen, CNS effects (dizziness, nausea), extended exposure can cause death, fetal studies not complete
	Carbon tetrachloride	Specific toxicity to liver and kidneys, suspected carcinogen, passes placental barrier to cause fetal liver damage in animals
	Petroleum solvents	Reproductive failure in both men and women
	Trichloroethylene	See above
	Benzene	See above
Textile and apparel	Carbon disulfide	Menstrual irregularities, decreased fertility, miscarriage, decreased sex drive and sperm abnormalities in men
	Dyes, aniline	Carcinogenic
	Chloroprene	Functional disruption of spermatogenesis in men, miscarriage rate increased three times in their wives, chemically related to vinyl chloride
	Cotton dust	Chronic lung disease (byssinosis, brown lung) with reduced fetal oxygenation
	Benzene	See above
	Toluene	See above
	Asbestos	See above
	Trichloroethylene	See above
	Perchlorethylene	See above
Electronic workers, rubber workers	Nitrosamides	100% incidence of nervous system tumors in animal studies in offspring
	Lead	Sterility, birth defects, prematurity, mental retardation, chromosomal aberrations, menstrual disorders

(continued)

T A B L E   2 2 - 2   *(continued)*

Occupation	Potential Hazard	Known or Suspected Effects on Reproduction
	Polychlorinated biphenyls (PCB)	"Cola-colored babies" with high frequency of growth retardation, gingival hyperplasia, spotted skull calcification, stillbirths, liver cancer, and reduced fertility in animals
	Arsenic	Carcinogenic; can cause death
	Mercury	See above
	Trichloroethylene	See above
Agricultural workers	Pesticides (chlorinated hydrocarbons)	Carcinogenic, abnormalities in offspring and infertility in animals, kepone causes decreased sex drives and sterility in human males
	Dioxin (2,4,5T)	Miscarriages in humans; mutations, birth defects, and miscarriages in animals
	Heptachlor and chlordane	Carcinogenic in animals; possibly cause neuroblastomas and leukemia in prenatally or postnatally exposed children
	Chloroprene	See above

Outdoor work
  Toll booth workers
  Traffic controllers
  Airline stewardesses
	Carbon monoxide	Acute exposure has caused fetal and fetal–maternal deaths; chronic exposure causes decreased birth weight and increased neonatal mortality in animals

Hairdressers and cosmetologists	Hair dyes	Mutations in bacterial lab cultures, possibly carcinogenic, chromosomal damage in women using hair dyes
	Vinyl chloride (aerosol sprays)	Documented carcinogen, linked to angiosarcoma of the liver, possible chromosomal aberrations of sperm, increased miscarriage rate and birth defects in humans
	Asbestos (hair dryers)	See above
	Benzene, toluene	See above

Arts and crafts
  Painters
  Printers
  Potters
  Silkscreen, woodwork, stained glass
	Benzene, toluene	See above

	Lead	See above
	Mercury	See above
	Lithium, barium	Heavy metal poisoning
	Chromium	Suspected carcinogen
	Benzidine dyes	Suspected carcinogen
Various	Cadmium	Implicated in bronchogenic and prostatic cancer, testicular damage, sterility, teratogenic effects, low birth weight in animals, cigarette smoke high in cadmium and heavy smoking increases risk
	Manganese	Impotence and decreased sex drive in exposed males

(After Greenberg J: Implications for primary care providers of occupational health hazards on pregnant women and their infants. J Nurse–Midwifery 25(4):21–30, July/August 1980)

recreation at proper intervals help to keep the pregnant mother well and happy in an environment conducive to her well-being.

Traveling

Even though there is little restriction on travel from a medical point of view, it should be discussed with the mother, so that any of her concerns or misinformation may come to light. Pregnant women are generally advised to avoid any trip that will cause undue fatigue, since they are prone to tiring easily. For traveling long distances, the railway or airplane is safest and provides greatest comfort. If travel is by private automobile, rest periods of 10 to 15 minutes ought to be planned at least every 2 hours. This not only helps to avoid fatigue, but also benefits the general circulation by providing the chance to stretch and walk.

The pregnant woman should be advised to use seat

belts because they have been found to decrease mortality in severe car accidents. Seat belts should be worn low and comfortably under the abdomen and in conjunction with the shoulder strap if one is available. Both belts can be adjusted so that they are not pressing tightly against the neck and abdomen.

While traveling in general is not usually contraindicated during pregnancy, each expectant mother should seek individual consultation concerning the advisability of extensive travel at any time during the period of pregnancy.

Immunizations and Vaccinations

Another important topic that is interrelated with travel is that of immunization and vaccination protection for the pregnant woman. The diseases that she will be exposed to during her travels, as well as in the course of her daily life, must be considered. The American College of Obstetricians and Gynecologists has reviewed vac-

cinations and made the recommendations indicated in Immunizations and Vaccinations for Traveling.

As there is at least somewhat of a risk with many of these vaccinations, it is important to counsel clients regarding the spacing of conception well after receiving these injections. The client also can be counseled to plan vacations and travels during pregnancy to minimize the opportunity for disease exposure and the consequent need for *post hoc* vaccination. In addition, all clients should be advised to report any illness, no matter how trivial, to their physician so that appropriate follow-up can be done.

Skin Care

The glands of the skin may be more active during pregnancy, and there may be increased or decreased perspiration, resulting in irritation or dryness. Since the skin is one of the organs of elimination, bathing is obviously important. A bath or a shower should be taken daily because it is stimulating, refreshing, and relaxing. Elimination through the skin is an important method of removing body waste products. The old idea that tub baths should be avoided because the wash water enters the vagina and thereby carries infection to the uterus now is believed to have little validity. However, tub baths should not be taken after rupture of the membranes. The only objection to tub baths during the last trimester of pregnancy is that the heavy weight of the large abdomen may put pregnant women off balance and make climbing in and out of the tub awkward. Therefore, the likelihood of slipping or falling in the bathtub is increased.

Chilling the body should be avoided; thus, cold baths, sponges, or showers should be avoided if they produce this sensation.

Breast Care

Special care of the breasts during pregnancy is an important preparation for breast-feeding. During the antepartal period the breasts often have a feeling of fullness and become larger, heavier, and more pendulous. A well-fitted supporting brassiere that holds the breasts up and in may relieve these discomforts. It may also help to prevent the subsequent tissue sagging so often noticeable after delivery owing to the increased weight of the breasts during pregnancy and lactation.

Early in pregnancy the breasts begin to secrete colostrum. The breasts are to be bathed daily with a clean washcloth and warm water. Some studies have demonstrated that the use of soap, alcohol, and other such materials during the antepartal period tends to be detrimental to the integrity of the nipple tissue because

---

Immunizations and Vaccinations for Traveling

Cholera. This is a killed bacterial vaccine and should be given only if there is danger of infection such as with travel where there is a great risk of exposure.

Mumps and measles (rubeola). These are live viruses and should never be given to pregnant women.

Poliomyelitis. Immunization during pregnancy is rarely indicated except when epidemics could occur.

Rubella. Pregnancy is a contraindication for administration of the live rubella vaccine. This virus has been shown on occasion to infect both the placenta and the fetus and for this reason is avoided.

Hepatitis A. This may be given after exposure or when traveling in developing countries. In the United States, there usually is no need.

Smallpox. Vaccinia virus administered during pregnancy occasionally infects the fetus. This fetal vaccinia has almost always been associated with primary vaccination. Hence, primary vaccination should be given only to pregnant women who have been exposed to an endemic area.

Yellow fever. Since this is a live virus, it should be given to pregnant women only if there has been an exposure or if there is a great risk of exposure, such as with travel.

Other vaccines and immunizations. Tetanus and diphtheria toxoids are considered safe and the tuberculin and histoplasmin test are also permitted.[5]

Typhoid. This is recommended if traveling in endemic areas.

they remove the protective skin oils and leave the nipple more prone to damage. Rubbing the nipples with a rough towel during the last trimester of pregnancy may be helpful in attempting to toughen them.

Some specialists advise the use of nipple cream, a hydrous lanolin preparation, to prepare the nipples for nursing. This can be applied after the breasts are bathed. First, a small quantity of cream is placed on the thumb and the first finger; then the nipple is grasped gently between the thumb and this finger. With a rolling motion, the cream is worked into the tiny creases found on the surface of the nipple. The position of the thumb and finger should be gradually shifted around the circumference of the nipple until a complete circuit has been made. See the illustrations and directions for nipple preparation.

Clothing

During pregnancy the clothes should be comfortable and nonconstricting. Most women are able to dress in their usual manner until the enlargement of the abdomen becomes apparent. Maternity specialty shops and department stores carry a wide variety of maternity fashions.

Designers have given consideration to the pregnant mother's clothing, making it easy to dress attractively and feel self-confident about appearance. Maternity clothes are designed to be comfortable and "hang from the shoulders," thus avoiding any constriction; they are made in a variety of materials. The expectant mother can dress according to the climate and the temperature for her comfort.

Abdominal Support

If the mother's abdomen is large or if previous pregnancies have caused her abdominal musculature to become lax or pendulous, a properly made and well-fitting maternity girdle gives support and comfort. The purpose of the garment is support, not constriction of the abdomen. When putting the girdle on, the women should lie on the bed rather than stand and should fasten it from the bottom upward, so support is provided to the uterus from below. Abdominal support provided by a maternity girdle can help relieve backache, prevent fatigue, and assist in maintaining good posture.

Avoidance of Constricting Clothing

Pregnant women should avoid any type of clothing or accessories that constrict movement or circulation. Tight belts, garters, knee socks, knee-high stockings, panty girdles, garter belts, stretch pants, and such should not be worn. Particularly dangerous are round garters, rolled stockings, and tight knee-high stockings that might re-

strict circulation in the lower extremities. These can aggravate varicose veins, cause edema of the lower legs and feet, and produce venous stasis.

Clothing that fits snugly in the perineal area, such as tight pantyhose and stretch pants, can contribute to vaginal infections and heat rash (miliaria). Pantyhose are preferable to hose held up by garters or tight waist garter belts, but should not be constricting and should have cotton crotches.

Breast Support

It is advisable that every pregnant woman wear a well-fitted brassiere to support the breasts in a normal uplifted position. Proper support of the breasts is conducive to good posture and thus helps to prevent backache.

The selection of a brassiere is determined by individual fitting and is influenced by the size of the breasts and the need for support. It is important to see that the cup is large enough and that the underarm is built high enough to cover all the breast tissue. Wide shoulder straps afford more comfort for the woman who has large and pendulous breasts. Again, the size of the brassiere is determined by the size of the individual, but in most instances the brassiere is approximately two sizes larger than that usually worn. The mother who is planning to breast-feed finds it practical to purchase nursing brassieres with drop flaps over the nipples, which can be worn during the latter months of pregnancy, as well as during the postpartal period for as long as she is nursing her baby.

Shoes

A comfortable, well-fitting shoe is essential for the expectant mother. The postural changes that occur as the mother's abdomen enlarges may be aggravated by wearing high-heeled shoes and create backache and fatigue. It is advisable that low-heeled shoes be worn during working hours and for busy daytime activities. For evening or more fashionable afternoon attire, a 2-inch heel is acceptable if the client does not develop backache from the increased lordosis induced by the heels, and if she can maintain adequate balance. Platform shoes contribute to precarious balance and are not advised.

The height of the heel is but one consideration; the support that the shoe gives the foot adds materially to the mother's comfort. Many flat-heeled shoes give little or no support to the feet and thus may cause fatigue and aching legs and back. A simple method to check the support of a shoe is to place the shoe flat on the floor, and press the thumb down on the inner sole against the shank (the part that would come under the arch of the foot). If the shoe gives under pressure, it will give weak support to the foot.

C L I E N T   E D U C A T I O N

Techniques Used During Pregnancy to Prepare Nipples for Breastfeeding

Nipple Rolling. The nipple is placed between thumb and fingers and rolled gently. This helps toughen the nipple surface.

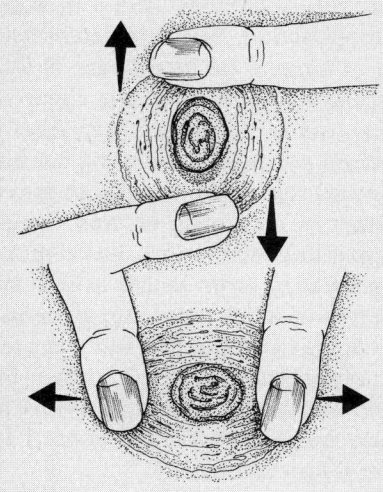

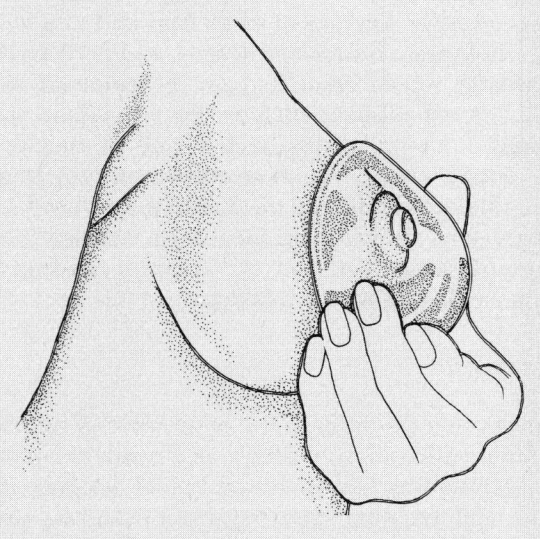

Nipple Stretching. The fingers or thumbs are placed close to the nipple and pressed firmly into the breast tissue. Gradually the fingers are pushed away from the nipple toward the edge of the areola and beyond. Stretching is done vertically and horizontally and repeated several times. This helps to evert nipples that are flat or inverted.

Nipple Cup. Plastic cups can be used to help correct inverted nipples. These cups apply a constant, gentle pressure around the areola and push the nipple forward through a central opening in the inner shield. They can be worn for several hours a day toward the end of pregnancy.

Care of the Teeth

Good dental care is necessary because the teeth are important for adequate mastication of food. The teeth should be brushed carefully on arising, after each meal, and before retiring at night. An alkaline mouthwash may be used if desired. It is advisable for the expectant mother to visit her dentist at the very beginning of pregnancy and follow any recommendations made. Any extensive elective work is better postponed until after the pregnancy. The most favorable period for routine, minor procedures is from the fourth to the seventh month. The mother is usually less nauseated and, in general, feeling well.

Diagnostic dental roentgenograms should be postponed until the latter half of pregnancy. A lead apron over the abdomen gives sufficient protection.

The old saying, "For every child a tooth," based on a belief that the fetus takes calcium from the mother's teeth, has no real scientific basis. An adequate diet during pregnancy supplies the baby with calcium and phosphorus in sufficient amounts to build his bones and teeth. Therefore, this old adage need not be true if proper attention is given to the care of the teeth and nutrition during pregnancy.

Bowel Habits

The pregnant woman with regular elimination habits often experiences little or no change in the daily routine. Those who have a tendency toward constipation become noticeably more irregular during pregnancy because of decreased physical exertion, relaxation of the bowel smooth-muscle systems, and pressure of the enlarging uterus. The presenting part of the fetus exerts pressure on the lower bowel, especially during the latter part of pregnancy. Iron supplementation during pregnancy is an additional contributing factor to constipation.

Constipation may be prevented or alleviated by maintaining regular bowel elimination, drinking a large amount of fluids daily, and maintaining a diet that contains several daily servings of fresh fruit and raw vegetables, whole grain breads and cereals, and particularly products with whole bran. If these measures are not effective, a stool softener such as dioctyl sodium sulfosuccinate or a mild laxative such as milk of magnesia may be recommended. Harsh laxatives and purgatives are contraindicated. Mineral oil should not be used because it prevents absorption of fat-soluble vitamins from the gastrointestinal tract. Lack of vitamin K can lead to hemorrhagic disease of the newborn.

Hemorrhoids

Pregnancy often precipitates the occurrence of hemorrhoids (anal varicosities), partially as a result of constipation. Maintaining regular bowel habits, keeping the stool soft, and avoiding straining at stool can help prevent or minimize hemorrhoids. Standing for long periods of time and wearing constricting clothing are aggravating factors. Passage of hard fecal material can injure the rectal mucosa and cause bleeding from fissures or hemorrhoids. Hemorrhoids may become thrombosed or protrude through the anus. The little bumps and nodules seen in a mass of hemorrhoids are the distended portions of the affected vessels. As varicosities in other areas, they are caused by pressure interfering with return venous circulation and are aggravated by constipation. They often cause great discomfort to the pregnant woman and, due to pressure at the time of delivery, may cause great distress during the postpartal period.

The prevention and the treatment of constipation can minimize the severity of hemorrhoids. When internal hemorrhoids protrude through the rectum, the mother can be instructed to replace them carefully by pushing them gently back into the rectum. Usually the client can manage this quite well, after a thorough explanation or demonstration. She lubricates her finger with petrolatum or mineral oil to aid ease of insertion and to avoid trauma to the veins. If the client wishes, a finger cot can be used to cover her finger. Also, taking either the knee–chest position or elevating her buttocks on a pillow facilitates replacement through gravity.

The application of an icebag or cold compresses wet with witch hazel or Epsom salts solution gives great relief. The physician may order tannic acid in suppositories, or compresses of witch hazel and glycerin. If the hemorrhoids are aggravated the first few days after labor, the same medications usually give relief. Surgery is seldom resorted to during pregnancy. Doing Kegel's exercises regularly helps prevent and control hemorrhoids (see Client Education insert).

Douches and Vaginal Hygiene

Vaginal douching, a common practice of feminine hygiene by some women, should be kept at a reasonable minimum or avoided during pregnancy. If excessive vaginal secretion or infection exists, then a douche may be prescribed. In the absence of excessive secretions or infection, the nurse can instruct the client that a washcloth and soap and water are quite adequate for general cleanliness, emphasizing washing anteriorly first, and the rectal area last. The use of moist towelettes that are sold in foil packages is not usually recommended, as many are perfumed or medicated and may cause rash or contribute to vaginitis.

Deodorant "feminine hygiene" sprays are contraindicated as they have been found to cause severe perineal irritation in many women, as well as urethritis and cystitis. During pregnancy, the sebaceous glands in the genital area are quite active and there may be a characteristic odor that some women find quite unpleasant. Plain soap and water are very effective agents to keep this odor under control.

Specific instructions about douching are to be given if the woman so desires. Having copies of the instructions for douching that agree with the philosophy of the office or clinic is an effective method of conveying this information. The instructions should be clear enough for the client who has never douched and knows nothing about it (see Client Education insert).

(see Chap. 13 for a full discussion of this area).

CLIENT EDUCATION

Kegel's Exercises

Tightening and relaxing the pubococcygeal muscle keeps the vagina toned, increases the strength of the perineum, and helps prevent or control hemorrhoids. This contributes to the strength of the pelvic sling in supporting the fetus, increases sexual pleasure, and enhances urinary control.

The muscle that is used to stop the flow of urine is the pubococcygeal muscle. Practice stopping urine by squeezing this muscle several times to become familiar with it. When lying down, insert one finger into the vagina and contract the pubococcygeal muscle; note the feeling of the contraction around your finger.

Exercises:

1. Squeeze the pubococcygeal muscle for 3 seconds, relax for 3 seconds, and squeeze again. Begin with 10 three-second squeezes per day, and increase gradually until you are doing 100 twice daily.
2. Squeeze and release, then squeeze and release alternately as rapidly as you can. This is called the "flutter" exercise.
3. Bear down as during a bowel movement, but concentrate on the vagina instead of the rectum. Hold for 3 seconds.

Kegel's exercises can be done anywhere and anytime. The increased control gained over the pubococcygeal muscle is useful throughout pregnancy, during labor, during intercourse, and to prevent loss of vaginal tone with aging. This exercise, done regularly, is useful for the rest of your life.

Sexual Relations

The nurse should be prepared to provide counseling about sexual activity and act as a resource person to pregnant couples.

It is important to understand the anatomical, physiological, and psychological aspects of sexual response and sexuality during pregnancy (see Chaps. 10 and 13). The approach here is extremely important and requires adroit use of communication skills, especially those of listening, reflecting, and gentle probing. Finally, one's own feelings and attitudes about sexuality, pregnancy, and motherhood need to be examined to understand and better empathize with the client's situation.

While sexuality has become a more open topic in today's society, there is a wide variety of views among people of different cultural backgrounds. Nonetheless, there is a growing expectation on the part of clients that health professionals will offer counseling related to sexuality as an integral part of health care. Particularly in maternity nursing, sexual concerns are close to the surface, providing a ready situation for intervention and satisfying sexual adjustments. Being willing to explore and respond to a client's sexual concerns and having knowledge of appropriate sources of referral for sexual counseling are part of the function of the maternity nurse (see Chap. 13 for a full discussion of this area).

Smoking

The Surgeon General's report, as well as other recent studies, has indicated that cigarette smoking is a health hazard of sufficient importance in this country to warrant remedial action. Lung cancer, vascular thrombotic problems, and heart disease have been linked significantly with cigarette smoking. With respect to pregnancy, several studies have found a relationship between smoking and lower birthrates, higher rates of prematurity, and higher neonatal mortality.

CLIENT EDUCATION

Douching During Pregnancy

It is a 4-minute procedure (after the initial few times).

It can be done while sitting on the toilet.

A gravity bag must be used (never a hand bulb syringe).

The douche tip should not be inserted more than 3 inches.

The frequency and the solution are prescribed according to the needs of the client.

The douche bag may be placed (hung or held) no higher than 2 feet above the level of the vagina.

The douche tip should be held at about the 3-inch length and inserted in the vagina, and the labial tissue in that area should be held around the douche tip with the same hand.

The solution is allowed to run in until there is a slight feeling of fullness, then it is expelled (the douche bag holds enough solution to do this four or five times).

The bag and the tube should be rinsed and hung to dry with a towel underneath.

For comfort, the solution should only be barely warm to the hand. Holding the labial tissue around the douche tip allows the water to flow in without flowing out immediately, and this, along with rapid expelling, enables the solution to get into the folds of the wall of the vagina. In the nonpregnant woman there is no contraindication to inserting the entire douche tip or as much of it as the vagina can accommodate.

Adverse effects of maternal smoking have been confirmed in recent studies. Smoking during pregnancy is related to increased spontaneous abortions, stillbirths, premature infants, placental abruptions, placenta previa, early and late bleeding in pregnancy, and premature and prolonged rupture of the membranes. An increased incidence of Rh disease and anomalies of the heart and other organs has also been found. Women who smoke deliver small-for-gestational-age infants almost twice as often as women who do not smoke. These newborns (weighing less than 2500 g) are at increased risk for hypoglycemia, which can result in permanent brain damage. Small-for-date infants have more learning disorders, mental retardation, and lower IQ, and are more prone to neurologic deficits such as cerebral palsy and epilepsy.[6]

Smoking prevents efficient assimilation of essential vitamins and minerals in the mother. The fetus can be adversely affected by inadequate maternal nutrition. Smoking causes rapid calcium mobilization, which can reduce calcium stores, reduces vitamin B_{12} levels, causes significantly lower vitamin C levels (one cigarette depletes vitamin C levels by 25 mg, the amount from an average orange), and may cause deficiencies of vitamins B_6, B_1, and A. There is also evidence that components of tobacco smoke interfere with placental processes involved in metabolization of hormones and transport of amino acids, vitamins, and other nutrients.

Data from the United States Collaborative Perinatal Project indicate that the negative effects of smoking continue even if the woman quits before becoming pregnant. Placenta previa and the presence of abnormally large areas of dead tissue on the placenta are common for smoking mothers and could be related to past smoking (measured as cigarettes per year over a period of time). It is unclear how long these effects of smoking continue. This study also found a direct link between smoking and sudden infant death syndrome. Although prematurity and respiratory and prenatal infections are the greatest risk factors in crib death, smoking alone increases the risk by 52%.[7]

The mechanism by which smoking affects fetal well-being is somewhat obscure, but it is thought that the nicotine in the cigarettes causes peripheral vasoconstriction, with subsequent changes in the heart rate, blood pressure, and cardiac output that appear to have a detrimental effect on the development and the health of the fetus. Carbon monoxide also is found in higher concentrations in smokers, with a consequent decrease of oxygen, which also affects the fetus. The lack of key nutrients is believed important, and even mild maternal undernutrition in the last few weeks of gestation may compromise the intricate process of brain cell division.

Data from a large perinatal mortality study revealed that birth weight distributions shifted downward as maternal smoking level increased. However, maternal weight gain distributions were the same for smokers and nonsmokers, indicating that smoking does not reduce maternal weight gain. Within each level of maternal weight gain, from below 5 pounds to over 40 pounds, the more the mothers smoked, the greater percentage of neonates weighing less than 2500 g. Evidence supports a direct effect of maternal smoking on infant birth weight, possibly due to hypoxic effects of carbon monoxide, rather than an effect mediated through eating. Thus, efforts to prevent smoking should have greater benefits than efforts to increase maternal food intake.

Some disturbing observations from long-term studies indicate that low-birth-weight babies of smokers are small-for-date at birth and continue to grow at low percentiles for height and weight after birth.[8] When all major contributing factors to intrauterine growth retardation other than smoking were eliminated, infants of smokers had low birth weights independent of pregravid maternal weight and weight gain during pregnancy.[9] Newborns of smokers were significantly smaller than newborns of nonsmokers, even though pregnancy weight and dietary intake during pregnancy were equivalent in both groups.[10]

On the first prenatal visit, assessment of whether and how much the woman smokes is important. Previous obstetric history and presence of other risk factors are taken into consideration to inform the woman of problems that might occur as a result of smoking. It is strongly advised that smoking be stopped, ideally as early before conception as possible. The nurse can discuss whether the woman has ever quit smoking before and if she thinks she could quit now. Pregnancy can be a motivation to stop smoking based on concern about harming the baby. Information about quitting smoking is available from several sources, and smoking clinics or support groups are common. On follow-up visits, if the mother has not been successful in quitting smoking, she can be encouraged further or provided more direct guidance. As a minimum, she can be advised to reduce the number of cigarettes smoked daily. Women who continue smoking during pregnancy need careful nutritional teaching to ensure adequate intake of nutrients. Their pregnancy is then considered high risk and is followed accordingly (Table 22-3).

Alcohol

Alcohol consumption during pregnancy is now recognized as a major health problem. In 1973 the fetal alcohol syndrome (FAS) was first identified as a distinct clinical entity caused by maternal alcohol consumption. Infants born with this syndrome have altered patterns of growth and morphogenesis, having characteristic facies, growth deficiencies, and mental retardation (see

Chap. 45). The severity of FAS depends on the amount of alcohol consumed and the time during pregnancy it is consumed. About 40% of women who drink heavily during pregnancy give birth to infants with FAS. Maternal alcohol consumption may be related to a number of other neurologic, behavioral, and psychosocial disorders and may possibly cause abortion and stillbirth. Alcohol may be the most common fetal teratogen, and intrauterine alcohol damage may be the leading cause of mental retardation in this country.[11]

No minimum safe level of alcohol consumption during pregnancy has been established. Therefore, it is recommended that the mother abstain from alcohol while pregnant. It is important for the nurse to assess alcohol use early in pregnancy. A decrease in consumption at any time, however, even in the third trimester, may limit fetal damage. Counseling and education about FAS are important in assisting women to understand the risk involved and in helping her make informed choices (see Table 22-3).

Alcoholism is often a difficult problem to identify and remedy. The nurse may need to be alert to indirect cues, such as missed clinic appointments, women with isolated life-styles, or women in lower-status jobs than their educational level indicates. Problems brought up by the client about behavior problems with children, sexuality, and family conflicts may be symptoms of alcoholism. The history may be suggestive, especially if there has been a previous failure-to-thrive infant or an unexplained neonatal death. Women with a family history of either alcoholism or teetotalism seem more prone to have alcohol problems. Avoidance of discussion of drinking may be a cue to alcoholism, since people who drink socially are usually not defensive or elusive when discussing drinking habits.

Mothers with mild to moderate drinking problems may respond to education and encouragement to stop or limit intake. Specific suggestions for avoiding drinking or limiting the amount of alcohol in drinks or times of consumption can be helpful. Depending on the client's response, and when alcoholism is severe, referral to an alcohol counselor or program may be necessary. Detoxification procedures must be carefully selected because of potential effects on the fetus. Disulfiram (Antabuse) is contraindicated during pregnancy because of its inhibitory action on several enzymes.

Nursing Management of Minor Discomforts

The minor discomforts of pregnancy are the common complaints experienced by most expectant mothers, to some degree, in the course of a normal pregnancy. However, all mothers do not experience all of these discomforts, and, indeed, some mothers pass through the entire antepartal period without any complaints of this type. Although the discomforts are not serious in themselves, their presence detracts from the mother's feeling of comfort and well-being. In many instances they can be avoided by preventive measures or can be entirely overcome by common sense in daily living once they do occur.

TABLE 22-3

Smoking and Alcohol Risks

	Fetal Risks	*Maternal Risks*
Smoking	Abortion, stillbirth, prematurity	Hemorrhage (from abruptio placentae and placenta previa)
	Placenta previa and abruptio placentae	
	Premature rupture of membranes	Sepsis (from ruptured membranes)
	Low birth weight (brain damage, mental retardation, learning disorders, neurologic deficits, lower IQ)	Vitamin and mineral deficiencies
		Bronchitis, emphysema, bronchiectasis
	Deficiency in key nutrients	Lung cancer
	Sudden infant death syndrome	Hypertension and cardiovascular disease, heart attacks
Alcohol	Fetal alcohol syndrome (developmental defects, mental retardation)	Cirrhosis
	Withdrawal after birth	Malnutrition, vitamin and mineral deficiencies
	Neurologic, behavioral, and psychosocial disorders	Withdrawal (delirium tremens)
	Abortion, stillbirth (results tentative)	Chronic brain syndrome
		Family and social disruption
		Sexual problems

Frequent Urination

One of the first signs the woman may notice to make her suspect she might be pregnant is the frequent desire to empty her bladder. This is caused by the pressure of the growing uterus against the bladder and subsides about the second or the third month, when the uterus expands upward into the abdominal cavity. Later, during the last weeks of pregnancy, the symptoms recur.

Gastrointestinal Problems

Nausea

Nausea and vomiting to mild degree, called morning sickness, constitute the most common disorder of the first trimester of pregnancy. Symptoms usually appear about the end of the fourth or sixth week and last until about the 12th week. Nausea occurs in about one half of all pregnanct women; of these, about one third experience some vomiting. Usually, it occurs in the morning only, but a small percentage of women may have nausea and vomiting throughout the entire day.

Altered hormonal status, with high levels of hCG and progesterone, is involved in producing these symptoms through effects upon gastrointestinal smooth musculature. Changes in carbohydrate metabolism and other metabolic processes may also contribute.

For many years it was thought that this condition has an emotional basis. In all life's encounters, there are probably few experiences that are as anxiety provoking as the realization of being pregnant. At first there is the anxious uncertainty before the woman can be sure of the diagnosis. Then, there are numerous adjustments that have to be made and responsibilities that may seem to be overwhelming. Emotionally, the implications of pregnancy extend far back into her childhood. It is understandable that women who cannot adjust to all these new circumstances could have problems. Moreover, whether causative or not, the stress of pregnancy and all its ramifications can contribute to the symptoms caused by the metabolic changes associated with pregnancy.

Manifestations.   The typical sign of morning sickness starts with a feeling of nausea when the woman is getting out of bed in the morning. She is unable to retain her breakfast but by noon she has completely recovered and has no further episodes until the next morning. The nausea does not always occur in the morning but may happen in the afternoon or in the evening. In a small percentage of women the nausea and vomiting may persist throughout the day and even be worse in the afternoon. With the majority of women this problem lasts from 1 to 3 months and then suddenly ceases.

There may be a slight loss of body weight but no other signs or symptoms.

Nursing Care.   Often this condition can be controlled or at least relieved. Various before-breakfast remedies are used often. Taking a dry piece of toast or a cracker a half hour before getting out of bed may produce relief. In some instances sips of hot water (plain or with lemon juice), hot tea, clear coffee, or hot milk have been tried and found successful. However, the dry carbohydrate foods seem to be more effective. After remaining in bed for about a half hour after taking these rememdies, the woman gets up and dresses slowly (meanwhile sitting as much of the time as possible). After this she is usually ready for her breakfast.

Greasy foods and those known to cause disagreeable aftereffects should be avoided in the diet. Other suggested remedies include eating an increased amount of carbohydrate foods during this period of disturbance or eating simple and light food five or six times a day instead of three regular full meals. Unsweetened popcorn during the morning is sometimes advised. Another helpful remedy is sweet lemonade, about half a lemon to a pint of water sweetened with milk sugar. Such a drink is usually welcome following a bout of vomiting. Small amounts of ginger ale or cola drink or spearmint, raspberry, or peppermint tea also may be helpful.

Once nausea and vomiting are established, they are difficult to overcome; therefore, it is especially desirable to prevent the first attack, or at least to control this condition as soon as possible after it develops. Vomiting can deplete the system of necessary nutrients at a time when daily health should be maintained. Eating high-protein meals (*e.g.*, eggs, cheese, meat), fruit, and fruit juices may help prevent morning sickness by avoiding hypoglycemia, which is a cause of nausea. Taking 10 mg of vitamin B_6 at bedtime may be helpful also.

Pregnancies differ, and what may help one person may not benefit another. The trial-and-error method often is necessary to obtain results. If persistent vomiting develops, as it does with a small number of women, the condition is no longer considered to be a minor discomfort but a serious complication called hyperemesis gravidarum (see Chap. 36).

Heartburn

Heartburn is a neuromuscular phenomenon that may occur any time throughout gestation. As a result of the diminished gastric motility that normally accompanies pregnancy, reverse peristaltic waves cause regurgitation of the stomach contents into the esophagus. It is this irritation of the esophageal mucosa that causes heartburn. It may be described as a burning discomfort diffusely localized behind the lower part of the sternum, often radiating upward along the course of the esophagus. Although it is referred to as heartburn, it really has nothing to do with the heart. Often it is associated with other gastrointestinal symptoms, of which acid regurgitation, belching, nausea, and epigastric pressure are most troublesome. Nervous tension and emotional disturbances may be a precipitating cause. Worry, fatigue, and improper diet may contribute to its intensity.

Very little fat should be included in the diet. Although fatty foods are especially aggravating in this disturbance, strangely enough, the taking of some form of fat, such as a pat of butter or a tablespoon of cream, a short time before meals acts as a preventive because fat inhibits the secretion of acid in the stomach. However, this does not help if the heartburn is already present. Coffee and cigarettes tend to make heartburn worse because they stimulate acid secretion in the stomach and irritate the mucosa.

Eating several small meals daily instead of three large ones may help prevent heartburn. Wearing clothes that are loose around the waist may also be helpful. When heartburn occurs, it may be relieved with small sips of water, milk, or a carbonated drink. Lying down makes regurgitation worse, so it is best to sit upright. Relaxing and breathing deeply for several minutes may help. The "flying exercise" is also suggested: sitting tailor fashion, the arms are raised and lowered quickly, bringing the hands together over the head; this is repeated several times.

When antacids are used, those with an aluminum or magnesium base should be taken. Many over-the-counter remedies contain sodium, which promotes water retention and could lead to serious problems. Women are advised to avoid Alka-Seltzer, Fizrin, and baking soda (sodium bicarbonate), which are high in sodium ions. Equally effective medications are aluminum compounds, such as aluminum hydroxide gel, or this medication in tablet form with magnesium trisilicate.

Flatulence

Flatulence is a somewhat common and often disagreeable discomfort. Usually it is due to undesirable bacterial action in the intestines, which results in the formation of gas. Eating only small amounts of food and masticating it well may prevent this feeling of distress after eating. Regular daily elimination is of prime importance, as is the avoidance of foods that form gas (*e.g.*, beans, parsnips, corn, sweet desserts, fried foods, cake, and candy). If these measures fail to relieve the condition, the physician should be consulted.

Backache

Most pregnant women experience some degree of backache. As pregnancy advances, the woman's posture changes to compensate for the weight of the growing uterus. The shoulders are thrown back as the enlarging abdomen protrudes, and, for body balance to be maintained, the inward curve of the spine is exaggerated. The relaxation of the sacroiliac joints, in addition to the postural change, causes varying degrees of backache following excessive strain, fatigue, bending, or lifting.

The woman can be advised early in pregnancy how to prevent such strain through measures such as good posture and body mechanics in everyday living and avoidance of fatigue. Appropriate shoes worn during periods of activity and a supporting girdle may be helpful (see Clothing).

The key to good posture is to sit, stand, walk, and lie in a way that minimizes the hollow or curvature of the lower back. To do this, the abdominal and gluteal muscles are contracted and those of the lower back are relaxed, while the pelvis is tilted slightly upward and forward. The pelvic tilt exercise brings the pelvis into this alignment (see Chap. 20). Sitting posture can be improved by using armrests, foot supports, and a pillow for the back. The tailor position or lotus position used for yoga is useful for relief of back pain. The mother should always bend from the knees rather than the back when lifting, keeping the spine straight. Avoiding forward leaning while doing chores helps prevent strain on the back and is facilitated by adjusting the height of the work surface or the mother's position to maintain proper posture when standing or sitting.[12]

Daily exercises such as walking, swimming, and stretching are effective ways of preventing backache. The knee–chest twist is a particularly beneficial exercise. When backache occurs, it may be relieved by applying a heating pad or hot water bottle to the lower back, by having a back rub, or by sitting in a Jacuzzi that is not too hot.

Dyspnea

Difficult breathing or shortness of breath occasionally results from pressure on the diaphragm by the enlarged uterus and may interfere considerably with the client's sleep and general comfort during the last weeks of pregnancy. Usually it is not a serious condition, but unfortunately it cannot be wholly relieved until after lightening (the settling of the fetus into the pelvic cavity with relief of the upper abdominal pressure) or after the birth of the baby, when it will disappear spontaneously. It is most troublesome when the client attempts to lie down, so that her comfort may be greatly enhanced by propping her up in bed with pillows. In this semi-sitting posture she can sleep better and longer than with her head low. It is well for the nurse to demonstrate how these pillows may be arranged comfortably so that the client's back is adequately supported.

In clients with known heart disease, shortness of breath, especially of rather sudden onset, may be a sign of oncoming heart failure and should be reported at once to the physician.

Varicose Veins

Varicose veins or varices may occur in the lower extremities and, at times, extend up as high as the external genitalia or even into the pelvis itself. A varicosity is an enlargement in the diameter of a vein due to a thinning and stretching of its walls. Such distended areas may occur at short intervals along the course of the blood vessel; they give it a knotted appearance. Varicosities generally are associated with hereditary tendencies and are enhanced by advancing age, multiple pregnancy, and activities that require prolonged standing.

During pregnancy the pressure in the pelvis due to the enlarged uterus, which presses on the great abdominal veins, interferes with the return of the blood from the lower extremities. Added to this, any debilitating condition favors the formation of varicosities in the veins because of the general flabbiness and lack of tone in the tissues.

Naturally, the greater the pressure in the abdomen, the greater the chance of varicose veins of the lower extremities and the vulva. Therefore, any occupation that keeps a client constantly on her feet, particularly in the latter part of pregnancy, causes an increase in abdominal pressure and so acts as an exacerbating factor.

Symptoms. The first symptom of the development of varicose veins is a dull aching pain in the legs due to distention of the deep vessels. Inspection may show a fine purple network of superficial veins that cover the skin in a lacelike pattern, although this does not always appear. Later, the true varicosities appear, usually first under the bend of the knee, in a tangled mass of bluish or purplish veins, often as large as a lead pencil. As the condition advances, the varicosities extend up and down the leg along the course of the vessels, and in severe cases they may affect the veins of the labia majora, the vagina, and the uterus.

Nursing Care. Treatment for varicose veins begins by promptly abandoning any constricting garters, stockings, or other clothing that causes pressure, particularly on the legs or thighs. If varicosities persist in spite of this precaution, the client can be taught to take the right-angle position, that is, to lie on the floor with her legs extended straight into the air at right angles to her body, with her buttocks and heels resting against the wall (see Chap. 20). At first, this position is taken for 2 to 5 minutes several times a day. For some clients this position is very uncomfortable at first, but if it is explained, and the discomfort is therefore anticipated, the client is less likely to discontinue the exercise. Late in pregnancy this position may be too difficult to assume because of pressure against the diaphragm.

To give support to the weak-walled veins, either an elastic stocking or an elastic bandage often is recommended. The initial cost of elastic stockings is somewhat more than that of bandages, but they are easier to put on, are more effective, and have a neater appearance and a longer usefulness than bandages. A regular nylon stocking put on over the elastic hose further improves

FIGURE 22-11

Sims' position for varicosities of the vulva and rectum.

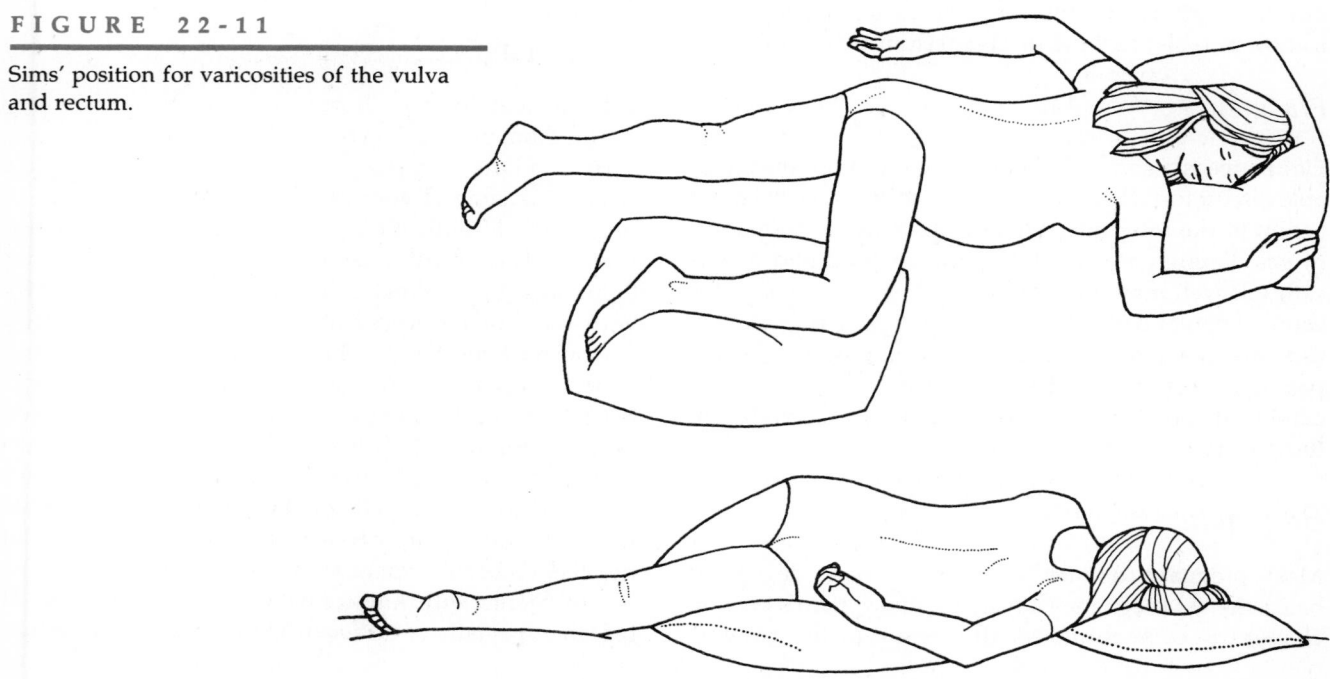

the appearance. Many hosiery companies are manufacturing "support" hose that do not have the strength of the elastic stockings but are very effective in giving a moderate amount of support. This type of stocking is useful in cases in which the varicosities are very mild or may not even be apparent peripherally but are suspected because of the ache they produce. Many women who must be on their feet a great deal and do not have the opportunity to rest frequently wear these stockings during working hours as a prophylactic measure. The nurse can be very helpful in apprising mothers of the varieties of hose now available to meet the needs of individual clients.

The client also must be told that the stocking or the bandage should be removed at night for greater comfort and reapplied in the morning after the legs have been elevated so that the vessels will be less dilated. The longer stockings or bandage is more satisfactory when the varicosities are above the knee. Both the elastic stocking and the bandage are washable, which helps to maintain their original elasticity. However, mild soap rather than detergent should be used.

Varicosities of the vulva may be relieved by placing a pillow under the buttocks and elevating the hips for frequent rest periods or by taking the elevated Sims' position for a few moments several times a day (Fig. 22-11). Clients suffering from this condition should not stand when they can sit, and they should not sit when they can lie down.

More important than the treatment of this condition is its prevention. Every pregnant woman should be advised to sit with her legs elevated whenever possible. When the legs are elevated, care should be taken to see that there are no pressure points against the legs to interfere with the circulation, particularly in the popliteal space. Tight constricting garments, round garters, constipation, standing for long periods of time, and inadequate rest all tend to aggravate this condition.

A *varicose vein in the vagina* may rupture during the antepartal or intrapartal period, but this is rare. The hemorrhage is venous and can be controlled readily by pressure. The foot of the bed can be markedly elevated.

Cramps

Cramps are painful spasmodic muscular contractions in the legs. They may occur at any time during the pregnancy but more generally during the later months owing to pressure of the enlarged uterus on the nerves affecting the lower extremities. Other causes have been attributed to fatigue, chilling, tense body posture, and insufficient or excessive calcium in the diet. They are commonly noted after the use of diuretics.

A quart of milk in the daily diet has been generally recommended to meet the calcium needs during pregnancy. However, studies show that large quantities of milk or dicalcium phosphate predispose to muscular tetany and leg cramps as a result of the excessive amount of phosphorus absorbed from these products. Some authorities suggest that small quantities of aluminum hydroxide gel be taken with the quart of milk because it removes some of the dietary phosphorus from the intestinal tract. Immediate relief may be obtained by forcing the toes upward and by putting pressure on the knee to straighten the leg. Elevating the feet and keeping the extremities warm are preventives.

Cramps, while not a serious condition, are excruciatingly painful for the duration of the seizure. Regular exercise to keep circulation good in the legs helps prevent cramps. Taking a warm bath before bedtime can improve circulation at night. Cramps are often brought on by pointing the toes when stretching; the woman needs to be reminded to avoid this. Massaging the cramped muscle, soaking it in warm water, using a heating pad, and standing and walking when able relieve cramps.

Edema

Swelling of the lower extremities is very common during pregnancy and is sometimes very uncomfortable. It is especially likely to occur in hot weather. Often it may be relieved by a proper abdominal support or by resting frequently during the day. Elevating the feet or taking the right-angle position often gives relief (Fig. 22-12).

Edema may be prevented by avoiding highly salted foods, eating high-protein foods, and avoiding tight clothing. Women who work or must remain standing or sitting for long periods need to rest two to three times daily with legs raised for about 20 minutes. When edema occurs, elevating the legs as much as possible reduces swelling and discomfort.

Although edema of the ankles, feet, and even hands is common, particularly in late pregnancy, the nurse must always be alert for possible complications. *Edema is one of the signs of preeclampsia and must not be overlooked.* Sudden weight gain of more than 2 lb per week needs careful evaluation. The nurse should look for distribution of edema on the face and sacrum as additional indices of preeclampsia. This must be brought to the physician's attention. The prevention of various minor discomforts of pregnancy, medications to avoid, and safe natural remedies are described in Table 22-4.

Vaginal Discharge

In pregnancy there is increased vaginal secretion so that a heavier discharge at this time usually has no particular significance. However, it is wise to instruct the client to call to the attention of the physician any copious or yellow or greenish foul-smelling or irritating discharge. For instance, a profuse yellow discharge may be re-

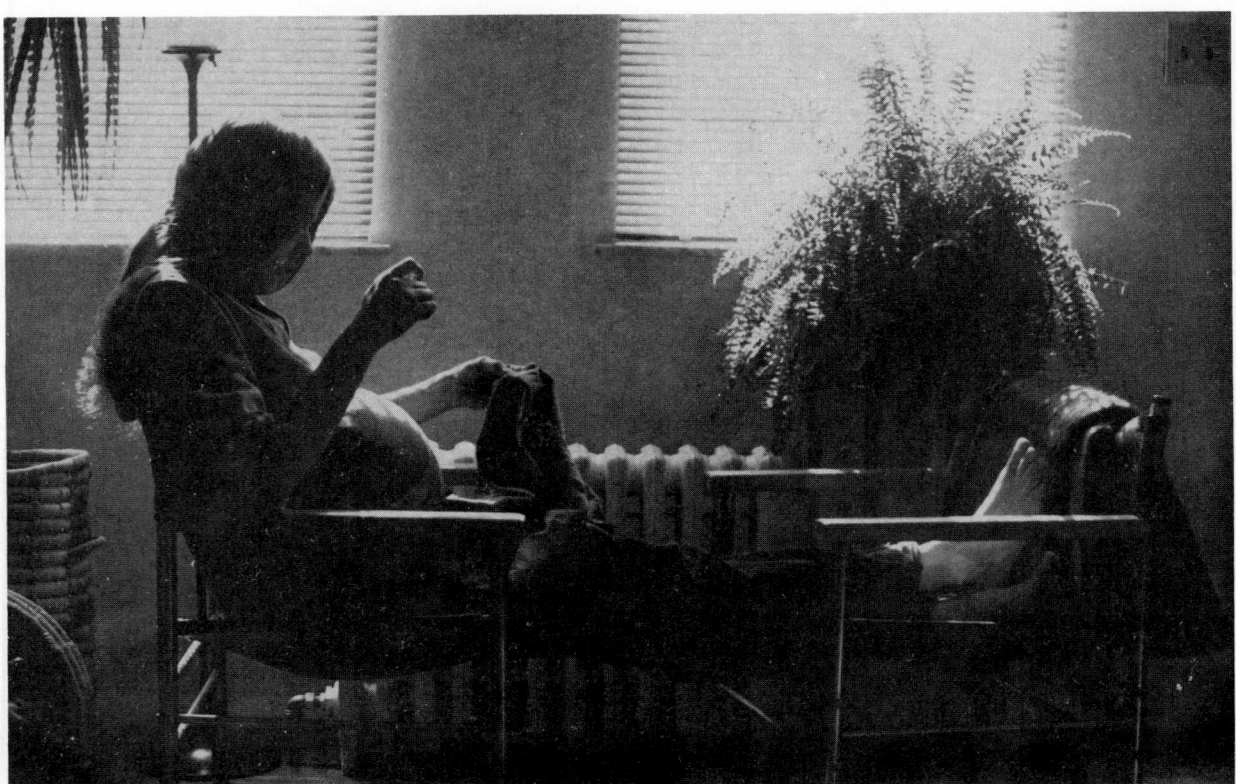

FIGURE 22-12

Elevate legs to relieve edema. Swelling and discomfort are reduced if the legs can be elevated as much as possible, even at work.

garded as possible evidence of gonorrhea or trichomoniasis (see Chap. 37), especially when it is accompanied by such symptoms as vaginal itching or burning or by such urinary manifestations as burning on urination and frequency. The microscopic result of a smear or culture indicates whether or not definite treatment is necessary. The two most common vaginal discharges occurring during pregnancy are listed in Table 22-5.

If any discharge becomes irritating, the client may be advised to bathe the vulva with a solution of sodium bicarbonate or boric acid. The application of KY jelly after bathing often relieves the condition entirely. Instructing a client to wear a perineal pad is sometimes all the advice that is needed. A douche should never be taken unless prescribed by the physician.

Trichomoniasis

A particularly stubborn form of leukorrhea in pregnancy is caused by the parasitic protozoan known as *Trichomonas vaginalis*. It is characterized not only by a profuse frothy discharge (yellow green in color), but also by irritation and itching of the vulva and the vagina. The diagnosis is easily made by taking a small quantity of the fresh vaginal discharge and examining it under the microscope in a hanging-drop or wet prep. Here the spindle-shaped organisms, somewhat larger than leukocytes, with whiplike processes attached, can be seen in active motion.

Trichomonas vaginitis is treated with sulfanilamide, aminacrine hydrochloride, and allantoin (AVC cream), aminoacridine hydrochloride, polyoxyethylene nonyl phenol, sodium edetate, sodium dioctyl sulfosuccinate (Vagisec suppositories), or trichofuron cream. Although oral metronidazole (Flagyl) is highly effective, it is contraindicated during pregnancy because of its potential for fetal abnormalities.[13] Simultaneous treatment of the sexual partner is recommended, usually with orally administered Flagyl, because the infection is transmitted through sexual contact, although males are generally asymptomatic.

Candidiasis

Candidiasis, a yeast infection caused by *Candida albicans*, is another common cause of profuse vaginal discharge. The organism is frequently present in the vaginal canal without producing symptoms, but during pregnancy the physical changes in the vagina produce con-

(text continued on page 418)

TABLE 22-4

Natural Remedies for Minor Discomforts of Pregnancy

Prevention	Natural Remedies	Medicines Not to Be Used*
Nausea and vomiting		
Eat high-protein meals and fruit and drink fruit juices to avoid hypoglycemia	Eat dry bread or crackers	Antihistamines (contained in most antinausea medicines)
Eat several small meals daily	Sip soda water	
Avoid fried foods	Take a walk in fresh air	
Drink liquids between meals rather than with meals	Drink spearmint, raspberry leaf, or peppermint tea	
Get out of bed slowly, avoid sudden movements		
Eat dry bread or crackers before rising (keep by bed)		
Eat yogurt or drink milk at night or before rising		
Headache		
Get enough sleep at night and enough rest during the day	Apply a cool, wet washcloth to forehead and back of neck (some prefer warm cloth)	Narcotic analgesics
Do not go for long periods without eating	Massage neck, shoulders, face, scalp, forehead	Aspirin, Excedrin, Percogesic, Cope
Drink plenty of fluids	Take a walk in fresh air	
Avoid things that contribute to headaches (*e.g.*, eye strain, stuffy rooms, cigarette smoke, rushing around)	Take a warm bath	
	Find a quiet place and relax	
	Meditate or do yoga	
Difficulty sleeping		
Exercise daily	Relax and do not worry about not sleeping; even lying in bed is restful to the body	Sleeping aids (Sleep-Eze, Nytol, Sominex, Compoz, etc)
Take a warm bath at bedtime	Read for a while	Sedatives
Drink hot water with lemon, or warm milk, at bedtime	Follow suggestions under prevention	Tranquilizers
Do not eat a large meal within 2–3 hr of bedtime		
Decrease noise and lights		
Do relaxation exercises		
Use pillows under knees, back, or abdomen		
Avoid caffeine		
Stuffy nose and allergies		
Avoid allergens	Breathe steam from hot shower, pot of boiling water, or vaporizer/humidifier	Antihistamines (in most cold remedies—Contac, Coricidin, Allerest, Dristan, etc)
Do not smoke cigarettes, avoid smoke-filled rooms	Drink plenty of liquids	
	Use salt-water nose drops (¼ tsp salt in 1 cup warm water)	
	Use warm, moist towel on sinuses; massage sinuses	

(continued)

416 UNIT IV : *Assessment and Management in the Antepartum Period*

T A B L E   2 2 - 4   (*continued*)

Prevention	Natural Remedies	Medicines Not to Be Used*
Heartburn		
Avoid foods known to cause gastric upset	Take small sips of water	Sodium base antacids (*e.g.*, Alka-Seltzer, Fizrin, Soda Mint, baking soda)
Avoid greasy, fried foods	Sip carbonated beverage	
Avoid highly seasoned foods	Sit upright	
Eat several small meals daily	Relax and breathe deeply for several minutes	
Avoid coffee and cigarettes	Do the flying exercise	
Wear loose clothes at waist	Use aluminum base antacids	
Drink 6–8 glasses water daily		
Fatigue		
Get enough sleep and rest	Take the time to rest when the body demands it	Caffeine (*e.g.*, coffee, tea, cola drinks, stay-awake pills)
Take naps during the day	Sit with feet up whenever possible	Amphetamines
Pace daily life to provide for extra rest	Use suggestions under Prevention	
Eat well-balanced meals		
Exercise regularly		
Leg Cramps		
Get enough calcium (milk, dark green leafy vegetables, supplements)	Sit down, straighten the leg, point or pull toes upward toward the knees	Quinine
Exercise regularly	Massage the cramped muscle	Muscle relaxants
Keep the legs warm	Walk around when able	
Take a warm bath at bedtime	Soak cramped muscle in warm water or use heating pad	
Do not point the toes when stretching		
Constipation		
Drink plenty of fluids (6–8 glasses of water daily)	Drink either hot or very cold liquid on an empty stomach	Laxatives that are other than bulk producing (best to avoid all laxatives; at least use only twice per week; taking too many laxatives causes more constipation)
Exercise regularly	Follow suggestions under Prevention	
Eat raw vegetables, cooked fruit (*e.g.*, prune juice), 3 tbsp bran daily, whole grain bread and cereal, oatmeal, brown rice	Use bulk-producing laxatives (*e.g.*, Metamucil, Effersyllium)	
Caution—raw apples and coffee increase constipation		
Chew food thoroughly		
Have good bowel habits (do not force bowel movements, go when having the urge, take time for bowel movements, raise feet on stool to reduce strain)		
Varicose veins		
Exercise regularly	Lie with feet raised several times daily	No medications
Avoid tight or binding clothes (especially garters, knee-length stockings)	Lie with feet against wall	
Wear full-length support hose when standing or walking for a long time	Wear elastic support hose (put on before rising)	

(*continued*)

TABLE 22-4 *(continued)*

Prevention	Natural Remedies	Medicines Not to Be Used*
Avoid sitting or standing for a long time		
Wear shoes with well-padded soles to absorb shock		
Hemorrhoids		
Prevent constipation and straining during bowel movements	Sit in warm tub for 15–20 min 3–4 times daily	Local anesthetic creams (Preparation H, Americaine, Anusol)
Follow good bowel habits	Apply dilute lemon juice or vinegar compresses, use Tucks or witch hazel compresses	
Do not sit for a long time on the toilet		
Do Kegel's exercises regularly	Use bulk-producing laxatives to keep stool soft	
Backache		
Maintain good posture	Do prenatal exercises (especially the pelvic tilt and knee–chest twist)	Analgesics
Bend from knees when lifting		Aspirin, Tylenol
Wear supportive shoes with low heels	Apply heat to the lower back	
Exercise regularly	Have a back rub or back massage	
Do prenatal exercises or yoga	Rest the back	
Maintain normal weight gain		
Edema		
Eat high-protein foods	Sit with legs raised as much as possible	Diuretics (prescriptions and over-the-counter water pills)
Avoid highly salted foods	Follow suggestions under Prevention	
Avoid standing for long periods		
Avoid tight clothing and constrictions of legs		
Rest and elevate legs 2–3 times daily for 20 min		

* In severe cases, the physician may prescribe a medication after weighing the benefits to the mother and risks to the fetus.

TABLE 22-5

Vaginal Discharge Caused by Infections

Type	Causative Organism	Signs and Symptoms	Treatment
Candidiasis	*Candida albicans*, yeast	Thick, white, cottage-cheese or curdy discharge on cervix and vagina	Fungicidal creams or suppositories (Nystatin, Mycostatin, Nilstat)
		Pruritus (itching) of perineum, labia, thighs	
		Erythema of labia, perineum	
		Edema of genitalia if severe	
Trichomoniasis	*Trichomonas vaginalis*, protozoan	Copious yellow green, frothy discharge	AVC cream, trichofuron cream or suppositories, Vagisec suppositories
		Pruritus (itching) of perineum, labia, thighs	Note. *Flagyl (metronidazole), although highly effective, is contraindicated during pregnancy owing to its teratogenic effects*
		Erythema of labia, perineum	
		Petechiae of cervix and vagina	

(text continued from page 414)

ditions that foster development of infection. It is characterized by white patches on the vaginal mucosa and a thick cottage-cheese-like discharge that is extremely irritating, so that burning or pruritus is present. Even the external genitalia often become inflamed, and occasionally extensive edema is observed. Bleeding may accompany the other symptoms if the patches on the mucosa are removed.

Specific fungicidal suppositories, such as Mycostatin, are used to treat this condition. Although this treatment is effective, the infection is stubborn and likely to recur and require repeated treatment during the pregnancy. The *pruritus,* or itching of the skin, may be relieved to a marked degree if proper hygienic measures are employed to keep the area free of the irritating discharge being deposited on the skin surface.

The woman who has this infection may transmit it to her infant during the process of delivery. *Thrush* develops when the organisms colonize the mucous membrane of the infant's mouth.

Nursing Management of Drug Use During Pregnancy

The use of all medication is to be minimized during pregnancy. Evidence regarding the adverse effects of many chemical substances when taken by a pregnant woman continues to accumulate. Because of the rapid formation of fetal organ systems and development of cellular functions, the first trimester is a particularly susceptible time. However, ingestion of drugs at any time during pregnancy holds potential for fetal damage. The impact of a drug on the developing fetus may range from no measurable effect to such marked toxicity that the embryo is killed (aborted). Sublethal doses of drugs may result in gross anatomical defects or a permanent subtle metabolic or functional deficit.

The effects of drugs and other substances, such as toxic chemicals used in industry or agriculture, upon the embryo or fetus can be grouped into three classes:

- *Mutagens* are chemicals or substances that cause a change in gene structure; they alter genetic information. When sperm or ova are affected, such mutations can cause miscarriage, congenital defects, mental retardation, and other mental and physical abnormalities in the infant. Radiation is one classic cause of mutations, but many other substances are known or suspected causes of mutagenic action.
- *Carcinogens* are chemicals or substances that can induce or promote cancer. Transplacental carcinogens are often difficult to identify because of the long latency period in development of tumors. In prenatally exposed females, vaginal adenomas caused by administration of diethylstilbestrol to their mothers do not appear in the daughters for some 18 to 20 years. Many agents have been identified as carcinogenic in either humans or animals. It is suggested that the recently discovered rise of cancer in children may be due to chemical exposures during pregnancy.
- *Teratogens* are chemicals or substances that interfere with fetal development after conception. This is an acute toxicologic event that requires only short or instantaneous exposure. The pathologic results are seen within a relatively short time. Many drugs are known to have teratogenic effects on the fetus if taken during pregnancy, causing such anomalies as bone and limb deformities, deafness, cardiac defects, growth retardation, prematurity, and metabolic abnormalities.

A drug's potential for teratogenesis or other adverse effects depends upon the degree to which it enters fetal circulation, dosage, duration of administration, stage of pregnancy, and physical condition of mother and maturity of infant at birth. Most drugs cross the placenta by simple diffusion. Diffusion of a substance depends on its concentration, degree of ionization, lipid solubility, and molecular weight. Nonionized and highly lipid-soluble compounds diffuse more readily across the placenta; substances with molecular weights greater than 1000 do not pass by diffusion. The fetus and infant are particularly susceptible to drugs because they have a limited ability to metabolize and excrete drugs, and there may be inefficiency in the blood–brain barrier and increased affinity of various receptor sites.[14]

Over-the-Counter Drugs

About half of all drugs taken during pregnancy are over-the-counter (OTC) products used to relieve symptoms of physiological changes of pregnancy. Most commonly used are preparations for nasal congestion, backache, constipation, hemorrhoids, and heartburn. Despite longstanding and continuing use, there is little information about possible harmful effects of these drugs during pregnancy. Aspirin and acetaminophen, used as analgesics, have not been shown to be associated with an increased risk of fetal malformation. Aspirin in substantial doses might prolong gestation or labor (owing to prostaglandin synthesis inhibition) or contribute to bleeding problems in the newborn (owing to reduced platelet aggregation and prolonged bleeding time).

Cold and allergy preparations have not been associated clearly with fetal malformations, although some animal data suggest possible teratogenic effects of antihistamines and sympathomimetic amines (deconges-

Precautions Concerning Drug Use During Pregnancy

Drugs Contraindicated Throughout Pregnancy

Antineoplastic agents

Diethylstilbestrol

Oral hypoglycemics

Radioactive iodine

Tetracycline

Metronidazole (Flagyl)

Oral contraceptives

Quinine

Corticosteroids

Thalidomide

Sedatives and tranquilizers (*i.e.*, Librium, Valium, Meprobamate, Tofranil)

Diphenylhydantoin (Dilantin)

Trimethoadione (Tridione)

Lasix

Propylthiouracil

Indomethacin (Indocin)

Streptomycin

Chloramphenicol (Chloromycetin)

Chloroquine (Aralen)

Dextroamphetamines

Vitamins A, C, D, or K in excess

Drugs Used with Caution During Pregnancy

Diuretics

Antihypertensives

Anticonvulsants

Oral anticoagulants

Phenothiazines

Antithyroid drugs (except those contraindicated above)

Antibiotics (except those contraindicated above)

Antihistamines

Theophylline

Caffeine (anomalies, abortion with more than 600 mg/day)

Salicylates

Laxatives (other than bulk producing)

Local anesthetics

Nicotine

Drugs to Avoid Near Term or During Delivery

CNS depressants

Narcotic analgesics

Nitrofurantoin

Oral anticoagulants

Salicylates

Sedatives

Sulfonamides

Vitamin K

Lithium

Some authorities recommend that drugs not be used at all during pregnancy. A pregnant woman should not take any drugs unless prescribed by her physician.

---

tants such as pseudoephedrine). There is no good OTC antinausea drug for use during pregnancy; most contain an antihistamine and are mainly for use in preventing motion sickness. Antacids have not been shown to cause fetal malformations, although they can interfere with intestinal absorption and renal clearance of other drugs. Stool softeners containing dioctyl sodium sulfosuccinate have not been linked with congenital defects or metabolic derangement.

OTC vitamins do not supply enough elemental iron or folic acid to meet minimum requirements during pregnancy. Pregnant vegetarians may need additional supplementation (above prenatal vitamins) of vitamin B_{12}. Vitamin B_6 has been used to treat nausea, in combination with other measures. Excessive doses of vitamins A and D should be avoided; prolonged use can cause gastrointestinal symptoms, kidney stones, hypercalcemia, and renal failure.

Used occasionally in small doses, adverse effects of most OTC products on mother or fetus are unlikely. However, most studies of these drugs have been on animals given high-dose exposures, and there have been very few human investigations.[15] The safest approach is to avoid OTC drugs and to discuss their use with the physician if symptoms cannot be relieved by natural remedies.

Caffeine

The Food and Drug Administration (FDA) recommends that pregnant women avoid or limit consumption of coffee, food, and drugs containing caffeine.[16] Caffeine intake of 600 mg or more per day has been associated with decreased fertility, increased chromosomal breakage, animal teratogenicity, and increased risk of spontaneous abortion and low birth weight. There is no documentation of caffeine-caused human malformations, however.[15]

The average cup of coffee contains 120 mg caffeine. Many OTC drugs have caffeine as one ingredient, but in doses usually less than 120 mg. Soft drinks often contain caffeine, such as Coca-Cola, Mountain Dew, Pepsi, and others. Caffeine does cross the placenta and can be detected in the serum and urine of newborns. Breast-fed infants receive caffeine through their mother's milk.

Studies of adverse effects of caffeine on mother or fetus are usually confounded by other covariables, such as alcohol use, smoking, and demographic characteristics. As with OTC drugs, reliable data are largely missing, and the safest approach is to avoid caffeine use.

Substance Abuse

Alcohol and smoking were discussed earlier in this chapter. Recreational drugs and their abuse are discussed in Chapter 8.

Nursing Care

Prenatal counseling stresses the importance of avoiding use of self-medication and prescription medication. The vast majority of drugs have not received adequate clinical testing to establish their safety during pregnancy. Those drugs with known or suspected toxicity should be avoided. All other drugs must be given very cautiously to pregnant women, with the benefits of administering the drug weighed against the potential risk to the fetus. The nurse assesses medication and street-drug use during the prenatal history and discusses the risks involved if the mother is taking drugs. When the physician does prescribe a drug for a necessary treatment, the smallest dosage for the shortest period of time is given.

When assisting the pregnant woman in finding relief from the minor discomforts of pregnancy, the nurse can suggest natural remedies that do not rely upon medications. The safest course for the baby is to avoid taking any drugs at all (see Table 22-4).

Preparations for the Baby

As the time of delivery nears, parents become involved in planning for the baby's homecoming. The baby's layette and equipment are of special interest. The nurse should be familiar with clothing and equipment needed and should advise parents accordingly. Costs should be in keeping with the family's economic circumstances.

Layette

The mother can be advised to prepare a very simple layette. As she sees how fast her baby grows, and what is needed, the additional items can be secured. The complete layettes that can be purchased often contain unnecessary items and are costly. Also, many articles may be received as baby gifts. Therefore, it is wise to choose only those things that are necessary for immediate use.

Baby clothing should have the following characteristics. It should be comfortable, lightweight, and easy to put on and launder. Any clothing that comes in contact with the infant's skin should be made of soft cotton material. Wool should be avoided because it can irritate an infant's skin. Knitted materials are preferred because they are easy to launder and can stretch sufficiently to allow more freedom in dressing the baby. Caution should be taken that the materials are fire resistant. Garments that open down the full length and fasten with ties or grippers are easier to put on. Ties or grippers are also safer than buttons.

The geographic location and climate greatly influence the selection of the infant's clothing. Size 1 shirts and gowns are recommended, since the infant grows rapidly in the first 6 months and quickly outgrows garments. It is important to remember that clothing should not inhibit the baby's normal activities. The complete outfit of clothes that the baby wears need not weigh more than 12 oz to 16 oz.

Some further suggestions in relation to the selection of specific items are as follows.

Shirts, Gowns, and the Like. The sleeves should have roomy armholes, such as the raglan-type sleeve. If a pullover-type garment is used, the neck opening should be so constructed that it is large enough to be put on easily over the feet or the head.

Diapers. The selection of diapers should be considered from the standpoint of their comfort (soft and

---

Layette

Layette Necessities

Five or six shirts

Three to four dozen diapers (if diaper service is not used)

Four to six receiving blankets (These are very versatile items and can be used in various ways. For instance, they can be rolled firmly and used to support the back when the infant is on his side; in emergencies, they can be used as bath towels, diaper pads, and sheets.)

Three to six nightgowns, kimonos, or sacques

Six cotton-covered waterproof diaper pads (11″ × 16″)

Two waterproof protectors for under diaper pads

Two afghans or blankets

One bunting } (if climate is cold)

Two to four soft towels (40″ × 40″)

Two to four soft washcloths

Nursery Equipment

Basket, bassinet, or crib

Mattress (firm, flat, and smooth)

Mattress protector (waterproof)

Sheets or pillowcases for mattress

Chest or separate drawer

Cotton crib blankets

Bathtub

Diaper pail

Equipped toilet tray

Absorbent cotton or cotton balls

Baby soap (bland, white, unscented)

Rustproof safety pins

Soapdish

Bath apron (for mother)

Table for bathing or dressing

Chair (for mother)

Additional Suggestions for Layette and Equipment

Sweaters

Crib spreads

Bibs

Clothes drier

Chest of drawers

Nursery stand

Footstool

Diaper bag (for traveling)

Disposable diapers

Nursery light

Carriage or stroller

Car seat

---

light in weight), absorbency, cost, and washing and drying qualities. The mother who plans to use a commercial diaper service may use either the company's diapers or her own. Disposable diapers are frequently used, but they may be more expensive in the long run than cloth diapers or a diaper service.

Receiving Blankets. Receiving blankets should be made of cotton flannelette, 1 yard square. This square is used to fold loosely about the baby. If the blanket is properly secured, the baby may lie and kick and at the same time keep covered and warm. In the early weeks these squares take the brunt of the service and in this way save the finer covers from becoming soiled so quickly.

Afghans or Blankets. Afghans or blankets can be of very lightweight cotton or polyester material. The temperature and the weather will determine the amount of covering needed.

Sheets. Crib sheets are usually 45 by 72 inches and are available in muslin, percale, and knitted cotton materials. The knit sheets are practical for bottom sheets and do not need to be ironed. Pillowcases are very usable for the carriage or the basket mattress. Receiving blankets may be used for top sheets.

Waterproof Sheeting. Various waterproof materials are suitable to protect the mattress and to be used under the pads. Even though the mattress may have a protective covering, it is necessary to have a waterproof cover large enough to cover the mattress completely—something that can be removed and washed.

Waterproof Pants. Waterproof pants offer protection for special occasions. If the plastic variety is used, they should not be tight at the leg or the waist. For general use, a square of protective material such as Sanisheeting or a cotton quilted pad can be used under the baby next to the diaper.

Bath Apron. The bath apron is a protection for both mother and baby and may be made of plastic material covered with terry cloth.

Nursery Equipment

In choosing the equipment, again the individual circumstances should be considered. Expense, space, and future plans all influence the selection. Most nurseries are planned for the satisfaction of the parents. Eventually the baby's room becomes the child's room; if economy must be considered, furniture should be selected that will appeal to the child as he grows and develops.

Bed. A basket, bassinet, or crib may be used as the baby's bed. The trimming on the basket or the bassinet should be such that it can be removed easily and laundered. A bed may be improvised from a box or a bureau drawer, placed securely on a sturdy table or on chairs that are held together with rope. Many parents may have a carriage that may be used as a bed. However, after about the first 2 months, the baby needs a crib. The crib should be constructed so that the bars are close enough together to prevent the baby's head from being caught between them. If it is painted, a nonleaded paint that is "safe for babies" should be used.

Mattress. The mattress is to be firm (not hard) and flat. All mattresses, including the waterproof-covered type, can be protected by a waterproof sheeting to prevent the mattress from becoming stained and from absorbing odors. The waterproof sheet is easily washed and dries quickly.

Bathtub. The plastic tub is safe and easy to keep clean. Some mothers adapt the kitchen or bathroom sink for the baby's bath.

Diaper Pail. The diaper pail should be large enough for at least the day's supply of soiled diapers. It may be used also for boiling the diapers.

References

1. Gordon M: Nursing Diagnosis: Process and Application. New York, McGraw-Hill, 1982
2. Woodward SL: How does strenuous maternal exercise affect the fetus? A review. Birth Fam J 8(1):17–24, Spring 1981
3. Shearer MH: Teaching prenatal exercise: Part 1. Posture. Birth Fam J 8(2):105–108, Summer 1981
4. Greenberg J: Implications for primary care providers of occupational health hazards on pregnant women and their infants. J Nurse–Midwifery, 25(4):21–30, July/August 1980
5. Pritchard JA, MacDonald P: Williams Obstetrics. 16th ed, p 321. New York, Appleton–Century–Crofts, 1980
6. Deibel P: Effects of cigarette smoking on maternal nutrition and the fetus. JOGN Nurs 9(6):333–336, November/December 1980
7. New smoking risk found: Quitting before pregnancy no safeguard. J Nurse–Midwifery 24(2):24, March/April 1979
8. Meyer MB: How does maternal smoking affect birth weight and maternal weight gain? Am J Obstet Gynecol 131:888–893, August 15, 1978
9. Naeye RL: Influence of maternal cigarette smoking during pregnancy on fetal and childhood growth. Obstet Gynecol 57(1):18, January 1981
10. Haworth JC et al: Fetal growth retardation in cigarette smoking mothers is not due to decreased maternal food intake. Am J Obstet Gynecol 137:719, July 1980
11. Stephens CJ: The fetal alcohol syndrome: Cause for concern. MCN 6:251–256, July/August 1981
12. Cooper SB: Preventing back abuse in young mothers. MCN 2(4):260–263, July/August 1977
13. Is Flagyl dangerous? Med Lett Drugs Ther 17:53–54, 1975
14. Gullekson DJ, Temple AR: Maternal drug use during the perinatal period. Family and Community Health 1(3):31–41, November 1978
15. Rayburn WF: OTC drugs and pregnancy. Perinatology and Neonatology 8:21–27, September/October 1984
16. Dri EA, Cheddie M: Substance abuse and the prenatal employee: A Nursing diagnosis perspective. Occup Health Nurs 32:485–488; 497, September 1984

Suggested Reading

Baruffi G, Dellinger WS, Strobine DM et al: A study of pregnancy outcomes in a maternity center and a tertiary care hospital. Am J Public Health 74(9):973–978, September 1984

Bracken MB, Holford TR: Exposure to prescribed drugs in pregnancy and association with congenital malformations. Obstet Gynecol 58:336, 1981

Bullsard JA: Exercise and pregnancy. Can Fam Physician 27:977, 1981

Carter-Jessop L: Promoting maternal attachment through prenatal intervention. MCN 6:107, March/April 1981

Dale E et al: Exercise during pregnancy: Effects on the fetus. Can J Appl Sport Sci 7:98, June 1982

Erikson MP: Trends in assessing the newborn and his parents. MCN 3(2):99–103, March/April 1978

Fisher ES, LoGerfo JP, Daling JR: Prenatal care and pregnancy outcomes during the recession: The Washington State experience. Am J Public Health 75(8):866–870, August 1985

Hammer RM, Bower EJ, Messina LJ: The prenatal use of

Rh₀D immune globulin. MCN 9:29–31, January/February 1984

Jopke T: Pregnancy: A time to exercise judgment. Phys Sportsmed 11:139, July 1983

Kotelchuck M, Schwartz JB et al: WIC participation and pregnancy outcomes: Massachusetts Statewide Evaluation Project. Am J Public Health 74(10):1086–1092, October 1984

Leap TL: Equal employment opportunity and its implications for personnel practices in the 1980s. Labor Law J 31:669, 1980

Luke B: Does caffeine influence reproduction? MCN 7:240, July/August 1982

McKay S: Smoking during the childbearing years. MCN 5:46, January/February 1980

Makinson C: The health consequences of teenage fertility. Fam Plann Perspect 17:132–139, May/June 1985

Martin LM: Health Care of Women. Philadelphia, JB Lippincott, 1978

Over-the-Counter-Drug Committee of the Coalition for the Medical Rights of Women: Safe natural remedies for discomforts of pregnancy. 1638B Haight Street, San Francisco, CA 94117

Rush D: Further evidence on the value of the WIC program. Am J Public Health 75(8):828–829, August 1985

Singh S, Torres A, Forrest JD: The need for prenatal care in the United States: Evidence from the 1980 National Natality Survey. Fam Plann Perspect 17:118–124, May/June 1985

Smith JC, Hughes JM, Pekow PS et al: An assessment of the incidence of maternal mortality in the United States. Am J Public Health 74(8):780–783, August 1984

Snyder C et al: New findings about mothers' antenatal expectations and their relationship to infant development. MCN 4:354, November/December 1979

Trotter R et al: The pregnancy disability amendment: I. What the law provides. Personnel Admin 27(2):47, 1982

Wilsnack RW, Wilsnack SC, Klassen AD: Women's drinking and drinking problems: Patterns from a 1981 national survey. Am J Public Health 74(11):1231–1238, November 1984

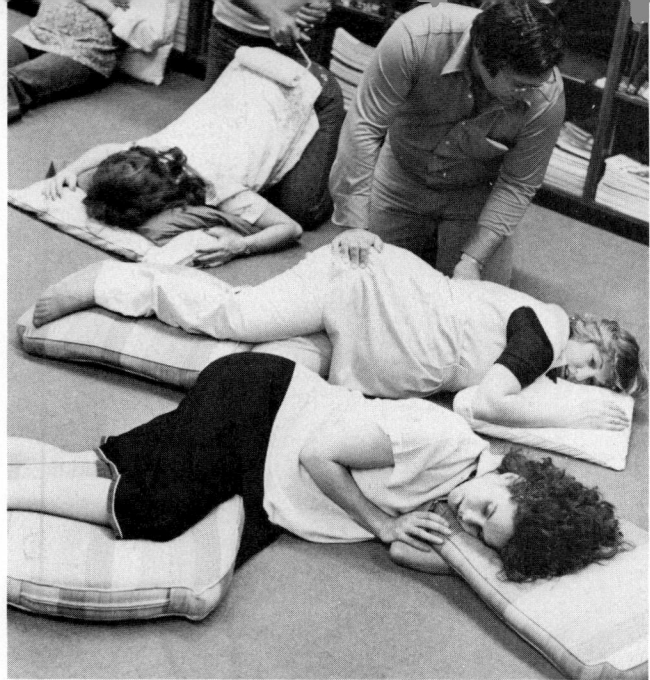

Unit IV:
Assessment and Management in the Antepartum Period

Conference Material

1. A mother in her first trimester of pregnancy is undergoing a difficult divorce. She appears very anxious and upset and tells you that she sometimes feels like she is losing her mind. What do you know about the psychological and physiological effects of anxiety during pregnancy? What specific interventions would you plan to help this mother?

2. A couple comes to childbirth education classes and the husband complains that he had symptoms of morning sickness during the first trimester and is now experiencing low back pain and aching legs. What might your counseling be for this couple?

3. A young husband complains to you that his wife's sexual desire has changed since she has become pregnant. When he tells you, you note that his wife becomes flushed and tense. What would you tell this couple to reassure them about their apparent problem?

4. What childbirth education classes are available in your community? How do they compare to the "variables to consider in selecting a childbirth class?" (See display box in Chap. 20.)

5. What community resources are available for prenatal and postpartum exercise classes and parenting classes?

6. A 34-year-old woman delivered her first baby a few hours ago. She and her husband attended childbirth classes.

The woman requested and received 50 mg demerol during her labor. She tells you how guilty she feels because she needed medication for pain, since she and her husband had hoped to have a "natural birth." How would you respond to this patient?

7. Examine several women on their third postpartum day for diastasis recti. Depending on the results of your findings teach each woman an appropriate exercise to strengthen her abdominal muscles.

8. A 15-year-old mother from a low-income family will be going home with her baby in 2 days. She will be living with her mother and father. What specific teaching measures would you include in discharge planning for this patient?

9. Dorothea W. is a 28-year-old married mother of two, presently in the seventh month of her third pregnancy. Her husband Sam works as a printer; the children are both boys, ages seven and four. Dorothea quit her secretarial job last month, and plans not to work until the new baby is about 2 years of age. Her pregnancy has been progressing normally; she has experienced recent discomfort with hemorrhoids and heartburn. At her prenatal visit, you notice that she has gained 8 lb since the last visit 1 month ago, and she has moderate edema of the ankles and hands. The couple will begin childbirth classes in 2 weeks; both previous deliveries have been conscious and participative, without complications. In conducting Dorothea's prenatal visit, discuss how you would approach and manage the following areas:

- Assessment of potential occupational hazards to the fetus
- Counseling her about prevention and control of hemorrhoids and heartburn
- Evaluation of her weight gain and edema
- Assessing the family's economic situation
- Determining her educational and informational needs at this stage of pregnancy

10. Sally S. has come to the clinic for her first antepartal visit. She is 20 years old, unmarried, and is 16 weeks pregnant. She is presently unemployed and is receiving welfare assistance; she lives at home with her divorced mother and two siblings. Sally is in good general health, but is 30% overweight and smokes one and one half packs of cigarettes per day. She wants to keep the baby, and relates that her mother will help her care for it. In your antepartal assessment, what areas will receive particular attention, both psychosocial and physical? What types of problems and complications are potentially present in Sally's situation? Based upon the information given, what risks can you identify for Sally, and what risks for the baby? How will you counsel Sally about weight gain during pregnancy? How will you counsel her about cigarette smoking? What types of community agency or specialist referrals might be appropriate for Sally?

11. One of the patients you have been following in the prenatal clinic, Mrs. Scott, has missed several appointments.

She is a 43-year-old multipara with several moderately severe physical problems, including vulvar varicosities and gestational diabetes. Because of her missed appointments, a thorough antepartal assessment has not been done. However, the history does reveal that her last pregnancy, 3 years ago, ended in an unexplained stillbirth. Today Mrs. Scott has kept her appointment. When discussing the missed appointments, she mentions that she has been preoccupied with family troubles and difficulties with the children. She appears distracted and has a hard time keeping focused in the discussion. What specific problems will you consider as potential causes of Mrs. Scott's behavior? How will you further assess these problems? What risks are present for the fetus with each problem? What nursing intervention is appropriate, and what types of referrals might be indicated?

Multiple Choice

Read through the entire question and place your answer on the line to the right.

1. Below are some signs, symptoms, and conditions commonly associated with pregnancy. Those that the patient might notice and describe in the first trimester of pregnancy are
   A. Amenorrhea
   B. Enlargement and tenderness of breasts
   C. Enlargement of uterus
   D. Frequent micturition
   E. Goodell's sign
   Select the number corresponding to the correct letters.
   1. A and C
   2. A, B, and D
   3. B, D, and E
   4. All of the above   ——

2. In pregnancy, morning sickness is most common during which of the following periods?
   A. First month
   B. First 6 weeks
   C. Sixth week to twelfth week
   D. First 4 months
   E. Eighth week to sixteenth week   ——

3. A pregnant woman seen for the first time in the antepartal clinic has a hemoglobin of 10 g. The nurse should understand that this condition is
   A. A true anemia
   B. Caused by increased blood volume
   C. Dangerous to the baby's development
   D. Predisposing to postpartal hemorrhage   ——

4. Active fetal movements are usually first perceived by motion
   A. In the third month of gestation
   B. Toward the end of the fifth month
   C. Between the sixth and seventh months   ——

5. Which of the following placental hormones is detected by immunologic tests for pregnancy?
   A. Estrogens
   B. Progesterone

C. Human placental lactogen (HPL)
D. Human chorionic gonadotropin (hCG)   ——

6. During her first visit to the clinic the mother confides to the nurse that she is afraid to have a baby. The most appropriate response of the nurse might be
   A. "Modern obstetrics makes having a baby so safe that you have absolutely nothing to fear."
   B. "Perhaps if you discussed this with a psychiatrist he would help you to overcome this feeling."
   C. "Many women feel this way, so I wouldn't be concerned about it if I were you."
   D. "I can understand that you might feel this way. What is it in particular that you are worried about?"   ——

7. Pregnancy has been referred to as a critical event in the lives of parents. Which of the following descriptions best describes pregnancy?
   A. Pregnancy is always a crisis.
   B. Pregnancy is a role transition.
   C. Pregnancy is just a normal developmental stage people go through.   ——

8. Current research on pregnancy demonstrates that
   A. Men as well as women experience changes in body image during pregnancy
   B. Men often have the physiological symptoms of pregnancy that their mates experience
   C. Men do not identify with their mates very well during pregnancy
   Select the number corresponding to the correct letter or letters.
   1. All of the above
   2. A and B
   3. A and C
   4. B and C
   5. C only   ——

9. Several psychological tasks have to be accomplished by the mother during pregnancy. Which of the following is *not* a usual task?
   A. Preparation for physical separation from the infant
   B. Belief that she is pregnant and incorporation of the fetus into her body image
   C. Working through the anger that usually accompanies pregnancy
   D. Resolution of the identity confusions that accompany role transition   ——

10. Certain specific psychological tasks of pregnancy seem to occur at specific times during gestation. Which one is not evident during later stages of pregnancy?
    A. Perception of the fetus as a separate object
    B. Readiness to assume the care-taking relationship with the baby
    C. Incorporation and integration of the fetus
    D. Preparation for labor   ——

11. Expectant parents should consider which of the following variables when selecting a childbirth class?
A. Class size
B. Instructor's age
C. Whether or not the instructor has given birth
D. Professional credentials of instructor and type of training as a childbirth educator
E. Amount of class hours for the fee
Select the number corresponding to the correct letters.
1. A, C, D, and E
2. D and E
3. A, D, and E
4. A, B, D, and E
5. All of the above ____

12. The purpose of breathing techniques for labor is to
A. Increase pain perception
B. Provide oxygenation
C. Aid in relaxation
D. Obviate the need for analgesics
Select all that are correct. ____

13. Which exercise can help relieve low backache in pregnancy?
A. Shoulder circling
B. Back massage
C. Calf stretching
D. Pelvic rocking or pelvic tilt ____

14. Both prenatal and postpartum exercises are concerned with which of the following?
A. Improving circulation
B. Strengthening abdominal muscles
C. Improving tone of pelvic floor muscles
D. Strengthening leg muscles
E. Improving posture
F. Developing an awareness of relaxation of pelvic floor muscles
Select all that are correct. ____

15. Relaxation is
A. A learned activity
B. A passive process
C. An active process
D. Requires awareness and concentration
E. A natural reaction
Select the number corresponding to the correct letters.
1. A, B, D, and E
2. A, C, D, and E
3. A, D, and E
4. A, C, and D
5. A, B, and D ____

16. Which of the following statements is true regarding weight gain during pregnancy?
A. Excessive weight gain is a cause of preeclampsia.
B. The obese client should be advised to limit her weight gain to 10 lb or less.
C. Inadequate weight gain during pregnancy is related to an increased incidence of low-birth-weight infants.

D. A weight gain of 20 lb is sufficient for most women during pregnancy. ____

17. Protein needs
A. Are decreased during pregnancy
B. Can be met by a combination of foods from plant and animal sources
C. Require inclusion in the diet of 20 essential amino acids
D. Are more important than the need for other nutrients. ____

18. Which of the following questions would be helpful in the dietary assessment of a pregnant woman?
A. Where are you from?
B. Who purchases the food for your household?
C. Are there any foods you cannot eat?
D. All of the above ____

19. Two physical examination procedures done during antepartal visits that assess the condition of the fetus are
A. Leopold's maneuvers and fetal heart beat
B. Chadwick's sign and fundal height
C. Fetal heart beat and fetal presentation
D. Fundal height and fetal heart beat ____

20. Information provided by Leopold's maneuvers includes
A. Fetal presentation
B. Fetal position
C. Fetal growth status
D. Fetal heart beat
Select the number corresponding to the correct letters.
1. A and B
2. B and C
3. C and D
4. A, B, and C ____

21. Return visits for uncomplicated pregnancies routinely include
A. Fetal heart beat
B. Leopold's maneuvers
C. Measurement of fundal height
D. Pelvic examination
E. Examination for edema
F. Urinalysis for glucose and protein
Select the number corresponding to the correct letters.
1. A, B, C, and D
2. C, D, E, and F
3. A, B, C, E, and F
4. All of the above ____

22. Danger signs that should be reported immediately to the physician during pregnancy include
A. Bleeding from vagina
B. Loss of amniotic fluid
C. Persistent blurred vision or light flashes
D. Severe headache
E. Abdominal pain and cramping
F. Pain and swelling of calf

Select the number corresponding to the correct letters.
1. A, B, C, and F
2. A, B, C, D, and F
3. A, B, C, E, and F
4. All of the above   _____

23. What is considered an acceptable weight gain during pregnancy for a woman at ideal body weight?
A. 20 lb
B. 30 lb
C. 40 lb
D. 50 lb   _____

24. Which statement is true regarding pregnant women who are obese?
A. Weight gain should be limited to 20 lb.
B. Weight gain should be about as much as for nonobese women.
C. Weight loss of about 10 lb should be sought.
D. Weight should be monitored carefully but no limits set.   _____

25. Hemorrhoids may be prevented or minimized during pregnancy by which measures?
A. Adequate dietary roughage to avoid constipation
B. Adequate fluids to prevent dehydration
C. Regular bowel habits to evacuate colon
D. Avoiding long periods of standing or sitting
E. Adequate exercise for muscle tone
Select the number corresponding to the correct letters.
1. A, B, and C
2. A, C, and D
3. A, B, C, and D
4. All of the above   _____

26. Risks to the fetus from maternal smoking include
A. Low birth weight
B. Premature labor and delivery
C. Hypoxia from bleeding problems (placenta previa, abruptio)
D. Congenital defects (cleft palate, heart, anencephaly)
Select the number corresponding to the correct letters.
1. A and B
2. A, B, and C
3. All of the above   _____

27. What advice should be given to pregnant women regarding alcohol consumption?
A. There is no safe level of alcohol consumption during pregnancy.
B. Less than 1 to 2 drinks per week are safe.
C. Less than 3 to 5 drinks per week are safe.
D. Less than 1 drink per day is safe.   _____

28. What is the danger of a boggy uterus?
A. Urinary retention
B. Hemorrhage
C. Severe afterpains
D. Hematomas   _____

29. Early ambulation after delivery promotes maternal health and comfort by
A. Reducing the risk of thrombophlebitis
B. Improving bladder function
C. Improving bowel elimination
D. Reducing abdominal distention
E. Reducing the incidence of postspinal headache
Select the number corresponding to the correct letters.
1. A, B, and C
2. A, B, C, and D
3. B, C, and D
4. All of the above   _____

30. How may leg cramps be prevented during pregnancy?
A. Regular exercise
B. Warm bath at bedtime
C. Not pointing toes when stretching
D. Aluminum hydroxide gel
Select the number corresponding to the correct letters.
1. A and B
2. A, B, and C
3. A and C
4. A, B, C, and D   _____

31. In evaluating edema in later pregnancy, what signs would raise your suspicion of preeclampsia?
A. Weight gain >2 lb in one week
B. Edema over sacrum
C. Edema of face
D. Pretibial edema
Select the number corresponding to the correct letters.
1. A and B
2. A, B, and C
3. A, C, and D
4. A, B, C, and D   _____

32. Vaginal infection during pregnancy characterized by thick, white, curdy discharge, itching, and inflammation of the vulva is due to
A. *Candida albicans*
B. *Trichomonas vaginalis*
C. *Gardinerella*
D. *Chlamydia trachomatis*   _____

33. What general advice is given to pregnant women about use of drugs?
A. All medications are to be minimized during pregnancy.
B. The fetus is particularly susceptible to teratogenic effects during the first trimester.
C. Ingestion of drugs at any time during pregnancy has potential for fetal damage.
D. Many over-the-counter drugs have not been thoroughly investigated for their fetal effects; the safest approach is to avoid them.
E. Medications prescribed by the physician are safe during pregnancy.
Select the number corresponding to the correct letters.
1. A, B, and C
2. B, C, and D

3. A, B, C, and D
4. All of the above   ____

34. Which of the following immunizations are contraindicated during pregnancy?
   A. Rubeola
   B. Mumps
   C. Rubella
   D. Tetanus toxoid
   Select the number corresponding to the correct letters.
   1. A and B
   2. A, B, and C
   3. A and C
   4. A, B, C, and D   ____

35. Natural remedies to prevent or control nausea during pregnancy include
   A. Dry toast, plain popcorn
   B. Frequent, light meals
   C. Separate liquids from dry foods
   D. Spearmint, raspberry, or peppermint tea
   E. High-protein meals and fruit
   Select the number corresponding to the correct letters.
   1. A, B, and C
   2. A, B, C, and D
   3. A, B, C, and E
   4. All of the above   ____

36. Backache during pregnancy may be prevented or relieved by
   A. Pelvic tilt while sitting, standing, and walking
   B. Sitting in tailor or lotus positions
   C. Avoiding fatigue
   D. Using proper body mechanics in lifting and moving
   E. Daily exercise such as walking, swimming, or stretching
   Select the number corresponding to the correct letters.
   1. A, B, and C
   2. B, C, and D
   3. C, D, and E
   4. All of the above   ____

37. Varicose veins during pregnancy may be treated by
   A. The right angle position for 5 minutes several times per day
   B. Wearing elastic support stockings daily
   C. Avoiding constricting clothing
   D. Sclerosing injections into the veins
   E. Anticoagulants to prevent thrombosis
   Select the number corresponding to the correct letters.
   1. A, B, and C
   2. B, C, and D
   3. B, C, and E
   4. All of the above   ____

38. When can the postpartal mother take tub baths?
   A. In 1 week
   B. In 2 weeks
   C. In 3 weeks
   D. In 4 weeks   ____

39. How can the nurse determine that the patient is adequately emptying the bladder?
   A. The amount of voiding is 100 ml or more.
   B. The uterus is not displaced.
   C. The mother fails to report suprapubic discomfort.
   D. Lochia is normal in amount.
   E. The bladder is not palpable.
   Select the number corresponding to the correct letters.
   1. A, B, and C
   2. A, B, C, and D
   3. A, B, D, and E
   4. All of the above   ____

40. Signs and symptoms of thrombophlebitis include
   A. Unilateral calf swelling
   B. Unilateral erythema and tenderness of calf
   C. Pain in calf on flexion of foot (Homan's sign)
   D. Reduced or absent pulses in foot on affected side
   Select the number corresponding to the correct letters.
   1. A and B
   2. A, B, and C
   3. A, B, C, and D   ____

41. Contraceptive counseling for nonlactating postpartal mothers includes
   A. Although unlikely, ovulation can occur before 6 weeks
   B. Short-term contraception using foam or jelly and condom is preferred.
   C. IUD insertion or oral contraceptives should be delayed until 6 weeks.
   D. There is no reason to delay intercourse after lochia has ceased and there is no perineal discomfort.
   E. There are often emotional benefits for couples by resuming intercourse early following birth.
   Select the number corresponding to the correct letters.
   1. A, B, and C
   2. A, B, C, and D
   3. All of the above   ____

Discussion

42. Why is regular exercise so important during pregnancy? What are some exercises the nurse could advise the mother to do?

43. Name three occupational hazards to which women are frequently exposed, and describe the dangers to the fetus or mother from these.

44. Describe preventive measures in breast care during pregnancy that help mothers avoid nipple cracking and infection later while nursing.

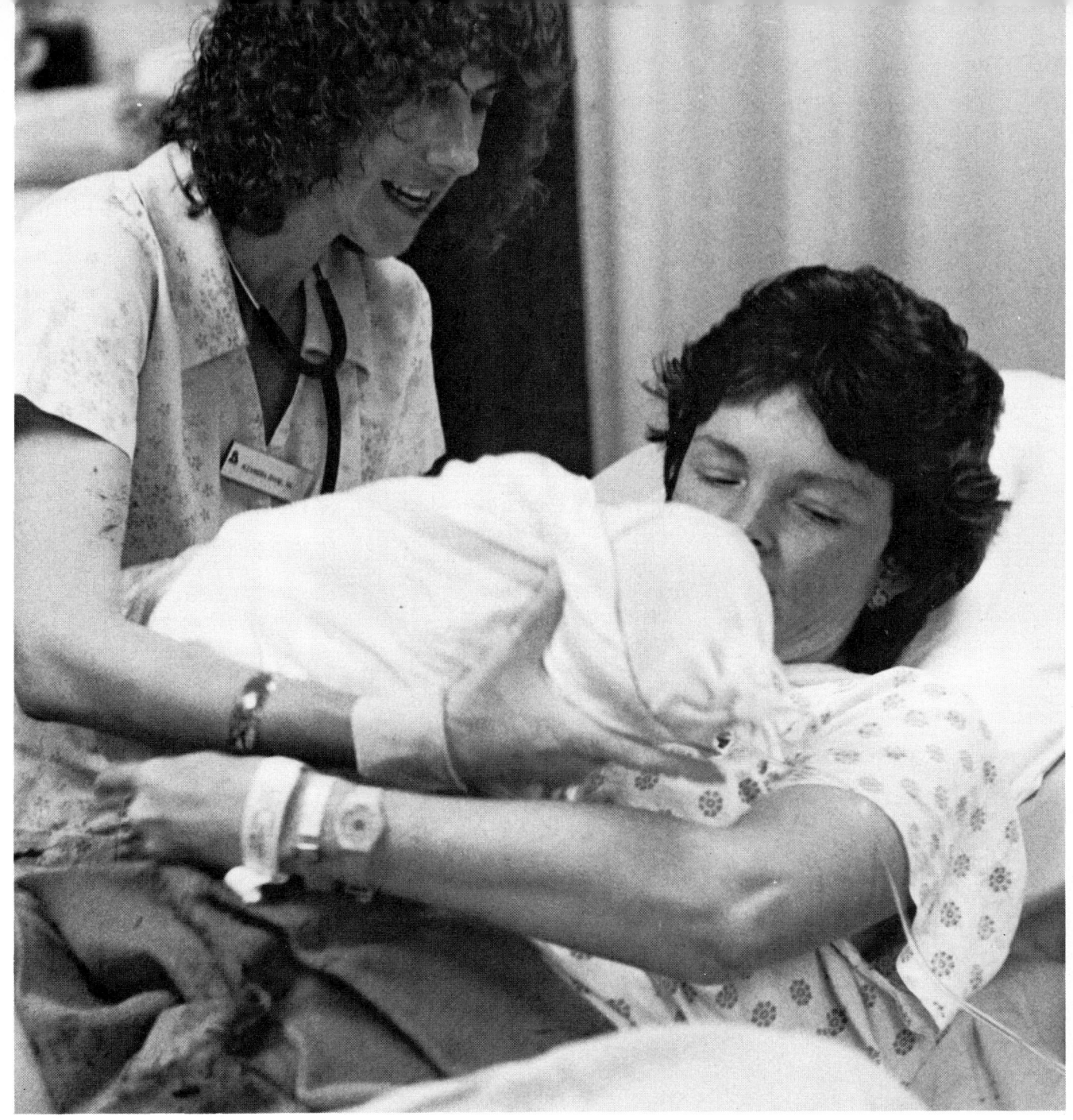

UNIT V

Assessment and Management in the Intrapartum Period

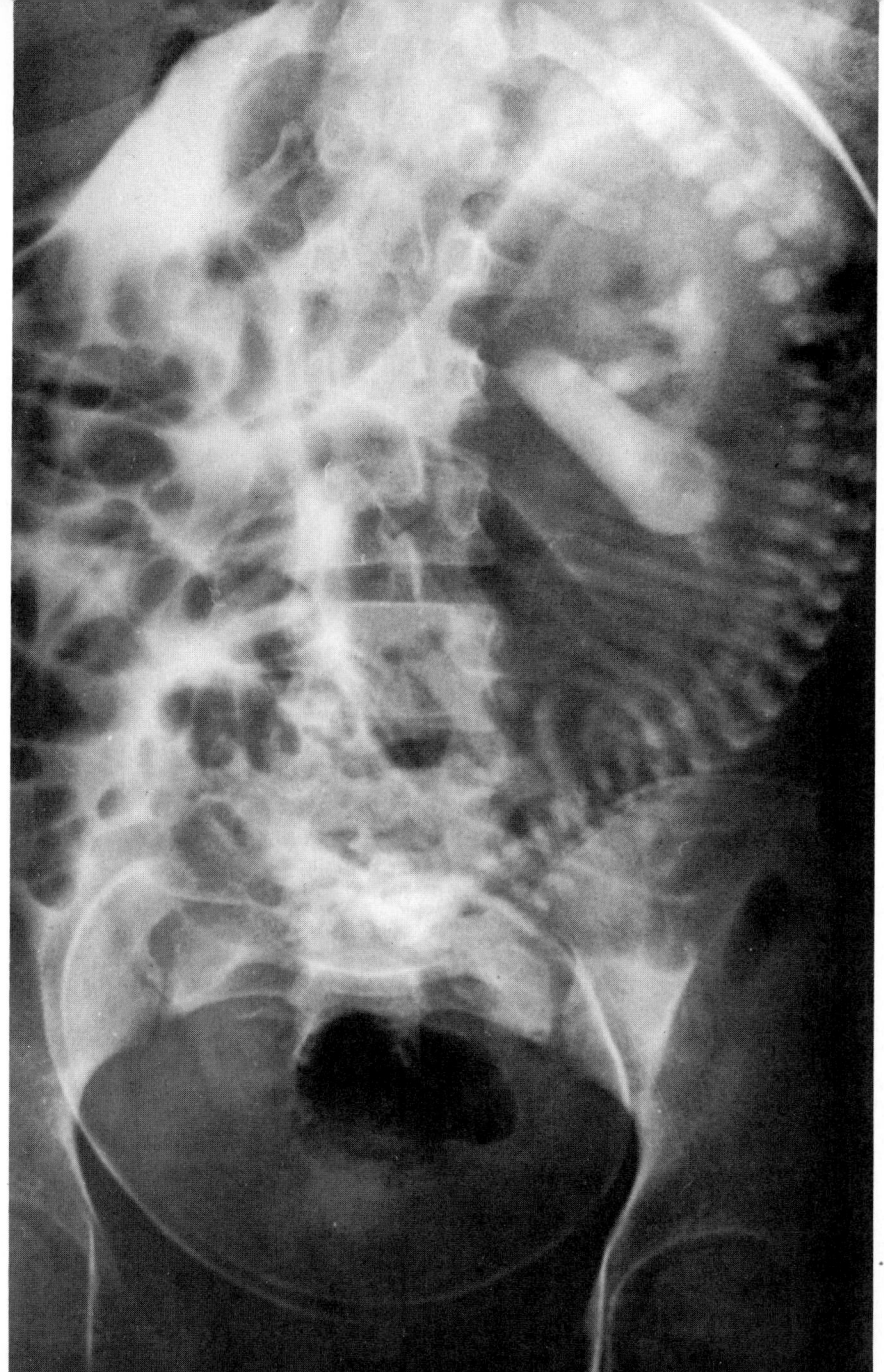

CHAPTER 23

Assessment of the Passageway and Passenger

The process of labor can be thought of as divided into three components, each of which must be normal for progress to be made and birth to occur. These components may be described as the powers (forces) of labor, the passenger, and the passageway. The powers, including uterine contractions with the addition of maternal "bearing down" during the second stage, must be of adequate strength with coordination of muscle activity. These forces propel an irregular object, the infant or *passenger*, through the birth canal or *passageway*. The passenger must be of appropriate size and shape and able to undergo the necessary maneuvers to pass through the different dimensions of the birth canal. The passageway must also be of normal size and configuration, not presenting any undue obstacles to the descent, rotations, and expulsion of the baby. The passageway and passenger are discussed in this chapter, and the powers are discussed in the next chapter concerning the phenomena of labor. When nature tries to propel the fetus through the birth canal and fails to do so, there are problems in the powers, the passenger, or the passageway. These problems are discussed in Chapter 38.

The Passageway

The entire childbirth process centers on the safe passage of the fully developed fetus through the pelvis. Slight irregularities in the structure of the pelvis may delay the progress of labor, and any marked deformity may render delivery through natural passages impossible.

True Pelvis

True and false pelves were discussed briefly in Chapter 9. The difference between the two is illustrated in Figure 23-1. It is the true pelvis that concerns us here.

The true pelvis, or lower part, forms the bony canal through which the fetus must pass during parturition. For descriptive purposes it is divided into three parts: an inlet or brim, a cavity, and an outlet.

Pelvic Inlet

Continuous from the sacral promontory and extending along the ilium on each side in circular fashion is a ridge called the *linea terminalis*, or brim (Fig. 23-1*A*). This bounds an area or plane, the *inlet*, so named because it is the entryway or inlet through which the fetal head must pass to enter the true pelvis.

The pelvic inlet, sometimes called the pelvic brim or superior strait, divides the false pelvis from the true pelvis. It is heart shaped, and the promontory of the sacrum forms a slight projection into it from behind (Fig. 23-1*B*). Generally, it is widest from side to side and narrowest from back to front (*i.e.*, from the sacral promontory to the symphysis). It should be noted that the fetal head enters the inlet of the average pelvis with its longest diameter (anteroposterior) in the transverse diameter of the pelvis (Fig. 23-2*A*). In other words, as shown in Figure 23-2*B*, the greatest diameter of the head accommodates itself to the greatest diameter of the inlet.

Because the inlet is entirely surrounded by bone, it cannot be directly measured with the examining fingers in a living woman. However, the measurements of its anteroposterior diameter can be estimated on the basis

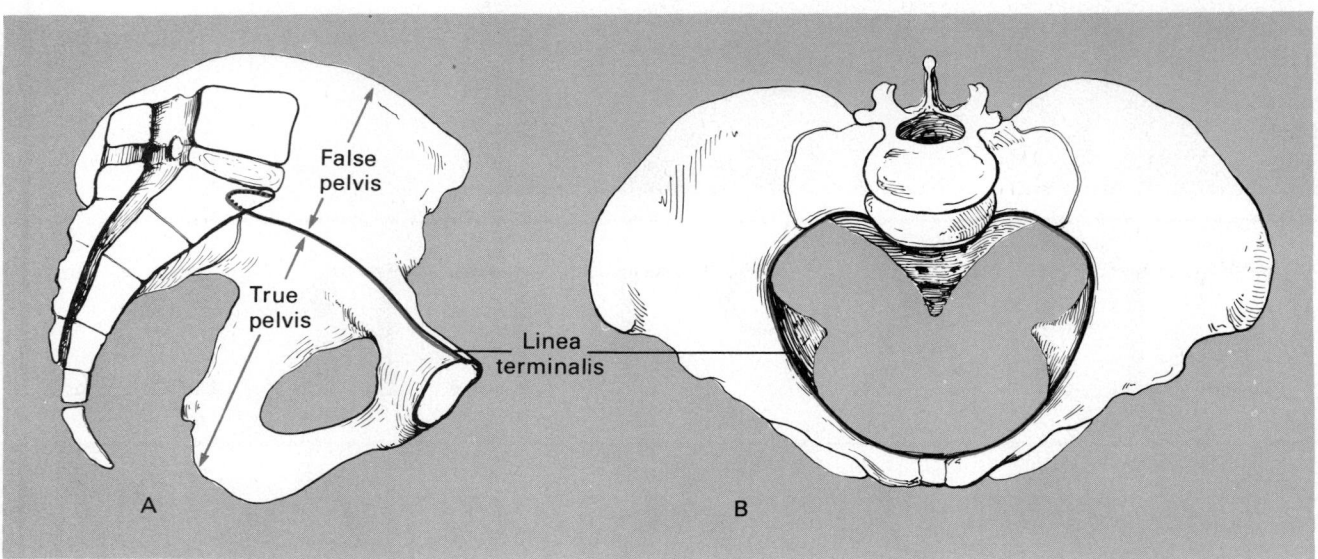

F I G U R E   2 3 - 1

(*A*) Side view of true and false pelvis. (*B*) Front view showing linea terminalis (pelvic brim).

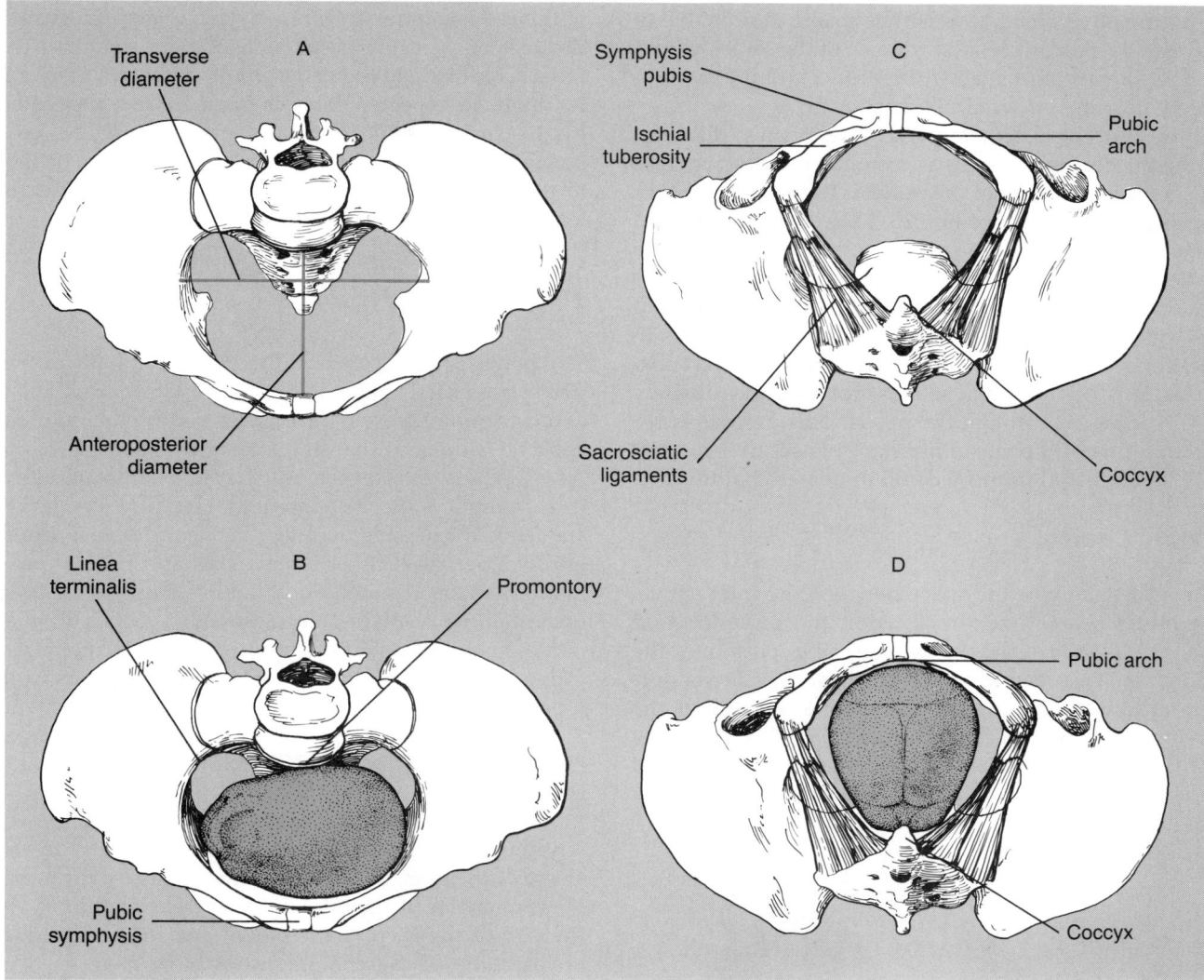

FIGURE 23-2

Views of pelvic inlet and outlet with fetal head in place. (*A*) Inlet of normal female pelvis showing transverse and anteroposterior diameters. (*B*) Largest diameter of the fetal head passing through the largest diameter of the inlet; therefore, it enters transversely. (*C*) Pelvic outlet and sacrosciatic ligaments. (*D*) Largest diameter of the fetal head passing through the largest diameter of the outlet; therefore, it passes through anteroposteriorly.

of the diagonal conjugate diameter (see Fig. 23-6). The measurement of the diameters is very important, because variations from the normal (*e.g.,* smaller in size or flattened) may cause grave difficulty at the time of labor (see Chap. 25).

Pelvic Outlet

When viewed from below, the *pelvic outlet* is a space bounded in front by the symphysis pubis and the pubic arch, at the sides by the ischial tuberosities, and behind by the coccyx and the greater sacrosciatic ligaments (Fig. 23-2C). The front half of the outlet resembles a triangle, the base of which is the distance between the ischial tuberosities, and the other two sides of which are represented by the pubic arch. From an obstetric point of view, this triangle is of great importance because the fetal head must use this space to exit from the pelvis and the mother's body (Fig. 23-2D). Nature has provided a wide pubic arch in females, whereas in males it is narrow (see Fig. 23-5). If the pubic arch in women were as narrow as it is in men, vaginal delivery would be extremely difficult because the fetal head, unable to traverse the narrow anterior triangle of the outlet, would be forced backward against the coccyx and the sacrum, where its progress would be impeded.

In the typical female pelvis, the greatest diameter of the inlet is the transverse (from side to side), whereas the greatest diameter of the outlet is the anteroposterior (from front to back, see Fig. 23-2A and C). As the fetal head emerges from the pelvis, it passes through the outlet in the anteroposterior position, again accommodating its greatest diameter to the greatest diameter of the passage. Since the fetal head enters the pelvis in the transverse position and emerges in the anteroposterior, it is obvious that it must rotate approximately 90° as it passes through the pelvis. This process of rotation is one of the most important phases of labor and will be discussed in more detail in a later chapter.

Pelvic Cavity

The *pelvic cavity* is the space between the inlet above, the outlet below, and the anterior, the posterior, and the lateral walls of the pelvis. The upper portion of the pelvic canal is practically cylindrical, and the lower portion is curved. It is important to note the axis of the cavity when viewed from the side (Fig. 23-3). During delivery, the head must descend along the downward prolongation of the axis until it almost reaches the level

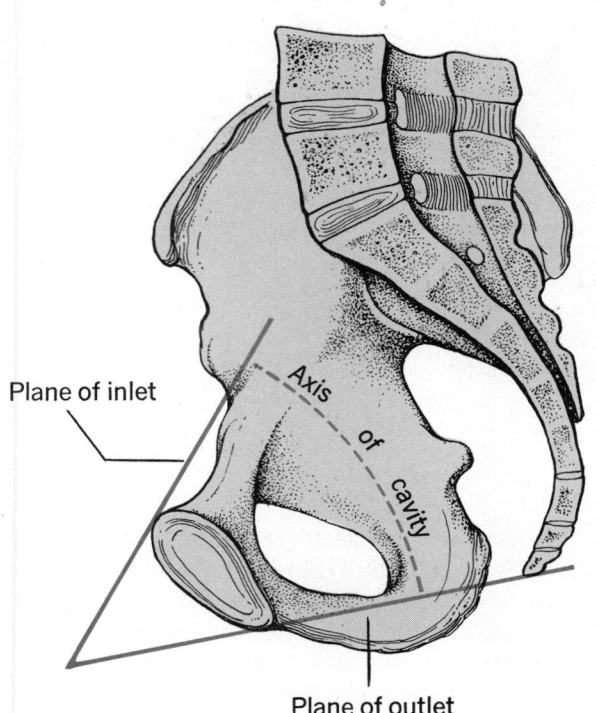

Plane of inlet

Axis of cavity

Plane of outlet

FIGURE 23-3

Pelvic cavity showing plane of inlet and outlet. The direction the fetus takes through the pelvis is determined by the axis of the cavity.

of the ischial spines and then begins to curve forward. The axis of the cavity determines the direction that the fetus takes through the pelvis in the process of delivery. As might be expected, labor is made more complicated by this curvature in the pelvic canal because the fetus has to accommodate itself to the curved path as well as to the variations in the size of the cavity at different levels.

Pelvic Variations

The pelvis presents great individual variations: no two pelves are exactly alike. Even clients with normal measurements may present differences in contour and muscular development that influence the actual size of the pelvis. These differences are due in part to heredity, disease, injury, and development. Heredity may be responsible for passing on many racial and sexual differences. Diseases such as tuberculosis and rickets cause malformations. Accidents and injuries during childhood or at maturity result in deformities of the pelvis or other parts of the body that affect the pelvis. Adequate nutrition and well-formed posture habits and exercise have much influence on the development of the pelvis.

Also, the pelvis does not reach the final stages of maturity until the age of 20 to 25, when ossification is completed.

There are several types of pelves. Even pelves whose measurements are normal differ greatly in the shape of the inlet, in the proximity of the greatest transverse diameter of the inlet to the sacral promontory, in the size of the sacrosciatic notch, and in their general architecture. These characteristics have been used in establishing a classification of pelves that has been of great interest and value to obstetricians. The four main types according to this classification are shown in Figure 23-4. The manner in which the fetus passes through the birth canal and, consequently, the type of labor vary considerably in each pelvic type.

In addition, there are many pelvic types that result from abnormal narrowing of one or the other diameters. These contracted pelves are described in Chapter 38.

In comparing male and female pelves, several differences are observed (Fig. 23-5). The most conspicuous difference is in the pubic arch, which has a much wider angle in women. The symphysis is shorter in women, and the border of the arch probably is more everted. Although the female pelvis is more shallow, it is more capacious, much lighter in structure, and smoother. The male pelvis is deep, compact, conical, and rough in texture, particularly at the site of muscle attachments. Both males and females start life with pelves that are identical in type; the major differences do not appear until puberty and are created by sex hormones. (For the definition and description of the sex hormones see Chap. 9.)

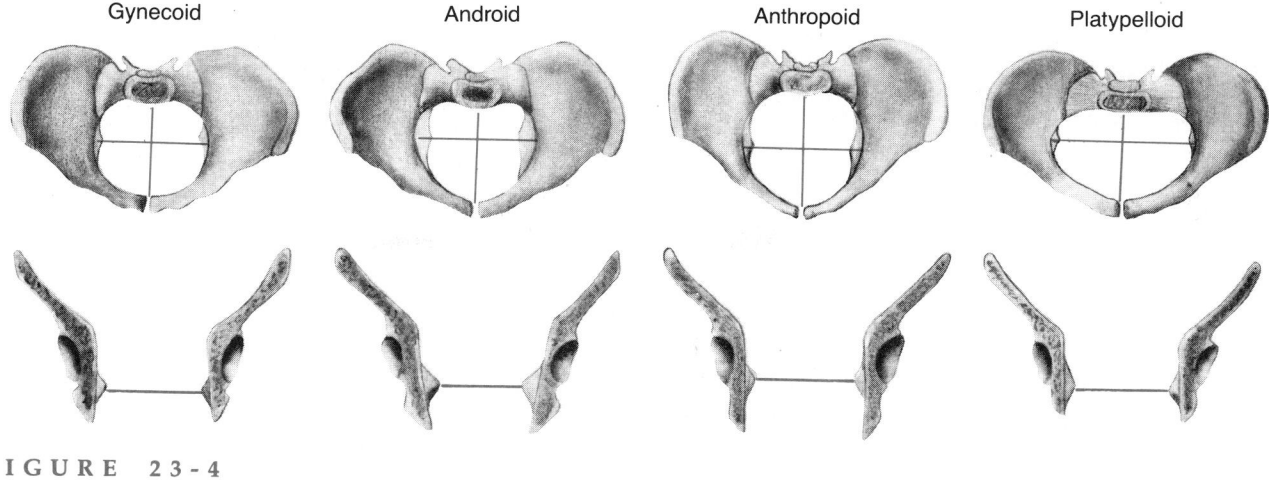

Gynecoid   Android   Anthropoid   Platypelloid

FIGURE 23-4

Caldwell–Maloy classification of pelvic types. (*Top*) The typical shape of the inlet for each type is shown. A line has been drawn through the widest transverse diameter, dividing the inlet into an anterior and posterior segment. The longitudinal line illustrates the anteroposterior diameter of the inlet. (*Bottom*) The typical interspinous diameter of each type is depicted.

Assessment: Pelvic Measurements

The pelvis of every pregnant woman should be measured accurately in the antepartal period to determine whether or not there is anything about the condition of the mother's pelvis that may complicate the delivery. This examination is a part of the antepartal evaluation. It is most useful to know in advance whether there are any abnormalities in the size or configuration of pelvis,

and this information is most readily and appropriately obtained well in advance of the onset of labor.

Types of Pelvic Measurements

Internal pelvic measurements, made manually, are an important means of estimating the size of the pelvis. In the past, a number of external pelvic measurements

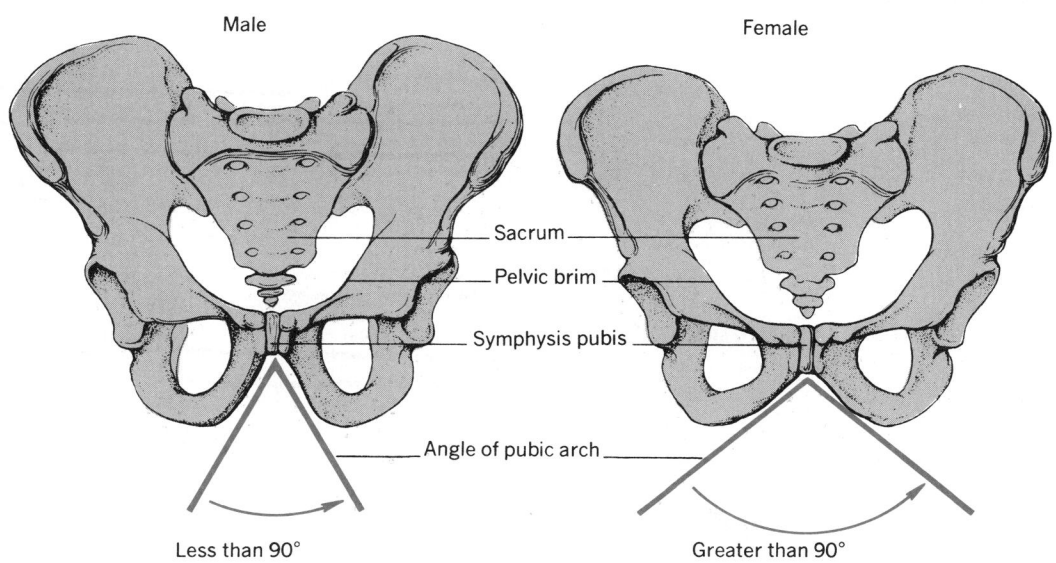

Male   Female

Sacrum
Pelvic brim
Symphysis pubis
Angle of pubic arch

Less than 90°   Greater than 90°

FIGURE 23-5

Comparison of the male and female pelvis. (*Left*) The male pelvis is narrow and compact; the pelvic arch is less than a right angle. (*Right*) The female pelvis is broad and capacious; the pubic arch is greater than a right angle.

were recorded. Except for measurement of the outlet, these are of dubious value in evaluating the true pelvis; thus, they are no longer used. In the majority of abnormal pelves, the most marked deformity affects the anteroposterior diameter of the inlet.

Diagonal Conjugate.

Internal pelvic measurements are made to determine the actual diameters of the inlet. The chief internal measurement taken is the *diagonal conjugate,* or the distance between the sacral promontory and the lower margin of the symphysis pubis. The client should be placed on her back on the examining table, with her knees drawn up and her feet supported by stirrups. Two fingers are inserted into the vagina and, before the diagonal conjugate is measured, the contour of the pelvis is evaluated by palpation. Included in this evaluation are the height of the symphysis pubis, the shape of the pubic arch, the motility of the coccyx, the inclination of the anterior wall of the sacrum and the side walls of the pelvis, and the prominence of the ischial spines.

To obtain the length of the diagonal conjugate, the two fingers passed into the vagina are pressed inward and upward as far as possible until the middle finger rests on the sacral promontory. The point on the back of the hand just under the symphysis is marked by putting the index finger of the other hand on the exact point (Fig. 23-6). Then the fingers are withdrawn and measured. The distance from the tip of the middle finger to the point marked represents the *diagonal conjugate measurement.* This distance may be measured with a rigid measuring scale attached to the wall or with a pelvimeter. If the measurement is greater than 11.5 cm,

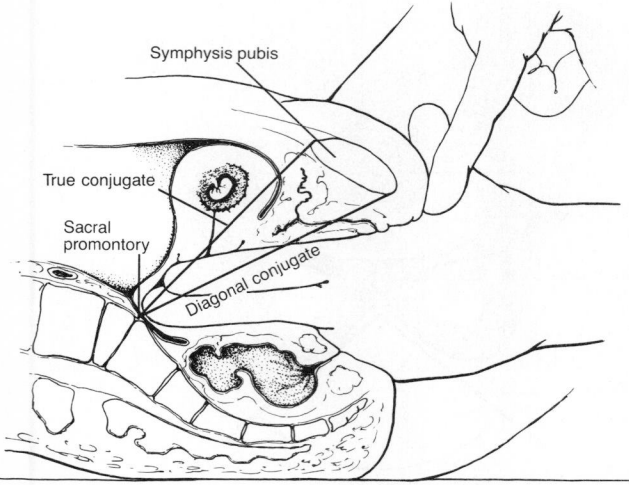

Symphysis pubis

True conjugate

Sacral
promontory

Diagonal conjugate

FIGURE 23-6

Method of obtaining diagonal conjugate diameter.

it is justifiable to assume that the pelvic inlet is of adequate size for childbirth.

True Conjugate.

An extremely important internal diameter is the *true conjugate* or, in Latin, the conjugata vera, which is the distance between the posterior aspect of the symphysis pubis and the promontory of the sacrum. However, direct measurement of this diameter can be made only by means of an x-ray study; consequently, it has to be estimated from the diagonal conjugate measurement. It is believed that if 1.5 cm to 2 cm, according to the height and the inclination of the symphysis pubis, is deducted from the length of the diagonal conjugate, the true conjugate is obtained. For example, if the diagonal conjugate measures 12.5 cm and the symphysis pubis is considered to be "average," the conjugata vera may be estimated as about 11 cm. In this method, the problem consists of estimating the length of one side of a triangle, the conjugata vera; the other two sides, the diagonal conjugate and the height of the symphysis pubis, are known. If the symphysis pubis is high and has a marked inclination, the examiner takes this into consideration and may deduct 2 cm.

The length of the conjugata vera is of utmost importance, because it is about the smallest diameter of the inlet through which the fetal head must pass. Indeed, the main purpose in measuring the diagonal conjugate is to give an estimate of the size of the conjugata vera.

Obstetric Conjugate.

Students sometimes are confused when they are confronted with the term *obstetric conjugate.* This term identifies a diameter that begins at the sacral promontory and terminates on the inner surface of the symphysis pubis, a few millimeters below its upper margin. The obstetric conjugate is in reality the shortest diameter through which the fetal head must pass as it descends into the true pelvis. A distinction is rarely made between the conjugata vera and the obstetric conjugate, except in x-ray pelvimetry.

Biischial Diameter.

Next to the diagonal conjugate, the most important clinical dimension of the pelvis is the transverse diameter of the outlet, the diameter between the ischial tuberosities. This is sometimes called the biischial diameter or intertuberous diameter. This measurement is taken while the client is in the lithotomy position, well down on the table and with the legs widely separated. The measurement is taken from the innermost and lowermost aspect of the ischial tuberosities, on a level with the lower border of the anus. The instruments usually used are the Williams's pelvimeter (Fig. 23-7) or the Thoms's pelvimeter. The intertuberous diameter may also be estimated by inserting the closed fist between the tuberosities. The known di-

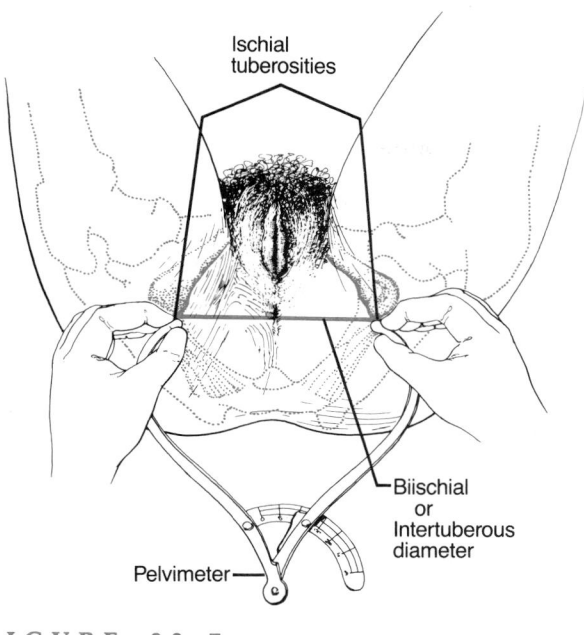

FIGURE 23-7

Method of measuring biischial or intertuberous diameter of the outlet.

ameter of the hand can then be used as a reference. A diameter of more than 8.0 cm is considered adequate.

X-Ray Pelvimetry

X-ray pelvimetry is the most accurate means of determining pelvic size. The method subjects the maternal ovaries and fetal gonads to a certain amount of radiation. Although the amount involved is minimal, exposure of pregnant women to radiation should be avoided unless the procedure is absolutely necessary. X-ray pelvimetry is no longer used prior to labor, except in cases in which there are sound reasons for suspecting pelvic contraction, such as small manual measurements or a history of previous injury or disease that could have affected the bony pelvis.

Pelvimetry may be indicated to evaluate pelvic size in breech presentations when vaginal delivery is anticipated. The head is the largest part of the fetus, and the adequacy of the pelvis is not really tested until the body has already been delivered. It may also provide helpful information when there is a face or other abnormal presentations.

A variety of pelvimetry techniques have been developed. These provide views of the inlet and the interischial spinous diameter of the midpelvis (Fig. 23-8), as well as the anteroposterior dimensions of the pelvis including the obstetric conjugate (Fig. 23-9). When x-ray films are made late in pregnancy or in labor, it is

also possible to gain an impression of the size of the fetal head. When this is considered in relation to pelvic structure, helpful information may be obtained in forecasting whether or not the pelvis is large enough to allow the fetus to pass through.

The Passenger

Even in an adequately sized pelvic outlet, there may be difficulties in delivery if the passenger, the fetus, is too large or in a difficult position. There are various means of assessing the fetal head, fetal lie, fetal attitude, fetal presentation, and fetal position.

Fetal Head

From an obstetric viewpoint the head is the most important part of the fetus. If it can pass through the pelvic canal safely, there is usually no difficulty in delivering the rest of the body, although occasionally the shoulders may cause trouble.

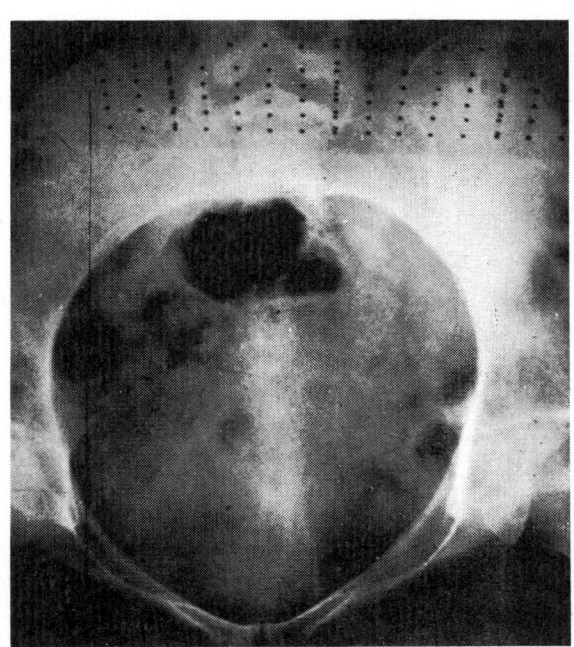

FIGURE 23-8

Pelvic inlet roentgenogram. The scale represents corrected centimeters for various levels of the pelvic canal. The top line is used for measuring the diameters of the inlet. The other levels are established on the lateral roentgenogram. Pelvic morphology is readily established by viewing both lateral and inlet views. This is known as Thoms's technique.

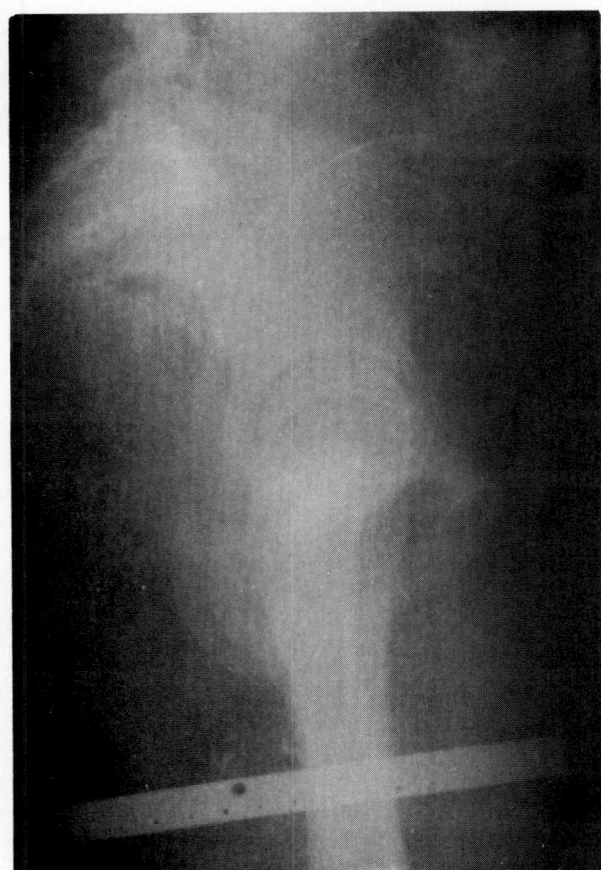

FIGURE 23-9

Lateral roentgenogram. The scale represents corrected centimeters in the midplane of the body. The various diameters may be measured with calipers. The lateral morphologic aspects are readily visualized.

The cranium, or skull, is made up of eight bones. Four of the bones—the sphenoid, the ethmoid, and the two temporal bones—lie at the base of the cranium, are closely united, and are of little obstetric interest. On the other hand, the four bones forming the upper part of the cranium—the frontal, the occipital, and the two parietal bones—are of great importance. These bones are not knit closely together at the time of birth but are separated by membranous interspaces called *sutures.* The intersections of these sutures are known as *fontanels* (Fig. 23-10).

By means of this formation of the fetal skull, the bones can overlap each other somewhat during labor and so diminish materially the size of the head during its passage through the pelvis. This process of overlapping is called "molding," and after a long labor with a large baby and a snug pelvis, the head often is so definitely molded that several days may elapse before it returns to its normal shape.

The most important sutures are the sagittal, between the two parietal bones; the frontal, between the two frontal bones; the coronal, between the frontal and parietal bones; and the lambdoid, between the posterior margins of the parietal bones and the upper margin of the occipital bone. The temporal sutures, which separate the parietal and the temporal bones on either side, are unimportant in obstetrics because they are covered by fat parts and cannot be felt on the living baby.

The important fontanels are the anterior and the posterior. The anterior fontanel is large and diamond shaped and is located at the intersection of the sagittal and the coronal sutures, while the small triangular posterior fontanel lies at the junction of the sagittal and the lambdoid suture. The sutures and the posterior fontanel ossify shortly after birth, but the anterior fontanel re-

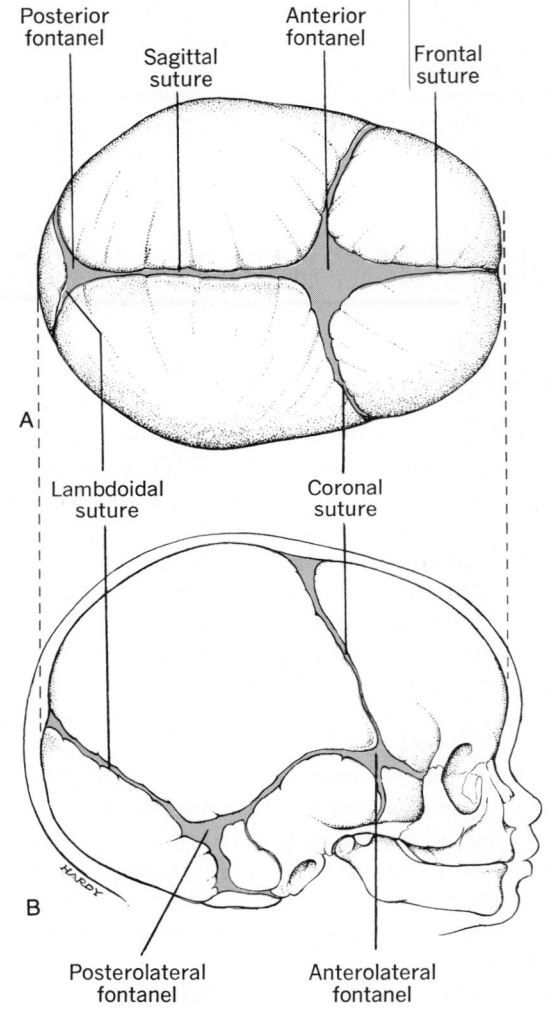

FIGURE 23-10

Fetal skull showing fontanels and sutures. (*A*) Superior aspect. (*B*) Lateral aspect.

mains open until the child is over a year old, constituting the familiar ''soft spot'' just above the forehead of an infant.

By feeling or identifying one or another of the sutures or fontanels and considering its relative position in the pelvis, one is able to accurately determine the position of the head in relation to the pelvis.

Fetal Skull Measurement

The principal measurements of the fetal skull are shown in Figure 23-11. The most important transverse diameter is the biparietal; it is the distance between the biparietal protuberances and represents the greatest width of the head. It measures, on an average, 9.25 cm.

There are three important anteroposterior diameters: the suboccipitobregmatic, which extends from the undersurface of the occiput to the center of the anterior fontanel and measures about 9.5 cm; the occipitofrontal,

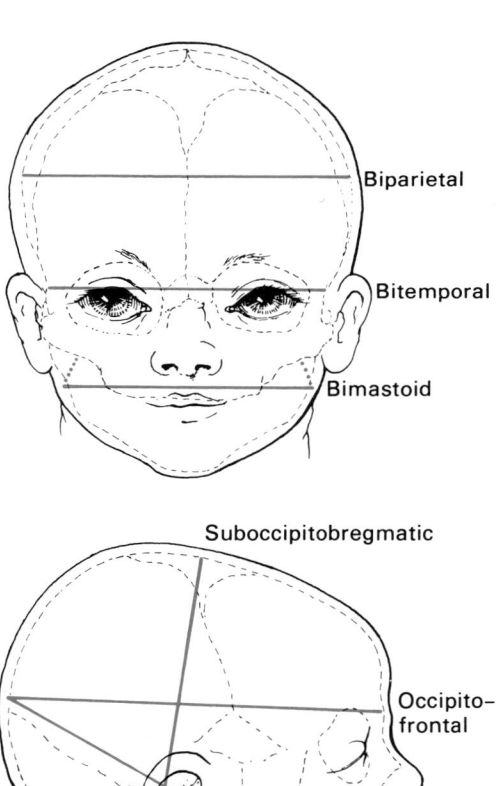

FIGURE 23-11

Fetal skull showing various diameters.

which extends from the root of the nose to the occipital prominence and measures about 12 cm; and the occipitomental, which extends from the chin to the posterior fontanel and averages about 13.5 cm.

In considering these three anteroposterior diameters of the fetal skull, it is important to note that with the head in complete flexion and the chin resting on the thorax, the smallest of these, the suboccipitobregmatic, enters the pelvis, whereas if the head is extended or bent back (which no flexion whatsoever), the greatest anteroposterior diameter presents itself to the pelvic inlet. Herein lies the great importance of flexion; the more the head is flexed, the smaller is the anteroposterior diameter that enters the pelvis. This basic principle is shown in diagrammatic form in Figure 23-12.

Fetal Lie

The lie of the fetus refers to the relation of the long axis of the fetus to that of the mother. When the long axis of the fetus is approximately perpendicular to that of the mother, the condition is referred to as a transverse lie. When it forms an acute angle in relation to the axis of the mother, it becomes an oblique lie. An oblique lie is usually converted during the course of early labor to either a longitudinal or a transverse lie. The common causes of the transverse lie are abnormal relaxation of the abdominal wall due to grand multiparity, pelvic contraction, and placenta previa.

Fetal Attitude

The attitude of the fetus means the relation of the fetal parts to one another. The most striking characteristic of the fetal habitus is flexion. The spinal column is bowed forward, the head is flexed with the chin against the sternum, and the arms are flexed and folded against the chest. The lower extremities also are flexed; the thighs are on the abdomen, and the calves are against the posterior aspect of the thighs. In this state of flexion the fetus assumes a roughly ovoid shape, occupies the smallest possible space, and conforms to the shape of the uterus. In this attitude it is about half as long as if it were completely stretched out. However, there are times when the fetus assumes a different position.

Fetal Presentation

The term *presentation* or *presenting part* is used to designate that portion of the infant's body that lies nearest the internal os, or, in other words, that portion that is felt by the examining fingers when they are introduced

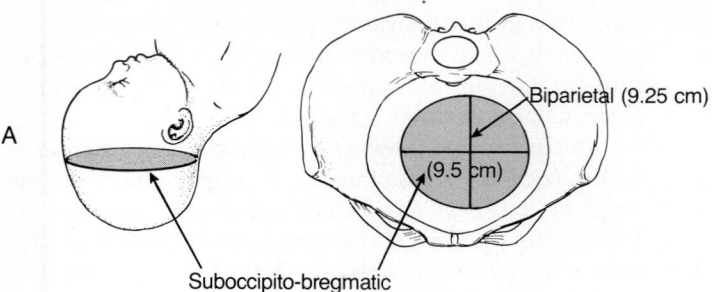

A

Biparietal (9.25 cm)

(9.5 cm)

Suboccipito-bregmatic

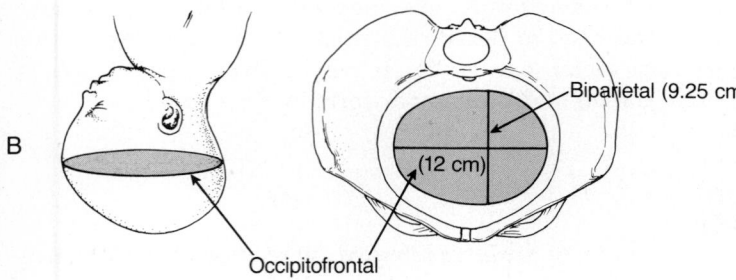

B

Biparietal (9.25 cm)

(12 cm)

Occipitofrontal

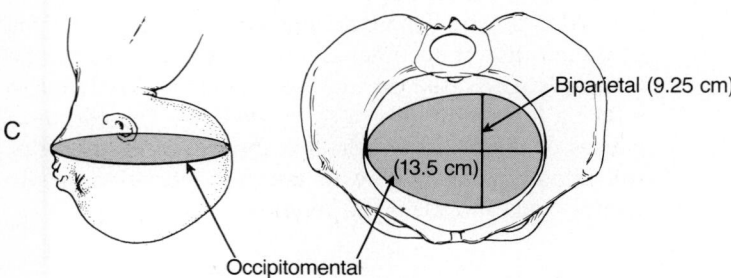

C

Biparietal (9.25 cm)

(13.5 cm)

Occipitomental

FIGURE 23-12

(*A*) Complete flexion allows the smallest diameter of the head to enter the pelvis. (*B*) Moderate extension causes the larger diameter to enter the pelvis. (*C*) Marked extension forces the largest diameter against the pelvic brim, but the head is too large to enter the pelvis.

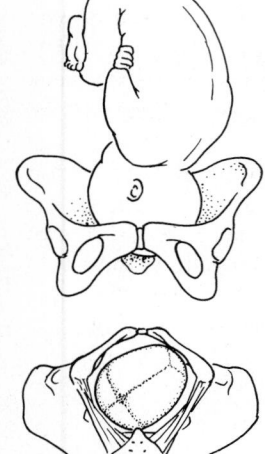
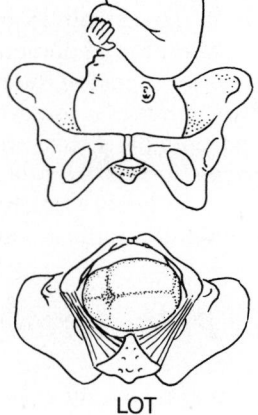
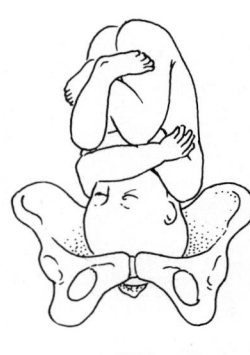
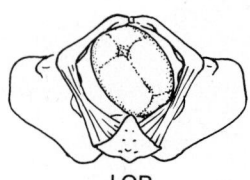

LOA

LOT

LOP

Vertex Presentations

FIGURE 23-13

Fetal presentations. (Redrawn from Benson, RC: Handbook of Obstetrics and Gynecology, 7th ed. Los Altos, CA, Lange Medical Publications, 1980) into the cervix. When the presenting part is known, by abdominal palpation, it is possible to determine the relation between the long axis of the baby's body and that of the mother (Fig. 23-13).

Head or *cephalic presentations* are the most common; they are seen in about 97% of all cases at term. Cephalic presentations are divided into groups, according to the relation of the infant's head to its body. The most common is the *vertex presentation,* in which the head is sharply flexed so that the chin is in contact with the

thorax; thus, the vertex is the presenting part. The *face presentation*, in which the neck is sharply extended so that the occiput and the back come in contact, is more rarely observed.

Breech presentation is the next most common; it is present in about 3% of cases. In breech presentations the thighs may be flexed and the legs extended over the anterior surface of the body (*frank breech presentation*), or the thighs may be flexed on the abdomen and the legs on the thighs (*full breech presentation*), or one or

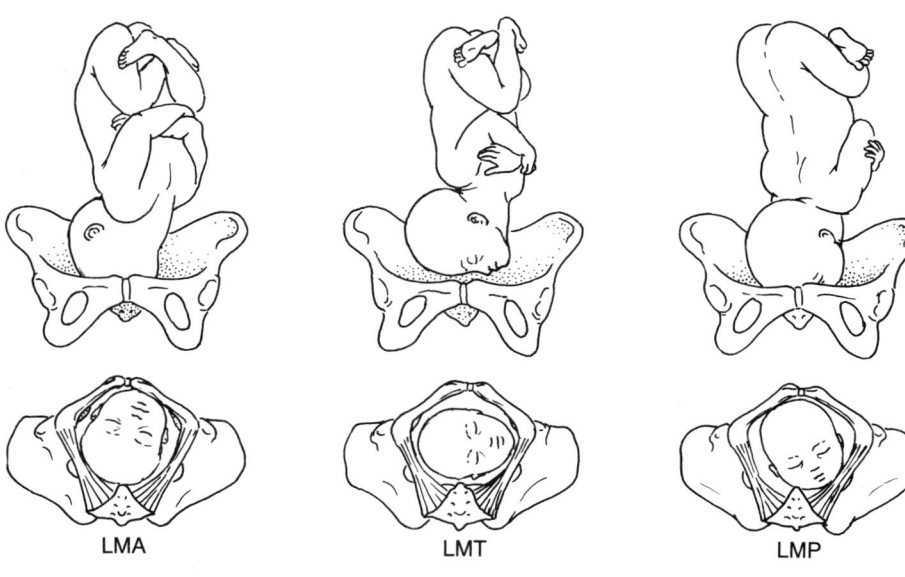

LMA   LMT   LMP

Face Presentations

F I G U R E   2 3 - 1 3 (*continued*)

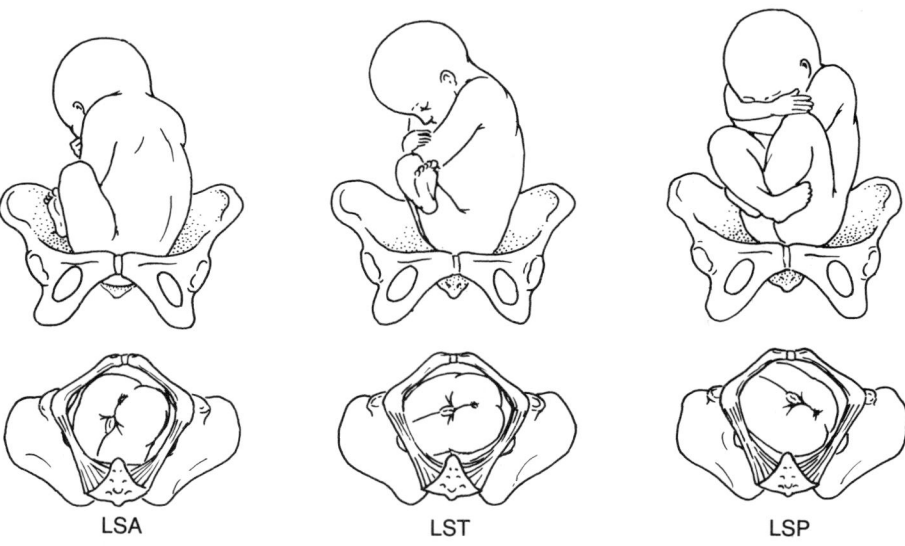

LSA   LST   LSP

Breech Presentations

-

both feet may be the lowest part (*foot* or *footling presentation*).

When the fetus lies crosswise in the uterus, it is in a transverse lie and the shoulder is the presenting part—*shoulder presentation.* Shoulder presentations are relatively uncommon, and, with very rare exceptions, the spontaneous birth of a fully developed child is impossible in a "persistent transverse lie."

Fetal Position

In addition to knowing the presenting part of the baby, it is important to know the exact position of the presenting part in relation to the pelvis. This relationship is determined by finding the position of certain points on the presenting surface and relating these to the four

---

Abbreviations for Fetal Presentations

Positions—Vertex Presentation

L.O.A.—Left occipitoanterior
L.O.T.—Left occipitotransverse
L.O.P.—Left occipitoposterior
R.O.A.—Right occipitoanterior
R.O.T.—Right occipitotransverse
R.O.P.—Right occipitoposterior

Positions—Breech Presentation

L.S.A.—Left sacroanterior
L.S.T.—Left sacrotransverse
L.S.P.—Left sacroposterior
R.S.A.—Right sacroanterior
R.S.T.—Right sacrotransverse
R.S.P.—Right sacroposterior

Positions—Face Presentation

L.M.A.—Left mentoanterior
L.M.T.—Left mentotransverse
L.M.P.—Left mentoposterior
R.M.A.—Right mentoanterior
R.M.T.—Right mentotransverse
R.M.P.—Right mentoposterior

Positions—Shoulder Presentation

L.A.D.A.—Left acromiodorso-anterior
L.A.D.P.—Left acromiodorso-posterior
R.A.D.A.—Right acromiodorso-anterior
R.A.D.P.—Right acromiodorso-posterior

---

imaginary divisions or regions of the pelvis. For this purpose the pelvis is considered to be divided into quadrants: left anterior, left posterior, right anterior, and right posterior. These divisions aid in indicating whether the presenting part is directed toward the right side or the left side and toward the front or the back of the pelvis.

Certain points on the presenting surface of the baby have been arbitrarily chosen as points of direction in determining the exact relation to the presenting part of the quadrants of the pelvis. In vertex presentations, the occiput is the guiding point; in face presentations, the chin (mentum); in breech presentations, the sacrum; and in shoulder presentations, the scapula (acromion process).

Position, then, has to do with the relation of some arbitrarily chosen portion of the fetus to the right or the left side of the mother's pelvis. Thus, in a vertex presentation, the back of the head (occiput) may point to the front or to the back of the pelvis. The occiput rarely points directly forward or backward in the median line until the second stage of labor, but usually it is directed to one side or the other.

The various positions are usually expressed by abbreviations made up of the first letter of each word that describes the position (see Abbreviations for Fetal Presentations). Thus, left occipitoanterior is abbreviated L.O.A. This means that the head is presenting with the occiput directed toward the left side of the mother and toward the front part of the pelvis. If the occiput is directed straight to the left with no deviation toward front or back of the pelvis, it is termed left occipitotransverse, or L.O.T. The occiput might also be directed toward the back or posterior quadrant of the pelvis, in which case the position is left occipitoposterior, or L.O.P. There are also three corresponding positions on the right side: R.O.A., R.O.T., and R.O.P.

The occipital anterior positions are considered the most favorable for both mother and baby, and of these, the L.O.A. position is most common.

The same system of terminology is used for face, breech, and shoulder presentations, as indicated in Abbreviations for Fetal Presentations.

Although it is customary to speak of all "transverse lies" of the fetus simply as shoulder presentations, the examples of terminology sometimes used to express position in the shoulder presentation are listed. Left acromiodorso-anterior (L.A.D.A.) means that the acromion is to the mother's left and the back is anterior.

Assessment

Assessment of fetal position is made in five ways: abdominal palpation, vaginal examination, combined auscultation and examination, ultrasound, and, in certain doubtful cases, the roentgenogram. The first three are discussed here. Ultrasound and roentgenogram are discussed in Chapter 42.

Palpation. It is extremely helpful to palpate the abdomen before listening to the fetal heart tones. The region of the abdomen in which the fetal heart is heard varies according to the presentation and the extent to which the presenting part has descended. The location of the fetal heart sounds by itself does not give very important information as to the presentation and the position of the child, but it sometimes reinforces the results obtained by palpation. To obtain satisfactory information by adominal palpation for the determination of fetal position, the examination should be made systematically by following the four *Leopold maneuvers* (Fig. 23-14).

The client should empty her bladder before the procedure begins. This not only contributes to her comfort but also aids in gaining more accurate results in the latter part of the examination. The first three maneuvers are conducted at the side of the bed, facing the client; during the last maneuver the examiner stands to the side, facing the client's feet.

Although a diagnosis should not be made on the basis of inspection, actual observation of the client's abdomen should precede palpation. For the examination

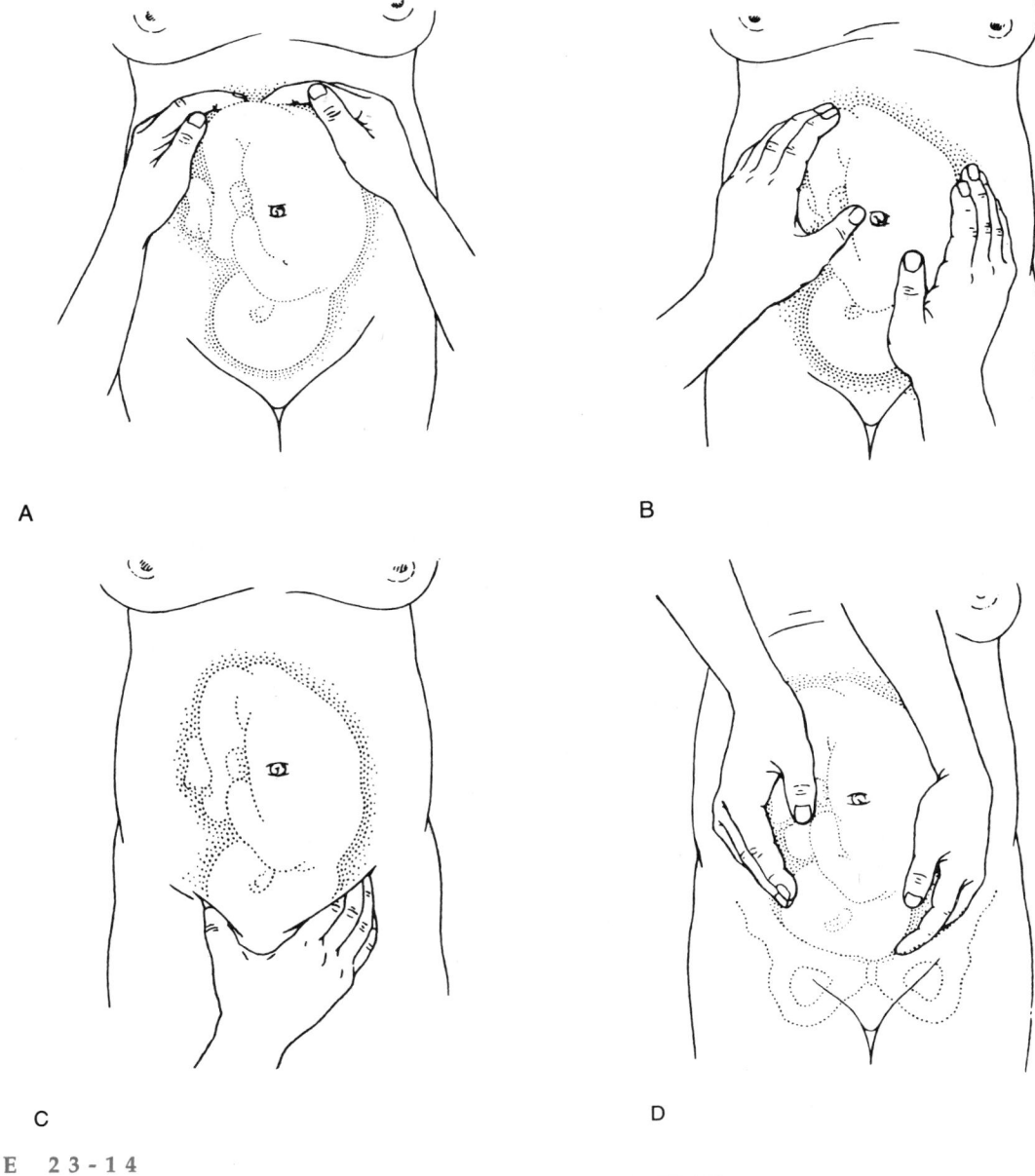

FIGURE 23-14

Leopold maneuvers, or palpation of fetal position. (*A*) First maneuver. (*B*) Second maneuver. (*C*) Third maneuver. (*D*) Fourth maneuver.

the client should lie flat on her back, with her knees flexed to relax the abdominal muscles. The examiner should lay both hands gently and, at first, flat upon the abdomen. If done in any other manner than this, or if the hands are not warm, the stimulation of the fingers will cause the abdominal muscles to contract. One should become accustomed to palpating the uterus in a definite, methodical way.

First Maneuver.   The examiner should ascertain what is lying at the fundus of the uterus by feeling the upper abdomen with both hands (Fig. 23-14*A*). Generally, one will find that there is a mass, which is either the head or the buttocks (breech) of the fetus. The pole of the fetus can be ascertained by observing the following three points:

1. Its relative consistency. The head is harder than the breech.
2. Its shape. The head is round and hard, and the transverse groove of the neck may be felt; the breech has no groove and usually feels more angular.
3. Mobility. The head moves independently of the trunk, but the breech moves only with the trunk; the ability of the head to be moved back and forth against the examining fingers is spoken of as ballottement.

Second Maneuver.   Having determined whether the head or the breech is in the fundus, the next step is to locate the back of the fetus in relation to the right and left sides of the mother. Still facing the client, the examiner places the palmar surfaces of both hands on either side of the abdomen and applies gentle but deep pressure (Fig. 23-14*B*). If the hand on one side of the abdomen remains still to steady the uterus, a slightly circular motion with the flat surface of the fingers on the other hand can gradually palpate the opposite side from the top to the lower segment of the uterus to feel the fetal outline. Then, to palpate the other side, the functions of the hands are reversed (*i.e.*, the hand that was used to palpate now remains steady and the other hand palpates the opposite side of the uterus).

A smooth, hard, resistant plane, the back, is felt on one side, while on the other, numerous angular nodulations are palpated, the knees and the elbows of the fetus.

Third Maneuver.   The third maneuver is an effort to find the head at the pelvic inlet and to determine its mobility. It should be conducted by gently grasping the lower portion of the abdomen, just above the symphysis pubis, between the thumb and the fingers of one hand and then pressing together (Fig. 23-14*C*). If the presenting part is not engaged, a movable body is felt, which is usually the head.

Fourth Maneuver.   The fourth maneuver is conducted while facing the client's feet. The tips of the first three fingers are placed on both sides of the midline about 2 inches above Poupart's ligament. Pressure is now made downward and in the direction of the birth canal, the movable skin of the abdomen being carried downward along with the fingers (Fig. 23-14*D*). The fingers of one hand meet no obstruction and can be carried downward well under Poupart's ligament; these fingers glide over the nape of the baby's neck. The other hand, however, usually meets an obstruction an inch or so above Poupart's ligament; this is the brow of the baby and is usually spoken of as the "cephalic prominence." This maneuver gives several kinds of information, such as the following:

1. If the findings are as described above, it means that the baby's head is well flexed.
2. Confirmatory information is obtained about the location of the back, as naturally the back is on the opposite side from the brow of the baby, except in the uncommon cases of face presentation, in which the cephalic prominence and the back are on the same side.
3. If the cephalic prominence is very easily palpated, as if it were just under the skin, a posterior position of the occiput is suggested.
4. The location of the cephalic prominence tells how far the head has descended into the pelvis. This maneuver is of most value if the head has engaged, but may yield no information with a floating, poorly flexed head.

Vaginal Examination.   During a vaginal examination, the fontanels and the suture lines of the fetal skull are identified. Prior to the onset of labor, the vaginal examination gives limited information concerning the position of the fetus because the cervix is closed and the landmarks on the fetal head are not palpable. However, during labor, after dilatation of the cervix, important information about the position of the fetus and the degree of flexion of its head can be obtained, by pal-

---

The Four Maneuvers of Leopold

1. Palpate the upper abdomen to determine contents of fundus.
2. Locate the fetal back in relation to the right and left sides.
3. Locate the presenting part at the inlet and check for engagement by evaluating mobility.
4. Palpate just above the inguinal ligament on either side to determine the relationship of the presenting part to the pelvis.

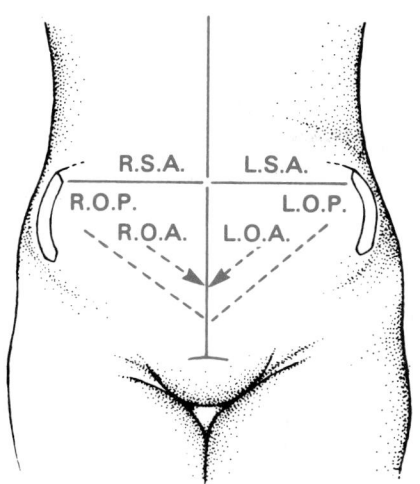

R.S.A. | L.S.A.
R.O.P. | L.O.P.
R.O.A. | L.O.A.

FIGURE 23-15

Fetal heart tone locations on the abdominal wall indicate possible corresponding fetal positions and the effects of the internal rotation of the fetus.

presentation the fetal heart sounds usually are heard loudest at the level of the umbilicus or above.

Suggested Reading

Pritchard JA, MacDonald PC, Gant NF: Williams' Obstetrics, 17th ed. New York, Appleton-Century-Crofts, 1985

pating and identifying the fontanels through the dilated os. When the head is well flexed, the posterior fontanel is easily identified by palpating the junction point of the sagittal suture and the two lambdoid sutures. When the fetal head is well flexed, the anterior fontanel is located well within the birth canal. It is diamond shaped and has four sutures that lead to it: the sagittal posteriorly, two coronal laterally, and the frontal. One can easily develop skill at identifying these landmarks on the fetal skull by palpating the skull of the newborn after delivery, first with eyes closed and then confirming their location visually. The steps in a vaginal examination and an illustration are given in Chapter 25.

Auscultation.   The location of the fetal heart sounds, as heard through the stethoscope, yields helpful information about fetal position, but it is not wholly dependable. Certainly, it never should be relied on as the sole means of diagnosing fetal position. Ordinarily, the heart sounds are transmitted through the convex portion of the fetus, which lies in intimate contact with the uterine wall, so that they are heard best through the infant's back in vertex and breech presentations and through the thorax in face presentation.

In cephalic presentations the fetal heart sounds are heard loudest midway between the umbilicus and the anterior superior spine of the ilium (Fig. 23-15). In general, in L.O.A. and L.O.P. positions the fetal heart sounds are heard loudest in the left lower quadrant. A similar situation applies to the R.O.A. and R.O.P. positions. In posterior positions of the occiput (L.O.P. and R.O.P.) often the sounds are heard loudest well down in the flank toward the anterior superior spine. In breech

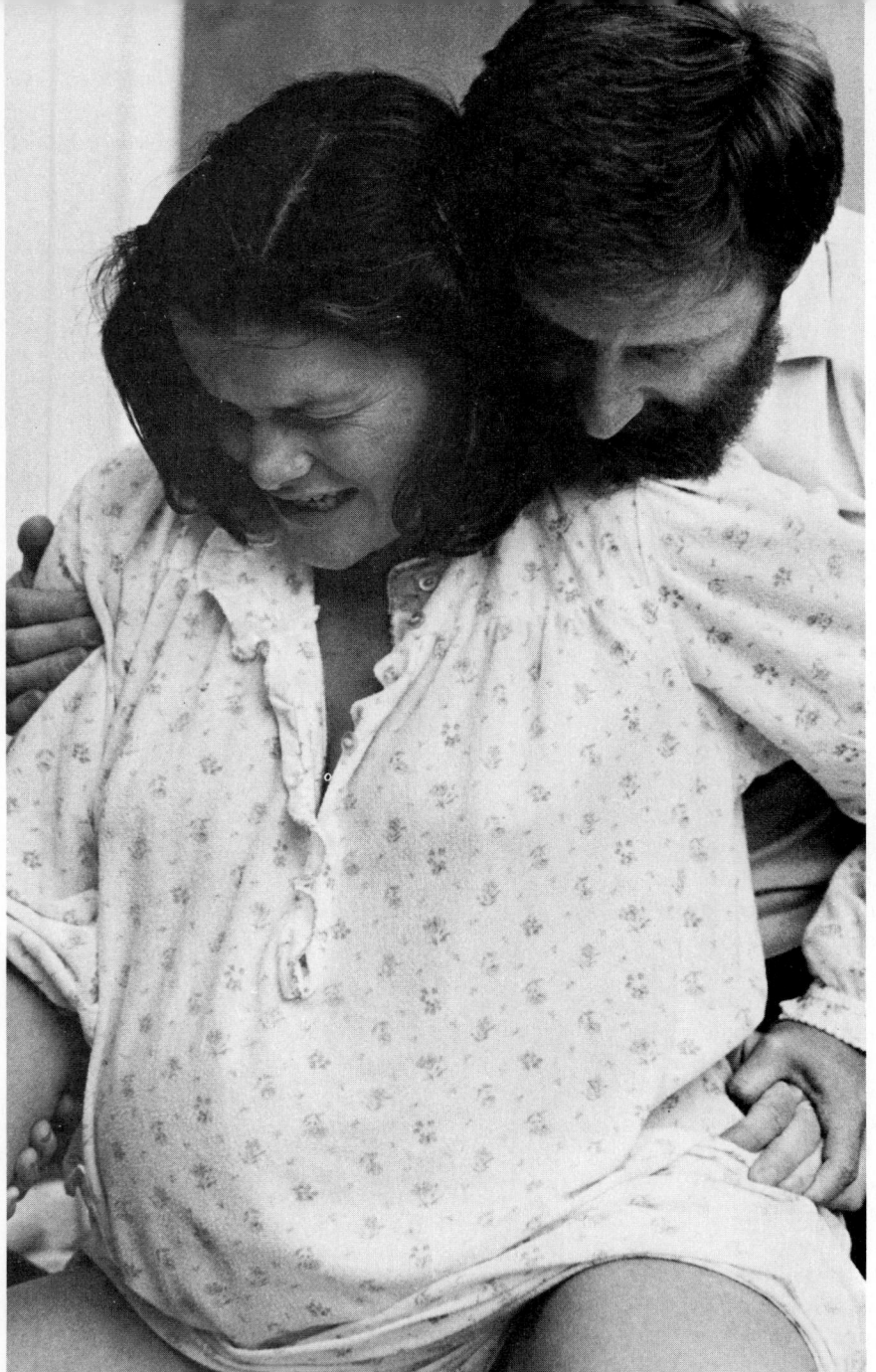

CHAPTER 24

Phenomena of Labor

Labor refers to the series of processes by which the products of conception are expelled by the mother. It implies physical exertion applied to attaining a specific goal. Other terms for these processes are childbirth, parturition, accouchement, and confinement. The actual birth of the baby is called *delivery*.

In mammalian species, whether the fetus weighs 2 g at the end of a 21-day pregnancy, as with the mouse, or whether it weighs 200 pounds at the end of a 640-day pregnancy, as with the elephant, labor usually begins at the right time for that particular species, namely, when the fetus is mature enough to cope with extrauterine conditions but not yet large enough to cause mechanical difficulties in labor. The process responsible for this beautifully synchronized achievement has not yet been clearly identified.

Causes of Onset of Labor

During pregnancy the uterus consists of a large number of greatly hypertrophied smooth-muscle cells. Each cell is activated by a series of chemical reactions to begin rhythmic contractions in a highly coordinated way and with such force that the cervix is dilated and the baby is expelled. The fundamental question is what stimulates these uterine cells, at a precise time in most pregnancies, to begin labor contractions. Various theories have been advanced to explain the onset of labor. It appears that several mechanisms are involved in initiating and maintaining labor, each having varying importance depending upon individual circumstances.[1]

Progesterone Deprivation Theory

Progesterone, secreted first by the corpus luteum and then by the placenta, is essential in maintaining pregnancy. Since the uterus is composed of smooth muscle and most smooth-muscle organs will contract when stretched, it is significant that the uterus remains quiescent throughout the greater part of pregnancy. This suggests that some substance, most likely progesterone, is acting to inhibit uterine contractility. The role of a "progesterone block" in the maintenance and termination of pregnancy has been upheld by some investigators for many years. In several animal species, this theory is well supported by studies that show a drop in maternal progesterone with a rise in estrogen, which has opposite effects on uterine musculature, before labor begins. This could not be documented in humans until recently, when new methodology was able to identify a fall in circulating progesterone with a continuing increase of estrogen in a study population of women during the 5 weeks preceding labor.[2] The onset of labor in humans might result from withdrawal of progesterone at a time of relative estrogen dominance.

Oxytocin Theory

It has been clearly demonstrated that the human uterus is increasingly sensitive to oxytocin as pregnancy advances. Oxytocin is an effective stimulant of uterine contractions in late pregnancy and is commonly used to induce or augment labor. Although oxytocinlike activity in the blood has been found in women during labor, with the highest concentration during the second stage, it is also present in both males and females having surgery. It is possible that any stress may release this hypophyseal hormone. Also, blood contains an enzyme that promptly inactivates oxytocin. Studies of blood oxytocin levels before labor and through the first stage have not revealed increases.[3] Humans as well as several other mammals still go into labor normally when the hypophysis has been removed or destroyed. While oxytocin alone seems unlikely as initiator of the labor process, it may well be significant in combination with other substances.

Fetal Endocrine Control Theory

At the appropriate time of fetal maturity, it appears that the fetal adrenals secrete cortical steroids that are felt to trigger the mechanisms leading to labor. Shortly before labor, the sensitivity of the fetal adrenal to adrenocorticotropic hormone (ACTH), produced by the pituitary, increases. As a result, the production of cortisol increases. In laboratory studies with sheep, destruction of the fetal pituitary or hypothalamus (which would interfere with ACTH production) leads to prolonged pregnancy. In contrast, administration of ACTH or cortisol directly to the fetus leads to premature labor.[4]

Corticosteroids are released during periods of stress, which suggests one cause of premature labor in the instance when the fetus is compromised. Conditions that cause decreased blood flow to the uterus, such as preeclampsia or uterine overdistention due to multiple pregnancy or polyhydramnios, are known to be related to premature labor. These conditions also compromise the fetus and thus could be implicated in fetal release of corticosteroids. The suggested mechanism of action is that fetal steroids stimulate the release of precursors to prostaglandins which in turn produce uterine labor contractions.[5]

Prostaglandin Theory

Research has shown prostaglandins to be very effective in inducing uterine contractions at any stage of gestation. Prostaglandins are formed by the uterine decidua, and their concentration in the amniotic fluid and blood of women increases during labor. Study of the mechanisms of prostaglandin synthesis has shown that arachidonic acid, the obligatory precursor to prostaglandin, increases markedly in comparison to the other fatty acids in the amniotic fluid of women in labor. Arachidonic acid injected into the amniotic sac during the second trimester is highly effective in producing abortion, while other fatty acids do not induce labor. It is hypothesized that initiation of human labor results from a sequence of events including the release of lipid precursors possibly triggered by steroid action, release of arachidonic acid from these precursors perhaps at the site of the fetal membranes, increased prostaglandin synthesis from the arachidonic acid, and increased uterine contractions as a consequence of prostaglandin action on the uterine muscle.

The Powers of Labor

In Chapter 23 the three necessary elements in labor and birth are described: the passageway, the passenger, and the force or powers. The first two are discussed in that chapter. As part of the phenomena of labor, the powers are discussed here.

Uterine Contractions

To expel the contents of conception, the uterus goes through a series of contractions (the intermittent shortening of a muscle). Each contraction presents three phases, a period during which the intensity of the contraction increases (increment), a period during which the contraction is at its height (acme), and a period of diminishing intensity (decrement). The increment, or crescendo phase, is longer than the other two combined.

The contractions of the uterus during labor are intermittent, with periods of relaxation between, resembling, in this respect, the systole and the diastole of the heart. The interval between contractions diminishes gradually from about 10 minutes early in labor to about 2 or 3 minutes in the second stage. These periods of relaxation not only provide rest for the uterine muscles and for the mother, but are also essential to the welfare of the fetus because unremitting contractions may so interfere with placental functions that the resulting lack of oxygen produces fetal distress.

Another characteristic of labor contractions is that they are quite involuntary; their action is not only independent of the mother's will but also of extrauterine nervous control.

During labor, the uterus is soon differentiated into two identifiable portions, the upper and lower uterine segments. The upper segment is the active, contractile portion of the uterus. Its function is to expel the uterine contents. It displays a decreasing gradient of intensity of contractions from the fundus downward. As labor progresses, a passive lower segment is developed. With each contraction, the muscle fibers of the upper segment retract, becoming shorter as the fetus descends. The upper segment, therefore, becomes thicker. Fibers of the lower segment stretch, and consequently it becomes thinner. The distinct boundary between the upper and lower uterine segments is called a physiological retraction ring.

The degree of discomfort during labor varies considerably from client to client. The woman who anticipates a painful experience generally has more pain than the woman who is properly prepared for what can be a good experience. To allay preexisting fear, one should refer to uterine contractions as *contractions*, not *pains*.

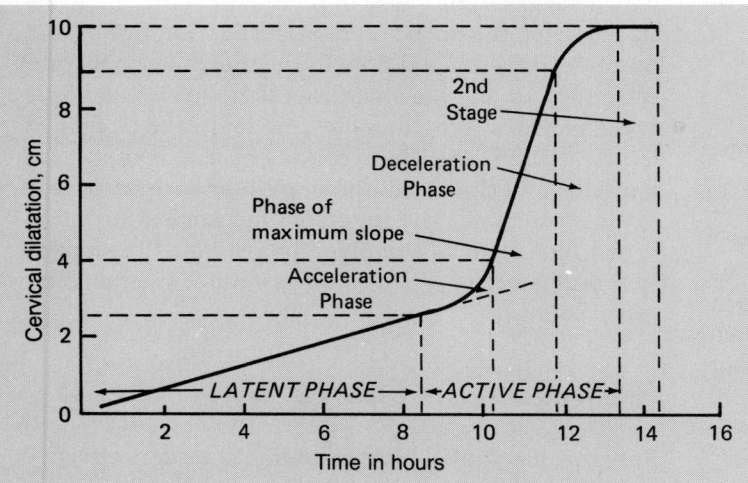

FIGURE 24-1

Composite of the average dilatation curve for nulliparous labor. The first stage is divided into a relatively flat latent phase and a rapidly progressive active phase. The active phase has three identifiable component parts: an acceleration phase, a linear phase of maximum slope, and a deceleration phase. (Friedman: Labor and Clinical Evaluation and Management, 2nd ed. New York, Appleton–Century–Crofts, 1978)

The duration of these contractions ranges from 45 to 90 seconds, averaging about 1 minute.

Duration of Labor

Although there is usually some degree of variation in all labors, an estimate of the average length of labor can be based on studies of records of some several thousand primigravidas and multiparas.

The average duration of first labors is about 14 hours, approximately 12½ hours in the first stage, 1 hour and 20 minutes in the second stage, and 10 minutes in the third stage.

The average duration of multiparous labors is approximately 6 hours shorter than for first labors (*e.g.*, 7 hours and 20 minutes in the first stage, ½ hour in the second stage, and 10 minutes in the third stage).

During the first stage of labor full dilatation of the cervix (10 cm) is accomplished, but for the greater part of this time the progress of cervical dilatation is slow (Fig. 24-1). This has been clearly demonstrated in Friedman's study of 500 labors of primigravidas. From his study, the first stage of labor is divided into the latent phase and the active phase. The *latent phase*, from the onset of uterine contractions, takes many hours and accomplishes little cervical dilatation. But with the beginning of the *active phase*, cervical dilatation proceeds at an accelerated rate and then reaches a deceleration phase shortly before the second stage of labor.

The first 4 cm of cervical dilatation occurs during the slow, latent phase. The remainder of cervical dilatation is accomplished much more rapidly in the active phase. Hence, 5 cm of dilatation has taken the client well past the halfway point in labor, even though 10 cm represents full dilatation. In fact, at that point the average labor is more than two thirds over.

Premonitory Signs of Labor

During the last few weeks of pregnancy a number of changes indicate that the time of labor is approaching. Lightening occurs about 10 to 14 days before delivery, particularly in primigravidas. This alteration is brought about by a settling of the fetal head into the pelvis. This may occur at any time during the last 4 weeks, but occasionally does not occur until labor actually begins. Lightening may take place suddenly, so that the expectant mother arises one morning entirely relieved of the abdominal tightness and diaphragmatic pressure that she had experienced previously.

But the relief in one direction often is followed by signs of greater pressure below, such as shooting pains down the legs from pressure on the sciatic nerves, an increase in the amount of vaginal discharge, and greater frequency of urination due to pressure on the bladder. In mothers who have had previous children, lightening is more likely to occur after labor begins.

True Labor vs False Labor

False contractions may begin as early as 3 or 4 weeks before the termination of pregnancy. They are merely an exaggeration of the intermittent uterine contractions that have occurred throughout the entire period of gestation, but now, they may be accompanied by discomfort. They are confined chiefly to the lower part of the abdomen and the groin and do not increase in intensity, frequency, or duration. The discomfort is rarely intensified if the mother walks about, and it may even be relieved if she is on her feet. Examination reveals no changes in the cervix.

Premonitory Signs of Labor

"Lightening" or descent of fetal head into pelvis
Sciatic nerve pressure
Increased vaginal discharge
Greater frequency of urination

False Labor	True Labor
No change in cervix	Progressive cervical dilatation
Discomfort, usually in low abdomen and groin	Discomfort in back and abdomen
Contractions occur at irregular intervals	Contractions occur at regular intervals
No increase in frequency and intensity of contractions	Progressive increase in frequency and intensity of contractions

The signs that accompany true labor contractions present a contrasting picture. True labor contractions usually are felt in the lower back and extend in girdlelike fashion from the back to the front of the abdomen. They have a definite rhythm and gradually increase in frequency, intensity, and duration. In the course of a few hours of true labor contractions, a progressive effacement and dilatation of the cervix is apparent.

Show

Another sign of impending labor is pink "show." After the discharge of the mucous plug that has filled the cervical canal during pregnancy, the pressure of the descending presenting part of the fetus causes the minute capillaries in the cervix to rupture. This blood is mixed with mucus and therefore has the pink tinge. It must be differentiated from substantial discharge of blood, which may indicate an obstetric complication.

Rupture of the Membranes

Occasionally, rupture of the membranes is the first indication of approaching labor. It was once thought that this was a grave sign, heralding a long and difficult dry labor, but present-day statistics show that this is not true. Nevertheless, the physician must be notified at once; under these circumstances, the client may be advised to enter the hospital immediately.

After the membranes rupture there is always the possibility of a prolapsed cord if the presenting part does not adequately fill the pelvic inlet. This is more likely if the infant presents as a footling breech, or by the shoulder, or in the vertex presentation when the fetal head has not descended far enough into the true pelvis prior to the rupture of the membranes.

Three Stages of Labor

The process of labor is divided into three distinct stages.

The *first stage of labor,* or the dilating stage, begins with the first true labor contraction and ends with the complete dilatation of the cervix. This stage may be further subdivided into the latent phase and the active phase.

The *second stage of labor,* or the stage of expulsion, begins with the complete dilatation of the cervix and ends with the delivery of the baby.

The *third stage of labor,* or the placental stage, begins with the delivery of the baby and terminates with the birth of the placenta.

First Stage of Labor

At the beginning of the first stage the contractions are short, slight, and 10 or 15 minutes or more apart and may not cause the woman any particular discomfort. She may be walking about and is generally quite comfortable between contractions. Early in the first stage the sensation is usually located in the small of the back, but, as time goes on, it sweeps around, girdlelike, to the anterior part of the abdomen. The contractions recur at shortening intervals, every 3 to 5 minutes, and become stronger and last longer.

When labor has progressed to the active phase, the woman usually prefers to remain in bed; ambulation is no longer comfortable. She becomes intensely involved in the sensations within her body and tends to withdraw from the surrounding environment.

As cervical dilatation progresses to 8 cm to 9 cm, the contractions reach peak intensity. This phase, between 8 and 10 cm dilatation, is called *transition* and is frequently the most difficult and painful time for the woman. At this time, there is usually a marked increase in the amount of show owing to rupture of capillary vessels in the cervix and the lower uterine segment.

As the result of uterine contractions, two important changes occur in the cervix during the first stage of labor: *effacement* and *dilatation.*

Cervical Effacement

Cervical effacement is the shortening of the cervical canal from a structure 1 or 2 cm in length to one in which no canal at all exists, except a circular orifice with almost paper-thin edges. As may be seen in Figure 24-2, the edges of the internal os are drawn several centimeters upward, so that the former endocervical canal becomes part of the lower uterine segment. In primigravidas, effacement is usually complete before dilatation begins, but in multiparas it is rarely complete; dilatation proceeds with rather thick cervical edges.

The terms *obliteration* and *taking up* of the cervix are synonymous with effacement. Effacement is measured during pelvic examination by estimating the percentage by which the cervical canal has shortened. For example, in a cervix 2 cm long before labor, 50% effacement has occurred when the cervix measures 1 cm in length.

Dilatation of the Cervix

This means the enlargement of the cervical os from an orifice a few millimeters in size to an aperture large enough to permit the passage of the fetus (*i.e.,* a diameter of about 10 cm). When the cervix can no longer be felt, dilatation is said to be complete.

Although the forces concerned in dilatation are not well understood, several factors appear to be involved.

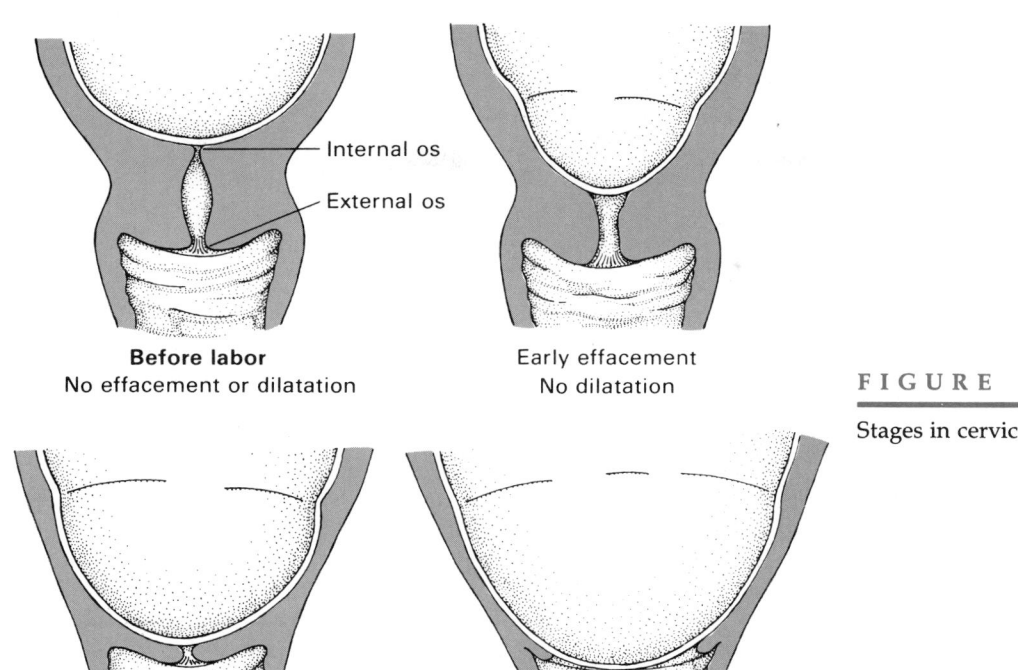

Internal os

External os

Before labor
No effacement or dilatation

Early effacement
No dilatation

Complete effacement
No dilatation

Complete dilatation

FIGURE 24-2

Stages in cervical effacement and dilatation.

The muscle fibers about the cervix are so arranged that they pull upon its edges and tend to draw it open. The uterine contractions cause pressure on the amniotic sac and this, in turn, burrows into the cervix in pouchlike fashion, exerting a dilating action (see Fig. 24-2). In the absence of the membranes, the pressure of the presenting part against the cervix and the lower uterine segment has a similar effect.

Measurement of cervical dilatation is done during pelvic examination through digital estimation of the diameter of the cervical opening. It is expressed in centimeters, and often tactile charts are available in labor rooms to help the examiner translate the mental picture obtained during this "blind" examination into centimeters.

Dilatation of the cervix in the first stage of labor is solely the result of involuntary uterine contractions. In other words, there is nothing that the mother can do, such as bearing down, that can help to expedite this period of labor. Indeed, bearing-down efforts at this stage serve only to exhaust the mother and cause the cervix to become edematous.

Second Stage of Labor

The contractions are now strong and long, last 50 to 70 seconds, and occur at intervals of 2 or 3 minutes. Rupture of the membranes usually occurs during the early part of this stage of labor, with a gush of amniotic fluid from the vagina. Sometimes, however, membranes rupture during the first stage and occasionally before labor begins. In rare cases the baby is born in a *caul*, which is a piece of the amnion that sometimes envelops the baby's head. According to superstitious beliefs, this is considered to be a good omen.

During this stage, as if by reflex action, the muscles of the abdomen are brought into play, and when the contractions are in progress the woman strains, or "bears down," with all her strength so that her face becomes flushed and the large vessels in her neck become distended. As a result of this exertion she may perspire profusely. During this stage the mother directs all her energy toward expelling the contents of the uterus. There is a marked pressure in the area of the perineum and rectum, and the urge to bear down is usually beyond her control.

Toward the end of the second stage, when the head is well down in the vagina, its pressure causes the anus to become patulous and everted (Fig. 24-3), and often small particles of fecal material may be expelled from the rectum with each contraction. This should receive careful attention to avoid contamination. As the head descends still further, the perineal region begins to bulge, and the skin over it becomes tense and glistening. At this time the scalp of the fetus may be detected through a slitlike vulvar opening. With each subsequent contraction the perineum bulges more and more and the vulva becomes more dilated and distended by the head, so that the opening is gradually converted into an ovoid and at last into a circle. With the cessation of each contraction the opening becomes smaller and the head recedes from it until it advances again with the next contraction.

The contractions now occur very rapidly, with scarcely any interval between. As the head becomes increasingly visible, the vulva is stretched farther and finally encircles the largest diameter of the baby's head. This encirclement of the largest diameter of the baby's head by the vulvar ring is known as *crowning*. An episiotomy is usually done at this time, while the tissues surrounding the perineum are supported and the head is delivered. One or two more contractions are normally enough to effect the birth of the baby.

Whereas in the first stage of labor the forces are limited to uterine action, during the second stage two forces are essential, namely, uterine contractions and intra-abdominal pressure, the latter being brought about by the bearing-down efforts of the mother. (The force exerted by the mother's bearing down can be likened to that used in forcing an evacuation of the bowels.) Both forces are essential to the successful spontaneous outcome of the second stage of labor: uterine contractions without bearing-down efforts are of little avail in expelling the infant, while, conversely, bearing-down efforts in the absence of uterine contractions are futile. As explained in Chapter 25, Management of Normal Labor, these facts have most important practical implications.

Mechanism of Labor

In its passage through the birth canal, the presenting part of the fetus undergoes certain positional changes that constitute the mechanism of labor. These movements are designed to present the smallest possible diameters of the presenting part to the irregular shape of the pelvic canal, so that it will encounter as little resistance as possible.

The mechanism of labor consists of a combination of movements, several of which may be going on at the same time. As they occur, the uterine contractions bring about important modifications in the attitude of the fetus, especially after the head has descended into the pelvis. This adaptation of the baby to the birth canal involves four processes: flexion, internal rotation, extension, and external rotation (Fig. 24-4).

For purposes of instruction, the various movements are described as if they occurred independently.

Descent.   The first requisite for the birth of the infant is descent. When the fetal head has descended such that its greatest biparietal diameter is at, or has passed, the pelvic inlet, the head is said to be *engaged*. This provides a clear indication that the pelvic inlet is large enough to accommodate the widest portion of the fetal

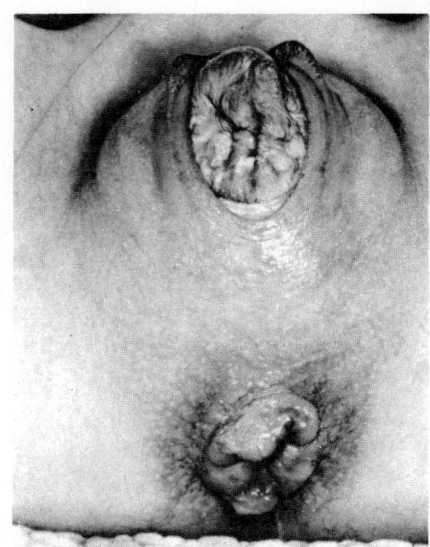

F I G U R E   2 4 - 3

Extreme bulging of the perineum showing a patulous and everted anus.

head and is, therefore, of adequate size. For the average fetal head, the linear distance between the occiput and the plane of the biparietal diameter is less than the distance between the pelvic inlet and the ischial spines. Thus, when the occiput is at the level of the spines, its biparietal diameter has usually passed the pelvic inlet, and the vertex is therefore engaged. However, one cannot assume that engagement has occurred simply because the vertex is at the spines. When the fetal head has been molded markedly, with consequent increase in the distance between the occiput and the biparietal diameter, the vertex may be felt at the spines, but its greatest diameter may still be above the pelvic inlet.

The ischial spines are used as a landmark to describe the relative position of the fetal head in the pelvis (Fig. 24-5). When the vertex is at the level of the spines, it is at 0 station. One cm below is a +1 station; 2 cm below is a +2 station; 3 cm below is a +3 station. When the vertex is 1 cm above the spines, it is a −1 station; 2 cm above is a −2 station; 3 cm above is a −3 station. This relationship is evaluated during the course of each pelvic examination and recorded, along with the assessment of cervical dilatation and effacement.

With primigravidas, engagement often precedes the onset of labor. This is the process of lightening, described earlier. Because the vertex is frequently deep in the pelvis at the onset of labor, further descent does not necessarily begin until the second stage of labor. In multiparas, on the other hand, descent often begins with engagement. Once having been inaugurated, descent is inevitably associated with the various movements of the mechanism of labor.

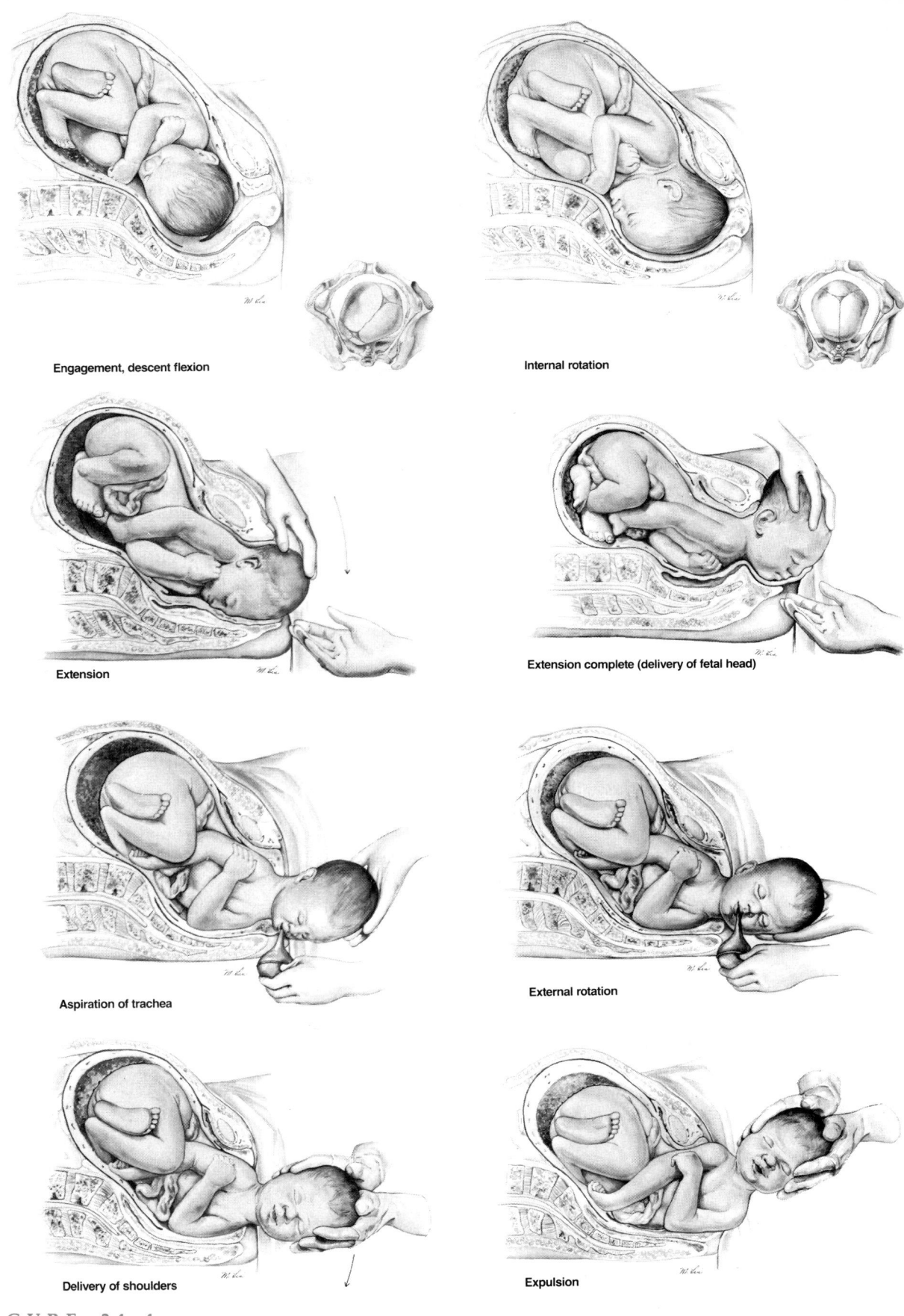

Engagement, descent flexion

Internal rotation

Extension

Extension complete (delivery of fetal head)

Aspiration of trachea

External rotation

Delivery of shoulders

Expulsion

FIGURE 24-4

Mechanism of delivery for a vertex presentation (Whitley N: A Manual of
Clinical Obstetrics. Philadelphia, JB Lippincott, 1985)

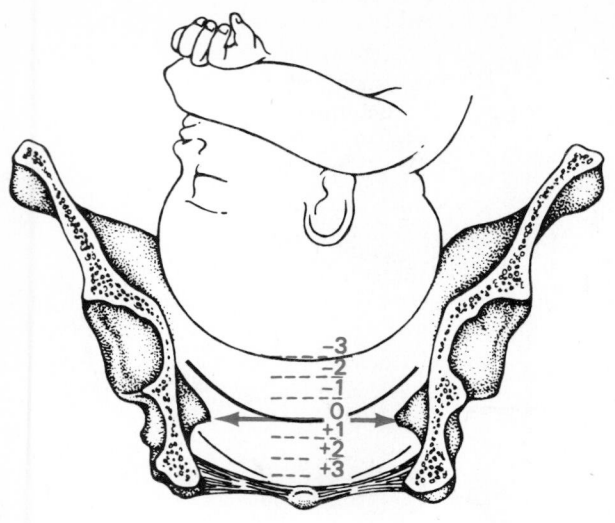

Stations of the fetal head.

Flexion.   Very early in the process of descent the head becomes so flexed that the chin is in contact with the sternum; as a consequence, the very smallest anteroposterior diameter (the suboccipitobregmatic plane) is presented to the pelvis.

Internal Rotation.   The head enters the pelvis in the transverse or diagonal position. When it reaches the pelvic floor, the occiput is rotated and comes to lie beneath the symphysis pubis. In other words, the sagittal suture is now in the anteroposterior diameter of the outlet. Although the occiput usually rotates to the front, on occasion it may turn toward the hollow of the sacrum. If anterior rotation does not take place at all, the occiput usually rotates to the direct occiput posterior position, a condition known as persistent occiput posterior. Because this represents a deviation from the normal mechanism of labor, it will be considered in Chapter 38, in the section on abnormal fetal positions.

Extension.   After the occiput emerges from the pelvis, the nape of the neck becomes arrested beneath the pubic arch and acts as a pivotal point for the rest of the head. Extension of the head now ensues, and the frontal portion of the head, the face, and the chin are born.

External Rotation.   After the birth of the head, it remains in the anteroposterior position only a very short time, then turns to one or another side of its own accord, *restitution*. When the occiput originally has been directed toward the left of the mother's pelvis, it then rotates toward the left and to the right when it originally has been toward the right. This is known as external rotation and is due to the fact that the shoulders, having entered the pelvis in the transverse position, undergo internal rotation to the anteroposterior position, as did the head; this brings about a corresponding rotation of the head, which is now on the outside.

The shoulders are born in a manner somewhat similar to that of the head. Almost immediately after the occurrence of external rotation, the anterior shoulder appears under the symphysis pubis and becomes arrested temporarily beneath the pubic arch to act as a pivotal point for the other shoulder. As the anterior margin of the perineum becomes distended, the posterior shoulder is born, assisted by an upward lateral flexion of the infant's body. Once the shoulders are delivered, the infant's body is quickly extruded (*expulsion*).

Third Stage of Labor

The third stage of labor is made up of two phases, *the phase of placental separation* and *the phase of placental expulsion.*

Immediately following the birth of the infant, the remainder of the amniotic fluid escapes, after which there is usually a slight flow of blood. The uterus can be felt as a firm globular mass just below the level of the umbilicus. Shortly thereafter, the uterus relaxes and assumes a discoid shape. With each subsequent contraction or relaxation the uterine shape changes from globular to discoid until the placenta has separated, after which time the globular shape persists.

Placental Separation

As the uterus contracts down at regular intervals on its diminishing content, the area of placental attachment is greatly reduced. The great disproportion between the reduced size of the placental site and the size of the placenta brings about a folding or festooning of the maternal surface of the placenta, and separation takes place. Meanwhile, bleeding takes place within these placental folds, which expedites separation of the organ. The placenta now sinks into the lower uterine segment or upper vagina as an unattached body. The following are signs that indicate that placental separation has occurred:

Signs of Placental Separation

Globular and firmer uterus

Rise of uterus in abdomen

Descent of umbilical cord

Sudden gush of blood

---

1. The uterus becomes globular and firmer.
2. The uterus rises upward in the abdomen.
3. The umbilical cord descends 3 inches or more farther out of the vagina.
4. A sudden gush of blood often occurs.

These signs usually occur within 5 minutes after the delivery of the infant.

Placental Expulsion

Actual expulsion of the placenta may be brought about by the mother bearing down if she is not anesthetized. If this cannot be accomplished, it is usually effected through gentle pressure on the uterine fundus. Excessive pressure should be avoided to obviate the rare possibility of inversion of the uterus (see Chap. 38).

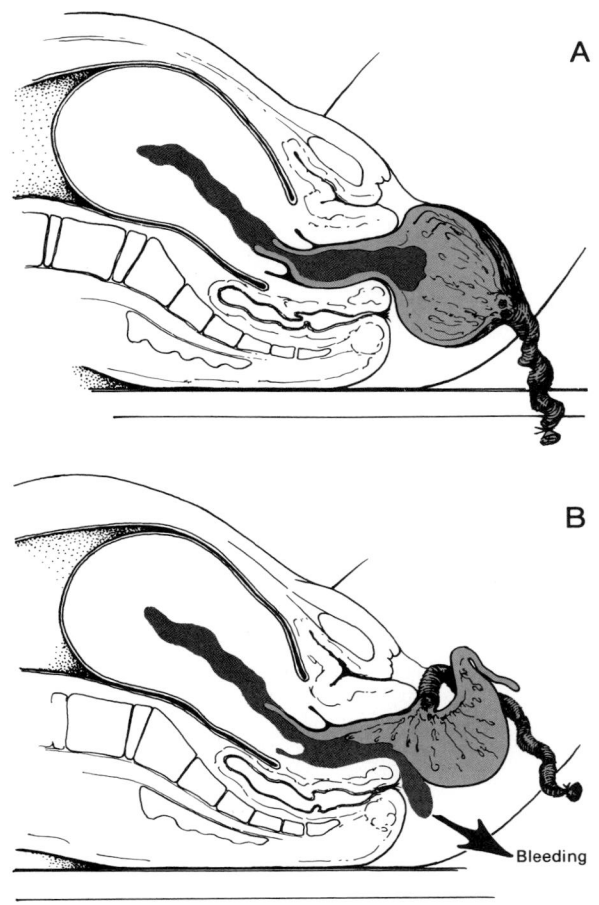

FIGURE 24-6

Expulsion of the placenta by (*A*) Schultze's mechanism, whereby the placenta is turned inside out within the vagina and is delivered with the glistening fetal surfaces to the outside, and by (*B*) the Duncan mechanism, whereby the placenta is rolled up in the vagina and is delivered with the maternal surface to the outside.

The extrusion of the placenta may take place by one of two mechanisms. First, it may become turned inside out within the vagina and be born like an inverted umbrella with the glistening fetal surfaces presenting. This is known as Schultze's mechanism and occurs in about 80% of cases. Second, it may become somewhat rolled up in the vagina, with the maternal surface outermost, and be born edgewise. This is known as the Duncan mechanism and is seen in about 20% of deliveries. It is believed that Schultze's mechanism signifies that the placenta has become detached first at its center, and usually a collection of blood and clots is found in the sac of membranes. The Duncan mechanism, on the other hand, suggests that the placenta has separated first at its edges, and it is in this type that bleeding usually occurs at the time of separation (Fig. 24-6). No clinical significance has been ascribed to either mechanism.

The contraction of the uterus following delivery serves not only to produce placental separation but also to control uterine hemorrhage. As the result of this contraction of the uterine muscle fibers, the countless blood vessels within their interstices are clamped shut. Even then, a certain amount of blood loss in the third stage is unavoidable, commonly amounting to 500 ml or more. It is one of the aims of the conduct of labor to reduce this bleeding to a minimum.

Summary of Stages of Labor

First Stage—Dilating Stage

Definition—Period from first true labor contraction to complete dilatation of cervix

What Is Accomplished—Effacement and dilatation of cervix

Forces Involved—Uterine contractions

Second Stage—Expulsive Stage

Definition—Period from complete dilatation of cervix to birth of baby

What Is Accomplished—Expulsion of baby from birth canal; facilitated by certain positional changes of fetus (descent, flexion, internal rotation, extension, external rotation, and expulsion)

Forces Involved—Uterine contractions plus intra-abdominal pressure

Third Stage—Placental Stage

Definition—Period from birth of baby through birth of placenta

What Is Accomplished—Separation of placenta; expulsion of placenta

Forces Involved—Uterine contractions; intra-abdominal pressure

Fourth Stage of Labor

The first hour post partum is sometimes referred to as the fourth stage of labor. During this time *restoration of physiological stability* occurs, following the tumultuous events of labor. It is a period of potential crisis, with increased incidence of hemorrhage, urinary retention, hypotension, and side-effects of anesthesia; it requires careful monitoring of uterine contraction, vital signs, and other physiological indices.

The first hour after the baby's birth is also considered critical for initial formation of the mother–child relationship and consolidation of the family unit. The process of maternal–child attachment is still under study, but it is possible that early parental interactions with the new baby and each other set the tone for the quality of their relationships later. If so, this is a key time for nursing care, which includes assessment of potential problems and support of satisfying interactions for the new family.

References

1. MacDonald PC, Porter JC (eds): Fourth Ross Conference on Obstetric Research. Columbus, Ohio, Ross Laboratories, 1983
2. Casey ML, Winkel CA, Porter JC et al: Endocrine regulation of parturition. Clin Perinatol 10:709, 1983
3. Chard T: The role of the posterior pituitaries of mother and fetus in spontaneous parturition. In Camline KS, Cross KW, Dawes GS (eds): Fetal and Neonatal Physiology. New York, Cambridge University Press, 1973
4. Ligging GC, Fairclough RJ, Grieves SA et al: The mechanism of initiation of parturition in the ewe. Recent Prog Horm Res 29:111, 1973
5. Casey ML, MacDonald PC: Initiation of labor in women. In Hugzar G (ed): The Biochemistry and Physiology of the Uterus and Labor. Cleveland, CRC Press, 1985

Suggested Reading

Friedman EA: Labor and Clinical Evaluation and Management, 2nd ed. New York, Appleton-Century-Crofts, 1978
Pritchard JA, MacDonald RC, Gant NF: Williams' Obstetrics, 17th ed. New York, Appleton-Century-Crofts, 1985

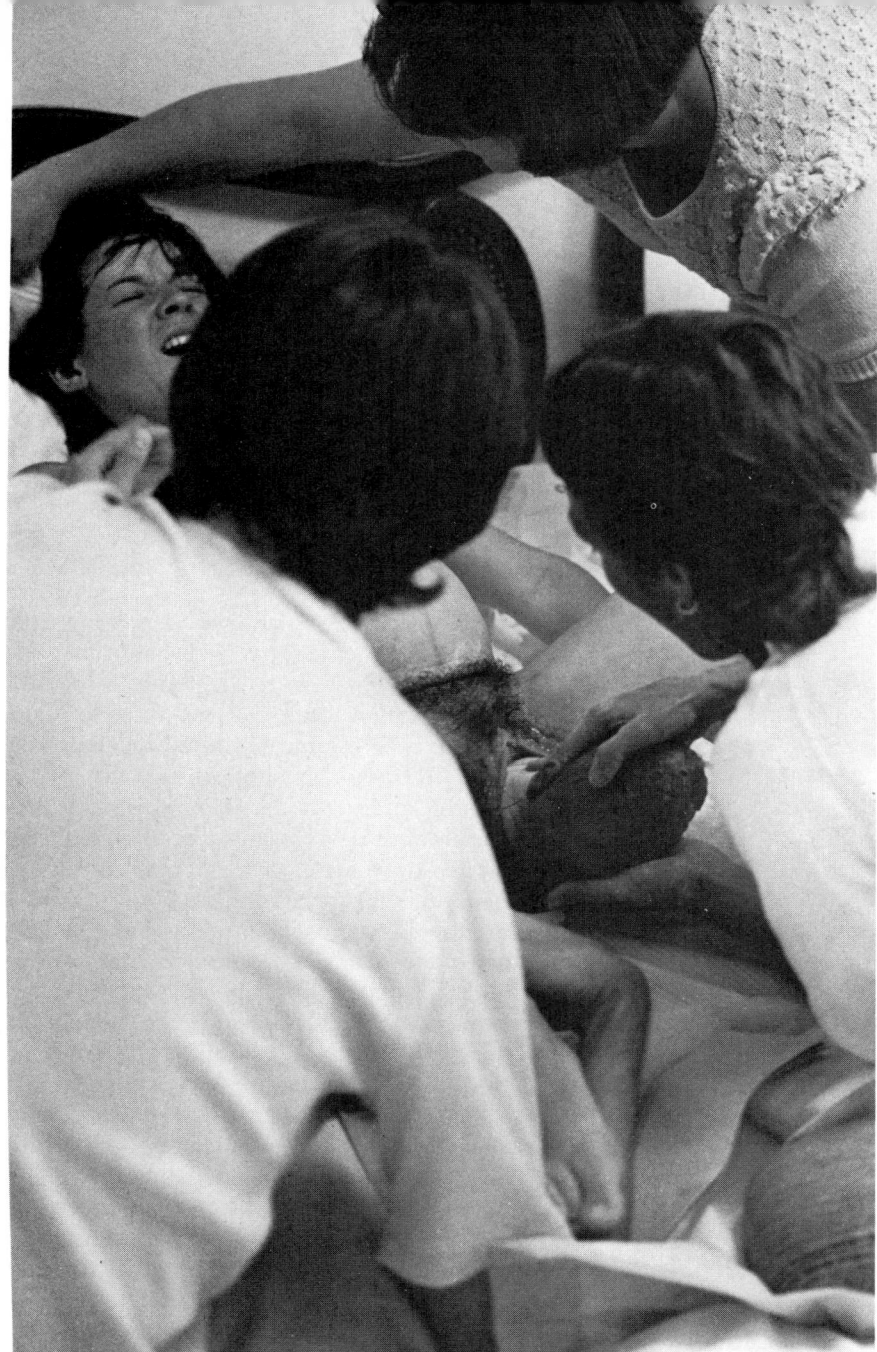

CHAPTER 25

Management of Normal Labor

Parturition is a unique and humbling experience not only for the mother and the father, the main participants, but also for the health-care staff who shares this experience. From the couple's point of view, labor looms as a critical period in the process of childbearing; often it is considered by them, and especially by the mother, as the end of a long drawn out process rather than the beginning of a new role. Hence, they attribute enormous significance to events and people who are necessary and helpful to them at this time.

Dimensions of Effective Nursing Care

The goal of nursing during the birth process is to instill maximum physical and emotional well-being in both the woman and the fetus. This goal extends to include the transitions of woman to mother and fetus to newborn. At the same time the nurse should facilitate the participation of the father or support persons in the birth. The nursing interventions used to achieve this goal are purposeful but flexible, based on thorough assessments and nursing diagnoses to meet the individual needs of the mother, newborn, and family. To implement such care the nurse must be familiar with the normal physiology of labor, deviations from the norm (both discussed in other chapters of this book), and the judgment, self-confidence, and skills required to cope with the stressful and emergency conditions. Additional attributes include a mastery of certain technical and communicative skills, which can be applied appropriately to meet the exigencies of the situation. These skills are used both with the client and in participating as a member of the health team in the labor and delivery unit. However, knowledge and technical ability are not sufficient in themselves; the nurse must also address the psychosocial aspects of care, by conveying warmth and empathy. The empathic nurse is able to enter into the feelings of the client and at the same time retain a sense of separateness. Thus, objectivity is maintained, which contributes to more effective care. Yet the worth and the individuality of each mother are always recognized.

The labor nurse is concerned with two clients, and this concern is reflected in the assessments, nursing diagnoses, interventions, and evaluation of care done on

The author recognizes that those professionals providing prenatal care and delivering babies within the hospital setting can be either physicians or nurse–midwives. For clarity within this chapter, the person delivering the infant will be referred to as a physician, with the clear understanding that in some instances a nurse–midwife could be the delivery attendant. In addition, within the text the primary support person for the mother will be referred to as the father or woman's partner. This may not hold true in some instances; the mother may be a single parent or the father may not be available and a relative or friend may assume that role.

each individual client. The ability of the nurse to assume these responsibilities is contingent upon competent guidance and instructions. To help the student or new graduate prepare for these responsibilities, we focus on both the woman and the nurse as they move through the successive stages of labor. Although it is the woman who truly delivers her infant, the other important people in this event—the father, the nurse, the physician or nurse–midwife, and ancillary personnel—are not to be forgotten; they also play important roles.

In this chapter we describe the environment and care that accompany a labor and delivery that is carried out in a conventional labor and delivery unit within a hospital setting. A discussion of the environment and care found in alternate birth facilities is given in Chapter 47. The care given in a conventional setting varies depending on each facility's policies and procedures, but tends to be accompanied by more technological interventions and more restriction on the client's activity. However, medical-center personnel must look at the traditional procedures and determine whether they are based on sound scientific research and are in the best interest of the client and her family.

Professional organizations are publishing documents supporting changes in perinatal care to incorporate family-centered care concepts in every aspect of perinatal service.[1,2] Above all, the family should not lose their rights when the enter the hospital. They have choices and options in care, and the professional is there to support those choices that are not life threatening.

The nursing-service personnel within the medical centers who are responsible for perinatal care need to work with the medical staff in the revision of protocols. The combined efforts of the professionals who deliver perinatal care should provide quality health care while recognizing both physical and psychosocial needs of the mother, the family, and the newborn.

Labor

Prelude to Labor

The prodromal signs that herald the onset of labor begin several weeks before true labor commences. As indicated in Chapter 24, lightening may occur any time during the last 4 weeks of pregnancy; in primigravidas it usually occurs about 10 to 14 days prior to labor. This phenomenon causes a sensation of decreased abdominal distention produced by the descent of the presenting part of the baby into the pelvis. In multigravidas, this may not occur until the labor has begun. The usually painless Braxton Hicks contractions that have occurred intermittently throughout the latter part of pregnancy

may increase so much that they become annoying. They may cause the mother many restless or sleepless nights that contribute to her gradually increasing tension and fatigue. Since the rise in the anxiety level contributes to heightened awareness, the mother becomes more sensitive to various stimuli—if the fetus is generally less active, she may worry; if the baby moves more than usual, she may worry. She wonders about the 2- to 3-pound weight loss that may occur 3 to 4 days before the onset of labor. Ordinarily this might be an occasion of great rejoicing, but now it may give her some concern. Even the increased vaginal mucous discharge may have an ominous significance for her. The spurt of energy that may occur 1 to 2 days before labor begins often leads her into activities that are overfatiguing. She needs anticipatory guidance from the nurse and the physician to help her to set limits on activity.

This is the time for the mother to finish packing her suitcase and to simplify her housekeeping duties. She may want to complete meal preparations for the family's use when she is in the hospital; if this is done daily, little by little, it should not become bothersome. Last-minute details for the care of the other children or the functioning of the household can be taken care of at this time. Walks in the fresh air are a good way to release extra tension without overfatigue. The mother should be encouraged to achieve a happy balance between activity and rest. As term approaches it is wise for the nurse to explore with the mother her preparations for coming to the hospital. The parents should know approximately how long it takes them to reach the hospital and what alternate means of transportation are available if the father is not able to take her. What entrance to the hospital they should use and what admission procedures they must go through also are important. A tour of the ward for the parents can be arranged during the antenatal period so that they can become more familiar with the surroundings.

Onset of Labor

Early in the third trimester the client should be apprised of what to do when labor starts and of certain situations that would necessitate a visit to the hospital for evaluation. The client should be encouraged to report early in labor and not wait at home to see if it is true or false labor. Most physicians instruct their clients to notify them if the labor contractions become regular. A primigravida, for instance, may be given instructions to wait at home until contractions are every 5 minutes for 2 hours, whereas the multigravida would be instructed to come to the hospital much sooner. Other situations of which the mother needs to be advised include breaking of the bag of waters and any vaginal bleeding. Further instruction needs to be given to clarify the breaking

Client needs to go to the hospital for evaluation when the following occur:
- There is a regular uterine contractions pattern, increasing in intensity
- The bag of water breaks
- There is bright-red vaginal bleeding
- There is a decrease in fetal movement (less than three movements per hour)

of the amniotic sac, in which the woman may experience anything from only a small intermittent leak to a gush of fluid from her vagina. However, in either situation the physician should be notified and the mother should come to the hospital. (See chart above.)

When the mother first becomes aware of the contractions, they may be 15 to 20 minutes apart and may last perhaps 20 to 30 seconds. Since these are of mild intensity, she usually can continue with whatever she is doing, except that she must be alert to time the subsequent contractions in order to have specific information when she calls the physician. It is important for the client to know when it is appropriate to go to the hospital in relation to her uterine contraction pattern.

Admission to the Hospital

As previously stated, the mother who has been given adequate antepartal care has also received instruction on what to anticipate when she comes to the hospital to have her baby. If this is the mother's first hospital experience, it will be much easier for her if she has been told about the necessary preliminary procedures, such as any vulvar and perineal preparation, the methods of examination employed to ascertain the progress of labor, and the usual routines exercised for her care in the course of labor.

If the mother has not had adequate antepartal care to prepare her, her labor may be rather advanced upon admission and she may not know what to expect. It then falls to the nurse to reassure this mother and orient her as quickly as possible to the process of labor and the physical environment. In these instances, the ability to make decisive clinical judgments, especially with regard to establishing priorities of care, is extremely helpful and necessary.

The preparation for delivery varies in different hospitals, since every hospital has its own admission procedure. Many of the details of management may be accomplished in a number of ways. Very few institutions employ precisely the same technique in preparing a mother for delivery. Actually, the differences are in details only, for the principles are the same everywhere,

namely, asepsis and antisepsis, together with careful observation of the mother for any deviations from the normal, and meticulous supportive care.

Admission Information

After making the mother comfortable in the labor room, the nurse needs to proceed with the admission as quickly as possible. It must be remembered that the mother's labor usually becomes progressively stronger; therefore, when admitting procedures are done early in labor, while she can be more responsive with relative ease, the client's comfort and well-being are enhanced. Also, there are generally several other people concerned with the care of the mother (*i.e.*, physician, nurse–midwife, and laboratory technician). Often they cannot carry out their duties until the client has been fully admitted.

The nurse initiates the admitting process with information that needs to be determined quickly in order to evaluate the following:

1. Is the client in true labor and if so how far has she progressed?
2. What is the general condition of mother and fetus?
3. What preparation has she done for childbirth and what are support systems to assist her through labor?

Each one encompasses those nursing skills specific to labor and delivery that take time for the new nurse to master.

As part of the admission procedure, determined by hospital policies and physician orders, the nurse may be doing perineal shaves, enemas, and electronic fetal monitoring, starting intravenous therapy, and ordering laboratory tests (*i.e.*, hematocrit, hemoglobin, type and screens, and urine analysis). A detailed look at admitting the laboring woman follows.

Assessment

Nursing History

Nursing practice is governed by standards, and in the course of admitting the laboring woman the nurse must document the name of the client, the reason for admission, the date and time of arrival, the time the physician was notified, and the time the client was seen by the physician.[1,2] The prenatal record is sent from the doctor's office or clinic to the labor and delivery unit at approximately 36 weeks and should be looked at by the admitting nurse. The following pertinent information is usually transcribed from the prenatal record to the admission form: blood group and Rh factor, irregular antibody detection, serology, and any diagnostic or therapeutic measures.

By taking a good nursing history and physical the admitting nurse evaluates the client in relation to high-risk factors. If any factors are found that place the mother or fetus at risk, the physician is notified, because they may alter the type of labor and delivery experience the client desires. (Refer to other chapters for further discussion of high-risk factors and how they influence perinatal outcome.) Clients who are not at high risk should have a more directed history, obtaining the following information: onset of contractions, status of membranes, bleeding, fetal activity, history of allergies, time and content of last ingestion, and current medications. The fetus is also evaluated by noting the gestational age, fetal position, and heart rate. Trained nursing personnel may perform the initial pelvic examination (first noting that there is no abnormal bleeding, status of membranes, and fetal position) to determine cervical dilatation, effacement, and fetal position and station. These were discussed in Chapters 23 and 24. See the sample admitting form for general information required.

The nurse, as the person who spends a great deal of time with the client after admission, is expected to report on the general character of the labor contractions as well as the other manifestations of labor. First, it must be determined whether the client is actually in labor. Friedman has pointed out that there are no fixed or uniformly applicable rules that can be used at the bedside. We can assume that the client is in true labor if her contractions continue uninterruptedly and result in dilatation of the cervix.[3] In practice, however, a variety of types of contractions may be apparent; thus, the following differential points between true and false labor are to be used only as *guidelines* for assessing the state of the mother's labor (Table 25-1).

Characteristics of Contractions

The frequency, duration, and intensity of the contractions should be watched closely and recorded whether a monitor is used or not.

The *frequency* of contractions is timed from the beginning of one contraction to the beginning of the next.

The *duration* of a contraction is timed from the moment the uterus first begins to tighten until it relaxes again (Fig. 25-1).

The *intensity* of a contraction may be mild, moderate, or strong at its acme. Since this is a relative factor if measured without the aid of the internal uterine pressure catheter, intensity is difficult to interpret unless one is at the mother's bedside palpating the uterus during contractions. The nurse uses the palmar surface of the fingertips, palpating different parts of the uterus during the contraction, to judge intensity.

TABLE 25-1

Differential Factors In True and False Labor

True Labor	False Labor
Contractions	
Occur at regular intervals	Occur at irregular intervals
Start in the back and sweep around to the abdomen	Located chiefly in abdomen
Increase in intensity and duration	Intensity remains the same, or is variable
Intervals gradually shorten	Intervals remain long
Intensify by walking	Walking has no intensifying effect; often gives relief
Show	
Usually present; pink tinged mucus released from the cervical canal as labor starts	Usually not present or if present is usually brownish. May be due to recent pelvic examination by her doctor or to intercourse
Cervix	
Becomes effaced and dilated	No change
Ambulation	
Increases the intensity of contractions	No change
Sedation	
Does not stop contractions	Tends to decrease number of contractions

During a *mild* contraction, the uterine muscle becomes somewhat tense, but can be indented with gentle pressure. During a *moderate* contraction the uterus becomes moderately firm and a firmer pressure is needed to indent. During a *strong* contraction, the uterus becomes so firm that it has the feel of woodlike hardness, and at the height of the contraction, the uterus cannot be indented when pressure is applied by the examiner's finger.

General Physical Condition

Chief Complaint. The client should be asked why she came to the hospital. The nurse should not assume that it was the onset of regular contractions that made her come in, because it could be a complaint of leaking amniotic fluid or decrease in fetal activity that prompted her to come to the unit. The mother should be given time to express in her own words to the nurse her reason for admission. The use of open-ended questions to elicit

A S S E S S M E N T   T O O L

Admitting Form: Labor/Delivery Unit

MEMORIAL MEDICAL CENTER OF LONG BEACH

DATE	TIME		DATE	TIME	
		How Arrived:			Additional Nursing Observations and Comments
		T P R B/P FHT			
		Allergies:			Rm: S/NS
		Grav: Para: EDC:			Breast Formula
		Chief Complaint and Nursing Observation:			WT: GAIN HT:
					Classes: FIDR
					Anesthesia:
					Peds.
					Blood type: VDRL
					Doctor's Comments:
		Examination Findings:			
					Medications:
		Dr. Notified:			
		Seen by Dr.:			
		To X-Ray: Amb. WC Guerney			
					Disposition:
		Lab. Tests: CBC VA			Signed & Recvd. Outpt. Instructions
		Other:			Name
				☐	Address
					Age Birth date:

LABOR-DELIVERY OUT-PATIENT RECORD
Form #1124/2 part NCR paper: White = Med. Records/Yellow = Labor Delivery Dept.

(Courtesy of Memorial Medical Centers of Long Beach, Long Beach, CA)

Dr.
Case No.
Nurse:

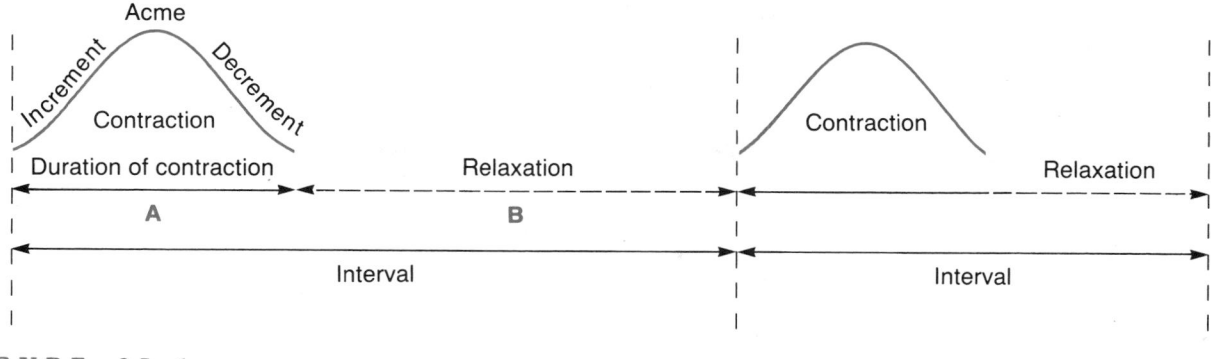

FIGURE 25-1

The interval and the duration of uterine contractions. The frequency of contractions is the interval timed from the beginning of one contraction to the beginning of the next contraction. The interval consists of two parts: (*A*) the duration of the contraction and (*B*) the period of relaxation. The broken line indicates an indeterminate period, because the time (*B*) is usually of longer duration than the actual contraction (*A*).

this information is beneficial, although more direct questions may be necessary later to clarify information.

Vital Signs

Temperature, Pulse, and Respiration.   The temperature and respiration should be normal. If there is an elevation in temperature over 99.6°F (37.2°C) orally or if the pulse and respiration become rapid, the physician is to be notified. The temperature and respiration rates are taken every 4 hours, or more frequently, if indicated.[2] Conditions that warrant closer observation are rupture of the membranes and the presence of a fetal tachycardia.

The pulse in normal labor is usually in the 70s or 80s and rarely exceeds 100. Sometimes the pulse rate on admission is slightly increased because of the excitement of coming to the hospital, but this returns to normal shortly thereafter. A persistent pulse over 100 suggests exhaustion or dehydration. Pulse rates are recorded every 4 hours.[2]

Blood Pressure.   There are significant hemodynamic occurrences observed during labor and delivery that affect the blood pressure value. With the contraction of the uterus, approximately 300 ml to 500 ml of blood is shifted to the central blood volume, causing increases in cardiac output.[4] Other conditions leading to significant increase in cardiac output are anxiety and pain, especially in the primigravida. Hendricks and Quilligan have shown that pain and anxiety alone can increase cardiac output by 50% to 60%.[5]

To obtain accurate blood pressure the nurse needs to be aware of the hemodynamic alterations involved with contractions and must work with the client to relieve her pain and anxiety as much as she is able. Blood pressures start to rise approximately 5 to 8 seconds preceding a contraction, returning to resting level when the contraction subsides.[6] Hence, the nurse should be taking the client's blood pressure and pulse after a contraction, well before the next one starts.

There are no recommendations that are based on research to help the nurse with the position of choice when obtaining a blood pressure. Most experts agree that the blood pressure taken with the client on her left side is the one to use for clinical diagnosis and management. If the nurse gets a blood pressure reading initially that needs to be reevaluated, either higher or lower than expected, the cuff should be deflated and a waiting period of 2 minutes observed. At this time the nurse would want to assess factors that may be contributing to the reading. Is the reading elevated owing to pain or anxiety, or is it low owing to regional anesthesia, supine position, or hemorrhage? The second reading can be taken in the same arm, and if the deviation from the expected norm still exists, this information is reported. The student needs to begin to realize that the person told the information, physician or staff nurse, will want other information to best evaluate the client. For instance, for an elevation in blood pressure the experienced nurse will evaluate the client for signs and symptoms of pregnancy-induced hypertension, knowing that a certain number of women will be asymptomatic during their pregnancy but will develop the disease when in labor.

For the most part, the minimal requirement for taking blood pressures during labor are every hour for the client without recognized high-risk factors and just prior to the delivery. When epidural anesthesia is given in labor, blood pressures are evaluated every 5 minutes for the first 15 to 20 minutes, or until stable. The client may then be on an every-30-minutes blood pressure schedule or as directed by the Department of Anesthesia at that particular hospital. The minimal requirements for evaluating a client following epidural anesthesia are usually present in the labor and delivery policy book, which guides the nurse in giving care.

Fetal Evaluation

It cannot be stressed enough that when caring for the pregnant woman, the nurse is treating two clients, mother and fetus. This is especially important to remember when admitting the laboring woman. The nurse must assess fetal health as well as maternal health. The assessments to establish fetal well-being are as follows:

1. Determine the estimated date of confinement (EDC).
2. Measure the fundal height of the uterus and correlate the height with the gestational age.
3. Determine fetal position by abdominal palpation.
4. Auscultate fetal heart tones to determine the baseline and any periodic changes.

Estimated Date of Confinement. The EDC can be obtained from the prenatal record. A term pregnancy is one that has achieved 37 weeks of gestation and has not exceeded 42 weeks. As explained in an earlier chapter, the date of the client's last normal menstrual period allows the nurse to calculate the EDC by using Nägele's rule. The EDC is truly an estimate, influenced by factors such as nutrition, cultural differences, and climate; fewer than 5% of the pregnancies deliver on the due date.[7]

Fundal Height. Even though determination of fundal height using a tape measure is not a common practice on admission, the labor and delivery nurse should be able to perform this measurement and know its significance (see Chap. 22). Another method used by experienced nurses is to palpate the fundal height and to be cognizant of the relationship of fundal height to gestational age. Finding an abnormally low or excessively high fundal height does not necessarily indicate an unhealthy fetus, but cues the nurse to look for the reason of the deviation from the norm.

Abdominal Palpation: Leopold Maneuvers. Confirmation of fetal position prior to the initial vaginal examination is a recommended practice.[1,2,8] Performing Leopold maneuvers in a systematic manner enables the nurse to assess fetal position and makes locating the fetal heart tone easier. In the cephalic and breech presentations the fetal heart is best heard through the back, since it is the fetal part in closest contact with the uterine wall (see Chap. 23 for procedure and illustrations).

Fetal Heart Rate. Determination of fetal heart rate (FHR) should be done early in the admission process.

Under normal circumstances, the heart rate of a term fetus, determined by the atrial pacemaker, usually ranges between 120 and 160 beats per minute.[9] The evaluation of the fetal heart rate in labor is of great importance. If the nurse works in a facility where electronic fetal monitoring is available, obtaining a 15- to 20-minute fetal monitoring strip prior to administering an enema or ambulation of the client gives her time to evaluate fetal health status.

The heart rate can be monitored in a number of ways. The simplest, and still an effective method, is by frequent auscultation using a specialized head stethoscope (Fig. 25-2). The widely used DeLee–Hillis stethoscope and the Leff fetal heart stethoscope are satisfactory for this purpose.

When checking the fetal heart sounds with a head fetoscope, the nurse listens and counts the rate for 1 full minute. Checking the rate before, during, and after a contraction is important so that any slowing or irregularities may be detected.

It may be difficult to hear the sounds during a contraction because the uterine wall is tense, and, in addition, it is more difficult for the mother to lie still during

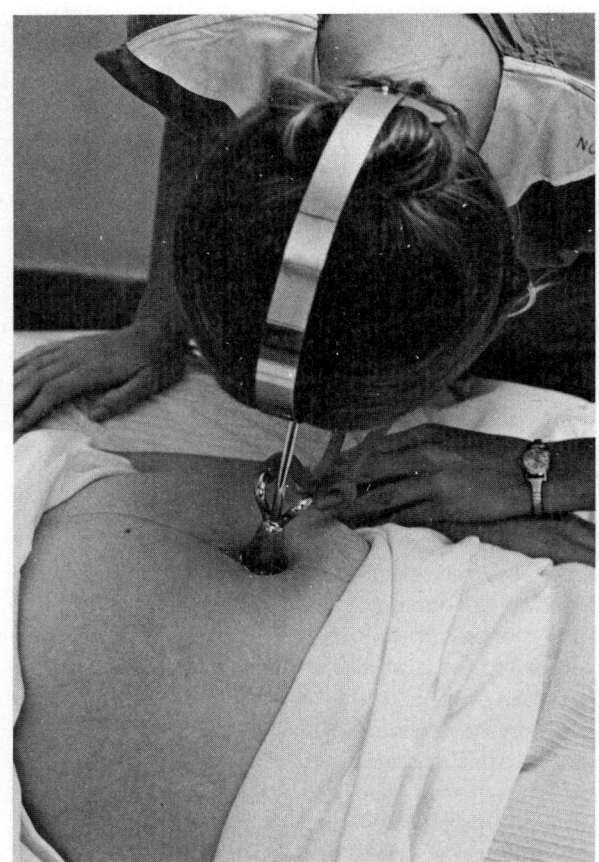

FIGURE 25-2

Auscultation of the fetal heartbeat using the fetoscope.

this period. But it is particularly important to listen at this time because these observations inform the listener on how the fetus reacts to the contraction.

The student in the clinical area should be working with a staff nurse and not be totally responsible for evaluation of the fetal heart rate. To learn interpretation of fetal monitor strips the registered nurse usually attends a separate class on fetal monitoring, with periodic updates to maintain clinical skill. If the student nurse notices a slowing of the fetal heart rate, the student should notify the staff nurse for further evaluation of the fetus, and the staff nurse will determine if the pattern warrants notification of the physician. The passage of meconium can also indicate fetal distress; its presence, color, and consistency are documented in the nursing notes, and the physician is notified. Interpretation of fetal heart rate patterns and appropriate nursing interventions for decelerations are covered in Chapter 43.

Amniotic Fluid Status

It is important to establish whether the mother's membranes are intact or not. Ruptured membranes are significant for the following three reasons:

- If the presenting part is not fixed in the pelvis, the possibility of prolapse of the cord and consequent cord compression is maximized.
- Labor is likely to occur quite soon after rupture if the pregnancy is at or near term.
- If the fetus remains in the uterus 24 hours or more after the membranes rupture, there is an increased probability of intrauterine infection that is especially harmful to the fetus even though the mother is given antibiotics.

Ruptured membranes are often difficult to diagnose unless the fluid is seen escaping from the vagina. Moreover, there are no tests that are completely reliable. Those most widely employed involve testing the acidity or alkalinity of the vaginal fluid. The amniotic fluid pH is generally 7 to 7.5, whereas vaginal secretions are in the range of 4.5 to 5.5. The nitrazine tests use test papers similar to the Clinitest. These papers are impregnated with a dye that reacts with the vaginal material and can be compared to a standard color chart. Color changes can be interpreted as in the chart below. Bloody show can confound the reading, giving a false reading of ruptured membranes when in fact the membranes are intact, since blood, like amniotic fluid, is not acidic.[8]

Some clients will come in wearing a peripad or wet underclothing that may be tested with the nitrazine. If the client presents to the unit with a term gestation and a history of leaking fluid from the vagina and is not in obvious labor, the choice procedure is a sterile speculum examination for the determination of ruptured membranes.

Nitrazine Test Color Interpretations	
Membranes Probably Intact	
Yellow	pH 5.0
Olive yellow	pH 5.5
Olive green	pH 6.0
Ruptured Membranes	
Blue green	pH 6.5
Blue gray	pH 7.0
Deep blue	pH 7.5

The nurse may be assisting the physician with this procedure, or if instructed properly on the technique the nurse may be incorporating it into his or her practice. The procedure uses a sterile speculum inserted into the vagina and visualization of the cervix. At this time sterile cotton swabs are used to take samples of vaginal secretions from the cervical os to test with nitrazine and make a slide to check for ferning. The practitioner also looks for fluid leaking from the cervix, vaginal pooling, color of the fluid, and any cervical dilatation. When the procedure is over the woman is made comfortable. The slide prepared for the fern test needs to dry for 5 to 7 minutes before it is examined under the microscope. Owing to the sodium chloride content in amniotic fluid, the dried specimen, if truly amniotic fluid, will look like clusters of fern leaves. The client and support person should be informed of the test results; if the membranes are ruptured the report will be a positive fern test, and if they are not ruptured, the report will be a negative fern test.

Some physicians may wait, up to a certain time, for labor to start on its own, while others may desire the starting of an oxytocin infusion. In either management, delaying or minimizing the number of vaginal examinations can lower the chance of introducing bacteria into the uterine cavity.[10]

Initial Vaginal Examination

Abdominally assessing fetal position, assessing for abnormal vaginal bleeding, and assessing amniotic fluid status are all recommended nursing practices prior to the initial vaginal examination. Historically, rectal examinations were the primary method used to assess the pregnant woman, but almost universally the vaginal examination is now the preferred method. In many teaching institutions the physician or resident primarily assumes this responsibility of examination, but in any other facility it is common for the nurse to perform the vaginal examination.

For this procedure the client lies on her back with her knees flexed and heels together; her knees then fall outward laterally. The nurse drapes the client so that she is well protected, leaving the perineal region exposed. Sterile gloves are donned by the examiner. Before the fingers are introduced into the vagina, the labia are opened widely to minimize possible contamination of the examining fingers if they should come in contact with the inner surfaces of the labia and the margins of the hymen. The index and middle fingers are lubricated with K-Y jelly; it is important not to touch the lubricant tube with the fingers. An assistant can squeeze the lubricant onto the examiner's fingers. Then the index and second fingers of the examining hand are gently introduced into the vagina (Fig. 25-3). Vaginal examination is more reliable than rectal because the cervix, the fontanels, and other structures can be readily palpated.

Nursing Diagnosis

Admission process is the time the nurse starts assessing the client and initiates the care plan. The following is a list of potential nursing diagnoses that may be used:

1. Alteration in comfort: acute pain related to uterine contractions
2. Fear related to hospital surroundings
3. Fear related to impending labor and birth
4. Alteration in tissue perfusion: placental perfusion to fetus decreased due to supine position
5. Sleep pattern disturbance
6. Knowledge deficit related to expectations in labor
7. Knowledge deficit related to hospital procedures
8. Knowledge deficit related to the process of labor and appropriate relaxation techniques
9. Ineffective individual coping related to lack of support systems

The birth of a baby is viewed as a major event in life so that the labor and delivery nurse may be addressing the care plan not only for the mother and fetus but for other family members such as father, grandparents, aunts, uncles, and friends. From the above list of diagnoses, numbers 2, 3, 5, 6, and 7 might apply to the other family members.

Planning/Intervention

Psychosocial Consideration

Because contact with the client during the labor and delivery process is short term, the nurse is faced with the problem of providing high-quality care in a short space of time. The key appears to be the ability to use whatever time is available, whether it be 5 minutes or

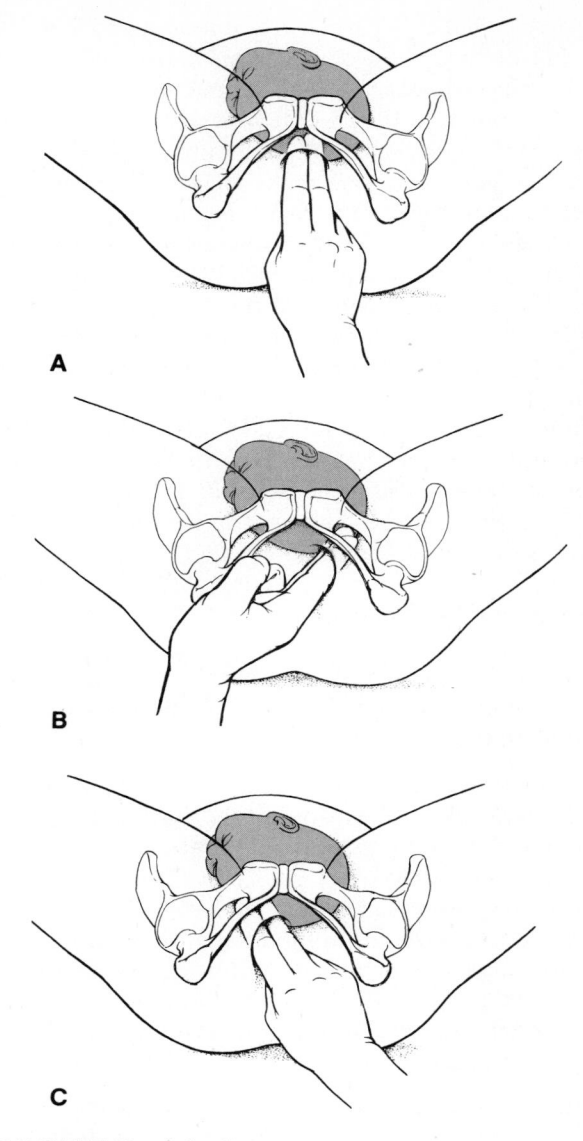

A

B

C

F I G U R E   2 5 - 3

Vaginal examination. (*A*) Determining the station and palpating the sagittal suture. (*B*) Identifying the posterior fontanel. (*C*) Identifying the anterior fontanel.

an hour, to provide an atmosphere of receptivity to the client's needs. The ability to determine needs lies in the perceptions that underlie the assessment and diagnosis portions of the nursing process. When effective care is implemented, the nurse's facility with therapeutic communication plus technical understanding and skill are key issues.

There has been a good deal of time and effort spent in nursing research to determine the needs of clients, especially the needs above and beyond those related directly to physiological and pathologic conditions. These needs have generally been classified as "emotional" or "psychosocial." Whatever their label they are especially important for consideration with the maternity client and support system.

Support Person.

Rarely do we see women having their babies without some sort of support person present. This person can be the father of the baby, a family member (*i.e.*, mother or sister), or a close friend. This person may have attended prepared childbirth classes with the client and may be ready to assume the role of coach during the labor and delivery. The converse is also true; the support person may not have attended classes and will need, as will the client, teaching on ways to relax and cope with labor.

Culture may dictate the amount of involvement the father is to have in the birth experience. Nursing needs to assess the family and be respectful of their choice and not judgmental if it differs from what the staff feels is the appropriate way for the father and family to act.

First Impressions.

The kind of greeting the client receives as she enters the labor and delivery unit is extremely important and sets the tone for future interaction with the health team. Some institutions permit the father to accompany the mother to the area. Others prefer to admit the mother first and then let the father join her. When the father is present, the nurse should be mindful that he is to be considered and welcomed in an appropriate way, as is the mother.

The mother needs to be made to feel welcomed, expected, and necessary. More hospitals are allowing not only the father to accompany the mother but also other support persons whom the mother may want to have with her during labor and delivery.

Orientation.

The mother and the father need to know what is expected of them and what they in turn can expect. The mother can then be helped, if necessary, to change to the hospital gown and can be made comfortable in a chair or, if she wishes, in bed.

The nurse can begin an orientation to the process of labor as well as to the general environment. There is no set form or content for this orientation and no set time for the introduction and the continuation of this process; rather the nurse must first explore what the parents do know about the environment and the labor process, in order to judge what needs to be introduced, reinforced, and so on, and when the most appropriate time to do this would be. An easy conversational manner may be employed rather than a rapid-fire explanation of dos and don'ts.

The rationale for any procedures or restrictions is always given. The client must not be overloaded with too many stimuli at one time and should be allowed to absorb any new information and explanation before additional material is presented. The nurse can structure the situation to allow the client to "feed back" information, so as to reveal how much the mother really understands.

Generally, the mother and the father need to know what procedures and activities will be performed and the reason for them. In addition, the couple should know the limits of the mother's activity and what restrictions of food and fluids there will be. What the client and the father can expect regarding the progress of labor should be included also (*i.e.*, what will be happening physically, how the mother will be feeling, and how she and her partner can participate in the labor experience).

As implied, this orientation continues throughout the entire course of labor and delivery. The nurse determines when and how each phase is to be instituted, according to the cues given by the mother and father.

Establishment of the Nurse–Client Relationship.

For many young women in labor, admission to the maternity unit may mark her first acquaintance with hospitals as a patient. Her immediate reaction may be one of strangeness, loneliness, and homesickness, particularly if the father is not permitted to stay with her in the labor room. Regardless of the amount of preparation for this event, whether she is happy or unhappy, whether she wants the baby or not, every mother enters labor with a certain amount of normal tension and anxiety. Moreover, some mothers are thoroughly afraid of the whole process. This may be attributed in part to the fact that the mother's preparation for childbearing has been limited, or she may have been reared in an environment fraught with mysteries and old wives' tales about childbirth. If she has had children previously, she may have had unfortunate and fear-producing experiences. All these factors make her fear understandable.

Rapport, Empathy, and Identification.

One of the most often talked about, yet not well understood, concepts deemed essential to an effective nurse–client relationship is *rapport*. Rapport may be thought of as a relationship consisting in interrelated thoughts and feelings that include empathy, compassion, interest, and respect for each individual as a unique human being.

One of the crucial components of this type of relationship is *empathy*. This is the ability to enter into the life of another person, to accurately perceive her *current* feelings and their meanings.[11] The idea of currency is an important one here. Empathy must involve understanding the current feelings of a client, not her feelings of sometime in the past. Previous perceptions based on earlier experiences with a client or clients similar to her can be misleading if they block understanding of what the client is currently experiencing.

Identification has been described as the mechanism that enables a person to take up any attitude toward another's mental life. Certain changes take place in the ego structure when this mechanism is employed, resulting in an expansion of ego boundaries to include the attitude once observed in the other and now made a part of one's self. This type of identification is seen in children as they learn their various social roles.

However, in the therapeutic relationship, the altered ego structure is only a temporary experience and remains "ego segregated" but available for reality testing and further thought. Certainly to be able to identify and share with another and then revert to one's own identity requires flexibility of the ego boundaries, and this flexibility can become enhanced with repeated use of the mechanism.

After attempting to experience the client's feelings, the nurse must be able to step back, that is, reestablish normal ego boundaries related to reality. Intellectual processes can then be used to review what has occurred from three perspectives: what is known about the client, what is known about herself, and what is known from theory. Thus, subjectivity is converted into objectivity and permits valid assessment of needs and problems.

For effective nursing therapy to be instituted, empathy must operate within a sound conceptual framework, backed by theoretical knowledge and clinical experience. It is a valuable aid in designing the implementing care, but is not to be considered a substitute for careful planning and rational evaluation. Unfortunately, we do not know if and how empathy can be taught or learned. We do know that the ability to use the identification mechanism has something very vital to do with the empathy process. More research needs to be directed to the identification-empathy-rapport linkage.[3]

Physical Preparation

Vulvar and Perineal Preparation. The aim in shaving or clipping and washing the vulva is to cleanse and disinfect the immediate area around the vagina, to visualize the perineal area better, and to prevent any contamination from entering the birth canal. During labor, pathogenic bacteria can ascend the birth canal; thus, every effort is made to protect the client from intrapartum infection. Research over the years has demonstrated that shaving the perineum actually enhances the possibility of infection, probably owing to the myriad of nicks that can occur in the shaving process. When clipping the hair is compared with not clipping, data indicate no difference in infection rates.[12-17] Nevertheless, in many institutions, shaving or clipping the perineal hair continues. Some physicians do not require that the mons pubis be shaved because of the discomfort that the regrowth of the hair causes; they feel that clipping the hair suffices. Other physicians do not order the perineum shaved and simply have the area washed well with a bacteriostatic soap.

When the perineum is to be shaved a pad is placed under the buttocks and the client assumes the same position she was in for the vaginal examination. Lighting must be optimal, and the nurse asks the woman if she has any warts or moles that she should be made aware of prior to shaving. The nurse may want to put on gloves for this procedure.

The vulvar hair is lathered prior to shaving to facilitate the procedure and to make it more comfortable for the client. An ordinary safety razor is used. The shave is started at the top of the labia majora. The direction of the stroke goes from above downward as the area of the vulva is shaved. The skin can be stretched above each downward stroke and the razor permitted to move smoothly over the skin without undue pressure.

When the entire area anterior to an imaginary line drawn through the base of the perineal body has been shaved, the client can turn to her side to allow the anal area to be completely shaved. With the upper leg well flexed, the anal area is lathered and shaved, again with a front to back stroke. It must always be remembered that anything that has passed over the anal region must not be returned near the vulvar orifice. If an enema is to be given it is at this time, with the client positioned on her left side (see next section).

In washing the genitals, the nurse first thoroughly cleanses the surrounding areas, using sterile sponges or disposable washcloths for each area, and gradually works in toward the vestibule. The strokes must be from above downward and away from the introitus. Special attention should be paid to separating the vulvar folds to remove the smegma that may have accumulated in the folds of the labia minora or at the base of the clitoris. Finally, the region around the anus is cleansed. The client is instructed not to touch the genital area after being cleansed.

Enema. Until recently, an enema was a routine admission procedure. It was deemed a necessity to prevent the presence of stool in the rectum, which might impede the descent of the presenting part, and also to ensure that no stool would be expelled during delivery, which might contaminate the sterile field. It was also thought to enhance the strength of the contractions. However, experience and research indicate that the enema is not as necessary as once believed. In some institutions, the decision to give an enema is left to the nurses on the basis of their clinical judgment. In other hospitals an enema is still required as prescribed. In any case, it is wise for the nurse to ascertain, during the history taking, if the client has had a recent bowel movement. If she had had a normal evacuation that day, an enema is probably not necessary. If the client is constipated, an enema can be helpful. However, if she is having diarrhea, the procedure is certainly not necessary and the possibility of an infection must be considered.

The type of enema may vary from warm tap water using an enema can or bag to a disposable type that

Admission of the Woman Into Labor Unit

Nursing Objectives

1. Assess the client for maternal and fetal well-being.
2. Make the client, father, and other support persons welcome in the labor and delivery unit during admission procedures.
3. Explain physical surroundings, procedures, and expectations to them.

Assessment	Potential Nursing Diagnosis	Planning/Intervention	Evaluation
Assess knowledge of: Preparation for labor process Hospital procedures Hospital surroundings	Knowledge deficit related to: Expectations during labor Hospital procedures and surroundings Preparation for labor relaxation methods Fear	Establish relationship with client and father Find out how client wants to be referred to (*e.g.*, first name) Provide an orientation to unit and labor process Convey that the couple is expected and welcomed Individualize teaching plan to cover expectations and restrictions of the environment, review or teach relaxation methods, answer questions	Client and father are familiar with the new environment and settle in Client understands equipment, procedures, expectations Client uses appropriate relaxation methods for stage of labor Client and family feel rapport with staff
Maternal			
Frequency, duration, intensity of contractions Status of bag of waters Character and amount of show Vital signs Bowel/bladder patterns Allergies to medication Time of last ingestion	Alteration in comfort: acute pain related to uterine contractions	Take nursing history Record and report findings as appropriate Begin to provide comfort measures as needed Discuss choice of anesthesia for delivery and use of analgesia in labor	Client understands use of analgesia and anesthesia Client chooses type to be used Appropriate comfort measures are provided
Fetal			
EDC, fundal height Fetal position, FHR		Document EDC and appropriateness of fundal height to gestational age, record FHR/fetoscope/Doppler/fetal monitor	Fetus at term, vertex position, appropriate fundal height, FHR within normal limits
Admission Procedures			
General physical assessment Vaginal exam, perineal clip or enema, if ordered	Alteration in tissue perfusion: placental perfusion to fetus decreased secondary to maternal supine position Sleep pattern disturbance Ineffective individual coping related to lack of support systems	Discourage supine position Perform physical assessment Complete admitting procedures, as indicated Provide quiet environment for resting, if indicated Encourage presence of support person(s), if none available, provide support	Client avoids supine position and FHR is maintained Client rests, if needed Support person is at bedside

comes with the solution prepared and with a prelubricated tip. The nurse uses the same principles in administering the enema as for any other client. However, it may be more difficult to insert the tube because of the pressure of the presenting part of the fetus or because of hemorrhoids that may accompany pregnancy.

Hemorrhoids or the strength of the contractions may make the enema uncomfortable for the client, and it is essential that she be informed that the nurse is aware of the possible discomfort. To aid in comfort the nurse can stop the enema infusion during the contractions by simply pinching the tubing or ceasing to squeeze the disposable enema container. The client is encouraged to hold the enema as long as possible before expelling. The nurse then will need to chart that the procedure has been done and the results of the enema.

The nurse needs to be aware that soapsuds enemas should not be used and have been associated with acute colitis, bowel perforation, gangrene, and even anaphylaxis.[18]

First Stage of Labor

The first stage of labor (dilating stage) begins with the first symptoms of true labor and ends with the complete dilatation of the cervix. The physician examines the client early in labor and sees her from time to time throughout the first stage but may not be in constant attendance at this time.

During labor, assessments of the fetal heart rate and vaginal examinations determine whether the fetus is in good condition and that the mother is making steady progress. Furthermore, the rate of progress often gives some indication as to when delivery is to be expected. During this stage, the nurse is in constant attendance, safeguarding the welfare of the mother and fetus and notifying the physician of the progress of labor.

Assessment

Vaginal Examinations

The frequency with which vaginal examinations are required during labor depends on the individual case; often one or two such examinations are sufficient, while in some instances more are required. The nurse who stays with the mother constantly becomes increasingly skillful in the ability to follow the progress of labor to a great extent by careful evaluation of the character of the uterine contractions, the amount of show, the progressive descent of the area on the abdomen where fetal heart sounds are heard, and the mother's overall response to her physical labor.

Uterine Contractions

Even today many young women approach childbirth with fear of pain. It is no easy task to dispel this age-old fear, but throughout the childbirth experience a conscious effort must be made to instill a wholesome point of view in the mother. The nurse will want to avoid the use of the word *pain* whenever possible because of the very connotation of the word.

Sociocultural factors play an important part in the meaning and interpretation and expression of pain for clients. While pain is basically a physiological phenomenon, the meaning pain has and the kinds of responses to pain that are deemed appropriate are partly matters of cultural prescription. Cultural orientations, social conditioning, and sociocultural sanctioning play a large part in molding patterns of response to painful experiences which are modal (*i.e.,* occur most frequently) in a group, and these modal patterns are meaningful in terms of the values and beliefs of a particular group. Therefore, the culture or subculture from which a person comes conditions the formation of her particular reaction patterns to pain, and a knowledge of a group's attitudes toward pain is extremely important to the understanding of the reaction of a particular member of that group.

It is important to remember, however, that as labor progresses, the contractions become increasingly painful. Therefore, it is the nurse's responsibility to help the mother distinguish between the *fear and anticipation* of pain and the *discomfort or actual pain* that she may be experiencing, and to help her cope effectively.

Timing the Contractions.   Frequency, duration, and intensity of the contractions should be watched closely and recorded whether or not an electronic fetal monitor is used. As labor progresses, the character of the contractions changes. They become stronger in intensity, last longer (a duration of 30 sec–60 sec), and come closer together (at a frequency of every 2 min–3 min). If the monitor is not being used, one effective method the nurse can employ to time contractions is to keep her fingers lightly on the fundus. The fingers are recommended because they are more sensitive than the palm. However, for some people the whole hand is helpful. It should be emphasized that enough of the fingers should be used to ensure adequate contact with the abdomen; too slight a contact does not enable the nurse to ascertain the contractions accurately.

Assessing contractions in this manner enables the nurse to detect the contraction, as it begins, by the gradual tensing and rising forward of the fundus and to feel the contraction through its three phases until the uterus relaxes again. The inexperienced nurse can get some idea of how a contraction feels under her fingertips by contracting her own biceps. First, the forearm should be extended and the fingertips of the hand on the opposite side placed on the biceps. Then the arm is gradually flexed until the muscle becomes very hard, held a few seconds, and gradually extended. This should take about 30 seconds to simulate a uterine contraction.

It is not reliable to rely on the mother to indicate when a contraction begins, because often she is unaware of it for perhaps 5 or 10 seconds, sometimes even until the contraction reaches its acme. It is important to observe the frequency and duration of the contractions and to be assured that the uterine muscle relaxes completely after each contraction.

As the labor approaches the transition, the contractions become very strong, last for about 60 seconds, and occur at 2- to 3-minute intervals.

If any contraction lasts longer than 90 seconds and is not followed by a rest interval with complete relaxation of the uterine muscle, this should be reported to the physician immediately. The implications for both the mother and her infant can be severe (see Chap. 38).

Show

Show is a mucoid discharge from the cervix that is present after the mucous plug has been dislodged. As progressive effacement and dilatation of the cervix occur, the show becomes blood tinged owing to the rupture of the superficial capillaries. The presence of an increased amount of bloody show, blood-stained mucus and not actual bleeding, suggests that rapid progress may be taking place and the client should be assessed. Often in conjunction with the increase in bloody show are strong uterine contractions and the urge to push. If by vaginal examination the woman is found to be close to delivery, the physician is notified.

Vital Signs

It is recommended that blood pressure be evaluated every hour and temperature, pulse, and respiration rate every 4 hours, or more frequently as necessary, depending on the clinical situation.

Fetal Heart Tones

Repeated auscultation of the fetal heart sounds constitutes one of the most important responsibilities during the first and second stages of labor if a monitor is not used. During the early period of the first stage of labor, the nurse records the fetal heart rate every hour; once good labor is established, this rate is recorded every half hour or even more often if indicated. During the second stage the fetal heart rate is checked and recorded every 5 minutes. The fetal heart rate is checked immediately following the rupture of membranes, regardless of whether they rupture spontaneously or are artificially ruptured by the physician. With the gush of water that ensues, there is a possibility that the cord may be prolapsed, and any indication of fetal distress from pressure on the umbilical cord can thereby be de-

tected by a decrease in the fetal heart rate. In the past decade, the electronic fetal monitor has been introduced and is widely used in the hospital setting for the assessment of fetal well-being and evaluation of uterine contractions during labor. A thorough discussion of this device can be found in Chapter 43.

Nursing Diagnosis

Updating the nursing-care plan is an ongoing process that is done in correlation with the client's progress in labor. Attending to the immediate needs of the client, assuring comfort, and maintaining maternal and fetal well-being may be the primary areas the nurse is addressing, whereas other identified diagnoses may not be readdressed until the fourth stage of labor or during the postpartum period. Below is a list of potential nursing diagnoses; nursing interventions and evaluation criteria are found in the nursing care plan on pages 276 and 277.

1. Alteration in comfort: pain related to uterine contractions
2. Fear related to impending labor and birth
3. Alteration in tissue perfusion: placental, decreased, secondary to maternal position
4. Sleep pattern disturbance
5. Fluid volume deficit related to decreased fluid intake
6. Alteration in oral mucous membrane related to mouth breathing
7. Alteration in nutrition: less than body requirements related to onset of labor and need to decrease oral intake
8. Self-care deficit related to immobility during labor (toileting, hygiene)
9. Ineffective individual/family coping related to hospitalization
10. Ineffective individual coping related to inappropriate relaxation/breathing patterns
11. Ineffective individual coping related to lack of support systems
12. Ineffective family coping related to client being in pain
13. Knowledge deficit related to the process of labor and appropriate relaxation techniques

Planning/Intervention

Psychosocial Considerations

As already emphasized, it is important for the nurse to have an empathic supportive attitude toward the mother in order to interpret the progress of labor and perform certain technical procedures skillfully. It should be pointed out that "supportive care" includes not only emotional support but also aspects of physical care that, in the total context of care, contribute to the well-being and the comfort of the mother and hence to her emotional equilibrium. Thus, a sponge bath, oral hygiene, a back rub, an explanation before a procedure, and so on all enhance the mother's comfort and help her to feel that she is a special, worthwhile person. The nursing staff must not just walk into the labor room, review the fetal monitor, and walk out.

The Effective Use of Touch.

Many of the physical-care activities that nurses perform consist, in part at least, in "laying on of hands," which is known to be necessary and helpful to clients in maintaining or reachieving good health. These activities can be valuable entrées in establishing and maintaining rapport and an effective relationship. Even the intrusive procedures that are so often painful or distasteful, if done with gentleness and skill, show the client that her dignity and integrity are respected.

Related to this laying on of hands is the effectiveness of the use of touch. Although this has not been explored to any great degree scientifically, its importance was recognized as far back as the mid-19th century. More recently, research indicates that the client's ability to work effectively with her labor contractions increased when extensive physical contact was introduced and then decreased when physical contact was withdrawn.[19] This contact can take the form of a back rub, allowing the client to grasp the nurse's hand, stroking the client's brow, and so on. Indeed, many of the relaxation techniques practiced in the prepared childbirth classes rely on the use of this sense.

However, touch need not be used indiscriminately; excessive or inappropriate touching is offensive to many people. The need varies from person to person, and the woman indicates which type of touch is helpful and who is the most appropriate person to give it. The nurse must use professional judgment regarding its use, and rapport with the client helps to indicate a correct decision. This type of communication can be a way of demonstrating the nurse's concern and empathy; especially when verbal communication is difficult or impossible. It is also an effective means of incorporating the partner into the care and the support of his mate.

Providing Assurance.

The mother who has attended antepartal classes that have included exercise and relaxation techniques is usually better prepared for labor, but nevertheless she needs to be coached in using the techniques that enable her to cooperate with the natural forces of labor. During early labor the client usually prefers to move about the room and frequently is more at ease sitting in a comfortable chair. She can be permitted and encouraged to do this and whatever else seems to be most relaxing and pleasant to her.

Once labor is well established, the mother should not be left alone. The morale of women in labor is sometimes hopelessly shattered, regardless of whether or not they have been prepared for labor during pregnancy, when they are left by themselves over long periods. During labor the mother is more sensitive to the behavior of those about her, particularly in relation to her perception of how much concern the personnel about her show for her safety and well-being. As labor progresses, there is a normal narrowing of the phenomenal field, an "inward turning," which results in easy distortion of stimuli and perception. For instance, careless remarks dropped in conversation often are misinterpreted as indicative of negligence or lack of feeling. It is important to remember that comments and laughter overheard in the corridor outside the client's room may contribute to her uneasiness. Therefore, the nurse must be on guard against unfortunate happenings of this kind.

The nurse will want to be aware that her own anxieties in the situation may be communicated to the client. The process of labor and the forthcoming delivery produce normal anxieties that are no more than a healthy anticipation of the events to come (in both client and nurse). *Thus, most clients tolerate their labor better if they are told the kind of progress that is being made and are assured that they are doing a good job working with their contractions.* This is part and parcel of the continuing orientation to the labor process that was mentioned earlier.

Another point that is apropos here is the usefulness and the effectiveness of suggestion for the mother in labor. The nurse can use this suggestibility to great advantage in her supportive care, since the mother responds very readily to suggestions, especially in early labor. The groundwork can be laid at this time for the more complicated instructions that may be necessary later in labor concerning relaxation, breathing techniques, and the management of pain.

Psychosocial Support During Contractions.

Particularly during the late active phase there is a need for human contact—someone to hold onto—during the severe contractions. The mother responds less well to other physical contact, stroking, sponging, and so on; she may even say, "Leave me alone," meaning, of course, "Don't disturb me." However, if it is helpful for her to have someone's hand to hold, she should be allowed to do this if she indicates the need.

Physical Comfort

Positioning.

Since the introduction of the electronic fetal monitors many hospitals attach the monitor to the client routinely for fetal assessment during labor. The mother must be in bed for this equipment to function appropriately. This, of course, limits the mother's mobility. The reason for the use of the monitor needs to be explained to the client so that she can understand why her activity is restricted and will not become unduly alarmed. If the client is requesting to ambulate it is important to get an order from the physician. Most facilities allow ambulation if the presenting part is engaged or the bag of waters is intact. The mother should come back to the labor room for periodic auscultation of the fetal heart rate (*i.e.*, every 30 minutes). It should be noted that the newer fetal monitors with improved electronics allow for better tracings on the external mode and allow more maternal movement to positions of comfort. Changes in position and transducer adjustments are noted on the strip chart.

If monitors are not employed, the client can be encouraged to assume any position that is comfortable for her, such as side, squatting, all fours, sitting (Fig. 25-4). A woman should not labor on her back. These other positions have been found to enhance the efficacy of the labor contractions, whereas in the supine position there is less uteroplacental perfusion, causing contractions to be more frequent but less intense (Fig. 25-5).[9,20,21]

Dealing with Contractions.
The contribution that the nurse can make in the management of pain during labor and delivery is discussed in Chapter 26. However, we would like to reiterate a few of the major points here to reinforce them. We know that studies of pain have demonstrated that the anticipation of pain can raise the anxiety level significantly so as to lower pain tolerance. Thus, the client reacts sooner to even minimal pain stimuli. The pain is subjectively intensified and

even a slight amount of pain seems to be much greater. Furthermore, other sensations may be misinterpreted as pain (*e.g.*, pressure, stretching), which explains why the digital examinations and even the pressure of the nurse's fingers on the abdomen as she manually times contractions "hurt." Therefore, "everything" is painful, and the heightening of the anticipation of pain in turn increases the response to pain, and soon a vicious cycle is established.

The nurse can help to break this cycle or prevent it from becoming established by intervening at the anticipation–anxiety junction. This is done by reminding the client that a contraction is over (and the pain is gone) and that since another contraction is not expected for several minutes this is the time for her to rest and to relax. The anxiety related to the anticipation of pain is then lowered or eliminated (the mother knows that she will be free from pain for several minutes and can rest), and the subjective intensification is diminished. It is obvious that the nurse or some other reliable person must be in continuous attendance to do this.

Breathing Techniques.
Since during the first stage of labor the uterine contractions are involuntary and uncontrolled by the client, it is futile for her to "bear down" with her abdominal muscles, because this only leads to exhaustion. The mother who has been prepared for childbirth has been schooled in breathing techniques, such as diaphragmatic breathing or rapid, shallow costal breathing, and with coaching from her partner or her nurse is usually able to accomplish conscious relaxation.

The Unprepared Mother.
A different situation exists with the unprepared mother. These mothers are

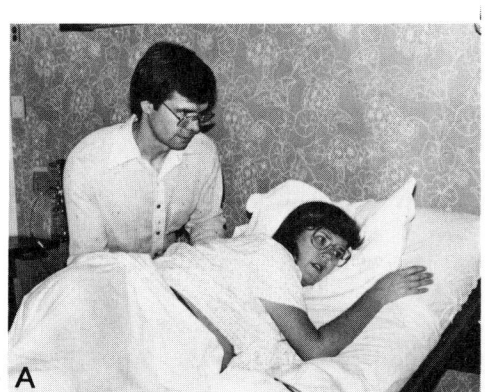
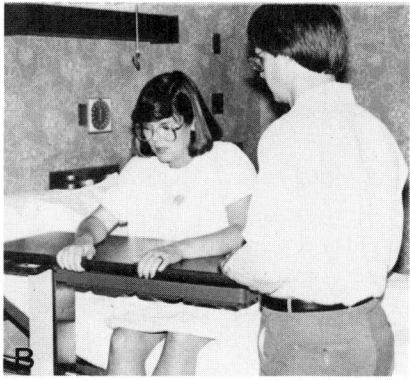
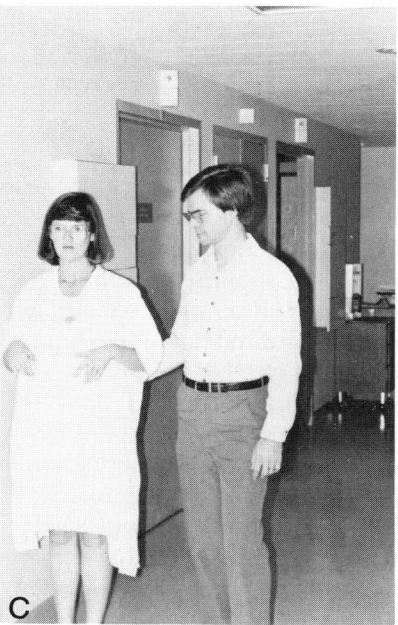

FIGURE 25-4

Examples of three types of positions that may be assumed during labor. Each couple chooses the best position for them. (Courtesy of Memorial Medical Center of Long Beach, Long Beach, California)

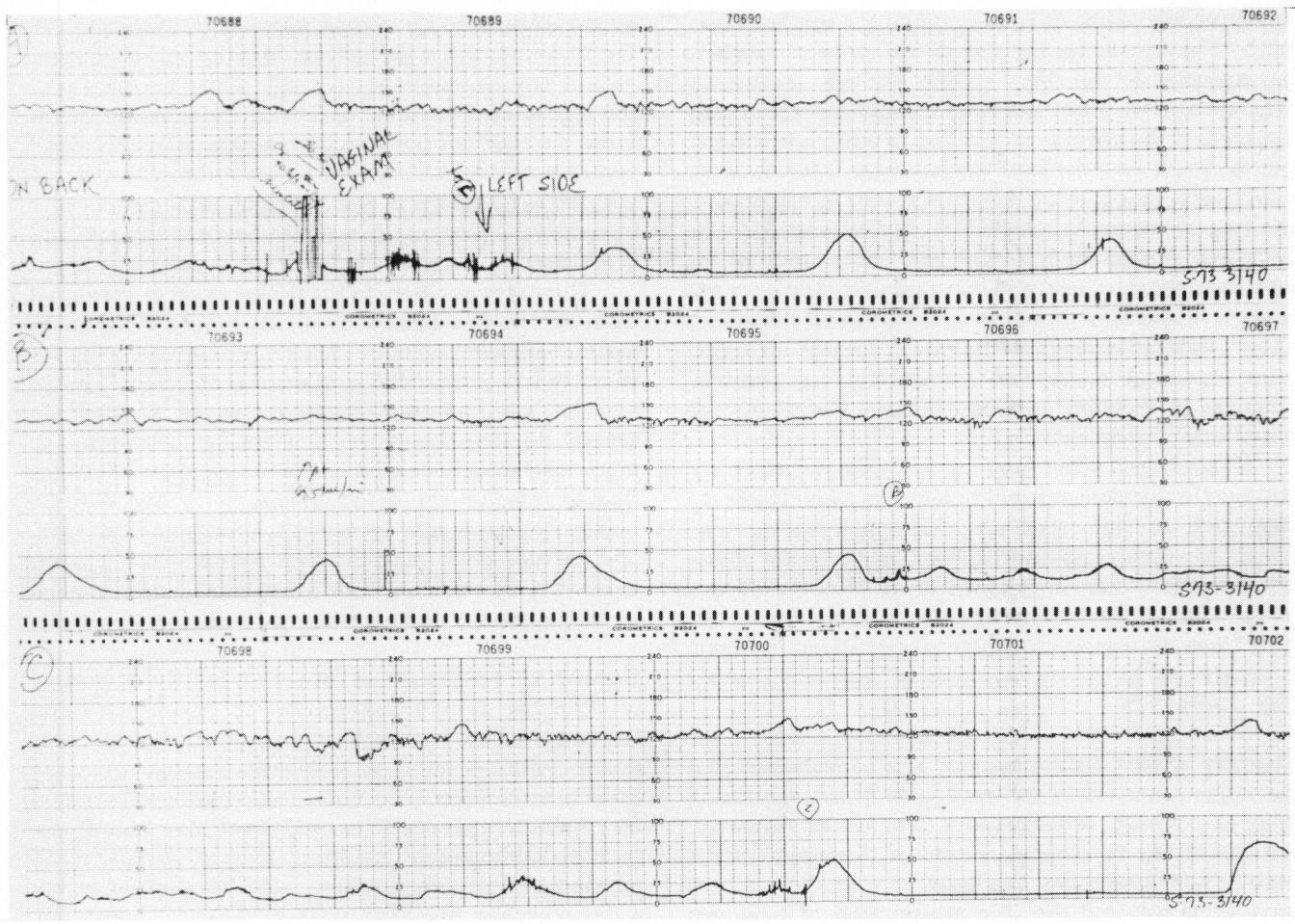

FIGURE 25-5

Uterine contractions. (*A*) Frequent uterine contractions are occurring. When the client is turned to her left side, the contractions become less frequent and increase in strength. (*B*) The woman has turned and is lying on her back; the contractions have become frequent and smaller. (*C*) Again on her left side, the contractions are spaced out as before, in *A*. (Freeman R, Garite T: Fetal Heart Rate Monitoring. Baltimore, Williams & Wilkins, © 1981)

often best helped to relax by encouraging and coaching them to keep breathing slowly and evenly during the early contractions and then to assume a pattern of more rapid and shallow breathing that is most comfortable to them during the late active phase. They very often need to be reminded not to hold their breath during the contractions.

One cannot expect perfection in breathing techniques with these clients; however, this activity gives the inexperienced mother a point of concentration, and her feeling that she is actually participating and "controlling" her labor to some degree is helpful to her. Most mothers in labor, whether they are "prepared" or not, want to cooperate, and the calm, kind, firm guidance of an interested nurse can do much to help the mother use her contractions effectively.

Fluid and Food Intake. The practice regarding the intake of fluid and food varies greatly. Therefore, the wishes of the physician in charge need to be ascertained before proceeding.

In the hospital setting, it is customary to limit oral intake to ice chips. If the client is admitted in the latent phase of labor the physician may order a clear liquid diet. The client in active labor is not given solid or liquid foods, since digestion is delayed during labor. The nurse may increase client comfort by providing frequent mouth care, using a washcloth or prepared swabs to moisten the mouth and lips. The use of a lip balm is also encouraged. Hydration and nourishment in prolonged labor should be provided by intravenous solutions (*e.g.*, 5% dextrose in lactated Ringer's), which also minimize acidosis and electrolyte imbalance.

Bladder. The client can be asked to void at least every 2 to 3 hours. The mother laboring often attributes all of her discomfort to the intensity of uterine contractions and therefore is unaware that it is the pressure of a full bladder that has increased her discomfort. In addition to causing unnecessary discomfort, a full bladder may be a serious impediment to labor or the cause of urinary retention in the puerperium. If the distended bladder can be palpated above the symphysis pubis and the client is unable to void, the physician is to be so informed. Straight catheterization may be prescribed in such cases.

Progression of Active Phase of Labor. As labor progresses into the active phase the woman's mood changes and she "gets down to business." She begins to concentrate on her breathing techniques and needs assistance from the father. She will need help to get in a position of comfort. Regardless of how diligently the mother has practiced the various breathing and relaxing techniques during pregnancy, or the level of her understanding about the physiology of labor, the situation is changed somewhat during active labor. Encouragement should be given to both the mother and the father. The nurse remains with the client, providing care in an organized, calm manner; instructions need to be short and direct. Nursing-care measures include mouth care, keeping ice chips available, placing a cool washcloth on the mother's forehead, keeping the perineum clean and dry, lowering the lights and keeping the environment quiet, providing counterpressure on the sacral area during contractions, and updating the physician and family members on the progress. Also the nurse may also want to suggest that the father take some nourishment for himself before the actual birth. As labor progresses (*i.e.*, 8 cm–10 cm) the nurse should continue to encourage correct breathing techniques and assist the client not to bear down prematurely. The client should be reassured that she will shortly be completely dilated and will then be ready to start to push.

Second Stage of Labor

The second stage of labor begins with complete dilatation of the cervix and ends with delivery of the baby. The complete dilatation of the cervix can be definitely confirmed only by a vaginal examination. However, the experienced nurse is often able to suspect complete dilatation by observing changes in her client's behavior, particularly if these findings are correlated with knowledge of the client's parity, the speed of any previous labors and the present labor, and the anticipated size of the baby. The median duration of the second stage of labor has been shown to be 50 minutes for the primigravida and 20 minutes for the multipara.[8] The length of the second stage can vary considerably.

Assessment

There are certain signs and symptoms, both behavioral and physical, that herald the onset of the second stage of labor. These are to be watched for carefully (see Signs and Symptoms of Second Stage). Reporting any or all of these manifestations promptly allows enough time to prepare the mother for the delivery without rushing and provides an opportunity to cleanse and drape the mother properly. If these signs are overlooked, a precipitous delivery may occur without benefit of medical attention. In the traditional setting, in which different rooms are used for labor and the delivery, the primigravida is usually not taken to the delivery room when the cervix is fully dilated and in fact may push in the labor room for some time before transfer. In contrast, the multipara should be taken to the delivery room much sooner, often at 7 cm to 8 cm of dilatation. The use of epidural anesthesia during labor usually delays transfer of the multipara also and she may even push in the labor room for awhile, much like the primigravida.

Nursing Diagnosis

As the client begins the second stage of labor she begins to realize that the dilatation phase of labor is done. Now the final part of labor, the pushing stage, is about to begin. Below is a list of potential nursing diagnoses.

1. Ineffective individual coping related to physical exhaustion in response to labor
2. Alteration in comfort: increased pain related to lower fetal position and uterine contractions
3. Fear related to new surroundings.

Nursing interventions and evaluation criteria are found in the nursing care plan, The Woman During Second Stage of Labor.

Planning/Intervention

Methods for Bearing Down

During this period the client will be requested to exert her abdominal forces and bear down. In most cases bearing-down efforts are reflexive and spontaneous in the second stage of labor, but occasionally the mother does not employ her expulsive forces to good advantage, particularly if she has had epidural anesthesia.

Positions and Pushing Efforts. The positions used during the second stage of labor must be such that the presenting part is in alignment with the axis of the pelvis. The student may find that in the hospital setting the semi-Fowler and lateral positions are frequently used. Other positions, such as squatting, kneeling, standing, and semisetting, are becoming more popular

(text continued on page 479)

The Woman/Family During First Stage of Labor

Nursing Objectives
1. Keep the client informed of her progress in labor.
2. Keep the client comfortable through comfort measures done by the nurse and support person(s).
3. Make sure the support person/family is oriented to hospital environment and expectations.
4. Keep the support person/family informed of progress in labor.
5. Give support to the family as indicated.

Assessment	Potential Nursing Diagnosis	Planning/Intervention	Evaluation
Monitor labor, contractions, FHR, vital signs	Alteration in tissue perfusion: placental, secondary to maternal position	Check vital signs regularly per hospital policy and clinical needs Attach fetal monitor or time contractions Check FHR for rate, accelerations, variability, decelerations Avoid supine position	Woman has vital signs within normal limits FHR maintains normal rate Woman's labor progresses
Monitor intake and output	Fluid volume deficit related to decreased fluid intake Alteration in oral mucous membrane related to mouth breathing Alteration in nutrition less than body requirement related to restriction of intake during labor	Give ice chips prn Maintain adequate parenteral intake (125 ml/hr) Encourage voiding q2–3 h; catheterize if needed Record intake and output Encourage use of lip balm Provide mouth care Instruct/reinforce proper breathing techniques	Woman's mouth and lips are moist Woman's bladder remains normal
Determine which comfort measures are most helpful	Alteration in comfort; acute pain related to labor contractions Self-care deficit related to immobility during labor (toileting, hygiene)	Rub back and change client's position and linen as necessary Apply cool washcloth to face Encourage rest Encourage frequent voiding, giving assistance to bathroom or with bedpan Give analgesia if client requests and as ordered by physician	Client breathes appropriately with contractions Client relaxes between contractions Client states what comfort measures are most helpful
Determine client's need for explanations and emotional support as indicated	Sleep pattern disturbance related to labor Ineffective individual coping related to inappropriate relaxation/breathing patterns	Keep explanations and instructions short and simple Encourage mother to sleep/rest between contractions Decrease environmental stimulus	Couple changes breathing patterns to coincide with stage of labor Couple follows instruction with minimum of difficulty Client rests when able

(continued)

Assessment	Potential Nursing Diagnosis	Planning/Intervention	Evaluation
Determine support person's ability to coach and support the client	Knowledge deficit related to coaching role	Allow couple time together	Support person assists mother in coping with labor
Determine support person's needs	Ineffective individual/family coping related to hospitalization for the onset of labor	Encourage support person's participation in care	Support person feels a part of the labor process
	Ineffective family coping related to client being in pain	Explain labor process as things progress to client and support person	Client benefits from support person's presence and support
		Keep support person(s) in waiting room up to date	
		Assist client in changing breathing techniques as labor progresses	
		Identify and reinforce adaptive coping behavior	
		Provide support to the coach (refreshments, breaks) and reinforce appropriate behavior	

Signs and Symptoms of Second Stage

1. The client begins to bear down of her own accord; this is caused by a reflex when the head begins to press on the perineal floor.

2. Her mood of increasing apprehension, which has been building since the contractions began, deepens; she becomes more serious and may appear bewildered by the force of the contractions.

3. There is usually a sudden increase in show, which is more blood tinged.

4. The client may become increasingly irritable and unwilling to be touched; she may cry if disturbed.

5. The mother thinks that she needs to defecate. This symptom is due to pressure of the head on the perineal floor and consequently against the rectum.

6. Although she has been "working" successfully with her contractions during most of her labor, the uncertainty that she has been experiencing (since 6 cm–8 cm cervical dilatation) as to her ability to cope with the contractions may become overwhelming; she is frustrated and feels unable to manage if left alone.

7. The membranes may rupture, with discharge of amniotic fluid. This, of course, may take place any time but occurs most frequently at the beginning of the second stage.

8. The mother may be saying at this time that she wants to be "put to sleep" or have a cesarean section owing to the increased pain and the desire for labor to be done. It is important to remember that the mother's consciousness is somewhat altered because of the pain, her enforced concentration, and possibly medication; therefore, any coaching needs to be short and explicit and may need to be repeated with each contraction. The nurse also must be firm but gentle in setting limits with the mother, so that she can conserve her energy for the second stage. Thrashing about and continued crying only lead to exhaustion, and the mother needs the firm guidance of a skillful person to help her to maintain control.

9. The perineum begins to bulge and the anal orifice begins to dilate. This is a late sign, but if signs numbered 1, 3, 5, and 7 occur, it should be watched for with every contraction. Only a vaginal examination or the appearance of the head can definitely confirm the suspicion.

The Woman During Second Stage of Labor

Nursing Objectives

1. Help the client continue to make progress in labor as evidenced by descent of the presenting parts.
2. Help the client maintain control by pushing effectively and resting between contractions.
3. Provide for delivery of a healthy infant under aseptic conditions.

Assessment	Potential Nursing Diagnosis	Planning/Intervention	Evaluation
Continue to monitor client's labor	Ineffective individual coping related to physical exhaustion in response to labor	Record and report as before; monitor FHR every 15 minutes	Client continues with stable blood pressure and FHR
Determine appropriateness of bearing down		Monitor maternal blood pressure	Support person(s) participate actively
Assess client/support person's present coping status		Position client for pushing	Client relaxes her body between contractions
		Encourage active participation of support system	Client stays in control through the support given to her by the nurse and support person
		Praise client's pushing efforts	Client pushes effectively
		Promote complete rest between contractions	
		Assist in promoting constructive coping behaviors	
		Provide quiet environment	
Transfer to delivery room	Fear related to new surroundings	Explain procedures	Client understands and verbalizes her role and upcoming procedures
		Instruct support person in delivery room procedures and policies	Support person understands delivery room procedures and policies and coaches mother correctly
Assist with anesthesia	Alteration in comfort: increased pain related to lower fetal position and uterine contractions	Help with positioning for anesthesia, if necessary	Client experiences a decrease in pain
		Assist with supplies	Client expresses comfort
		Monitor vital signs and intravenous infusions	
Assist with delivery		Continue coaching of client in pushing and panting, when appropriate	Client positions herself appropriately for birth
		Prepare delivery room	Client delivers a healthy infant
		Position client for delivery	
		Do perineal prep	
		Monitor FHR at no more than 15-minute intervals	
		Take blood pressure immediately prior to delivery	
		Prepare warm environment for newborn	
		Check resuscitation equipment	

(text continued from page 475)

but require the staff to be flexible in their delivery of care.

Previously, the bearing-down efforts were thought to be best when the client used long and sustained pushes with no audible sounds made. This methodology is now being changed in conjunction with research showing the disadvantage on mother and fetus with repetitive Valsalva maneuvers. Caldeyro-Barcia's recommendations include the following:[22]

- Short pushes of no longer than 6 to 7 seconds
- Physiological pushing: pushing only with the urge to push or approximately three to five times during each contraction
- Pushing with an open glottis and slight exhale

The woman should be encouraged to listen to her body. Caregivers may treat all clients the same in this stage, but it is incorrect to assume that all labors are the same. It is the uterus that decides the amount of effort and the timing of that effort during the second stage.[23] The nurse should review with the couple the type of pushing method they learned in prepared childbirth classes and adapt as necessary. The nurse should facilitate a quiet environment and encourage total relaxation between contractions. Muscular cramps in the legs are common in the second stage because of pressure exerted by the baby's head on certain nerves in the pelvis. To relieve these cramps, the leg can be straightened and the ankle dorsiflexed by exerting pressure upward against the ball of the foot until the cramp subsides. Meanwhile, the knee is stabilized with the other hand. These cramps cause excruciating pain and must never be ignored.

The following is a description of how the nurse can assist the client during second stage in the semi-Fowler position:

1. The mother's head and shoulders can be raised to a 45° angle and supported firmly during the contraction. The father is of great help in this regard and can provide the strength needed for this physical support.
2. The mother's thighs are then flexed on the abdomen, with hands grasped just below the knees when a contraction begins.
3. The client can be encouraged to work with the urge to push, using short, 5-second pushes, with glottis open. She should be instructed that the action is similar to straining during a bowel movement. The long breath-holding pushes may be used if needed to hasten delivery, but should be avoided if possible.
4. Pulling on the knees at this time, as well as flexing the chin on the chest, is a helpful adjunct to maintain downward pressure of the diaphragm and to stabilize the chest and the abdominal musculature.
5. In addition, maintaining the legs flexed as for the

"push" position deters the mother from pushing her feet against the table or bed. Avoiding such pressure on the feet is important because it discourages tensing of the gluteal muscles and contributes to further relaxation of the pelvic floor.

Psychosocial Support

When the mother is ready to be transferred to the delivery room, it is helpful if the nurse who attended her in labor accompanies her. This transfer means a new environment for the client to cope with under very stressful circumstances. Great physical and mental exertion may be called for with little preparation or practice. To the mother in labor who is unfamiliar with such surroundings, the "sterile" atmosphere of the delivery room can be strange, cold, and uninviting, with its obstetric furnishings and supplies that become even more foreboding as they reflect the glittering lights of the room. Under such circumstances the sight of familiar faces and the sound of familiar voices, even though partially concealed and muffled by the surgical caps, masks, and gowns, do give the client some sense of continuity and security. Furthermore, by this time the nurse and the client have established a communication pattern, each able to pick up the other's more covert cues. Thus, the coaching, guidance, and follow-through necessary in the second stage of labor is expedited if the same person continues with the care even though the father may be the primary coach.

The nurse will notice that the mother has become increasingly involved in the whole birth process. The seemingly panicky frustration of the late active phase subsides a bit (with appropriate coaching and reassurance), and the client may experience a sense of relief that the expulsive stage has begun. The desire to push and to bear down is very strong now—uncontrollable, in fact—and the client generally gets enormous satisfaction with each push. Some clients, however, experience acute pain and need all available help and encouragement to continue bearing down. The nurse will note that in most instances there is complete exhaustion after each expulsive effort, and the mother often drops off to sleep, only to be roused by the next contraction. Because consciousness is still altered, it may be difficult for the mother to follow directions readily even though she may want to. Again, repeated, short, explicit directions are required to encourage her to rest or to work, but especially to prepare the mother for the expulsive effort if she is sleeping between contractions and awakens abruptly.

Preparation for Delivery

As the second stage progresses the nurse will notice changes in the perineum such as bulging and anal orifice dilatation; if a fetal scalp electrode is in place, the wire will be coming out as the presenting part descends. Transfer to the delivery room can be a stressful time for the mother; contributing factors include temperature, environmental, bed, and potential staff changes. Maternity centers are now changing delivery methods and are using one room for labor, delivery, and recovery. This change is being referred to as the labor, delivery, recovery concept, or as LDR rooms. In this setting, labor, delivery, and recovery of both the mother and the infant occur in the same room with the same nurse. This type of delivery system avoids the transfer to the delivery room and facilitates the family's presence during the entire childbirth process.

Regardless of the type of delivery system, the nurse at this time has certain responsibilities:

- Notifying the delivery attendant
- Setting up for the delivery
- Providing a warm environment for the newborn
- Checking to see that infant resuscitation equipment is present and functioning
- Checking that the adult emergency equipment is available
- Preparing for the type of anesthesia the client is requesting
- Assisting the father and other support persons to get ready for the delivery; this includes changing into scrub clothes, washing hands, getting camera or video equipment prepared, and setting out eyeglasses for the client if she needs them for the delivery.

All of this is done in addition to being supportive of the efforts of the client and father, pointing up the multifaceted role of the labor and delivery nurse. Preparation for delivery demands the closest teamwork among the physician, nurse, and anesthetist, if required, to best meet the needs of the client, newborn, and support person. By previous understanding, or more often by established hospital routine, each has his or her own responsibilities in the delivery room.

Up to now, the primary focus for the nurse has been on direct client care. Now she must enlarge her focus to include the physician and other allied professionals (*i.e.*, there will be more activities that will require the actual assistance of these persons than was necessary during the first stage of labor). Thus, the nurse must be sensitive not only to the cues sent by the mother but also to those relayed by the other personnel.

Preparation of the Delivery Room

There are no two hospitals in which the delivery room setup or the procedure for delivery is precisely the same. Therefore, observation and experience in a particular institution serves as the basis for becoming acquainted with the physical layout and the method of care offered.

The following, however, gives a general idea of the equipment and materials used in the typical setting.

The delivery table is designed so that its surface is actually composed of two adjoining sections, each covered with its own mattress. This permits the client to lie on her back in the supine position or with her head and back elevated by using the table's hand crank, if the bed model has that feature; if that is not possible, a large wedge-type pillow or regular bed pillows can be used until she must put her legs up into stirrups or the lithotomy position. A word of caution: the mother is still at risk for hypotension due to compression of the gravid uterus on the inferior vena cava. To avoid this the nurse may want to wedge or tilt the woman using folded towels or a sandbag under her right hip to shift

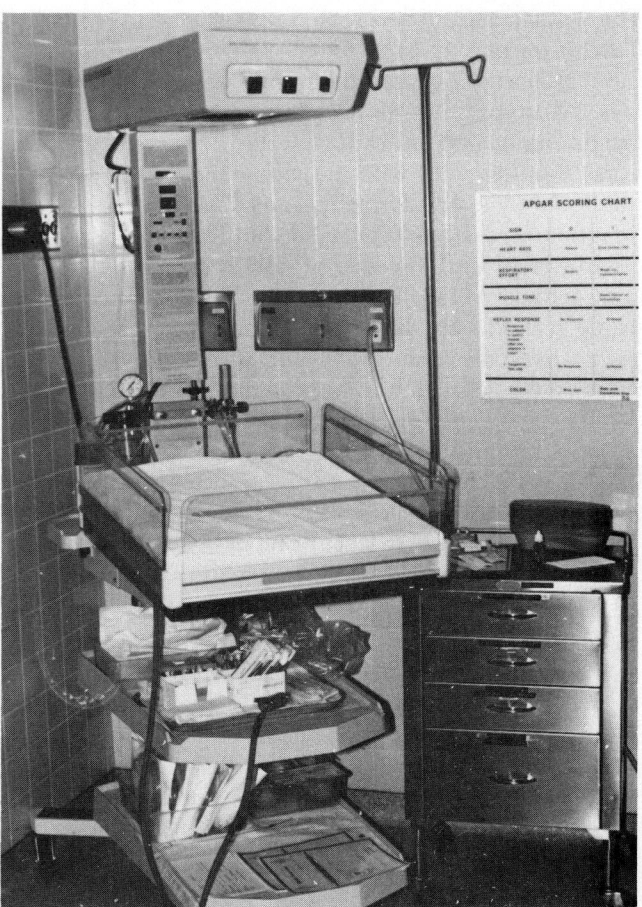

F I G U R E   2 5 - 6

An infant resuscitation cart with an overhead radiant warmer for use in the delivery room. The overhead radiant heater provides a thermal environment for the infant and allows access to and full visualization of the infant. The lower shelves and metal cabinet to the side of the resuscitation cart are used to store infant supplies that include equipment and drugs needed in an infant resuscitation. (Courtesy of Memorial Medical Center, Long Beach, Long Beach, California)

the uterus off the vein and maintain venous return. The table is "broken" by a mechanical device. The retractable or lower end of the table drops and is rolled under the main section of the table. Thus, ready access is given to the perineal region. Or, if it is desired to deliver the client in the dorsal recumbent position, the lower portion of the table can remain in place.

The table opposite the foot of the delivery table, referred to as the back table, contains the principal sterile supplies and instruments needed for normal delivery, including sterile gowns, drapes, towels, sponges, basins, and cord set. The cord set is a group of instruments used for clamping and cutting the umbilical cord: two Kelly clamps, a pair of bandage scissors, and a cord clamp. Other instruments often are included because it may be necessary for the birth attendant to perform an episiotomy or to repair lacerations. Other instruments frequently included are two Kelly clamps, two Allis clamps, one mouse-tooth tissue forceps, two sponge sticks, two tenacula, one needle holder, and straight scissors. The nurse will add to this setup sterile gloves of the correct size, bulb syringe, syringe with large-bore needle for cord blood sample, and, if needed, local anesthesia tray with anesthetic solution, catheter, and suture.

A single- or double-bowl solution stand or basin rack will be used to hold warm sterile water or normal saline. Depending on the birth attendant's preference, the nurse may be asked to put into the basin an antimicrobial solution. If the double-bowl stand is used the other basin may be used to place the placenta; again, this depends on the facility's preference. A prep set used to prepare the perineal area needs to be set up. Prep sets range from a small basin with sponges, to which the nurse must add antimicrobial solution and warm sterile water, to a prep set that the manufacturer prepares, requiring only that the nurse open it, put on the sterile gloves, and do the prep. To prepare for the newborn a radiant warmer and a resuscitator are present with the necessary emergency equipment (Fig. 25-6).

Asepsis and Antisepsis

Persons who have a communicable disease or persons who have been in contact with a communicable disease should be excluded from maternity service until examined by a physician. Only after a physician has certified that the employee is free from infections should he or she be allowed to return to duty. Personnel with evidence of upper respiratory tract infections or open skin lesions, diarrhea, or any other infectious disease also should be excluded. Furthermore, it is recommended that all persons working in the maternity area should have a preemployment physical examination and rubella titers and such interim examinations as may be required by the hospital.

Of prime importance in the conduct of the second stage of labor are strict asepsis and antisepsis throughout the entire delivery. To this end everyone in the delivery room wears clean scrubs, cap, and mask and those actually participating in the delivery are in sterile attire. Masking includes both nose and mouth, but some facilities are reevaluating the need for a mask for a normal delivery. Caps are to be adjusted to keep *all* hair covered. If the nurse scrubs to assist the doctor, the strict aseptic technique is observed. The hands are scrubbed as carefully as for a surgical operation. Scrubbing the hands should be started sufficiently early to allot full time for the scrub, as well as to don gown and gloves.

Transfer of the Mother to the Delivery Room

When birth appears imminent, the mother is transferred to the delivery room and prepared for delivery. If the father has chosen not to accompany the mother to the delivery room, time is allowed for them to bid each other a temporary goodbye. This kind of planning not only is supportive but also enables both to cooperate more fully. If the father is going to the delivery room he should be changed in appropriate scrubs, cap, and mask, if needed, and ready with camera equipment, if appropriate.

Care should be taken to have only one person instruct or coach the mother at any one time. When delivery is imminent, her attention is limited, as already illustrated, and the sound of several voices at one time is confusing.

Prior to the actual transfer to the delivery room, the nurse finds out what type of anesthesia will be used. Since the immediate positioning of the client in the delivery room depends on the type of anesthesia used, this preplanning expedites activities during delivery and promotes smoother functioning of the team.

Positioning

For Anesthesia. If regional anesthesia is to be administered, the client is usually turned on her side. If she is given a saddle block, she may be placed on her side or assisted to a sitting position on the side of the delivery table, with her feet supported on a stool and her body leaning forward against the nurse. Her back should be toward the operator and bowed (the position requires flexion of the neck and the lumbar spine). This principle of cervical and lumbar flexion is used also in the side-lying position (see Chap. 27). A caudal or epidural anesthesia may be started in the labor room.

Although the positioning and the administration of the anesthesia take only a few minutes, the mother may be extremely uncomfortable owing to the severity of the contractions at this time; she can be assured that this discomfort is only temporary. The fetal heart rate and the maternal blood pressure are checked frequently, every 5 minutes or so. In addition, the mother's head should be elevated with at least two pillows to help prevent the anesthetic level from rising beyond the desired height. To allow the anesthetic level to stabilize, the nurse waits for instructions from the anesthetist before putting the mother's legs in stirrups or performing any other manipulations.

Local or pudendal anesthesia is administered with the mother in the lithotomy position.

As previously stated, anesthesia should be administered by a qualified physician or a nurse–anesthetist. This entire subject is discussed in more detail in Chapter 27.

During the time that the anesthesia is being administered, the circulating nurse can uncover the sterile tables, check the resuscitator, and attach a sterile suction catheter and oxygen mask and perform other duties for which she is responsible. Once the anesthesia has been administered, the nurse resumes recording the fetal heart rate every 5 minutes.

For Delivery.   Some hospitals and physicians do not require that the mother be placed in the lithotomy position for delivery. She simply grasps her legs at the knees as she did during the pushing phase of the second stage. This position allows visualization of the perineum and adequate prepping and draping of the area. Before the mother's legs are placed in stirrups or leg holders of some type, cotton flannel boots that cover the entire leg are put on. When the legs are placed in the stirrups or holders, care is taken not to separate the legs too widely or to have one leg higher than the other. Both legs are raised or lowered at the same time, with a nurse supporting each leg if the mother is unable to help in the positioning. Failure to observe these principles may strain the ligaments of the pelvis, with consequent discomfort in the puerperium. Care should be taken to avoid pressure on the popliteal space and to angle the stirrups so that the feet are not dependent.

If stirrups are used during the delivery, the mother can be given handles to grip and pull on, which aid her in her bearing-down efforts.

Preparing the Perineum

After the client is placed in the lithotomy position, the nurse carries out the procedure for cleansing the vulva and the surrounding area (Fig. 25-7). If the delivery is to be conducted with the mother in the recumbent position, this may be carried out with the knees drawn up slightly and the legs separated. Once the physician has scrubbed and donned sterile gown and gloves, the client is draped with towels and sheets appropriate for the purpose.

After the client has been prepared for delivery, catheterization, if needed, is carried out by the physician. Sometimes it is difficult to catheterize a client in the second stage of labor because the fetus's head may compress the urethra. If the catheter does not pass easily, it should not be forced. The mirror may now be positioned for viewing of the delivery by the couple.

Delivery

As the infant descends the birth canal, pressure against the rectum may cause fecal material to be expelled. Sponges (as a rule with saline solution) may be used to remove any fecal material that may escape from the rectum.

Fundal pressure should not be used to accomplish spontaneous delivery or to bring the head deeper into the birth canal. Severe fundal pressure may cause uterine damage or rupture.

As soon as the head distends the perineum to a diameter of 6 or 8 cm (crowning—Fig. 25-8), a towel may be placed over the rectum while forward pressure is exerted on the baby's chin with one hand, at the same time that downward pressure is applied to the occiput by the other hand. This technique, called the Ritgen's

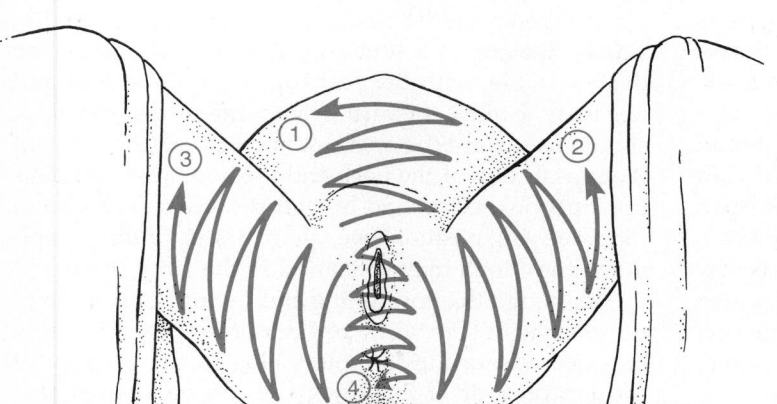

FIGURE   25-7

Perineal preparation. A recommended method when cleansing the perineum. Use a new sponge or gauze square for each numbered area; clean the rectal area last. To finish the procedure blot the perineum dry with a sterile towel or rinse with warm sterile water.

maneuver (Fig. 25-9), provides control of the head as it is emerging and directs the extension phase of delivery so that the head is born with the smallest diameter presenting. The head is usually delivered between contractions and as slowly as possible. At this time the mother may complain about a ''splitting'' sensation caused by the extreme vaginal stretching as the head is born. Birth is illustrated in Figure 25-10.

Control of the head by Ritgen's maneuver, extension, and slow delivery between contractions help to prevent lacerations. If a tear seems to be inevitable, an incision that is called an episiotomy may be made in the perineum. This not only prevents lacerations but also facilitates the delivery.

Immediately after the birth of the infant's head the mouth and nose are suctioned with the bulb syringe, then a finger is passed along the occiput to the infant's neck to feel whether a loop or more of umbilical cord encircles it. If such a coil is felt, it should be gently drawn down and, if loose enough, slipped over the infant's head. This is done to prevent interference with the infant's oxygen supply, which could result from pressure of its shoulder on the umbilical cord. If the cord is too tightly coiled to permit this procedure, it must be clamped and cut before the shoulders are delivered; then the infant must be extracted immediately before asphyxiation results. The anterior shoulder is usually brought under the symphysis pubis first and then the posterior shoulder is delivered, after which the remainder of the body follows without particular mechanism. The exact time of the baby's birth should be noted. The infant usually cries immediately, and the lungs gradually become expanded. The pulsations in the umbilical cord begin to diminish about this time.

Clamping the Cord

The cord usually is clamped before pulsations cease to prevent transfusion from the placenta and, consequently, hyperviscosity in the infant. The cord is then cut between the two Kelly clamps, which have been placed a few inches from the umbilicus; the umbilical clamp is then applied (Figs. 25-11 and 25-12). There are several types of umbilical clamps, such as the Kane, the Hollister, and the Hesseltine, which are used extensively in many institutions. With these the possibility of hemorrhage is minimized. The delivery room nurse must assess and document the numbers of vessels present in the cord.

Psychosocial Considerations

If the mother is awake, she is usually eager to have a closer look at her baby and hold it. The nurse should remember that, although she is quite tired, she is usually elated, proud of her accomplishment of giving birth, and eager to share this with the baby's father. Whenever

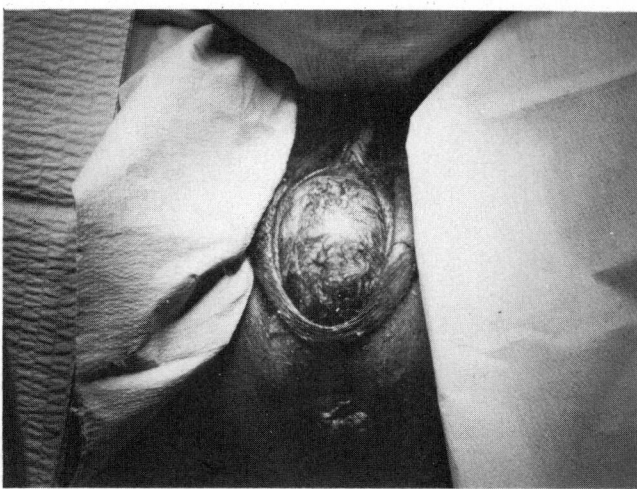

FIGURE 25-8

Note crowning, encirclement of the largest diameter of the baby's head by the vulvar ring.

possible, all efforts should be made to allow the mother, father, and infant to share this momentous time together if they so desire. More hospitals are allowing the mother to hold her infant immediately after delivery and put it to breast if she is breast-feeding. Other institutions have the mother wait to hold the infant or nurse it until she has been transferred to the recovery room. These kinds

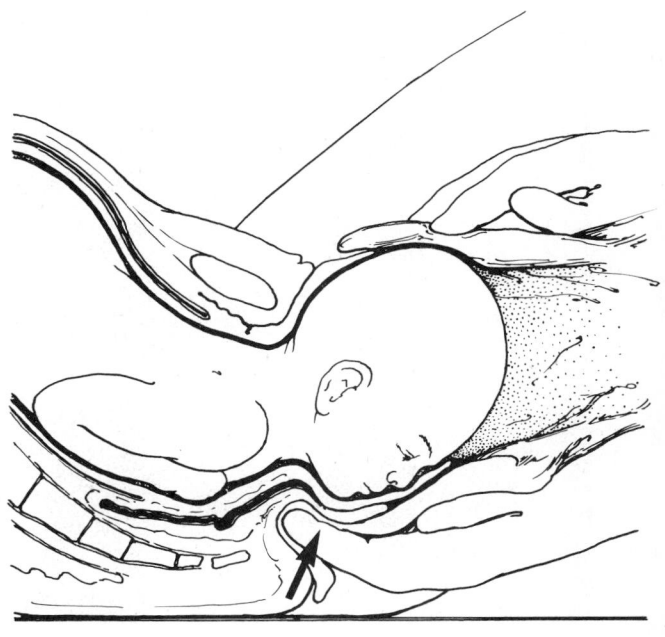

FIGURE 25-9

Ritgen's maneuver as it appears in median section. Arrow shows direction of pressure.

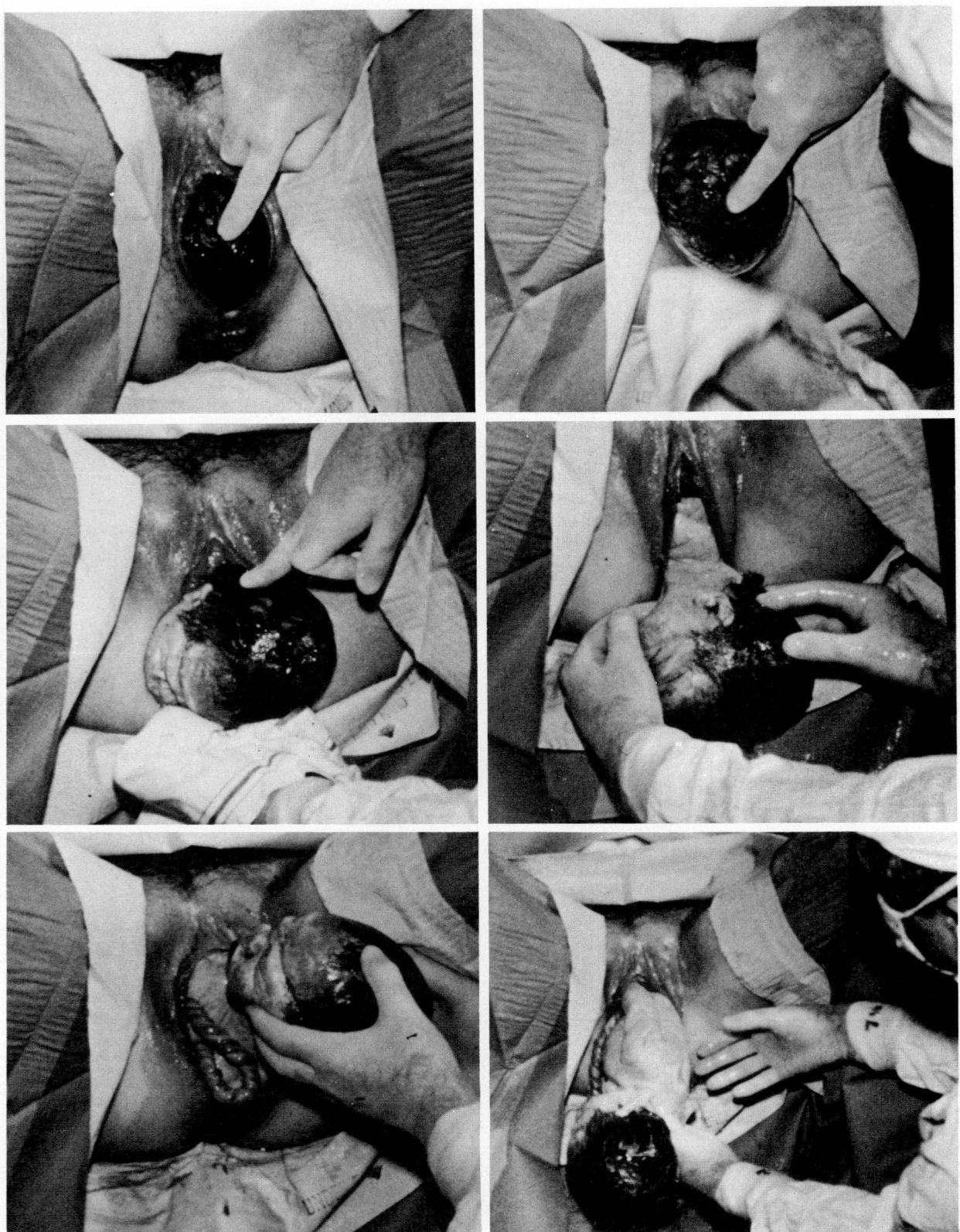

FIGURE 25-10

The normal birth process. (From the film Human Birth, published by J. B. Lippincott, Philadelphia.)

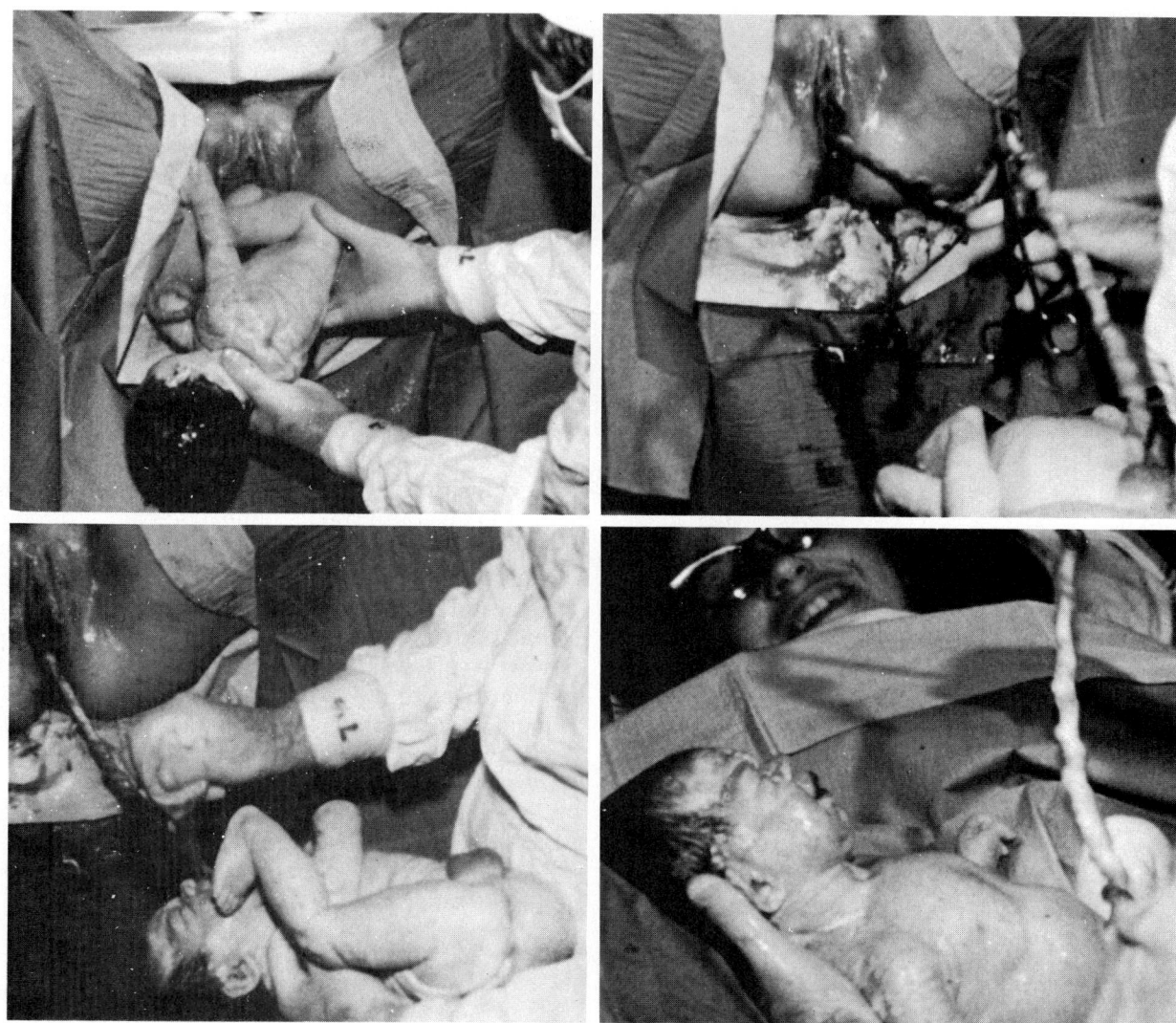

FIGURE 25-10 (*continued*)

Leboyer Method of Delivery

of arrangements provide more opportunities for the parents to have a close, thorough look at their baby and to let the triad begin the necessary process of bonding and integrating the new member into the family constellation.

Leboyer Method of Delivery

In recent years a newer method of delivery has been advocated by a French obstetrician, Frederick Leboyer, who suggests that delivery room procedures be changed to make birth less a traumatic event for the newborn. In his book and lectures he has described a method of handling infants during birth that includes a dimly lit and quiet delivery room, placing the infant on the mother's abdomen and stroking (massaging) it gently, delaying the clamping of the cord, and immersing the infant in a warm bath until it is relaxed and quiet.[24,25] Leboyer contends that the traditional method of delivery with all of its harsh, sudden sensory stimulation can be detrimental to the infant. The shock of birth produces jitteriness, interferes with eye contact between the mother and infant, and may even prevent optimal bonding with the mother given the other restrictive practices followed in some hospitals.

There has been some controversy about this type of "gentle" birth mainly because of questions concerning possible threats to infant safety from undue chilling, placental transfusion, and possible infection. There has been no definitive research to either prove or disprove the efficacy of this method. Preliminary data do indicate that infants delivered by this technique do not tend to tremble or shudder as much and have more relaxed hand muscles than other infants. Moreover, they spend

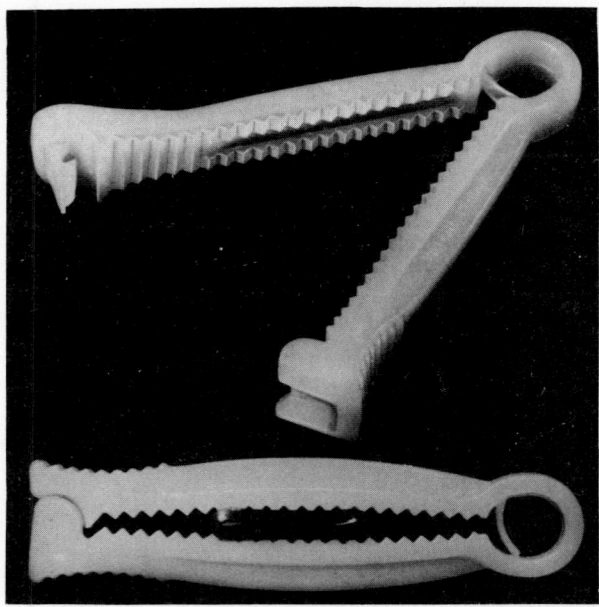

Umbilical cord clamp. A double-grip cord clamp in the opened and closed positions. (Courtesy of Hollister, Inc., Chicago, IL)

more time with their eyes open in the period immediately subsequent to delivery. In addition, no greater risk for mother or infant of infection or chilling was found.[26] Many hospitals are offering at least a modified version of this technique.

Third Stage of Labor

The third stage of labor, the placental stage, begins after the delivery of the baby and terminates with the birth of the placenta. Immediately after delivery of the infant the height of the uterine fundus and its consistency are ascertained by palpating the uterus through a sterile towel placed on the lower abdomen. The physician will place his hand on top of the sterile drape and hold the uterus very gently, with the fingers behind the fundus and the thumb in front. So long as the uterus remains hard, and there is no bleeding, the policy is ordinarily one of watchful waiting until the placenta is separated. No massage is practiced; the hand simply rests on the fundus to make certain that the organ does not balloon out with blood.

Placental Separation and Delivery

Since attempts to deliver the placenta prior to its separation from the uterine wall are not only futile but may be dangerous, it is most important that the signs of pla-

cental separation be well understood. The signs that suggest that the placenta has separated are as follows:

1. The uterus rises upward in the abdomen because the placenta, having been separated, passes downward into the lower uterine segment and the vagina, where its bulk pushes the uterus upward.
2. The umbilical cord protrudes 3 inches or more farther out of the vagina, indicating that the placenta also has descended.
3. The uterus changes from a discoid to a globular shape and becomes, as a rule, more firm.
4. A sudden trickle or spurt of blood often occurs.

These signs are apparent sometimes within a minute or so after delivery of the infant and usually within 5 minutes. When the placenta has separated and the uterus is firmly contracted, the client is asked to bear down so that the intra-abdominal pressure so produced may expel the placenta. If this fails, or if it is not practicable because of anesthesia, gentle pressure is exerted downward with the hand on the fundus and the placenta is gently guided out of the vagina. This procedure, known as placental *expression*, must be done gently and without squeezing (Figs. 25-13 and 25-14). It never should be attempted unless the uterus is hard; otherwise, the organ may be turned inside out. This is one of the gravest complications of obstetrics and is known as inversion of the uterus. Once the placenta is expelled, it is carefully inspected to make sure that it is intact (Fig. 25-15); if a piece is left in the uterus, it may cause subsequent hemorrhage.

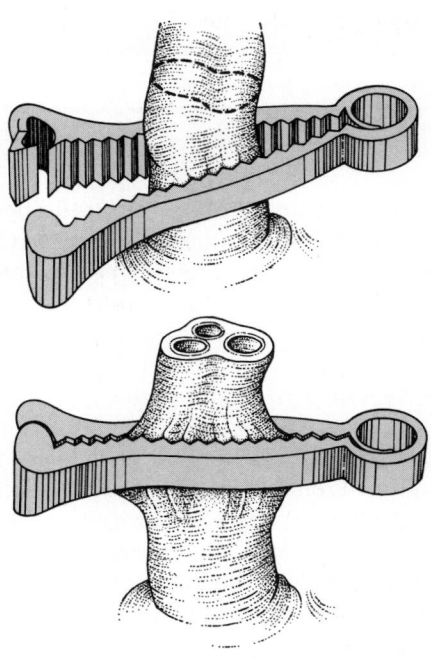

Clamp applied to cord.

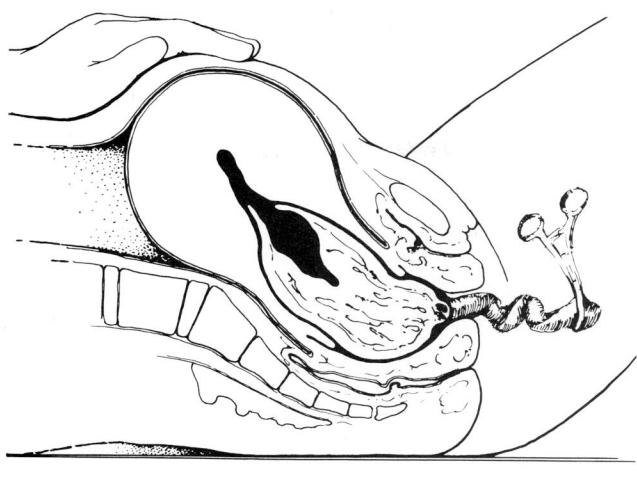

FIGURE 25-13

Placental expression.

Use of Oxytocics

With the separation and delivery of the placenta in the third stage of labor, hemostasis is achieved at the placenta site by vasoconstriction of the myometrium. Oxytocin (Pitocin, Syntocinon), ergonovine maleate (Ergotrate), and methylergonovine maleate (Methergine) may be administered, at the physician's request, to stimulate uterine contractions and control bleeding. These agents are employed widely in the conduct of the normal third stage of labor, but the timing of their administration differs greatly in various hospitals. These oxytocics are not necessary in most cases, but their use is considered ideal from the viewpoint of minimizing blood loss and the general safety of the mother.

The oxytocic fraction separated from posterior pituitary extract is called oxytocin; it is widely used because it does not possess the strong vasopressor effects of Pituitrin, which was used more extensively in former years.

Oxytocin causes marked uterine contractions for the first 5 to 10 minutes, after which normal rhythmic contractions of amplified degree return with intermittent periods of relaxation. It is the most frequently used drug, and is given either when the shoulders are delivered or after the delivery of the placenta, but it may be administered only on the order of the physician.

Oxytocin's most important side-effect is its antidiuretic effect, which can cause water intoxication if administered intravenously in a large volume of electrolyte-free aqueous dextrose solution. Fortunately, the antidiuretic effect disappears within a few minutes after the infusion is discontinued.

On the physician's order the nurse administers oxytocin intramuscularly or adds the medication to the intravenous fluid. The average dose is as follows: 10 units (1 ml) IM or 20 units added to 1000 ml intravenous solution.

Ergonovine is an alkaloid of ergot and is a powerful oxytocic; it stimulates uterine contractions and exerts an effect that may persist for several hours. When it is administered intravenously, the uterine response is almost immediate, within a few minutes of intramuscular or oral administration. This response is sustained with no tendency toward relaxation. *However, this drug does cause an elevation in blood pressure.* Intravenous route should be considered only with emergencies.

More recently a semisynthetic derivative of ergonovine, *methylergonovine maleate*, has been employed. It is thought to cause less elevation in blood pressure when given parenterally.

Both drugs when given intravenously may cause transient headache and, to a lesser extent, temporary chest pain, palpation, and dyspnea. These side-effects are less likely to occur with intramuscular administration of the drug, which is the usual route of administration.

The usual doses are ergonovine, 0.2 mg ($^1/_{320}$ gr) IM or IV, and methylergonovine, 0.2 mg ($^1/_{320}$ gr) IM or IV. Various institutions use the drugs separately or in conjunction, as is necessary to produce the desired results.

The choice of the oxytocic usually depends on the anesthetic agent administered. Oxytocin is contraindicated for use with drugs that have a sympathomimetic action.

Lacerations of the Birth Canal

During the process of a normal delivery lacerations of the perineum and the vagina may be caused by rapid and sudden expulsion of the head, excessive size of the infant, and very friable maternal tissues. In other circumstances they may be caused by difficult forceps deliveries, breech extractions, or contraction of the pelvic outlet in which the head is forced posteriorly. Some tears are unavoidable, even in the most skilled hands, but control of the head is extremely important to deter perineal lacerations.

Perineal lacerations usually are classified in three degrees, according to the extent of the tear.

- *First-degree lacerations* are those that involve the fourchette, the perineal skin, and the vaginal mucous membrane without involving any of the muscles.
- *Second-degree lacerations* are those that involve (in addition to skin and mucous membrane) the muscles of the perineal body but not the rectal sphincter. These tears usually extend upward on one or both sides of the vagina, making a triangular injury.
- *Third-degree lacerations* are those that extend completely through the skin, the mucuous mem-

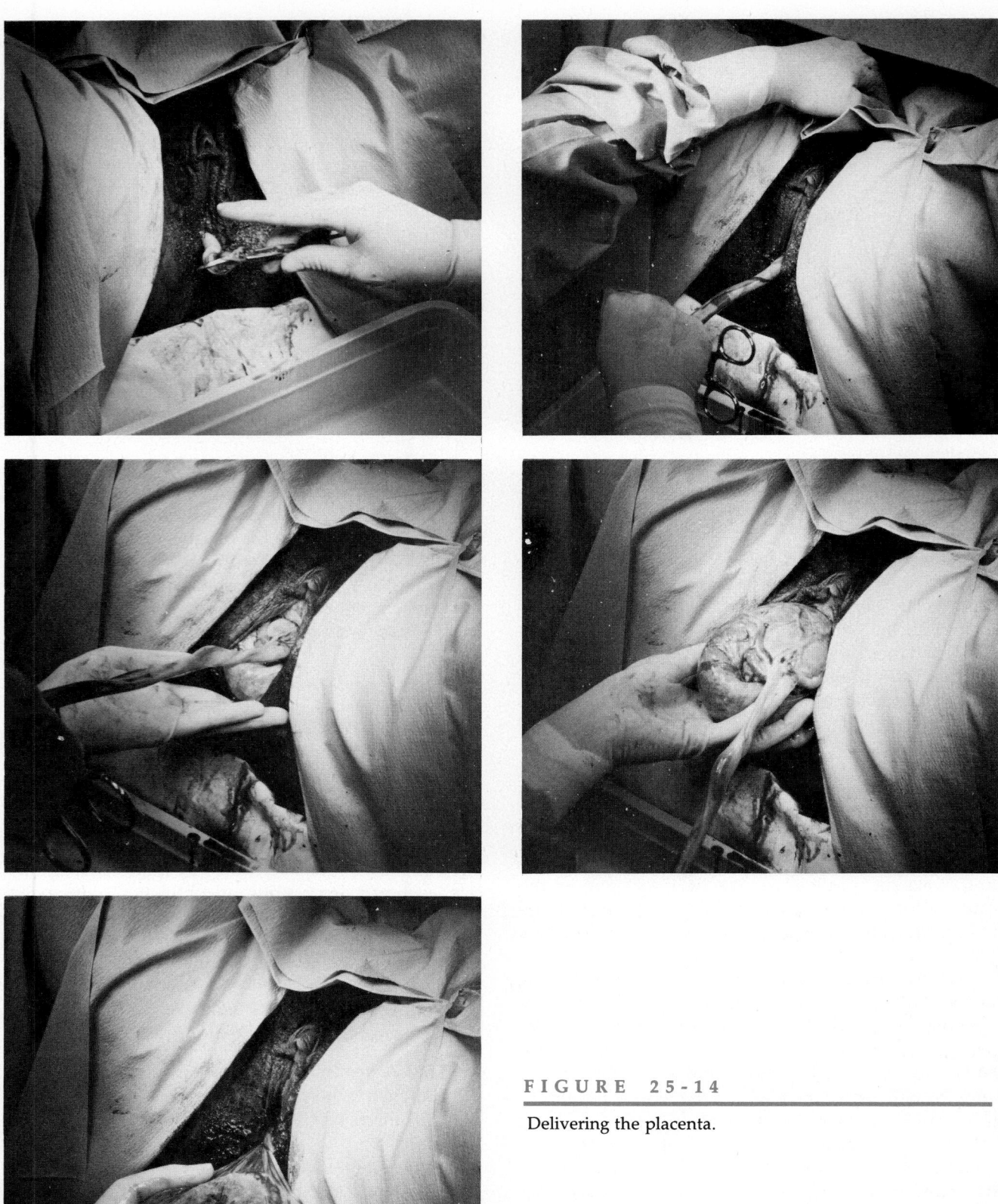

FIGURE 25-14

Delivering the placenta.

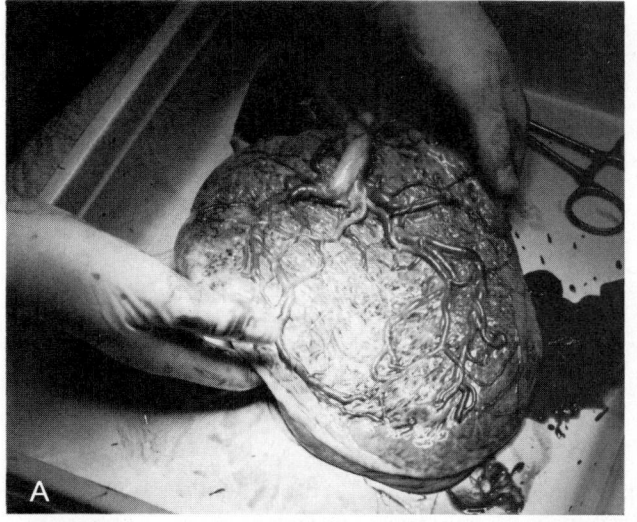

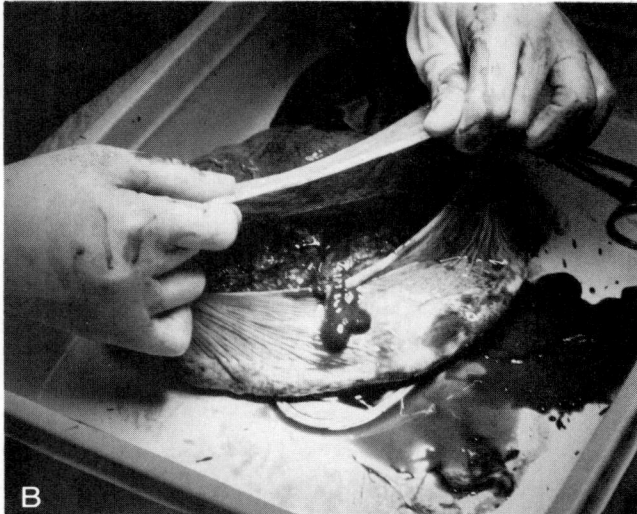

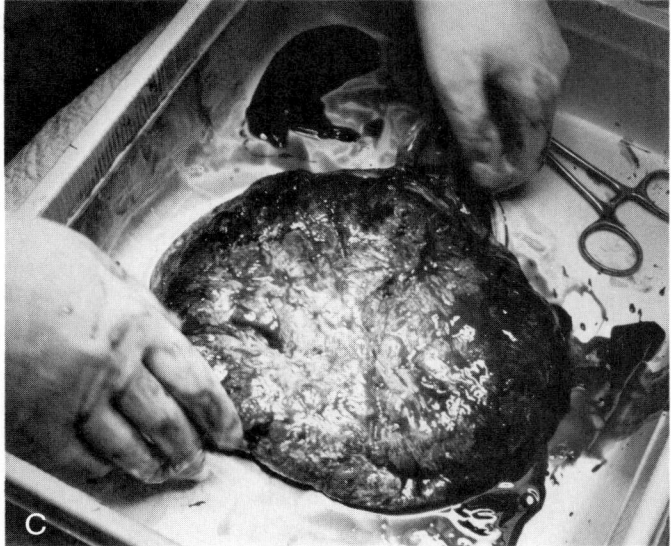

FIGURE 25-15

Inspecting the placenta. (*A*) Fetal surface. (*B*) The placenta is carefully turned inside out. (*C*) Maternal surface.

brane, the perineal body, and the rectal sphincter. This type is often referred to as a complete tear. Frequently these third-degree lacerations extend a certain distance up the anterior wall of the rectum.

Some classifications refer to a laceration that extends into the rectum as a fourth-degree tear.

First- and second-degree lacerations are extremely common in primigravidas; their high incidence is one of the reasons that episiotomy is widely employed. Fortunately, third-degree lacerations are far less common. All three types of lacerations are repaired by the physician immediately after the delivery to ensure that the perineal structures are returned approximately to their former condition. The technique employed for the repair of a laceration is virtually the same as that used for episiotomy incisions, although the former is more dif-

ficult to do because of the irregular lines of tissue that must be approximated.

Episiotomy and Repair

An episiotomy is an incision of the perineum made to facilitate delivery (Fig. 25-16). The incision is made with blunt-pointed straight scissors about the time that the head distends the vulva and is visible to a diameter of several centimeters. The incision may be made in the midline of the perineum, a median episiotomy, or it may be begun in the midline and directed downward and laterally away from the rectum, a mediolateral episiotomy. In the latter instance the incision may be directed to either the right or the left side of the mother's pelvis.

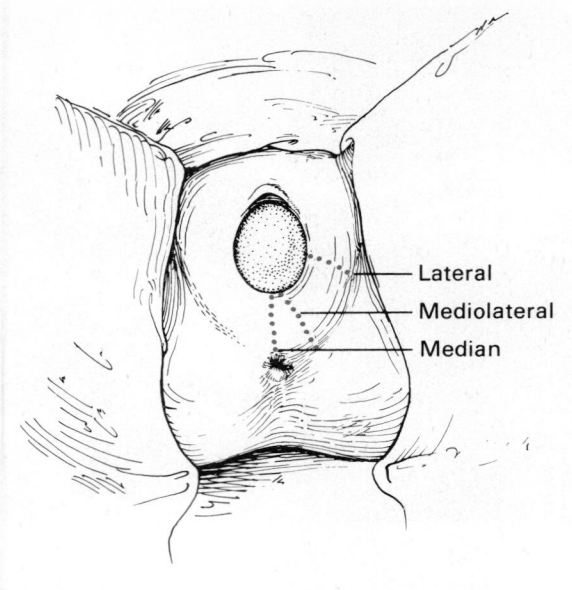

FIGURE 25-16

Types of episiotomies.

If a laceration seems to be inevitable as the infant's head distends the vulva, the physician undoubtedly chooses to incise the perineum rather than allow that structure to sustain a traumatic tear. This operation serves the following purposes:

- It substitutes a straight, clean-cut surgical incision for the ragged, contused laceration that otherwise may ensue; such an incision is easier to repair and heals better than a tear.
- The direction of the episiotomy can be controlled, whereas a tear may extend in any direction, sometimes involving the anal sphincter and the rectum.
- Inordinate stretching and tearing of the perineal musculature is avoided, and the incidence of subsequent perineal relaxation with cystocele-rectocele may be reduced.
- The operation shortens the duration of the second stage of labor.

In view of these advantages many physicians employ episiotomy routinely in the delivery of the primigravida.

There are many equally satisfactory methods that are used for episiotomy repair (Fig. 25-17). The suture material ordinarily used is a fine chromic catgut, either 2-0 or 3-0.

A round needle and continuous suture are used to close the vaginal mucosa and fourchette; the continuous suture is then set aside while several interrupted sutures are placed in the levator ani muscle and the fascia. Then the continuous suture is again picked up and used to unite the subcutaneous fascia. Finally, the round needle is replaced by a large, straight cutting needle, and the

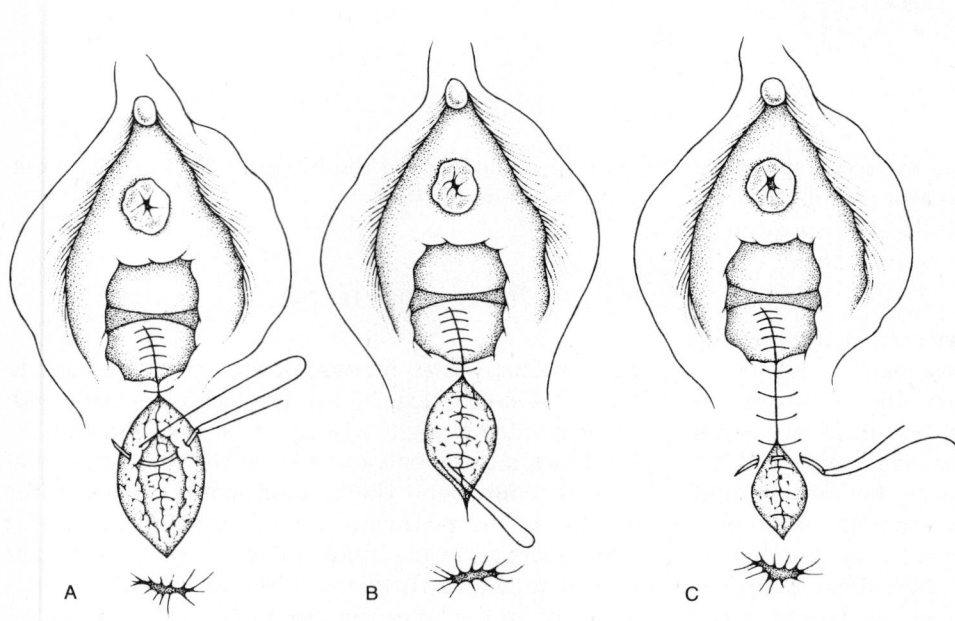

FIGURE 25-17

Repair of median episiotomy. (*A*) Chromic catgut 2-0, or preferably 3-0, is used as a continuous suture to close the vaginal mucosa and submucosa. (*B*) After closing the vaginal incision and reapproximating the cut margins of the hymenal ring, the suture is tied and cut. Next, three or four interrupted sutures of 2-0 or 3-0 catgut are placed in the fascia and muscle of the incised perineum. (*C*) Repair of complete perineal tear. The rectal mucosa has been repaired with interrupted, fine chromic catgut sutures. The torn ends of the sphincter ani are next approximated with two or three interrupted chromic catgut sutures. The wound is then repaired, as in a second-degree laceration or an episiotomy.

running suture is continued upward as a subcuticular stitch.

Fourth Stage of Labor

The fourth stage can be defined as starting after the delivery of the placenta and ending when the mother's physical status has stabilized. This usually occurs within 1 to 2 hours. The weary work of labor is completed now, and the mother and father should be commended by the nurse on the good job they did. Questions can be answered, and any labor occurrences can be clarified. This may not be adequate, and at a later time the couple may still need their delivery nurse to clarify the labor and birth process. This stage is a transitional period for the new parents, and many important physical and psychosocial tasks begin at this time. A couple making the transition to a three-member family is shown in Figure 25-18.

After the delivery has been completed and the episiotomy, if needed, repaired, the drapes and the soiled linen are removed and the lower end of the delivery table is replaced. If stirrups have been used, the mother's legs are lowered simultaneously to prevent cramping or twisting of the extremities. A sterile perineal pad is applied, and the mother is given a clean gown and covered with a warm blanket to avoid chilling. Usually mother, infant, and father then go to the postpartum recovery area (Fig. 25-19). Some institutions still require that all infants be taken to the nursery at this time, and mother and infant are recovered separately.

Assessment

Postpartum care begins immediately after the delivery; both mother and newborn are making adjustments that need to be assessed. If problems arise, actions need to be taken promptly to assure well-being. Care of the newborn will be addressed in Chapter 28. The first maternal assessment is to be done in the delivery room prior to transfer. If the delivery has taken place in the LDR, as soon as the mother's legs are down and the warm blanket has been placed the assessment is done. The immediate postpartum checks, done every 15 minutes, include blood pressure, pulse, respirations, massaging the fundus and observing the vaginal flow, inspecting the perineum, and assessing for bladder distention. A temperature reading is usually taken within the first hour.

To be assured of well-being, scrupulous assessment needs to be done, since the mother is at great risk at this time for postpartum hemorrhage and development of a hematoma. If a change in nursing staff occurs, in that the labor and delivery nurse is not the recovery room nurse, a complete report is given. The report includes name of the physician who delivered, method of delivery, presence of an episiotomy, presence of lacerations, type of anesthesia, IV bottle solution and number, amount of oxytocin in the bottle (or if not used,

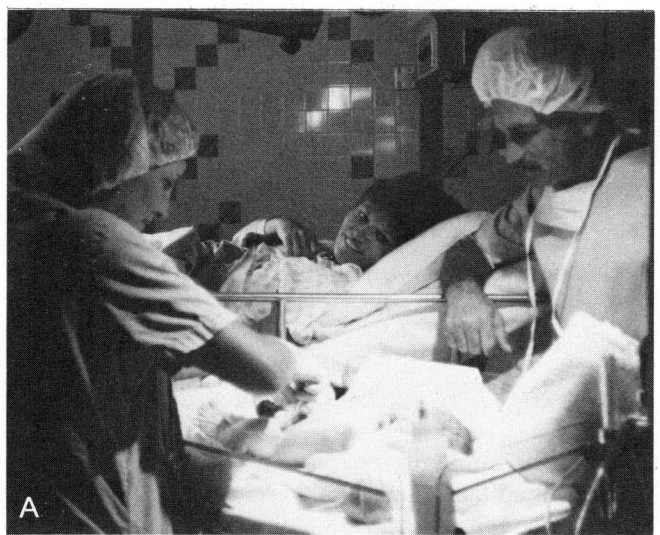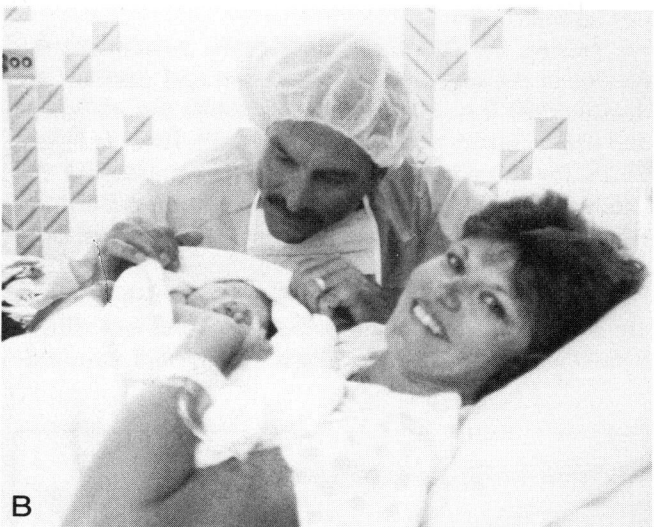

FIGURE 25-18

Psychosocial tasks begin after birth. (*A*) Both parents watch intently as the nurse cares for the newborn. (*B*) The father gazes fondly at the newborn while the mother shows pride in her accomplishment. (Courtesy of Memorial Medical Center, Long Beach, Long Beach, California)

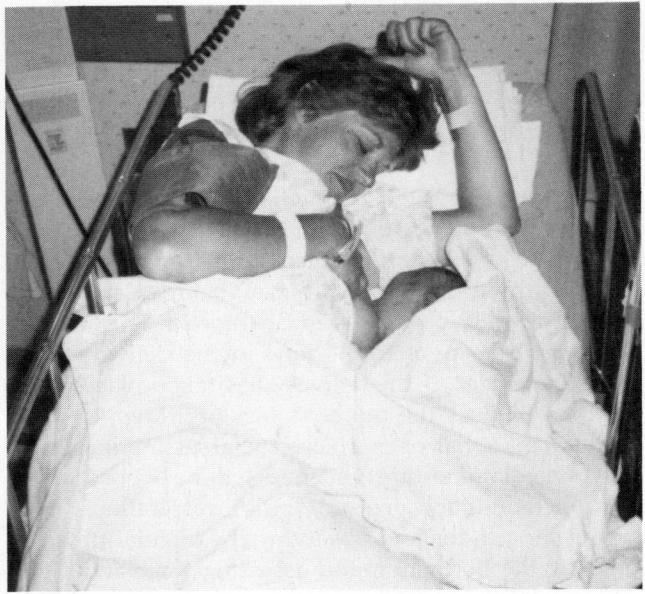

FIGURE 25-19

In the recovery area the mother and newborn have quiet time together during breast-feeding, while the father announces the birth to family and friends. (Courtesy of Memorial Medical Center, Long Beach, Long Beach, California)

any medications she received to decrease bleeding), method of infant feeding, time of last voiding, sex of the infant, summary of the labor, any pertinent items that need to be observed for and any pertinent medical history, and any medical orders that need to be carried out immediately.

During the first hour, with every assessment the fundus is massaged and its condition and position are documented (*i.e.,* 1 fingerbreadth above the umbilicus and firm or boggy and massaged to firm). Refer to Figure 25-20 for the correct procedure when massaging the fundus. Vaginal bleeding is assessed in relation to amount, color, and presence of clots or foul odor. Documentation of the amount of bleeding is done: scant, light, moderate, or heavy. Problems arise when amounts are not standardized and when measurement differs between nurses. The following is a suggested standard-

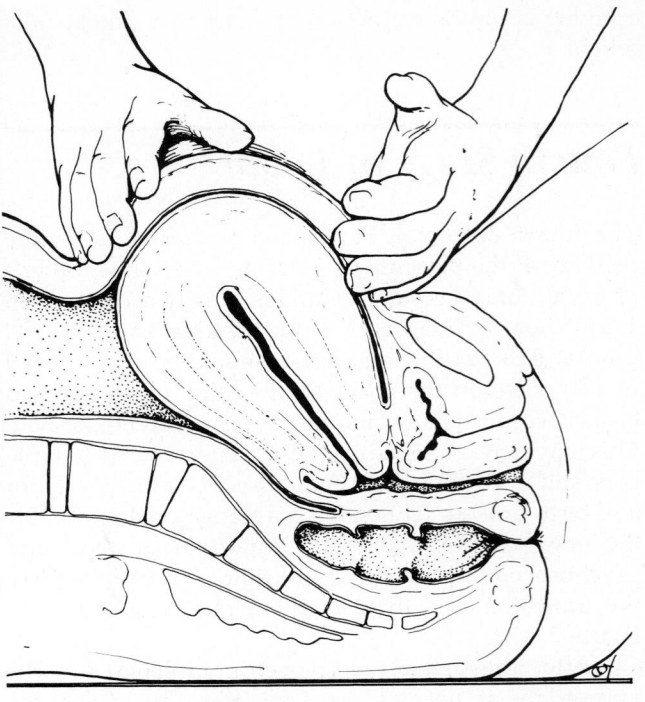

FIGURE 25-20

Proper method of palpating fundus of uterus during first hour after delivery to guard against relaxation and hemorrhage. The right hand is placed just above the symphysis pubis to act as a guard; meanwhile the other hand is cupped around the fundus of the uterus.

ized method to record vaginal flow. It can be implemented to ensure accurate documentation of the flow and reflection of the client's condition.[27]

- Scant: blood on tissue only when wiped, or less than 1-inch stain on peripad
- Light: less than 4-inch stain on peripad
- Moderate: less than 6-inch stain on peripad
- Heavy: saturated peripad within 1 hour

The subject is discussed further in Chapter 31, with an illustration of peripads.

Nursing Diagnosis

During the third and fourth stages of labor the nursing goal of maintaining maternal and now newborn well-being is ongoing. At this time the nurse may be able to address and plan for some of the diagnoses identified in the admitting process that she was unable to attend to during the actual labor and birth of the newborn. Assuring her that physical systems are stabilized and providing comfort prepare the client for the new role of mothering.

Fourth-Stage Assessments

- Vital signs
- Fundus
- Amount of lochia, presence of clots
- Perineum
- Bladder distention
- Family interaction

1. Alteration in comfort/discomfort related to involution of uterus, episiotomy
2. Sleep pattern disturbance
3. Alteration in nutrition: less than body requirements
4. Potential alteration in parenting related to inexperience, lack of role models
5. Potential grieving related to labor and delivery not occurring the way client wanted it to be, baby not desired sex, pregnancy over
6. Potential for infection: vaginal, perineal, related to bacterial invasion secondary to trauma during labor and delivery and episiotomy
7. Potential alteration in parenting related to inexperience, lack of role models
8. Potential knowledge deficit related to infant care, infant behavior, self-care, normal postpartum physiological occurrences

Planning/Intervention

Management of Potential Complications

Hypothermic Reactions. Chilling accompanied by uncontrollable shaking often occurs in this early period after delivery. It is uncomfortable and sometimes embarrassing or frightening for the client, but it is self-limiting (usually not over 15 min) and is not considered an ominous sign. The exact etiology of this chilling has not been determined, although several explanations have been offered, which include sudden release of intra-abdominal pressure after delivery, nervous and exhaustion responses related to the stress of childbirth, disequilibrium in the internal and external body temperature resulting from the waste products of muscular exertion, break in aseptic technique (which predisposes to infection), minute circulatory amniotic fluid emboli, and previous maternal sensitization to elements of fetal blood.

Clean, dry, warm gowns and blankets and a warm, nondrafty environment help in the prevention and control of this phenomenon. Warm fluids by mouth can be given and are much appreciated for their hydrating and energy-giving effects.

Postpartum Hemorrhage. Constant massage of the uterus during this period immediately after delivery is unnecessary and undesirable. However, if the organ shows any tendency to relax, it is to be massaged immediately with firm but gentle circular strokes until it contracts effectively. *Relaxation of the uterus is a prime cause of postpartum hemorrhage, and surveillance of the uterus and the amount of bleeding is of extreme importance at this time.*

Since the prevention of postpartum hemorrhage is such a crucial factor in the health and well-being of the mother, those clients at risk to develop this condition should be identified quickly. The following are the most predictive factors associated with postpartum bleeding.

Advanced maternal age and high parity
Rapid labor
Prolonged first and second stages of labor
Operative delivery (*i.e.*, forceps extraction)
Overdistention of the uterus (polyhydramnios, multiple pregnancy, overly large infant)
Previous uterine atony or associated previous postpartum hemorrhage
Other hemorrhagic complications such as abruptio placentae or placenta previa
Induced labor
Heavy medication during labor or general anesthesia
Preeclampsia and eclampsia

The nurse will have an intravenous infusion with an oxytocic for immediate administration ready in the event that the attendants suspect hemorrhage is imminent.

Psychosocial Considerations

Emotional Reactions. Immediately after delivery, or perhaps later, the parents, particularly the mother, may relieve tension by giving way to some emotional displays such as laughing, crying, talking incessantly, or expressing anger (if all has not gone well or as expected). These emotions often are quite unexpected and may shock and embarrass those involved. A calm, accepting, nonjudgmental attitude on the part of the nurse is very effective in allaying any embarrassment and in helping the client to gain control.

The nurse must remember that the client is beginning a period that is enormously important; she is, in fact, now a "mother" with all its concomitant responsibilities. This is not the end but only the beginning of a whole new role. In addition, she is physically and emotionally exhausted from the labor and birth and is at risk for potential sleep/rest disturbance.

Several comfort measures can be employed to restore calm and to help the mother relax enough to get some much needed rest and sleep. A soothing back rub, change of gown and linen, a quiet conversation with the nurse or the father in which the client is allowed to ventilate her feelings, an environment conducive to rest—all are helpful. In addition, if she is stable after the first hour, a warm beverage can be offered to help relaxation. Since the mother is apt to be extremely hungry and thirsty, this is welcome nourishment as well as a therapeutic soporific.

Many mothers do not have an emotional outburst *per se*, although the majority do experience some degree

NURSING CARE PLAN

The Woman/Family During Third and Fourth Stages of Labor

Nursing Objectives

1. Help client achieve stabilization of physical systems by the second hour post partum.
2. Guide family with initial interactions.

Assessments	Potential Nursing Diagnosis	Planning/Intervention	Evaluation
Observe post delivery Fundus Flow Bladder Vital signs Perineum Complications Hemorrhage Hematoma Infection	Alteration in comfort: pain related to: Involution of uterus Episiotomy Potential for infection: vaginal, perineal, related to bacterial invasion secondary to trauma during labor and delivery and episiotomy	Administer oxytocin after delivery of placenta as ordered Gently massage fundus; if boggy express clots as necessary Wash hands when doing pericare Take pad off front to back Record and report amount and character of flow, vital signs, hematoma/bleeding from episiotomy Record temperature	Client maintains normal temperature and vital signs
Determine need for comfort, rest, and nourishment	Sleep pattern disturbance Alteration in nutrition: less than body requirements	Reposition mother as needed: give warm, dry gown and blanket Provide adequate explanations, answers to questions; provide quiet environment for rest; provide light nourishment as indicated	Client is warm and comfortable Client takes nourishment Client rests
Assess family interaction	Alteration in parenting related to: Inexperience Lack of role models Grieving related to: Labor and delivery not the way client wanted it to be Infant not the desired sex Pregnancy over	Facilitate family interaction in the delivery and recovery rooms Answer any questions parents have about newborn Refer to Chapters 28 and 30 for more interventions Allow woman to ventilate feelings over loss Clarify when necessary	Client verbalizes feelings to nurse Client satisfied with outcome

of excitement and elation when the delivery is accomplished. Any of the above nursing activities are also suitable for them. Some clients experience a great need for sleep and drop off as soon as they know that the baby is normal and healthy. If the client is sleeping continuously or intermittently, she should be allowed to do so, being disturbed only for those nursing observations that are necessary. When she indicates readiness, her baby can be presented and she can be allowed to examine and to explore it to her heart's content.

Mothers who have not been conscious during the delivery may have rather different reactions from those who have participated in the birth process. Often they do not seem to believe that delivery has taken place or that the baby shown to them is really theirs. They question again and again, "Is it really all over?" "Tell me again, is it a boy or a girl?" "Did I have the baby?" The apparent alteration in awareness seems to be related to the anesthesia and the unconsciousness. These mothers may need more firm reassurance and contact with their infants to help them realize that they have had a baby. Even though the repeated questioning may become annoying, the nurse must recognize that this is necessary for the mother to begin the important process of disengagement from the symbiotic relationship that she had with her infant during pregnancy. She must now establish the baby as a real entity outside her body rather than inside. All mothers have this task to perform, but it may be harder for the mother who has been delivered under heavy anesthesia, for as far as she is concerned, she was not "there" when it all happened.

Family Interactions. As we know, the couple's attachment for the new infant does not spring unbound at the time of delivery. At the birth there may be excitement over the sex, the color and amount of hair, and other physical characteristics, but attachment develops over time, as in any other relationship. Attachment is defined as a "unique relationship between two people which is specific and endures through time."[28] Parental attachment may have started prior to conception and continued through the pregnancy; it is enhanced with the actual birth and will be intensified during the next weeks.[28]

The nurse attending the delivery and giving care in recovery can assist the couple with the first interactions. The nurse may help the mother with her first breastfeeding or the father as he holds the infant the first time. These interactions are important as the beginning foundation for their family relationship continues to develop.

Assessment of Family Integration. Rising has pointed out that there is a certain openness about the fourth stage of labor that may not occur again during the postpartum period. This openness allows the nurse to make assessments regarding the couple's ability to proceed with integrating the infant smoothly into the family.[29] If family units are identified for potential alteration in parenting, the nurse will want to set aside more time to be with the couple to reinforce any positive responses that they might demonstrate and to give encouragement. Listening attentively as the couple relive their recent experience and encouraging verbalization of these feelings can be helpful. Most importantly, the nurse will want to pass on the client's care plan to ensure continuity in care. The postpartum nursing staff can work closely with community-health nurses or arrange for other follow-up care to encourage appropriate adjustment for the family. This is a time when the nurse needs to use all the observational skills, time, and laying on of the hands to foster initial integration and to begin prescribing future care aimed at consolidating the family unit. The topic of parent–infant attachment is discussed more thoroughly in Chapter 30, Psychosocial Aspects of the Postpartum Period.

References

1. Nurses Association of the American College of Obstetricians and Gynecologists: Standards for Obstetric, Gynecologic, and Neonatal Nursing, 2nd ed, 1961
2. American Academy of Pediatrics, The American College of Obstetricians and Gynecologists: Guidelines for Perinatal Care, 1983
3. Friedman EA: Labor, Clinical Evaluation and Management, 2nd ed. New York, Appleton-Century-Crofts, 1978
4. Adams JQ, Alexander AM: Alterations in cardiovascular physiology during labor. Am J Obstet Gynecol 12:542–549, 1958
5. Hendricks CH, Quilligan EJ: Cardiac output during labor. Am J Obstet Gynecol 71:953–972, May 1956
6. Elkayam V, Gleicher N (eds): Cardiac Problems in Pregnancy. New York, Alan R Liss, 1982
7. Martin J, Miller J, Heins H et al (eds): Intrapartum Assessment and Management Module, Perinatal Education Program for Community Hospital. Charleston, Medical University of South Carolina, 1982
8. Pritchard JA, MacDonald PC, Gant NF: Williams' Obstetrics. Norwalk, CT, Appleton-Century-Crofts, 1985
9. Freeman RF, Garite TJ: Fetal Heart Rate Monitoring. Baltimore, Williams & Wilkins, 1981
10. Garite TJ: Achieving good outcomes when membranes rupture prematurely. Contemp OB/GYN 25:96–105, February 1985
11. Kalish BJ: What is empathy? Am J Nurs 73:1548–1552, September 1973
12. Kantor HI et al: Value of shaving the pudendal–perineal area in delivery preparation. Obstet Gynecol 25:509–512, April 1965
13. Johnston RA, Sidall RS: Is the usual method of preparing patients for delivery beneficial or necessary? Am J Obstet Gynecol 4:645–650, December 1922
14. Sweeney WJ, III: Perineal shaves and bladder catheterization: Necessary and benign or unnecessary and potentially injurious? Obstet Gynecol 21:291–294, March 1963
15. Long AE: Unshaved perineum at parturition. Am J Obstet Gynecol 99:333–336, October 1, 1967
16. Seropian R, Reynolds BM: Wound infections after preoperative depilatory versus razor preparation. Am J Surg 121:251–254, March 1971
17. Landry KE, Kilpatrick DM: Why shave a mother before she gives birth? MCN 2(3):189–190, May/June 1977
18. Mahan CS, McKay S: Preps and enemas: Keep or discard? Contemp OB/GYN 22(5):241, November 1983
19. Saltenes SJ: Physical Touch and Nursing Support in Labor. Master's thesis, Yale University, 1962
20. Liu YC: Effects of the upright position during labor. Am J Nurs 74:2202–2205, December 1974
21. Roberts JE: Maternal positions for childbirth: A historical review of nursing care practices. JOGN Nurs 8:24–32, January/February 1979
22. Caldeyro-Barcia R: The influence of maternal bearing-down efforts during second stage on fetal well-being. Birth Fam J 6(1):17–21, Spring 1979

23. Carr KC: Management of the second stage of labor. NAACOG Update Series Lesson 9(1), 1983

24. Leboyer F: Birth Without Violence. New York, Alfred A Knopf, 1975

25. Oliver M, Oliver GM: Gentle birth, its safety and effect on neonatal behavior. JOGN Nurs 7:35–40, September/October 1978

26. Barnett CR, Leiderman H, Grobestein R et al: The maternal side effects of interactional deprivation. Pediatrics 45:197, 1970

27. Jacobson H: A standard for assessing lochia volume. MCN 10:174–175, May/June 1985

28. Klaus M, Kennell J: Parent-Infant Bonding. St Louis, CV Mosby, 1982

29. Rising S: The fourth stage of labor: Family integration. Am J Nurs 74:870–874, May 1974

Suggested Reading

Carpenito LJ: Nursing Diagnosis Application to Clinical Practice. Philadelphia, JB Lippincott, 1983

Carr KC: Management of the second stage of labor. NAACOG Update Series, Lesson 9(1), 1983

Cronenwett LR, Newmark LL: Father's responses to childbirth. Nurs Res 23:210–217, May/June 1974

Henson D: Natural childbirth in the year, 0. Nurs Forum 17(3):228–244, 1978

Highley BL, Mercer RT: Safeguarding the laboring woman's sense of control. MCN 3(1):39–41, January/February 1978

Huprich PA: Assisting the couple through a Lamaze labor and delivery. MCN 2(4):245–253, July/August 1977

Jacobson H: A standard for assessing lochia volume. MCN 10:174–175, May/June 1985

McDonough M, Sheriff D, Zimmel P: Parents' responses to fetal monitoring. MCN 6(1):32–34, January/February 1981

Malinowski J: Nursing Care of the Labor Patient. 2nd ed. Philadelphia, FA Davis, 1983

Martin J, Miller J, Heins H et al (eds): Intrapartum Assessment and Management Module, Perinatal Education Program for Community Hospital. Charleston, Medical University of South Carolina, 1982

Moore ML: Potential alterations in attachment: Maternal and/or neonatal illness. NAACOG Update Series, Lesson 7(1), 1983

Newel NJ: Grandparents: The overlooked support system for new parents during the fourth trimester. NAACOG Update Series, Lesson 21(1), 1984

Roberts JE: Maternal positions for childbirth: A historical review of nursing care practices. JOGN 8:24–32, January/February 1979

Shannon-Babitz M: Addressing the needs of fathers during labor and delivery. MCN 4(6):378–382, November/December 1979

Walker MM: Siblings in the childbearing experience. NAACOG Update Series, Lesson 17(1), 1984

Wheeler L: Intrapartal measurement of blood pressure. NAACOG Update Series, Lesson 20(1), 1984

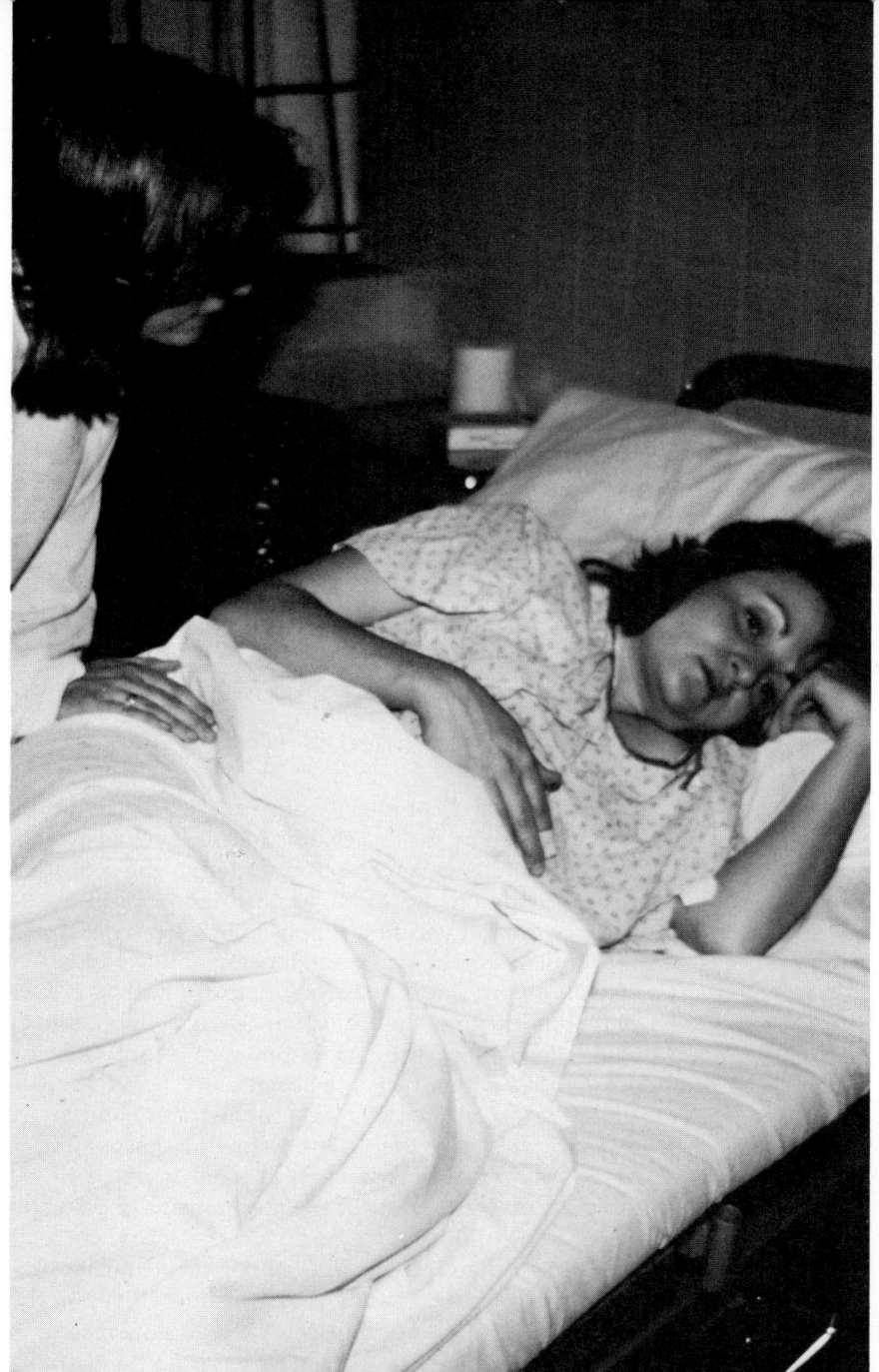

CHAPTER 26

The Nurse's Contribution to Pain Relief During Labor

The relief of pain and suffering is a humane and moral act. However, pain relief is often given a low priority by health-team members, especially in regard to childbirth. It has been pointed out that during childbirth the two primary tasks of the mother and the staff are "to deliver a 'good' baby and to conclude that process with an unimpaired mother . . . each takes precedence over the relief of pain."[1] Information about nonpharmacologic pain relief measures is now more readily available to parents and health professionals. Thus, pain relief can be a priority without harming the mother or child. In fact, pain relief may contribute to their physiological and emotional well-being (see Table 26-4).

Pain Mechanisms

Gate Control Theory

The mystery and complexity of pain are especially well demonstrated by the fact that no one really knows what neurophysiological mechanism underlies the sensation of pain. Among the more recent theories is the *gate control theory.* It was first proposed in 1965 by Melzack and Wall and has since been debated and expanded.[2-5] Like all theories, it is not absolute truth. Rather, it uses available information to explain the phenomenon of pain, suggesting reasons for known facts and offering possibilities where facts are absent.

There are numerous facets to the theory and many ways to categorize them. The following discussion focuses only on those aspects that seem most pertinent to a basic understanding of the mechanisms of pain and its relief in childbirth.

As its name implies, the gate control theory proposes that there is a gating mechanism involved in the transmission of pain impulses. A closed gate results in no pain; an open gate results in pain; and a partially open gate results in less pain. This gating mechanism is probably located in various places throughout the central nervous system. When the gate is closed, the transmission of pain impulses is stopped and pain does not reach the level of awareness.

The transmission of pain impulses to the level of cortical awareness can be affected in the following three ways:

- *The activity in large and small sensory nerve fibers.* The gate is opened by excitation of small-diameter fibers that carry pain impulses. However, these pain signals can be blocked (*i.e.,* the gate can be closed to prevent or decrease their transmission to the cortex) by stimulation of large-diameter fibers. Since many cutaneous fibers are large-diameter fibers, stimulation of the skin by rubbing or other means may result in pain relief (Fig. 26-1).

- *Projections from the brain stem reticular formation.* The reticular activating system regulates or adjusts incoming and outgoing signals, including the amount of sensory input. Somatic inputs from all parts of the body, as well as visual and auditory inputs, are monitored by the reticular system. Although it is not well understood, it appears that a

sufficient amount of sensory input may cause the reticular system to project inhibitory signals to the gate (*i.e.*, the reticular formation may cause the gate to be closed to the transmission of pain impulses). Hence, pain signals would not reach the level of cortical awareness (no pain), or fewer pain signals would reach the brain (less intense pain). Thus, distraction, for example, may inhibit pain impulses, whereas monotony (unvarying sensory input) would increase pain.

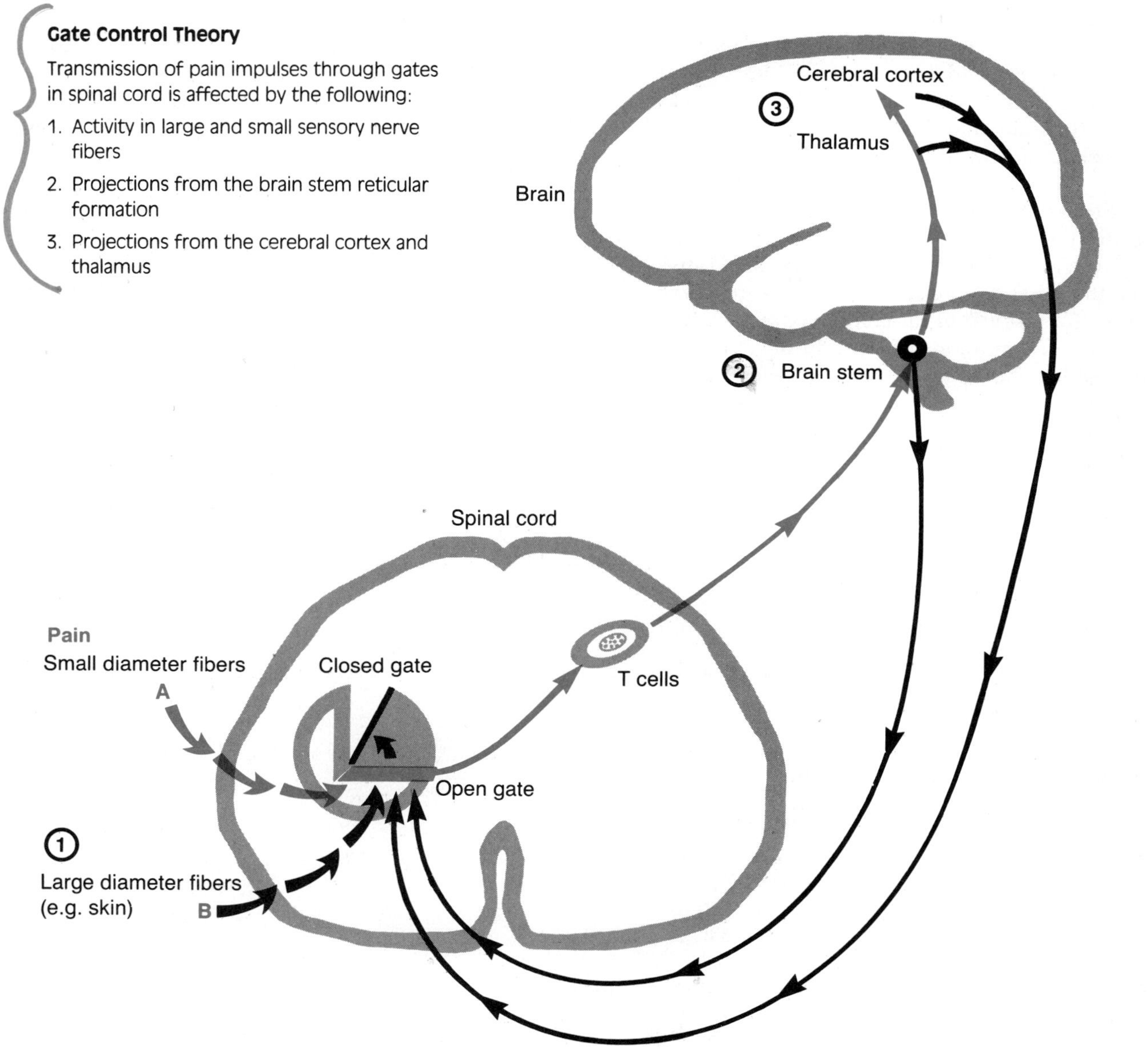

Gate Control Theory

Transmission of pain impulses through gates in spinal cord is affected by the following:

1. Activity in large and small sensory nerve fibers
2. Projections from the brain stem reticular formation
3. Projections from the cerebral cortex and thalamus

FIGURE 26-1

One influence on the gating mechanism is the ratio of large/small fibers activated. (*A*) Impulses traveling on small-diameter nerve fibers cause the gate to be held open. (*B*) Impulses traveling on large-diameter fibers generate feedback to the gate, almost closing it. (Hassid P: Textbook for Childbirth Educators. New York, Harper & Row, 1978)

- *Projections from the cerebral cortex and thalamus.* Signals from the cortex or thalamus can open or close the gate to transmission of pain impulses, either indirectly by projecting through the reticular formation or directly by projecting to the gate. Cognitive and affective processes are subserved at least in part by neural activity in the cortex and thalamus. Therefore, the individual's own unique thoughts and feelings can influence the transmission of pain impulses from the gate to the level of cortical awareness. Such thoughts and feelings may include the meaning of the pain, the person's beliefs, anxieties, memories of past painful experiences, and any number of other factors. Thus, input to the gating mechanism is evaluated by the individual *before* it is felt as a sensation as well as afterward.

Perhaps the most important contribution of the gate control theory is the possible explanation it offers for the individuality of the pain experience (Table 26-1). One thing has been clear for many years: comparable stimuli (or lesions) in different people do not produce comparable sensations of pain. In other words, when comparable stimuli are applied to several people, one person may perceive intense pain, another moderate pain, and still another no pain at all. The gate control theory suggests mechanisms by which a myriad of factors may determine the existence of pain and influence the nature of a painful experience. In summary, these factors may include not only stimulation of pain fibers but also cutaneous stimulation, other sensory input, thoughts, and feelings.

The gate control theory also provides a basis for understanding and devising pain relief measures.

Endorphins

It has recently been discovered that opiatelike substances occur naturally within the body.[6] These substances have been called endorphins, a combination of the words endogenous and morphine. To date several have been isolated, but it is clear that many more exist. Their role in the cause and alleviation of pain has not yet been clarified. An overview of the possible ways endorphins affect pain such as that felt in labor and delivery follows.

Endorphins influence the transmission of impulses interpreted as painful. Endorphins may possibly act as either neurotransmitters or neuromodulators that inhibit the transmission of pain messages. Thus, the presence of endorphin at the synapse of nerve cells results in a decrease in the sensation of pain. Failure to release en-

T A B L E 2 6 - 1
___

Nursing Practice Aspects of the Gate Control Theory of Pain
___

Major contributions

1. An integrated conceptual model for appreciating the many factors that contribute to individual differences in the experience of pain
2. Conceptualization of categories of activity that may form a theoretical base for developing various pain relief measures

Nature of the gate

The transmission of potentially painful impulses to the level of conscious awareness may be affected by a gating mechanism, possibly located at the spinal cord level of the CNS.

Structures Involved	*No Pain or Decreased Intensity of Pain*	*Pain*
Spinal cord (?)	Results from closing the gate in one of the following ways:	Results from opening the gate in one of the following ways:
Nerve fibers	1. Activity in the *large-diameter nerve fibers* (*e.g.,* caused by skin stimulation)	1. Activity in the *small-diameter nerve fibers* (*e.g.,* caused by tissue damage)
Brain stem	2. Inhibitory impulses from the *brain stem* (*e.g.,* caused by sufficient or maximum sensory input arriving through distraction or guided imagery)	2. Facilitory impulses from the *brain stem* (*e.g.,* caused by insufficient input from a monotonous environment)
Cerebral cortex and thalamus	3. Inhibitory impulses from the *cerebral cortex* and *thalamus* (*e.g.,* caused by anxiety reduction based on learning when the pain will end and how to relieve it)	3. Facilitory impulses from the *cerebral cortex* and *thalamus* (*e.g.,* caused by fear that the intensity of pain will escalate and will be associated with death)

(McCaffery M: Nursing Management of the Patient With Pain, 2nd ed. Philadelphia, JB Lippincott, 1979)

dorphin allows pain to occur. Opiates, such as morphine or endorphin (sometimes referred to as enkephalin), probably inhibit transmission of pain messages by attaching to opiate receptor sites (Fig. 26-2) of nerves in the brain and spinal cord.[7]

Endorphin levels differ from one individual to another, explaining in part why some people feel more pain than others. Persons with a high endorphin level obviously feel less pain. Also, it has been found, for example, that persons with a low endorphin level prior to surgery require more analgesia postoperatively than persons with a higher level of endorphin. Differences in endorphin levels may be inherited and may thereby explain cultural differences in pain sensitivity.[8]

Certain situations such as stress and pregnancy cause an increase in endorphin levels. Therefore, the endorphin level varies within the individual from one situation to another. During pregnancy and birth both mother and infant may have a decreased sensitivity to pain because of increased endorphin levels.[8]

Various pain relief measures may be dependent upon the endorphin systems. For example, it is possible that certain kinds of client teaching or stimulation of the skin, such as massage, can cause an increase in endorphin, which in turn relieves pain.[9]

Uniqueness of Pain During Childbirth

The discomfort and pain of childbirth are unique. Hence, the childbirth experience has a high potential for the achievement of satisfactory pain relief. Studies suggest that anxiety is reduced if the person knows when a painful event will occur and how long the discomfort will last. Ordinarily the mother knows the approximate date of confinement, and she has some idea of the approximate length of labor. In other words, she knows labor will occur, she knows the expected date

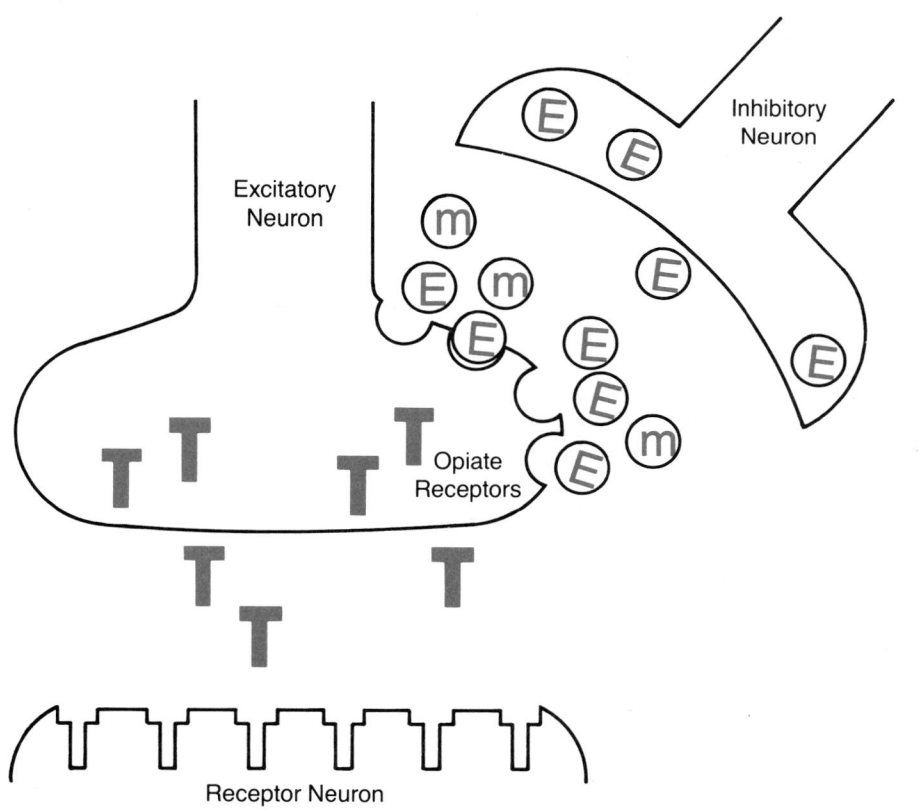

FIGURE 26-2

The opiate receptor is thought to be located on the endings of excitatory neurons. Binding of endorphin, or enkephalin (*E*), or opiates such as morphine (*M*) may inhibit release of transmitter (*T*) and thereby lead to alteration in pain perception. (Adapted from Pittman AW, Rudd GD: Analgesic Therapy, Part 2: Analgesia for Severe Pain, p 8. Chapel Hill, NC, Health Sciences Consortium, 1980)

within a few weeks, and she knows labor usually lasts a matter of hours, not days.

Even more helpful is the information the mother has once labor has actually begun. With the assistance of a watch she can determine the usual length of her contractions and predict when the next one will occur. In addition, she knows that contractions generally become more intense and more frequent as labor progresses. Further, although her discomfort may increase in intensity, she is not usually in constant discomfort. Between contractions there are periods of relative comfort even during the final phase of labor contractions.

The mother also knows the cause of her discomfort. At least she knows it is a normal process that has something to do with the expulsion of her baby and that parts of her body are contracting and stretching to accomplish this event. Most mothers recognize the onset of labor and do not fear that something harmful or life threatening is happening.

The discomfort of labor is also unique in that there is a tangible end product, the baby. The birth of the baby is something in which there has been deep personal involvement, both emotional and physiological. The involvement may have been positive and desirable or unpleasant and unwanted. Nevertheless, when the baby is born, the discomfort of labor subsides markedly and the event is characterized by physical and psychological closure. Few episodes of pain end so dramatically.

Nursing Assessment

To assess pain during labor and delivery the nurse needs an understanding of the various aspects of experiencing pain. For example, the following definitions will demonstrate that the mother's manner of expressing pain may not clearly reflect the intensity of pain she feels or the degree to which she is willing to tolerate the pain.

Definitions of Pain

Pain

Pain defies definition. It is a personal and subjective experience, differing from one person to another and varying within the same person from one time to the next. Quite simply, pain is a localized sensation of hurt. However, for both the nurse and the client, who work together to relieve pain, it seems more productive for the nurse to adopt the client's definition of pain.

The definition of pain may then be stated as whatever the experiencing person says it is, existing whenever she says it does.[10] A crucial aspect of this definition

---

Definitions Concerning Pain

Pain—a localized sensation of hurt; whatever the experiencing person says it is, existing whenever he or she says it does

Pain experience—all aspects surrounding the sensation of pain, before, during, and after it is felt, including the client's responses and external events of which the client is aware

Pain expressions—the client's observable responses to pain, both behavioral and physiological

Pain intensity—the severity of the pain sensation

Pain tolerance—the intensity or duration of pain the client is willing to endure without making further efforts to relieve it

Suffering—the agonizing or bothersome component of pain

---

is that the nurse believes what the client tells her. Of course, the client may communicate the pain experience in any number of ways besides verbalization. For example, in some clients a marked increase in rate and depth of respirations may alert the nurse to the intensification of discomfort.

Pain Experience

The phrase *pain experience* encompasses all the client's sensations, feelings, and behavioral responses, including physiological activities such as blood pressure changes. The pain experience may also refer to any or all of the three phases of pain: anticipation, presence, aftermath. It may include not only the client's actions, but also the impact that others have upon the client during the pain experience.

Pain Expressions

The manner in which an individual responds to pain is dependent upon numerous and varied factors, such as the culture in which the person lives, the personal meaning of the pain, and the intensity of the pain. Hence, pain expressions may be absent or minimal or not easily observed. For example, a slight and momentary frown may be the only sign that the client is experiencing pain. Or the client may be more expressive and engage in prolonged moaning.

Expressions of pain are usually observed in one or more of the following categories of behavioral response: physiological, verbal, vocal, facial, body movement, physical contact with others, and general response to the environment.[10]

Pain Intensity

The intensity of pain refers to the severity of the sensation itself. To determine this the client may be asked to rate the intensity of pain on a numerical scale such as zero to ten, with zero being no pain at all and ten being the worst possible pain. An alternative is a series of words for rating pain intensity, such as none, mild, moderate, severe, and very severe.

When a client does not exhibit many expressions of pain, it is very helpful to ask her to use a rating scale to convey the intensity of pain, since it cannot be easily observed. If this is explained early in labor, the mother may be able to use the scale throughout labor and delivery whenever she is requested to do so.

Pain Tolerance

It is very important to differentiate between the presence and intensity of a pain sensation, as indicated by expressions of pain, and the client's tolerance for that pain. Pain tolerance may be defined as the duration or intensity of pain that the client is willing to endure without pain relief.

Pain tolerance differs markedly from one person to another. Some clients state that the pain sensation is severe, yet they are willing to tolerate the pain and do not request pain relief. Other clients request pain relief measures when they rate the pain as mild. The latter group may be said to have a low tolerance for pain. While a high pain tolerance is valued by many people, the nurse should realize that a client's tolerance for pain is not a matter of good or bad, or right or wrong. Indeed, none of the client's responses to pain are to be judged in this way.

During childbirth, the mother is expected to endure or tolerate a certain amount of pain to ensure her own and her baby's good health. However, some mothers have a low pain tolerance, and it is especially important for the nurse to help these mothers find a way to cope with their discomfort. Admonishing the mother to cope with the discomfort or leaving the room when she complains certainly is not helpful. Other techniques can be called upon in such instances. The nonpharmacologic measures discussed in this chapter are especially appropriate for the mother with a low pain tolerance.

Suffering

Suffering is an affective state that may accompany pain. Copp, a nurse–researcher in the field of pain, pointedly uses the term *suffering* in reference to pain and defines it as "the state of anguish of one who bears pain, injury, or loss."[11] When pain cannot be eliminated, it is imperative that the client receive whatever assistance is necessary to prevent or diminish feelings of suffering. While a painful experience is at best only unpleasant, in most cases it need not be unrelenting agony.

Assessment of Pain

Before the nurse assesses the individual mother's expectations about pain or her actual experience with pain during childbirth, it is helpful to know the wide range of beliefs and experiences that may be encountered.

Prejudices That Hamper Assessment of Pain

Precautions must be taken to avoid certain prejudices that may hamper the nurse's assessment of the pain experience.

Signs of Acute Pain. There is a tendency to recognize the existence of pain only in those clients who show signs of acute pain, such as perspiration, muscle tension, or moaning. The absence of these expressions of pain, as noted previously, does not necessarily mean the client is not in pain. In fact, the client may suffer greatly but exhibit only minimal pain expression.[10]

In childbirth there appear to be two major reasons for minimal pain expressions: (1) the mother may have learned that minimal pain expressions are the expectations of the culture or (2) activities learned from a method of prepared childbirth may preclude expressions of pain. For example, practicing relaxation techniques may preclude muscle tension as a sign of acute pain; use of a breathing pattern or mouthing the words of a song may preclude the behavior of moaning.

It is often quite difficult, if not impossible, to rely upon signs of acute pain in assessing the laboring mother who is using one of the methods of prepared childbirth. Usually she simply is too busy to show signs of acute pain.

Physical Cause of Pain. We also tend to be prejudiced in favor of believing clients only when we know the physical cause of pain.[10] This hampers our understanding of the subjective pain experience. Hence, when the mother states, for instance, that she feels severe pain, her statement must be believed even if there seems to be no physical cause for such a painful labor. The temptation to judge the mother's discomfort by the results of electronic monitoring of intrauterine pressure must also be avoided.

Values of Mother or Father. The mother or father may also harbor prejudices or values that make it difficult for the nurse to assess the pain experience. Either or both of the parents may feel that responses to pain should be minimized. The only appropriate response may be a verbal description of the pain. Some mothers may not even volunteer this much, so they have to be questioned directly and at regular intervals. Still other mothers may want to avoid using the word *pain* or resist any tendency to say they feel pain. They may prefer to use other terms, which may be deceptive if taken at face value. For example, the mother may verbalize feeling "enormous pressure" but refuse to call it painful. Yet the mother may need assistance in coping with this sensation, so that measures designed to relieve severe pain may be very appropriate.

Still another type of problem may arise with a father who forcefully tries to impose his own goals upon the mother who does not share his values. In the situation in which the father does not want the mother to admit pain or to seek assistance with pain relief measures, the nurse may find that she obtains more accurate information when the father is absent from the room. Of course, the opposite type of situation may exist. The mother may feel perfectly capable of handling the pain and discomforts of labor, but the father may become insistent that she be "put out of this misery."

Rating by Health-Team Members. There is a tendency for health-team members to rate the mother's pain as less intense than the mother rates her pain. This is particularly true of the first stage of labor. Health-team members also tend to agree with each other about the degree of the mother's pain.[12,13] In other words, the staff observing the mother may agree with one another that her pain is not as severe as the mother actually experiences it. We must guard against letting agreement among ourselves about the mother's pain cause or reinforce any doubts about the intensity of the pain.

Variability in Beliefs and Facts

Most laypersons expect pain to occur during childbirth. This expectation may evolve from a variety of sources, such as television, movies, books, comments from one's own parents, and reports from friends who have had babies. However, information about childbirth in general may be incomplete, if not inaccurate. Hence, fear of pain may be anticipated by expectant parents as a result of their overall lack of knowledge about labor.

The fear of pain is second only to the fear of death. Understandably, then, some expectant parents are eager to examine and accept any information suggesting that childbirth need not be associated with pain. Such information may be forthcoming from several sources.

Reports of how childbirth is handled in some other cultures, especially the more primitive ones, often emphasize the lack of any expression of pain. Some women are noted to have their babies in the fields and resume work immediately following delivery. Other women are observed to remain quiet with relaxed facial expressions during childbirth. However, *lack of expression of pain does not necessarily mean that pain is absent.* Indeed, a study of Samoan women revealed that while their expressions of pain were minimal during labor, they admitted afterward in interviews that they did experience pain or discomfort.[14]

Some methods of prepared childbirth may also suggest that labor is painless. Most methods of prepared childbirth inadvertently insinuate lack of pain in their films on childbirth and in the written narratives of couples who use the organization's particular method of childbirth. These films and reports focus on the techniques of a particular method and on the "peak experience" or ecstasy of giving birth while fully conscious. While one study showed that childbirth education did consistently result in lower levels of pain during labor, the reduction in pain was not dramatic. Most women still experienced severe pain.[15]

Factually, probably only 9% to 14% of untreated labors are painless or minimally uncomfortable.[15,16] In one study of both multiparas and primiparas, the women were asked how painful childbirth was in comparison to other pain they had experienced. Ninety-seven percent said it was the most painful experience they had ever had.[17] In another study of both multiparas and primiparas using the McGill Pain Questionnaire, the intensity of labor pain showed a wide variation but was found to rank among the most intense of pains. Further, pain intensity was significantly higher for primiparas than for multiparas.[18] In a study of primiparas only, 35% rated their pain as intolerable; 37% rated it as severe; and 28% rated it as moderate. Various studies of both primiparas and multiparas reveal that anywhere from about 35% to 61% of the women report pain that is intolerable or severe.[12,15]

Variability is probably the most striking feature of pain during labor. Not only does overall intensity vary, as noted above, but also the progression of pain intensity during labor and the location of pain. In one study some women showed the expected rising curve of pain intensity, but others experienced increases and decreases in pain intensity throughout labor, some had high levels early in labor, and still others had a low level pain up to the time of delivery. Location of pain also varied; some women had widespread pain over a large part of the abdomen, back, and perineum, while others had very localized areas of pain (Fig. 26-3).[15]

Description of Painful Sensations

While no two labors are alike, the following is a description of the painful or uncomfortable sensations often felt during normal labor (Table 26-2). Considerably

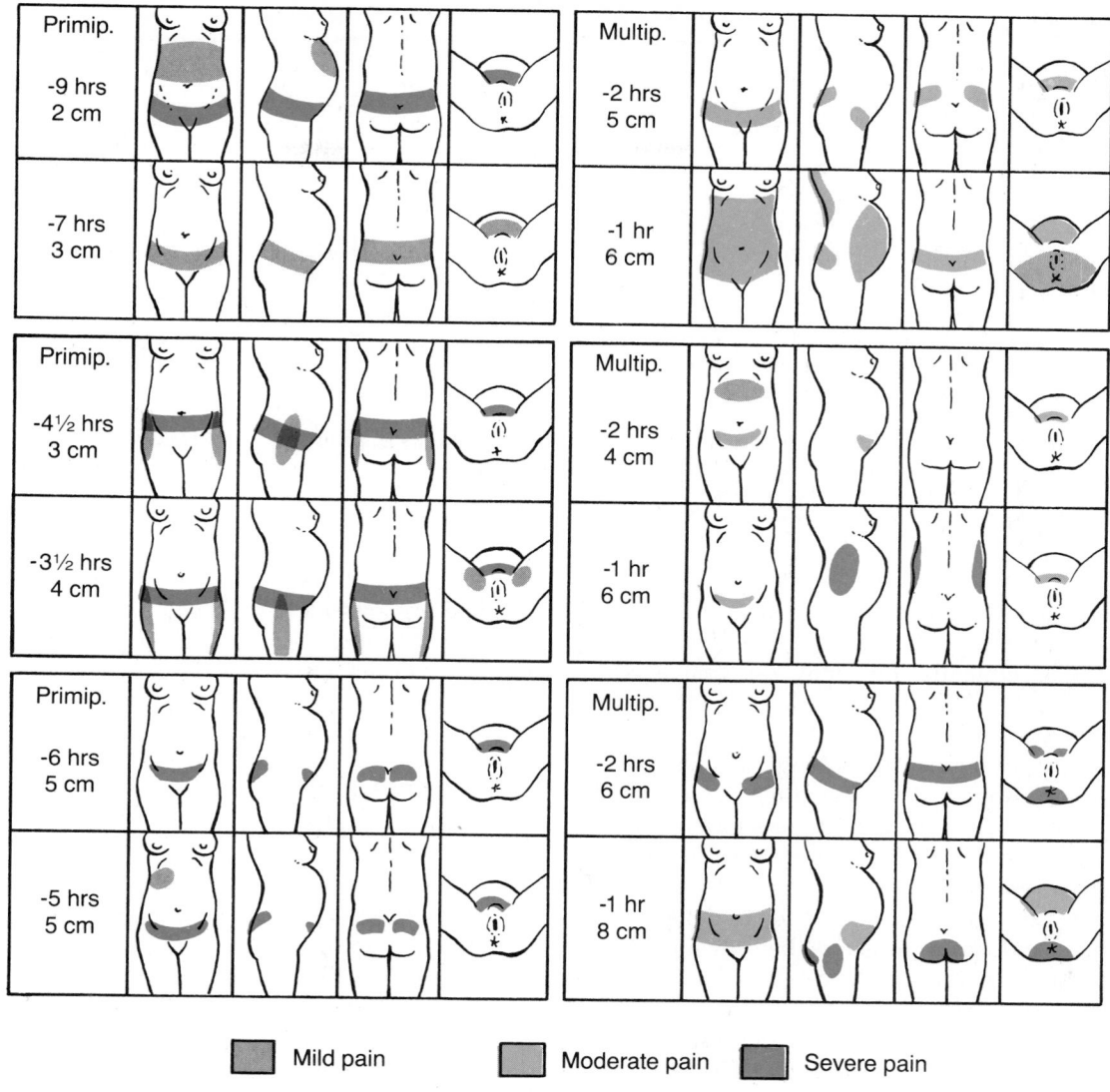

Mild pain ▢   Moderate pain ▢   Severe pain ▢

FIGURE 26-3

Distribution and intensity of pain during labor. Shaded areas show the distribution of pain in six women at various points during labor prior to delivery. Pain intensity is indicated as follows: stipple, mild pain; crosshatch, moderate pain; black, severe pain. (Adapted from Melzack R et al: Severity of labour pain: Influence of physical as well as psychological variables. Can Med Assoc J 130: 579–584, 1984)

more pain may be experienced with certain complications of labor, such as hypertonic uterine dysfunction, delivery of an oversized baby, or a contracted pelvis.

Uterine Contractions. During the first stage of normal labor, pain or discomfort may result from the involuntary contraction of the uterine muscle. The contraction tends to be felt in the lower back at the beginning of labor. As labor progresses the sensation encircles the lower torso, covering both back and abdomen.

Contractions are frequently described as wavelike: they come and go rhythmically, each one increasing to a certain height or intensity and then decreasing and, finally, disappearing. Contractions last from about 45 to 90 seconds. In early labor the contractions are not necessarily uncomfortable. As labor progresses the intensity of each contraction increases, resulting in a greater possibility or intensity of discomfort.

The quality of the discomfort is difficult to describe and certainly is varied. Basically there appear to be three

T A B L E 2 6 - 2

Common Painful Sensations During "Normal" Childbirth

	Uterine Contractions	Back Labor	Delivery
Site	Initially, lower back; as labor progresses, encircles lower torso	Lower back	Vagina, perineum
Pain Intensity	Progresses throughout labor from no discomfort to mild to moderate, perhaps severe; may be severe, especially during transition	Severe	Less than during transition
Quality of Pain	"Wavelike"; each one increases to a certain intensity and decreases, usually over a 45- to 90-second period	Deep pressure, aching	Pressure, stretching, splitting, sometimes burning

possible qualities to any painful sensation: burning, pricking, and aching. Also, pain can be either deep or superficial. Consequently, one may say that a labor contraction is felt as deep aching. Words commonly chosen by women in labor to describe their pain are sharp, cramping, aching, throbbing, stabbing, hot, shooting, heavy, tiring, exhausting, intense, and tight.[15]

The intervals between contractions shorten as labor proceeds. Early labor contractions are about 20 minutes apart. Then for several hours they occur 3 to 5 minutes apart. During about the last hour prior to delivery the intervals between contractions may be only a few seconds long. This period, when the cervix is dilating from about 7 cm to 10 cm, is referred to as transition.

Uterine contractions are at their highest intensity and greatest frequency during transition. This is usually when the mother experiences the most discomfort and has the most difficulty handling her discomfort.

Back Labor. In addition to uterine contractions, approximately 25% of women in labor also have to cope with the discomfort of *back labor*. This occurs when the fetus is in an occipitoposterior position (see Chap. 38). With each contraction the occiput presses on the mother's sacrum, causing extreme discomfort as the intensity of contractions increases. Back labor is considerably more painful for the mother than labor in which there is an anterior occipital position.

Delivery. Of course, the mother certainly may experience discomfort during delivery, but it is generally much less intense than what she felt during transition. Apparently the mother's more noisy behavior during expulsion efforts has been interpreted by observers as indicative of more pain.[19]

The predominant sensations during delivery occur in the vaginal and perineal area and can be described

as pressure, stretching or splitting, and sometimes burning. Most of the time the mother has an overwhelming desire to push. Pushing may relieve whatever discomfort is felt. Also, the pressure of the baby's head causes a degree of numbness in the perineum.

Assessment of the Individual Mother's Contractions

When labor is discussed with the mother, the sensations should be referred to as contractions, not pains. The initial contractions are not necessarily uncomfortable, and pain is usually a misnomer. Later in labor the contractions may be uncomfortable but not unbearable. Most mothers probably are not so suggestible that they would actually feel unbearable pain during contractions simply because the nurse used the term *pains* rather than *contractions*. But the use of the term *pains* may generate needless anxiety.

When assessing the characteristics of uterine contractions (onset, frequency, duration, intensity, description of sensation, and attitude toward contractions) it is important to note the time when labor begins (*onset*), since prolonged labor intensifies the painful experience. Not only is a longer time spent in discomfort, but a lengthy labor often fatigues and discourages the parents, making it more difficult to cope with labor (see Part I of the Assessment Tool).

Regularity and increasing *frequency* of contractions, along with increasing intensity of contractions, indicate a normal labor. Such information can be used to assure the parents that progress is being made.

To obtain more detailed and useful information about *intensity of contraction*, the nurse may ask the mother to rate the contraction on a scale of mild, moderate, intense (strong), or very intense (very strong).

It is also helpful to encourage the mother to *describe*

Factors in Assessing the Pain Experience During Labor

I. Contractions
   Onset
   Frequency
   Duration
   Intensity
   Description of sensation, location
   Attitude toward contractions

II. Pain Relief Methods Employed by Parents for Labor
   Persons to assist or be present during labor
   Positioning
   Relaxation techniques
   Distraction (or concentration) methods
   Breathing patterns
   Physical activities
   Medication

III. Current Discomforts of Mother Other Than Labor
   Pregnancy
   Chronic illness
   Recent illness or injury
   Methods of handling above; effectiveness of methods

IV. Parents' Current Concerns Other Than Labor
   Activities or plans interrupted by labor
   Care of children at home
   Financial arrangements
   Condition of mother or unborn child
   Plans for care of infant
   Unexpected change in childbirth plans
   Plans and needs for assistance regarding above

V. Parents' Goals and Expectations Regarding Labor
   Presence and intensity of pain
   Provisions for pain relief (if any)
   Father's (coach's) presence
   Episiotomy
   Differences between mother and father regarding above
   Which of the above not possible or not discussed with physician

other characteristics of the contraction, such as where the sensation begins and where it is felt most intensely. This information often suggests the need for specific pain relief measures. For example, if the contraction begins in the lower back and is felt most intensely there, rubbing that area and applying pressure may provide considerable comfort.

At the same time that the mother is discussing her contractions she may reveal her *attitude* toward labor in general. The degree of fear or anxiety experienced is of special importance, since these feelings have a profound effect upon pain. They decrease pain tolerance

and increase the perceived intensity of pain. Anxiety or fear also increases muscle tension and may increase painful stimuli during labor by interfering with contractions.

Anxiety or fear during labor may be related to worry about how pain will be managed and how labor is progressing. To alleviate such anxiety, the nurse may inform the mother of the various pain relief measures that may be employed. Concern over the progression of labor, or the effectiveness of the contractions, may be partially diminished if the nurse keeps the mother informed of signs of progress, such as increasing cervical dilatation or regularity of contractions. It is sometimes helpful to assure the mother that it is possible to stop or correct ineffective or dysfunctional uterine contractions.

Assessment of Pain Relief Methods Employed by Parents

Since a thorough assessment of the mother in labor is inextricably related to intervention, some pain relief measures are mentioned in this discussion of assessment. Actually, the manner in which the nurse assesses the client is often a pain relief measure. When the nurse conveys to the mother that she believes the mother and that she desires to understand the mother's experience as completely as possible, anxiety may be reduced and the pain thereby relieved.

Method of Childbirth Preparation

The nurse questions the parents about how they have handled the discomforts of labor thus far and what their plans are for the remainder of labor. There are many methods of preparation for childbirth in the United States. Some of the techniques and pain relief methods may seem odd. Sometimes mothers feel foolish doing them, and nurses may be surprised to observe such techniques. However, a woman should be encouraged to use whatever method works for her. Some mothers intuitively devise their own special way of handling childbirth.

It is difficult to keep abreast of the constant changes taking place within each method, but the nurse can be reassured by the fact that in any single hospital labor suite one or two basic methods are used. This is partially because physicians using one particular method of childbirth tend to congregate at the same hospital where they can share ideas and know that the nursing staff is reasonably familiar with the method. Also, certain methods tend to be popular only in certain geographic areas. Thus, the nurse is likely to be able to quickly identify which methods are most common and can then study them in greater depth.

Part II of the Assessment Tool lists some common

pain relief methods employed during childbirth. They are discussed briefly below, additional examples are given under Nonpharmacologic Pain Relief, and a complete discussion is given in Chapter 19.

Persons Present During Labor

The father almost always is the support person during labor if the couple has attended classes on one of the methods of prepared childbirth. Sometimes the couple's children are allowed an occasional and brief visit to the labor room. When the father is absent or does not want to attend labor, or when the mother is unwed, the person in attendance may be a childbirth educator, the mother's friend, or a relative. After identifying the support person the nurse finds out if he has been with the mother prior to hospital admission and if the mother wants him to remain with her in the labor and delivery rooms. She also assesses the attending person's attitude and desires. It is possible, for instance, that the mother might want the father to remain with her, but the father may be quite reluctant and fearful. (For convenience, the person the mother brings to the hospital to be with her during labor henceforth will be referred to as the father.)

In addition, the nurse determines what the father has done for the mother prior to admission, what is planned for the remainder of labor, what (if any) preparation the mother and father have had, and, whether they have practiced what they plan to do. Sometimes the father simply stays near the mother, touching her gently and offering verbal encouragement. In other cases the father is expected to take a very active role in pain relief measures, such as massaging the back or abdomen or applying counterpressure.

Positioning

When the mother is admitted to the labor room the nurse asks her which positions have been comfortable and which have not and which positions she may wish to consider later in labor. Some positions require additional pillows, which the nurse can then obtain in advance. Positioning is discussed in Chapter 25.

Relaxation

Numerous techniques are used to achieve and maintain total skeletal muscle relaxation. A pillow may be placed between the mother's legs when she is on her side to support the limbs. For general relaxation, the mother may smile, yawn, or take deep breaths at regular intervals. The father may aid by giving tactile or verbal cues to induce relaxation.

Again, the nurse finds out what techniques are used for relaxation so she can accurately interpret the mother's behavior. Knowing that the mother intends to keep her eyes closed, for example, prevents the nurse from mistakenly concluding that this laboring mother is sleeping most of the time. See Chapter 20 for a review of relaxation as it is taught by the nurse–educator and Appendix A for the technique.

Distraction

Distraction and concentration are frequently used for coping with pain. Distraction techniques are also the most individualized and therefore the most varied of all the techniques a mother may employ during childbirth. For example, some women bring with them a personal "concentration point," an object to be stared at during a contraction. Other examples of distraction are breathing patterns, which are discussed below (see also Distraction, later in this chapter).

Breathing Patterns

Controversy and change are characteristic of many of the breathing patterns employed in the various methods of prepared childbirth. The two basic types of breathing are chest breathing and abdominal or diaphragmatic breathing (see Chap. 20 and Appendix A).

The nurse may be able to obtain information about the breathing patterns from some mothers simply by asking. Others may not be aware of the breathing pattern they are using. In such cases the mother should be observed closely to ascertain the breathing patterns being used. (A thorough assessment of breathing patterns helps the nurse anticipate the needs of the mother.) If a breathing pattern is not helpful, the nurse can suggest another. If the mother uses rapid breathing, the nurse can remind her to report any tingling in the hands and other initial signs of hyperventilation, or carbon dioxide insufficiency.

Physical Activities

Physical activities other than those that fall into the above categories may be used during labor. During a contraction the mother or father may rhythmically massage the abdomen, using some preparation such as talcum powder to keep the skin smooth. The father may rub her lower back between and during contractions. The mother may rock her pelvis while standing or lying on her side. The latter appears to be particularly helpful during back labor. Counterpressure is also useful. To achieve this the father may place tennis balls, a rolling pin, his knee, or his fist against the lower back.

Medications

When the mother is admitted, the nurse also asks whether or not she has taken medication or any other substance for pain relief, such as aspirin, codeine, an alcoholic beverage, or even paregoric, which is prescribed for false labor. If medication was taken, the nurse notes the time, type, and amount.

It is always possible that the mother has taken some illegal drug such as marijuana, heroin, or a black-market drug of unknown composition. The mother who uses illegal drugs may fear legal action against her or disdain from the health team. Therefore, to increase the likelihood of obtaining an honest answer from a mother who has used an illegal drug, the nurse should always stress that the questions about medication are asked for important reasons, such as determining what other medication can be used safely.

It is also important to inquire about what analgesics and anesthetics are being considered for use during labor. The mother may have no knowledge at all about medication, or she and the father may have discussed several possibilities with the physician.

Assessment of Problems Other Than Labor

Current Discomforts

The process of labor may not be the only source of discomfort for the mother. Indeed, there are other diseases or symptoms that may be much more irritating and painful than the concurrent labor. Such discomforts may be associated with the pregnancy itself or may represent a chronic illness or a recent illness or injury (see Part III of the Assessment Tool presented earlier in this chapter). For example, pregnancy may cause or increase heartburn, hemorrhoids, or varicose veins in the legs or vagina, all of which can be extremely uncomfortable.

As for chronic illness, any one of a number of disorders (*e.g.*, arthritis, allergy) may result in pain and discomfort. The same is true of a recent illness or injury, such as influenza or an accident resulting in a broken bone, lacerations, or a sprained ankle.

The nurse assesses sources of discomfort extraneous to labor so that appropriate actions can be taken to provide relief. At the same time, any treatment instituted prior to the onset of labor should be identified. If the mother has found effective means of handling discomforts, it obviously is expedient for her to use the same methods during labor whenever possible.

Current Concerns

Since the precise time for the onset of labor is rarely predictable, significant activities or plans may be interrupted by labor (see Part IV of the Assessment Tool). For example, the onset of labor may interfere with the requirements of the father's occupation and cause him to worry over the possibility of losing his job if he does not report to work. If the parents have other children,

they may be anxious about what will happen to them during their absence. The parents may also be concerned about financial arrangements related to hospitalization and the physician's fee, particularly if complications arise.

For some reason, realistic or not, the parents may be fearful about the condition of the mother or the unborn infant. The mother or father may be considering giving up the baby for adoption. Onset of labor may precipitate many feelings about this.

There may have been an unexpected change in some aspect of the parents' plans for childbirth. Their physician may be out of town, or labor may have progressed so rapidly that they were unable to reach the hospital of their choice.

It is important for the nurse to realize that such concerns can stir anxiety and interfere with the parents' ability to concentrate on handling discomforts, responding to directions, cooperating with examinations, and dealing with all the other aspects of labor. Any of these should be noted on the assessment.

Assessment of Goals and Expectations Regarding Labor

Parents generally have certain expectations regarding labor. The nurse may encounter extremes in parents' expectations related to pain and pain relief. One mother may expect severe pain and desire that the physician render her practically unconscious throughout labor. Another mother may expect no pain at all and, therefore, no pain relief measures. When discomfort and pain are expected, the parents may believe that the techniques they have been taught to use during labor, such as breathing patterns, are sufficient assistance for the mother. Their goal may be a completely unmedicated labor. Or, the parents may expect to use the methods they were taught in combination with some type of medication if they desire it.

In some cases the father remains with the mother from the beginning of labor, during delivery, and through the recovery period following delivery. In other instances the mother does not want the father present. Parents' expectations of the nurse and physician also need to be determined.

Some parents, particularly mothers, want very much to observe the effects of their pushing and the delivery of the baby. Many delivery rooms have mirrors for this purpose. The parents may have brought a camera to take pictures in the labor room and in the delivery room. They may also want someone to take a picture of them with their baby immediately after delivery. Some parents want to tape record the delivery.

A fully conscious mother almost always wants to touch the newborn as soon as possible. The mother may plan on holding the baby before the cord is cut. She may also expect to be allowed to breast-feed the baby on the delivery table.

In helping the parents express their goals and expectations the nurse is alert to differences between the desires of the mother and father. For example, the father may not want to witness the delivery although the mother wants him in the delivery room. Or the father may think the mother is unrealistic in her plans for little or no medication. When the nurse observes such differences she helps the parents become aware of them and formulate compatible goals.

In her assessment of the parents' goals the nurse also notes whether or not these goals have been discussed with the physician. Some goals may be contraindicated for medical reasons. Other goals may require the awareness and cooperation of the physician. In addition, hospital policy sometimes places limitations on the parents. For instance, some delivery rooms are so small that the hospital must have a policy of excluding the father.

As labor progresses the nurse continues to monitor the client for any changes in the items listed in Part V of the Assessment Tool. Some aspects of the labor situation may change dramatically, such as the nature of the contractions. There may be a sudden need for modification of pain relief methods. Also, the discomforts and concerns extraneous to labor may be resolved or suddenly may appear when none had existed before.

Nursing Diagnoses

Because we are concerned with pain in this chapter, nursing diagnoses are related to pain and its relief. Two possible diagnoses, then, are alteration in comfort (pain) related to contractions and knowledge deficit of methods to relieve back pain related to nonparticipation in childbirth classes.

Planning/Intervention

Goals and Principles of Pain Relief

Good pain relief does not necessarily mean the total elimination of painful sensations. In fact, complete abolition of pain is rarely a realistic goal. It is significantly helpful to the mother and often more reasonable to aim at a decrease in the intensity of pain or a decrease in the degree to which pain bothers the mother. The latter is closely related to another possible goal of increasing the mother's tolerance for pain.

Two important principles that underlie the accom-

plishment of these goals are decreasing the pain impulses that reach the cortex of the brain, and managing anxiety. The transmission of pain signals may be interrupted in a number of ways, such as decreasing the source of noxious stimuli or closing the gate (see Gate Control Theory, earlier in the chapter). Likewise, there are numerous ways of managing anxiety.

The interaction between anxiety and pain may become a spiraling process. Pain may cause anxiety, which may increase the intensity of pain by causing muscle tension or by opening the gate to pain impulses. In this way mild pain and anxiety can eventually become severe pain and panic.

Pharmacologic Pain Relief

Analgesia and anesthesia for pain relief are discussed in the following chapter. Implications for nursing related to care of the mother receiving pharmacologic pain relief are included in that chapter.

Nonpharmacologic Pain Relief

There are pain relief methods that may be used either instead of or in addition to analgesics and anesthetics. The focus here is purposefully limited to what the nurse may do for the mother or what she may assist the mother or father to do. Nursing activities related to the use of pharmacologic agents are discussed in Chapter 27.

Support During Labor

From the beginning of labor the mother needs to have someone with her at increasingly frequent intervals and to know that someone is available at all times. Toward the end of labor she needs to have someone with her constantly. The presence, actions, and words of this person can be very supportive to the mother. This person may be the nurse, the father, or someone else. At times the nurse's greatest contribution is to support the father so that he can in turn support the mother.

Giving Information

As mentioned previously, part of the uniqueness of labor pain is that the mother may possess anxiety-reducing knowledge. If the mother does not obtain this information for herself, the nurse can supply it. For example, the nurse may tell the mother approximately how long it will be before the next contraction and how long that contraction will last. During intense contractions the nurse may "count down" at 15-second intervals until the end of the contraction, telling the mother

The Woman With Increased Pain During Labor

Nursing Objectives

1. Provide information and assistance with methods to decrease the perceived intensity of pain during labor.
2. Provide information and assistance with methods to increase the tolerance for pain (make pain more bearable).

Assessment	Potential Nursing Diagnosis	Planning/Intervention	Evaluation

Identify or describe the presence or absence of:
 	
  Consistent person for support during labor
 	
  Mother's statement about intensity, tolerability, or other characteristics of discomfort from contraction and other sources
 	
  Concerns other than labor
 	
  Ability to fulfill goals and expectations regarding labor
 	
Use:
 	
  Positioning
 	
  Relaxation
 	
  Breathing patterns
 	
  Physical activities
 	
  Medications
	Alteration in comfort: pain related to contractions
	
	Knowledge deficit of methods of relieving back labor related to nonattendance of childbirth classes
		Identify one person who will remain with mother for support throughout remainder of labor
		
		Keep mother and support person informed of progress of labor
		
		Determine whether abdominal or chest breathing is most comfortable, and teach an appropriate breathing pattern
		
		Perform abdominal lifting
		
		Try position other than supine (e.g., 30° upright, up-on-all-fours)
		
		Give deep back massage; apply cold, heat, or firm pressure to lower back
		
		Suggest abdominal massage by mother or support person
		
		Encourage active listening with music and headset
		
		Teach simple relaxation technique
			Client's back pain decreases with use of cold
			
			Client's back pain is more bearable when active listening is used and support person is present

how long it will be until the contraction is over. Or the nurse may time the contraction so she can reassure the mother by telling her when the contraction has reached its peak and will begin to subside. Information about the progress of labor, such as cervical dilatation and descent of the baby, is also important. It serves as a reminder that there is a purpose to labor, that labor does end, and that the end is getting closer and closer.

Such information not only reduces anxiety but may also motivate the mother to tolerate pain. Especially toward the end of labor when discomfort increases, the knowledge that the ordeal is almost over may enable the mother to tolerate an intensity of pain that she would otherwise find unbearable.

Knowing that she and her baby are not in danger also reduces anxiety. Sometimes the mother finds the forces of labor so unexpectedly powerful that she is fearful of harm. The nurse should periodically reassure the mother that she and her baby are doing well (provided, of course, that this is true). She may say, for example, that the baby's heartbeat is strong and regular. Remembering that discomfort is associated with a normal process and not a life-threatening illness may be helpful to the mother. Briefly and in simple terms the nurse can remind the mother of what is happening (e.g., that each contraction enlarges the opening for the baby).

Understanding what is happening during labor seems to increase the mother's sense of control over the event. Feelings of powerlessness can provoke anxiety, so it is important to further feelings of control. This may be done through instructions and explanations that help the mother cooperate with examinations and with the

T A B L E   2 6 - 3

Summary of Pain Relief Measures Used by Lamaze-Trained Parents During Labor

Approximate Progress of Labor	Position	Relaxation	Mother's Activities During Massage
Onset to 3 cm, or contractions 5 min–20 min apart	Supported comfortably sitting or lying on side; may walk between contractions; may stand and lean on object during contractions	Inhales deeply at beginning of contraction and relaxes totally upon exhalation; takes a deep breath at end of each contraction	Hands move slowly from pubic area up to umbilicus and out around abdomen down to pubic area, or other body areas such as thighs may be massaged
Dilates from 4 cm–7 cm, or contractions 2 min–4 min apart	Same as above	Same as above	Same as above

process of labor, such as effective pushing. In particular the mother's feelings of control can be strengthened by teaching her about pain relief measures as early as possible. When this has not been done prior to labor the nurse can begin in early labor to explain certain of the following pain relief measures. The mother then knows that pain relief is available, that there are several possibilities, and that to some extent she may choose from among them.

Prepared Childbirth

The method of prepared childbirth growing most rapidly throughout the United States is the psychoprophylactic method (PPM), or Lamaze. Table 26-3 summarizes those activities the nurse generally might expect to be used by Lamaze-trained couples during labor for the purpose

of handling discomfort or pain. The nurse encounters variations in these activities because instructors are always making efforts to improve the method and because each mother may adapt the method to her own particular needs.

Sometimes the nursing staff tends to spend very little time with Lamaze-trained or otherwise prepared couples. While it is true that some couples may manage quite well on their own, most couples need some type of assistance. Knowledge of how a mother and father may attempt to cope with pain and discomfort enables the nurse to provide appropriate help. For example, when a breathing pattern has ceased to be effective, the Lamaze-trained mother may need assurance that labor has progressed sufficiently to warrant changing to the next breathing pattern. Or when the father must leave the labor room the nurse knows how to assume some

Eye Focus	Each Contraction in Relation to Breathing Pattern	Thoughts	Father's Activities Either During or Between Contractions
Eyes open and focused on one particular object ("concentration point," "focal point"), or eyes may be closed while doing guided imagery during contractions	Slow paced breathing, inhale through nose, exhale through nose or mouth. *Maximum* rate is half individual woman's resting respiration rate	On inhalation, "In, 1, 2" On exhalation, "Out, 1, 2" or Concentrate on imagery	Times frequency of each contraction Helps mother get in comfortable positions, changing positions at least hourly As need arises, may give signals to help increase relaxation, do abdominal massage for her, or rub her lower back Reminds her to urinate—a full bladder can slow labor progress
Same as above	Modified paced breathing, accelerates as contraction intensifies, decelerates as contraction subsides; breathing is maximum rate of twice woman's resting respiration rate Breathing may be inhale nose, exhale nose; inhale nose, exhale mouth; or inhale mouth, exhale mouth. Breathing may be in 4/4 rhythm	Counts each breath in 4/4 rhythm, emphasizing count of 1 (*e.g.*, "1, 2, 3, 4, 1, 2, 3, 4," etc or silently sings Yankee Doodle, a 4/4 song) or Concentrate on imagery	Same as above plus the following: During contractions at 15-sec intervals he calls off time that elapses (*i.e.*, "15 seconds, 30 seconds, 45 seconds, 60 seconds") until contraction is over As need arises, may breathe in rhythm with her, count aloud in rhythm to her breathing, or sing song in rhythm, remind her of eye focus, remind her to breathe deeply at end of contraction If back labor or backache may try deep counterpressure to lower back and position changes Reminds her to urinate

(continued)

of his responsibilities, such as counting or breathing with the mother.

Guidelines to Using Pain Relief Measures During Labor

Pain relief measures are aimed at reducing either anxiety or pain impulses. Some guidelines to the effective use of these pain relief measures are listed.

Some of the pain relief methods discussed later are not possible or acceptable in conventional labor rooms or when external monitoring is used. However, there is growing public demand for more natural childbirth and nonpharmacologic methods of pain relief during childbirth. Alternative Birth Centers (ABCs) are one response to that demand. Thus, in the future the following low-risk, nonpharmacologic pain relief measures may be in-

Nursing Guidelines for Pain Relief Measures

- Use a variety of pain relief measures.
- Use pain relief measures *before* pain becomes severe. (It is easier to prevent severe pain and panic than to alleviate them once they occur.)
- Include those pain relief measures that the client believes will be effective.
- Take into account the client's ability to be active or passive in the application of the pain relief measure.
- Regarding the potency of the pain relief measure needed, rely on the client's experience of the severity of pain rather than the known physical stimuli.
- If a pain relief measure is ineffective the first time it is used during a contraction, encourage the mother to try it at least one or two more times before abandoning it.

T A B L E   2 6 - 3   (continued)

Approximate Progress of Labor	Position	Relaxation	Mother's Activities During Massage
Dilates from 8 cm–10 cm, or contractions 1 min apart	Same as above	Same as above	Omitted unless feels good
Birth (fully dilated)	Same as above, except when pushing For pushing in labor room, ABC room, or LDR may conserve energy during pushing by elevating and supporting legs on pillows or by lying on side with back curved and top knee pulled up. Other positions: squatting on all fours (see Chap. 20 for illustrations) For pushing in delivery room, ABC room, or LDR, semipropped position with back curved, head and shoulders supported by pillows, head forward; if legs not in stirrups, she may hold leg under knees with elbows out or may give birth on her side	Same as above, except omitted when pushing	Omitted

creasingly acceptable to both health professionals and expectant parents.

Breathing Methods

Pressure may also be prevented by either abdominal breathing or chest breathing. While there is controversy as to which breathing method best relaxes abdominal muscles, the fact seems to be that it depends largely upon the individual mother.

Between contractions the nurse can assist the mother to differentiate between abdominal and chest breathing and to learn to use one or the other of the methods. While the mother is lying on her back, she places one hand on her chest and the other on her abdomen. The nurse points out that during an abdominal breath, the abdomen rises as air is inhaled. During a chest breath, the chest rises as air is inhaled. The nurse can have the mother practice each breathing method several times. Then the mother can choose the method that seems the most comfortable or the easiest. However, there may be no need for the nurse to assist the mother to differentiate between chest and abdominal breathing as long as the abdominal muscles are not contracted and the mother finds breathing easy and comfortable.

Eye Focus	Each Contraction in Relation to Breathing Pattern	Thoughts	Father's Activities Either During or Between Contractions
Same as above or focuses eyes on father	Patterned paced breathing through mouth or nose (rhythm of 1–6 breaths and then one blow), may accelerate and decelerate with intensity of contraction; breathing is maximum rate of twice woman's resting respiration rate If not allowed to push but feels urge to push, blows repeatedly If uncomfortable between contractions, uses slow paced breathing	Counts each breath according to rhythm selected (*e.g.,* "1, 2, 3, 4, 5, 6, blow")	Between contractions offers encouragement; wipes face with cool, wet cloth; moistens lips and mouth with water, ice chips, or lollipop
Same as above, except when pushing For pushing may focus on mirror or perineum, if visible, to see results of pushing	Same as above, except when pushing For pushing: 2 deep breaths, inhale, hold breath, lean forward, hold 5 sec–7 sec, release breath; repeat inhalation and continue as before until contraction is over or until instructed to stop pushing Alternate method: 2 deep breaths, on 3rd breath blow out slowly and bear down; repeat as necessary Making grunting noises is OK	Same as above, except when pushing For pushing may visualize baby slowly coming out of uterus and through birth canal	Same as above, except when pushing For pushing may stand at mother's back to support her in pushing position if no back rest Counts aloud 5 sec–7 sec during each breath holding, tells her to take a deep breath and hold it, then counts to 10 again Reminds her to relax pelvic floor and "push through vagina" or "bulge" pelvic floor

Abdominal Lifting

Another obvious method of reducing abdominal pressure is simply to lift the abdominal wall (Fig. 26-4). The nurse may do this for the mother, or the father may be taught how to do this maneuver. A hand must be kept on the uterus to identify the beginning of the contraction. The instant the uterus begins to contract, the nurse places both hands at waist level with the fingers pointing toward the spine. She quickly slides her hands down and under the mother's back until the fingertips meet at the spine. The nurse then firmly and gently *lifts* until her hands rest between the pelvic bone and rib cage.

As the hands are drawn from underneath the back, the hands are turned gradually (without releasing the upward lift) until the fingertips point toward the rib cage. The upward lift must be completed before the contraction reaches its peak. There should be lifting only and *no inward pressure.* When the contraction is over, the upward lift is released slowly.[20]

A more simple method of abdominal lifting is possible, but it is equally strenuous for the nurse or father. At the beginning of the contraction the fingers are hooked under the ribs and the distended abdomen is lifted as the mother inhales. In both methods of abdominal lifting it is important that the mother not arch

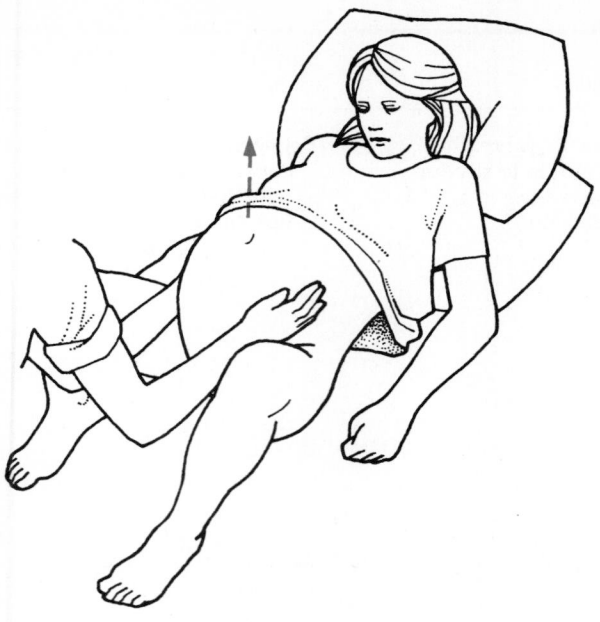

F I G U R E 2 6 - 4

Abdominal lifting. One approach to lifting the abdominal wall begins at the onset of the contraction with hands on the back at waist level, fingers pointing toward the spine. Firmly and gently turn hands and bring to the position shown here with pressure that lifts. Use no inward pressure.

her back, since this would cause discomfort. Depending upon the amount of pressure exerted by the hand, the latter method may also result in lifting the baby, thus removing the pressure of the uterus on the back.[21]

Position

Positioning is an especially important and effective pain relief measure when the mother experiences back labor (*i.e.*, when the occiput of the fetus presses on the mother's sacrum). Regardless of the position of the fetus, a mother in normal labor is probably more comfortable if she avoids the supine position.

One study compared the 30° upright position with the recumbent position during labor. The upright position was recommended for several reasons. Although the intensity of contractions was higher in this position, the contractions did not last any longer, the uterus relaxed more completely between contractions, and the first two stages of labor were shorter.[22] Thus, the duration of discomfort may be shortened by the upright position. In another study ambulation shortened labor and reduced the mother's discomfort.[23]

Unless there are complications such as a prolapsed cord, the mother should be allowed to choose the position she finds most comfortable. However, if she wants to lie on her back, the head of the bed should be somewhat elevated and her thighs slightly flexed.

Besides the 30° upright or semisitting position, other positions that may provide comfort during labor are the lateral Sims and the tailor sitting position. An unusual but increasingly popular position for mothers with back labor is the up-on-all-fours position. This position may even succeed in rotating the baby's head to an anterior position. If the baby's head is not in the posterior position, this crawl position may still relieve pain, especially during transition, when labor is so often felt in the back.

Pushing

As delivery approaches, most mothers feel the urge to push. However, unnecessary noxious stimuli can be eliminated if the mother understands that it is futile to push early in labor. Painful stimuli may also be avoided during delivery if the mother obeys instructions as to when she should and should not push. The urge to push can be almost irresistible. Thus, the mother may need some techniques such as blowing or rapid breathing to help her refrain from pushing.

Relieving External Pressure

When external electronic monitoring is used, the transducer may be a source of discomfort if it is secured in the same position over a period of time. The sensations of discomfort or heaviness may be decreased by moving the transducer as little as ¾ inch.

Distraction

Distraction is an effective method of pain relief; the gate control theory may provide a possible explanation for this. When the cerebral cortex is involved in activity (cortical excitation), the gate may be closed to pain. The cortex may signal a decreased attention to pain impulses. Or the reticular system in the brain stem may register that there is sufficient incoming stimuli and therefore signal the gate to be closed to further stimuli, painful stimuli in this case.

Regardless of the theoretical mechanism, common sense suggests that pain is more tolerable if the client becomes less aware of it—in short, distracted from it. Distraction places pain on the periphery of awareness. A person may be distracted from pain in an almost limitless variety of ways.

When the nurse wishes to assist the laboring mother with pain relief measures in the form of distracters, it is only reasonable to approach the mother between, not during, contractions. The nurse can describe briefly one or two possibilities. The mother should be asked to decide which one she would like to try first. It usually is most helpful if the nurse first demonstrates the pattern and then has the mother do it. If a song or counting is to be used, it is often much easier for the mother if the nurse counts or sings for her during the first contractions in which the pattern is used. If the mother does not like any of the distracters discussed in this section, the nurse may creatively invent some others or simply ask the mother for suggestions. Some mothers prefer a form of distraction that involves an inward focus rather than the outward focus of the distracters described here. For example, the mother may stare into space or close her eyes and focus on the forces of her body, concentrating on the contraction being a wavelike force, which she envisions herself on top of.

Variety of Distracters. We have not yet begun to uncover and understand fully the various strategies people use to cope with pain. These strategies include much more than distraction, but within the area of distraction there are numerous approaches.

The nurse needs to be familiar with a variety of distracters that she may suggest to the mother. What is sufficiently distracting for one mother may not be for another. A mother may need assistance with distracters even if she has attended prepared childbirth classes. Instructors of methods of prepared childbirth have devised and taught many means of distraction for use during contractions. It is interesting to note that a large number of these are rhythmic, such as "riding the wave," tapping out the rhythm of a song, rhythmic head movements, and rhythmic breathing.

Emphasis is placed on distracters that are of some proven effectiveness and are also relatively easy to teach the mother. Most of the techniques taught in the Maternity Center Association (MCA) method and the Lamaze method meet these criteria. A brief comparison of the Lamaze method and the MCA method reveals some of the ideas common to most methods of prepared childbirth: concentration on relaxation and a rhythmic breathing pattern during contractions. (A review of the information in Chapter 20 and Table 26-3 will assist the reader in the following discussion of these distracters.) Some distracters used in the various methods of prepared childbirth are extremely distracting but difficult to teach quickly once labor is in progress.

Table 26-3 provides examples from the Lamaze method of activities that may serve as distracters. Many of these activities serve double purposes. The breathing rhythms and purposeful thoughts undoubtedly serve as distracters, but maintenance of rhythmic breathing is also thought to relieve pain by providing adequate oxygenation of the uterus.

While relaxation serves such purposes as anxiety reduction and prevention of abdominal pressure, the mother may find that her concentrated efforts to relax provide a significant distraction. Changing positions and massaging the abdomen require both motor and cognitive effort and therefore may be distracting. Keeping the eyes open and focused on a particular point is perhaps the purest and simplest distracter. Altogether, the Lamaze-trained mother consciously performs several varied activities with the end result of distraction from pain.

Other breathing patterns for use during contractions are suggested by the MCA and are described in Chapter 20; guided imagery is also discussed in Chapter 20.

Whatever type of distracters the mother may choose to use during a contraction, the nurse and others must take care not to prevent her from using them. Early in labor it may be a helpful distraction to the mother to have someone to talk with during a contraction, but later she may find this irritating because it interferes with other strategies for coping with pain. In any event, the nurse needs to find out from the mother what, if anything, she wants the nurse to do for her during a contraction.

Active Listening. Another type of distraction strategy that is becoming more popular in many clinical areas, including labor, is active listening, or auditory stimulation through a headset or earphone. The equipment required is a battery-operated tape recorder or cassette player, headset or earphone, and one or more cassettes of music chosen by the mother. The music may be relaxing, soft, and familiar, or it may be fast and lively. Some may use a combination of both. Usually during the contraction, but sometimes between contractions, the mother listens to the preselected music through the earphone or headset. This provides a demanding auditory stimulus very difficult to ignore. For visual input she may focus on an object or close her eyes and imagine something suggested by the music. Often the mother taps out the beat to the music to help increase her concentration on the distraction. As the contractions become more uncomfortable or during the rising discomfort of a single contraction, the mother may increase the volume to provide more distraction from the increasing discomfort.

The equipment for active listening is usually brought by the mother. However, this is such a simple and effective distraction that hospitals might well consider making the equipment available to mothers, especially if many mothers come to the hospital in labor and without previous childbirth education.

Method Changes as Labor Progresses. The method of distraction tends to change as labor progresses, seemingly taking into account the increasing intensity of pain and the increasing effort the mother must exert to engage in any activity not related to labor. Thus, as demonstrated by the Lamaze method (see Table 26-3), abdominal massage is eliminated and a relatively more easy breathing pattern is adopted during transition. As a rule, the more intense the pain, the more involved the mother must become in the distraction to achieve pain relief. However, the involvement must be compatible with the mother's ability.

First Stage of Labor. Early in labor the mother may be able to distract herself by "walking and talking" through a contraction. As labor progresses, some form of rhythmic breathing pattern is usually helpful. Slow rhythmic breathing is both relaxing and distracting, examples being either the "complete breathing" of the MCA or the "slow paced breathing" of Lamaze. If this is not effective, the nurse may suggest adding some of the distracters of the Lamaze method, such as a concentration point, counting during inhalation and exhalation, and abdominal massage.

Intensification. When discomfort intensifies and a more powerful form of distraction is needed, the nurse may teach the mother the "modified complete breathing" of the MCA or the accelerating and decelerating "modified paced breathing" of the Lamaze method. Either of these may result in hyperventilation. Hyperventilation may be treated by having the mother breathe into a paper bag and suggesting that henceforth she breathe more slowly. Again, more distraction may be added to these breathing patterns by incorporating one or more of the distracters of the Lamaze method: the concentration point, abdominal massage, silent counting, or singing in rhythm with breathing. Another effective and relatively easy distracter to employ is finger tapping the rhythm to a 4/4 song, coordinating the rhythm with breathing.

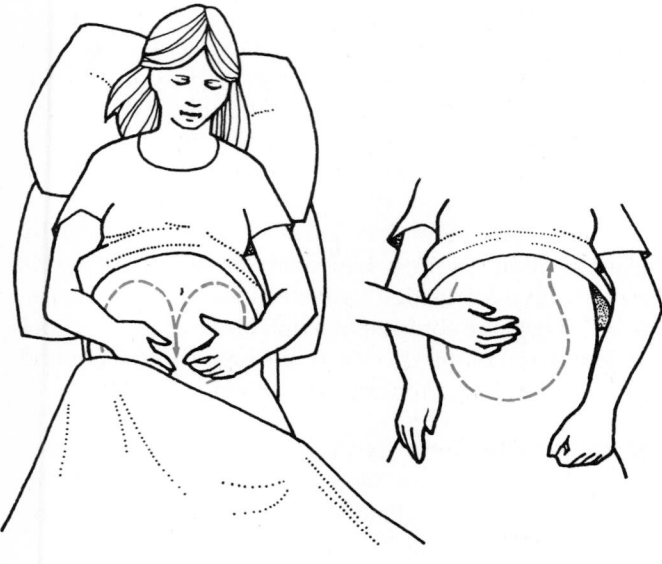

FIGURE 2 6 - 5

Two types of effleurage, or abdominal massage.

Transition. During transition the mother's focus tends to become extremely narrow because of the great increase in the intensity of contractions. Whereas earlier in labor the distracters could be suggested and taught between contractions, there is little time now and it is difficult for the mother to focus on anything but labor. Therefore, distracters used during transition should be more simple and must be taught prior to the onset of transition. The Lamaze method suggests patterned paced breathing with blowing. Although this breathing pattern includes acceleration and deceleration with the intensity of the contraction, it is an easy breathing pattern to learn and to use. The MCA suggests "modified complete breathing" with the further modification of puffing out gently upon exhalation of every third or fourth breath. Simple additions to these breathing rhythms include coordinated and silent counting and use of a concentration point.

Cutaneous Stimulation

Rubbing a painful body part is a universal means of relieving pain. The gate control theory provides a possible reason for the effectiveness of this and other forms of cutaneous stimulation. As discussed previously, the theory suggests that stimulation of large-diameter nerve fibers may partially or completely close the gate to the transmission of pain impulses to the cortex. Because many cutaneous (skin) fibers are large-diameter fibers, stimulation of the skin may result in pain relief.

Several types of cutaneous stimulation may be used during labor and may prove to be effective pain relief measures. One of the more common of these is effleurage, or abdominal massage (Fig. 26-5). Rubbing the lower back is also common (Fig. 26-6). The Lamaze method describes a type of abdominal massage. The application of heat or cold (with the physician's permission) may be especially comforting to the client with back labor. Creams or gels containing menthol may also be rubbed on the lower back for pain relief.

The above are examples of relatively moderate stimulation of cutaneous fibers. Mild to moderate stimulation is ordinarily more effective than intense stimulation. However, one notable exception is the use of intense pressure over the sacrum during a contraction. The pressure may be applied with the knee or fist, or the mother may lean back (in a semisitting position) on a tennis ball or rolling pin (Fig. 26-7). It has been estimated that applying pressure during a contraction is equivalent to the pain relief potential of 50 mg to 100 mg of meperidine.[24]

Rubbing of any part of the body, even between contractions, possibly may contribute to pain relief. This not only encourages relaxation, but experimentation with cutaneous stimulation shows that it may help close the gate to painful impulses long after its use and that

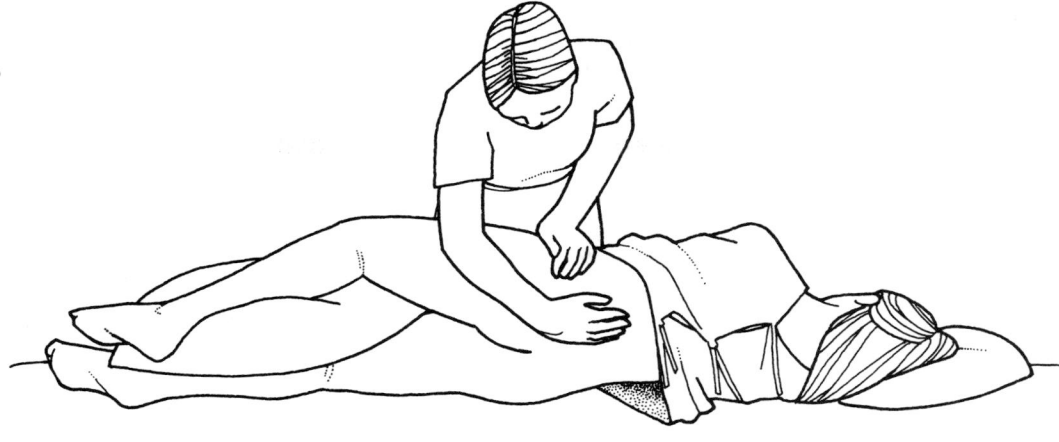

FIGURE 26-6

Deep back massage, while the mother lies on her side, relieves back pain between contractions.

the painful area need not always be the area of stimulation.[10] For example, if an external monitor prevents abdominal massage, the thighs may be massaged instead. Some mothers find that foot massage by the father or nurse brings considerable comfort.

Transcutaneous electric nerve stimulation (TENS) is a newer form of cutaneous stimulation that has been used successfully for pain relief during the first stage of labor. A mild electric current is applied to the skin by way of electrodes connected to a battery-operated device with controls to regulate the sensation. The client usually feels a buzzing, tingling, or vibrating sensation. In one study of labor pain, two pairs of electrodes were placed

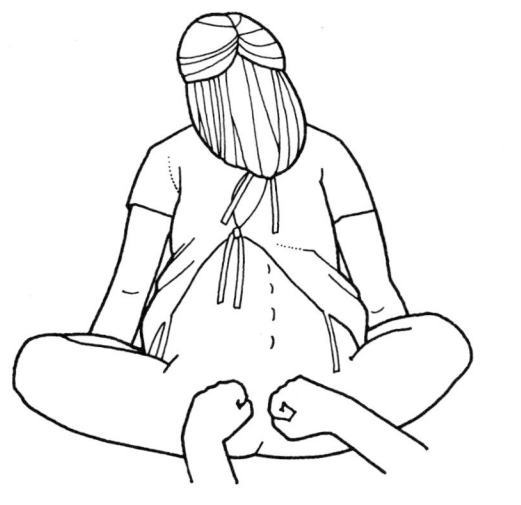

FIGURE 26-7

Firm counterpressure of the fists on the lower back, while the mother is in the tailor sitting position, effectively relieves back labor.

on either side of the spinal column over the sacral and thoracic regions. Low-intensity stimulation was provided continuously, and the mother increased the stimulation during a contraction. No complications occurred except that in a few cases sacral stimulation interfered with monitoring the fetal heart rate. The researchers recommended TENS as a primary method of pain relief during labor, noting that it is a low-risk, nonpharmacologic method that can be interrupted at any moment.[25] Comparable results have been obtained in studies of Egyptian and Italian mothers during childbirth.[26,27]

Nursing responsibilities when TENS is used might include placing and securing the electrodes, explaining the use of the controls to the mother, and evaluating the effectiveness of TENS in relieving pain.

Relaxation

Virtually every method of prepared childbirth heavily emphasizes total skeletal muscle relaxation during labor. Relaxation relieves pain by interrupting the spiraling process of pain and anxiety. Muscle tension is a response to pain and anxiety. Since relaxation is the opposite of muscle tension, it prevents or diminishes tension. The behavioral response of relaxation, therefore, is incompatible with pain–anxiety responses. Some research suggests that a person's evaluation of the intensity of pain is in part a function of her evaluation of her own overt behavioral response to pain.[28] Possibly, when the client observes herself relaxed instead of tense, she evaluates her pain as less intense, or relaxation may cause the cortex to send signals to close the gate to the transmission of pain impulses.

Relaxation undoubtedly provides pain relief for other reasons, depending upon the individual client. For some mothers efforts to relax can serve as a distraction from pain. In other mothers a state of relaxation may increase suggestibility, causing her to accept explicit and implicit suggestions of comfort.[29] The teaching of relaxation is discussed in Chapter 20, and techniques for relaxation are presented in Appendix A.

How can the client achieve total skeletal muscle relaxation? Possibly the most frequently used but most unproductive method is for the nurse to say, "Relax." The verbal cue *relax* may be used effectively with mothers who have been trained in relaxation, but to the untrained mother such a command often sounds impossible, if not absurd. The mother's inability to follow such an instruction may engender feelings of powerlessness, failure, and more tension.

When the nurse encounters a mother who has been trained in relaxation techniques, she simply finds out how best to assist her. It is particularly helpful to identify cues that will encourage relaxation if the mother becomes tense. These cues may be verbal, such as "relax," or tactile-kinesthetic, such as touching or moving the tense body part.

If the mother has not been trained in relaxation, the nurse may use some simple techniques that can make a significant difference in the mother's level of relaxation. The nurse first explains to the mother that relaxing during a contraction is very important because it can decrease abdominal pressure on the uterus and also help her feel more calm and generally comfortable. The quickest and easiest way to promote relaxation is to instruct the mother to take a deep breath or to yawn and to "go limp" or relax as she exhales. The nurse suggests that the mother try one or both of these at the beginning and end of contractions and anytime during contractions that she feels the need to relax. (The client who chooses to yawn may find it becomes spontaneous and more frequent.)

These techniques are effective because they take advantage of conditioned responses. Both a big sigh (deep breath) and a yawn are associated with relaxation.

Relaxation may be furthered by providing support to comfortably positioned and slightly flexed extremities. Also, the nurse may gently move extremities and the head to test for the degree of relaxation. This slight movement enables the mother to feel tense muscles and helps her to relax them.

Assistance With Change in Expectations and Goals

During the relatively brief and rapidly moving events of labor, any unexpected change in the parents' goals or expectations must be handled quickly. Otherwise anxiety may persist or increase, resulting in an increased intensity of pain. Some items listed in Part V of the Assessment Tool given earlier are examples of areas in which a disturbing change may occur. Several examples of changes are the following: because of unforeseen circumstances there is a physician unknown to the parents in attendance at labor and delivery or the father is unable to attend the birth; crowding of the labor section at this time limits use of planned facilities; internal or external monitors may be used, which may signify complications or limit movement; and pain relief methods may be necessary.

When a situation occurs that disturbs the parents, the nurse encourages them to express their feelings and indicates an appreciation of their disappointment. She then explains the reasons for any rules, policies, or circumstances that prevent them from achieving their goals or expectations.

One of the more difficult problems is assisting the parents who are not able to achieve their "ideal" of labor and delivery. This ideal may vary considerably from one couple to another. Inability to achieve this ideal labor may cause profound feelings of failure in the mother or father. Also, they may refuse or be very reluctant to accept measures incompatible with their ideal.

Clients who have specific expectations or goals associated with an ideal labor may have arrived at these in a number of ways. But these parents seem most often to be a product of classes that prepare them in a specific method of childbirth. One of the most common criticisms of methods of prepared childbirth is that the mother and father are taught to strive for a particular kind of labor and delivery experience, such as medication-free delivery or ecstasy over the delivery. Not all childbirth educators state such goals. Yet parents, especially mothers, tend to adopt these goals and feel a sense of failure if they are not achieved.

How does the nurse help the mother and father minimize feelings of failure and accept a change in their goals? Throughout childbirth, and particularly when goals must change, the nurse praises the mother and father for their efforts and abilities to handle labor. This promotes feelings of success. For example, the mother may have the goal of an unmedicated labor, but she may find the discomfort intolerable and request medication. If medication is given, the nurse can say that she knows medication was not planned. She can allow the mother to express her feelings and then praise the mother for the success of her efforts up to now and for the length of time medication was not necessary. She may add that the mother's continuing efforts may reduce the amount of medication required. She may also stress to the father that his approval and support are extremely valuable.

The mother may, however, choose to handle the above situation in a different manner. She may decide it is in the best interests of herself and her baby for her not to request medication, in spite of how intolerable she finds the pain. Such pain may cause her to become extremely tense and unable to cooperate with exami-

NURSING CARE PLAN

The Woman in the Process of Aftermath Assimilation of Labor

Nursing Objectives

1. Identify the mother who has negative feelings about any aspect of physical discomfort during her labor and delivery.
2. Provide the mother with an opportunity to explore and clarify the experience of discomfort in terms of her own behaviors and feelings, as well as those of others, so that she can intellectually and emotionally assimilate the childbirth experience.

Assessment	Potential Nursing Diagnosis	Planning/Intervention	Evaluation
Encourage the mother to talk about all aspects of any discomfort experienced during labor	Disturbance in self-concept related to guilt about her perception that she was unable to use breathing methods to handle discomfort during the latter portion of labor	Assist the mother to relive those moments when she felt unable to be effective in using breathing methods	Mother talks less about negative feelings related to handling pain during labor
Identify the presence of any feelings of guilt, lack of information, anxiety, or failure		Praise her ability to resume use of breathing method after she occasionally failed to use the method	Mother shares with nurse and others about how hard she worked at breathing methods when pain increased
		Give information about reasons for increased pain at that time	Mother expresses pride in how she handled labor
		Point out positive attitude of others toward her efforts	
		Remind her that she successfully delivered a healthy baby	

nations or the forces of labor. This may prolong labor and increase the possibility of complications. If medication seems highly desirable, the nurse may find it necessary to use a direct approach with the mother to modify her perceptions of the situation. This may be accomplished by stating how the health team views the situation and by pointing out differences in this view and the mother's perceptions. One thing the nurse may point out is that the mother wants to avoid both medication and complications, but the two goals are now incompatible.

This direct approach tends to cause unpleasant psychological tension, called cognitive dissonance. In other words, the mother's goals are at odds with one another and with the knowledge received from the nurse. Cognitive dissonance may motivate a person to change. One way the mother may reduce dissonance in this case is to adjust her thinking so that she accepts other pain relief measures.[30]

Another approach to this type of situation is to employ analogy. This may disrupt the mother's denial of what is actually happening, assist her with a clearer understanding of the situation, or foster feelings of normality about her childbirth experience. Explaining the situation by comparing it with something else allows the mother to distance herself from the actual situation. She is able to understand the problem but avoid the anxiety associated with looking directly at the problem.[31] For example, the nurse may compare labor to a menstrual cycle. She may say that no two labors are exactly alike, just as no two women have exactly the same menstrual cycle. She may add that some women normally experience more pain than others. Or she may cite some other symptom or sign that explains the need for a change in the mother's goal.

Aftermath Assimilation

After anticipation of pain and the presence of pain, a third and final phase of the pain experience occurs, the aftermath. The pain experience does not end with the cessation of the painful sensations. The client does not necessarily immediately forget about the pain, especially if it was severe, frightening, or in any way disconcerting.

On the maternity unit it is a common observation that mothers talk a great deal about their childbirth experiences. It is a frequent topic of conversation regardless of whether the mother experienced "ecstasy," "failure," or simply relief mixed with satisfaction. Not only may the mother want to talk about the pain, but a variety of feelings resulting from the pain may be present, such as nausea, vomiting, chills, anger, or embarrassment. The mother may even have nightmares about the pain.

Clearly, at least some mothers need assistance during the aftermath phase of the pain experience. The most appropriate nursing action may be to assist the mother with the intellectual and emotional assimilation of her childbirth experience. In a sense the nurse helps the mother relive her labor. The nurse can ask the mother questions that help her discuss her discomforts, emotions, thoughts, and overt responses and the reactions of others during her labor. The nurse needs to be particularly alert and responsive to the mother's needs for support, such as praise, confirmation that her perceptions of discomfort are believed by others, or reassurance that her behavior was acceptable. Some mothers need information to help them fill in memory gaps or to correct understandings that are inaccurate and anxiety provoking.[10]

It is particularly important to encourage assimilation in mothers who may harbor feelings of failure about childbirth. But assimilation may help maintain or restore a positive self-concept for any mother and aid in her ability to deal with mothering and other impending tasks.

Evaluation

Identifying whether or not certain emotional and physiological benefits have occurred is one way of evaluating the success of the nurse, mother, and others involved in efforts to provide as much comfort as possible during labor.

Emotional Benefits

Control or relief of pain potentially allows the significant step toward becoming parents to be a positive experience for the mother and father (Table 26-4). Ultimately one or both parents may be able to witness that moment that remains miraculous and awesome even to many obstetricians, the emergence of a new human being into the world. Even when the parents do not observe the delivery, there are other desirable outcomes. If the mother and father can handle the discomforts during childbirth, they can feel they are active participants in the actual birth of their own child. When people jointly plan for an event such as childbirth and are then able to carry through with these plans, the event will probably foster growth in the relationship between them. In the case of childbirth, a satisfying labor experience for both parents probably also fosters their relationship with their baby (Fig. 26-8).

At least a childbirth experience in which pain is adequately controlled does not impede these relationships. Pain has the potential for eliciting anger and aggression, often referred to as the fight or flight response. Such feelings resulting from a miserably painful childbirth experience sometimes are projected onto the infant or the father. The mother temporarily may express hatred toward the infant or father, and she may withdraw from these relationships for a while. During and following very painful labors mothers have been quoted as saying they despise their partners. Fathers have been known to say they felt angry toward the baby because its birth caused the mother pain. One mother even commented that her labor was so painful it took her a year to forgive her child and establish a warm relationship with him.

It does not seem likely, however, that pain and suffering during labor could be the sole reason for permanent or prolonged impairment of mother–father–child relationships. Labor may be a convenient scape-

T A B L E 2 6 - 4

Benefits of Pain Control in Labor and Delivery

Emotional Advantages	Physiological Advantages
Positive experience with a significant step toward parenthood	Mother can cooperate with examinations
Feeling of actual participation in birth of own child	Mother can work with contractions
Fostering growth of relationship between parent and child	Mother is less fatigued after labor and delivery
Fostering growth of relationship between parents	Successful use of nonpharmacologic pain relief reduces risk to infant
	Complications, such as pain-related decrease in oxygen, can be avoided in the fetus already at risk

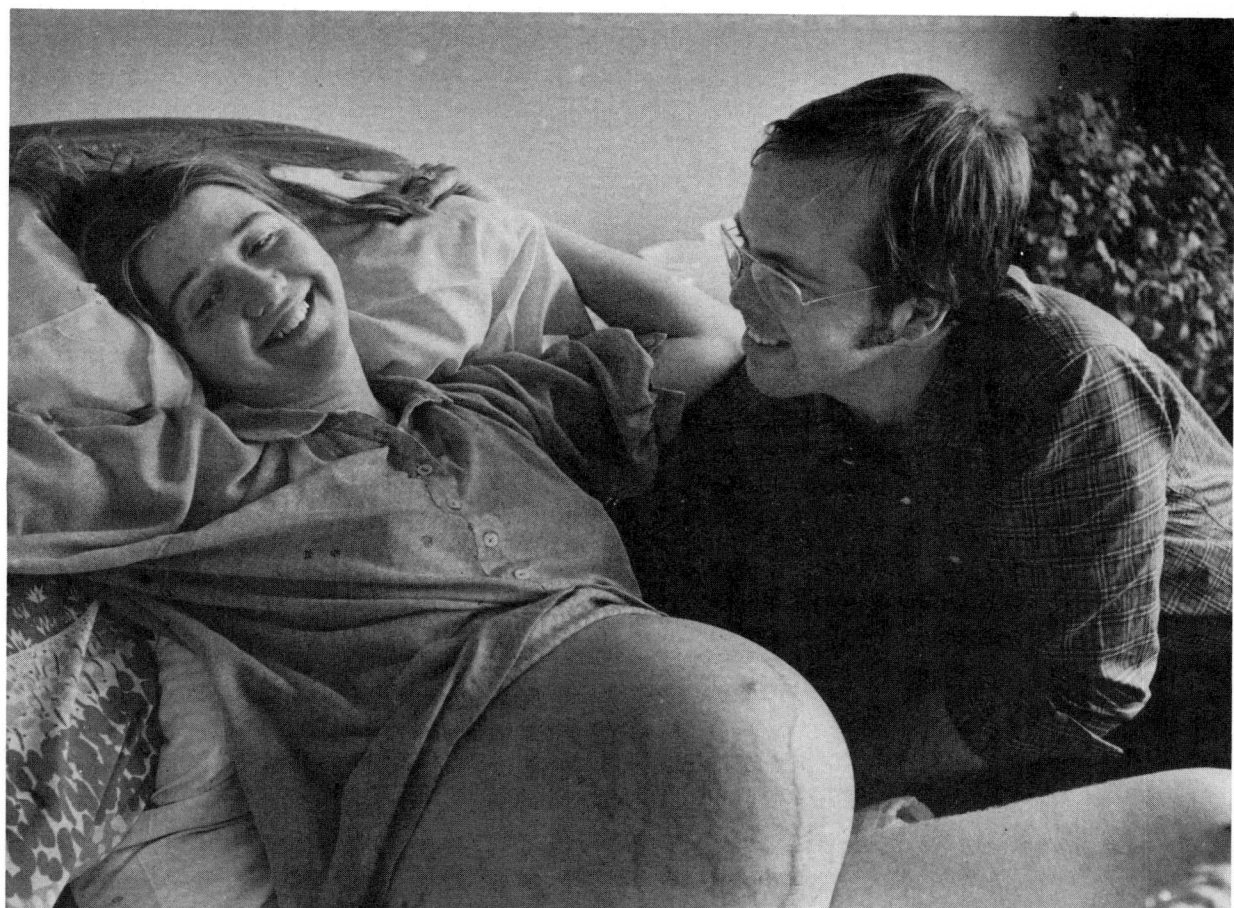

FIGURE 26-8

This mother and father work together throughout labor and delivery in an alternative birthing center. Such experiences can foster a closer relationship between the parents and contribute significantly to successful parental–infant attachment.

goat. Other more significant factors operating over a long period of time have probably affected the relationships.

Physiological Benefits

The adequate relief of pain also results in physiological benefits (see Table 26-4). The mother who experiences tolerable discomforts in labor is able to cooperate with examinations and to work with her contractions. Consequently, she facilitates efforts of the health-team members to obtain information and she avoids prolongation of labor. After childbirth she is less fatigued.

If she is able to use pain relief measures other than medication, she may eliminate the need for medication or reduce the amount necessary. This is of enormous physiological benefit to the infant because many anal-gesics and anesthetics, including regional anesthesia, have untoward effects on the fetus, such as respiratory depression and bradycardia. There simply is no drug that has been proven entirely safe for the unborn child.

Pain and stress may cause exaggerated effects on ventilation, circulation, endocrine function, and other body functions. Further reasons to minimize pain during labor and delivery are to avoid the following specific problems that Bonica believes could occur as a result of severe pain during labor:[32]

- Severe respiratory alkalosis. The pain of uterine contraction may cause a fivefold to 20-fold increase in ventilation.
- A 50% to 150% increase in cardiac output and a 20% to 40% increase in blood pressure. This is due to a significant increase in sympathetic activity and norephinephrine release.

- Significant increases in metabolism and oxygen consumption.
- Decrease in gastrointestinal and urinary bladder motility and at times in uterine contractility.
- Progressive metabolic acidosis that may be deleterious to mother and fetus. This is due to increased oxygen consumption, loss of bicarbonate from the kidney as compensation for respiratory alkalosis, and possible reduction in carbohydrate intake.
- Increased risk of aspiration of gastric contents. This is due to decreased gastrointestinal motility and retention of fluid and food in the stomach.

Healthy mothers and newborns may tolerate the above well. However, mothers with heart disease may have problems. If the fetus is already at risk because of obstetric complications, reduction of oxygen from intermittent impairment of placental blood gas exchange may be critical.

References

1. Fagerhaugh SY, Strauss A: Politics of Pain: Staff-Patient Interaction, pp 223–224. Menlo Park, CA, Addison–Wesley, 1977
2. Melzack R, Wall PD: Pain mechanisms: A new theory. Science 150:971–979, 1965
3. Melzack R: The Puzzle of Pain, pp 153–190. New York, Basic Books, 1973
4. Nathan PW: The gate-control theory of pain: A critical review. Brain 99:213–258, 1976
5. Wall PD: Modulation of pain by nonpainful events. In Bonica JJ, Albe-Fessard D (eds): Advances in Pain Research and Therapy, Vol 1, pp 1–16. New York, Raven Press, 1976
6. Snyder SH: Opiate receptors and internal opiates. Sci Am 236:44–56, March 1977
7. Pittman AW, Rudd GD: Analgesic Therapy, Part 2: Analgesia for Severe Pain. Chapel Hill, NC, Health Sciences Consortium, 1980
8. Terenius L: Endorphins and pain. Front Horm Res 8: 162–177, 1981
9. West A: Understanding endorphins: Our natural pain relief system. Nursing 81(11):50–53, February 1981
10. McCaffery M: Nursing Management of the Patient with Pain, 2nd ed. Philadelphia, JB Lippincott, 1979
11. Copp LA: The spectrum of suffering. Am J Nurs 74: 491, March 1974
12. Nettelbladt P, Fagerstrom C-F, Uddenberg N: The significance of reported childbirth pain. J Psychosom Res 20:215–221, 1976
13. Winsberg B, Greenlick M: Pain response in Negro and white obstetrical patients. J Health Soc Behav 8:222–227, September 1967
14. Clark AL, Howland R, Affonso D et al: MCH in American Samoa. Am J Nurs 74:700–702, April 1974
15. Melzack R: The myth of painless childbirth. Pain 19: 321–337, 1984
16. Potter H, MacDonald RD: Obstetric consequences of epidural analgesia in nulliparous patients. Lancet 1: 1031–1034, 1971
17. Davenport-Slack B, Boylan CH: Psychological correlates of childbirth pain. Psychosom Med 36:215–223, May/June 1974
18. Melzack R, Taenzer P, Kinch RA: Labor pain: Nature of the experience and the role of prepared childbirth training. Pain (Suppl) 1:S271, 1981
19. Cogan R: Comfort during prepared childbirth as a function of parity, reported by four classes of participant observers. J Psychosom Res 19:33–37, July 1975
20. Gamper M: Preparation for the Heir Minded, p 48. Illinois, Margaret Gamper, 1971
21. Bean CA: Methods of Childbirth, pp 103–104. New York, Dolphin Books, 1974
22. Liu YC: Effects of an upright position during labor. Am J Nurs 74:2202–2205, December 1974
23. Flynn AM, Kelly J, Hollins G: Ambulation in Labor. Br Med J 2:591–593, August 1978
24. Pace JB: Psychophysiology of pain: Diagnostic and therapeutic implications. J Fam Pract 1:4, May 1974
25. Augustinsson L-E, Bohlin P, Bundsen P et al: Pain relief during delivery by transcutaneous electrical nerve stimulation. Pain 4:59–65, October 1977
26. Tawfik MO, Badraoui MHH: The value of transcutaneous nerve stimulation (TNS) during labour in Egyptian mothers. Pain (Suppl) 1:S146, 1981
27. Piva L et al: Transcutaneous electrical stimulation as a safe and useful method for pain relief in labour. Pain (Suppl) 1:S142, 1981
28. Bandler RJ Jr, Madaras GR, Bem DJ: Self-observation as a source of pain perception. J Pers Soc Psychol 9:205–209, July 1968
29. Chertok L: Motherhood and Personality: Psychosomatic Aspects of Childbirth, pp 13–16. Philadelphia, Tavistock Publications and JB Lippincott, 1969
30. Miller J: Cognitive dissonance in modifying families' perceptions. Am J Nurs 74:1468–1470, August 1974
31. Wacker MS: Analogy: Weapon against denial. Am J Nurs 74:71–73, January 1974
32. Bonica JJ: Obstetric Analgesia and Anesthesia. Amsterdam, World Federation of Societies of Anaesthesiologists, 1980

Suggested Reading

Bean CA: Methods of Childbirth. New York, Dolphin Books, 1982

Bing E: Six Practical Lessons for Easier Childbirth. New York, Grosset and Dunlap, 1982

Bonica JJ: Principles and Practice of Obstetric Analgesia and Anesthesia, Vol I. Philadelphia, FA Davis, 1967

Bonica JJ: Principles and Practice of Obstetric Analgesia and Anesthesia, Vol II. Philadelphia, FA Davis, 1969

Bonica JJ: Obstetric Analgesia and Anesthesia. Amsterdam, World Federation of Societies of Anesthesiologists, 1980

Bonnel AM, Boureau F: Labor pain assessment: Validity of a behavioral index. Pain 22:81–90, 1985

Bradley RA: Husband-Coached Childbirth, 3rd ed. New York, Harper & Row, 1981

Dick-Read G: Childbirth Without Fear, 5th ed. New York, Harper & Row, 1984

Emrich HM (ed): The role of endorphins in neuropsychiatry. In Ban TA et al (eds): Modern Problems of Pharmacopsychiatry. Basel, Werner Druck, 1981

Hassid P: Textbook for Childbirth Educators, 2nd ed. New York, Harper & Row, 1983

Hollingsworth AO, Brown LP, Brooten DA: The refugees and childbearing: What to expect. RN 43:44–48, November 1980

Liu YC: Effects of an upright position during labor. Am J Nurs 74:2202–2205, December 1974

McCaffery M: Nursing Management of the Patient With Pain, 2nd ed. Philadelphia, JB Lippincott, 1979

McCaffery M: Relieving pain with noninvasive techniques. Nursing 80 10:55–57, December 1980

McCaffery M: When your patient's still in pain don't just do something: Sit there. Nursing 81(11):58–61, June 1981

McKay SR: Second stage labor: Has tradition replaced safety? Am J Nurs 81:1016–1019, May 1981

Meinhart NT, McCaffery M: Pain: A Nursing Approach to Assessment and Analysis. New York, Appleton-Century-Crofts, 1983

Melzack R: The myth of painless childbirth. Pain 19:321–337, 1984

The Pregnant Patient's Bill of Rights. Distributed by Committee on Patient's Rights, Box 1900, New York, NY 10001

Reading AE, Cox DN: Psychosocial predictors of labor pain. Pain 22:309–315, July 1985

Wilson RW, Elmassian BJ: Endorphins. Am J Nurs 81:722–725, April 1981

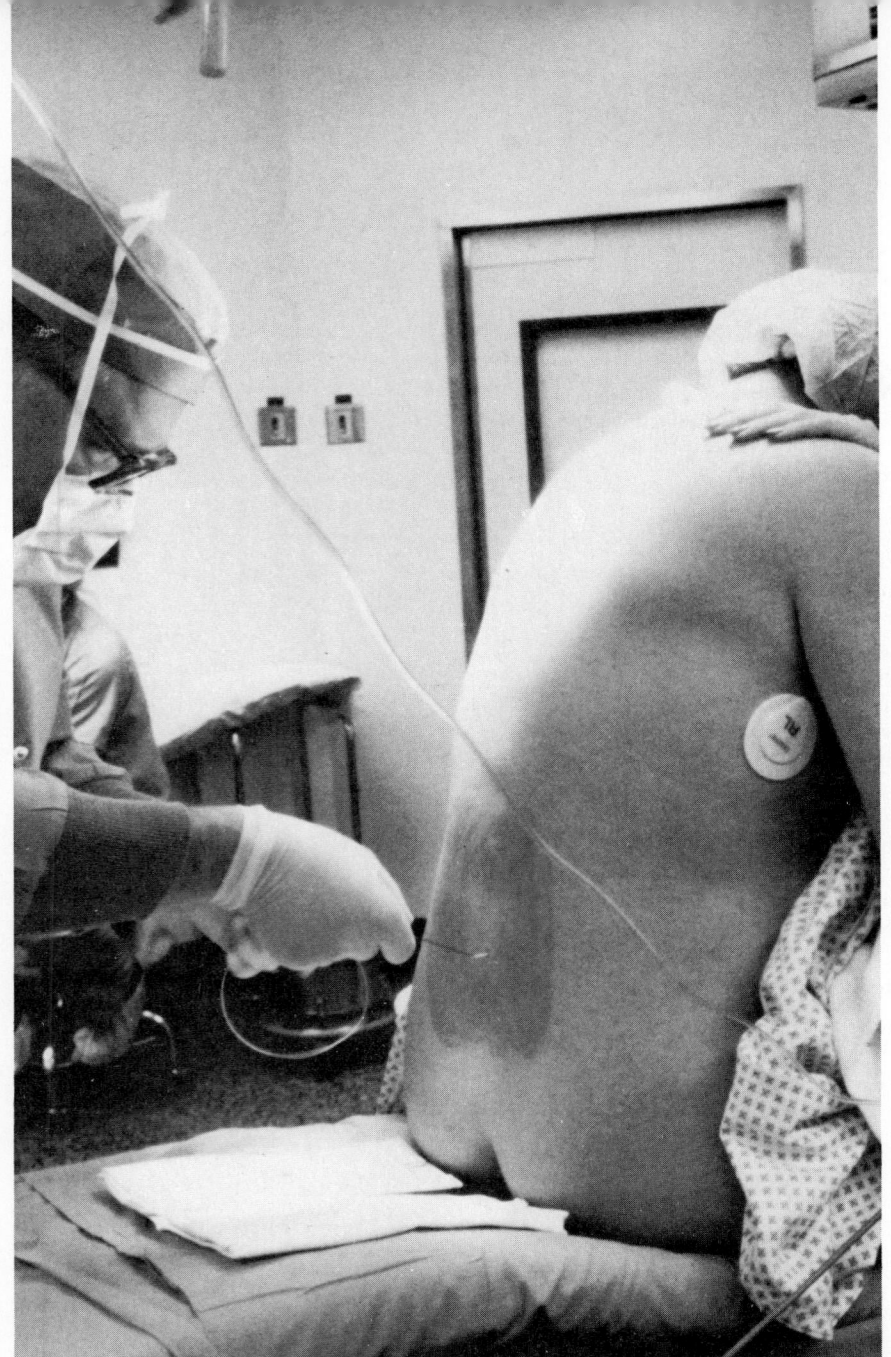

CHAPTER 27

Analgesia and Anesthesia During Childbirth

526

It is impractical to have qualified anesthesiologists or nurse–anesthetists remain in the labor room; however, the parturient deserves constant, competent observation and support throughout labor and delivery and in the immediate postdelivery period. The administration of any form of anesthesia or analgesia demands constant observation if anesthetic morbidity and mortality are to be minimized. The maternity nurse in the labor and delivery room plays an important and active role.

Overview

Historical Significance

The discomfort and suffering endured by women during childbirth has been recounted in historical records. In colonial America and in Europe women were imprisoned and even put to death for either seeking or providing pain relief during parturition. In 1847, a courageous 36-year-old obstetrician, James Young Simpson, reported on the efficacy of chloroform to alleviate the pain associated with childbirth. He was harshly criticized on theological grounds.

It was not until 1853 that obstetric anesthesia was accepted and respectable. John Snow, the first fulltime physician anaesthetist, introduced "chloroform à la reine" when he attended the birth of Queen Victoria's eighth child, Prince Leopold. Chloroform analgesia was administered for 53 minutes during labor. Snow again used chloroform for the anesthetic needs of his queen at the birth of Princess Beatrice in 1857. The monarch herself ended the need for women to suffer in childbirth by saying, "Dr. Snow gave that blessed chloroform and the effect was soothing, quieting and delightful beyond measure."

During the following 100 years, pain relief during childbirth was administered by persons untrained in the art and science of anesthesia. Anesthetic practices varied tremendously from area to area. Little thought was given to tailoring the anesthesia or analgesia to the specific needs of the laboring mother and the welfare of the fetus. New drugs producing analgesia, sedation, and anesthesia were often used for the first time in the parturient after few, if any, controlled studies. The concept of "twilight sleep," in which the mother was drugged to the state of oblivion (oftentimes lasting hours if not days into the postpartum period), came into vogue. To this, general anesthesia was frequently added at the time of delivery, primarily for the convenience of the obstetrician. The labor floor nurse or the nearest medical student, who was completely untrained and unaware of the dangers associated with general anesthesia, usually administered it. In some more "enlightened" centers, conduction or regional anesthesia was used by farsighted obstetricians who lacked training and support from their colleagues in anesthesia. Indeed, as late as 1962, it was estimated that in the United States 100 women died each year from pulmonary aspiration of stomach contents during the administration of general anesthesia for childbirth.

In the early 1950s, Dr. Virginia Apgar, then the Director of Anesthesia at Columbia Presbyterian Hospital in New York City, effectively addressed this problem. Although Apgar is better known for her evaluation of the newborn with the Apgar score, her realization that trained anesthesia personnel had as important a role to play on the labor floor as in the operating room is a greater contribution. Apgar's labors resulted in the first effective multidisciplinary teaching and research program devoted to obstetric anesthesia. Her program provided the impetus for other well-known teaching institutes to establish similar full-time anesthesia coverage for the labor floor and adequate training in obstetric anesthesia for both nurses and physicians specializing in anesthesia.

In the past three decades there have been great improvements in obstetric anesthesia. The parturient can be offered a wide range of methods for pain relief. Knowledge of these choices places the maternity nurse in the best possible position to counsel and advise on these matters. The importance of psychological support systems and the advantages of nonpharmacologic pain relief measures are increasingly recognized (see Chap. 26). Regional anesthesia, particularly continuous lumbar epidural block, is more readily available than in the past. This method, when initiated once active labor commences, can lead to a nearly painless labor and delivery and avoids the need for drugs that are potentially depressant to mother and fetus. It also may improve the intrauterine environment and provide ideal conditions for the delivery of the high-risk fetus. General anesthesia, useful in certain emergency situations, can be induced rapidly and maintained with little depressing effect on the fetus and newborn if special techniques are used. Regional and general anesthesia require special skills and a team effort if they are to be used effectively and safely. Although there has been substantial recent progress, even today in many centers anesthesia on the labor floor is not yet on a par with that in the operating room.

General Principles

Many guidelines covering anesthesia for the surgical patient have little applicability for the parturient. The psychological status of the laboring woman is different from that of her surgical counterpart. Furthermore, the parturient usually wishes to be an active participant and

---

Pregnancy's Physiological Implications for Anesthetic Techniques

- Pregnancy is associated with an increased sensitivity to most anesthetics, analgesics, and tranquilizers, which makes overdose more likely.
- Because of the edema of the upper airway normally present in late pregnancy, the possibility of airway obstruction is increased.
- Changes in pulmonary function and an increased oxygen requirement predispose the parturient to the rapid development of hypoxia, particularly in the second stage of labor or during induction of anesthesia. A 40% increase in pulmonary minute ventilation at term, which may increase further to 300% in the second stage of labor, makes induction of anesthesia with inhalation drugs rapid.
- Gastrointestinal tract changes are brought about by pregnancy and labor; the effects of many drugs used in labor, which increase nausea and vomiting and prolong gastric emptying time; and the fact that the maternity client may have recently eaten subject her to an increased risk of pulmonary aspiration of gastric contents with its devastating morbidity and mortality.
- Changes in the cardiovascular system, particularly those associated with aorta caval compression by the gravid uterus, predispose the obstetric client to sudden hypotension and cardiovascular collapse and her fetus to hypoxia and acidosis at the time of general or major conduction anesthesia.

---

her cooperation is needed in a vaginal delivery. Most important, the administration of anesthetic and analgesic drugs affects not only the mother but also the fetus and newborn.

Despite the fact that pregnancy, labor, and delivery are considered normal physiological processes, the changes wrought by these physiological processes have profound implications.

Pregnancy alters, and often exacerbates, the pathophysiology of many disease states, particularly those involving the cardiovascular and endocrine systems. Obstetric emergencies, especially fetal distress and maternal hemorrhage, demand the rapid induction of anesthesia. Thus, although the parturient is usually considered a healthy young female undergoing a physiological process, she becomes a high anesthetic risk requiring markedly different considerations from those applied to the surgical patient. Failure to take these factors into account can result in a disaster for the mother and her fetus.

It has been stated that pregnancy is the only normal physiological state in which all of the physiological parameters are abnormal (see Pregnancy's Physiological Implications for Anesthetic Techniques).

Selection of Anesthesia / Analgesia

Ideal analgesia or anesthesia for labor and delivery satisfies the following conditions:

- It provides satisfactory alleviation of pain for the individual parturient.
- It does not interfere significantly with the normal mechanics or progress of labor and delivery.
- It is not associated with undue risk to the mother.
- It is associated with minimal fetal and newborn depression.
- It provides safe and satisfactory conditions for the delivery.
- It allows early interaction between the mother and her newborn, preferably in the delivery room.

No single technique of pain relief fulfills all of the above objectives for every mother.

Anesthesia is best tailored to the conditions surrounding the labor of each parturient. However, it is unwise for the obstetrician or the delivery room nurse to promise any particular type of analgesia. Routine use of a particular type of pain relief is also to be discouraged. The mother should be encouraged to approach her labor with an open mind toward anesthesia. The expectant mother should be aware that intervention with pharmacologic analgesia at times may be necessary in the best interest of both her and her fetus.

When the woman arrives on the labor floor in early labor, she should be visited by those who will be responsible for her analgesia and anesthetic needs. They should give further counseling and reassurance that her needs will be met as much in accordance with her own desires as possible.

Four factors, then, should play a major role in deciding on the anesthetic management of labor and delivery (see list). The form of pain relief should be individualized and tailored to the needs of the parturient.

Nonpharmacologic Methods of Analgesia

Sometimes fetal and maternal needs come in conflict during labor. The mother's needs may involve relief of pain, but the fetal needs or problems may preclude medication. Nonpharmacologic methods have developed to meet coexisting needs. Techniques such as psychoprophylaxis, hypnosis, acupuncture, biofeedback, relaxation, therapeutic touch, imagery, and distraction are useful in labor. These techniques provide control of pain rather than elimination of pain. The laboring woman who can control her pain requires less medi-

---

Factors in Choosing Anesthetic Management

- The desires of the mother
- The amount of discomfort experienced during labor and delivery
- Anesthesia personnel and facilities at hand
- Needs of the obstetrician or midwife to accomplish a safe delivery

---

cation. Several examples are given here. However, further discussion is found in Chapter 26. The nurse as educator in these methods is discussed in Chapter 20.

Natural Childbirth

Both health professionals and the lay public have come to realize that heavy sedation and narcose during labor may have prolonged and pronounced deleterious effects on the neonate. Prepared or natural childbirth has become popular because mothers wish to experience the birth process fully and to be able to relate to their newborn shortly after birth. The various approaches to natural childbirth and the variety of techniques employed are discussed in detail in Chapters 20 and 26. Suffice it to say here that prepared or natural childbirth classes seek to minimize the need for the use of medications that can decrease the mother's awareness and cause newborn depression.

Unfortunately, these methods are not applicable to all clients. Clearly the key to successful experience in natural childbirth is motivation, but, at times, in spite of the best preparation, a mother who undertakes natural childbirth will require pharmacologic analgesia or even anesthesia.

Hypnosis

Hypnosis has been used sporadically for pain relief in both obstetric and surgical patients. Enthusiasts claim that its use results in better maternal cooperation, reduces or eliminates the need for depressant drugs, decreases blood loss, provides postpartum analgesia, and aids in milk letdown in nursing mothers.

The use of formal hypnosis requires preparation by a medical hypnotist well before the onset of labor. It may require the therapist's presence throughout parturition, although some clients may be taught autohypnosis or self-induction of trance.

Hypnosis requires that the subject enter a state of trance, which is essentially a state of altered and focused attention and hypersuggestibility. The trance state is not associated with sleep but rather with increased attention, whereas narcotics, sedatives, and tranquilizers decrease the ability to reach a state of trance by decreasing the ability to concentrate. The depth of the hypnotic or trance state varies tremendously from individual to individual. A rare individual may be placed sufficiently deep to allow surgery with no other anesthesia. In others, the depth of trance state is minimal or nonexistent.

While formal hypnosis may not be available, informal hypnosis or hypnoidal techniques involving suggestion, encouragement, and reassurance are most valuable and can be safely used by both nurses and physicians responsible for the care of the parturient. Examples of such techniques include using the term uterine *contractions* rather than uterine *pains*, reassuring the mother that she can relax and rest between contractions, and having concerned and experienced personnel present throughout labor and delivery. The injection of one's understanding presence and encouragement may do far more than the injection of pharmacologic substances to alleviate anxiety and pain.

Acupuncture

The use of acupuncture for analgesia during labor and vaginal delivery has met with little success. Classic Chinese medicine has never advocated its use for this purpose, and it is not employed for labor and vaginal delivery in the People's Republic of China. Two studies in the United States using Chinese acupuncturists failed to demonstrate significant or satisfactory pain relief during normal labor. A later study from Japan found that acupuncture gave partial but incomplete analgesia to some parturients during labor. In some women, acupuncture has been used successfully for cesarean delivery, but, like hypnosis, it is not effective in the majority of mothers undergoing abdominal delivery.

Pharmacologic Methods of Analgesia and Anesthesia

The pharmacologic techniques that are used to relieve pain during labor and delivery fall into four general categories:

- Regional or conduction anesthesia (*i.e.*, nerve block with local anesthetics)
- Systemic medications with narcotics, sedatives, tranquilizers, and amnestics
- Inhalation analgesia with subanesthetic concentration of inhalation drugs
- General anesthesia

Regional Anesthesia

The primary neuropathways of pain and methods of effectively blocking them with local anesthetics are illustrated in Figure 27-1. Uterine pain, resulting from dilatation and effacement of the cervix and from uterine contractions, is conveyed by small nerve fibers that pass from the cervix diffusely through the pelvis, join the sympathetic chain at L2–L5, and enter the spinal cord at T10–T12. These pain fibers can be blocked effectively by a paracervical block at the cervix, by a bilateral lumbar sympathetic block at L2, or by a segmental lumbar epidural block from T10–T12. Vaginal and perineal pain, associated with the second and third stages of labor, are mediated primarily through the pudendal nerve originating from S2–S4. There is additional perineal innervation from the genitofemoral, ilioinguinal, and lateral femoral cutaneous nerves. Pudendal nerve block, true "saddle block" (subarachnoid or "spinal" block, S1–S5), and low caudal epidural block (S1–S5) will alleviate most of the vaginal and perineal pain. A combination of blocks or a subarachnoid, lumbar epidural, or caudal epidural block from T10–S5 will provide complete relief of pain throughout labor and delivery. These medications are discussed in Table 27-1.

Advantages.   Regional or conduction anesthesia is ideally suited to vaginal delivery. If the complications of hypotension and local anesthetic toxicity are avoided, it is associated with no newborn depression and with a mother who is awake, free from pain, and capable of relating to her newborn baby immediately following birth. Awake, she is unlikely to aspirate gastric contents and can cooperate with the obstetrician. Except when uterine relaxation is required, regional analgesia can provide complete pain relief and suitable conditions for both vaginal and abdominal delivery.

Disadvantages.   Despite its many advantages, regional anesthesia has disadvantages and requires constant observation of the mother if it is to be both safe and effective. A former investigation suggested that both the local anesthetics lidocaine (Xylocaine) and mepivacaine (Carbocaine) were associated with minimally depressed neonatal tone at birth, which resolves rapidly. More recent studies have indicated that lidocaine is free from this depression. This has not been observed with the use of the local anesthetics bupivacaine (Marcaine) and 2-chloroprocaine (Nesacaine).

The newer amide local anesthetics lidocaine, mepivacaine, and bupivacaine have a prolonged half-life in maternal and neonatal blood owing to their slow metabolism by the liver. This causes no difficulty in routine use, since levels usually remain well below toxic levels. However, repeated injection of these drugs, as

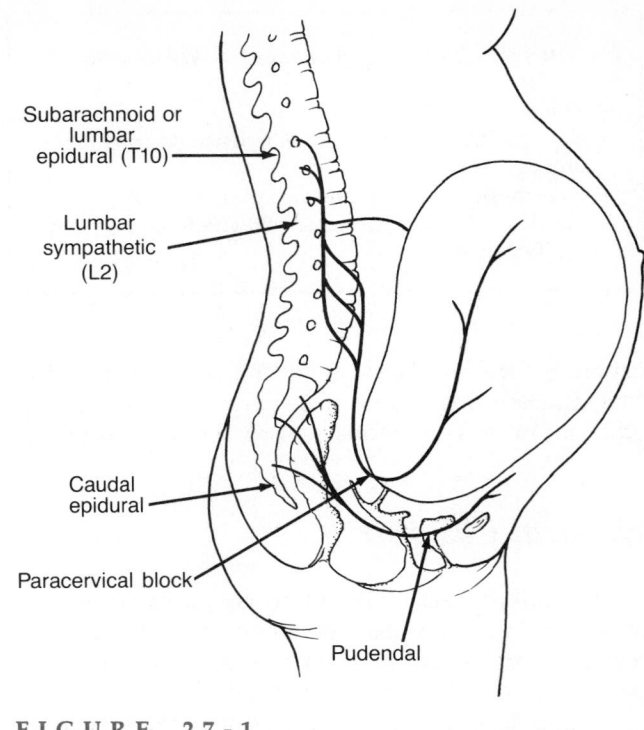

FIGURE 27-1

Pain pathways during labor and appropriate techniques of nerve block. (After Bonica JJ: *Principle and Practice of Obstetric Analgesia and Anesthesia.* Philadelphia, FA Davis, 1967)

in the case of continuous lumbar and caudal epidural anesthesia, can result in toxic blood levels in both mother and fetus, particularly when the repeated drug doses are high and the block is maintained for a prolonged period of time. This is not a problem with the older ester-type local anesthetics, such as procaine and 2-chloroprocaine, which are rapidly metabolized to nontoxic products by the enzyme pseudocholinesterase, normally found in both maternal and fetal blood.

Local anesthetics administered during labor may decrease fetal heart rate beat-to-beat variability, making fetal heart rate evaluation more difficult. This action of local anesthetics has not been associated with deleterious effects on the newborn and is shared by other drugs, including the narcotics, tranquilizers, anticholinergics, and magnesium.

Pudendal Block

Of all the regional anesthetic blocks for vaginal delivery, bilateral pudendal nerve block is perhaps the safest and one of the most useful available. Although pudendal block provides no relief of uterine pain and no analgesia for cervical or uterine manipulations, it does alleviate most of the vaginal and perineal pain associated with delivery. It produces adequate analgesia for episiotomy and repair and allows most uncomplicated outlet forceps deliveries. When supplemented with inhalation analgesia, it usually produces adequate analgesia for other types of forceps deliveries. Since pudendal block does not completely anesthetize the perineum, it does not completely abolish the bearing-down reflex of the second stage of labor. It is relatively painless to administer, and when local anesthetic toxicity is avoided, it has essentially no ill effects on the mother or her newborn. Pudendal block is not associated with maternal hypotension and is the only technique of conduction anesthesia that does not affect autonomic innervation of the uterus.

The pudendal nerve runs just lateral to the tips of the ischial spines, the obstetric landmarks that determine the station of the presenting part. It may be blocked either from the transvaginal approach (Fig. 27-2), most commonly used in obstetrics, or from the transcutaneous route. A bilateral block requires only 10 ml to 20 ml of a dilute local anesthetic solution, such as 1% lidocaine or 1% to 2% chloroprocaine hydrochloride, and is usually administered by the obstetrician or midwife who is delivering the baby.

Spinal Block (Subarachnoid Anesthesia)

Advantages. Subarachnoid or "spinal" block is one of the most useful blocks for obstetrics and is technically easy to administer (Fig. 27-3). The amount of drug needed is less than that required for any other block used in obstetrics: about one fifth that required to produce the same level of anesthesia by the epidural route. Thus, local anesthetic toxicity in both mother and fetus is not a problem. Onset of anesthesia is very rapid, usually complete within 5 minutes. Essentially every obstetric procedure not requiring depression of uterine activity can be accomplished with subarachnoid block. Late in labor a true saddle block of the perineum (S1–S5) allows forceps delivery and repair of episiotomy. If a modified saddle block (T10–S5) is produced, both uterine as well as perineal discomfort are completely abolished. Long-acting local anesthetics such as tetracaine (Pontocaine) with epinephrine produce 3 hours of pain relief when injected into the subarachnoid space, permitting elimination of all pain in the latter part of labor and for delivery. Increasing the level of block to T4 or higher produces satisfactory anesthesia for cesarean birth (Fig. 27-4).

Disadvantages. The major disadvantages of subarachnoid block are its potential for causing maternal hypotension, total spinal block, postspinal headache, the abolishment of the reflex urge to bear down in the second stage of labor, and early relaxation of the perineal musculature, which can result in persistent occiput posterior presentation.

Maternal Hypotension. Severe and sudden maternal hypotension that leads to fetal distress and maternal cardiovascular collapse due to vasodilatation, secondary to sympathetic block, is still a significant cause of maternal mortality. Prophylaxis includes left uterine displacement and hydration with a liter or more of balanced salt solution administered intravenously 15 to 30 minutes before the block is instituted. Treatment of hypotension includes these two steps as well as the use of a central-acting vasopressor, such as ephedrine (10 mg–15 mg given intravenously), and the administration of high concentrations of oxygen. Potent peripheral vasoconstrictors such as norepinephrine (Levophed), phenylephrine (Neo-Synephrine), and methoxamine (Vasoxyl) rapidly correct maternal hypotension but are to be avoided because they cause further decline in uterine perfusion, resulting in additional fetal distress.

Total Subarachnoid Block. Total or dangerously high levels of subarachnoid block usually result when the subarachnoid injection is made just before or during a uterine contraction or when too large a dose of local anesthetic is used. The same level of block can be obtained in the obstetric client with only two thirds of the amount of drug required to produce a given level in her nonpregnant counterpart. Treatment of a high block consists of immediate correction of hypotension, support of maternal ventilation with positive-pressure oxygen, and, if necessary, protection of the upper airway with a cuffed endotracheal tube. With proper therapy a high or total spinal need not delay delivery and should not be associated with increased maternal or fetal morbidity or mortality.

Postspinal Headache. The incidence of postspinal headache is highest in the postpartum woman. An incidence of over 40% can be expected when the subarachnoid space is entered with a 20-gauge or larger-bore needle. The headache usually occurs within 24 to 72 hours of the subarachnoid block, may last a few days to several weeks, and can be mild to incapacitating. The headache inevitably resolves. It is positional and is characteristically exacerbated in the upright position and relieved by assuming the supine position or by increasing abdominal pressure. It is caused by loss of cerebrospinal fluid through the hole made in the dura mater and pia-arachnoid by the spinal needle. Steps to prevent postspinal headaches include using small-gauge needles (25-gauge or less), providing adequate hydration during the postpartum period, and using a tight abdominal binder when the client is in the upright position. Treatment consists of appropriate analgesics, bed rest (preferably in the prone position with the head down), hydration, a tight abdominal binder, and reassurance. When the headache is incapacitating, epidural blood patch is initiated. This consists in sealing the hole in the

TABLE   27-1

Characteristics of Local Anesthetics Commonly Used in Obstetrics

Local Anesthetic and Trade Name	Characteristics	Maximum Safe Initial Dose (mg)		Epidural	
		Without Epinephrine	With Epinephrine	Dose* Vaginal Delivery	Dose* C-section
Procaine (Novocain)	Low toxicity, rapid metabolism with little accumulation, poor spread, short duration, slow onset	500	750	1%–2% 8 ml–12 ml	2%–3% 20 ml–25 ml
2-chloroprocaine (Nesacaine)	Very low toxicity, most rapidly metabolized with little accumulation, rapid onset but poor spread	600	1000	1%–2% 8 ml–12 ml	3% 15 ml–25 ml
Tetracaine (Pontocaine)	Five times toxicity but 10 times potency of procaine. Today used only for spinal and topical. Poor spread, very slow onset	100	200	Not available	
Lidocaine (Xylocaine)	Most versatile local anesthetic, moderate toxicity, rapid onset, moderate duration, excellent spread	300	500	1%–1½% 8 ml–12 ml	1½%–2% 15 ml–25 ml
Mepivacaine (Carbocaine)	Rapid onset, moderate duration, moderate toxicity, but very slow metabolism, marked accumulation with repeated dosage	300	500	1%–1½% 8 ml–12 ml	1½%–2% 15 ml–25 ml
Bupivacaine (Marcaine, Sensorcaine)	Slow onset, long duration, marked cardiac toxicity, low concentrations give excellent sensory and little motor block, ideal for obstetrics	175	225	⅛–½% 8 ml–12 ml	½% 20 ml–25 ml
Etidocaine (Duranest)	Rapid onset, long duration, marked cardiac toxicity. Produces profound motor block and often poor sensory block, making it a poor drug for obstetrics	300	400	Not recommended for vaginal delivery	1%–1½% 15 ml–25 ml

* Doses are given as suggested concentration and milliliters required.
† Duration: lower dose represents minimum duration without epinephrine; upper dose represents maximum duration using epinephrine.
‡ All solutions described have a higher specific gravity than cerebrospinal fluid, since they are weighted with local anesthetic and dextrose.
§ Dose given as concentration of solution and milligrams of local anesthetic used. Note the low dose of local anesthetic required for subarachnoid block as compared with epidural block.
‖ Addition of epinephrine to subarachnoid bupivacaine does not significantly prolong the duration of block.

dura by injecting the client's own nonanticoagulated blood into the epidural space. In well over 90% of clients, there is a dramatic cure within a few minutes to hours.

Loss of Urge to Bear Down.   Abolishment of the reflex urge to bear down in the second stage of labor results from the complete perineal analgesia produced by subarachnoid block. It does not prevent the parturient from bearing down voluntarily with each contraction. In cases of occiput posterior presentation, the tone in the muscles of the perineum causes the occiput to rotate to the anterior presentation. Because subarachnoid block does produce profound relaxation of

Block Duration† (min)	Bilateral Pudendal Block Dose*	Duration† (min)	Hyperbaric Subarachnoid (Spinal)‡ Dose§ Vaginal Delivery	C-section	Duration† (min)	Comments
30–60	1%–2% 10 ml–20 ml	30–60	5% 50 mg	5% 100 mg–150 mg	30–60	Rarely used today; replaced by lidocaine for spinal and nerve block and 2-chloroprocaine for epidural
30–60	1%–2% 10 ml–20 ml	30–60	Not available			Large inadvertent subarachnoid injection associated with neurologic residual. Its rapid onset and metabolism make it an ideal drug for epidural in the obstetric client. Extremely low maternal and fetal toxicity
	Not available		0.2%–0.5% 3 mg–6 mg	0.3%–0.5% 6 mg–10 mg	120–200	In past was used for epidural and local infiltration, but has been replaced by others owing to poor spread and slow onset. Now manufactured only for subarachnoid block
60–90	1% 10 ml–20 ml	60–90	1.5% or 5.0% 15 mg–50 mg	5% 60 mg–90 mg	60–120	Epidural use in past was thought to be associated with depressed neonatal muscle tone. Recent studies question this.
75–120	1% 10 ml–20 ml	75–120				Epidural use associated with minimal decrease in temporary neonatal muscle tone
90–180	¼% 10 ml–20 ml	180–720	0.75% 4 mg–6 mg	0.75% 7 mg–12 mg	100–150‖	Inadvertent intravascular injection associated with cardiovascular collapse
120–240	½% 10 ml–20 ml	180–720	Not available			Inadvertent intravascular injection associated with cardiovascular collapse

the perineum, an increased incidence of persistent occiput posterior presentations can be expected with its use. Since perineal relaxation occurs, the occiput can usually be easily rotated manually or delivery can be accomplished in the occiput posterior position. Another alternative is to prevent perineal relaxation by employment of a lower concentration of local anesthetic adequate to produce sensory block, but not motor block (*e.g.*, 5% lidocaine produces both sensory and motor block, while 1.5% lidocaine results in sensory block alone).

Technique. Because of its rapid onset, subarachnoid block is usually given just prior to delivery in the de-

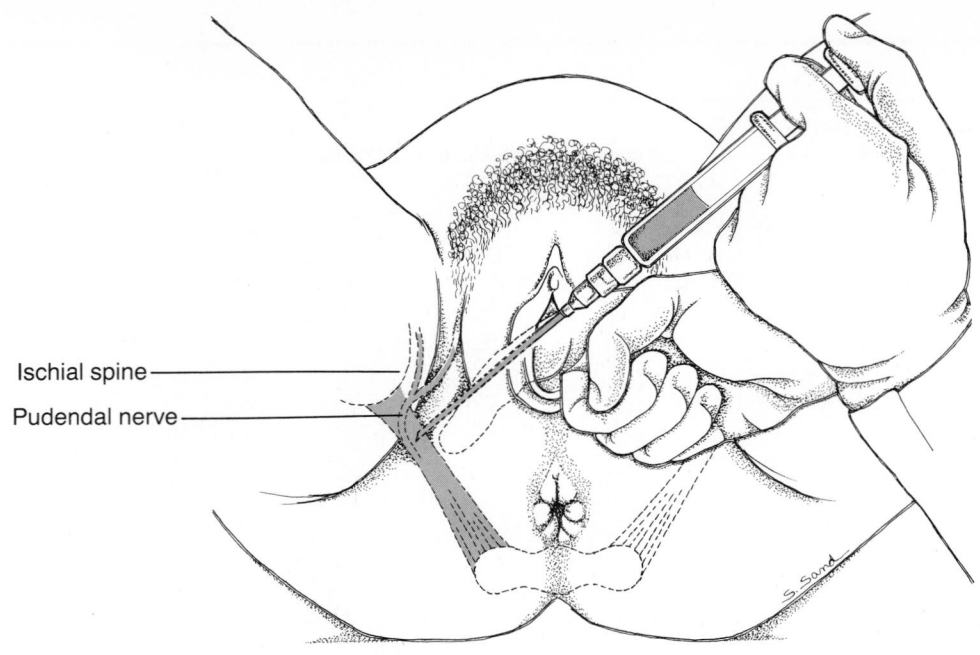

FIGURE 27-2

Pudendal block technique by the transvaginal approach. The examiner's fingers guide the needle to the ischial spine; the pudendal nerve is lateral to the spine at its tip.

livery room. A modified saddle block to provide a T10 sensory level provides ideal conditions for forceps delivery and allows uterine exploration or curettage. Lidocaine 5% (40 mg–50 mg) in 7.5% dextrose gives the necessary T10 level, with anesthesia lasting over an hour. Bupivacaine is now available for subarachnoid block. Like tetracaine, bupivacaine, 5 mg to 6 mg, produces a modified saddle block, but with a duration of

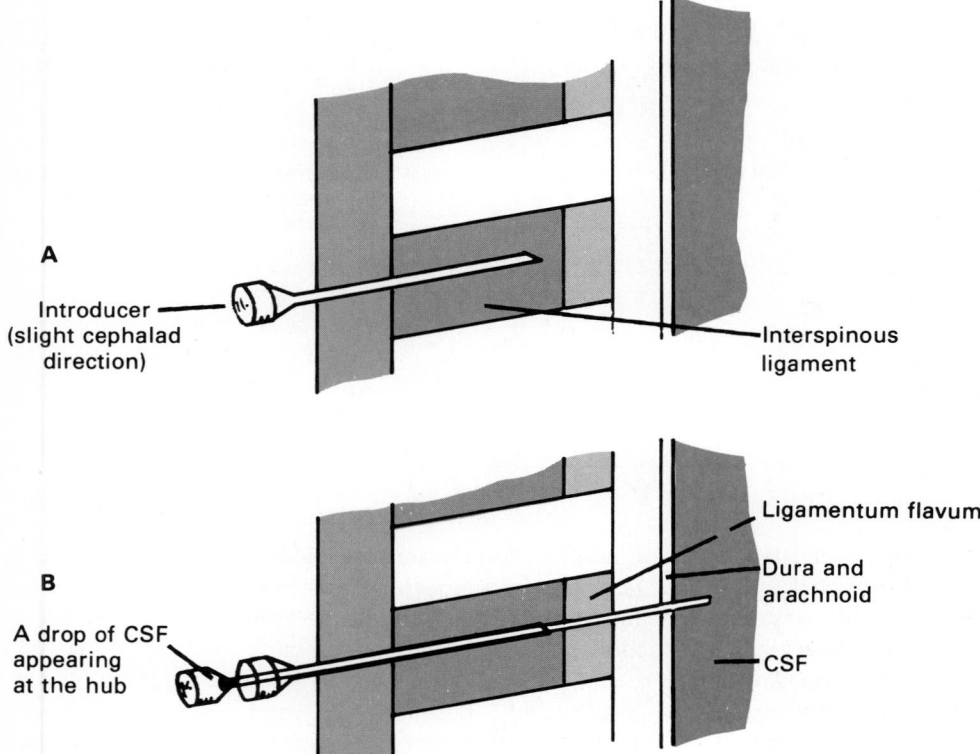

FIGURE 27-3

Technique of subarachnoid (spinal) block. The small 25- or 26-gauge spinal needle traverses the epidural space and pierces the dura and arachnoid to enter the subarachnoid space, which contains the cerebrospinal fluid (*CSF*). Local anesthetic injected subarachnoidally acts on the spinal nerve roots within the subarachnoid space.

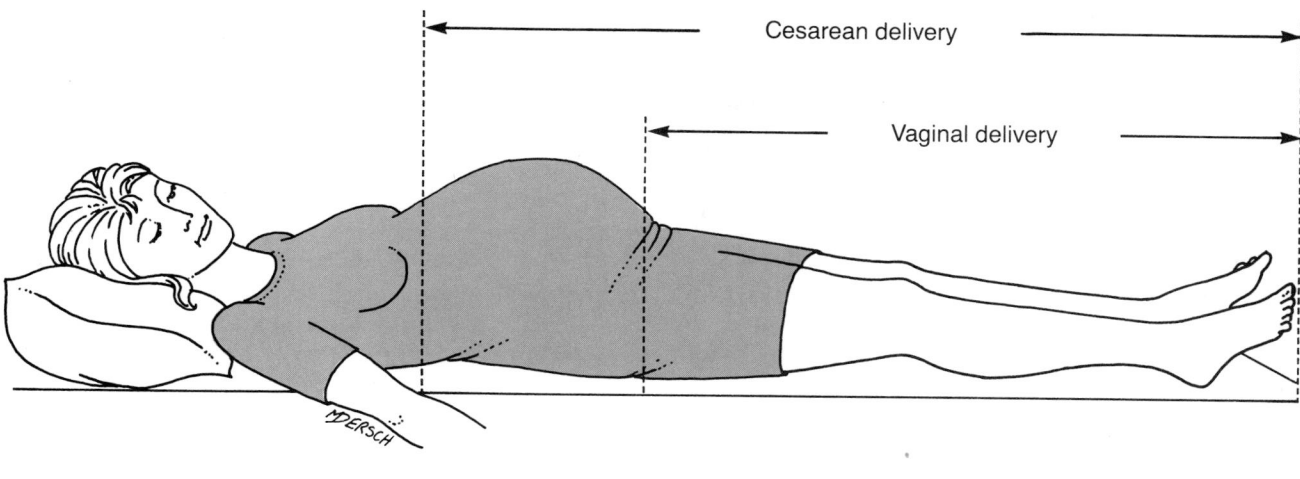

FIGURE 27-4

Levels of anesthesia required for vaginal and cesarean deliveries.

about 2 hours. Tetracaine (5 mg–6 mg) in dextrose with epinephrine added provides more than 3 hours of effective analgesia. The subarachnoid injection is usually made at the L3–4 or L4–5 lumbar interspace.

Epidural Anesthesia

Lumbar epidural analgesia has achieved great popularity in both the United States and Great Britain. Using a continuous catheter technique, a segmental block with an upper level of T10 can be established with the onset of painful contractions and then maintained throughout the first stage of labor. In the second stage of labor, the block can be extended to give perineal analgesia. If a cesarean section becomes necessary, the level of the block can be elevated to T4. Thus, as with subarachnoid block, lumbar epidural block can provide adequate analgesia for all obstetric procedures not requiring depression of uterine activity. Its use allows a pain-free labor in an alert and cooperative mother who will require no additional medications for pain. Since it follows the logical sequence of labor, lumbar epidural anesthesia

has largely replaced caudal epidural anesthesia. The latter (injection of local anesthetic through the sacral hiatus) provides perineal analgesia initially, requires about twice as much drug, and cannot be reliably extended to provide adequate analgesia for cesarean section. Caudal epidural is technically more difficult and more painful to perform and produces less reliable results than does lumbar epidural.

The epidural space is a potential space filled with loose fatty tissue and a marked plexus of veins (Fig. 27-5). It is the space in the vertebral canal surrounded by the ligamentous and bony structure of the vertebral canal on the outside and the dura containing the cerebrospinal fluid and the spinal cord on the inside. The uppermost limit of the epidural space is the foramen magnum at the base of the skull; inferiorly, it ends at the sacral hiatus at the base of the sacrum. It may be entered at any of the intervertebral spaces from the cervical area C1–2 to the L5–S1 interspace or through the sacral hiatus.

In obstetrics, the epidural space is usually entered at L2–3, L3–4, or L4–5 where it is largest and most

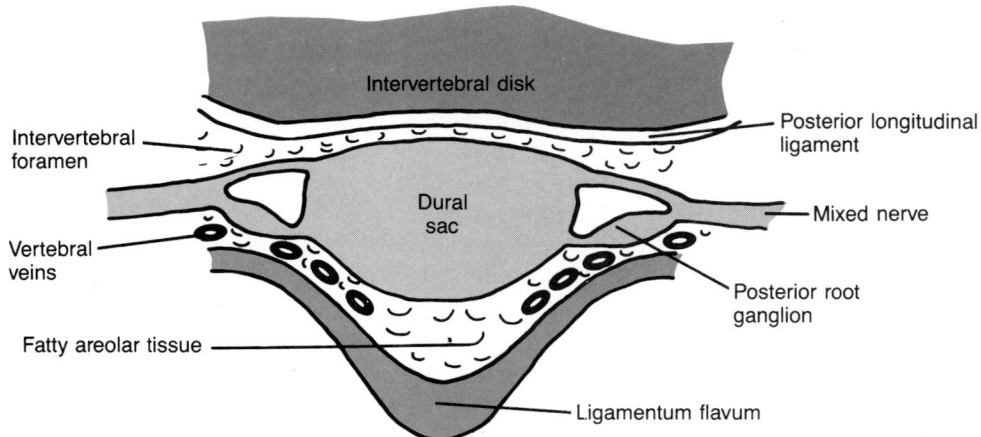

FIGURE 27-5

Diagrammatic cross section of the vertebral canal showing the contents of the epidural space. Note the prominent epidural veins. Local anesthetic injected into the epidural space primarily blocks conduction of nerve roots as they traverse the epidural space.

easily identified. Once the needle is properly placed, a catheter can be threaded through it. The needle is then withdrawn, leaving the catheter in place in the epidural space. Local anesthetic solution is introduced through the catheter as needed to initiate, maintain, or extend the level of analgesia. Recently a technique of continuous infusion of dilute local anesthetics, such as 10 ml to 12 ml per hour of ⅛% to ¼% bupivacaine, has been described. This technique maintains a continuous level of sensory block with minimal motor block and low dosage of local anesthetic. As the nerve roots leave the spinal cord, they pass through the epidural space and hence are exposed to a local anesthetic injected in the epidural space.

Advantages.
There are two primary advantages of lumbar epidural analgesia over subarachnoid analgesia. Since the dura is normally not entered, the problem of postspinal headache is avoided. However, since the needle used for epidural block is much larger in diameter than that used for subarachnoid block (18 versus 25 gauge), inadvertent puncture of the dura will result in a very high incidence of postspinal headache. The second advantage of the epidural technique is that it allows the placement of a catheter for reinjection of local anesthetic drug as required.

Disadvantages
Amount of Drug.   The major drawback of epidural block as compared with subarachnoid block is that close to five times the amount of drug is required with the epidural technique. As an example, 150 mg to 200 mg of lidocaine is required by epidural injection to provide complete anesthesia for vaginal delivery, whereas by the subarachnoid route only 40 mg to 50 mg of lidocaine is needed. Epidural anesthesia necessitates careful control of the amount of local anesthetic drug used, particularly when the slowly metabolized amide-type drugs (*e.g.*, lidocaine, bupivacaine) are employed to avoid local anesthetic toxicity. When it is necessary to use large amounts of local anesthetic drug with epidural technique, one can employ the rapidly metabolized ester-type local anesthetics, such as procaine and 2-chloroprocaine.

Maternal Hypotension.   Like subarachnoid block, epidural block does block sympathetic outflow and can result in vasodilatation and maternal hypotension. Although the onset of hypotension is slower with the epidural technique, it can be as serious as with subarachnoid block if unrecognized and untreated. Prevention and treatment of hypotension resulting from epidural block are the same as for subarachnoid block and include left uterine displacement, intravenous hydration with non-dextrose-containing balanced salt solutions, the use of small intravenous doses of ephedrine, and

oxygen administration. As the onset of hypotension is slower with epidural block, so also is the onset of analgesia. The onset of analgesia following subarachnoid injection occurs within a minute and is usually complete in 5 minutes, whereas the onset of analgesia with epidural block requires about 5 minutes and is not complete for 15 to 20 minutes. This slow onset of block can be partially overcome by initiating the block with a short-acting rapid-onset local anesthetic such as 2-chloroprocaine and then using longer-acting local anesthetics such as bupivacaine through the epidural catheter for later injections.

Loss of Urge to Bear Down.   Like subarachnoid block, epidural block, by providing complete perineal analgesia, eliminates the urge to bear down in the second stage of labor. If low concentrations of local anesthetics are used, such as 0.25% bupivacaine or 1% lidocaine, the mother may sense perineal pressure during contractions and retain some urge to bear down in the second stage. In addition, perineal muscle tone will be maintained, causing rotation of the fetal head to an occiput anterior position when dilute solutions of local anesthetics are used.

Permanent Damage.   Since the amount of local anesthetic required for epidural block is five times greater than that required for subarachnoid block, accidental subarachnoid injection of the epidural drug will produce a sudden, extremely high or total spinal. The undetected injection into the subarachnoid space of large doses of local anesthetics, particularly 2-chloroprocaine, for epidural block has resulted in prolonged recovery and even permanent neurologic deficits such as footdrop and bowel and bladder incontinence.

High Blood Levels.   In pregnancy the epidural veins are dilated, since they serve as a collateral pathway for blood returning to the heart to bypass the inferior vena cava, which is partially obstructed by the gravid uterus. In the performance of an epidural block these veins are not infrequently inadvertently entered by the needle or the epidural catheter. Catheters properly placed in the epidural space have also been documented to migrate into epidural veins and even the subarachnoid space. Since these veins are thin walled and tortuous, blood frequently will not flow nor can be aspirated from the needle or catheter. Obviously local anesthetics injected into the epidural veins will not produce a block, but more seriously can result in sudden high blood levels in the mother, causing local anesthetic toxicity characterized by grand mal convulsions. In addition to causing convulsions, sudden high blood levels of bupivacaine have been associated with sudden ventricular fibrillation and cardiovascular collapse that is resistant to standard methods of cardiopulmonary resuscitation.

As of 1983 there were over 30 maternal deaths associated with inadvertent intravascular injection of bupivacaine, most of which occurred when 0.75% solution was used. Both the anesthesiologist initiating epidural block and those responsible for maintaining the level and monitoring the mother must have the knowledge to effectively treat these complications of high or total spinal and local anesthetic toxicity. They require immediate access to the equipment and drugs necessary for treatment. Failure to be so prepared can rapidly result in irreversible harm and even death of both the mother and her fetus.

Prevention of Serious Complications.
The prevention of these potentially serious complications is desirable and possible. It consists of (1) gently aspirating before, during, and following each epidural injection, (2) giving a test dose (or doses) before each therapeutic injection, (3) slowly injecting through either the epidural needle or the catheter while observing and asking for signs and symptoms of a reaction, and (4) never injecting a potentially lethal dose of local anesthetic in a single bolus, but rather in interspaced incremental doses.

A test dose has two purposes, to detect a subarachnoid or an intravascular injection. Initially, an amount of local anesthetic is injected that if placed in the subarachnoid would produce a rapid, definite, but safe level of analgesia. To this may be added 15 mcg to 20 mcg epinephrine, which would normally produce maternal tachycardia if injected intravascularly. If 3 to 5 minutes after the test dose no signs of subarachnoid block or intravascular injection occur, the remainder of the calculated dose of local anesthetic is given slowly in appropriate increments.

Initiation of Block.
Lumbar epidural block is usually initiated in the first stage of labor when uterine contractions become uncomfortable. While the onset of discomfort varies considerably from client to client, it is usually seen with the onset of active labor, which occurs at 5 cm to 6 cm dilation in the primigravida and at 4 cm to 5 cm dilation in the multipara. Despite controversy, there is little evidence to suggest that epidural block initiated after onset of active labor slows labor. Indeed, more recent studies have indicated that alleviation of maternal pain by effective epidural block may actually hasten cervical dilation.

Lumbar epidural analgesia has revolutionized obstetric anesthesia. In hospitals with adequate personnel, its use has become widespread because of its ability to alleviate all maternal pain associated with labor and delivery while maintaining an alert, cooperative mother and avoiding the risk of neonatal depression. If complications are to be avoided, the same expertise is required in its administration, maintenance, and monitoring as would be afforded the surgical patient. If this

care is not available, epidural anesthesia should not be used, because improperly administered and monitored it can cause serious consequences.

Paracervical Block

Paracervical block is produced by injection of small quantities of dilute local anesthetic solution into the parametrium at sites in the cervix at the 3- and 9-o'clock positions or at the 4- and 8-o'clock positions (Fig. 27-6). It provides rapid complete relief of uterine pain with minimal maternal side-effects. Paracervical block does not affect vaginal and perineal sensation and therefore does not interfere with the bearing-down reflex of the second stage of labor. Unfortunately, paracervical block has been associated with fetal bradycardia, fetal acidosis, and even fetal death. These untoward fetal effects are thought to be caused by the local anesthetic passing rapidly through the placenta to the fetus secondary to absorption through the uterine artery. There is also evidence that proximity of the local anesthetic to the uterine artery may result in vasoconstriction of the uterine artery with decreased uteroplacental

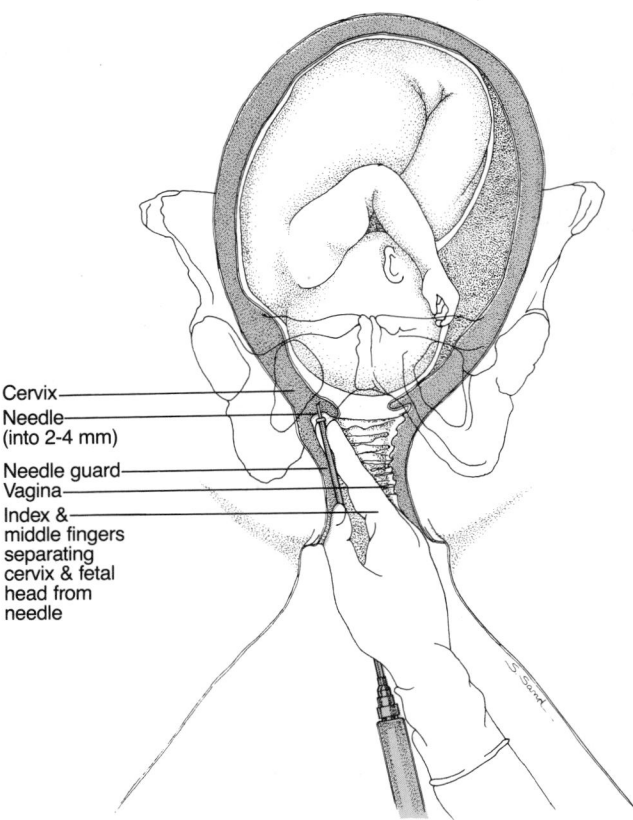

Cervix
Needle
(into 2-4 mm)

Needle guard
Vagina

Index &
middle fingers
separating
cervix & fetal
head from
needle

F I G U R E   2 7 - 6

Technique of paracervical block. Five milliliters of dilute local anesthetic solution is injected superficially into the vaginal fornix at 3 and 9 o'clock *or* at 4 and 8 o'clock.

perfusion. The danger to the fetus can be minimized by using minimal doses of the less toxic local anesthetics such as 2-chloroprocaine and by injecting them superficially and laterally into the parametrium.

Because of the unpredictable occurrence of fetal bradycardia associated with paracervical block, many obstetricians and anesthesiologists avoid its use entirely when a viable fetus is present. A premature or a high-risk fetus definitely contraindicates its use. When used in the presence of a viable fetus, electronic monitoring of the fetal heart rate and uterine contractions is required. Following delivery of the baby or in the presence of a nonviable fetus, paracervical block is a safe technique to provide analgesia for cervical or uterine manipulation (*e.g.*, repair cervical laceration, D&C).

Lumbar Sympathetic Block

Like paracervical block, a bilateral lumbar sympathetic block at L2 abolishes uterine pain only. While this mode of anesthesia is associated with maternal hypotension, such a reaction is usually minimal and can be avoided by providing adequate hydration and left uterine displacement. Lumbar sympathetic block is associated with minimal, if any, fetal and newborn depression, which makes its use acceptable in the high-risk pregnancy. Bilateral sympathetic block may result in improved uterine contraction because it interrupts the sympathetic innervation of the uterus, which inhibits uterine activity. Since the block is rather complicated and somewhat painful to administer, it has not been used widely in maternal care.

Systemic Medication

Systemic medications, given intravenously or intramuscularly, are frequently used to decrease the pain and anxiety of the first stage of labor (Table 27-2). In the past, this form of pain relief was selected because it is simple to administer. Small doses of systemic medications can be used with relative safety for the mother, although certain aspects of newborn neurobehavior may be modified for several days following their use in labor.

Narcotics

Narcotics or analgesics are the keystone of systemic medications. In general, equal analgesic doses of various narcotics produce equal amounts of depression in both mother and newborn. The major difference among the various narcotics is in the duration of their action. Knowledge of the duration of action allows the rational selection of the appropriate narcotic. If prolonged duration is desired, for example, in early labor, narcotics such as meperidine (Demerol) or morphine are indicated. If the narcotics are administered late in labor, when only a short duration of action is desired, short-acting narcotics such as fentanyl (Sublimaze) or alphaprodine (Nisentil) are appropriate.

While narcotics, such as meperidine, administered in reasonable doses for labor may have some mild neurobehavioral depressant effects on the newborn, these are of short duration and are usually dissipated by the second day of life. Contrary to claims by some, there is little to support the contention that narcotics used in moderate amounts for labor pain are associated with decreased learning abilities, decreased IQ, or delayed development.

Both the analgesic and the depressant properties of all the narcotics can be rapidly antagonized in mother and newborn by the use of naloxone (Narcan), a specific narcotic antagonist. Unlike the previous narcotic antagonists nalorphine (Nalline) and levallorphan (Lorfan), naloxone has no narcotic or depressive activity of its own. It is useless in antagonizing depression from causes other than narcotics. The effective duration of naloxone is only about 1 hour. After its use, both the newborn and the mother must be carefully observed for signs of renarcotization, which can be treated with additional doses of the drug.

Naloxone should not be used in the mother to treat narcotic depression in the fetus shortly before birth unless another form of analgesia is first instituted because it rapidly antagonizes the analgesic activity of the narcotic. Furthermore, the effects of its use in a client who has received a narcotic are unpleasant; its use is often associated with dyspnea as well as nausea and vomiting. It must be used with great caution in mothers who take narcotics chronically or habitually and in their newborns, since it can cause sudden and severe narcotic withdrawal. The usual dose of naloxone in the adult is 0.4 mg intramuscularly or intravenously and in the newborn, 0.01 mg/kg similarly given.

Tranquilizers and Sedatives

Frequently a tranquilizer or sedative is administered with a narcotic. These drugs may produce sedation and alleviate anxiety. However, they add little, if any, analgesia and, if given in the presence of pain without adequate alternative analgesia, they produce confusion, disorientation, delirium, and uncontrollable behavior during contractions. Tranquilizers and sedatives also add to the depressant effects of narcotics in both mother and newborn. Finally, many of the commonly used tranquilizers, particularly the phenothiazines such as promethazine (Phenergan), have a long duration of action (6 hr–8 hr) and should not be repeated each time a narcotic is used. The benzodiazepines, diazepam (Valium) and, more recently, lorazepam and medazolam, have also been used in conjunction with narcotics.

TABLE 27-2

Common Medications Used for Analgesia During Labor

Drug	Category	Dosage and Route	Actions	Comments

Meperidine hydrochloride (Demerol)	Narcotic: Nonopiate addicting analgesic	IM: 50 mg–100 mg, repeated 3 hr–4 hr prn
		IV: 25 mg, repeated 1 hr–2 hr prn
			Peaks
			IM: Onset 10 min
			  Peaks 60 min
			  Duration 2 hr–3 hr
			IV: Onset 5 min
			  Duration 1 hr–2 hr
				Maternal effects: analgesia, sedation, nausea, vomiting
				Fetal effects: Loss of variability of fetal heart tone (FHT)
				Can cause respiratory depression at birth
				Can cause decrease muscle tone at birth

Alphaprodine hydrochloride (Nisentil)	Similar to meperidine	SC: 40 mg, repeated 2 hr–3 hr prn IV: 20 mg, repeated 1 hr–2 hr prn	IM: Onset 2 min Duration 60 min–90 min SC: Onset usually within 10 min (ranging from 2 min–3 min) Duration 1 hr to over 2 hr	Maternal effects: Fast onset of analgesia very effective in labor Fetal effects: Loss of variability of FHT; benign sinusoidal-type pattern has been reported after parenteral Nisentil; severe newborn respiratory depression
Hydroxyzine hydrochloride, USP (Atarax, Vistaril)	Antianxiety agent (minor tranquilizer) antihistamine, antiemetic	IM: 25 mg to 100 mg, repeated 4 hr–6 hr prn	Sedative, antiemetic	Can reduce the narcotic requirement needed Never given by SC, intra-arterial, or IV injection
Promethazine hydrochloride, USP (phenergan)	Antihistaminic, antiemetic	Sedation early labor: 12.5 mg–50 mg Sedation active labor: 25 mg–50 mg with 25 mg–75 mg of meperidine; may be repeated Nausea and vomiting: 12.5 mg–25 mg, repeated 4 hr–6 hr prn	Antihistaminic effects occur within 20 min following IM Duration of action 4 hr–6 hr	

The buterophenones (droperidol), long-acting major tranquilizers and very potent antiemetics, are occasionally used in the obstetric client. In small doses these drugs have minimal effects on the newborn, but in larger doses they are associated with depressed muscle tone, decreased alertness, and impaired temperature regulation with a tendency to hypothermia. All of the above tranquilizers, even when used in small dose, are associated with a decreased fetal heart rate beat-to-beat variability.

The anticholinesterase physostigmine antagonizes the maternal sedation and delirium associated with the use of scopolamine. It has also been claimed to antagonize these effects associated with the use of other tranquilizers, such as the phenothiazines (*e.g.*, promethazine) and benzodiazepines. Physostigmine is usually administered to the mother intravenously in 1.0-mg doses until the desired effect is obtained or the maternal heart rate falls below 70 beats per minute. Its efficacy and safety in the newborn have as yet to be determined. Scopolamine, a belladonna alkaloid and an anticholinergic, may produce sedation and amnesia. In the past it was frequently used with morphine or other narcotics to produce twilight sleep. It is rarely used in obstetrics today owing to the frequently observed delirium, excitement, and even hallucinations associated with its use.

Ketamine, a dissociative analgesic and anesthetic, given in doses of 0.25 mg/kg (10 mg–20 mg), produces profound somatic analgesia without loss of consciousness. Used in these quantities, the dosage may be repeated as needed, but not exceeding a total of 1.0 mg/kg before the birth of the baby. In these small doses it is associated with minimal newborn depression, no appreciable effects on uterine activity, and few bad dreams or hallucinations. When ketamine is given alone or in combination with inhalation analgesia in doses of 0.25 mg/kg, the mother remains awake with upper airway reflexes intact. Larger doses are associated with newborn depression and loss of maternal consciousness, which predisposes the mother to the catastrophe of pulmonary aspiration of gastric contents unless her airway is protected with a cuffed endotracheal tube. Ketamine in analgesic doses is most often indicated at the time of delivery. Its use in combination with a pudendal block will frequently allow the obstetrician to employ low forceps without the use of general anesthesia. Low-dose ketamine does not produce analgesia for visceral pain and hence does not provide effective analgesia for manipulation of the cervix or uterus.

Inhalation Analgesia

Inhalation analgesia requires that the mother breathe subanesthetic concentrations of inhalation anesthetics. Properly administered, the mother remains conscious, yet has profound analgesia. Numerous inhalation anesthetic drugs have been used, including chloroform, ether, nitrous oxide, ethylene, cyclopropane, trichloroethylene (Trilene), methoxyflurane (Penthrane), and, more recently in this country, enflurane (Ethrane). Today in the United States the drugs used for inhalation analgesia are limited to nitrous oxide and enflurane. The other drugs mentioned are no longer manufactured for anesthetic use in the United States. Previously, inhalation analgesia was often given in the labor room for the first stage of labor. Potent inhalation drugs such as methoxyflurane and trichloroethylene were usually self-administered during contractions by hand-held devices in which the drug was vaporized with room air. Today this practice largely has been abandoned because it causes air pollution that subjects those who work in the area to prolonged exposure to trace amounts of the anesthetic gases. While not conclusive, recent evidence indicates that such exposure may be associated with teratogenesis and spontaneous abortion. Hence, inhalation analgesia now is usually limited to the later first stage and second stage of labor, in which it is administered in the delivery room using an anesthetic gas machine equipped with a scavenger device that avoids atmospheric pollution.

Nitrous Oxide. Since nitrous oxide is a gas at atmospheric conditions, it is stored under pressure in steel gas cylinders and must be administered through a calibrated anesthesia machine with oxygen by a trained physician or nurse. As 30% to 50% nitrous oxide is required to produce analgesia, it is given in a mixture of 50% to 70% oxygen. During labor and delivery in the United Kingdom, midwives often give a 50% nitrous oxide, 50% oxygen mixture called Entonox that has been premixed in cylinders. In the United States, nitrous oxide analgesia is usually administered in the delivery room by a nurse– or physician–anesthetist during the latter part of the first stage of labor, for delivery of the baby and the placenta, and during the immediate postpartum examination. While intermittent administration of nitrous oxide analgesia during contractions is still used, nitrous oxide is more effective when administered continuously in a 30% to 50% concentration with oxygen.

Enflurane. Enflurane is a very potent inhalation drug that at room temperature is a volatile liquid. It must be administered with an accurate vaporizer and an anesthetic machine. Concentrations in excess of 1.5% are associated with loss of consciousness and general anesthesia. Given in concentrations of 0.5% to 1.25% in oxygen it provides good analgesia without loss of consciousness. In lower concentrations it may supplement 30% to 40% nitrous oxide analgesia. Because enflurane is relatively insoluble and potent, general anesthesia with loss of consciousness, loss of protective airway reflexes, depression of the maternal cardiovascular system, and fetal depression can be rapidly induced during maternal hyperventilation that occurs with contractions. Inhalation analgesia with enflurane requires administration by a skilled physician or nurse trained in anesthesia.

Halothane and Isoflurane. There are two other potent inhalation drugs commonly used for the production of general anesthesia: halothane and isoflurane. Halothane in subanesthetic concentrations does not reliably produce analgesia; thus, it is not suitable for inhalation analgesia. Isoflurane is the newest potent inhalation anesthetic; its structure is closely related to enflurane, and it shares many similar properties with it. Presently its efficacy in producing inhalation analgesia in the obstetric client requires further investigation.

Advantages and Disadvantages. Inhalation analgesia provides profound but not complete analgesia for labor and delivery. Used alone, it often produces adequate pain relief for labor and uncomplicated vaginal delivery without episiotomy. If an episiotomy is to be performed and repaired or use of forceps is anticipated, the obstetrician should supplement inhalation analgesia with local infiltration of the perineum or, better still, a bilateral pudendal block. In addition to analgesia, inhalation analgesia often provides amnesia, particularly for painful events.

If inhalation analgesia is properly administered, it has many advantages and is safe for mother and newborn. Maternal and newborn depression is not produced in measurable degree by subanesthetic concentrations of inhalation drugs, regardless of the duration of their administration. The mother remains awake with upper airway reflexes intact and is protected from catastrophe of pulmonary aspiration of gastric contents without the need for intubation. The mother's reflex urge and ability to bear down in the second stage of labor are little affected. The onset of inhalation analgesia is rapid, and the degree of analgesia can be altered quickly by changing the inspired concentration of the inhalation drug. It can be given safely to nearly every parturient and may be used to supplement other forms of analgesia, particularly regional or conduction anesthesia.

Despite its advantages, however, inhalation analgesia does have drawbacks. The amount of inhalation drug required for adequate analgesia varies from mother to mother and indeed for the same mother throughout the various phases of labor. She may pass from the stage of analgesia and amnesia (first stage of anesthesia) into the stage of delirium and excitement (second stage of anesthesia) or even into the stage of surgical anesthesia (third stage of anesthesia), with loss of protective airway reflexes, subjecting her to the danger of pulmonary aspiration and her fetus to newborn anesthetic depression. *It is imperative that a fully trained nurse or physician always be present when inhalation analgesia is used.*

Inhalation analgesia does not produce complete analgesia. Except for the uncomplicated vaginal delivery, it must be supplemented. Even then, adequate analgesia and client cooperation may not be satisfactory. Increasing the concentration of the inhalation drug often results in excitement and activity or general anesthesia with its attendant problems. When a client receiving inhalation analgesia is delirious and uncooperative, it is often an indication that too much inhalation drug is being administered; this can be corrected rapidly by decreasing the concentration of the inhalation drug.

General Anesthesia

General anesthesia is rarely, if ever, indicated for uncomplicated vaginal delivery. Indeed most vaginal deliveries are more safely performed with other forms of analgesia or anesthesia. Obstetricians today are coming to realize that vaginal delivery with general anesthesia is fraught with many serious complications. Fortunately, women of the childbearing age are now less inclined to request that they be "put under" for delivery. Rather, they want to take part in the delivery and frequently wish the baby's father to be present in the delivery room to share the joy of birth. These changing attitudes deserve to be encouraged and supported by all those involved in the care of the mother-to-be.

Disadvantages. The disadvantages of general anesthesia in obstetrics are many. General anesthesia prevents the mother from participating in the birth of her baby and relating to her newborn at birth. When used for vaginal delivery, it cannot be administered until the baby is deliverable because it immediately stops the bearing-down reflex of the second stage of labor. In addition, the newborn, like the mother, is depressed by the anesthetic. While this depression from general anesthesia is usually rapidly overcome by ventilatory support of the newborn, it may compound depression from other sources. In addition to neonatal depression resulting from the anesthetic drugs themselves, general anesthesia may have further deleterious effects on the fetus and newborn by depression of the maternal cardiovascular system causing a decreased uterine and placental perfusion.

General anesthesia predisposes the parturient to the dreadful complication of pulmonary aspiration of gastric contents. Every parturient is at risk of this catastrophe because her stomach is rarely empty, the gastroesophageal junction may not function as a result of changes in gastric position caused by the gravid uterus, and the gravid uterus and lithotomy position increase intragastric pressure.

General anesthesia for any woman in the third trimester of pregnancy necessitates intubation with a cuffed endotracheal tube. The endotracheal tube should be inserted either before induction or immediately after a rapid induction during which cricoid pressure (Sellick's maneuver) is applied from the time of the loss of consciousness until intubation (Fig. 27-7). General anesthesia for the parturient without endotracheal intubation is unacceptable anesthetic practice.

Indication for General Anesthesia. Despite the numerous disadvantages and problems associated with the use of general anesthesia for delivery, its proper use with rapid induction by a skilled anesthetist may result in the delivery of a healthy baby and the prevention of maternal morbidity and mortality. In certain circumstances, general anesthesia is the only form of anesthesia that can provide adequate conditions for the obstetrician to deliver the newborn rapidly and safely. The immediate availability of a skilled anesthetist who is provided with proper equipment and assistance in the obstetric suite is a primary requirement for good obstetric care.

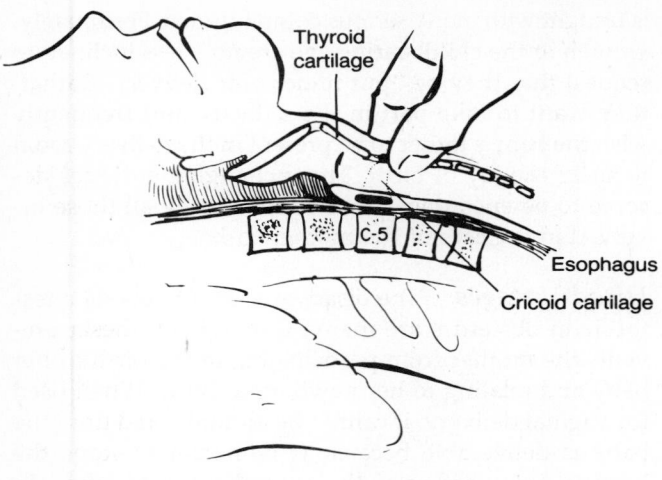

FIGURE 27-7

The technique of cricoid pressure (Sellick's maneuver) prevents pulmonary aspiration of gastric contents during anesthesia induction. The esophagus is compressed and occluded between the cricoid ring of the trachea and the bodies of the cervical vertebrae. Pressure is applied as soon as the patient loses consciousness and is maintained until the trachea is intubated with a cuffed endotracheal tube.

The indications for general anesthesia for vaginal delivery are listed on this page.

Depression of uterine activity may be indicated to abolish a tetanic uterine contraction, which is usually the result of too large a dose of oxytocin given during induction or augmentation of labor. It may also be required to allow intrauterine manipulation for the extraction of a distressed second twin or removal of a retained placenta. Although ether and all of the halogenated inhalation anesthetic drugs can depress uterine activity, halothane, given initially in a 2% concentration, or enflurane, given initially in a 3% concentration, is usually favored because the onset of its effect is rapid and its action is predictable.

If the mother has satisfactory regional analgesia (epidural or subarachnoid block), tocolysis may be rapidly obtained by inhalation of amyl nitrite or intravenous infusion of a β_2-agonist, either of which avoids the problems of general anesthesia.

Techniques for General Anesthesia. While the scope of this chapter does not allow a discussion of techniques of general anesthesia, certain points concerning its use should be emphasized.

1. Clients beyond the first trimester of pregnancy who require general anesthesia need to be intubated during anesthesia to protect against the risk of pulmonary aspiration of gastric contents. The time interval from the last ingestion of food or the onset of labor to the time of induction of general anesthesia is of no value in determining the risk of aspiration. The use of oral antacids during labor does not lessen the need for intubation when general anesthesia is needed.

2. The extent of newborn depression is directly proportional to the induction-to-delivery interval. General anesthesia is induced only when the obstetrician is ready. Delivery should be accomplished as rapidly thereafter as is in keeping with good obstetric principles. Nothing is gained by delaying delivery after induction to allow the drug to be removed from the fetus. Such delay will only expose the fetus to more depressant anesthetic drug.

3. The plane of anesthesia sought before delivery is that which will provide maternal analgesia and amnesia. Favorable surgical conditions and prevention of movement are provided by the use of skeletal muscle relaxants such as succinylcholine, curare, and pancuronium. If used in large doses, nondepolarizing relaxants such as curare and pancuronium may cross the placenta in amounts sufficient to depress newborn skeletal muscle activity. The newer nondepolarizing relaxants, atracurium and vecuronium, when used in reasonable doses may also be used to provide satisfactory conditions for delivery.

4. Oxygen should make up greater than 50% of the inspired maternal anesthetic mixture before birth, to ensure a more vigorous and better oxygenated newborn. Maternal analgesia and amnesia is provided by the addition of low concentrations of potent inhalation drugs such as 0.5% halothane, 1% enflurane, or 0.75% isoflurane added to 30% to 40% nitrous oxide.

Indications for General Anesthesia in Vaginal Delivery

- Fetal distress, which demands immediate delivery and which can be safely accomplished by the vaginal route; usually the use of inhalation analgesia supplemented by local infiltration of the perineum or pudendal block provides satisfactory conditions for such a delivery
- A parturient who becomes uncontrollable during delivery
- A parturient who presents an indication for an operative delivery but refuses regional or other forms of analgesia or anesthesia, or a parturient in whom these alternative forms of pain relief are contraindicated
- The need for rapid depression of uterine activity

5. While adequate maternal ventilation is to be ensured, marked maternal hyperventilation as regulated by the anesthetist must be avoided until birth of the newborn, since hyperventilation is associated with decreased uterine blood flow, fetal acidosis, and fetal hypoxia.
6. Left uterine displacement (L.U.D.) must be maintained at all times until the birth of the newborn to avoid aortocaval compression with its associated decreased maternal cardiac output and hence depressed uterine blood flow.
7. Following delivery, the depth of maternal anesthesia may be increased by increasing the concentration of nitrous oxide and giving narcotics. The concentration of the potent inhalation drugs should not be increased, since this may depress uterine contractions and be associated with increased maternal blood loss.
8. The same quality of anesthetic care available to the surgical patient must be available to the parturient. This includes adequate monitoring during anesthesia and adequate postoperative observation.
9. When general anesthesia is required in an emergency, it is in the mother's interest to wait until qualified anesthesia personnel are available. Nurses and physicians not fully trained and competent in anesthesia must not attempt the administration of general anesthesia.

Anesthesia for Cesarean Birth

Cesarean delivery can be performed under major conduction anesthesia (subarachnoid or epidural block), general anesthesia, or local infiltration.

Major Conduction Anesthesia

Major conduction anesthesia is now widely used for cesarean birth, particularly when trained anesthesiologists are available.

Advantages. One advantage of major conduction anesthesia is the absence of associated newborn depression. In addition, there is evidence that the induction-to-delivery interval is not as important with conduction anesthesia in causing newborn depression, provided normal maternal physiology is maintained. The pressure for a quick delivery is eliminated. Major conduction anesthesia allows the mother to be wide awake, to be comfortable, and to see and relate early with her baby. Provided hypotension and local anesthetic toxicity are avoided, the risk of pulmonary aspiration is minimal.

Disadvantages. The disadvantages of conduction anesthesia for cesarean birth are that (1) it provides inadequate analgesia, (2) it involves the risk of maternal hypotension, (3) the time required for its onset may delay urgent surgical intervention, and (4) it is contraindicated in certain maternal conditions. Inadequate analgesia is usually the result of low level of block, compounded by traction on the perineum. A minimum of solid T4 sensory block is required to avoid maternal discomfort unless the obstetrician is extremely gentle and quick. Sensory levels of less than T4 frequently allow delivery, but then general anesthesia or heavy sedation is required for closure. Without proper prophylaxis, such high levels of block, particularly in the parturient, will uniformly result in significant maternal hypotension. Such hypotension is associated with fetal and newborn acidosis secondary to a depressed uterine perfusion. The prevention and treatment of this hypotension has been dealt with in the section on regional anesthesia.

Despite the fact that subarachnoid block produces complete analgesia in less than 5 minutes, performing the block requires several minutes even in the most skilled hands. General anesthesia can be induced in less time. The minimal time required to induce general anesthesia is extremely important when an emergency cesarean birth is indicated. As the anesthetist is preparing the client for general anesthesia, the abdomen can be prepared and draped. In clients who have a functioning epidural catheter in place, injection of a rapid-acting local anesthetic such as 2-chloroprocaine will usually produce an adequate level of sensory block in about 3 to 5 minutes. Thus, if the mother's condition is stable, an epidural block can often be used for emergency cesarean section. However, in a true emergency situation, one should not delay the cesarean section while waiting for the onset of adequate epidural analgesia.

Contraindications. There are several conditions that contraindicate major conduction analgesia. An unstable maternal personality or cases in which the newborn is to be given for adoption constitute relative contraindications. Maternal fear and refusal to have major conduction analgesia are absolute contraindications. Maternal hypovolemia or shock from any cause is a contraindication because these conditions are exacerbated by the sympathetic block associated with subarachnoid or epidural analgesia. Sepsis or localized infection at or near the site of injection is an absolute contraindication because of the danger of causing an epidural abscess or arachnoiditis. Abnormal coagulation of maternal blood contraindicates the use of conduction analgesia because of the risk of forming an epidural hematoma. Certain neurologic conditions, such as meningomyelocele and spina bifida, may contraindicate the use of major conduction analgesia.

Uses.   In general, major conduction analgesia is ideal for elective cesarean section or cesarean section that is urgent but not emergent. It provides ideal conditions for the father to be present with the mother in the delivery room. If an adequate level of block is obtained, ensuring freedom from pain, nearly all mothers will opt for major conduction for repeat cesarean deliveries.

The injection of small amounts of narcotics into the epidural space following the conclusion of a cesarean section has been found to produce prolonged and profound analgesia without the concomitant motor and sympathetic block and the associated maternal hypotension. The epidural injection of 5 mg preservative-free morphine provides excellent analgesia lasting 15 to 25 hours. While not as yet reported in the postpartum client, the use of epidural morphine and other narcotics has been associated only rarely with mild respiratory depression and not with severe depression nor apnea. This has been rapidly antagonized by intravenous naloxone without loss of analgesia. Therefore, women receiving epidural narcotics require frequent observations to ensure adequate respirations. Other side-effects of epidural narcotics include nausea and vomiting, itching, urinary retention, and, rarely, somnolence. As is true of respiratory depression, these side-effects are rapidly antagonized by naloxone. These latter adverse effects, commonly seen with morphine, are much less common when the narcotic fentanyl is used in a dose of 50 mcg. This dose of fentanyl provides equivalent degrees of analgesia, but with a duration of only 3 to 5 hours. Other narcotics, including the agonists/antagonists, have been and are currently being investigated.

General Anesthesia

General anesthesia, properly administered, can be used safely for almost every cesarean birth. Unlike major conduction anesthesia, there are few absolute contraindications for its use. It is possible to induce anesthesia and to allow the obstetrician to commence surgery in less than 1 minute if the mother has a functioning intravenous line and the anesthetist has drugs and equipment ready. It is the method of choice in cases of hypovolemia, shock, abnormal blood coagulation, septicemia, and a fearful mother or mother who refuses major conduction anesthesia. For anesthetists not trained or allowed to use major conduction anesthesia, it is the method of choice for cesarean birth anesthesia.

Disadvantages.   General anesthesia for cesarean section has three major disadvantages. It denies the mother immediate contact with her baby at birth. Second, it is associated with a higher incidence of newborn depression. With modern techniques of light balanced general anesthesia, however, the obstetrician usually has at least 10 minutes from induction to delivery of the baby before depression from anesthesia is significant. Further, even when the baby is depressed from general anesthesia alone, there is no associated acidosis, provided that the mother has been maintained in good physiological balance during the anesthesia. Resuscitation of anesthetic-depressed babies is usually easy and consists largely of support of the respirations and maintenance of the airway until the anesthetic gases and vapors can be eliminated through the newborn's lungs.

The third disadvantage is that general anesthesia exposes the mother to the potentially lethal complication of pulmonary aspiration of gastric contents. However, proper protection of the airway with cricoid pressure (Sellick's maneuver, see Fig. 27-7) from the time consciousness is lost until the trachea can be intubated with a cuffed endotracheal tube essentially eliminates this catastrophe. There is also evidence that the risk of pulmonary aspiration may be further decreased by elevating gastric pH with soluble solutions of antacids (*e.g.*, 0.3 Molar sodium citrate), decreasing gastric volume and acid content with the H_2 blockers (cimetidine, ranitidine), and using of gastric emptiers, which increase gastroesophageal tone (metoclopramide).

Local Infiltration

Local infiltration was used widely in the past because of the apparent lack of depression in the newborn. Unfortunately, local infiltration seldom produces complete and satisfactory maternal anesthesia, and frequently the mother required supplemental general anesthesia following delivery. Other problems with local infiltration include the time required to produce analgesia and the large amount of local anesthetic drug required. With the refinements in major conduction anesthesia and general anesthesia, there is seldom justification for using local infiltration unless no skilled anesthetist is available.

Applying the Nursing Process to Use of Analgesia

Expectant mothers, as active consumers, are usually aware of the negative effects of drugs used during labor and birth. They want specific information before they will agree to the administration of analgesics. Therefore, health-care professionals must be knowledgeable about the medications that are used in labor and delivery.

Prior to the date of confinement, information should be given to the pregnant woman about possible medications, alternative methods of pain relief, and the necessity to use drugs occasionally even when alternative methods are used. The woman should be encouraged to discuss these freely and to ask questions. She chooses from her options accordingly.

Nursing Assessment

One of the most important responsibilities of the nurse in labor and delivery is the careful observation and monitoring of maternal and fetal status. This is especially true when medications are being used or there is a potential for their use.

While generally not responsible for administering most forms of analgesia or anesthesia, the maternity nurse must appreciate the complications of various techniques of pain relief, be able to recognize the signs and symptoms of the complications early, and know what action to take until an anesthesiologist or anesthetist is available. Without this kind of support, conduction anesthesia cannot be safely used during labor.

An accurate record of vital signs must be kept. Figure 27-8 shows an anesthesia record for a woman with a history of seasonal asthma and moderate obesity who is delivering. Note the frequency of recordings of maternal vital signs.

Continuous recorded electronic fetal monitoring of fetal heart rate and uterine contractions should be considered when regional anesthesia is used in the first stage of labor. Such monitoring is indicated in the high-risk pregnancy or when regional anesthesia is used for the mother receiving oxytocin stimulation.

Nursing Diagnosis

The following diagnoses are related specifically to the material covered in this chapter: ineffective airway clearance related to regional anesthesia; anxiety related to ability to cope with childbirth; alterations in comfort (pain) related to contractions; ineffective individual coping related to amount of pain; knowledge deficit related to use of analgesia for labor and delivery.

Planning/Intervention

The parturient and her coach need to know the progress of the labor and the steps being taken by health-care personnel to assist in the labor and to alleviate pain. Before administering the medication prescribed to promote analgesia, the nurse informs the mother that she is about to receive medication that will make her more comfortable and help her in labor. The mother should be encouraged to rest and should be given reassurance that she will not be left alone. It may also be wise to remain quietly at the bedside and keep conversation to

the very minimum to allow the medication to take maximum effect.

The mother may be asked to empty her bladder prior to receiving the drug, the fetal heart tones and the mother's vital signs are recorded before and after such medication is given. Once analgesic therapy has been instituted, the mother should not receive fluids or food by mouth and should remain in bed. The environment needs to be conducive to rest. Most institutions require that side rails be applied when the client is medicated, even though there is someone in attendance. The necessity of this can be explained to both the client and her partner to avoid any undue fears or misinterpretations. The father, especially, can be alerted to the importance of keeping the rails up if he is attending to any of his mate's needs.

The maternity nurse may have to assist the anesthesiologist in the performance of regional anesthetic techniques. The nurse may be asked to administer various drugs under supervision, to apply cricoid pressure for the intubation of a mother who requires general anesthesia, and to evaluate the newborn and take initial appropriate steps in its resuscitation in the delivery room. Post partum, the maternity nurse may have to observe and support the client until the effects of anesthesia have dissipated.

With regional anesthesia, a reliable intravenous infusion must be maintained at all times. The personnel and means to ensure a clear airway and apply positive-pressure ventilation with oxygen and the ability to treat local anesthetic reactions, high levels of block, and maternal hypotension must be immediately available if serious problems to both mother and fetus are to be avoided. In all situations the nurse must know what actions to take until the physician or anesthetist is available.

In some cases, even when natural childbirth methods are being used, some form of supplementary pharmacologic analgesia becomes desirable in the best interest of the fetus or mother. It is important that the maternity nurse provide reassurance in these circumstances that this should not be looked upon either as lack of motivation or as a failure in life. Here the maternity nurse plays a pivotal role in bringing the parturient to an understanding of the reasons for the necessity for intervention, in dispelling any perceived notion that this represents a failure on the part of the parturient, and in giving assurance that potential hazards to the fetus can be minimized entirely through skillful anesthetic management.

Comfort measures (discussed in Chap. 26) lessen the parturient's anxiety, fear, and tension. The prepared mother can be supported by the nurse who helps by "talking through" the contraction, or the nurse can encourage the parturient's coach to talk through the contractions. The need for medications will be relieved.

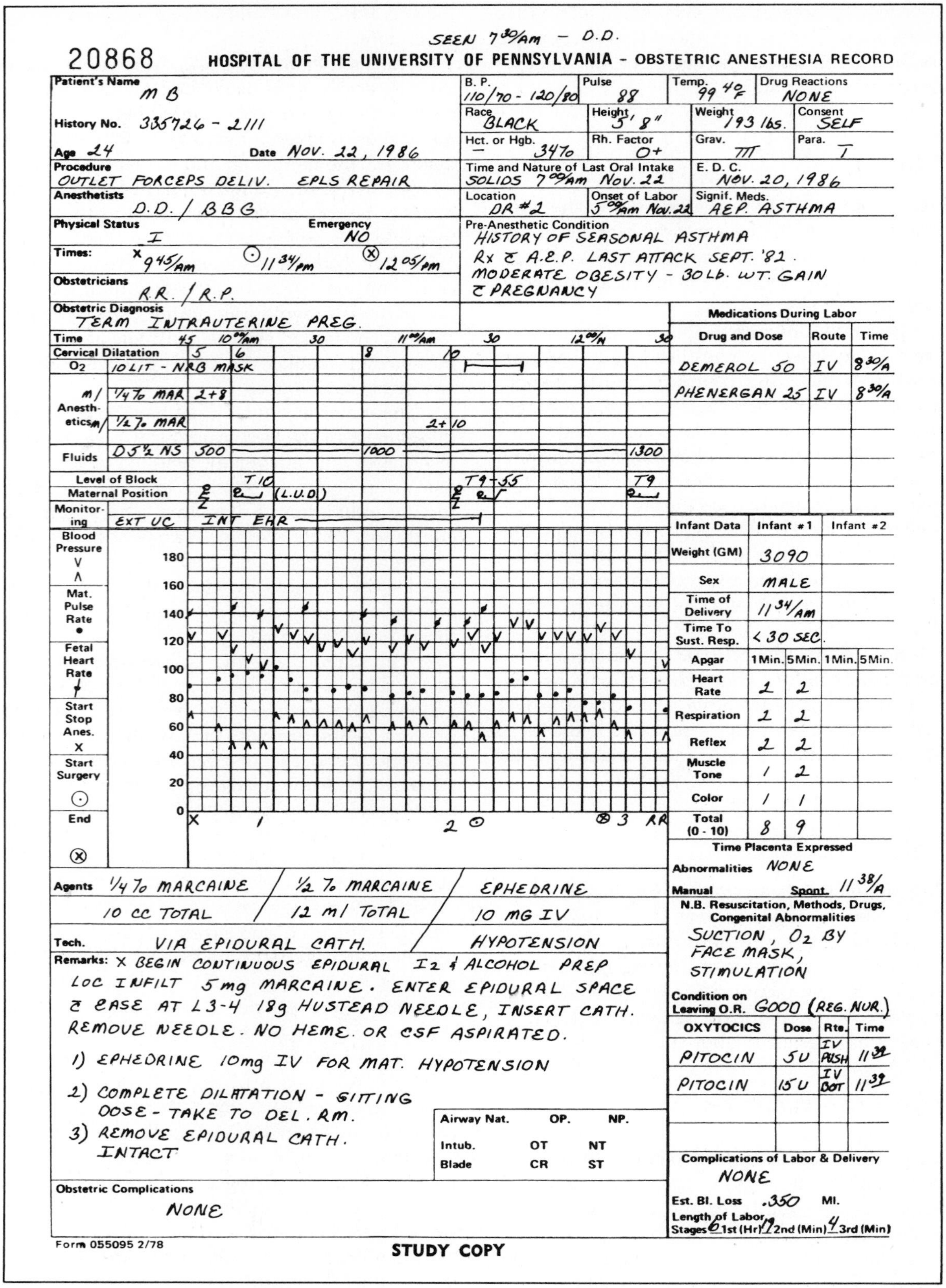

SEEN 7³⁰/AM — D.D.

20868   HOSPITAL OF THE UNIVERSITY OF PENNSYLVANIA - OBSTETRIC ANESTHESIA RECORD

Patient's Name M B	B.P. 110/70 - 120/80 Pulse 88 Temp. 99 4° F	Drug Reactions NONE
History No. 335726 - 2111	Race BLACK Height 5' 8" Weight 193 lbs.	Consent SELF
Age 24 Date NOV. 22, 1986	Hct. or Hgb. — 34% Rh. Factor O+ Grav. III Para. I	

Procedure OUTLET FORCEPS DELIV.   EPLS REPAIR

Time and Nature of Last Oral Intake SOLIDS 7⁰⁰ AM NOV. 22   E.D.C. NOV. 20, 1986

Anesthetists D.D. / BBG

Location DR #2   Onset of Labor 5⁰⁰ AM NOV. 22   Signif. Meds. AEP. ASTHMA

Physical Status I   Emergency NO

Pre-Anesthetic Condition HISTORY OF SEASONAL ASTHMA Rx c̄ A.E.P. LAST ATTACK SEPT. '82. MODERATE OBESITY - 30 Lb. WT. GAIN c̄ PREGNANCY

Times: X 9⁴⁵/AM   ⊙ 11³⁴/PM   ⊗ 12⁰⁵/PM

Obstetricians R.R. / R.P.

Obstetric Diagnosis TERM INTRAUTERINE PREG.

Time	45	10⁰⁰ AM	30	11⁰⁰ AM	30	12⁰⁰ N	30
Cervical Dilatation	5	6		8	10		
O₂	10 LIT - NRB MASK						

Anesthetics m/ 1/4% MAR 2+8 m/ 1/2% MAR   2+10

Fluids D5½ NS 500 — 1000 — 1300

Level of Block T 10   T9-S5   T9

Maternal Position ⚢ (L.U.D.)

Monitoring EXT UC   INT EHR —

Medications During Labor

Drug and Dose	Route	Time
DEMEROL 50	IV	8³⁰/A
PHENERGAN 25	IV	8³⁰/A

Blood Pressure V ∧ / Mat. Pulse Rate • / Fetal Heart Rate ↓ / Start Stop Anes. X / Start Surgery ⊙ / End ⊗

(graph: 180, 160, 140, 120, 100, 80, 60, 40, 20, 0)

X   1   2 ⊙   ⊗ 3 RR

Infant Data	Infant #1	Infant #2
Weight (GM)	3090	
Sex	MALE	
Time of Delivery	11³⁴/AM	
Time To Sust. Resp.	< 30 SEC.	

Apgar	1 Min.	5 Min.	1 Min.	5 Min.
Heart Rate	2	2		
Respiration	1	2		
Reflex	2	2		
Muscle Tone	1	2		
Color	1	1		
Total (0 - 10)	8	9		

Time Placenta Expressed Abnormalities NONE Manual   Spont. 11³⁸/A

Agents	1/4% MARCAINE	1/2% MARCAINE	EPHEDRINE
	10 CC TOTAL	12 ml TOTAL	10 MG IV
Tech.	VIA EPIDURAL CATH.		HYPOTENSION

N.B. Resuscitation, Methods, Drugs, Congenital Abnormalities SUCTION, O₂ BY FACE MASK, STIMULATION

Condition on Leaving O.R. GOOD (REG. NUR.)

Remarks: X BEGIN CONTINUOUS EPIDURAL   I₂ & ALCOHOL PREP LOC INFILT 5 mg MARCAINE. ENTER EPIDURAL SPACE c̄ EASE AT L3-4 18g HUSTEAD NEEDLE, INSERT CATH. REMOVE NEEDLE. NO HEME. OR CSF ASPIRATED.

1) EPHEDRINE 10 mg IV FOR MAT. HYPOTENSION

2) COMPLETE DILATATION - SITTING DOSE - TAKE TO DEL. RM.

3) REMOVE EPIDURAL CATH. INTACT

OXYTOCICS	Dose	Rte.	Time
PITOCIN	5 U	IV PUSH	11³²
PITOCIN	15 U	IV BOT	11³²

Airway Nat.	OP.	NP.
Intub.	OT	NT
Blade	CR	ST

Complications of Labor & Delivery NONE

Obstetric Complications NONE

Est. Bl. Loss .350 ML.

Length of Labor Stages: 1st (Hr) 6 2nd (Min) 12 3rd (Min) 4

Form 055095 2/78   **STUDY COPY**

FIGURE   27-8

Obstetric anesthesia record during the course of continuous epidural anesthesia for labor and delivery.

Sometimes the intervention is needed during the postpartum period. The new mother may feel disappointment, anger, or loss of self-confidence. One mother may have demanded a pain-free, amnesiac birth, but the health status of her infant may have made that impossible. Another mother may have wanted a drug-free experience, with herself fully in control, but fetal or maternal emergencies may have required drugs. In either instance, the nurse can assist the mother in exploring her feelings. Most importantly, the mother may need a great deal of help so that she is not angry at the infant for what has happened.[1]

Evaluation and Reassessment

The nurse assesses the emotional significance of having used analgesia as discussed above in the section on intervention. The nurse determines if further care is needed to work through these emotional problems.

Reference

1. Lipkin GB: Drug therapy in maternal care. In Spencer RT et al: Clinical Pharmacology and Nursing Management, 2nd ed. Philadelphia, JB Lippincott, 1986

Suggested Reading

Albright GA: Anesthesia in Obstetrics: Maternal, Fetal, and Neonatal Aspects, 2nd ed. Menlo Park, CA, Addison-Wesley, 1986 (A text devoted to the problems and their solutions in obstetric anesthesia. Good chapter on psychoanalgesia)

Bonica JJ: Obstetrical Analgesia and Anesthesia, 2nd ed. Amsterdam, World Federation of Societies of Anesthesiologists, 1980

Gutsche BB: Obstetrical anesthesia, why? Clin Perinatol 9: 215, 1982

James FM, III, Wheeler AS: Obstetric Anesthesia: The Complicated Patient. Philadelphia, FA Davis, 1982 (A concise text dealing with the anesthetic management of the complicated parturient or high-risk pregnancy)

Joyce TH, III: Symposium on Obstetric Anesthesia and Analgesia. Philadelphia, WB Saunders, 1982

Kenepp NB, Gutsche BB: Continuous infusion epidural block for analgesia in labor. Anesthesia 53:S295, 1980

Moir DD: Obstetric Anaesthesia and Analgesia, 2nd ed. London, Baillière, Tindall, 1980 (A short, concise English text on obstetric anesthesia and analgesia)

Schneider SM, Abboud T, Artal R et al: Maternal autogenous catecholamines decrease during labor after lumbar epidural anesthesia. Anesthesia 53:S299, 1980

Shnider SM, Levinson G: Anesthesia for Obstetrics, 2nd ed. Baltimore, Williams & Wilkins, 1986 (Best overall text on subject of obstetric analgesia and anesthesia. New edition currently in preparation)

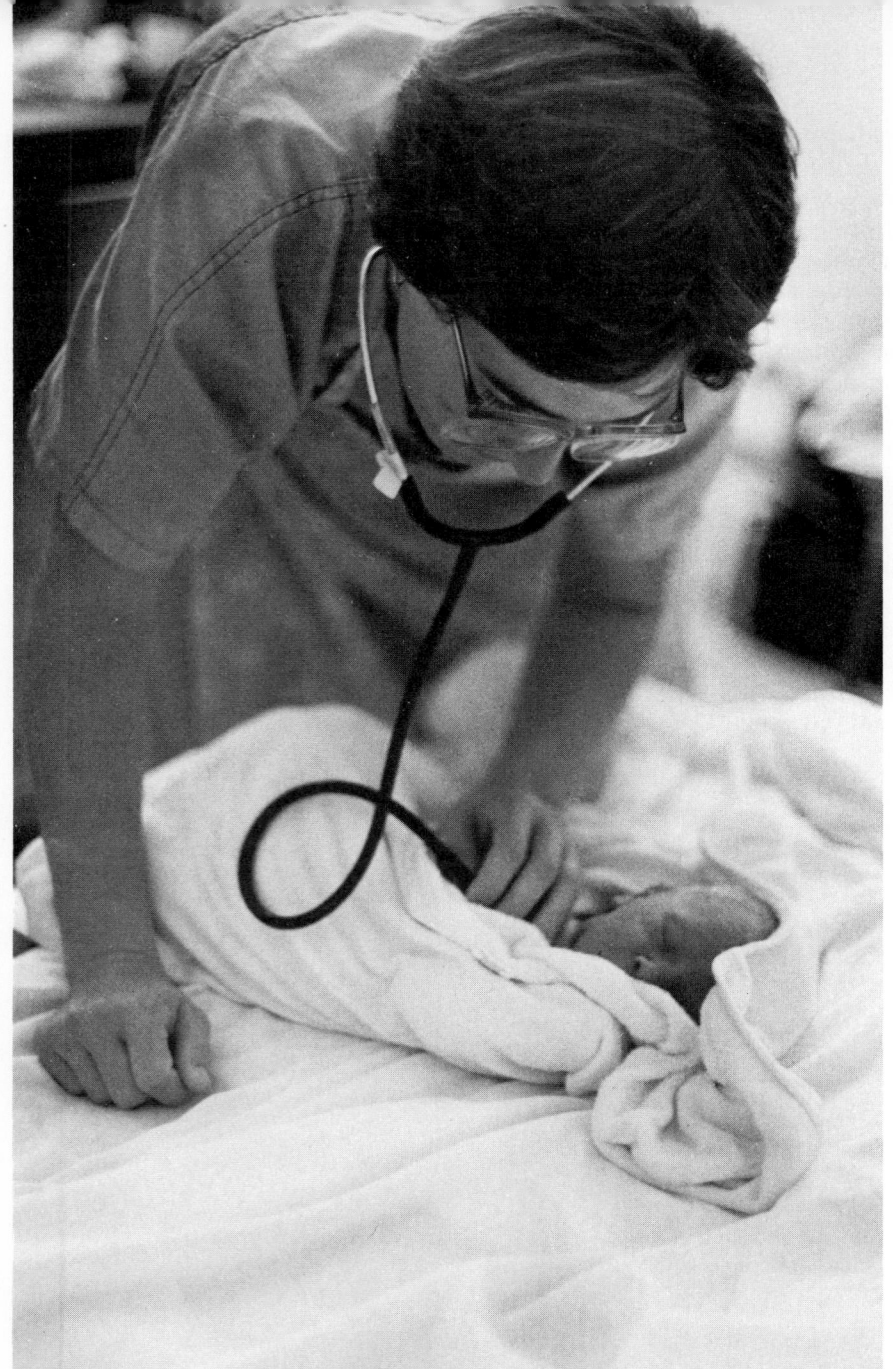

CHAPTER 28

Immediate Care of the Newborn*

During the first and second stages of labor the mother has been the primary center of attention, while the fetus has been assessed and cared for only indirectly. As the newborn emerges into the outside world the term *fetus* no longer applies. The newborn *infant* receives direct attention as the doctor and nurse care for its immediate needs and the mother and father ask, "Is it a boy or a girl?", "Is it OK?", and other questions to identify its characteristics and to verify its well-being.

A typical hospital birth of a normal full-term newborn might proceed as follows: The physician uses a bulb syringe to suction the infant's mouth and nose as the head is born. When expulsion of the infant is complete, the nurse notes and records the time and the sex and sets the 1-minute timer. The physician holds the infant at about the level of the uterus, with the head slightly dependent, to facilitate drainage of fluid and mucus from the nose and mouth while he continues to use the bulb syringe. He then places two clamps on the cord and cuts between them. By this time the infant is crying vigorously and the physician holds him up for the parents to see. When the timer goes off at 1 minute, the nurse assesses and records the infant's 1-minute Apgar score and resets the timer for the 5-minute score.

The nurse picks up a sterile blanket and places it across her chest and arms, making sure the side away from her remains sterile. The doctor places the infant in her outstretched arms and she then brings the infant in close to her body to hold him securely, grasping one leg through the blanket. She shows the infant to his parents, and the mother may hold him for a few minutes; he is then placed under the preheated radiant warmer. When he has been dried off well, the nurse places a clean, dry, warm blanket under him and leaves him uncovered, with the temperature probe on his abdomen to regulate the radiant heat. She places a cord clamp on the cord, ½ to 1 inch from the umbilicus, and cuts off the excess cord with sterile scissors. Identification bands are made up. Two are placed on the infant's extremities, and one is placed on the mother's wrist. Erythromycin ointment might be placed in the infant's eyes and an injection of vitamin K given at this time, or these procedures might be deferred until the infant is in the nursery.

While caring for the infant, the nurse does a brief physical examination to detect any problems or defects and continues to keep his airway clear by suctioning as necessary. The 5-minute Apgar score is done at the appropriate time and recorded. When initial care of the infant is completed, the nurse places a stockinette cap on his head and wraps him in a warm blanket before giving him to one of his parents to hold. By the time

---

* This chapter covers briefly the immediate care of the newborn. Various aspects of this care are discussed in more detail in Chapters 32 and 33, Assessment of the Newborn and Nursing Care of the Newborn.

the infant leaves the delivery room, the nurse should have the newborn record completed, with all pertinent information recorded. The nurse who takes the infant to the nursery gives the record and a verbal report to the nursery nurse and checks the infant's identification bands with her.

Most newborns adapt readily to extrauterine life, as in the above example, and the infant can soon be shown to or placed in the arms of the new parents. However, because this transitional period can be very hazardous for the newborn, the nurse must be aware of the potential problems and alert to the infant's changing condition, to intervene appropriately when necessary.

Goals for Immediate Care

To assist the infant in this transition, goals for the initial care of the newborn include the following:

- Establish and maintain an airway and respiratory effort.
- Provide warmth and prevent hypothermia.
- Provide safety from injury or infection.
- Identify actual or potential problems that might require immediate attention.

How these goals are accomplished may vary according to the setting, agency policy, parents' wishes, and condition of mother and infant. The delivery room nurse uses the nursing process and her knowledge of the newborn's transitional changes to play an important role in meeting these goals.

Assessment of the Newborn

The importance of accurate assessment of the newborn immediately after birth and continued observation during the first critical hours cannot be stressed enough. The information about the infant's condition and responses that the nurse gathers at this time provides valuable baseline data for subsequent care in the nursery. All assessment and care should be well documented and should be reported to those caring for the infant after he leaves the birth area.

Risk Assessment

Ongoing risk assessment plays an important part in the newborn's care by alerting the health-care professionals to potential problems and allowing them time to prepare for these problems. Although nurses often are aware of risk factors and their significance, knowledge of the risk is not always transmitted from one health-care giver to the next. Many hospitals have adopted standardized risk assessment systems. These use forms that follow the obstetric client throughout her antepartal, intrapartum, and postpartum course and include copies to go on the newborn's chart also. Some hospitals have developed their own forms.

Most factors that cause the mother to be identified as high risk will also place the fetus/newborn at increased risk. The mother's age, marital status, family history, and previous obstetric history are some of the

general factors to be considered. Factors that should be noted from the present pregnancy and the intrapartum period are shown in Table 28-1. Examples are given of specific conditions or situations that would alert the nurse to the need to call a special resuscitation team or additional people to assist with resuscitation.

Of special importance as a risk factor after the delivery is information about analgesia or anesthesia given to the mother during the first and second stages of labor. The timing and amount of medication used influences the infant's responses immediately and for some time after birth. Ahls and Brazelton have made the point

TABLE 28-1

Perinatal Risk Assessment

Areas to be Assessed	Conditions Associated With Increased Risk	Areas to be Assessed	Conditions Associated With Increased Risk
Antepartal Course			*Difficult labor
General prenatal information	Lack of prenatal care		Cephalopelvic disproportion
	Weight gain ≤15 lb or ≥ 35 lb	Maternal conditions	Preexisting problems (see antepartal course)
Maternal health	Medical conditions:		Progressive hypotension
	Diabetes		Progressive hypertension
	*Insulin-dependent		*Excessive bleeding
	Heart disease		Signs of infection
	Habits:		*Severe
	Smoking		
	Substance abuse		
	Infections during pregnancy:	Fetal presentation and position	*Breech
	Rubella		*Transverse lie
	Venereal disease		
	Complications of pregnancy:	Events indicating possible fetal distress	Fetal monitoring
	Pregnancy-induced hypertension		*Persistent late decelerations
	*3rd-trimester bleeding		*Severe variable decelerations
	Rh sensitization		Heart rate <120 or >160 for >30 min
	*Severe		*Poor beat-to-beat variability
	*Multiple fetuses		*Scalp $pH \leq 7.25$
Results of antepartal tests	Estriol levels: ↓ or no ↑ after 36 wk		*Meconium-stained fluid
			*Prolapsed cord
	Ultrasound: growth retardation ≥2 wk	Analgesia	Large or repeated doses of analgesia
	Amniocentesis:		IM analgesia within 1 hr of delivery
	Bilirubin or meconium present		
	L/S ratio < 2:1		IV analgesia within ½ hr of delivery
	Nonstress test: nonreactive		
	Stress test: positive	Anesthesia	General anesthesia
Intrapartum Course			Conduction anesthesia with maternal hypotension
Length of pregnancy	≤37 wk; ≥42 wk; *< 34 wk	Method of Delivery	*Cesarean delivery
Duration and character of labor	*Prolonged 1st or 2nd stage		*Mid forceps or high forceps delivery
	Precipitous labor or delivery		*Failed vacuum extraction
	PROM > 24 hr		

* Conditions usually requiring presence at delivery of someone skilled in resuscitation.

that infants whose mothers have been heavily pre-medicated may respond at delivery with excellent function and optimal Apgar scores. However, these same infants, about 30 minutes later, may be in a dangerously depressed state and require special nursing care to help them keep their airways clear of mucus.[1]

Apgar Scoring System

The *Apgar score*, developed by the late Dr. Virginia Apgar, provides a valuable index for assessing the newborn's condition at birth. The score is usually determined for each infant at 1 and 5 minutes after birth. If the 5-minute Apgar is less than 7, it is suggested by the American Academy of Pediatrics that additional scores be obtained every 5 minutes for up to 20 minutes, unless there are two successive scores of 8 or greater.[2] It is helpful for all nurses who are responsible for the care of newborns, not merely those in the delivery room, to be familiar with the principles set forth by Apgar for infant assessment. These provide a simple, accurate, and safe means of quickly appraising the infant's condition.

The Apgar scoring system focuses attention on the following five signs ranked in order of importance. Each sign is evaluated according to the degree to which it is present and is given a score of 0, 1, or 2 (Table 28-2). The scores of each of the signs are then added to give a total score, with 10 being the maximum.

Heart Rate. The heart rate is the most important sign and the last to be absent when the infant's condition is grave. It may be evaluated by palpating the pulsation of the cord or by observing the pulsation where the cord joins the abdomen. Listening to the heartbeat with a stethoscope is the most accurate method of ascertaining the beat. The beat may range from 150 beats per minute to 180 beats per minute during the first few minutes of life; later, within the hour, it usually slows to between 130 beats per minute and 140 beats per minute. Crying or increased activity will increase the number of beats. If the rate is 100 per minute or under, asphyxia is present and resuscitation is indicated.

Respiratory Effort. An infant who is responding well cries vigorously and has no difficulty in breathing. ''Regular'' respiration usually is established in a minute or so. Slow, irregular respiration or apnea indicates that respiratory difficulty or depression is present, and these signs should be reported immediately so that prompt treatment may be instituted.

Muscle Tone. An infant who has excellent tonus will keep his extremities flexed and resist efforts to extend them. An infant who does not keep his extremities flexed consistently usually has only moderate tonus; one who is flaccid is in extremely poor condition.

Reflex Irritability. Although there are several ways to test reflex irritability, the one most frequently used is a gentle slap on the sole of the infant's foot. This sign can be observed when a vigorous infant is suctioned for mucus by the way in which it resists the catheter. A newborn who is in excellent condition will respond with a vigorous cry. An infant is judged to have a poor response if it cries weakly or merely makes a grimace. If there is a good deal of central nervous system depression, the infant does not respond at all.

Color. Cyanosis is seen in almost all infants at the moment of birth. As the infant's circulation makes the change from fetal to extrauterine existence and breathing begins, the body of a healthy infant usually becomes pink within 3 minutes. Since acrocyanosis usually is present for a short while, even in infants who are in excellent condition, those who have scored 2 for each of the other signs may receive only a score of 1 for this part of the evaluation.

Interpretation. An Apgar score of 7 to 10 indicates that the infant's condition is good. If the infant breathes and cries (or coughs) seconds after delivery, there are

T A B L E   2 8 - 2

The Apgar Scoring Chart

Sign	0	1	2
Heart rate	Absent	Slow (less than 100)	Over 100
Respiratory effort	Absent	Slow, irregular	Good, crying
Muscle tone	Flaccid	Some flexion of extremities	Active motion
Reflex irritability	No response	Weak cry or grimace	Vigorous cry
Color	Blue, pale	Body pink, extremities blue	Completely pink

usually no special procedures necessary other than those of routine close observation, maintaining a clear airway, and supplying warmth as necessary.

A score of 4 to 6 means that the infant is in fair condition. There may be moderate central nervous system depression, some muscle flaccidity, and cyanosis; respiration is not readily established. *These infants must have the air passage cleared and be given oxygen promptly.* Sometimes directing a stream of oxygen toward the infant's face while suctioning is being done will be sufficient, but administration of oxygen can best be done by mask, and the flow should not exceed 4 liters. Gentle patting and rubbing with the receiving blanket to dry the infant's body usually acts as an additional stimulus.

A score of 0 to 3 denotes an extremely poor condition. Resuscitation is needed immediately (see Chap. 44). If an infant is obviously depressed at birth, resuscitative measures should begin even before the 1-minute evaluation. For the depressed neonate, scores repeated at intervals provide an index of recovery.[3]

General Assessment

Initial assessment of the newborn should include a brief general physical assessment. Hospitals may have different policies as to what is to be checked in this brief initial physical examination, but the following basic areas should be covered:

1. Inspection
   a. Head and face, anterior of body, posterior of body, or extremities: for any obvious defects or evidence of trauma
   b. Skin: for color, staining, peeling
   c. General appearance: for anything unusual
   d. Nostrils: for patency
   e. Cord: for three vessels

2. Auscultation
   a. Heart: for rate and quality of sounds
   b. Lungs on each side: for comparison and to evaluate efficiency of respiratory exchange
3. Palpation
   a. Liver: for enlargement
   b. Chest: for position of maximum impulse of heart

Although not of critical importance for immediate intervention, checking the cord for three vessels should be done as soon as possible after the cord is cut, since the edges of the vessels are more difficult to see as the cord begins to dry. When first cut, the edges of the arteries are seen as two white papular structures, which usually stand out slightly from the surface. The vein is larger, often gaping, so that the lumen and thin wall are easily seen. The presence of only one artery is suggestive of congenital abnormalities.

Prompt detection of congenital anomalies or other problems is important to facilitate early treatment, and knowledge that there are no problems allows more leisurely time for parents and infant to get acquainted. Some congenital anomalies would be obvious, but others require some knowledge of what to look for. The practice of dimming the delivery room lights for a Le Boyer-type birth would increase the need to look more closely at the infant at birth. Newborn physical assessment is covered in more detail in Chapter 32, and congenital anomalies are covered in Chapter 45.

Gestational Age Assessment

Estimation of gestational age during the prenatal period is usually based on the mother's expected date of delivery as calculated from her last menstrual period. After birth, a more accurate estimation can be made by phys-

T A B L E   2 8 - 3

Rapid Estimation of Gestational Age of the Newborn

	Gestational Age		
Sites	*36 Wk or Less*	*37–38 Wk*	*39 Wk or More*
Sole creases	Anterior transverse crease only	Occasional creases anterior two-thirds	Sole covered with creases
Breast nodule diameter	2 mm	4 mm	7 mm
Scalp hair	Fine and fuzzy	Fine and fuzzy	Coarse and silky
Earlobe	Pliable, no cartilage	Some cartilage	Stiffened by thick cartilage
Testes and scrotum	Testes in lower canal, scrotum small, few rugae	Intermediate	Testes pendulous, scrotum full, extensive rugae

(Pritchard JA, MacDonald PC, Gant NF: Williams Obstetrics, 17th ed. Norwalk, CT, Appleton-Century-Crofts, 1985)

ical examination of the infant. The complete gestational age assessment is usually done in the nursery (see Chap. 32), but it is often helpful to use a shorter version during the immediate newborn period, especially if the infant appears smaller or larger than expected from the mother's dates. A rapid estimation of gestational age as suggested by Pritchard includes examination of sole creases, breast nodules, scalp hair, earlobes, and, in the male infant, testes and scrotum (Table 28-3).[4]

Nursing Diagnosis

By using the previously noted assessment methods, the nurse is able to assist in identifying problems and potential problems that require early intervention. In the immediate care of the newborn, certain potential nursing diagnoses are kept in mind during assessment to assist with early identification and intervention if problems are present or developing. Problems that are possible during this early neonatal period include: ineffective breathing patterns related to alteration in response to extrauterine life; ineffective airway clearance related to excess mucus; impaired gas exchange; potential for injury (hypothermia) related to newborn status; potential for infection related to immature immune system; potential for alteration in parenting (maternal–infant attachment process).

Planning/Intervention

While caring for the infant immediately after birth the nurse uses her assessment of the preceding areas and her nursing diagnoses to plan and implement care to meet the stated goals.

Establishing and Maintaining an Airway

At birth the neonate undergoes profound and rapid physiological changes as the fetoplacental circulation ceases to function. The infant's survival depends on the rapidity and efficiency of these changes. The fluid-filled alveoli of the infant's lungs must fill with air, and respiratory motion must occur to exchange that air.

As soon as the infant is born, measures are taken to promote a clear air passage. As the head is delivered, the mucus and fluid are wiped or suctioned from the infant's nose and mouth to avoid aspiration of more fluid and mucus into the lungs with the first breath. A bulb syringe is usually used for this purpose. The infant

is then observed to make sure respiratory efforts begin and are maintained. The first cry is eagerly awaited, since crying is one way the infant demonstrates its respiratory effort. The infant may not cry at once, but the removal of the mucus and the stimulation provided by the suctioning usually elicit a gasp or cry.

Some infants cry very little, but are alert, active, and breathing well. Others seem to need to cry to force mucus from the nose and throat. If it is necessary to stimulate the infant to cry, this should be done with care. Vigorous external irritants, including spanking, forcible rubbing of the skin along the spine, alternate hot and cold tubbing, and dilatation of the anal sphincter, are no longer considered necessary or effective and can be dangerous and shocking to the infant. Drying the infant with the blanket or gentle rubbing of the back or soles of the feet is usually sufficient stimulus to initiate crying (Fig. 28-1).

At first the infant should be kept in a modified Trendelenburg position to facilitate drainage of mucus. An exaggerated Trendelenburg position should be avoided, because the relatively large amount of abdominal contents will press against the diaphragm and the partially expanded lungs and may impede the infant's respiratory efforts. The bulb syringe should be used as

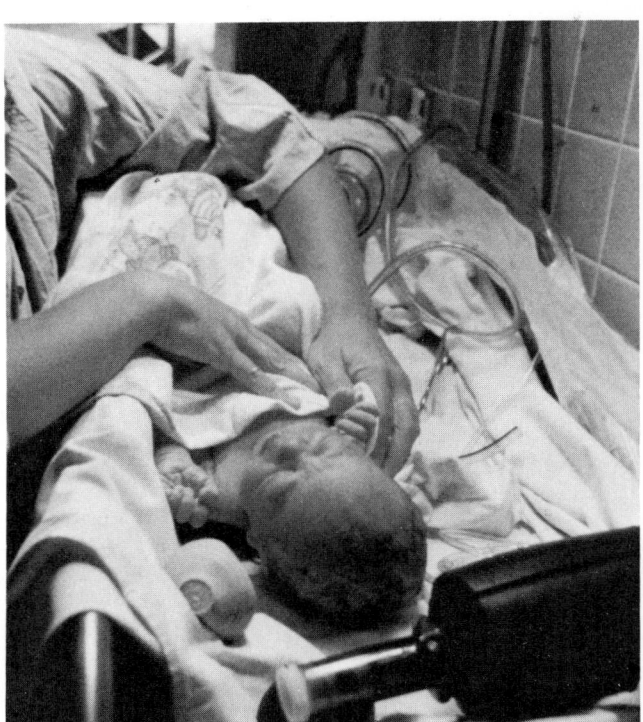

FIGURE 28-1

The baby may be stimulated to cry by rubbing it gently with a blanket. (Courtesy of Booth Maternity Center, Philadelphia)

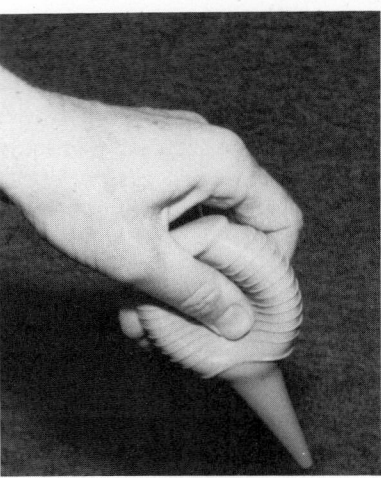

FIGURE 28-2

To prevent mucus from being forced into the bronchi and lungs, the bulb syringe is collapsed before it is inserted into the newborn's nostrils and mouth.

needed. Collapsing the bulb before inserting it into the baby's mouth will prevent the material in the oropharynx from being forced into the bronchi and lungs when the bulb is squeezed (Fig. 28-2). If the bulb syringe is not adequate to remove the mucus, the nurse may use a suction catheter attached to mechanical suction, or to a DeLee mucus trap, which uses the nurse's mouth to provide suction for aspirating the mucus (Fig. 28-3). It is important not to oversuction, because this may deprive the infant of oxygen by interfering with breathing. Deep, prolonged suctioning can also cause vagal stimulation, which can result in bradycardia.[2] Care should be taken not to traumatize the tissues of the oropharynx with the tip of the catheter or bulb syringe or with forceful suction. The mouth should be suctioned before the nose. If it is necessary to remove mucus through the nostrils, force should be avoided and the catheter should not be inserted far back. If the catheter is directed horizontally, as if passing over the roof of the mouth, instead of directed upward as for the adult patient, it usually slips into the tiny infant nostril with more ease.

Resuscitation

For the majority of normal newborns, there is little need for resuscitative measures beyond clearing the airway and applying warmth and gentle tactile stimulation. A small percentage of newborns do require assistance, and

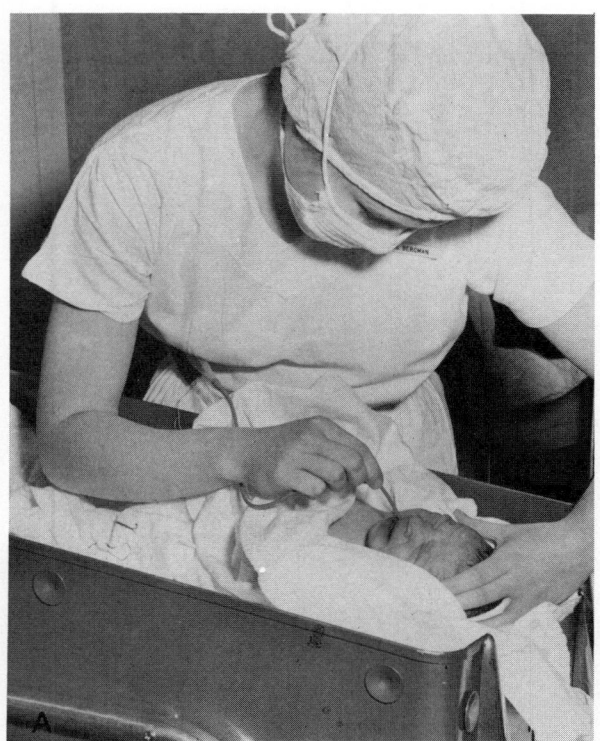
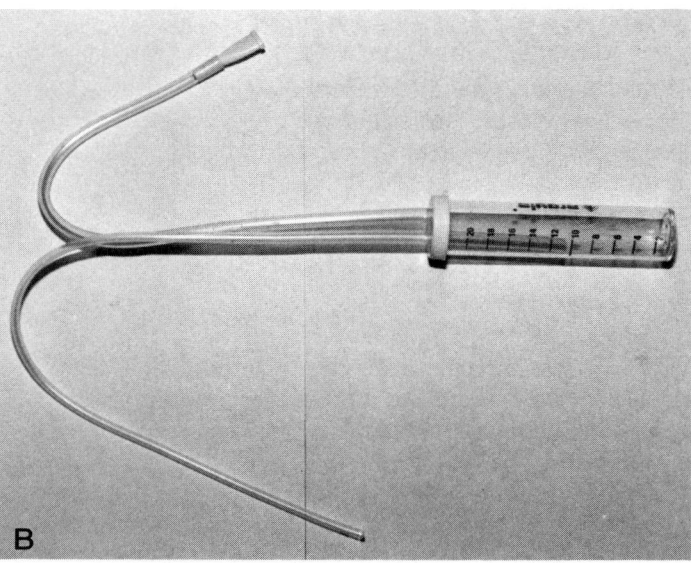

FIGURE 28-3

Suctioning the newborn in the delivery room. (*A*) The suctioning may be done mechanically. (*B*) A DeLee mucus trap in which the nurse's mouth provides suction for aspiration.

for them the immediate availability of this assitance may be lifesaving. Successful active resuscitation requires skilled personnel who have been trained in the procedures, an adequate work area that is warm and well lighted, and appropriate equipment (Fig. 28-4), including the means to deliver oxygen by positive pressure (see Fig. 25-6). It is important for any facility where births occur to have a plan that can be implemented immediately when emergency resuscitation of a newborn is anticipated or needed.[2] Part of this plan should be a list of maternal and fetal conditions that, when identified, would require someone specifically trained in newborn resuscitation to be present at the birth. The items starred in Table 28-1 are samples of conditions that might be included on the list. An additional item might be "request by the pediatrician or obstetrician."

Respiratory depression, the inability to initiate respirations, is the most common cause of perinatal asphyxia. Maternal analgesia and anesthesia are among the most frequent contributors to respiratory depression, since they can reduce the responsiveness of the respiratory center in the brain of the neonate. Inadequate respirations that persist beyond a minute severely compromise the infant by leading to a falling heart rate, decreased muscle tone, and greater possibility of acidosis.[3] A schematic approach for resuscitation is presented in Figure 28-5. Before beginning resuscitative efforts with positive-pressure oxygen, the airway must

be cleared well by suctioning, because oxygen delivered under pressure may force any foreign material present in the airway deep into the infant's lungs. A well-fitting mask is placed over the infant's mouth and nose, and oxygen is adminstered by bag and mask ventilation at a rate of 40 to 60 breaths per minute to deliver the oxygen into the bronchi. If this procedure (called "bagging") does not promptly stimulate breathing and correct the evidence of hypoxia, endotracheal intubation will be necessary under direct visualization with a laryngoscope.[5] Further details of resuscitative measures can be found in Chapter 44.

When resuscitative measures are needed and used in the delivery room, it can be a very frightening time for the parents. In the rush to resuscitate the infant, it is important not to ignore the parents and their concern. The nurse should explain what is happening, as much as possible, and assure the parents that, although the baby has a problem, measures are being taken to correct it.

Maintaining a Neutral Thermal Environment

An important aspect of the newborn's immediate care is the prevention of hypothermia. The environmental temperature in the delivery room is much cooler than

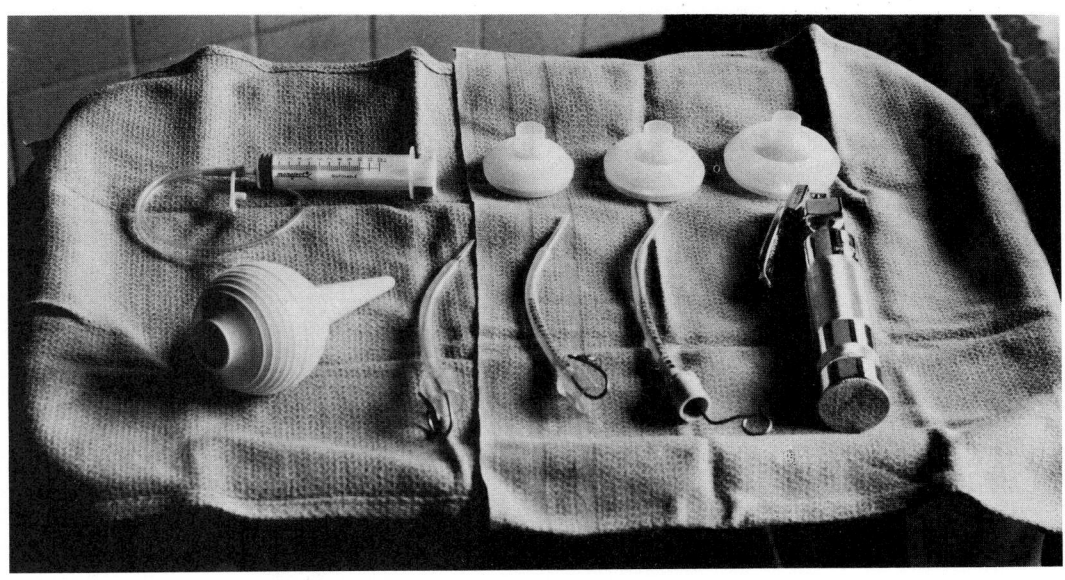

FIGURE 28-4

Close-up view of a sterile tray for management of the airway. Counterclockwise from top left are a sterile, disposable syringe and tube for suctioning the stomach; a bulb syringe for suctioning the mouth; Cole endotracheal tubes (three sizes); an infant laryngoscope; and Bennet masks (three sizes).

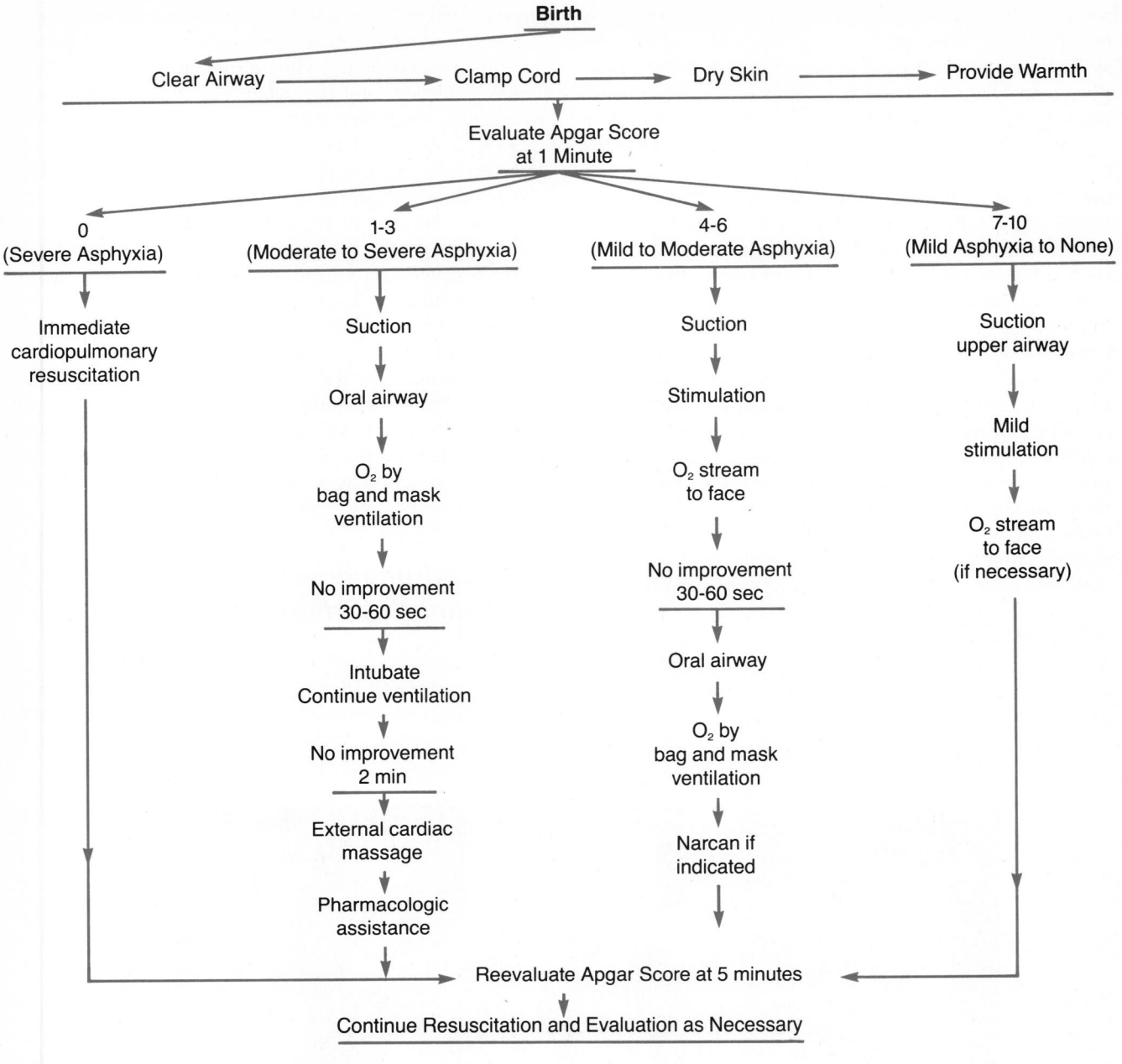

Schematic approach for resuscitation based on 1-minute Apgar score.

the intrauterine temperature and the infant is wet, which further increases the chilling effects of the transition to the outside world. Wiping the amniotic fluid from the newborn's head and body as soon as possible will help to minimize heat loss by evaporation. A stockinette cap is often placed on the infant's head to help prevent heat loss from this area. Use of a radiant warmer and a prewarmed mattress for the infant's initial care provides a heat-gaining rather than a heat-losing environment. Prevention of hypothermia and cold stress in the neo-

nate is related to the amount of oxygen needed by the infant and to the control of apnea and the acid–base balance (see Chap. 32).

Providing a Safe Environment

Safety for the newborn is not always considered as a separate entity and is sometimes taken for granted. The newborn is very vulnerable to environmental hazards, including infection or physical harm. When handling the infant immediately after birth, the nurse should be aware that newborns are slippery and that a firm grip is essential. The infant should be placed in a safe area for care. Following initial care, the nurse will need to observe the infant frequently for any change in condition.

Infection control in the delivery room is important for both mother and infant. The newborn has an immature immune system and is susceptible to acquiring an infection when exposed to a variety of organisms. The nurse should consider hand washing an integral part of the procedure before handling the baby. Personnel who are ill should stay out of the delivery room. The umbilical cord stump is a potential portal of entry for infection, especially while still moist. Although it should be left uncovered, care should be taken that it is not contaminated. Further measures to prevent infection of the cord are usually implemented in the newborn nursery (see Chap. 33).

Care of the Eyes

Another aspect of preventing infection is eye care. The eyes of the newborn are at risk for becoming infected by a variety of infectious agents that might be present in the mother's vagina. For about 100 years, instillation of silver nitrate solution into the eyes of newborns has been used as a preventive measure against gonococcal ophthalmia neonatorum, or infectious conjunctivitis of the newborn (Fig. 28-6). In the United States the use of some form of prophylaxis against eye infections is required by law. Although silver nitrate was used almost

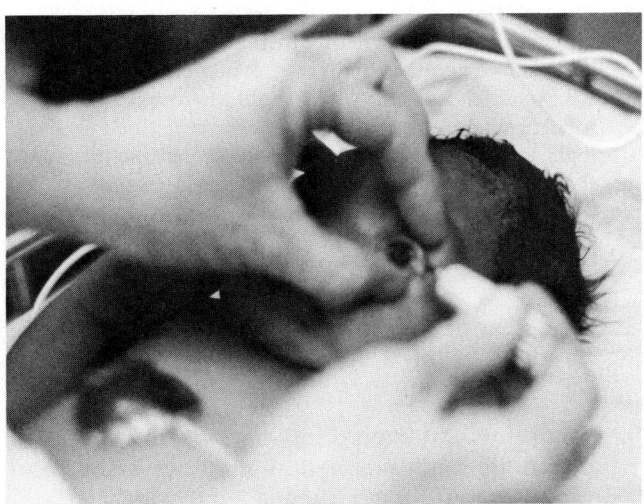

FIGURE 28-6

Ointment is applied to the eyes to prevent infection.

exclusively for years, other anti-infective agents are now acceptable. Two of the reasons for replacing silver nitrate as the agent of choice are that it often causes a chemical conjunctivitis and that it is not effective against *Chlamydia*, another infectious agent sometimes responsible for ophthalmia neonatorum.[2]

The Committee on Ophthalmia Neonatorum of the National Society to Prevent Blindness states that the prevention of both gonococcal and chlamydial infections must be considered (see Recommendations for Prevention and Treatment of Ophthalmia Neonatorum).

Although both tetracycline and erythromycin are acceptable for use, erythromycin ointment is usually the drug of choice, since it is less expensive than tetracycline and is more effective against *Chlamydia*.[7] It is recommended that infants born by cesarean delivery also receive eye prophylaxis. Even though they did not pass through the vagina, it is possible that these infants have been infected by ascending organisms.[2]

Eye prophylaxis may be done in the delivery room or may be delayed until the infant is taken to the nursery. This allows the parents to see the infant with his eyes open, since he is less likely to open his eyes for awhile after having drops or ointment instilled.

Other Aspects of Care

Prophylaxis Against Hypoprothrombinemia

A single 0.5-mg to 1.0-mg dose of phytonadione solution (AquaMEPHYTON) is administered intramuscularly to the newborn in the delivery room or on admission to the nursery (see Fig. 33-5). This water-soluble form of vitamin K_1 acts as a preventive measure against neonatal hemorrhagic disease. Amounts of the medication in excess of 1 mg may predispose to the development of hyperbilirubinemia and are to be avoided (see Chap. 32).

Identification Methods

While the newborn is still in the delivery room, it is the nurse's responsibility to prepare and apply some means of identification. Most hospitals use flexible plastic bands that come in sets of three with identical numbers on them. The mother's name and admission number, the physician's name, the date, the time of birth, and the sex of the baby are written on a special insert, which is put into each band. Two bands are placed on the infant, usually one on a wrist and one on an ankle, and the other band is placed on the mother's wrist. The number on the bands should be entered on the infant's record,

Recommendations for Prevention and Treatment of Ophthalmia Neonatorum

1. A prophylactic agent should be instilled in the eyes of all newborns.
2. Acceptable prophylactic agents that prevent gonococcal ophthalmia neonatorum include the following:
   a. Silver nitrate solution (1%) in single-dose ampules
   b. Erythromycin (0.5%) ophthalmic ointment or drops in single-use tubes or ampules
   c. Tetracycline (1%) ophthalmic ointment or drops in single-use tubes or ampules
3. Acceptable prophylactic agents that prevent chlamydial ophthalmia neonatorum include the following:
   a. Erythromycin (0.5%) ophthalmic ointment or drops in single-use tubes or ampules
   b. Tetracycline (1%) ophthalmic ointment or drops in single-use tubes or ampules
   Silver nitrate does not prevent chlamydial infections.
4. Prophylactic agents should be given shortly after birth. A delay of up to 1 hour is probably acceptable and may facilitate initial maternal–infant bonding.
5. The importance of performing the instillation so the agent reaches all parts of the conjunctival surface is stressed. This can be accomplished by careful manipulation of the lids with fingers to ensure spreading of the agent. If medication strikes only the eyelids and lid margins, but fails to reach the cornea, the instillation should be repeated. Prophylaxis should be applied as follows:
   a. Silver nitrate
      (1) Carefully clean eyelids and surrounding skin with sterile cotton, which may be moistened with sterile water.
      (2) Gently open infant's eyelids and instill two (2) drops of silver nitrate on the conjunctival sac. Allow the silver nitrate to run across the whole conjunctival sac. Carefully manipulate lids to ensure spread of the drops. Repeat in the other eye. Use two (2) ampules, one for each eye.
      (3) After 1 minute, gently wipe excess silver nitrate from eyelids and surrounding skin with sterile water. Do not irrigate eyes.
   b. Ophthalmic ointment (erythromycin or tetracycline)
      (1) Carefully clean eyelids and surrounding skin with sterile cotton, which may be moistened with sterile water.
      (2) Gently open infant's eyelids and place a thin line of ointment, at least ½ inch (1-2 cm), along the junction of the bulbar and palpebral conjunctiva of the lower lid. Try to cover the whole lower conjunctival area. Carefully manipulate lids to ensure spread of the ointment. Be careful not to touch the eyelid or eyeball with the tip of the tube. Repeat in other eye. Use one tube per baby (Fig. 28-6).
      (3) After 1 minute, gently wipe excess ointment from eyelids and surrounding skin with sterile water. Do not irrigate eyes.
   c. Ophthalmic drops (erythromycin or tetracycline). Apply as silver nitrate.
6. The eye *should not* be irrigated after instillation of a prophylactic agent. Irrigation may reduce the efficacy of prophylaxis and probably does not decrease the incidence of chemical conjunctivitis.
7. Infants born to mothers infected with agents that cause ophthalmia neonatorum may require special attention and systemic therapy, as well as prophylaxis. A single dose of aqueous crystalline penicillin G, 50,000 units/kg body weight for term and 20,000 units for low-birth-weight infants, should be administered intravenously to infants born to mothers with gonorrhea.
8. The detection and appropriate treatment of infections in pregnant women, which may result in ophthalmia neonatorum, are encouraged.
9. All physicians and hospitals should be required to report cases of ophthalmia neonatorum and etiologic agent to state and local health departments so that incidence data may be obtained to determine the effectiveness of the control measures.[6]

(After Committee on Prevention and Treatment of Ophthalmia Neonatorum: Prevention and treatment of ophthalmia neonatorum. New York, National Society to Prevent Blindness, 1981)

and the information on the bands should be verified with the mother as soon as possible. The bands are checked with the nursery nurse when the infant is admitted to the nursery and are rechecked with the mother's band each time the infant is brought to her, to make sure they match.

Footprints and fingerprints are sometimes used and have at times been required as methods of newborn identification. Although they are no longer recommended as a universal practice, many individual hospitals may still use them. If the infant's footprints are to be made, care should be taken to get a good print.

The infant's foot should be clean and dry and must be pressed firmly against the ink pad and then gently on the footprint form, "walking it on" beginning with the heel. The excess ink should be wiped from the infant's feet.

A newer alternative to the ink pad for footprinting is a disposable cardboard frame with squares of ink-coated plastic to press the infant's feet and mother's thumb against. The frame, with ink side down, is placed over the identification form on a clipboard (see Fig. 28-7). As with the ink pad method, the feet must be clean and dry and each foot "walked" onto the form with gentle pressure, beginning at the heel. The nurse must be careful not to move the infant's foot while pressing it down on the frame. Because the ink does not come in contact with the infant's feet, no clean-up is required.

Promotion of Early Maternal–Infant Attachment

It is important for the new mother to see and hold her infant as soon as possible after he is born. Many women will be eager to do this and will ask. Others may want to hold the infant but will not know that it is permitted and may hesistate to ask. Still others may be too tired or too uncomfortable or for some other reason may not

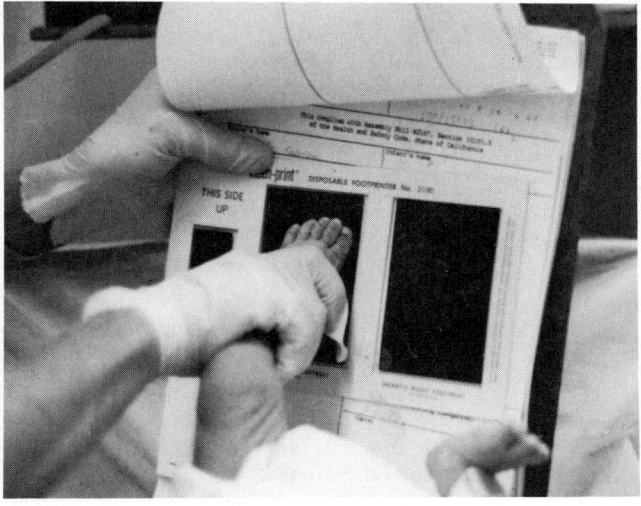

FIGURE 28-7

A newer method of footprinting includes a disposable plastic frame with the ink side away from the infant's foot. The foot is "walked" across the form just as it is when using the ink pad style. By using this new method the infant's foot does not get ink on it.

be as eager for contact with the baby. Although the reluctant mother should not be forced to hold her baby, by bringing the newborn to the mother's side and showing it to her, the nurse may help to initiate the attachment process. When desired, and the condition of mother and infant are favorable, allowing the mother to breast-feed or have skin-to-skin contact with the infant in the delivery room is an excellent way to promote attachment.[8] Provision for warmth should be made by using a radiant warmer or warm blanket. Allowing time for parents and infant to be alone together, with the nurse near enough to provide assistance if needed, is another way of getting the new family off to a good start.

When there are problems with mother or infant and early contact is not possible, it is particularly important that the infant be shown to the mother before being taken from the delivery room and that she be given information about the infant's condition.

Baptism of the Infant

If there is any probability that the infant is in imminent danger and may not live, the question of baptism should be considered if the family is Roman Catholic; this also applies to some of the other denominations of the Christian church. This is an essential duty and means a great deal to the families concerned, and thoughtfulness in this matter will never be forgotten by them. (It is to be understood that such baptism would be reported to the family.)

The following simple instructions, issued by a member of the clergy, may be followed:

> The Catholic church teaches that in case of emergency, anyone may and should baptize. It is important to make the intention of doing what the Church wishes to do and then to pour the water on the child (preferably the head) saying at the same time, "I baptize thee in the name of the Father and of the Son and of the Holy Ghost." The water may be warmed if necessary but it must be pure water and care should be taken to make it flow. If there is any doubt whether the child is alive or dead, it should be baptized, but conditionally (*i.e.*, "If thou art alive, I baptize thee . . .").

In the Book of Common Prayer of the Protestant Episcopal church, it is stated, "In cases of extreme sickness, or any imminent peril, if a Minister cannot be procured, then any baptized person present may administer holy Baptism, using the foregoing form" (*i.e.*, the form given above).

Immediate Care of the Newborn

Nursing Objectives

1. Provide nursing support to assist the infant to
   (a) maintain stable vital signs and
   (b) attain an Apgar score of between 7 and 10 at 1 and 5 minutes.
2. Keep the infant's airway clear.
3. Protect the infant from cold stress.
4. Identify the infant with appropriate identification methods.
5. Provide prophylaxis against ophthalmia neonatorum and hypoprothrombinemia.
6. Promote early parent–infant interaction.

Assessment	Potential Nursing Diagnosis	Planning/Intervention	Evaluation
Apgar score Heart rate Respiratory effort Muscle tone Reflex irritability Color	Ineffective breathing patterns related to alteration in response to extrauterine life	Have resuscitation equipment available and in good working order Alert resuscitation team when problems anticipated and summon when necessary Place infant in a modified Trendelenburg position	Newborn scores 7 to 10 at 1 and 5 minutes
Ongoing general assessment of airway and responsiveness	Ineffective airway clearance related to excess mucus	Gently bulb suction mouth and nose Use other suctioning methods as needed Proceed with resuscitation measures if necessary	Infant breathes without difficulty
	Impaired gas exchange	Gently stimulate by rubbing body with towel. Use O₂ or resuscitative measures as needed	Infant is reactive, is pink, and cries lustily when stimulated
Continuous temperature monitoring	Alteration in temperature: (hypothermia) related to newborn status	Dry head and body well Place stockinette cap on head Place in radiant warmer on top of warm blanket Tape temperature probe on abdomen for monitoring heat regulation	Newborn maintains stable temperature
Determine general status Size Maturation Normality of body systems Vital signs		Weigh; measure length and head circumference Perform gestational age assessment Examine body systems by thorough observation, inspection, auscultation, and palpation Record, report as appropriate	Infant adapts to extrauterine life with minimal trauma Infant has good color and good muscle tone Infant remains free of trauma
Recognize needs of newborn	Potential for infection related to immature immune system	Use good hand-washing and aseptic technique when caring for newborn	Infant remains free of infection

(continued)

Assessment	Potential Nursing Diagnosis	Planning/Intervention	Evaluation
Protection from infection		Provide prophylaxis against ophthalmia neonatorum	Infant's clotting time is normal
Protection from hypo-prothrombinemia		Administer vitamin K	
Proper identification		Apply matching identification bands to infant and mother	Mother has correct infant
		Check numbers and information with mother	
Family interaction	Potential for alteration in parenting (maternal–infant attachment process)	Encourage father or support person to be with mother	Family interacts favorably
		Allow couple to hold and explore infant as soon as possible	
		Point out infant's features; explain normal variations	
		Observe for inappropriate behaviors (e.g., reluctance to touch baby, lack of eye contact, inappropriate remarks)	

References

1. Ahls H, Brazelton TB: Comprehensive neonatal assessment. Birth Fam J 2:3–9, Winter 1974–1975
2. Brann AW Jr, Cefalo RC (eds): Guidelines for Perinatal Care. Evanston, Illinois, American Academy of Pediatrics and American College of Obstetrics and Gynecology, 1983
3. James LS: Emergencies in the delivery room. In Fanaroff AA, Martin RJ (eds): Behrman's neonatal-perinatal medicine, pp 179–195. St Louis, CV Mosby, 1983
4. Pritchard JA, MacDonald PC, Gant N: Williams Obstetrics, pp 379–388. Norwalk, CT, Appleton-Century-Crofts, 1985
5. Ehrenkranz RA: Delivery room emergencies and resuscitation. In Warshaw JB, Hobbins JC (eds): Principles and Practice of Perinatal Medicine, pp 209–225. Menlo Park, CA, Addison-Wesley Publishing Co, 1983
6. Committee on Ophthalmia Neonatorum: Prevention and treatment of ophthalmia neonatorum, New York, National Society to Prevent Blindness, 1981
7. Bryant BG: Unit dose erythromycin ophthalmic ointment for neonatal ocular prophylaxis. JOGN Nurs 13(2):83–87, March/April 1984
8. Klaus MH, Kennell JH: Care of the mother, father and infant. In Fanaroff AA, Martin RJ (eds): Behrman's neonatal-perinatal medicine, pp 240–253. St Louis, CV Mosby, 1983

Suggested Reading

Brodish MS: Perinatal assessment. JOGN Nurs 10(1);42–46, January/February 1981

Korones SB: High Risk Newborn Infants: The Basis for Intensive Nursing Care, 3rd ed. St Louis, CV Mosby, 1981

Lum Sister B, Lartz R, Barnett E: Reappraising newborn eye care. AJN 80(9):1602–1603, September 1980

Taylor PM, Hall BL: Parent–infant bonding: Problems and opportunities in a perinatal center. Semin Perinatol 3(1):73–84, January 1979

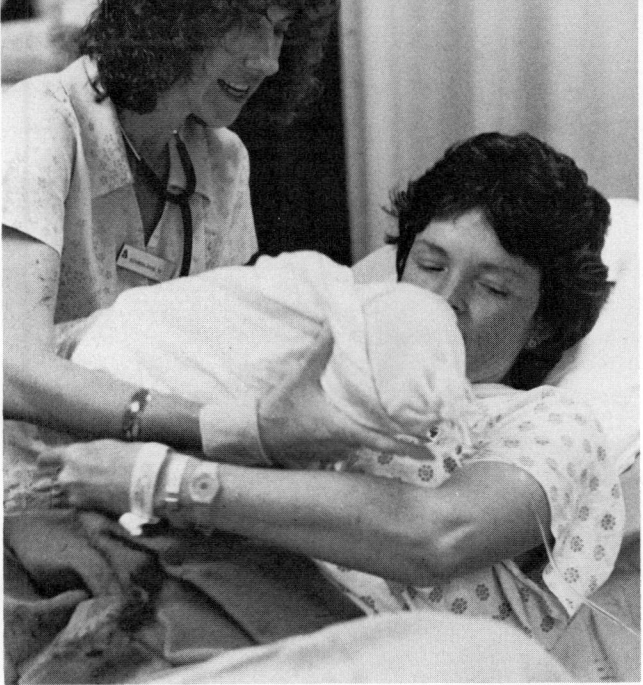

Unit V: Assessment and Management in the Intrapartum Period

Conference Material

1. Your client is a gravida 1, para 0, who is now dilated to 9 cm and 100% effaced, and the presenting part is at 0 station. Her husband is present and assisting well with her relaxation in labor. In the waiting room are both grandparents and the client's sister, who have visited the couple during labor but now decided it best to wait and not disturb the couples' concentration. Describe what the nurse's responsibilities are as delivery approaches.

2. An 18-year-old woman who is having her first baby is admitted to the hospital in early labor. It is obvious from her behavior that she has no preparation for this experience and is frightened and apprehensive. What are your nursing diagnoses and what interventions would you include in your nursing plan for her care?

3. The nurse has two clients to assess and to determine the well-being of both mothers and fetuses upon admission to the labor and delivery unit. Discuss the nursing actions done to assess for fetal well-being upon admission.

4. A couple who have attended Lamaze childbirth education classes find that all patients must be monitored externally during labor at the hospital they have chosen for delivery. What explanation would you give the couple for this practice? What specific measures would you include in your care plan to help the couple practice their relaxation and concentration and still maintain monitoring?

5. Why is prophylaxis for the eyes of the newborn required by law in all states? How would you go about securing the desired information concerning such legislation in the various states of the United States?

6. A 21-year-old mother at term who attended prepared childbirth classes for a previous pregnancy comes to the hospital on her birth attendant's instructions because her membranes have ruptured. She is apologetic because no contractions have started and states that she "should not really be here yet." Discuss your nursing care plan if this were your client, outlining how you would document the rupture of membranes, rule out infection, and establish both maternal and fetal well-being, and describe the explanation you would give in response to her statement about coming to the hospital when contractions have not started.

7. Your hospital does not permit the infant to stay with the mother during recovery. What specific steps might you take to help get this policy changed. Who would you have to talk to in order to implement the change?

8. What arguments might you put forth to institute a policy of putting the newborn to breast immediately after birth?

9. You are attending a mother in the recovery room who was heavily medicated immediately before delivery. She has her infant in the bed with her. What precautions should you take to ensure the safety of *both* the mother and infant? What signs should you be especially alert for in the couple?

10. A mother is dilated 6 cm and states that she is experiencing severe discomfort in the lower back during contractions and some discomfort in that area between contractions. What comfort measures can you consider using to relieve the discomfort?

Multiple Choice

Read through the entire question and place your answer on the line to the right.

1. After a protracted labor and a difficult delivery, the mother, upon seeing her baby, was shocked at the elongated appearance of the infant's head. The nurse could correctly reassure the patient by saying
   A. "The baby's head is molded during delivery and will return to normal in a few days."
   B. "All newborn babies' heads are shaped this way."
   C. "The child's head shape was changed during delivery, and it will take 6 months for it to return to normal."
   D. "After the 'soft spot' closes, the head will return to normal." _____

2. The character and the frequency of uterine contractions and the location of the discomfort experienced by the mother during labor often provide pertinent information regarding the labor.

Situation No. 1: In the case of a multipara who is having discomfort but is not in true labor, which of these symptoms would most probably serve to identify false labor contractions?

 A. Discomfort may begin as early as 3 weeks or 4 weeks before the onset of true labor.
 B. Discomfort occurs 3 days or 4 days before the onset of true labor.
 C. Contractions occur at regular intervals.
 D. Contractions occur at irregular intervals.
 E. Discomfort is confined to the lower abdomen and the groin.
 F. Discomfort is felt in the upper abdomen and the back.

Select the number corresponding to the correct letter or letters.

 1. A only
 2. A and C
 3. A, D, and E
 4. All of the above   _____

Situation No. 2: In the case of a primigravida in the beginning of the first stage of labor, which of the following symptoms would most probably describe her labor contractions?

 A. Contractions occur at regular intervals.
 B. Contractions occur at irregular intervals.
 C. Discomfort is confined to the lower abdomen and the groin
 D. Discomfort is located in the lower back and the abdomen.
 E. Contractions occur at intervals of from 2 minutes to 3 minutes.
 F. Contractions occur at intervals of from 10 minutes to 15 minutes.

Select the number corresponding to the correct letters

 1. A and C
 2. A, D, and F
 3. B, C, and E
 4. All of the above   _____

Situation No. 3: In the case of a primigravida approaching the end of the first stage of labor, which of the following symptoms would most probably give an accurate description of her labor?

 A. Contractions occur at regular intervals.
 B. Contractions occur at irregular intervals.
 C. Contractions occur at 1-minute to 1½-minute intervals.
 D. Contractions occur at 2-minute to 3-minute intervals.
 E. Duration of contraction is from 35 seconds to 50 seconds.
 F. Duration of contraction is from 50 seconds to 70 seconds.

Select the number corresponding to the correct letters.

 1. A, C, and E
 2. A, D, and F
 3. B, D, and E
 4. All of the above   _____

3. Labor is divided into the first, the second, and the third stages.

 A. When is the first stage of labor considered to be terminated?
  1. When contractions occur at 10-minute to 15-minute intervals.
  2. When the cervix is completely dilated.
  3. When the baby is delivered. _____

 B. When is the second stage of labor considered to be terminated?
  1. When the cervix is completely dilated.
  2. When contractions occur at 2-minute to 3-minute intervals.
  3. When the baby is delivered. _____

 C. When is the third stage of labor considered to be terminated?
  1. When the baby is delivered.
  2. When the placenta is delivered.
  3. After the uterus has remained firm for 1 hour. _____

4. In the typical vertex presentation, the sequence of events by which the fetal head adapts to the birth canal during descent is

 A. Flexion, external rotation, internal rotation, and extension
 B. External rotation, internal rotation, extension, and flexion
 C. Flexion, internal rotation, extension, and external rotation
 D. External rotation, extension, flexion, and internal rotation _____

5. The signs that suggest that the placenta has separated include

 A. The uterus becomes firmer and globular in shape.
 B. The umbilical cord descends further out of the vagina.
 C. There is often a sudden gush of blood.
 D. The mother exhibits deep respirations.

Select the number corresponding to the correct letter or letters.

 1. A only
 2. A and D
 3. A, B, and C
 4. All of the above   _____

6. The nurse is caring for a mother in the active phase of labor who is being internally monitored both for fetal heart rate and uterine pressure. She is 42 weeks' gestation with suspected fetal distress, and meconium staining is present in the amniotic fluid. Which of the following observations would you report promptly to the birth attendant?

 A. Minimal variability with periodic late decelerations
 B. Reactive fetal heart rate baseline that is fluctuating more than 5 beats per minute with periodic accelerations

C. Minimal amount of bloody show
D. Increasing thickness in the meconium-stained amniotic fluid
E. Uterine contraction frequency of every 70 seconds, with rising resting tone

Select the number corresponding to the correct letters.
1. A and C
2. A, C, and E
3. B, D, and E
4. A, D, and E   ____

7. Why is an enema sometimes ordered for a mother during the early part of the first stage of labor?
A. To obtain a stool specimen
B. To avoid straining as the mother bears down with contractions
C. To cleanse the lower bowel   ____

8. Often it is the nurse's responsibility to decide when the mother is ready to be moved from the labor room to the delivery room. Which of the following signs would signify to the nurse that the time of delivery is near?
A. Mother has a desire to defecate
B. Increase in frequency, duration, and intensity of uterine contractions
C. Mother begins to bear down spontaneously with uterine contractions
D. Bulging of the perineum
E. Increase in amount of blood-stained mucus from the vagina

Select the number corresponding to the correct letter or letters.
1. D only
2. A, C, and E
3. B, D, and E
4. All of the above   ____

9. Which of the following are indications that the placenta is beginning to separate?
A. Gradual descent of the uterus into the pelvis
B. Protrusion of several more inches of umbilical cord
C. Uterus becomes more firm and rounded
D. A sudden gush of blood from the vagina
E. Large clots of blood coming out of the vagina

Select the number corresponding to the correct letters.
1. A and C
2. B, C, and D
3. B, C, and E
4. All of the above   ____

10. The nurse who is caring for the mother during the fourth stage of labor would include which of the following in her nursing care plan?
A. Keep the mother warm and out of drafts
B. Massage the uterus every 15 minutes or more often if needed
C. Massage the uterus continuously
D. Administer oxytocin medication, as ordered
E. Check maternal vital signs every 15 minutes during the first hour after delivery

Select the number corresponding to the correct letter or letters.
1. B
2. A and C
3. A, B, D, and E
4. All of the above   ____

11. The most common cause of postpartal hemorrhage is atony of the uterus. What is the first thing to do as a preventive measure if the uterus appears to be atonic?
A. Take a firm grasp on the uterus.
B. Massage the uterus firmly.
C. Administer an oxytocic drug.   ____

12. Soon after delivery, a new mother complains of feeling cold. Which of the following are common practices that should occur after every delivery and will assist this mother from feeling cold?
A. Changing the client's gown
B. Giving oxygen per mask
C. Placing a warm blanket on the client
D. Removing the linen wet from the delivery
E. Placing the mother in Trendelenburg position

Select the number corresponding to the correct letter or letters.
1. A
2. A and C
3. A, B, and C
4. A, C, and D   ____

13. Which of the following are reasons to place the infant in the mother's arms right after delivery?
A. Prevent chilling in the infant
B. Allow the bonding process to begin in the sensitive period
C. Prevent infection in the mother and infant
D. Allow the mother to begin identifying her infant

Select the number corresponding to the correct letter or letters.
1. A, C, and D
2. A and B
3. B and D
4. B, C, and D
5. All of the above   ____

14. After the physician clamps and cuts the umbilical cord and hands the infant to the nurse, which of the following acts would the nurse perform in the immediate care of the infant?
A. Suction mucus from the infant's mouth with a bulb syringe
B. Hold the infant up by the heels to allow gravity to assist in removal of mucus
C. Slap the infant's back and soles of the feet sharply to stimulate crying
D. Dry the infant's body and head with the receiving blanket

Select the number corresponding to the correct letter or letters.
1. A only

2. A and B
3. A and D
4. B, C, and D
5. All of the above   ____

15. Which of the following may relieve pain during labor contractions by distracting the mother from pain?
  A. Walking and talking
  B. Slow rhythmic breathing
  C. Focusing eyes on an object
  D. Firm pressure to the lower back
  Select the number corresponding to the correct letter or letters.
  1. A only
  2. B only
  3. A, B, and C
  4. D only   ____

16. One method of helping a mother who is untrained in relaxation to relax quickly at the beginning or end of a contraction is to suggest that she
  A. Stare at an object
  B. Count backwards from 100
  C. Take a slow, deep breath
  D. Massage her abdomen   ____

17. What is the main objective in prophylactic eye care in the newborn?
  A. To enhance and protect the infant's vision in the immediate period after birth
  B. To prevent candidiasis neonatorum
  C. To prevent ophthalmia neonatorum
  D. To prevent staphylococcus colonization
  Select the number corresponding to the correct letter or letters.
  1. A only
  2. B only
  3. C only
  4. A, B, and C
  5. B, C, and D
  6. All of the above   ____

18. Which of the following are needed for successful resuscitation of the newborn immediately after birth?
  A. Skilled personnel trained in resuscitation
  B. Well lighted area
  C. Equipment to deliver O_2 by positive pressure
  D. Drug therapy
  E. Intubation as necessary
  Select the number corresponding to the correct letter or letters.
  1. A, C, and E
  2. A, B, C, and D
  3. A, C, and D
  4. C only
  5. All of the above   ____

19. The factors that should be considered in selection of an anesthetic for labor and delivery include
  A. The amount of discomfort experienced
  B. Experience of the personnel available and the facilities available
  C. The desires of the mother
  D. The dictum that no anesthesia is the safer course of action in all circumstances
  Select the number corresponding to the correct letters.
  1. A and B
  2. A, B, and C
  3. A and D
  4. All of the above   ____

20. The discomfort caused by uterine contractions and cervical dilatation is conveyed to the spinal cord
  A. At levels T10 to T12
  B. At L3 to L5
  C. At S1 to S4
  D. At T8 to T10   ____

21. Identify and match the most important risks of the various methods of obstetrical anesthesia listed below:
  A. General anesthesia   ____
  B. Conduction anesthesia   ____
  C. Paracervical block   ____
  1. Aspiration of stomach contents
  2. Fetal bradycardia
  3. Maternal hypotension

Completion

22. On admission of the mother to the labor suite, which of the following procedures are usually carried out on every client and which procedures are done in relation to the client's birth attendant's specific orders? Fill in the appropriate answer.
  A. Check mother's vital signs _____
  B. Take the mother to the bathroom to void _____
  C. Do a perineal shave _____
  D. Listen to the fetal heart rate _____
  E. Prepare the mother for vaginal examination _____
  F. Give an enema _____

23. Indicate the abbreviations that might be used on a patient's chart to represent each of the positions and the presentations described.
  A. Back of head directed straight to the left   ____
  B. Back of head directed toward the left side and the front quadrant of the pelvis   ____
  C. Back of head directed toward the right side and the back quadrant of the pelvis   ____
  D. Breech presentation, buttocks at the left back quadrant
  E. Face presentation, chin at the right front quadrant   ____

24. Give the term or the phrase that best fits each of the following statements.
  A. Enlargement of the external os to 10 cm in diameter   ____
  B. Maximum shortening of the cervical canal   ____
  C. A condition caused by failure of the uterine muscle to stay contracted after delivery   ____

    D. A surgical incision of the perineum during second stage of labor   _____

    E. Settling of the baby's head into the brim of the true pelvis   _____

25. In each of the following write the term or the phrase by which the pelvic measurement described is commonly called.

    A. From the lower margin of the symphysis pubis to the sacral promontory   _____

    B. The posterior portion of the symphysis pubis to the promontory of the sacrum   _____

    C. From the inner aspects of the ischial tuberosities   _____

26. By using the letter of the measurements described in question 25, indicate the following:

    A. The one that must be estimated rather than measured directly   _____

    B. The one that represents the most important measurement   _____

    C. The one that represents a transverse diameter   _____

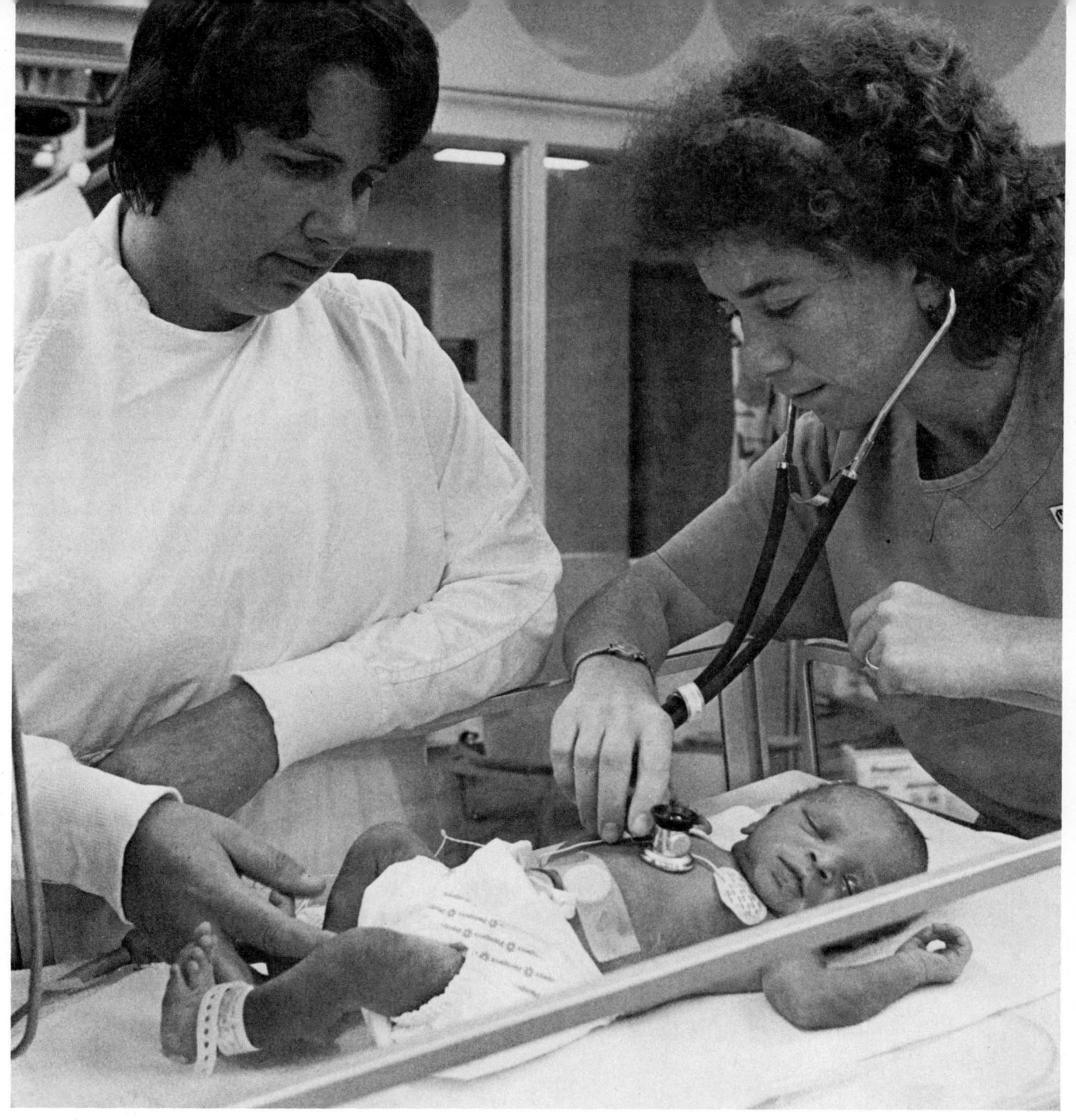

UNIT VI

Assessment and Management in the Postpartum Period

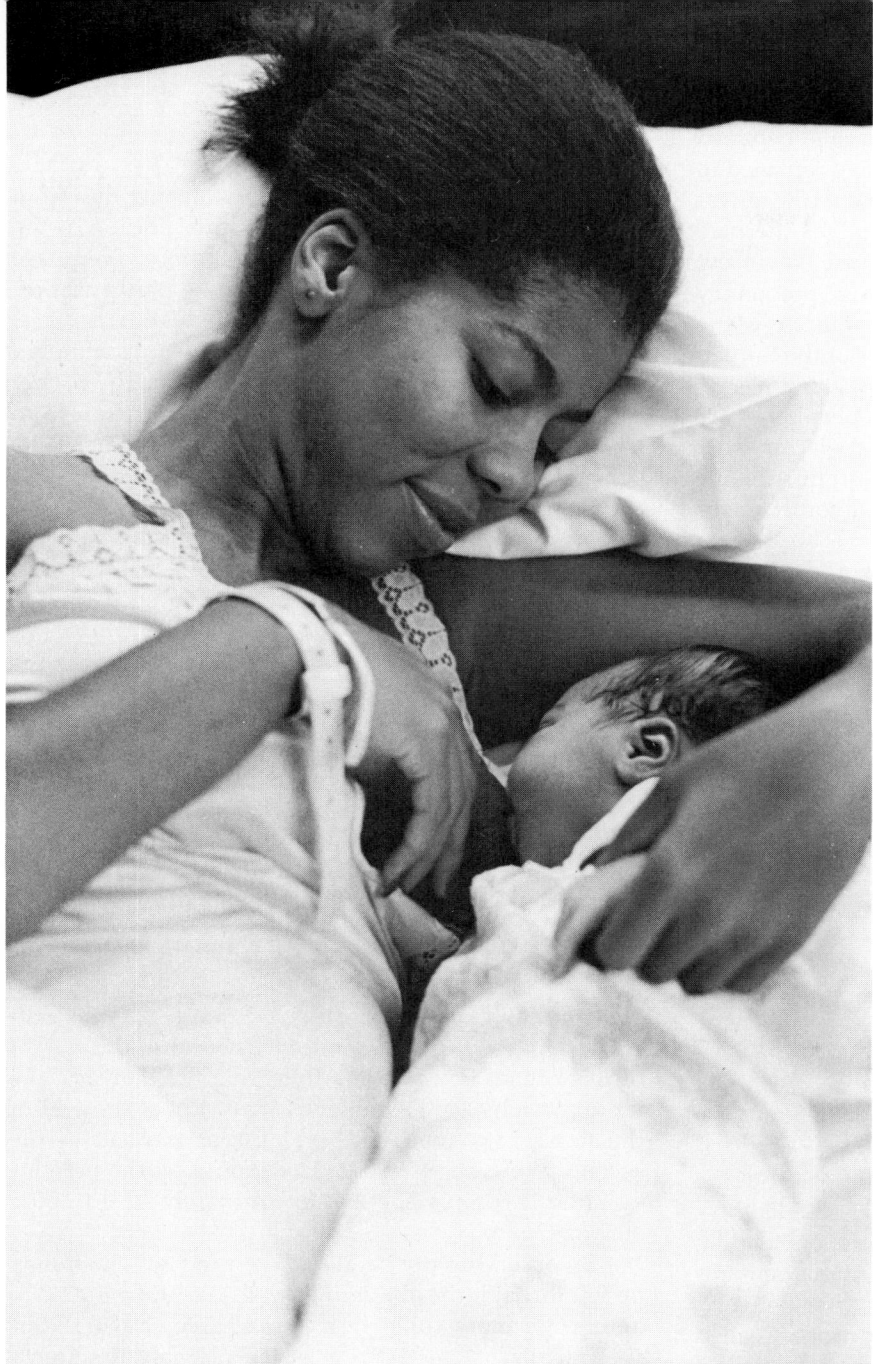

CHAPTER 29

Biophysical Aspects of the Postpartum Period

569

The postpartum period encompasses the time between delivery until the reproductive organs have returned to their prepregnant state. Marked anatomical and physiological changes occur during this period, as the processes undergone during pregnancy are reversed. Knowledge of the reproductive process in pregnancy and labor serves as a basis for understanding how the generative organs and the various systems of the human body adapt following the delivery.

The term *puerperium* (*puer,* a child, plus *parere,* to bring forth) refers to the 6-week period elapsing between the termination of labor and the return of the reproductive organs to their normal condition. This includes both the *progressive changes* in the breasts for lactation and *involution* of the internal reproductive organs. Although the changes brought about by involution are considered normal physiological processes, they are remarkable in that under no other circumstances does such marked and rapid involution of tissues occur without a departure from a state of health. For this reason, the quality of the mother's care at this time is important to ensure her immediate as well as her future health. The text of this chapter provides a basis for understanding these changes. Chapter 31 covers postpartum nursing care.

Anatomical and Physiological Changes

Uterus

Immediately following the delivery of the placenta the uterus becomes an almost solid mass of tissue. Its thick anterior and posterior walls lie in close opposition, leaving the center cavity flattened. The uterus remains about the same size for the first 2 days after delivery, but then rapidly decreases in size by a process called involution. This is effected partly by the contraction of the uterus, with decrease in size of individual myometrial cells, and partly by autolytic processes in which some of the protein material of the uterine wall is broken down into simpler components that are then absorbed.

Constriction and occlusion of underlying blood vessels occur at the placental site. This accomplishes hemostasis (to control postpartal bleeding) and causes some endometrial necrosis. Involution occurs by the extension and downward growth of marginal endometrium and by endometrial regeneration from the glands and stroma in the decidua basalis. Except for the placental site, where involution is not complete until 6 weeks after delivery, the process is completed in the remainder of the uterine cavity by the end of the third postpartum week.

Process of Involution

The separation of the placenta and the membranes from the uterine wall takes place in the outer portion of the spongy layer of the decidua, and, therefore, a remnant of this layer remains in the uterus to be partly cast off in a vaginal discharge called the lochia. Within 2 or 3 days after labor, this remaining portion of decidua becomes differentiated into two layers, leaving the deeper or unaltered layer attached to the muscular wall from which the new endometrial lining is generated. The layer adjoining the uterine cavity becomes necrotic and is cast off in the lochia. The process is very like the healing of any surface; blood oozes from the small vessels on this surface. The bleeding from the larger vessels is controlled by compression of the retracted uterine muscle fibers.

The process of regeneration is rapid, except at the site of former placental attachment, which requires 6 or 7 weeks to heal completely. Elsewhere, the free surface of the endometrium is restored in half that time.

Progress of Involution

The normal process of involution requires 5 or 6 weeks, and at the end of that time the uterus regains its normal size, although it never returns exactly to its nulliparous state.

One can realize more fully the rapidity of this process by comparing the changes that occur in the weight of this organ. Immediately following the delivery, the uterus weighs approximately 1 kg (2 lb); at the end of the first week, about 500 g (1 lb); at the end of the second week, about 350 g (12 oz); and by the time involution is complete, only approximately 40 g to 60 g (1½ oz–2 oz).

By observing the height of the fundus, which may be felt through the abdominal wall, the nurse is able to appreciate more fully these remarkable changes. Immediately after the delivery of the placenta the uterus sinks into the pelvis and the fundus is felt midway between the umbilicus and the symphysis, but it soon rises to the level of the umbilicus (13 cm–14 cm, 5 in–5½ in, above the pubes); 12 hours later, it is probably found a little higher (Figs. 29-1 and 29-2).

Lochia

A knowledge of the healing process by which the lining of the uterus becomes regenerated is valuable in understanding and interpreting the lochial discharge. At first the discharge consists almost entirely of blood with a small amount of mucus, particles of decidua and cellular debris that escape from the placental site. It should not contain large clots or membrane or be excessive in

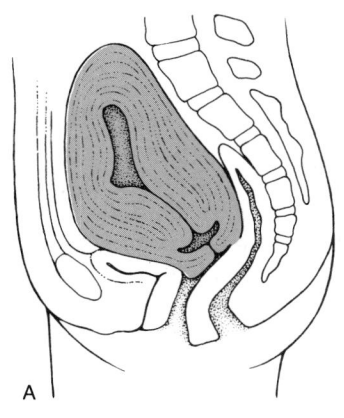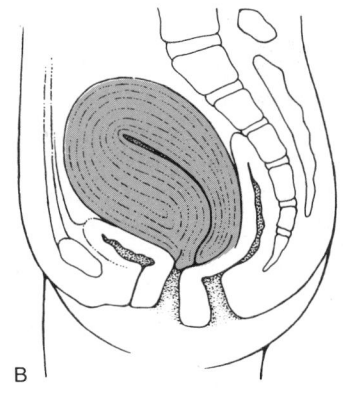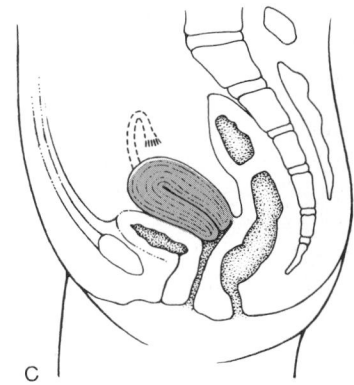

FIGURE 29-1

Changes in uterus size and shape following delivery. (*A*) Uterus after delivery.
(*B*) Uterus at sixth day. (*C*) Nongravid uterus.

amount. The discharge lasts about 3 days and is called
lochia rubra.

As the oozing of blood from the healing surface
diminishes, the discharge becomes more serous or watery and gradually changes to a pinkish color; this discharge is called *lochia serosa.* Toward the tenth day the
lochia is thinner, greatly decreased, and almost colorless;
this is called *lochia alba.* By the end of the third week
the discharge usually disappears, although a brownish
mucoid discharge may persist a little longer. Lochia
possesses a peculiar animal scent that is quite characteristic and should never, at any time, have an offensive
odor. Standards for assessing lochia character and volume are described in Chapter 31.

Organs and Structures of Reproduction

Cervix

Immediately following delivery the cervix collapses and
has little tone; it appears soft and edematous and has
multiple small lacerations. It can admit two fingers and
is about 1 cm thick. Within 24 hours it rapidly shortens
and becomes firmer and thicker. The cervical os closes
gradually to 2 cm to 3 cm after a few days and by 1
week is only about 1 cm dilated. Histologic examination
immediately after birth reveals almost universal edema

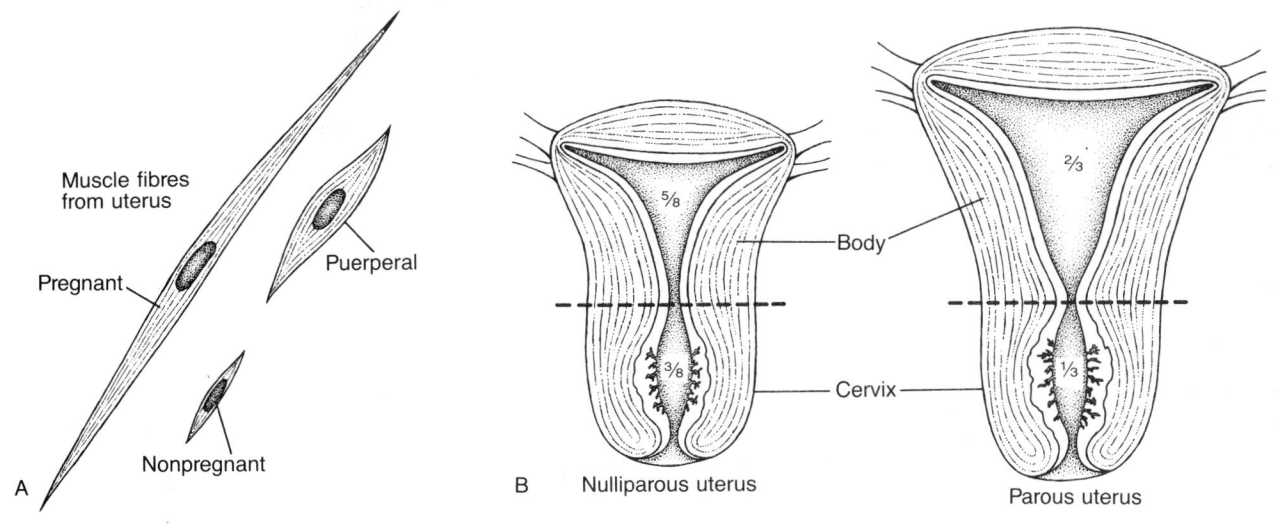

FIGURE 29-2

(*A*) Changes in the size and shape of myometrial cells during the nonpregnant,
pregnant, and puerperal states. (*B*) Size and relationship of the cervix and fundus
in the nulliparous and parous uterus.

and hemorrhage. The endocervical epithelium remains generally intact, with occasional areas of partial denudation. As early as the fourth day, there is regression of glandular hypertrophy and hyperplasia seen during pregnancy, and reabsorption of interstitial hemorrhage. Cervical involution is still proceeding beyond 6 weeks, however, with edema and round cell infiltration persisting as long as 3 to 4 months.

Examination of the cervix with a colposcope (a viewing instrument similar to a microscope, with low magnification and binocular viewing, designed to fit a speculum for close viewing of the cervix) shows ulceration, laceration, bruising, and yellow areas within several days of delivery. These lesions, which are usually smaller than 4 mm, are seen more often in primiparas. Repeat examination 6 to 12 weeks later usually shows complete healing; this indicates rapid reepithelialization of the injured tissue.[1] There is variable retraction of everted columnar epithelium (ectropion) beginning early in the postpartum period. Not every cervix regains its prepregnant appearance; some have more ectropion, and the os is generally wider, shaped in a transverse slit, and may gape if there have been lacerations of clinical significance (Fig. 29-3).

Vagina and Introitus

The vagina is smooth and swollen and has poor tone following delivery. After 3 weeks the vascularity, edema, and hypertrophy resulting from pregnancy and birth are markedly decreased. When vaginal cells are examined microscopically on a smear, the epithelium appears atrophic by the third to fourth week, but regains its proper estrogen index by 6 to 10 weeks post partum. This relative estrogen deficiency contributes to poor vaginal lubrication and decreased vasocongestion, which leads to a diminished sexual response in the weeks following delivery. The lower vagina usually has multiple superficial lacerations after birth, but these are resolved by 6 weeks post partum.

Vaginal rugae reappear by the fourth week post

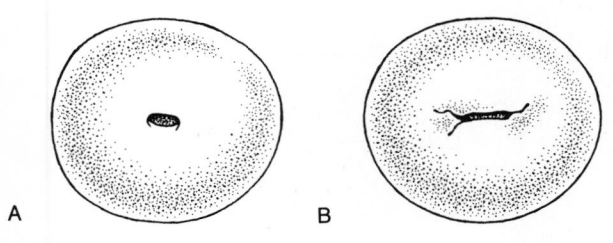

FIGURE 29-3

The perfectly round os of the nulliparous cervix becomes elongated after childbirth. The cervical os may gape if there have been significant lacerations during delivery. (*A*) Round os of nulliparous cervix. (*B*) Transverse slit of os in parous cervix.

partum, but many remain permanently flattened. After birth, rugae are not as thick as in nulliparas. The vaginal mucosa thickens when ovarian function returns and often remains atrophic in lactating women until they begin to menstruate.

Immediately following delivery, the introitus is edematous and erythematous. If lacerations or an episiotomy is present, this condition may be exaggerated in the area of repair. In the absence of infections or hematomas, the introitus heals rapidly. By 2 weeks post partum, most women are relatively free of perineal pain and the introitus has returned to its prepregnant configuration. Perineal and introital integrity can be decreased by large lacerations or inadequate repairs, however.

Other Pelvic Organs

Histologic changes in the *fallopian tubes* reveal reduction in the size of secretory cells, decrease in size and number of ciliated cells, and atrophy of the tubal epithelium. After 6 to 8 weeks, the epithelium reaches the condition of the early follicular phase of the menstrual cycle. There is transient nonbacterial inflammation of the tubal lumina appearing about the fourth day.

The *ligaments* that support the uterus, the ovaries, and the tubes, which have also undergone great tension and stretching, are now relaxed, but it takes them a considerable amount of time to return almost to their normal size and position.

Pelvic Muscular and Fascial Support

The muscular and fascial support structures of the uterus and vagina may be injured during childbirth. This can lead to pelvic relaxation, the weakening and lengthening of support structures for the uterus, vaginal wall, rectum, urethra, and bladder. Although relaxation of pelvic structures can occur in women who have not experienced childbirth or sexual activity, it is most often a delayed result of injuries during the birth process. Symptoms and signs of pelvic relaxation usually appear around menopause, when atrophic changes in fascia occur and the tonic effects of estrogens on pelvic tissues decrease.

The most common types of pelvic relaxation include rectocele, enterocele, uterine prolapse, urethrocele, and cystocele. These defects are due to distention and separation of muscle bundles, fascial lacerations, and stretching and tearing of support structures. They tend to be progressive over time and are often not responsive to exercise or rest.

Kegel's exercises (see Chap. 22) are recommended soon after delivery to assist restoration of vaginal and pelvic muscle tone and function. These exercises also aid healing by increasing pelvic circulation after delivery. While a strong pubococcygeal muscle helps prevent urinary incontinence and pelvic relaxation, exercises alone are often not sufficient when there is enough disruption of muscular–fascial integrity.

Abdominal Wall

The abdominal wall recovers partially from the overstretching but remains soft and flabby for some time. The striae, due to the rupture of the elastic fibers of the cutis, usually remain but become less conspicuous because of their silvery appearance. The process of involution in the abdominal structures requires at least 6 weeks. Provided that the abdominal walls have retained their muscle tone, they gradually return to their original condition. However, if these muscles are relaxed because they have lost their tone, there may be a marked separation or *diastasis of the recti muscles*, so that the abdominal organs are not properly supported (Fig. 20-7). Rest, diet, prescribed exercises, good body mechanics, and good posture may do much to restore the tone of these muscles.

Hormonal Changes: Ovulation and Menstruation

Circulating levels of *estrogen* and *progesterone* decline rapidly after delivery. Follicle-stimulating hormone (FSH) levels are low in postpartum women for 10 to 12 days, then increase to follicular phase concentrations by the third week. Estrogen reaches follicular phase levels in about 3 weeks in nonlactating women, and it takes longer in those who are lactating. Ovulation and menstruation following childbirth are influenced by whether or not the woman is breast-feeding. Menses that occur within the first 6 weeks are rarely ovulatory; the longer after delivery the first menses occur, the greater the likelihood that they will be ovulatory. Once menstruation begins, the percentage of subsequent menses that are ovulatory rises rapidly.

The first ovulation after delivery in nonlactating women occurs, on an average, at 10.2 weeks. Among women lactating for at least 3 months, the first ovulation occurs at 17.0 weeks, on an average. With increased duration of lactation, the average time of ovulation rises, and among women lactating for 6 months, ovulation occurred at 28 weeks. Nonlactating women may ovulate as early as 27 days after delivery.

The return of menstruation after delivery follows a linear pattern. By 12 weeks post partum, 70% of nonlactating women will have their first menses; over the next 24 weeks this rises to 80%. In lactating women menses return more gradually, with 55% to 75% menstruating by 36 weeks. The average time until the first menses in nonlactating women is 7 to 9 weeks, and in women who breast-feed the average time until menstruation is greater than in women who are not breast-feeding, depending upon the length of nursing (Table 29-1).

The basis for postdelivery amenorrhea is not completely understood. The hormone *prolactin* (associated with lactation) reaches peak concentration around delivery, then declines erratically over the next 2 weeks in nonlactating women. In nursing mothers it increases in the early puerperium, then diminishes. Levels of luteinizing hormone (LH) and human chorionic gonadotropin (hCG) decline rapidly after delivery to low follicular phase by 2 weeks and do not change again until ovulation occurs. FSH levels are low until they reach normal levels by 3 weeks. This return of gonadotropins occurs whether or not the woman is lactating, although return to normal estrogen levels is delayed by lactation. This is interpreted to mean that lactation causes a temporary refractory state of the ovaries to pituitary gonadotropins.

Breasts

During pregnancy, progressive changes occur in the breasts in preparation for lactation. The breast lobules have developed under the stimulation of the estrogen and progesterone produced by the placenta, and the lactiferous ducts have undergone further branching and elongation. Prolactin, released from the anterior pitui-

T A B L E   2 9 - 1

Return of Menstruation

	Average Time of First Ovulation	Average Time of First Menstruation
Nonlactating women	10.2 weeks	7–9 weeks‡
Lactating women	17.0 weeks* 28.0 weeks†	30–36 weeks§

* Lactating for 3 months.
† Lactating for 6 months.
‡ First menses usually anovulatory.
§ Depends upon duration of lactation.

tary, cortisol from the maternal adrenal, and insulin, all of which appear in increasing amounts during gestation, also contribute to breast changes. Although all of the essential factors are more and more available as gestation progresses, milk production *per se* is held in abeyance. Its appearance is delayed until 3 or 4 days after delivery, when estrogen and progesterone levels have decreased.

Physiology of Lactation

At least six pituitary hormones play a role in mammary development and lactation. These include prolactin, adrenocorticotropic hormone (ACTH), human growth hormone (hGH), thyroid-stimulating hormone (TSH), FSH, and LH. In addition, human chorionic somatotropin (hCS), human placental lactogen (hPL), and steroid hormones secreted by the adrenal glands, the ovaries, and the placenta play a part, as does pancreatic insulin. Prolactin has a central role in preparation of the breasts for lactation. It is involved in the increase in breast size and in the number and complexity of the ducts and alveoli that occur during pregnancy. As pregnancy progresses, prolactin stimulates secretion by mammary alveolar cells, and estrogen and progesterone stimulate ductal and alveolar growth, but these latter two paradoxically inhibit milk secretion.

With the delivery of the placenta, the source of most estrogen and progesterone during pregnancy, as well as of all hPL, is suddenly removed. The blood levels of these hormones falls rapidly, but the secretion of prolactin by the anterior pituitary gland continues. The appearance of milk postpartally has been demonstrated to coincide with falling estrogen and progesterone levels in the presence of elevated prolactin. The synthesis and secretion of milk is thus initiated when the inhibitory effects of estrogen and progesterone are removed, and under the continuing effects of prolactin.

The secretion of milk begins at the base of the alveolar cells, where small droplets are formed and migrate to the cell membrane; these are extruded into the alveolar ducts for storage. Milk ejection is the process by which contraction of myoepithelial cells in the breasts propels milk along the ducts into the lactiferous sinuses. These sinuses are located beneath the areola, and milk is removed from them by infant suckling. A neurohormonal reflex controls milk ejection and works through afferent nerve pathways to the hypothalamus. Suckling is the primary afferent stimulus, but the ejection reflex can be activated by auditory (infant crying) and visual (seeing the infant) stimuli. The efferent limb of this pathway is clearly hormonal, since oxytocin that is released from the posterior pituitary causes contraction of the myoepithelial cells of the breasts.[2]

The importance of higher cortical centers in the brain is demonstrated by the sensitivity of the ejection reflex to various noxious stimuli. Anxiety and tension,

severe cold, and pain inhibit the ejection reflex and decrease milk ejection. This points to the need for the mother to have a comfortable, relaxed setting in which to breast-feed her infant. Chronic stress in life situations contributes to an ineffective lactation response. The nurse needs to assess the mother's psychosocial situation carefully and to plan approaches to alleviate factors that increase stress if successful breast-feeding is to be accomplished.

Prolactin appears to be more critical for initiation of lactation than for its maintenance once it is established. With continued nursing, levels of prolactin released in response to suckling increase less dramatically than in the beginning. Eventually prolactin levels may not rise at all with suckling. The pathways by which lactation and milk ejection are brought about are illustrated in Figure 29-4.

Lactation Suppression

The production and ejection of milk may be suppressed at the level of the breast, the pituitary, or the hypothalamus. The most simple, natural method is to avoid stimulation of the breast, which reduces the milk ejection reflex and decreases the stimulation of prolactin required for continuation of milk production. When the milk ejection reflex is inhibited in this way, over the course of several days the distended alveoli suppress lactation. However, some women experience engorged breasts during this time and have considerable discomfort. Lactation can be suppressed with natural methods in about 60% to 70% of postpartum women by wearing a tight brassiere and avoiding stimulation of the nipples and breasts.

Hormonal methods are also frequently used to suppress lactation. Estrogens can successfully inhibit milk production in another 10% of women. Adding an androgen to the estrogen increases the success rate of hormonal suppression of lactation to about 90%. However, the use of these hormones is not infrequently associated with rebound lactation (resurgence of milk production some time after administration of hormones) and is implicated in postpartum thromboembolic disorders. Inhibiting prolactin secretion with synthetic ergot alkaloids, such as bromocriptine, is a safe and highly effective approach to lactation suppression, but the drug must be administered for a 2-week period. A single injection of testosterone enanthate and estradiol valerate is equally effective, and it is not associated with significant risk in young women with normal vaginal deliveries.

Colostrum

On delivery, the breast produces increased amounts of a thin yellow fluid, colostrum. Women who carry out special breast-care preparation during the last weeks of

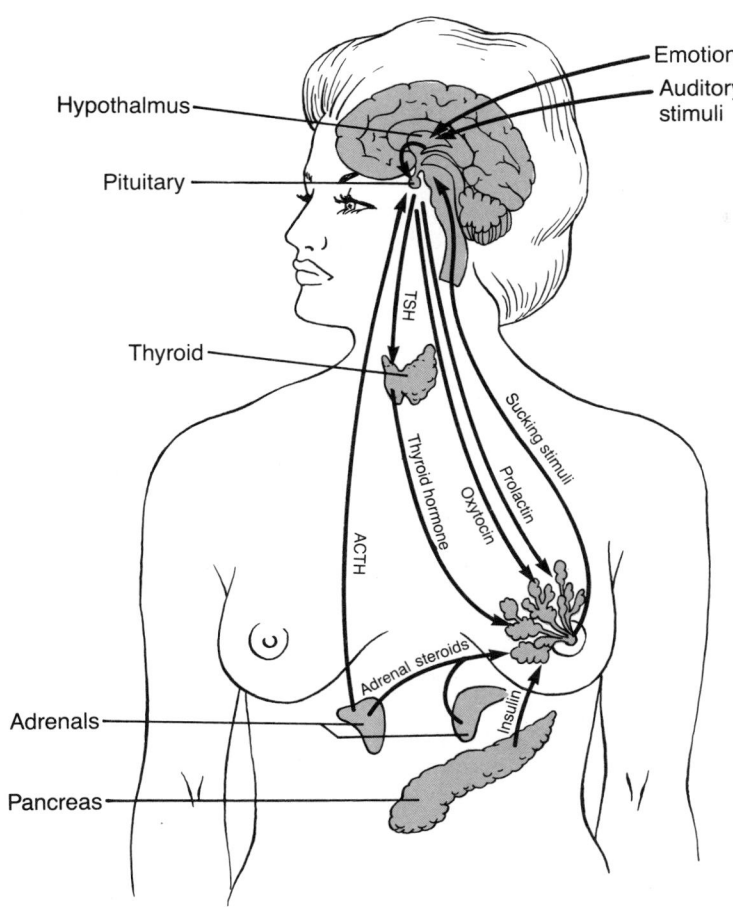

FIGURE 29-4

Neurohormonal pathways influencing lactation and milk ejection. (Redrawn from Hytten FE, Leitch I: The Physiology of Human Pregnancy, 2nd ed. Oxford, Blackwell Scientific Publications, 1971)

pregnancy often are able to express manually small amounts of it before birth. Colostrum contains more protein and inorganic salts, but less fat and carbohydrate, than does breast milk. It also contains demonstrable levels of antibodies, and its immunoglobulin content (IgA) may offer the newborn protection against enteric infections. The nutritive value of colostrum is lower than that of breast milk.

Lactation

On the third or fourth postpartum day the breast milk usually "comes in." There is an obvious change in the color of the secretion from the nipples; it becomes bluish white, the usual color of normal breast milk. At this time the breasts suddenly become larger, firmer, and more tender as lacteal secretion is established, causing the mother to experience throbbing pains in the breasts that extend into the axillae. This congestion, which usually subsides in 1 or 2 days, is caused in part by pressure from the increased amounts of milk in the lobules and the ducts but even more by the increased circulation of blood and lymph in the mammary gland, producing tension on the very sensitive surrounding tissues. This is sometimes referred to as *primary engorgement* (see Chap. 35).

The efficiency and maintenance of milk production is, in large measure, controlled by the stimulus of repetitive nursing. The neurohormonal mechanism involving prolactin and oxytocin release, which triggers the milk ejection reflex, has been discussed previously. The oxytocin released by suckling also stimulates uterine contractions, which explains the mild abdominal cramps often associated with the initiation of breast-feeding.

Supply of Breast Milk

Breast milk varies markedly in its quality and quantity, not only in different individuals, but also in the same individual at various times. In general, the amount of breast milk increases as the infant's need for it increases. Nature seems to have carefully coordinated the mother's need for rest and the infant's need for food during the first 2 days, when only colostrum is secreted. But during this time, lactation is definitely stimulated by the infant's suckling, and, although the secretion of breast milk would occur naturally, without this stimulation and the complete emptying of the breasts the secretion of breast milk would not continue for more than a few days.

If the infant is put to breast consistently, by the end of the first week a healthy mother usually has about 200 ml to 300 ml (6 oz–10 oz) of breast milk a day. By the end of 4 weeks this amount almost doubles, so that she produces about 600 ml (20 oz) a day. Breast milk is produced on the basis of "supply and demand" (*i.e.*, the amount secreted gradually adjusts in relation to what the baby takes at an average feeding). In time, as the baby grows, the mother may have about 900 ml (30 oz) of breast milk a day.

The supply of breast milk is dependent on several factors, such as the mother's diet, the amount of exercise and rest she gets, and her level of contentment. An adequate diet for lactation requires increased amounts of protein, calcium, iron, and vitamins, as well as an ample fluid intake. The mother who is breast-feeding needs a good night's sleep, a rest period in the middle of the day, and normal exercise. Worry, emotional tension, and too much activity (overexertion and fatigue) have an adverse effect on lactation (see Chap. 35).

In relation to lactation, the actual size of the breast is not as important as the amount of glandular tissue, since the secreting tissues of the mammary gland produce the breast milk and not the fat. It has been verified that if large doses of salicylates, certain cathartics, iodides, bromides, quinine, atropine, or opium are administered to the lactating mother, they are excreted in the breast milk.

Various Systems

Cardiovascular Changes

After delivery there often is a transient bradycardia, with a pulse rate as low as 40 to 50 beats per minute, lasting for 24 to 48 hours. This is caused by hemodynamic changes and a vagal hyperreactivity in response to the increased sympathetic nervous system activity during labor. The 40% increase in blood volume that occurs during pregnancy gradually undergoes reduction until it reaches normal levels by about 2 weeks post partum. However, it is important to note that there is an increase of 15% to 30% in circulating blood volume in the first 2 to 3 postpartal days, due to the elimination of placental circulation and an increase in venous return. This process is responsible for the profound diuresis that occurs in the early puerperium. It also explains the fall in hematocrit, which is a hemodilutional phenomenon. Cardiac output increases by 35% as a result of these combined hemodynamic changes, making the early postpartum period the time of greatest risk of heart failure in women with heart disease and limited cardiac reserve.[3]

The pregnant total blood volume of 5 to 6 liters decreases to 4 liters by the fourth postpartum week. There is a loss of about 400 ml of blood in a normal vaginal delivery, although this varies considerably. By the third to seventh postpartal day, the hematocrit usually rises unless there has been substantial blood loss

at delivery. The leukocytosis that occurs during pregnancy and labor continues for the first several postdelivery days, with values up to 20,000 WBC/ml to 25,000 WBC/ml, and is characterized by increased neutrophils and eosinophils and decreased lymphocytes. There is a rapid but short-lived reticulocytosis as a result of sudden blood loss. Sedimentation rate, fibrinogen, and thromboplastic factors remain elevated after delivery and return to normal in 2 to 3 weeks. These increased clotting factors may interact with immobility, sepsis, or trauma to predispose women to postpartum thrombosis.

Blood pressure undergoes little change under normal conditions. Bradycardia is frequent after delivery, whether or not anesthesia was used. This is a result of increased cardiac output and stroke volume in the immediate postpartal period. By 2 to 3 weeks after delivery, cardiac output has returned to nonpregnant levels. The pulse returns to its nonpregnant rate by about 3 months post partum.

Serum electrolytes are altered following delivery. A negative chloride balance results from rapid excretion of extracellular fluid during the phase of diuresis. Serum sodium rises in part because of falling steroid levels (mainly plasma progesterone) and relatively greater water than sodium loss. Increased serum potassium levels are probably due to catabolism of tissues during involution.

Respiratory Changes

Changes in abdominal pressure and thoracic cage capacity after delivery result in rapid alterations of pulmonary function. Increases are found in residual volume, resting ventilation, and oxygen consumption. There are decreases in inspiratory capacity, vital capacity, and maximum breathing capacity. By 6 months post partum, pulmonary functions return to nonpregnant levels. During this time, however, women have less efficient responses to exercise.

Acid–base balance changes during labor and in the early postpartum period. Progesterone during pregnancy creates a type of hyperventilation at the alveolar level (without changing respiratory rate). Pregnancy is characterized by respiratory alkalosis (due to decreased carbon dioxide concentration in alveoli) and a compensated metabolic acidosis. During labor, these begin to change with rising blood lactate, falling *p*H, and hypocapnia (<30 mm Hg) toward the end of the first stage. These conditions continue into the early puerperium, but more normal nonpregnant values (PCO_2 35 mm Hg–40 mm Hg) appear within a few days. Falling progesterone levels affect this postpartum hypercapnia, which is accompanied by elevated base excess and plasma bicarbonate. Gradually the *p*H and base excess increase until normal values are reached, about 3 weeks after delivery. The basic metabolic rate remains increased for 1 to 2 weeks following delivery.

Oxygen saturation and PO$_2$ are higher during pregnancy than in nonpregnant women. In labor, women may experience decreases in oxygen saturation, especially when supine. This may be a result of decreased cardiac output in this position. Oxygen saturation rises rapidly after delivery, to 95% during the first postpartal day. An oxygen debt in the postdelivery period may occur, apparently related to the length and difficulty of the second stage of labor. There is increased resting oxygen consumption during this time, which may also be affected by lactation, anemia, and emotional and psychological factors.

Urinary and Renal Changes

The bladder mucosa following delivery shows varying degrees of edema and hyperemia, with diminished bladder tone. This results in decreased sensation to increased pressure, increased capacity, overdistention with overflow incontinence, and incomplete emptying of the bladder. It is important that postpartum nursing care include careful monitoring of the condition of the bladder, as distention and urinary retention are common occurrences and can cause discomfort as well as predispose to infection. With adequate emptying of the bladder, tone is usually restored within 5 to 7 days.

Reversal of the water metabolism of pregnancy results from decreased steroid hormones and the involutional processes of the puerperium. Catabolic processes contribute to increased values for blood urea nitrogen, proteinuria, and, occasionally, acetonuria. Changes in blood volume and hormone levels affect postpartum diuresis, the glomerular filtration rate (GFR), and serum electrolytes.

The GFR remains elevated during the first postpartum week, and combined with increased blood volume, it causes marked diuresis of up to 3000 ml/day for the first 4 to 5 days. Fluid is lost from the body tissues; combined with involutional changes, this contributes to a loss of about 9 lb of weight during the puerperium. Glycosuria occurs about 20% of the time, and proteinuria for a day or two occurs up to 50% of the time. The ureters and renal pelvis of the kidneys remain dilated after delivery and return to normal in 3 to 6 weeks, although this may occasionally take as long as 8 to 12 weeks. This must be kept in mind in interpreting intravenous pyelography (IVP) during this time. By 6 weeks post partum, the renal plasma flow, GFR, plasma creatinine, and nitrogen usually return to nonpregnant levels.

Gastrointestinal Changes and Weight Loss

The motility and tone of the gastrointestinal system usually returns to normal within 2 weeks after delivery. Most women are quite thirsty the first 2 to 3 days, probably because fluids are restricted during labor and be-

TABLE 29-2

Sources and Amount of Weight Loss During the Postpartum Period

Source of Weight Loss	Amount of Weight Loss	
	Pounds	Kilograms
Fetus and placenta; amniotic fluid and blood loss at delivery	12–13	5.5–6.0
Perspiration and diuresis during the first postpartum week	5–8	2.5–4.0
Uterine involution and lochia	2–3	1
Total weight loss	19–24	9–10

cause fluid shifts within the body are associated with diuresis. Constipation is common during the early postpartum period. Physiological processes are exacerbated by effects of the predelivery enema, restriction of fluids during labor, and drugs given during labor and delivery. Pain from the episiotomy and from hemorrhoids may further deter defecation. Most postpartum clients are given stool softeners or laxatives such as DOSS, Dulcolax, or milk of magnesia to aid elimination.

Weight loss after delivery totals about 22 lb; this includes loss of the fetus and placenta, amniotic fluid, and blood at the time of delivery; perspiration and diuresis during the first postpartum week; and involution of the uterus as well as lochial discharge (Table 29-2).

Neuromuscular Changes

After delivery there is reversal of neurologic adaptations caused by pregnancy. Discomforts due to nerve compression disappear as mechanical pressure from the enlarged uterus and pressure from fluid retention are relieved. Numbness of the thighs due to compression of nerves against the pelvic sidewall or beneath the inguinal ligament during pregnancy improves. Periodic numbness and tingling of the fingers, which affect 5% of pregnant women as a result of brachial plexus traction, are relieved. Elimination of edema and reversal of physiological changes in fascia, tendons, and connective tissue during pregnancy relieve pressure on the median nerve and improve carpal tunnel syndrome (pain, numbness, and tingling in sides of hands and fingers). Depending upon their cause, leg cramps may improve after delivery.

Endocrine effects on fibrocartilage during pregnancy are gradually reversed during the postpartum period. The relative relaxation and increased mobility of pelvic articulations are restored to nonpregnant stability by about 6 to 8 weeks after delivery. This often relieves backache characteristic of pregnancy, although a new source of strain from lifting the infant may confound symptomatic improvement. Postural changes caused by the enlarged uterus are reversed, improving lumbar lordosis and compensatory dorsal kyphosis. However, enlarged lactating breasts and weakened abdominal wall muscles may contribute to poor posture after delivery.

Integumentary Changes

The increased melanin activity of pregnancy causing hyperpigmentation of nipples, areola, and linea nigra gradually decreases after delivery. Although darker coloration of these areas regresses, color may not return to prepregnant character, and some women have persistent darker pigment. Chloasma (mask of pregnancy) usually improves, although it may not disappear completely.

Vascular effects during pregnancy causing spider angiomas, darker nevi, palmar erythema, and epulis regress as estrogen levels decline rapidly following delivery. Spider angiomas, which occur in 10% to 15% of women, may become permanent although smaller. Increased fine hair distribution seen in pregnancy usually disappears; coarse bristly hair usually remains. Pruritus due to hyperestrogen states improves postpartum.

Clinical Considerations

Temperature

Slight rises in temperature may occur without apparent cause following the delivery, but, in general, the mother's temperature should remain within normal limits during the puerperium, that is, below 38°C (100.4°F) when taken orally. Any mother whose temperature exceeds this limit in any two consecutive 24-hour periods of the puerperium (excluding the first 24 hours post partum) is considered to be febrile.

It was formerly believed that an elevation in temperature naturally occurred with the establishment of lactation on the third or the fourth day after delivery; the so-called *milk fever* was considered a normal accompaniment of this process. At the present time this is considered to be a fallacy. On rare occasions a sharp peak of fever for several hours may be caused by extreme vascular and lymphatic engorgement of the breasts, but this does not last longer than 12 hours.

In judging the significance of a rise in temperature, the pulse rate is a helpful guide because a slow pulse and a slightly elevated temperature are not likely to signify a complication. Nevertheless, any sustained rise in temperature in the puerperium should excite the suspicion of endometritis (see Chap. 40).

Pulse

In the early puerperium a pulse rate somewhat slower than normal is a favorable sign. The rate usually averages between 60 and 70, but may even become a little slower than this (*e.g.*, 40–50) in 1 or 2 days after the delivery. This is merely a transient phenomenon, so that by the end of 7 to 10 days the pulse returns to its normal rate. On the other hand, a rapid pulse after labor, unless the mother has cardiac disease, may be an indication of shock or hemorrhage.

Blood and Blood Pressure

Most of the vascular and metabolic alterations characteristic of normal pregnancy disappear within the first 2 weeks of the puerperium. Blood pressure should not change significantly from levels during pregnancy and labor.

Afterpains

Normally, after the delivery of the first child, the uterine muscle tends to remain in a state of tonic contraction and retraction. However, if the uterus has been subjected to any marked distention or if tissue or blood clots have been retained in the cavity, active contractions occur in an effort to expel them, and these contractions may be painful. In multiparas a certain amount of the initial tonicity of the uterine muscle has been lost, and these contractions and retractions cannot be sustained. Consequently, the muscle contracts and relaxes at intervals, and these contractions give rise to the sensation of pain called afterpains.

These afterpains are more noticeable after a pregnancy in which the uterus has been greatly distended, as with multiple births or hydramnios. They are particularly noticeable in the breast-feeding mother when the infant is put to breast (because suckling causes release of oxytocin from the posterior pituitary, which stimulates the uterus to contract). They may last for days, although ordinarily they become almost unnoticeable in about 48 hours after delivery. They also occur with increased intensity following the administration of oxytocic agents such as ergotrate. Often afterpains become so sharp that the administration of a sedative is necessary. Any time that they are severe enough to disturb the mother's rest and peace of mind, the physician should be notified.

Digestion

Although the mother's appetite may be diminished the first few days after labor, the digestive tract functions normally early in the puerperium. Thirst is considerably increased at this time owing to the marked diuresis and diaphoresis associated with involution. Moreover, the fact that the mother may have gone without fluids for some hours in labor undoubtedly increases her thirst.

Intestinal Elimination

The mother is nearly always constipated during the first few days of the puerperium. This is because of the relaxed condition of the intestines (adynamic ileus) and the inability of the abdominal wall to aid in the evacuation of the intestinal contents. Predelivery enema or diarrhea and dehydration contribute to this constipation. In addition, if hemorrhoids, episiotomy, or lacerations are present, the mother often is afraid to pass stools because of discomfort.

Kidneys

The amount of urine excreted by the kidneys in the puerperium is of particular sigificance. During pregnancy there is an increased tendency of the body to retain water, so that now the tremendous output of urine represents the body's effort to return its water metabolism to normal. Diuresis regularly occurs between the second and the fifth day after delivery, sometimes reaching a daily output of 3000 ml, as discussed previously. After the delivery, in particular, the bladder may distend without any awareness on the part of the mother, especially if she has received any form of analgesia. *Therefore, it becomes a major responsibility of the nurse to be alert to signs of a full bladder and thus to prevent distention from occurring.*

During the first few days after labor there may be an increase in the amount of nitrogen in the urine. This excretion is due to the breakdown of endometrial proteins during involution. The presence of acetone in the urine, related to the incomplete metabolism of body fat, occurs when the woman has gone a long period without food. Occasionally, during the first weeks of the puerperium the urine contains substantial amounts of glucose prior to full restoration of normal glucose metabolism. This glycosuria has no relationship to diabetes. Lactose (milk sugar) is present in the urine, especially in lactating women, but is not detected by standard dipstick urinalysis.

Perspiration

Elimination of waste products by way of the skin is accelerated in the early puerperium, often to such a degree that the mother is drenched with perspiration. These episodes of profuse sweating, which frequently occur in the night, gradually subside and do not require any specific treatment aside from protecting the mother from chilling when they occur and ensuring adequate skin cleansing.

Early Ambulation

The normal client should be encouraged to get out of bed as soon as practical, and certainly within the first 24 hours post partum. In general, clients feel stronger and psychologically better as a result of early limited activity, and constipation and bladder complications are less frequent. Most important, the incidence of thrombophlebitis and pulmonary embolus has been decreased materially as a result of early ambulation.

References

1. Monheit AG, Cousins L, Resnik R: The puerperium: Anatomic and physiologic readjustments. Clin Obstet Gynecol 23(4):973–984, December 1980
2. Kochenour NK: Lactation suppression. Clin Obstet Gynecol 23(4):1045–1059, December 1980
3. Frisoli G: Physiology and pathology of the puerperium. In Iffy L, Kaminetzky HA (eds): Principles and Practice of Obstetrics and Perinatology, p 1659. New York, John Wiley & Sons, 1981

Suggested Reading

Auerbach KG et al: Maternal employment and breastfeeding. Am J Dis Child 138(10):958–960, October 1984
Benson R: Current Obstetric and Gynecologic Diagnosis and Treatment, 5th ed. Los Altos, CA, Lange Medical Publications, 1984
Danforth DN: Textbook of Obstetrics and Gynecology, 5th ed. New York, Harper & Row, 1982
Metheny NM: Fluid Balance. Philadelphia, JB Lippincott, 1984
Tilkian SM: Clinical Implications of Laboratory Tests, 3rd ed. St Louis, CV Mosby, 1983
Willson JR et al: Obstetrics and Gynecology, 7th ed. St Louis, CV Mosby, 1983
Zuspan F, Quilligan E: Practical Manual of Obstetrical Care. St Louis, CV Mosby, 1982

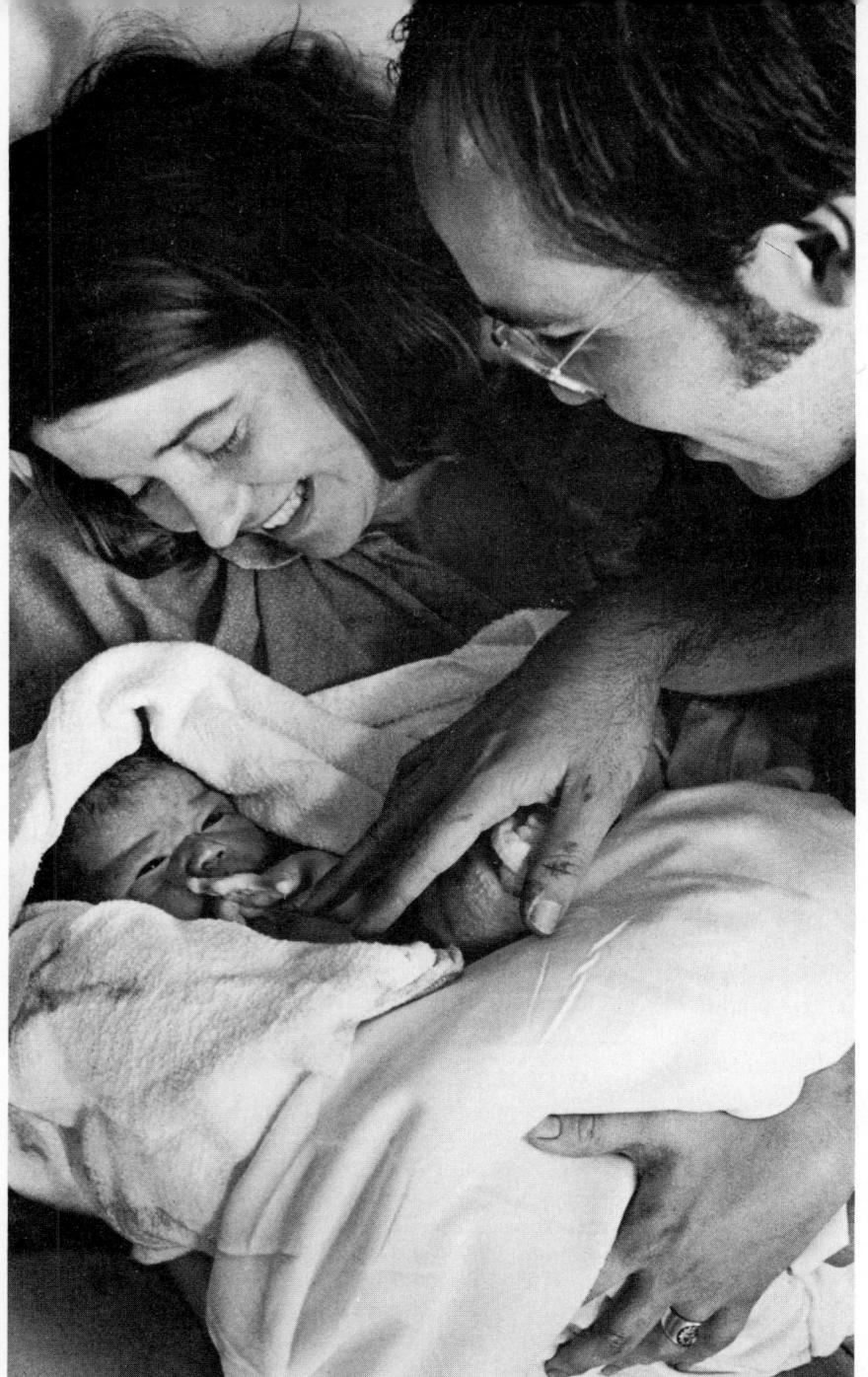

CHAPTER 30

Psychosocial Aspects of the Postpartum Period

In discussing psychosocial aspects of pregnancy in Chapter 19, we made the point that pregnancy and parenthood can be thought of as a role transition. We noted the tremendous change that comes with childbirth and the assumption of the new role and the concomitant instability that can occur until new roles are allocated and the new member is integrated. In this chapter we continue our exploration of the psychosocial needs of the new, expanded family as they assume their responsibilities as parents.

The present discussion is based on the underlying assumption that the degree of ease and satisfaction with which individuals make the transition to parenthood depends in a large part how successfully they have defined and accepted their relationship with each other. If they have developed an ability to see each other as they are (not as they ought to be) and if they can allow for divergence of values and behaviors, work collaboratively toward a flexible power base for each, and develop norms that allow for mutual growth, then they are more likely to move smoothly into the new role.[1] Moreover, the transition to parenthood is viewed as a process rather than a state.[2]

These assumptions are identified specifically here because much of the literature on parenting singles out either the content of the parent–child relationship *per se* or the parents' own childhood relationships as the primary determinants of the family's progression through this phase. This neglects three other vital areas: (1) the needs of each person within the system as an individual, (2) the needs of the parents as a couple, and (3) the influence of the couple's (and the infant's) interaction over time. Use of these assumptions does not negate the importance of the parent–child relationship or the parents' own background, but it does provide some focus on the marital couple as an entity. In reality it is the balancing of the three areas of needs within the family that is the ultimate task of the new family. Moreover, it is these areas that the nurse must be aware of and respect when working with families undergoing the transition to parenthood.[3]

According to Meleis, one integrative conceptual framework for the care and support of couples experiencing role transition to parenthood is role supplementation.[4,5] By using this framework, health providers can help the parents and their significant others gain the necessary information or experience to bring them to a full awareness of the anticipated behavior patterns, sensations, and goals involved in the complementary roles of mother and father. In essence, this approach assists the parents-to-be in moving to role mastery of parenthood. The student will recall that we previously said that pregnancy is the anticipatory phase of the transition to parenthood. The impending role must be at least partly rehearsed, modeled, and clarified through a process of communication with significant others. In so doing, the role expectations become clearer and the couple begin to put themselves into the role of parents (role take). As this is done, there is a better "fit" to the impending role, with increased confidence leading to role mastery. A schematic drawing of the role mastery process is shown in Figure 30-1. Ideally this process should be begun during pregnancy. However, a similar modified process can be instituted or reinforced in the crucial early postpartum period. Thus, the parents are not entirely separated from providers during this critical

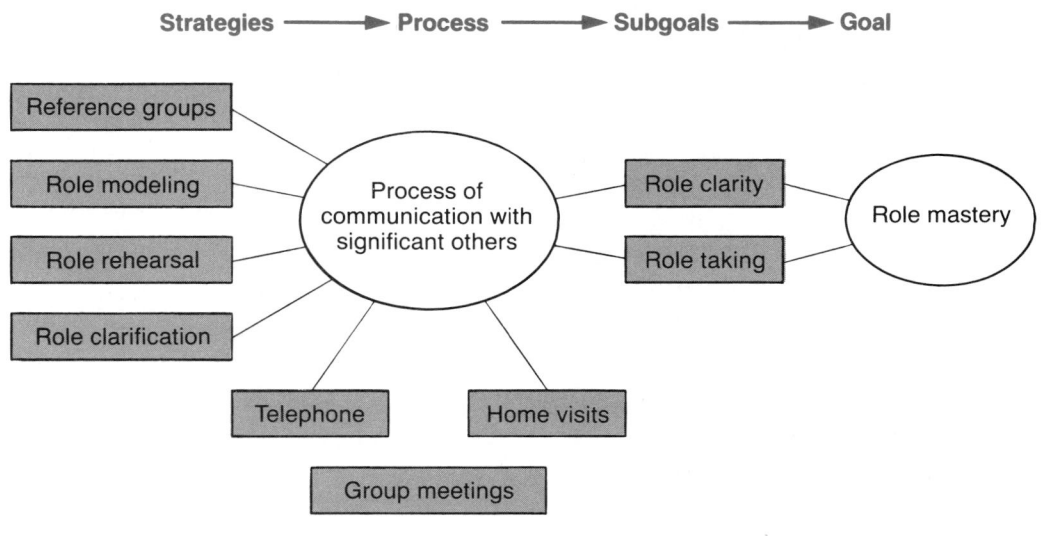

FIGURE 30-1

A conceptual framework of preventive role supplementation leading to role mastery. (After Swendsen LA, Meleis A, Jones D: Role supplementation for new parents—A role mastery plan. MCN 3(2):84–91, March/April 1978)

fourth period in their reproductive cycle. The student is referred to the article by Swendsen and co-workers in the Suggested Reading for details in the implementation of the process.[5]

Parenthood as Crisis vs Transition

La Rossa and La Rossa have pointed out that the majority of studies on the assumption of the parenting role focus on how the quality of personal or marital life changes after the birth of a child.[2] Moreover, these studies tend to perceive and define quality of life in individualistic terms. An individualistic measure of the quality of life focuses on the degree to which an individual succeeds in accomplishing his desires and goals despite the constraints placed on him by a variety of forces, including an indifferent or hostile nature and the social order.[2,6] An individualistic measure of health care, for instance, would focus on how personally inconvenienced persons feel who have to be hospitalized periodically for illness. The less the inconvenience, the better the health care. This formulation suffers from three major flaws. First, the individualistic approach stresses attitudes at the expense of behavior; thus, interaction patterns are often ignored altogether. Second, the approach looks at the variable under study (*e.g.*, health, parenthood) as a "status" rather than a process and therefore fails to consider the reciprocal relationship between it and other aspects of the individuals' lives. Third, the individualistic approach is laden with administrative bias that dictates that researchers be more concerned with bureaucratic efficiency: if complaints can be reduced, then the best goal has been achieved.[2,6]

Probably the best-known series of studies on the assumption of the parenting role is the "parenthood as crises" series. This line of research began with the Le Masters article in 1957 and continued with Dyer, Russell, and the various reports of Hobbs and his colleagues.[7-13] The principal question that these studies have pursued has been: To what extent does the transition to parenthood constitute a "crisis"? With the exception of the Le Masters and Dyer papers, the only criterion for answering this question has been a 23-item checklist developed by Hobbs in his first paper.[2,10] Moreover, the checklist did not focus on the patterns (or changed patterns) of interaction between the couple; rather it stressed *coping ability* of the parents. For instance, the parents were not asked if there *was* an interruption of routine, a *change* in their sex life and sleeping patterns, and the like. Instead, they were asked to indicate the *extent to which* each item in the checklist *bothered* them; they had to choose from three choices: "not at all," "somewhat," and "very much." Thus, if either marked "not at all" to "decreased sexual respon-

siveness of spouse," for instance, the reader could not know whether there had been no change in the couple's sexual pattern or whether they simply were not bothered by such a change. From an individualistic standpoint, those using the checklist have been interested in how well their subjects were doing in spite of the *assumed* crisis brought on by the constraints of parenthood.[2] In 1969, Jacoby called attention to the conceptual limitations of this formulation by pointing out that this body of research allowed little opportunity or stimulus for the reporting of affectively positive (or neutral) attitudes toward the adjustments required by parenthood.[14] In addition, there was no attempt to delineate any behavioral changes as distinct from attitudes that might accompany the behavioral changes. This criticism obtains today.

We have already pointed out some methodological problems inherent in this research, namely, small skewed samples and the lack of sophisticated analyses. While this body of research has limitations, it is important to remember that it was "pioneering" in a sense. Current difficulties arise from the *use* to which it is put, that is, by its uncritical acceptance and application by many health providers who proceed on the faulty assumption that parenthood for everyone is a time of crisis. In future research, there needs to be greater attention to determining the social processes and patterns involved in the transition and a teasing out of attitudes toward the phenomena as opposed to behavior associated with the transition.

Transition to Parenthood

The student will recall that we have used Rossi's formulation of phases in the process of role transition. Specifically, these were the anticipatory phase, the honeymoon phase, the plateau phase, and the disengagement phase (see Chap. 19). In the puerperium, it is the honeymoon phase of the transition that has the most bearing on the nursing care that the maternity nurse must render. However, we shall also review briefly the anticipatory phase, since we previously focused primarily on its relevance to pregnancy rather than to parenthood (see Nursing Care Plan: Couples in Transition to Parenthood, p 591).

Anticipatory Phase

We noted previously that pregnancy is an anticipatory stage to becoming a parent and we outlined tasks that the parents must accomplish during this time. We spoke of decision making and expectations that have bearing on later parenting. Another aspect is the division of labor in the family. This becomes extremely crucial when the baby arrives. The mundane activities of family maintenance are often indicative of how comfortable the parents are in accepting their changing roles. This also gives a clue as to what later role assignments the child may have in the family. It is important that the nurse note whether there is any negotiation for task assignment or some indication of a flexible allocation and sharing of tasks. If one partner unilaterally appoints the other to a responsibility or if there is a rigid "his work, her work" attitude, there may be subtle sabotage or task overload as responsibilities mount with the addition of the infant.[15] Thus, how the family uses the time of pregnancy to work out or rework their division of labor in the family has a large impact on their transition.

Overall, couples in the anticipatory phase experience many intense feelings, challenges, and responsibilities. If used correctly, this can be an opportune time to test skills in preparing to accept and integrate the new family member into the system. The nurse can be very helpful in aiding the couple to examine and understand what they are experiencing by providing accurate information and feedback of perceptions and offering validation of the dynamics that are emerging.[3]

Honeymoon Phase

The honeymoon phase refers to the postchildbirth period during which, through prolonged contact and intimacy, an attachment between the parents and child is achieved.[16] It should be noted that this is a "psychic honeymoon" and not necessarily a time of romanticized peace and joy. Rather, it is a period of intensity when both the mother and the father are exploring the new family member and where they stand in relation to him or her. The couple's personal relationship is no less important at this time, but with the limited energy, emphasis is often placed on development of the new relationship.

Bonding and Attachment

Much has appeared in the literature regarding the fourth stage of labor, the time immediately after delivery when there appears to be an optimum time for close contact between parents and child to initiate the process of bonding the trio together. The terms *bonding* and *attachment* are often used interchangeably to describe this process of parent–child affiliation. Brazelton has pointed out, however, that there is a difference in the connotation of these terms. Bonding refers to the initial attraction and desire to "make it" with another person. Attachment, on the other hand, is the long, hard work of staying in love.[17] Thus, bonding can be thought of as the initial step in a process, the mutual attractiveness and response *between parents and child* that paves the way for the later development of love and affiliation.

In everyday use, however, the two terms are interchangeable.

Until quite recently health providers and the public in general have viewed the newborn as essentially passive. Many medical schools still teach that the newborn has limited perceptual abilities, as if only the midbrain is functioning. This misconception has directly and indirectly affected the delivery of maternity care at all levels. If, instead of using the "lump of clay" model of the infant, we think of the child as organizing around various positive stimuli and experiences, we can readily see that the present tendency toward overstimulating and noncontingent care (care-taking timed *asynchronously* with the infant's responses) is not conducive to the organization of the infant's central nervous system and hence to expeditious positive parent–infant interaction. Care for the newborn needs to be timed to his activity and responses, not to schedules preordained by professionals.[17–19]

As we explore more carefully the amazing newborn, research indicates that neonates are very adaptive, not only able to survive in an often unwelcoming or uncomfortable environment but also to capture the important adults around them. For instance, they demonstrate a marked ability to habituate to different stimuli. If a light is flashed repeatedly into the eyes, the baby startles the first two or three times, then gradually settles down and no longer responds. The same response occurs with the stimuli of a rattle, bell, and pinprick. Moreover, there are definite auditory and visual orienting responses. It one talks and begins to play with the baby, he becomes alert and searches for a face (Fig. 30-2). When he finds it, he softens, and as long as the face moves, the baby follows it. If it becomes still, however, the infant frowns and averts his face. The immobile face has no attraction for the newborn.[17]

Responses to auditory stimuli also demonstrate the ability of the neonate to make choices. If a man and woman stand on opposite sides of the baby and begin to talk, the infant stops moving, his face knits, and he turns toward the female's voice again and again. There is also a differential response to human and nonhuman, machine sounds even if their qualities are exactly alike. When you present a baby who is sucking with a nonhuman sound, he stops sucking and then quickly resumes. If, however, he is offered a human sound, he stops and then resumes with a pattern of suck, suck, pause, suck, suck, pause, indicating by this different, complex pattern a preference for the human sound.[17]

These manifestations of the infant's ability to control and console himself are powerful reinforcers for parents who are ready to move beyond the initial bonding and continue their attachment. The nurse, during both the immediate and the later postpartum period, can be very helpful to parents and facilitate bonding by pointing out and *reinforcing parents' perceptions* of their infant's ability to interact with them. One reinforcer

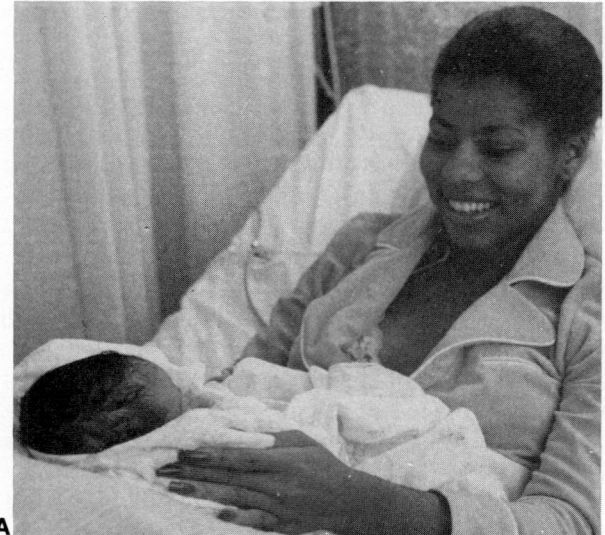

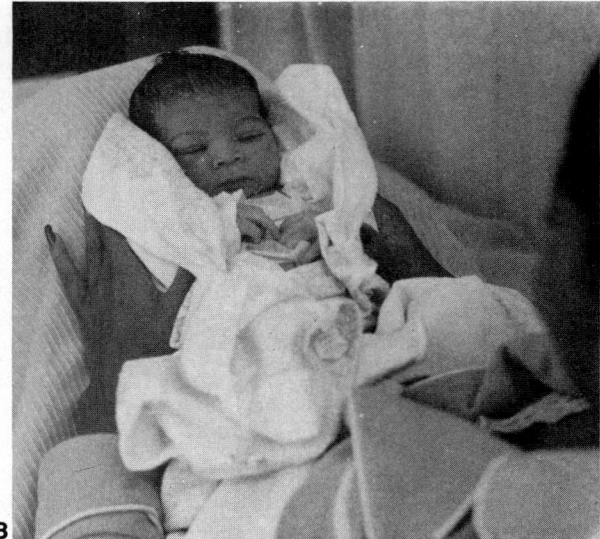

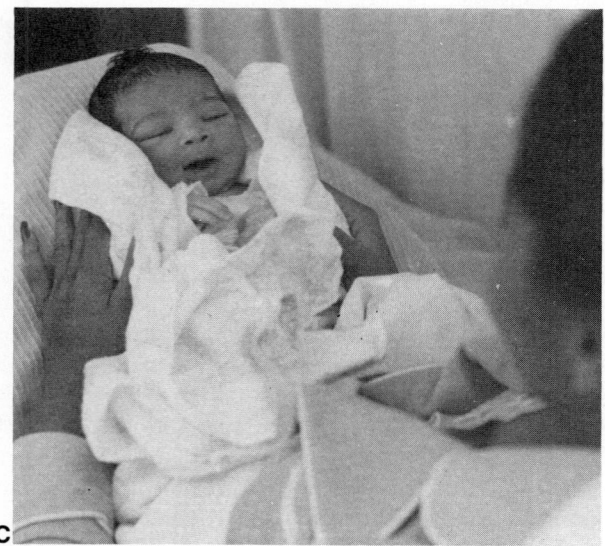

F I G U R E   3 0 - 2

(*A*) An infant responds to an animated smiling face. (*B*) The infant establishes eye contact with the mother. (*C*) The infant begins to move his mouth as the mother smiles and talks.

to attachment that can be shown to the mother and father is the manner of consoling the baby. When a baby is crying, even at the top of his voice, he can be quieted by insistently saying "baby, baby, baby. . . ." Simply by using the voice, one can get the infant to turn his head, put his fist in his mouth and start looking for you.[17]

Principles of Bonding

The work of Robson, Rubin, Moss, Brazelton, Klaus, Korsch, Kennell, Bowlby, and many others has begun to shed light on the fascinating subject of how infants and parents first develop their acquaintance. While we still do not have many of the answers and while some of the information that we do have must still be considered tentative, there appear to be several general principles of the bonding process. Again, these are not

to be regarded as definitive; rather, they reflect the state of the art in thinking and research in the area. The work of Klaus and Kennell, in particular, has undergone revision over time.[20,21] Various researchers have attempted to replicate or test some of the principles specified by Klaus and Kennell and have come up with equivocal or inconsistent results.[22–25] If there are generalizations to be made, it is that much of the findings are hampered by small, self-selected samples. Moreover, there should not be a clear extrapolation made from animal behavior studies to parental–infant behavior. Finally, health providers should not instill guilt in parents by insisting that parents "participate" in the birth process and "bond" immediately with their infants (with the implied threat of irrevocable damage to the infant if they don't). Keeping these caveats in mind, we will review the principles of bonding that Klaus and Kennell have adapted over time:

- There may be a sensitive period in the first hours or days after birth when it seems advantageous for the mother and father to have close contact with their infant for later attachment to proceed optimally.
- There appear to be species-specific responses to the infant in the human mother and father when the infant is first given to them.
- The attachment process seems to be structured so that the parents become attached to only one infant at a time. In 1958, Bowlby stated this principle as *monotropy*.
- For attachment to occur appropriately, it is necessary for the infant to respond to the mother and father by some signal such as body or eye movements. This principle has been called the "You can't love a dishrag" phenomenon.
- Witnessing the birth process may be an enhancement for some parents.
- It is difficult (but not impossible) to simultaneously go through the processes of attachment and detachment. Thus, it is difficult (but not impossible) for parents to attach to an infant while mourning the loss or threatened loss of another person.
- Some early events *may* have long-term effects. For instance, anxiety over an infant with a temporary disorder in his or her early days may result in long-term concerns or behavior that may have implications for future development.[20,21]

Assumption of the Parental Role

As the parents continue in their transition, certain behaviors become apparent. It is important to note that there is much more information on maternal behavior than on paternal behavior. Again, as with attachment principles these observations and findings are not to be considered definitive.

Paternal Behavior

While most researchers agree that more studies need to be done regarding paternal behavior, we are still in the very early stages of this type of research. Parke, a pioneer in this area, has concluded in his studies that there are no significant behavioral differences between fathers alone with their infants and mothers alone with their infants. If, however, the trio are together, the father tends to hold the infant twice as much as the mother, to vocalize more, and to touch the infant slightly more, but he smiles significantly less. Thus, the father plays a far more active role than the passive cultural stereotype suggests.[26]

The term *engrossment* has been used by Greenberg and Morris to describe the behavior pattern noted in fathers when they are involved and interacting with their newborn (Fig. 30-3). They conclude that there are identifiable aspects of paternal bonding similar to maternal bonding that are enhanced by newborn behavior and normal reflex activity.[27]

A study by Bowen and Miller tends to substantiate this contention.[28] These researchers compared three groups of fathers: those who had attended childbirth classes and were present during delivery, those who were present at delivery but had not attended childbirth classes, and those who did not attend either childbirth classes or delivery. Fathers who attended the birth demonstrated significantly more attachment behavior to their infants than fathers who were not present. Interestingly, attendance at childbirth education classes was not correlated with better attachment scores. Moreover, sleeping infants elicited significantly less attachment behavior from the father than did alert infants. These results lend support for the theory of a sensitive period shortly after birth in the development of parental bonding for the father as well as the mother.[28]

May, on the other hand, refutes these findings and suggests that there are a wide range of paternal behaviors that reflect personality factors and antecedent life experiences.[23]

Lamb and Howells contend that mothering and fathering are separate entities and may be dissimilar. Lamb proposes the following thesis: (1) the mother–child relationship is originally based on the infant's dependence and helplessness and gradually diminishes in importance as the child becomes older and more independent and (2) the father–child relationship revolves around

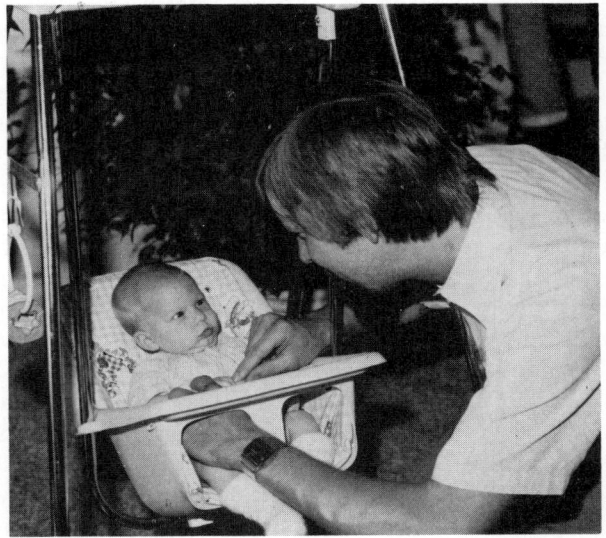

FIGURE 30-3

Fathering. Paternal involvement is engrossing and can be satisfying to everyone.

not only caretaking activities but also many outside enjoyable activities. Hence, the father introduces and socializes the child to the world outside the home. Female parents could function in the paternal role but would have to dissociate from the mothering and nurturing tasks. This, therefore, is the reason for the dissimilarity of the two roles.[29] Why the father can caretake and socialize outside the home at the same time and the mother cannot is not clear in Lamb's formulation.

Howells also believes that both fathering and mothering are equally important but may have dissimilar components. According to his formulation, the relationship of both parents to a child is unique and is dependent on the sum total of the variables that make up the psychosocial dynamics of each family.[30]

In view of the similarities found in the better research studies and society's recent trend toward a more flexible masculine–feminine role definition, the utility of breaking apart maternal and paternal behavior may well be called into question.

Maternal Behavior

A pioneer in delineating parental behavior was Reva Rubin, who focused on the mother and identified various phases of maternal behavior, particularly relating to maternal touch and the infant.[31] She contends that mothering is composed of a set of interpersonal and production skills designed to foster the emotional, intellectual, and physical development of the child. Thus, Rubin described the tasks of mothering as (1) identifying the new child, (2) determining one's relationship to the child, and (3) guiding and reconstructing the family constellation to include a new member. In general, this formulation is still used.[31] However, Martel and Mitchell caution that Rubin's sample was very small and her methodology not as explicit as it might be, thus making replication difficult.[32] In their research (again with an admittedly small sample) they found similar "phases" during the postpartum period as Rubin had described, but they did not seem to be as time bound as those found by Rubin in her work in 1961. The authors attribute this to a changed philosophy surrounding maternity care and to changed hospital practices that involve the mother and parents in the infant's care immediately, as well as to much shorter hospital stays. The main thrust of their argument is that we should not uncritically hold on to old concepts without attempting to validate them under existing new conditions. That is certainly an important and worthwhile admonition.

Rubin maintained that certain behaviors have been found to accompany these various tasks and the assumption of the maternal role. These behaviors have also been found to be related to three phases that Rubin also classified. As previously mentioned, the time spans

for these phases may vary, particularly if the parents are permitted immediate contact with the newborn. The following discussion derives primarily from Rubin's classification.[33]

Taking-In Phase

In the taking-in phase the mother is oriented primarily to her own needs. She may be quite passive and dependent. Rubin found that this phase may last a day or two, although Martel and Mitchell found this time span hardly existent. The mother might not initiate contact with the infant. This is not out of disinterest, but rather because of her own immediate dependency. Although she may not indicate much interest in assuming responsibility for the baby's care, she is taking in information that helps her identify the infant. In this phase, *fingertip touch* with the infant can be observed (Fig. 30-4). The mother may lay the infant on her lap or bed and gently explore him or her with her fingers. This is one of the first steps in the identification process and an indication of awakening interest in the newborn. One may also note that she holds the baby facing her, so that they mutually explore each other's faces. This has been called the *en face* position.

Gottlieb has pointed out that beginning attachment is accompanied by a *discovery* process. The mother must ask herself, "Who is this infant? What is he able to do?" and so on. She accomplishes this discovery during the taking-in phase by means of *identification, relating,* and *interpreting* with the infant.[34] In *identification* she points out various physical aspects or features of the infant so as to have a frame of reference. From there she *relates* actions and characteristics to some familiar person, object, or fantasy (*e.g.,* "Face like daddy; hiccups like I used to have"). Finally, in *interpreting* she gives a meaning to the infant's actions and perceived needs. For instance, if the infant is crying and is difficult to quiet, She may say, "He's going to be a holy terror, I just know it." All of these behaviors help the mother realize the infant as a separate entity.

Sleep and Food.   Sleep and food play an important part during this phase. The mother is far more able to begin the activities required of her if she is allowed to have a well-earned refreshing sleep. If this necessary rest is disrupted, the mother may experience a "sleep hunger" that may last for several days; this results in irritability, fatigue, and general interference with the normal restorative process. Thus, the necessity of appropriate intervention by the nurse to allow the mother to get adequate sleep cannot be stressed enough.

The nurse should also note if the mother usually has a good appetite and, in fact, may talk a good deal about either the adequacy or the inadequacy of her meals. Between-meal nourishment is appreciated and needed, especially by nursing mothers. The concern

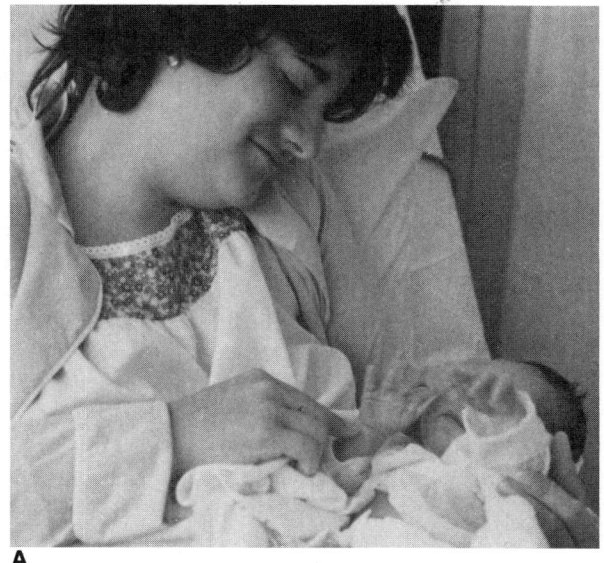

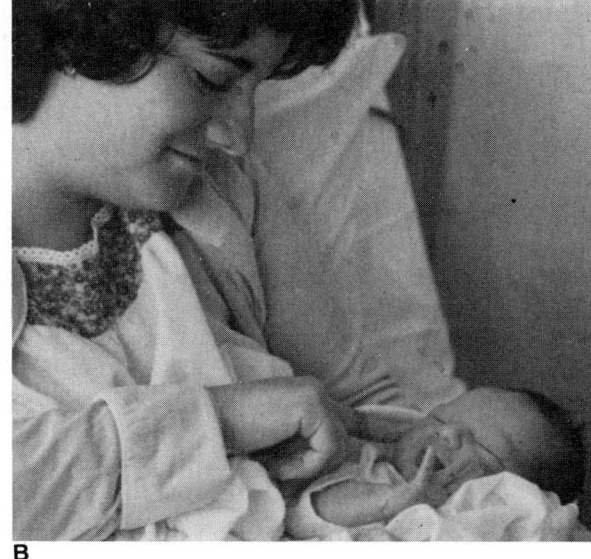

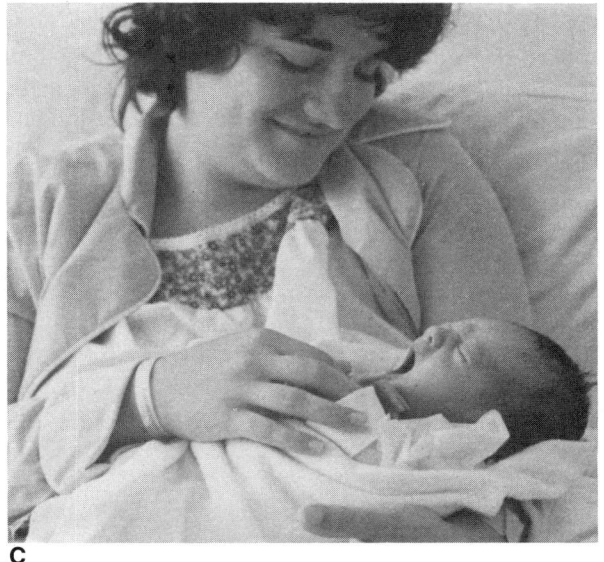

FIGURE 30-4

Identification process through maternal touch. (*A*) Exploring the infant with fingertip touch. (*B*) The mother continues her exploration progressing to the infant's face. (*C*) The baby is finally enfolded by the mother.

about food seems to be a part of the mother's general need to be restored. Food, as we know, has tremendous psychological significance for care asking and care giving. The nurse should be especially cognizant of the mother's need for hearty meals and should expedite extra nourishment whenever possible. Moreover, she should be aware that a poor appetite often is one of the first symptoms that all is not proceeding normally in the puerperal period.

Integrating the Experience. During the taking-in phase the mother begins to relive the delivery experience in order to integrate it fully into reality. She is apt to be very talkative at this time, and she may want to know certain specifics and details so that she can form a total picture of what "really happened" during delivery. As she obtains this information, she is able to realize more fully that the pregnancy and the delivery are truly over

and that her baby now is born and is an individual outside of and separate from herself. This is a considerable task and involves rather profound changes in attitudes and feelings. The symbiotic relationship between mother and infant during pregnancy is at an end, and the mother now must identify her child as a separate individual.

Taking-Hold Phase

The second phase in the puerperal period has been described as a taking-hold phase; the mother strives for independence and autonomy and finally begins to be the initiator. One of her main concerns at this point seems to be her ability to control her bodily functions; her bowels and bladder must perform well, and she takes an active part in seeing that they do. If she is nursing her infant, she is concerned about producing an acceptable quantity and quality of milk. She cannot have enough explanation and reassurance that she is "performing" well at this time. She wants to walk, to sit, to move as she did before delivery and is very anxious and impatient if she cannot make her body behave as it once did. It is as though she is thinking, "How can I possibly assume all my responsibilities for others if I cannot control my own body?"

Her first mothering tasks are especially important to her, and "failures" (inability to elicit a bubble from her infant, poor suckling response on the part of the baby, her awkwardness in handling her child), no matter how small and expected (by the staff), can send her to the depths of despair. Even the skillful intervention of the nurse seems only to point up her "inadequacy" as a mother. She often voices her feelings with an "Oh, I'll never be able to bathe her as easily as you do." Or another mother may say, "He always seems to take his milk better when *you* feed him." Conversely, when she succeeds at a task, her delight and relief are wonderful to behold. It is difficult to imagine (for anyone other than a new mother) how thrilling a hearty bubble from a small infant can be.

Since there is a good deal of anxiety as well as activity in this phase, fatigue and exhaustion may occur if the mother is not helped to set realistic expectations and limits for herself. Rubin found that the "taking-hold" phase lasted approximately 10 days. Thus, much of it will take place at home. Also, with the short hospital stay, this phase may be telescoped.

The nurse can be invaluable in giving the mother, as she appears able and ready to accept it, anticipatory guidance about what to expect and how to manage. During the hospital stay the mother profits greatly from reassurance and explanation regarding the various processes and hour-by-hour events. She finds guidance and reinforcement of appropriate behavior particularly

helpful when she attempts to perform her mothering tasks.

When assisting the mother, the nurse must be careful not to impose herself between the mother and her baby (no matter how awkward or maladroit the mother seems). Rather, the nurse should allow the mother to perform the actual task (after necessary demonstration or instruction) and then encourage or reinforce whatever behavior was appropriate. This is one way of demonstrating confidence in the mother's ability to cope with new tasks. To gain skill and confidence in her mothering ability, the mother needs the opportunity to make decisions about the baby's needs as well as guidance regarding his or her physical care. When she is allowed to find answers to her questions (again with guidance as necessary) and is reassured that her judgment is correct, she is able to feel confident in her ability to perceive needs accurately and to make decisions. Thus, she is better able to meet problems in the future.

As the mother becomes more comfortable with her infant, she moves to the second stage of maternal touch, *total hand contact,* and finally the third stage, *enfolding* (Fig. 30-4*B* and *C*). In general, the more competent she feels and the more satisfying her relationship with the infant, the greater the enfolding. These touching behaviors can be observed in fathers also if they are given the opportunity to handle and care for the infant. They, too, can be observed placing the infant in the *en face* position.

The mother who remains distant and aloof may not be attaching to her infant as optimally as she should. The nurse will want to be alert for such signs.

Letting-Go Phase

As her mothering functions become more established, the mother enters the letting-go phase. This generally occurs when the mother returns home. In this phase

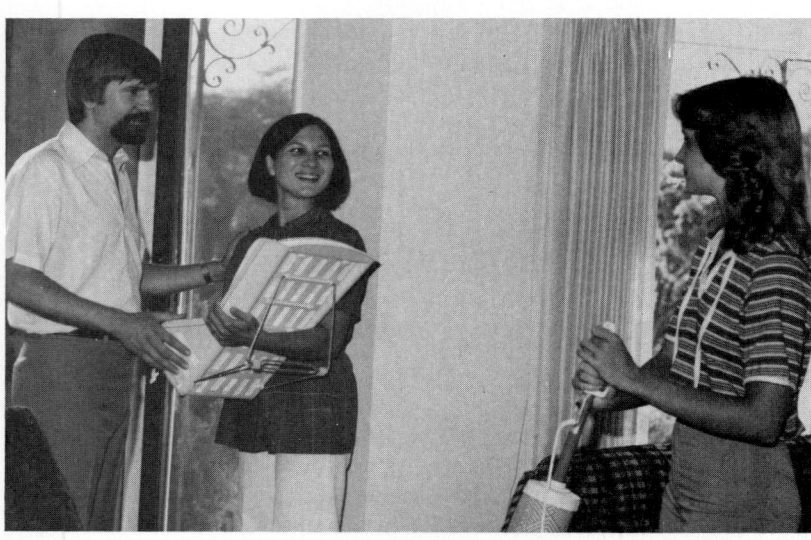

FIGURE 30-5

Teenage "mother's helpers" allow parents more time to enjoy an outing with their infant.

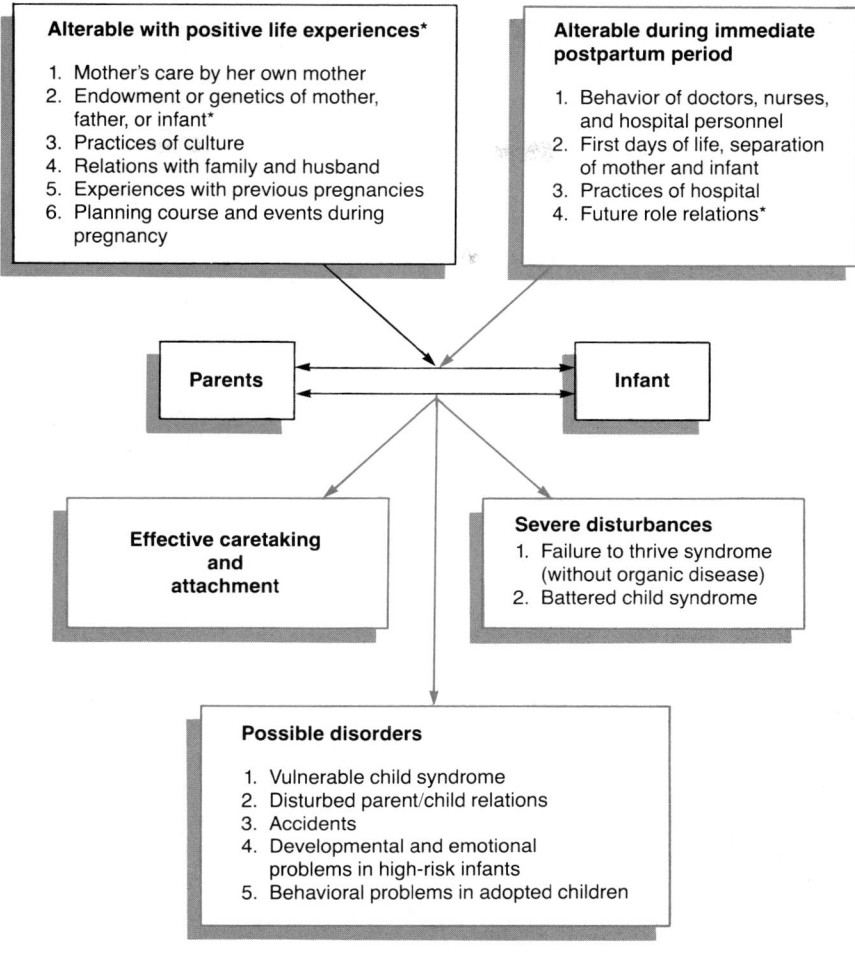

*Not in original Klaus/Kennell diagram.

FIGURE 30-6

Hypothetical diagram of the major influences on maternal behavior and the resulting disturbances. (After Klaus MH, Kennell JH: Maternal-Infant Bonding. St Louis, CV Mosby, 1976)

there are two separations that the mother must accomplish. One is to realize and accept the physical separation from the baby and the other is to relinquish her former role of childless person. As we pointed out in Chapter 19, she will never again be childless until the death of those whom she has borne. The implications are enormous. She must now adjust her life to the relative dependency and helplessness of her child. If she stops working, she must adapt, at least temporarily, to less freedom, autonomy, and social stimulation. If she does continue working, she and the father will have to handle the complex details of finding mother substitutes and other household caretakers (Fig. 30-5). Her work load is such that there is almost always some role strain and overload even when the father is helpful or outside help is found. This can be managed by appropriate antici-

patory guidance from the nurse, but nearly all mothers find the adjustment at least somewhat difficult.

Postpartum Blues. Thus, during the puerperium (for no apparent reason, the mother thinks) she may experience a letdown feeling accompanied by irritability and tears. Occasionally her appetite and sleep patterns are disturbed. These are the usual manifestations of the postpartal or "baby" blues. This depression is usually temporary and may occur in the hospital. It is thought to be related in part to hormonal changes and in part to the ego adjustment that accompanies role transition. Discomfort, fatigue, and exhaustion certainly contribute to this condition if not cause it. Crying often relieves the tension, but if the parents are not knowledgeable about the condition, the mother, especially, may feel rather guilty for being depressed. Understanding and anticipatory guidance help the parents become aware that these feelings are a normal accompaniment to this role transition. (This aspect of postpartal care is explored more extensively in Chap. 31.)

Influences on Parental Behavior

A schematic diagram of the major influences on parental behavior and their outcomes, including some disorders that have been hypothesized but not definitely concluded to arise from them, is presented in Figure 30-6. The diagram has been adapted from the earlier work of Klaus and Kennell.[20] We note that, at the time of the infant's birth, some of the influences are felt to be alterable with positive subsequent life experiences (black line), such as the genetic endowment of the parents, the type of mothering they received, previous pregnancies, and the like. Other determinants are more alterable in the immediate postpartum period (blue line), such as practices of hospital personnel, separation of infant and mother, and future parental relations. Klaus and Kennell felt that many of the disturbances and disorders could be directly attributed to separation of the infant from the mother after birth and the consequent interference with the bonding process. They point out that the separation of mother and infant is the one variable that is most easily manipulated and urge that hospitals reexamine their policies to bring them in line with more current findings regarding bonding and attachment.[20] In an earlier work Klaus and Kennell said the determinants in the first box were fixed or unalterable.[20] In a later work they state that the "fixed" determinants may, in fact, be mutable and can be influenced by positive life experiences. We show them here as "alterable with positive life experiences" to indicate to the student that these may be a little more difficult to change and not easily attained in the first days post partum.[21]

Once again, it is important to note that new parents face a major decision regarding the enactment of their sex roles in addition to the myriad of other large and small decisions they must make. For instance, will the woman assume the more traditional role of total homemaker/mother or will she attempt to combine a career with parenthood? Similarly, will the father extend his role to active involvement in homemaking and child-rearing or choose the traditional "breadwinner" role (Fig. 30-7)? The choice of either of the nontraditional parental roles is accompanied by a certain amount of stress. There is little support for either mother or father from employers, and there may be little support from significant others. On the other hand, assuming the traditional parental roles can also be stressful because this course of action may be thwarting the potential and

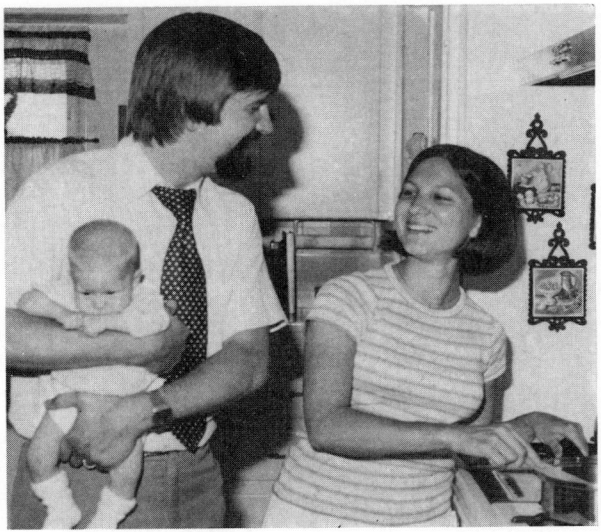

F I G U R E   3 0 - 7

The extension of the paternal role is often helpful for new parents.

actualization of the parents.[35] Zaslow and Pedersen found that in the case of fathers' adjustment to parenthood, it does not matter so much whether they choose a traditional fathering role or nontraditional fathering role, but rather whether they assume the role in a consistent and coherent manner.[35] As more research is done on this fascinating topic, we should gain more insight into how we can better help the family make the parental role transition more smoothly.

Applying the Nursing Process to the Developing Family

Assessment and nursing diagnosis are based on careful observation and interviewing. Knowledge deficit may be a primary diagnosis.

One key element of nursing intervention with the expanding family is the teaching of parenting skills that promote the child's maturity, autonomy, and competence. If the parents have a realistic conception of the infant's needs and their resources, they need not expend all their energy on their parenting responsibilities at the expense of their own personal needs and growth.

Nursing's involvement in the recent trend toward health maintenance and promotion has set the stage for classes that include information and skill development needed after the infant is born. Teaching styles and format for parenting classes resemble those in prenatal instruction.[36]

Learning needs of the parents can be determined by assessing the following areas: expectations of chil-

Couples in Transition to Parenthood

Nursing Objectives

1. Promote parent–child attachment.
2. Determine learning needs for parenting skills.
3. Identify families at risk for potential transition to parenthood difficulties.

Assessment	Potential Nursing Diagnosis	Intervention	Evaluation
Quality of parent–child interaction: Appropriate holding Talking to infant Synchronous touch, care giving	Ineffective individual coping related to parenthood	Identify potential and actual stressors relating to attachment Identify sources of social and maternal support for the parents; encourage their utilization Reduce knowledge deficit Identify sources of asynchrony in the parent–child relationship Teach alternate synchronous methods of interaction Provide for role modeling, group discussions, and so forth, as necessary	Parents identify stressors and accept methods of reducing them Parents identify sources of support and use them to reduce stressors Parents learn the sources of their asynchrony and reorganize their behavior to become effective in caretaking
Additional learning needs of parents relating to parenting: Parental perceptions of the infant's present level of maturity; autonomy needs, level of competence Parental perceptions of future expectations for children's performance Feelings about developmental lags Parental perceptions of their parental responsibilities, personal needs, growth needs and resources	Knowledge deficit of infant performance related to unrealistic expectations Knowledge deficit of infant's and own present and future needs related to unrealistic perception	Identify parents' expectations regarding levels of growth and development patterns for infants Identify their perceptions of their infant's present and future growth and development patterns; clarify misconceptions through individual counseling, group discussions, and so forth Identify parental perceptions of their own individual and family needs; support positive perceptions, provide alternate methods for achieving needs as necessary	Perceptions regarding growth and development become more realistic Parents utilize groups and other supports as necessary Perceptions and behavior relating to parenting become more realistic
Presence or absence of social isolation (the amount if it exists)	Social isolation related to constraints of new parenthood	Support social integration through the use of social supports; clarify misconceptions regarding parental responsibilities	Social isolation or role overload (if present) diminishes. Time managed more efficiently. Social supports used appropriately)
Presence or absence of role overload (the amount if it exists)	Anxiety related to mismanagement of time or misuse of support systems	Reduce role overload through helping parents manage time more efficiently, appropriately use social supports	Couple expresses a diminish in their social isolation or role overload Couple manages time more efficiently Couple uses social supports appropriately

dren's performance ability, lags in development task fulfillment, social isolation, immobilization due to role overload, and ability to set limits and carry them out. When these learning needs are diagnosed, the nurse can develop a teaching plan aimed at preventing and alleviating problems in these areas. Strengths of the couple should always be delineated and worked with. When deficits are found, verbal and behavioral skills can be developed to cope with the problem. If the deficit is related to outside institutions, the nurse will want to be aware of community institutions and agencies to which she can refer the parents.[36] These factors are further discussed in Chapters 20 and 31.

It is impossible to teach all of the skills necessary to parenting. However, if the nurse can help parents sort out problems, examine options and resources, and negotiate outcomes, she has accomplished a great deal and has been instrumental in this momentous role transition. A care plan for nursing during this transition is included in this chapter.

References

1. Broom BL: Consensus about the marital relationship during transition to parenthood. Nurs Res 33(4):223–228, July/August 1984
2. La Rossa R, La Rossa MM: Transition to Parenthood: How Infants Change Families. Beverly Hills, Sage Publications, 1981
3. Hrobsky DM: Transition to parenthood: A balancing of needs. Nurs Clin North Am 12:457–468, September 1977
4. Meleis AI: Role inefficiency and role supplementation: A conceptual framework. Nurs Res 24:264–271, July/August 1975
5. Swendsen LA, Meleis A, Jones D: Role supplementation for new parents. MCN 3:84–91, March/April 1978
6. Gerson EM: On "quality of life." Am Soc Rev 41:793–806, October 1976
7. Le Masters EE: Parenthood as crisis. Marr Fam Living 19:352–355, November 1957
8. Dyer ED: Parenthood as crisis: A re-study. Marr Fam Living 25:196–201, May 1963
9. Russell C: Circumplex model of family systems: III. Empirical evaluation with families. Fam Process 18:29–46, March 1979
10. Hobbs DF Jr: Parenthood as crises: A third study. J Marr Fam 27:367–372, August 1965
11. Hobbs DF Jr: Transition to parenthood: A replication and extension. J Marr Fam 30:413–417, August 1968
12. Hobbs DF Jr, Cole SP: Transition to parenthood: A decade of replication. J Marr Fam 38:723–731, November 1976
13. Hobbs DF Jr, Wimbish JM: Transition to parenthood by black couples. J Marr Fam 37:677–689, November 1977
14. Jacoby AP: Transition to parenthood: A reassessment. J Marr Fam 31:720–727, November 1969
15. Turner RH: Family Interaction. New York, John Wiley & Sons, 1970
16. Rossi A: Transition to parenthood. J Marr Fam 30:26–39, February 1968
17. Brazelton TB: The remarkable talents of the newborn. Birth Fam J 5:187–191, Winter 1978
18. Jannson P: Early postpartum discharge. AJN 85:547–550, May 1985
19. Roberts FB: Infant behavior and transition to parenthood. Nurs Res 32:213–217, July/August 1983
20. Klaus MH, Kennell JH: Maternal-Infant Bonding. St Louis, CV Mosby, 1976
21. Klaus MH, Kennell JH: Parent-Infant Bonding, 2nd ed. St Louis, CV Mosby, 1982
22. Korsch BM: More on parent-infant bonding. J Pediatr 102:249–252, February 1983
23. May KA: Father participation in birth: Fact and fiction. J Can Perinatal Assoc II:41–43, Fall 1982
24. Curry MA: Maternal attachment behavior and the mother's self-concept: The effect of early skin-to-skin contact. Nurs Res 31:73–78, March/April 1982
25. Tulman LJ: Theories of maternal attachment. Adv Nurs Sci 4:7–14, July 1981
26. Parke R: The father's role in infancy: A reevaluation. Birth Fam J 5:211–213, Winter 1978
27. Greenberg M, Morris N: Engrossment: The newborn's impact on the father. Am J Orthopsychiatry 44:520–531, July 1974
28. Bowen SM, Miller BC: Paternal attachment behavior as related to presence of delivery and preparenthood classes: A pilot study. Nurs Res 29:307–311, September/October 1980
29. Lamb ME: Fathers: Forgotten contributors to child development. Hum Dev 18:245–266, 1975
30. Howells JG: Fathering. In Howells JG (ed): Modern Perspectives in International Child Psychiatry. Edinburgh, Oliver & Boyd, 1969
31. Rubin R: Basic maternal behavior. Nurs Outlook, 683–686, November 1961
32. Martel LK, Mitchell SK: Rubin's "puerperal change" reconsidered. JOGN Nurs 13:145–149, May/June 1984
33. Rubin R: Puerperal change. Nurs Outlook 753–755, December 1961
34. Gottlieb L: Maternal attachment in primiparas. JOGN Nurs 7:39–44, January/February 1979
35. Zaslow MJ, Pedersen FA: Sex role conflict and the experience of childbearing. Prof Psych 12:47–55, February 1981
36. Perdue BJ et al: Mothering. Nurs Clin North Am 12:491–503, September 1977

Suggested Reading

Celotta B: New motherhood? A time of crises? Birth 9:21–23, Spring 1982
Crawford G: A theoretical model of support network conflict experienced by new mothers. Nurs Res 34:100–102, March/April 1985

Croft CA: Lamaze childbirth education: Implications for maternal-infant attachment. JOGN Nurs 11:333–336, September/October 1982

Hock E, Gneda MT, McBride SL: Mothers of infants: Attitudes toward employment following birth of the first child. J Marr Fam 46:425–431, May 1984

La Rossa R: The transition to parenthood and the social reality of time. J Marr Fam 45:579–589, August 1983

Mercer RT: Factors impacting on the maternal role and the first year of motherhood. Birth Defects XVII:233–252, 1981

O'Donnell L: The social world of parents. Marr Fam Rev 5: 9–36, Winter 1982

Torrey L: The effects of holding the newborn at delivery on paternal bonding. Nurs Res 32:16–19, January/February 1983

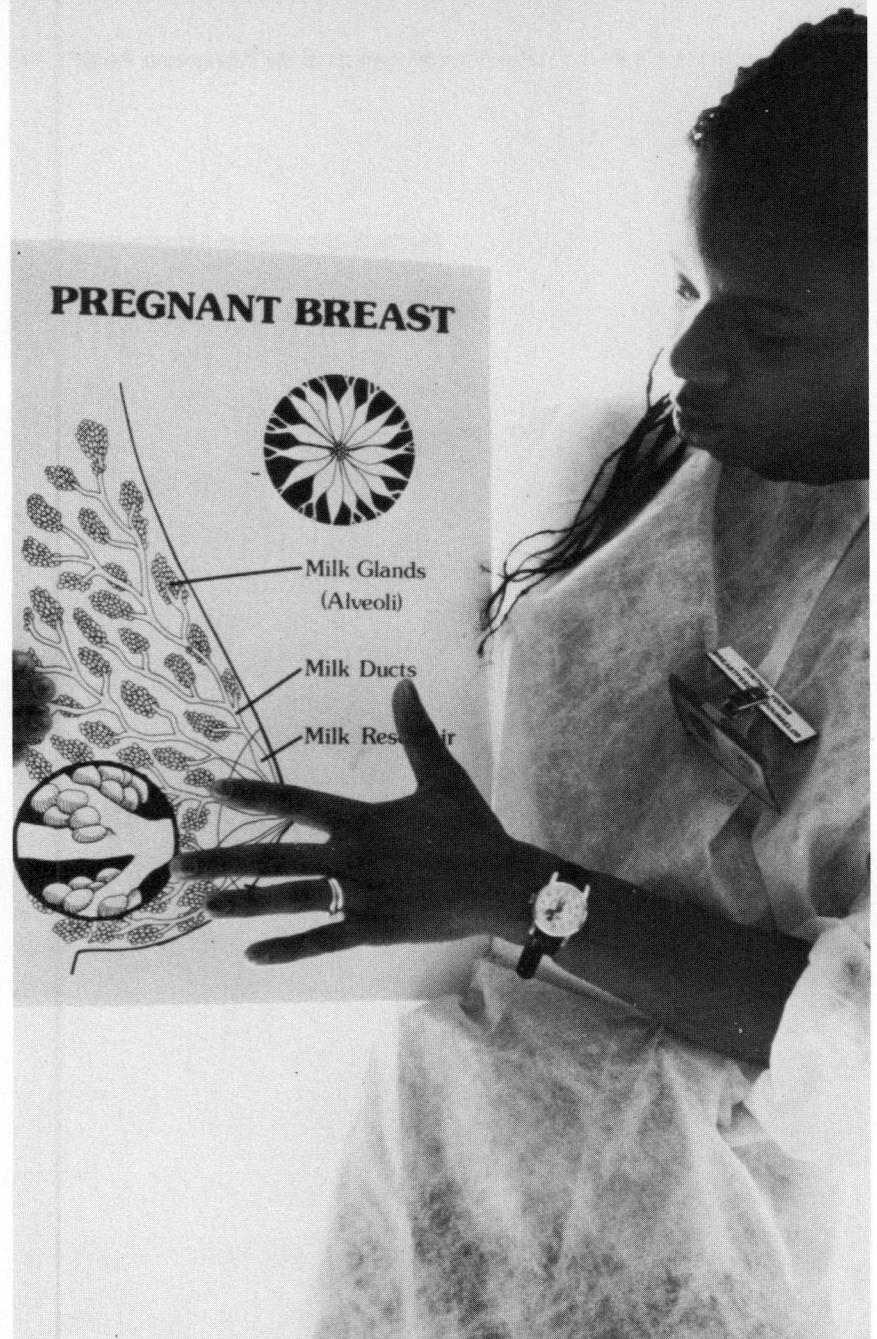

CHAPTER 31

Nursing Care in the Postpartum Period

The postpartum period is a time of major physical and psychological transition for the new mother, as discussed in Chapters 29 and 30. The father also experiences similar psychological processes in initiating and developing his relationship with the newborn. Both parents must adapt to a new family structure, integrate the newborn into their family, and develop different interactional patterns within the family unit. The postpartum period usually is stressful, and sensitive professional care is helpful to new parents.

Nursing care takes both the physical and the psychological needs of mothers and families into consideration. The mother's physiological functioning must be observed accurately, her dependency needs must be met, anticipatory guidance and health teachings must be given according to the mother's readiness to learn, and the developing relationship between mother and infant should be appropriately observed, guided, and nurtured.

In today's highly organized hospitals, the needs of the mother and her newborn do not always coincide with hospital policy or routine. Increased awareness of the importance of the first few days after birth for development of appropriate bonding and attachment between mother and baby has led many hospitals to alter routines. Modified rooming-in procedures and other family-centered approaches generally provide mother and infant with longer time periods together, during which the identification and claiming phases of maternal–infant attachment may occur. Progressive policies for visits by fathers and other family members in many hospitals encourage integration of the new infant into the family.

Immediate Postpartum Care

Immediately after labor, the mother usually experiences a sense of complete fatigue comparable to that which would normally follow any strenuous muscular activity. At the same time, she may be so exhilarated by the experience and the feeling of relief that accompanies it that she is not aware of being exhausted. She is interested in seeing and holding her baby and visiting with the father. Within the first hour of delivery, the mother, the father, and the infant ideally should be provided the opportunity for a private session together, in which the parents can get to know the infant by holding and exploring the nude infant in skin-to-skin contact. Since the infant is in the quiet, alert state for 45 to 60 minutes following birth, his eyes are generally wide open and he can respond to his environment. He is ideally equipped for the critical first encounter with parents, an important phase in bonding and attachment (see Chap. 30). Silver nitrate eye drops can be withheld while the baby is in this alert state and can visually relate to his parents.[1] Following the parents' session with their

---

Nursing Guidelines for Postpartum Assessment, Care, and Teaching

I. Postpartum Observations
  A. Vital signs
  B. Condition of fundus
  C. Lochia (character, amount, type)
  D. Perineum (sutures, edema, pain)
  E. Urinary system (first voiding, amount, color, character)
  F. Intestinal elimination (hemorrhoids, perineal sutures, stool softeners or laxatives)
  G. Breasts (lactation or lactation suppression, engorgement, condition)
II. Personal Care and Comfort
  A. Ambulation
  B. Shower or bathing
  C. Perineal care (solutions, Tucks, anesthetic sprays, etc)
  D. Sitz bath
  E. Perineal heat lamp
  F. Breast support and comfort (milk expression, ice packs, etc)
  G. Rest and exercise (postpartum exercises, Kegel's exercises)

H. Nutrition
I. Emotional adjustment

III. Family Relations
  A. Visitors (father, relatives, friends, etc)
  B. Children at home
  C. Sexuality and birth control
  D. Family adjustments to the new baby
  E. Adapting family routines

IV. Infant Care
  A. Feeding (formula, breast)
  B. Positioning and handling
  C. Bathing
  D. Clothing and diapering
  E. Cord and circumcision care
  F. Temperature and thermometer use
  G. Suctioning and use of bulb syringe
  H. Infant behavior (crying, fussing, neuromuscular, eye movements, etc)
  I. Recognizing signs of illness
  J. Infant safety (car seats, poisons, physical environment)

newborn baby, every effort should be made to help the
mother rest. With a little encouragement she usually
falls into a sound natural sleep. The discomforts and
activities that may interfere with sleep should be expedited or mitigated as much as possible.

Many mothers complain of feeling chilled immediately after labor; some actually shake with the chill.
Some authorities believe that the "chill" may be due
partly to the sudden release of intra-abdominal pressure
that results as the uterus is emptied at delivery. This
reaction may be alleviated if the mother is made comfortable in a warm bed and given a warm beverage
when possible. If her body does begin to quiver, an
extra cotton blanket should be placed over her or tucked
close around her body for comfort. Many mothers (and
their partners) are frightened or disturbed by the chill;
thus, reassurance by the nurse that this is not an unusual
occurrence following delivery is extremely helpful.

Assessment

Initial assessment after delivery focuses on physiological
processes, including the status of the uterus, amount of
bleeding, status of the bladder, vital signs, and condition
of the perineum. Early interaction between mother and
infant and between mother, father, and infant provides
cues concerning parental bonding and family relationships.

Hemorrhage is the major danger to the mother, and
the condition of the uterus must be carefully monitored
and bleeding assessed. Considerable information can
be gained by palpating the fundus through the abdominal wall to be assured that the uterus remains firm,
round, and well contracted. At the same time it is also
important to inspect the perineal pad for obvious signs
of bleeding, as well as to take the pulse and the blood
pressure. During the first hour these observations should
be made at least every 15 minutes, or more often if
indicated.

Although excessive postpartum bleeding can happen to any mother, the nurse can identify those at increased risk. A multipara who has had several deliveries
has an increased tendency for heavy postpartum bleeding, as does the woman whose uterus was excessively
distended by hydramnios, multiple pregnancy, or a large
infant. Operative deliveries with lacerations of the cervix, vagina, or perineum also predispose toward hemorrhage. Clients with a history indicating increased risk
require more frequent observation for bleeding.

If the mother's bladder becomes distended, this can
interfere with uterine contraction and produce atony,
which leads to heavy bleeding. With each 15-minute
check of the condition of the uterus, the bladder should
also be assessed. It is not unusual for the mother to
need to void within the first 4 hours after delivery. If
she is unable to void spontaneously and there is bladder
distention, catheterization is necessary to prevent both
bladder and uterine atony.

Observations of the perineum and vulva are made
to detect hematomas or continued bleeding from lacerations. As perineal pads are changed, the amount of
saturation is noted and a careful pad count is kept to
estimate blood loss (see Fig. 31-3).

At the end of the first hour after delivery, if the
uterus remains well contracted, bleeding is normal, and
vital signs are stable, observations can be made less
frequently, usually every 4 hours. Temperature is taken
at this time also. The mother is allowed to rest as much
as possible and kept comfortable. Liquids are usually
provided if the mother's condition is stable.

Intervention

As long as the bleeding is minimal and the uterus remains firm and well contracted and does not increase
in size, it is neither necessary nor desirable to stimulate
it. However, it the uterus becomes soft and boggy because of relaxation, the fundus should be massaged immediately until it becomes contracted again. This can
be best accomplished by placing one hand just above
the symphysis pubis to act as a guard, as the other hand
is cupped around the fundus and rotated gently. It
should be remembered that the uterus is a sensitive organ that, under normal circumstances, responds quickly
to tactile stimulation.

Care must be taken to avoid overmassage, because,
in addition to causing the mother considerable pain,
this may stimulate premature uterine contractions and
thereby cause undue muscle fatigue. Such a condition
would further encourage uterine relaxation and hemorrhage.

If the uterus is atonic, blood that collects in the cavity should be expressed with firm but gentle force in
the direction of the outlet, but only after the fundus has

> ### *Nursing Guidelines: Procedure for Fundus Check*
>
> 1. Explain procedure and rationale to client.
> 2. Position client on back, with feet together and knees apart.
> 3. Remove perineal pad, note amount of saturation, and record pad count.
> 4. Have client empty bladder if necessary.
> 5. With one hand supporting the lower fundus just above the symphysis pubis, cup the other hand around the fundus and rotate gently.
> 6. If the uterus is boggy (atonic), blood that has collected in the cavity is expressed with firm but gentle pressure downward. Only do this procedure to express blood *after* the fundus has been first massaged to increase its contraction.
> 7. Observe the vulva for passage of blood clots and for development of hematomas or bleeding from lacerations.
> 8. Remove bloody pads, cleanse perineum, and apply fresh perineal pad.
> 9. Provide comfort, such as sips of water and helping the client find a comfortable position.
> 10. Record findings related to fundus, bleeding, and perineum.

been first massaged (see Fig. 25-19). Failure to see that the uterus is contracted before pushing downward against it could result in inversion of the uterus, which is an extremely serious complication.

Family Interactions

The immediate postpartum period, also called the fourth stage of labor (see Chap. 25), is important for the development of parent–infant relations as well as for the mother's physiological status (Fig. 31-1). When there is no contraindication due to the infant's condition, the infant is usually placed in the mother's arms and the two are allowed to visit with the father in a private area. The infant's state of alertness immediately after birth facilitates eye contact with parents and is felt to be important in establishing the parental bond.[2]

After the excitement and strain of labor and delivery, the parents also appreciate this quiet time together. Needs for information or support vary during this time, and care must be individualized. People of various cultural backgrounds respond differently during the immediate postdelivery period. In some cultures, the mothers' female relatives assume the major supportive role during childbirth and thus want to be with her after delivery. The extent of the father's involvement can vary considerably even among families in which fathers have a significant part in the childbearing pro-

cess. Flexible policies in hospitals permit the nurse to respond individually to these different cultural practices and family structures.

Ongoing Postpartum Care

The daily routine procedures for the postpartum client vary in different hospitals, but the principles of care are essentially the same.

Assessment

Physiological assessment continues during the postpartum period as reproductive organs undergo involution and lactation is either instituted or suppressed. Psychosocial assessment focuses upon family interactions and mother–infant interactions, particularly the development of mothering relations and skills and integration of the infant into the family.

Certain observations should be made and recorded daily. These would include such findings as temperature, pulse, and respiration; urinary and intestinal elimination; and the physical changes that occur normally in the puerperium. One should note the changes in the breasts; the height and consistency of the fundus; the character, amount, and color of the lochial discharge; and the condition of the perineum and episiotomy. It is equally important for the nurse to be alert to the mother's general comfort and well-being: how she rests and sleeps, her activity, her appetite, her emotional status, and particularly, because of its vast influence, how she is adjusting to her role as a new mother.

Temperature, Pulse, and Respiration

The temperature is carefully observed during the first few days of the puerperium, since fever is usually the first symptom of an infectious process. The pulse rate provides a helpful guide in determining the significance of a rise in temperature. These observations are usually made and recorded every 4 to 8 hours for the first few days after delivery, omitting the 2 AM observations, which would disturb the mother's sleep.

Temperatures up to 38°C (100.4°F) can be due to dehydration in the first 24 hours after delivery, to the onset of lactation or breast engorgement, or to normal postpartum leukocytosis. Persistent or recurring fever higher than this may signify infection, especially if other signs are present. A rapid, thready pulse (above 100) and hypotension could signify hemorrhage, shock, or embolization. However, postpartum clients can experience orthostatic hypotension because their cardiovascular system has not yet readjusted to its nonpregnant

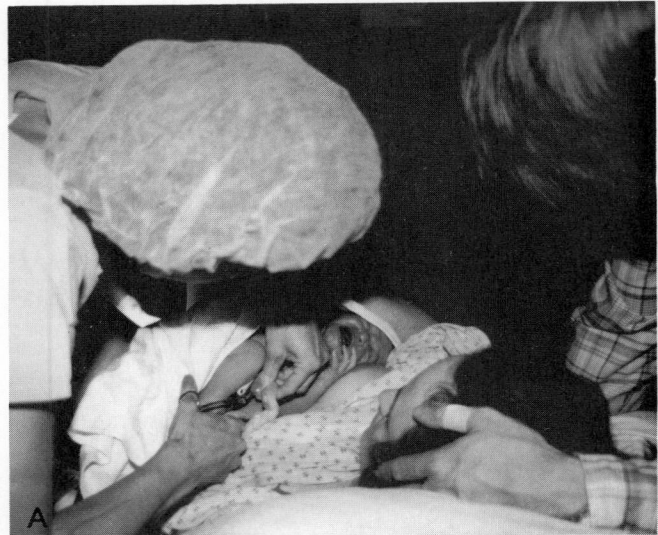

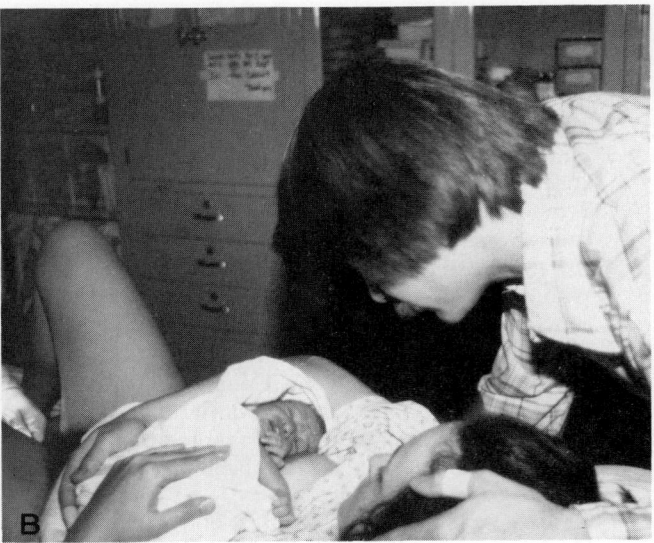

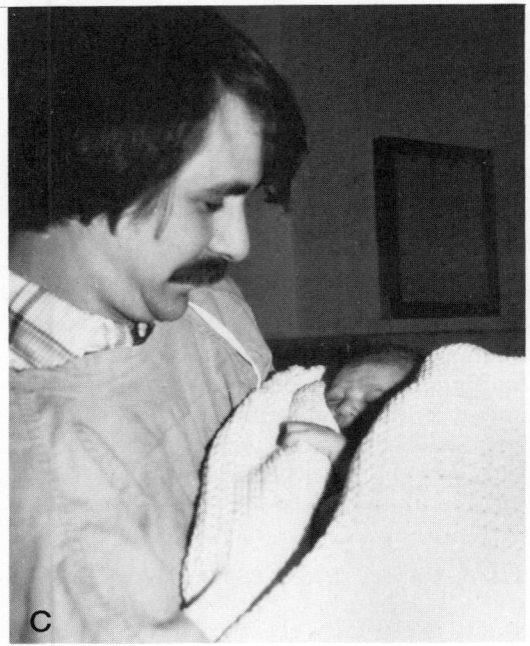

F I G U R E   3 1 - 1

Parents should be given the opportunity to hold the infant soon after birth. (*A*) The naked newborn is placed on the mother's abdomen while the midwife cuts the cord. (*B*) Wrapped with a blanket for warmth the newborn remains on the mother's abdomen while the placenta is delivered, and the parents can begin their bonding. (*C*) After the baby has had its initial assessment, the father holds the baby. (Courtesy of Booth Maternity Center, Philadelphia)

state. Elevated blood pressure may indicate preeclampsia, which can develop up to 72 hours after delivery.[3] Blood pressure is checked every 4 to 8 hours until stable, then daily unless problems are present.

Involution

Careful daily measurements show that the uterus diminishes in size (Fig. 31-2), and by about 10 days it cannot be detected by abdominal palpation.

The approximate rate of decrease in the height of the fundus is a little over a centimeter (½ in) or 1 fingerbreadth a day. Observation of this rate of involution is very important; the physician should be kept informed

about any marked delay, especially if it is accompanied by suppression of the lochia or retention of clots. In measuring the height of the uterus, care should be taken that the observations are made after the bladder is emptied, because a full bladder raises the height of the fundus.

The following are indications that the involution is not occurring satisfactorily:

- The uterus fails to decrease progressively in size
- The uterus remains poorly contracted (flabby)
- Pelvic discomfort or backache persist
- Bleeding remains heavy (see Subinvolution in Chap. 40)

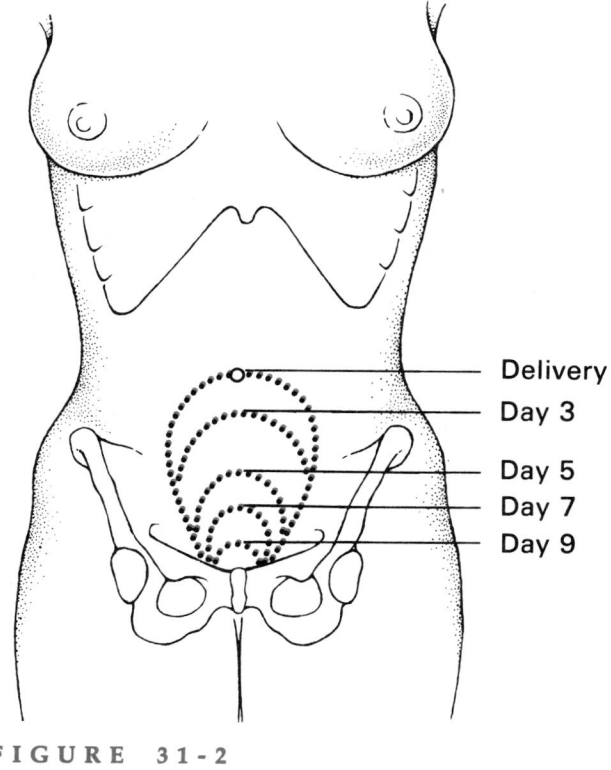

FIGURE 31-2

Involution of the uterus.

Lochia

The quantity of lochia varies with individuals, but generally it is more profuse in multiparas. It is to be expected that when a mother is out of bed for the first time there

TABLE 31-1

Characteristics of Lochia

Rubra	Serosa	Alba
Bright red, bloody, may have small clots	Pink to pink brown, serous, no clots	Cream to yellowish, may be brownish
Characteristic fleshy odor (animallike scent)	Usually no odor (unless poor hygiene)	Usually no odor (unless poor hygiene)
1–3 days post partum	5–7 days post partum	1–3 weeks post partum
Heavy to moderate flow	Decrease in flow	Scant flow

may be a definite increase in the amount of discharge. *Nevertheless, the recurrence of fresh bleeding after the discharge has become dark and diminished in amount, or the persistence of bright blood in the lochia, or the suppression of the discharge should be reported to the physician.* The daily observation of the amount and the character of the lochia is of the greatest importance as an index of the progress of healing of the endometrial surface. To accurately assess the volume of lochia, a standard for measurement is needed.[4] Such standards are given in Table 31-1 and Figure 31-3.

Lochia smells similar to normal menstrual flow and should not have a foul odor. Heavy, persistent, and malodorous lochia rubra, especially if accompanied by

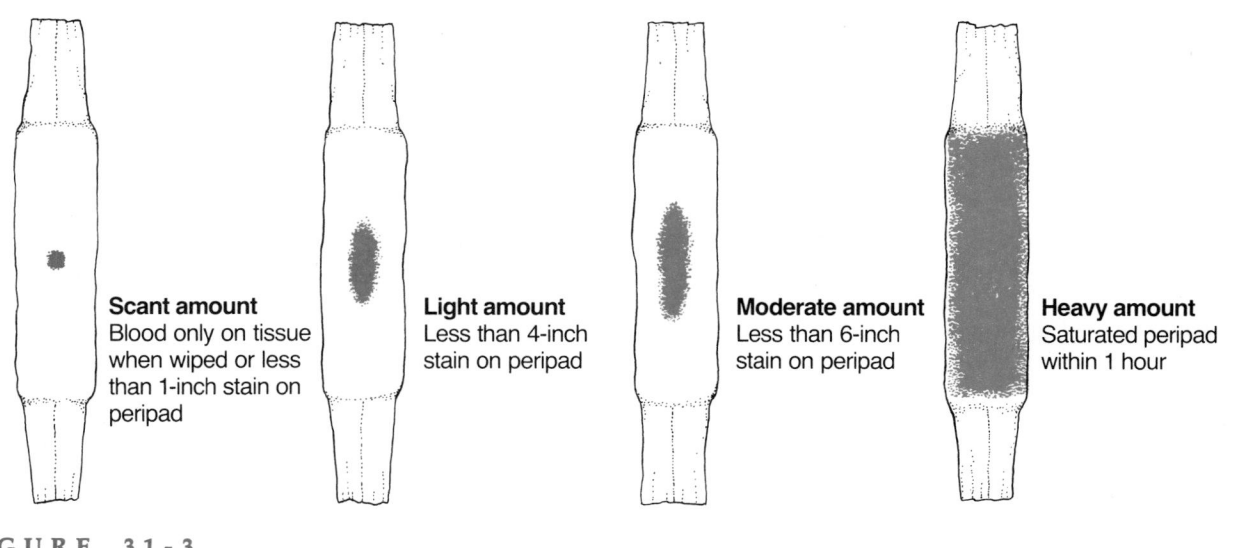

Scant amount
Blood only on tissue when wiped or less than 1-inch stain on peripad

Light amount
Less than 4-inch stain on peripad

Moderate amount
Less than 6-inch stain on peripad

Heavy amount
Saturated peripad within 1 hour

FIGURE 31-3

Assessing the volume of lochia by peripad saturation.

fever, indicates a potential infection or retained placental fragments. A sudden gush of lochia as the client first gets out of bed is normal; however, the fundus should be assessed for contraction. Persistent lochia serosa or alba, beyond normal time ranges, may indicate endometritis, particularly when the discharge is brown, malodorous, and accompanied by fever or abdominal pain.

Urinary Assessment

The newly delivered mother may not express a desire to void, in part because the bladder capacity is increased as a result of reduced intraabdominal pressure. In addition, if the mother has received analgesia or anesthesia during labor, the sensation of a full bladder may be further diminished. The mother should be encouraged to void within the first 6 to 8 hours following the delivery.

Bladder Distention.   The nurse should rely on assessment indicating the degree of bladder distention. It is important to keep in mind that there is an increased urinary output during the early puerperium. Mothers who have received intravenous fluids are very likely to develop a full bladder. As the bladder fills with urine, it gradually protrudes above the symphysis pubis and can be observed bulging in front of the uterus (Fig. 31-4). If the bladder is markedly distended, the uterus may be pushed upward and to the side and may become relaxed. When a hand is cupped over the fundus to massage it and to bring the uterus back to its midline position, the bladder protrudes farther. When the hand is removed, the uterus returns to its displaced position.

Further evidence of bladder distention can be gained by palpation and percussion of the lower abdomen, which reveals a difference in consistency between the uterus and the bladder. The latter is ballotable and filled with liquid in contrast to the uterus, which has a firm tone. Such observations are of extreme importance and demand immediate attention.

A full bladder is one cause of postpartum hemorrhage, and if the bladder is permitted to become distended, urinary retention will inevitably follow.

Perineum

Observations of the condition of the vagina, perineum, and perianal area are made regularly. The perineum is observed for healing and signs of complications, such as hematoma, bruising, swelling, and tenderness. If an episiotomy has been done, the status of the stitches is assessed, particularly for infection and hematoma. The anal area is inspected for hemorrhoids and fissures.

Following a spontaneous vaginal delivery without laceration, mothers usually do not experience perineal discomfort. It is most likely to be present if an episiotomy has been performed or if lacerations have been repaired, particularly if the perineum is edematous and there is tension on the perineal sutures. Almost all primigravidas experience some degree of discomfort from an episiotomy, depending largely on the extent of the wound and the amount of suturing done.

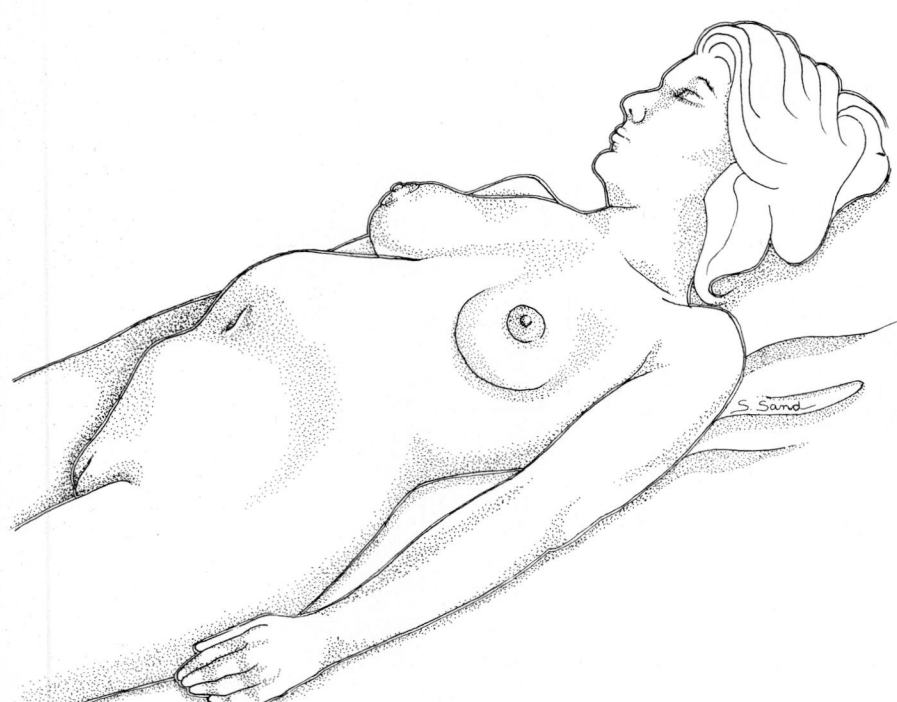

F I G U R E   3 1 - 4

Full bladder displacing uterine fundus. (Redrawn from Ruben D: De Lee's Obstetrics for Nurses, 18th ed. Philadelphia, WB Saunders, 1966)

Breast Engorgement

Breast discomfort several days after delivery that mothers experience in relation to initiation of lactation is termed engorgement. The mechanism underlying breast engorgement and its prevention and management are fully discussed in Chapters 29 and 35.

Nursing Diagnosis

Various needs or problems may be identified as a result of the nurse's assessments. Physiological complications such as hemorrhage, urinary retention, or hematomas may occur. Potentials for genital and breast infections, constipation, altered urinary elimination, and sleep disturbances may be present. Mothers often experience alterations in comfort, such as perineal pain, hemorrhoids, and engorged breasts. Knowledge deficits can occur in many areas, including infant care, nutritional requirements, self-care, adaptation to parenting, emotional changes, and household management (to name a few). Alterations in parenting can be related to inexperience, feeling incompetent, disappointment or conflict related to the child, or a sense of powerlessness. The new mother may have a disturbance in self-concept related to body changes persisting after delivery (*i.e.*, weight gain, lack of muscle or skin tone).

Planning/Intervention

Based on the assessment and diagnosis, plans are made to alleviate the problem and nursing interventions are carried out. Interventions can include providing direct care, teaching, supporting the mother in carrying out self-care and infant care, providing a supportive and health-promoting environment, coordinating care, and making referrals for other medical or social services.

Goals of Postpartum Nursing Care

- Promote normal involution
- Prevent or minimize complications
- Promote comfort and healing
- Assist in restoration of normal body functions
- Increase client understanding of physiological and emotional changes
- Support self-care
- Promote family adaptation and integration of the infant
- Support parenting abilities and parent–infant relationships

Nursing Guidelines for Care in Bladder Distention

Step One

Communicate with the client about the distended bladder, and assess urge to void. Provide support for spontaneous voiding:
1. Assist client to ambulate to bathroom.
2. Run water in sink.
3. Have client dip fingers in warm water or drink warm beverage.
4. Position client comfortably on bedpan (if unable to ambulate).
5. Pour warm water over perineum.
If the client empties the bladder completely (voids at least 100 ml and bladder feels empty by palpation), teach the importance of voiding every 3 to 4 hours.

Step Two

If the client is unable to void spontaneously or does not empty the bladder completely, assess perineal discomfort. If this is a factor:
1. Employ comfort measures (ice pack to perineum, moist heat, reposition peripad).
2. Administer analgesic medication as ordered.
Wait a suitable amount of time and have the client try to void again spontaneously.

Step Three

If the client is still unable to void or does not empty the bladder completely, then:
1. Use intermittent catheterization to empty the bladder completely, measure urine, and note color and characteristics.
2. Use indwelling catheter (per physician's order) if client has repeated urinary retention and measures to encourage spontaneous voiding are consistently unsuccessful.

Bladder Distention

Because bladder distention can create a serious problem, the nurse is responsible for careful management, involving nursing assessment and intervention and implementing medical treatments as designated in the chart Nursing Guidelines for Care in Bladder Distention.

Voiding. Some mothers have difficulty in voiding at first. As a result of the labor itself, the tone of the bladder wall may be temporarily impaired, or the tissues at the base of the bladder and around the urethra may be edematous. When the mother is able to go to the bathroom early, urinary elimination may present no problem. On the other hand, some efforts may be needed to stimulate normal urination. Running water so that the mother can hear it, letting the mother dabble her fingers in warm water, or offering a warm beverage may help to initiate voiding.

If the mother must be on bed rest, the nurse can facilitate voiding by helping her assume a comfortable position on the bedpan, providing privacy and giving her assurance that she will soon be able to urinate. The nurse should offer the mother a bedpan at 2- to 3-hour intervals, and measure the urine at each voiding during the first day (or days) until the mother is emptying her bladder completely. A voiding must measure 100 ml to be considered satisfactory.

At the first voiding, the bladder may not be entirely emptied. If the bladder is not distended, the mother is allowed to wait for an hour or so; the second voiding usually empties the bladder. If, however, the mother continues to void small amounts frequently, the nurse may suspect that there is residual urine and these voidings are the result of the overflow of a distended bladder. If all attempts fail and the mother cannot void a sufficient quantity, catheterization is necessary. Because of the risk of hospital-induced infection, it is very important to avoid this procedure unless the mother is absolutely unable to void despite astute and persistent nursing intervention.

Catheterization.   Although the procedure for catheterization varies to some degree in different hospitals, the principles involved are essentially the same. Aseptic technique must be maintained throughout to avoid introducing bacteria into the bladder or contaminating the birth canal. If the mother is given routine perineal care prior to the catheterization procedure, the potential danger of infection is further reduced.

Because there is a certain amount of soreness of the external genitalia, it is important to proceed with extreme gentleness and convey an awareness of the additional tenderness. As the labia are separated to expose the vestibule, care should be exercised so as not to pull on the perineal sutures. The meatus may be difficult to locate owing to the edema and consequent distortion of the tissues; therefore, a good light is imperative.

The urinary meatus and surrounding area are cleansed prior to the insertion of the catheter. The cleansing procedure is carried out in a gentle manner with just enough friction to allow proper cleansing of the area. None of the cleansing solution is permitted to run into the vaginal orifice because of the danger of contaminating the birth canal. Immediately following the cleansing, a dry cotton ball can be placed at the introitus to prevent excretion from the vagina (*i.e.,* blood or lochia) from spreading upward to the urinary meatus, from which it can be carried into the bladder when the catheter is inserted.

A small gauge flexible catheter is then gently inserted until urine flow begins. The catheter is held in

---

CLIENT EDUCATION

Perineal Care

1. The perineal pad is removed from front to back, to avoid dragging microorganisms from the rectum across the vaginal opening and perineum.
2. The perineal area is flushed with warm water or a mild antiseptic solution, using a pitcher, squeeze bottle, or applicator such as the surgitator.
3. The perineal area is patted dry with clean paper wipes (using a wiping motion should be avoided to provide comfort and to prevent contamination).
4. A fresh perineal pad is applied, again using a front to back motion, and secured with a belt to prevent its moving back and forth between the rectum and vaginal opening.

---

place until the flow of urine stops and then is carefully withdrawn. The urine is measured, and its color and character are noted. Specimens are sent for examination if indicated.

Intermittent catheterization is preferred to an indwelling catheter for postpartum women with continuing urinary retention. Even though any catheterization presents the risk of introducing infection, the risk is less with careful aseptic technique in intermittent catheterization than with a closed-system indwelling catheter. If an indwelling catheter is used, it is usually removed in 48 hours and a urine specimen is sent for culture and sensitivity. An antibiotic may be ordered and continued for 7 to 10 days, after which the urine is recultured. Indwelling catheters should be used for the shortest possible time.

Perineal Care

Self-care.   Usually some method of perineal cleansing is used after voiding and defecation, with the client instructed in the method and the proper removal and application of perineal pads (see Perineal Care). Cotton balls, soap and water, or medicated wipes may be used, or a method may be used such as the surgitator, which directs a spray of solution onto the perineum while the client sits on the toilet (Fig. 31-5).

The woman is instructed to cleanse and wipe from front to back in one motion, to prevent contamination of the vagina and urinary meatus with fecal material. She should wash her hands before applying a perineal pad and should not touch the inner surface of the pad before applying it from front to back. Pads should also be removed with this motion.

Cold and Heat Therapy.   *Cold therapy* may be used immediately following delivery when there has been

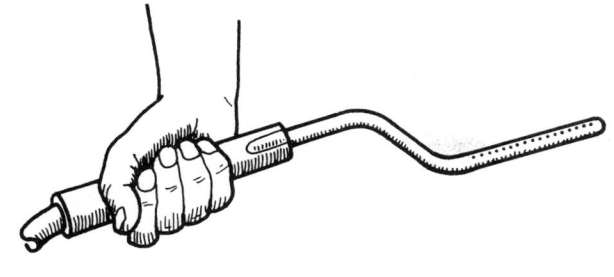

FIGURE 31-5

Surgitator for perineal care. With client seated on toilet, hold nozzle several inches from perineum, start flow, and direct against perineum. Do not touch nozzle to perineum; use a new nozzle for each client. Dry perineum with gentle front-to-back blotting motion.

significant perineal trauma or a large episiotomy. An ice pack is applied to the perineum to diminish edema and provide anesthesia. This is continued for several hours. *Moist heat therapy* is used after the woman has begun ambulating, to relieve discomfort and promote healing by increasing circulation to the perineum. Sitz baths are a common form of this therapy. The woman sits in a specially constructed tub in water maintained at 38°C to 43.2°C (100°F–110°F) two to three times per day for 20 minutes. The call bell should be within reach, and assistance should be provided to sit down and get up from the sitz bath tub. *Dry heat therapy* may be used also to promote comfort and healing. A lamp is positioned about 15 to 20 inches from the perineum while the woman is lying down and draped for privacy and warmth. The lamp is used for 20 minutes three times per day. At home, mothers can use a desk lamp with a 40-watt bulb, being careful to keep it at a comfortable distance from the perineum.

Medication.   Anesthetic sprays or ointments or witch hazel pads (Tucks) may be applied directly to sutured areas on the perineum. These relieve pain and promote comfort. Analgesic medications are sometimes needed when pain is severe. Women with extensive perineal repair may need medication every 4 hours for the first 1 or 2 postpartum days. If medications are needed, they should be given about 30 to 40 minutes before the infant's feeding period. This relieves the mother's pain and allows her to concentrate her energies and attention on the infant.

Sitting.   Mothers who have discomfort from perineal sutures usually find it uncomfortable to sit for the first few days. Many of them are observed sitting in a rigid position, bearing their weight on one side of the buttocks or the other, with obvious discomfort to the back as well as the perineum. Therefore, it is important to teach the mother how to sit comfortably with her body erect.

In the sitting position, the perineum is suspended at the lowermost level of the ischial tuberosities, which bear the weight of the body. Thus, to achieve a greater measure of comfort, the mother must bring her buttocks together to relieve pressure and tension on the perineum, in the same manner as that described in the exercise for contraction and relaxation of pelvic floor muscles (Kegel's exercises). After assuming a sitting position the mother is instructed to raise her hips very slightly from the chair, only enough to permit her to squeeze her buttocks together and contract the muscles of the pelvic floor, and to hold her muscles this way momentarily until after she has let her full weight down again. This exercise is also helpful to the mother when she is reclining in bed.

Breast Care

Routine breast care is directed at maintaining cleanliness and adequate breast support necessary for the normal function of the breasts and the comfort of the mother. The breasts should be handled gently and precautions taken to avoid rough rubbing, massage, or pressure on these organs.

If the mother is breast-feeding, her nipples may be cleansed with clear water. Under normal circumstances the best nipple care is provided by the body itself, without outside interference.[5] Further care of nipples and breasts in the breast-feeding mother is covered in Chapter 35.

The mother who is bottle-feeding her infant can bathe her breasts daily with mild soap and water; this is done most conveniently at the time of the daily shower or bath. No other special care need be given except that of breast support with a well-fitted brassiere. Usually these mothers are given some type of lactation-suppressing hormone to help the breasts dry up, and engorgement is not a problem. Occasionaly, however, they do suffer this phenomenon and may experience throbbing pains in the breasts that extend back into the axillae. During this time, analgesic medication may be required for pain relief until the condition subsides in 1 or 2 days. Ice bags to the breasts and axillae also are often helpful.

Other Postpartum Concerns

Nutrition.   Very shortly following the delivery, after having gone without food or fluids for some hours, the mother may express a desire for something to eat. Unless she has received a general anesthetic or is nauseated, there is usually no contraindication to giving her some nourishment. She usually enjoys a normal diet.

The two factors to bear in mind when considering the mother's diet are as follows: (1) providing for her general nutrition and (2) providing enough nourishing

604 UNIT VI: Assessment and Management in the Postpartum Period

foods to supply the additional calories and nutrients required during lactation. If these nutritional requirements are provided for, the mother's convalescence is more rapid, her strength is recovered more quickly, and the quality and quantity of her milk is better. She is also more able to resist infections.

Intervention. Mothers in general, and particularly mothers who are breast-feeding, usually have good appetites and become hungry between meals. For this reason it is advisable to see that they receive a nourishing beverage or a snack three times a day. If the nourishment is in the form of a glass of milk or some milk product, this helps to incorporate the additional milk requirement for the nursing mother (see Chap. 35).

Rest and Sleep. During the puerperium the mother needs an abundance of rest and can be encouraged to relax and sleep whenever possible. This can best be accomplished if she is comfortable and free from worry and other anxiety-producing situations. The need for rest has even more significance for the mother who is breast-feeding, because worry and fatigue inhibit her milk supply. With the exception of the father, visitors should be limited during the first few days because they can be tiring. A mother who is not getting sufficient rest is usually anxious and worries over minor things that otherwise might cause her little concern. Furthermore, many emotional problems are often precipitated by sleeplessness and fatigue.

Intervention. It becomes the nurse's responsibility to adjust the hospital routine whenever possible to provide the mother with uninterrupted periods of rest. Routine procedures can be delayed or rearranged to meet the mother's needs. A bottle-fed infant may be fed occasionally by the nurse if the mother is sleeping and does not want to be awakened. If the mother is unable to nap during the day (and she may not, due to excitement and fatigue), she can be encouraged to rest as quietly as possible for certain periods. The need for rest and sleep may have to be explained and reiterated, especially during the "taking-hold" phase, as she is eager to be up and about and may tend to overdo things.

Early Ambulation. Early ambulation has intrinsic health-promoting value for the newly delivered mother. With this increase in exercise, circulation is stimulated, and there are fewer complications of thrombophlebitis. Moreover, bladder and bowel functions are improved; therefore, bladder complications leading to catheterization are greatly reduced. Abdominal distention and constipation occur less frequently.

If the mother has had a conduction anesthesia that involves entering the dura, she may be kept in a recum-

bent position for about the first 8 hours. Many physicians feel that keeping the mother flat in bed for this time helps to prevent the occurrence of a postspinal headache, since headache is precipitated and aggravated when the head is elevated. Postspinal headache is thought to be caused by a leakage of the spinal fluid through the puncture hole of the dura, with subsequent decrease in cerebrospinal fluid volume and pressure. Therefore, having the client in a recumbent position while the puncture hole is sealing and encouraging her to force fluids (to hasten fluid replacement) may help this condition. The majority of healthy mothers are encouraged to be out of bed in 4 to 8 hours.

The first time that any mother is out of bed she can "dangle" for a short time before actually getting up. Then usually she can walk a few steps from the bed and sit in a chair for a brief period. On succeeding times up, she can increase her activity gradually. The newly delivered mother needs someone to assist her in and out of bed and to go with her when she walks to the bathroom. The nurse should remain close at hand while the mother is in the bathroom so that she can give immediate assistance if the mother becomes weak or faint.

It is important that the nurse explain the purposes of early ambulation to the mother and help her to learn how she can achieve an effective combination of sitting, walking, and lying in bed.

Bathing. The mother is prone to have marked diaphoresis in the early puerperium, so that a daily shower is refreshing and a source of comfort. When the mother showers for the first time, the nurse usually gives the self-care instructions for breast care, perineal care, and other aspects of physical care. The nurse is guided by the mother's readiness to learn as well as by the realization that the mother can absorb only so much information at one time. As the mother is able to absorb the information, the nurse can explain about breast care, perineal hygiene, elimination, general activity, and hospital routines.

Showers usually are permitted as soon as the client becomes ambulatory. The first time or two that the mother takes a shower, the nurse or the attendant should remain nearby for safety. Tub baths usually are allowed in 2 weeks.

Intestinal Elimination

Constipation. Because the bowel tends to remain relaxed in the early puerperium (as in pregnancy), intestinal elimination may be a problem. In view of the sluggishness of the bowels during this time, constipation can be anticipated unless measures are instituted to prevent it. It is common to give a stool softener each night after delivery or a laxative on the evening of the first or second day following delivery. If a bowel evacuation has not occurred by the morning of the second or third day, a cleansing enema or a suppository may be prescribed. The latter is very effective and less traumatic for most clients.

If there has been no elimination and especially if the mother has had extensive perineal repair done, an oil retention enema, followed some hours later by a cleansing enema, sometimes is prescribed.

The mother who is breast-feeding is advised to follow her physician's prescription if laxatives are required to encourage proper elimination after she is discharged from the hospital. Certain laxatives are excreted in breast milk and therefore affect the infant (see Chap. 35). In addition, the usual measures employed to encourage good bowel habits (*i.e.,* adequate fluid intake, roughage foods in the diet, establishing a habit time, and so on) are to be included in the health teaching. Prevention of constipation is discussed in Chapter 22.

Hemorrhoids. Hemorrhoids are a common problem for women during the postpartum period, as a result of pressure extered on the pelvic floor by the presenting part and the straining of the expulsive phase of labor. They are most painful during the first 2 to 3 days after delivery, then gradually reduce in size and regress. Painful hemorrhoids are treated with sitz baths, anes-

thetic sprays, and cool astringent compresses (such as witch hazel or Tucks). Comfort is promoted by wearing perineal pads loosely and lying on the side in Sims's position while in bed. Prevention of constipation is the main measure to relieve ongoing difficulties with hemorrhoids.

Lower Extremities. The lower extremities are observed for varicosities, symmetry, edema, shape, size, temperature and color, and range of motion. Signs of thrombophlebitis include unilateral swelling, erythema, tenderness, and pain in the calf when the foot is flexed with the leg extended (*Homan's sign*) (Fig. 31-6). Pulses in the lower extremities may be absent in thrombophlebitis. The mother is advised to avoid constricting garters or clothing that interferes with circulation.

Afterpains. Uterine contractions following delivery continue as part of involution and in some instances are felt as cramps similar to that of a menstrual period. Intermittent uterine contractions with subsequent afterpains occur more frequently in multiparas than in primiparas, because in primiparas the uterus remains tonically contracted. Afterpains are also more common and severe when there has been excessive distention of the uterus due to a large baby, hydramnios, or multiple

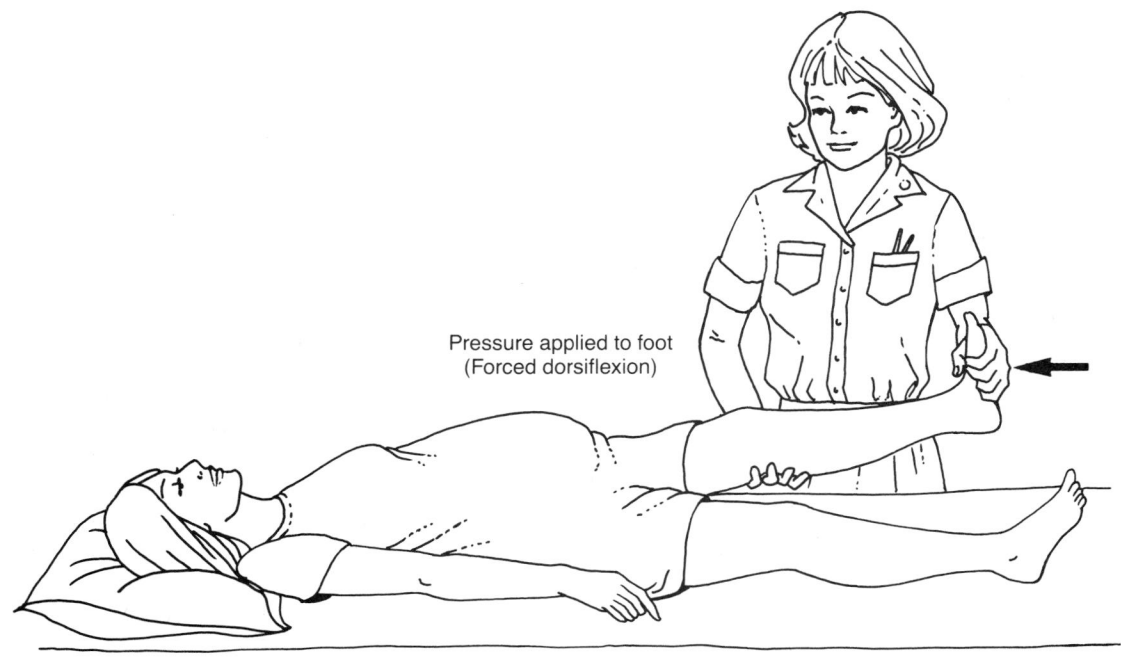

Pressure applied to foot
(Forced dorsiflexion)

Pain experienced behind calf
or in calf when thrombosis is present

FIGURE 31-6

Homan's sign—method to identify presence of thrombosis in the calf.

pregnancy. Breast-feeding mothers notice afterpains occurring when the infant nurses, because suckling stimulates release of oxytocin, which increases uterine contractions. These cramps gradually diminish and are usually quite mild within 48 hours of delivery. Often simply explaining the cause of afterpains and their functional purpose enables the mother to tolerate them. If afterpains are severe, an analgesic is usually ordered to provide relief.

Postpartum Depression ("Blues").   Many mothers experience a transitory depression beginning the second or third day after birth. Severe depressive psychosis occurs in only 1% to 2% of all normal childbirths. Symptoms of transitory depression include crying easily, feelings of despondency, loss of appetite, poor concentration, difficulty sleeping, feeling let down, and anxiety. These usually disappear within 1 to 2 weeks, although some women remain mildly depressed much longer. Causes of postpartum blues are discussed in Chapter 30.

Intervention.   Mild postpartum blues usually respond to empathy, support, and acceptance by the nurse. The nurse can provide opportunities for the mother to express her anxiety, despondent feelings, and other concerns. Sharing these with an empathetic listener is often therapeutic in itself. Helping the mother put her responses in perspective and understand that this is a common experience can help alleviate her concerns about having an inappropriate or abnormal reaction to childbirth. It is also helpful to encourage adequate rest and nutrition and to assist the mother to be successful in early mothering tasks. Seldom are psychotropic drugs necessary in transitory depression. However, persistent and severe depression requires psychotherapy.

Postpartum Exercises

Exercises may be initiated postpartally to hasten recovery, prevent complications, and strengthen the muscles of the back, pelvic floor, and abdomen. By toning the muscles, these exercises assist the mother to restore her figure and can be psychologically beneficial. Exercises can be started on the first postpartum day and increased gradually. The mother must take care not to overexercise and to allow slow progression in adding to the routine. A new exercise can be added daily, with each done five to ten times per day for at least 6 weeks after delivery (see Appendix A for postpartum exercises).

Kegel's exercises can be taught to increase vaginal tone, which may be flaccid and distended following delivery. This exercise consists of contracting the muscles of the perineum with enough force to stop a stream of urine. The contraction is held for a few seconds and

then released. The exercise is repeated 50 to 100 times and can be done several times per day. Kegel's exercises facilitate perineal healing and help restore muscle tone by increasing circulation and through isometric muscle activity. The pubococcygeal muscle is strengthened, which helps prevent urinary stress incontinence and pelvic relaxation and enhances orgasmic capacity.

Parental Guidance and Instruction

Each mother's understanding and ability in providing infant care varies, depending largely on her background and previous experiences. Undoubtedly, the primipara who has not been accustomed to infants has much to learn about the care and handling of her new baby. On the other hand, the multipara may feel uncertain about the response of an older child to the new baby and thus require guidance in understanding and dealing with sibling rivalry. Many mothers need to know more about their own care; others need to know how to facilitate certain adjustments within the home or the family group. If the mother knows what she can expect and what to do, she usually can handle simple problems that might otherwise cause fear or apprehension.

Proper care for the mother during the puerperium emphasizes the need for rest and nourishing food and protection from worry. Parents, as a rule, seem to be under the impression that once the delivery is over, things return to "normal," allowing them to resume their usual activities immediately. However, it takes several weeks before the generative organs have returned to normal size and position and the emotional and endocrine adjustments are made. (Postpartum teaching is further discussed in Chap. 20.)

Help with the Household.   One of the most important points to be emphasized is that the mother should proceed *as slowly as possible* in the postpartum period at home. The general feeling of well-being and the excitement of having the baby, together with the emotions aroused in the taking-hold phase, provide such an intense stimulus that the mother has a tendency to overdo things.

If possible, the major responsibilities of housekeeping should be taken over by a "helper," so that the mother can be more relaxed and devote herself primarily to caring for her new infant and spending more time with the immediate family. Family relationships can be strengthened if the mother is not overwhelmed with apprehension and fatigue. The subject of household assistance needs to be explored thoroughly with the mother (and if necessary, the father).

Resources.   By discharge, the mother should have at least a basic understanding of her own condition and know what physical and emotional changes to expect. In addition, she should be familiar with the daily care of her baby and know infant behavior and other important details related to infant care. Parents also need to know how and where to contact the physician if any medical problem of the mother or the infant should arise before the next scheduled visit.

Since the maternity stay is rather short, follow-up service often is desirable. Parents need information about the public-health nursing agency in the community and how they may use these services. In cases of obvious need, a referral to an agency should be instituted before the client leaves the hospital.

Individual Teaching. Each mother should be given individual help to learn how to handle and care for her infant while she is in the hospital, particularly if this is her first baby. Many new mothers are timid at first because they do not know what to expect of their infants, or they are afraid of harming them because of their own feelings of inadequacy. A mother who has had no previous experience with infants needs some guided practice in changing diapers, dressing her baby, and handling the infant. Rooming-in units provide an environment in which the mother can have such an experience over an extended period of time. However, even in situations in which the infants are kept in a central nursery, the nurse should plan to spend some time with the mother, in addition to the regular feeding periods, to help her learn to care for her baby. Demonstration of the infant bath by the nurse, in the client's room, is often an important step in the mother's gaining infant care skills. Providing the mother with written brochures on infant care is another effective way of offering information that can be used at a time when she is more receptive and feels the need directly.

Sexuality and Contraception. Postpartum sexuality is affected by the degree to which the mother's steroid hormones have been depleted following delivery. This is discussed more fully in Chapter 13. Postpartum instructions are given regarding resumption of intercourse, with the couple advised that sex is appropriate after lochia has ceased and the perineum has healed to the point that intercourse is not painful, and as long as there are no contraindicating factors such as hematoma or infection.

Sexual adjustment following birth of a baby is a major concern of new parents, and it is often a source of conflict and confusion. The mothers' interest in intercourse is usually less than her partner's in the first month or so after delivery, and her physiological responses diminish[6] because of low hormonal levels, the adjustment to the maternal role, and fatigue due to lack of sleep and rest. Lochia has generally ceased or progressed to the alba stage by 2 to 4 weeks post partum,

and the perineal area and episiotomy are well healed and not painful. If intercourse causes discomfort, the couple is advised to wait somewhat longer or use noncoital sexual practices if they find this acceptable. Positions for intercourse that avoid the penile shaft pressing posteriorly on the perineum can also alleviate discomfort. In addition to the emotional benefits to the parents' relationship, intercourse after childbirth can promote perineal healing by softening the episiotomy scar.[7]

For most couples, intercourse is resumed before the 6-week checkup, so it is important to provide contraceptive information before the mother leaves the hospital. Although it is unlikely that she will ovulate and become fertile before 6 weeks, it is possible. Menses usually resume by about 9 weeks in the nonlactating woman and by 30 weeks to 36 weeks in the lactating woman. However, the time of return of fertility is unpredictable, and all postpartum women are counseled to use contraception if they desire to avoid pregnancy (see Chaps. 14 and 29). Many hospitals provide a supply of contraceptive vaginal cream and condoms and nurses instruct the parents on their use before discharge.

Evaluation and Discharge

Most mothers are discharged home on the second day (or after 24 hours in some hospitals, when mother and infant are considered low risk). Regardless of the day of discharge, mothers need to be cautioned to proceed slowly at home during the puerperium, resting a large part of the time. If teaching about "getting back to routine gradually" was begun early in the antepartal period, the mother is better prepared during the puerperium.

The condition of the mother is confirmed before she is discharged from the hospital to make sure that her progress has been satisfactory during the early puerperium. In addition to verifying her vital signs and

---

Nursing Guidelines for Discharge Planning

- Assistance with household tasks and functions
- Equipment and supplies for mother and baby
- Adjustments during the first few weeks at home
- Continuing maternal needs for rest, nutrition, and recovery
- Sibling relations and rivalry
- Self-care at home
- Review of prescribed medications
- Return of ovulation and menstruation
- Signs and symptoms of maternal complications
- Six-week checkup
- Community resources and referrals

present weight, observations are made to determine the condition of her breasts, the progress of involution, and the healing of the episiotomy. A pelvic examination is deferred, since findings made by palpation of the uterus and inspection of the lochia give satisfactory evidence as to the progress of involution at this time.

Early Postpartum Discharge

Low-risk mothers and infants may be discharged from the hospital as early as 6 to 24 hours after birth. Mothers interested in early discharge usually are concerned with optimal bonding, developing family relations with the new baby, privacy and comfort in self-care and infant care, and avoiding physical and emotional risks presented by the hospital environment. Other advantages include reduced hospital costs, early presence of extended family, and personalized feeding schedules.

Careful prenatal screening is used to be certain that the pregnancy and labor are low risk. In some programs, a prenatal home visit is made to determine that necessary supplies and equipment are available and to assess the home environment. Home-visit nurses may meet parents at prenatal office visits and assess suitability for early discharge. Public-health nurses or nurses employed by the maternity service or clinic are responsible for parent evaluation and home visits.

Following a normal pregnancy, labor, and delivery, the new mother and infant are carefully evaluated during the first several hours. Birth may take place in a hospital delivery suite or in an alternate birth center. Written protocols or guidelines are used to assess mother

---

Factors Related to Transition to Parenthood

Factors Contributing to Difficulty in the Transition to Parenthood in Contemporary United States Society

1. Minimal role preparation. Few American parents enter parenthood with sufficient previous childcare experience to give them a comfort level with care of their infant.
2. Limited role preparation during pregnancy. There is little opportunity to develop skills and make adjustments to ease transition to parenthood during pregnancy, when the focus of education is on childbearing.
3. Abruptness of transition. There is no gradual taking on of responsibility for the infant as there is in assuming a work role.
4. Lack of guidelines for successful parenthood. Childrearing advice can include general recommendations, but it is not possible to tell new parents exactly what they must do to achieve a specific end result with their infant.

Factors Positively Related to Adaptation to Motherhood in Women

1. The capacity to visualize oneself as a mother in the first and second trimesters of pregnancy
2. The personality characteristics of being high in nurturance and having ego strength
3. A retrospective recall of one's own mother as being warm, empathetic, close, and happy with her role
4. Having interest in and experience with children
5. The existence of a high-quality marital relationship
6. Physical health during pregnancy

Factors Positively Related to Adaptation to Fatherhood in Men

1. Previous experience with children
2. Enjoyment of taking care of young children in the past
3. Knowledge of baby care
4. Knowing the number of children desired before marriage
5. Knowing the number of children desired after baby's arrival
6. Planning this pregnancy

(After Jennings B, Edmundson M: The postpartum period: After confinement: The fourth trimester. Clin Obstet Gynecol 23(4):1093–1103, December 1980)

and infant. The mother's physical condition must be stable, including normal temperature and blood pressure, normal blood loss, ambulation without difficulty, and ability to completely empty the bladder. Fundus and perineum must be in normal postdelivery condition, without undue pain. Homan's sign is usually performed and must be negative.

The infant must be healthy, must weigh more than 2500 g, and must have normal cry and reflexes. A complete physical examination is done, which must be normal. Temperature, heart and respiratory rates, skin color, and condition of umbilical cord and circumcision (if done) must be in the normal range. Initial feeding is assessed, and the infant should be sucking well. Required laboratory tests (phenylketonuria, or PKU; bilirubin) are done before discharge.

A home visit by the nurse is scheduled for 1 to 2 days after discharge. Further assessment of mother, baby, and family takes place on this visit. Teaching about self-care and infant care, feeding, family adaptation, physical and emotional changes and needs, and birth control is included. The nurse identifies potential problems and takes appropriate preventive action, or institutes referrals. Further testing is reinforced, such as the second PKU test and thyroid screening. Additional home visits are made as needed.[8]

Early discharge programs are feasible when the family is well-prepared, both mother and infant are observed intensively in the postdelivery period, low-risk discharge criteria are followed carefully, skilled nurses provide home visits for assessment and teaching, and physician backup is available.[9] Problems must be identified early and action taken to prevent further complications. Skilled nurses can handle many common problems, particularly related to inadequate knowledge, comfort, and self- or infant-care needs. Only a small number of mothers and infants will need physician attention within the first several days of delivery, if careful prenatal screening for early postpartum discharge is carried out.

First Weeks at Home

The process of integration of a new baby into the family is a stressful period and one in which there is little professional help available. Many parents have no contact with health providers during the time between discharge from the hospital and the 6-week checkup, although they are contending with major changes and adjustments in what is often a new experience in their lives. In contrast to the cultural ideals of joyful parenthood and fantasies of blissful motherhood, many women find the first few weeks of their child's life to be extremely disillusioning.[10] The household is often disorganized and untidy, with greatly increased work related to diapers, feeding, and care of the new baby, while the mother copes with fatigue and frustration in trying to learn the baby's patterns and ways of communicating. Within the first 6 weeks, many mothers find that they have yelled at and spanked their infants, that they cannot cope with or understand the baby's crying, that they feel trapped spending the greatest part of their lives caring for the baby, and that they wish they had not had the baby because they feel unsuited for such responsibility.[11]

The concerns of new mothers in the first weeks after delivery cover a wide range, and there seem to be few resources to assist them in coping with problems and providing information and support. The most common concerns expressed by new mothers are in the following areas: changes in their figures, fatigue and lack of sleep, infant care, changing roles and life-styles, and nursing care.

Changes in Body Image

One of the most frequently expressed concerns of the postpartum period involves return of the figure to normal. This concern appears to be more than just a minor anxiety. Although new mothers are initially delighted when their abdomens decrease in size after delivery, this positive feeling turns to dismay in the days and weeks following, when the abdominal wall remains soft and flabby and part of the weight gained during pregnancy is retained, making it impossible to wear clothes that fit before pregnancy. Frequently, the mother feels as though she is still several months pregnant.

Although mothers may want to lose weight and tighten up muscles, they often find that the baby's demands and their own fatigue interfere with these attempts. A flabby postpartum figure and the feeling that one lacks the control or ability to improve it can be depressing.[12] Fathers, too, are often disappointed because of the time it takes for the figure to become slim again, and both partners may fear that the figure changes are permanent. Another source of concern is the lack of tone in the vaginal introitus, which carries many implications for the couple's sexual relationship.

The first few weeks at home can also be a time of continued physical discomfort, much to the woman's dismay, especially if she has anticipated a quick return to normal. Persistent discomforts—from episiotomy pain, which lasts about 2 to 3 weeks, breast engorgement, which is a source of discomfort for both breast-feeding and non-breast-feeding mothers, nipple soreness, and the annoyance of leaking milk—all are troubling in themselves and a drain on energy at a time when added strength is needed to respond to the infant's constant demands. The continued discharge of lochia may also be disconcerting, particularly if it is compared to a menstrual period.

Fatigue and Lack of Sleep

Fatigue appears to be a consistent problem for new mothers. Labor and delivery are hard, exhausting work, followed immediately by the demands of caring for a totally dependent infant. The short stay in the hospital is insufficient to restore energy levels, since excitement, the strange environment, and physical discomforts often interfere with rest and sleep. Most women have also not slept well during the last weeks of pregnancy. This leaves them with a tremendous deficit of energy and sleep, which increases sharply during the first weeks at home with the baby.

Sleep deprivation is to some degree a part of living for all new mothers, and it can be severe. The mother's sleep needs are curtailed by the baby's needs for food and attention. It may be difficult for new mothers to obtain more than 30 to 45 minutes of uninterrupted sleep per night, particularly if there are other small children who frequently need attention at night. Increased bodily tension as a result can lead to insomnia when there is the opportunity to sleep. Mothers may find themselves resenting their partner's ability to sleep uninterrupted. Sleep deprivation can also produce changes in mood and mental functioning, with the mother experiencing increased anxiety, apathy, depression, withdrawal, irritability, illogical thought patterns, mental confusion, and aggression and decreased sociability.[10]

Infant Care

Concerns about caretaking activities for the infant vary. Many primiparas have had little previous contact with infants and possess little knowledge of procedures and the common behaviors expected. Often care is learned by trial and error because there are few sources of expert advice. Infants are quite different in their patterns, so even multiparas may find that their prior experience does not apply to the new infant. Babies range from quiet to active and respond in different ways to attempts to console and comfort them. A new mother must learn her baby's particular patterns and why he cries and fusses at various times. The greatest part of this learning occurs during the first few weeks after birth, and the difficulty is compounded by such concerns and problems as fatigue, discomforts, and worries about restoration of the figure.

Mothers are concerned about how normal their infant's behaviors are, particularly in the areas of weight gain and loss, crying, bowel movements, feedings, and sleeping patterns.[13] There is little written information that can help identify "normal" ranges, and health professionals often do not discuss specific changes that may occur during the first months of life. Parents are often surprised at the range of behaviors among infants.

Conflicting advice regarding how frequently the baby should be fed, when to add solid food, when to pick up a crying baby, what clothes to put on the baby, who should be allowed to visit and when, and so forth, leads to further confusion.

The processes for successful mothering have apparently been set in motion by the end of the first month following birth. The way a mother perceives her 1-month-old infant is an indication of the child's subsequent growth and development and reflects the degree to which the mother is satisfied with her interaction with the infant. If she feels rewarded, she has a more positive perception of the infant and reinforcement of her own identity as a mother. This, in turn, fosters a nurturing relationship.[14] Clearly, nursing intervention before maternal perception is set should be aimed at increasing the mother's sense of mastery and satisfaction in infant care, thereby promoting healthier infant development.

Changing Roles and Life-styles

Few parents are prepared for the amount of change required in their roles, relationships, and life-styles as the infant is integrated into the family. Many parents may actually "grieve" over the passing of former life patterns. The mother particularly may have to make major changes in career and other activities, although the gratifications of motherhood may be enough to compensate for these relinquishments. Changes occur in the family constellation, with problems related to jealousy among the other children and marital problems between spouses arising from relative neglect of their relationship. With less time for each other, and possible strain in their sexual relations, many couples report stress in their relationship following the birth of a new baby. Social isolation, lack of recreational activities, and financial concerns can compound family stresses.

Nursing Intervention

The first few weeks at home represent a gap in health-care services. However, the nurse can provide anticipatory care during the prenatal period and during the hospital stay post-partally. During the third trimester the expectant mother has increased interest in caretaking activities, so that teaching related to infant behavior and infant care can be productive at this time. The nurse can include such topics as preparing other children for the new baby, exploring ways to meet the increased demands of a new baby for attention and continuous care, and considering sources of potential stress to the marital and family relations and ways of coping with these problems.

Reinforcing the importance of help with household tasks during the first few postpartum weeks at home may encourage the mother to make arrangements. This can help to alleviate fatigue and sleep deprivation. Knowing that she will need time to regain her energy levels will help the mother to be more realistic in her expectations. Also knowing that her figure will take time to return to its prepregnant form and that physical discomforts will exist for a time after delivery will prepare the parents and reduce stress from unrealistic expectations.

Mothers can be assisted to recognize and respond appropriately to their baby's unique patterns and ways of communicating and to identify various states of consciousness of the infant and its particular needs for stimulation, sleep, and feeding. When able to respond more smoothly to her infant, the mother's satisfactions are increased and the development of a healthy relationship is encouraged.[14]

Community-health nurses may be available to visit new mothers and provide teaching and support during the first few weeks at home. For many mothers, however, there is no clearly identifiable resource and they are often reluctant to call the hospital or physician's office with their concerns. Providing professional contact by telephone as part of postdischarge care would be helpful. Parental guidance and instruction were discussed in a previous section. Various methods and groups for postpartum teaching were referred to in Chapter 20.

Six-Week Checkup

The reproductive tract should return to its nonpregnant condition within 6 to 8 weeks after delivery. To assess the general physical condition of the mother, determine the progress of the involutional process, and evaluate the woman's and family's adaptation to the new baby, a follow-up visit in the physician's office or clinic is usually scheduled for 6 weeks after delivery. A postpartum visit may be scheduled at 2 to 4 weeks for early evaluation as indicated by the mother's condition.

Assessment

During the visit the weight and the blood pressure are taken and a urinalysis and a complete blood count may be done. The condition of the abdominal walls is observed, and the breasts are inspected. If the mother is breast-feeding, the condition of the nipples and the degree of lacteal secretion are a significant part of the observation. If the mother is not breast-feeding, the breasts should be observed to see that physiological readjustments have occurred.

Content of the 6-Week Postdelivery Checkup

Vital signs and weight

Perineal examination
    Amount and character of lochia
    Condition of episiotomy or lacerations
    Condition of anus, hemorrhoids

Pelvic examination
    Size and position of uterus and cervix
    Condition of vagina (musculature, lacerations)
    Pap smear

Breast examination
    Condition of breasts and nipples
    Whether lactating or not

Growth and development of baby
    Infant behavior
    Patterns of feeding, sleep, and elimination
    Crying
    Weight gain

Family response to new baby
    Father's response and involvement in care
    Reactions of siblings
    Relatives' and friends' visits or assistance
    Mother's response to caretaking, feeding, and reactions of others

Mother's physical condition and recovery
    Rest and exercise
    Weight loss
    Diet
    Energy level
    Recreation and activities
    Returning to work
    Physical discomforts and remedies

Sexual relations
    Resumption of intercourse
    Concerns or difficulties
    Responses of father
    Responses of mother

Contraception
    Current contraceptive practice (if any)
    Desires for regulating fertility and family planning
    Contraceptive methods and selection of best-suited method for couple

---

A thorough pelvic examination is carried out to investigate the position of the uterus, the healing of the episiotomy or perineal lacerations, the support of the pelvic floor, and whether involution is complete. The presence, amount, and character of lochia are assessed. The family's response to the new baby is discussed, and questions related to behavior, patterns of feeding, sleep and elimination, crying, weight gain, and so forth are explored (see Nursing Care Plan: The Woman Receiving Postpartum Care).

(text continued on page 614)

The Woman Receiving Postpartum Care

Nursing Objectives

1. Assist in bringing about involution and effective restoration of nonpregnant body functions.
2. Provide early detection of complications and prevent complications.
3. Promote comfort and healing of pelvic, perineal, and perianal tissues.
4. Guide in appropriate balance of rest and activity.
5. Assist in appropriate nourishment for lactation and restorative needs.
6. Give pertinent and timely education for mother and family to promote recovery, self-care, infant care, and family adaptation.
7. Provide effective discharge planning with coordination and referral to community-health resources.

Assessment	Potential Nursing Diagnosis	Planning/Intervention	Evaluation
Postdelivery observations			
Fundal checks Bleeding Status of bladder Vital signs Condition of perineum	Potential for injury: hemorrhage, uterine atony, hematoma, retained placental fragments, lacerations, urinary retention related to childbirth trauma Alteration in comfort: pain related to perineal trauma, uterine involution, muscular effort in labor	Give gentle massage of fundus if boggy Express clots from fundus Report and record amount and character of bleeding Report and record increase in pulse rate or decrease in blood pressure and elevation of temperature Encourage voiding if bladder becomes filled; catheterize if distended and unable to void Report development of hematoma or bleeding from episiotomy	Mother maintains a well contracted fundus Mother bleeds normal amount without clots Mother maintains stable vital signs Mother empties bladder as needed
Family interactions			
Comfort and rest Mother–infant contact Contact with partner or companion	Alteration in parenting related to disappointment with infant, unwanted child, separation from infant, lack of partner involvement, postdelivery pain or complications	Provide comfort measures (position, keep clean and dry, provide fluids as appropriate, encourage rest by doing observations efficiently) Enable mother to hold and explore infant if condition permits Enable partner or companion to visit mother and infant Respond to questions about labor and delivery, status of infant, postpartum status	Mother rests well between observations Mother holds and explores infant Partner or companion visits and interacts satisfactorily

(continued)

Assessment	Potential Nursing Diagnosis	Planning/Intervention	Evaluation
Hospital postpartum observations Vital signs Fundal checks Lochia Condition of perineum Elimination Ambulation and rest Nutrition Comfort Breast care	Potential complications: hemorrhage, uterine atony, hematomas, lacerations, retained placenta related to childbirth trauma Potential alteration in patterns of urinary elimination related to retention of urine or incomplete voiding Potential complications: infection related to milk production or breast-feeding trauma; or uterine, vaginal, or perineal trauma for childbirth Potential alteration in bowel elimination: constipation related to decreased peristalsis, inactivity, dehydration, or perianal pain Alteration in comfort: pain related to perineal trauma, hemorrhoids, engorged breasts, uterine involution Potential sleep pattern disturbance related to exhaustion, routines, demands of newborn Knowledge deficit of postpartum routines, breast and perineal hygiene, exercises, nutritional needs, sleep/rest requirements, managing discomforts, signs of complications related to being a primigravida	Record of progress of involution: report signs of hemorrhage, infection, hematoma, thrombophlebitis Instruct in perineal and breast care Administer stool softeners and laxatives as needed Provide supportive measures to enjoy nutritious diet, snacks Measure first voiding, check for bladder residual, catheterize as needed Assist mother to ambulate and shower first time Plan procedures to provide rest times without interruptions	Mother's uterus involutes normally without complications Mother maintains bowel and bladder elimination Mother performs breast and perineal care Mother rests and sleeps well
Development of mothering relation	Knowledge deficit of infant care, feeding routines, infant behavior related to first child Potential alteration in parenting related to inexperience, feeling incompetent, powerlessness, lack of role models, discomforts	Provide opportunity for extended mother–infant contact Answer questions about infant behavior and care, and feeding Provide specific instruction in areas of infant care as needed	Mother cares for infant satisfactorily

(continued)

Assessment	Potential Nursing Diagnosis	Planning/Intervention	Evaluation
Integration of infant into family	Knowledge deficit of family adaptation, parenthood stresses, sibling rivalry, parent–infant bonding, household management, community resources, social requirements related to lack of support persons Potential alteration in parenting related to inexperience in family adaptations, lack of supports, conflicts in family	Discuss family adaptation to new baby, changes in routines, response of father and other children Provide information, referrals as appropriate to individual needs Assist in planning for care of infant at home, management of tasks and sources of assistance	Family states concerns and is satisfied with responses Family adapts to new baby Family asks for sources of help Family follows through on referrals
Sexuality and contraception	Potential disturbance in self-concept related to persisting body changes (skin, weight, fatigue) Sexual dysfunction: dyspareunia, decreased vaginal lubrication, lack of arousal related to hormonal disequilibrium Knowledge deficit of sexuality after childbirth, postpartum emotional responses, contraception related to social background	Discuss postpartum sexual responses and alterations Instruct on when to resume intercourse, signs of problems Advise on contraceptive method until 6-week checkup	Couple understands changes in sexual response, when to resume intercourse, use of contraception Couple uses contraceptive measure successfully
6-week checkup Progress of involution Family adaptation to new baby Contraception	Potential complications: infection, subinvolution, delayed healing related to childbirth trauma Potential alteration in parenting related to inadequate family adaptation, conflicts, infant behavior difficulties, lack of support, fatigue, postpartum complications Knowledge deficit of contraception, sexuality, emotional responses related to lack of resources	Examine reproductive organs, provide specific treatment for problems Discuss routines of infant care, responses of family, concerns and problems, resumption of activities Discuss contraceptive methods, benefits and risks	Mother's reproductive organs return to prepregnant condition Family adapts and functions as a unit Couple practices contraception

(text continued from page 611)

Nursing Diagnosis

Potential postpartum complications such as infection, subinvolution, or delayed healing, may be medical diagnoses with associated nursing diagnoses (*e.g.,* knowledge deficits, alterations in comfort). An inexperienced mother may indicate anxiety or a disturbance in self-concept related to care of the infant. Ineffective individual coping related to emotional responses (postpartum blues) may become apparent at this time. Knowledge deficit related to contraception and sexuality may also be problems of this transitional stage, as may alterations in parenting related to a variety of stressors.

Planning/Intervention

Problems with healing or infection are treated, if present, and arrangements are made for further examinations and treatments as necessary. This return examination provides an opportunity to discuss any other problems or concerns relating to the birth experience. The mother's concerns about rest and exercise, weight, diet, her energy level, household tasks, relations with relatives and friends, sexual relations, and physical needs or discomforts are discussed. If weight continues to be a problem, a suitable weight reduction diet and other measures can be started. If desired, the woman can resume full employment or activities at this time, if there are no complications and she feels psychologically ready. The need for further care or referrals is identified.

Contraception is discussed at this visit, and a suitable method is decided upon if the parents wish to prevent another pregnancy. The method is instituted at this time, and the couple is instructed in its uses and risks.

The postpartum visit is an ideal time to emphasize the importance of periodic examinations for continued health care and to give advice on family planning.

Evaluation

The effectiveness of nursing care is determined by outcomes for the mother and family. Physiological outcomes, such as normal progression of lochia and healing of the episiotomy, can be observed. Satisfactory interaction between mother and infant and development of mothering abilities signify effective outcomes in mother–infant relationships. The mother, father, and family express comfort and harmonious adaptation to the new infant; new routines are developed and stabilized. Referrals and other sources of assistance are used and provide effective help. The mother and family feel their questions have been answered and feel capable of managing their new family processes.

References

1. Jenkins RL, Westhus NK: The Nurse Role in Parent-Infant Bonding. JOGN Nurs 10:114–118, March/April 1981
2. Klaus MH, Kennell JH: Maternal–Infant Bonding, pp 12–14, 50–66. St Louis, CV Mosby, 1976
3. Quistad C: How to smooth Mom's postpartum path. RN, 47:40–43, April 1984
4. Jacobson H: A standard for assessing lochia volume. MCN 10:174–175, May/June 1985
5. Countryman B: Breast care in the early puerperium. JOGN Nurs 2:36–40, September/October 1973
6. Kyndely K: The sexuality of women in pregnancy and postpartum: A review. JOGN Nurs 7:28–31, January/February, 1978
7. Clark AL, Hale RW: Sex during and after pregnancy. Am J Nurs 74:1430, 1974
8. Jansson P: Early Postpartum discharge. Am J Nurs 85(5):547–550, May 1985
9. Regan K: Early obstetrical discharge: A program that works. Can Nurse 80:32–35, October 1984
10. Roberts F: Perinatal Nursing, pp 165–167. New York, McGraw–Hill, 1977
11. Clark AL: Recognizing discord between mother and child and changing it to harmony. MCN 1:100–106, March/April 1976
12. Gruis M: Beyond maternity: Postpartum concerns of mothers. MCN 2:182–188, May/June 1977
13. Brown MS, Hurlock JT: Mothering the mother. Am J Nurs 77:439–441, March 1977
14. Clark AL, Affonso DD: Infant behavior and maternal attachment: Two sides to the coin. MCN 1:95–99, March/April 1976

Suggested Reading

Benson R: Current obstetric and gynecologic diagnosis and treatment, 5th ed. Los Altos, CA, Lange Medical Publications, 1984
Carr KC, Walton VE: Early postpartum discharge. MCN 6:53, 1981
Donaldson NE: The postpartum follow-up nurse clinician. JOGN Nurs 4:249, 1981
Harr B, Hastings J: Parturition care planning. JOGN Nurs 10:54, 1981
Harvey K: Mother–baby nursing. Nurs Management 13(7):22, 1982
Ketter DE, Shelton BJ: In-hospital exercises for the postpartum woman. MCN 8:120, 1983
Mansell KA: Mother–baby units: The concept works. MCN 9:132, 1984
Sheehan F: Assessing postpartum adjustment: A pilot study. JOGN Nurs 10:19–23, January/February 1981

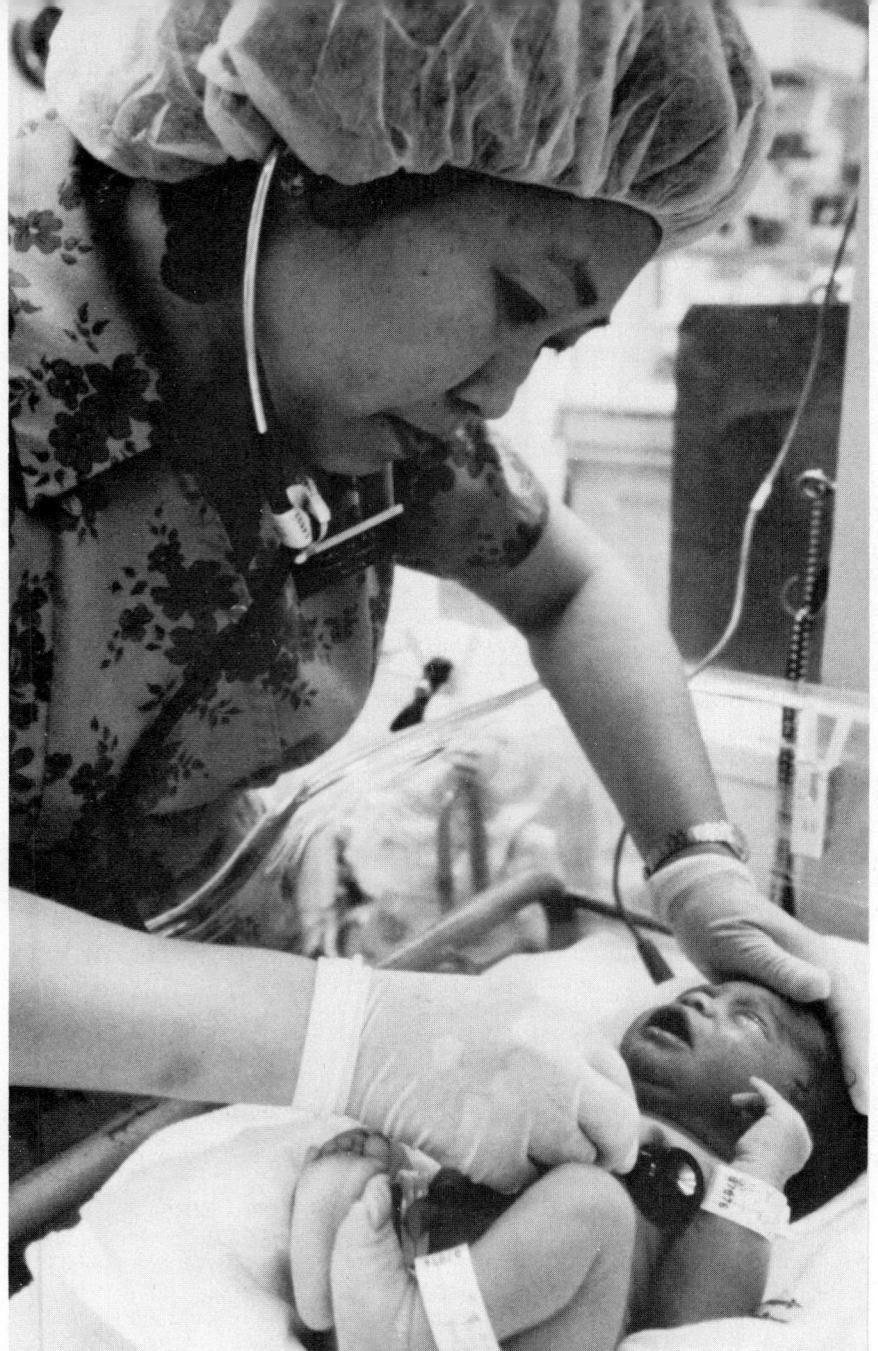

CHAPTER 32

Assessment of the Newborn

During the first few days of life, the newborn undergoes more profound physiological changes than at any other time in his life. Frequent assessments of the infant help to determine how well he is coping with the many changes that are occurring. The types of assessments that are done, and who does them, depend on the setting and the infant's condition. The registered nurse is usually the health-care professional who has closest contact with the newborn during this period of transition to extrauterine life. She needs to possess the knowledge and skills to comprehensively evaluate the newborn's status during this period.

Assessments continue to be made throughout the infant's hospital stay. Vital signs, general activity, color changes, feeding status, elimination, and the condition of skin, eyes, and cord are usually checked at least once each shift, and the infant is usually weighed daily. Although the infant's physical condition is of great importance, increasing attention is now placed on assessment of other areas, such as the infant's behavior and the interaction between the parents and the infant.

Physiological Basis of Assessment

While undergoing the changes that lead to adaptation to extrauterine life, the infant passes through several phases. This transitional period must be negotiated successfully if the infant is to survive and develop normally. The transition begins with labor when the fetus is stimulated by uterine contractions and pressure changes due to the rupture of the membranes. At birth a variety of foreign stimuli are encountered, such as light, sound, heat, cold, and gravitation. Breathing then must start and profound changes and reorganization in the functioning of the organ systems and metabolic processes begin. Respiration must be initiated, circulation must shift from fetal to neonatal, hepatic and renal function must be altered, and meconium must be passed. The final phase of the transition involves further reorganization of the metabolic processes to achieve a viable, steady state. This includes changes in blood oxygen saturation, reduction of enzymes, diminution in postnatal acidosis, and recovery of the neurologic tissues from the trauma of labor and delivery. Since these changes take time, it is no wonder that the infant's natal day is so crucial to his life and future well-being.

Respiratory Changes

Prior to birth, the oxygen needs of the fetus are met by the placenta. While the fetal lungs do not function as organs of respiration, it has been confirmed in recent years that respiratorylike movements do occur. The function of this "fetal breathing" is not known, but some of the hypotheses are that it is "prenatal practice" for later breathing; may aid in the development of alveolar and bronchial structures; or might have some relationship to the synthesis, release, and distribution of surfactant.[1]

For the newborn to survive extrauterine life, adequate maturation of the lungs is essential. The lungs are in a continuous state of development structurally throughout fetal life and early childhood. About the 20th week of gestation, canals begin to develop in the bronchial tree and primitive air sacs begin to form. By the 28th week, these are in close enough proximity to the developing blood vessel structures for gas exchange to be possible and surface-active lipoproteins (surfactant) to be detected for the first time, so there is a potential for independent survival. However, if the infant is born this early, he is at high risk for respiratory problems as a result of the limited amount of surfactant and the incomplete development of the alveoli.[2] (See Chap. 44 for discussion of respiratory problems of the preterm infant.)

At the time of birth, the normal, full-term fetus is ready for the initiation of effective breathing. For example, fetal respiratory movements have prepared the lungs for this activity and the complex interrelationships of swallowing and breathing have been developed. With everything in readiness, the question is often asked, "What keeps the fetus from taking real breaths before it is born?" Some important inhibitory mechanisms have been identified. One of these is facial immersion. Another is the inhibition of respiration by the presence of fluid in the laryngeal area. This emphasizes the importance of clearing fluid from this area after birth. Also, the fetal lungs are constantly filled with fluid that is thought to be secreted by the alveolar cells, and this fluid in the deep respiratory tracts stimulates inhibitory stretch receptors.[2]

Initiation of Respiration

A multiplicity of factors is probably involved in stimulating the infant's initial respirations. This would seem to provide a margin of safety for the infant. Physical, sensory, and chemical factors are involved, but precisely how each of these influences the other and to what degree is not known exactly. There is some evidence to indicate that the change in pressure from intrauterine to extrauterine life may produce enough physical stimulation to prompt respiration.

Of the sensory stimuli that have been thought to play a role, such as cold, pain, touch, light, sound, and gravity, cold seems to be the most important. In animal studies, cold stimulation has induced breathing in fetal sheep.[2] This should not be taken to mean that the infant

needs to be in a cold environment. Just being in normal room air of about 22°C (72°F) is a drop of more than 15°C (25°F) below the mother's normal body temperature that the neonate has been used to.

The chemical changes that occur in the blood as a result of the transitory asphyxia during delivery seem to be of paramount importance. These include a lowered oxygen level, an increased carbon dioxide level, and a lowered pH. If the asphyxia is prolonged, depression of the respiratory center ensues rather than stimulation, and resuscitation is usually necessary (see Chap. 44). A vigorous infant often breathes seconds after birth and certainly within 1 minute of delivery.

A great effort is required to expand the lungs and to fill the collapsed alveoli. Surface tension in the respiratory tract, as well as resistance in the lung tissue itself, the thorax, the diaphragm, and the respiratory muscles, must be overcome. Moreover, any obstruction (*i.e.*, mucus, and so on) in the air passages has to be cleared. The first active inspiration comes from a powerful contraction of the diaphragm, which creates a high negative intrathoracic pressure, causing a marked retraction of the ribs because of the pliability of the baby's thorax.

This first inspiration distends the alveolar spaces, and on expiration a residual volume of nearly 20 cc of air remains as molecules of pulmonary surfactant diminish surface tension. Therefore, the second breath takes less effort than the first, and the third breath even less, since by this time most of the small airways are open. Fluid is rapidly removed from the lungs by drainage, swallowing, evaporation, and pulmonary, capillary, and lymphatic circulation. After several minutes of breathing, lung expansion is usually complete.[3]

Respiration in First and Second Periods of Reactivity

A healthy infant begins life with intense activity. This phase has been designated by some authorities as the first period of reactivity. In this phase the infant exhibits outbursts of diffuse, purposeless movements that alternate with periods of relative immobility. At this time respiration is rapid (reaching as high as 80 breaths per minute), and there may be *transient* flaring of the nostrils; retraction of the chest and grunting are not uncommon. Tachycardia also is present at times, and the heart rate may reach 180 beats per minute in the first minutes of life. Thereafter it falls to an average of 120 to 140 beats per minute.

After this initial response, the baby becomes relatively quiet and does not respond intensely to either internal or external stimuli. He relaxes and may fall asleep. His first sleep occurs, on an average, at 2 hours after birth and may last anywhere from a few minutes to several hours.

Initiation of Respiration

Factors in stimulation of first breath

Physical—Changes in pressure

Sensory—Cold, pain, touch, light, sound, gravity

Chemical—Changes in blood (decrease in O_2 level, increase in CO_2 level, decrease in pH)

Expansion of alveoli

Must overcome the following:
    Surface tension in respiratory tract
    Resistance in lung tissue, thorax, diaphragm, and respiratory muscles
Must clear air passages of mucus

Fluid removed from lungs by the following

Drainage

Swallowing

Evaporation

Pulmonary capillary circulation

Lymphatic circulation

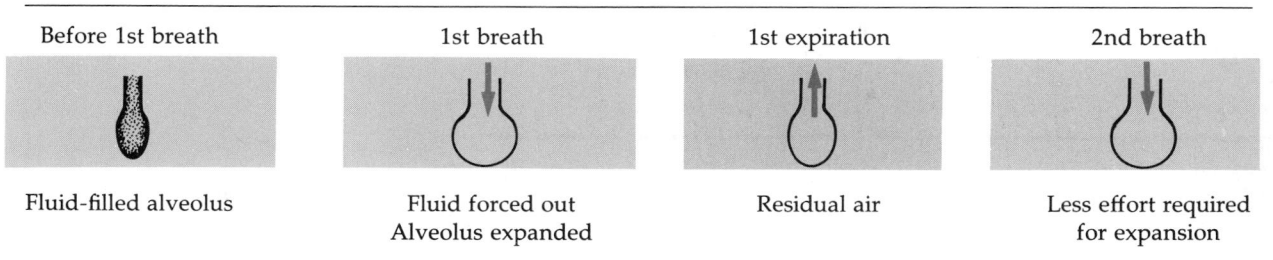

Before 1st breath	1st breath	1st expiration	2nd breath
Fluid-filled alveolus	Fluid forced out Alveolus expanded	Residual air	Less effort required for expansion

When he awakes, he is again hyperresponsive to stimuli, and he begins his second period of reactivity. His color may change rapidly (from pink to moderately cyanotic), and his heart rate responds to stimulation and becomes rapid. Oral mucus may be a major problem in respiration during this period. Choking, gagging, and regurgitation alert the nurse to the presence of mucus, and appropriate intervention must be taken (see Chap. 44). Since the length of the second period of reactivity is variable, the nurse must be particularly alert for the first 12 to 18 hours of the infant's life[4] (Fig. 32-1).

Circulatory Changes

The anatomical changes that occur with birth have been discussed previously in Chapter 12. It will be recalled that a rapid change takes place with closure of several fetal structures and with the redistribution of oxygenated blood to a circulation similar to that of an adult. Since all changes are not immediately complete, this time of conversion may be called a period of *transitional circulation.*

Total Blood Volume

It is difficult to give accurate values for the total blood volume of the newborn because of the variables involved, such as time of clamping the umbilical cord, weight and gestational age of the infant, type of delivery (vaginal or cesarean), and time after delivery the determination is made.

For example, an additional 50 ml to 100 ml of blood may be added to the circulation if the infant is placed below the level of the placenta and the clamping of the cord is delayed several minutes until the cord stops pulsating. Many studies have been done to help decide the issue of early or late clamping, but it is still unclear whether this placental transfusion that occurs with late clamping is advantageous for the infant. The rapid increase in blood volume might stress the heart and pulmonary vasculature, but according to some reports, the incidence of neonatal respiratory distress is decreased with delayed clamping. The infants who receive this extra blood gain an increased storage supply of iron, resulting from the breakdown of the additional hemoglobin. This may contribute to hyperbilirubinemia

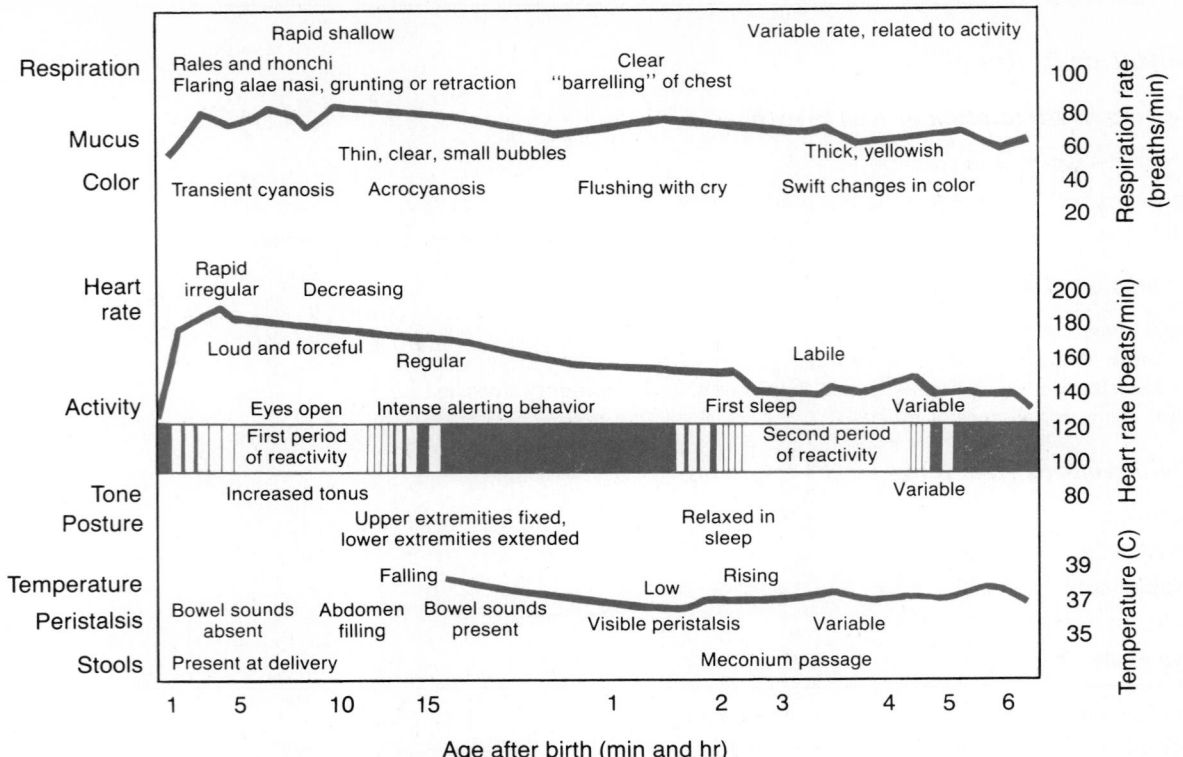

FIGURE 32-1

Periods of reactivity. (After Arnold HW, Putman NJ, Barnard BL et al: Transition to extrauterine life. Am J Nurs 65(10):78, 1965)

during the first week of life, but the iron stores may be used to good advantage later when iron is needed for rapid growth or when the dietary intake of iron is inadequate.[5]

Peripheral Circulation

Peripheral circulation in the newborn is somewhat sluggish. It is felt that this accounts for the residual cyanosis of the infant's hands, feet, and circumoral area. These areas often remain mildly cyanotic for 1 or 2 hours after delivery. The general circulatory lability probably accounts for the mottled appearance of the baby's skin when it is exposed to air and for the "chilliness" of the infant's hands and feet.

Pulse Rate

Like the rate of respiration, the pulse rate also is labile and generally follows a pattern similar to that of the respiration. When the respiration is rapid, the pulse tends to be rapid; similarly, when the respiration slows down, so does the pulse. Since the pulse is affected by both internal and external stimuli, taking the *apical* pulse rate while the baby is quiet provides a more accurate

evaluation of the infant's heart rate. The normal rate is usually 120 to 150 beats per minute, but it may rise to 180 beats per minute for short periods with crying and other intense activity, or drop to 100 beats per minute during deep sleep.

Blood Pressure

Accurate indirect assessment of arterial blood pressure is more difficult in the newborn; therefore, it has not always been checked routinely in the normal infant. Invasive methods using an arterial catheter for direct recording of the blood pressure are usually limited to the sick neonate who has an arterial line in place for other reasons (see Chap. 44). Indirect, noninvasive methods consisting of auscultation, palpation, and the color change (flush) method usually result in only the systolic pressure or the mean pressure and are not very precise. The advent of the Doppler reflected ultrasound technique has made the estimation of systemic blood pressure more accurate, and taking the blood pressure has become part of the routine procedure in many normal newborn nurseries.

Blood pressure in the neonate is characteristically low, averaging 71/49 at birth and rising slowly during the first week.[6] Pressure also varies according to the size and activity of the infant, with lower averages for the small, preterm infant and with the blood pressure rising when the infant is crying and active. The width of the cuff used in the procedure should be 25% greater than the diameter of the arm or leg where the blood pressure is being taken.[7] Too small a cuff will give too high a reading. Either the arm or the leg can be used in obtaining the blood pressure. Leg pressure will be slightly higher, but should be within 20 mm Hg of the arm pressure.[8]

Erythrocyte Count and Hemoglobin Concentration

The newborn has a much higher erythrocyte, hemoglobin, and hematocrit level than an adult. The erythrocyte level ranges between 5,000,000 and 7,000,000/μl, the hemoglobin level is usually 15 g to 20 g/dl of blood, and the hematocrit values average about 55%.[5]

The following factors influence these values:

1. *Duration of gestation.* During the final weeks of intrauterine life, hemoglobin concentration rapidly increases. The infant born before term does not have the benefit of this increase and has a low concentration compared with the full-term infant.
2. *Time of cord clamping.* In infants who receive the additional blood that is added to the circulation with delayed cord clamping, increased hemoglobin and hematocrit levels can be demonstrated for at least 3 or 4 days.
3. *Site of blood sample.* In the first week of life, owing to peripheral venous stasis, capillary blood samples usually show markedly higher hemoglobin and hematocrit values than venous samples drawn at the same time. The venous samples are considered to be more accurate. If only heel sticks are used for assessing blood values, anemia could go undetected. Warming the infant's heel before the stick is suggested as a way of decreasing the difference between the two values.[5]

The higher blood values are needed by the fetus *in utero* for adequate oxygenation. After birth, the need no longer exists, since the lungs are functioning, and a gradual decrease takes place. Immediately after birth there is an increase in erythrocyte count from cord blood levels because of a decrease in plasma volume. This reaches a maximum level 2 to 6 hours after birth. Then it decreases to cord blood levels when the infant is about 1 week of age. Red blood cell production (erythropoiesis) is suppressed for several months after birth and this, added to the increased blood volume caused by the infant's rapid growth, results in a progressive decline in the hemoglobin concentration. A low point of 11 g/dl ($\pm$2.0) may be reached after 2 to 3 months, producing a physiologic anemia that does not represent any abnormality or nutritional deficiency in the infant and is not affected by giving iron or other hematinics. Active erythropoiesis resumes about this time and, if the iron supply is adequate, the hemoglobin concentration gradually increases to an average of 12.5 g/dl, where it stays during early childhood.

Physiologic Jaundice

In the newborn period there is a rise in the serum concentration of unconjugated bilirubin from approximately 2 mg/dl in cord blood to a mean peak of 6 mg/dl between 60 and 72 hours of age. Then there is usually a rapid decline to 2 mg/dl by the fifth day of life and a slower decline until normal adult levels of less than 1 mg/dl are reached by about the tenth day. Jaundice is the visible evidence of this rise in serum concentration of unconjugated bilirubin to levels of 5 mg to 7 mg/dl or above.[9] Approximately 40% to 60% of full-term newborns (and a higher number of preterm infants) develop jaundice between the second and fourth days of life, and in the absence of disease or specific causes, this has been called "physiologic" jaundice. Bilirubin levels greater than 5 mg/dl or the appearance of jaundice during the first 24 hours, or bilirubin levels greater than 12 mg/dl at any time are indications that the condition might be pathologic jaundice and that further investigation is needed to attempt to find the cause.[9] (See Chap. 45 for a discussion of pathologic jaundice and its treatment.)

The etiology of physiologic jaundice is not fully understood, nor are the hypotheses agreed upon. The following are possible mechanisms in the development of this condition: (1) The newborn's high erythrocyte count and the shorter mean red blood cell life span lead to an increased breakdown of red blood cells, which contributes to the increased bilirubin load presented to the liver in the first days of life. Bilirubin from other sources such as myoglobin, a protein found in muscle, is also produced in increased amounts in the newborn. (2) The unconjugated, fat-soluble form of bilirubin that is produced when hemoglobin is broken down is usually changed in the liver to the conjugated, water-soluble

---

Course of Hyperbilirubinemia in Normal Newborn

Unconjugated bilirubin in cord blood = approximately 2 mg/dl

Mean peak between 60 and 72 hours = 6 mg/dl

Rapid decline by 5th day to 2 mg to 3 mg/dl

Slower decline by about 10th day to <1 mg/dl

Possible Mechanisms Related to Development of Physiologic Jaundice

Increased production of bilirubin due to increased breakdown of red blood cells

Decreased clearance of bilirubin by the liver cells probably secondary to inhibition of glucuronyl transferase

Immaturity of the liver

Recirculation of increased amounts of bilirubin reabsorbed from the intestine

---

form that can be excreted. In the newborn, there is interference with this conjugation, possibly owing to inhibition of the activity of the enzyme glucuronyl transferase. (3) Uptake of bilirubin from the plasma by the liver cells may be decreased because of immaturity of the liver. (4) Owing to the lack of intestinal bacterial flora in the newborn, bilirubin may be reabsorbed from the intestine and recirculated to the liver, rather than being excreted. Retention of meconium, which has a high bilirubin content, may add to the amount of bilirubin reabsorbed.[10]

There seem to be some genetic and ethnic influences on the incidence of physiologic jaundice. Oriental infants and some other isolated groups have mean maximal serum unconjugated bilirubin levels between 10 mg and 14 mg/dl, which is approximately double that of nonoriental populations. Kernicterus is also significantly increased in Oriental neonates. The reasons for these increases are not known, but there may be a genetic predisposition to slower maturation of hepatic bilirubin metabolism or a possible relationship to ethnic food or herbal medicines.[9]

The nurse should not be lulled into a false sense of security by the term *physiologic*. Any baby who develops observable jaundice should be closely watched for symptoms of other possible problems.

Blood Coagulation

At birth the vitamin K–dependent blood-clotting factors (Factors VII, IX, X, and prothrombin) are significantly decreased. The intestinal tract of the newborn does not harbor the bacteria necessary to help synthesize vitamin K; thus, the infant has a transitory deficiency in blood coagulation occurring between the second and the fifth postnatal days. This deficiency is sometimes severe enough to cause clinical bleeding. As a preventive measure, 0.5 mg to 1 mg of vitamin K is administered to the neonate during the first day of life.[5]

White Blood Cells

There is a wide range of normal for the leukocyte count at birth; the average is approximately 20,000 cells per microliter. Neutrophils comprise about 70% of this total. During the first few days after delivery there is a considerable decrease in the total count, as well as a shift in the type of predominant cell. The neutrophils decrease, and the lymphocytes increase, so that by the end of the first week the lymphocytes predominate and continue to do so until the child is 4 or 5 years old.[5]

T A B L E   3 2 - 1

Thermal Regulation in the Newborn

Mechanisms of Heat Loss	Prevention
Evaporation—loss of heat to air by way of moisture from skin or lungs	Dry well after delivery, especially head; protect from exposure while wet during bath; avoid very low humidity
Radiation—loss of heat to cool objects not in contact with infant	Avoid placing infant near cold outside walls or windows
Conduction—loss of heat from infant to cold surface	Do not place on cold surface; use warmed blankets in delivery room
Convection—loss of heat to air by way of drafts	Keep infant out of air flow currents

Mechanisms of Heat Production and Conservation	Effects
Nonshivering thermogenesis (metabolism of brown fat)	Increased metabolic consumption of calories Increased oxygen consumption Increased glucose consumption
Increase in voluntary muscular activity (shivering is rare in the newborn)	
Peripheral vasoconstriction	Conserve heat for body core Hands and feet may be blue, mottled, or cold to touch
Assumption of fetal position	Decreased surface area for loss of heat

Temperature Regulation and Metabolic Changes

The infant is born into an environment that is considerably cooler than the one encountered in the uterus. Because of this rapid change in environmental conditions, the newborn's temperature may drop several degrees after birth. In recent years attention has been focused on the effects of hypothermia on the newborn, and increasing efforts have been made to prevent this temperature drop in the delivery room and in the nursery. Neonates are predisposed to heat transfer between themselves and the environment because they have a limited supply of subcutaneous fat and a large surface area in relation to body weight.

Heat Loss. Evaporation, conduction, convection, and radiation are four ways in which the newborn can lose body heat to the environment. Excessive loss by *evaporation* occurs most often in the delivery room when the infant is wet (see Chap. 28), but it can also occur when the infant is being bathed. Heat evaporation may also occur from the lungs if the infant has tachypnea or if the humidity is low. Heat loss by *conduction* involves the transfer of heat from a warm object to a cooler one by direct contact and can occur when the infant is placed on a cold surface or when cool blankets or clothing are used. Through *convection*, the transference of heat is from a body to the surrounding air; the infant's temperature is affected by the air currents in the environment, such as those caused by air conditioners. The fourth mechanism, *radiation*, occurs when heat is transferred from a warm object to a cooler one when the objects are not in direct contact. This type of heat loss can occur in infants if the walls of an incubator are cool or if the crib is placed close to a cool outside wall or window. Each of these mechanisms with the exception of evaporation can be responsible for an increase in the infant's temperature as well as the losses described (Table 32-1).

Heat Production. To maintain a normal temperature when exposed to a cool environment the newborn increases his rate of heat production in an attempt to replace what is lost (see Table 32-1). Shivering is the most common mechanism of heat production in an adult, but the neonate rarely shivers, although there may be an increase in voluntary muscular activity. The primary mechanism of heat production in the newborn is nonshivering thermogenesis whereby a chemical reaction occurs in brown fat, which breaks down triglycerides into glycerol and fatty acids and thereby produces heat. Brown fat cells contain many small fat vacuoles in contrast to the single large vacuole of white fat. There is also a richer blood supply, which helps to account for its darker color and aids in the distribution of the heat produced. Brown fat is usually not found in adults, but in the newborn it accounts for 2% to 6% of the total weight and can be found between the scapulae, at the nape of the neck, in the axillae, in the mediastinum, and around the kidneys and adrenals.[11]

Heat Conservation. Conservation of body heat in the infant occurs through peripheral vasoconstriction and through assumption of a flexed or fetal position, which decreases the surface area from which heat may be lost.

Effects of Cold Stress on the Newborn. The increased metabolic rate associated with nonshivering thermogenesis necessitates an increase in both oxygen and calorie consumption. To replace the heat lost during a temperature drop of 3.5°C (6.3°F), it has been found that the infant requires a 100% increase in oxygen consumption for more than 1½ hours.[12] Even vigorous full-term infants may develop metabolic acidosis if allowed to become hypothermic. It is obvious that cold stress can be detrimental or even fatal to an infant who is having difficulty with metabolism or oxygenation.

Efforts should be made to keep an infant in a neutral thermal environment, which means an environment where the infant's metabolic rate, and therefore oxygen consumption, is minimal but the body temperature remains within the normal range.

Neurologic Changes

The nervous system of the newborn is immature, that is, it is neither anatomically nor physiologically fully developed. Although all neurons are present, many remain immature for several months and some for years. Thus, the infant is uncoordinated in his movements, is labile in his temperature regulation, and has poor control over his musculature—he "startles" easily, is subject to tremors of the extremities, and so on. However, during the neonatal period, development is rapid, and as the various nerve pathways controlling the muscles are used, the nerve fibers connect with one another. Gradually, more complex patterns of behavior emerge, and the higher cerebral levels begin to function.

Reflexes. The reflexes are important indices of the baby's normal development. Their presence or absence at certain times reflects the extent of normality in the functioning of the central nervous system (individual reflexes are discussed in Neurologic Assessment).

Gastrointestinal Changes

The gastrointestinal (GI) tract functions in a very limited capacity during fetal life. The fetus is known to swallow amniotic fluid, and a fecal material called meconium is formed, but the GI tract is not responsible for the digestion or absorption of nutrients. By 36 to 38 weeks, though, it is mature enough to adapt readily to extrauterine life. The various enzymes necessary for digestion are active, and the muscular and reflex development provide the capability of transporting the food.[13]

For the infant to swallow, food must be placed well back on the tongue, since the infant does not have the ability to transfer food from the lips to the pharynx. This means that the nipple should be placed well inside the infant's mouth. Sucking is facilitated by strong sucking muscles and ridges or corrugations in the anterior portion of the mouth. In addition, the *sucking pads* (deposits of fatty tissue in each cheek) prevent the collapse of the cheeks during nursing and further make sucking effective. This fatty tissue remains (even when fat is lost from the rest of the body) until sucking is no longer essential to the baby as a method of obtaining food. The salivary glands are immature at birth and manufacture little saliva until the infant is about 3 months old.

The newborn's intestinal tract is proportionately longer than that of an adult. Although it contains a large number of secretory glands and a large surface for absorption, its elastic tissue and supporting musculature are poor and not fully developed. This increases the likelihood of distention. Furthermore, nervous control is variable and inadequate. Nevertheless, the infant digests and absorbs a tremendous amount of food in proportion to body weight.

Most of the digestive enzymes seem to be present and adequate, with the exception of pancreatic amylase and lipase, which are somewhat deficient for several months but eventually reach a normal amount. The infant can digest simple foods easily, but has a difficult time with the more complex starches. Protein and carbohydrates are easily absorbed, but fat absorption is poor.

Changes in Kidney Function and Urinary Excretion

The kidneys become functional during fetal life, as evidenced by the presence of urine in the bladder as early as the fourth month of gestation. Even at full term, however, the level of kidney function in the newborn is low. The full number of nephrons are present, but the surface area of the glomerular capillaries and the tubule length are about one tenth of adult size.[14]

Owing to the relatively low rate of glomerular filtration at birth, excess water and solute cannot be disposed of rapidly and efficiently. The limitations in tubular reabsorption that are also present may cause inappropriate substances from the glomerular filtrate, such as certain amino acids and bicarbonate, to appear in the urine.[14] In the healthy neonate these limitations do not have a detrimental effect, but they do restrict the ability of the newborn to respond to stress. As the kidneys grow and mature, function increases.

Ninety-two percent of healthy infants void within 24 hours, but the first voiding may occur shortly after delivery and not be noticed. Voidings during the first days after birth may be scanty and somewhat infrequent unless the infant was edematous at birth, but as the fluid intake increases so does the output. Frequency usually increases from 2 to 6 times on the first and second day to 5 to 20 times per 24 hours after that until the infant begins to develop bladder control and the number of voidings per day decreases.

The urine of the newborn may appear cloudy owing to high mucus and urate content, but with increased fluid intake the urine becomes clear, straw colored, and nearly odorless. Uric acid crystals in the urine may cause a reddish "brick-dust" stain on the diaper that is sometimes confused with blood in the urine.

Changes in Hepatic Function

During fetal life, the liver performs an important role in blood formation, and it is thought that it continues this function to some degree after birth. Later in the neonatal period the liver produces substances that are essential in the coagulation of the blood. If the mother's iron intake has been adequate during pregnancy, enough iron is stored in the infant's liver to carry him over the first months of life when his diet (primarily milk) is iron deficient. About the fifth month, however, the baby's iron reserve is depleted, and unless foods containing iron are given, a deficiency will ensue.

Physical Assessment

The physical examination was traditionally done by the physician. In recent years many nurses have learned physical assessment skills, and in some hospitals a pediatric nurse practitioner has the responsibility for part of the newborn physical examinations. Although all nurses do not possess practitioner skills, they should be able to do a basic assessment and recognize deviations from normal.

The Newborn Physical Assessment Guide can be used in learning to assess the newborn. The discussion of newborn characteristics that follows and Table 32-2 are helpful in using the guide. Practice and experience also improve the nurse's ability to recognize the range of normal. Discussion of abnormalities is found in Chapters 44 to 46.

The format of the Newborn Physical Assessment Guide can be used for an admitting assessment or a later one. It is not intended to be a complete physical examination, but should give the nurse a good idea of the status of the infant. The examiner can use any system of notation that is helpful to fill in the spaces on the form. A suggestion is to use a "check" to indicate "within normal limits" and a "plus" or "minus" to indicate whether something is present or absent. When appropriate, description can be written in the spaces or under "comments."

Methods used in physical examination are inspection, auscultation, palpation, and percussion, usually in that order. Percussion is not specifically used in this form. The examination is written for use in evaluating the infant in a cephalocaudal direction, but it may be best to begin with items, such as auscultation of the chest, that require the infant to be quiet, before performing procedures that might cause the infant to cry. Each examiner should establish a definite pattern and follow it each time so that nothing is missed.

When any assessment of the newborn is carried out, the parents should be included as much as possible. If they cannot be present for the examination it should at least be discussed with them. Being there, though, is a good way to help them get better acquainted with their infant (see Fig. 32-8). Also, it is important for the nurse to look at the baby from the parents' viewpoint. The healthy newborn has many characteristics that momentarily may look unusual to them. The nurse should be ready to talk with the parents about their baby and to answer their questions.

Physical assessment of the neonate begins at birth when the delivery room nurse observes the infant to assign the Apgar score and to detect any anomalies or problems (see Chap. 28). When the infant is brought to the nursery, pertinent information concerning the mother's antepartal history, the course of labor and delivery, the condition of the infant at and following birth, and any care given to the infant is reported to the nursery nurse.

After confirming the report by looking at the newborn's record, the next step is the nursery nurse's initial evaluation of the infant's general condition, including the following:

1. Observe the infant's appearance. Is the color ruddy, pale, cyanotic, or jaundiced? Is the color evenly distributed? The infant usually is in a flexed position with good muscle tone. A "floppy" baby or a very tense baby needs careful observation.

2. The infant's cry can also be an indicator of general condition. A lusty cry is usually a good sign, but a weak or shrill cry can be indicative of central nervous system problems, and grunting sounds mean that the infant is having to work harder to get oxygen.
3. Other signs of increased respiratory effort such as retractions, gasping, or flaring of the nostrils should also be noted.
4. The vital signs should be taken.

From the foregoing observations the nurse can make a decision about whether the infant needs immediate treatment, if time is needed for the temperature to stabilize, or if the assessment can continue.

It is important to remember that certain symptoms that might be cause for concern in an older child (*e.g.,* rapid rate and irregular rhythm of respirations) may merely represent normal physiology in a newborn (see Newborn Physical Assessment Guide).

Assessment of Head and Neck

The infant's head is large, comprising about one quarter of his size, and with cephalic presentations may initially appear to be asymmetrical because of the molding of the skull bones during labor (Fig. 32-2). If there has been extended pressure on the head, caput succedaneum (a swelling of the soft tissues) or cephalhematoma (an accumulation of blood between the bone and the periosteum) might be present (see Chap. 46).

The suture lines between the skull bones and the anterior and the posterior fontanels can usually be palpated easily (see Fig. 23-10). The fontanels should feel soft and be neither bulging nor depressed. The diamond-shaped anterior fontanel is normally about 2 cm to 3 cm wide and 3 cm to 4 cm long at birth. It may feel smaller for the first day or two when there is marked overriding of the skull bones. Closure usually takes place by 12 to 18 months. The posterior fontanel is triangular and is located between the occipital and the parietal bones. It is smaller than the anterior fontanel and may be almost closed at birth and completely closed by the end of the second month.

The circumference of the head is measured by placing a nonstretchable tape measure just above the eyebrows and over the most prominent part of the occiput (Fig. 32-3). Normally the head circumference is 2 cm larger than the chest circumference, but an accurate measurement may not be obtained at first if molding is present. The normal range is 33 cm to 37 cm (13 in–14½ in), depending on the general size of the infant.

The face is small and round, and the lower jaw appears to recede. Facial asymmetry is sometimes seen, especially of the chin and mandible. This can be the

(*text continued on page 630*)

Newborn Physical Assessment Guide

Baby's Name _____ Date and Time of Birth _____

Mother's Name _____ Date and Time of Exam _____

Initial Evaluation

1. General Appearance: Color _____ Muscle tone _____
2. Respiratory Effort: Retractions _____ Gasping _____
   Grunting _____ Quality of cry _____
3. Temperature: _____
Comments: _____

Assessment of Head and Neck

1. Observe and palpate the infant's head for symmetry; note absence or presence of:
   Molding _____ Caput succedaneum _____ Cephalhematoma _____
2. Palpate the fontanels and sutures for: Fullness _____ Depression _____
   Overriding _____ Shape _____ Size _____
3. Measure circumference of head: _____
4. Evaluate ears: Position _____ Shape _____ Location _____
5. Evaluate symmetry of face: _____
6. Observe eyes for: Shape _____ Position _____ Size _____
   Appearance of pupils _____ Presence of hemorrhage _____ Red reflex _____
7. Evaluate mouth for: Clefts _____ Teeth _____ Frenulum linguae _____
8. Observe neck for: Length _____ Relationship to body _____
   Mobility _____ Presence of webbing or fat pad _____
9. Observe skin of scalp, face and neck for: Abrasions or contusions _____
   Other breaks or marks _____
10. Observe nose for: Symmetry _____ Septum _____ Flaring _____
Comments: _____

Assessment of Body

General Appearance
1. Measurements: Weight _____ Length _____ Circumference of chest _____
2. Observe throughout evaluation for: General activity _____
   Posture _____ Responsiveness _____
3. Observe skin for: Lanugo _____ Vernix _____ Meconium staining _____
   Texture _____ Hydration _____ Color _____ Rashes _____
   Pigmentation _____ Lesions _____
Comments: _____

Thorax

1. Palpate clavicles for masses and intactness: _____
2. Inspect thorax for: Size _____ Symmetry _____ Shape _____
3. Auscultate for: Breath sounds _____ Heart sounds _____ Rhythm _____
4. Count: respiratory rate _____ Apical pulse _____
Comments: _____

Abdomen

1. Inspect shape of abdomen: _____
2. Palpate: Liver _____ Spleen _____ Kidneys _____

(continued)

3. Observe cord for number of vessels: _____
4. Palpate: Femoral pulses _____
Comments: _____
_____

Genitals

1. Observe visible genitals for: Appropriateness with stated sex _____
2. Observe female infant for: Maturation of labia _____ Vaginal discharge _____
3. Observe male infant for: Position of urethral opening _____
   Maturation of scrotum _____ Presence of testes _____
4. Note elimination: (should occur within 24 hours)
   Urine _____ Color _____ Amount/24 hours _____
   Stool_____ Color _____ Type _____ Number/24 hours _____
Comments: _____
_____

Posterior of Body

1. Palpate and inspect spinal column for: Masses _____
   Symmetry of vertebrae _____ Intactness _____
2. Determine patency of anus: _____
3. Observe pilonidal dimple for intactness: _____
Comments: _____
_____

Extremities

1. Note for all extremities: Symmetry _____ Abnormalities _____
   Ability to move _____
2. Count digits on: Hands _____ Feet _____
   Observe for polydactyly _____ Syndactyly _____
3. Evaluate rotation of hips: Abduct thighs to bed _____
   Rotate hips through full range of motion _____
   Observe leg length, front and back (Are they equal?) _____ Knee height _____
   Observe symmetry of leg creases _____
4. Note position of feet _____
   Can they passively be returned to normal? _____
Comments: _____
_____

Assessment of Neurologic Function—Reflexes—Elicit and Evaluate:

1. Rooting and sucking: _____
_____
2. Grasp: Palmar _____ Plantar _____
_____
3. Traction: (Pull to sitting position, note head and arm position) _____
_____
4. Moro: _____
_____
5. Stepping: _____
_____
Comments: _____
_____
_____

Items that require manipulation, such as palpation of the abdomen and abduction of the hips, require care in performance to avoid injury to the infant and should not be attempted for the first time without supervision by a trained examiner.

(After NAACOG Technical Bulletin Number 2, "Physical Assessment of the Neonate")

TABLE 32-2

Summary of Newborn Physical Assessment

Assessment Area	Usual Findings	Deviations
General observations		
Muscle tone	Flexed position; good tone	"Floppy"; rigid or tense
Skin		
Color	Pink tone to ruddy when crying; appropriate to ethnic origin; acrocyanosis	Pallor; cyanosis; jaundice; ecchymosis; petechiae
Texture	Smooth; dryness with some peeling; lanugo on back; vernix	Excessive peeling or cracking; roughness
Rashes and pigmentation	Erythema toxicum; milia; mongolian spots	Impetigo; hemangiomas; nevus flammeus (port-wine stain)
Hydration	Skin pinch over abdomen immediately returns to original state	Skin maintains "tent" shape after pinch
Cry	Lusty	Shrill; weak; grunty
Measurements		
Weight	2700 g–4000 g (6 lb–9 lb)	
Length	48 cm–53 cm (19 in–21 in)	
Head circumference	33 cm–37 cm (13 in–14.5 in)	
Chest circumference	31 cm–35 cm (12.5 in–14 in)	
Vital signs		
Temperature	Axillary (preferred method)—36.5°C–37°C (97.7°F–98.6°F) Rectal–36.5°C–37.2°C (97.7°F–99°F)	Hypothermia; fever
Respirations	40 respirations/min–60 respirations/min; quiet and shallow; diaphragmatic; occasional periods of rapid breathing, alternating with short periods of apnea	Prolonged rapid breathing; apnea lasting longer than 10 sec; grunting; retractions; persistent slow rate
Heart rate (apical pulse)	120 beats/min–160 beats/min; faster when crying (up to 180 beats/min); slower when sleeping (down to 100 beats/min)	Tachycardia—greater than 160 beats/min at rest Bradycardia—less than 120 beats/min when awake
Head	Vaginal delivery—elongated (molding) Breech or cesarean birth—round, symmetrical Size within normal range	Caput succedaneum; cephalhematoma; hydrocephaly; microcephaly
Fontanels	Flat; soft; firm	Bulging; sunken
Anterior	Diamond shaped; 2 cm–3 cm wide; 3 cm–4 cm long; smaller at birth with molding	Small; almost closed; closed (craniostenosis); widened
Posterior	Triangular shape; small; almost closed	Enlarged
Face	Small; round; symmetrical; fat pads in cheeks; receding chin	Asymmetrical; distorted
Eyes	Edematous lids; usually closed; blue or slate gray color; no tears; red reflex present; pupils equal, round, react to light Common variations—subconjunctival hemorrhages; chemical conjunctivitis; occasional slight nystagmus or convergent strabismus	Elevation or ptosis of lids; epicanthal folds; absence of red reflex; unequal, dilated, or constricted pupils Purulent discharge; frequent nystagmus; constant, divergent, or unilateral strabismus

(continued)

T A B L E 3 2 - 2 *(continued)*

Assessment Area	Usual Findings	Deviations
Mouth	Intact lips, gums, palate; epithelial pearls; "sucking blisters" on lips; tongue midline, mobile, appropriate size for mouth; can extend to alveolar ridge	Cleft lip or palate; white, cheesy patches on tongue, gums, or mucous membrane; large or protruding tongue
Nose	In midline; even placement in relation to eyes and mouth; nares patent; septum intact, midline	Flattened or bruised; unusual placement or configuration; obstructed nares; deviated or perforated septum
Ears	Well-formed cartilage; appropriate size for head; upper attachment on line extended through inner and outer canthus of eye; external auditory canal patent	Floppy, large and protruding; malformed; low set; obstruction of canal
Neck	Short; thick; full range of motion; no masses	Webbing; abnormal shortening; limitation of motion; torticollis; masses
Clavicles	Straight; smooth; intact	Knot or lump; decreased movement of extremity on one side
Thorax	Round; symmetrical; protruding xiphoid process	Asymmetrical; funnel chest
Breath sounds	Loud; bronchial; bilaterally equal	Decreased breath sounds; increased breath sounds
Heart sounds	Regular rate and rhythm; first and second sounds clear and distinct	Murmurs; arrhythmias
Breasts	Symmetrical; flat with erect nipples; enrgorgement 2nd or 3rd day not unusual	Redness and firmness around nipple
Abdomen	Symmetrical; slightly protuberant; no masses	Scaphoid or concave shape; distention; palpable masses
Liver	Palpable 2 cm–3 cm below right costal margin	Enlargement
Spleen	Tip may be palpable in left upper quadrant	Enlargement
Kidneys	May be palpable at level of umbilicus	Enlargement
Femoral pulses	Bilaterally equal	Unequal or absent
Umbilicus	No extensive protrusion or herniation; no signs of infection	Umbilical hernia; omphalocele; redness; induration; foul-smelling discharge
	Cord—bluish white, moist → black, dry; 3 vessels; no oozing or bleeding	Two vessels; bleeding or oozing from stump
Genitalia	Appropriate for gender	Ambiguous genitalia
Female		
Labia	Edematous; labia majora cover labia minora; vernix in creases	Hematoma; lesions; fusion of labia
Vagina	Mucus discharge, possibly blood tinged	
Male		
Foreskin	Adherent to glans penis	
Urethra	Opening at tip of penis	Opening below tip of penis (hypospadias) Opening above tip of penis (epispadias)
Testes	Palpable in each scrotal sac	Palpable in inguinal canal; not palpable

(continued)

TABLE 32-2 *(continued)*

Assessment Area	Usual Findings	Deviations
Posterior of body		
Spinal column	Straight, flexible; intact; no masses	Exaggerated curves; spina bifida; any masses; pilonidal cyst
Anus	Patent	Imperforate anus; anal fissures
Extremities	Symmetrical in size, shape, and movement	Unequal or abnormal size or shape; asymmetrical or limited movement of one or more extremities
Digits	Five on each hand and foot; appropriate size and shape	Missing digits; syndactyly (webbing); polydactyly (extra digits)
Hips	Even leg length, knee height, gluteal folds; no resistance or limitation to abduction	Uneven leg length, knee height, or gluteal folds; uneven or limited abduction; hip "click" or "clunk" on abduction
Feet	Straight, or postural deviation easily corrected with gentle pressure	Structural deformities—talipes equinovarus (clubfoot); metatarsus adductus
Reflexes		
Rooting and sucking	Turns toward object touching cheek, lips, or corner of mouth; opens mouth; begins sucking movements; strong suck, pulls object into mouth May be diminished or absent after eating	No rooting; weak, ineffective, or absent suck
Grasp Palmar	Fingers grasp object when palm stimulated and hang on briefly	Weak or absent
Plantar	Toes curl downward when soles of feet are stimulated	Weak or absent
Moro	Symmetrical response to sudden stimulus—lateral extension of arms with opening of hands, followed by flexion and adduction	Asymmetrical; absent; incomplete
Stepping	Stepping movements when infant held upright with sole of foot touching surface	Asymmetrical or absent

(text continued from page 625)
result of posture *in utero* when the flexed head is tilted to one side and presses against the shoulder. The nose may also be asymmetrical or have a deviated septum from intrauterine pressure. It is important that the nose not be obstructed, since infants are nose breathers and have difficulty breathing through their mouths.

The scalp, face, and neck should be observed carefully for any abrasions, contusions, or breaks in the skin. These can result from application of internal fetal monitor electrodes, forceps, or other instruments used in delivery. Any opening in the skin is a potential site for bacterial invasion and should be watched for signs of infection.

Eyes. The eyes are closed much of the time but may open spontaneously if the infant's head is lifted or rocked gently (a valuable point to remember when one wants to inspect the eyes). From birth the infant can see and discriminate patterns as the basis for form perception. This capacity is rather limited by imperfect oculomotor coordination and inability to accommodate for varying distances. Moreover, the eye, the visual pathways, and the visual part of the brain are poorly developed at birth. Nevertheless, although the baby's vision is much less acute than an adult's, a good deal of visual experience is possible for him.

Many mothers do not realize that their infants can see as well as they do, and they appreciate being informed of this fact. In addition, some mothers become exceedingly anxious when they observe strabismus or nystagmus in their infants, but they should be reassured that this lack of coordination is normal during the first few months of life.

Most babies' eyes are blue or a slate-gray color at birth. By the time the infant is 3 months old, most have

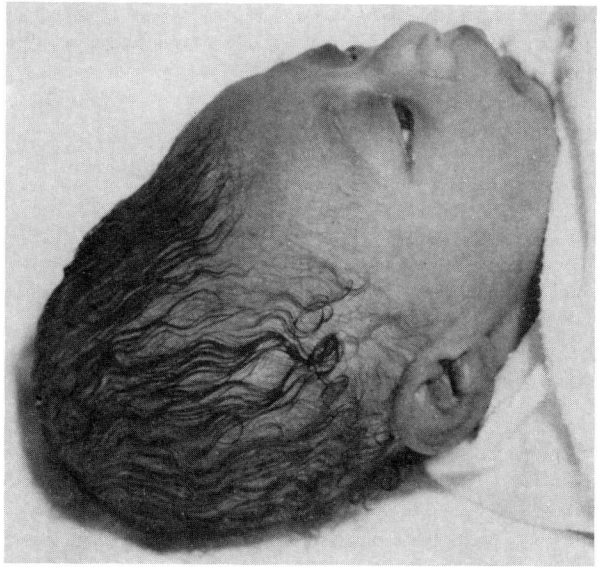

FIGURE 32-2

Molding of the head.

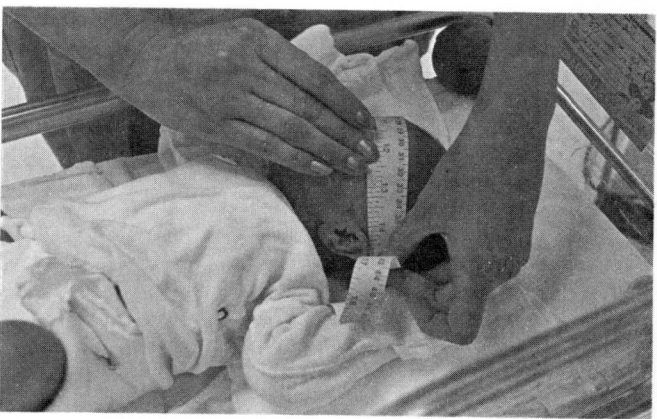

FIGURE 32-3

The circumference of the head is measured by placing a nonstretchable tape just above the eyebrows and over the most prominent part of the occiput.

achieved their permanent color, although complete pigmentation of the iris does not occur until the infant is about a year old. Since the lacrimal glands may not be functioning at birth, the baby does not usually shed tears when he cries. Tears may not appear for several weeks and sometimes for several months. There may be some edema of the lids or purulent discharge caused by the silver nitrate if it was used. The changes in the vascular tension of the eyes during delivery sometimes cause small areas of subconjunctival hemorrhage. These areas disappear spontaneously in 1 or 2 weeks and are not significant.

If an ophthalmoscope is used in examining the eyes, the pupil should appear as a small red orange circular spot when the light is directed at it. This is the red reflex, which is caused by the light shining on the retina, and any opacities of the lens or other obstructions would be visible if present.

Ears and Hearing. The ears should be inspected for size, shape, position, and anomaly. The point where the top of the ear is attached to the scalp should fall on or above an imaginary line drawn from the inner through the outer canthus of the eye (Fig. 32-4). Abnormal positioning of the ears is frequently associated with certain chromosomal abnormalities or kidney anomalies.

Otoscopic examination of the ear establishes the patency of the external auditory canal, but the tympanic membranes are usually difficult to visualize for the first 2 or 3 days of life owing to accumulated vernix caseosa.

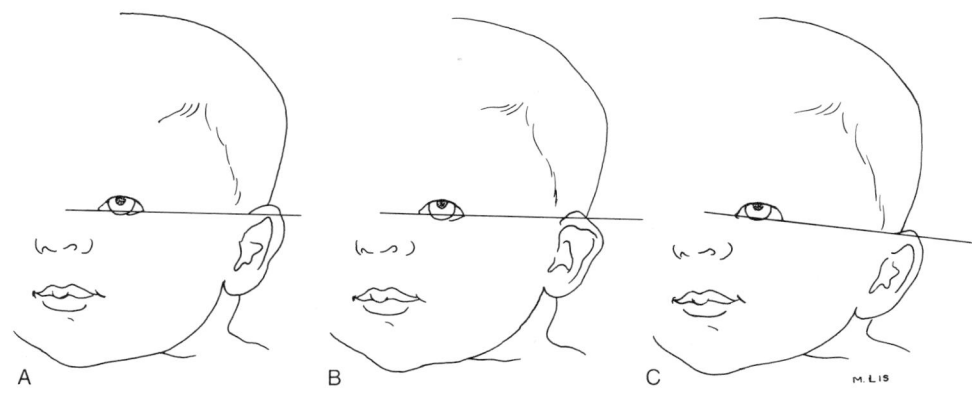

FIGURE 32-4

(A) Normal ear. (B) Abnormally angled ear. (C) Low-seated ear.

Phibbs suggests, however, that visualization should be attempted in the infant suspected of having an infection because otitis media can occur during these first days.[15] During the first few months the light reflex is diffuse, rather than cone shaped as it is later.

The ear and the nerve tracts for hearing are anatomically mature at birth, and the newborn can hear after his first cry. Hearing apparently becomes acute within several days as the eustachian tubes become aerated and the mucus in the middle ear disappears.

Hearing can be tested by sounding a bell or rattle near the baby's head but out of eyesight. Hearing the sound causes blinking of the eyes, momentary cessation of activity, or a startle response. This is not an accurate test, but it may be helpful in alerting the examiner to a possible problem.

Neck. The newborn generally appears to have a short neck, which sometimes makes it difficult to tell if webbing or other problems are present. The head should be gently rotated to determine the range of motion of the neck, and the muscles should be palpated for any masses.

Lips, Mouth, and Cheeks. The rounded, thickened areas often present on the lips (particularly on the center of the upper lip) are known as labial tubercles or "sucking blisters," although they are not true blisters since there is no fluid in them. Sucking (fat) pads are usually present in the cheeks. The lips, gums, and palate should be examined to see that they are intact. Epstein's pearls, small white cysts that may be seen on the hard palate or gums, are not abnormal. Occasionally a tooth is present, which may be pulled to avoid the possibility of its being aspirated.

At this early age, the tongue does not extend far beyond the margin of the gums because the frenulum is normally short. A mother's concern that her baby is tongue-tied is usually unwarranted.

Assessment of Body

General Appearance. The average term infant weighs 3500 g (7½ lb), and 95% weigh between 2500 g (5½ lb) and 4250 g (9½ lb). There is usually some weight loss in the first 3 to 5 days, possibly as much as 10% of the infant's birth weight. This is usually regained by the eighth to 12th day.

Length should also be measured soon after birth to serve as a baseline from which to judge future growth. The average length of a full-term infant at birth is 51 cm (20 in), with 95% between 46 and 56 cm (18 and 22 in). Since the newborn usually assumes a somewhat flexed position, it can be difficult to get an accurate measurement from the top of the head to the heels. Measurement is more accurate when done on a firm surface, and it is helpful to have an assistant hold the infant's head.

Color. The infant's color should be assessed early in the examination. The color may be pink, reddish, or pale, becoming more ruddy when the baby cries. The skin tends to be less pigmented in the neonatal period than later in life, so color changes may be noted even in darker-skinned babies. Initially the hands and feet are usually blue (acrocyanosis) owing to the sluggish peripheral vascular circulation, but this cyanosis of the extremities is transient and often disappears in a few hours. If more generalized cyanosis is present, the extent and circumstances of its appearance should be noted. The infant who is cyanotic at rest and pink only when crying may have choanal atresia. Cardiac or pulmonary problems may be suspected if crying increases the cyanosis. The infant who continues to be ruddy or plethoric even at rest should have a hematocrit done to rule out polycythemia. The very pale infant may be anemic or hypotensive and should be checked for these conditions.[16]

Frequent assessment of the newborn for jaundice is an important nursing responsibility, to help detect significant hyperbilirubinemia as early as possible. The red color of the blood or the pigment in the skin of dark-complected babies sometimes hides the yellow color. Blanching the skin over a bony area such as the chest or forehead by pressing with a finger and observing the area before the color comes back often allows the yellow to be seen. The sclera and the buccal mucosa are also good places to look.

Skin. The skin of the normal full-term newborn is soft, velvety, and wrinkled. At birth it is covered to varying degrees with vernix caseosa, a white, cheesy material made up of sebum and desquamating cells. The vernix serves as a protection for the skin *in utero* and at term is found primarily in the body creases. After the vernix is removed or disappears, the skin is often dry and peeling. A fine downy hair called lanugo may be found on the face, brow, and shoulders, especially in preterm infants.

A variety of rashes and discolorations of the skin are considered to be normal variations in the newborn period. Small, flat hemangiomas may be apparent on the nape of the neck, on the eyelids, or over the bridge of the nose. These clusters of small capillaries are sometimes called "stork bites." They usually disappear spontaneously during infancy, but some, especially those on the nape of the neck, may persist into adulthood.

Gray blue pigmented areas are seen most often in dark-skinned infants, especially in the lumbosacral area, although other sites are not uncommon. These

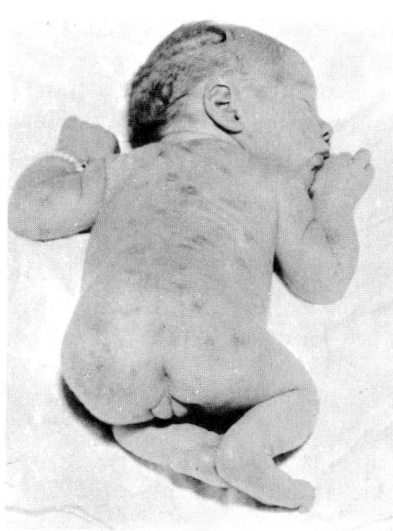 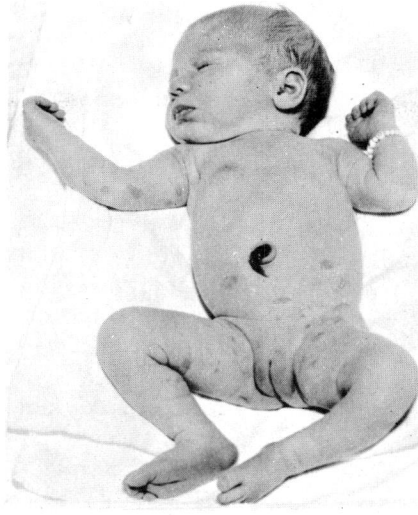

FIGURE 32-5

Erythema toxicum. This "newborn rash" develops more frequently on the back, the shoulders, and the buttocks. (Courtesy of MacDonald House, The University Hospitals of Cleveland, Cleveland, Ohio)

"mongolian spots" have no relationship to mongolism and usually disappear spontaneously during late infancy or early childhood.

Erythema Toxicum. Erythema toxicum is a blotchy erythematous rash that may appear in the first few days of life (Fig. 32-5). It is sometimes referred to as the newborn rash or as "flea-bite" dermatitis (although no fleas are involved). The erythematous areas, which develop most frequently on the back, shoulders, and buttocks, have a small blanched wheal in the center. The cause of this skin disturbance is obscure, and no treatment is necessary. The rash is transient, is likely to change appreciably within a few hours, and usually disappears entirely within a day or so.

Milia. Milia are pinpoint-sized, pearly white spots that occur commonly on the nose, forehead, or chin of the newborn. When touched gently with the tip of the finger, these spots feel like tiny, firm seeds. They are

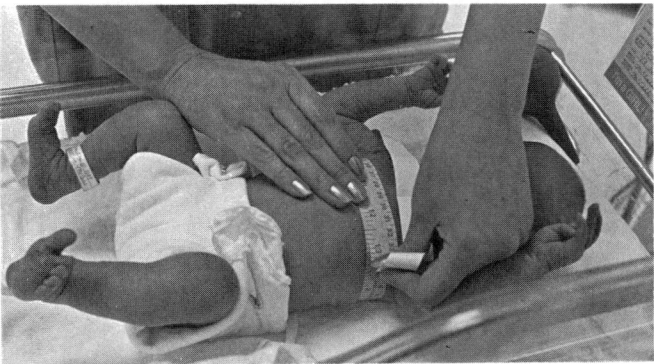

FIGURE 32-6

Measuring the infant's chest.

due to retention of sebaceous material within the sebaceous glands and, if they are left alone, usually disappear spontaneously during the neonatal period. Mothers often mistake milia for "whiteheads" and may attempt to squeeze them if the nurse or the physician has not warned them against such practice.

Café au lait spots. Café au lait spots or patches are flat, brown areas that are lighter in light-skinned individuals and darker in those with more pigmentation. Single small lesions are not unusual in newborns and are of no significance, but if the spots are greater than 1.5 cm in length or more than six are present, they may be indicative of neurofibromatosis or certain genetic syndromes.[17]

Thorax. The infant's chest is round with a transverse diameter that is approximately equal to the anteroposterior diameter. The circumference, measured just above the nipple line, is slightly smaller than the head (Fig. 32-6). The thorax is relatively short compared to the abdomen. The chest wall is thin with little musculature, and the rib cage is very soft and pliant. The tip of the xiphoid process often protrudes visibly.

Engorgement of the breasts is common during the neonatal period in both male and female infants (Fig. 32-7), owing to endocrine influence. The breasts have been acted on throughout pregnancy by the estrogenic hormone that passes to them through the placenta from the mother. This is the same hormone that prepares the mother's breasts for lactation. When it is withdrawn after birth, changes in the infant's breasts, similar to those in the mother, take place. Mammary engorgement in the newborn subsides without treatment, but may persist for 2 or 3 weeks.

Sometimes a small amount of fluid that has been called "witches' milk" is secreted. Mothers should be

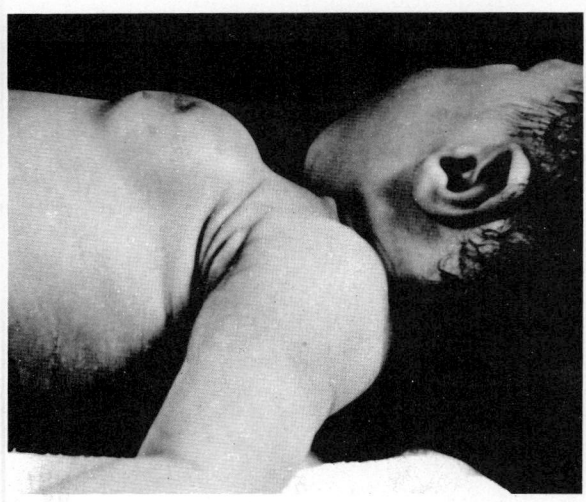

FIGURE   32-7

Hypertrophy of breast developing in the neonatal period.

cautioned against massaging the infant's breasts or trying to express the fluid because this could lead to an infection such as breast abscess or mastitis.

Assessing Respiration.   As the infant adapts successfully to extrauterine life, the respiratory rate usually ranges from 40 to 60 breaths per minute and is easily altered by internal and external stimuli. Counting respirations in the newborn can be very frustrating, since the infant may have periods of rapid breathing alternating with short periods of apnea. Intermittent crying may also interfere with counting. Respirations should be counted for 1 full minute or longer if necessary. Since the infant primarily uses diaphragmatic breathing, it is easier to count abdominal rather than chest excursions. An alternate method is to count respirations by auscultation (Fig. 32-8).

The respiration is normally quiet and shallow, with the chest and abdomen moving together. Although retractions, mild expiratory grunting, and nasal flaring may be considered normal during the first few minutes after birth, presence after that time leads one to suspect obstruction or abnormality.

In auscultation of the infant's chest, it is best to use the bell or small diaphragm of the stethoscope, since the adult-sized diaphragm may not make complete contact with the small chest wall. Auscultation should be done in both upright and supine positions because breath sounds may be altered with changing positions. Bronchial breath sounds are normally heard over most of the chest and sound louder and harsher because they are closer.

Periods of dyspnea and cyanosis may occur suddenly in an infant who is breathing normally, even after the transition period is over. This *may* indicate some anomaly or other pathologic condition and should be reported promptly. The nurse should notify the physician if the respiratory rate is persistently below 40 respirations per minute or if it increases beyond 60 res-

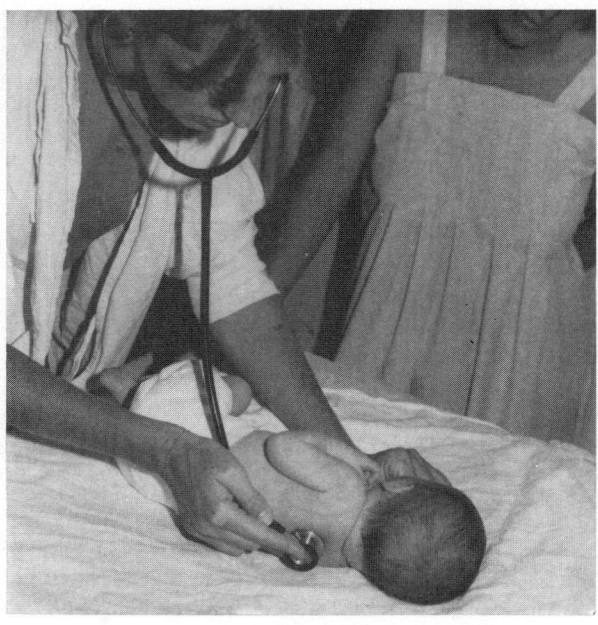
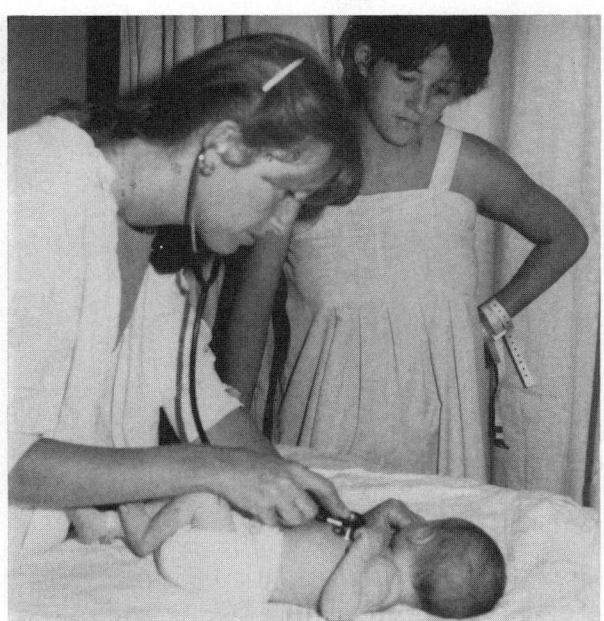

FIGURE   32-8

Auscultation of the newborn. The nurse practitioner performs a discharge physical examination while the mother observes.

pirations per minute when the infant is at rest, or if dyspnea or cyanosis occurs.

Heart. The heart rate is determined by counting the apical pulse (Fig. 32-9). It is normally between 120 and 160 beats per minute and, like the respiratory rate, changes with the infant's activity. It beats faster when he is crying, active, or breathing rapidly, and it beats more slowly when he is quiet, especially during the short periods of no breathing.

The first and second heart sounds should be clear and well defined. Murmurs may be present in the newborn period. They may be heard more easily with the bell of the stethoscope held lightly against the chest wall. The areas of cardiac auscultation where murmurs are most likely to be heard are the right sternal border, the upper left sternal border, the lower left sternal border, and the apex. Any murmurs should be reported, recorded, and followed but may be less significant in the newborn period than at other times, since a closing ductus arteriosus may cause a loud murmur that soon disappears, while a serious heart anomaly may cause no murmur at all.

Early experiences in listening to the newborn's chest can be confusing because both the heart rate and respirations are so much faster than an adult's and the infant often wiggles and fusses. With practice the student will learn how to quiet the infant and to be able to distinguish between the different sounds.

Abdomen. The abdomen is round and slightly protuberant owing to the relative size of the abdominal organs and weak muscular structures. Superficial veins are often visible. Observation can be a valuable part of the examination of the abdomen, since outlines of the anterior organs may sometimes be seen. An abdomen that is asymmetrical, scaphoid (sunken), or grossly distended is suggestive of abnormalities and should be checked carefully.

Palpation should begin with gentle pressure or stroking of the abdomen upward, then deeper palpation may be done. The liver edge is usually palpable just below the right rib margin, but it is not sharp and may be missed if palpation is too high or too forceful. The tip of the spleen may sometimes be palpated in the left upper quadrant. The kidneys can usually be palpated during the first 4 to 6 hours after birth, but they are more difficult to locate after this. If palpable, the lower edges are usually located approximately at the level of the umbilicus, about half way between the infant's side and the midline.

The umbilical cord stump should be checked for bleeding or oozing (Fig. 32-10), and the number of vessels noted if not already recorded (see Chap. 28). The umbilicus and surrounding area should also be inspected carefully. Redness, induration, skin warmth, and foul-

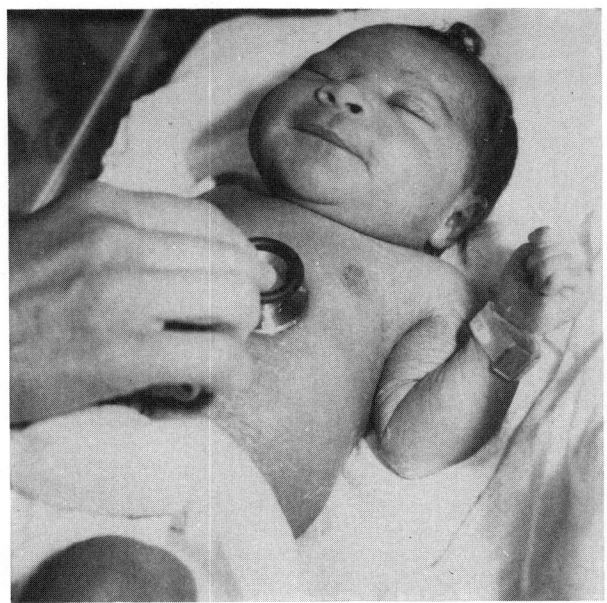

F I G U R E   3 2 - 9

Taking an apical pulse.

smelling discharge are signs of infection that should be reported. Infection in this area is potentially dangerous in the newborn because it can spread up the open arteries into the peritoneum. Serous or serosanguineous discharge continuing after separation of the cord stump may indicate a granuloma. This has the appearance of a small red button deep in the umbilicus. It can be cauterized by the physician with a silver nitrate stick.[18]

Genitals. Female genitalia should be inspected for presence and size of the labia majora, labia minora, clitoris, and vaginal opening. Enlarged labia or vaginal discharge may be present due to *in utero* stimulation by maternal hormones. The discharge is sometimes blood tinged but need cause no special concern. The swelling and discharge disappear spontaneously.

In male babies the scrotum usually appears relatively large and may have increased pigmentation at birth owing to maternal hormones. At term the testes usually can be palpated in the scrotum or can be easily brought down. The prepuce (foreskin) covers the glans penis and is usually adherent at birth. When the opening in the foreskin is so small that it cannot be pulled back at all, the condition is called *phimosis*. If it is tight enough to interfere with urination, circumcision may be recommended. The penis should be inspected to determine the location of the urinary meatus. It is usually located at the tip of the penis. When it is located on the underside of the penis the condition is known as *hypospadias*; location on the dorsum of the penis is called *epispadias*. If the meatus is covered by the foreskin, ob-

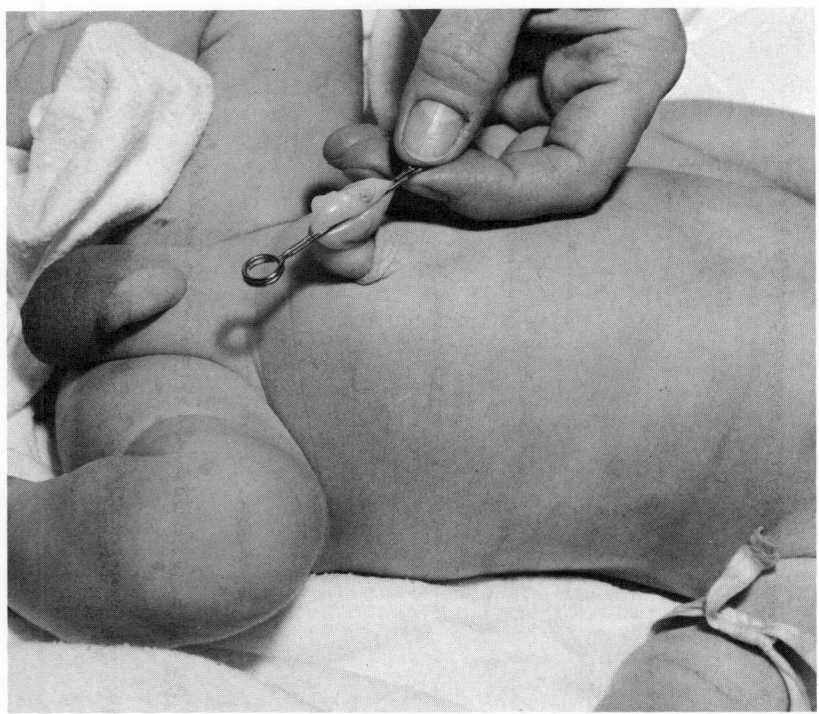

F I G U R E   3 2 - 1 0

Inspection of cord stump.

servation of the infant during voiding will help to determine its placement.

Posterior. With the infant in the prone position, the entire posterior surface of the body should be inspected and palpated. Any masses or abnormal curvatures of the spine should be noted. Tufts of hair or small indentations, especially in the sacral area, may be an indication of spina bifida occulta.

The perineal area should be inspected to determine the patency and location of the anus. A pilonidal "dimple" resulting from an irregular fold of skin is sometimes seen in the midline over the sacrococcygeal area. It should be examined for intactness to make sure no sinus is present.

Extremities. Throughout the examination, the infant's ability to move all four extremities is evaluated and the limbs are compared as to size, shape, and movement. Webbing (syndactyly) or extra digits (polydactyly) should be noted also.

To check for congenital problems of the hip, the infant is placed in the supine position and the legs are flexed on the abdomen and then abducted laterally toward the bed. With congenital dislocation, there may be uneven or limited abduction or uneven leg length or knee height, or a "hip click" might be felt (Fig. 32-11). Asymmetrical skin folds on the posterior aspect of the thigh are not diagnostic but may alert the examiner to this condition. Unusual positions of the feet can indicate

congenital clubfoot or other foot and ankle deformities. If the foot can be moved to the normal position with ease, the condition may just be due to intrauterine malposition.

Neurologic Assessment

The neurologic assessment deals with the functioning of the infant's nervous system. Some of the items assessed in the physical, gestational age, and behavioral assessments are also indicators of nervous system functioning. For example, vital signs are part of the physical assessment, but could also be included in the neurologic assessment because extreme lability of the temperature and blood pressure reflects immaturity of the autonomic neuromuscular mechanisms.[19] The focus in this section will be on the character of the infant's movements and on the reflexes that are usually present at birth.

Movements

At the beginning of the examination the infant's movements should be observed before he is touched. The spontaneous movements of the normal newborn usually involve all extremities and are random and symmetrical but not stereotyped. Sometimes jitteriness or tremors will be noted and might be interpreted as seizures. It is

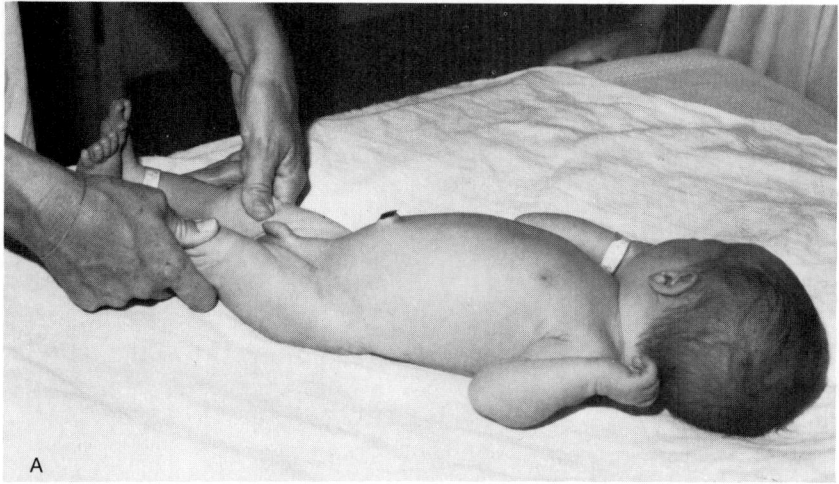

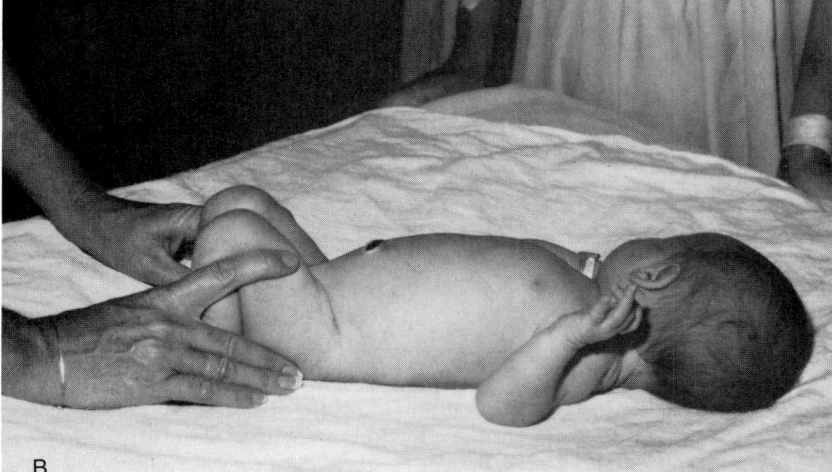

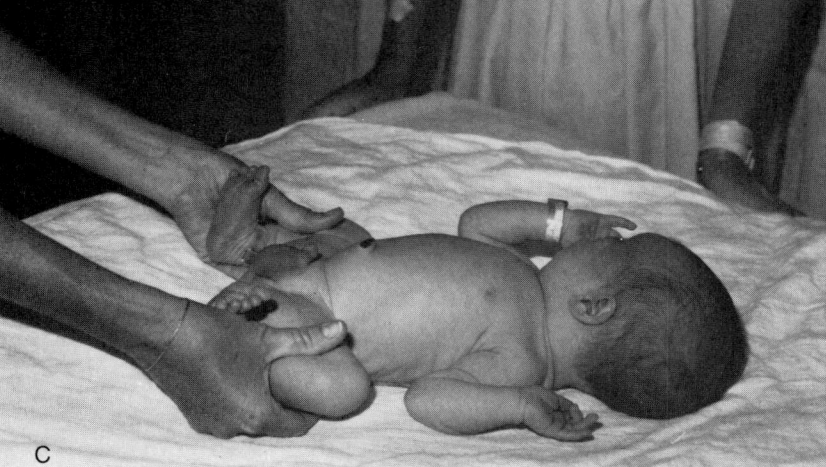

FIGURE 32-11

Assessment of the lower extremities.
(*A*) Comparing the length of the legs.
(*B*) Comparing the height of the knees.
(*C*) Hip abduction.

important to differentiate seizures from other movements, since neonatal seizures are usually treatable and brain damage might be avoided if they are identified early. The following clinical features are helpful in differentiating between tremors or jitteriness and seizures.[20]

- The rhythmic movements of jitteriness or tremors are equal in amplitude, but seizures have a fast and slow component to the movements.
- Jitteriness or tremors are provoked by external stimuli such as noise or handling, but this is not true of seizures.

- The examiner can usually stop the movements that are due to jitteriness or tremors by passively holding the affected limb still.

Reflexes

Rooting and Sucking

Gently stroking the infant's cheek or corner of the mouth with a sterile nipple or clean finger causes the baby to open his mouth and turn toward the stimulus (Fig. 32-12). This is known as the *rooting reflex*. The *sucking reflex* can be evaluated by placing the nipple or finger in the baby's mouth and noting the strength of the sucking response. These reflexes may not be too active if the infant has eaten recently.

It is well known that during the first 2 months of life the newborn has a great need to suck and usually sucks on anything that comes in contact with his lips. Newborns can suck while sleeping, and nonnutritive sucking can have a quieting effect on excitable babies.

Grasp Reflex

The *grasp reflex* is present at birth in both the hands and the feet (Fig. 32-13). The infant grasps any object placed in his hands, clings briefly, and then lets go.

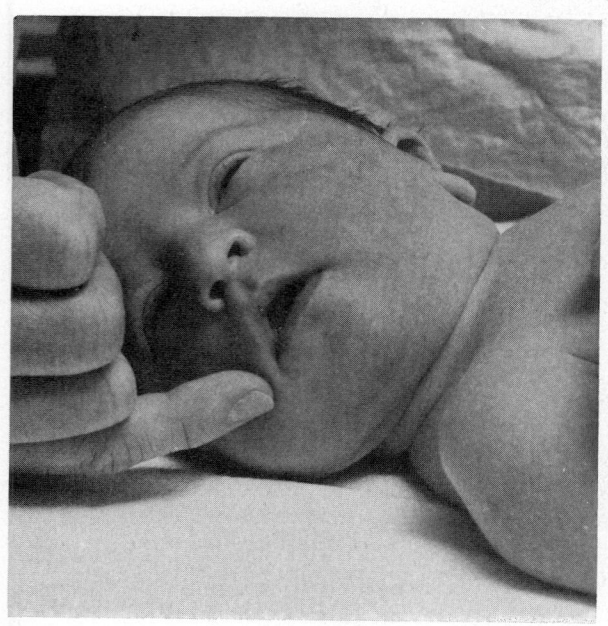

FIGURE 32-12

Rooting reflex. (Sullivan R, Foster J, Schreiner RL: Determining a newborn's gestational age. MCN, American Journal of Maternal/Child Nursing, January/February, pp 38–45, 1979)

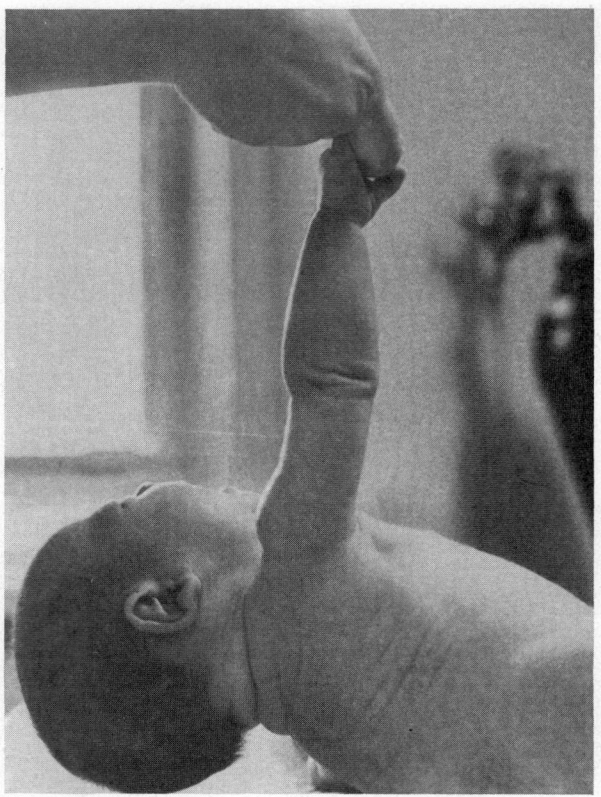

FIGURE 32-13

Grasp reflex. (A clinical review of concepts and characteristics in infant development. In Reflexes, Vol 2. Evansville, Indiana, Mead Johnson and Company. Copyright 1974.)

Even at birth he may be able to hold onto an adult's forefinger so securely that he can be lifted to a standing position. Although the baby cannot actually grasp with his feet, stroking the soles causes the toes to turn downward as though trying to grasp. The grasping movements are a reflex action at birth, but with practice and experience the hand grasp soon becomes voluntary and purposeful.

By grasping the infant's hands and arms, the examiner can gently pull the infant to a sitting position. The infant flexes the elbows to resist extension (traction response). The strength of the neck muscles can be assessed by noting the amount of head lag. The normal term newborn is able to support his head momentarily.

Moro Reflex

The *Moro* or *startle reflex* indicates an awareness of equilibrium in the newborn (Fig. 32-14). The preferred method of eliciting this reflex is to hold the infant with his head supported, then allow the head to drop backward a short distance. Alternately, the infant can be

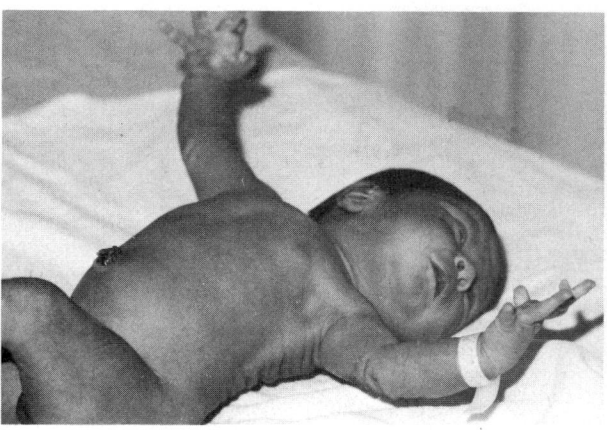 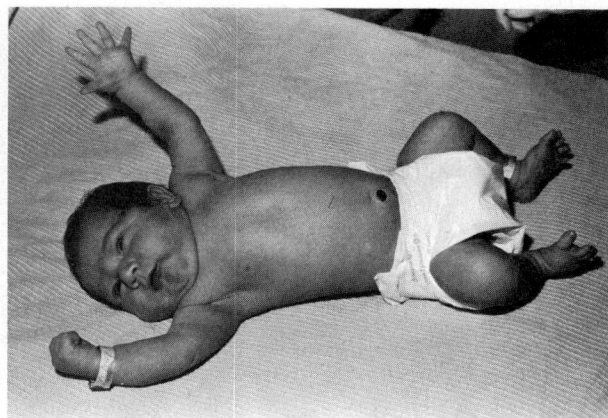

FIGURE 32-14

Moro reflex.

lying quietly and the mattress struck, or the head lifted a few inches and allowed to drop back. The reaction should consist of lateral extension of the upper extremities and opening of the hands, followed by anterior flexion and adduction of the arms in an embracing motion. The movements should be symmetrical. If they are not, injury to the part that lags should be suspected.

The Moro reflex should be present at birth; normally it disappears by 3 months of age. If it cannot be elicited at birth, edema of or injury to the brain may be present. As the edema subsides, the reflex returns, and it should be demonstrable on the day following delivery. If frank brain damage has occurred, the reflex is absent for several days; if the damage is not too severe, the reflex returns in 3 or 4 days. Occasionally, the reflex is present at birth but disappears over the first days. Increasing cerebral edema or slow intracranial hemorrhage then is suspected.

Tonic Neck Reflex

When the *tonic neck reflex* is elicited, the infant assumes a "fencing" position (*i.e.*, he lies on his back with his head rotated to one side). The arm and the leg on the side toward which he is facing are partially or completely extended, and the opposite arm and leg are flexed (Fig. 32-15). This reflex also disappears in a few months, since it is another manifestation of the immaturity of the newborn's nervous system.

Stepping Reflex

The *stepping* or *dancing reflex* is another action that is present at birth but soon disappears. This reflex causes the infant to make little stepping or prancing movements when he is held upright with his feet touching a surface

(Fig. 32-16). After this reflex diminishes, the infant does not attempt stepping motions until he is ready to stand and walk. However, he does exercise the leg muscles a great deal and seems to derive much enjoyment from waving and kicking his legs about.

Other Reflexes

The next group of reflexes might be termed protective, since they are necessary and at times essential to the preservation of the newborn's safety. The *blinking reflex* occurs when the infant is subjected to a bright light. The *cough* and the *sneeze reflexes* clear his respiratory passages. The *yawn reflex* draws in additional oxygen. These, together with the infant's ability to cry when uncomfortable, to withdraw from painful stimuli, to resist restraint, and so on, are all defensive measures. As the baby grows and develops, these together with the other reflexes mentioned either diminish or become more highly developed according to the need. Thus, the infant's behavior patterns become more complex and highly developed.

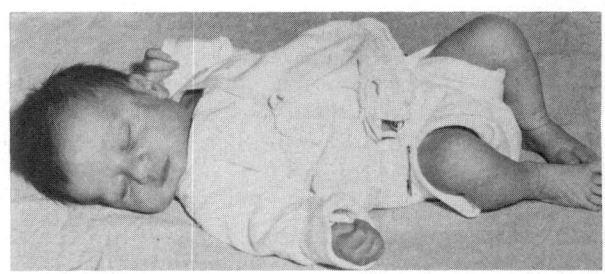

FIGURE 32-15

Tonic neck reflex.

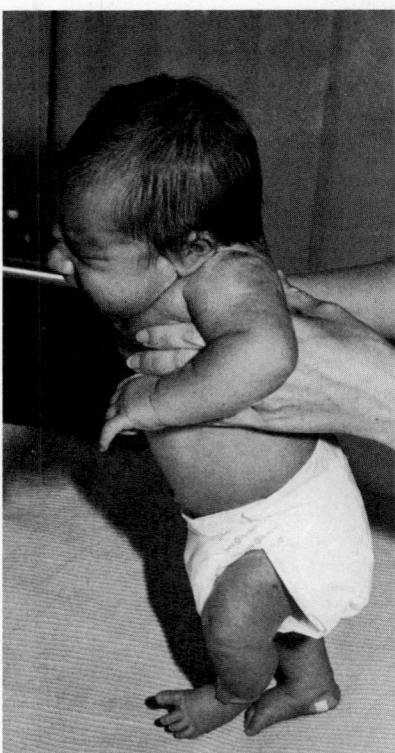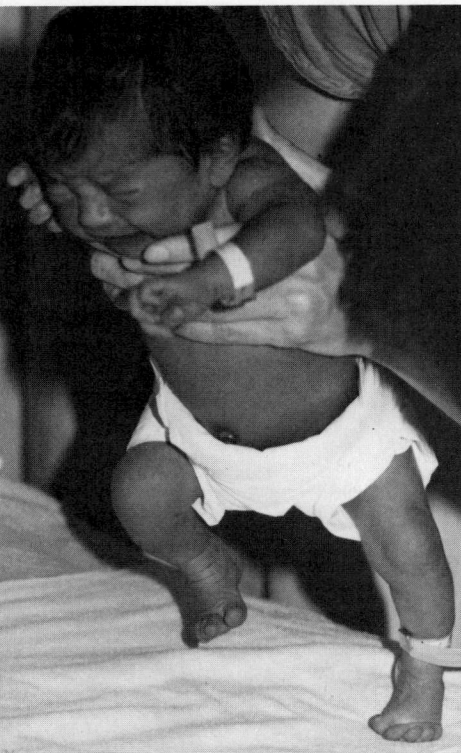

FIGURE   32-16

Stepping reflex.

Gestational Age Assessment

Accurate assessment of an infant's gestational age is another important aspect of newborn assessment. *Gestational age* is the estimated age of the fetus or newborn, expressed in weeks, counting from the first day of the mother's last menstrual period. During the prenatal period, a variety of techniques can be used in the estimation of gestational age (see Chap. 42). Following the infant's birth, assessment of certain external physical characteristics and neurologic signs can result in a more accurate estimate. Knowing the approximate gestational age helps to determine whether the infant was born early (preterm), born on time (term), or born late (post term), when compared with the expected gestation of 40 weeks. When gestational age is considered together with birth weight, infants can be designated as small, appropriate, or large for gestational age. Chapter 44 gives a more complete discussion of these categories, the potential problems they suggest, and the part they play in planning care for the newborn.

Assessment of gestational age by examination should be done in the first days of life, because the extrauterine environment leads to rapid changes in the characteristics of the newborn. The physical characteristics that are assessed are independent of the baby's health and ideally are evaluated within a few hours of the birth. The neurologic criteria can be altered by the infant's physical condition, and this part of the examination is deferred until later.[19]

The physical and neurologic criteria that have been identified as being useful in gestational age assessment are used in a variety of combinations in the different scoring systems that have been suggested. The Dubowitz scoring system uses a combination of physical, neurobehavioral, and reflex criteria to arrive at a gestational age (see Assessment Tool). This has the disadvantage of being rather long. An abbreviated system using seven physical and six neurologic signs, developed by Ballard and her colleagues, is more widely used (see Estimation of Gestational Age by Maturity Rating). Other combinations of criteria may be used in different settings. When learning to do the examination it may be helpful at first to check only five of the criteria, such as the breasts, ears, genitalia, sole creases, and posture, and then to expand to other areas as proficiency is achieved.[21]

Physical Characteristics

During the growth and development of the fetus, certain external physical characteristics develop and progress in an orderly manner. The presence, absence, or degree of development of these characteristics at birth is used to help determine gestational age.

(text continued on page 643)

ASSESSMENT TOOL

Dubowitz Scoring System

NAME	D.O.B./TIME	WEIGHT	E.D.D. L.N.M.P.	E.D.D. U/snd.	STATES
HOSP. NO.	DATE OF EXAM	HEIGHT			1. Deep sleep, no movement, regular breathing. 2. Light sleep, eyes shut, some movement. 3. Dozing, eyes opening and closing.
RACE SEX	AGE	HEAD CIRC.	GESTATIONAL ASSESSMENT	SCORE WEEKS	4. Awake, eyes open, minimal movement. 5. Wide awake, vigorous movement. 6. Crying.

Columns on the right: STATE | COMMENT | ASYMMETRY

HABITUATION (≤state 3)

LIGHT
Repetitive flashlight stimuli (10) with 5 sec. gap.
Shutdown = 2 consecutive negative responses

| No response | A. Blink response to first stimulus only. B. Tonic blink response. C. Variable response. | A. Shutdown of movement but blink persists 2-5 stimuli. B. Complete shutdown 2-5 stimuli. | A. Shutdown of movement but blink persists 6-10 stimuli. B. Complete shutdown 6-10 stimuli. | A. Equal response to 10 stimuli. B. Infant comes to fully alert state. C. Startles + major responses throughout. |

RATTLE
Repetitive stimuli (10) with 5 sec. gap.

| No response | A. Slight movement to first stimulus. B. Variable response. | Startle or movement 2-5 stimuli, then shutdown | Startle or movement 6-10 stimuli, then shutdown | A. B. Grading as above C. |

MOVEMENT & TONE
Undress infant

POSTURE (At rest — predominant) *

(figures) | (figures) | (figures) (hips abducted) | (figures) (hips adducted) | Abnormal postures: A. Opisthotonus. B. Unusual leg extension. C. Asymm. tonic neck reflex

ARM RECOIL
Infant supine. Take both hands, extend parallel to the body; hold approx. 2 secs. and release.

| No flexion within 5 sec. | Partial flexion at elbow >100° within 4-5 sec. | Arms flex at elbow to <100° within 2-3 sec. | Sudden jerky flexion at elbow immediately after release to <60° | Difficult to extend; arm snaps back forcefully |

ARM TRACTION
Infant supine; head midline; grasp wrist, slowly pull arm to vertical. Angle of arm scored and resistance noted at moment infant is initially lifted off and watched until shoulder off mattress. Do other arm.

| Arm remains fully extended | Weak flexion maintained only momentarily | Arm flexed at elbow to 140° and maintained 5 sec. | Arm flexed at approx. 100° and maintained | Strong flexion of arm <100° and maintained |

LEG RECOIL
First flex hips for 5 secs, then extend both legs of infant by traction on ankles; hold down on the bed for 2 secs. and release.

| No flexion within 5 sec. | Incomplete flexion of hips within 5 sec. | Complete flexion within 5 sec. | Instantaneous complete flexion | Legs cannot be extended; snap back forcefully |

LEG TRACTION
Infant supine. Grasp leg near ankle and slowly pull toward vertical until buttocks 1-2" off. Note resistance at knee and score angle. Do other leg.

| No flexion | Partial flexion, rapidly lost | Knee flexion 140-160° and maintained | Knee flexion 100-140° and maintained | Strong resistance; flexion <100° |

POPLITEAL ANGLE
Infant supine. Approximate knee and thigh to abdomen; extend leg by gentle pressure with index finger behind ankle.

| 180-160° | 150-140° | 130-120° | 110-90° | <90° |

HEAD CONTROL (post. neck m.)
Grasp infant by shoulders and raise to sitting position; allow head to fall forward; wait 30 sec.

| No attempt to raise head | Unsuccessful attempt to raise head upright | Head raised smoothly to upright in 30 sec. but not maintained | Head raised smoothly to upright in 30 sec. and maintained | Head cannot be flexed forward |

HEAD CONTROL (ant. neck m.)
Allow head to fall backward as you hold shoulders; wait 30 secs.

| Grading as above | Grading as above | Grading as above | Grading as above | |

HEAD LAG *
Pull infant toward sitting posture by traction on both wrists. Also note arm flexion.

VENTRAL SUSPENSION *
Hold infant in ventral suspension; observe curvature of back, flexion of limbs and relation of head to trunk.

HEAD RAISING IN PRONE POSITION
Infant in prone position with head in midline.

| No response | Rolls head to one side | Weak effort to raise head and turns raised head to one side | Infant lifts head, nose and chin off | Strong prolonged head lifting |

ARM RELEASE IN PRONE POSITION
Head in midline. Infant in prone position; arms extended alongside body with palms up.

| No effort | Some effort and wriggling | Flexion effort but neither wrist brought to nipple level | One or both wrists brought at least to nipple level without excessive body movement | Strong body movement with both wrists brought to face, or 'press-ups' |

SPONTANEOUS BODY MOVEMENT
during examination (supine). If no spont. movement try to induce by cutaneous stimulation.

| None or minimal Induced | A. Sluggish. B. Random, incoordinated. C. Mainly stretching. | Smooth movements alternating with random, stretching, athetoid or jerky | Smooth alternating movements of arms and legs with medium speed and intensity | Mainly: A. Jerky movement. B. Athetoid movement. C. Other abnormal movement. | COMMENT: 1 2 |

TREMORS Mark: Fast (>6/sec.) or Slow (<6/sec.)

| No tremor | Tremors only in state 5-6 | Tremors only in sleep or after Moro and startles | Some tremors in state 4 | Tremulousness in all states |

STARTLES

| No startles | Startles to sudden noise, Moro, bang on table only | Occasional spontaneous startle | 2-5 spontaneous startles | 6+ spontaneous startles |

ABNORMAL MOVEMENT OR POSTURE

| No abnormal movement | A. Hands clenched but open intermittently. B. Hands do not open with Moro. | A. Some mouthing movement. B. Intermittent adducted thumb | A. Persistently adducted thumb B. Hands clenched all the time | A. Continuous mouthing movement. B. Convulsive movements. |

(continued)

A S S E S S M E N T   T O O L   *(continued)*

					STATE	COMMENT	ASYMMETRY
REFLEXES							
TENDON REFLEXES Biceps jerk Knee jerk Ankle jerk	Absent		Present	Exaggerated	Clonus		
PALMAR GRASP Head in midline. Put index finger from ulnar side into hand and gently press palmar surface. Never touch dorsal side of hand.	Absent	Short, weak flexion	Medium strength and sustained flexion for several secs.	Strong flexion; contraction spreads to forearm	Very strong grasp. Infant easily lifts off couch			
ROOTING Infant supine, head midline. Touch each corner of the mouth in turn (stroke laterally).	No response	A. Partial weak head turn but no mouth opening. B. Mouth opening, no head turn.	Mouth opening on stimulated side with partial head turning	Full head turning, with or without mouth opening	Mouth opening with very jerky head turning			
SUCKING Infant supine; place index finger (pad towards palate) in infant's mouth; judge power of sucking movement after 5 sec.	No attempt	Weak sucking movement: A. Regular. B. Irregular.	Strong sucking movement, poor stripping: A. Regular. B. Irregular.	Strong regular sucking movement with continuing sequence of 5 movements. Good stripping.	Clenching but no regular sucking.			
WALKING (state 4, 5) Hold infant upright, feet touching bed, neck held straight with fingers.	Absent		Some effort but not continuous with both legs	At least 2 steps with both legs	A. Stork posture; no movement. B. Automatic walking.			
MORO One hand supports infant's head in midline, the other the back. Raise infant to 45° and when infant is relaxed let his head fall through 10°. Note if jerky. Repeat 3 times.	No response, or opening of hands only	Full abduction at the shoulder and extension of the arm	Full abduction but only delayed or partial adduction	Partial abduction at shoulder and extension of arms followed by smooth adduction A. Abd>Add B. Abd=Add C. Abd<Add	A. No abduction or adduction; extension only. B. Marked adduction only.	J S		
NEUROBEHAVIOURAL ITEMS							
EYE APPEARANCES	Sunset sign Nerve palsy	Transient nystagmus. Strabismus. Some roving eye movement.	Does not open eyes	Normal conjugate eye movement	A. Persistent nystagmus. B. Frequent roving movement C. Frequent rapid blinks.			
AUDITORY ORIENTATION (state 3, 4) To rattle. (Note presence of startle.)	A. No reaction. B. Auditory startle but no true orientation.	Brightens and stills; may turn toward stimuli with eyes closed	Alerting and shifting of eyes; head may or may not turn to source	Alerting; prolonged head turns to stimulus; search with eyes	Turning and alerting to stimulus each time on both sides	S		
VISUAL ORIENTATION (state 4) To red woollen ball	Does not focus or follow stimulus	Stills; focuses on stimulus; may follow 30° jerkily; does not find stimulus again spontaneously	Follows 30-60° horizontally; may lose stimulus but finds it again. Brief vertical glance	Follows with eyes and head horizontally and to some extent vertically, with frowning	Sustained fixation; follows vertically, horizonally, and in circle			
ALERTNESS (state 4)	Inattentive; rarely or never responds to direct stimulation	When alert, periods rather brief; rather variable response to orientation	When alert, alertness moderately sustained; may use stimulus to come to alert state	Sustained alertness; orientation frequent, reliable to visual but not auditory stimuli	Continuous alertness, which does not seem to tire, to both auditory and visual stimuli			
DEFENSIVE REACTION A cloth or hand is placed over the infant's face to partially occlude the nasal airway.	No response	A. General quietening. B. Non-specific activity with long latency.	Rooting; lateral neck turning; possibly neck stretching.	Swipes with arm	Swipes with arm with rather violent body movement			
PEAK OF EXCITEMENT	Low level arousal to all stimuli; never > state 3	Infant reaches state 4-5 briefly but predominantly in lower states	Infant predominantly state 4 or 5; may reach state 6 after stimulation but returns spontaneously to lower state	Infant reaches state 6 but can be consoled relatively easily	A. Mainly state 6. Difficult to console, if at all. B. Mainly state 4-5 but if reaches state 6 cannot be consoled.			
IRRITABILITY (states 3, 4, 5) Aversive stimuli: Uncover Ventral susp. Undress Moro Pull to sit Walking reflex Prone	No irritable crying to any of the stimuli	Cries to 1-2 stimuli	Cries to 3-4 stimuli	Cries to 5-6 stimuli	Cries to all stimuli			
CONSOLABILITY (state 6)	Never above state 5 during examination, therefore not needed	Consoling not needed. Consoles spontaneously	Consoled by talking, hand on belly or wrapping up	Consoled by picking up and holding; may need finger in mouth	Not consolable			
CRY	No cry at all	Only whimpering cry	Cries to stimuli but normal pitch	Lusty cry to offensive stimuli; normal pitch	High-pitched cry, often continuous			

NOTES ✳ If asymmetrical or atypical, draw in on nearest figure

Record any abnormal signs (e.g. facial palsy, contractures, etc.). Draw if possible.

Record time after feed:

EXAMINER:

Reprinted from *The Neurological Assessment of the Preterm and Full-term Newborn Infant,* by Lilly and Victor Dubowitz. © 1981 Spastics International Medical Publications, 5A Netherhall Gardens, London NW3 5RN.

ASSESSMENT TOOL

Estimation of Gestational Age by Maturity Rating

Symbols:　X - 1st Exam　O - 2nd Exam

NEUROMUSCULAR MATURITY

	0	1	2	3	4	5
Posture						
Square Window (Wrist)	90°	60°	45°	30°	0°	
Arm Recoil	180°		100°-180°	90°-100°	< 90°	
Popliteal Angle	180°	160°	130°	110°	90°	< 90°
Scarf Sign						
Heel to Ear						

Gestation by Dates _____ wks

Birth Date _____ Hour _____ am / pm

APGAR _____ 1 min _____ 5 min

MATURITY RATING

Score	Wks
5	26
10	28
15	30
20	32
25	34
30	36
35	38
40	40
45	42
50	44

PHYSICAL MATURITY

	0	1	2	3	4	5
SKIN	gelatinous red, transparent	smooth pink, visible veins	superficial peeling &/or rash, few veins	cracking pale area, rare veins	parchment, deep cracking, no vessels	leathery, cracked, wrinkled
LANUGO	none	abundant	thinning	bald areas	mostly bald	
PLANTAR CREASES	no crease	faint red marks	anterior transverse crease only	creases ant. 2/3	creases cover entire sole	
BREAST	barely percept.	flat areola, no bud	stippled areola, 1–2 mm bud	raised areola, 3–4 mm bud	full areola, 5–10 mm bud	
EAR	pinna flat, stays folded	sl. curved pinna, soft with slow recoil	well-curv. pinna, soft but ready recoil	formed & firm with instant recoil	thick cartilage, ear stiff	
GENITALS Male	scrotum empty, no rugae		testes descending, few rugae	testes down, good rugae	testes pendulous, deep rugae	
GENITALS Female	prominent clitoris & labia minora		majora & minora equally prominent	majora large, minora small	clitoris & minora completely covered	

SCORING SECTION

	1st Exam=X	2nd Exam=O
Estimating Gest Age by Maturity Rating	_____ Weeks	_____ Weeks
Time of Exam	Date _____ Hour _____ am/pm	Date _____ Hour _____ am/pm
Age at Exam	_____ Hours	_____ Hours
Signature of Examiner	_____ M.D.	_____ M.D.

(text continued from page 640)

Skin and Vernix.　The skin of premature infants is thin, pink, smooth, almost transparent (with blood vessels visible), and thickly covered with vernix. Presence or absence of blood vessels is usually observed over the abdomen. The skin becomes thicker and more opaque with increasing age, until by 40 weeks it is pale with few vessels visible and sparse vernix often occurring only in skin creases. In the postmature infant, there may be extensive desquamation of skin and absence of vernix (Fig. 32-17).

Lanugo.　Fine lanugo hair covers the infant's body at 20 weeks' gestation and begins to disappear first from

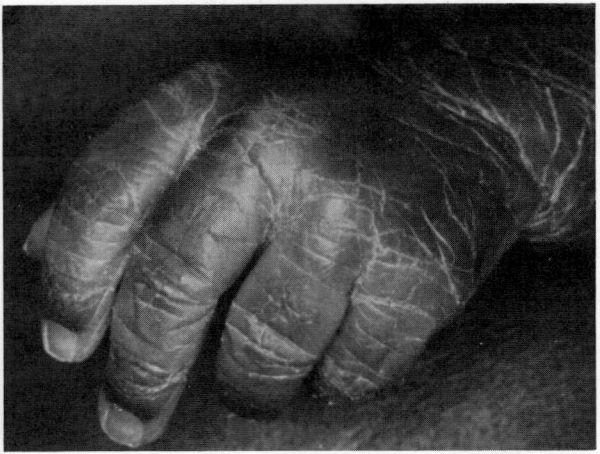

FIGURE   32-17

Postterm infant's hand. Note dry, peeling, cracked skin. (Sullivan R, Foster J, Schreiner RL: Determining a newborn's gestational age. MCN, American Journal of Maternal/Child Nursing, January/February, pp 38–45, 1979)

the face, then the trunk, and then the extremities (Fig. 32-18). At term, hair, if present, tends to be located only over the shoulders.

Sole Creases.

The soles of the feet become wrinkled first on the anterior portion and then in the area extending toward the heel as gestation progresses. At 32 weeks, one or two creases can be seen; they become more numerous, crisscrossed, and deeper, covering the anterior two thirds of the sole by 37 weeks. The entire sole, including the heel, is covered at 40 weeks (Fig. 32-19). In the post-term infant, creases are deeper and there may be desquamation of the soles.

Breast Tissue and Areola.

The nipples are present early in gestation, but the areola is barely visible until 34 weeks. After this time, the areola becomes raised and hair follicles become evident. Infants of less than 36 weeks' gestation have no breast tissue. At 36 weeks, a 1-mm to 2-mm nodule of breast tissue becomes palpable. This increases with gestational age under hormonal stimulation until it reaches 7 mm to 10 mm at 40 weeks (Fig. 32-20).

Ear Form and Cartilage.

Infants less than 33 weeks' gestation have relatively flat ears. After 34 weeks, the upper pinnae begin to curve inward. By 38 weeks, the upper two thirds of the pinnae are incurved; this extends to the earlobe by 39 to 40 weeks. Since ear form can vary widely from one individual to another, cartilage is more reliable than ear form in estimating gestational age. Owing to the absence of cartilage, the extremely premature infant's ear remains folded over if pressed. Cartilage begins to appear at 32 weeks, so the ear slowly returns to its original position when folded over. By 36 weeks, the pinnae spring back when folded, and at term they are firm, with the ear standing erect away from the head (see Fig. 32-18).

Genitalia.

The characteristics of both male and female genitalia change with gestational age. In the female, the clitoris is prominent at 30 to 32 weeks, while the labia majora are small and widely separated. The labia majora increase in size and fullness with age, and at term they completely cover the labia minora and clitoris (Fig. 32-21).

In the male, the testes are high in the inguinal canal at about 30 weeks, gradually descend to be felt high in the scrotal sac at 37 weeks, and are well descended into the lower scrotal sac by 40 weeks. Rugae first appear on the scrotum anteriorly at 36 weeks and extend to cover the entire sac by 40 weeks. The post-term infant often has a pendulous scrotum covered with numerous rugae (Fig. 32-22).

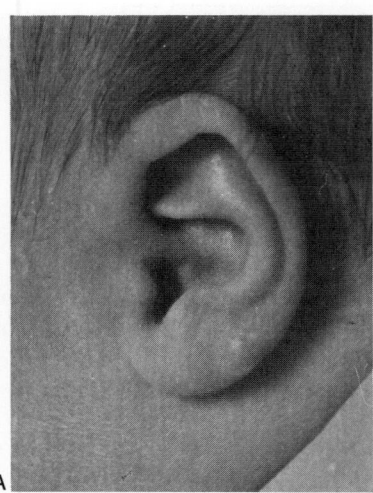

A

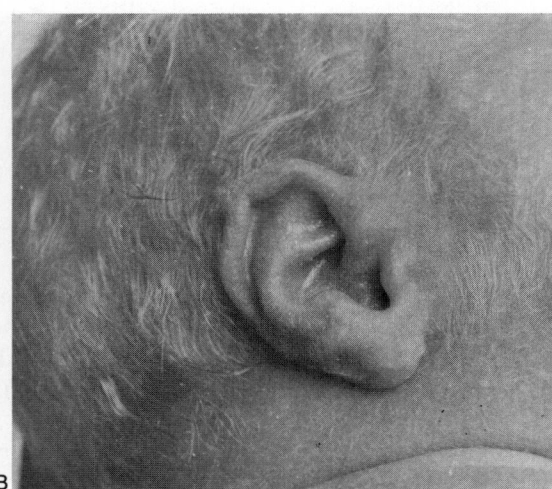

B

FIGURE   32-18

Cartilage is well developed in the term infant (*A*) and the ear is erect, away from the head, whereas the ears of the preterm infant (*B*) lie flat against the head. Also note the matted hair of the preterm infant. (Sullivan R, Foster J, Schreiner RL: Determining a newborn's gestational age. MCN, American Journal of Maternal/Child Nursing, January/February, pp 38–45, 1979)

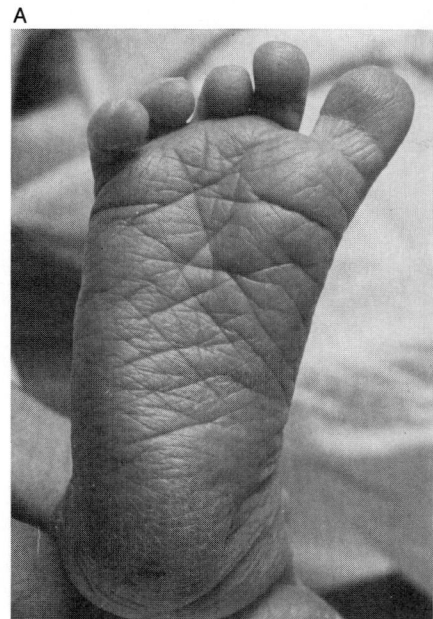
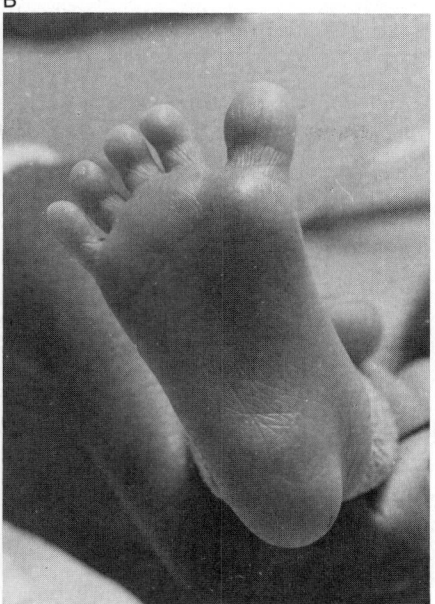

FIGURE 32-19

A comparison of the sole creases on the foot of a term infant (A) with those of a preterm infant (B). At 40 weeks' gestation, the entire foot, including the heel, is crisscrossed with creases. (Sullivan R, Foster J, Schreiner RL: Determining a newborn's gestational age. MCN, American Journal of Maternal/Child Nursing, January/February, pp 38–45, 1979)

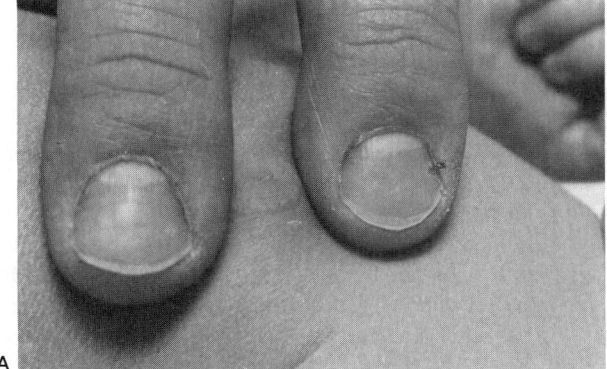
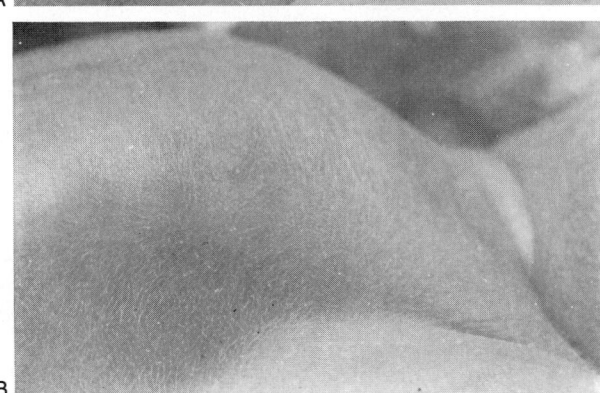

FIGURE 32-20

Note the relatively distinct areola of the term infant (A) as compared to the preterm infant (B). Also note the abundance of the fine hair, lanugo, on the body of the preterm infant. (Sullivan R, Foster J, Schreiner RL: Determining a newborn's gestational age. MCN, American Journal of Maternal/Child Nursing, January/February, pp 38–45, 1979)

Hair.   Strands of hair are very fine in early gestation and tend to mat together like wool, with small bunches sticking out from the head. The full-term infant has silky hair that lies flat in single strands. In the post-term infant the hairline may recede. Important considerations to take into account when using hair as an assessment criterion are that hair varies in texture and characteristics with race and must be free of vernix before it is observed (see Fig. 32-18).

Nails.   At about 20 weeks the nails appear and gradually grow to cover the nail bed. At term, the nails extend beyond the fingertips slightly, but long nails well beyond the fingertips are characteristic of postmature infants.

Skull Firmness.   The preterm infant has soft skull bones, particularly near the fontanels and sutures. The bones become firmer as gestation progresses, and at term the sutures are not easily displaced.

Neurologic Development

Gestational age may be assessed according to a number of neuromuscular responses of the newborn within the first few days of life. The infant's posture, the passive range of motion of certain parts, righting reactions, and various reflexes are evaluated.

The neurologic examination requires that the infant be in a quiet, rested state, although this may not be possible immediately after delivery. Most infants can be examined during the latter part of the first day of

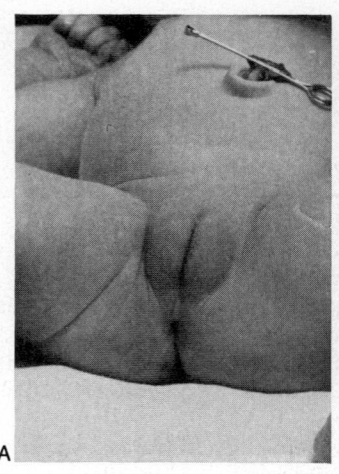
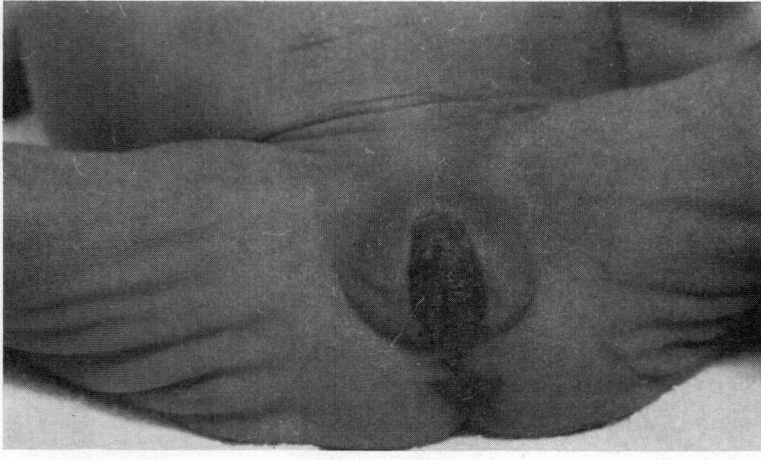

FIGURE   32-21

The labia majora of the term infant (*A*) completely cover the labia minora and clitoris. However, in the preterm infant (B) they are small and widely separated. Also note the loose skin folds on the posterior thighs of the preterm infant. (Sullivan R, Foster J, Schreiner RL: Determining a newborn's gestational age. MCN, American Journal of Maternal/Child Nursing, January/February, pp 38–45, 1979)

life, but others may not be ready until the second or third day. A shortened neurologic examination including posture, tonicity, and recoil may be done during the first few hours after birth, with the more extensive examination delayed. Charts and scoring systems are also used for these parameters. The development of muscle tone begins in the lower extremities and progresses in a cephalad direction.

Resting Posture and Extremity Recoil.
Resting posture and extremity recoil give a reasonable estimation of neurologic development in the first hour after birth. The remainder of the neurologic examination is better

carried out a day or two later to confirm the original findings. The resting posture of the premature infant is characterized by very little flexion of the upper extremities and only partial flexion of the lower. At about 30 weeks, there is slight flexion of the feet and knees. Flexion of the hips and thighs resulting in the characteristic frog position of the legs occurs at 34 weeks, but the arms are extended. At 36 to 38 weeks, the resting posture of the infant is one of complete flexion of all four extremities (Fig. 32-23).

Recoil of extremities lags behind flexion by about 2 weeks. At 36 to 37 weeks, the extremities remain extended, but there is prompt recoil at 40 weeks.

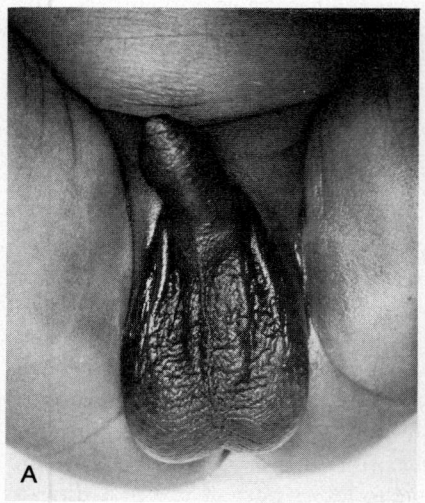
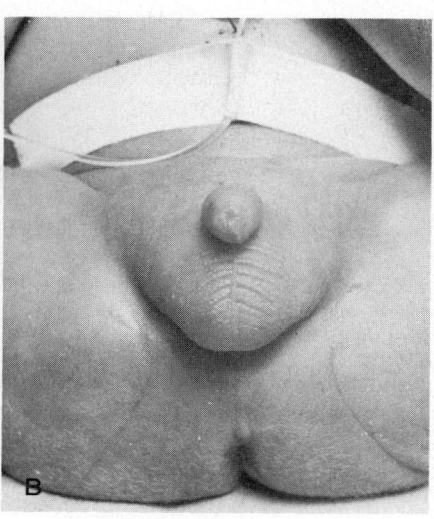

FIGURE   32-22

The testes are well descended into the scrotal sac and the scrotum is covered with numerous rugae in the term infant (*A*), whereas the testes remain high in the inguinal canal and the rugae are largely undeveloped in the preterm infant (*B*). (Sullivan R, Foster J, Schreiner RL: Determining a newborn's gestational age. MCN, American Journal of Maternal/Child Nursing, January/February, pp 38–45, 1979)

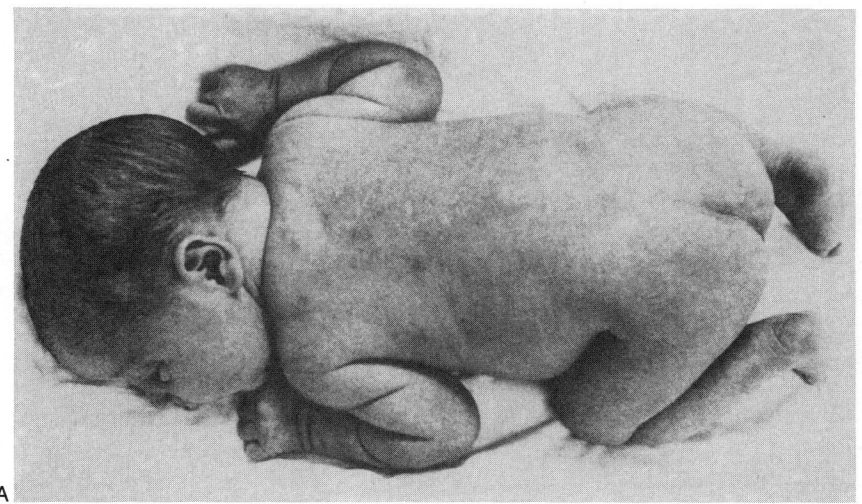

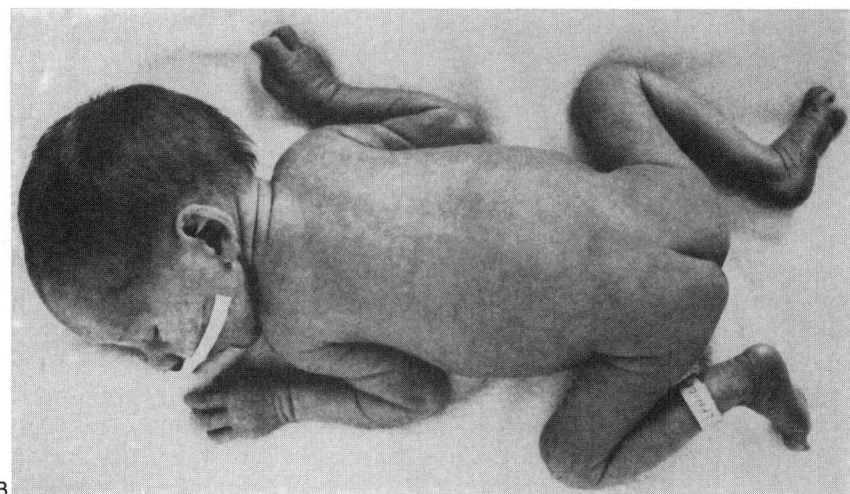

FIGURE 32-23

Resting posture. Note the flexion of the extremities in the term infant (*A*) as compared to the partial flexion in the preterm infant (*B*), resulting in a froglike resting posture. (A Clinical Review of Concepts and Characteristics in Infant Development, In Reflexes, vol. 2. Evansville, Indiana, Mead Johnson and Company, Copyright 1974)

To test recoil, one should flex the extremity and hold for 5 seconds, then extend for 30 seconds, and release. Brisk return to the flexed position indicates a full-term infant.

Ankle and Wrist Flexion. Pressure is applied to the foot to push it onto the anterior aspect of the leg, and the angle between the dorsum of the foot and the leg is measured. In premature infants this angle is 45° to 90°, whereas in the full-term infant the foot can be flexed until it touches the leg (Fig. 32-24). Similarly, the wrist is flexed with enough pressure to bring the hand as close to the forearm as possible (square window). The angle between the hypothenar eminence of the wrist and the ventral aspect of the forearm is measured, with care taken not to rotate the wrist. In the premature infant this angle is 90°. In the full-term infant the wrist can be flexed on the arm (Fig. 32-25).

Popliteal Angle. Passive movement of the leg reveals an inverse relationship between muscle tone and popliteal angle, with a smaller angle associated with greater tone. Premature infants have larger popliteal angles than full-term infants (see Fig. 32-27).

Scarf Sign. The infant's arms are drawn across the neck as far across the opposite shoulder as possible (like a scarf). In the premature infant, there is less resistance and a greater draping (or scarf) effect. This maneuver is best carried out by lifting the elbow across the front of the body. Note how far across the chest the elbow will go. In the premature infant, the elbow reaches near or across the midline, whereas in the full-term infant it does not reach the midline (Fig. 32-26).

Heel to Ear. With the infant supine and hips flat, the foot is drawn as close to the ear as possible without forcing. In a premature infant, there is very little resistance and the foot may approximate the ear, with the leg well extended. There is marked resistance in the full-term infant, and it is impossible to draw the foot to the ear and extend the leg well (Fig. 32-27).

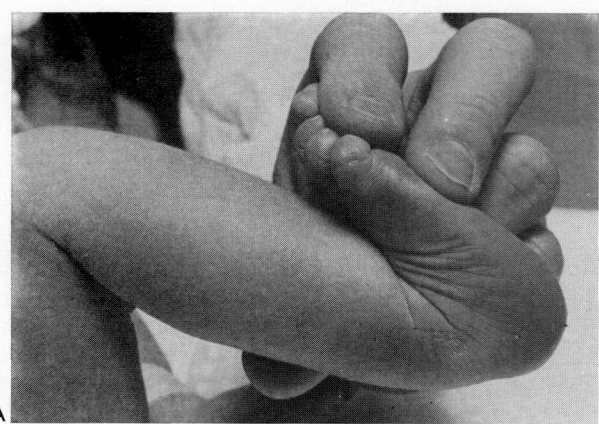
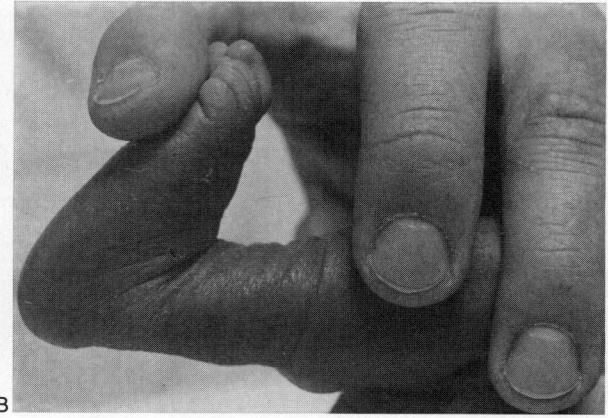

FIGURE   32-24

Dorsiflexion of the ankle. In the term infant (*A*) the foot can be flexed until it touches the leg, but in the preterm infant (*B*) the foot can be flexed only to an angle of 45° to 90°. (Sullivan R, Foster J, Schreiner RL: Determining a newborn's gestational age. MCN, American Journal of Maternal/Child Nursing, January/February, pp 38–45, 1979)

Ventral Suspension. The infant is suspended in the prone position with the hand of the examiner supporting it under the chest (two hands may be used for a large infant). The degree of extension of the back and head, as well as the degree of flexion of the arms and legs, are noted. The premature infant hangs limply with arms and legs almost straight and back rounded. The full-term infant extends the head, straightens the back, and flexes the arms and legs (Fig. 32-28).

Head Lag. With the infant supine, the hands or arms are grasped and he is pulled slowly to a sitting position. The position of the head should be observed in relation to the trunk. The premature infant has no flexion of the neck. A gradual increase in flexion can be noted as ges-

tation progresses. The full-term infant holds the head erect while being pulled to a sitting position (Fig. 32-29).

Reflexes

Although there are differences in reflexes according to the infant's gestational age, these are not as age specific as the other signs described above and are less useful in determining gestational age. The reflexes of the normal newborn are discussed under Neurologic Assessment.

In the premature infant, the rooting reflex is less developed, as evidenced by the slower response in turning the head toward the stimulus. The sucking reflex

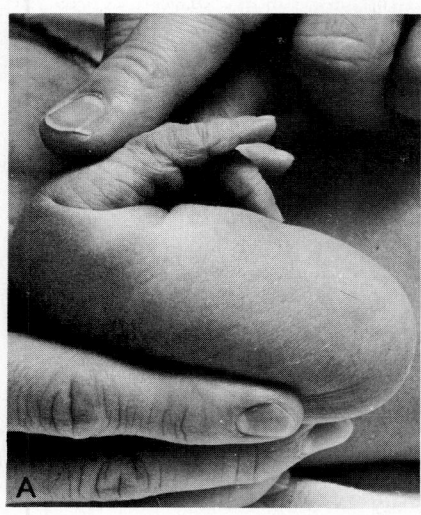
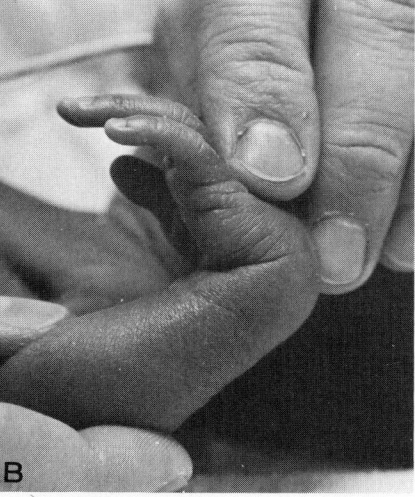

FIGURE   32-25

Wrist flexion. In the term infant (*A*) the wrist can be flexed onto the arm, but the wrist can only be flexed to an angle of about 90° in the preterm infant (*B*). (Sullivan R, Foster J, Schreiner RL: Determining a newborn's gestational age. MCN, American Journal of Maternal/Child Nursing, January/February, pp 38–45, 1979)

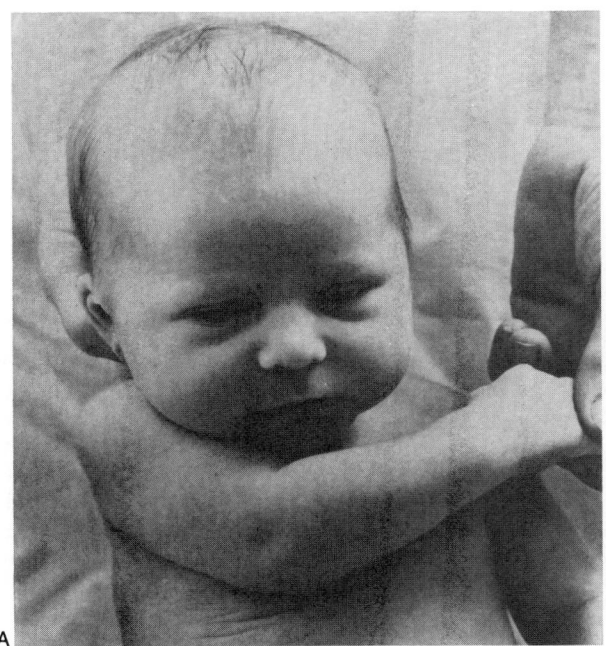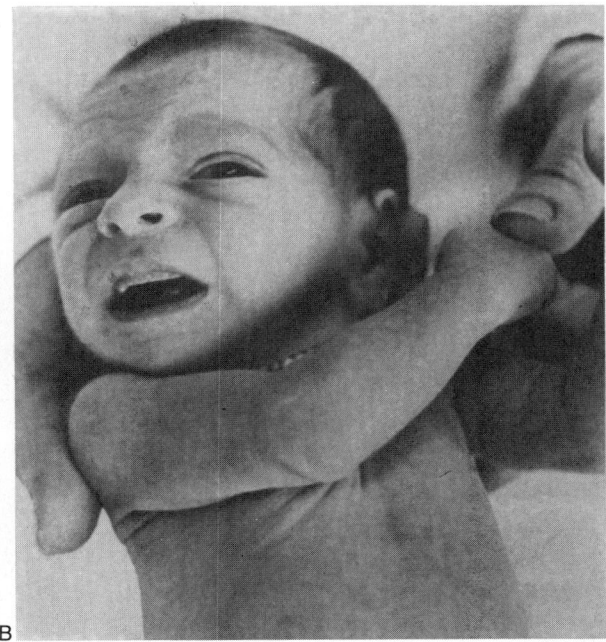

A   B

FIGURE 32-26

Scarf sign. In the term infant (*A*) the elbow will not reach the midline, but in the preterm infant (*B*) the elbow will reach across the midline. (A Clinical Review of Concepts and Characteristics in Infant Development, In Relfexes, Vol 2. Evansville, Indiana, Mead Johnson and Company, Copyright 1974)

is weak or absent, depending upon prematurity and condition. The grasp reflex is weak, and the infant cannot be lifted off the bed while grasping the examiner's finger. The Moro reflex is also weak, and the walking reflex is often absent. The sucking reflex, which is of particular importance because it is related to the ability to take adequate nourishment with nipple feedings, occurs at about 34 weeks.

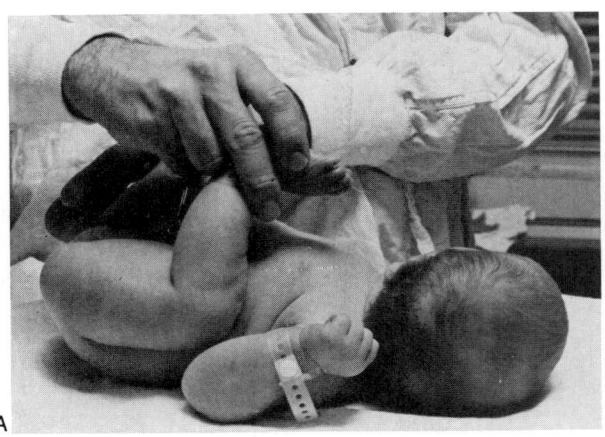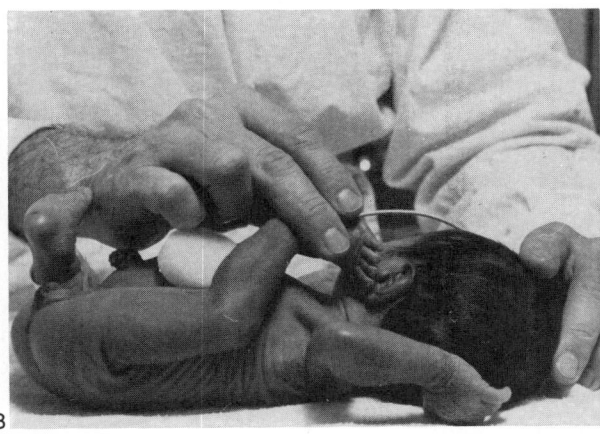

A   B

FIGURE 32-27

Heel to ear. In the term infant (*A*) there is a marked resistance in the leg as the foot is gently drawn toward the ear, whereas in the preterm infant (*B*) very little resistance is noted. Note the difference in the popliteal angle. (Sullivan R, Foster J, Schreiner RL: Determining a newborn's gestational age. MCN, American Journal of Maternal/Child Nursing, January/February, pp 38–45, 1979)

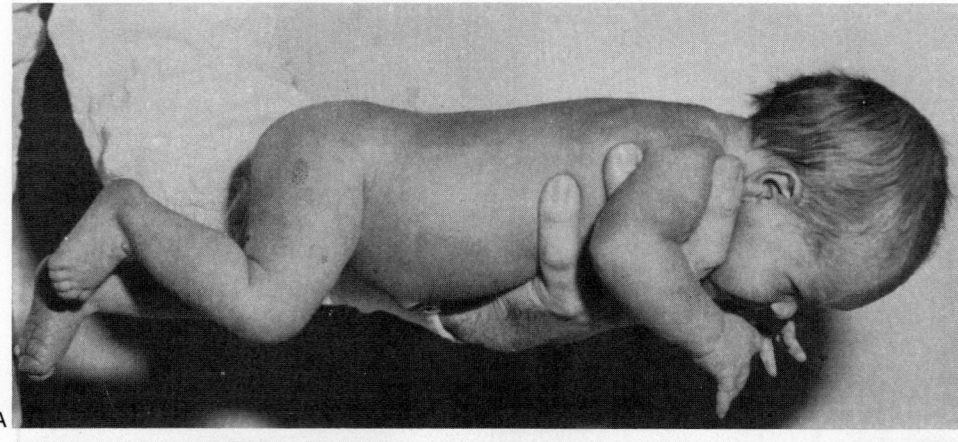

A

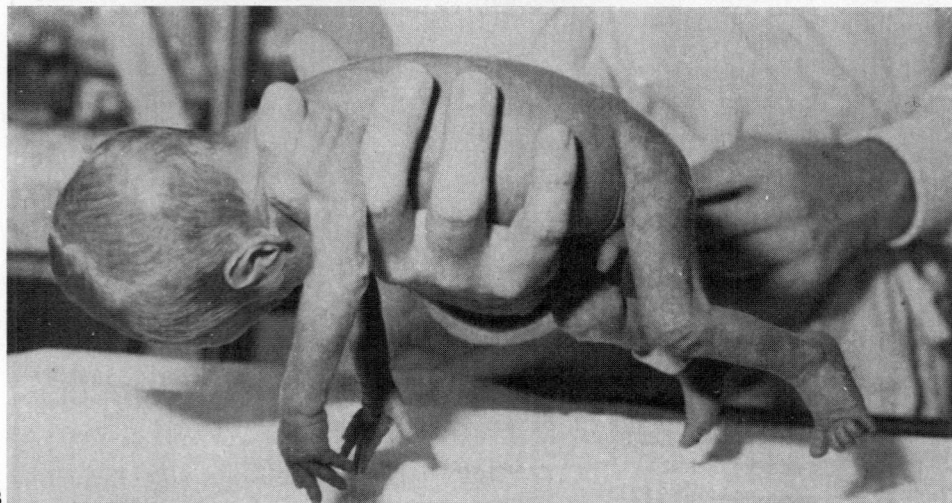

B

FIGURE 32-28

Ventral suspension. When suspended in the prone position the term infant's (*A*) head extends, the back is straight, and the arms and legs flex; however, the preterm infant (*B*) hangs limply with the arms and legs almost straight.

Behavioral Assessment

Although the newborn used to be thought of as essentially passive, we now recognize that the infant interacts actively with his environment from birth. To evaluate this interaction, a behavioral assessment can be conducted.

The Neonatal Behavioral Assessment Scale, developed by T. Berry Brazelton, includes both physical and behavioral assessment of the newborn.[22] According to Brazelton, the scale can be used both in clinical practice, as a predictive tool, and in research. Use of the scale for its intended purposes requires a trained examiner and considerable time, but some aspects of the scale and some of the findings can be useful to anyone working with newborns.

Essential to an understanding of the infant's behavior is the concept of the state of consciousness or "state." Brazelton recognizes the following six states.[22]

Sleep States

1. Deep sleep—regular breathing, eyes closed, no spontaneous activity except startles or jerky move-

ments at quite regular intervals; external stimuli produce startles with some delay; suppression of startles is rapid, and state changes are less likely than from other states; no eye movements

2. Light sleep—eyes closed, rapid eye movements can be observed under closed lids; low activity level, with random movements and startles or startle equivalents; movements are likely to be smoother and more monitored than in state 1; responds to internal and external stimuli with startle equivalents, often with a resulting change of state; irregular respirations; sucking movements occur off and on

Awake States

3. Drowsy or semidozing; eyes may be open or closed, eyelids fluttering; activity level variable, with interspersed, mild startles from time to time; reactive to sensory stimuli, but response often delayed; state change after stimulation frequently noted; movements are usually smooth

4. Alert, with bright look; seems to focus attention on source of stimulation, such as an object to be sucked, or a visual or auditory stimulus; imping-

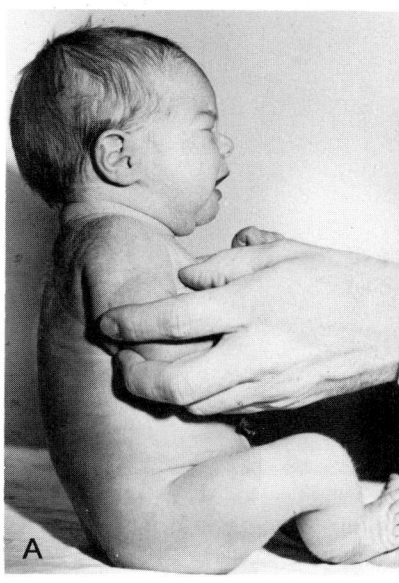
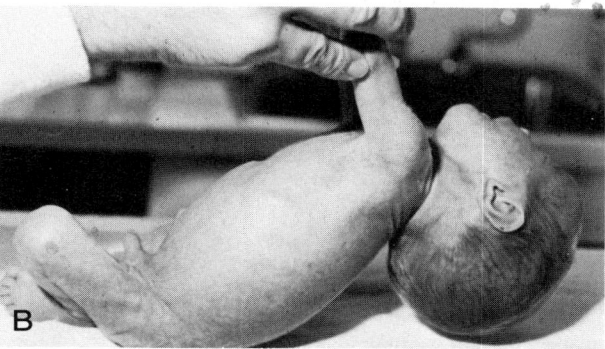

FIGURE 32-29

Head lag. As the infant is slowly pulled from a supine to a sitting position, the term infant (*A*) holds the head erect, but the preterm infant (*B*) has no flexion in the neck.

ing stimuli may break through but with some delay in response; motor activity is minimal (Fig. 32-30)

5. Eyes open; considerable motor activity, with thrusting movements of the extremities and even a few spontaneous startles; reactive to external stimulation with increase in startles or motor activity, but discrete reactions difficult to distinguish because of general high activity level

6. Crying; characterized by intense crying that is difficult to break through with stimulation (Fig. 32-31)

Babies vary greatly in the amount of time they spend in the various states and in the ease or difficulty with which they make the transition from one state to another. The concept of state is often helpful to parents

in interacting with their baby. If they can learn to recognize the various states and the individuality of their infant, they are better able to use the infant's timetable rather than their own in giving care and have a better understanding of when the infant will respond to them.

The Neonatal Behavioral Assessment Scale measures a total of 27 items (see Brazelton Scale Criteria). Each item is scored on a scale of one to nine and is based on the infant's best rather than his average performance. The infant's state at the time any given item is tested is important. Some items require that the infant be in a certain state for valid testing.

The items can be divided into the following six categories:[23]

1. Habituation—how soon the neonate diminishes his responses to specific repeated stimuli

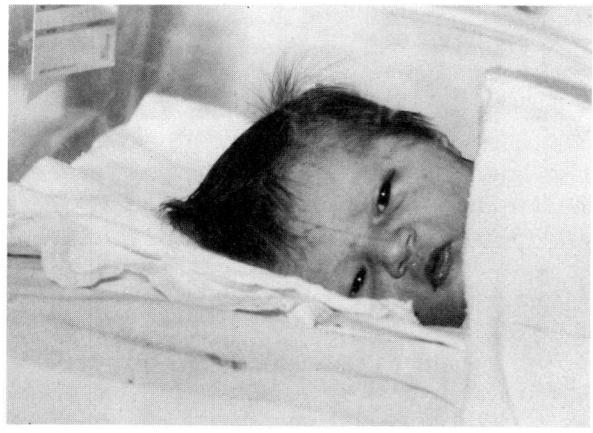

FIGURE 32-30

Quiet alert state.

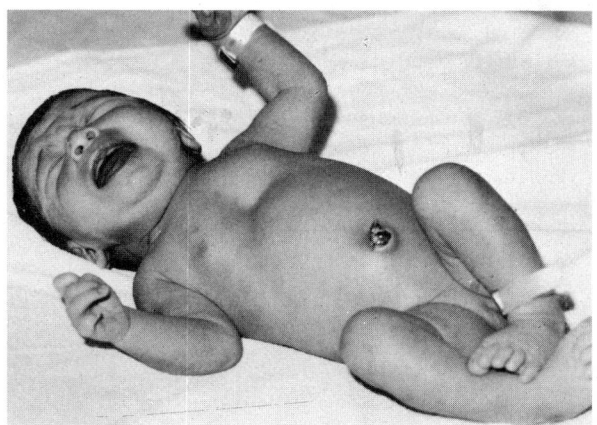

FIGURE 32-31

Active crying state.

2. Orientation—how often and when he attends to auditory and visual stimuli
3. Motor maturity—how well the infant coordinates and controls motor activities
4. Variation—how often he exhibits alertness, state changes, color changes, activity, and peaks of excitement
5. Self-quieting abilities—how often, how soon, and how effectively the neonate can use his own resources to quiet and console himself when upset or distressed
6. Social behaviors—how often and how much the newborn smiles and cuddles

A better understanding of the scale may be obtained from the booklet[22] or the films prepared by Dr. Brazelton. The discussion here is limited to a few items of particular interest.

Use of information from the Neonatal Behavioral Assessment Scale for anticipatory guidance when teaching parents about their newborn can be very helpful. Most parents are interested in what kinds of stimuli their infant will focus attention on. Some parents dis-

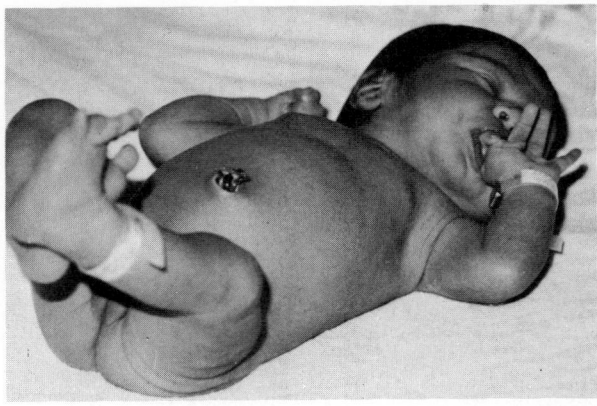

FIGURE 32-32

Self-consoling activity according to the Brazelton behavioral assessment scale: hand-to-mouth and sucking activity.

---

cover these things for themselves. Others need to be told that most infants will focus on a bright red ball and follow it briefly when they are in the quiet alert state (state 4) or that the infant particularly likes to follow a moving human face or a high-pitched voice.

Many people think that all infants are cuddly and that if an infant does not cuddle when held there is either something wrong with them or with the infant. In fact, infants respond in many different ways to being cuddled. Scores on "cuddliness" range from (1) "actually resists being held, continuously pushing away, thrashing or stiffening," to (9) "molds into arms and relaxes, turns toward examiner's body when held horizontally, or leans forward when held on the examiner's shoulder, all of the body participates and baby grasps examiner to cling to him."[22]

Infants also vary in their ability to be consoled or to console themselves. These items are scored when the infant is upset (state 6). Some babies only quiet down when they are dressed and left alone. Others need restraint to help them inhibit the startle reflex. These babies are the ones that usually do best when swaddled in a blanket.

Possible self-consoling activities that are counted in the assessment are hand-to-mouth efforts, sucking on fist or tongue (Fig. 32-32), or using visual or auditory stimuli from the environment to quiet self. Finding out ways in which their particular infant can console himself or be consoled can be very helpful to the parents.

Babies often smile even in the first days, but the statement is usually made that it is just a reflex or "gas." Brazelton comments that he has "seen close replicas of 'social smiles' in the newborn period" and that, although they are hard to be sure of, "they surely are the precursors of such smiling behavior and a mother reinforces them as such."[22]

Brazelton Scale Criteria

1. Response decrement to light
2. Response decrement to rattle
3. Response decrement to bell
4. Response decrement to pinprick
5. Orientation response—inanimate visual
6. Orientation response—inanimate auditory
7. Orientation—animate visual
8. Orientation—animate auditory
9. Orientation—animate visual and auditory
10. Alertness
11. General tonus
12. Motor maturity
13. Pull-to-sit
14. Cuddliness
15. Defensive movements
16. Consolability with intervention
17. Peak of excitement
18. Rapidity of buildup
19. Irritability (to aversive stimuli—uncover, undress, pull-to-sit, prone, pinprick, tonic neck response, Moro, defensive reaction)
20. Activity
21. Tremulousness
22. Amount of startle during exam
23. Lability of skin color
24. Lability of states
25. Self-quieting activity
26. Hand-to-mouth facility
27. Smiles

References

1. Manning FA, Platt L, LeMay M: Fetal breathing. In McNall L, Galeener J (eds): Current Practice in Obstetrics and Gynecologic Nursing, vol 2, pp 108–119. St Louis, CV Mosby, 1977
2. Harned H Jr: Respiration and the respiratory system. In Stave U (ed): Perinatal Physiology, pp 53–101. New York, Plenum Press, 1978
3. Nelson NM: Respiration and circulation after birth. In Smith CA, Nelson NM (eds): The Physiology of the Newborn Infant, 4th ed, pp 117–262. Springfield, IL, Charles C Thomas, 1976
4. Arnold HW, Putman NJ, Barnard BL et al: Transition to extrauterine life. Am J Nurs 65(10):77–80, October 1965
5. Gross S, Shurin SB, Gordon EM: The blood and hematopoietic system. In Fanaroff AA, Martin RJ (eds): Behrman's Neonatal-Perinatal Medicine, 3rd ed, pp 709–752. St Louis, CV Mosby, 1983
6. Hernandez A, Meyer DA, Goldring D: Blood pressure in neonates. Contemporary OB/GYN 5:34–37, March 1975
7. Cabal LA, Bijan S, Hodgman J: Neonatal clinical cardiopulmonary monitoring. In Fanaroff AA, Martin RJ (eds): Behrman's Neonatal-Perinatal Medicine, 3rd ed, pp 119–132. St Louis, CV Mosby, 1983
8. Lees MH, Sunderland CO: The cardiovascular system. In Fanaroff AA, Martin RJ (eds): Behrman's Neonatal-Perinatal Medicine, 3rd ed, pp 536–631. St Louis, CV Mosby, 1983
9. Gartner LM, Lee KS: Jaundice and liver disease. In Fanaroff AA, Martin RJ (eds): Behrman's Neonatal-Perinatal Medicine, 3rd ed, pp 753–784. St Louis, CV Mosby, 1983
10. Gartner LM: Hyperbilirubinemia In Pediatrics, 16th ed, p 1077. New York, Appleton-Century-Crofts, 1977
11. Sinclair JC: Metabolic rate and temperature control. In Smith CA, Nelson NM (eds): The Physiology of the Newborn Infant, 4th ed, pp 354–415. Springfield, IL, Charles C Thomas, 1976
12. Roberts FB: Perinatal Nursing. New York, McGraw-Hill, 1977
13. Sunshine P, Sinatra FR, Mitchell CH et al: The gastrointestinal system—development. In Fanaroff AA, Martin RJ (eds): Behrman's Neonatal-Perinatal Medicine, 3rd ed, pp 477–482. St Louis, CV Mosby, 1983
14. Spitzer A, Bernstein J, Edelman CM Jr: The kidney and urinary tract. In Fanaroff AA, Martin RJ (eds): Behrman's Neonatal-Perinatal Medicine, 3rd ed, pp 785–814. St Louis, CV Mosby, 1983
15. Phibbs RH: The newborn infant. In Rudolph AM (ed): Pediatrics, 16th ed, p 147. New York, Appleton-Century-Crofts, 1977
16. Gagliardi JV: Initial assessment of the newborn. In Warshaw JB, Hobbins JC (eds): Principles and Practice of Perinatal Medicine, pp 197–208. Menlo Park, CA, Addison-Wesley Publishing, 1983
17. Easterly NB, Solomon LM: The skin. In Fanaroff AA, Martin RJ (eds): Behrman's Neonatal-Perinatal Medicine, 3rd ed, pp 939–966. St Louis, CV Mosby, 1983
18. Alexander MM, Brown MS: Pediatric Physical Diagnosis for Nurses, p 156. New York, McGraw-Hill, 1974
19. Farwell J: Maturational and neurobehavioral assessment of the newborn. In Warshaw JB, Hobbins JC (eds): Principles and Practice of Perinatal Medicine, pp 226–247. Menlo Park, CA, Addison-Wesley Publishing, 1983
20. Brann AW Jr, Schwartz JF: Central nervous system disturbances. In Fanaroff AA, Martin RJ (eds): Behrman's Neonatal-Perinatal Medicine, 3rd ed, pp 347–403. St Louis, CV Mosby, 1983
21. Sullivan R, Foster J, Schreiner RL: Determining a newborn's gestational age. MCN 4(1):38–45, January/February 1979
22. Brazelton TB: Neonatal Behavioral Assessment Scale. Clinics in Developmental Medicine, No. 50. Philadelphia, JB Lippincott, 1973
23. Erickson MP: Trends in assessing the newborn and his parents. MCN 3(2):99–103, March/April 1978

Suggested Reading

Als H, Brazelton TB: Comprehensive neonatal assessment. Birth Fam J 2(1):3–9, Winter 1974–1975
Binzley V: State: Overlooked factor in newborn nursing. Am J Nurs 77:102–103, January 1977
Simpkin P, Simpkin PA, Edwards M: Physiologic jaundice of the newborn. BFJ 6(1):23–40, Spring 1979
Smith CA, Nelson NM (eds): The Physiology of the Newborn Infant, 4th ed. Springfield, IL, Charles C Thomas, 1976
Stave U (ed): Perinatal Physiology. New York, Plenum Medical Book, 1978
Waechter EH, Phillips J, Holaday B: Assessment and care of the newborn. In Nursing Care of Children, 10th ed. Philadelphia, JB Lippincott, 1985

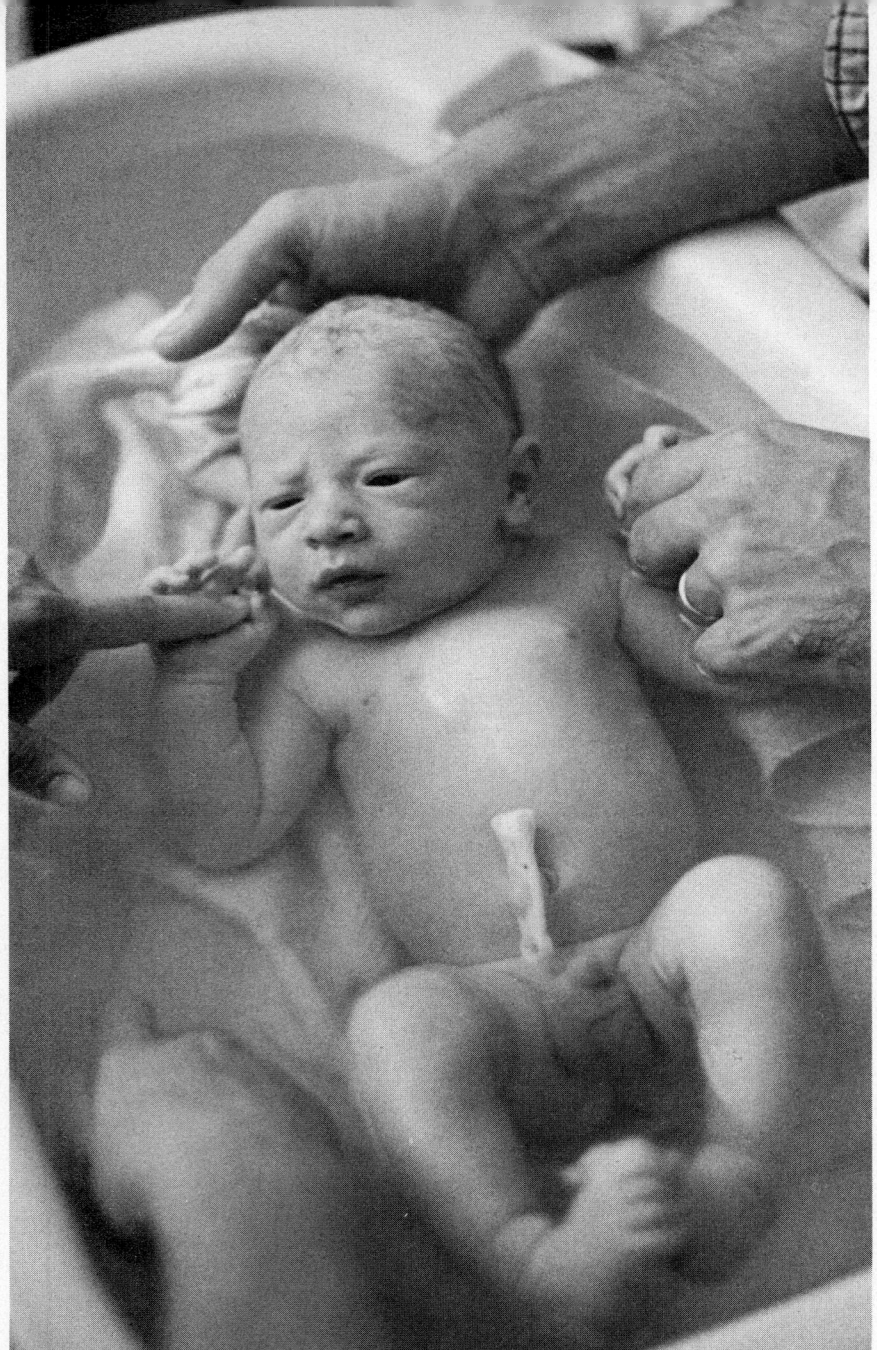

CHAPTER 33

Nursing Care of the Normal Newborn

The care of the newborn presents an interesting challenge to those in maternity nursing. In a very short period of time, usually a matter of seconds, the fetus, who has been completely dependent on the mother to supply all his physiological needs, suddenly becomes an "independent" being.

Although independent of the mother for vital functions, the newborn is, of course, still very dependent in other ways. He could not survive long without a caretaker. In the immediate postnatal period this caretaker is often the nurse.

Since these first days and weeks are so critical, the care given by the nurse is very important. The nurse must use the utmost care in handling the infant, keeping him warm and protecting him from exposure and injury, at the same time making accurate observations and recording and reporting them. Communication and teaching skills are used in contributing to the infant's future well-being by helping the parents to develop an understanding of their baby's needs and to acquire skill in his care. In this way their concept of themselves as adequate parents is reinforced. The nurse must also be aware that some parents need assistance in developing healthy attitudes regarding childrearing practices, so that the infant can make a satisfactory emotional and social adjustment. Opportunity must be provided in the hospital environment for the beginning development of a close parent–infant relationship. Also of importance is the maintenance of communication between the nurse and the parents.

Providing a Safe Environment

As in the immediate newborn period (Chap. 28), protection from injury and infection continues to be a major goal of nursing care throughout the infant's hospital stay. Policies are formulated by hospitals and communities in an effort to provide safe, individualized care for each newborn.

Prevention of Infection

The prevention of infection is of paramount importance in caring for the newborn. Although the immune system begins to develop during fetal life, it is still very immature at birth. The neonate has come from a highly protected environment *in utero* to the outside world, with its exposure to a wide variety of microorganisms. It is not surprising that organisms generally considered to be of low pathogenicity may cause infections in the neonate.[1] Areas to be considered in protecting the infant from infection include minimizing the number of or-

ganisms introduced into the infant's immediate environment and using specific prophylactic measures for the newborn.

Minimizing Exposure to Organisms

Nursing staff working in the newborn nursery should have preemployment and yearly physical examinations to detect any unrecognized infections that might possibly be passed on to the infants they care for. In addition, a staff member who contracts *any* type of infection (*i.e.*, respiratory, gastrointestinal, skin lesions) should not work in the nursery or be in contact with the infants until the infection is *completely* gone. Everyone who is in contact with the newborn, including parents and personnel, should assume responsibility for protecting the infant from infection. Parents may need help in reminding family and friends to postpone their visits if they are not well.

Hand Washing. The basis for prevention of infection when handling the newborn is thorough washing of the hands with an antiseptic detergent or soap. Some institutions require that the hands be scrubbed initially with a brush; others feel that detergent, water, and friction are sufficient. Whichever the procedure, meticulous washing of the hands is essential, whether the infant is cared for in the nursery or in a rooming-in situation. The scrub at the beginning of a shift should last 2 minutes and should cover all areas of the hands, including between the fingers.[2] Staff should be especially careful to wash their hands vigorously for 15 seconds before a feeding, after a diaper change, before going from one infant to another, and after touching anything that is not clean, such as a cabinet door or their own face or hair. The parents also need instruction about the importance (and technique) of proper hand washing, and reinforcement should be given as necessary during the hospital stay.

Nursery Dress Code. Protecting the infant from infection has traditionally involved a dress code for those coming in contact with the newborn in the hospital. Most nursery nurses (and in many hospitals where rooming-in is practiced, the postpartum nurses as well) change to scrub suits or dresses when they come to work. These should be short sleeved, so hands, forearms, and elbows can be washed more readily. An advantage of scrub clothes is the ease with which they can be changed when soiled, thus making the spread of infection from one infant to another less likely.

Other hospital personnel and visitors are usually expected to put cover gowns on over their street clothes before coming into the nursery or into the mother's room if the infant is there. If they are going to touch the baby, they should wash their hands and arms before putting on the gown. There are those who question whether cover gowns are necessary. Some studies have shown that bacterial colonization of the infant's nares or umbilicus has not increased when cover gowns were no longer used. In one study, colonization actually decreased significantly without the use of cover gowns for visitors.[3] The researchers speculated that the gowns may have provided a false sense of security for visitors and that without them better hand-washing technique may have been used.

Caps, beard covers, and masks are no longer considered necessary for routine activities in the nursery.[2] Hair should be worn short, however, or long hair should be pulled back, to avoid allowing the hair to come in contact with the infant or equipment. If circumstances arise necessitating masks, they should cover the nose and mouth, should be changed frequently, and, when removed from the face, should be discarded, not pulled down around the neck. Masks can become a reservoir for bacteria when not applied properly or changed regularly.

Maternal Infection. Special problems are created when the mother has an infection. Which maternal infections would the infant be most likely to acquire if the two are not separated? Hospital policies vary in this matter. In many hospitals the mother and infant are routinely separated if the mother is febrile. Some of the suggestions offered by the American Academy of Pediatrics and the American College of Obstetricians and Gynecologists are as follows:[2]

- Maternal genital infections are rarely spread to the infant postnatally. A mother who is febrile without a specific diagnosed site of infection may usually handle and feed her newborn if she feels well enough and uses good hand-washing technique. Additionally, she should wear a clean cover gown and protect the infant from potentially contaminated items such as her nightgown, bedclothes, and peri-pads.
- When a respiratory infection is present, the mother should be informed that these infections can be spread by hands or contaminated articles. She should also be instructed in careful hand-washing techniques and appropriate handling of tissues and other items contaminated by secretions. Wearing a mask may be helpful in reducing the droplet spread of infection.
- A woman with a communicable disease that may be transmitted to her baby should be separated from the baby until the disease is no longer communicable.

The mother who must be separated from her infant needs special attention from the nurse (see Chap. 40). Sometimes arrangements can be made for the mother to see the baby through the nursery window, but if this is not possible, the nurse should bring her frequent reports about the infant to let her know how he is eating and sleeping and so on. These mothers also appreciate and benefit from having a picture of their baby. Many nurseries have some type of instant camera available so they can provide these pictures for the mothers.

The mother who is breast-feeding may need assistance in pumping her breasts to ensure stimulation and continued milk supply (see Chap. 35).

If the mother with an infection is allowed to care for her infant, and is instructed to wear a mask, the nurse should make certain that the mother understands the underlying principles for applying and wearing the mask. She should be made especially aware of how her hands can be contaminated in adjusting and tying the mask. A clean mask should be worn on each occasion that a mask is needed, and the mother should be instructed to wash her hands each time after she adjusts it.

Specific Prophylaxis Against Infection

Several procedures routinely done for the newborn are directed toward prevention of specific types of infection. Within the first few hours after birth, a prophylactic agent is placed in the eyes to prevent ophthalmia neonatorum (see Chap. 28). Initial skin and cord care is done to help prevent colonization of the skin and umbilical area with potentially pathogenic bacteria. In choosing an agent to cleanse the skin, care must be taken that the agent does not have an adverse effect on the skin, is not toxic if absorbed, and does not give rise to new infection problems by altering the skin flora.[2] For cord care, triple dye or antimicrobial agents such as bacitracin ointment or sulfadiazine cream are currently recommended to prevent colonization.[2] Alcohol, which has been used for years to care for the cord, hastens drying of the stump, but is probably not very effective in preventing cord colonization or umbilical infection.[2]

Newborn-Care Areas

Current interest in family-centered maternity care has led to having infants spend increasing amounts of time in their mother's room and less time in central nurseries. Either location requires attention to environmental aspects of safe care.

Rooming-In

Rooming-in is a term applied to the plan of having the new infant share the mother's hospital unit so that mother and baby may be cared for together. This type of arrangement has come to mean much more than caring for the mother and the infant in the same unit of space. Rather, it implies an attitude in maternal and infant care that supports parental education and is based on recognition and understanding of the needs of each mother, infant, and family. Some authorities feel that the separation of mother and baby (and father) results in an unnatural fragmentation of the family at an important time for building family unity.

Rooming-in often is discussed as if it were a modern innovation. Historically, however, all mothers back to Paleolithic times "roomed-in" until the central nursery was instituted during the first 2 decades of the 20th century. Nevertheless, rooming-in as it is practiced today does represent a departure from the concept of the traditional central nursery.

Attitudes in maternal and infant care have changed, in part because of increased insight into the needs of the mother, her baby, and the family as a unit. Rooming-in plays an important part in the family-centered approach to maternity care, for it not only provides an environment that fosters a wholesome, natural mother–child relationship from the very beginning, but it also affords unlimited opportunities for both parents to learn about the care of their baby (Fig. 33-1).

Some hospitals have special rooming-in units with adjoining nurseries and workrooms. Although this is an ideal arrangement, it is not always possible, and the benefits of rooming-in should not be denied the family because of the physical setup of the hospital. Many hospitals allow rooming-in if the mother has a private room and keeps the baby in the room all the time. Some women are discouraged by this arrangement because of the expense of a private room or their desire to have more contact with other people. Perhaps a good compromise is the modified program used in many hospitals which allows a mother to have her infant in the room for long periods of time and in the central nursery the rest of the time.

The newborn must be protected from sources of infection regardless of where he is cared for. The same basic principles for asepsis employed in the nursery must be followed in infant care in the rooming-in unit.

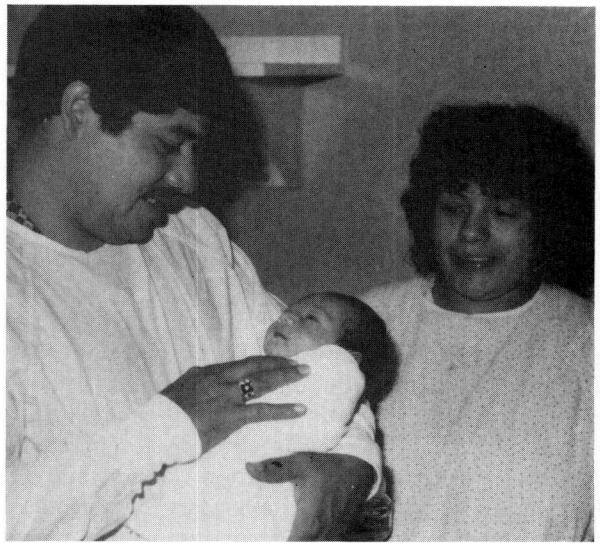
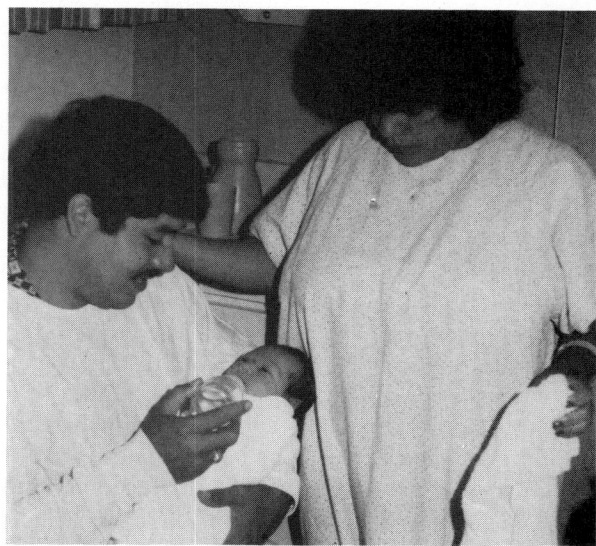
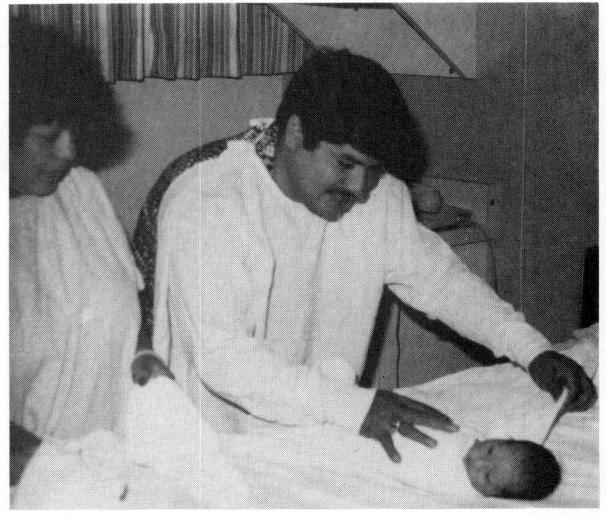

FIGURE 33-1

In the rooming-in unit the father has the opportunity to gain experience holding and caring for the new baby while the mother observes.

Central Nursery System

The central or general newborn nursery on the postpartum division is designed for the care of a variable number of healthy newborns (Fig. 33-2). In this system the infants are brought to their mothers at certain specified times during the day, generally for feeding or visiting. The staff assumes the responsibility for all the care of the babies. Some type of central nursery is usually found in most hospitals.

With the emergence of the many drug-resistant organisms that abound in the hospital environment, the danger of epidemics (whenever a large aggregate of persons collect) is enhanced. Control of the physical facilities and stringent personnel policies provide a good deal of protection for the newborn. For instance, the area should be well lighted, have a large wall clock, and be equipped for emergency resuscitation. Hand-washing facilities and materials should be readily available. Cribs should be placed at least 2 feet apart with 3-feet-wide aisles between the cribs. Limiting the number of infants in a nursery to between 8 and 12 is also suggested.

The precautions previously mentioned, such as hand washing, wearing scrub clothes, and following other aspects of nursery aseptic technique, afford additional protection.

The central nursery is a so-called clean nursery. However, it must be understood that there is a difference in nursery technique between what is considered to be nursery clean and what is considered to be baby clean (*i.e.*, what is clean for an individual baby). There should be no common equipment, such as a common bath table, used in providing care for the babies. There should be provisions in the nursery for individual technique to be followed. Each infant should have his own crib and general supplies, so that he can be given such care as his daily inspection bath or be diapered or dressed in his own bed.

Most cribs are constructed with a built-in cabinet or drawers to hold clean diapers, shirts, and linens and small items such as the thermometer, lubricant, cotton balls, and applicators. When such cribs are not available something should be improvised so that individual care techniques can still be carried out.

The Cohort Nursery System.

In hospitals in which the nursery area is comprised of more than one normal newborn nursery room, the cohort system is sometimes used to reduce cross-contamination between groups of newborns. All infants born during a designated time period are placed in one nursery room and, ideally, cared for by a group of personnel who do not care for infants from other nurseries during that shift. Mothers of the infants are placed with roommates who have infants in the same nursery. That particular nursery is closed to new admissions until all the cohort babies have been discharged. It is then cleaned and a new cohort is started.

Nurses must be alert for infants who show signs of, or are at increased risk for developing, an infection, so that isolation procedures can be implemented if necessary. Infants who are born at home or on the way to the hospital should be bathed and observed for signs of infection, but separate isolation facilities are not required.[2]

Isolettes are sometimes used for isolating infants within the central nursery. This may be helpful in keeping the infant separate and as a reminder of the isolation status, but it should not be assumed to provide adequate isolation for infected neonates. Although the air coming

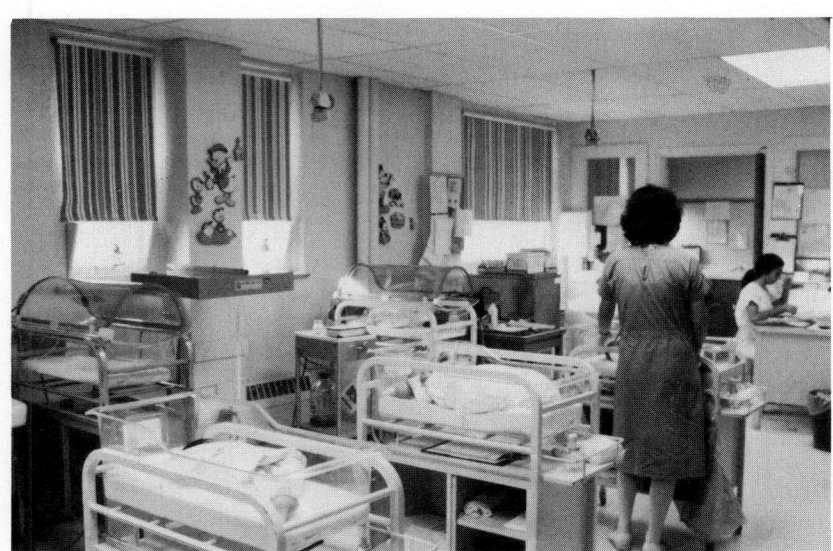

FIGURE   33-2

Term newborn nursery.

into the incubator is filtered, the air being discharged into the nursery is not. Also, the surface and portholes of the incubator are easily contaminated with organisms from the infected infant, so the hands and forearms of personnel are likely to be colonized.[2]

Observation/Isolation Nursery

Most maternity units have separate rooms in the nursery area for infants who are suspected of or are known to have infections. Whether the infected neonate is placed in one of these rooms, kept in the central nursery, allowed to room-in with his mother, or transferred to a pediatrics unit will depend on the type and manifestations of the infection, the staffing available, and hospital policy. Decisions are often made on an individualized basis. Infants segregated from the other neonates may require closer observation and additional care related to the infection, but they continue to need the usual care given to the healthy newborn. Also their need for human contact, holding, and cuddling should not be forgotten.

Transition Period

In the delivery room initial care has been given to the infant and any early problems have been dealt with (see Chap. 28). From the delivery room the infant may be taken to the recovery room and remain with the mother and father for a while, go to a transitional nursery, or be admitted directly to the regular nursery. Of course, if the infant has serious problems, a special-care nursery is indicated (see Chap. 43).

Since the day of birth is the most hazardous time for the infant, it is important that continuing observations be made during the first 24 hours. A receiving or transition nursery in the labor or nursery section provides an excellent physical environment for the extensive observations that are necessary, similar to that of recovery room care for adults. An infant whose mother has been heavily medicated during labor and delivery is particularly in need of this recovery care. If this kind of setup is not available, the new babies should be placed in an area of the regular nursery where they can be easily observed. Low-risk babies whose mothers had little or no medication can probably be safely left with their mothers for a time under close supervision of a nurse in case of presence of mucus or other sudden changes in the infant's condition. If the mother plans to have rooming-in, it is often delayed for several hours until the infant is considered stable, with no signs of excessive mucus.

Initial Assessment

When the infant is admitted to the nursery, the nursery nurse receives a report from the delivery room nurse, checks identification bands according to hospital policy, and checks the infant's record to note any additional important information. She then does an initial assessment of the infant (see Chap. 32). It is of particular importance at this time to check the infant's respiratory status and temperature and to observe for any congenital anomalies that might have been missed at birth but need immediate care.

The vital signs should be checked every half hour until they are stable or as indicated by hospital policy. Apical heart rate and respirations should each be counted for a full minute. The pulse may vary with the infant's activity, but a persistent rate below 120 beats per minute or above 150 beats per minute should be reported. The infant's temperature is checked on admission, then usually monitored frequently until the axillary reading reaches about 36.6°C (97.8°F). Axillary temperature (Fig. 33-3) is preferred because it eliminates the potential danger of perforation of the rectum with the rectal thermometer. In some settings, however, an

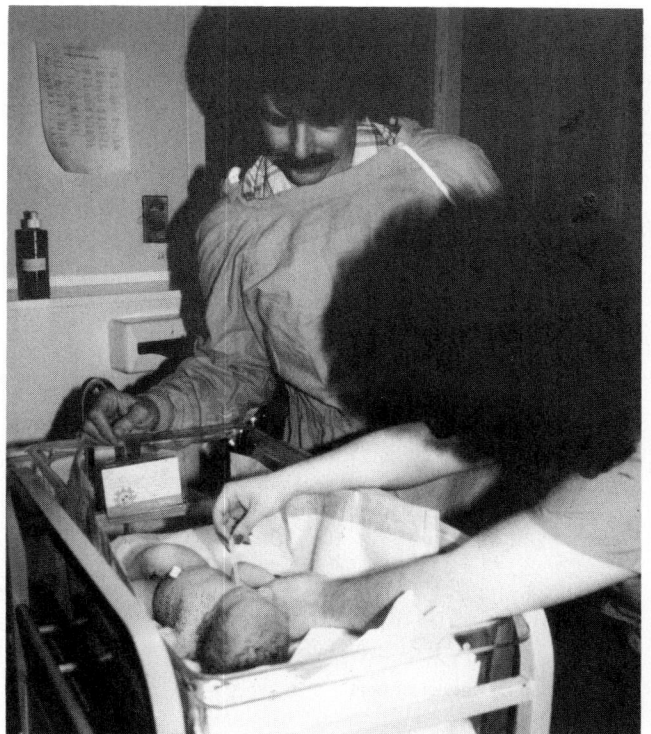

FIGURE 33-3

The newborn's axillary temperature is checked upon admission to the newborn nursery. (Courtesy of Booth Maternity Center, Philadelphia)

initial rectal temperature is taken to determine rectal patency. The axillary reading is usually slightly lower than the rectal temperature, but occasionally, if the infant has been chilled and brown fat stimulated, it may be higher[4] (see Chap. 32).

The infant's color and respiratory pattern are good indices of whether or not the newborn is experiencing respiratory insufficiency. Dyspnea, rapid respiration exceeding 50 breaths per minute, and persistent cyanosis should be reported. Since mucus in the nasopharynx often causes respiratory distress, the nurse should be particularly watchful for its presence. Gagging, vomiting, breath holding, retraction of the head, choking, and cyanosis all may be signs of the presence of mucus, which is particularly prone to develop in the second period of reactivity following the first sleep.

Breathing difficulties or excessive mucus may also be evidence of congenital anomalies, such as choanal atresia or tracheoesophageal fistula. Observing for the timing of the breathing difficulties will help determine the cause. Some nurseries, especially those with high-risk populations, gastric contents are routinely aspirated to screen for anomalies of the gastrointestinal tract. Others do this only when there is evidence of a problem.

Testing for Hypoglycemia

Many infants are at risk for becoming hypoglycemic in the first few hours after birth. Assessment for this condition can now be done by the nursery nurse using the Dextrostix to estimate blood sugar levels. The test, using blood from a heel stick, is done routinely on all newborns in some nurseries. In others it is done according to a protocol defining infants most likely to become hypoglycemic soon after birth, such as infants of diabetic mothers or those who are large or small for gestational age. If routine testing is not done, the nurse should be aware that such central nervous system symptoms as poor muscle tone, weakness, tremors, eye rolling, high-pitched cry, and, as a late symptom, even convulsions may be indicative of low blood sugar levels.

When a heel stick is to be done for a Dextrostix or to obtain blood for other tests, surface blood flow should first be improved by warming the infant's foot. This can sometimes be done by holding the infant's heel in the palm of the nurse's hand[5] or by wrapping the foot in a warm, moist compress for 3 to 5 minutes. After cleaning the heel with alcohol and allowing it to dry, a quick, clean stick is made in the outer surface of the heel with a disposable lancet (Fig. 33-4). The area is then wiped off with a sterile gauze square and when the blood starts to flow again it is dropped on the Dextrostix or collected in a capillary tube, depending on the intended purpose.

For the Dextrostix it is important to follow the package directions precisely, especially in regard to the 60-second lapsed time before wiping or washing off the blood. Care should be taken not to squeeze the foot too vigorously when obtaining the sample, since this may dilute the blood with tissue fluid or cause hemolysis. If the blood flow diminishes or stops before an adequate amount is obtained, wiping the area with a sterile gauze square will sometimes result in increased blood flow. Positioning the infant with the foot in a dependent position (lower than the body) may also increase blood

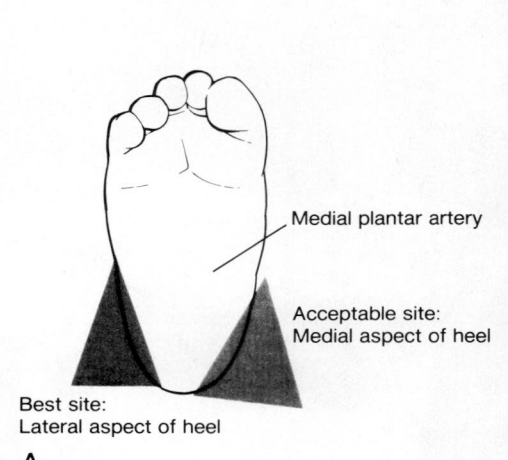

Medial plantar artery

Acceptable site:
Medial aspect of heel

Best site:
Lateral aspect of heel

A

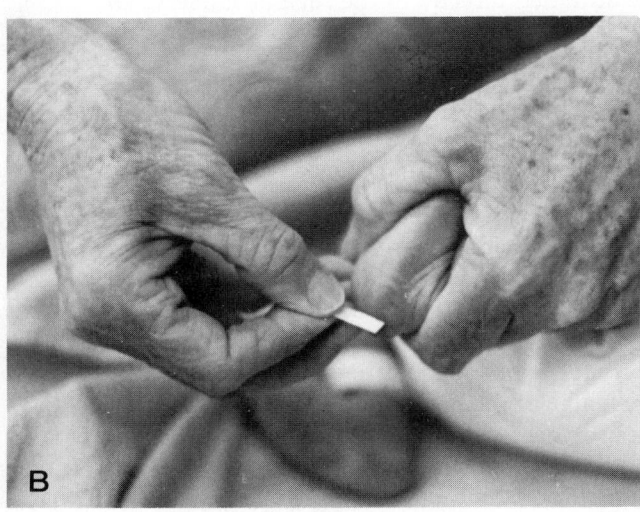

B

F I G U R E   3 3 - 4

The heelstick procedure is used to test for blood glucose. (*A*) Appropriate sites for the heelstick procedure. (*B*) After the site is punctured with a pediatric microlancet and following elimination of the first drop of blood, the nurse holds the Dextrostix under the heel to collect the second drop of blood.

flow. Following the procedure, a small sterile bandage is usually applied to the area.

Stools and Urine

The time of the infant's first stool and voiding should be noted to indicate proper excretory function. It is sometimes necessary for the nursery nurse to check the delivery record or check with the delivery room nurse to see whether the infant voided or defecated before being brought to the nursery.

Condition of the Cord

The cord should be checked periodically. Any oozing or bleeding should be reported immediately and the cord should be reclamped or retied as indicated. Oozing occurs most often between the second and sixth hour of life and is frequently associated with crying or the passage of meconium.

Nursing Diagnosis

Following initial assessment of the newborn the nurse will be able to develop a number of potential or actual nursing diagnoses. Examples of these would be alteration in airway clearance related to excess mucus; alteration in body temperature: hypothermia related to cooler environmental temperature and large body surface area; alteration in vital signs related to transition through the periods of reactivity; potential for complication of hypoglycemia secondary to mother's diabetic condition. Through the use of nursing diagnoses the nurse is able to plan care that is individualized for each infant.

Planning/Intervention

Nurseries vary as to what is included in routine admission care. Certain procedures such as eye prophylaxis (see Chap. 28) and vitamin K injection (see Chap. 32) are done in the nursery if they are not included in the delivery room care. The injection technique is shown in Figure 33-5. Results of the assessment procedures noted in the previous section guide the planning and intervention for each individual infant. Equipment for suctioning and resuscitation must be on hand, and someone who is trained in its use should be immediately available. A bulb syringe should be in each infant's bassinet.

Preventing hypothermia is a major concern. When a radiant warmer is used, the servo-control should be set to maintain the abdominal skin temperature at 36.5°C. The skin probe (thermistor) should be taped

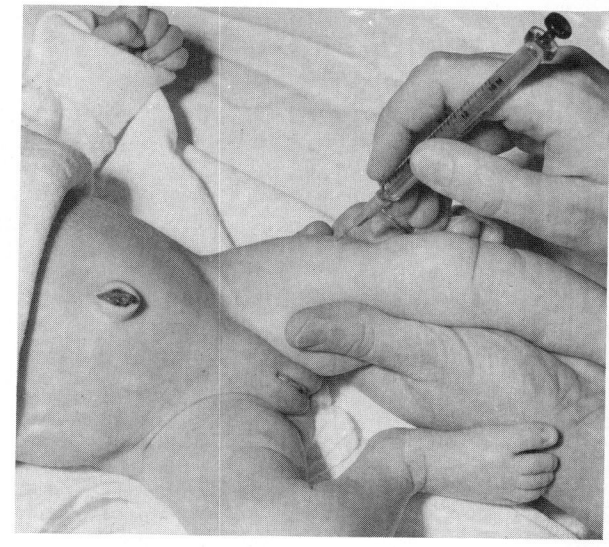

FIGURE 33-5

IM injection for infant.

securely to the anterior abdominal wall and covered with an aluminum patch to shield it from the radiant heat source.[2] The patch used in many nurseries is heart shaped, with gold-colored aluminum on one side and adhesive to hold the probe in place on the other. The skin probe should be checked periodically to make sure it is in contact with the skin. A probe not touching the skin causes the warmer to misinterpret the infant's temperature and continue to radiate heat after the desired infant temperature is reached. The infant can become overheated or possibly even burned. Hyperthermia, like hypothermia, increases the infant's metabolic requirements and oxygen consumption.[6] The temperature of an isolette being used as a warmer should also be checked periodically, because it also can rise higher than expected and cause overheating.

The first bath is usually delayed until after the temperature has stabilized. Bathing is often done under the radiant warmer, since wetting the skin can cause heat loss by evaporation. The temperature should be rechecked following the bath, and the infant should remain under the warmer if the temperature has dropped. Cord care may be done following the bath. Triple dye is usually done as a one-time treatment, applied over the junction between the cord stump and the skin. It leaves a temporary purple stain on the abdomen that may last several days. This should be explained to the parents so they don't worry about the stain. If an ointment such as bacitracin is used, it should not be applied until the infant no longer needs to be under the radiant warmer. The oily substance tends to concentrate the heat and could possibly cause a burn.

In a vigorous, normal infant, the cry should be lusty

NURSING CARE PLAN

Care of the Newborn During the Transition Period

Nursing Objectives

1. Keep infant's airway clear.
2. Protect infant from cold stress.
3. Protect infant from infection.
4. Identify problems or potential problems in infant's physical condition.

Assessment	Potential Nursing Diagnosis	Planning/Intervention	Evaluation
Respiratory status	Alteration in airway clearance related to excess mucus	Observe infant frequently during transition period Keep bulb syringe in bassinet and use as necessary	Newborn remains free of respiratory difficulties
Temperature	Alteration in body temperature: decreased related to newborn status	Place in radiant warmer and monitor temperature continuously until stable Delay bath until temperature stable Dry well after bath and place back in warmer until temperature is again stable	Newborn's temperature stabilizes Infant does not develop hypothermia

General status:
  Size
  Maturation
  Normality of body systems
  Vital signs
	Alteration in vital signs related to transition through periods of reactivity	Weigh; measure length and head circumference
		
		Perform gestational age assessment
		
		Examine body systems by thorough observation, inspection, auscultation, and palpation; monitor vital signs
		
		Record, report as appropriate
			Newborn adapts to extrauterine life with minimal problems
			
			Newborn shows no evidence of trauma or abnormalities
			
			Newborn has good color and muscle tone
			
			Newborn retains stabilized vital signs

Blood sugar levels	Potential complication: hypoglycemia secondary to maternal diabetes, cold stress, or infant large or small for gestational age	Observe for signs of hypoglycemia: jitteriness, tremors, eye rolling, weakness, high-pitched cry, poor muscle tone Use Dextrostix: report to doctor if less than 40 mg/dl Feed infant: glucose water, formula, or breast, according to hospital policy	Newborn does not develop symptoms of hypoglycemia Newborn has blood glucose level above 40 mg/dl

and will occur especially when the baby is handled or moved. If the infant doesn't cry at all when disturbed or seems unusually sleepy or depressed, or if the pulse and respiratory rate are slow, the condition should be reported. It may be necessary to stimulate him to cry periodically by rubbing his back, head, or feet or changing his position. Brief tremors and twitching are not unusual in the transition period, but if they are prolonged or occur frequently, they may indicate a problem and the physician should be notified (see Chap. 32).

Continuing Care and Parent Teaching

Assessment

Ongoing assessment during the newborn's hospital stay varies according to hospital policy (see Chap. 32). The nurse will be expected to assess not only the infant's physical condition, but also his behavioral patterns, his interaction with his parents, and the parents' need for information about the newborn and his care. Early detection of problems in any of these areas is of primary concern. Besides using the routine checklists found in most nurseries, the nurse should be alert to any changes she might notice while giving care. For example, subtle changes in color or vital signs in the newborn can indicate beginning infection or possible abnormalities.

Screening for Inborn Errors of Metabolism

Certain disorders related to inborn errors of metabolism have been found to be detectable by blood tests soon after birth. Early detection and appropriate treatment can often prevent or decrease permanent defects resulting from these disorders. Although a number of tests have been developed, not all are used in mass screening. To be most useful, the test should be sensitive and specific, and there should be effective intervention available for those who have positive tests.[7] Phenylketonuria (PKU), congenital hypothyroidism, and galactosemia meet these criteria and are the conditions most often tested for in government-funded neonatal screening programs. Tests for additional conditions may be done on the blood of infants at risk by family history.

The nurse is often the person responsible for obtaining the blood for the tests. This is usually done by heel stick with the blood being dropped on absorbent paper to fill premarked circles (see the discussion earlier in this chapter). The circles must be completely saturated for best results. The blood sample for the test should be taken before the infant leaves the hospital. Although the usual recommendation is to wait 24 hours, if the infant is discharged before this time it is better to get the blood early than to risk missing the test altogether in case the mother doesn't bring the infant back. It is suggested that infants initially screened before 24 hours of age be rescreened for PKU during the first 2 weeks of life for better reliability of this test, since results are thought to be related to food intake by the infant.[2] Recent information indicates, however, that most infants with PKU have an elevated blood phenylalanine concentration during the first day of life and probably will not be overlooked by early testing.[8]

Nursing Diagnosis

Awareness of potential nursing diagnoses, based on areas of assessment, will assist the nurse in planning care for the newborn. Examples of these would be potential for infection related to vulnerability of infant and lack of normal flora; potential alteration in skin integrity related to lack of normal skin flora and possible peeling and cracking of skin; potential alteration in par-

enting related to new parents' inexperience and feelings of incompetence. From her assessment the nurse would also identify actual nursing diagnoses for the individual infant. Examples include alteration in elimination: lack of stool in first 24 hours related to possible imperforate anus; alteration in urinary elimination: decreased related to insufficient fluid intake; maternal knowledge deficit regarding infant care (handling, bathing, feeding) related to mother having first baby.

Planning/Intervention

During the infant's hospital stay, the nurse is responsible for planning and providing daily care. The mother should be involved with as much of this care as possible to help her prepare for taking over the responsibility when she gets home. This is easiest if there is a rooming-in or modified rooming-in arrangement, but it is possible even with central nursery care.

It is important that the nurse assess the mother's understanding and her skill in caring for her infant. Any basic principles or procedures related to infant care that the mother finds necessary and useful should be part of the nurse's teaching plan for the mother during her hospital stay. A written plan or checklist of what the mother wants to learn and what teaching has been done is helpful in providing continuity between health-care providers. Consistency in what is taught is necessary to avoid confusing the parents. The following principles of care can be conveyed easily to the mother (and to the father when he is present).

Handling and Positioning the Infant

Although they are small, newborns are not as fragile as they sometimes seem. They should be treated gently, of course, but firm, smooth handling helps them feel secure. There is no one right way of turning, lifting, or holding a newborn, but the following points should be kept in mind:

- The head and buttocks need to be supported.
- Babies are wiggly and can push themselves out of your grasp.
- It is easier to pick an infant up from the supine position than from the side-lying or prone position.

A suggested way to lift an infant is to place one hand under the neck to support the head and shoulders and the other hand under the buttocks to grasp the opposite thigh (Fig. 33-6). The infant can then be lifted up to a holding position or moved from one place to another. A useful position for holding or carrying is the "football hold" (Fig. 33-7). Mothers appreciate learning about

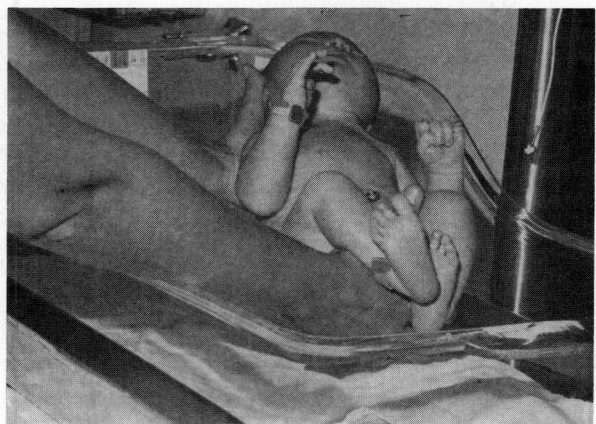

FIGURE 33-6

One method of lifting the baby is to place one hand under the infant's neck and the other under the buttocks.

this position, because, like the nurse, they often have times when they need to hold the baby and still have one hand free.

Feelings of confidence in dressing and undressing the baby come with practice. When putting on a shirt or gown, it is helpful to reach through the sleeve with your fingers and pull the infant's hand through. Diapering is fairly simple if disposable diapers that fasten with tapes are used. If pins are needed they should be inserted pointing toward the infant's back so there is less danger to the infant if they come open. The infant is usually wrapped snugly in a blanket (swaddling) be-

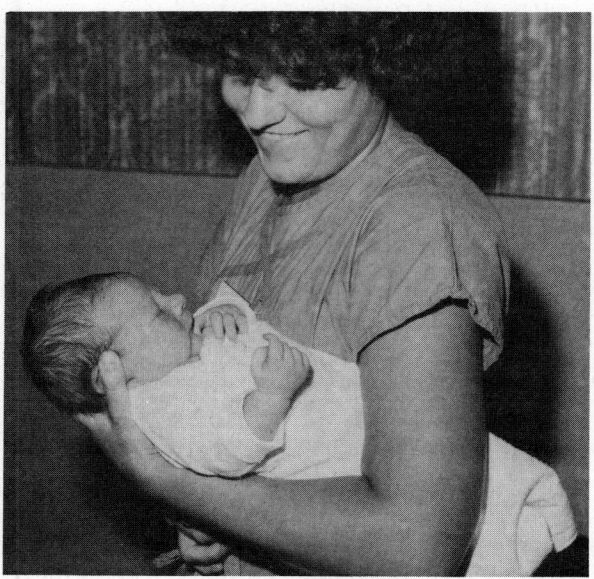

FIGURE 33-7

Football hold for carrying the infant.

fore he is taken to his mother or placed in his crib. Some infants seem happier with their arms inside the blanket, and others like their arms free. Positioning in the crib is usually on the side with a blanket roll at the infant's back for support. This should extend from shoulder to hip. If it is behind the infant's head, it pushes the head forward.

An alternate position would be to place the infant on his abdomen. Both of these positions allow for drainage of secretions such as mucus or regurgitation of milk from the infant's mouth. The back-lying position makes drainage of secretions difficult and should be avoided as a sleeping position or when the infant is unattended, to reduce the danger of aspiration.

Bathing and Hygiene

The daily cleansing of the infant affords an excellent opportunity for making the observations that are necessary during the immediate postnatal period. How frequently a bath is given and what materials are used may vary from institution to institution.

CLIENT   EDUCATION

Basic Principles in Bathing an Infant

1. All equipment, clothing, and supplies should be assembled. Safety pins, if used, should be closed and placed out of the reach of the baby. Receptacles for soiled clothing, cotton balls, and so on should be available.
2. Care should be taken so that the environment is free from drafts and warm enough (*i.e.,* 24°C–27°C or 75°F–80°F). The bath should not have to be interrupted to close a door or a window. The water for the bath should be about 37°C to 38°C (98°F–100°F). Water that feels warm to the elbow is approximately that temperature.
3. Proceed from the "cleanest" areas to those that are "most soiled." Thus, the eyes are bathed first, then the face, ears, scalp, neck, upper extremities, trunk, lower extremities, and finally the buttocks and the genitals (Fig. 33-8). Each of these in turn are washed, *rinsed well,* and dried. Particular attention should be paid to cleansing and drying the scalp and all creases at the neck, behind the ears, under the arms, the palms of the hands and between the fingers and the toes, under the knees, and in the groin, the buttocks, and the genitals.
4. *The infant never should be left unattended,* even on a large work area; one hand should be kept on him at all times. If it is necessary to leave the area, even for a second, he should be taken along or placed in the crib.

Several decades ago the daily soap and water and oil baths were replaced with merely wiping off excess vernix with dry or slightly moist cotton balls. The diaper area was cleansed as necessary. Recently, there has been a return by many hospitals to the practice of bathing the baby daily or every other day while in the hospital. In view of the increase in staphylococcal infections in newborn nurseries, many nurseries give an initial sponge bath with a liquid detergent containing 3%

hexachlorophene with special attention to the cord and genital areas. It is particularly important to rinse the baby well after the use of hexachlorophene. Daily use is no longer recommended because of suggestive evidence of central nervous system damage following prolonged exposure.

For the remainder of the infant's stay in the hospital, a mild soap and plain warm water can be used for cleansing purposes. The use of strong soap, oil, and

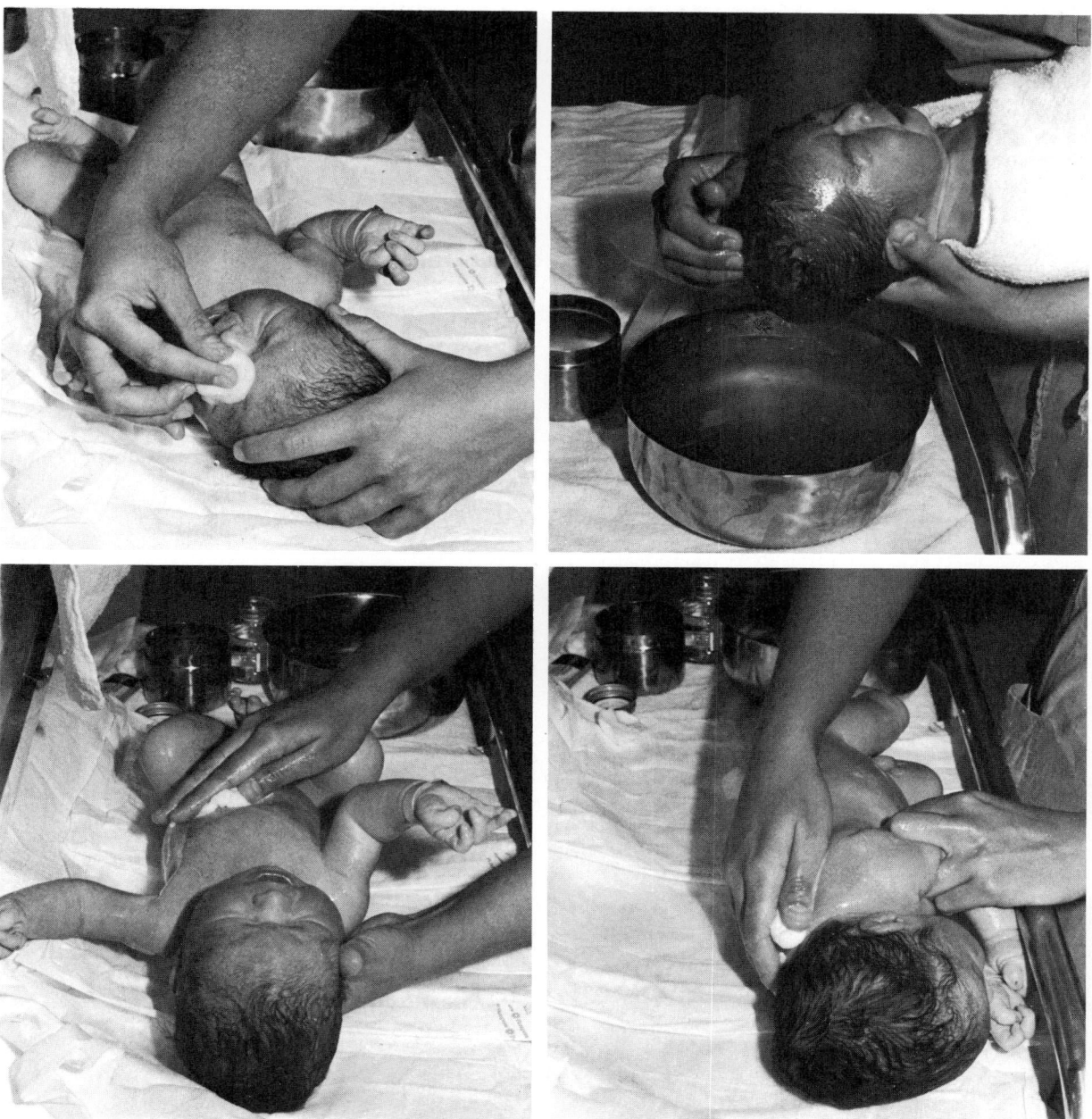

FIGURE 33-8

The cleanest areas of the infant are bathed first (eyes, head) before the chest and back.

baby powder is discouraged because of the sensitivity of the newborn's skin.

Blood is removed from the skin after the delivery, but no attempt is made to thoroughly remove the vernix caseosa unless it is stained with blood or meconium. The vernix caseosa serves to protect the skin and disappears spontaneously in about 24 hours. If it remains in the creases and folds of the skin longer than 2 days, it is apt to cause irritation. In this case gentle wiping usually removes it sufficiently.

Demonstration and Practice.   Each mother should have an opportunity to observe a demonstration of a sponge bath and, if at all possible, to give a bath to her infant. If there is an opportunity for only one bath with the mother present, the nurse can combine the demonstration and return demonstration by discussing the bath with the mother first and then letting her give the bath with the nurse there for moral support and assistance as necessary (Fig. 33-9). If the father can be present and encouraged to participate, it is an added benefit.

The basic principles of bathing should be conveyed to the mother, for safety's sake, but she should not be made to feel that there is only one way to bathe the baby. Each mother develops her own manner of bathing the newborn according to her manual dexterity, the size and the activity of the infant, and the facilities available. By discussing with the mother what she already knows or has heard about bathing the baby, the nurse can make her teaching more meaningful for the individual client.

The nurse should also explore with the mother what equipment and facilities are available in the home and instruct her in how the use of these might differ from what is available in the hospital. Usually the necessities can be met without undue expense or difficulty. For instance, a large drainboard that can be washed and padded adequately (and is a comfortable height for handling the infant) can be used as the bath area. A large pan or basin serves very well for the bathtub in the early weeks; it should be kept only for the baby's use. Thus, the extra expense of special equipment can be minimized. A soft towel and washcloth, for the baby's use only, and a mild soap is also needed.

The mother should not be made to feel that she has to give the baby a bath at the same time every day or that she can't skip a day of bathing. Some mothers and babies enjoy the bath as a daily routine, but others do not or cannot always find the time. For these, as long as the face, neck creases, and diaper area are washed as needed, giving a bath every other day should be sufficient. The mother should be advised that the sponge bath should continue to be the type of bath given until the cord stump has fallen off and the area has healed. After this, a tub bath can be given.

Suggestions for Care of Specific Areas

Eyes.   The eyes should be wiped from the inner corner to the outer corner, using a clean cotton ball or clean area of the washcloth for each eye. No care, other than this cleansing with clean water, is necessary unless there is evidence of inflammation or infection. There may be some reaction from the medication used for prophylaxis against ophthalmia neonatorum beginning in the first few hours, and this condition does not usually require treatment. However, any redness, swelling, or discharge should be reported and recorded so that the eyes can be observed more closely and tests to rule out infection can be done if necessary.

Nose and Ears.   Cotton-tipped applicators should not be used to clean inside the infant's nose or ears

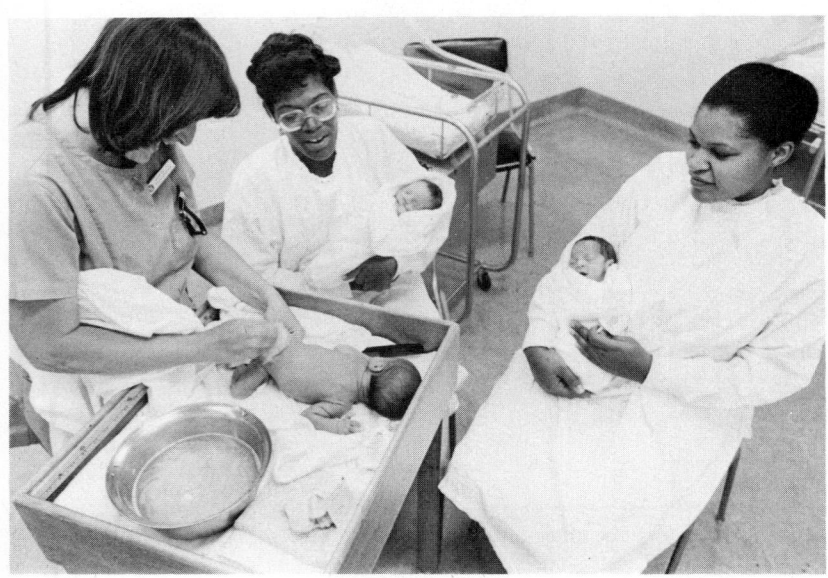

F I G U R E   3 3 - 9

Basic care methods such as bathing the baby are taught by the nurse either individually or as a demonstration class for a small group (Photo by Kathy Sloane).

because of danger of injuring the delicate tissues. The nose usually does not need cleaning because the infant sneezes to clear the nasal passages. If some dried mucus does need to be removed from the nose, a small twisted piece of cotton moistened with water may be used. Only the outer ear should be cleaned. Nothing should be put inside the ear.

Hair. The head should be washed each time the baby is bathed. Swaddling the baby in a blanket or towel and using the football hold makes the job easier. The same soap the baby is washed with or any brand of baby shampoo can be used. Oil should not be put on the hair, as it may predispose to cradle cap.

Skin. The newborn's skin is often dry and peeling within a few days after birth, and dry cracks may appear in the wrist and ankle areas. This is sometimes a cause of concern to mothers and they want to put oil or some other preparation on the skin to get rid of the dryness. They can be reassured that the flakiness and cracks will disappear in a few days and that oil and some lotions may make matters worse by causing a rash.

The skin is thin, delicate, extremely tender, and very easily irritated. Since the skin is a protective covering, breaks in its surface may initiate troublesome infection; hence, skin disturbances constitute an actual threat to the infant's well-being.

The newborn does not usually perspire until after the first month. Warm weather or excessive clothing may cause the infant to develop prickly heat, a closely grouped pinhead-sized rash of papules and vesicles, on the face, the neck, and wherever skin surfaces touch. Fewer clothes and some control over the room temperature help to relieve the discomfort.

Buttocks. Sometimes, despite good nursing care, the infant's buttocks become reddened and sore. A diaper rash that is caused by the reaction of bacteria with the urea in the urine may occur. This in turn causes an ammonia dermatitis. The most important prophylaxis is to keep the diaper area clean and dry. Sometimes petroleum jelly, baby oil, a bland protective ointment (such as Vitamin A and D), or a commercial ointment is used to protect the area. Pastes may not be advised, because they are much more adhesive than ointments and thus create cleansing problems.

A simple treatment that is often effective is merely to expose the infant's reddened buttocks to air (Fig. 33-10) and light several times a day, using care to keep the infant covered otherwise. Air may be all that is necessary, although the use of a *lamp* treatment is more effective and at the same time provides a measure of warmth. An ordinary gooseneck lamp with a screened bulb (no stronger than 40 watts) can be placed on the table so that it is a foot or more away from the infant's

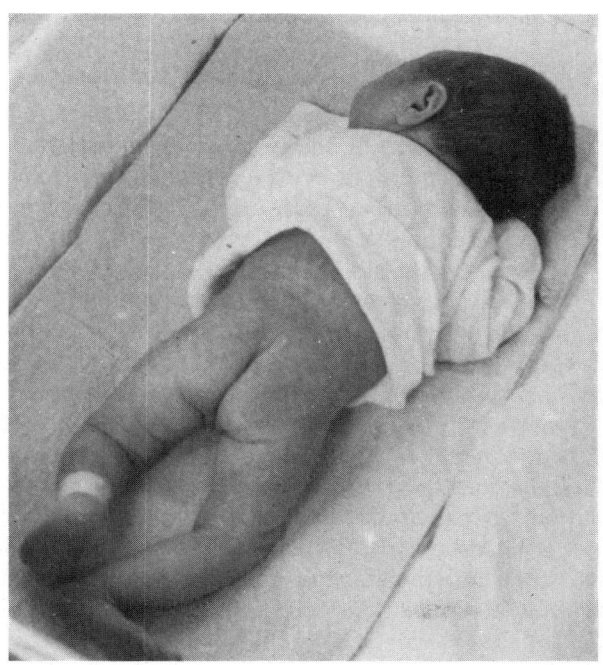

FIGURE 33-10

Exposing buttocks to air.

exposed buttocks. The light may be used for 30 minutes at a time. Because the already irritated skin is very sensitive, care should be exercised so that it is not burned by too strong a bulb or by placing the light too close.

If the condition occurs at home, the treatment described above also is appropriate, and the mother can be so instructed. Boiling the diapers is another effective measure, since this destroys the bacteria. However, many of the detergents and conditioners used today have antibacterial agents in them, and these may be effective in washing the diapers. Care should be taken to rinse the diapers thoroughly, since the residue of the detergent in itself can be irritating. In this respect, the modern diaper services have very effective facilities; many sterilize diapers and entire layettes as part of the service. Disposable diapers are less likely to cause diaper rash, but some brands may contain substances that are irritating to some babies.

Cord Care. The cord clamp is removed when the umbilical stump has dried sufficiently. This is usually in about 24 hours, but it might take more time for a cord that is cut long or that is thick and gelatinous. Depending on the initial care of the area, ongoing care of the umbilicus usually consists of cleaning around the junction between the cord stump and the skin with alcohol at each diaper change to encourage drying. In some hospital settings an antibiotic is used instead of alcohol, but alcohol is still recommended for home use.

The mother should be taught how to care for the infant's cord (Fig. 33-11) while in the hospital so she will feel comfortable with the procedure when she gets home.

To further promote drying of the cord, infants do not receive a tub bath until the cord has separated and the umbilicus has healed. A cord dressing is considered to be unnecessary since exposure to the air enhances drying of the cord.

No attempt should be made to dislodge the cord before it separates completely. If there is a red inflamed area around the stump or any discharge with an odor, this condition should be recorded and reported immediately. The cord usually becomes detached from the body between the fifth and the eighth day after birth, but it may not detach until the 12th or the 14th day. When the cord drops off, the umbilicus should be free from any evidence of inflammation. No further treatment is necessary, except to keep the area clean and dry. When inflammation or discharge is present, the physician gives specific orders for care.

Genitalia.   For the uncircumcised male it has often been recommended that the foreskin be retracted for cleansing purposes beginning a few days after birth. Since in most newborn males the still-developing prepuce is continuous with the epidermis of the glans, it is therefore nonretractable.[9] Forced retraction may cause adhesions to develop. If retraction is done, the foreskin should not be pushed any farther than it will go easily, and it must be replaced over the glans after cleaning or edema may occur.

Current recommendations are to wait until separation occurs naturally with further growth and development, sometime between the age of 3 years and puberty, before trying to retract the foreskin.[10] Most foreskins are retractable by 3 years of age and should be pushed back gently for cleaning about once a week. As the child learns to do more for himself, he should be taught to retract the foreskin and wash the penis, as he is taught to wash other areas of his body. As he gets older, cleaning should be done daily.[11]

In female infants, a curdy secretion, smegma, may accumulate between the folds of the labia and should be carefully cleansed with moistened cotton balls, using the front-to-back direction and a clean cotton ball for each stroke. When demonstrating this technique to the mother the nurse can underscore the importance of teaching a little girl to wipe herself from front to back to help prevent urinary tract infections.

Circumcision

Circumcision, the surgical excision of the end of the prepuce (foreskin) of the penis, is an elective procedure quite often performed in the neonatal period. Although almost routine in many American hospitals, it is done

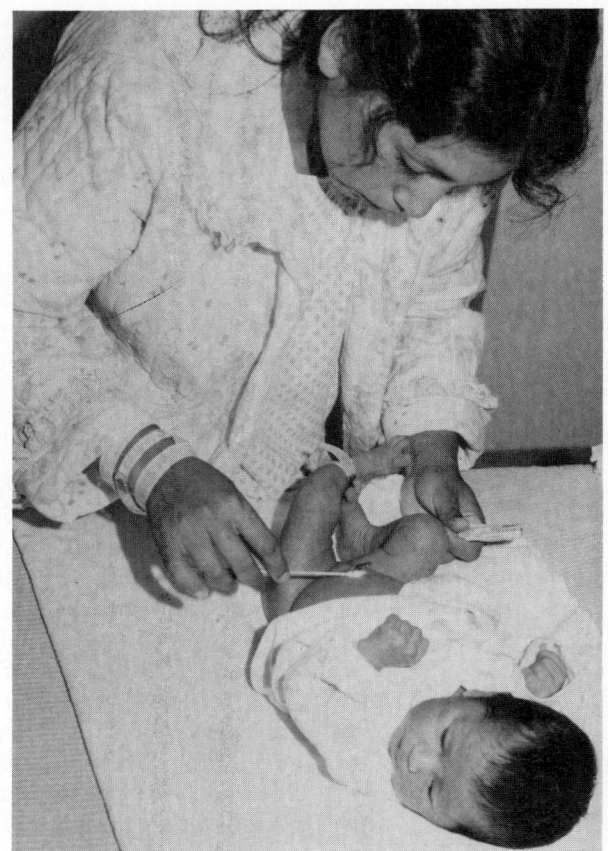

F I G U R E   3 3 - 1 1

The mother can be encouraged to give cord care to her infant.

less frequently in other parts of the world. The value of circumcision is controversial. Some of the advantages that have been stated by advocates of the procedure are that circumcision promotes better hygiene, prevents inflammation and infection of the penis, and decreases the incidence of cancer of the penis. Those who are opposed to routine circumcision contend that good personal hygiene practices by uncircumcised males can also prevent these problems. The Committee on Fetus and Newborn of the American Academy of Pediatrics has stated that there is "no absolute medical indication for circumcision."[12] Opponents of circumcision also list potential hazards of the procedure, such as pain, hemorrhage, infection, and mutilation, as reasons for discouraging its routine use.[10]

Making a Decision and Giving Consent.   The parents of the male infant are asked to make the decision about circumcision. Traditional, cultural, and religious factors may be involved in deciding whether or not the procedure should be done. Studies have shown that major influences on the decision are the physician's opinion and whether or not fathers and older brothers of the infant are circumcised.[10] Some mothers are concerned about having to clean the penis and retract the foreskin if circumcision is not done, and they choose circumcision for that reason. Receiving information during the prenatal period about the pros and cons of circumcision and about cleaning the circumcised and uncircumcised penis can be helpful to parents and can give them more time to make the decision. If not already given to them, however, the information should be made available soon after the baby's birth.

The decision concerning circumcision is becoming more of a dilemma for some parents. When it was a recommended procedure it was easier for the parents to justify the possible risks and discomforts by saying, "It's the best thing to do." Now that the procedure is not encouraged by many doctors, the parents have to take more responsibility. The final decision is up to them and a consent must be signed by one of them before the circumcision is done. "Informed consent" often means listening to a long list of possible undesirable side-effects of the procedure. Some mothers feel very guilty after deciding to have it done. It is important for the nurse to give the parents factual answers to their questions, then support them in their decision, whichever it is.

Care During Circumcision. If the decision is made to circumcise the infant, the procedure is usually delayed

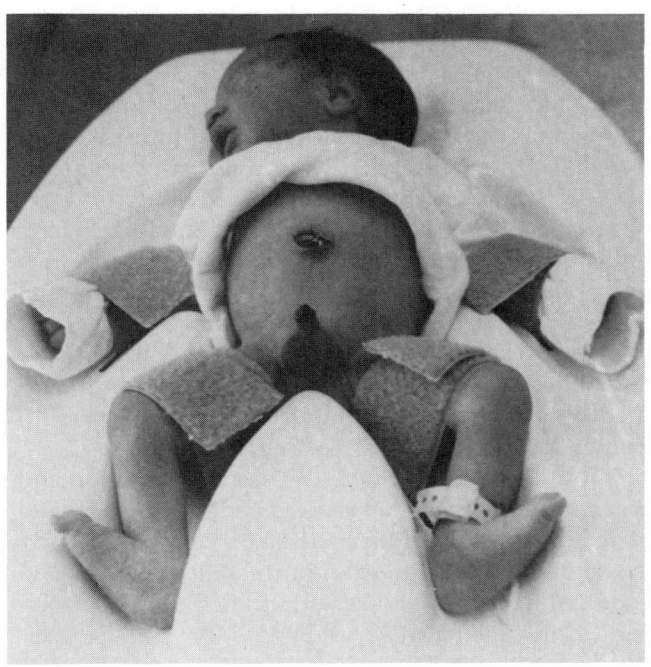

FIGURE 33-12

The infant is placed on a plastic restraining form to restrict movements during the circumcision procedure.

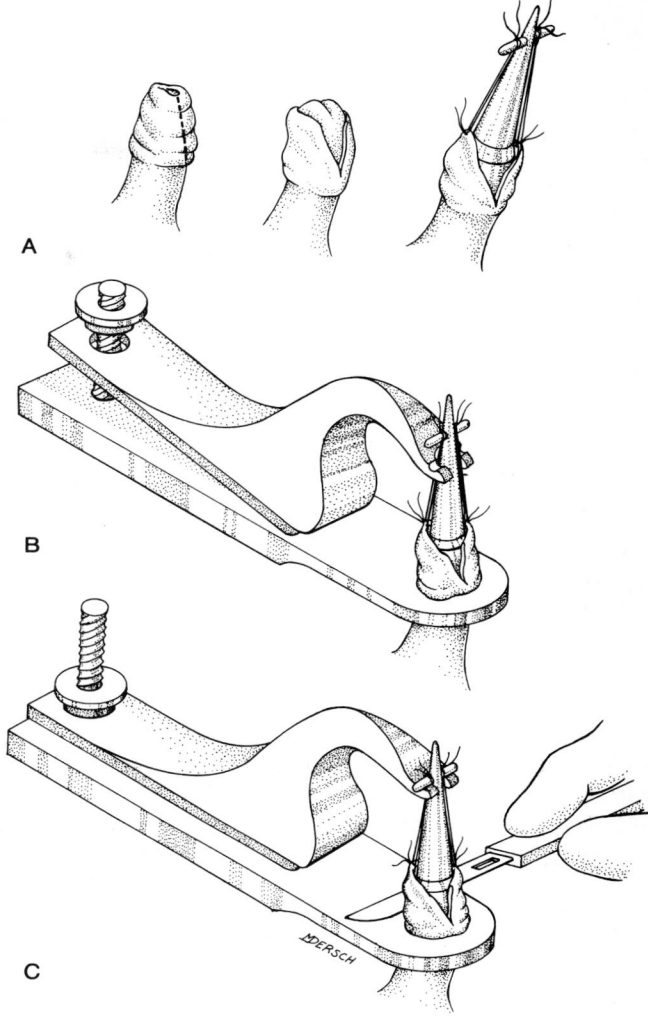

FIGURE 33-13

Circumcision using Gomco clamp. (*A*) Prepuce is slit and drawn over cone. (*B*) Clamp is applied and pressure is maintained for 3 to 5 minutes. (*C*) Excess prepuce is then cut away.

for 12 to 24 hours until the infant has had time to stabilize. Since the infant will be restrained in a supine position for some time, it is best if he is not fed just prior to the circumcision, to avoid regurgitation. After checking to be sure the permit has been signed, the nurse prepares for the procedure by placing the infant on the restraint board (Fig. 33-12) and setting out the sterile gloves, instruments, and drapes that the physician will use.

Several techniques have been devised for circumcising newborns. The most common methods currently in use are the Gomco (Yellen) clamp or the Plastibell. Further explanation of these techniques is given in Figures 33-13 and 33-14. The nurse should assess the in-

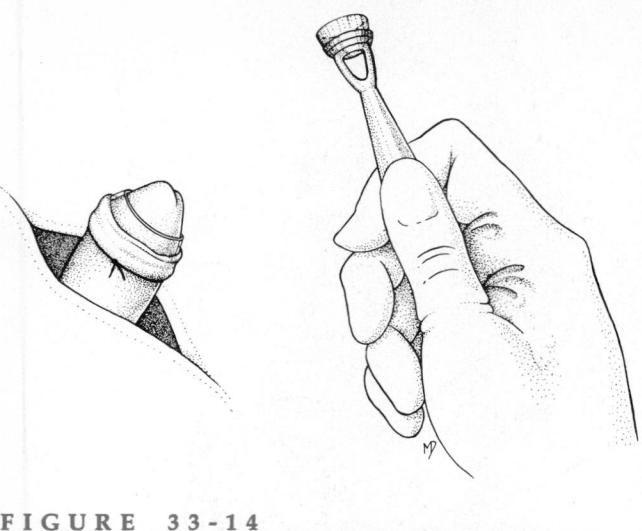

FIGURE 33-14

Circumcision using the Plastibell. The bell is fitted over the glands. Suture is tied around the rim of the bell. Excess prepuce is cut away. The plastic rim remains in place until it falls off, after healing has taken place.

fant's condition periodically during the procedure and be alert for any changes. Comfort measures, such as talking to him or stroking his head, may have a calming effect. Although the infant undoubtedly feels pain during the procedure, it is difficult to tell how much of the crying is due to pain and how much to being restrained.

Care Following Circumcision. When the newborn is circumcised, the main principles of postoperative care are to keep the wound clean and to observe it closely for bleeding (Fig. 33-15). For the first 24 hours the area is covered with a sterile gauze dressing to which a liberal amount of sterile petroleum jelly has been added. If the circumcision is done with the Plastibell, no dressing or petroleum jelly is used.

Mothers are naturally anxious about their babies at this time, so as soon as it is feasible after the circumcision has been done, the nurse should take the baby to his mother for a brief visit. It may be helpful to show her what the circumcision looks like and explain how it will look when healing, so that she can recognize any deviations from normal. With the Plastibell, there is a plastic ring and suture in place, which drops off with the foreskin in about 7 to 10 days.

Occasionally, a local anesthetic is used, but generally the procedure is performed without it. The infant may be fed immediately after the circumcision, and both mother and baby seem to enjoy the comfort that the feeding and cuddling bring. If the infant is left in the mother's room for an extended length of time, the nurse should go in periodically to check the circumcision for bleeding.

In changing the infant's diaper the nurse should hold his ankles with one hand so that he cannot kick against the operative area. Unless the physician orders otherwise, the circumcision dressing can be removed postoperatively when the infant voids for the first time. Cleansing must be done gently but can be accomplished as necessary with cotton balls moistened with warm tap water. A fresh sterile petroleum jelly dressing is usually applied to the penis each time the diaper is changed for the first day. The penis must be observed closely for bleeding and should be inspected every hour during the first 12 hours. It is advisable to place the infant's crib where he can be watched conveniently. Moreover, to keep all the nursing personnel alerted, some signal, such as a red tag, can be attached to the identification card on the crib. If bleeding occurs it can usually be controlled with gentle pressure. If bleeding persists, the physician should be notified immediately.

Since the length of the maternity stay has been considerably shortened, circumcision may be done on the day of discharge; therefore, the nurse should ascertain the physician's wishes for aftercare and make certain that the mother knows how to care for her newly circumcised infant. Generally, the care is the same as that described.

Other Areas of Concern

Weight. The infant should be weighed on the day of birth and then daily or every other day while in the hospital. If the infant remains in the hospital longer than 5 days, he should be weighed at intervals prescribed by the medical staff. His weight should be recorded accurately.

During the first few days after birth the infant may lose 5% to 10% of his birth weight. This is due partly to the minimal intake of nutrients and fluid and partly to the loss of excess fluid.[13] About the time the meconium begins to disappear from his stools, the weight begins to increase, and in normal cases does so regularly until about the tenth day of life, when it may equal the birth weight. Many infants regain their birth weight in a shorter period of time. During the first 5 months, the weight gain should be from 4 oz to 6 oz per week. After this time the gain is from 2 oz to 4 oz per week. At 6 months of age, the infant has usually doubled his birth weight, and by his first birthday it has tripled.

This is one way to note the infant's condition and progress. When the infant is not gaining weight it should be reported to the physician. Besides gaining regularly in weight and strength, the infant should be happy and good-natured when awake and inclined to sleep a good part of the time between feedings.

Sleeping. If the infant is well and comfortable, he usually sleeps much of the time and wakes and cries when he is hungry or uncomfortable. He may sleep as much as 20 out of 24 hours (although this varies con-

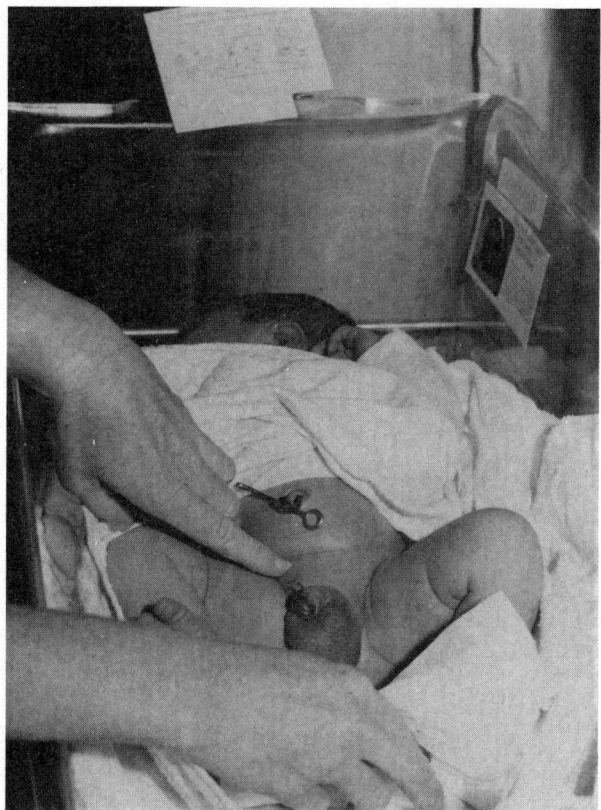

FIGURE 33-15

Postcircumcision inspection.

siderably from infant to infant). It is not the sound sleep of the adult; rather, he moves a good deal, stretches, and at intervals awakens momentarily. Since he responds so readily to external stimuli (and this may make him restless), his clothing and coverings are important. They should be light in weight and warm, but not too warm. His position should be changed each time he is put down in his crib. He can be placed on either side or his abdomen, especially when he is ready for sleep. If he is positioned on his back, someone should be present, for if the infant regurgitates, he is more likely to aspirate in this position. The importance of avoiding the back as a sleeping position should be emphasized to parents. As he gets older and learns to roll over, he will assume the position that he likes most for sleep.

Crying. After the infant is dressed and placed in a warm crib he usually does not cry unless he is wet, hungry, ill, or uncomfortable for some reason, or is moved. One learns to distinguish an infant's condition and needs from the character of his cry, which may be described as follows:

- A fretful, hungry cry, with fingers in the mouth and flexed, tense extremities, is easily recognized.

- A fretful cry, if due to indigestion, is accompanied by green stools and passing of gas.
- A loud, insistent cry with drawing up and kicking of the legs usually denotes colicky pain.
- A whining cry is noticeable when the baby is ill, premature, or very frail.
- A peculiar, shrill, sharp-sounding cry suggests injury, especially to the central nervous system.

Every effort should be made to recognize any deviation from the usual manner in which a baby announces his normal requirements. Moreover, this information should be conveyed to the mother, since it is essential that the mother learn to interpret her infant's cues. The newborn has only his posture and his voice at this time to inform others of his needs.

Hypertonic Babies. Occasionally, the nurse finds an infant that seems to be fussy from birth. He appears very active, startles easily, cries readily and more frequently (and apparently for no reason), is alert and awake much of the time, and in general does not fit the usual pattern of activity, feeding, and sleeping described. These babies may be described as *hypertonic* (*i.e.*, they do not seem to be able to relax as well as other infants).

The parents of hypertonic infants may find it difficult to adjust to their new baby and may experience a great deal of anxiety until they are informed (or learn by trial and error) that this is "normal behavior" for this child. Too often they assume they must be doing something "wrong," since despite their efforts, their baby remains fussy, tense, and crying. The nurse can be very helpful to the parents in giving them anticipatory guidance about their baby's behavior and helpful ways in which he can be soothed. The physician should also be informed of the nurse's observations in order to give appropriate advice to the parents.

These infants usually respond favorably to being held securely. Thus, wrapping them snugly with a receiving blanket, cuddling them securely, and changing their position slowly and surely rather than quickly all help to allay undue tenseness. Rocking the baby and walking with him are particularly successful measures, but no parent can or should do this over protracted periods of time.

An automatic baby swing with a music box is often soothing, and even a young infant can be placed in one for a short period of time supported by pillows. Recorded heartbeat sounds and various types of music are also soothing to many infants. The parents should be encouraged to experiment to find out which sounds have the best effect on their infant.

Any new activity or procedure should be introduced slowly to infants with this type of personality. For instance, when a tub bath is given for the first time,

Continuing Care of the Newborn

Nursing Objectives

1. Protect infant from infection.
2. Identify problems or potential problems in infant's physical condition.
3. Provide safe care for infant's hygiene and comfort.
4. Provide instruction for parents regarding infant care and newborn characteristics.
5. Promote parent–infant interaction.

Assessment	Potential Nursing Diagnosis	Planning/Intervention	Evaluation

General status:
  Vital signs
  Color
  Responsiveness
  Activity
	Potential for infection related to vulnerability of infant and lack of normal flora
	
	Potential alteration of skin integrity related to lack of normal flora and possible peeling and cracking
		Make observations according to hospital policy
		
		Note any changes in infant's condition and report and record as appropriate
		
		Use good hand-washing and individual clean technique when caring for newborn
			Newborn has stabilized vital signs
			
			Newborn does not develop hypothermia nor hyperthermia
			
			Newborn remains free of evidence of jaundice or cyanosis
			
			Newborn alternates sleep and activity
			
			Newborn's skin remains intact

Elimination: stools and urine	Alteration in bowel elimination: lack of stool related to possible imperforate anus Alteration in patterns of urinary elimination: decreased related to insufficient fluid intake	Record passage of first and subsequent stools: describe color, consistency, and amount Report if no stool in first 24 hours Record number of wet diapers Report if number decreases Encourage more frequent feedings	Newborn passes meconium stool within first 24 hours Newborn voids within first 24 hours and has at least 6 to 10 wet diapers per day after first 24 hours

(continued)

the infant should be placed very slowly in a small amount of water, and each lower extremity immersed gradually in order not to frighten or startle the infant too much. The parents should not consider an occasional evening out a luxury; it should be considered a necessary item in the care of their baby. These infants do place greater demands on their parents than do infants of a more placid nature, and a short time away from the baby does wonders in restoring the perspective and good humor of the parents.

Urinary Elimination. Urinary activity of the fetus is evidenced by the presence of urine in the amniotic fluid. The baby usually voids during delivery or immediately after birth, but the function may be sup-

pressed for several hours. However, if the baby does not void within 24 hours, the condition should be reported to the physician; retention of the urine may be due to an imperforate meatus. After the first 2 or 3 days the infant voids from 10 to 15 times a day. When the urine is concentrated, red or rusty stains on the wet diaper may be due to uric-acid crystals in the urine.

Intestinal Elimination. During fetal life the content of the intestines is made up of greenish black tarlike material called meconium. It is composed of epithelial and epidermal cells and lanugo hair that probably were swallowed with the amniotic fluid. The color of the meconium is due to the bile pigment. Before birth and for the first few hours after birth, the intestinal contents

Assessment	Potential Nursing Diagnosis	Planning/Intervention	Evaluation
Condition of umbilical cord stump and umbilicus	Potential for infection related to moist umbilical cord	Observe umbilical area for inflammation or odor and cord stump for dryness	Newborn remains free of infection
		For long, moist cord, obtain permission to cut shorter	
		Apply anti-infective agent (tripple dye, antibiotic ointment, or alcohol) according to hospital policy	
Behavioral patterns	Alteration in comfort related to hypertonic disposition, manifested by excessive crying	Observe for individual infant's behavior patterns	Newborn cries normally
		Provide comfort measures: holding, swaddling, gentle touch	
Family interactions	Potential alteration in parenting related to inexperience and feelings of incompetence	Provide opportunities for parents to handle and get acquainted with infant	Parents express their comfort in handling the infant
		Provide assistance as needed without taking over	
Knowledge of infant care	Possible knowledge deficit about infant care related to being new parents	Develop teaching plan for individual couple, based on assessment of knowledge	Parents express and demonstrate ability to care for infant before discharge from hospital
		Provide information, demonstrations, practice opportunities, and other teaching modalities as appropriate	

are sterile. Apparently, there is no peristalsis until after birth, because normally there is no discoloration of the amniotic fluid.

The newborn passes meconium stools for the first day or two of life (Fig. 33-16). After this, the stools gradually begin to change to greenish brown and then to yellowish brown. These "transitional stools" are less sticky than meconium and contain some milk curds. Following the transitional stools, the characteristics depend on whether the infant is fed breast milk or formula. The stools of the breast-fed infant tend to be a golden yellow color with a distinctive odor, sometimes described as "sweet." Their consistency varies from loose to mushy, and they may be frequent or infrequent. If the infant is formula-fed the stools may be pale yellow to light brown and of firmer consistency and may have a slightly offensive or foul odor.

Most newborns pass the first stool within 12 hours of birth; nearly all have a stool in 24 hours. If an infant has not passed a stool by this time, imperforate anus or intestinal obstruction must be considered as a possible reason for the delay, and the baby must be observed closely.

The daily number of stools on about the fifth day of life is usually four to six. As the infant grows, this number decreases to one or two each day. The type of stool of the breast-fed baby may be influenced by the mother's diet. However, there may be slight variations from the normal, which may have little significance if the baby appears to be comfortable and sleeps and

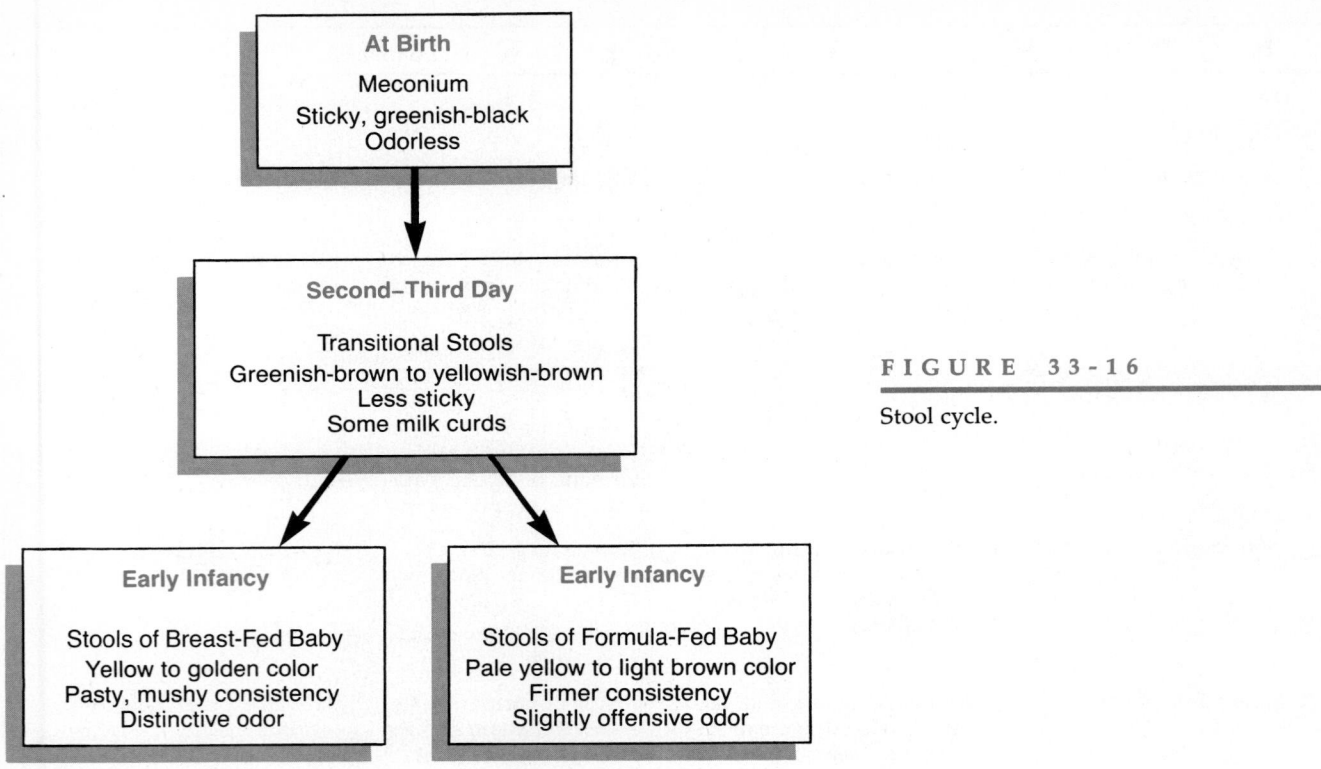

FIGURE 33-16

Stool cycle.

nurses well. If the baby's stools have a watery consistency, are of a green color, and contain much mucus, and flatus is being passed, the condition may be evidence of some digestive or intestinal irritation and should be reported to the physician.

The number, color, and consistency of stools should be recorded daily on the baby's record.

Discharge from the Hospital

Discharge planning for the new mother and baby may begin in the prenatal class or clinic when discussions are held about planning for "what happens after the baby comes home?" During the hospital stay the nurse continues to assess the family's needs for assistance in planning for care of the baby at home. Early discharge (less than 24 hr) for mothers and babies without complications is a reality in many places, owing either to the parents' desire or to hospital policy. Observations and care traditionally done by hospital personnel is now the responsibility of the new parents. This increases the need for adequate instruction, but decreases the time available for teaching. Giving the parents a phone number they can call at any hour if they need help or further information after they get home is often very helpful. For some new mothers, especially the inexperienced, a referral to a community-health agency for a home visit may be appropriate for follow-up. Some families with financial problems may need to be referred to a family-service agency.

As part of the plan for taking the infant home, the nurse should find out if the parents have and plan to use a car seat for the infant. Car seats, even in the states where they are mandatory, are not being used consistently by many parents. Nurses should be well informed about the use of car seats and should take the opportunity to advocate their use whenever possible. New parents are usually very receptive to information that will help them provide good care for their baby, so discussing car seats is particularly appropriate at this time. A space on the discharge chart form to indicate the use of a car seat will encourage staff members to include this in their discharge planning and teaching.[14]

Plans for health-care follow-up of the infant should be discussed with the mother. A follow-up appointment should be made with a private physician or at a well-baby clinic. Most new mothers appreciate an opportunity to talk to the nurse regarding their concerns about taking the baby home. Taking time for such a talk is well worth the nurse's effort, since it can help make those first few days at home less frightening and more enjoyable for the new parents.

References

1. Polmar SH, Sorenson RU, Pittard WB, III: Immunology. In Fanaroff AA, Martin RJ (eds): Behrman's Neonatal-Perinatal Medicine, 3rd ed, pp 632–649. St Louis, CV Mosby, 1983
2. Brann AW Jr, Cefalo RC (eds): Guidelines for Perinatal Care. Evanston, IL, and Washington, DC, American Academy of Pediatrics and American College of Obstetricians and Gynecologists, 1983
3. Renaud MT: Effects of discontinuing cover gowns on a postpartal ward upon cord colonization of the newborn. JOGN Nurs 12(6):399–401, November/December, 1983
4. Phibbs RH: The newborn infant. In Rudolph AM (ed): Pediatrics, 16th ed, p 153. New York, Appleton-Century-Crofts, 1977
5. Roberts FB: Perinatal Nursing. New York, McGraw-Hill, 1977
6. Scopes JW: Thermoregulation in the newborn. In Avery GB (ed): Neonatology, 2nd ed, p 178. Philadelphia, JB Lippincott, 1981
7. Nicholson JF: Inborn errors of metabolism. In Fanaroff AA, Martin RJ (eds): Behrman's Neonatal-Perinatal Medicine, 3rd ed, pp 816–817. St Louis, CV Mosby, 1983
8. Avery ME, Taeusch HW Jr: Schaffer's Diseases of the Newborn, 5th ed, p 60. Philadelphia, WB Saunders, 1984
9. NAACOG Committee on Practice: Nurse's Role in Neonatal Circumcision (pamphlet). Washington, DC, NAACOG, August 1985
10. Kaplan G: Circumcision: An overview. Curr Probl Pediatr 7:1–33, March 1977
11. Poole CJ: Neonatal circumcision. JOGN Nurs 5:207–211, July/August 1979
12. Committee on Fetus and Newborn, American Academy of Pediatrics: Report of the ad hoc task force on circumcision. Pediatrics 56:610–611, October 1975
13. Kaplan S: Normal and abnormal growth. In Rudolph AM (ed): Pediatrics, 16th ed, p 107. New York, Appleton-Century-Crofts, 1977
14. Nachem B, Bass RA: Children still aren't being buckled up. MCN 9(5):320–323, September/October, 1984

NAACOG Committee on Practice: Nurse's Role in Neonatal Circumcision (pamphlet). Washington, DC, NAACOG, 1985
Nachem B, Bass RA: Children still aren't being buckled up. MCN 9:320–323, September/October 1984
Newton LD: Helping parents cope with infant crying. JOGN Nurs 12:199–204, May/June 1983
Renaud MT: Effects of discontinuing cover gowns on a post-partal ward upon cord colonization of the newborn. JOGN Nurs 12:399–401, November/December 1983

Suggested Reading

Bryant BG: Unit dose erythromycin ophthalmic ointment for neonatal ocular prophylaxis. JOGN Nurs 13:83–87, March/April 1984
Care of the Uncircumcised Penis (pamphlet). Elk Grove, IL, American Academy of Pediatrics, 1984
Circumcision: A Personal Choice (pamphlet). Washington, DC, American College of Obstetricians and Gynecologists, 1984

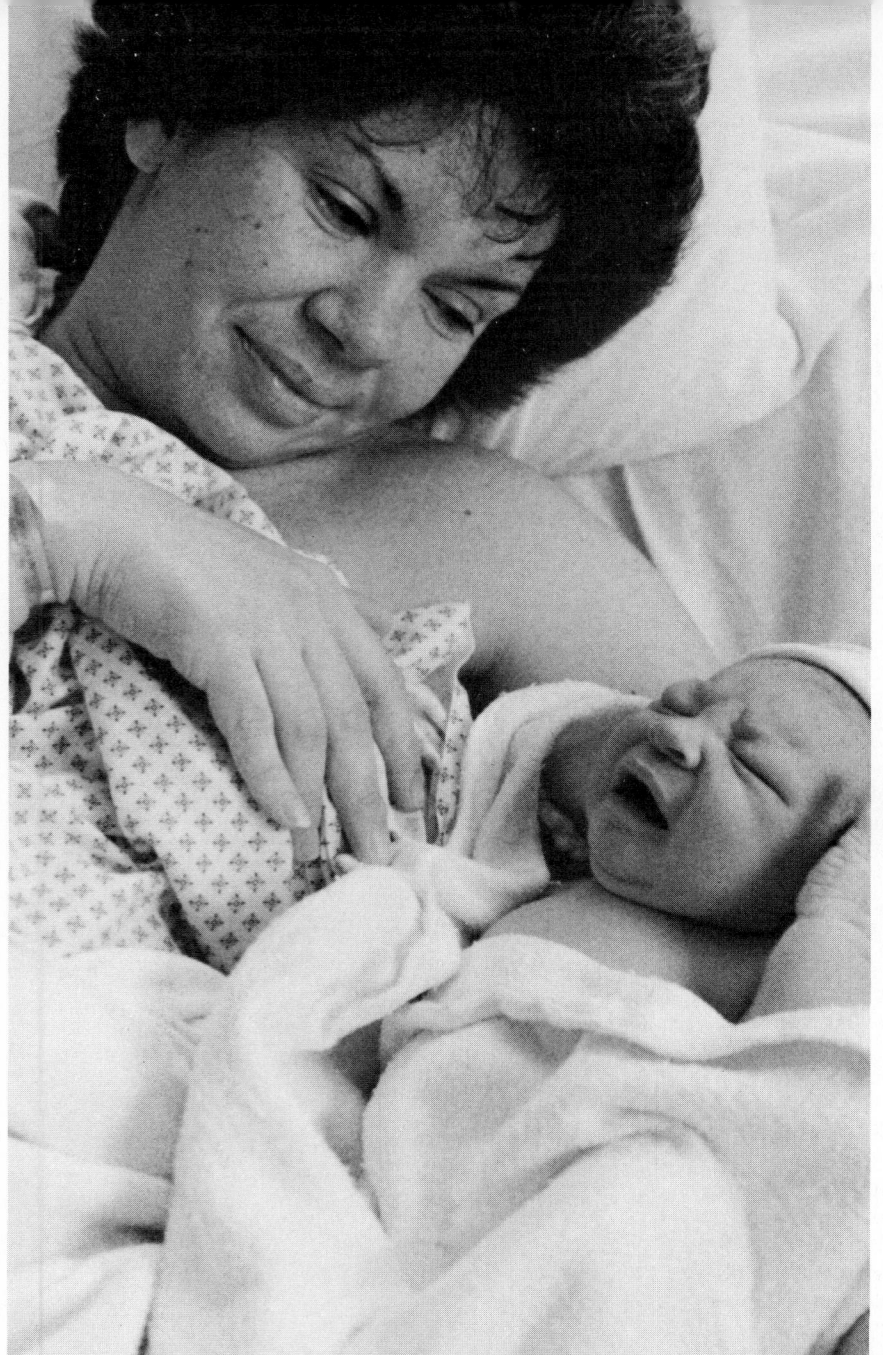

CHAPTER 34

Sensory Enrichment With the Newborn

The senses are the primary source of information for the neonate brain until intentional thought develops 8 or 9 months later. Intentional thought is the deliberate creation of thoughts, which can in turn stimulate the mind.[1] All learning prior to this time is a result of sensory enrichment, using and challenging each sense. In this first year of life, the sensory and motor systems are used to navigate through the environment. Once thoughts are formed, the infant no longer relies solely upon his senses and motor abilities to learn and solve problems.

Sensory Enrichment

As soon as an infant is born he is capable of sensing and responding to all that he experiences. At birth he can sense the brightness of the room, the drop in ambient temperature, and the presence of a warm embrace, and he listens to the familiar sound of his mother's heartbeat and his parents' voices. As he is cuddled, he relaxes his body and assumes a posture of contentment. As he is spoken to, his face brightens and he gazes intently, conveying interest and pleasure in this contact.

A certain amount of sensory stimulation, such as feeding and swaddling for warmth, is necessary for proper maturation. Sensory experiences that transcend satisfaction of shelter, nutrition, warmth, and protection needs are enrichment experiences.

Enrichment experiences are designed to provide the infant with pleasure and empower him to achieve mastery and self-esteem as he progresses through infancy. Once an infant has seen a human face and established eye-to-eye contact, he learns to build up a repertoire of gestures that keep the caregiver entrained upon him, thereby being provided with additional sensory experiences. An empowered infant, then, is one who is able to precipitate and encourage caregiving and social interactions, not just passively receive enrichment.

Sensory enrichment is an important corollary to physical care of the newborn. Supervising and supporting the parents in their enrichment endeavors is an important maternal–newborn nursing intervention, especially if supervision can prevent an overzealous and inadvertent bombardment with multiple stimuli in hopes of accelerating the infant's development. Overstimulation and "pushing" an infant is always a potential risk when educating parents about sensory enrichment.

Support of the parent ultimately impacts upon the infant, enhancing his development. To support the parent the nurse must first have an understanding of the rationale for sensory enrichment, the development of the central nervous system, the effects of sensory enrichment, maternal and infant assessments to prevent overstimulation, principles guiding active sensory en-

richment interventions, and safe sensory enrichment interventions that can be incorporated into previously existing caregiving strategies with the newborn.

Rationale for Sensory Enrichment

There are three reasons for recommending incorporation of sensory enrichment in maternal–newborn nursing care:

- Sensory enrichment facilitates satisfaction with the maternal role.
- Sensory enrichment promotes positive interactions between parent and infant.
- Sensory enrichment is an integral force influencing infant development.

Satisfaction with Maternal Role

Parents are driven by a desire to please their infant. This desire is fueled by the biologic drives known as maternal and paternal instincts, attachment and affection for the infant, and the extreme dependency of the infant upon his caregivers. New parents often find their time is consumed by the feeding, changing, consoling, and cuddling needs of their infant. Overwhelmed by the demands, a perceived inequity in the giving and receiving of the parent–infant relationship may occur. When reciprocal giving and receiving is not present, either in reality or perception, mutual gratification is denied and maternal stress, anger, frustration, anxiety, and dissatisfaction with the maternal experience ensue.[2] Sensory enrichment offers the caregiver a repertoire of approaches that foster pleasure in the infant, an emotional response that the caregiver can then observe. When the mother is buttressed by knowledge and the ability to recognize her infant's cues, this positive feedback promotes satisfaction with the maternal experience.

Positive Interactions Between Parents and Child

Sensory enrichment fosters the positive interaction cycle demonstrated in Figure 34-1. In observing maternal reactions to her alert infant once she has called his name, it may be noticed that the mother comes back with smiles, inflected vocalization, and caressing that brings the infant into a face-to-face orientation. The infant's behavior in response to her call has been detected, altering the mother's behavior into a pattern that is congruent with the infant's manifestations, changing the frequency, duration, intensity, and quality of the stimulation.

Infants actively participate in interactions. Babies initiate and regulate behavioral exchanges and com-

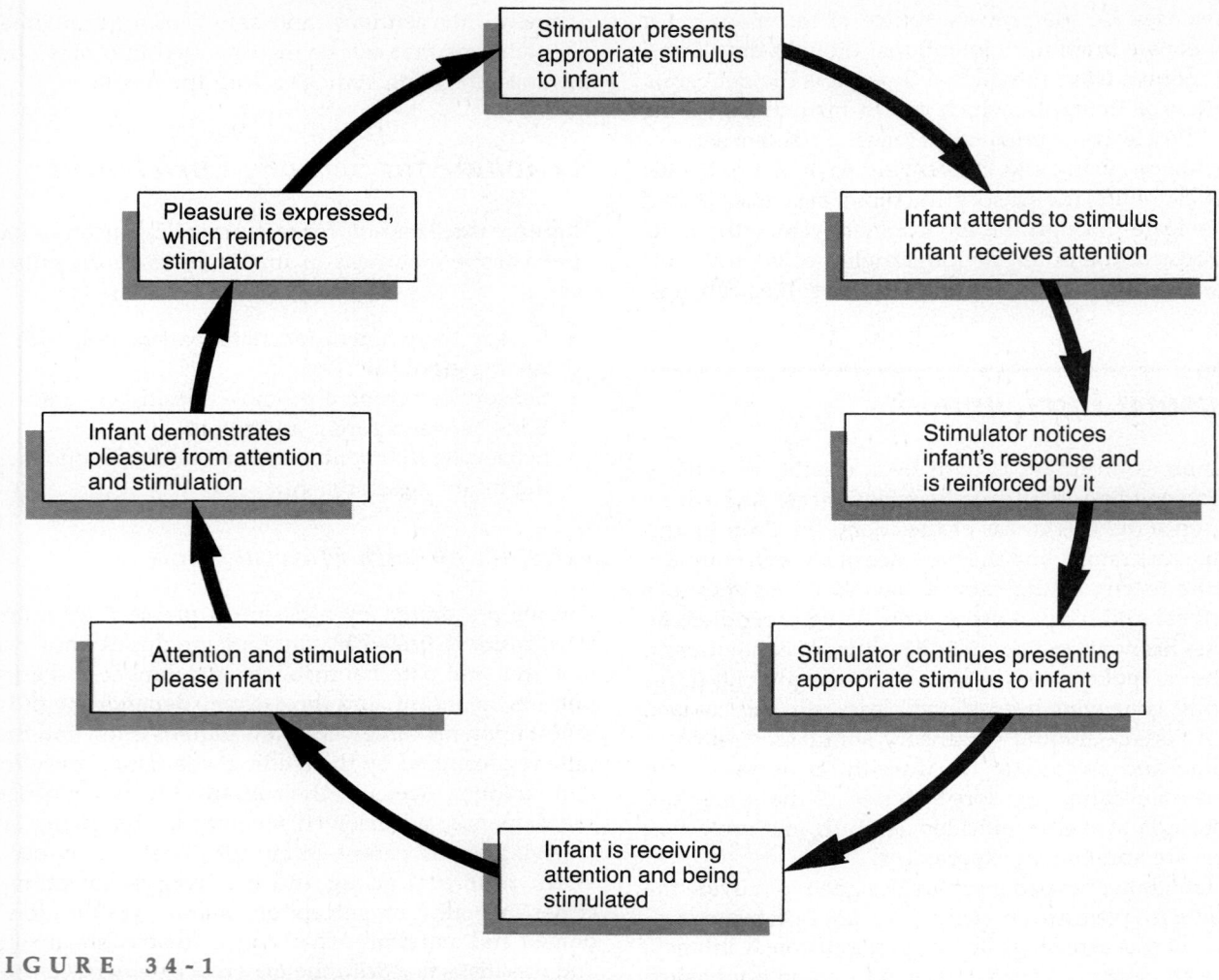

FIGURE   34-1

Sensory enrichment interaction cycle. (Copyright 1982, 1986, Infant Stimulation Education Association, ISEA)

municate in accordance with rules.[3] They do so using gestures and prespeech movements and sound known as protoconversations.[4] Newborns effectively communicate in burst–pause patterns, expecting alternating interchanges with the caregiver. Communication begins with random movements at birth, and by 6 weeks of age, facial expressions and hand gesturing are employed to indicate "greeting" and withdrawal responses to both people and objects.

Many researchers support the precept that "mutually enjoyable interactions between caregiver and infant constitute the foundation of optimum development."[5-7] Other researchers have found that stability and constancy of maternal stimulation of the infant are major factors in his cognitive development.[8] Even in mothers who have expressed concern about their mothering skills, maternal education and enrichment strategies have been instrumental in aiding normal infant development in potentially detrimental situations.[9]

It is crucial to note that gratification and the beneficial effects of this interaction cycle can be thwarted if inappropriate or overstimulating activities occur. Cautious assessment to prevent their appearance is recommended and discussed as a nursing assessment.

Forces Influencing Development

Barnard and co-workers propose an interactional model in which characteristics of the environment, mother, and child are forces that interact to influence the infant's development.[10] Brazelton postulated that the infant is equipped with reflexive responses that are organized into complex patterns of behavior, attention, and interaction with his world. The organization occurs once the infant reaches a state of homeostatic control (physiological balance and stability) and then devotes his energies to a *quest for social stimuli*.[11] This system, including the sensory enrichment provided, increases the infant's availability to his world. Once available and interested in the environment, the infant responds in such a way that he learns more about himself.

Development of the Central Nervous System

In the first year of life the brain grows faster than it will at any other time. The infant has obtained 25% of adult brain weight by birth, 50% by 6 months, and 70% by 1 year; this period is known as the brain growth spurt period.

This accelerated central nervous system development is influenced by three factors: *genetic endowment,* which may account for 25% to 70% of a child's optimal capabilities; *good nutrition,* especially a well-balanced diet with 20 g to 40 g of extra protein per day during pregnancy if renal function is adequate;[12] *environmental factors* such as adversity or enrichment.[13]

The rapid growth period is thought to be one of increased vulnerability to nutrition restriction and environmental conditions, particularly adversity (*e.g.*, drug and radiation exposure). Malnutrition is associated with a decreased number of brain cells, diminished size of the brain cells, and a reduction in the branching and synapses formed by each cell. Each of these conditions contributes negatively to mental function.

Environmental enrichment during the brain growth spurt period also has dramatic effects. Enriched environments have conclusively been shown to alter the actual structure and function of brains of many mammals.[14] Animal studies strongly support the belief that there are critical and sensitive periods for brain development. Critical periods are those in which certain types of stimuli must be present for a particular structure or function to develop. Sensitive periods are those in which the brain's continuing function is particularly vulnerable to internal and external environmental conditions. It is postulated that the brain growth spurt is a critical and sensitive period in humans, but this can never be confirmed, since information about brain responses to environmental conditions can be derived only from animal studies.

Development of the Senses

Each of the six senses (visual, auditory, tactile, gustatory, olfactory, and vestibular proprioceptive) is receptive to sensory enrichment at birth. This capability is based upon prenatal growth and development.

The senses are known to be functional by 25 weeks' gestation. It is not unreasonable to expect that the senses are capable of detecting changes in the intrauterine environment after 17 weeks of gestation. Mothers commonly report that the fetus kicks more when music is played or quiets down when she starts rocking. Verny reports that fetuses behave in a particular manner when classical music is played over the abdomen. Bright lights and sounds induce specific heart rate changes in the fetus as he becomes aware of their presence. It is evident that the newborn is capable of perceiving environmental events at birth. The senses may be exquisitely sensitive at birth, as in the olfactory sense, or they may be relatively immature, as in the visual and auditory senses; however, even the immature senses perform well within their limitations.

Scientists now realize that infants can see at birth with good acuity within 10 to 12 inches of their face, fixate longer on patterned than unpatterned stimuli, accommodate more easily to big items (3 inches high by 3 inches wide), and seek out high-contrast geometric shapes rather than pastel bunnies, butterflies, and balloons.[15,16] Head-turning devices and suck meters are used to analyze infant choices for various sensory stimuli and reactions to others. Babies selectively respond to the human voice and soft, rhythmical sounds.[17] The "mass of buzzing confusion," as infants were characterized prior to 1960, has become a competent infant who, in fact, thinks he is a human being.[18]

Brain Growth Time Chart

10–18 weeks' gestation. Phase 1 (hyperplasia phase): number of brain cells is set

20 weeks' gestation to 2 years of age. Phase 2 (brain growth spurt): neuron cells increase in size; nerve fibers insulated; dendrites develop

20 weeks' gestation to 4 years of age. Nerve fibers are insulated (myelinated) at rapid rate; process slows down after 4 years of age

8 months' gestation. Brain undergoes extra spurt of growth

8th and 9th months of pregnancy. Brain doubles in weight from 183 g to 365 g to 392 g

Birth. Brain has attained 25% of its adult brain weight

6 months of age. Brain has doubled its weight again from 392 to 870 g; brain has attained 50% of its adult brain weight; brain growth after 6th month slows considerably

1 year of age. Brain weighs 1000 g; brain has attained 70% of its adult brain weight; majority of DNA in brain cells has been set down

3 years of age. Brain has attained more than 90% of its maximum size

The majority of brain growth occurs in the first year of life!

Adapted from Ludington-Hoe SM. Foundations of Infant Stimulation (Los Angeles: Infant Stimulation Education Association), p. 12, 1981

Effects of Sensory Enrichment

Common patterns of parenting are usually sufficient to guarantee normal development in a healthy, full-term infant. Yet, the role of sensory enrichment in this development should not be negated.

According to Piaget, the first stage of infant development and cognitive growth is the sensorimotor period, spanning the period from birth to age 2. This is a reflex stage in which the infant learns to adapt to the sensory stimuli coming to him. This adaptation occurs through *assimilation*, acquisition of new knowledge from the environment, and *accommodation*, adjusting to the assimilated knowledge. Each sensory stimulus is a schema that will be joined with other schema to form schemata, units of thought that direct the infant's cognitive or physical reaction to his environment. In this way programs for the anticipation, thinking, reasoning, logic, and problem-solving aspects of cognition are formed quite early. For example, following a few days of conditioning by being placed in a feeding position, newborns engaged in anticipatory sucking, having successfully been conditioned, which is a rudimentary form of learning.[19]

The role of early sensory enrichment in acceleration and broadening of cognitive ability in normal infants is not conclusively known. Sensory stimulation programs to date rarely report success in helping a normal infant achieve significantly higher IQ scores; instead, infants in early intervention programs acquire distinct mental and motor development advantages compared with infants who were not in the early intervention program.[20,21] A "number" of intelligence is not as important as a "profile" of intelligence, an infant's ability to master some tasks and feel powerful in influencing his immediate environment.

The positive cognitive effects of early sensory enrichment may be limited by a genetic ceiling. The genetic ceiling, or what is commonly called a child's potential, is not a definitive cutoff. It is instead a range of potential such as encountered when one has a gene for medium-to-tall height. A study investigating the long-term effects of daily skin-to-skin stroking and placement upon a rocking hammock with simulated heartbeat sounds during the first 3 months of life found that the "enriched" infants performed similarly to the "unenriched" infants on mental and motor tests at birth, 1 month, and 4 months of age.[22] In another study, full-term infants who were exposed to extra stimulation or handling have not shown evident acceleration, only an increased variability of performance within the accepted normal range, with perhaps more of them functioning at the upper limits of normal range than unstimulated full-term infants.[23] The genetic ceiling may have been ex-

erting influence in these experiments, or development measurements may have been taken too early, since most cognitive gains from sensory enrichment do not appear until 24 months of age.[24] This means that manifestations of enhanced cognition may not appear until the child is at least 2 years old.

Many parents misinterpret enrichment to mean approaches to increase their offspring's IQ. This is not correct. Sensory enrichment is designed to foster development of a well-rounded, well-balanced baby, one who is equally comfortable, competent, and accomplished in mental, motor, social, and emotional skills. The "enhancing intelligence" motive has recently been associated with clinical observations that children who are "pushed" to improve their intelligence lose an inherent interest in learning[25] and suffer emotional setbacks.[26]

Assessment

Prior to the initiation of sensory enrichment with any infant, several assessments need to be made to determine the extent of knowledge, supervision, and support the parents need. These assessments prevent oversimplified, nonindividuated enrichment programs that may do more harm than good. Individuated programs have the potential of interacting with each infant in ways that address his unique needs and will make him feel special.

Awareness of an infant's characteristic rhythm of interaction, maternal reciprocity, and signs of infant attention, habituation, fatigue, and engagement/disengagement cues ensures personalization of enrichment interventions and avoidance of overstimulation. Overstimulation is the threat or presence of physiological and alert-state compromise due to enrichment interventions that are too much, too intense, and poorly timed. Recognition of the signs of overstimulation can assist in the early reversal of this condition, should it occur.

In addition to assessments designed to personalize sensory enrichment interventions, there are some principles of enrichment that are applicable to all infants as a measure of safety. These principles are used to foster positive responses in the infant and apply interventions in nonirritating, physiologically supportive ways.

Infant Rhythms

In the first 2 days following delivery there will be many opportunities to observe the neonate display his rhythm of interaction. Each infant moves through the rhythm at his own rate, lingering at some stages while traversing others with such swiftness that its manifestations escape observation except in the most vigilant and astute nurse; however, the pattern is relatively similar. It is best to pick a peaceful interlude in which the infant is quietly lying in his crib with eyes open and an expression of interest on his face. This is the period of alert inactivity. At this time he is most receptive to the presentation of sensory stimuli and will demonstrate the stages of his rhythm.

- *Presentation.* The stimulus is presented by softly calling the infant's name. As the stimulus reaches his brain, there will be an alerting response and slight movements in the trunk, legs, and head as acknowledgment of the stimulus.
- *Orientation.* Once the stimulus has been received and recognized as something different from what existed a minute before its presentation, the infant makes attempts to orient toward the stimulus. Orientation is marked by trunk straightening, slight head righting or raising, head turning toward the stimulus, and fanning motions of the fingers and toes. Orientation is the infant's attempt to get the stimulus into his visual field and capture all of its sensory modalities.
- *Attentiveness.* The infant pays attention to the stimulus for the length of his attention span, which, in normal newborns, is about 4 to 10 seconds. Attention is different from arousal and alertness. Arousal is the change from a less alert state to a more alert state, such as going from drowsiness to alert inactivity. Alertness refers to eyes open rather than shut or half closed. An infant can have his eyes open and be inattentive, just as adults can go into a stare. Attentiveness, on the other hand, is an active process that makes demands on the infant's energy and concentration abilities. Pupil dilation; slowing of heart rate (by six to eight beats per min), respiratory rate (by four to six per min), and sucking rate; cessation of gross arm and leg movements; and quiet gazing characterize this stage of rhythm, as does change in affect.[27]
- *Acceleration.* As the infant reaches the end of his attention span and exhausts his attentional energy supply and concentration ability, he accelerates his body movements, initially squirming and later flailing his arms and legs about, extending his fingers and toes and twisting his torso. The acceleration of random, uncontrolled movements adds sensory input, driving the infant toward sensory overload.
- *Peak of Excitement.* The input from attentiveness and aggressive movements surges toward the infant's threshold, the level at which no more input can be tolerated without jeopardizing his physiological status or behavioral balance. The only alternative left for this infant is withdrawal if sensory enrichment continues rather than subsiding.
- *Withdrawal.* The infant attempts to shut out the sensory stimuli, to get away from it by turning his head away, averting his gaze, drowning out the sounds with his own wailing, or physically distancing himself from the source. It is often best to allow the infant to console himself rather than adding to the sensory input with active consoling (cooing, rubbing, talking) by the mother.
- *Refractory.* This is a period of recovery that varies in duration for each infant but is generally 10 to 20 seconds long. The infant needs some time to regroup his resources and organize himself for another interaction. He will stop his crying, slow his movements, regain his posture and flaccid expression, and eventually become alert as he gains control over his autonomic functions, motor movements, state of alertness, and interactional faculties. Sustained human presence accompanied by silence will facilitate rapid recovery, making the infant available for another rhythmic interaction.

These stages should be highlighted for the parent and family members so that overstimulation can be avoided and interactions remain mutually gratifying.[28] Most mothers are relatively synchronous with their infant's rhythm within 3 months of delivery.

Reciprocity

The infant actively engages in interaction, but his ability to interact is marked by bursts and pauses. A neonate may undergo three or four cycles of attentiveness/recovery/attentiveness prior to fatiguing or reaching the point at which rest is advised. If the infant is still fascinated by his eye contact with mother, then mother can be reciprocal to the infant by maintaining her intent gaze. When the infant reaches acceleration, mother should gradually withdraw the intensity and number of stimuli involved in the interaction. Maternal responses that enable the infant to regain attentiveness and control over his movements and physiological status are reciprocal behaviors. Reciprocity with the infant is to be reinforced whenever observed.[29]

Habituation

Habituation is the progressive decrease in response by an organism when repeatedly stimulated. Although this is a rudimentary form of learning and indicates intact central nervous system function,[30] it is also a potent indicator of the infant's waning interest or ability to attend. Each time an infant is shown the same picture, the intensity and extensiveness of his response decrease, undergoing diminution until the response is entirely extinguished. If one is timing the neonate's attention span for a stimulus, when the attention span starts to fall off, habituation or fatigue may be coming on. Habituation is very individual and may even vary within each infant depending upon his interest and state.[31]

Fatigue

Fatigue as a result of sensory enrichment can be successfully prevented when its signs are recognized early. The infant will signal that he is tiring and cannot engage in further interaction. Sagging cheeks, closing eyelids, drooping chin, limp extremities, and yawning are all signs of fatigue that can accompany sensory overload. Mother should modify the sensory components of the environment accordingly and permit the infant some quiet time.

Engagement/Disengagement Cues

Eye-to-eye contact is a potent nonverbal communication between infant and parent, one that acknowledges the existence of the other person and conveys a sense of worth to the person. As long as the infant gazes, his mother pays attention to him and a dialogue of eye movements, facial twitches, and sound emissions transpires. This cascade of interactions effectively keeps both parent and infant engaged, learning about each other's likes, dislikes, and needs. An infant who smiles receives attention in the form of a smiling face, a gentle rock, cooing noises, and engulfing arms. This infant eventually learns that smiles result in many pleasing sensory experiences. These behaviors are known as *cues*, little segments of nonverbal or verbal communication designed to influence the environment to which the infant is exposed, creating an interaction between infant, caregivers, and environment. Infants use engagement cues to initiate and sustain interactions and disengagement cues to detach from interactions. Examples of subtle disengagement cues are lip compression or grimace, pucker face, eyes clinched, gaze aversion, tongue show, and immobility. Examples of potent disengagement cues are crying, whining, fussing, spitting, vomiting, and pushing away.[32] The disengagement cues are activated when an infant is reaching his sensory threshold or desires to withdraw from sensory stimulation. Each of these behaviors, when considered singly, may not indicate a need for disengagement, but when followed or accompanied by others, the message should be clear.

Sensory interactions need to be gradually withdrawn if overstimulation is to be avoided. Enraptured mothers who desire to engage the infant may not recognize the disengagement cues. Astute observation and gentle comment can improve a mother's sensitivity to her infant's communication. Two easily identified signs of disengagement are a furrowed brow and tightly fisted hands that may or may not be in the mouth.

Using these signals, the infant is a socially competent individual.[33] Interactions with people and objects refine his competency and enable him to seek out pleasing experiences, shut out unpleasant ones, and keep people fascinated with him while he is dependent upon them for his physical, cognitive, and emotional growth.

Overstimulation

Babies can be overstimulated. It is important that the nurse use her keen observation skills to identify behaviors before this physiological, attentive, and behavioral compromise occurs. Distress, crying, skin color change, sudden dramatic alteration in respiratory or cardiac rates, flaccid extremities, arching of the head, neck, and back, tongue thrusting, and a painful expression of the infant's face are all signs heralding the onset of overstimulation. If these signs fail to convey the message, the infant may be forced to close his eyes and drop off to sleep to shut out the relentless bombardment of his senses. This bombardment commonly occurs during medical procedures, nursing and medical rounds, and physical examinations.

Nursing Diagnosis

Based upon the foregoing, several nursing diagnoses are possible. The most common one encountered in sensory enrichment nursing practice is that of the parents' and grandparents' knowledge deficit. The science of infancy has expanded so greatly in such a short time that the consumer is not always familiar with infants' sensory capabilities and the need to use these senses for learning in the first year of life. Parents require information about an infant's individual overtures and responses to interaction as well as sensory interventions. Other problems involve lack of reciprocity and potential for overstimulation. Inappropriateness of stimuli may occur if individuation of sensory enrichment does not exist. Individuation can be learned best if it is modeled by the nurse in her interactions with the infant, as well as modeled by the environment of the hospital nursery. Nursing diagnoses are stated in accepted terms in the nursing care plan at the end of the chapter.

Intervention

Each sense can be appropriately stimulated to use and expand sensory capabilities. Sensory capabilities and appropriate enrichment strategies for each modality are enumerated in the following text.

Principles Influencing Nursing Interventions

Sensory stimulation may be actively and passively provided by the environment. Active provision means that deliberate efforts to stimulate each sense are being made; passive infant stimulation occurs spontaneously without conscious intent. Fortunately, caregivers offer a plethora of passive stimulation, ensuring infant development within the normal range. Most of the unconscious sensory stimulation occurs during changing and feeding.[34] These instinctual presentations of sensory stimuli are to be encouraged if they are in accordance with the principles of sensory enrichment.

Briefly, these principles are as follows:

1. All newborns have right-sided preferences during the first 3 months. The infant's right side is more sensitive to touch than his left, the right side conducts messages to the brain faster than the left, and infants turn their heads to the right more reliably than to the left. Stimulating experiences encourage more infant attention if they are begun on the infant's right side, regardless of the infant's eventual handedness.

2. If newborn attention or concentration is desired, it is best to present the stimulus during periods of alert inactivity, when the infant is awake with his eyes open, but his legs and arms are still. During this restive phase the newborn can attend to and track with ease and sustained interest. The alert inactive state characterizes the infant for an hour or two immediately after birth and for 5 to 10 minutes before and after feedings.

3. Newborns become alert for longer periods if they are in upright positions and being held. Sitting in this manner increases infant gazing by 70%. When an infant looks around he receives visual stimulation, which helps him learn how to relate to his environment.

4. Stimulating an infant to the point of agitation may not be wise, since agitation causes increased heart rate, increased respiratory rate, and prolonged inspiratory phases, which can induce aspiration. Some types of sensory stimulation will agitate

some infants and please others. Each infant should be the guide, and his particular rhythm and readiness for stimulation, as manifested by engagement cues, should be respected.

Once these principles are used to guide nursing interventions, administration of sensory enrichment will be beneficial to the infant. Since the nurse cannot provide continuity of enrichment once the infant goes home, it is vital that the mother be exposed to sensory enrichment techniques and given opportunities to practice them.

Visual Interventions

Visual Capabilities. The normal newborn has very good visual abilities. At 9 minutes of life, infants can turn their eyes and head significantly to follow schematic (black-and-white) faces.[35] An infant can see items with great clarity as long as they are within his visual field, which is 20 cm to 22 cm (9 in–12 in), the same distance from the breast-feeding infant's eyes to his mother's eyes.[15] Within this visual field, he can see items distinctly (known as acuity), without blurriness, and can search the field to 30° either side of midline before deciding the item of preference upon which to gaze.[36] Gazing can be deliberately prolonged, depending upon the amount of interest an item holds for the infant. Newborns have individual preferences and differences, so it is necessary to allow for variation.

Visual Strategies. The newborn prefers visual items that provide contrast between figure and background.[16] The greatest contrast occurs when black is placed against a white background. The newborn loves faces, especially eyes. Until he realizes they are not the real thing, two big black dots on a white background will appeal to him.

Moving objects are more fascinating to an infant than are stationary ones, and newborns prefer to maintain their gaze (fixate) on circular items because of their immature ocular movement ability.[37]

The newborn searches the visual field by moving across it with little jumps (saccades) rather than rolling both eyes simultaneously in the same direction. Eye-to-eye contact in the face-to-face position facilitates eye fixation for both parent and infant. If the mother's or the father's face is not available, black-and-white schematic faces or black-and-white glossy photos are the next best thing.

Infants also like to look at geometric figures, and they prefer cylinders and circles to rectangles and squares.[38] The geometric figures should be sharp rather than blurry and in a black-and-white configuration to

CLIENT EDUCATION

What Your Infant Likes to Look At in the First Month of Life

AGE	STIMULATOR (Held 10 in–13 in from baby's face)
Newborn to 2 weeks	• Your animated face, smiling and talking • Your eyes • The breast as he nurses • Simple black-and-white drawing of your smiling face on a paper plate • Black stripes (8 inches long by 2 inches high) pasted or drawn on white 8 × 11 cardboard background • A 4-square black-and-white checkerboard, each square 3 × 3 inches • One black dot, 3 inches in diameter, pasted on white 8 × 11 background
2 to 4 weeks	Add (held 10 in–13 in from baby's face): • Simple bold drawing of two round faces, each at least 6 inches in diameter—one male and one female—done in heavy black ink on white 11 × 14 background • A 4- to 6-square checkerboard, each square 2½ × 2½ inches • Black or red stripes (3 inches long by 1½ inches high) pasted or drawn on white 8 × 11 cardboard background or crocheted • Two black dots, 3 inches in diameter, pasted or drawn on 8 × 11 white background • Simple black-and-white bull's eye: one 3-inch black dot in the center, surrounded by a 2-inch white band and a 1-inch black outline at the edge drawn on a paper plate • Simple two-dimensional mobile made from 4 dessert-size paper plates with drawings of stripes, 4-square checkerboard, a black dot, and a simple bull's-eye, hung so that the plates face down 10 to 13 inches from baby's eyes • Simple drawing of face on paper plate glued onto Popsicle stick (Popsicle face)

Ludington-Hoe SM, Golant S: How to Have a Smarter Baby. New York, Rawson Associates, © 1985

enthrall the newborn. Newborns do not like to look at plain-colored walls or walls with little figures on them. Animals and cartoon characters are inappropriate visual stimuli for the full-term newborn. These patterns are not appreciated until the infant is more than 1 year of age. In the first 6 months of life, infants prefer to look at big geometric figures (2 × 2 in) rather than small ones (½ × ½ in).[39] After the first 3 weeks of life, the size of the geometric figures can be decreased to accommodate the newborn's preference for increasing complexity and visual information processing. Stripes (especially good for the first 3 wk–4 wk of life), black-and-white checkerboards, bull's-eyes, dots, and triangles are appealing geometric shapes. Cards containing these items can be used separately as stimuli or used in mobiles and crib hangings. Black-and-white geometric-shaped mobiles may be made from other materials also (Fig. 34-2).

Auditory Interventions

Auditory Capabilities. The newborn has the capacity to hear all sounds greater than 55 decibels,[40] with slightly higher sensitivity to the lower frequencies. This sensitivity may be a reflection of the smaller degree of attenuation of low-frequency sounds during transmission through the amniotic sac. Immediately after birth, infants may alert to their father's voice more readily than to their mother's for this reason. The infant can learn to discriminate his mother's and father's voices from all others within the first 2 weeks of life and has at that time a distinct reaction pattern established to the voice he hears.

Speech Strategies. Although slightly more sensitive to the low-frequency male voice, newborn behavior

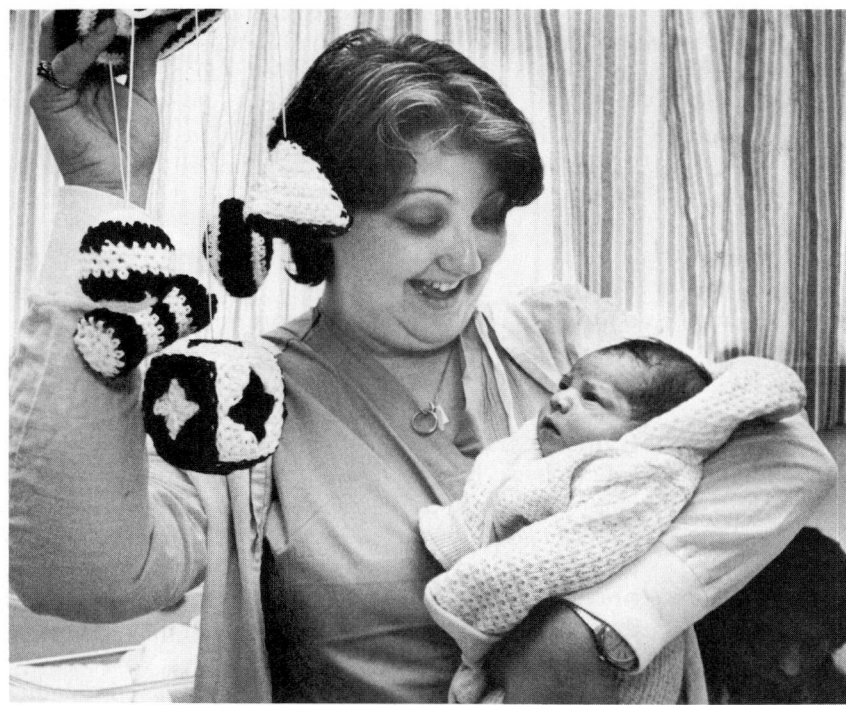

suggests a preference for the female voice. The gleeful response to the female voice is based primarily on the pitch, tone, and inflection pattern women demonstrate when speaking to infants. Women tend to exhibit cooing behaviors, which are various-pitched musical sounds. Instinctual maternal speech uses exaggerated intonation. Higher-pitched sounds are attention-getting sounds, while low, bass sounds are consoling and quieting. Monotonous speech and monotone sounds are boring to the newborn, who prefers modulating auditory input.[41] The infant accustoms to monotone quickly and does not attend to it. Some fathers have a tendency to speak in bass, monotone speech patterns and should be encouraged to use more inflection and exaggerated tone. Slow speech, 55 words per minute or less, is easier for the infant to discern than faster speech.[42]

Talking to an infant is very important. The more speech he hears, the sooner he will learn language. The more speech he is exposed to, the more likely he is to reach his potential for mental skills. Gorski and coworkers have suggested that maternal speech is the single most important aspect of the newborn's sensory environment, and desirable maternal speech can ameliorate anticipated delays and handicaps in risk infants.[43]

Talking in a face-to-face orientation is especially important. This position conveys nonverbal cues and facial expressions that relate emotion to the infant.[3]

Sound Strategies. Speech stimulates the development of the left hemisphere of the brain; music stimulates the right hemisphere.[42] Therefore, parents may provide musical stimulation for their infant also. Newborns have demonstrated less agitation in the presence of classical music than rock and roll music.[44] However, individual preference may very well be for the music the neonate was exposed to while *in utero*. If mother played jazz during her pregnancy, her newborn will probably enjoy jazz more than unfamiliar classical music. Mothers have much latitude in choice of music, but true, pure tones are preferred to synthesized music.

Tactile Interventions

Tactile Capabilities. The skin is the largest sense organ in the infant. Infants are very sensitive to touch, especially around the mouth, in the palms, over the soles of the feet, and around the genitals. Tactile stimulation, or touching, is instrumental in helping the neonate adjust to life outside the womb. Skin-to-skin touch in a rhythmic, stroking pattern has been found to reduce the birth weight loss from 10% of birth weight to 3% of birth weight.[45] This is accomplished because skin-to-skin stroking stimulates the haptic nerve pathways, which in turn stimulate gastrointestinal and genitourinary system function. As a result, feces and urine are passed through the system more quickly and with better utilization of digested food.[46]

Tactile Strategies. Skin-to-skin touch is to be encouraged at all times. Newborns cannot be spoiled by too much caressing. The closer they are held and the more often they are patted, the more secure they become. Observe the power of touch on the newborn: it can make him either quiescent or aroused. Reassuring parental touch makes crying subside, extremities flex, and the eyes open—if he doesn't fall asleep.

It is wise to provide skin-to-skin stroking in a head-to-toe fashion. Nerve myelinization occurs in this sequence, and touch may positively influence the process if it is provided in a similar direction. Stroking in this manner, at a rate of 12 to 16 times per minute, may decrease the incidence of apnea and encourage even, regular respirations in the neonate.[47] As one strokes, it is wise to give extra strokes of slightly more pressure to the most sensitive tactile areas, outlined above. Stroking that is begun on the right should continue on the infant's left, to encourage midline awareness.[48] Stroking the head is very comforting to the neonate, especially if the hand proceeds from the forehead to the occiput. Slow repetitive strokes over the top of the head can calm a colicky infant, as do finger strokes across the forehead.

Many infants become quite fond of stroking and never tire of it. For these infants it becomes a relaxation technique and is widely used as such in Australia and India. Touch is believed to help relieve the unspent tensions infants accumulate throughout the day, as well as accelerate neuromuscular development.[48] Two tools are available for mothers who desire to continue with a stroking treatment. *Loving Hands* by Frederick Leboyer has many pictures and is found in most bookstores. A scientifically validated stroking protocol called "Loving Touch," which is accompanied by a tape that contains appropriate music stimulation, is also available.*

Many mothers collect swatches of different textures with which to stroke the infant. These tactile experiences will be especially valuable if the texture is experienced within context (*e.g.,* fur on a panda bear, rough on daddy's face, smooth on the mirror, etc). Caution should be exercised so that the infant is not assaulted by multiple sensations.

Vestibular Interventions

Vestibular Capabilities.
Vestibular stimulation refers to movement, and the term is derived from the vestibule of the ear, which perceives alterations in fluid pressure as movement occurs. Movement stimulation begins *in utero* as the fetus moves about in weightless space, stretching and rotating. The sucking that originates around the eighth to 11th week of gestation is a form of movement stimulation that is necessary if the fetus's chin and buccal pads are to develop sufficiently

* Cradle Care Incorporated, 6455 Meadow Road, Dallas, Texas 75230.

for suckling. All babies exhibit individual patterns of spontaneous activity, some quite active and others calm. Activity patterns may be an early index of a child's temperament, but we are not yet able to say with any significance what active babies will be like when they are older.[49] Movement stimulation, especially rotary movements, has been associated with enhanced motor development.[50]

Vestibular Strategies.
Following delivery, it is important for infants to have opportunities to move about and stretch and pull and push. These activities are best facilitated by "tummy time," being placed on the tummy in a safe place for self-initiated, unstructured movement. If infants are accustomed to always sleeping on their side or back, tummy time may be upsetting. Having a parent on the floor, in a face-to-face orientation, may alleviate some of the stress of this new position. It is important to try to get a baby to enjoy this position, since the freedom of movement afforded by it enables the child to crawl within normal time limits rather than significantly later.[51]

Rocking is the most common vestibular stimulation that is passively given, providing excellent opportunities for vestibular sensations that aid in weight gain[52] and neuromuscular coordination. There is no recommended rate of rocking or frequency, but a little each day can be encouraged. Parents may prefer to provide vestibular stimulation by carrying infants in chest wraps. No detrimental effects have resulted from this. In fact, infants who accompany their mother in a pouch appear to fall into deep levels of sleep more smoothly and awaken less irritable.[53]

Baby exercises provide opportunities for vestibular stimulation. Extension and flexion of all extremities followed by tummy tickles, pressure against the kicking foot, circular swinging of the well-supported infant, and relaxation techniques are possibilities. Levy's book is a useful resource for additional motor games.[54]

Olfactory Interventions

Olfactory Capabilities.
Olfaction in the newborn is quite sensitive. Shortly after birth, newborns will change their breathing and activity rates in response to strong artificial odors.[55] At 5 days of age the infant can differentiate the odor of his mother's breast pad from that of a stranger. If mother's nipples have been smeared with petroleum jelly, the neonate will violently refuse approaching the noxiously scented nipple. This ability to perceive maternal odor originates at birth, when the infant is held close. By 2 weeks of age, infants are able to recognize their mother's axillary odors.[56] At this time

his olfactory sensitivity is instrumental to the bonding/parental recognition process and emotional development in infants.[57] The importance of olfactory markers for emotional development is revealed when one considers that olfaction is the only sense that is not mediated by the reticular activating system, going instead *directly* to the limbic center of the brain. The limbic center is the seat of emotions.

Olfactory Strategies. The most potent stimulus is breast milk, followed only by the body scents of both parents. Actively providing various smells such as cherry juice, nutmeg, cinnamon, and honey is not really necessary, but may be enjoyable. The newborn detects these scents when in the kitchen environment without special attention to them for the first 6 months of life. After that, smelling can become a stimulating game. Various "scratch and sniff" books are available in toy stores.

Gustatory Interventions

Gustatory Capabilities. The fetus demonstrates a preference for sweet fluids as early as 20 weeks' gestation. When glucose water is injected into the amniotic fluid, the fetus accelerates his swallowing actions. This preference would not be manifested if gustatory sensitivity were not possible. It is known that the nerve tracts for taste sensation are operational by the 20th week of gestation and that the entire oral cavity is covered with taste receptors during gestation. Just prior to birth, some of these receptors are lost, leaving the tongue as the only source for taste sensitivity.

Gustatory Strategies. The most prevalent taste sensation the newborn is exposed to is breast milk (or formula). As the nipple is compressed against the hard palate, the milk spurts onto the bitter receptors in the back of the tongue. With repetitive stimulation of the bitter receptors, the infant grows quite fond of the bitter-tasting foods. Yet they always like sweet tastes as well and can smile with sweet and frown with sour tastes. Breast milk is the preferred gustatory stimulus for newborns. Mothers should be encouraged to avoid sour tastes that might pass into breast milk (*e.g.*, lemon juice,

cranberry juice) so that the newborn does not associate his caregiver with unpleasant stimuli.

Evaluation

The goal of sensory enrichment is a happy, secure, well-rounded infant, one who is loved by his caregivers and lives in a reciprocal environment. The first signs of goal achievement may be visible prior to discharge, but final evaluation is many months, maybe even years, down the road.

Resources for Sensory Enrichment

Family-centered maternity care recommends involvement of all family members in the care of the newborn. Siblings are eager to make simple designs to show to the newcomer, and fathers can set aside 5 minutes per day of special time with the infant to help develop a positive father–infant relationship. All nursing interventions (except breast-feeding) are suitable for the infant's various caregivers, so grandparents should be allowed an opportunity to demonstrate their sensory enrichment skills too.

As parents become involved with their amazing newborn, additional knowledge and support services may be sought. In addition to numerous consumer publications (a list is available from the Infant Stimulation Education Association [ISEA]* and the Center for Parent Education†), infant stimulation classes and support groups are conducted around the nation by certified infant stimulation instructors (a directory is maintained by ISEA). Many educational materials, such as videotapes, films, and care plans and posters, are available to health professionals and parents through the national clearing house for infant sensory enrichment, the ISEA.

* Infant Stimulation Education Association, % Dr. S. Ludington, School of Nursing, UCLA Center for Health Sciences, Factor 5-942, Los Angeles, CA 90024. Phone (213) 206-1038.
† Center for Parent Education, 55 Chapel Street, Newton, MA 02150. Phone (617) 964-2442.

(*text continued on page 691*)

The Parents and Infant Participating in Sensory Interactions

Nursing Objectives	
	1. Instruct parents concerning infant's capabilities, individual sensitivity to enrichment, and individual preferences in each sensory modality.
	2. Identify and, when appropriate, reinforce positively each woman's spontaneously occurring sensory enrichment activities.
	3. Explain the newborn's signs of attention to and detachments from sensory activities and indicate when observed.
	4. Identify and correct overstimulation signs immediately.

Assessment	Potential Nursing Diagnosis	Intervention	Evaluation
Parental Assessment Factors			
Visual			
Eye-to-eye contact between mother and infant within 10–13 inches of infant's face	Knowledge deficit of infant stimulation strategies	Provide education on the potency of eye-to-eye contact and depth of newborn's visual field	Mother and infant maintain short-duration eye-to-eye contact
Face-to-face experiences with infant	Diversional activity deficit related to inappropriate stimuli or lack of individuation	Provide education on the appeal of human face to the infant	Parents aware of allure of the human face
	Alteration in parenting (bonding) related to separation of high-risk newborn and parents	Demonstrate attentiveness on infant's part to motionless, noiseless face and then to animated face	Parent repeats demonstration
	Noncompliance to sensory enrichment related to disinterest, misinformation		
Experiences with visual targets		Provide opportunities for infant to visually search high-contrast geometric shapes	Parent observes the appeal of such items
Auditory			
Inflected, modulating tone of parent used with attentive infant in face-to-face vocalizations		Demonstrate pleasing, higher-pitched vocalizations with alert, attentive infant	Infant is attentive
		Provide education on the type of tone that appeals	Mother uses appealing tone of voice
Soothing cooing or humming with agitated infant		Provide education on individual infant's response to auditory enrichment when upset	Mother uses soothing approach
		Provide parent with a repertoire of auditory approaches to soothe agitated infant	
Little or no conversation with newborn during early breast-feeding experiences		Provide education about the fascination of human voice and its supremacy over breast-feeding for an infant who is still learning how to breast-feed	Mother allows infant to breast-feed
Speech and music (humming, singing) or other nonspeech sounds are provided		Provide education on benefits of speech and nonspeech sounds	Mother initiates mother–infant dialogue

(continued)

Assessment	Potential Nursing Diagnosis	Intervention	Evaluation
Tactile			
Skin-to-skin contact between parent and infant is allowed		Provide education on human need for touch and special need for parental touch	Mother sees positive signs in infant in response to touch
		Provide skin-to-skin opportunities for both parents in a warm room	Mother expresses infant individuality that she sees
Quality of touch		Demonstrate firm, gentle touch for parents on their skin; allow return demonstration on infant's skin	Parent comments upon infant's signs of pleasure or sensitivity to the type of touch experienced
		Encourage rhythmic, short stroking	Parent uses short, rhythmic strokes
Parents' holding patterns		Demonstrate swaddling of an infant who is flailing about	Parent holds infant securely, swaddling or embracing him as determined by infant's cues
Observe use of pacifiers and nonnutritive sucking		Provide education on importance of sucking and hand–mouth activity for self-consolation and self-control	Parent encourages/permits hand-to-mouth activity and sucking
Vestibular			
Observe linear movement		Provide education on role of movement in motor development and proprioception	Parents provide linear movement of infant by lifting/lowering and walking with infant
Observe for violent, sudden, or accentuated movements of infant that cause exaggerated, independent head movement		Provide education on need to keep head from swinging about, which throws the brain against a hard, potentially bruising cranium	Parents hold infant securely and maintain head alignment
Gustatory			
Provision of breast milk or formula to satiety		Provide appropriate supervision and support of chosen feeding method	Mother expresses satisfaction with feeding experience
Olfactory			
Opportunities for close skin contact with parents are provided		Provide education on the influence of olfactory markers of the parent on helping an infant learn to whom he belongs	Parents are aware of reaction of infant to their olfactory markers
Infant Assessment Factors			
Signs of Attention	Knowledge deficit of infant attention signs related to lack of experience in interaction	Provide education on differentiating alertness from attentiveness; on importance of frequent, short-duration enrichment episodes rather than infrequent, long-duration epi-	Parents determine length of infant's attentiveness
Face brightens			
Pupils dilate			
Head orients toward stimulus	Sensory perceptual alteration related to separation of newborn and parents		

(continued)

Assessment	Potential Nursing Diagnosis	Intervention	Evaluation
Arm and leg movements cease Sucking rate decreases Heart rate decreases Respiratory rate decreases		sodes; and that length and quality of attentiveness will increase as the infant matures	
Signs of Fatigue Yawning Eyes closing, drooping Cheeks sagging Chin dropping Extremities limp Body collapses, doubles over	Activity intolerance related to overstimulation	Provide education for early recognition of fatigue	Parents can read the infant cues
Interaction Pattern* Initiation—orientation—attention—acceleration—peak of excitement—withdrawal—recovery—reorganization		Provide education on each infant's ability to create and alter his own pattern Point out infant's behaviors and pattern during a social interaction; reinforce parent's ability to recognize infant's cues	Parents reciprocate to the infant's pattern
Engagement Behaviors Alerting, eyes opening Hands opening Head raising Babbling, cooing, clicking, giggling noises Smiling Mutual gazing Cyclic movements of the extremities	Knowledge deficit of engagement behaviors related to lack of experience in interaction	Provide education on their infant's engagement behaviors; supervise an enrichment interaction, verbally acknowledging each behavior as it is observed	Parents verbally acknowledge these behaviors when they appear
Disengagement Behaviors Arching Fussing Crying Head turning away Gaze shifting Head shaking Arms and legs flailing Fingers extending Facial grimacing Facial swiping Hands clasping each other Hands in prayer position	Knowledge deficit of disengagement behaviors related to lack of experience in interaction	Provide education of these cues that convey the idea that it is time to slow down and cease the interaction Verbally identify the behaviors when demonstrated by the infant Provide education on the importance of acknowledging these behaviors and acting accordingly	Parents able to read their infant's cues and respond appropriately

* This paradigm is explained by Ludington-Hoe (1977) and derived from Brazelton TB: Early Infant Reciprocity. In Vaughan VC, Brazelton TB (eds): The Family—Can It Be Saved?, pp 133–142. Chicago, Year Book Medical Publishers, 1975

References

1. Segal J, Segal Z: The infant: Ready and able to learn. Children Today 19–22, April 1985
2. Zabielski MT, Guring T: Giving and receiving in the neomaternal period: A case of distributive inequity. MCN 13:19–45, 1984
3. Tronick E, Als H, Brazelton TB: Monadic phases: A structural descriptive analysis of infant–mother face-to-face interaction. Merrill-Palmer Quarterly 26:3–24, 1980
4. Trevarthen C: Communication and cooperation in early infancy: A description of primary inter-subjectivity. In Bullowa M (ed): Before Speech: The Beginnings of Interpersonal Communication. New York, Cambridge University Press, 1979
5. Belsky J: Experimenting with the family in the newborn period. Child Dev 56:407–414, April 1985
6. Magnusson D, Allen VL: An interactional perspective for human development. In Magnusson D, Allen VL (eds): Human Development: An Interactional Perspective, pp 3–27. New York, Academic Press, 1983
7. Parmelee AH, Beckwith L, Cohen SE et al: Early intervention and experience with preterm infants. In Brazelton TB, Lester BM (eds): New Approaches to Developmental Screening of Infants, pp 77–85. New York, Elsevier, 1983
8. Barnard KE, Bee HL, Hammond MA: Development changes in maternal interactions with term and preterm infants. Infant Behav Dev 7:101–113, 1984
9. Fineman JB, Boris M: Outcome of early intervention: A summary of an on-going follow-up study. In Call JD, Galenson E, Tyson RL (eds): Frontiers of Infant Psychiatry, pp 231–234. New York, Basic Books, 1983
10. Barnard K, Eyres S, Lobo M et al: An ecological paradigm for assessment and intervention. In Brazelton TB, Lester BM (eds): New Approaches to Developmental Screening of Infants, pp 199–218. New York, Elsevier, 1983
11. Brazelton TB: Early intervention: What does it mean? In Fitzgerald HE, Lester BM, Yogman MW (eds): Theory and Research in Behavioral Pediatrics, pp 1–15. New York, Plenum Press, 1984
12. Crnic LS: Effects of nutrition and environment on brain biochemistry and behavior. Dev Psychol 16(32):129–145, 1983
13. Ferry PC: On growing new neurons: Are early intervention programs effective? Pediatrics 67:38–44, 1981
14. Diamond M: Cortical change in response to environmental enrichment and impoverishment. In Brown CC (ed): The Many Facets of Touch, pp 22–28. New Brunswick, NJ, Johnson & Johnson, Roundtable No. 10, 1984
15. Ludington-Hoe SM: What can newborns really see? Am J Nurs 1286–1289, September 1983
16. Apostolakis E, Cha C: Visual preference of preterm and term neonates. J Calif Perinatal Assoc 11(1):62, May 1982
17. Ludington-Hoe SM, Golant S: How to Have a Smarter Baby. New York, Rawson Associates, 1985
18. Gluck L: The cutting edge. Calif J Perinatol 50–55, Fall 1983
19. Brazelton TB: Behavioral competence of the newborn infant. In Avery GB (ed): Neonatology: Pathophysiology and Management of the Newborn, 3rd ed. Philadelphia, JB Lippincott, 1986
20. White B: Missouri's new parents as teachers project: Report on the final evaluation. Center for Parent Education Newsletter 7(6):1–5, 1985
21. Derevensky JL, Wasser-Kastner E: The Effects of an interdisciplinary stimulation-parent intervention program upon infant development. Infant Mental Health J 5(1):3–13, 1984
22. Koniak DK, Ludington-Hoe SM: Effects of multisensory stimulation upon full-term infant development. Presented at the International Conference of Infant Studies, Beverly Hills, California, April 11–13, 1986
23. Touwen BCL: The preterm infant in the extrauterine environment: Implications for neurology. Early Hum Dev 4(3):287–300, 1980
24. Barnard KE, Bee HL, Hammond MH: Home environment and cognitive development in a healthy low-risk sample: The Seattle study. In Gottfried AW (ed): Home Environment and Early Cognitive Development, pp 117–147. New York, Academic Press, 1984
25. Brazelton TB: Do you really want a super baby? Family Circle, pp 74, 76, 77, December 1985
26. Zigler E, Lang ME: The emergence of "super baby": A good thing? Ped Nurs 11:337–340, 1985
27. Adamson LB, Baheman R: Affect and attention: Infants observed with mothers and peers. Child Dev 56(3):582–593, 1985
28. Springer LW, Boyce WT, Gaines JA: Family–infant congruence: Routines and rhythmicity in family adaptations to a young infant. Child Dev 56(3):564–572, 1985
29. Anderson JC: Enhancing reciprocity between mother and neonate. Nurs Res 30(2):89–93, 1981
30. Bornstein MH, Benasich AA: Infant habituation: Assessments of individual differences and short term reliability at five months. Child Dev 57(3):1–10, 1986
31. Power TG, Hildebrandt KA, Fitzgerald HE: Adults' responses to infants varying in facial expression and perceived attractiveness. Infant Behav Dev 5:33–44, 1982
32. Barnard K: NCAST Learning Resource Manual, pp 50–59. Seattle, University of Washington, 1979
33. Temeles MS: The infant: A socially competent individual. In Call JD, Gelenson E, Tyson RL (eds): Frontiers of Infant Psychiatry, pp 178–187. New York, Basic Books, 1983
34. Day S: Mother-infant activities as providers of sensory stimulation. Am J Occup Ther 36(9):579–585, 1982
35. Goren CG, Sarty M, Wu PYK: Visual following and preterm discrimination of facelike stimuli by newborn infants. Pediatrics 56:544–549, 1976
36. Maurer D, Maurer C: Newborn babies see better than you think. Psychology Today, pp 85–88, October 1976
37. Haith MM: The response of the human newborn to movement. J Exp Child Psychol 31:235–243, 1980
38. Fantz RL, Miranda SB: Newborn infant attention to contour. Child Dev 46:224, 1975
39. Fantz RL, Fagan JF: Visual attention to size and number

of pattern details during the first 6 months. Child Dev 46(1):3–18, 1975

40. Dunkle T: The sound of silence. Science 82, pp 48–51, April 1982
41. Eimas PD: The perception of speech in early infancy. Sci Am 25(2):46–52, 1985
42. Morse PA: The discrimination of speech and non-speech stimuli in early infancy. J Exp Child Psychol 14: 477–492, 1972
43. Gorski PA, Davison MF, Brazelton TB: Neurobehavioral organization of the high risk neonate. Semin Perinatol 3(1):61–72, 1979
44. Klaus MM, Fanaroff AA: Bach, Beethoven, or rock—and how much. J Pediatr 88:300, 1976
45. Ludington SM: Vaginal and Cesarean Infants' Responses to Extra Tactile Stimulation, Ph.D. dissertation, p 74, Texas Woman's University, 1976
46. Rausch P: Effects of tactile and kinesthetic stimulation on premature infants. JOGN Nurs 10:34–40, 1981
47. Kattwinkel T et al: Apnea of prematurity and effects on CPAP, cutaneous stimulation and levels of urinary biogenic amines. Pediatr Res 8:468, April 1974
48. Rice RD: The effects of sensorimotor infant stimulation treatment on the development of high risk infants. Birth Defects 15:7–26, 1979
49. Korner AF: Individual differences in neonatal activity. In Call JD, Galenson E, Tyson RL (eds): Frontiers of Infant Psychiatry, pp 379–387. New York, Basic Books, 1983
50. Ottenbacher KJ, Petersen P: The efficacy of vestibular stimulation as a form of specific sensory enrichment: Quantitative review of the literature. Clin Pediatr 23(8): 428–433, 1983
51. Menzies A: Effect of infant temperament and prone position on motor development. Aust J Adv Nurs 2(1):24–29, 1981
52. Frieman DG et al: Effects of kinesthetic stimulation on weight gain and on smiling in premature infants. Paper read at the annual meeting of the American Orthopsychiatric Association, San Francisco, April 15, 1979
53. Kennell JH, Klaus MH: Early events: Later effects on the infant. In Call JD, Galenson E, Tyson RL: Frontiers of Infant Psychiatry, pp 7–16. New York, Basic Books, 1983
54. Levy J: The Baby Exercise Book. New York, Pantheon Books, 1975
55. Engen T: The Perception of Odors. New York, Academic Press, 1982
56. Cernoch JM, Porter RH: Recognition of maternal axillary odors by infants. Child Dev 56:1593–1598, 1985
57. Porter RH, Cernoch JM, Perry S: The importance of odors in mother-infant interactions. Matern Child Nurs J 12(3):147–154, 1983

Brazelton TB: Introduction: Many Facets of Touch, p vii. Skillman, New Jersey, Johnson & Johnson, Roundtable No. 10, 1984
Burns KA, Hatcher RP: Developmental intervention with preterm infants. In Burn WJ, Lavigne JV (eds): Progress in Pediatric Psychology, pp 47–78. New York, Grune & Stratton, 1984
Donate-Bartfield E, Passman RH: Attentiveness of mothers and fathers to their baby's cries. Infant Behav Dev 8: 385–393, 1985
Frye D, Rawling P, Moore C et al: Object-person discrimination and communication at 3 to 10 months. Dev Psychol 19(3):383–389, 1983
Lester BM, Hoffman J, Brazelton TB: The rhythmic structure of mother-infant interaction in term and preterm infants. Child Dev 56:15–27, 1985
Yogman MW: Development of the father-infant relationship. In Fitzgerald HE, Lester BM, Yogman MW (eds): Theory and Research in Behavioral Pediatrics, pp 221–280. New York, Plenum Press, 1984

Suggested Reading

Aslin RN, Pisoni DB, Jasczyk PW: Auditory development and speech perception in infancy. Hearing 20:573–670, October 23, 1985

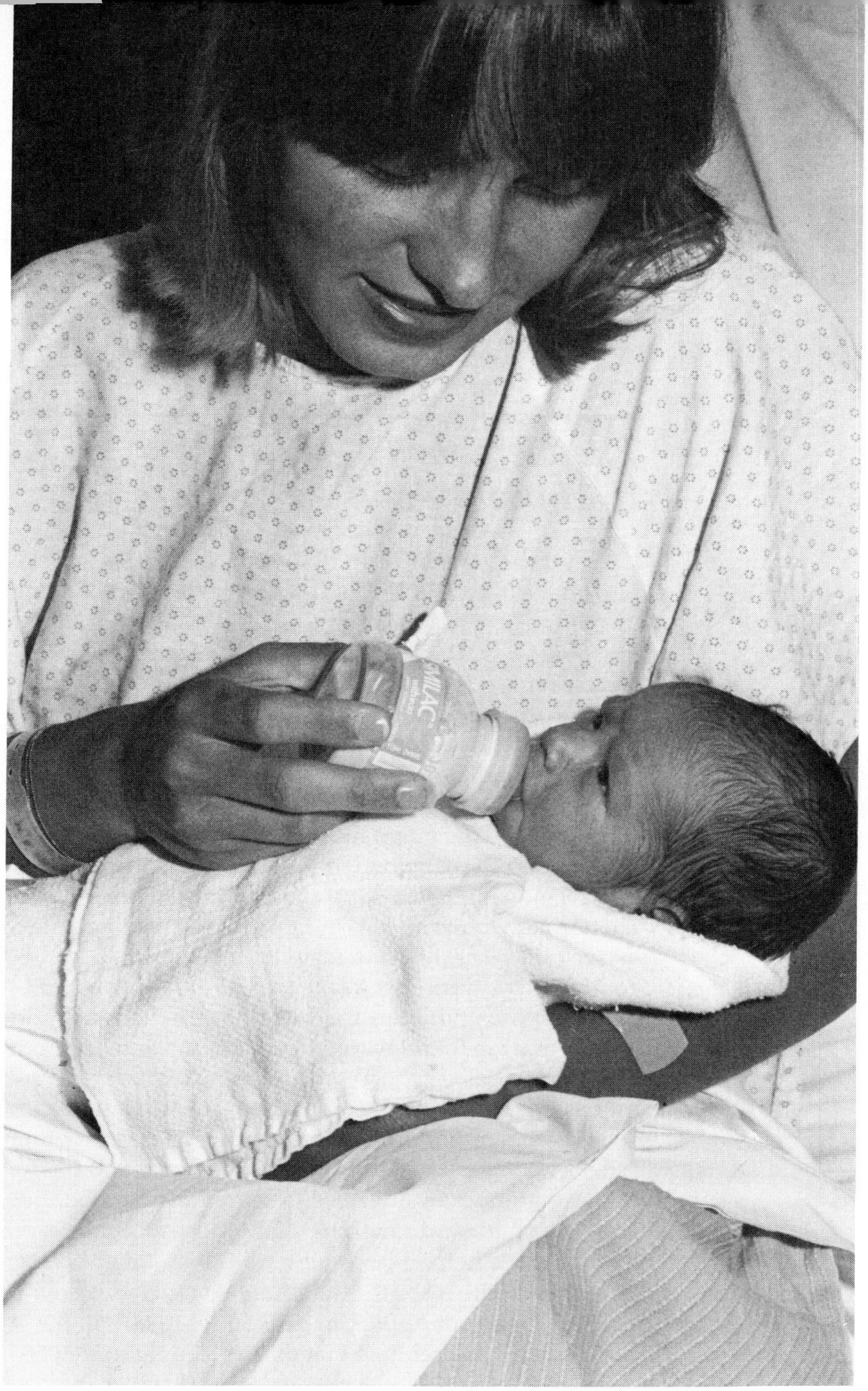

CHAPTER 35

Nutritional Care of the Infant

Nutrition is very important in preserving health throughout the life cycle. It is particularly important during the rapid growth phase of infancy. The long-term effects of feeding practices in early infancy are gaining increased recognition. According to Neumann and Jelliffe, infant feeding is more than just "nutrient refueling"; it is also a "social, psychological and educational interaction between caretaker and baby."[1]

The Newborn's Ability to Handle Food

Up until the time of birth, the nutritional needs of the fetus have been met through placental circulation. One of the major physiological adaptations that the infant must make in the transition from intrauterine to extrauterine life is to adjust to the change in the source of nourishment and to take food into the body orally, digest it, and assimilate it.

Following birth, the gastrointestinal tract begins abruptly to process a rather large amount of food. At the same time the infant must begin to suck and swallow as a means of taking food into the stomach. The sucking and swallowing reflexes are already present at birth and are normally quite strong. In fact, the swallowing reflex, as well as peristaltic movements in the stomach, becomes active during the last two months of fetal development, as noted in the bits of vernix caseosa and lanugo that are found with other debris in the meconium stool. In the delivery room, the infant will often swallow mucus or suck on anything that gets near his mouth.

Another important instinctive reaction is the rooting reflex, which enables the newborn to find food. The human infant does not have to search for its food, but it does turn toward anything that touches its cheeks or lips. This is a help in latching onto the bottle or breast.

At the time of birth, the infant's stomach is small, with a capacity of approximately 50 ml to 60 ml. But it can dilate considerably so that during feeding it stretches to at least three or four times its approximate capacity. It is distended not only by the amount of food taken in (*i.e.,* milk) but also by the amount of air swallowed as the infant sucks the milk or cries. In the act of crying, the infant tends to gulp in air.

The glandular structures in the gastric mucosa are present at birth, although they are shallow in comparison to those of the adult. The gastric musculature is somewhat deficient. This, plus the relatively greater length of the intestinal tract and the weakness of the abdominal musculature, which serves as a supporting structure, explains in part why considerable distention of the stomach is possible.

Studies on gastric motility have demonstrated wide individual differences in the emptying time of the stomachs of newborns. The major portion of the feeding usually leaves the stomach in less than 3 or 4 hours; however, in some instances, the emptying time is more than 8 hours. It was found also that the introduction of a second feeding before the stomach was empty caused portions of the first feeding to remain somewhat longer in the stomach than if the stomach was emptied before the next feeding was offered. Another important finding is that human milk leaves the stomach somewhat more rapidly than cow's milk, although a formula made of cow's milk that has been boiled leaves the stomach more rapidly than that which is fed without being boiled.[2]

Choosing the Method of Feeding

Choosing the method of infant feeding is an important decision for parents to make. Their ultimate choice will be influenced by a variety of factors, physical and psychological as well as social. Ideally, the subject of infant feeding will be raised during the antepartal period, thereby providing an opportunity to guide the parents in making a decision that is most suitable for them. The nurse should explore with the mother (and the father, if possible) mutual attitudes concerning this subject.

In the past, breast-feeding, by the mother or a "wet nurse," was essential for the survival of the infant. This is still true to some extent in underdeveloped countries, but in most of the world modern methods of artificial feeding have offered women an alternative. Although the production of infant formulas has become a big business and the choice of artificial feeding is now safe for the infant and convenient for the mother, there are still many advantages to breast-feeding.

One should avoid being so overzealously in favor of breast-feeding that it is forced on a reluctant mother. Those women who do not want to breast-feed their infants should not be made to feel guilty about their choice. On the other hand, the nurse should not hesitate to inform expectant parents of the differences between the various milks available (including human) and of the advantages of breast-feeding to both mother and infant (Table 35-1). Many women are uninformed about the differences in the available methods and may base their decision on how their mothers fed them or what a friend has said. For these women, information can be very useful in helping them to make a decision based on facts.

Advantages of Breast-Feeding

For many years, the saying "breast is best" has been used when talking about the relative merits of breast- or bottle-feeding. At the same time reassurances have been given that formula is also fine for babies. In the past two decades, research studies from many disciplines have focused attention on the uniqueness of human milk and other favorable aspects of breast-feeding. Though knowledge is still incomplete, certain advantages of breast-feeding can be identified.

Biochemical/Nutritional Considerations

Although literature promoting proprietary formula stresses similarities and often states that modern formula is "almost like mother's milk," in reality the constituents of cow's milk and human milk are dissimilar in almost every way except for water and lactose.[3] For example, whey protein, which accounts for more than 60% of the total protein in human milk, constitutes only 20% of cow's milk. Even when the formula has been "modified" or "humanized" by altering the protein, there are still many differences. Substances, such as zinc, that are found in approximately the same amounts in both milks may have different absorption rates. The human infant absorbs zinc more effectively from human milk because human milk has a different zinc binding factor than is found in cow's milk.[3] Formulas also have added substances such as emulsifiers, thickening agents, *p*H adjusters, and antioxidants, the effects of which are unknown and which are "not found in the original product for human infants."[3]

Another difference of unknown consequence is the rigidly consistent composition of formula compared with the variability of mother's milk. Besides the changes that occur in the progression from colostrum to mature milk, there is variation in the composition of mother's milk within each nursing period. The foremilk, which accumulates in the alveoli between nursings, has a higher concentration of lactose and whey protein (lactalbumin), while the hindmilk, which is secreted during the nursing period, is higher in fat and casein.[4] There are also differences in composition of breast milk according to the time of day of the nursing period.

Immunologic and Antiallergenic Factors

Human milk and colostrum have been found in many recent studies to be rich in defense factors, such as immunoglobulins, lactoferrin, enzymes, macrophages, lymphocytes, and *Lactobacillus bifidus* (a growth enhancer of lactobacilli).[5] Research in a variety of populations has indicated that the most effective protection offered by breast-feeding is against diarrhea and secondly against upper respiratory tract infection. The protection against diarrhea is apparently related to the difference in intestinal flora of breast-fed infants compared with those on formula. The gut flora of breast-fed babies consists mainly of lactobacilli and bifidobacteria, which are nonpathogenic and, owing to fermen-

T A B L E   3 5 - 1

Composition of Mature Breast Milk, Cow's Milk, and a Routine Infant Formula*

Composition/dl	Mature Breast Milk	Cow's Milk	Routine Formula With Iron†
Calories	75.0	69.0	67.0
Protein (g)	1.1	3.5	1.5
Lactalbumin (%)	80	18	
Casein (%)	20	82	
Water (ml)	87.1	87.3	
Fat (g)	4.0	3.5	3.7
CHO (g)	9.5	4.9	7.0
Ash (g)	0.21	0.72	0.34
Minerals			
Na (mg)	16.0	50.0	25.0
K (mg)	51.0	144.0	74.0
Ca (mg)	33.0	118.0	55.0
P (mg)	14.0	93.0	43.0
Mg (mg)	4.0	12.0	9.0
Fe (mg)	0.1	Tr.	1.2
Zn (mg)	0.15	0.1	0.42
Vitamins			
A (IU)	240.0	140.0	158.6
C (mg)	5.0	1.0	5.3
D (IU)	2.2	1.4	42.3
E (IU)	0.18	0.04	0.83
Thiamin (mg)	0.01	0.03	0.04
Riboflavin (mg)	0.04	0.17	0.06
Niacin (mg)	0.2	0.1	0.7
Curd size	Soft Flocculent	Firm Large	Mod. firm Mod. large
pH	Alkaline	Acid	Acid
Anti-infective properties	+	±	−
Bacterial content	Sterile	Nonsterile	Sterile
Emptying time	More rapid		

* Composite of a number of sources.
† Enfamil.
(Avery GB, Fletcher AB, Nutrition. In Avery GB (ed): Neonatology, 3rd ed. Philadelphia, JB Lippincott, 1987)

tation of sugars and production of acetic acid, produce feces with a pH of 5 to 6. This low pH inhibits growth of bacteria such as *Escherichia coli* and *Streptococcus faecalis,* which are the predominant flora of formula-fed infants who have a higher fecal pH.[6]

One known advantage of the immunoglobulin secretory IgA, which is present in human milk, is the protective antiabsorptive effect it has in keeping protein molecules from passing through the intestinal walls. During the first 6 months of life, foreign proteins are more likely to be absorbed through the intestinal wall than they are in later life, which can lead to allergies. The protein in cow's milk is one of the most common food allergens encountered in infancy. Human milk proteins, on the other hand, are virtually nonallergenic to humans.[7]

Psychological Aspects

The psychological advantages of breast-feeding are not as easily documented, and sometimes it is said that bottle-feeding and breast-feeding are interchangeable for the emotional well-being of mother and child. However, breast-feeding, by establishing a more direct and intimate biologic relationship between infant and mother, may very well influence the quality of the mother–child interaction.[3]

Other Aspects

For the baby, breast milk can be safer because it is not subject to incorrect mixing or contamination. The baby does not have to wait to eat—if mother is nearby the milk is always available and at the right temperature. The action of sucking at breast is different from sucking on a bottle and may help the mouth and jaw to develop better (see Fig. 35-6).

For the mother, an early benefit is promotion of uterine involution stimulated by the release of oxytocin when the infant sucks. The mother also has the convenience of not having to prepare bottles or incur the added expense of buying formula. When a woman breast-feeds her infant, she is less likely to conceive again during the first 8 to 10 months of lactation. As a means of birth control, this, of course, is not as reliable as modern contraceptive measures, but it can be helpful for those who cannot afford or accept artificial contraception.[7] (See References and Suggested Reading for a more complete discussion of advantages of breast-feeding.)

Choosing to Bottle-Feed

Throughout recorded history, women have sought alternatives to breast-feeding their infants. Although the most popular alternative was the use of a wet nurse, attempts at artificial feeding were widespread, as can be seen from the remains of spouted feeding pots, artificial teats, and other mechanical feeding devices. Historical writings show that women were often urged to breast-feed their own children, but many ignored these admonitions for various reasons.[8]

Women still give a variety of reasons for choosing artificial feeding. Some feel that breast-feeding is too tiring or confining or is simply distasteful; others may be afraid that it will disfigure their breasts; and still others fear that they will fail at breast-feeding, especially if previous attempts to breast-feed a child were unsuccessful.

The mores and pressures of the mother's socioeconomic class and peer group also are important. Bottle-feeding may be the accepted practice in the community or neighborhood; relatives, friends, and others may be either very much for or against breast-feeding. Return to employment for the mother may be a very significant factor.

Certain conditions in both the mother and the infant also can have a bearing on the decision and outcome. There are very few absolute contraindications to breast-feeding. Galactosemia in the infant is one, since it is imperative for these infants to have a lactose-free diet and breast milk is rich in lactose.[9] The mother with certain diseases or infections, such as active pulmonary tuberculosis, might be advised not to breast-feed. Some other conditions and infections in the infant might also preclude breast-feeding, at least temporarily. Generally the decision can be made on an individual basis, and in many cases, if the mother is determined to breast-

feed, she can pump her breasts and keep up her milk supply until it is possible for her to begin nursing the baby. Breast infection or painful, cracked, or fissured nipples might require changes in the breast-feeding routine and discontinuance of sucking on the affected breast for a while, but the breast should continue to be emptied by some means. Becoming pregnant is usually an indication for weaning because of the physiological strain that it places on the mother, although some women have breast-fed through a subsequent pregnancy.

Breast-Feeding

If breast-feeding is the method of choice for a new mother, the degree to which she perseveres in this endeavor is often influenced by her care in the hospital. A consistent approach to assisting with breast-feeding is important. A "breast-feeding protocol," as suggested by Dutton, can be developed in a hospital setting to help "standardize teaching and eliminate contradictory guidance."[10]

Recent studies have shown that many breast-feeding mothers perceive nurses as being negative or neutral toward breast-feeding.[11] After returning home, many mothers encountered problems that they felt could have been prevented if they had been given more anticipatory guidance by the nurses in the hospital about possible problems.[12] In light of these findings, it seems safe to say that support from knowledgeable nursing personnel, permissive hospital policies, and anticipatory teaching can do much to make breast-feeding a more pleasant and successful experience for mother and infant.

Mechanisms of Lactation

A working knowledge of how the breasts function in the lactation process can help the nurse with the guidance she gives the new mother. The anatomy of the breasts and the physiology of lactation have been discussed previously in Chapter 29, but are reviewed briefly here. The student is referred to Chapter 29 for a renewal of background understanding of the subject. Figure 35-1 reviews the anatomical structures of the breast. Two major mechanisms are involved in lactation: the secretion of milk and the milk-ejection reflex. Figure 29-4 illustrates these mechanisms.

Secretion of Milk

The secretion of milk is of course a prerequisite for successful breast-feeding. During pregnancy major changes occur in the mammary glands in preparation for milk

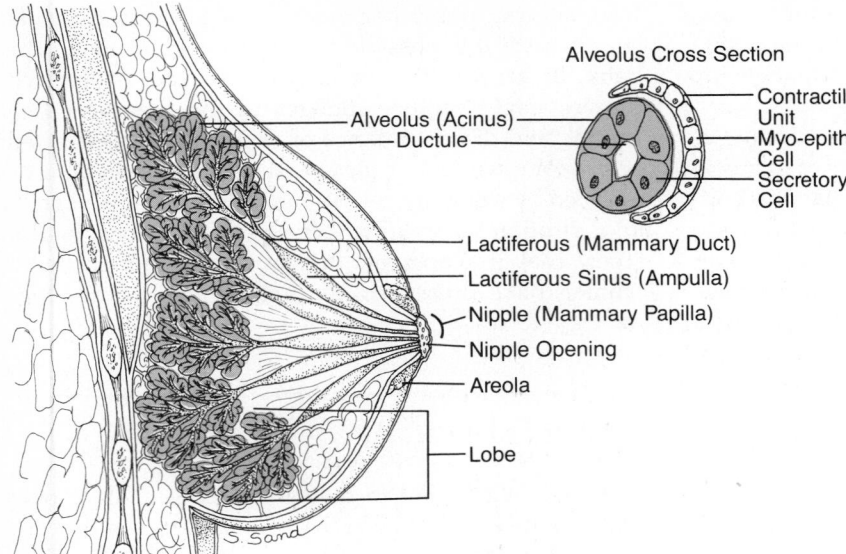

Alveolus Cross Section

Alveolus (Acinus)
Ductule

Contractile
Unit
Myo-epithelial
Cell
Secretory
Cell

Lactiferous (Mammary Duct)
Lactiferous Sinus (Ampulla)
Nipple (Mammary Papilla)
Nipple Opening
Areola
Lobe

S. Sand

F I G U R E   3 5 - 1

Schematic diagram of the breast. (Redrawn from Riordan J, Countryman BA: Basics of breast-feeding, part II: The anatomy and psychophysiology of lactation. JOGN Nurs 9(4):210, July/August 1980)

production. From the second trimester on, a secretion with fairly stable composition (precolostrum) can be found in the breasts. With the birth of the baby and the expulsion of the placenta, the secretion enters a transitional phase, which begins with colostrum and changes, over the following 10 days to a month, to mature milk. It is believed that increased levels of the hormone prolactin and decreased levels of estrogen and progesterone are at least partly responsible for the changes in the mammary secretion following birth, which includes an increase in both the volume of milk secreted and the total output of nutrients.[13] The release of prolactin from the anterior pituitary is enhanced by the stimulation of afferent nerves in the nipple when the infant suckles at the breast.[14]

Colostrum is higher in protein and lower in fat and lactose than mature milk. It also contains greater amounts of other substances, such as sodium chloride and zinc, and is rich in antibodies. Besides its nutrient purpose and anti-infective function, colostrum also may act as a laxative in facilitating the passage of meconium.[15] As the prolactin levels continue to increase and the estrogen and progesterone levels drop, newly secreted milk is progressively mixed with the colostrum until the mature milk stage is reached. During this time there is a decrease in the concentration of immunoglobulins and total protein and an increase in lactose, fat, and total calories.[16]

In the early stages of lactation, milk secretion can be stimulated by having the infant nurse from both breasts at each feeding and by increasing the frequency of the feedings. Milk production begins slowly in some mothers, but it can be stimulated by allowing the infant to nurse both breasts every 2 to 3 hours. Although prolactin stimulates the synthesis and secretion of milk into the alveolar spaces, it is thought that the amount of

milk produced is regulated by the amount left in the alveolar spaces after a feeding.[14] Therefore, frequent emptying of the breasts is very important, especially in the early stages of lactation. Both the production of milk and the quantity produced are dependent on frequent and complete emptying of the breasts. If the breasts are not entirely emptied, and the back pressure in the alveoli is not relieved, milk secretion decreases and eventually stops.

Possible Consequences of an Inadequate Let-Down Reflex

1. Let-down reflex doesn't occur. (Mother may be tense, nervous, in pain, and so forth.)
   ↓
2. Milk is not propelled into ducts by contraction of myoepithelial cells.
   ↓
3. Insufficient milk available to infant = hungry baby.
   ↓
4. Mother afraid she doesn't have enough milk → further inhibits let-down → gives infant formula → less sucking stimulation → decreased milk production.
   ↓
5. Engorgement due to inadequate emptying of breasts → more difficult for infant to suck → may lead to infection from stasis of milk.
   ↓
6. Termination of breast-feeding—reasons given:
   "I didn't have enough milk." Or,
   "My breasts were too sore." Or,
   "My breasts were infected so the doctor told me to stop."

Milk-Ejection Reflex

The second mechanism involved in lactation is the milk-ejection or let-down reflex. Initiated by the infant's sucking, oxytocin released from the posterior pituitary stimulates the myoepithelial cells in the alveoli to contract and eject the milk through the ducts into the lactiferous sinuses. This reflex affects the quantity of milk the infant is able to obtain because the milk has to be in the sinuses before it can be removed by the infant's sucking. The quality of milk is also affected because the fat-containing hindmilk is not secreted until the foremilk is removed. Failure of the let-down reflex may be a direct or indirect cause of early termination of breast-feeding in many women (see Possible Consequences of an Inadequate Let-Down Reflex).

Initiation of Breast-Feeding

The first hours after birth are generally an excellent time for the initiation of breast-feeding. The newborn usually is awake and alert for the first hour or so and will often be seen trying to suck on his fist. Taking advantage of this heightened sucking reflex will give an opportunity for a successful initial breast-feeding experience.[11] In their "Guidelines for Perinatal Care," the American Academy of Pediatrics and the American College of Obstetricians and Gynecologists recommend that breast-feeding begin as soon as possible after delivery.[17] If the mother has been heavily medicated or the labor has been long or difficult, the mother and infant may be sleepy and need very close supervision during the breast-feeding attempt. Even if the baby is too sleepy to nurse well at this time, the closeness to mother and the contact with the nipple may still be enough to stimulate release of oxytocin and prolactin.

Some hospital policies still call for the infant to receive a water feeding before beginning breast-feeding, with the explanation that this will help clear out excess mucus and help detect congenital anomalies such as tracheoesophageal fistula. The alternate view is that colostrum can serve the same purpose as water and, because it is a physiological secretion, would be safer and less irritating than water in case of aspiration.[18] Those advocating early breast-feeding also point out that an observant nurse would be quick to detect a problem such as tracheoesophageal fistula in the initial breast-feeding sessions and could then obtain help quite readily.

Assessment

When working with a mother–baby couple to help them establish or continue breast-feeding, the nurse can use the nursing process to good advantage. Adequate assessment is essential before beginning. Use of an assessment tool or checklist is helpful in determining the mother's level of knowledge and detecting any problems or potential problems. It is important to know whether the mother has breast-fed an infant before and what her previous experiences were. It is sometimes erroneously assumed that if the mother has other children she must have nursed a baby before and therefore will probably need less help. There are a number of reasons why a mother might not have nursed her previous infants and why even if she did, nursing this baby might be quite different.

After assessing the available information and talking with the mother, the nurse should also assess the interaction between mother and infant. The mother's questions and the way she handles the baby will give the nurse clues to possible problems. Even after the infant appears to be nursing well, periodic observation of a feeding is important to assess positioning and the infant's suckling behavior.[19]

Nursing Diagnosis

Observation and assessment of the mother's ability to feed the infant properly and of her knowledge pertaining to her anatomy and that of the infant will aid the nurse in making diagnoses concerning situations that may cause problems or concerns for the mother. The general nursing diagnosis "knowledge deficit about breast-feeding related to lack of experience" (or lack of information) could be made more specific by including the particular areas this new mother needs help with (*e.g.*, "knowledge deficit about positioning infant for breast-feeding related to lack of experience with breast-feeding following a cesarean delivery").

If problems were detected during the assessment, there would be nursing diagnoses related to the particular problems. For the mother this might be "alteration in comfort: pain related to sore nipples." A problem for the infant might be "alteration in nutrition, less than body requirements, related to ineffective sucking technique."

Planning/Intervention

After gathering information about this particular mother and baby and formulating nursing diagnoses, the nurse can plan her individualized interventions, using as much of the following information as necessary.

Initial Supervision

When assisting the new mother with breast-feeding it is important to remember that *both* mother and baby must learn how to work as a team during the breast-

A S S E S S M E N T   T O O L

Breast-Feeding

Initial Assessment

1. Mother's previous experience with breast-feeding
   Has she breast-fed before? _____
   If yes, what was her experience with it? _____
   If no, has she had close contact with anyone who was breast-feeding? _____
2. Mother's knowledge about breast-feeding
   Has she taken prenatal classes? _____
   Has she attended La Leche meetings or other breast-feeding classes? _____
   What books has she read about breast-feeding? _____
   Pamphlets? _____
   Other sources of information? _____
3. Assessment of mother's current condition
   Number of hours post delivery? _____
   Type of delivery? _____
   Apparent mood: anxious, eager, uncomfortable, tired, cheerful? _____
   Breasts: soft, firm, engorged, large, small _____
   Nipples: size, protractility _____
4. Assessment of infant's current condition
   Size: appropriate for gestational age? _____
   Physical condition: _____
   Activity: alert, sleepy, crying, sucking on fist _____
5. Maternal–infant interaction
   Position mother holds infant in spontaneously: _____
   Confidence mother demonstrates in handling infant: _____

Follow-up Assessment:

1. Positioning
   Mother finds comfortable position for herself _____
   Holds infant correctly: supports head and body, brings baby in close, supports breast with other hand using "C" hold _____
   Makes sure infant has jaws over areola _____
2. Sucking
   Infant is sucking correctly _____
   Tongue is under nipple and is coming out over lower gum during sucking (check by pulling down lower lip)
   _____
3. Nipples
   Appearance: no bruises, cracks, abrasions _____
   Sensation: no tenderness or pain _____

feeding process. Hence, practice is essential. Even though the mother may have breast-fed before, there is a wide range of nursing behaviors among infants, and the experience of breast-feeding each infant can be somewhat "new." The mother will need to learn how to handle the infant appropriately, how to interpret cues of hunger and satiety, and how to help the infant to grasp the nipple to withdraw the milk. The infant, in turn, must learn to associate the nipple with food and to coordinate grasping of the nipple with sucking and swallowing in such a way as to get food successfully. No wonder that mother and baby often take a few days to become adept at this process!

An interested and experienced nurse should be immediately available to mothers in their first experiences with their new babies. Maternity nurses in the hospital can play a major role in facilitating the mothers' efforts to breast-feed their babies (Fig. 35-2).

Many of the problems associated with unsuccessful breast-feeding experiences can be prevented or solved through purposeful nursing action. Nurses need to accept the responsibility of helping mothers gain the knowledge and skill necessary to successfully breast-feed their babies.[20]

Preparing the mother *before* the actual breast-feeding experience plays a large part in giving effective care. This includes instructions about hand washing, sterile technique procedures, and other rituals associated with the feeding of the infant in the hospital. If these tasks have to be carried out when the hungry infant is brought to the mother for feeding, the delay can be frustrating and stress producing for both mother and baby.

Whenever it is indicated, the mother should be informed about the feeding reflexes of her infant. During the actual nursing period the nurse can reinforce this information (as necessary) and *show* the mother how to elicit these responses. It is essential that the mother be able to evoke these reflexes herself, since she ultimately must assume total responsibility. Too often the nurse takes over these aspects and the mother does not get sufficient practice to acquire skill during these first days in the hospital. It is not easy to "stand by" and watch the inexperienced mother trying to breast-feed her baby without offering too much interference. But it is necessary to be careful not to disrupt the learning process.

Whether the first nursing is done in the delivery room, in the recovery room, or in the patient's room later, the nurse who assists the mother should record the type of instruction given and the response of the mother and infant to the experience. This information can help other staff members working with the mother to provide needed assistance and consistency.

Positioning the Mother

Assisting the mother to experiment with various positions during breast-feeding is another important facet of care. The mother is sometimes asked whether she wants to nurse the baby sitting up or lying down. An inexperienced mother may be unaware of the options and should be given an opportunity to try various po-

sitions while help is available. If the mother is shown only one position, she may think there is only one "right" way to do it.

The best positions for any given mother and infant depend on several factors, including the size and shape of the breast, the size of the infant, and the condition of the mother, who may have a sore perineum or tender incisional area from a cesarean section. However, it is a good idea to encourage the mother to avoid using the same position at each feeding. The area of the nipple in line with the infant's nose and chin is subjected to the greatest stress. Varying the nursing positions from one feeding to the next can be helpful because it changes the position of the infant's mouth on the nipple. This allows the breast to empty more completely and prevents the nipples from becoming tender and the ducts from becoming plugged.[21]

If the mother is lying down (Fig. 35-3), the nurse can suggest that she be on her side with her arm raised and her head comfortably supported. The baby lies on his side, flat on the bed or supported so that he can grasp the breast easily. Tucking the baby's feet close to the mother's body will help give him room to breathe. If the mother prefers to sit up to nurse, she may be most comfortable in a chair, with a stool to support her feet, if necessary (Fig. 35-4). If she stays in bed, the high Fowler's position is probably best. For the mother following a cesarean delivery, it is usually more comfortable if the knees are bent and abducted, with pillows to support them on each side and something, such as an overturned washbasin, at the end of the bed for her

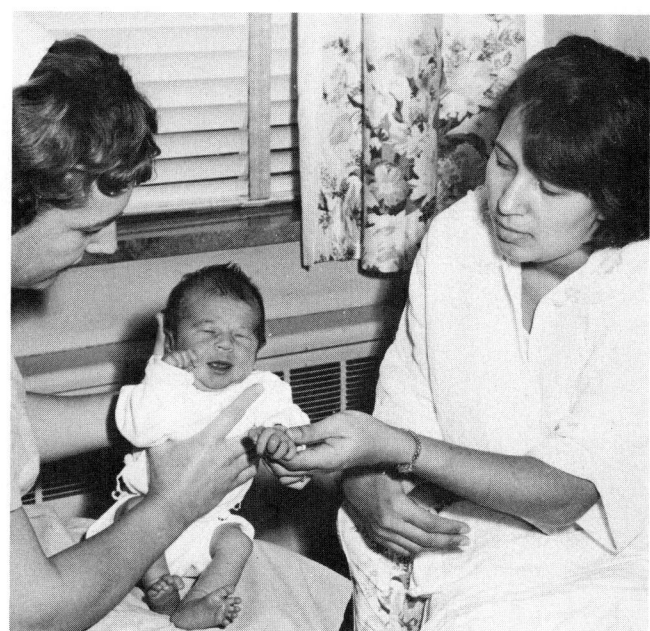

FIGURE 35-2

The nurse demonstrates methods of handling the baby prior to feeding.

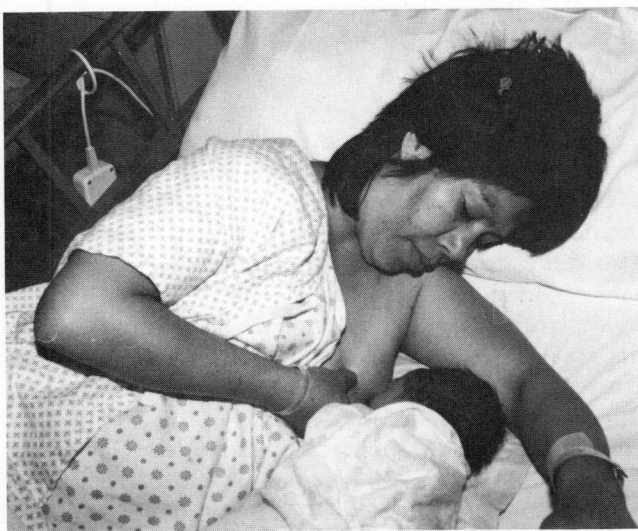

FIGURE 35-3

The mother who breast-feeds her newborn while lying down turns her baby toward her and curves her arm around him.

to brace her feet against.[22] It is often helpful to place a pillow under the arm that is supporting the infant, to reduce the tension on the muscles, or to place a pillow under the baby to raise him to a sufficient height to reach the breast easily. An alternate position for the baby is facing the breast with his body supported on a pillow along the mother's side and under her arm in the "football hold" (Fig. 35-5). This is especially helpful for the mother who has delivered by cesarean section or the mother who wants to nurse twins simultaneously.

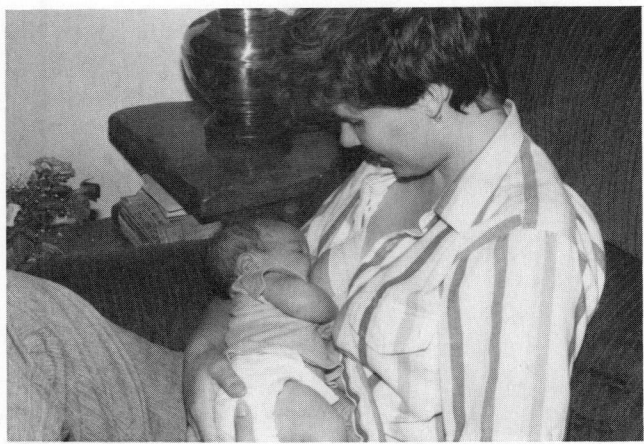

FIGURE 35-4

The mother may prefer to assume a sitting position while nursing. She should prop her feet or legs so she is comfortable and can comfortably hold the baby.

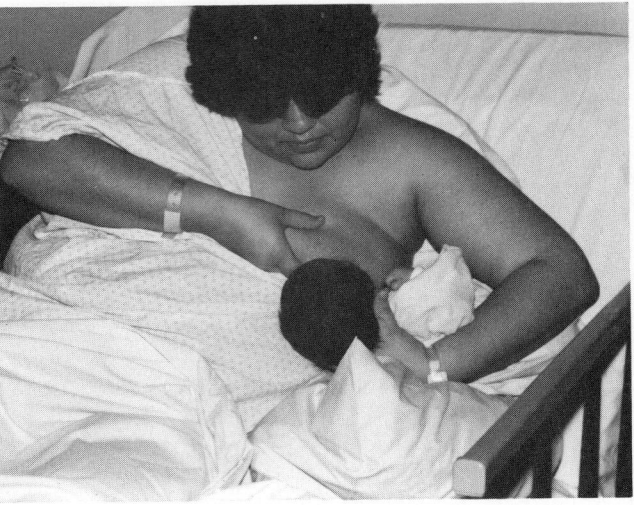

FIGURE 35-5

The mother may position the newborn in a football hold. The baby is supported by a pillow. The side rail is up for added security.

Some mothers will improvise positions that work well for them and their baby, but the nurse may have to work with other mothers to be sure they find a comfortable position.

Often, in their eagerness to get the baby on the breast, mothers become very tense and assume quite uncomfortable positions (although they assure the nurse they are "comfortable"). Patience and gentle reminding on the part of the nurse encourage these mothers to relax more readily.

Positioning the Infant

After the mother is comfortable, the nurse can assist her in positioning the infant so that he can "latch on" to the breast correctly (Fig 35-6).

To nurse satisfactorily, the infant needs to be held properly by the mother. Although some mothers seem to know how to support a baby at the breast, many are awkward at first and need definite instructions. The following are some helpful teaching points:

- The mother and baby must be comfortable.
- The baby should be at the level of the breast so his weight does not pull on the breast.
- The baby must be able to grasp the nipple and most of the areola. If only the nipple is grasped, the baby will not be able to draw out the milk because the milk sinuses will not be compressed. Possible damage to the nipple may occur, along with pain to the mother.

If the mother is in the sitting position, cradling the infant in her arms, the following steps described by

Frantz[23] have proven to be helpful in positioning the baby and preventing or decreasing nipple soreness:

- The baby's head should be in the bend of the mother's arm with her hand holding on to his buttocks or leg, turning his body completely toward her with his mouth at the level of the nipple. His lower arm should be around the mother's waist.
- The mother can help the baby grasp the nipple by supporting her breast with her hand, four fingers below and thumb above, with all fingers behind the areola.
- The mother then tickles the baby's lips very gently with the nipple, waits for him to open his mouth *wide*, centers the nipple, then brings him in close to her body so that his nose and chin just touch her breast and the nipple is in his mouth, past the gums.

Critical points seem to be that the infant is well over on his side facing the mother, so he doesn't have to turn his head to grasp the nipple, and that his whole body is pulled tightly against her with his shoulder and hip in alignment. These points also apply when the mother chooses the side-lying or football position.

Use of the second and third fingers to "shape" and introduce the nipple into the infant's mouth is an alternate technique that has been advocated for several years. Using this technique has often proved to be counterproductive because the mother's fingers are frequently placed on the areola, where the infant's gums should be, and thus prevent the infant from getting

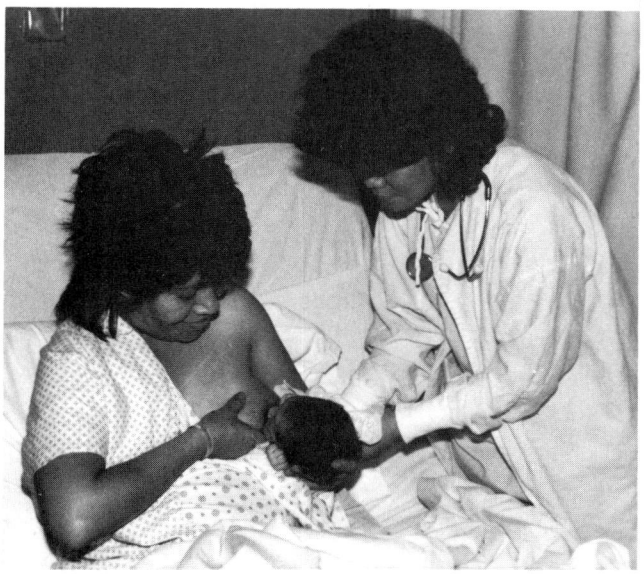

FIGURE 35-6

The nurse assists the mother in positioning the newborn.

enough of the areola into his mouth. Also, depression of the breast by the mother's index finger to allow breathing space may inadvertently result in removing the nipple from the baby's mouth.

Advice to get "all of the areola" into the baby's mouth is misleading and often impossible to follow, since many areolae are quite large. The important thing to remember is that the baby needs to get enough of the areola into his mouth so that his jaws can compress the sinuses, which are behind the nipple and under the areola.

Instructions About Sucking Behavior

To extract milk from the breast, the infant uses more than just suction. He must draw the nipple well back into his mouth, close his lips tightly around the areola, and squeeze the nipple against his palate with his tongue. The breast is emptied through a combination of compression and suction. As the baby nurses he moves his jaws up and down to compress and empty the sinuses; his tongue, as it draws the nipple back against the palate, suctions the milk from the nipple. Swallowing occurs when enough milk has been obtained to induce the swallowing reflex. This activity is carried on rhythmically, interspaced with periods of rest, until the infant is satisfied (Fig. 35-7).

Sometimes the let-down reflex is so active that the milk literally streams out of the nipple. The baby may almost have to stop sucking and may have difficulty in swallowing fast enough to keep up with the stream. Placing the baby in a more upright position temporarily may help him handle the milk and prevent choking. He may have to nurse a bit, stop, and then continue as he learns to cope with the increased flow.

When assisting the mother, the nurse should be sure that the baby has the nipple on top of his tongue and that enough of the areola is in his mouth to prevent damage to the nipple. If he has a good grasp, his jaws

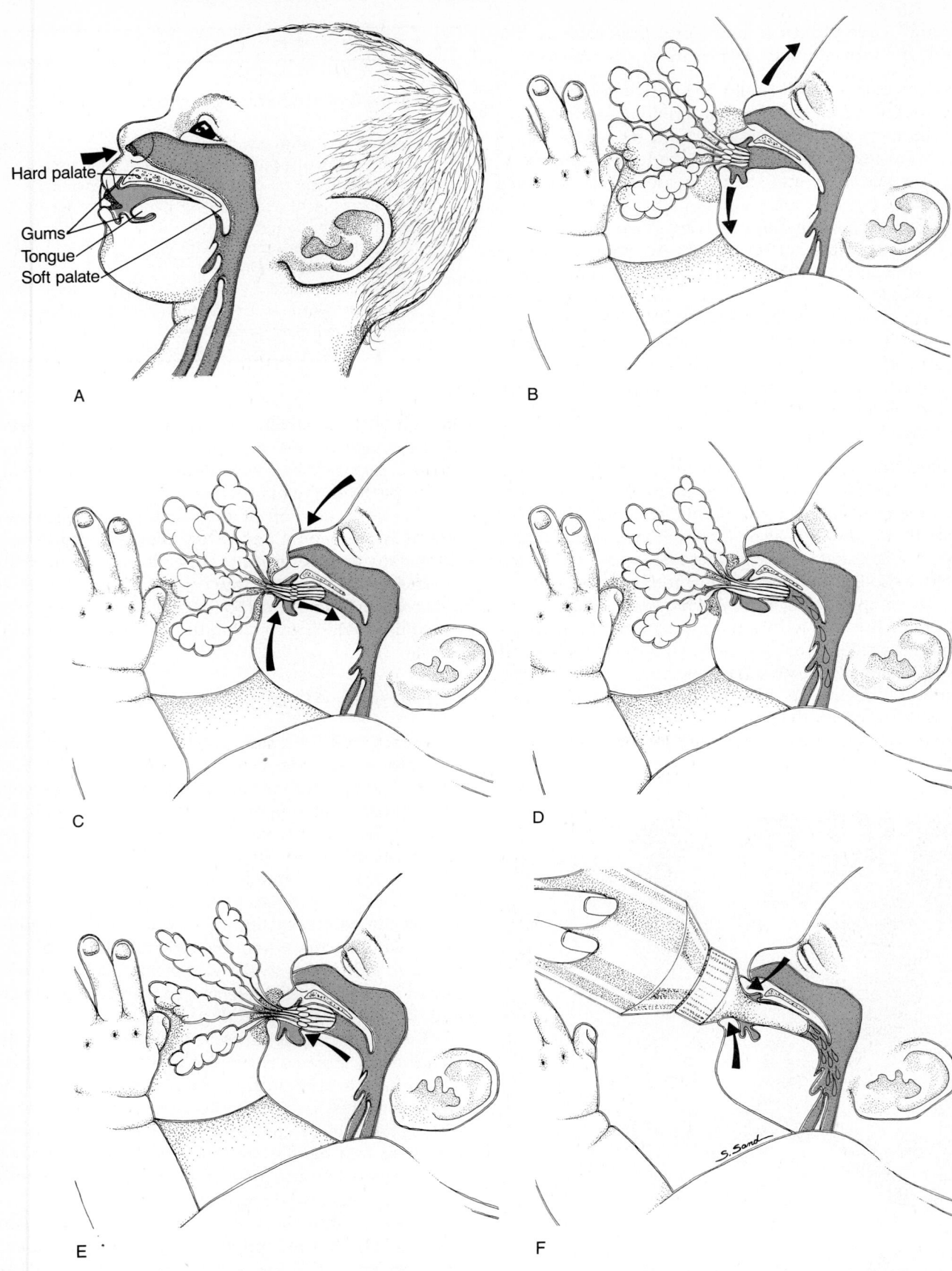

Hard palate

Gums
Tongue
Soft palate

A

B

C

D

E

F

will move up and down regularly, and sucking and swallowing movements can be seen in his cheeks and throat. If his grasp is poor, sucking and swallowing may be infrequent or absent, although his jaws may continue to move. Ineffective sucking should not be allowed to continue. The infant should be removed from the breast and encouraged to start again with a better grasp.

Any time the infant needs to be removed from the breast, the mother will need to break the suction first. Failure to do this can result in pain or trauma to the nipple. To break the suction, a clean little finger can be placed in the corner of the infant's mouth or the infant's chin can be pulled down. Sometimes the mother needs to pull away a little at the same time so the infant does not grasp the nipple again.

Breast tissue pressing against the infant's nose may obstruct his breathing and cause him to stop sucking. Pulling his buttocks and legs in closer to the mother's body may help by changing his head position slightly and allowing more air space. Lifting the breast slightly to allow more air space is another suggestion. Depressing the breast tissue with the thumb is more likely to dislodge the breast from the mouth.[19]

Babies exhibit a wide variety of sucking behaviors. Some, after finding the nipple, suck vigorously without stopping until they are satisfied. Others may suck vigorously for a time, appear to sleep or to rest, and then resume sucking. Still others mouth the nipple before actually sucking, but eventually nurse well. Others seem rather disinterested in the whole thing and dawdle throughout the nursing period. When the milk comes in, however, a change usually is noted, and even the

FIGURE 3 5 - 7

(A) Normal breathing for a young baby is through the nose; the back of the mouth is closed by contact of tongue and palate. (B) Infant opens mouth to receive the breast, and the tongue comes forward to grasp nipple and areola. (C) Nipple is sucked far back into mouth. The gums close on the areola while elevation of the tongue, traveling from front to back, presses nipple against hard palate, squeezing milk out of sinuses. Note how lips curl in around areola, forming an airtight seal. (D) When milk reaches the back of the throat the swallowing reflex is initiated. (E) The gums then open, allowing sinuses to refill. The tongue comes forward, and the cycle is repeated. Enough suction is maintained to keep nipple back in the mouth, and the infant continues to breathe through the nose, one breath to one or two swallows. (F) Rubber nipple is less pliable, reaches farther into mouth, and may strike soft palate, interfering with normal tongue action and sometimes causing gagging. Milk comes more freely and tongue is thrust forward against gums to control overflow. Note the lips flaring outward from pressure of widened area of nipple.

seemingly disinterested infants begin to nurse more in earnest.

The important point here is that individual differences do exist in infants, apparently from birth; hence, care must be taken to allow for these differences. To try to force the infant into a style or speed that is not natural for him will only result in screaming, resistance, and refusal; the nursing period should be adapted to the infant and not the infant to the nursing period.

Mothers, especially, are appreciative of learning about this; often they think there is "a way to nurse" and do not realize that infants have different eating behaviors. Giving mothers anticipatory guidance and instruction in this aspect of nursing a baby is a very important component of nursing care.

Bubbling Baby. Mothers often have questions about bubbling or burping the infant. This may be done when the infant is changed to the other breast and at the end of the feeding period. If the infant was crying hard before the feeding, she may want to bubble him before beginning. For the infant who has difficulty getting started, it might be better to bubble him only at the end of the feeding. Breast-fed babies tend not to swallow as much air as bottle-fed infants, hence the need for bubbling usually does not present much of a problem.

"Disinterested" Baby. Usually, getting the nipple into the mouth and tasting the milk seem to increase the baby's interest and ability to nurse. If the infant does not seem too interested or adept, moistening the nipple by expressing a few drops of colostrum or milk often encourages sucking.

Sometimes a baby will continue to be sleepy and difficult to arouse. If the mother unwraps him, plays with his hands, sings to him, or uses some other type of loving stimulation, it may be enough to awaken him. If it does not, the mother should be reassured that the baby will nurse when he is hungry. The nurse should then make sure that the baby is brought to the mother as soon as he awakens and is not given any feeding in the nursery. If possible, the infant should be left at the mother's bedside, so that she is available when the baby is ready to eat.

Nipple Confusion. If breast-feeding has not begun early and the infant has had experience with a rubber nipple, he may be "nipple confused." The sucking behavior required to obtain milk from the bottle is quite different from that of breast-feeding, described below. The milk from the bottle comes into the infant's mouth with very little effort on his part, and instead of using his tongue to help extract the milk, he has to thrust his tongue forward to control the flow of milk (see Fig. 35-7F). It is not surprising that many infants have some difficulty in switching from bottle to breast, but with a little time they usually do well. It is helpful for the mother to know about these sucking differences so she doesn't become frustrated.

Giving Support and Supervision

Once the infant has taken the breast without difficulty and has been sucking well for several minutes, the nurse probably does not need to remain in constant attendance at the bedside. The mother needs some opportunity to feel that she can manage on her own. Letting her have reasonable periods of managing breast-feeding by herself will help to instill some confidence. However, she should never be left without adequate instruction and reassurance. The nurse might find something else to do in the room or can place a call-bell within easy reach so that the mother can ring for help if need be. The nurse should make a point of looking in occasionally to observe the progress. The reassurance that the nurse is readily available may be all the encouragement the mother needs.

Since some infants do not nurse well during the first few days, the nurse will want to remind the mother that the first week is a time of learning for both the nursing mother and the child. Many mothers feel that all infants are born knowing how to suck and that if their infant does not latch on immediately, it must be because of something the mother is doing wrong. Some mothers even have a feeling of being rejected, stating, "The baby doesn't like me," or "The baby doesn't want my milk." Actually, taking milk from the breast is more than just a simple act of sucking, and some infants do need help in learning how. If the mother is helped to understand this, she will be less inclined to blame herself and more able to enjoy the nursing experience.

Because hospital stays are so short, there is less time available to provide professional assistance for the new mother. Most women still need support after leaving the hospital. In some cases the father fills this need, but in others another support person is needed. In the past, information and positive feelings about breast-feeding were passed from mother to daughter. However, since breast-feeding has not been a universal practice recently, grandmothers or other relatives may not have breast-feeding experiences to relate. Also, in our mobile society and with the trend toward nuclear families, female family members are not always available to give support to the new mother. To fill this void, nursing mothers' groups have been started across the country. One particularly popular group is La Leche League International, which holds classes about breast-feeding for women either before or after the baby is born. This organization also publishes a book about breast-feeding (*The Womanly Art of Breast Feeding*) along with other pamphlets, including one called "How the Nurse Can Help the Breast-Feeding Mother." In many communities there are 24-hour phone numbers that nursing mothers may call if they are having problems with breast-feeding.

Another source of help for the nursing mother is the lactation educator or consultant. These individuals have special training and experience in the area of assisting mothers with breast-feeding. The lactation educator presents prenatal classes specifically on breast-feeding and is available to the mother for counseling and advice after the baby is born. The lactation consultant is a health professional who has additional training and experience, is prepared to assist mothers with more serious breast-feeding problems, and usually works in a clinic setting or in private practice.

The mother may also be referred to a public-health agency if necessary. Some hospitals are now encouraging mothers to call the nursery or obstetric unit if they need support or help with problems. While many mothers are reluctant to call, they welcome the chance to ask questions if the nurse makes the call or a home visit. Some hospitals and some private doctors are hiring nurses to make follow-up visits after the woman leaves the hospital.

Feeding Schedule

A self-regulatory or self-demand schedule is the usual accepted practice today, especially for breast-fed babies (*i.e.*, the baby is fed when he indicates hunger by crying and body posture). The infant cries when he is hungry because actual contractions in his stomach cause him pain. If he is fed when he cries and is experiencing pain, he learns to associate food with the relief of pain. Thus, food and the mother who supplies it become pleasant factors in his life. If, on the other hand, he is made to wait until "time" for feeding, he may not nurse well because he is exhausted from crying or has lost his feeling of hunger. Similarly, if a baby is "sleepy" and not allowed to wake up sufficiently by himself, he also will not nurse well and will soon resent efforts to wake him up. Slapping the soles of his feet, spanking his bottom, and the like generally are not effective.

Problems of this type can often be avoided in a rooming-in situation, because with the mother and baby together most of the time, the mother knows when the infant is awake for a feeding. She also has the opportunity to learn to recognize the cry and behavior that indicate that her baby is hungry.

Most breast-fed babies will want to nurse every 2 to 3 hours at first. This is helpful in stimulating milk production and in satisfying the infant's sucking needs. The nursing pattern will vary greatly in the early weeks of life. Each time the infant has a growth spurt he will want to nurse more frequently for a few days until the supply catches up with his increased demand. The mother will be encouraged to know that her baby will gradually go longer between feedings and that his eating pattern will become less varied.[24]

Length of Nursing Time

Limitation of sucking time during the initial stages of breast-feeding, as a means of preventing sore nipples, is an idea that is still practiced in many hospitals. Most recent studies, however, have shown that this is not effective. Whitley found that women who restricted nursing time during the first few days of breast-feeding did have a lower incidence of sore nipples while in the hospital, but more of them developed soreness at home when they allowed the infant to suck longer.[25] If positioning and attachment are correct, unlimited nursing has not been found to increase nipple soreness.

Time limitations can actually cause some problems for the breast-feeding mother. With severe limitation, such as starting with 1 or 2 minutes on each breast at each feeding, the let-down reflex will not have a chance to function before the baby is removed from the breast. Even with 4 or 5 minutes per side there may be increased incidence of breast engorgement and reduction in the infant's fluid intake. Another disadvantage is that the mother may become too involved in clock watching to have a pleasant, relaxed time with her baby.[19]

It is best to offer both breasts at each feeding to provide maximum stimulation for the mother and an adequate supply of milk for the infant. The infant should be encouraged to nurse for at least 5 to 7 minutes on each side to allow time for the let-down reflex to occur and the ducts to be emptied. As the infant's thirst and hunger increase he will probably want to nurse 10 to 15 minutes on the first breast and a little less on the second. If the mother does develop severe nipple problems, she might need to shorten the time on the affected breast and to complete the emptying by expressing the milk.

When the breasts are full and the let-down reflex is functioning well, the baby usually gets most of the milk in the first 5 to 10 minutes of sucking. Therefore, the mother need not worry that the baby is not getting enough milk if she has to limit nursing time for a short period due to nipple soreness. Nursing should begin on the side used last at the previous feeding. A safety pin on the bra strap will help the mother remember which breast to start with.

Not Enough Milk

Many mothers worry that they will not have enough milk. The mother can be assured that the baby is probably getting an adequate amount of milk if he is wetting four to six diapers a day, sleeping fairly well, and gaining weight at a steady rate. The wet diapers may be the best guide, because "colicky" babies cry for reasons other than hunger and usually gain well, and some breast-fed babies are slow weight gainers even when the milk supply is adequate.

If the mother thinks her baby is not getting enough milk, putting the baby to breast more often will usually increase the supply. The concept of supply and demand, that the more milk the baby takes from the breast, the more the mother will produce, is important for the mother to remember. Sometimes women mistakenly think that they can "save" their milk and have more for the next feeding if they give the baby a bottle at one feeding. Getting more rest and increasing fluid and protein intake may also help increase the milk supply.

Some mothers fear that they are losing their milk at the time when engorgement subsides because their breasts go back to a more normal size and feel less full. An explanation that this might happen and that it is just the swelling that has gone down, not the milk supply, helps prevent worry.

If the mother's breasts seem full but the infant does not seem to be getting enough, there could be a problem with the let-down reflex. It may be helpful to the mother to learn how to recognize whether or not the let-down reflex is occurring. Mothers usually feel the let-down as a kind of tingling or drawing sensation in the nipple, followed by a fuller, heavier feeling of the breasts. Since let-down occurs bilaterally, another sign is dripping of milk from one breast while the infant is sucking on the other. Also there is often a change in the infant's sucking as the milk begins to flow more freely and he doesn't have to work as hard.

The let-down reflex can be influenced profoundly by psychic factors and the mother's emotions. If let-down is not occurring, the nurse can help the mother determine and eliminate disturbing factors. The mother may need to lie down, have a warm drink, or discover other ways of relaxing before the feeding time. A relaxed atmosphere, adequate assistance, effective pain relief, and a supportive attitude on the part of the nurse and family are important to the establishment of the let-down reflex.

Sometimes mothers are concerned that their milk isn't "rich enough" because they compare the thin, bluish white color of breast milk with the creamy color of cow's milk. They need to know that human milk is naturally different from cow's milk in many ways, including color. They may be interested in the fact that the milk of each animal species has a characteristic color. For example, buffalo's milk is completely white and kangaroo's milk is pink.[15]

Supplementary or Complementary Feedings

A bottle given instead of a breast-feeding is called a *supplementary feeding*, while one given in addition to the breast-feeding is called *complementary* (Fig. 35-8).

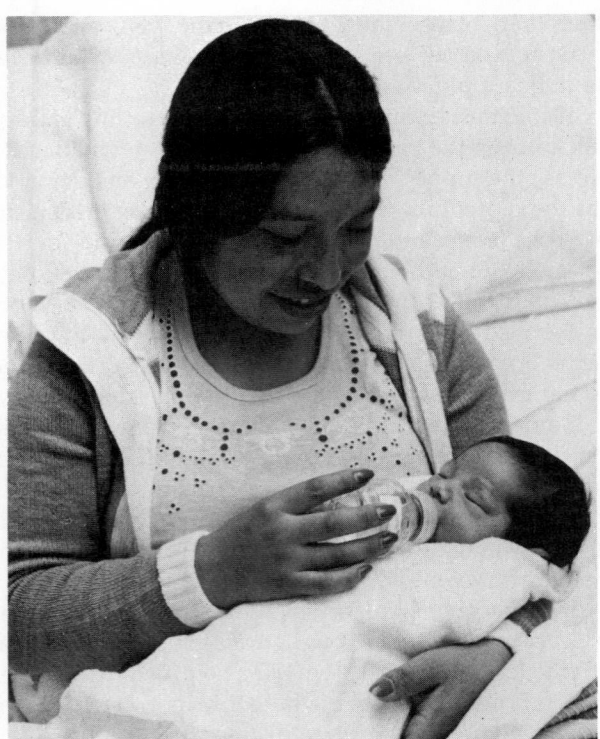

F I G U R E   3 5 - 8

A mother cuddling her infant while giving a complementary bottle of water.

This subject has long been controversial. Some physicians (and mothers) feel that giving the infant any artificial feedings diminishes the success of breast-feeding and is extremely detrimental to establishing and maintaining lactation (see References and Suggested Reading). Others feel that there are legitimate indications for an occasional artificial feeding. A variety of feedings may be used (*i.e.*, plain water, glucose water, dilute formula, full-strength formula). It is sometimes suggested that these be given by spoon or dropper to avoid the use of a rubber nipple.

If the mother is to use supplemental or complementary feedings when she returns home, the nurse will want to be sure that the mother understands how to prepare these feedings, the kind and the amount of feedings, and the indications for their use.

Care of the Nipples

To facilitate breast-feeding, it is important to discuss nipple care with the new mother. Cleanliness is important in breast-feeding, but it is the hands that need washing, not the nipples. There is a natural antisepsis provided in the oils secreted by the nipple and by enzymes in the milk.[21] Washing the breasts with plain water at the time of the daily bath or shower is thought to be enough. The use of soap should be avoided, because it is drying and can lead to cracking. There are many commercial nipple ointments and creams available, but hydrous lanolin has also been found to be soothing to tender nipples. Whatever is used should be safe for mother and baby and not have to be washed off before nursing. The nipples should be dried and the ointment or cream applied lightly so air circulation will not be obstructed and the nipples won't become clogged. Keeping the nipples dry is another important aspect of their care. Air drying after each nursing period and leaving the bra flaps down for 15 to 30 minutes several times a day are suggested.[21] Some women find a hair dryer helpful. Also, plastic liners of any kind in the bra should be removed because they hold the moisture in. In case of some milk leakage, especially in the first days after the milk comes in, something absorbent, such as a breast pad or a clean, folded, man's handkerchief, can be used to keep the nipples drier and prevent the outer clothing from getting wet. They should, of course, be changed frequently when they get damp.

Addressing Common Concerns and Problems

Painful Nipples. Nipple pain is frequently a reason mothers give for discontinuing breast-feeding. Although it may not be possible to prevent or eliminate this problem completely, it can be minimized with good care. Measures to prevent nipple trauma include the following:

1. Make sure most of the areola is in the infant's mouth so that he does not just chew on the nipple.
2. Change nursing positions with each feeding so that different areas of the nipple are subjected to the greatest stress from sucking.
3. Do not allow the breasts to become engorged so that the infant has difficulty grasping the breast.
4. Feed the infant on demand so that he does not become overly hungry, causing him to suck the nipple too vigorously.
5. Start each feeding on alternate breasts so that both breasts are subjected to the vigorous sucking that occurs at the beginning of the feeding.

The mother should also avoid allowing the infant to suck on empty ducts. Before the let-down reflex is established, she can manually express a few drops of colostrum or milk to fill the ducts prior to allowing the baby to begin nursing.

The mother can probably benefit from some anticipatory guidance about nipple soreness. She needs to know that it is not unusual and is usually self-limiting. The discomfort is often most noticeable as the baby begins to suck but diminishes rapidly as the let-down reflex occurs. The discomfort with the first few sucks can last for several days or weeks and does not mean that there is anything wrong.

It is possible, of course, for the nipples to develop fissures, erosions, or blisters, which can serve as entryways for bacteria and possible infection. If any of these do develop, the nurse should check with the mother to be sure she is carrying out proper nipple care. The nipples may be exposed to a lamp with a 40-watt bulb for 15 to 20 minutes. Grassley and Davis also suggest that an application of cold tea to the nipples can aid healing because of the tannic acid it contains.[26]

If symptoms of mastitis or breast abscess develop, such as localized increased warmth, tenderness, or redness, the physician should be consulted so that treatment can be started immediately. Since these problems usually occur after the woman has left the hospital, she should be given some guidance prior to discharge and instructed to observe her breasts for signs of infection. Antibodies are usually the treatment of choice. Most physicians now feel that it is best for the woman to continue breast-feeding even when these difficulties develop.[4] (See Chapter 40.)

Engorgement. When the milk "comes in," the breasts suddenly become larger, firmer, and more tender. New mothers experience varying degrees of discomfort at this time. Two factors thought to be involved in causing this discomfort are venous and lymphatic congestion and the filling of the alveolar cells with milk. The lymphatic and venous engorgement is usually transitory. Ideally, with early, frequent sucking by the infant, establishment of the let-down reflex, and periodic emptying of the alveoli, painful engorgement will not occur.

In some women, probably at least partly due to delayed emptying, the breasts do become distended or "engorged," sometimes so much so that the skin appears shiny. The tissue surrounding the nipple may also become taut to the extent that it actually retracts the nipple, making it extremely difficult for the baby to grasp the nipple and the areola adequately. The breasts may be reddened and warm to the touch, but engorgement is *not* an inflammatory process, so if fever occurs, some other cause should be suspected. With severe engorgement, the breasts can become very painful, especially when touched or moved, and throbbing pains sometimes extend into the axilla.

Although this condition is transitory and usually disappears in 24 hours to 48 hours, prompt treatment is to be instituted, not only for the mother's comfort but also to prevent the condition from progressing. If engorgement is allowed to become marked, emptying of the breasts (which is the basis of treatment) becomes very difficult because the ducts become occluded by the surrounding congested tissues and the thick and tenacious character of the retained secretions. Secondary

lymphatic and venous stasis may occur because the milk cannot be emptied.

Prevention of engorgement is preferable to treatment and is generally possible with good management. Early and regular nursing is considered by many to be the best preventive measure. When the mother and infant are together around the clock as in rooming-in, engorgement tends to occur less often because the baby can nurse in response to the mother's needs as well as his own. If rooming-in is not available, the infant can be taken to the mother as soon as her breasts begin to fill and as often thereafter as is necessary to maintain her comfort.

If engorgement does occur, management is directed toward removing the milk and relieving the discomfort. To assist in moving the milk from the alveoli to the sinuses where the baby can obtain it, Murdaugh and Miller suggest that the breasts be massaged before nursing.[27] This helps to open the lacteal ducts and relieve breast tightness by increasing circulation, thus making the breast softer and the nipple area easier to grasp. The mother can be instructed to place both hands at the upper part of the breast near the clavicle. With continuous downward pressure the fingers move out and around on opposite sides of the breast until they encircle it, then slide smoothly over the tip. Some lubrication, such as lotion, should probably be used for this procedure. When the beasts begin to soften, the infant can be placed at the breast.[27]

The use of an oxytocin nasal spray by the mother before the baby nurses may facilitate the removal of milk by encouraging the let-down reflex. Some mothers find that the use of hot packs or a hot shower before nursing also improves the flow of milk.

Another aid to emptying the breast and further relieving engorgement is alternate massage. To do this, the infant's sucking movements should be observed during nursing. When they become short and choppy instead of long and rhythmic, it indicates that the milk is no longer flowing as freely. Without removing the infant from the breast, the mother can alternately massage different areas of the breast to bring more milk down into the ducts where the infant can remove it by sucking.[27]

For relief of discomfort, ice packs applied between nursing periods may be useful. The use of a bra for good uplift support should be stressed. Analgesics such as aspirin, acetaminophen, or codeine may be needed for pain relief. They should be given in adequate dosage and with appropriate timing so that the mother can be relatively comfortable during nursing.

Expression of Milk. There are some instances in which the mother wishes to breast-feed, but for certain reasons the infant cannot be "put to breast." There are also situations in which the breast-fed infant is not able to empty the breast completely. At such times it becomes necessary to empty the breasts of milk by artificial means. Otherwise, if this condition is allowed to persist for several days, lacteal secretion is inhibited, and the future milk supply may be jeopardized. Before attempting to empty the breast by hand or pump, the mother may find it helpful to use measures to facilitate the let-down reflex, such as taking a warm shower, having a warm drink, or gently massaging the breasts.[21]

Manual Expression.   It is helpful if a woman can learn the technique of manual expression before the baby is born, but it can be taught afterward if necessary. The mother should have the opportunity to try it in the hospital, where she can have guided practice under the supervision of the nurse, so that she will be able to do it with more confidence when she returns home.

A sterile glass or wide-mouthed container should be ready before beginning, and if the milk is to be fed to the infant, a sterile bottle and cap also will be needed. It may be desirable first to massage the breast for a few seconds to stimulate the flow of milk, as described in the section on engorgement.

The hands of the person expressing the milk should be washed thoroughly with warm water and soap and dried with a clean towel. Since the daily care of the breast is designed to maintain cleanliness, the same cleansing ritual required before putting the baby to breast would be used here.

1. One hand is used to support the breast and to express the milk; the other is used to hold the container that will receive the milk. Although some authorities advocate that the right hand be used to milk the left breast, the decision as to which hand is used should depend on how the mother can accomplish this with the greatest ease.
2. The forefinger is placed below and the thumb above the outer edge of the areola. The first action is gentle but firm pressure toward the chest wall and the second is movement of the finger and thumb toward each other, then drawing forward with a slight milking motion. The forefinger is kept straight so that pressure can be exerted between the middle of this finger and the ball of the thumb. As the finger and thumb are alternately brought together and released, compressing the area of the lactiferous sinuses between them, milk is forced out in a stream (Fig. 35-9).

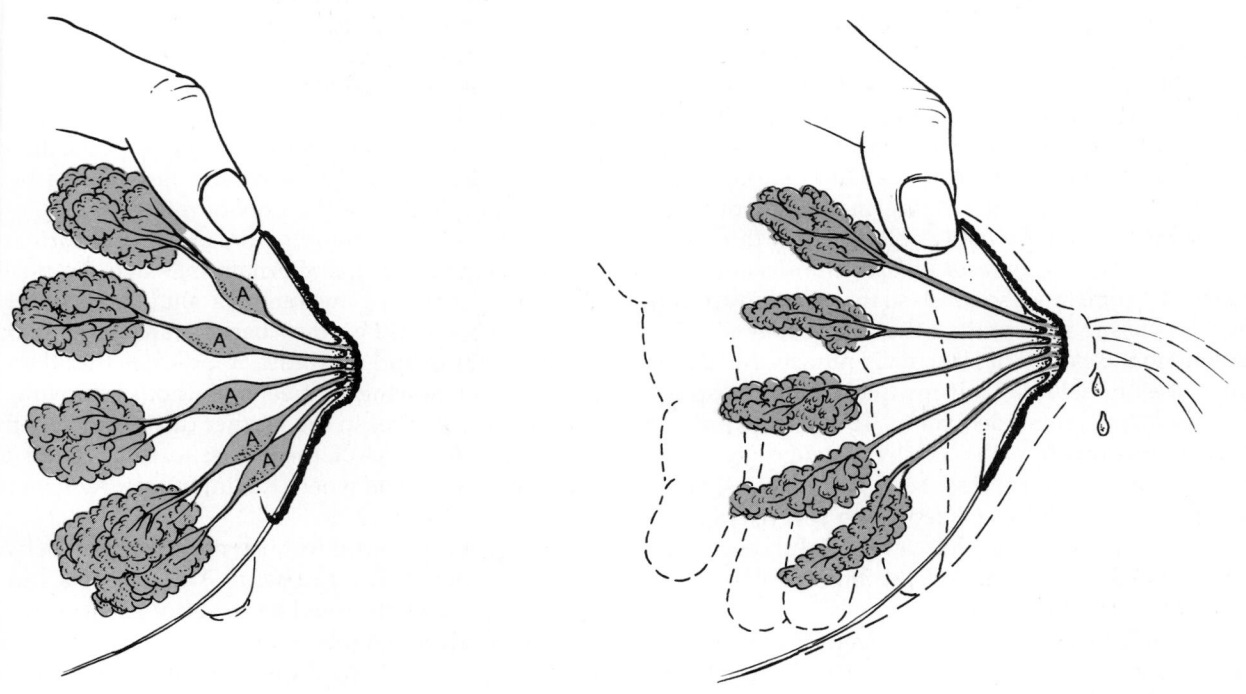

FIGURE   3 5 - 9

A lateral view of the left breast showing the method of expressing milk from the breast. The thumb and forefinger are placed on opposite sides of the breast just behind the areola. The lactiferous sinuses (ampulla, *A*) are compressed and milk is forced out as the thumb and forefinger are brought together. See text for complete explanation.

3. The fingers should not slide forward on the areola or the nipple during the milking process. It is of paramount importance to avoid pulling, pinching, or squeezing movements, since these can possibly bruise and damage the breast tissue.
4. The position of the thumb and forefinger should be changed as the sinuses are emptied, moving in a clockwise direction, so that milk can be removed from all the sinuses.

Many authorities advocate this method of emptying the breast rather than using the breast pump, because the action more nearly simulates the action of the infant's jaws as he nurses. Furthermore, since no mechanical equipment is required, it is a method that can be readily used when necessary after discharge from the hospital.

Electric-Pump Expression. When an electric pump is used, there is always the potential danger of traumatizing the breast tissue. This was particularly true of the older-style electric pumps that were originally designed for other purposes and then modified for use as a breast pump. The more recently introduced electric breast pumps have been specifically designed for pumping the breast and have a physiological sucking action, which decreases the danger of trauma (Fig. 35-10). Mothers using these pumps have found them efficient and easy to use.

Before using any pump, the mother should be given explanations about why it is used, how it works, and how to use it. If this information is not offered, the mother may experience fear and anxiety, which could retard the flow of milk. The nurse should stay with the mother and assist her the first few times until she feels confident to use the pump alone.

It takes approximately 5 to 12 minutes to empty a breast completely, depending on the stage of lactation, but pumping should be stopped as soon as milk ceases to flow. A breast should never be pumped longer than 10 minutes at any one time. One method is to change breasts every 5 minutes until the milk no longer flows freely. If the mother experiences back or chest pain, an indication that the breast is dry, the pumping should be stopped immediately.

The breast milk obtained is measured and the amount recorded. When only one breast is pumped at a time, the record should indicate whether it was the right or the left breast, so that the next time the other breast can be pumped. If the milk is to be fed to the infant, it can be poured into a sterile nursing bottle, labeled with the infant's name and the time and the date, and refrigerated immediately.

The electric breast pump may be used for more than one mother and thus should be washed with soap or detergent each time that it is used. In addition, certain removable parts, such as the breast-pump bottle and cap, the breast funnel, and the rubber connection tubing, must be washed thoroughly, wrapped, and autoclaved immediately after use.

Hand-Pump Expression. A variety of new hand breast pumps have been introduced. The old-style pump that looks a little like a bicycle horn, although probably still the least expensive, is no longer the most popular. The newer pumps are more efficient and less trauma-

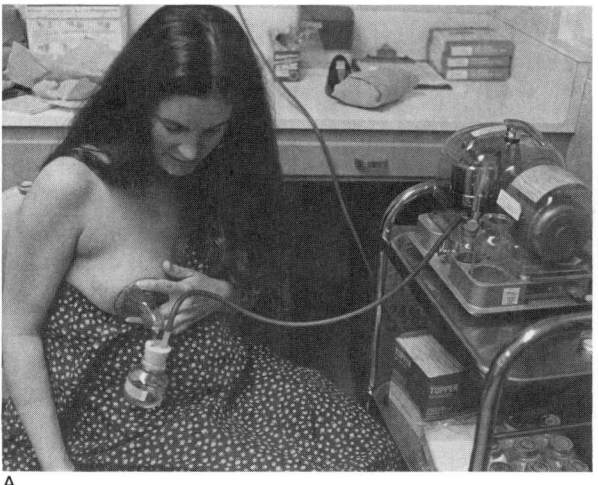
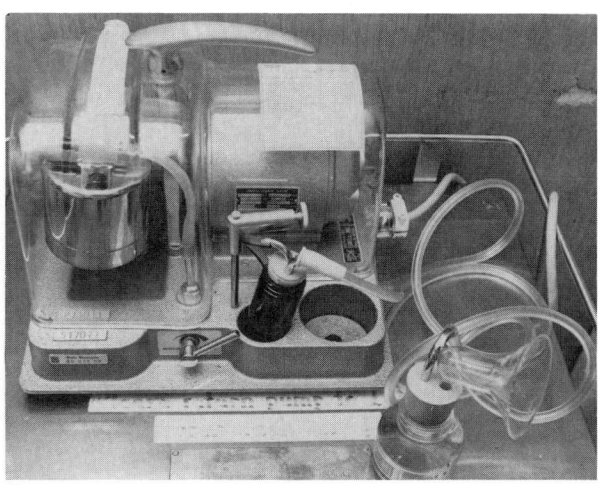

A   B

FIGURE 35-10

Electric breast pump. (*A*) Mother using electric breast pump. (*B*) Close-up of electric breast pump.

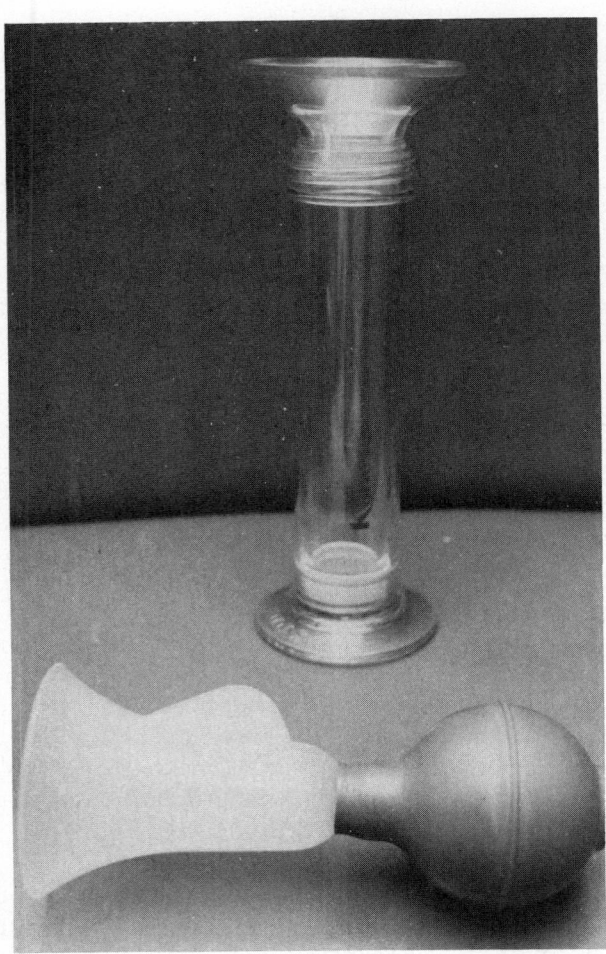

FIGURE 35-11

Hand breast pumps. (*Top*) Kaneson Breast Milking Unit. (*Bottom*) Bicycle horn pump.

tizing to the nipple. The Kaneson Breast Milking Unit (Fig. 35-11) uses a piston-type action to remove the milk. It is small and portable and has been found by many women to be effective and comfortable to use. One complaint is that its straight line makes it difficult to use in anything but a sitting position. Some newer pumps have solved this problem by attaching the cone at an angle. Two pumps that use different mechanisms for suction are the Loyd-B and Ora'Lac. The Loyd-B hand pump operates with a trigger action that creates a vacuum that can be controlled by the mother, and the Ora'Lac pump operates by suction from a tube that the mother puts in her mouth.[21]

Instructions for Hygiene

Rest.   Rest is one of the most important considerations for the lactating mother. The detrimental effects of fatigue and worry already have been discussed. In the hospital the nurse is able to act as a buffer between the mother and some of these problems. In addition, the mother is relieved of household responsibilities and is able to have meals served to her. When she leaves the hospital, she no longer has this somewhat protected environment. Thus, it is important for the nurse to make sure that the parents understand the importance of rest for the mother and that they have made adequate plans to provide for it. If it is at all possible, the mother should have help at home. Her main energies then can be directed to the care of the infant and other family members. Housekeeping chores will have to be simplified and the mother's activity restricted so that she will get sufficient rest. Since her sleep will be broken at night, naps during the day become particularly *essential*—they should not be considered a luxury. Without adequate rest, the milk supply will soon decrease. If heretofore the woman has been very active, she may need special help to realize the importance of naps and rest periods. It is helpful, also, if visitors (including relatives) are restricted at first. They can become fatiguing to the mother, and they may be a source of potential infection to the newborn.

Diet.   The daily diet of the lactating mother should be similar to that recommended during pregnancy (see Chap. 21) except that, according to the Food and Nutrition Board of the National Research Council, the need for calories, vitamin A, vitamin C, niacin, riboflavin, and iodine is greater than during pregnancy. It is hoped that the new mother has become more aware of good nutrition during her pregnancy and will be able to incorporate the proper foods into her diet to meet these increased needs. The nurse should discuss the recommendations with her, assess her knowledge, and give instruction as necessary.

If the mother's diet was adequate during pregnancy, additions rather than changes are all that will be necessary. Often nursing mothers, not realizing that their nutritional needs increase even over the needs of pregnancy, go back to their prepregnant diet or limit their intake in the hope of losing weight. Dieting should be discouraged during lactation. Any limitation of maternal nutrient intake during lactation can interfere with the quantity of milk produced and, if the limitation is severe, with the composition of the milk.

Individual caloric needs will vary with the body size of the woman and with the quantity of breast milk produced. Since it is difficult to determine exactly how much milk is being produced, a caloric intake of 800 to 1000 calories over that recommended for a nonpregnant woman is usually suggested. The mother's weight is one of the best criteria in determining adequate caloric intake: it should remain stationary. Wide fluctuations will require that the diet be adjusted, most likely in the amount of carbohydrates and fats consumed, assuming that protein intake is adequate.

The value of protein in the diet should be stressed. The efficiency of converting the dietary protein into milk protein is about 75%, so that about three fourths of the extra protein taken in by the lactating woman is secreted in the milk she produces.[28]

Increasing the milk intake to at least 1½ quarts daily will meet the additional protein, thiamine, riboflavin, calcium, phosphorus, and niacin needs. Supplementing the citrus fruit recommendations in pregnancy with generous servings of other fruits and vegetables will meet the vitamin C requirements. To further ensure optimum vitamim and mineral intake, many physicians will prescribe that the vitamin supplement capsules taken during pregnancy be continued.

A high fluid intake also is necessary for milk production. Between 2500 and 3000 ml is recommended for the mother engaged in usual activity under pleasant environmental conditions. More may be required in hot weather or with physical exertion. This fluid intake should include a good deal of water as well as other beverages. Many mothers find that taking a beverage prior to nursing facilitates the let-down reflex. Concentrated urine or constipation may be indications of inadequate fluid intake.

Mothers have often heard that there are foods that should be avoided during lactation. Although some babies are bothered by certain foods that their mothers eat, this is not universally true. Most mothers can eat any nutritious food without causing the baby any distress. However, because many babies do seem to be upset after the mother eats large quantities of certain foods, such as chocolate or cabbage, moderation should be the rule when eating these foods. If the mother herself is bothered by a particular food, she would be wise to avoid it because it could have an effect on the baby also. In addition, some babies seem to have more sensitive taste buds and object to certain flavors that come through in the milk by being reluctant to nurse.

Drugs. Most drugs ingested by the mother while she is lactating are secreted in the milk, but in varying amounts and with differing effects on the infant. Concentration of the drug in the breast milk depends on several factors, including the concentration in the mother's blood, the lipid solubility of the drug, the degree of ionization, and the composition of the milk. Usually the amount of drug in the milk is small, but the cumulative effect over a 24-hour period may give the infant a fairly large dose. Some drugs seem to have highest concentrations shortly after they are ingested; therefore, taking them after breast-feeding rather than before might help to minimize the infant's exposure.[29] Delayed excretion or inactivation of drugs due to the immaturity of the infant's renal and hepatic functions can be a factor in the concentration of the drug in the infant's body. Decreased renal function in the mother

can also lead to increased concentrations of drugs in the milk.

Interpreting the data concerning concentration of drugs in breast milk is hampered by the fragmentary and contradictory nature of the information available. Most drug companies state in their inserts that "Safety in pregnancy and lactation has not been established and the benefits of the drug must be weighed against possible risks." When drugs are prescribed for a nursing mother, she should remind the physician that she is breast-feeding. If she is taking drugs for a chronic condition, she should discuss their possible effects with the physician during pregnancy, before she decides on the method of feeding her infant.

Drugs that have been shown to have adverse effects on some infants are usually avoided. (See the table in Appendix B for further information on drugs.) If any of these drugs are given to the mother, the infant should be kept under close observation.

Some nonprescription medications also contain drugs that can be harmful to the infant when passed through the breast milk. Mothers need to be warned to read the label of any medication they are going to take to determine the presence of any potentially dangerous components. The following examples are given by Rothermel and Faber.[30] Bromo-Seltzer and some over-the-counter sleeping aids contain bromides, which are contraindicated during lactation. Laxatives containing cascara or senna may cause diarrhea in the infant. Some preparations for migraine headaches contain ergot, which can cause vomiting, diarrhea, a weak pulse, and unstable blood pressure in the nursing infant.

Contaminants in Breast Milk. Ever since investigators first discovered DDT in breast milk in the 1950s, people have been asking if breast milk is still safe for babies. A variety of contaminants are now known to be present in breast milk, including DDT, pesticides, and other chemicals. Pesticides are stored in body fat from whence they are mobilized and enter into milk fat. Toxic chemicals, such as PCB (polychlorinated biphenyls) and PBB (polybrominated biphenyls), have also been detected in human milk. None of these substances has yet been shown to have damaging effects on human infants as a result of ingestion from mother's milk, but newborn rats were shown to have a higher mortality when their lactating mothers were heavily dosed with DDT.[31] Lead, another contaminant of human milk, is found in larger amounts in other forms of milk. More research is needed to determine the possible long-term effects of contaminated breast milk. The benefits of breast-feeding still seem to outweigh the possible dangers in most cases. Women who have had excessive exposure to contaminants should be encouraged to have their milk analyzed to aid them in making a decision about the method of feeding. Nurses should join with others in attempts to rid the environment of pollutants as a more permanent solution to the problem.

Counseling Concerning Weaning

When it comes to initiating breast-feeding, many mothers receive advice and counseling. However, frequently, little is said about how or when they should stop nursing. Although stopping abruptly at a time set by the physician has sometimes been the accepted method of weaning, this can be very uncomfortable and distressing to both mother and baby. Most recent professional advice advocates that the infant be weaned slowly at a time chosen by either mother or infant. The mother should be helped, from the beginning, to feel comfortable with any length of time she chooses, even if it is considerably longer or shorter than usual.

The mother can begin to wean her infant by omitting either the feeding the infant is least interested in or the one that is least convenient for her. Parsons suggests substituting the feeding with another comforting experience that the baby enjoys, such as rocking, singing, or sucking on a pacifier.[32] Anywhere from a week to a month later, when both mother and baby are ready, another feeding may be dropped. This can be continued with periodic omissions until the child is completely off the breast. Additional omissions should be avoided when there are stressful situations in the family, such as illness, traveling, or guests. The child can be weaned to a cup or to a bottle depending on age and sucking needs.

Weaning is as likely to be traumatic to the mother as it is to the baby, especially if nursing has been a satisfying experience. Support from the father or another significant person may help guide her through this difficult time.

Sudden weaning is seldom necessary because the mother can express milk for a short time if she and the baby must be separated because of illness or absence for some other reason. If weaning does become necessary, a good supportive bra and mild analgesics for discomfort will probably be helpful for the mother. The medications that are given to inhibit lactation during the early puerperium are not used for weaning because they are not effective if started after lactation has begun.

Guidance for Working Mothers

An increasing number of women are choosing to breast-feed even though they plan to return to work. The new mother may ask the nurse for her opinion of whether it is possible to breast-feed if she must return to work soon after the baby is born. There are many factors involved in this decision and its outcome for the individual mother. Answers to the following questions can help the nurse assess what information the mother needs to help her in the decision-making process:

1. How soon will she start working? Waiting at least 6 weeks until breast-feeding is well established is preferable.
2. How flexible is her job? Can she come home to feed during the day or have the baby brought to her? If not, is there time and a place to pump her breasts at work? The answers to these questions will determine the arrangements she will need to make before starting work.
3. How much support does she have? Are family and friends supportive? Is her employer or supervisor supportive? Support from those around her will make it easier for her to continue with her dual roles.

The average working mother will probably need to be away from the baby during the entire working day. Her breasts will continue to fill at the regular feeding times when she first goes back to work. She can empty them each day by hand, manual pump, or electric pump to keep up the supply and have breast milk to be fed to the baby when she isn't there, or she can allow the daytime milk supply to dwindle by not pumping and have the baby receive formula during the day. Before going back to work she will need to make these decisions and practice the method of expression she chooses. She will also need to arrange for refrigeration facilities for the breast milk at work.

Some mothers find that their milk supply diminishes when they first return to work. Factors involved here may be inadequate rest, reduction of intake of food and fluids, and temporary inhibition of the let-down reflex related to the tension involved with starting back to work.[33] The working, breast-feeding mother has to pay particular attention to obtaining enough food and rest. She also should be aware that those who pump their breasts during the day can usually keep the milk supply at a higher level than those whose breasts are only emptied by the baby in the morning and evening.[34]

Studies have shown that most mothers who have breast-fed babies after returning to work have felt it was worthwhile and would do it again. They often reported how much they enjoyed the special closeness that breast-feeding promoted between them and the baby, even though they didn't have a lot of time to spend with the baby.[34]

Evaluation

The nurse's interest and assistance can play a major role in the successful outcome of the breast-feeding experience for the new mother and baby. To increase the effectiveness of her interventions, it is important for the nurse to evaluate these outcomes and to implement additional interventions when indicated. After a teaching session, the nurse evaluates whether or not the mother

Infant and Mother Who Are Breast-Feeding

Nursing Objectives

1. Identify mother's needs for information and assistance with breast-feeding.
2. Provide information and assistance to ensure a satisfying experience for mother and baby.
3. Maintain infant's hydration and nutritional status by encouraging adequate breast-feeding experiences.
4. Identify potential problems

Assessment	Potential Nursing Diagnosis	Planning/Intervention	Evaluation

Mother's past experiences	Knowledge deficit about breast-feeding related to lack of experience and prior information	Review with mother her prenatal preparation for breast-feeding
		
		Provide information as needed regarding:
		  Lactation process
		  Let-down reflex
		  Nutrition for lactation
			Mother expresses understanding of breast-feeding process

Mother's handling of infant		Assist mother with breast-feeding:	

Infant's reflexes (rooting, sucking, swallowing) and responsiveness	Alteration in nutrition, less than body requirements, related to infant's lack of effective sucking technique or lack of responsiveness	Comfortable positioning of mother
		  Positioning of infant
		  Demonstrate newborn reflexes
		  Verify correct position of nipple in infant's mouth
		  Encourage frequent (every 2–3 hours) feeding
		Provide further information:
		  Terminating feedings
		  Burping
		  Manual expression or use of pumps
		  Determination of adequate amount of milk (4–6 wet diapers/day, sleeping well, gaining weight)
		  Breast and nipple care
		  Answer questions
		Refer to support groups or lactation counselor as appropriate
		Provide literature
			Mother assumes comfortable position and infant "latches on" to breast without difficulty
			
			Infant experiences minimal weight loss
			
			Infant remains well hydrated
			
			Mother and infant experience satisfaction from the breast-feeding experience

(1) verbalizes understanding of the breast-feeding process, (2) assumes a comfortable position, and (3) uses the suggested techniques for positioning the infant on the breast.

The infant's weight and hydration may also be used as criteria for evaluation. The infant will (1) have at least four to six wet diapers a day, (2) have good skin turgor, and (3) begin to regain birth weight by 1 week

T A B L E   3 5 - 2

Types of Formula

Type	Packaging Available	Comments
Ready-to-Feed	Small cans, large cans, bottles	Most convenient; most expensive; should not be diluted
Concentrate	Large or small cans	Less expensive; must be diluted 1:1 with water from safe source
Powder	Large cans	Least expensive; simple to prepare individual bottles with warm water from safe source; sometimes difficult to dissolve

of age. Other evaluations would be made depending on the situation. If the criteria are not met, the nurse might need to assess for further problems or provide the mother with additional information or demonstrations.

Artificial Feeding

The mother who chooses to bottle-feed her infant may have as many concerns about feeding as the breast-feeding mother, especially if this is her first child. She may feel a little uncertain about her choice and become defensive if questioned. She may also have heard about formulas disagreeing with some infants or causing allergies so that it becomes necessary to switch from one formula to another. By keeping up to date on the latest information about infant nutrition, the nurse can help allay the mother's fears about the adequacy of formulas, instruct her in safe preparation, and give guidance about when to seek medical assistance.

Comparison of Formulas

In today's hospital nursery the infant will probably receive ready-to-feed formula in a disposable bottle. However, since formula in disposable bottles is expensive, one of the other packaging methods will be rec-

T A B L E   3 5 - 3

Composition of Frequently Used Milks and Formulas

Milk or Formula	Cal/dl	Percentage Composition			mmol/dl		mg/dl		Type of Carbohydrate	Type of Protein	Remarks
		Pro	Fat	CHO	Na	K	Ca	P			
Human milk	74	1.1	4.5	6.8	0.7	1.3	34	121	Lactose	Human	
Cow's milk	67	3.5	3.7	4.9	2.2	3.5	117	92	Lactose	Cow	
Goat's milk	67	3.2	4.0	4.6	1.5	4.5	129	106	Lactose	Goat	Insufficient folate
Enfamil	67	1.5	3.7	7.0	1.2	1.8	55	56	Lactose	Cow	
Enfamil With Iron	67	1.5	3.7	7.0	1.2	1.8	55	46	Lactose	Cow	
Similac	67	1.6	3.6	7.2	1.1*	2.0*	51	39	Lactose	Cow	
Similac With Iron	67	1.6	3.6	7.2	1.1*	2.0*	51	39	Lactose	Cow	
Similac PM 60/40	67	1.6	3.5	7.6	0.7	1.5	40	20	Lactose	Casein, whey	60/40 lactalbumin; casein
S-M-A	67	1.5	3.6	7.2	0.6	1.4	44	33	Lactose	Whey from cow, cow	60/40 lactalbumin; casein
Advance	54	2.0	2.7	5.5	1.3	2.2	51	39	Corn syrup, lactose	Cow, soy	16 cal/oz
Isomil	67	2.0	3.6	6.8	1.3	1.8	70	50	Corn syrup, sucrose, corn starch	Soy, methionine	
Soyalac-i	67	2.1	3.8	6.7	1.4	1.9	63	52	Sucrose, tapioca	Soy, methionine	
Nursoy	67	2.3	3.6	6.8	0.9	1.9	64	44	Sucrose	Soy, methionine	
ProSobee	67	2.5	3.4	6.8	1.8	1.9	79	53	Corn syrup solids	Soy, methionine	
Soyalac	69	2.2	3.8	6.6	1.5	2.0	63	52	Dextrose, maltose, sucrose	Soy, methionine	
Meat base	67	2.8	3.3	6.3	0.8	1.0	99	66	Sucrose, tapioca	Beef	High protein, low sodium

* Slightly higher if made from powder.
(After Avery GB (ed): Neonatology, 3rd ed. Philadelphia, JB Lippincott, 1987)

ommended once the baby is ready to go home (Table 35-2). Formula is available in various sized cans in ready-to-use, concentrated, or powdered form.

The model usually used in planning a formula is human milk. Companies that manufacture infant formula are continually making adjustments to match new discoveries concerning the composition of human milk (Table 35-3).

To provide adequate nutrition for an infant, a formula must meet the following criteria: it must have an appropriate distribution of calories from protein, fat, and carbohydrate; it must meet the infant's need for water, energy, vitamins, and minerals; and it must be readily digestible. Recommended standards for calories, protein, fat, vitamins, and minerals in formulas have been published by the Committee on Nutrition of the American Academy of Pediatrics.[35]

Cow's milk has more protein, sodium, and calcium and less carbohydrate than human milk, but is about the same in fat, calories, and the ratio of water to solids. The protein in cow's milk is quite different from that in human milk and contains much more casein and less whey protein. The approximate whey/casein ratios are 20:80 in cow's milk and 60:40 in human milk. The increased casein leads to a tougher curd, which is more difficult to digest. Boiling or pasteurizing fresh milk, and using the process employed in making evaporated milk, will soften the curd and make it more digestible. Adding water to the milk also softens the curd and dilutes the composition, bringing it closer to human milk. However, since the dilution lowers the proportion of carbohydrate, corn syrup or dextromaltose is usually added.

Before commercially prepared formulas became widely available, evaporated milk formulas were most commonly used. They are still less expensive than the commercial formulas but are no longer recommended for infant feeding. Evaporated milk contains adequate amounts of vitamins A, B, and K and is usually fortified with vitamin D, but, along with fresh whole milk, it fails to meet current recommendations for vitamin C, vitamin E, and essential fatty acids.

Many ingredients and processes are used in an effort to make commercial formulas meet the recommended nutritional standards and come as close as possible to the composition of human milk. Formulas generally use a nonfat cow's milk base with added vegetable oil and carbohydrate. Another type of formula, called "humanized," attempts to duplicate the 60:40 whey/casein ratio of human milk by using dialyzed whey. The dialysis removes electrolytes, bringing the formula closer to the lower-electrolyte human milk. Similac, Enfamil, and S-M-A all now have formulas with the 60:40 ratio.

Some infants are not able to tolerate formulas based on cow's milk. Many formulas have been developed to try to meet the nutritional needs of these infants. Some of these, such as meat-based formulas, may be difficult for the mother to accept, since they do not look like

milk. Soybean-derived products are commonly used as the protein source in these artificial formulas. Soy protein isolate has a lower biologic value than casein and whey, so slightly larger amounts are needed to meet the infant's nutritional needs.

Sometimes an infant will be given milk other than a formula. In our weight-conscious society it might seem that *nonfat milk* would be a good choice for an infant who was gaining weight too rapidly. Or nonfat dry milk may seem desirable for economic reasons. But nonfat milk is not recommended for infants under 1 year because it provides an excessive intake of protein with inadequate calories. To meet energy requirements and growth needs, body fat is mobilized. The infant may look healthy but have little reserve for illness. Nonfat milk also lacks an adequate content of iron, ascorbic acid, and essential fatty acids. *Low-fat* (2%) milk is midway between nonfat and whole milk in fat content, but probably would not meet all the infant's energy needs.[36]

Commercial milk substitutes such as filled milk or imitation milk are also available. *Filled milks* consist of a combination of true milk solids and a nonmilk fat. They usually have all the nutrients of regular milk but may have more carbohydrate. Depending on which nonmilk fat is used, one or more of the essential fatty acids may be missing, along with the fortified vitamins that are usually found in regular milk. Thus they usually are not recommended for infants. *Imitation milk* is available in a few states. Although it may be cheaper than regular milk, it is also nutritionally inferior and should not be given to infants or children as a substitute for milk.[37]

Assessment

Assessing maternal concerns and knowledge about infant feeding techniques and formula is an important part of nursing care, especially for the first-time mother. If these concerns have not been addressed antepartally, the nurse needs to help her adjust in the postpartum period. The nurse should talk with the mother to assess her level of knowledge and her previous experience with infant feeding. She should also observe the mother and infant during feeding to assess the mother's handling of the infant and the infant's feeding reflexes, responsiveness, and amount of intake.

Nursing Diagnosis

A possible nursing diagnosis might be "maternal knowledge deficit related to lack of information or experience with infant feeding." For the infant who is taking too little formula at a feeding or who is feeding infrequently, the nursing diagnosis might be "alteration in nutrition, less than body requirements, related to inadequate caloric intake" or "potential fluid volume deficit related to inadequate fluid intake." The infant who is taking more formula than expected would have the potential for "alteration in nutrition, more than body requirements, related to excessive caloric intake."

Planning/Intervention

Feeding in the Hospital

Most hospitals have a routine for when the bottle-fed baby will receive the first water feeding and when the formula feedings will start. In some hospitals it is the rule that the first water is given by the nurse in the nursery. Other hospitals are more permissive and allow the mother to give the first water. If this is the case, the nurse should show the mother how to use the bulb syringe because the water often causes the infant to bring up mucus. The nurse should also stay nearby to observe the infant's responses to the water.

The first feeding experiences can be very important for mother and infant. The mother begins to learn how the infant communicates his wants and needs, while the infant, besides learning to coordinate his feeding behaviors, begins to find out how the discomfort from hunger is relieved and who provides the relief. The nurse can help the mother and infant with these tasks by being available during initial feeding periods to observe their behaviors, assess the interaction, and intervene with suggestions or demonstrations as necessary. When intervening, the nurse should be careful not to make the mother feel as though she is incompetent or inadequate.

Before feeding begins, the mother should be helped to get into a comfortable position. She may want to sit up in a chair instead of in the bed. Holding the baby

in a semireclining position will allow any air that is swallowed to rise to the top of the infant's stomach, where it is more easily expelled. To minimize the amount of air swallowed, the bottle should be tilted enough to keep the nipple filled with milk (Fig. 35-12).

The mother may need some help in getting the infant started on the bottle. If the infant does not open his mouth readily, gently stroking the lips with the nipple might help. Some babies elevate their tongue when opening their mouths, and an inexperienced mother may not recognize that the nipple is under the tongue. Stimulating the baby to open his mouth wide enough so that the tongue can be seen usually helps in placing the nipple in the right position. Also, care should be taken that the nipple is not pushed too far into the mouth, since it may cause gagging if it strikes the soft palate.

As the baby sucks, air bubbles rise in the bottle, indicating that the baby is getting milk. If air bubbles do not appear, the nipple should be checked to see if the hole is clogged or too small. If the milk is coming too fast the nipple holes may be too large. Nipple holes can be checked by holding the bottle upside down. The

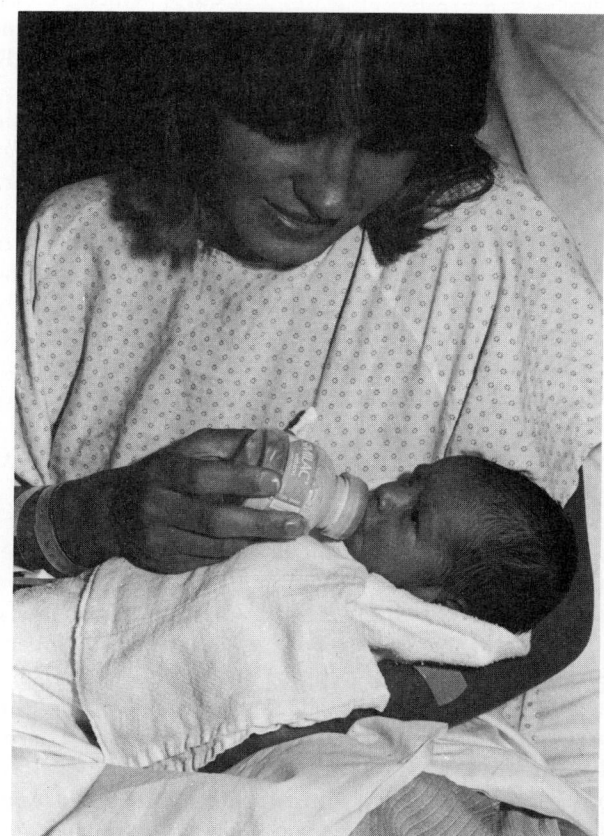

FIGURE 35-12

When bottle-feeding her infant, the mother tilts the bottle in such a way that the nipple is filled with milk.

milk should drop freely but not run in a stream. If milk is coming at the right speed a feeding should take 15 to 20 minutes. If it takes much longer the infant may get too tired, but if it is much shorter the infant may not meet his sucking needs.

Babies have many different feeding behaviors, some of which may not correspond to the mother's expectations. Identifying the infant's individual behavior patterns and interpreting the baby's individuality to the mother can help to avert potential problems.[38]

If the mother is concerned that the baby is not taking enough milk, it may help her to know that babies are often sleepy the first few days after birth but that they are born with reserves of fat and water and do not really need many calories until the second or third day.[36] The bottle-fed baby, like the breast-fed baby, should have the opportunity to be on a self-demand schedule. Some babies get hungry more frequently than every 4 hours, and some will want to wait longer than that between some feedings.

Anticipatory Guidance

Before the mother and baby leave the hospital, the mother should be given some anticipatory guidance in how much formula the infant may take and how to prepare it.

According to the Recommended Dietary Allowances established by the Food and Nutrition Board of the National Academy of Sciences in 1973, infants from birth to 5 months need approximately 117 calories/kg (51 calories/lb) each day. From 6 months to a year the need decreases to 108 calories/kg (47 calories/lb).[39] Using this as a guide, the nurse can help the mother

calculate the infant's daily caloric needs. Most formula contains 20 calories per ounce, so a 7-pound baby would need about 17½ ounces a day, or a little less than 3 ounces at each of six feedings. As the infant grows, he will increase his consumption. At times of particularly fast growth, he will want to eat more at each feeding or more frequently. Again, the reminder should be given that each baby is an individual and that babies of the same age and weight may have different needs.

Counseling Concerning Preparation of Formula at Home

Bottles and Nipples. With the wide variety of bottles and nipples available, selection depends on the parents' preference. Some will prefer glass bottles with plastic nipple caps; others will opt for the boilable plastic bottles that are nonbreakable. There are also kits that have a hollow plastic holder in which a disposable plastic bag containing the milk is suspended. Supposedly less air will be swallowed with this method because the bag collapses rather than filling with air when the milk is sucked out. However, the infant can still swallow air around the nipple.

Nipples also come in several shapes and sizes. One supposedly resembles the mother's breast in appearance; another (Nuk) is supposed to elicit sucking responses more like the breast. The number of bottles and nipples needed will depend on the method of preparation. (For examples of bottles and nipples available, see Fig. 35-13).

Methods of Preparation. Strict sterilization procedures for preparing formulas have been considered a

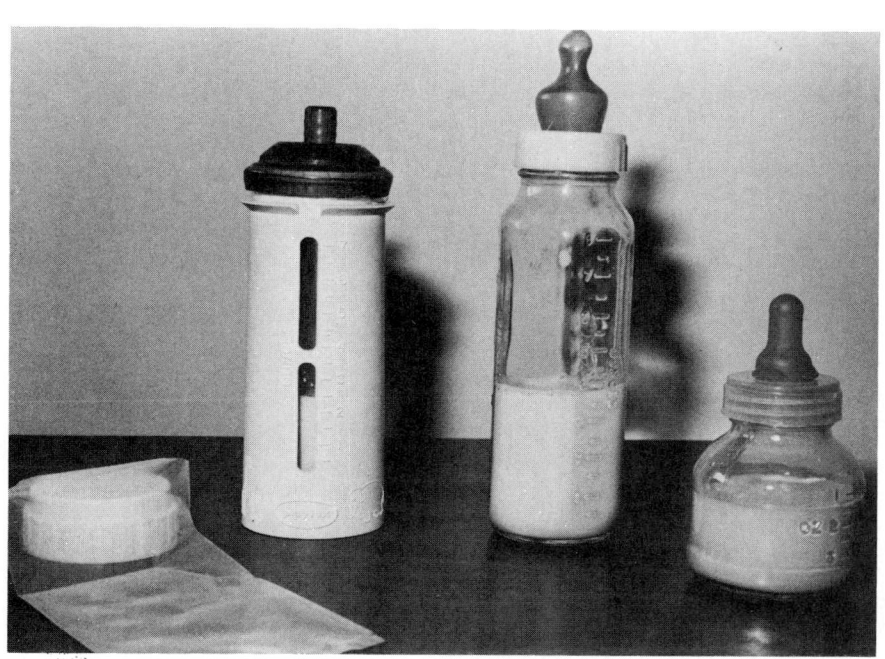

FIGURE 35-13

Types of bottles and nipples. (*From left to right*) A disposable bag and nipple cover; the bottle and nipple that are used with the disposable bag; regular bottle with Nuk nipple; and ready-to-feed bottle with standard nipple.

must in the past. Some recent studies have shown that formulas that are prepared at home and sterilized are frequently contaminated.[40] Many physicians are no longer insisting that bottles or formulas be sterilized if there is an uncontaminated water source and good refrigeration, and if hands and equipment are cleaned properly, since this clean technique is proving to be as safe as sterilization. There was no higher incidence of illness or infection when infants were fed formula prepared by the clean technique than when infants were fed formula prepared by terminal sterilization.[41]

There are four basic methods of formula preparation (Table 35-4). Points common to all methods of preparation are the following:

1. Hands should be washed well before starting.
2. If canned milk is used, the top of the can should be washed with soap and water using friction and then rinsed thoroughly. Hot water can be poured over the top just before opening.
3. All equipment should be washed thoroughly in warm soapy water. A bottle and nipple brush should be used and water should be squeezed through the nipple to make sure no milk particles or residue remain. Equipment should be rinsed thoroughly so all soap or detergent is gone.
4. Opened cans of formula or milk should be covered with fresh foil or plastic wrap, placed in the refrigerator, and used within 48 hours.

One Bottle Method. The one bottle method is the method recommended in the pamphlet *Infant Care*, put out by the Children's Bureau of HEW.[42] According to these recommendations, a concentrated prepared infant formula is poured directly into the bottle once the four steps mentioned above are carried out. One half of the total amount of formula desired is measured according to the markings on the bottle. For example, if 4 ounces of formula are needed, 2 ounces of concentrated formula would be used. Assuming a safe water supply, an equal amount of fresh tap water is added. The formula in the bottle should be fed to the infant within 30 minutes of the time it is made. If it is not used within an hour, it should be discarded.

Clean Method. The major difference between the clean method and the one bottle method is that in the former the whole day's formula is prepared at one time. The bottles should be refrigerated immediately after preparation.

Since some physicians still recommend sterilization and since some people still live under conditions in which sterilization is necessary, the aseptic method and terminal sterilization are included in this discussion.

Aseptic Method. In this method, the bottles, nipples, nipple caps, and equipment used in making the formula are sterilized before the formula is prepared. The mother will need a glass or enamel pitcher in which

TABLE 35-4

Formula Preparation Using Concentrated Formula

One Bottle Method	Clean Method	Aseptic Method	Terminal Sterilization
1. Open can of concentrated formula, pour ½ of total amount desired into bottle.	1. Same as one bottle method, but prepare day's supply at one time.	1. Equipment includes glass or enamel pitcher, measuring cup and spoons, mixing spoons, funnel, can opener, tongs.	1. Prepare as in clean method.
2. Add equal amount of fresh tap water from safe source.	2. Refrigerate immediately after preparation.	2. Sterilize bottles, nipples, nipple caps, and equipment by boiling for 10 minutes in pan or sterilizer half full of water.	2. Apply nipples and caps loosely.
3. Feed within 30 minutes of preparation.		3. Mix formula in pitcher.	3. Place in sterilizer with water in bottom and cover with tight-fitting lid.
4. Discard if not used within 1 hour.		4. Pour into bottles.	4. Boil for 25 minutes.
		5. Put on nipples and caps. Refrigerate until needed.	5. Tighten nipple collars.
			6. Refrigerate until needed.

For all methods start by washing hands, formula can top, bottles, nipples, and equipment well.
Ready-to-feed and powdered formula can be prepared by any of the above methods.
Ready-to-feed formula needs no water or mixing.
For powdered formula follow directions on can for proportions.

Infant and Mother Who Are Bottle-Feeding

Nursing Objectives

1. Identify mother's needs for information and assistance with infant feeding.
2. Provide information and assistance to promote a satisfying feeding experience for mother and baby.
3. Maintain infant's hydration and nutritional status.

Assessment	Potential Nursing Diagnosis	Planning/Intervention	Evaluation
Mother's past infant feeding experiences Decision to bottle-feed Mother's handling of infant Infant's feeding reflexes and responsiveness	Knowledge deficit about infant feeding related to lack of information and experience	Provide information as needed regarding: Newborn sucking reflexes Handling infant during feeding Assist mother with feeding process:	Mother expresses understanding of infant feeding process
	Alteration in nutrition, less than body requirements related to inadequate caloric intake Alteration in nutrition, more than body requirements related to excess caloric intake Potential fluid volume deficit related to inadequate fluid intake	Comfortable positioning of mother and infant Placing nipple in baby's mouth Checking flow of milk Keeping nipple full Provide anticipatory guidance: How much formula infant needs Types of formula, bottles, nipples Preparation of formula Answer mother's questions regarding: Hunger cries Burping Regurgitation Hiccups Constipation Introduction of solid foods Distribute literature as appropriate	Infant receives appropriate amount of formula at appropriate rate with minimal amount of air Infant's weight gain is appropriate Infant is well hydrated and well nourished

to mix the formula, a measuring cup, measuring spoons, tablespoon (to mix the formula), funnel (depending on the size of the bottle mouth), can opener (if canned milk is used), and some kind of tongs that can be sterilized. The tongs will be used as a forceps to handle the equipment. These items, together with the bottles, caps, and nipples, are placed in a large pan or sterilizer half full of water and boiled vigorously for 10 minutes. The equipment and the bottles, nipples, and so on may be done separately if the sterilizer cannot accommodate such a large load. Care should be taken to place the forceps in such a way that the mother can reach the handles easily after sterilization without burning her hand and contaminating the water when she picks them up. After sterilization the formula is made according to directions. A specific amount of the formula is put into each bottle. The bottles are then nippled, capped, and refrigerated.

Terminal Sterilization. In this method, the formula is prepared under a clean but not aseptic technique. The equipment, bottles, nipples, and nipple caps are washed thoroughly but are not sterilized. The formula is prepared and poured into the bottles, and the nipples and the caps are applied loosely. They then are placed in the sterilizer, covered with a tight-fitting lid, and sterilized by having the water boil rapidly in the bottom of the sterilizer for 25 minutes. In this method, formula, bottles, nipples, and protectors are all sterilized in one operation. Before the formula is refrigerated, the screw collar should be made secure.

Evaluation

To evaluate nursing care of the formula-fed infant, the nurse might ask the mother to verbalize her understanding of the infant feeding process. She would observe whether or not the mother holds the infant for feeding and assumes a comfortable position. She would also evaluate the infant's response to feeding and verify that the infant receives an appropriate amount at an appropriate rate without swallowing a large amount of air.

Nursing Care Related to Common Concerns in Infant Feeding

There are several topics related to infant feeding that are of concern to the new mother regardless of the method of feeding.

Hunger

The mother may wonder how she can tell if her infant is getting enough to eat. She can be told that most babies when awakened from sleep by hunger "pains" will fuss and cry and make sucking movements with their mouths, but that at first the infant may have difficulty distinguishing between hunger and other discomforts. If the baby awakens a short time after a feeding, the mother should try other comfort measures, such as holding, changing the diaper, and bubbling, before assuming he is hungry. Occasionally a baby appears hungry when in reality he is only thirsty and will be satisfied with a small amount of water. If he is obviously hungry and crying, refuses water with apparent disgust, and when a feeding is offered seizes the nipple ravenously and nurses with great vigor, he may need to eat more frequently for a while if he is breast-fed or be offered more in his bottle at each feeding if he is bottle-fed.

Bubbling (Burping)

After 5 minutes or so, or in the middle and at the end of each feeding, the infant should be held in an upright position and his back *gently* patted or stroked (Fig. 35-14). Pounding the baby on the back vigorously is neither effective for bubbling him nor conducive to his well-being. The change in position (from semi-reclining to upright) is an important factor in eliciting a bubble. Often holding the infant upright and pressing him against the breast is all that is necessary.

An alternate position is for the mother to sit the infant up on her lap, with his chest resting on her hand and his chin supported by her thumb and index finger, while she pats him with her other hand. A third position is to place the infant prone over her knees with the knee nearest the infant's head elevated slightly. The last two positions are sometimes preferred by nurses in the newborn nursery because they keep the infant away from the nurse's face and hair (Figs. 35-15 and 35-16).

Because the new infant's gastrointestinal tract is labile, milk may be eructated with the gas bubbles. A diaper is usually kept in front of the infant while he is being bubbled, in case this occurs (see Fig. 35-14). If there is doubt about whether or not the infant has brought up all the air when he is placed in his crib, putting him on his right side or in a prone position will help bring up the air and also prevent the infant from choking on any milk that might be regurgitated with the air.

Regurgitation

Regurgitation, which is merely an overflow and often occurs after nursing, should not be confused with vomiting, which may occur at any time, is accompanied by other symptoms, and usually involves a more complete emptying of the stomach. This regurgitation is the means of relieving the distended stomach and usually indicates that the baby either has taken too much food or has taken it too rapidly.

Hiccups

Some mothers need reassurance that hiccups are not unusual for infants and really do not seem to bother them. If the mother is disturbed, she can try giving the infant a few sips of water, but the hiccups go away by themselves without treatment.

Constipation

Constipation is almost nonexistent in breast-fed babies and is uncommon in those fed commercially prepared formulas, but mothers frequently express concern about possible constipation. Many parents believe that an infant is constipated if he misses having a bowel movement one day. The nurse can explain that it is quality

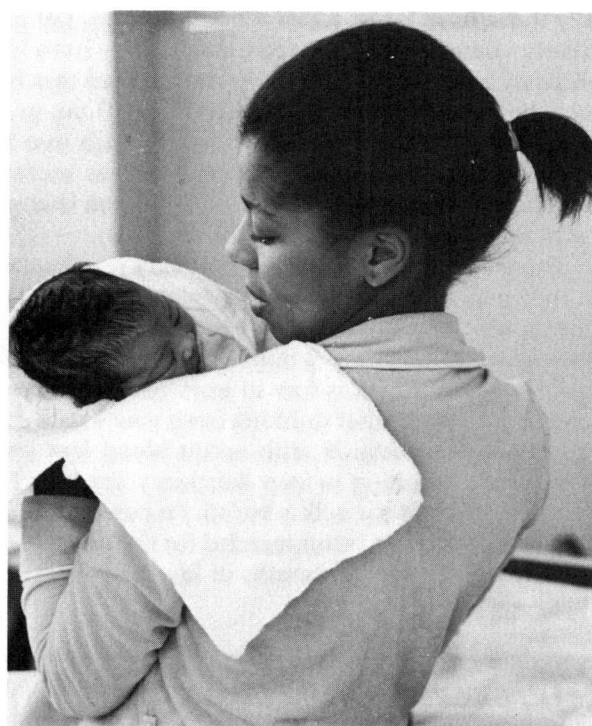

FIGURE 35-14

One method of bubbling or burping an infant is to place him in an upright position over the shoulder where he can be pressed against the breast.

not frequency of the stool that indicates the presence of constipation. An infant is considered to be constipated when the stools are hard, formed, and difficult to pass.

Nutritional Considerations During the First Year

Diets for infants are sometimes based on temporary scientific fashions or local customs. Long-term effects of infant diets are not known. Standards for formulas and baby foods are based on infant growth, but it is not known whether a diet that is optimum for growth in infancy will offer freedom from allergy, obesity, arterial disease, or cancer later in adult life.

During the first year of life the infant's growth exceeds that of any future period. In the first 4 months he usually doubles his birth weight and may triple it by 1 year. Watching the infant grow is pleasing to the parents, and they often see the chubbiness of the infant as evidence of good health and their good parenting. This attitude can lead to overfeeding.

The infant's caloric needs per unit of body weight are relatively constant during the first year. This is because as he becomes more physically active from the

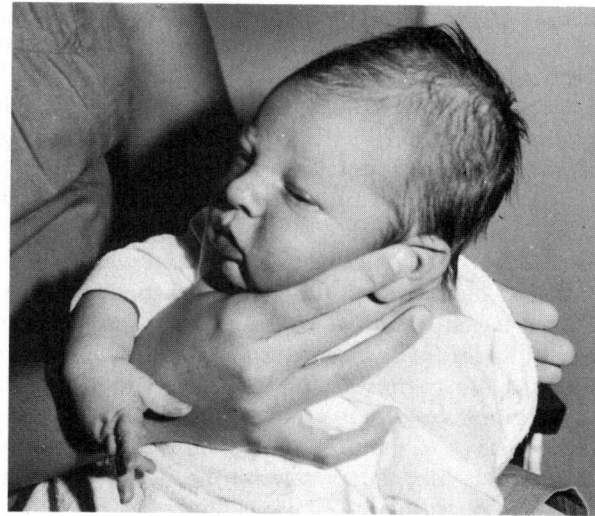

FIGURE 35-15

When bubbling the infant in the nursery, the nurse sits the infant up in her lap, with his chest resting on her hand and his chin supported by her thumb and index finger.

fourth month on, his rate of growth is slowing down, and energy is relocated from growth to activity.

Introduction of Solid Foods

The time for adding solid foods is an area in which recommendations in the literature and actual practice often differ markedly. Although an adequate amount of all essential nutrients can be provided during the first 6 months without the addition of solids, many babies in the United States are receiving solid foods before they are a month old.[43] This early feeding often occurs because the parents request it, thinking it will help the

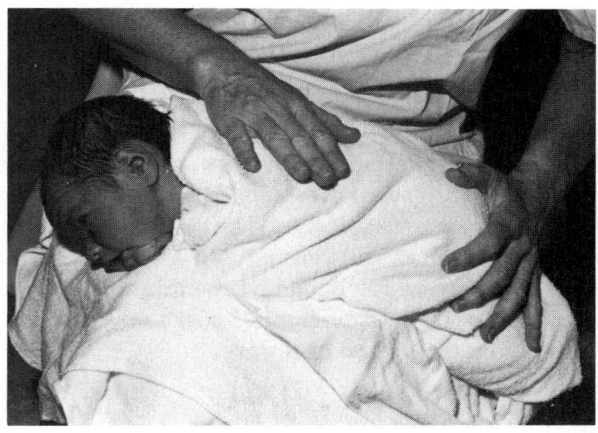

FIGURE 35-16

For an alternate method of bubbling, the infant is placed over the knees while his back is gently rubbed.

baby sleep through the night or considering it a sign that he is more advanced than infants who are "only taking milk."

There are many reasons suggested for delaying the introduction of solids until the infant is 4 to 6 months old. First, the baby is not developmentally ready to deal with nonliquid foods until about the end of the third month, and his tongue will usually push them out of the mouth. Also, the large protein molecules from the foods may pass through the mucosa of the infant's immature gastrointestinal tract and become antigens, sensitizing the infant and causing allergic reactions. After 6 months the gastrointestinal system is more mature and the infant's antibody production has reached a more desirable level. In the breast-fed infant, early introduction of solids may interfere with the desire for breast milk, decreasing the infant's sucking and subsequently decreasing the milk supply. Other drawbacks to early feeding of solids are the potential for not supplying the infant's nutritional needs, the relatively high cost of the food, and the possibility of overfeeding.

Infantile obesity has become a growing concern in recent years because of its possible relation to adult obesity. Growth during infancy is mostly due to cell hyperplasia (tissue growth involving increases in the number of cells). It is felt that the obese infant will have more fat cells than normal throughout life and therefore be more prone to continuing obesity.[44]

Some suggestions for avoiding infant obesity are as follows:

1. Help parents use factors other than weight gain to evaluate their role as parents.
2. Help mothers discover the infant's satiety behavior and avoid encouraging the infant to get down the last drop or bite.
3. Encourage practices that promote more physical activities in infants.
4. Avoid early introduction of solids.

Nutritional Supplements

Vitamins

Woodruff states that since both breast milk and prepared formulas contain adequate vitamins for normal infants, routine supplementation should be abandoned.[36] However, some sources still recommend a vitamin D supplement for breast-fed babies. If the infant is on a formula made of fresh or evaporated cow's milk, a vitamin C supplement might be necessary.

Iron

Iron deficiency anemia is currently the most common specific nutritional deficiency encountered. Infants and children between the ages of 6 and 30 months, especially those from lower socioeconomic groups, are particularly vulnerable. Breast-fed infants rarely have iron deficiency anemia and it is now recommended that formulas be fortified with iron at a level of 10 mg to 12 mg/liter. Infant cereal has been fortified with iron for a long time, but the form of iron used was recently found to be poorly absorbed and has now been changed to a more absorbable form in most cereals.

These sources of iron would probably be adequate, but they may not continue to be available to the infant as he grows older. By the age of 6 months many infants are switched to fresh cow's milk. This causes two problems. First, cow's milk is low in iron. Second, there is increasing evidence that drinking fresh cow's milk during infancy is associated with occult blood loss from the intestine, resulting in iron deficiency anemia. The latter is less likely if the milk is boiled. Prepared formulas fortified with iron are recommended for the non-breast-fed baby for the first 12 months of life.[36]

References

1. Neumann CC, Jelliffe DB: Foreword: Symposium on Nutrition in Pediatrics. Pediatr Clin North Am 24(1):1, February 1977
2. Smith C, Nelson N: The Physiology of the Newborn Infant. Springfield, IL, Charles C Thomas, 1979
3. Jelliffe DB, Jelliffe EFP: Current concepts in nutrition: Breast is best; Modern meanings. N Engl J Med 912–915, October 27, 1977
4. Nichols BL, Nichols VN: The biologic basis of lactation. Compr Ther 4(10):63–70, October 1978
5. Grams KE: Breast feeding: A means of imparting immunity? MCN 3(6):340–344, November/December 1978
6. Hayward AR: The immunology of breast milk. In Neville MC, Neifert MR (eds): Lactation-Physiology, Nutrition, and Breast-Feeding, pp 249–266. New York, Plenum Press, 1983
7. Gunther M: The value of breast feeding. In Early Nutrition and Later Development. Chicago, Year Book Medical Publishers, 1976
8. Gerard A: Please Breast-feed Your Baby, chap 7. New York, Hawthorn Books, 1970
9. Worthington-Roberts BS, Vermeersch J, Williams SR: Nutrition in Pregnancy and Lactation, 3rd ed, p 348. St Louis, Times Mirror/CV Mosby, 1985
10. Dutton MA: A breastfeeding protocol. JOGN 8(3):151–155, May/June 1979
11. Lawson B: Perception of degrees of support for the breast-feeding mother. BFJ 3:2, Summer 1976
12. Johnson NW: Breast feeding at one hour of age. MCN 121:12–16, January/February 1976
13. Neville MC, Allen JC, Watters C: The mechanisms of milk secretion. In Neville MC, Neifert MR (eds): Lactation-Physiology, Nutrition, and Breast-Feeding, pp 49–92. New York, Plenum Press, 1983
14. Neville MC: Regulation of mammary development and

lactation. In Neville MC, Neifert MR (eds): Lactation-Physiology, Nutrition, and Breast-Feeding, pp 103–133. New York, Plenum Press, 1983

15. Jelliffe DB, Jelliffe EFP: Human Milk in the Modern World, p 30. Oxford, Oxford University Press, 1978
16. Lawrence RA: Breastfeeding—A Guide for the Medical Profession, p 47. St Louis, CV Mosby, 1980
17. Brann AW Jr, Cefalo RC (eds): Guidelines for Perinatal Care. Chicago and Washington, American Academy of Pediatrics and American College of Obstetricians and Gynecologists, 1983
18. Countryman BA: Hospital care of the breastfed newborn. Am J Nurs 71:2365–2367, December 1971
19. L'Esperance C, Frantz K: Time limitation for early breastfeeding. JOGN Nurs 14(2):114–118, March/April 1985
20. Iffrig SM: Nursing care and success in breast feeding. Nurs Clin North Am 3:353, June, 1968
21. Nichols MG: Effective help for the nursing mother. JOGN 7(2):22–30, March/April 1978
22. Frantz KB, Kalmen BA: Breastfeeding works for cesareans, too. RN, pp 39–47, December 1979
23. Frantz KB: Managing Nipple Problems. LaLeche League International, Inc, Reprint No. 11, March 1982
24. Haire D, Haire J: The nurse's contribution to successful breast-feeding; and The medical value of breast-feeding. Implementing Family Centered Maternity Care with a Central Nursery, New Jersey, ICEA
25. Whitley N: Preparation for breastfeeding. JOGN 7(3): 44–48, May/June 1978
26. Grassley J, Davis K: Common concerns of mothers who breastfeed. MCN 3(6):347–351, November/December 1978
27. Murdaugh A Sr, Miller LE: Helping the breast-feeding mother. Am J Nurs 72:1420–1423, August 1972
28. MacKeith R, Wood C: Infant Feeding and Feeding Difficulties. Edinburgh, Churchill Livingstone, 1977
29. Horning MG et al: Identification and quantification of drugs and drug metabolites in human breast milk using GC-MS-COM methods. In Modern Problems in Paediatrics—Milk and Lactation, pp 73–79. Basel, S. Karger, 1975
30. Rothermel BS, Faber MM: Drugs in breastmilk—A consumer's guide. BFJ 2(3):76–88, Summer 1975
31. Doucette JS: Is breast feeding still safe for babies? MCN 3(6):345–346, November/December 1978
32. Parsons LJ: Weaning from the breast. JOGN 7(3):12–15, May/June 1978
33. Broome ME: Breastfeeding and the working mother. JOGN Nurs 10(3):201–202, May/June 1985
34. Auerbach KG: Employed breastfeeding mothers: Problems they encounter. Birth 11(1):17–20, Spring 1984
35. American Academy of Pediatrics, Committee on Nutrition: Commentary on breast feeding and infant formulas, including proposed standards for formulas. Pediatrics 57:278–285, February 1976
36. Woodruff C: The science of infant nutrition and the art of infant feeding. JAMA 240(7):657–661, August 18, 1978
37. Brown MS, Murphy MA: Ambulatory Pediatrics for Nurses. New York, McGraw-Hill, 1975
38. Scahill MC: Helping the mother solve problems with

feeding her infant. JOGN 4(2):51–54, March/April 1975
39. Slattery J: Nutrition for the normal healthy infant. MCN 2(2):105–112, March/April 1977
40. Kendall V, Kusakcroglu: A study of preparation of infant formulas. Am J Dis Child 122:215, 1971
41. Hargrove T, Hargrove C: Formula preparation and infant illness. Clin Pediatr 13:1057, 1974
42. Children's Bureau, U.S. Department of Health, Education, and Welfare: Infant Care, p 11. Washington, DC, US Government Printing Office, 1973
43. Anderson TA, Fomon S: Beikost. In Infant Nutrition, 2nd ed. Philadelphia, WB Saunders, 1974
44. Parham E: The effect of early feeding on the development of obesity. JOGN 3(3):58–61, May/June 1975

Suggested Reading

Arafat I et al: Maternal Practice and Attitudes Toward Breastfeeding. JOGN 10(2):91–95, March/April 1981

Avery GB, Fletcher AB: Nutrition. In Avery GB (ed): Neonatology, 2nd ed. Philadelphia, JB Lippincott, 1981

Broome ME: Breast-feeding and the working mother. JOGN 10(3):201–202, May/June 1981

Cadwell K: Improving nipple graspability for success at breast-feeding. JOGN 10(4):277–279, July/August 1981

Foman SJ (ed): Infant Nutrition. Philadelphia, WB Saunders, 1974

Giacoia GP, Catz CS: Drugs and pollutants in breast milk. Clin Perinatol 6(1):181–196, March 1979

Hambraeus L: Proprietary milk vs human breast milk in infant feeding. Pediatr Clin North Am 24(1):17–35, February 1977

Jelliffe DB, Jelliffe EFP: Human Milk in the Modern World. New York, Oxford University Press, 1978

Lawrence RA: Breast-Feeding: A Guide for the Medical Profession. St Louis, CV Mosby, 1980

Lawrence RA (ed): Counseling the Mother on Breast-Feeding. Report of the Eleventh Ross Roundtable on Critical Approaches to Common Pediatric Problems. Columbus, Ohio, Ross Laboratories, 1980

L'Esperance CM: Pain or pleasure: The dilemma of early breast-feeding. BFJ 7(1):21–26, Spring 1980

Markesbery BA, Wong WM: Watching baby's diet: A professional and parental guide. MCN 4(3):177–180, May/June 1979

Marmet C, Shell E: Training neonates to suck correctly. MCN 9(6):401–407, November/December 1984

Riordan J, Countryman BA: Basics of breast-feeding. Parts I and II, JOGN 9(4):207–213, July/August, 1980; Parts III and IV, JOGN 9(5):273–283, September/October, 1980; Parts V and VI, JOGN 9(6):357–366, November/December 1980

Waletzky LR (ed): Symposium on Human Lactation. Rockville, MD, US Department of Health, Education, and Welfare, Bureau of Community Health Services, 1976

Worthington-Roberts B et al: Nutrition in Pregnancy and Lactation, 3rd ed, chaps 7 and 8. St Louis, CV Mosby, 1985

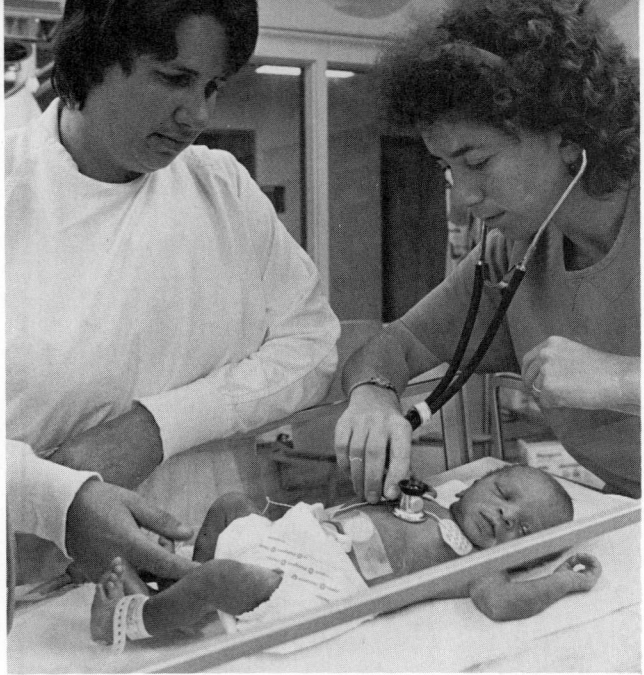

Unit VI:
Assessment and Management in the Postpartum Period

Conference Material

1. Discuss in detail the mechanisms by which lactation occurs, including hormonal preparation of the breasts, neurohormonal control of milk secretion and ejection, effects of noxious stimuli, and approaches to the suppression of lactation. What implications for nursing care can be found by understanding the physiology of this delicate mechanism?

2. Describe the patterns of return of menstruation and ovulation in nonlactating and lactating women. Include in your discussion anovulatory versus ovulatory menses, the influence of breast-feeding upon both ovulation and menstruation, and the risk of pregnancy with unprotected intercourse. How would you counsel a postpartum patient who was (a) not breast-feeding, and (b) one who was breast-feeding about what to expect regarding first menstruation and return of fertility?

3. A mother experienced a sudden postpartum hemorrhage after delivery and the infant had to be taken to the nursery immediately after birth. What assessments and interventions might you plan to aid in reinstituting the bonding process?

4. Rita R. delivered her second baby 3 days ago and is to be discharged home this afternoon. Mother and infant are healthy and have adapted well to each other during their hospital stay. Rita is breast-feeding and her milk just began to come in today. Her husband, who will take her home later, has been able to take 1 week off from work. Their child at home is 2½ years of age. You have set aside 30 minutes to counsel Rita about the first few weeks at home. What topics will you include in this discussion, and what key points will you make concerning each? How did you set priorities for these topics?

5. Elizabeth S. is an 18-year-old primipara who underwent a long but normal labor and delivery. She and her 20-year-old husband are fascinated with their new son, although neither have experience caring for children. On her second postpartum day, Elizabeth experiences severe discomfort from her large mediolateral episiotomy, to the point of not wanting to care for the baby. What measures will you initiate to promote her comfort? What will be the primary focus of your nursing care plans for the remainder of her hospital stay?

6. What approach would you use to help a mother who was undecided about whether or not to breast-feed her infant?

7. A mother tells the nurse that she wants to breast-feed her infant for 6 months to 8 months because she knows she can not become pregnant as long as she is nursing. What information should the nurse include in her reply?

8. A mother who is bottle-feeding tells the nurse she does not know anything about preparing formula so she thinks she will buy "ready-to-feed" formula that comes in bottles. What do you think about this plan? How can the nurse help her in choosing the type of formula to use and the method of preparation?

Multiple Choice

Read through the entire question and place your answer on the line to the right.
1. The principles found to be involved in bonding are
   A. There seems to be a species-specific response between the parents and infant when the infant is first given to them.
   B. The attachment process is structured around monotropy.
   C. The infant must give some signal with eye or body movements to the parents.
   D. Individuals who witness the birth process become strongly attached to the infant.
   E. There may be a sensitive period after the birth.
   F. It is difficult for parents to attach to an infant while mourning the loss or expected loss of another person.
   G. Some early events may have a long-lasting effect on the raising and caretaking of the infant.
   Select the number corresponding to the correct letter or letters.
   1. All but A
   2. All but B
   3. All but D
   4. All but E
   5. All of the above

2. Engrossment refers to
A. The infant becoming interested in moving objects and smiling faces
B. The parents' interest in their infant
C. The behavior noted in fathers when they are interacting with their infants
D. The behavior noted in mothers when they are interacting with their infants
Select the number corresponding to the correct letter or letters.
1. A only
2. B only
3. C only
4. C and D
5. A and B
6. All but A _____

3. Current research indicates that fathers who attend the birthing process
A. Feel a significant strengthening of the marital bond
B. Exhibit more loving behavior to their mates
C. Exhibit significantly more attachment behavior to their infants
D. Have significantly more desire to have more children
Select the number corresponding to the correct letter or letters
1. A only
2. C only
3. A and B
4. A and C
5. All of the above _____

4. Rubin's description of the tasks of mothering includes
A. Determining her relationship with her child
B. Identifying the child
C. Redefining her relationship with her husband
D. Guiding and restructuring the family constellation
Select the number corresponding to the correct letter or letters.
1. A only
2. B only
3. D only
4. All but D
5. All but C
6. All but A _____

5. To keep the nipples in good condition for breast-feeding, which of the following should be included in their daily care?
A. Wash with plain water once a day.
B. Air dry after each nursing period.
C. Wash with mild antiseptic solution prior to each feeding period.
D. Cover the nipples with clean plastic squares to avoid contamination.
E. If nipple is sore, discontinue breast-feeding until tenderness subsides.

Select the number corresponding to the correct letters.
1. A and B
2. A, C, and D
3. B, D, and E
4. All of the above _____

6. The young mother asks how she will know when her baby is hungry. Which of the following responses would be most appropriate for the nurse to give?
A. "All crying indicates hunger."
B. "Feed the baby whenever he is awake."
C. "He will cry, fret, and suck on anything in contact with his lips."
D. "Offer him water first; if he refuses the water, feed him." _____

7. How does the composition of mother's milk compare with cow's milk?
A. Human milk contains more whey protein.
B. Human milk contains more casein.
C. Human milk forms a tougher curd.
D. Human milk contains more carbohydrates.
E. Human milk contains less sodium.
Select the number corresponding to the correct letters.
1. A and C
2. A, D, and E
3. B, C, and D
4. All of the above _____

8. Which of the following is true of the let-down reflex?
A. It occurs unilaterally.
B. It is under voluntary control.
C. It is usually felt by the mother as a tingling or drawing sensation in the nipple.
D. It is not affected by external stimuli. _____

9. What is the principle underlying the concept of demand feedings for the newborn infant?
A. Maintaining a regular 4-hour schedule to establish eating habits
B. Feeding the infant every 2 hours to 3 hours to stimulate digestion
C. Fitting individual feedings to individual needs
D. Permissive feeding schedule causes less conflict with the mother's household activities
E. More frequent feedings ensure an adequate nutritional intake. _____

10. Identify the statement that *best* describes taste perception in the newborn.
A. Newborns possess fine taste acuity, which develops *in utero.*
B. Newborns possess an innate preference for sweet substances.
C. Newborns are unable to differentiate sweet taste from bitter taste. _____

11. The proliferation of human brain cells occurs during the
A. First half of pregnancy
B. Second half of pregnancy

C. First six months of life
D. Second six months of life   ____

12. The most important benefit of vestibular stimulation in the normal newborn is improvement of
A. Sucking capability
B. Tactile sensitivity
C. Motor coordination
D. Attention span   ____

13. The nurse is conducting a parenting class in the postpartum unit. Based on an understanding of the newborn's sensory needs, mothers could be advised to
A. Continuously rock their newborns during feeding
B. Stroke their newborns from toe to head daily
C. Provide auditory stimulation for 10 minutes each hour
D. Sing to infants in the *en face* position   ____

Discussion

14. The removal of the inhibitory effect of which two hormones, in the presence of continued secretion of which other hormone, are keys to the initiation of lactation?

15. Why is it important for mother, father, and newborn to spend some time together privately during the first hour after birth?

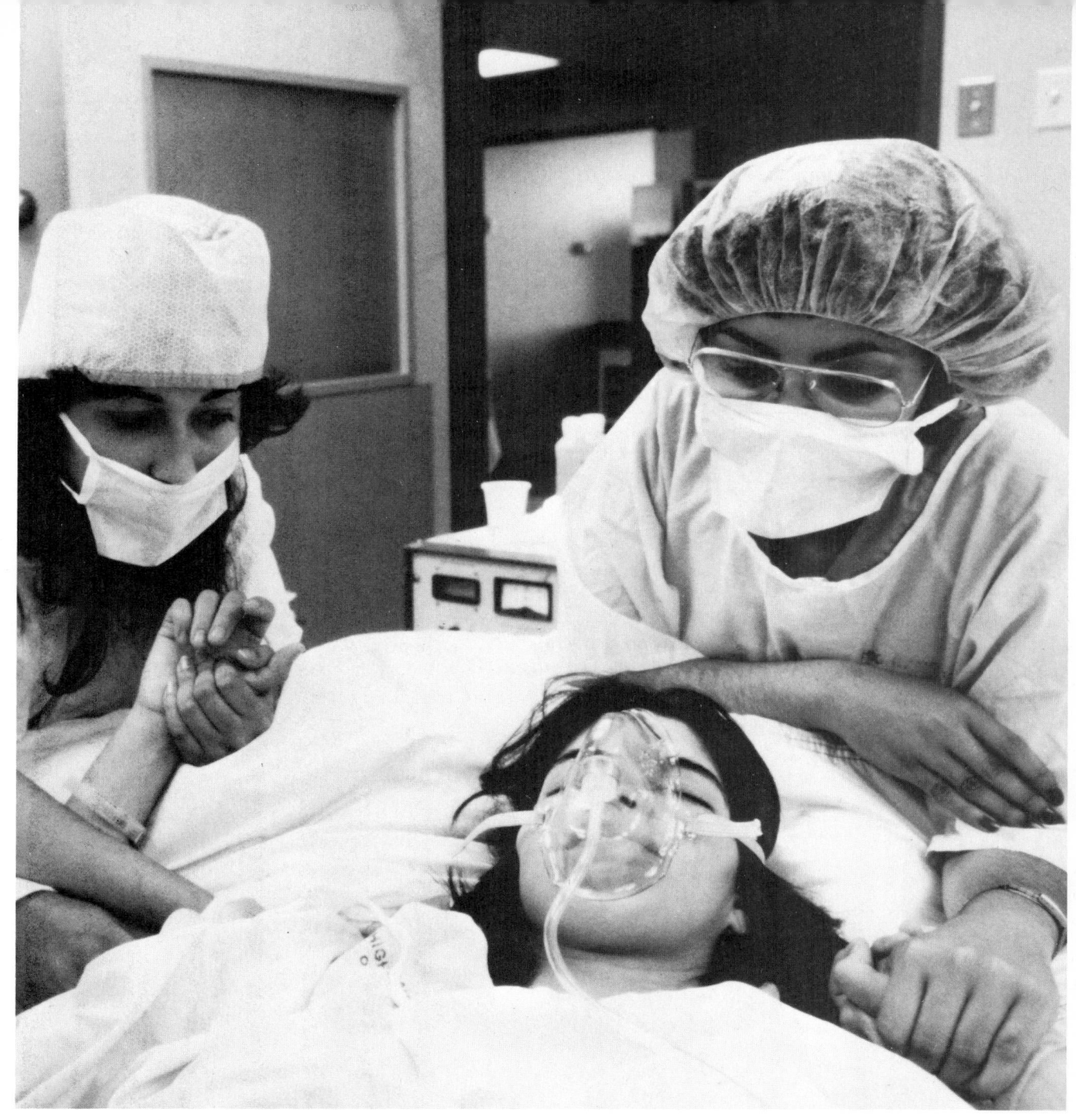

UNIT VII

Assessment and Management of Maternal Disorders

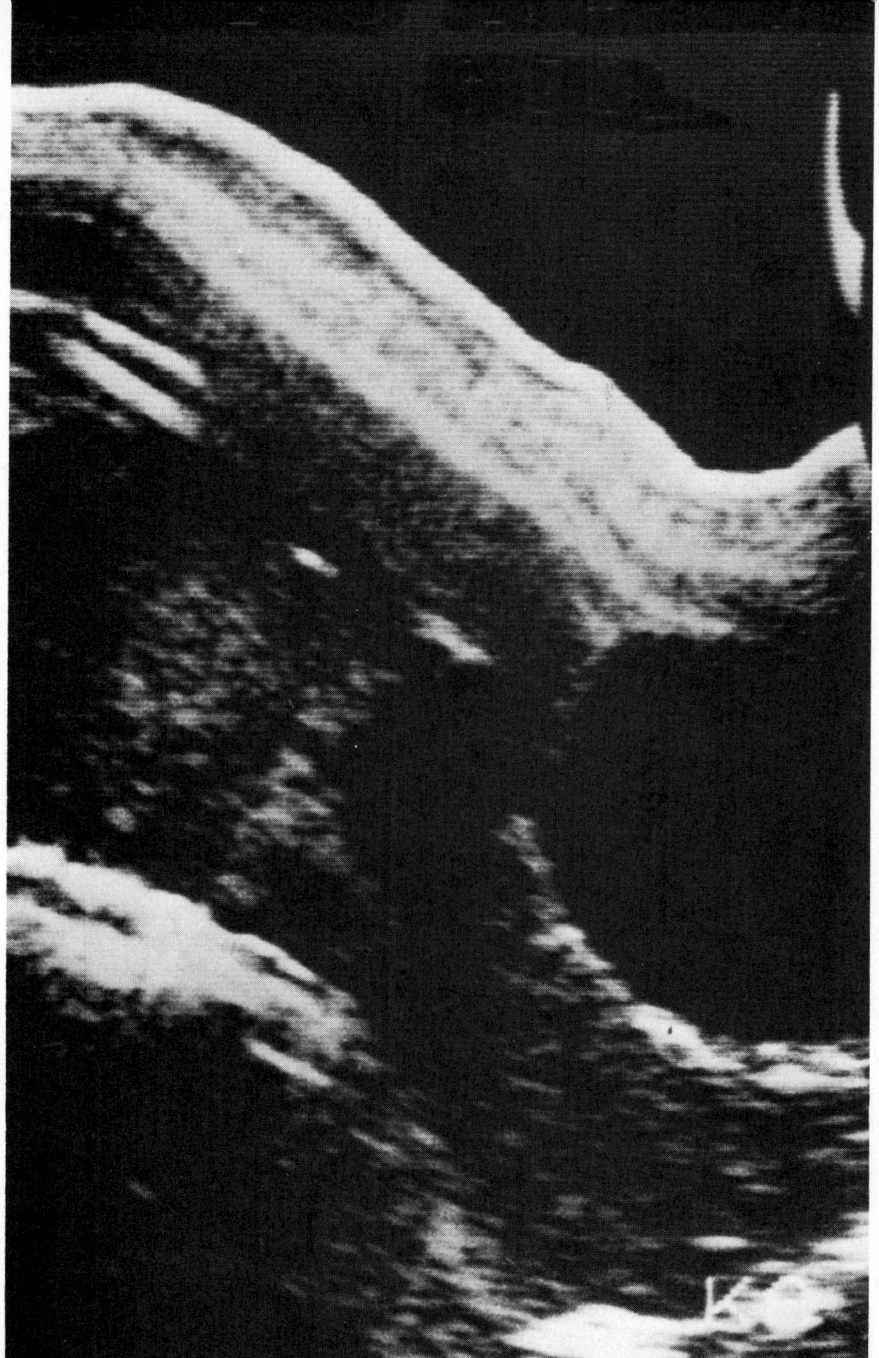

CHAPTER 36

Complications of Pregnancy

From a biologic point of view, childbearing is considered a normal process. Nevertheless, the borderline between health and illness is less distinct at this time because of the numerous physiological adaptations that occur during the course of pregnancy. The well-being of mother and unborn child is enhanced by the existence of a healthy maternal condition prior to conception and the early and continued provision of health supervision during pregnancy. Regular prenatal care is of paramount importance for achieving a good perinatal outcome, since it makes possible the early detection of the warning signals of potential, unexpected alteration from the normal course of pregnancy. Serious problems can be averted or controlled by preventive care, client education, and implementation of appropriate interventions.

Certain "common complaints" are experienced by most expectant mothers to some degree. These are the so-called minor discomforts of pregnancy, which in themselves are not serious but detract from the mother's feeling of well-being. Since these discomforts are usually related to physiological changes occurring within the mother's body and are not in themselves pathologic, they have been included in the chapter on antepartal care (see Chap. 22).

Pregnancy-related maternal disorders are divided into two broad categories: complications related to the pregnancy itself and not seen at other times, and diseases that are not pregnancy related but occur coincidentally. The latter may arise in the nonpregnant woman as well, but when they occur during pregnancy they may complicate the pregnancy and influence its course or may be aggravated by the pregnancy. Such conditions are considered in Chapter 37.

There are only a few major complications that result from pregnancy, but these may present serious health hazards. These complications, which will be considered here, include the following: hemorrhagic conditions of early pregnancy, hyperemesis gravidarum, hemorrhagic complications of placental origin in late pregnancy, and hypertensive disorders of pregnancy.

Hemorrhagic Complications of Early Pregnancy

The causes of bleeding in pregnancy are usually considered in relation to the stage of gestation in which they are most likely to cause complications. Frequent causes of bleeding during the first half of pregnancy are abortion, ectopic pregnancy, and hydatidiform mole. The two most common causes of hemorrhage in the latter half of pregnancy are placenta previa and abruptio placentae.

Abortion

Definitions

Abortion is the termination of pregnancy at any time before the fetus has attained a stage of viability (*i.e.*, before it is capable of extrauterine existence). The term *miscarriage* is commonly used by lay persons to denote an abortion that has occurred spontaneously rather than one which has been induced. Since *abortion* is the accepted medical term for either, this point should be clarified in discussions with clients, to avoid confusion or misinterpretation. In medical parlance the word miscarriage is rarely employed. Spontaneous abortions occur in about 10% to 20% of all pregnancies.

It is customary to use the weight of the fetus as an important criterion in abortion. Modern advances in the management and care of preterm infants have made it possible for smaller and smaller infants to survive, so it is now not uncommon for infants weighing less than 750 g (1 lb 10½ oz) to survive. For this reason many authorities now maintain that fetal weight of 1000 g or less but more than 500 g is classified as *immature* and that fetal weight of 500 g (about 20 weeks of gestation) or less constitutes an *abortion*. In many states a birth certificate is prepared for any pregnancy terminating beyond the 20th week of gestation or when the fetus weighs 500 g or more. It is obvious, therefore, that how the termination of pregnancy is classified in different hospitals depends wholly on the interpretation to which they subscribe.

A preterm infant is one born after the stage of viability has been reached but before it has the same chance for survival as a full-term infant. By general consensus, an infant that weighs 2500 g or less at birth is termed *preterm;* one that weighs 2501 g (5½ lb) or more is regarded as *full term.*

It is important to remember that preterm labor does not refer to abortion. *Preterm labor* is the termination of pregnancy after the fetus is viable but before it has attained full term. Although the cause of many preterm labors cannot be explained, the condition can be brought on by maternal diseases such as chronic hypertensive vascular disease, abruptio placentae, placenta previa, untreated syphilis, congenital uterine anomalies, or a mechanical defect in the cervix.

Types of Abortions. The term *abortion* includes many varieties of termination of pregnancy prior to viability but may be subdivided into two main groups, spontaneous and induced.

Spontaneous abortion is one in which the process starts of its own accord through natural causes. *Induced abortion* is one that is artificially induced whether for therapeutic or other reasons. Induced abortion has been considered in Chapter 15.

Threatened Abortion. An abortion is regarded as threatened if vaginal bleeding or spotting occurs in early pregnancy. This may or may not be associated with mild cramps. The cervix is closed. The process has presumably started but may abate. Some threatened abortions have resulted in actual abortion of one embryo from an undiagnosed twin gestation while the other embryo continued its growth and development.

Inevitable Abortion. Inevitable abortion is so called because the process has gone so far that termination of the pregnancy cannot be prevented. Bleeding is copious, and the pains are severe. The membranes may or may not have ruptured, and the cervical canal is dilating.

Incomplete Abortion. An incomplete abortion is one in which part of the products of conception has been passed, but part (usually the placenta) is retained in the uterus. Bleeding usually persists until the retained products of conception have been passed.

Complete Abortion. Complete abortion is the expulsion of all the products of conception.

Missed Abortion. In a missed abortion the fetus dies in the uterus but is retained. The woman often experiences a regression in uterine growth and breast changes. If 6 weeks or more elapse between fetal death and expulsion, the fetus may undergo marked degenerative changes. Of these, maceration, or general softening, is the most common. Occasionally it dries up into a leatherlike structure (mummification), and very rarely it is converted into stony material (lithopedion formation). Symptoms, except for amenorrhea, are usually lacking, but occasionally such clients complain of malaise, headache, and anorexia. Hypofibrinogenemia, a hemorrhagic complication, may result.

Missed abortions are often discovered when there is no increase in fundal height between prenatal visits or when fetal heart tones become absent.

Habitual Abortion. Habitual abortion is a condition in which spontaneous abortion occurs in successive pregnancies (three or more). This is a most distressing condition; some women have had six or eight spontaneous abortions.

Illegal Abortion. An illegal abortion is the termination of pregnancy outside of appropriate medical facilities (hospital or clinic), generally by nonphysician abortionists, regardless of the validity of the indication. Standards of abortion care are questionable and follow-up is often not provided. The frequency of such abortions is not precisely known, but has dropped precipitously in the United States following the Supreme Court decision of 1973.

Attempts at producing illegal abortion are generally made by the ingestion of drugs such as quinine or castor oil, which usually do nothing or, if taken in sufficient quantities to produce an abortion, place the woman in serious jeopardy.

Another common approach involves the placement of a foreign body, such as a urethral catheter, into the uterus with or without the instillation of toxic substances. Severe infection, often with shock and renal failure, is a common consequence of such crude efforts at pregnancy termination. Women so affected are some of the most critically ill that the nurse may ever have to care for, and, unfortunately, they sometimes die in spite of the best efforts of all concerned.

Manifestations and Causes

Clinical Picture.
About 75% of all spontaneous abortions occur during the second and third months of pregnancy (*i.e.*, before the 12th week). The condition is very common; it is estimated that about one pregnancy in every eight to ten terminates in spontaneous abortion. Almost invariably the first symptom is bleeding due to the separation of the fertilized ovum from its uterine attachment. The bleeding is often slight at the beginning and may persist for days before uterine cramps occur, or the bleeding may be followed at once by cramps. Occasionally the bleeding is torrential, leaving the woman in shock. The uterine contractions bring about softening and dilatation of the cervix and either complete or incomplete expulsion of the products of conception.

Causes.
The etiology of spontaneous abortion is varied and often is nature's way of extinguishing imperfect embryos. Indeed, careful microscopic study of the ma-

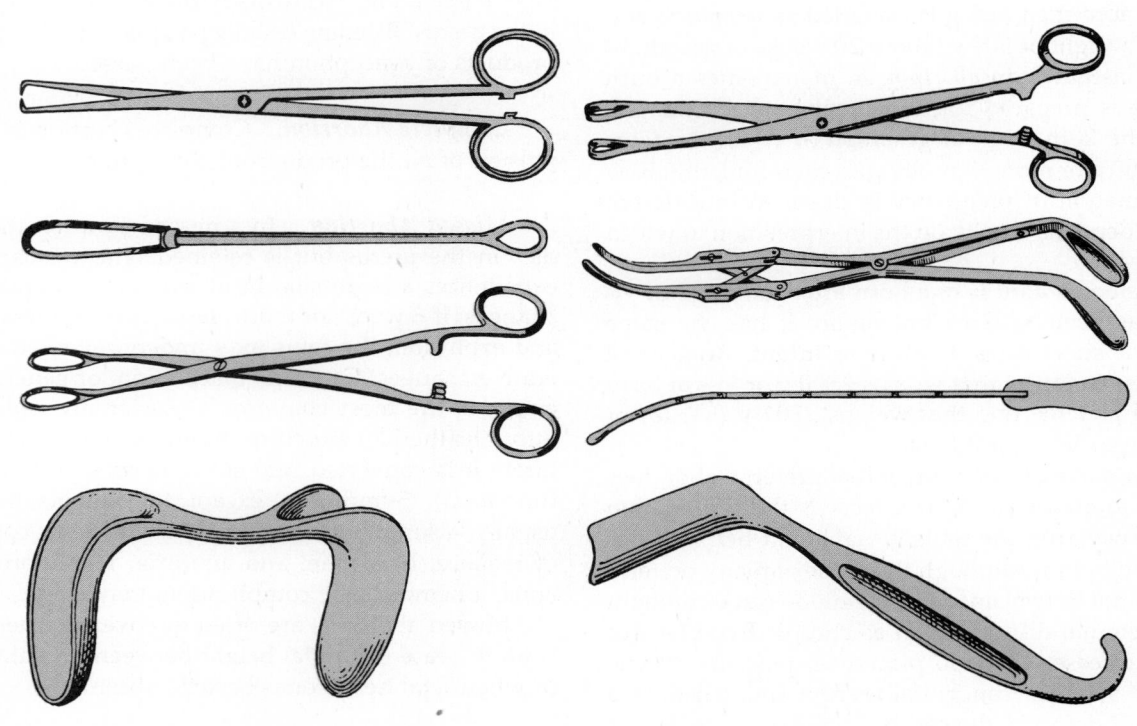

FIGURE 36-1

(*Left, top to bottom*) Bullet forceps used in grasping the lips of the cervix. Sims's sharp curet, a scraper or spoonlike instrument for removing matter from the walls of the uterus. Sponge holder. Sims's speculum for inserting into the vaginal canal so as to expose the cervix to view. (*Right, top to bottom*) Placental forceps with heart-shaped jaws. Modified Goodell–Ellinger dilator used for enlarging the canal of the cervix. Uterine sound. Schroeder vaginal refractor for drawing back the vulvar or vaginal walls during an operation.

terial passed in these cases shows that the most common cause of spontaneous abortion is an inherent defect in the products of conception. This defect may express itself in an abnormal embryo, an abnormal trophoblast, or both abnormalities.

In early abortions, 80% are associated with some defect of the embryo or trophoblast that is either incompatible with life or would result in a grossly deformed child. The incidence of abnormalities after the second month is somewhat lower but not less than 50%. It is usually difficult, if not impossible, to determine whether the germ plasm of the spermatozoon or the ovum is at fault in these cases.

Abortions of this sort are obviously not preventable; however, although they are often bitterly disappointing to the parents, they do serve a useful purpose.

Spontaneous abortions may result from causes other than defects in the products of conception. Severe acute infections, such as pneumonia, pyelitis, and typhoid fever, often lead to abortion. Endocrine disorders affecting progesterone and estrogen levels may alter the endometrial lining of the uterus and result in abortion. Occasionally, abnormalities of the generative tract, such as a congenitally short cervix or uterine malformations, produce the accident. Abortion is common in women whose mothers were treated with diethylstilbestrol (DES) during pregnancy. Retroposition of the uterus rarely causes abortion, as was formerly believed. Many women tend to explain abortion as a result of an injury or excessive activity. Women exhibit the greatest variation in this respect. In some the pregnancy may go blithely on despite falls from second-story windows and automobile accidents severe enough to fracture the pelvis. In others a trivial fall, anxiety, or overfatigue may appear to be related to abortion, but there is obviously no way to determine a cause–effect relationship.

Medical Diagnosis and Prognosis

Determination of the cause of vaginal bleeding in early pregnancy is essential for accurate diagnosis. The vagina and cervix are carefully inspected to ascertain possible causes of the bleeding and to determine if the cervix is dilated.

Through the use of ultrasound techniques it is now possible to differentiate between a live fetus and a pregnancy that will end inevitably in spontaneous abortion. Prognosis is evaluated by ultrasound markers that can explain bleeding and distinguish between harmless and ominous blood loss. The accompanying clinical symptoms of pelvic cramping and low back pain are suggestive of spontaneous abortion. Bleeding is usually observed first, and a few hours, sometimes days, later uterine contractions ensue.

In women in whom bleeding is scant and does not extend beyond 3 days and the ultrasound scan is normal, the risk of pregnancy failure is lower than in women who bleed for 3 days or more and have at least one abnormality on ultrasound examination.[1] Epidemiologic studies have revealed that the risk of spontaneous premature birth or the term delivery of a low-birth-weight infant is significantly correlated with threatened abortion.[2] Additional associated maternal complications incude preeclampsia, placenta previa, abruptio placentae, and breech delivery.

Medical Management

The pregnant woman should be instructed to contact her physician or midwife whenever bleeding occurs during pregnancy. The client may be kept at home, and bed rest and sexual abstinence are prescribed. Occasionally sedatives are ordered to promote relaxation. If bleeding becomes copious and is accompanied by cramps or uterine contractions, hospitalization is recommended. Intravenous therapy for fluid replacement or blood transfusions are prescribed as necessary.

In cases of incomplete abortion, efforts are ordinarily made to aid the uterus in emptying its contents. Since there is a danger of maternal hemorrhage, oxytocin may be administered, but if this is ineffectual, surgical removal of the retained products of conception should be done promptly. Active bleeding may make this urgently necessary. Many times the tissue is loose in the cervical canal and can simply be lifted out with ovum forceps; otherwise, dilatation and curettage of the uterine cavity or vacuum extraction may be necessary. The instruments commonly used in completing an incomplete abortion are shown in Figures 36-1 and 36-2. The suction curet may also be used.

In cases of missed abortion the products of conception are often spontaneously expelled within 4 to 5 weeks of fetal death. If this does not occur, hospitalization for surgical removal of the abortus is indicated. The administration of Rh₀D immune globulin (RhoGAM) within 72 hours following the abortion is indicated for Rh-negative women who have not been previously sensitized.

If evidence of infection is present (*e.g.*, fever, foul discharge, or suspicious history of illegal abortion), evacuation of the uterus should be delayed only long enough to obtain appropriate studies (especially smears and cultures) and to initiate antibiotic therapy. Such prompt and aggressive management of the woman with an infected abortion effectively reduces the incidence of more serious complications, such as septic shock, thrombophlebitis, and renal failure, and reduces morbidity and hospital stay as well.

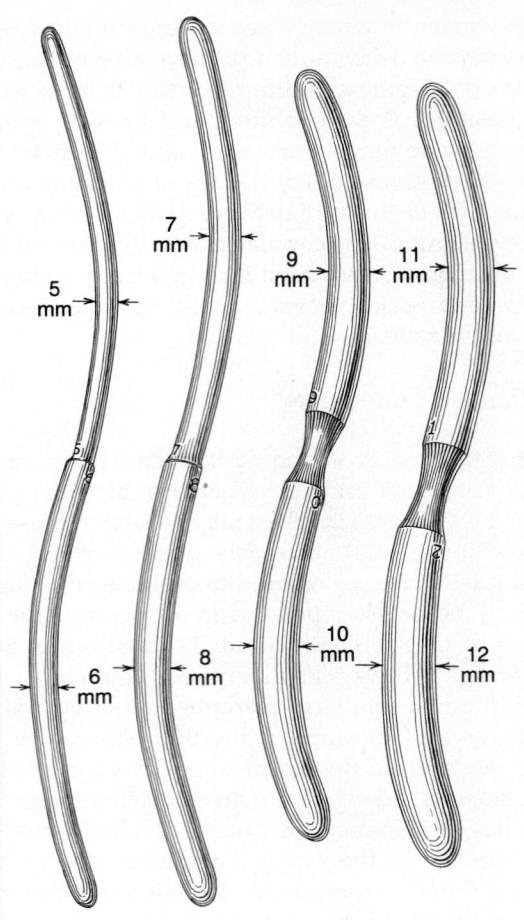

FIGURE 36-2

Hegar dilators of graduated diameters from 5 mm to 12 mm. Larger sizes are also used. (Mattingly RF: Telinde's Operative Gynecology, 5th ed. Philadelphia, JB Lippincott, 1977)

Nursing Assessment

Bleeding in the first half of pregnancy, no matter how slight, always must be considered as threatened abortion. The nurse must first obtain a detailed accurate history, including length of gestation, source of prenatal supervision, and the onset, duration, and intensity of the bleeding episode. The client should be asked to describe the quantity of bleeding in amounts that she can relate to (*e.g.*, a teaspoon, one half cup). The nature of the blood loss must similarly be assessed (*e.g.*, bright red or dark brown, with or without tissue fragments or mucus, malodorous, steady trickling of blood or intermittent spotting). The presence, nature, and location of accompanying discomforts such as cramping, dull or sharp pain, and dizziness are evaluated.

Assessment of blood loss for hospitalized women often includes weighing perineal pads before and after use and then subtracting the difference. When tissue is present on the pad, it is useful to examine the products of conception to ascertain whether or not the abortion is complete.

Nursing Diagnosis

As a result of the comprehensive assessment of the woman with hemorrhagic complications of early pregnancy, nursing diagnoses are formulated. The classification of diagnostic labels will vary depending upon the presenting nursing problems and is likely to focus upon the unexpected physiological alterations occurring in the reproductive system during the first trimester. An example of this type of potential or actual diagnosis is knowledge deficit related to physiological alterations occurring in the reproductive system. Other related diagnoses may include fluid volume deficit related to bleeding complication of early pregnancy; potential for infection related to excessive fluid volume deficit; grieving about actual or threatened loss of pregnancy. Additional diagnoses may be identified as new information about the client is gathered or as the client's condition changes owing to progressive alterations in physiological status or recovery.

Nursing Intervention

Interventions are planned based on the type of abortion, prognosis, and nursing diagnoses. The client at home is generally on restricted activity. If she is having only slight vaginal bleeding or even spotting, without pain, she should be instructed to stay in bed and eat a well-balanced diet. Some midwives and physicians may not recommend restricted activity, based on the concept that the uterus is well insulated from outside influences. Uniformly the client should be counseled to save all perineal pads, as well as all tissue and clots passed, for inspection. In cases in which bed rest has been prescribed, if the bleeding disappears within 48 hours, the woman may get out of bed but should limit her activities for the next several days. The nurse should counsel the client to avoid coitus for 2 weeks following the last evidence of bleeding or as otherwise recommended by the physician.

Psychosocial support is of prime importance since bleeding episodes are frightening and anxiety provoking for all pregnant women. Emotional reactions of shock and disbelief are normal responses experienced regardless of the category of abortion. The woman often searches for answers regarding the cause of her condition. She may express guilt and blame herself for behaviors that contributed to the situation. Verbalizations of feelings should be encouraged among all family members. The nurse should respond to concerns by offering accurate information on the cause of most spontaneous abortions and any facts specifically related to the actual case. False reassurance that "everything will be alright" should be avoided because in fact the client may lose her pregnancy.

Particular consideration is given to the special needs of the habitual aborter. Her prognosis for carrying a pregnancy to term decreases with each successive abortion. A complete diagnostic work-up is necessary to determine the cause and treatments indicated.

Incompetent Cervical Os

An incompetent cervical os is a mechanical defect in the cervix that causes it to dilate prematurely during pregnancy and cause late habitual abortion or preterm labor. Symptoms of this condition include painless dilatation, presence of bloody show, and premature rupture of the membranes. When repeated termination of pregnancy in the second trimester is due to an anatomical factor such as this, a surgical treatment known as cervical cerclage may make it possible to save the fetus.

Shirodkar Technique

One type of treatment used to prevent relaxation and dilatation of the cervix is the modified Shirodkar technique. In this, the vaginal mucous membrane is elevated and a narrow strip of some material such as Mersilene is carried around the internal os of the cervix and tied. Then the vaginal mucosa is restored to its original position and sutured. The procedure may be done between pregnancies, if the diagnosis is clearly established, or during pregnancy. When done during pregnancy, it is usually elected to wait until the early part of the second trimester (12 wk–14 wk) to avoid the possibility of having to remove the suture if a spontaneous first-trimester abortion occurs.

Postoperatively, the main concerns are monitoring fetal heart rate and uterine contractions. Observation should also be made for signs of rupture of the membranes. If the membranes rupture, the suture must be removed and the uterus emptied because of the risk of infection. If contractions ensue, the client should be placed at bed rest immediately, and a pharmacologic agent such as ritodrine hydrochloride may be given in an effort to control the contractions. Attempts to control contractions should not be persistent if they are not effective promptly, since there is a risk of uterine rupture. It is not uncommon for a woman to have bright-red vaginal spotting following this procedure.

Decisions regarding the type of delivery a client is to have are generally based on the position of the suture when the client reaches term or when labor begins. If the suture is in good position, with the cervical closure maintained, cesarean delivery may be elected to preserve the suture for future pregnancies. If the suture has loosened or rolled down on the cervix, it is not adequate for subsequent pregnancies. In that case, it is removed when labor begins and vaginal delivery is permitted.

McDonald Technique

A more simple procedure is the McDonald technique. This involves placing a nonabsorbable suture, such as No. 1 nylon, around the cervix high on the cervical mucosa while the woman is under anesthesia. The McDonald procedure is usually carried out during pregnancy when premature dilatation of the cervix is detected or electively in the fourth month. The suture is easily removed near term to allow spontaneous delivery.

Success rates with both the McDonald and the Shirodkar procedure are now approaching 85% to 90%.

Ectopic Pregnancy

An ectopic pregnancy is any gestation located outside the uterine cavity. The majority of ectopic pregnancies are tubal gestations located most frequently in the ampullar portion; the isthmus portion is the next most frequent site (Fig. 36-3). Other types, which make up about 5% of all ectopic pregnancies, are interstitial (in the interstitial portion of the tube), cornual (in a rudimentary horn of a uterus), cervical, abdominal, and ovarian gestations.

There has been a dramatic increase in the rate of ectopic pregnancy over the past decade.[3] No single factor has been identified as a cause of this increase; however, an association between rates of ectopic pregnancy and pelvic inflammatory disease, as well as age and race, has been suggested in many studies.[3] Although the majority of ectopic pregnancies occur in whites and Hispanic Americans, ectopic pregnancy rates are higher for black women. The incidence of the disease is particularly high in women between 35 and 44 years of age. Other factors that potentially contribute to the incidence of ectopic pregnancies include the use of intrauterine devices (IUDs), previous tubal sterilization, and the use of low-dose progestogen oral contraceptives.

About once in every 200 pregnancies the fertilized ovum, instead of traversing the length of the fallopian tube to reach the uterine cavity, becomes implanted within the walls of the fallopian tube. Since the wall of the tube is not sufficiently elastic to allow the fertilized ovum to grow and develop there, rupture of the tubal wall is the inevitable result. Rupture most frequently occurs into the tubal lumen, with the passage of the products of conception, together with much blood, out the fimbriated end of the tube and into the peritoneal cavity, so-called tubal abortion. Rupture may occur through the peritoneal surface of the tube directly into the peritoneal cavity; again, there is an outpouring of blood into the abdomen from vessels at the site of rupture. In either case, rupture usually occurs within the first 12 weeks.

Occasionally an ectopic pregnancy may develop in that portion of the tube that passes through the uterine wall, a type known as interstitial pregnancy. In very rare instances, the products of conception, after rupturing through the tubal wall, may become implanted on the peritoneum and develop to full term in the peritoneal cavity. This extraordinary occurrence is known as abdominal pregnancy. Surprisingly, living infants have been delivered in such cases by means of abdominal incision.

Manifestations and Causes

Clinical Picture. The clinical symptoms of ectopic pregnancy are likely to vary depending upon the site of implantation. In cases of unruptured ectopic pregnancy, vague and variable discomforts may develop. At first the woman exhibits the usual early signs of pregnancy and, as a rule, regards herself as being normally pregnant. Within 3 to 5 weeks after a missed menstrual period, pelvic pain often develops. The nature, duration, and intensity of pain vary considerably with the length of gestation, site of implantation, and extent of blood loss. Tubal rupture occurs in the majority of undiagnosed cases and is manifest by sudden knifelike pain, often of extreme severity, in one of the lower quadrants. This is usually associated with slight vaginal bleeding, commonly referred to as "spotting." Depending on the amount of blood that has escaped into the peritoneal cavity, the woman may or may not undergo a fainting attack and show symptoms of shock. In cases of shock, immediate medical intervention is necessary to treat the condition.

Causes. Tubal ectopic pregnancy may be caused by any condition that narrows the tube or brings about some constriction within it. Under such circumstances the tubal lumen is large enough to allow spermatozoa to ascend the tube but not big enough to permit the downward passage of the fertilized ovum (see Fig. 36-3). Among the conditions that may produce such a narrowing of the fallopian tube are previous inflammatory processes involving the tubal mucosa and producing partial agglutination of opposing surfaces, such as gonorrheal salpingitis; previous inflammatory processes of the external peritoneal surfaces of the tube, such as puerperal and postabortal infections; endo-

metriosis of the tubal wall and lumen; and developmental defects resulting in a segmental narrowing of the tubes.

Medical Diagnosis and Prognosis

Physical examination, a pregnancy test, culdocentesis, laparoscopy, and ultrasonography are diagnostic modalities for ectopic pregnancy. Simple differential diagnosis can be made through use of ultrasound techniques that demonstrate an empty uterine cavity. Unfortunately, if this test is not performed, the nonspecific signs and symptoms of ectopic pregnancy contribute to a high rate of misdiagnosis (salpingitis, appendicitis, ovarian cyst, ruptured corpus luteum) upon initial examination.

Ectopic pregnancy is a grave complication of pregnancy and is a significant cause of maternal death, especially in the first trimester. It accounts for 15% of all maternal deaths, 75% of which are estimated to be preventable.[4] Moreover, if a woman has had one ectopic pregnancy, she is more likely to have another in a subsequent pregnancy (10% chance).

Medical Management

In cases of ruptured ectopic pregnancy medical management is directed toward establishing homeostasis and combating shock. Most often a laparotomy and salpingectomy are performed to ligate bleeding vessels and to remove the involved tube.

Occasionally the ovary must be removed with the tube. Under certain circumstances in which subsequent fertility must be maintained, the tube may be preserved by removing the products of conception from the tube, either through a linear incision (salpingostomy) or by milking the conceptus out of the tubal lumen by external pressure applied with the fingers. This approach is applicable if the contralateral tube is badly diseased or has been previously removed and it is the client's wish to preserve fertility.

Rh_oD immune globulin should be prescribed postoperatively to protect against isoimmunization in the unsensitized Rh_o-negative woman.

Nursing Assessment

The initial assessment should focus upon the classic three symptoms of an ectopic pregnancy: missed menstruation followed by abdominal pain and vaginal spotting. Abdominal pain, the most common sign of ectopic pregnancy, is often described as "crampy," "dull," or "restricting to the shoulder and back." Shoulder pain is suggestive of intraperitoneal bleeding causing irritation of the diaphragm (phrenic nerve). The

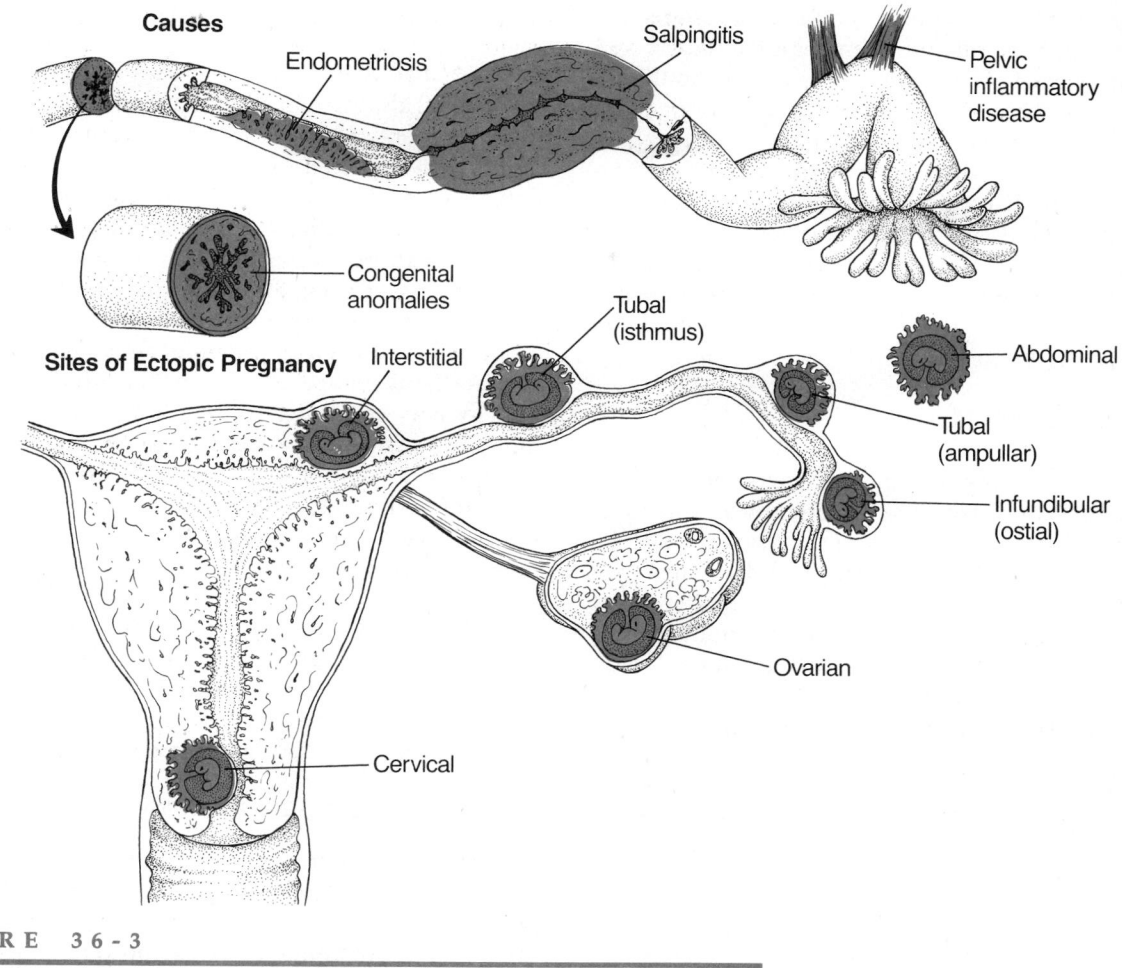

Causes

Endometriosis

Salpingitis

Pelvic inflammatory disease

Congenital anomalies

Sites of Ectopic Pregnancy

Interstitial

Tubal (isthmus)

Abdominal

Tubal (ampullar)

Infundibular (ostial)

Ovarian

Cervical

FIGURE 36-3

Causes and sites of ectopic pregnancy.

client should be questioned as to her contraceptive method, particularly the current use of an IUD. A woman who becomes pregnant with an IUD inserted has a tenfold greater chance that the pregnancy will be ectopic than if it were not being used.[5] A history of previous tubal damage caused by disease or developmental problems adds further support to the likelihood of a tubal pregnancy.

Upon pelvic examination the client is assessed for fullness in the cul-de-sac, cervical pain, and adnexal tenderness. The uterus is generally not enlarged beyond the 8 weeks gestational size. Laboratory analysis frequently reveals falling hematocrit (Hct) and hemoglobin (Hb) levels and leukocytosis.

The amount of bleeding evident may be a poor indicator of the severity of the situation, since blood loss may be concealed in the pelvic cavity. Extensive blood loss leading to hypovolemic shock may be revealed through a rapid, thready pulse, tachypnea, and hypotension. The umbilicus may display a blue tinge (Cullen's sign), indicating bleeding in the peritoneal cavity.

Nursing Diagnosis

Based upon the nursing assessment and differential medical findings, nursing diagnoses are identified. These are most likely to relate to the presenting problem of fluid volume deficit secondary to rupture at the implantation site. The potential for infection secondary to this hemorrhagic disorder is another nursing problem that should be given careful consideration. Similar to the woman experiencing a spontaneous abortion, the client with an ectopic pregnancy is also in a state of "grieving related to her actual or anticipated loss of the pregnancy."

Nursing Intervention

Nursing care is aimed at combating the shock that is frequently present in clients with a rupture. An intravenous infusion should be maintained so that blood or plasma expanders can be administered as needed to replace losses from the hemorrhage and surgery.

During the postoperative period vital signs are carefully monitored, fluid replacement is continued, and intake and output are recorded. The nurse should accurately record the perineal pad count. The surgical site may require special care and dressings.

Emotional care is directed toward facilitating effective coping through a critical complication of pregnancy, death of the fetus, and possibly altered fertility. The client is assisted in resolving feelings of guilt, self-blame, and despair as previously described for abortion patients.

Hydatidiform Mole

Hydatidiform mole is a benign neoplasm of the chorion in which the chorionic villi degenerate and become transparent vesicles containing clear, viscid fluid. The vesicles have a grapelike appearance and are arranged in clusters involving all or part of the decidual lining of the uterus (Fig. 36-4). Although there is usually no embryo present, occasionally there may be a fetus and only part of the placenta involved.

Hydatidiform mole is rather an uncommon condition, occurring about once in every 1500 to 2000 pregnancies in the United States and Europe. The incidence of this complication is much higher among Asian women.

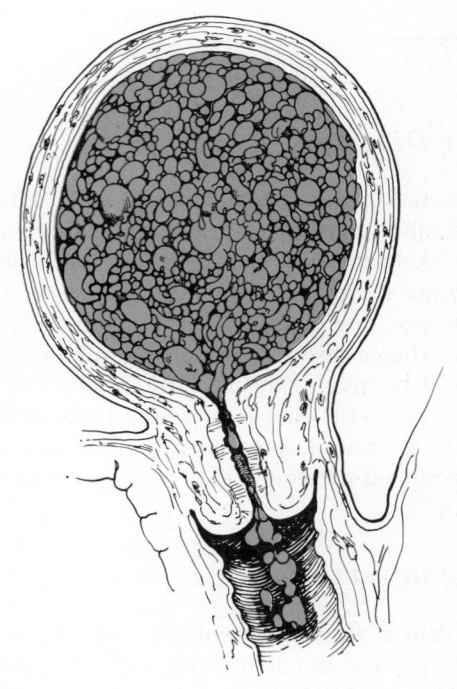

FIGURE 36-4

Hydatidiform mole.

Manifestations and Causes

Clinical Picture. The pregnancy appears to be normal at first, although in about 50% of women the uterus enlarges more rapidly than a normal pregnancy and is larger than expected for the duration of pregnancy by dates. Then bleeding, a usual sign varying from brownish-red spotting to heavy bleeding, occurs, so that one might suspect threatened or inevitable abortion. It may occur just prior to abortion or, more frequently, may persist intermittently for several weeks. If the woman does not abort, the uterus enlarges rapidly and profuse hemorrhage may occur, at which time these vesicles may be evident in the vaginal discharge. Vomiting in rather severe form may appear early. Preeclampsia, a complication that does not usually occur until the later months of pregnancy, may appear before the 20th week of gestation. Blood loss commonly leads to iron deficiency anemia.

Causes. The exact cause of hydatidiform mole is unknown. Age, multiparity, and dietary factors appear to be associated with hydatidiform mole. These suggest that an "at-risk" maternal host and abnormal gametogenesis may be important etiologic considerations.

Medical Diagnosis and Prognosis

When diagnosis of hydatidiform mole is suspected based upon persistent bleeding, a uterus larger than the expected size, and absence of fetal parts, it may be confirmed by sonographic examination (Fig. 36-5). Ultrasound techniques enable differential diagnosis to be made between the two types of molar growth: a *complete mole*, characterized by a large amount of edematous enlarged villi but no fetus or fetal membranes, and a *partial mole*, characterized by some normal villi and some fetal material or an amnionic sac. Tests for elevated levels of chorionic gonadotropin are also useful in diagnosis.

With appropriate therapy hydatidiform mole is generally not associated with maternal mortality. Approximately 10% to 20% of complete hydatidiform moles advance to invasive, potentially metastatic choriocarcinoma.

Medical Management

The first phase of medical management for hydatidiform mole consists in emptying the uterus. The approach used for evacuating the uterine contents depends on the size of the uterus at the time molar pregnancy is diagnosed. *If* the uterus is less than the size of a 10-week gestation, dilatation of the cervix, followed by suction curettage, is the usual procedure. This must be carried out with great care to avoid injury to the uterine wall, which is

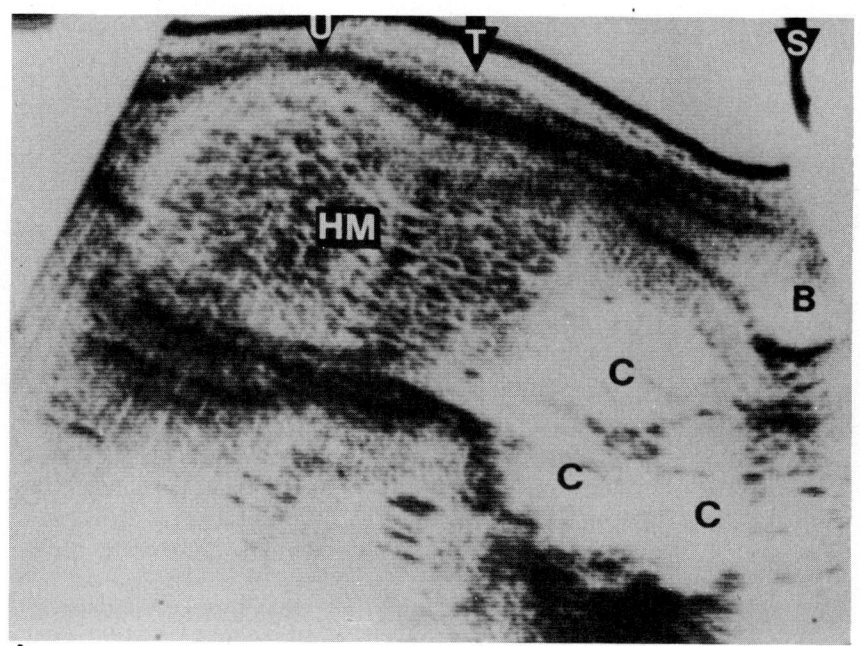

A

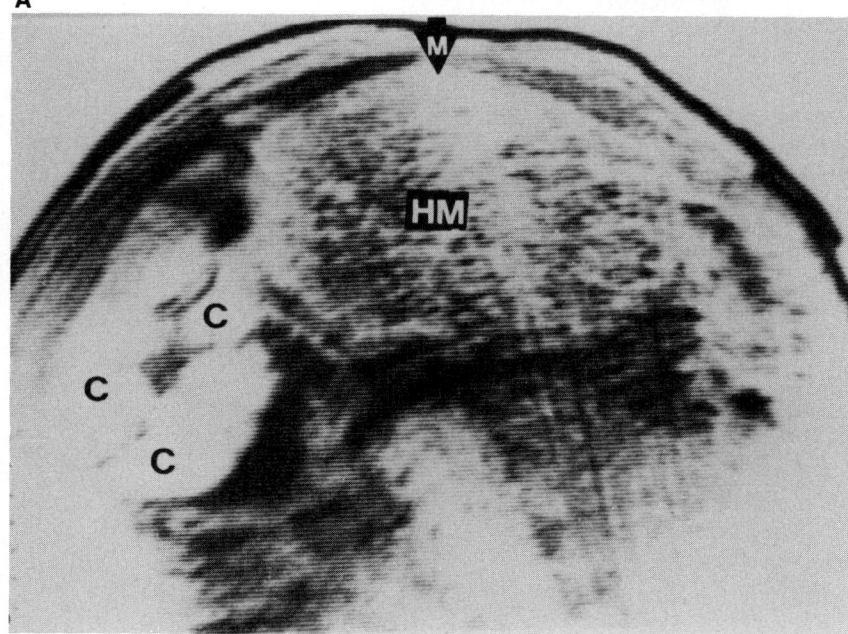

B

FIGURE 36-5

T, point at which transverse scan is obtained. Hydatidiform mole with theca-lutein cysts in a gravida, at 20 weeks' gestation, presenting with nausea and vomiting. (*A*) Longitudinal midline scan shows a complex multilocular cyst (*C*) in the cul-de-sac displacing the lower aspect of the uterus to the left side. The upper portion of the uterus is filled with echoes consistent with a hydatidiform mole (*HM*). (*B*) Transverse scan at T shows the echo pattern of hydatidiform mole and the cystic structure (*C*) (theca-lutein cysts) on the right side. (Sabbagha RE (ed): Diagnostic Ultrasound Applied to Obstetrics and Gynecology. Hagerstown, Harper & Row, 1980. Courtesy of Carlos Reynes, M.D., Loyola Hospital, Maywood, Illinois)

weakened and spongy from growth of the mole. If uterine size is larger, labor is stimulated with a continuous oxytocin infusion. After a portion of the uterine contents have been expelled, curettage is carried out to evacuate uterine contents completely.

The tissue obtained must be carefully evaluated by the pathologist, because, while a mole is a benign process, choriocarcinoma, an extremely malignant tumor, sometimes complicates the picture. For this reason, follow-up care, the second phase of intervention, is very important in cases of molar pregnancy. The main pur-

pose of follow-up is early detection of any changes suggestive of trophoblastic malignancy. Chorionic gonadotropin values are routinely evaluated for 1 year; negative human chorionic gonadotropin (hCG) levels should be evident within 6 weeks after evacuation.

The use of prophylactic chemotherapy for women who have had a hydatidiform mole remains controversial, since it may produce several adverse effects. Women receiving this drug therapy should be closely observed for blood dyscrasias and renal complications.

(text continued on page 744)

The Woman with Hemorrhagic Complications of Early Pregnancy

Nursing Objectives

1. Identify cause of early antepartal bleeding.
2. Provide appropriate interventions to support/terminate pregnancy.
3. Prevent complications of early antepartal bleeding.
4. Promote expressions of fear, grief, and anger to effectively cope with threatened/actual loss.

Assessment	Potential Nursing Diagnosis	Planning/Intervention	Evaluation

History
  Previous spontaneous abortion
  Multiple therapeutic abortions
  Pelvic inflammatory disease or previous tubal damage
  Previous ectopic pregnancy
  Current pregnancy confirmed
  Nausea and vomiting
  Lower abdominal pain or knifelike pain in lower quadrant (suggestive of ectopic pregnancy)
  Uterine cramping or contractions
  Previous bleeding/coagulation problems
  Contraceptive use, especially IUD
Physical examination
  Spotting or active bleeding (color, quantity, consistency)
  Relaxed or dilated cervix
  Fundal height (higher than expected with hydatidiform mole)
  Tenderness in adnexa
  Lower abdominal pain (right or left side)
  Blood pressure (elevated with hydatidiform mole)
  Vital signs
Laboratory studies
  Complete blood count
  Rh factor
  Hemoglobin, hematocrit
	Knowledge deficit related to physiological alterations in the reproductive system	Instruct client about "danger signals" in early pregnancy and appropriate actions indicated
		
		Maintain bed rest or limited physical activity
		
		Monitor vital signs and fetal heart tones (if indicated)
		
		Explain diagnostic ultrasound (or other prescribed procedures) and prepare for testing
		
		Provide client education on pathophysiology of condition and management
			Woman repeats danger signals in early pregnancy and what actions to take
			
			Woman complies with limited activity
			
			Woman's vital signs remain stable
			
			Woman acknowledges understanding of procedures
			
			Woman repeats accurate description of her condition

(continued)

Assessment	Potential Nursing Diagnosis	Planning/Intervention	Evaluation
Ultrasound to determine cause of bleeding			
Ectopic pregnancy			
Threatened abortion			
Incomplete abortion			
Hydatidiform mole			
Signs and symptoms of shock	Fluid volume deficit related to bleeding complications of early pregnancy	Draw blood, type, and cross match	
Rapid thready pulse		Observe, record, and report blood loss	
Tachypnea		Take pad count—note quantity, quality, and constituents of drainage	
Pallor, clammy skin			
Decreased blood pressure		Start and maintain intravenous infusion for administration of blood, antibiotics, or other medications as prescribed (use large-bore cannula)	Woman does not show signs of hypovolemic shock
Restlessness			
Decreased urine output			
Decreased level of consciousness		Replace fluids as prescribed intravenously	Woman's fluid and electrolyte balance are maintained
Laboratory screening for coagulation defect		Monitor intake and output (insert Foley catheter, if necessary)	Woman has her intake and output monitored
		Observe for signs and symptoms of shock—frequently assess vital functions, state of consciousness	
		Replace fibrinogen, if indicated	
		Institute nursing interventions for treatment of shock, if necessary; supine position often used, oxygen administered	Mother is stabilized
		Explain potential medical or surgical procedures that may be necessary (*e.g.,* dilatation and curettage, laparoscopy, salpingectomy, induction)	Woman demonstrates her knowledge of potential medical/surgical procedures in discussions
		Administer RhoGAM to Rh-negative client who aborts pregnancy	
Physical examination	Potential infection related to excessive fluid volume deficit	Provide client education on	Woman demonstrates proper cleansing technique after voiding
Fever			
Local tenderness		Perineal hygiene (*e.g.,* wipe perineal area from front to back after voiding)	
Malodorous vaginal discharge			

(continued)

743

Assessment	Potential Nursing Diagnosis	Planning/Intervention	Evaluation
Pain in lower abdomen, adnexa		Avoidance of tampons to control bleeding	
History		Observe for signs and symptoms of infection	Woman remains free of signs and symptoms of infection
Large amount of antepartal bleeding		Tenderness	
Illegal abortion		Swelling	
		Redness	
		Pain	
		Encourage fluid intake or administer parenteral fluids as ordered	Woman takes adequate amounts of fluid
		Administer antibiotics and pain medication as prescribed	
Signs and symptoms of anxiety	Grieving related to actual or threatened loss of pregnancy	Provide opportunities for expressions of grief, anger, self-blame	Woman expresses feelings of anger, grief, and self-blame
Jitteriness		Allow client to be with supportive family members	Family members offer each other mutual support
Restlessness			
Crying		Accept client's feelings of grief	Woman verbalizes fears related to future reproductive abilities
Nail biting			
Expresses		Provide factual information about abortion (or ectopic pregnancy or hydatidiform mole) and possible future reproductive capacities	Woman demonstrates understanding of potential loss of pregnancy
"Why me"			
Fear of losing baby			
Anger			
		Initiate referral for genetic counseling if appropriate	Woman complies with referral suggestions
		Initiate referral for religious support services if desired	

(text continued from page 741)

Nursing Assessment

Assessment of fundal height provides basic data about expected gestational age, which in the case of hydatidiform mole is beyond that expected by menstrual history but may be suggestive of multiple gestation. Careful auscultation for fetal heart sounds reveals no findings, while the pregnancy tests remain highly positive (owing to unusually high levels of hCG) beyond the time of usual decline in hCG levels. The client may also report intense nausea and vomiting.

Vital signs and blood pressure evaluation may reveal hypertension before the 20th week of pregnancy. Bleeding often develops in the second trimester. The blood should be carefully assessed by the nurse for clear, filled vesicles. Results of laboratory studies often reveal falling hemoglobin and hematocrit levels, as well as proteinuria.

Nursing Diagnosis

Several of the nursing diagnoses are similar to those of other hemorrhagic complications of early pregnancy; these include knowledge deficit of pathophysiological changes in the reproductive system; fluid volume deficit related to uterine bleeding; and grieving related to loss of pregnancy. There are several other nursing problems specific to hydatidiform mole, such as alteration in tissue perfusion related to pregnancy-induced hypertension

(PIH); alteration in nutritional status secondary to nausea and vomiting; and anxiety about potential malignancy.

Nursing Intervention

Once the diagnoses are made, the nurse plans interventions to prepare the client for evacuation of the uterus. Preoperative nursing care will vary depending upon the type of medical procedure required.

In providing client education, it is of paramount importance that the nurse emphasize that every woman who has had a hydatidiform mole must submit a urine specimen or have her serum tested for hCG each month for the course of an entire year. In addition, family-planning counseling should be offered to assist the women in selecting a desirable contraceptive. Pregnancy should be avoided for at least 1 year, after which time conception is permitted, if pregnancy tests remain negative.

Psychosocial support is also an important component of nursing care for the woman with a hydatidiform mole. Although the woman may never have experienced a "true pregnancy," her reactions following treatment frequently closely resemble those of women who have had a spontaneous abortion or an ectopic pregnancy. Further anxiety and despair may be created by the lengthy delay necessitated for future pregnancies and the risk of potential neoplasms. Opportunities should be provided by the nurse for the client to express her varying reactions to the situation, including extreme remorse, anger, and fear. Much understanding and guidance is needed by the client and her family to work through grief reactions and assess future plans (see Nursing Care Plan: The Woman with Hemorrhagic Complications of Early Pregnancy).

Choriocarcinoma

Choriocarcinoma is a highly malignant trophoblastic neoplasm that develops during or shortly after some form of pregnancy. Approximately one third to one half of choriocarcinomas are preceded by hydatidiform mole. The characteristic progression of this disease involves a rapidly growing mass invading both uterine muscle and blood vessels, causing hemorrhage and necrosis. The chorionic villi of hydatid moles are absent. Metastases to the lungs, vagina, brain, and blood vessels are early complications, often occurring before symptoms of the primary disease present.

Trophoblastic neoplasia is suspected in the presence of persistent or rising titers of gonadotropin when pregnancy is absent. Modern treatment of choriocarcinoma has greatly improved the prognosis. In the past, hysterectomy offered the only possible curative treatment. Currently, drugs such as methotrexate and actinomycin D offer much promise as successful chemotherapeutic agents that may be used alone or in combination with irradiation. If the disease is treated early an overall cure rate of about 90% can be achieved.

Hyperemesis Gravidarum

A mild degree of nausea and vomiting, morning sickness, is the most common complaint of women in the first trimester of pregnancy. This manifestation is considered in the realm of minor discomfort rather than a complication, and it usually responds to measures discussed in Chapter 22. It is uncommon today for this mild form of nausea and vomiting to progress beyond the first trimester and to such a serious extent that it produces systemic effects (*i.e.*, marked loss of weight and acetonuria), but when it becomes thus exaggerated, the condition is *hyperemesis gravidarum*, sometimes called pernicious vomiting. The incidence of this disease is approximately 3 in 1000 deliveries.

Because even the gravest case of hyperemesis starts originally as a simple form of nausea, all cases of nausea and vomiting should be treated with proper understanding and judgment, and none should be regarded casually.

Manifestations and Causes

Clinical Picture. The clinical picture of the pregnant woman suffering from pernicious vomiting varies in relation to the severity and the duration of the condition. In any event, the condition begins with a typical picture of morning sickness. The woman experiences a feeling of nausea, which may be most pronounced on arising in the morning but may occur at other times of the day. With the majority of these women this pattern persists for a few weeks and then suddenly ceases.

A small number of women who have morning sickness develop persistent vomiting that lasts for 4 to 8 weeks or longer. These women vomit several times a day and may be unable to retain any liquid or solid foods, with the result that marked symptoms of dehydration and starvation occur. *Dehydration* is pronounced, as evidenced by diminished urinary output and dryness of the skin. Hypovolemia with associated hypotension may result if dehydration is not corrected.

Starvation, which is regularly present, manifests itself in a number of ways. Weight loss may vary from 5 lb to as much as 20 lb or 30 lb. This is tantamount to saying that the digestion and the absorption of carbohydrates and other nutrients have been so inadequate that the body has been forced to burn its reserve stores of fat to maintain body heat and energy. When fat is burned without carbohydrates being present, the process of combustion does not go on to completion. Consequently, certain incompletely burned products of fat metabolism make their appearance in the blood and the urine. The presence of acetone and diacetic acid in the urine in hyperemesis is common. In severe cases considerable changes associated with starvation and dehydration become evident in the blood chemistry. There is a definite increase in the nonprotein nitrogen, uric acid and urea; a moderate decrease in the chlorides; and little alteration in the carbon dioxide combining power. Then, too, vitamin starvation is regularly present, and in extreme cases, when marked vitamin B deficiency exists, polyneuritis occasionally develops and disturbances of the peripheral nerves result.

Causes.   It is currently recognized that during pregnancy there are certain organic processes that are basic to all cases of vomiting, regardless of whether the symptoms are mild or severe. The endocrine imbalance created by a high level of chorionic gonadotropins, metabolic changes of normal gestation, fragments of chorionic villi entering the maternal circulation, and the diminished motility of the stomach might well give rise to clinical symptoms.

It has long been thought that hyperemesis gravidarum is in large measure a *neurosis*. The term *neurosis*, it will be recalled, is employed very loosely to designate a large array of conditions in which symptoms occur without demonstrable pathologic explanation, the symptoms being due, it is thought, to a disturbance of the woman's psyche. In hyperemetic women it is theorized that the disturbance is related to psychological adjustments of pregnancy and the role of mothering.

Medical Diagnosis and Prognosis

Appropriate diagnostic testing should be performed to detect underlying causes of nausea and vomiting, such as gastroenteritis, hepatitis, cholecystitis, or peptic ulcer, which may contribute to the hyperemetic status of the pregnant woman.

At present, grave cases of hyperemesis gravidarum are rare and recovery is usually rapid once fluid and electrolyte balance are restored.

Medical Management

Hospitalization is recommended for the pregnant woman who is unable to effectively remedy the symptoms of hyperemesis. The change in atmosphere and separation from relatives, as well as the availability of therapy provided in the hospital, may confer unusual benefits in this condition. The goals of intervention are (1) to treat the dehydration by liberal administration of parenteral fluids; (2) to reverse the starvation by administering glucose intravenously and thiamine chloride

subcutaneously and, if necessary, by feeding a high-caloric, high-vitamin fluid diet through a nasal tube or hyperalimentation method; and (3) to treat the emotional component with an understanding attitude, supportive measures, and sedatives if necessary. Oral intake of fluids is restricted until the nausea and vomiting subside.

Occasionally, the hyperemetic woman may be unable to successfully respond to treatment. In such rare circumstances total parenteral nutrition (TPN) may be prescribed through a subclavian line to restore a positive nitrogen balance.

Nursing Assessment

During the initial contact with the hyperemetic woman, the nurse should assess the particular pattern of nausea and vomiting experienced by the client (*e.g.*, onset, duration, frequency, predictability). Results of laboratory studies are carefully reviewed for evidence of hemoconcentration (elevated hemoglobin and hematocrit), fluid and electrolyte imbalance (decreased sodium, potassium, and chloride), and vitamin deficiency (B folate). The client's current weight is measured and compared with her nonpregnant weight. Selected questions are asked about activities for daily living and the client's life-style and attitudes about herself and the pregnancy. Nutritional habits are evaluated in detail and then compared with findings upon physical examination (*e.g.*, skin turgor, energy level, color of mucous membranes).

Nursing Diagnosis

Assessment of the client with signs and symptoms of hyperemesis gravidarum may lead the nurse to some of the following nursing diagnoses: alteration in nutrition related to pernicious vomiting; potential impairment in skin integrity related to excessive vomiting and dehydration; and ineffective individual coping with the psychological tasks of pregnancy and motherhood. In addition, the fetus is at risk for alteration in nutrition secondary to maternal malnourishment.

Nursing Intervention

The nurse must carefully monitor the client's intake and output during the course of hospitalization. Generally oral intake is restricted. However, once vomiting ceases oral feedings are started. Various approaches are used to restore oral intake. Small quantities of dry food (*e.g.*, crackers or toast) may be given hourly alternating with small quantities (1 oz) of water. This is followed by a progression of clear liquids. If clear liquids and dry food are tolerated well, the client may slowly advance to a soft diet and, finally, a normal diet. In preparing solid foods the nurse should arrange the portions at-

The Woman with Pernicious Vomiting (Hyperemesis Gravidarum)

Nursing Objectives

1. End pernicious vomiting.
2. Restore circulatory volume and fluid and electrolyte balance.
3. Protect fetal well-being by providing basic intrauterine needs for nourishment.
4. Promote effective coping abilities with psychological tasks of pregnancy and motherhood.

Assessment	Potential Nursing Diagnosis	Planning/Intervention	Evaluation

History
  Onset, duration, and frequency of vomiting episodes
  Prepregnancy weight
  Current weight
  Previous eating disorder
Laboratory studies
  Blood
    Electrolytes (decreased)
    Hemoglobin and hematocrit (elevated)
    pH (acidosis, alkalosis)
    BUN (increased)
    SGOT (elevated)
  Urine
    Ketones (present)
    Specific gravity (elevated)
  Other diagnostic tests
    Liver function
    Renal function
    Gastric function
	Alteration in nutrition: less than body requirements related to pernicious vomiting	Restrict or limit oral intake until vomiting ceases
		
		Initiate and maintain intravenous therapy to correct hypovolemia and electrolyte imbalance
		  Glucose
		  Vitamins
		  Sodium
		  Chloride
		  Potassium
		  Bicarbonate
		  Lactate
		
		Record intake and output, including emesis
		
		Record daily weights
		
		Begin alternatively giving water or dry food (*e.g.,* toast) in small quantities after vomiting has stopped
		
		Advance diet slowly to clear liquids, soft foods, and solid foods, respectively. Arrange food attractively in small quantities
		
		Initiate total parenteral nutrition (TPN) if unable to establish oral feedings for prolonged period
			Woman responds to restricted intake by ending her vomiting
			
			Woman's electrolyte imbalances and hypovolemia are corrected
			
			Woman's urine output remains greater than 30 ml/hr
			
			Woman ceases weight loss and begins to gain weight
			
			Woman retains food and liquid
			
			Woman receives diet that adequately meets nutritional demands of pregnancy

Personal hygiene
  Skin care
  Mouth care
Integrity of skin
  Pressure sores
  Turgor
  Color (jaundice, pallor)
  Dryness
  Thinness
	Potential impairment in skin integrity related to excessive vomiting and dehydration	Encourage ambulation (if appropriate) or frequent change in position
		
		Inspect mouth for irritation or lesions
		
		Assist with oral hygiene and offer frequent mouthwashes
		
		Maintain personal hygiene using mild soap and avoiding excessive moisture
			Woman ambulates or changes positions frequently
			
			Woman's mouth remains free of irritation and lesions
			
			Woman maintains good personal and oral hygiene

(continued)

Assessment	Potential Nursing Diagnosis	Planning/Intervention	Evaluation

Integrity of oral cavity
  Tenderness
  Redness
  Lesions
		Explain effects of condition on skin integrity and oral cavity; emphasize importance of preventive intervention	Woman's skin retains its integrity

History
  Planned vs unplanned pregnancy
  Financial difficulties
  Interpersonal conflicts in family
	Ineffective coping with the psychological tasks of pregnancy and motherhood	Control environment by restricting or limiting visitors as necessary	Woman relaxes and remains calm

		Demonstrate a calm and relaxed manner	

Communication patterns
  Ability to verbalize feelings
  Maintenance of eye contact
  Nonverbal behaviors
		Assess client's achievement of the tasks of pregnancy	

		Offer psychological support	Woman indicates her trust in the nurse
		Reduce anxiety by explaining all procedures necessary for diagnosis and treatment	

Achievement of the psychological tasks of pregnancy
  Denial
  Ambivalence
  Acceptance
  Future plans
		Provide positive reinforcement for concerns expressed about pregnancy and fetal well-being	Woman vebalizes feelings about pregnancy

		Maintain good ventilation in client's room and reduce odors from vomitus, food	
		Refer for mental health services if necessary	Woman accepts sources of assistance
		Refer to social worker for socioeconomic assistance if necessary	
Pregnancy test positive High level of hCG Fetal heart tones (Doppler) Fundal height	Alteration in fetal nutrition related to maternal malnourishment	Explain purposes and prepare for diagnostic tests as indicated (*e.g.,* sonography)	Woman indicates her understanding of diagnostic tests and follows instructions
		Monitor fetal heart tones with Doppler	Fetus retains normal heart beats
		Monitor fetal movement (if present)	Fetus moves normally
		Assess fundal height and compare measurements for growth	Woman shows growth in fundal height

tractively and in small amounts. A positive approach should be displayed when serving food. It is important for the nurse to be aware of the effects that food odors have upon the mother.

It is most important for the nurse to provide a hygienic environment for the client. Quick removal of emesis from the client's room and use of room deodor-izers will decrease noxious odors that may disturb appetite and diminish food appeal.

Psychological support is most effectively provided by the nurse who demonstrates an understanding and empathetic manner. A relaxed and tolerant attitude may facilitate the client's verbalizations of any psychological conflicts because of family, financial, or social difficulties. Visitors may have to be restricted or limited if they have an adverse effect upon the client.

Hemorrhagic Complications of Late Pregnancy

Placental disorders causing bleeding and possible hemorrhage during late pregnancy may seriously jeopardize fetal well-being and maternal health. Problems that develop may have originated either early or late in pregnancy as the placenta matures and becomes more vascular. The most common cause of bleeding and hemorrhage during the later months of pregnancy is placenta previa. Premature separation of the placenta (abruptio placentae) is another potentially serious condition associated with third-trimester bleeding. An overview comparison of these conditions is presented in Table 36-1.

Placenta Previa

Placenta previa is the development of the placenta in the lower uterine segment (instead of high up in the uterus as usual) so that it either wholly or partially covers the region of the cervix.

There are three types, differentiated according to the degree to which the condition is present (Figs. 36-6 and 36-7). *Total placenta previa* occurs when the placenta completely covers the internal os; *partial placenta previa* occurs when the placenta partially covers the internal os; and *low implantation of placenta* occurs when the placenta encroaches on the region of the internal os, so that it can be palpated by the physician on

TABLE 36-1

A Comparative Overview of Placenta Previa and Abruptio Placentae

	Placenta Previa	Abruptio Placentae
Etiology	Unknown	Unknown
Associated Risk Factors	Multiparity, multiple gestation, advancing age (especially over age 35), uterine incisions, previous cesarean birth	Maternal hypertension, grand multiparity, multiple gestation, hydramnios, external trauma (rare), short umbilical cord (rare)
Frequency	1:167 deliveries	1:77–1:200 deliveries
Symptoms	Painless bleeding appearing at the end of the second trimester or in the third trimester (usually bright red) Uterus is soft Observed blood loss comparable to signs of shock	Bleeding—may or may not be external (often dark brown) Uterine rigidity and tenderness Shock out of proportion to blood loss
Prognosis	Maternal mortality 0.1% Major problems: prematurity	Maternal mortality 0.5%–5% Major problem: prematurity Perinatal mortality 15%
Recurrence	1:17	1:6–1:18
Complications	Hemorrhage Hypovolemic shock Thrombocytopenia Anemia Premature rupture of membranes and labor Fetal malposition Air embolism Postpartum hemorrhage Uterine rupture	Hemorrhage Coagulation defects (*e.g.*, hypofibrinogenemia) Renal failure Anemia

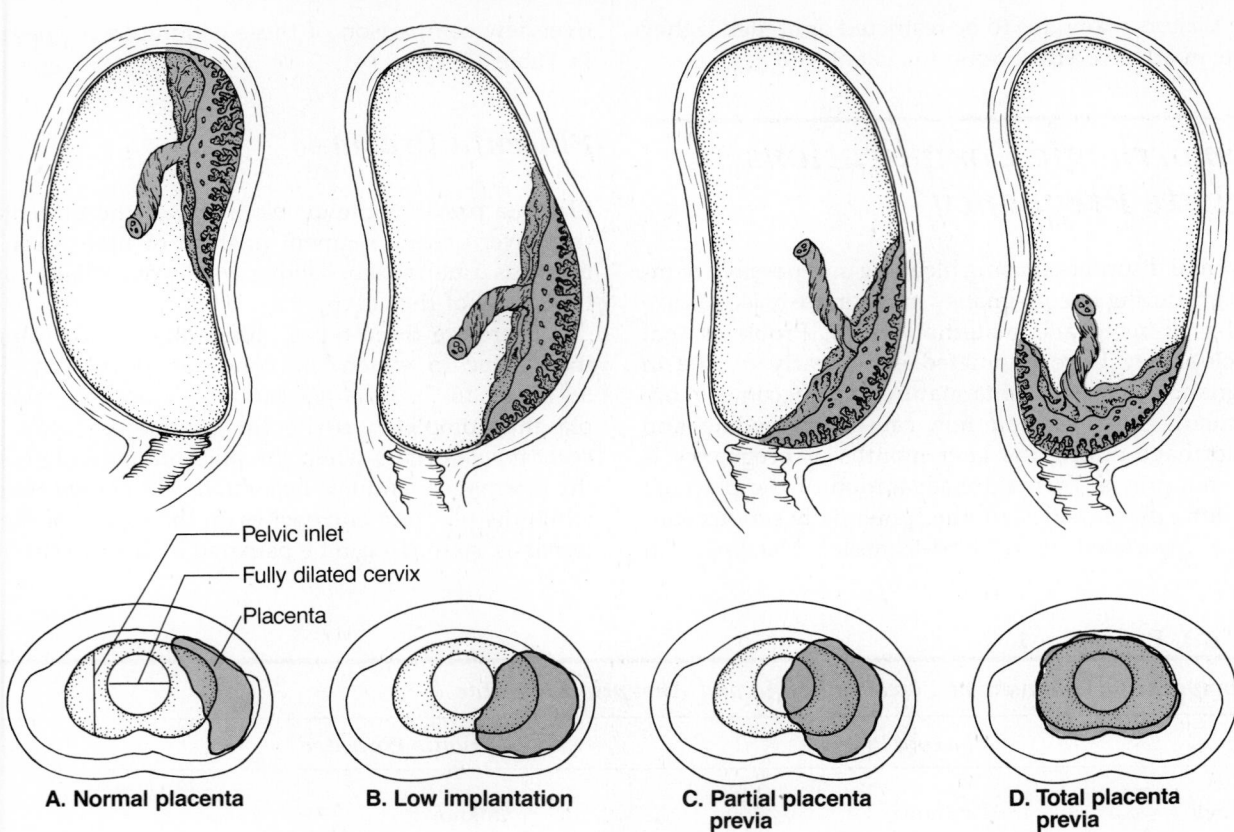

- Pelvic inlet
- Fully dilated cervix
- Placenta

A. Normal placenta   **B. Low implantation**   **C. Partial placenta previa**   **D. Total placenta previa**

FIGURE 36-6

Placenta previa. (*A*) Normal placenta. (*B*) Low implantation. (*C*) Partial placenta previa. (*D*) Total placenta previa. (Redrawn from Benson RC: Handbook of Obstetrics and Gynecology, 6th ed. Los Altos, CA, Lange Medical Publications, 1977)

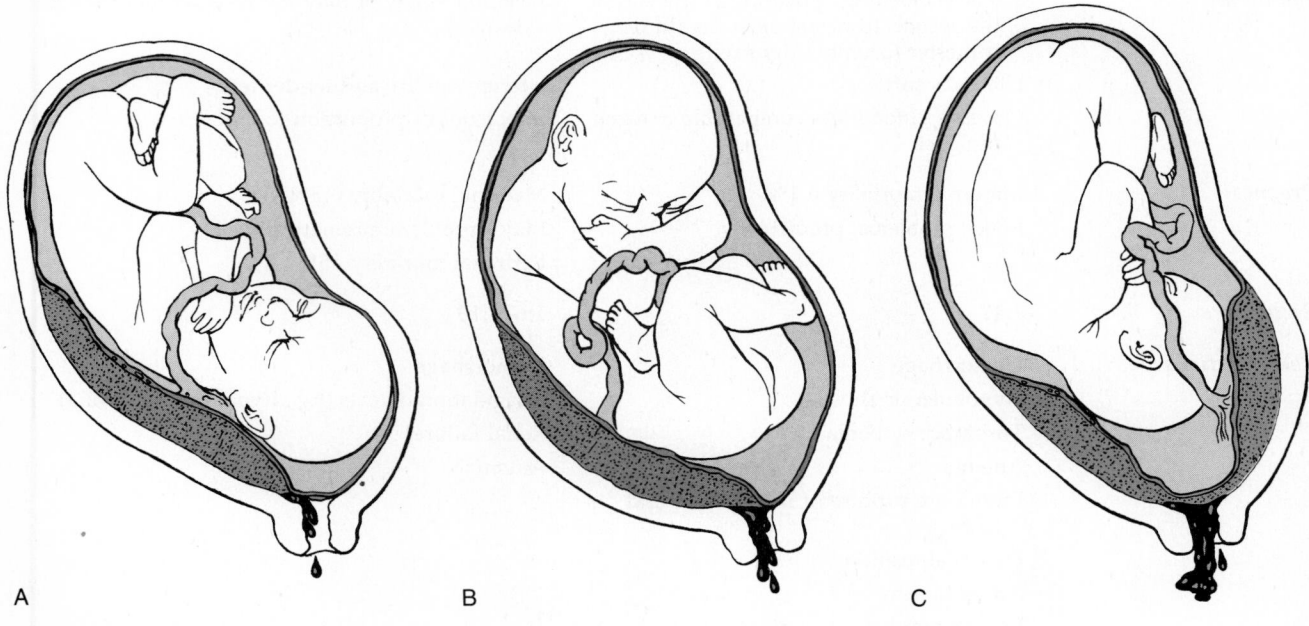

A   B   C

FIGURE 36-7

Placenta previa. (*A*) Low implantation. (*B*) Partial placenta previa. (*C*) Central (total) placenta previa.

digital exploration about the cervix, but does not extend beyond the margin of the internal os.

Fortunately, placenta previa is not a very common condition; it occurs about once in every 167 deliveries.

Manifestations and Causes

Clinical Picture.
Changes occurring in the lower uterine segment during the later months of pregnancy cause varying degrees of placental separation from its site of attachment. This separation opens up the underlying blood sinuses of the uterus from which the bleeding occurs. Painless vaginal bleeding during the second half of pregnancy is the main sign in the woman presenting with placenta previa. The bleeding usually occurs after the seventh month. It may begin as mere spotting, or it may start with profuse hemorrhage. The woman may awaken in the middle of the night to find herself in a pool of blood. Most commonly the natural history of placenta previa is such that uncontrolled bleeding is not likely to occur with the first episode. In fact, there may be several episodes of bleeding, starting early in the third trimester, before there is sufficient bleeding to force the obstetrician to intervene and terminate the pregnancy. The uterus usually remains soft in women with placenta previa.

Causes.
There is no known cause of placenta previa. Multiparity, advancing maternal age, multiple gestation, previous cesarean birth, and uterine incisions increase the risk of occurrence.

Medical Diagnosis and Prognosis

The possibility of placenta previa should always be suspected in women with uterine bleeding during the latter half of pregnancy. Diagnosis can be established clearly and simply by using sonographic techniques to locate the placenta (Fig. 36-8). Placental localization by ultrasound "B" scanning offers 95% accuracy. Other techniques of placental localization are useful in confirming the diagnosis. Such measures as isotope scans, amniog-

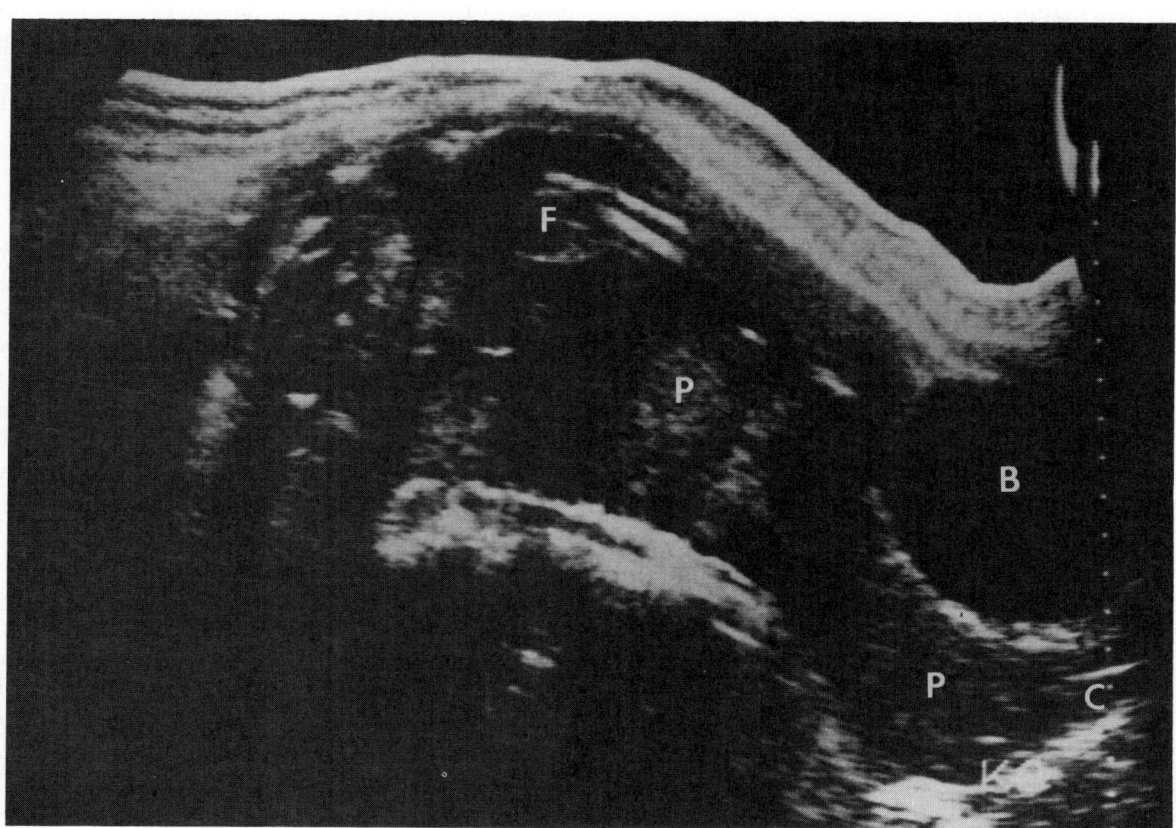

F I G U R E 3 6 - 8

Ultrasonogram of 25 weeks' gestation, showing placenta previa. The placenta (*P*) is located on the posterior wall of the lower uterine segment and extends anteriorly to cover the cervix (*C*). Bladder (*B*) is outlined in front. Fetal echoes (*F*) are seen in the upper part of the uterus.

raphy, and soft-tissue abdominal films have been used in the past with varying degrees of success. These have been largely supplanted by sonography. Physical examination of the cervix in cases of suspected previa is contraindicated unless the woman is in an operating room with all the preparations for immediate cesarean section, should severe hemorrhage result from mild manipulation. This examination is known as a *double setup procedure.*

Placenta previa must always be regarded as a grave complication of pregnancy. The presence of this condition creates two main problems for the mother: bleeding and obstruction of the birth canal. For the baby, the most significant concern is prematurity. Up until recent years placenta previa was associated with a maternal mortality rate of approximately 10%. Modern methods of management, plus the more liberal use of blood transfusion, have reduced this figure considerably. The fetus may be compromised not only because the placental separation interferes with the oxygen supply, but also because many of the babies are very premature when delivery must necessarily take place.

Medical Management

Medical interventions are planned based upon careful consideration of the mother's condition as primarily evidenced by the degree of obstetric hemorrhage and the fetal condition, particularly current status and gestational age. Conservative management is in order when the fetus is premature (by weight or dates) and the bleeding is not excessive. Under such circumstances, bed rest and observation often result in cessation of the bleeding and provide valuable days for the maturation of the fetus. To confirm fetal maturity, amniocentesis is often performed prior to planned delivery. An active approach is indicated if the fetus is at term by size and dates, if labor has begun, or if bleeding is sufficient to threaten the well-being of mother or fetus. Then the mother is taken to the operating room where the previously described double setup examination may be performed. Delivery must be performed irrespective of gestational age under emergency situations.

In all instances of total and partial placenta previa, and in most instances of low implantation of the placenta, cesarean birth is the approach of choice for delivery. In an occasional case of low implantation, especially if the baby is small and the cervix is already partially dilated, the obstetrician may elect to rupture the membranes in the hope that the presenting part may enter the pelvis and control the bleeding by compressing the area of placenta that has separated. If this does occur, vaginal delivery may sometimes be accomplished. By and large cesarean delivery is the procedure of choice, since it is generally associated with better fetal survival.

Nursing Assessment

Assessment of the woman with placenta previa is very similar in many ways to the approach employed for the woman with a spontaneous abortion, discussed earlier in the chapter.

Initial evaluation of the client by the nurse should include (1) baseline vital signs; (2) bleeding; (3) uterine activity and condition (size, contour, irritability, relaxation); (4) pain or tenderness, especially in the abdomen; (5) fetal heart tones and activity; and (6) level of consciousness. The client must be typed and cross matched so that necessary transfusions may be administered. She should be instructed to save all perineal pads; these are carefully examined by the nurse for blood loss. The client is also instructed to report if she feels any fluid escaping from her vulva. It is important to gently palpate the uterus periodically to detect contractions suggesting the onset of labor.

Since bleeding is from the uterine decidua, the amount of actual visible blood loss may be deceiving. Assessment should be performed for signs of shock (pallor, coldness, tachycardia) and fetal hypoxia secondary to inadequate oxygenation. Fetal heart tones and pattern are often evaluated continuously through application of an external monitoring system. Daily measurements of hemoglobin and hematocrit may also be done to assess blood loss.

Nursing Diagnosis

From her assessment the nurse formulates nursing diagnoses for the woman with placenta previa. Some of the potential nursing diagnoses may include fluid volume deficit (hypovolemia) related to bleeding secondary to abnormal placental implantation; alteration in tissue perfusion related to hypovolemic shock; potential for infection related to excessive blood loss; alteration in placental tissue perfusion; and ineffective maternal attachment related to disease.

Nursing Intervention

Plans for nursing intervention will vary depending upon whether conservative or active medical management is prescribed. The client who is being managed at home or is being discharged after an initial bleeding episode may require a referral for homemaking services and child care. Assistance in these areas is likely to facilitate client compliance with bed rest or restricted activities. In addition, ongoing assessments for changes in perinatal status may be performed by the community-health nurse. Client education should focus upon preoperative teaching to prepare the woman for a probable cesarean delivery and preparation of the family for a possible premature infant with special-care needs.

The client experiencing an excessive blood loss prior to or during delivery often requires blood replacement by transfusion. It may also be necessary to administer oxygen to prevent maternal and fetal hypoxia. The nurse should help the woman with a diagnosis of placenta previa to maintain her self-esteem by listening to her concerns and offering clear explanations about the situation and management approach. It is only natural for the woman and her family to have many fears about the infant's well-being, maternal dangers, and a possible cesarean delivery. Listening to fetal heart tones with a Doppler device may provide the prenatal client with some reassurance and reduce her anxiety.

Abruptio Placentae

Abruptio placentae (meaning that the placenta is torn from its bed) is a complication of the last half of pregnancy in which a normally located placenta undergoes separation from its uterine attachment. The condition is frequently called premature separation of the normally implanted placenta; other synonymous terms, such as *accidental hemorrhage* (meaning that it takes place unexpectedly) and *ablatio placentae* (ablatio meaning a carrying away), are sometimes used. The incidence is about 1 in every 77 to 200 pregnancies.

Manifestations and Causes

Clinical Picture. The clinical picture will vary depending upon the type of premature separation present (Fig. 36-9). *Covert* or *severe* abruptio placentae is characterized by central separation that entraps lost blood between the uterine wall and the placenta. In this situation there is a *concealed hemorrhage*, which often masks the seriousness of the problem. When a separation occurs at the margin, blood passes between the uterine wall and fetal membranes, creating an *external hemorrhage*. This type of abruptio is called *overt* or *partial*. Situations involving complete or almost total separation are known as *placental prolapse* and are associated with massive vaginal bleeding.

Premature separation of the normally implanted placenta is characterized not only by bleeding beneath the placenta but also by pain (often sudden and severe—"knifelike"). The pain is produced by the accumulation of blood behind the placenta, with subsequent distention of the uterus. The uterus also enlarges as the result of the accumulated blood and becomes distinctly tender and exceedingly firm. Because of the almost woody hardness of the uterine wall, fetal parts may be difficult to palpate. Shock is often out of proportion to blood loss, as manifested by a rapid pulse, dyspnea, yawning, restlessness, pallor, syncope, and cold, clammy perspiration.

Causes. Although the precise cause of the condition is unknown, it is frequently encountered in association with cases of hypertensive disorder of pregnancy and grand multiparity (five or more pregnancies). Other possible contributing factors include multiple gestation and hydramnios.

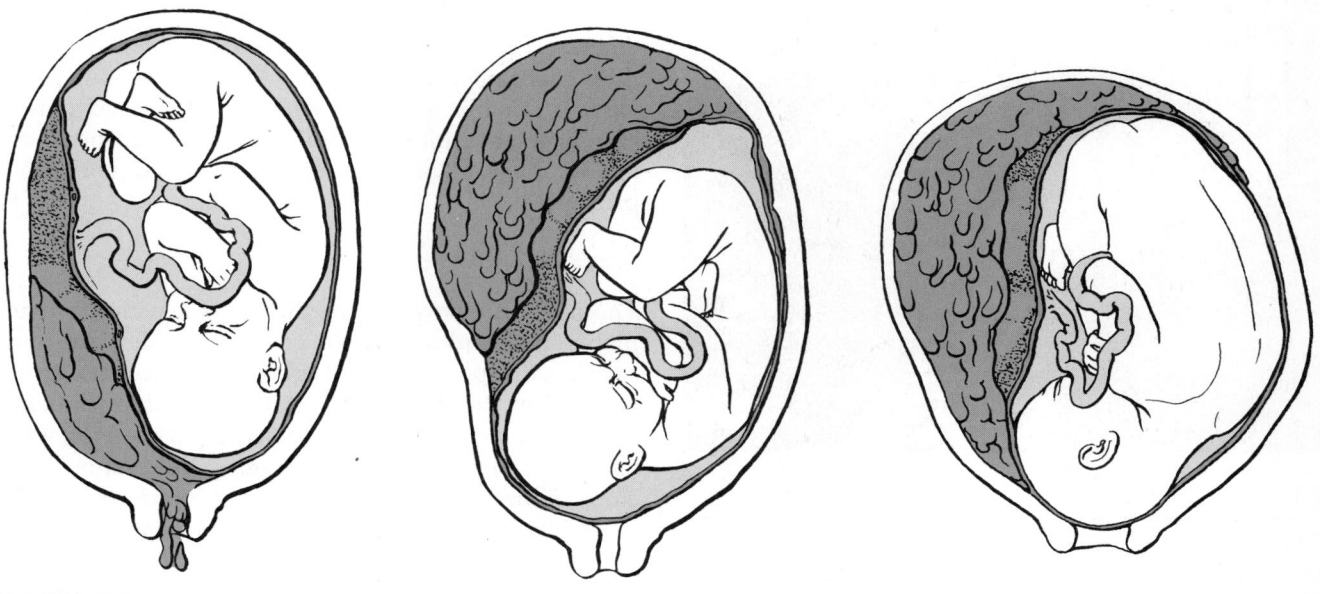

FIGURE 36-9

Abruptio placentae at various separation sites. (*Left*) External hemorrhage. (*Center*) Internal or concealed hemorrhage. (*Right*) Complete separation.

Medical Diagnosis and Prognosis

The physical signs and symptoms of placental abruption may vary greatly. Ultrasonography is often helpful in establishing the diagnosis (Fig. 36-10); however, negative sonography does not exclude life-threatening degrees of placental abruption.

Abruptio placentae may be classified according to the degree of placental separation (see classification).

Perinatal mortality rates vary greatly with the type of abruptio, ranging from 15% to approaching 100% for infants experiencing nearly total or complete abruptios. Assuming fetal survival, infant maturity at the time of delivery will also influence prognosis. Maternal mortality from abruptios has declined significantly and is now uncommon, although morbidity may be severe in some cases.[6]

Medical Management

Treatment is dependent upon the condition of the fetus and the mother at the time the diagnosis is made. If the fetus is alive and at or near term, prompt delivery is in order for moderate to severe abruptios and should be by cesarean birth, unless vaginal delivery can be accomplished quickly. If the fetus has already succumbed,

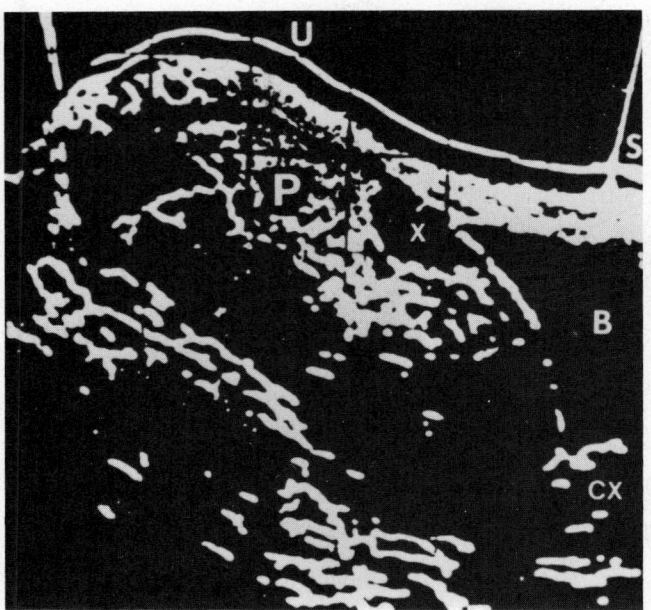

FIGURE 36-10

Ultrasonography of placental abruption at 27 weeks. The clear space, X, represents a retroplacental blood clot between the placental basal plate and the uterine wall. (Sabbagha RE (ed): Diagnostic Ultrasound Applied to Obstetrics and Gynecology. Hagerstown, Harper & Row, 1980)

Classification of Abruptio Placentae According to Placental Separation

Grade 0	No symptoms; diagnosed after delivery when placenta is examined and found to have a dark, adherent clot on its surface
Grade 1	Some external bleeding; uterine tetany and tenderness may not be noted; no signs of shock or fetal distress
Grade 2	External bleeding; uterine tetany and tenderness; fetal distress
Grade 3	Bleeding may be external or internal; uterine tetany; maternal shock and fetal death; complicating disseminated ultravascular coagulation (DIC)

---

this is usually an indication of an extensive placental separation. Vaginal delivery is preferred with fetal death except if hemorrhage cannot be successfully handled through blood replacement or if other complications arise. The risk of serious coagulation defects, to be described subsequently, is likely to be greater when delivery is performed transabdominally. In circumstances in which the fetus is immature and blood loss is occurring at a slow rate, delivery may be delayed. Ongoing assessment of fetal viability should be performed with ultrasonic Doppler devices to hear the fetal heart and with real-time ultrasound, which allows visualization of the heart movements.

Maternal hypovolemia and anemia may be corrected by administration of fresh whole blood plus electrolyte solution either prior to or during labor and delivery. Packed red cells and lactated Ringer's solution offer alternative replacements. A central venous pressure (CVP) line may be inserted for hemodynamic monitoring in critical cases. If the client is in shock, an arterial line may have to be inserted to monitor blood pressure.

Nursing Assessment

The nursing assessment of the woman with abruptio placentae includes all of the components described for clients with spontaneous abortion and placenta previa. In addition, the nurse must carefully assess for changes in fundal height because an increase is associated with concealed bleeding. Initial laboratory studies should include fibrinogen levels, fibrin split products (FDP), thrombin time, prothrombin time, and partial thromboplastin time.

It is important to note that on occasion a false alarm concerning hemorrhage may occur, when bleeding is actually normal show characteristic of early labor. This

(text continued on page 757)

The Woman with Hemorrhagic Complications of Late Pregnancy

Nursing Objectives

1. Identify early women at risk for hemorrhagic disorders in late pregnancy.
2. Prevent or detect early complications from third-trimester bleeding.
3. Maintain adequate tissue perfusion and oxygen to maternal–fetal unit.
4. Deliver a live and stable neonate at or near term.

Assessment	Potential Nursing Diagnosis	Planning/Intervention	Evaluation
Predisposing factors	Fluid volume deficit (hypovolemia) related to bleeding complication of late pregnancy	Assess maternal blood loss and vital signs q15min–q1h	Woman's blood loss is controlled
Grand multiparity			Woman's vital signs remain stable
Advanced maternal age			
Multiple gestation		Maintain bed rest in flat, lateral position	Woman rests comfortably in bed
Hydramnios		Initiate and monitor intravenous fluids to restore circulating volume (use at least 18-gauge needle)	Woman receives adequate fluid intake amounts
Hypertensive disorders of pregnancy			
History of previous bleeding disorder, blood coagulopathy		Type and cross match 2 (or more) units of whole blood	
Previous cesarean section			
Estimated gestational age		Monitor and record intake and output	Woman returns to normal urine output
Blood loss (color, quantity, consistency)		Count and weigh perineal pads, inspect contents for tissue	
Laboratory studies			
Blood: CBC, hematocrit, hemoglobin, electrolytes		Assess for further blood loss and integrity of maternal system	Woman's arterial blood gases and other laboratory tests remain within normal limits or are restored to within normal limits
		Serial CBC, hemoglobin, hematocrit	
		Arterial blood gases prn	
		Administer iron supplements as prescribed	
Vital signs and blood pressure	Alteration in tissue perfusion related to hypovolemic shock	Assess for signs of shock q15min–q1h	Woman is comfortable and free of signs of shock
Hypotension		Pallor	
Tachycardia		Clamminess	
Uterus		Irritability	
Pain		Decreased blood pressure	
Tenderness		Tachycardia	
Rigidity		Assess for abdominal tenderness, rigidity, pain (abruption) q30min–q1h	
Contour			
Height			
Contractions		Administer oxygen as necessary (6 liters–8 liters/min) to maintain adequate perfusion	
Arterial pulse quality (decreased or absent)			
Skin (color, pallor)			
Nausea or vomiting		Monitor vital signs q15min–q1h until stable	Woman's vital signs remain stable
Restlessness or irritability			

(continued)

Assessment	Potential Nursing Diagnosis	Planning/Intervention	Evaluation
Shortness of breath		Assess level of consciousness (LOC) and peripheral perfusion	Woman remains alert and well oriented; her extremities remain warm and pink
Level of consciousness (confusion)		Color	
Urinary output and fluid intake		Warmth	
Laboratory studies		Pulses	
Blood type and cross match		Prevent further bleeding by prohibiting vaginal and rectal exams, enemas	
Clotting time			
Prothrombin time		Administer transfusion as prescribed and observe for reaction (whole blood, frozen plasma, cryoprecipitate, as indicated)	Woman shows no adverse reaction to transfusion
Fibrinogen level			
Platelets			
FDP			
Thrombin time		Monitor CVP line for vital functioning	Woman maintains adequate blood return to the heart
Prothrombin time		Assess for sudden increase in fundal height (abruption)	
Partial thromboplastin time			
		Assess for associated blood coagulation problems (hypofibrinogenemia and DIC)	Woman remains free of blood coagulation complications
		Clot observation test	
		Coagulation studies	
		Prepare for emergency delivery (vaginal or cesarean section, as indicated)	Woman verbalizes understanding of need for possible emergency delivery and potential method to be used
		NPO	
		Double setup operating room (placenta previa only)	
		Preoperative teaching	
Understanding of hemorrhagic complication	Ineffective maternal attachment related to disease	Encourage client to verbalize anxieties, fears, and possible guilt feelings	Woman verbalizes concerns about situation
Grieving response		Demonstrate a caring and empathetic attitude	Woman expresses grief
Crying			
Grimacing		Support maternal–fetal bonding by:	Mother listens to normal fetal heart tones
Verbalizations of anger, denial, sorrow		Allowing mother to listen to normal fetal heart tones (FHTs) (if present)	
Feelings about pregnancy		Maintaining a positive but realistic attitude	
		Providing factual information on condition of fetus/neonate	
		Remain with mother at frequent intervals	

(continued)

Assessment	Potential Nursing Diagnosis	Planning/Intervention	Evaluation
		Involve supportive family members in discussions and provide them with information about problems	Family members offer each other mutual support
FHTs	Risk of fetal distress related to alteration in placental tissue perfusion	Monitor fetal heart rate, activity, and response to contractions by external monitor	Fetus remains reactive with normal FHTs
Rate (120 bpm–160 bpm)			
Variability (good)			
Reactivity (present)		Assess uterine activity for signs of labor	
Uterine activity			
Frequency of contractions		Turn on left side and administer oxygen if signs of fetal distress present	Woman changes position and restores normal FHT and rhythm
Length of contractions		Prepare client for and assist with amniocentesis if ordered	Woman is prepared for amniocentesis, as ordered
Irritability			
Palpation of fetal parts and movement		Assist with emergency delivery if indicated for fetal distress	

(text continued from page 754)

bleeding is slight and due to dilation of the cervix. No treatment is required except for reassurance and continued client observation of vaginal discharge.

Nursing Diagnosis

Assessment of the client for signs and symptoms of abruptio placentae may lead the nurse to some of the previously described nursing diagnoses for placenta previa. It should be noted that the identified problems of fluid volume deficit and alteration in placental tissue perfusion in this clinical condition are secondary to premature separation of the normally implanted placenta. The client is likely to experience fear/anxiety related to concern about bleeding as a life-threatening situation for herself and the fetus.

Nursing Intervention

Nursing interventions are planned based on the identified nursing diagnoses and on the medical plan of treatment. If the abruption is mild and the fetus is immature, careful and continuous nursing observation is necessary to detect evidence of progressive maternal blood loss or changes in fetal status (e.g., ominous decelerations, bradycardia). In more acute situations, intake and output are recorded hourly and oxygen may be administered by mask to prevent or minimize fetal

hypoxia. If a CVP line is in place, readings must be carefully obtained, recorded, and reported. Occasionally, CVP monitoring may be replaced by pulmonary artery wedge pressure (PAWP) monitoring with the Swan-Ganz catheter. Observation should be made for signs and symptoms of hypovolemia such as cough, abnormal respiratory sound, and shortness of breath. It is also essential for the nurse to assess the client for adverse reactions to blood transfusion.

In cases of moderate to severe abruption and a live fetus, the nurse should provide preoperative teaching about the possibility of a cesarean delivery and birth of a preterm infant. A realistic attitude about the client's health situation and factual reassurance are important aspects of the psychological support offered by the nurse to the family.

Following delivery the nurse should continue assessing fluid volume balance and vital signs. The uterus should be frequently palpated for atony and excessive blood loss.

Other Problems Associated with Bleeding

Bleeding may lead to hypovolemia and hemorrhagic shock unless vigorous treatment is implemented to control bleeding and replace lost blood. In most emergency situations the uterus must be expeditiously emptied of all contents. Delay may result in complications such as *hypofibrinogenemia* and *DIC*.

Hypofibrinogenemia

Fibrinogenopenia occurs in the childbearing woman who has depleted her blood fibrinogen in an attempt to control bleeding by clot formation. Following an abruption of the placenta, thromboplastin enters the circulation, causing small fibrin clots to form in the capillaries. As the level of fibrinogen decreases in the circulating blood, normal clotting mechanisms are impaired. This complication is also seen in other entities, such as amniotic fluid embolus, prolonged retention of a dead fetus, and septic abortion. Because of the danger of this complication, the client with abruptio placentae should receive laboratory analysis for fibrinogen levels (normal, 300 mg–500 mg/dl). The nurse can also perform a simple *clot observation test* by placing a small amount of fresh blood in a test tube and watching how quickly a clot is formed. A firm clot should rapidly form (normal time, 4 min–12 min).

Treatment for hypofibrinogenemia involves replacement of blood and fibrinogen and termination of the pregnancy. The administration of cryoprecipitate is generally effective in raising the fibrinogen concentration of plasma.

Another complication of impaired coagulation associated with severe abruption is *Couvelaire uterus* (uteroplacental apoplexy). In this condition the uterine muscle fills with blood and is therefore unable to contract well after delivery. The uterus feels hard and boardlike on palpation. Treatment consists in complete evacuation of the uterus and stimulation of contractions with intravenous oxytocin.

Disseminated Intravascular Coagulation

DIC is a paradoxical disorder with anticoagulation and procoagulation effects existing simultaneously.[7] In DIC, clotting is overstimulated throughout the circulatory system, possibly initiated by an abruption or other obstetric complication, such as PIH, retained products of conception, infection, or amniotic fluid embolism. These pathologic conditions act on either the intrinsic or the extrinsic pathways, creating increased formation of thrombin. The thrombin interacts with fibrinogen, resulting in formation of clots.

Figure 36-11 displays how the rapid and extensive formation of clots causes platelets and clotting factors to be depleted in clients with DIC. Concurrently, thrombin stimulates the fibrinolytic system to dissolve clots of fibrin, leading to the formation of fibrin degradation products (FDP), which have an anticoagulant effect. The overall result is bleeding diathesis and potential vascular occlusion of organs due to the formation of thromboemboli.

It is imperative that the nurse perform careful evaluation of women at risk for early signs of DIC. Clinical manifestations may be difficult to assess in the early stage, but become more obvious as the severity of the disease progresses. Symptoms include bleeding from the gums and injection sites, petechiae and purpura on the skin, restlessness, anxiety, and tachycardia. The results of laboratory assessment reveal several abnormalities; these are presented in Table 36-2. Plasma fibrinogen and platelets are decreased, whereas FDP, thrombin time, prothrombin time, and partial thromboplastin time are increased.

Intervention for DIC is directed toward correcting causative factors, including termination of pregnancy if there is a placental abruption or fetal demise and treatment of infection or amniotic fluid embolism. The need for further intervention may be unnecessary once the cause of DIC is removed. If physiological support is indicated it may be provided by (1) maintaining fluid and electrolyte balance with appropriate parenteral solutions; (2) administering oxygen to prevent or treat hypoxia; (3) replacing whole blood or its constituents (*e.g.*, frozen plasma, platelets, cryoprecipitate); and (4) carefully and continuously assessing vital functions through CVP monitoring or a pulmonary artery catheter.

The infusion of heparin to block DIC is controversial, since it has the potential to aggravate hemorrhage when there has been severe disruption of the vasculature.[6]

Hypertensive Disorders of Pregnancy

Hypertensive disorders include a variety of vascular disturbances that either antedate pregnancy or occur as a complication during gestation or the early puerperium. Because of the many cardiovascular alterations, pregnancy may induce hypertension in women who have been normotensive prior to gestation or may aggravate existing hypertensive conditions. Until recently *toxemia* was the term used to describe the type of hypertension peculiar to pregnancy, since it was believed that the condition was caused by toxins derived from the products of conception circulating in the blood. In 1972 the American College of Obstetricians and Gynecologists (ACOG) introduced a new classification system for hypertensive disorders of pregnancy that excluded the diagnosis of toxemia. The term *pregnancy-induced hypertension* (PIH) is the current diagnostic label being used

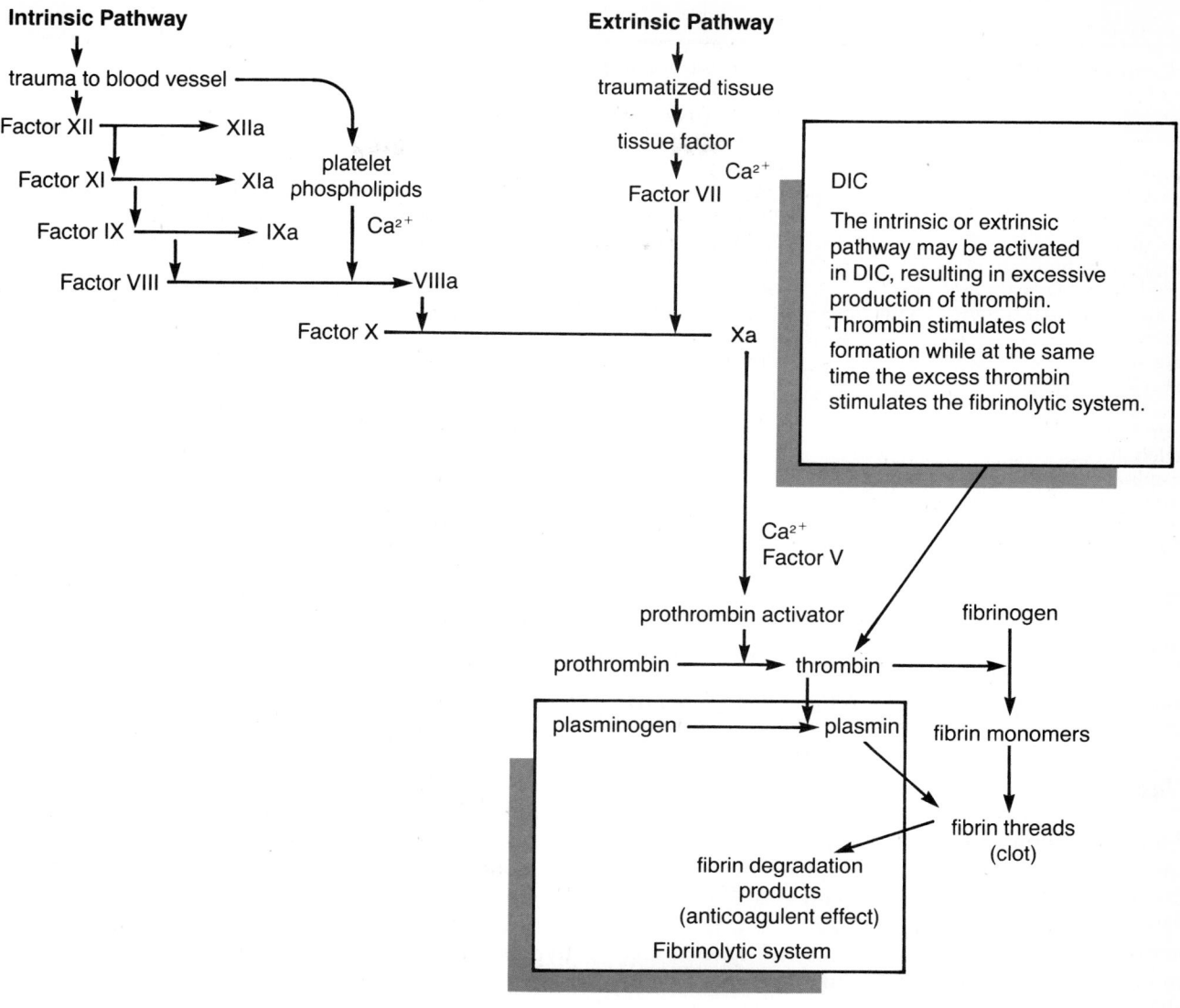

Intrinsic Pathway

trauma to blood vessel

Factor XII → XIIa

Factor XI → XIa

platelet phospholipids

Factor IX → IXa

Ca^{2+}

Factor VIII → VIIIa

Factor X → VIIIa

Extrinsic Pathway

traumatized tissue

tissue factor

Ca^{2+}

Factor VII

Xa

Ca^{2+}
Factor V

prothrombin activator

prothrombin → thrombin

fibrinogen

fibrin monomers

fibrin threads (clot)

DIC

The intrinsic or extrinsic pathway may be activated in DIC, resulting in excessive production of thrombin. Thrombin stimulates clot formation while at the same time the excess thrombin stimulates the fibrinolytic system.

plasminogen → plasmin

fibrin degradation products (anticoagulent effect)

Fibrinolytic system

FIGURE 36-11

Normal blood coagulation pathways, the fibrinolytic system, and DIC.

to describe the syndrome of hypertension, edema, and proteinuria evident in certain pregnant women. *Preeclampsia* and eclampsia are two categories of PIH that represent one and the same process, but the term *eclampsia* is used when the woman's clinical course has advanced to generalized convulsions or coma.

PIH is a very common complication; it is seen in 6% or 7% of all gravidas. The prevalence of the disease may be much higher among certain groups, including young primigravidas, women with chronic hypertension, and women from low socioeconomic backgrounds. PIH also tends to recur in up to one third of the women.[8]

In the United States, PIH ranks among the three major complications (hemorrhage and puerperal infection being the other two) responsible for the vast majority of maternal deaths and accounts for some 250 maternal deaths each year. As a cause of fetal death, PIH is even more important. It can be estimated conservatively that at least 25,000 stillbirths and neonatal deaths occur each year in the United States from hypertensive diseases of pregnancy, and those newborns who survive may suffer impairments that affect the quality of their lives. The great majority of perinatal deaths are related to prematurity.

TABLE 36-2

Laboratory Tests for Disseminated Intravascular Coagulation

Test	Nonpregnant Values	Normal Pregnancy	Result in DIC
Clotting time	6 min–12 min	Normal	Normal
Clot retraction	Good	Good	Poor (lyses in 15 min–60 min)
Fibrinogen	200 mg–400 mg/dl	300 mg–500 mg/dl	Usually depressed
Thrombin time	12 sec–18 sec	Shortened	Usually prolonged
Prothrombin time	11 sec–13 sec	Shortened	Usually prolonged
Partial thromboplastin time or	40 sec–60 sec	Shortened	Usually prolonged
activated partial thromboplastin time	25 sec–45 sec	Shortened	Usually prolonged
Factor assays		Normal	V, VIII, XIII reduced
Platelets	150,000–400,000/mm³	Normal	Usually decreased
Red cell morphology		Normal	Often abnormal (schistocytes, etc)
Fibrin split products (FDP)		Usually absent	Present
Euglobulin clot lysis		Normal	Usually shortened
Plasminogen		Normal	Usually depressed
Plasma protamine paracoagulation		Fibrin monomer absent	Fibrin monomer present
Ethanol gelation		Fibrin monomer absent	Fibrin monomer present
Protamine sulfate precipitation		Fibrin monomer absent	Fibrin monomer present
Staphylococcal clumping		Fibrin monomer absent	Fibrin monomer present

(Cavanagh D et al: Obstetric Emergencies. Philadelphia, Harper & Row, 1982.)

Classification

The classification system and definition of the hypertensive disorders of pregnancy, originally developed by Chesley[8] and later modified by Gant and Worley,[9] are presented in the accompanying outline. The term *pregnancy-induced hypertension* covers those specific conditions that develop as a direct result of pregnancy. Preeclampsia is characterized by hypertension with proteinuria or edema development after the 20th week of gestation. Severe preeclampsia exists when one or more of the symptoms listed in the outline are present.

When the preeclamptic woman develops convulsions or coma unrelated to other cerebral conditions, the term *eclampsia* is used. If hypertension develops without edema or proteinuria during labor or in the early postpartum period and then returns to normal within 10 days following delivery, it is described as *late* or *transient hypertension*. The term *superimposed preeclampsia and eclampsia* is used when the client who already has chronic hypertensive vascular or renal disease develops preeclampsia and possible eclampsia, which is heralded by a significant rise in blood pressure (systolic blood pressure 30 mm Hg or diastolic blood pressure 15 mm Hg to 20 mm Hg above baseline) with edema and/or proteinuria. The term *chronic hypertension* is used when the client has a concurrent hypertensive vascular disorder that is unrelated to pregnancy and was evident prior to gestation. For purposes of discussion, the hypertensive disorders of pregnancy are considered in two broad classifications: PIH, including preeclampsia and eclampsia, and hypertensive disorders not confined to pregnancy but that may exist during pregnancy and may be complicated by superimposed preeclampsia or eclampsia. The latter includes chronic hypertension.

Etiology and Pathophysiology of PIH

Although the exact mechanism underlying PIH remains unknown, several theories exist to explain the etiology. Since PIH is a *multisystem disease*, it is obvious that no single alteration or disturbance can explain the condition. PIH is characterized by an increase in arterial blood pressure and an increase in peripheral vascular resistance. The vasospasm existing in women with PIH is attributed to the extreme sensitivity of the vasculature to vasopressors. Unlike the normal pregnant woman who is resistant to the pressor effects of infused angiotensin II, women who will subsequently develop preeclampsia show an increased pressor responsiveness to angiotensin II several weeks prior to the appearance of clinical symptoms.[10] A similar receptivity is found in women who have chronic hypertension preceding the development of superimposed PIH.[11]

There is also a lower level of plasma renin activity, aldosterone, and angiotensin II in women with preeclampsia as compared with normal pregnant women.

Hypertensive Disorders of Pregnancy

A. Pregnancy-induced hypertension (PIH)
  1. Preeclampsia—hypertension with proteinuria and/or edema developing after the 20th week of gestation
     a. Symptoms may occur earlier with hydatidiform mole
     b. Occurs almost exclusively in primigravidas
     c. Affects women at extremes of reproductive age (less than 20 yr or more than 35 yr)
     d. May be seen in multigravidas with the following:
        (1) Uterine overdistention as with twins or hydramnios
        (2) Vascular disease, including essential chronic hypertension and diabetes mellitus
        (3) Chronic renal disease
     Hypertension: 140/90 or an increase of 30 mm Hg systolic or 15 mm Hg diastolic over baseline;
       observation of these criteria on at least two occasions 6 or more hours apart
     Edema: significant edema generally limited to the face and hands even after arising in the morning
     Proteinuria: 500 mg or more protein in a 24-hour urine collection or 2+ protein in a random sample; develops late in the course of PIH
     Severe preeclampsia:
       When one or more of the following are present:
       • Systolic blood pressure of 160 mm Hg or diastolic of 110 mm Hg on two occasions at least 6 hours apart while the client is on bed rest
       • Proteinuria of at least 5 g/24 hr or 3+ to 4+ by semiquantitative analysis
       • Cerebral or visual disturbances such as altered consciousness, headache, scotomata, or blurred vision
       • Pulmonary edema or cyanosis

     Signs of advancing disease:
       • Epigastric or upper quadrant pain
       • Thrombocytopenia or impaired liver function
  2. Eclampsia—extension of preeclampsia with grand mal seizure
       • One half the cases occur before labor
       • One fourth of the cases occur during labor
       • One fourth of the cases occur within 48 hours post partum

B. Chronic hypertension
  1. Blood pressure of 140/90 before pregnancy
  2. Blood pressure of 140/90 before 20th week gestation and/or persisting indefinitely following delivery
  3. For differential diagnosis after the 20th week of gestation:
     a. Hemorrhage and exudates seen on funduscopic examination
     b. Plasma urea nitrogen: 20 mg/dl
     c. Plasma creatinine levels: 1 mg/dl
     d. Presence of chronic disease, such as diabetes mellitus or connective tissue diseases

C. Chronic hypertension with superimposed preeclampsia—often a quick progression to eclampsia, which may develop before the 30th week of gestation
  1. Documented evidence of chronic hypertension
  2. Evidence of a superimposed, acute process
     a. Elevation of systolic blood pressure 30 mm Hg or of diastolic blood pressure 15 mm Hg to 20 mm Hg above baseline on two occasions at least 6 hours apart
     b. Development of proteinuria
     c. Edema as observed in women with preeclampsia

D. Late or transient hypertension—transient elevations of blood pressure are observed during labor or in early postpartum period, returning to normal within 10 days post partum

(Gant NF, Worley RJ: Hypertension in Pregnancy: Concepts and Management, pp 2–9. New York, Appleton–Century–Crofts, 1980)

Catecholamines, prolactin, vasopressin, and prostaglandins have all been cited as humoral substances having a possible role in the pathogenesis or maintenance of PIH. A hypothesized association of circulating antigen–antibody complexes with the development of PIH is currently being investigated.

Glomerular endotheliosis often develops in the kidneys of women experiencing proteinuria of PIH. This disturbance causes partial obstruction of capillary lumina and may be related to the release of placenta thromboplastin, which initiates intravascular coagulation and formation of fibrin deposits.[12] Other PIH-associated renal alterations that are atypical of pregnancy include a decrease in the plasma renal flow and glomerular filtration rate and increased serum uric acid, serum creatinine, and urea levels. The proteinuria that usually accompanies PIH is believed to be correlated with the severity of kidney involvement as the disease advances. Related changes in the clotting mechanism (thrombocytopenia and DIC) have also been postulated as causative factors of PIH; however, it is not clearly established whether these alterations are an effect of PIH or a contributing etiologic factor.

There is an overall fluid shift from the intravascular space to the intracellular space. Proteins and electrolytes similarly move into the intracellular space.

The uteroplacental manifestations of PIH include increased peripheral vascular resistance in the spiral and basal arteries with associated hypertensive lesions, poor placental perfusion resulting from decreased blood flow and vasospasm, and occasional decreased amniotic fluid volume. The effects of these changes can cause placental–fetal anoxia,[13] intrauterine growth retardation, and fetal death.[14] Uterine activity is increased both spontaneously and in response to oxytocin in women with PIH.

Preeclampsia

Manifestations

Preeclampsia is characterized by elevation in blood pressure, proteinuria, or edema in a gravida after the 20th week of pregnancy who previously has been normal in these respects. It is a forerunner or prodromal stage of eclampsia; in other words, unless the preeclamptic process is checked by treatment or by delivery it is likely that eclampsia (*e.g.*, convulsions or coma) will ensue. The rise in blood pressure may occur suddenly, or it may be gradual and insidious.

The earliest warning signal of preeclampsia is *sudden development of hypertension*. Accordingly, the importance of frequent and regular blood pressure readings during pregnancy cannot be emphasized too strongly. The absolute blood pressure level is probably of less significance than the relationship it bears to previous determinations and the time in gestation when these determinations were recorded. The healthy client often exhibits a lower than normal blood pressure in the midtrimester of pregnancy, and hence a baseline reading in midpregnancy may be misleading. For example, a pressure of 120/80 may actually indicate hypertension in a client whose midpregnancy pressure has been running in the 100/70 range.

The next most constant sign of preeclampsia is *sudden excessive weight gain*. If cases of preeclampsia are studied from the viewpoint of fluid intake and output, it is at once apparent that these sudden gains in weight are due entirely to an accumulation of water in the tissues. Such weight gains represent occult edema and almost always precede the visible face and finger edema that is so characteristic of the advanced stages of the disease.

The sudden appearance of *protein in the urine*, with or without other findings, should always be regarded as a sign of preeclampsia. A complete urinalysis, including a microscopic examination, helps to exclude infection as a cause of proteinuria. Usually it develops later than the hypertension and the gain in weight and for this very reason must be regarded as a serious omen when superimposed on these other two findings.

But the very essence of preeclampsia is the lightninglike fulminance with which it strikes. Although the above physical signs of preeclampsia usually allow ample time to institute preventive treatment, it sometimes happens that these derangements develop between antepartal visits, even if they are only a week apart.

There are several other clinical manifestations of PIH that when recognized by the client or health-team member necessitate immediate attention; these include the following:

- Severe, continuous headache, often frontal or occipital
- Swelling of the face or the fingers
- Dimness or blurring of vision
- Persistent vomiting
- Decrease in the amount of urine excreted
- Epigastric pain (a late symptom)

It should be emphasized that the three early and important signs of preeclampsia, namely, hypertension, weight gain, and proteinuria, are changes of which the client is usually unaware. All three may be present in substantial degree, and yet she may feel quite well. Only by regular and careful antepartal examination can these warning signs be detected. By the time the preeclamptic client has developed symptoms and signs that she herself can detect, such as headache, blurred vision, and puffiness of the eyelids and the fingers, she is usually in an advanced stage of the disease, and much valuable time has been lost.

Headache is rarely observed in the milder cases, but is encountered with increasing frequency in the most severe grades. In general, clients who develop eclampsia often have a severe headache as a forerunner of the first convulsion. The visual disturbances range from a slight blurring of vision to various degrees of temporary blindness. Although convulsions are less likely to occur in cases of mild preeclampsia, the possibility cannot be entirely eliminated. Clients with severe preeclampsia should always be considered as being on the verge of having a convulsion.

Medical Diagnosis and Prognosis

Detection of preeclampsia (or other hypertensive diseases) is facilitated by careful antepartal observation and early identification of women known to have predisposing risk factors. A large number of the risk factors may relate to preeclampsia; these include (1) the client's exposure to chorionic villi for the first time; (2) an excess of chorionic villi, such as in cases of hydatidiform mole, multiple gestations, or a large fetus; or (3) the presence of vascular disturbances.[15] Conditions predisposing to chronic hypertension should also be considered, since preeclampsia is a common complication of this preexistent disease. Examples of specific risk factors classified according to time of existence during the childbearing cycle are presented in Table 36-3.

Women with recognized risks for hypertensive disease should have antepartal health supervision scheduled at more frequent intervals, especially during the third trimester. The appearance of an upward trend in blood pressure in a normotensive woman or a rapid weight gain in the second or third trimester suggests a potential diagnosis of preeclampsia. Chronic hypertension should be suspected in pregnant women displaying elevated blood pressures before 24 weeks' gestation.

The *rollover test* is often useful for selectively screening women, particularly primigravidas between 28 and 32 weeks' gestation. It involves placing the woman at rest in the left lateral recumbent position until her blood pressure stabilizes (15 min–20 min). After rolling the woman on her back, her blood pressure is immediately taken, then reobtained in 5 minutes. A diastolic rise of 20 mm Hg is considered a positive response to the test. It should be noted that there is now some concern about the applicability of this test, owing to the high rate of false-positive readings.[16] However, in the experience of the investigators who originally developed the rollover test, it is a valid instrument for predicting PIH.

Determination of mean arterial pressure (MAP) may also be useful in predicting risk for developing hypertensive disease, since it reflects the resistance against which the heart works. To calculate MAP, the systolic blood pressure is added to twice the diastolic blood pressure, then the product is divided by three. An increase of 20 mm Hg in mean arterial pressure is considered ominous.

The prognosis for women with preeclampsia is dependent upon the maternal effects of hypertension on the body systems (*e.g.,* cardiovascular, central nervous system, renal) and the ability to prevent or control disease before eclampsia develops. The combination of proteinuria and hypertension dramatically increases the risk of perinatal mortality and morbidity. The only definitive cure for preeclampsia is delivery.

Medical Management

Medical management of all pregnant women is directed toward prevention and early detection of the development of preeclampsia through early and regular prenatal care. Every pregnant woman should be assessed each week during the last month of pregnancy and every 2 weeks during the 2 previous months.

If mild symptoms of the disease develop (*e.g.,* minor elevation of blood pressure with minimal or no signs of edema and proteinuria), the client may remain at home in the hope that symptoms will abate with proper treatment. During this period the client should be examined at least twice a week, and she should implement a regimen such as the following:

- Restriction of activities, including bed rest during the greater part of the day, and sexual abstinence
- Administration of prescribed sedative drugs as necessary to encourage rest and relaxation

T A B L E   3 6 - 3

PIH: Recognizing Risk Factors

Before Pregnancy	Possibly Before Pregnancy	During Pregnancy
Nulligravida	Diabetes mellitus*	Primigravida
Age extremes:	Preexisting hypertensive, vascular, or renal disease	Glomerulonephritis
≤20 yr		Multiple gestation
≥35 yr*		Hydramnios
Underweight		Large fetus
Obesity		Hydatidiform mole
Dietary deficiencies		Fetal hydrops
Family history of hypertension/ vascular disease*		
Diagnosis of PIH in previous pregnancy		

* Predisposes to chronic hypertension as well as PIH.
(Willis SE, Sharp ES: Hypertension in pregnancy: Prenatal detection and management. Am J Nurs 82(5):798, 1982)

• Ingestion of a well-balanced diet with ample protein, particularly lean meat, fish, and eggs

Although in the past some have suggested that sodium restriction and routine therapy with thiazide diuretics would prevent preeclampsia, in a group of high-risk women it has now been clearly established that this is not true. The value of diuretic therapy has been questioned because it has been shown to decrease both placental and renal clearance.

In the event that the client's condition does not respond promptly to restricted activity at home, hospitalization may be recommended. Hospitalization becomes mandatory if proteinuria appears. Medical care of the hospitalized preeclamptic woman is directed toward the prevention of eclampsia by decreasing blood pressure and reducing fluid retention, as well as promoting other aspects of perinatal well-being until the fetus reaches maturity.

The nature of drug therapy prescribed by the physician is dependent upon the client's condition. In mild cases of preeclampsia, medications may or may not be ordered. However, when severe preeclampsia develops, immediate and intensive therapy is imperative. Sedation is of major importance to forestall convulsions. The dosage of drugs employed should be regulated so that they produce drowsiness and sleep, from which the client can be easily awakened, and also suppress the client's hyperactive reflexes. Magnesium sulfate (MgSO$_4$) is most often used as a sedative and an anticonvulsant under these circumstances. In addition to being an excellent anticonvulsant, magnesium causes vasodilataton and, therefore, is also effective in lowering blood pressure. A complete assessment of the client's reflexes should be performed prior to and during the administration of MgSO$_4$ (see Nursing Assessment).

For rapid action, an intravenous dose of 20 ml to 40 ml of a 10% solution (2 g–4 g) is administered by way of an infusion pump. Very often the drug is given intramuscularly in doses of 10 ml to 20 ml of a 50% solution (5 g–10 g). The dose is divided, half given into each buttock, and often 1 ml to 2 ml of 1% procaine is added to the injection to minimize discomfort. The advantage of intravenous administration of MgSO$_4$ is that it allows titration and more careful regulation of the medication. Intramuscular injection is painful but requires less intravenous fluid.

A repeat dose of MgSO$_4$ should not be given unless the reflexes and respiratory rate are normal, since it depresses both.

Other sedatives, such as barbiturates, have long been used, the dose being larger (60 mg–120 mg every 4 hr–6 hr) than for mild cases, and they are administered parenterally. The possibility has been raised, however, of adverse effects such as depletion of fetal coagulation factors or delay of fetal lung maturation. Furthermore, if the client is in labor, barbiturates should be avoided because of their depressant effect on the fetus. Although many use morphine in the management of severe preeclampsia, it would seem best reserved for the client who has the added stimulus of pain (*i.e.*, labor). Minimizing this stimulus certainly reduces the likelihood of a seizure.

Another drug that is an effective anticonvulsant is diazepam (Valium) in 5-mg to 10-mg doses intramuscularly or, if the situation warrants, intravenously. Diazepam is usually reserved for severe cases and is discussed further in the management of eclampsia.

Agents that reduce peripheral blood pressure find occasional use in the treatment of the client with extreme degrees of hypertension. Opinions differ as to their general effectiveness, largely because they are known to decrease placental perfusion and hence may have an untoward effect on the fetus. Nevertheless, they are sometimes prescribed in cases of severe preeclampsia and eclampsia when the diastolic blood pressure exceeds 100 mm Hg to 110 mm Hg. They are used as a temporary measure to reduce blood pressure and thus decrease the possibility of a cerebrovascular accident. They have also been found to improve kidney function and are associated with some improvement in cardiac output. The most widely used antihypertensive agent at present is hydralazine (Apresoline). This is given intravenously (5 mg–10 mg) in a dilute solution by slow drip. The maternal blood pressure must be monitored every 2 to 3 minutes after the initial dose, then every 5 to 10 minutes until the hypertensive crisis is stabilized. The use of antihypertensive agents has not been shown in careful studies to improve either fetal or maternal survival, and their long-term use in preeclampsia is generally not recommended.

The administration of diuretics is usually not recommended for treatment of PIH because these drugs may further deplete the intravascular volume and worsen vasospasm. Diuretics directly stimulate the release of renin. Swan-Ganz catheterization is increasingly being performed in severe cases of preeclampsia and other hypertensive disorders for purposes of hemodynamic monitoring. Since there is a very diversified population of women with PIH, volume management must be individualized.

Monitoring of fetal well-being is of continuous concern in the medical management of the client with preeclampsia. Various prenatal assessment tests are used to ascertain adequacy of fetal oxygenation and functioning of the placenta. These tests are used in many high-risk situations and include the nonstress test, performed weekly or more often if indicated; the oxytocin challenge test (OCT); and 24-hour urinary estriol/creatinine (E/C) ratios, determined biweekly or daily. Serially increasing E/C ratios and reactive nonstress tests are favorable signs that may permit continued management until further *in utero* maturation occurs. If nonstress tests are unsatisfactory on two or more occasions and other indices of fetal well-being (such as OCTs) indicate potential fetal compromise, the pregnancy may not be allowed to continue. Amniocentesis is usually performed to determine fetal lung maturity prior to planned delivery. In such situations induction of labor may be most desirable for the welfare of mother and infant. If conditions for induction of labor are not favorable, cesarean delivery may be the procedure of choice. This most often occurs when preeclampsia is severe and fulminating.

The signs and symptoms of preeclampsia usually abate rapidly after delivery, but the danger of convulsions does not pass until 48 hours have elapsed post partum. Therefore, continuation of previously prescribed sedation throughout this interval may be indicated. In the majority of cases the elevated blood pressure as well as the other derangements have returned to normal within 10 days or 2 weeks. In about 30% of cases, however, the hypertension shows a tendency either to persist indefinitely or to recur in subsequent pregnancies. For this reason prolonged follow-up of these clients is highly important.

Nursing Assessment

The nurse's responsibility in the detection and care of cases of preeclampsia is manifold. Since this complication of pregnancy is common and may occur antepartally, intrapartally, or postpartally, it is important for the nurse to observe all maternity clients closely for the first indication of early symptoms and to report any evidence pointing to an aggravation of the process. The objective of assessment is for the nurse to recognize symptoms before they become obvious to the client. The early symptoms and the manifestations related to more severe preeclampsia, such as persistent headache, blurred vision, spots or flashes of light before the eyes, epigastric pain, vomiting, torpor, or muscular twitchings, are all vastly important. Data collected in relation to these symptoms, in addition to nutritional status, fluid intake and elimination, and attitudes about pregnancy, when accurately recorded, can be of great assistance in planning the course of therapy.

During the first prenatal examination it is particularly important to assess the woman for predisposing risk factors associated with hypertensive disease in pregnancy. Prepregnancy weight should be recorded and compared with current weight.

Subsequently the pattern of weight gain should be carefully followed and recorded by the nurse. Weight gain of 1 lb a week or so may be regarded as normal. Sudden gains of more than 2 lb a week should be viewed with suspicion; gains of more than 3 lb a week, with alarm. Weight increases of the latter magnitude call for more frequent blood pressure determinations, and if these latter are also abnormal, stricter medical management may be indicated.

As finger edema is a frequent forerunner of preeclampsia, which may precede the hypertension by several weeks, it is a most valuable warning signal for assessment. In investigating suspected edema, it is important to ask the client if her wedding ring is becoming tight. It is also essential to observe for facial edema, characterized by swelling of the eyelids and a marked coarseness of features. This condition generally does not become apparent in early disease states.

Initial assessment of the *hospitalized* preeclamptic woman should include all of the parameters described above plus several other components. Body weight should be obtained on admission and daily thereafter. Vital signs and blood pressure readings should be assessed every 4 hours except between midnight and morning, unless the midnight blood pressure has risen or vital signs are abnormal. Evaluations are made daily, or at more frequent intervals if indicated, for fluid intake and output. Urine specimens should also be sent to the laboratory daily for protein and casts analysis.

Results of laboratory studies should be assessed for baseline values and changes reflecting altered organ functioning. The effects of preeclampsia on the kidneys, liver, and fetoplacental unit and, in some cases, the presence of hematologic abnormalities may be evidenced through laboratory changes. In severe preeclampsia there are elevations in serum creatinine, blood urea nitrogen (BUN), and uric acid levels; decreases in creatinine clearance; proteinuria; and changes in the urinary sediment. Liver pathology may be revealed through marked elevations in SGPT, SGOT, and lactate dehydrogenase.

One of the most significant elements of the nurse's physical examination is assessment of reflexes, because abnormal findings may indicate central nervous system pathology. Signs of excessive nervous system irritability generally precede the onset of seizures in preeclamptic women. Assessment of deep tendon reflexes is performed most often in the patellar tendon of the quadriceps muscle; however, a comprehensive examination should also include the brachioradialis, Achilles, biceps, and triceps reflexes. Selected information on testing of deep tendon reflexes is presented under Nursing Guidelines for Administration of Magnesium Sulfate. It is important for the nurse to remember to observe the symmetry of the reflexes from one side of the body to the other. Clonus should be assessed by briskly dorsiflexing the foot while slightly flexing the knee. Involuntary oscillations may be seen between flexion and extension when continuous pressure is applied to the sole of the foot in the hyperreflexic client. If difficulty is encountered in producing muscle stretch reflexes, the nurse may find certain reinforcement techniques helpful, such as instructing the client to contract muscles other than the ones being evaluated.

It is particularly important for the nurse to observe the client with moderate to severe preeclampsia for changes in level of consciousness. Clinical appraisal includes assessing the client's awareness of external stimuli and internal state-mood, alertness and emotional expression. Observations are made for disturbances in orientation and attention span.

Nursing Diagnosis

The complexity of this disorder creates many potential associated nursing problems. Focus should be placed upon diagnosis related to alterations in tissue perfusion, namely, general, cerebral, cardiac, and uteroplacental. The client is also likely to experience a knowledge deficit of risks for PIH and potential injury secondary to seizures.

Nursing Intervention

During the antepartal period the nurse should instruct all women about the importance of maintaining a well-balanced diet high in protein intake. Calorie and fluid restrictions are generally not recommended at this time. It is believed that the development of preeclampsia may be related to poor nutritional status; therefore, dietary counseling is a most significant component of client education. In addition, all pregnant women should be informed, both orally and by some form of printed material, about the warning signs of preeclampsia, which they themselves may recognize and should immediately report to the nurse or physician.

The woman manifesting early symptoms of preeclampsia who is managed at home on modified activity or rest should be advised to position herself in the left lateral position to increase uterine and renal blood flow. The administration of prescribed sedatives or antihypertensive agents should be reviewed. Blood pressure should be monitored regularly by the community-health nurse or a trained family member.

If symptoms of preeclampsia remain evident or progress with these interventions, the client is likely to be admitted to the hospital. In establishing a therapeutic hospital atmosphere, the nurse should see that the environment is as comfortable and pleasant as possible. The client should be in a single room, free from noise and strong lights. The nurse must protect the client from needless traffic into the room; otherwise, the coming and going of personnel to the bedside may be so constant that it could interfere with the efficacy of the treatment being carried out. Every effort should be exerted to relieve the client's anxiety, which sometimes is brought about by apprehension regarding her illness or which may be due to concern for the welfare of her family at home.

The nurse should see that the equipment necessary for the safe and efficient care of the client is immediately available in the client's room and is in good working order. A padded mouth gag should always be ready for use at the bedside to prevent the client from biting her tongue if a convulsion develops. Trays for catheterization equipment and for the administration of special medications constitute part of the necessary equipment. Since water retention plays such a large role in the disease and urinary output is likely to be diminished, an indwelling bladder catheter may be ordered to ensure accuracy in obtaining output from the kidneys. To carefully monitor the client's urinary output it is imperative that the nurse promote proper drainage of the retention catheter at all times.

Other necessary supplies for the care of the preeclamptic woman may include suction apparatus for aspirating mucus and equipment for administering oxygen, should symptoms such as cyanosis or depressed respiration indicate the need.

When any treatment is ordered, the procedure is best carried out after sedation has been administered. Before heavy sedation is initiated, any removable dentures or eyeglasses should be stored in a secure place. If the client is not in labor, the nurse must be alert to watch for signs of labor, particularly after sedation has been given.

Regardless of the severity of the preeclampsia, certain responsibilities are carried out by the nurse. Complete bed rest is essential. Since rest and relaxation are major considerations in the care of the preeclamptic woman, the nurse should plan a schedule of activities so that the client is disturbed as little as possible. Medications, treatments, and nursing procedures should be administered at the same time as far as the physician's orders will permit, but only as much as will not overtire the client should be planned for any one time.

The hospitalized client is encouraged to eat the prescribed diet, which is ample in protein and caloric content. Sodium and fluid intake are usually neither restricted nor forced, but held to normal recommended dietary allowances (2.5 g–7.0 g of salt per day and 1500 ml–2000 ml of fluid per day). The client should be instructed by the nurse not to add salt to food and to avoid foods high in sodium, such as potato chips, pretzels, prepared luncheon meats, and hot dogs.

Frequent observations are made for progressive symptoms or changes in condition, with special attention for visual disturbances, headaches, and epigastric pain. Urine is tested for proteinuria using a clean-catch, midstream specimen. A 2+ or more reading of proteinuria is considered significant.

The administration of prescribed drugs to decrease blood pressure is an important nursing intervention for preeclamptic women in advanced stages of the disease. When $MgSO_4$ is ordered, the nurse must follow certain steps in preparing the medication and assessing the client (see Nursing Guidelines for Administration of Magnesium Sulfate). Intramuscular doses of $MgSO_4$ should be given deeply in the upper outer quadrant of each buttock, and the tissue should be massaged following the injection. Intravenous $MgSO_4$ should be carefully administered and regulated by an infusion pump. Calcium gluconate is an effective antidote, which should be kept readily available whenever administering $MgSO_4$. Since serious side-effects may occur, it is essential for the nurse to monitor urinary output, deep tendon reflexes, and respiratory rate prior to, during, and following $MgSO_4$ administration. The fetal heart rate should be carefully assessed through electronic monitoring, since $MgSO_4$ may decrease beat-to-beat variability. If intravenous hydralazine (Apresoline) is prescribed to lower blood pressure, the nurse should expect an almost immediate response. Blood pressure should be monitored every 5 minutes, and the client should be observed for common side-effects of this medication, such as tachycardia, flushing, and palpitations. Hydralazine may also induce additional reductions in uteroplacental blood flow; therefore, continuous fetal monitoring is mandatory.

Eclampsia

As indicated, the development of eclampsia is almost always preceded by the signs and symptoms of pre-eclampsia. An eclamptic episode is most likely to occur as term approaches and is rarely seen prior to the last 3 months. Eclampsia is particularly likely to present in twin pregnancies, the likelihood being about four times that in single pregnancies. Approximately 5% of women with preeclampsia develop eclampsia.

Manifestations

The onset of eclampsia is often sudden. A preeclamptic woman, who may have been conversing a moment before, is seen to roll her eyes to one side and stare fixedly into space. Immediately, twitching of the facial muscles ensues. This is the *stage of invasion* of the convulsion and lasts only a few seconds.

The client's whole body then becomes rigid in a generalized muscular contraction; the face is distorted, the eyes protrude, the arms are flexed, the hands are clenched, and the legs are inverted. Since all the muscles of the body are now in a state of tonic contraction, this phase may be regarded as the *stage of contraction;* it lasts 15 or 20 seconds.

Suddenly the jaws begin to open and close violently, and forthwith the eyelids also. The other facial muscles and then all the muscles of the body alternately contract and relax in rapid succession. The muscular movements are so forceful that the client may throw herself out of bed, and almost invariably, unless protected, the tongue is bitten by the violent jaw action. Foam, which is often blood tinged, exudes from the mouth; the face is congested and purple, and the eyes are bloodshot. This phase in which the muscles alternately contract and relax is called the *stage of convulsion;* it may last a minute or so. Gradually the muscular movements become milder and farther apart, and finally the client lies motionless.

Throughout the seizure the diaphragm remains fixed, with respiration halted. For a few seconds the client appears to be dying of respiratory arrest, but just when this outcome seems almost inevitable, she takes a long, deep, stertorous inhalation, and breathing is resumed. Then coma ensues. The client does not remember anything about the convulsion or, in all probability, events immediately before and afterward.

The coma may last from a few minutes to several hours, and the client may then become conscious, or the coma may be succeeded by another convulsion. The convulsions may recur during coma, they may recur only after an interval of consciousness, or they may never recur at all. Mild cases of eclampsia involve 1 or 2 convulsions; in severe cases there may be 10 to 20 convulsions. Convulsions may start before the onset of labor (antepartum), during labor (intrapartum), or anytime within the first 48 hours after delivery (postpartum). About a fifth of the cases develop postpartally, generally within 24 hours of delivery.

Upon physical examination, the findings of eclampsia are similar to those in preeclampsia, but exaggerated. Thus, the systolic blood pressure usually ranges around 180 mm Hg and sometimes exceeds 200 mm Hg. Proteinuria is frequently extreme, from 10 g/liter to 20 g/liter. Edema may be marked, but sometimes is absent. Oliguria, or diminution of urinary excretion, is common and may progress to complete anuria. Fever is present in about half of these women.

In favorable cases the convulsions cease, the coma lessens, and urinary output increases. However, it sometimes requires 1 or 2 days for clear consciousness to be regained. During this period eclamptic women are often in an obstreperous, resistant mood and may be exceedingly difficult to manage. A few develop actual psychoses. In unfavorable cases the coma deepens, urinary excretion diminishes, the pulse becomes more rapid, the temperature rises, and edema of the lungs develops. The last is a serious symptom and usually is interpreted as a sign of cardiovascular failure. Edema of the lungs is readily recognizable by the noisy, gurgling respiration and by the large quantity of frothy mucus that exudes from the mouth and the nose. Toward the end, convulsions cease altogether, and the final picture is one of vascular collapse, with falling blood pressure and overwhelming edema of the lungs.

Medical Diagnosis and Prognosis

The onset of convulsions in a preeclamptic woman indicates progression of the hypertensive disease to eclampsia. It is important for the obstetrician to differentiate diagnoses of epilepsy, encephalitis, and other

Nursing Guidelines for Administration of Magnesium Sulfate*

Preparation of the MgSO₄

1. IM dose
   MgSO₄, 10 g or 5 g
   a. 10 g of MgSO₄ in 20 ml of a 50% solution.
   b. Divide into 2 doses, 10 ml in 2 syringes.
   c. Add 0.5 ml of lidocaine to each 10 ml of MgSO₄ in the syringe.
2. IV dose
   MgSO₄, 2 g to 4 g, IV stat by soluset.
   a. 2 g to 4 g of MgSO₄ in 20 ml to 40 ml of a 10% solution.
   b. Add ordered grams of MgSO₄ to soluset, fill to 100 ml with IV fluid.
   c. Infuse medication over a 10-minute period.
   MgSO₄, 1g, IV by IMED
   a. 1 g of MgSO₄ in 2 ml.
   b. Add 10 g of MgSO₄ in 20 ml to a 500 ml of D₅/u.
   c. Infuse medication at 50 ml/hr by IMED to give MgSO₄ 1 g/hr.

Nursing Assessment of Client Receiving Magnesium Sulfate

1. Detection of the signs of magnesium intoxication
   a. Early signs mother may experience and you recognize are as follows:
      1. Hot all over   5. Depression of reflexes
      2. Flushing   6. Hypotension
      3. Thirsty   7. Flaccidity
      4. Sweating
   b. Later signs of hypermagnesemia are as follows:
      1. CNS depression
      2. Respiratory paralysis
      3. Circulatory collapse
2. Deep tendon reflexes should be checked hourly if the client is receiving continuous IV infusion or before each dose of intermittent therapy is administered. Disappearance of the patellar reflex is one of the most important clinical signs to detect increasing hypermagnesemia. However, if the client has received regional anesthesia (epidural) you will have to test the biceps or radial reflex.
3. CNS depression is at first characterized by anxiety. This changes to drowsiness, lethargy, slight slurring of speech, ataxic gait, and a tendency to fall sideward while standing erect. Constantly evaluate the client's orientation to person, place, and time.
4. Intake and output of the client are monitored carefully. Specific gravity should be obtained. Urine should be observed for color and volume. The volume should be 30 ml or more per hour; if not, the next dose of MgSO₄ should be withheld.
5. If the client is receiving an IV infusion, blood pressure (BP) and temperature-pulse-respiration (TPR) should be evaluated at least every 15 to 30 minutes. For the client on intermittent therapy of MgSO₄, a BP and TPR should be taken before and after each administration.
6. Do not administer MgSO₄ if the client's respirations are less than 12 to 14 per minute or there is a drop in pulse rate, BP or fetal, or any other sign of fetal distress.
7. a. Complaints the client may have are headache, malaise, nausea, and vomiting. The nurse must assess whether these signs are due to progression of toxemia or drug therapy.
   b. Another complaint that the mother may have if she is receiving MgSO₄ intramuscularly is pain at the site of the injection.
8. Calcium gluconate (10% solution) is kept at the client's bedside.
   a. This is the antidote for magnesium intoxication (usually reverses respiratory depression and heart block). The dosage should be 5 mEq to 10 mEq (10 ml–20 ml) given intravenously over a 3-minute period.

Testing Deep Tendon Reflexes

1. As outlined above, deep tendon reflexes should be tested hourly.
   a. Absence of or decrease in the patellar reflex indicates that a toxic blood level (7 mg/liter–10 mg/liter of Mg) has been reached.
   b. The reflexes that are tested besides the patellar reflex (knee jerk) are the biceps and radial reflexes. These

(continued)

(continued)

reflexes are tested by striking the tendon and watching for contraction of the appropriate muscle. The muscle need not contract forcefully enough to move the limb but must simply contract.
  c. These reflexes are difficult to elicit when the client is tense, so relaxation is important for proper testing.
  d. Reflexes are compared from one side to the corresponding side and expressed with an aribtrary scale.
    0 = Reflex absent
    +1 = Reflex hypoactive
    +2 = Normal reflex
    +3 = Reflex hyperactive
    +4 = Clonus
2. In testing a muscle reflex, it is actually the tendon that is stimulated, the reflex is involuntary. A sensory impulse is initiated when a stimulus is applied to the tendon and in return a motor response is elicited.
  a. When testing reflexes on a client who has recently received epidural or spinal anesthesia, motor responses will be diminished. An accurate response will not be elicited if the knee jerk is used. The biceps or radial reflex will have to be used.
3. Knee jerk reflex or patellar tendon reflex
  a. The knee should be positioned halfway between the longest and shortest positions.
  b. Support is given under the knee with the foot off the bed (45° angle).
  c. The patellar tendon is struck (tapped) just below the patella, and the quadriceps muscle group should be observed for contraction (slight movement). The lower leg should extend in response.
4. Biceps reflex
  a. The forearm should be resting on the client's trunk.
  b. Place your thumb firmly on the client's biceps tendon (antecubital space) and strike the thumbnail briskly with the reflex hammer.
  c. The biceps muscle will respond by slight movement. The lower arm should flex in response.
5. Radial reflex
  a. The client's hand and forearm should be resting on her trunk. Place a finger over the tendon and gently tap your finger with the reflex hammer.
  b. The brachioradial tendon is located on the lateral surface of the lower end of the radius. It is often difficult to feel this tendon. If the tendon cannot be felt, tap the lateral surface of the lower end of the radius. The brachioradial muscle will respond by a slight movement. The response consists of the hand jerking.
6. For relaxation
  a. If the client is having difficulty relaxing, two techniques can be tried.
    1. Testing the knee jerk—have the client lock her fingers together and pull in the opposite directions (monkey grip). This technique will help the client relax her leg by having her concentrate on a physical activity.
    2. Testing the biceps or radial reflexes—have the client bite down hard. This technique will help the client relax her arm by having her concentrate on doing something else.
  b. If it is necessary to try either of these techniques while testing the reflexes, it is likely that the reflexes are slightly depressed.
  c. *Clonus* is the sudden stretching of a hypertonic muscle, producing reflex contraction. If the stretch is maintained during subsequent relaxation, further reflex contraction occurs, and this may continue almost indefinitely, unless the stretch stimulus is released. It is demonstrated by dorsiflexion of the foot or by sharply moving the patella downward, but it may be present at any joint. Clonus represents an increase in reflex excitability and may be present in a very tense client.

* Used at the Hospital of the University of Pennsylvania.

central nervous system diseases during late pregnancy from PIH. This may be especially of concern in situations of absent prenatal care. Until eclampsia can be ruled out as a diagnosis, all pregnant women having convulsions should be considered eclamptic.

Eclampsia is one of the gravest complications of pregnancy; the maternal mortality rate in different localities and in different hospitals ranges from 0.4% to 17%. The outlook for the baby is particularly grave, since fetal mortality rates are reported to range from 13% to 30% or more. Although it is difficult in a given case to forecast the outcome, the following are unfavorable signs: oliguria, prolonged coma, a sustained pulse rate over 120, temperature over 39.5°C (103°F), more than ten convulsions, 10 g/liter or more of protein in the urine, systolic blood pressure of more than 200, and edema of lungs. If none of these signs is present, the outlook for recovery is good; if two or more are present, the prognosis is definitely serious.

Even though the client survives an attack, she may not escape unscathed, but may continue to have high blood pressure indefinitely. It is even more important to note that a still larger percentage of these women with PIH (about 35%) again develop hypertensive disease in subsequent pregnancies. This is known as recurrent or repeat PIH. These facts make it plain that careful, prolonged follow-up of those mothers who have suffered from preeclampsia or eclampsia is imperative. Moreover, the prognosis for future pregnancies must be guarded, although, as the figures indicate, such women stand at least a fairly good chance of going through subsequent pregnancies satisfactorily.

Medical Management

Since the cause of eclampsia is not known, there can be no "specific" therapy, and treatment must necessarily be empirical, which means use of those therapeutic measures that have yielded the best results in other cases. Empirical treatment is thus based on experience. The approaches employed and related interventions may vary from one hospital setting to another in respect to the drugs prescribed, availability of invasive hemodynamic monitoring, and standard nursing protocols. However, the general principles followed for client management are very comparable among institutions. These are enumerated as follows:

Prevention. Since eclampsia is largely preventable, it is essential to provide comprehensive and regular prenatal care and education directed toward early detection and treatment of PIH.

Termination of Pregnancy. Although the precise cause of preeclampsia and eclampsia is not known, it is quite clear that since they occur in pregnancy, the one sure "cure" is to render the woman nonpregnant. In almost all instances of eclampsia, efforts to effect delivery should be undertaken as soon as the client is stabilized. This involves control of seizures as well as hyperreflexia by using adequate doses of anticonvulsants and initiating diuresis. If is often helpful to monitor CVP in addition to urinary output in an attempt to optimize fluid balance.

Efforts to accomplish delivery before the client is stabilized may result in increased maternal morbidity and mortality. The method of delivery should be by the most expeditious route. Prolonged attempts at induction in the face of an unripe cervix are not indicated; however, the possibility of vaginal delivery should not be discounted even at early gestational age, since, for unexplained reasons, the cervix often quickly becomes

favorable for induction. Occasionally the obstetrician is faced with the dilemma of an eclamptic woman with an immature fetus. Although it is tempting to try to prolong the pregnancy in the interest of bringing about greater fetal maturity, such attempts are generally unsuccessful, with impaired placental function and failure of the fetus to prosper.

Sedation. The purpose of administering sedative drugs is to depress the activity of the brain cells and thereby stop convulsions. The drugs most commonly employed are described below:

Magnesium sulfate. This drug is an excellent central nervous system depressant and therefore an anticonvulsant and also a smooth-muscle relaxant that causes dilatation of peripheral blood vessels and thereby reduces blood pressure. For these reasons it is probably the most common drug used in eclamptic women. The routes of administration, doses, and precautions have already been discussed. The drug is most often given intravenously, at least initially, because the situation with the eclamptic woman is so urgent.

Diazepam (Valium). Intravenous diazepam is widely used for seizure control. Generally, 40 mg is diluted in 500 ml of 5% dextrose in water, and this is administered at a rate of 30 drops per minute. Diazepam can cause neonatal depression if more than 30 mg are used within 15 to 20 hours before delivery. For this reason, $MgSO_4$ remains the sedative drug of choice.

Hydralazine (Apresoline). Intravenous hydralazine is used to decrease marked elevations of blood pressure. This helps to decrease the likelihood of cerebral hemorrhage and left ventricular failure. If the diastolic blood pressure is 110 mm Hg or higher, 5 mg hydralazine is administered intravenously. If the diastolic blood pressure does not decrease to the desired range, the dosage of hydralazine is increased in 5-mg to 10-mg increments every 15 to 20 minutes until a therapeutic response (90 mm Hg diastolic) is achieved or a dose of 20 mg is administered.

Other Medication. Diuretics and hyperosmotic agents should be avoided because they may enhance maternal hypovolemia and have adverse effects on the fetus.

Nursing Assessment

The nurse's responsibilities in the assessment and management of clients with eclampsia are extensive and quite challenging. Although eclampsia is regarded as the climax to a mounting preeclampsia that has been present, it is occasionally observed as a fulminating case in an apparently normal woman who may develop severe symptoms in the span of 24 hours. In such circumstances the nurse and other health-team members may be unprepared for the emergency and must immediately intervene to restore maternal and fetal physiological integrity.

If the nurse is present at the onset of convulsions, several immediate assessments must be made and recorded, including events preceding the seizures, the exact time of onset, and the duration of each convulsive phase. When the client stops thrashing, the nurse must check maternal vital signs and fetal heart tones (usually continuously monitored). This assessment is repeated every 5 minutes until the client stabilizes and then every 15 minutes. The depth and duration of coma following seizure are observed. Chest auscultation is performed by the nurse to detect any signs of pulmonary edema or cardiac failure. Urinary output and parenteral fluid intake are also carefully monitored.

For more comprehensive assessment hemodynamic measurements may be obtained by inserting a Swan-Ganz catheter. Data should be collected on central volume status, including pulmonary capillary wedge pressure, cardiac output, and MAP.

Amidst all of the demands of this acute situation it is also important for the nurse to remember to assess for signs of labor or abruption in both the unconscious and the conscious antepartal client. In eclampsia, labor or placental separation may proceed with few external signs, and occasionally such a woman gives birth beneath the sheets before anyone knows that the process is under way. The nurse should be suspicious when the client grunts or groans or moves about at regular intervals, every 5 minutes or so. If this occurs, the consistency, texture, and height of the uterus should be assessed and observations made for show and bulging of the membranes or bleeding. Convulsions that occur during labor may speed up the labor process, and more rapid preparation for delivery should be made.

Nursing Diagnosis

Assessment of the eclamptic woman may lead the nurse to formulate the following diagnoses: potential for injury related to physiological deficit; potential adverse effects of medication; self-care deficit; and potential delivery of an immature/compromised fetus. Early recognition of these diagnoses provides a basis for appropriately planning nursing interventions.

Nursing Intervention

If eclampsia develops, the nurse must intervene immediately to protect the client from self-injury and further physiological decompensation. Nursing management is coordinated with medical therapy. The eclamptic woman must never be left alone for a second. When in the throes of a convulsion, she may crash her head against a bedpost or throw herself onto the floor, or she may bite her tongue violently. To prevent injury, the side rails of the bed should be padded or cushioned with pillows and some device that can be inserted between the jaws at the very onset of a convulsion should be kept within easy reach. A piece of heavy rubber tubing, a rolled towel, or a padded clothespin is often employed. The nurse must take care in inserting it not to injure the client (*e.g.*, lips, gums, teeth) and not to allow her own fingers to be bitten. If unable to gently insert the tongue blade, the nurse should abandon all further efforts.

Turning the client's head and body to the side when the seizure begins aids circulation to the uteroplacental unit and may prevent aspiration. Eclamptic women must never be given fluids by mouth unless they are thoroughly conscious. Failure to adhere to this rule may result in aspiration of the fluid and consequent pneumonia.

Since loud noises, bright lights, jarring of the bed, or sudden drafts may be enough to precipitate a convulsion, the nurse must protect the eclamptic woman from all extraneous stimuli. Light in the room should be eliminated except for a small lamp, so shaded that none of the light falls on the client. Although the room should be darkened, the light should be sufficient to permit observations of changes in condition, such as cyanosis or twitchings. Only absolutely necessary conversation should be carried out in the room, and this should be in the lowest tone possible.

During the coma that follows cessation of the convulsion, care must be taken to see that the client does not aspirate vomitus or mucus. An oral airway may be inserted into the client's mouth, and her nasopharynx is suctioned. Oxygen administration is initiated during or immediately following the seizure to prevent or treat maternal–fetal hypoxia. The position of the client in bed should be such that it promotes drainage of secretions and the maintenance of a clear airway. It may be necessary to raise the foot of the bed of the comatose client a few inches to promote drainage of secretions from the respiratory passage. When this measure must be resorted to, it is particularly important to watch for signs of pulmonary edema, which would be aggravated by this position. The head of the bed may need to be elevated to relieve dyspnea.

Although the nurse is not directly responsible for decisions related to pregnancy termination, her role encompasses direct intrapartum care and prenatal preparation of the client for labor and delivery. Therefore, it is most imperative that the nurse understand guidelines for decision making used by the obstetrician. Careful and continuous monitoring of maternal and fe-

(text continued on page 775)

The Woman with the Complication of Pregnancy-Induced Hypertension (PIH)

Nursing Objectives

1. Prevent or detect early the signs and symptoms of PIH through early and regular prenatal care.
2. Promote normal physiological adaptations in the woman with PIH by delivering optimum health care.
3. Prevent or detect early and manage progressive disease and complications of PIH.
4. Protect fetal well-being and deliver a healthy neonate at or near term.

Assessment	Potential Nursing Diagnosis	Planning/Intervention	Evaluation
History	Knowledge deficit of risks for PIH	Observe for early signs and symptoms of PIH each prenatal visit	Woman's blood pressure remains normal or returns to normal
Primigravida		Rising trend in blood pressure	
<20 or >35 years		Edema of feet and fingers	
Hypertensive disease in family			
Obesity or malnourishment		Collect urinary specimen for protein (clean midstream sample)	
Diabetes			
Chronic renal disease			
Physical examination		Provide client education of PIH	Woman repeats signs and symptoms of PIH
Blood pressure 140/90 *or* an increase in diastolic pressure of 15 and an increase in systolic pressure of 30		Signs and symptoms	
		Perinatal implications	
		Importance of rest and calmness	
Sudden weight gain of greater than 2 lb a week		Emergency actions	
Edema present in hands and face		Administer roll over test (28 wk–32 wk gestation)	
Obstetric factors		Instruct on importance of bed rest or modified activity (at home) if mild PIH is detected	Woman remains on bed-rest as instructed
Multiple gestation			
Past history of PIH		Side-lying position	
Hydramnios		Assess dietary history	
Hydatidiform mole			
Laboratory studies		Provide dietary counseling (often in collaboration with nutritionist)	Woman modifies her diet according to instructions
Proteinuria (trace, 1+ dipstick) on 2 specimens at least 6 hr apart		High protein	
		Low sodium	
		Fluid intake 6–8 glasses per day	
Physical examination	Alteration in tissue perfusion: general	Maintain bed rest in left lateral recumbent position while hospitalized	Woman maintains bed rest in left lateral recumbent position
TPR			
Coolness of skin		Monitor vital signs and blood pressure q4h or more frequently if indicated	
Pallor			
Cyanosis			
Pulse quality (decreased)			
Laboratory studies		Measure urine albumin q4h or more frequently	Woman shows no evidence of progressive renal involvement
Proteinuria (3+ or 4+ dipstick)		Monitor intake and output	

(continued)

Assessment	Potential Nursing Diagnosis	Planning/Intervention	Evaluation
Concentrated urine CBC Hematocrit (elevated) BUN (elevated) Serum creatinine (elevated)		Assess deep tendon reflexes q4h Assess extremities for edema Weigh daily	Woman's reflexes remain normal or mild hyperreflexia is present Woman avoids sudden weight gain as fluid retention is controlled
History 　Headaches 　Visual disturbances 　Epigastric pain Physical examination 　Elevated blood pressure (160/110 or higher) 　Edema of face, hands, lower extremities 　Hyperreflexia (3+ to 4+) 　Blurred vision 　Funduscopic changes Oliguria Laboratory studies 　Platelet (may be decreased) 　Prothrombin time (may be elevated) 　Partial thromboplastin (may be elevated)	Potential for injury secondary to seizure(s)	Assess for signs of severe PIH 　Increased edema 　Blood pressure (160/110) 　Headache 　Hyperreflexia 　Epigastric pain 　Decreased urinary output 　Visual disturbances Provide a calm and controlled environment with minimal external stimuli 　Limit visitors 　Darkened, quiet room Maintain seizure precautions 　Padded side rails 　Airway or padded tongue blade at bedside 　Emergency equipment accessible 　Oxygen and suction equipment at bedside Administer MgSO$_4$ (IM or IV) to prevent seizures Advise client about side-effects of MgSO$_4$ 　Burning 　Nausea 　Pain at injection site Administer sedatives and antihypertensives as prescribed Have antidote for MgSO$_4$ readily available (calcium gluconate) Insert Foley catheter for careful assessment of urinary output (hourly) and protein content If seizure should develop	 Woman remains calm and gets rest Woman rests in a bed with padded siderails and emergency equipment available Woman receives prescribed medication to prevent seizures and control hypertension Woman's urinary output is carefully monitored

(continued)

Assessment	Potential Nursing Diagnosis	Planning/Intervention	Evaluation
		Observe and record time of onset and duration of each phase	
		Protect from self-injury	Woman is protected from self-injury during seizure
		Promote adequate ventilation by suctioning	Woman is adequately ventilated
		Position to prevent aspiration	
		Administer anticonvulsants as prescribed	
Physical examination	Alteration in tissue perfusion: cerebral and cardiac	Maintain CVP monitoring	Woman becomes stabilized
Restlessness		or	
Confusion		Arterial pressure monitoring by Swan-Ganz if indicated	
Loss of motor or sensory function			
Memory losses		Continue administration of cerebral depressants as prescribed until stabilization is achieved	
Altered LOC			
		Assess cerebral function	Woman has normal cerebral function
		LOC	
		Restlessness	
		Memory	
		Sensory awareness	
		Motor function	
Fetal heart rate and pattern (early, late, or variable decelerations)	Alteration in tissue perfusion, uteroplacental	Assess and monitor fetal well-being by	Fetus retains normal fetal heart tone patterns
Fetal activity level		FHTs (auscultated or by external monitor)	Woman recognizes and reports changes in fetal activity
Nonstress testing		Record of fetal activity	
Laboratory studies		Report FHTs <120 or >180 or absence of fetal activity to obstetrician	
L/S ratio			
PG levels			
Fetal scalp sample		Explain procedures and prepare client for prenatal diagnostic testing	Woman understands and cooperates with prenatal diagnostic procedures
24-hr urine for estriol			
		Sonography	
		Amniocentesis	
		Estriol levels	
		Nonstress testing	
		OCTs	
		Assess for signs of labor or abruption	
		Prepare for vaginal delivery unless cesarean section necessitated by fetal compromise or other condition	Woman understands preparations for delivery

(text continued from page 771)
tal status, as well as direct interventions to support and educate the client, may prevent further aggravation of the client's hypertensive state and may promote a more positive perinatal outcome. The nurse should review and answer questions about the prescribed medical regimen. A complete discussion of nursing care during the intrapartum period is presented in Chapter 25.

Chronic Hypertension (With and Without Superimposed Preeclampsia)

As the name implies, chronic hypertension indicates the presence of high blood pressure before pregnancy. The etiology of this hypertension is usually related to vascular or renal disease. Difficulty is encountered in establishing a diagnosis of chronic hypertension because many women are not seen between pregnancies and blood pressures are, therefore, not recorded. Also, there is normally a decrease in blood pressure during the second trimester, which could mask a preexisting hypertension if the client does not report for care until the fourth or fifth month of gestation. The diagnosis is justified if hypertension (blood pressure is 140/90 or higher) is detected prior to the 20th week of gestation. Most often women with chronic hypertension are multiparae and usually over the age of 30. At least 75% of such women are able to complete their pregnancies successfully, with no significant change in the status of their hypertension. Fifteen percent develop superimposed preeclampsia, an occurrence that carries an ominous fetal prognosis (20% mortality) and even an increase in maternal mortality.

The treatment, then, for the majority of pregnant women with chronic hypertension is no different from treatment for the nonpregnant woman. Prepregnancy antihypertensive and diuretic medications are continued. Thiazides are the drugs of choice despite reports of neonatal thrombocytopenia. The antihypertensive drug most often recommended is hydralazine (Apresoline) or methyldopa (Aldomet). All medications should be titrated to the lowest possible effective dose.

The pregnancy is allowed to run its normal course, unless gestation aggravates the already existing hypertension. When the gravida with this chronic process develops a further elevation of blood pressure (systolic blood pressure 30 mm Hg or diastolic blood pressure 15 mm Hg–20 mm Hg above baseline), significant proteinuria, or edema, the condition is called *superimposed preeclampsia.*

In the case of superimposed preeclampsia, after 24 to 48 hours of intensive medical therapy, pregnancy termination is generally indicated. Even though the fetus may be preterm, its chances for survival under these circumstances are generally better outside the uterus.

In a small number of women the hypertension will be so severe, with evidence of kidney involvement, severe retinal changes, or cardiac involvement, that therapeutic abortion might be considered if the woman comes to medical attention in the first trimester. It is also important to consider the advisability of postpartum tubal ligation in this group of women, who are generally older, with established families, and for whom additional pregnancies may represent a serious health hazard. This of course can be only a recommendation; the final decision rests with the client.

References

1. Mantoni M: Ultrasound signs in threatened abortion and their prognostic significance. Obstet Gynecol 65(4): 471–475, 1985
2. Hert JD, Heisterberg I: The outcome of pregnancy after threatened abortion. Acta Obstet Gynecol Scand 64: 151–156, 1985
3. Ectopic pregnancy rate has doubled since 1980. American College of Obstetrics and Gynecology Newsletter 18(14):14, 1983
4. Demarest CB: When to think ectopic pregnancy. Patient Care 18:63–72, 1984
5. Edelin KC: Evaluation of female pelvic pain. Hosp Med 19:37–67, 1983
6. Pritchard JA, MacDonald PC, Gant NF: Williams' Obstetrics, 17th ed. Norwalk, CT, Appleton-Century-Crofts, 1985
7. Caplin M: Disseminated intravascular coagulation: A multisystem problem. Dimens Critical Care Nurs 3:76–83, 1984
8. Chesley LC: Hypertensive disorders in pregnancy. In Hellman LM, Pritchard JA: Williams Obstetrics, 14th ed, p. 685. New York, Appleton-Century-Crofts
9. Gant N, Worley RJ: Hypertension in Pregnancy, Concepts and Management, pp 1–10. New York, Appleton-Century-Crofts, 1980
10. Willis S: Hypertension in pregnancy: Pathophysiology. Am J Nurs 82:792–793, 1982
11. Worley RJ et al: Vascular responsiveness to pressor agents during human pregnancy. J Reprod Med 23: 115–128, 1979
12. Thompson D et al: The renal lesion of toxemia and abruptio placentae studied by light and electron microscopes. J Obstet Gynecol Br Commonw 79:311–320, 1976
13. Brosens IA et al: The role of spiral arteries in the pathogenesis of preeclampsia. Obstet Gynecol Annu 1:177–197, 1972
14. Page EW, Christianson R: The impact of mean arterial pressure in the middle trimester upon the outcome of pregnancy. Am J Obstet Gynecol 125:740–746, 1976
15. Willis SE, Sharp ES: Hypertension in pregnancy: Prenatal detection and management. Am J Nurs 82:798–808, 1982
16. Kasser NS et al: Roll over test. Obstet Gynecol 54:411–413, 1980

Suggested Reading

Cavanagh D, Woods RF, O'Connor TCF (eds): Obstetric Emergencies. Philadelphia, Harper & Row, 1982

Chesley LC: Hypertensive Disorders in Pregnancy. New York, Appleton-Century-Crofts, 1978

DeMarest CB: When to think ectopic pregnancy. Patient Care 18:63–72, 1984

Hankin GDV et al: Cardiovascular monitoring in high-risk pregnancy. Perinatology/Neonatology 7:29–32, 1983

Hertz DB, Heisterberg L: The outcome of pregnancy after threatened abortion. Acta Obstet Gynecol Scand 64: 151–156, 1985

Hoffmaster JE: Detecting and treating pregnancy-induced hypertension: A review. MCN 8:398–405, 1983

Mayberry LJ, Forte AB: Pregnancy-related disseminated intravascular coagulation (DIC). MCN 10:168–173, 1985

Weil S: The unspoken needs of families during high risk pregnancies. Am J Nurs 81:2047–2049, 1981

Willis S: Hypertension in pregnancy: Pathophysiology. Am J Nurs 82:792–797, 1982

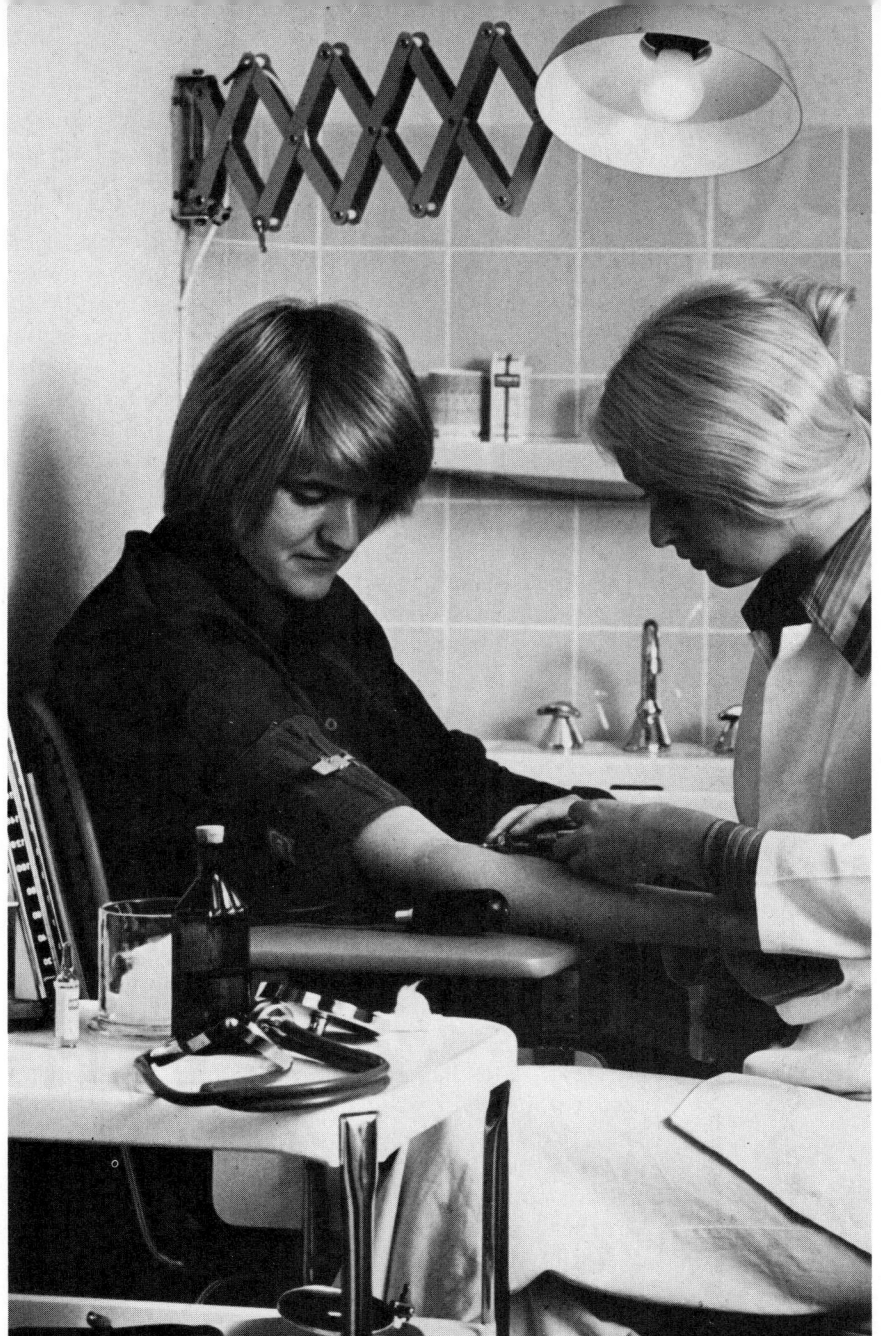

CHAPTER 37

Concurrent Diseases in Pregnancy

The pregnant woman can have any diseased state that her nonpregnant counterpart can have, except for infertility. Many disease states are modified by the physiological changes of pregnancy. Pregnancy may alter the classic clinical picture of a disease state, and some of the normal physiological changes of pregnancy mimic disease. Therapeutic approaches to diseases must be altered in some cases, especially with regard to possible effects on the fetus. For most coincidental diseases, the effects of pregnancy on the disease and of the disease on pregnancy are negligible and do not influence the management of either. Some diseases, however, have profound fetal effects, as discussed in Chapter 42; others have a predominantly maternal effect; and some, such as diabetes, affect both. The most common diseases in the latter two categories are discussed in this chapter.

Over the past decade advances in perinatology have contributed directly to decreases in perinatal mortality and morbidity for clients whose pregnancies are complicated by a variety of medical conditions.

Diabetes Mellitus

Diabetes mellitus is a major complication and illustrates the interplay between the altered physiology of pregnancy and the pathophysiology of disease. In contrast to the majority of disease states, which do not alter or are not affected by pregnancy, there is a significant change in the course of diabetes when pregnancy supervenes, and diabetes has a profound effect on the course of pregnancy as well as on the fetus. In addition to participating in the regular medical and prenatal care of the diabetic gravida, the nurse can serve a very important counseling role. Care involves an interdisciplinary team effort and necessitates cooperation among obstetrician, internist, pediatrician, nurse, social worker, and nutritionist.

Diabetes mellitus is an endocrine disorder of carbohydrate metabolism that results from a deficiency in insulin production by the cells of the islets of Langerhans in the pancreas. Insulin is an essential hormone required for glucose transfer into the muscle and adipose tissue cells. When glucose is unable to enter body cells because of deficient or inadequate quantities of insulin, fat and protein metabolism are altered. Protein catabolism, ketosis, and a negative nitrogen balance may result. As blood glucose levels steadily rise, cellular water is lost and glycosuria appears. Extracellular dehydration develops because of the high osmotic pressure and increased amount of glucose in the urine. As a result of these pathophysiological adaptations, the classic symptoms of diabetes manifest: polyuria, polydipsia, polyphagia, and weight loss. Degenerative vascular changes such as nephropathy and retinopathy are associated with long-term poorly controlled carbohydrate metabolism.

In recent years, the number of pregnant diabetics has increased, partly because with modern management, diabetics are now able to conceive and maintain pregnancies and partly because there is presently an increased recognition of the milder forms of gestational diabetes. Gestational or pregnancy-induced diabetes occurs in 1% to 2% of pregnancies and pregestational diabetes, in 0.1% to 0.2%.[1] Approximately 25% of women with gestational diabetes initially diagnosed during pregnancy will later develop insulin-dependent diabetes.[2]

Effect of Pregnancy on Diabetes

During the course of pregnancy, the placenta produces human placental lactogen (HPL), which is a powerful insulin antagonist. The rate of secretion is proportionate to the placental mass. The estrogen and progesterone produced by the placenta also counteract the influence of insulin, albeit to a less degree. The effects of these placental products on insulin increase the maternal requirement for insulin during the course of pregnancy. In other words, more insulin must be produced to make up for the antagonistic effect of these hormones. The placenta also produces placental insulinase, an enzyme that accelerates the degradation of insulin, and this further increases insulin requirements. The glomerular filtration rate of glucose in the kidneys is increased, resulting in a reduced renal threshold for glucose from normal nonpregnant levels. These physiological alterations occurring in insulin and carbohydrate metabolism render pregnancy a *diabetogenic* condition.

During the course of normal pregnancy, there is a lower fasting blood sugar level. There is, however, no difference between the pregnant and nonpregnant intravenous glucose tolerance test (GTT), and the degree of induced hyperglycemia is the same during the course of this test in both pregnant and nonpregnant states. When the oral GTT test is used, the hyperglycemia persists somewhat longer in pregnancy because of slower and more prolonged absorption of glucose from the gastrointestinal tract.

In the first trimester, the caloric intake may be decreased because of diminished appetite, anorexia, or vomiting. Concomitantly, there is a significant transfer of glucose and glucogenic amino acids to the embryo/fetus. These factors place the pregnant diabetic at risk for hypoglycemia or starvation ketosis.

During the second half of pregnancy due to the previously described progressively increasing insulin antagonist factors and rising insulin requirements, the client is prone to develop diabetic *ketoacidosis.* Insulin demands drop dramatically in the intrapartum and early postpartum periods because of the rapid clearance of HPL and the cessation of its production, as well as the temporary suppression of pituitary growth hormone. Insulin administration must be discontinued or greatly reduced in prescribed dosage to prevent hypoglycemia following delivery.

Effect of Diabetes on Pregnancy

Despite great gains achieved in modern obstetric management, perinatal mortality and morbidity remain significantly higher in diabetic pregnancies than in normal pregnancies. The risk factor for maternal fetal complication is increased for women with a longer duration of diabetes, especially if there is a history of poor control prior to conception.

Diabetes can have a deleterious effect on pregnancy in the following ways:

1. Infection, especially genitourinary tract infection, is more common and more serious. The presence of glycosuria places the pregnant diabetic at particular risk for monilial vaginitis, which may in some cases become intractable.
2. The fetus is often larger (macrosomia) owing to prolonged fetal hyperinsulinism and hyperglycemia, and if this occurs it can increase the possibility of a difficult vaginal delivery and postpartum hemorrhage.
3. There is a fourfold greater overall incidence of preeclampsia or eclampsia, with an increase even when there is no associated preexisting vascular disease.
4. There is an increased incidence of hydramnios, and if this is coupled with fetal macrosomia, it can cause cardiopulmonary symptoms.
5. The fetus and newborn can also be adversely affected. Reported mortality rates for the perinatal infant vary from as high as 10% to 30% to as low as 2% to 4% in major treatment centers.[3] There is a twofold to fourfold increase in congenital anomalies among infants of diabetic mothers. Mounting evidence suggests that uncontrolled diabetes during early pregnancy is a cause of fetal malformation.[4] Other neonatal problems encountered include intrauterine growth retardation, prematurity, hypoglycemia, and respiratory distress syndrome. These and other conditions are discussed in Chapter 44.

Medical Diagnosis

During the course of normal pregnancy, glucose may appear in the urine with blood sugars as low as 100 mg because of a lowered renal threshold to glucose excretion. Although the presence of glucose in the urine does not necessarily indicate high blood glucose levels, any client exhibiting glucosuria should be suspected of having diabetes, and the diagnosis should be established or ruled out by evaluation of glucose blood levels. The GTT administered orally (50 g or 100 g) or intravenously (25 g) is primarily used to screen potential diabetes during pregnancy. If a woman has already been identified as being diabetic prior to pregnancy, diagnostic GTTs are not required. In preparation for the GTT, the client is requested to fast overnight. The next morning a fasting blood glucose is drawn. The client is then given a carbohydrate load and 1-, 2-, and 3-hour postprandial venous blood samples are taken for glucose. O'Sullivan and Mahan have established criteria for comparative interpretations of GTTs in pregnant and nonpregnant women (Table 37-1).[2] It should be noted that the initial peak values are higher during pregnancy and remain elevated for the entire test. An oral GTT is considered abnormal if two of the client's blood glucose values are elevated or if one blood glucose value is exceeded in two successive tests.

A client initially diagnosed for diabetes during pregnancy may regress completely following delivery. In these circumstances the condition is referred to as *gestational diabetes*. It should be suspected on the basis of the following factors:

- Previous large infants (9 lb or more)
- Family history of diabetes mellitus
- Glucosuria on two successive occasions
- Obesity
- Unexplained pregnancy wastage (spontaneous abortions, stillbirths)
- Multiparity
- Presence of hydramnios
- Previous infant with a congenital anomaly

The 2-hour postprandial blood glucose test is occasionally employed for primary screening of pregnant women with known risk factors for diabetes. This test offers the advantage of being simpler to administer than the GTT; however, definitive diagnosis for the disease cannot be established without further evaluation. A blood glucose value of 145 mg/dl or above on the postprandial test is suggestive of diabetes and necessitates follow-up with a full GTT. When a potential diabetic obtains a normal value on the 2-hour postprandial blood glucose, the test should be repeated in the second or third trimester.

A special diagnostic problem occurs when a client is not suspected of being diabetic until after delivery, as might be the case if she has delivered an unusually large baby or an unexplained stillborn. Since the diabetogenic effects of pregnancy disappear quickly following delivery, a normal GTT 48 to 72 hours post partum is not necessarily reassuring. The so-called *steroid enforced GTT*, in which cortisone is administered prior to the testing, may bring out the abnormality.

Classification

Several methods for classifying diabetes are available in clinical practice. The National Diabetes Data Group[5] has developed the system in Table 37-2.

Another widely used classification scheme specific for pregnant women with diabetes was originally developed and recently modified by White.[6] The progressively severe categories A through T are represented in Table 37-2; in general, perinatal wastage can be related to class. The pregnancy outcome is invariably poor in those clients with vascular disease (Classes D through T), and better in Classes A, B, C. It should also be noted that mothers with significant vascular involvement often have small-for-date rather than large-for-date babies.

Nursing Process

The nursing process is designed to accomplish the major objectives of nursing care:

1. Identification of women at risk for diabetes and provision of appropriate perinatal care
2. Maintenance of blood glucose levels that mimic physiologic levels in pregnant diabetic women (*e.g.*, fasting blood sugar less than 90 mg/dl and 2-hour postprandial less than 145 mg/dl)
3. Provision of adequate client education for safe self-management of mother and fetus/newborn
4. Prevention or early detection of potential complications of diabetes during the entire childbearing cycle
5. Promotion of a positive psychosocial adjustment to childbearing through understanding and acceptance of pregnancy and diabetes.

The plan of nursing care is developed in cooperation with the client who may be initially encountered in the outpatient clinic or inpatient antepartum unit. Short-

T A B L E 3 7 - 1

Oral Glucose Tolerance Test

	Nonpregnant Glucose (mg/dl)		Pregnant Glucose (mg/dl)	
	Whole Blood	Plasma	Whole Blood	Plasma
Fasting	110	130	90	105
One hour	170	195	165	190
Two hours	120	140	145	170
Three hours	110	120	125	145

(Data from O'Sullivan JB, Mahan CM: Criteria for the oral glucose tolerance test in pregnancy. Diabetes 13(3):278–285, 1964)

T A B L E   3 7 - 2

Two Methods of Classification of Diabetes

Classification of Diabetes by the National Diabetes Data Group	White's Revised Classification of Diabetes in Pregnant Women*
A. Insulin-dependent type (type I)	A Chemical diabetes; abnormal GTT; initial onset during pregnancy

B. Non-insulin-dependent type (type II)
   1. Nonobese
   2. Obese
	B Maturity onset (age over 20 yr); duration under 10 years; no vascular disease

C. Other types (secondary diabetes)
   1. Pancreatic disease
   2. Hormonally induced
   3. Chemically induced
   4. Insulin receptor abnormalities
   5. Certain genetic syndromes
   6. Others
	C_1 Age at onset 10 to 19 years
	C_2 Duration 10 to 19 years
	D_1 Under age 10 years at onset
	D_2 Over 10 years' duration
	D_3 Benign retinopathy
	D_4 Calcified vessels of legs
	D_5 Hypertension

D. Impaired glucose tolerance (subclinical diabetes)	E Calcified pelvic arteries; no longer sought
E. Gestational diabetes (pregnancy-induced glucose intolerance)	F Nephropathy G Many failures H Cardiomyopathy R Proliferating retinopathy T Renal transplant

* (White P: Classification of obstetric diabetes. Am J Obstet Gynecol 130:229, 1978)

term hospitalization for the purpose of evaluation and regulation of disease state is often recommended for diagnosed diabetic women who become pregnant. During the hospitalization the health-team members collect a complete health and dietary history, perform a comprehensive assessment of body systems, and individualize care plans based upon knowledge of client needs.

Nursing Assessment

Prenatal assessment should include observations for the signs and symptoms of diabetes in all pregnant women; these include polydipsia, polyphagia, polyuria, blurred vision, orthostatic dizziness, and weight loss. The client's family and prenatal history should be carefully obtained and reviewed for predisposing factors.

All women with known risk factors for diabetes should receive the appropriate screening tests (see Medical Diagnosis section) early in their pregnancies. Knowledge of diabetes and the normal physiological–psychological adaptations of pregnancy are assessed. Baseline vital signs, blood pressure, and fetal heart rate should be recorded and subsequently compared with later readings. A steady rise in blood pressure or a sudden increase in weight may be a sign of pregnancy-related hypertension, a frequent complication of diabetes. Measurements of glycosylated hemoglobin (A_1 or A_{1c}) are obtained, since it is likely to be elevated in diabetes and the magnitude of the elevation generally correlates inversely with the degree of long-term control of plasma glucose concentration that has been achieved.[7] The average blood glucose level over the last 4 to 6 weeks is reflected by measuring the amount of glycosylated hemoglobin. The optic fundi should be examined to detect vascular disease at the time of the initial encounter with the pregnant diabetic and subsequently at least once per trimester. Urine analysis, culture, and sensitivity are important for detection of asymptomatic bacilluria, a precursor to overt pyelonephritis to which the diabetic is especially prone.

Results of blood glucose monitoring should be assessed to determine if hyperglycemia or hypoglycemia exists. Although urine testing is not an adequate determinant for management, most women with diabetes test their urine daily for glucose and acetone. Therefore, their knowledge of the basic testing procedures must be determined. Accurate assessment of gestational age is essential. Uterine size, fetal activity, and fetal heart rate sounds provide valuable information. To determine fetal well-being and exact gestational age, a variety of prenatal assessments may be performed (*e.g.*, sonography, nonstress tests, amniocentesis, estriol levels) (see Chap. 42).

Psychosocioeconomic factors are appraised, with special consideration given to the potential stress evoked by the high-risk pregnancy and high costs of possible hospitalizations and antepartal testing procedures. The existence of family support systems in the home or community is determined. The need for additional assistance for child care should also be assessed for multiparous women.

Nursing Diagnosis

As a result of the nursing assessment several potential nursing diagnoses may be identified that focus upon alterations in the life processes of the pregnant diabetic. These include alteration in carbohydrate metabolism related to diabetes; knowledge deficit related to diabetic self-care during pregnancy; disturbance in self-concept related to complications of pregnancy; alteration in tissue perfusion: uteroplacental; potential for infection: vaginal related to monilial infection; potential impairment in skin integrity related to skin stretching secondary to hydramnios.

Nursing Intervention

Adequate control of the pregnant diabetic is of primary concern in planning nursing interventions to prevent or lessen the incidence of perinatal mortality and morbidity. Major components of direct nursing care and client education relate to nutrition management, insulin administration, blood and urine glucose monitoring, and exercise. There are several obstetric considerations of which the nurse must also be aware in implementing care.

Nutrition. Ideally, diabetic women who anticipate pregnancy will follow a well-balanced prescribed dietary regimen before conception and will be in a state of good metabolic control. The caloric requirement for the normal-weight client is approximately 2200 to 2500 calories; at least 45% of the total calories are in the form of carbohydrates (200 g–300 g), 30% are in the form of fat (70 g–80 g), and 25% are in the form of protein (100 g–125 g). At least 30 g/day more protein is recommended in the second and third trimesters than in the nonpregnant state. Clients with nephropathy and proteinuria require additional protein. The caloric requirement should be evenly distributed (three meals and three snacks), with no less than 2000 calories consumed daily. The exact calorie intake is determined based on the client's prepregnant weight and daily activities. A weight gain of 22 lb to 27 lb at term is most desirable.

The diabetic pregnant woman should be specifically instructed to include complex carbohydrates in each meal to delay absorption of glucose. Similarly, adequate fat consumption delays gastric emptying and prevents hyperglycemia. An evening snack consisting of a complex carbohydrate and protein is effective in preventing hypoglycemic episodes during the night. Concentrated sweets should be avoided because they are likely to produce marked swings in blood glucose.

It is difficult to decrease caloric intake below 1800 calories and maintain adequate protein and carbohy-drate intake with a palatable formulation; therefore, weight reduction even for overweight women is generally not recommended. Diabetic women with deficient intake of carbohydrates are at risk for acidosis and ketonemia.

Insulin Administration. The goal of treatment with insulin is to keep blood glucose levels as near the normal range as possible. Maintaining optimal blood glucose levels requires careful regulation of medication, adherence to the prescribed diet, and carefully planned activity. Progressive insulin resistance is characteristic of pregnancy, and it is not unusual for insulin requirements to increase as much as fourfold. During the latter half of pregnancy, the effective half-life of insulin is reduced owing to increased placenta degradation. This commonly necessitates the use of evening as well as morning doses of insulin to achieve good control. Adjustment of insulin dosage is individualized according to the clinical picture and the results of blood glucose analysis. The daily dosage of insulin is frequently split, with about two thirds being administered in the morning and about one third after dinner. A small amount of fast-acting insulin (regular or Semilente) is often added to each dose of intermediate-acting insulin to control the 4- to 6-hour interval before the intermediate insulin begins to have a significant effect on blood glucose level. The combined insulins are administered approximately one half hour before meals. It is essential that the nurse teach the client about time interval peaks for insulin. As this information is discussed it should be related to the signs and symptoms of hypoglycemia and hyperglycemia.

The gestational diabetic may occasionally require insulin therapy despite nutritional management. Oral hypoglycemics are generally not recommended during pregnancy. Client education for the insulin-dependent gestational diabetic encompasses proper technique for injection, rotation of sites, storage of medication, and skin care.

The overt diabetic (Classes B through T) requires counseling about changes in her insulin demands due to pregnancy. Counseling sessions provide excellent opportunities to reinforce the client's acquired skills in self-management and to allay fears concerning new interventions.

In an effort to improve metabolic control some medical centers are using *portable insulin pumps* for pregnant diabetics. These electromechanical devices are implanted into the subcutaneous tissue of the woman's abdomen by way of a small-gauge needle, which continuously delivers a fixed small amount of insulin. A bolus of insulin may be self-administered by the client before meals. The dosage of insulin delivered by the pump is based on capillary blood sample levels drawn by the client or nurse. This type of system does not

(text continued on page 785)

The Pregnant Diabetic Woman

Nursing Objectives

1. Identify the woman at risk for diabetes and provide appropriate perinatal care.
2. Maintain blood glucose levels that mimic physiologic levels in the pregnant diabetic (*e.g.*, fasting blood sugar less than 90 mg/dl and 2-hour postprandial less than 145 mg/dl).
3. Provide comprehensive client education for safe self-management of mother and fetus/newborn.
4. Prevent or detect early potential complications of diabetes during the entire childbearing cycle.
5. Promote a positive psychosocial adjustment to childbearing through understanding and acceptance of pregnancy and diabetes.

Assessment	Potential Nursing Diagnosis	Planning/Intervention	Evaluation

Maternal factors
  Previous large infant (9 lb or greater)
  Family history of diabetes mellitus
  Glucosuria
  Obesity
  Unexplained pregnancy wastage (previous habitual abortions or unexplained stillbirth)
  Previous birth of infant with congenital abnormality
  Multiparity
	Alteration in carbohydrate metabolism related to diabetes	Screen for predisposing factors for diabetes
		
		Determine blood glucose levels by Dextrostix or Chemstik
		
		Check urine specimens for glucose and acetone as ordered
			Woman at risk for diabetes is identified

Fetal/newborn factors
  Hydramnios
  LGA infant
		Observe for signs and symptoms of hypoglycemia or hyperglycemia
		
		Administer 4 oz of orange juice for symptomatic hypoglycemia
			Woman has no signs and symptoms of hypoglycemia or hyperglycemia
			
			Woman maintains normal blood glucose level or restores to normal level after administration of orange juice

Signs of diabetes
  Polyuria
  Polydipsia
  Polyphagia
  Weight loss
		Chart blood glucose levels, treatments, and insulin administration
		
		Assist in preparing for 2-hour postprandial or oral GTT
			Woman repeats instructions to indicate understanding the purpose of testing; she follows instructions

Signs and symptoms of hypoglycemia (hunger, weakness, nausea, agitation, pallor, perspiration) and hyperglycemia (nausea and vomiting, flushed skin, deep rapid respirations, restlessness, thirst, acetone odor to breath)		Administer insulin as ordered Refer to community-health nurse for home follow-up and additional teaching as needed	Woman displays no insulin reaction Woman cooperates with follow-up referrals
Physical examination including assessment of optic fundi, cardiovascular system, vital signs, blood pressure, fundal height			

(continued)

Assessment	Potential Nursing Diagnosis	Planning/Intervention	Evaluation

Glucose tolerance test
  Fasting 90 mg/dl
  1 hr 165 mg/dl
  2 hr 145 mg/dl
  3 hr 125 mg/dl			

Knowledge of carbohydrate metabolism	Knowledge deficit related to diabetic self-care during pregnancy	Review normal carbohydrate and fat metabolism	Woman repeats explanations of effects of diabetes on pregnancy and effects of pregnancy on diabetes
Knowledge about pathophysiology of diabetes during pregnancy		Discuss pathophysiology of diabetes during pregnancy	
24-hour diet recall		Explain changes in insulin regulation throughout childbearing cycle	
Past experience managing diabetes (e.g., self-administration of insulin)		Request nutritional consultation	
Exercise schedule (predictability, length)		Review prescribed dietary plan (exchange lists)	Woman follows prescribed diet based upon knowledge of nutritional needs
Knowledge of complications of diabetes		Record dietary intake on appropriate record	Woman records dietary intake
		Teach newly diagnosed insulin-dependent diabetic the techniques for insulin preparation, administration	Woman repeats demonstration of safe procedure in preparation, self-administration, and storage of insulin
		Instruct in regulation and care of insulin pump prn	
		Instruct in blood glucose monitoring and importance of maintaining fasting blood sugar between 60 and 120 mg/dl	Woman shows proper technique in return demonstration of blood glucose monitoring
		Instruct in fractional urine testing for glucose and acetone levels by Tes-Tape or Diastix	Woman correctly checks urine for glucose and acetone levels
		Provide specific information on signs and symptoms of diabetic complications (e.g., ketoacidosis, insulin shock, hypertensive disorders of pregnancy, UTI)	Woman identifies signs and symptoms of diabetic complications during pregnancy
		Discuss activities for daily living and exercise schedule (prn)	Woman maintains safe level of activities and avoids hypoglycemia
Response to diabetes	Disturbance in self-concept related to complication of pregnancy	Discuss family adaptation to pregnancy and alterations necessitated by diabetes	Woman expresses fears, griefs, and concerns
Expectations about pregnancy			

(continued)

Assessment	Potential Nursing Diagnosis	Planning/Intervention	Evaluation
Achievement of maternal tasks of pregnancy		Define possible stressors and resources in family and community	
		Involve supportive family member(s) in education about complication	Family member(s) provide appropriate support
		Develop strategies for adjusting to complication	Family repeats demonstrations of effective problem-solving skills
Fetal Factors	Alteration in tissue perfusion: uteroplacental	Frequent monitoring of fetal heart rate (q2–4 h if stable)	Fetal heart rate remains within normal limits
Heart rate			
(Activity (*e.g.*, kicking)			
Prenatal diagnostic tests		Instruct mother to maintain fetal activity record and report any significant changes in fetal activity	Fetus shows no signs of distress
L/S ratio			
Nonstress test (NST)/ oxytocin challenge test (OCT)		Discuss importance of frequent prenatal evaluations during entire pregnancy	Woman follows through on prenatal visits
Sonography			
Estriol levels		Explain rationales and prepare for prenatal diagnostic tests (*e.g.*, amniocentesis, sonography, NST/OCT) and provide support during procedures	Woman remains relaxed for testing

(text continued from page 782)

include an integral glucose sensor or feedback mechanism and is called an *open-loop system*.

Approximately 24 to 48 hours before a planned delivery, an intravenous infusion with regular insulin may be started to titrate blood glucose levels accurately. A heparin lock is often inserted as a means of avoiding the repetitive venipunctures required for close blood glucose surveillance.

Blood and Urine Glucose Monitoring.
Until recent years control of diabetes was primarily monitored by the use of preprandial determinations of the percentage of glucose in the urine. Glucosuria is a poor indicator of the diabetic's metabolic regulation because there is an alteration in the renal threshold for glucose during pregnancy. An alternative and effective means being used to accomplish the normalization of maternal glucose levels during pregnancy is home blood glucose monitoring (HBGM).[8] There are now a variety of machines such as the Dextrometer available for use with blood glucose reagent strips. Clients are instructed to measure their blood glucose levels four times a day (before each meal and before their snack in the evening). All blood glucose levels should be entered by the client in her home record-keeping system, which also includes insulin doses, weight, and diet.

Exercise.
Pregnancy is not an optimum time to begin vigorous exercise. During exercise, glucose is absorbed into the muscle and the blood glucose level is lowered. The effect of exercise may last up to 12 hours.

Well-controlled diabetic women who regularly engage in exercise may continue and should be reminded to eat a snack consisting of carbohydrate or protein before activity. A consistent and structured program of activity should be followed rather than an irregular and unpredictable schedule. If signs of hypertensive complications arise, exercise programs should be discontinued.

Obstetric Considerations.
The timing of delivery is probably much more critical than the method, which depends on fetal condition, cervical condition, and, to a lesser extent, maternal medical stability.[1] Since the major target of diabetes is the small blood vessels, it is not surprising that the placenta may also be involved, and therefore placental insufficiency and even fetal death may occur. This result is far less common in gestational diabetics than in prepregnancy diabetics and is

the basis for the common practice of delivering diabetic mothers 3 to 4 weeks prior to the expected date of confinement. This is not, however, always necessary if one can identify the fetus at risk and accurately establish gestational age and well-being through amniocentesis, sonography, nonstress testing, and estriol levels.

Diabetic women are often hospitalized from 34 to 36 weeks gestation until delivery. In those women with no evidence of fetal compromise and who are otherwise stable (good diabetic control, absence of preeclampsia, and no significant hydramnios), pregnancy may be allowed to go to term, with careful surveillance. The method of delivery is a matter of obstetric judgment at the time. Vaginal delivery is carried out whenever possible. Cesarean section is indicated for cases of fetal compromise or an unfavorable cervix.

Cardiac Disease

Approximately 1% of all pregnant women have some type of cardiac disorder. Rheumatic heart disease has for some time been the most common type of heart disease seen in pregnancy. The mitral valve is most commonly affected, with stenosis resulting. Recognition of the role of streptococcal infection and its appropriate therapy has greatly reduced the frequency of rheumatic fever and its cardiac consequences. Congenital heart disease is now relatively more commonly encountered in pregnancy. Another new population of women has been added by cardiac surgeons. Surgically treated women, some with valve replacements, now often proceed through pregnancy uneventfully.

The likelihood of a favorable perinatal outcome for the pregnant woman with heart disease depends upon the functional capacity of her heart and the presence or absence of other complications that increase the cardiac load, as well as the quality of health services rendered and her psychosocial capabilities.[7] Overall, maternal–fetal prognosis for pregnancies complicated by cardiac disease is steadily improving.

Effect of Pregnancy on the Cardiovascular System

A complete discussion of cardiovascular adaptations normally occurring in pregnancy is presented in Chapter 18. As background for discussion on the perinatal effects of heart disease, a brief review follows. There is a progressive rise in cardiac output during pregnancy, with maximum output (30%–50%) reached between 28 and 32 weeks. Increases in both stroke volume and heart rate (10 bpm) contribute to the change. Blood volume expands approximately 40% by the 30th week of pregnancy and then remains fairly constant. Most of the increase in plasma volume occurs in the second trimes-

ter. Vascular resistance and blood pressure decrease during the course of pregnancy.

In normal pregnancy functional systolic murmurs are rather common. Upward displacement of the diaphragm and heart by the enlarging uterus moves the apex of the heart laterally. This may create a false impression of cardiac enlargement. Progesterone stimulates the respiratory center, accentuating breathing effort, which is reminiscent of the dyspnea sometimes seen in heart disease. Edema of the lower extremities that is commonly encountered in normal pregnancy is also a sign of cardiac failure. The normal changes must be considered when the cardiac status of the pregnant woman is evaluated.

The first stage of labor is associated with a modest increase in cardiac output, and there is an appreciable change related to the expulsive efforts of the second stage. The healthy woman has the ability to adapt to the stresses that pregnancy superimposes on the cardiovascular system; however, the woman with heart disease may not have the cardiac reserve to adjust to these new demands.

Effect of Cardiac Disease on Pregnancy

The pathophysiology of disease evident in pregnancy depends on the type of cardiac disorder present. For most types of heart disease, the major threat imposed by pregnancy is that the increasing blood volume will precipitate congestive heart failure. If maternal blood flow is severely compromised, signs and symptoms of right-sided, left-sided, or total failure may develop in the mother and placental circulation may diminish, resulting in a higher risk of prematurity and low birth weight.[9] Pregnant women who have successfully undergone surgical repair and have no residual effects of heart disease generally may experience pregnancy without complication. Unlike these women, women with cyanotic heart disease are at greater risk for perinatal morbidity and mortality. The incidence of congestive heart failure increases over the age of 30 and is further aggravated by parity.

A major problem in managing clients with artificial cardiac valves is that of coagulation. Clients with tissue valves usually do not require anticoagulants, unless they are experiencing other cardiac complications. Reports have revealed that such pregnancies are relatively uneventful; however, in women who were anticoagulated because of artificial heart valves the rate of fetal loss was 33%.[10] Pregnancy exposes women who have had previous valvuloplasty to three most common problems: thromboembolism, infective endocarditis, and myocardial decompensation. Several factors contribute to the risk of thromboembolism from either the valve site or the periphery: thrombogenicity of the valve, trauma to the formed elements of blood, increased clotting factors, and venous stasis.[11] The danger is increased if the pregnant woman discontinues oral anticoagulants to protect the fetus from teratogenic effects (as experienced with sodium warfarin and related drugs).

Other conditions that contribute to the severity of the effects imposed by cardiac disease during pregnancy include obesity, smoking, and anemia.

Medical Diagnosis

The most useful criteria in establishing a diagnosis of heart disease in pregnancy include a diastolic, presystolic, or continuous heart murmur; unequivocal cardiac enlargement; a harsh systolic murmur associated with a thrill; or a significant cardiac arrhythmia.[12] Serious heart disease is usually absent in pregnant women who do not fulfill the above criteria.

Classification

The American Heart Association has developed a classification system for heart disease (Table 37-3) based on the woman's functional capacity. With appropriate management, women in Classes I and II are generally able to experience a normal pregnancy with no or few problems, whereas women in Classes III and IV are at much greater risk for decompensation and other complications. Whenever possible, Class III and IV women with correctable lesions should be counseled to undergo cardiac surgery before conception. It is now the very rare cardiac patient (Class IV) who should be considered for therapeutic abortion on medical grounds.

Nursing Process

Appropriate therapy demands close cooperation between the obstetrician and the cardiologist, with the nurse playing a major role by coordinating information for the client, as well as providing day-to-day direct client care and education. Treatment is governed to a considerable extent by the functional capacity of the client.

Nursing Assessment

A thorough history is obtained on all women with heart disease. Questions should be asked about the client's ability to perform various types of physical activity before pregnancy and the associated cardiovascular effects (*e.g.*, dyspnea upon exertion, palpitations, coughing). A complete physical examination is performed, with special attention given to auscultation of heart and breath sounds. The extremities and more central body surfaces are carefully palpated for edema and tenderness. Baseline maternal vital signs, blood pressure, and fetal heart rate are determined at the initial assessment and then frequently compared with subsequent readings. Capillary filling time is assessed, and observations are made for venous distention.

Results of an electrocardiogram (ECG) or chest x-ray films are reviewed by the nurse, as are laboratory findings. Observations must always be made for arrhythmias. The onset of atrial fibrillation in pregnancy or the puerperium is particularly ominous, since the condition is often associated with various types of heart failure and pulmonary emboli.

Hemodynamic monitoring provides valuable information about the cardiac status of the acutely ill pregnant woman. The Swan-Ganz flow-directed pulmonary artery catheter allows continuous measurement of right atrial pressure (RAP), pulmonary artery pressure (PAP), pulmonary capillary wedge pressure (PCWP), and central venous pressure (CVP). It can effectively be used to assess cardiac output, as well as to administer fluids or drugs.

Nursing Diagnosis

As is true of all concurrent diseases of pregnancy, nursing assessment is an essential step in formulating nursing diagnosis. Examples of nursing diagnoses that specifically appertain to the woman with a pregnancy complicated by heart disease are activity intolerance related to increased metabolic requirements (pregnancy) in the presence of impaired cardiac function; risk of clotting disorder secondary to venous stasis; alteration

(text continued on page 790)

TABLE 37-3

Classification of Heart Disease

Class	Description
Class I	Cardiac disease with *no* limitation of physical activity. Absence of symptoms of cardiac insufficiency and anginal pain.
Class II	Cardiac disease with *slight* limitation of physical activity. Comfortable at rest. Experience fatigue, palpitation, dyspnea, or anginal pain with *ordinary* physical activity
Class III	Cardiac disease with *moderate* to *marked* limitation of physical activity. Comfortable at rest. Experience excessive fatigue, palpitation, dyspnea, or anginal pain with *less* than ordinary physical activity.
Class IV	Cardiac disease with *inability* to perform any physical activity without discomfort. Symptoms of cardiac insufficiency or of the anginal syndrome may occur *at rest* and with *any* physical activity.

(The Criteria Committee of New York State Heart Association: Nomenclature and Criteria for Diagnosis of Diseases of the Heart and Blood Vessels, 6th ed. Boston, Little, Brown & Co, 1964)

The Antepartum Woman with Heart Disease

Nursing Objectives

1. Maintain adequate cardiac functioning throughout the childbearing cycle by limiting cardiac demands.
2. Decrease risks of complications imposed by underlying cardiac disorder(s) and treatment.
3. Protect fetal/newborn well-being by maintenance of a safe intrauterine environment.
4. Promote a positive psychosocial adaptation to the stress of cardiac disease during pregnancy.

Assessment	Potential Nursing Diagnosis	Planning/Intervention	Evaluation
Physical examination	Activity intolerance related to increased metabolic requirements (pregnancy) in the presence of impaired cardiac function	Recommend 10 hours of sleep per night and frequent rest periods during the day as necessary	Woman sleeps a minimum of 10 hours per night and rests in morning and afternoon
Heart rhythm			
Bradycardia			
Tachycardia		Assist in modifying schedule to allow rest	
Murmurs			
Hypotension/hypertension		Instruct to perform a 24-hour dietary history	
Skin color		Provide nutritional counseling	Woman avoids food with high sodium content; consumes 2200-calorie diet with 125 g protein per day
Venous distention		Well-balanced, high-protein diet with no added salt	
Edema			
Rales		Identify foods high in sodium that should be avoided	
Cough			
History		Administer iron supplement as ordered	
Fatigue			
Arrhythmias		Discuss normal cardiovascular changes in pregnancy and how these interact with heart disease	Woman indicates her understanding in discussion of extra demands placed on cardiovascular system during pregnancy
Vertigo			
Angina			
Dyspnea			
Activity level			
Age		Counsel to avoid strenuous work (e.g., heavy housekeeping)	Woman limits her work activities
Parity			
Duration of heart disease			
Complications of heart disease		Review actions, side-effects and administration of each prescribed medication	Woman discusses actions, use, and side-effects of medications
Medications (digoxin, Coumadin, diuretics, antibiotics)			
Dietary history		Initiate referral to community agency for household help or assistance with child care	Family follows through on referral
Weight			
Sodium and fluid intake			
ECG and x-ray results			
Laboratory studies			
Hemoglobin, hematocrit, CBC			
Electrolytes			
Cholesterol			
Phospholipids			

(continued)

Assessment	Potential Nursing Diagnosis	Planning/Intervention	Evaluation
Physical examination	Risk of clotting disorder related to venous stasis during pregnancy*	Observe for signs and symptoms of thromboemboli and identify these for client	Woman identifies absent or early signs and symptoms of clotting disorder
Extremities (swelling, redness, numbness)		Numbness	
Laboratory studies		Tingling	
Prothrombin time		Color change of legs	
Partial thromboplastin time		Chest pain	
Thromboplastin generation test		Abdominal discomfort	
Bleeding time		Apply antiemboli stockings	
Platelet count		Administer anticoagulants as prescribed	
Fibrinogen level		Explain anticoagulant therapy and provide rationale for any medication changes	Woman discusses the actions, adverse effects and precautions of prescribed anticoagulants
		Actions	
		Adverse effects	
		Interactions	
		Warfarin: hematuria, epistasis, gingival bleeding, hematomas	
		Heparin: thrombocytopenia, alopecia, fever, osteoporosis	
		Note: Therapy is discontinued prior to delivery	
		Discuss importance of avoiding salicylates with heparin and verifying use of any medication before self-administering	
		Demonstrate heparin administration (if prescribed) including preparation, injection procedure, rotation of sites	Woman performs a return demonstration of heparin administration
		Observe for adverse effects of anticoagulation	
		Maintain schedule of regular anticoagulant studies during pregnancy (1-wk to 3-wk intervals)	Woman regularly returns to laboratory for blood studies
		Avoid intramuscular injections	
		Secure and store specific antidotes for anticoagulants:	
		Vitamin K—heparin	
		Protamine sulfate—Coumadin	

(continued)

Assessment	Potential Nursing Diagnosis	Planning/Intervention	Evaluation
Physical exam (signs of cardiac decompensation—heart failure)	Alteration in cardiac output and circulation related to cardiac decompensation during pregnancy	Maintain bed rest	Woman remains on bed-rest
Tachycardia (≥100 bpm)		Assist with physical care and personal hygiene as necessary	
S3		Administer digoxin and diuretics as prescribed	
Peripheral edema		Restrict sodium in diet as prescribed (0.5 g to 2 g/day)	Woman restricts sodium intake
Dyspnea			
Orthopnea		Observe for side-effects of diuretic therapy	
Tachypnea (>24 rpm)		Electrolyte imbalance	
Cough unrelated to respiratory disease		Water depletion	
Hemoptysis		Discuss "warning signals"	Woman understands warning signals
Rales at base of lung		Shortness of breath, dyspnea	
Excessive weight gain		Sudden change in ability to do activities	
Hepatomegaly		Extreme fatigue	
Laboratory studies (electrolytes)		Swelling	
		Monitor fetal well-being	Fetus shows no signs of distress
		Fetal heart rate, activity level	
		NSTs, sonography	
History	Infection related to bacterial invasion	Review signs and symptoms of infective bacterial endocarditis, UTIs, and other complicating infections	Woman identifies signs and symptoms of bacterial endocarditis and other complicating infections
Valve replacement (duration and procedure)			
Laboratory studies			
Culture and sensitivity of ordered specimens		Advise to immediately report signs and symptoms	Woman reports all possible infections

(continued)

(text continued from page 787)

in cardiac output and circulation related to cardiac decompensation; infection related to bacterial invasion; anxiety related to fears concerning perinatal outcome; knowledge deficit about signs and symptoms of complications; self-care deficit related to dyspnea, fatigue, and discomforts of pregnancy.

Nursing Intervention

Rest and Activity. Regardless of cardiac classification level, all women with heart disease require additional rest during pregnancy. A minimum of 10 hours of sleep per night plus additional morning and afternoon rest periods is recommended. Based upon knowledge of the client's functional capacity, the nurse and client explore the need for modification of and adjustments in activity level during pregnancy. Some women may need to terminate employment. Complete bed rest in the second half of pregnancy is necessitated by certain cardiac disorders and is required for all Class IV women. Elastic support stockings should be applied to all bed-ridden women to increase venous return.

Nutrition. It is recommended that the pregnant woman with cardiac disease eat a well-balanced nutritional diet (approximately 2200 calories), with large amounts of high-quality protein and no salt added to food (2 g sodium per day). If complications arise or the disease is severe, sodium may be restricted to 1 g to 1½ g/day. Of course, all women should avoid foods rich in sodium. Supplementary iron is often prescribed to

Assessment	Potential Nursing Diagnosis	Planning/Intervention	Evaluation
Platelets Anemia Leukocytes Erythrocyte sedimentation rate		of *any* infection, including UTIs, cold	
		Instruct about administration of prescribed prophylactic antibiotics	Woman correctly self-administers antibiotics
		Discuss importance of regular and frequent antepartal supervision	Woman attends clinic or visits physician as recommended
		Teach principles and techniques of perineal hygiene	Woman uses proper hygiene when voiding
		Caution against contact with "sick" individuals (colds, fever, etc)	Woman avoids interactions with individuals experiencing colds, fever, etc
Expectations of pregnancy Past obstetric history Support systems in home or community Knowledge about labor and delivery	Anxiety related to fears concerning perinatal outcome	Demonstrate acceptance of expressed concerns about pregnancy outcome	Woman verbalizes concerns about stressors of pregnancy
		Clearly explain purpose of all treatments and antepartal diagnostic tests	Woman demonstrates decreased anxiety about treatments
		Reinforce positive aspects of pregnancy (*e.g.,* normal fetal heart rate and activity level)	Woman displays positive reaction to fetal movement
		Offer reassurance for progress being made (*e.g.,* ability to tolerate activities and to manage components of self-care)	
		Involve family members or other supportive individuals in discussions, whenever possible and acceptable	Family demonstrates understanding of client's fears and offers support appropriately

* Prosthetic valves also contribute to risk.

prevent anemia. A weight gain between 22 and 27 pounds is desirable. Excess weight gain places additional strain on the heart and circulatory system. The lateral recumbent position is recommended for clients on bed rest or in labor.

Medications. Women who were receiving digitalis prior to pregnancy must continue use of the drug throughout the childbearing cycle. Changes in the cardiovascular system may also necessitate the initiation of digitalis treatment for previously nonmedicated women. Maternal and fetal heart rate are both slowed by the administration of digitalis, which crosses the placental barrier. If arrhythmias should develop during pregnancy, cardioversion may be safely accomplished through the use of quinidine.

Diuretic therapy is generally not recommended for Class I and II women during pregnancy. However, it may be prescribed for Class III and IV women. The woman on diuretic therapy should be observed for potassium depletion and postural hypotension.

Just prior to delivery some physicians prescribe prophylactic antibiotics for women with valvular heart disease and congenital defects because of their high susceptibility to bacterial endocarditis.

The use of sodium warfarin (Coumadin) as an anticoagulant for women who have had valve replacements is associated with an increased risk of congenital anomalies (nasal hypoplasia, stippling of bones, intrauterine growth retardation, and ophthalmologic abnormalities) in the first trimester and questionable safety factors in later pregnancy.[13–15]

Heparin, an alternative anticoagulant that does not cross the placental barrier, may be administered prior to conception and during early pregnancy. Specific information about the actions, side-effects, and self-administration of heparin is provided by the nurse to all women beginning therapy.

Prevention of Infection. Febrile episodes increase the cardiac demands and are often associated with tachycardia. The pregnant woman with cardiac disease should be cautioned against contact with individuals suffering from respiratory infections or other contagious diseases. The importance of using proper perineal care should be emphasized as a means of preventing urinary tract infections (UTIs) and pyelonephritis. Emphasis is also placed on the need to immediately report potential infections.

Obstetric Considerations. The diagnosis of cardiac disease is not an indication for early induction of labor. Clients are usually allowed to go into spontaneous labor. Hospitalization for a short period prior to the expected onset of labor is occasionally recommended. It is essential that the laboring woman with heart disease be relieved of discomfort and anxiety. Systemic analgesics combined with sedatives may be administered early in the first stage of labor. To facilitate cardiac circulation and maximum oxygenation, the client is placed in a side-lying or semi-Fowler's position. Oxygen may be administered if pulmonary complications arise. Continuous fetal heart rate monitoring is performed. Vaginal deliveries are preferable to cesarean births. In the second stage of labor forceps are commonly applied to avoid the stress of increased abdominal pressure created by maternal pushing. The use of high stirrups is inappropriate for women with cardiac disease. Caudal or epidural anesthesia is administered for delivery. Broad-spectrum antibiotics may be administered during the intrapartum and postpartum periods to prevent development of bacterial endocarditis and bacteremia.

Hematologic Disorders

Iron Deficiency Anemia

Iron deficiency anemia is the most common hematologic disorder in pregnancy. Several physiological alterations occurring in pregnancy contribute to the risk for this type of anemia. There is a pronounced increase in maternal plasma volume and a relatively lower increase in total red blood cells. These alterations increase the nutrient-carrying capacity of the plasma but reduce the viscosity of whole blood. The disproportionate rise in blood constituents causes hemodilution with a resultant fall in hemoglobin concentration unless the need is met by augmented hematopoiesis. These blood changes are unrelated to the pregnant woman's iron status; they occur whether the client is receiving iron supplementation or is not given iron.

There is, in addition, the fetal requirement for iron to contend with. Since many women have depleted iron stores as a result of regular menstrual blood loss, these added demands often result in the total depletion of storage iron and the development of overt anemia. The socioeconomically deprived woman with poor general nutrition is more susceptible to this condition.

Medical Diagnosis

A hemoglobin level below 11 g/dl or a hematocrit of less than 35% is generally considered suggestive of anemia, and further evaluation is indicated to determine the reasons for the condition. Erythrocyte indexes aid in assessing the cause of the low hemoglobin level. The red blood cells are characteristically found to be microcytic and hypochromic. There is a decrease in the mean corpuscular volume (MCV, size of the erythrocyte) and mean corpuscular hemoglobin (MCH, quantity of hemoglobin in the erythrocyte).

Effect of Iron Deficiency Anemia on Pregnancy

In most clients with mild to moderate anemia, the signs and symptoms (fatigue) are few and often indistinguishable from the normal symptoms of pregnancy. Such women are detected by frequent antepartal hemoglobin or hematocrit determinations. Iron deficiency anemia renders the pregnant woman particularly susceptible to infection and increases her risk of postpartum hemorrhage. Severely anemic women (hemoglobin < 8 g/dl) are symptomatic and in the most severe cases can even develop heart failure as a result of the anemia.

Chronic anemia limits the amount of oxygen available for fetal exchange. There is an increased risk for abortion and premature birth. Severe anemia is associated with increased frequency of neonates in the small-for-gestational-age (SGA) category.

Nursing Process

All pregnant women should have a complete blood count (CBC), including hemoglobin, hematocrit, and red blood cell indices early in the prenatal period. Oral administration of iron is commonly prescribed to prevent or cure iron deficiency. It should be noted that the prophylactic use of iron during pregnancy is somewhat controversial. Approximately 3 mg to 5 mg of iron per day is needed to supply the needs of mother and fetus, with demands for iron increasing in the last 5 months of pregnancy to as much as 3 mg to 7.5 mg/day. A number of oral preparations of organic and inorganic iron are available for treatment; most common compounds include ferrous sulfate (200 mg–300 mg tid) or ferrous gluconate (320 mg tid). These drugs should be ingested with meals, to decrease gastrointestinal side-effects. The absorption of iron and the metabolism of folic acid are enhanced by vitamin C (ascorbic acid). Injectable iron therapy is rarely required because absorption is generally not a limiting factor. More often a failure to respond to oral iron therapy is the result of failure to take the medication (iron tends to produce gastrointestinal symptoms) or a concurrent folic acid deficiency. It is important to assess the existence of side-effects in all pregnant women receiving iron supplementation. Constipation may be a particularly troublesome side-effect; it can be relieved by prescribing stool softeners such as dioctyl sodium sulfosuccinate (Colace).

An iron-rich diet is recommended for all pregnant women. Ideally, an extra 1000 mg of iron intake should be added to the daily diet.

Folic Acid Deficiency

Folic acid deficiency can produce severe anemia of the megaloblastic type in pregnancy. Megaloblastic anemia is much less common than iron deficiency anemia, occurring in fewer than 3% of gravidae. In its full-blown form there is also a reduction in white blood cells and platelets and the MCV is elevated. Symptoms of this type of anemia include glossitis, sore tongue, and anorexia. Perinatal outcome may be seriously threatened by folic acid deficiency, which is reportedly associated with higher early abortion and abruptio placentae.

Treatment consists of oral folic acid (1 mg administered orally once a day) and diet. Prevention is achieved by the inclusion of folic acid in prenatal vitamin–mineral supplements. All pregnant women should be instructed to eat foods that are high in folic acid. These include fresh vegetables, especially of the uncooked green leafy variety, red meats, fish, legumes, and poultry. Preparing vegetables by steaming them in small quantities of water will decrease folic acid loss.

Hemoglobinopathies

Hemoglobinopathies present special problems in pregnancy. The most commonly encountered of the hemoglobinopathies are sickle cell anemia (SS disease), sickle cell–hemoglobin C disease (SC disease), and sickle cell–β-thalassemia disease (S-thalassemia disease). These are recessively inherited diseases that are seen principally in the black population and are invariably associated with an increased maternal morbidity and mortality, perinatal mortality, and abortion.

In managing hemoglobinopathies, detailed counseling is called for. One must consider not only the impact of pregnancy in precipitating crises but also the genetic implications and the fact that women with sickle cell anemia have a limited life expectancy. Women with

sickle cell anemia might well wish to consider limiting childbearing or even avoiding pregnancy completely.

Sickle Cell Anemia (SS Disease)

Sickle cell anemia occurs when the gene for the production of S hemoglobin is inherited from both parents. When S hemoglobin is transmitted from one but not the other, the individual does not exhibit frank anemia but has *sickle-cell* trait. Between 8% and 10% of the black population have the sickling trait only or are heterozygous.[16] Pregnant women with sickle-cell trait have a predisposition to urinary tract infections and hematuria, but are otherwise normal. About 1 in 12 black individuals has sickle-cell trait, whereas 1 in every 576 black women has the disease.[17] The actual incidence of sickle cell anemia in pregnancy is about one third as high as in the general population, probably because many affected individuals do not survive to childbearing age or elect not to carry their pregnancies to term.

Individuals affected by sickle cell anemia have inherited a defect in the hemoglobin molecule that causes erythrocytes to become elongated and crescent shaped (sickle), particularly when they are exposed to temperature variations, lowered blood pH, or increased blood viscosity. Decreases in circulating oxygen levels resulting from exercise, anesthesia, high altitudes, and air pollution may also cause sickling.[18]

Sickle cell anemia has great impact throughout the childbearing cycle. The anemia is exacerbated during pregnancy, and life-threatening hemolytic crises can occur, especially during the intrapartum period. Maternal mortality rates are high (10%–20%) owing to the risk of pulmonary complications, infection, congestive heart failure, and hypertension. Other problems encountered by pregnant women with sickle-cell disease are severe anemia, kidney dysfunction, pneumonia, and pregnancy-induced hypertension. About one half of the pregnancies end in spontaneous abortion, neonatal death, or stillbirth. The risk for spontaneous premature labor is similarly high.

All black pregnant women not previously tested should be screened for sickle cell anemia at the time of their first prenatal visit. Women with diagnosed sickle cell anemia require the most meticulous of prenatal care. The main goal of therapy is to prevent conditions that cause sickling and to minimize the complications of sickling when it occurs. Antepartal diagnostic procedures are frequently performed to assess uteroplacental functioning and fetal well-being. Nonstress testing is particularly useful for identifying problems of placental dysfunction associated with placental infarction.[19]

Throughout pregnancy the diet of women with sickle cell anemia should be supplemented with folic acid because of the rapid turnover of red blood cells. Fluid intake should be well maintained to prevent dehydration. Regular screening of urine is recommended for early diagnosis of asymptomatic bacteriuria. Hemoglobin levels are frequently assessed for rapid decreases in value, which are suggestive of sickle-cell crisis. It is not unusual for pregnant women with sickle-cell disease to have hemoglobin levels in the range of 6 g to 9 g/dl. Multiple prophylactic transfusions of packed red cells are sometimes used to suppress the client's bone marrow from forming abnormal cells while at the same time permitting her to exist on transfused cells during the period of risk. All clients with sickle-cell disease should be advised to avoid contact with individuals suffering from infectious diseases.

Sickle Cell–Hemoglobin C Disease (SC Disease)

Sickle cell–hemoglobin C disease occurs when the gene for the production of hemoglobin C is inherited along with that for hemoglobin S. It is much less common and certainly less serious in the nonpregnant state. During pregnancy and the puerperium, however, mortality and morbidity are greatly increased, with a maternal mortality reported in some series as high as 2%. In contrast to sickle cell anemia, the perinatal mortality is increased only slightly.

Sickle Cell–β-Thalassemia Disease (S-Thalassemia Disease)

Sickle cell–β-thalassemia disease results from the inheritance of the gene for hemoglobin S from one parent and the allelic gene for β-thalassemia from the other parent. Perinatal mortality and morbidity of this disease are similar to sickle cell–hemoglobin C disease.[7] Although β-thalassemia has been reported among all populations, it is most common in people from the Mediterranean region, with a significant prevalence among African and Southeast Asians from Cambodia, Laos, and Vietnam.

Urinary Tract and Renal Disease

Almost all forms of acute and chronic renal disease have been reported in association with pregnancy. Not infrequently, specific diagnosis is difficult during pregnancy because proteinuria and hypertension may mimic preeclampsia and also because definitive studies such as renal biopsy and intravenous urography are relatively contraindicated.

The most common renal problem in pregnancy is urinary tract infection (UTI). Anatomical changes as well as hormonal effects cause narrowing of the lower ureter and renal pelvis, with dilation of the upper ureter. These changes result in stasis of urine, delayed emptying, and an increased risk of infection. The risk increases as pregnancy progresses and continues into the puerperium.

Approximately 3% to 8% of all pregnant women have asymptomatic bacteriuria, depending on parity, race, and socioeconomic factors. In pregnancy this condition is significant because of its high association with subsequent pyelonephritis; consequently, it should be treated. Association with other obstetric problems such as prematurity and congenital abnormality has been suggested, but it has not been clearly established. The presence of 100,000 (10^5/ml) organisms in a urine culture is diagnostic of bacteriuria.

Pregnant women with sickle-cell trait, multiple sex partners, and a past history of renal disease are at greater risk for bacteriuria and therefore must be frequently screened. Symptomatic UTI may result from failure to treat pregnant women with asymptomatic bacteriuria. As a precaution, nurses should routinely teach all pregnant women to recognize the symptoms of UTI.

Manifestations of UTI include dysuria, frequency, urgency, chills, low-grade fever, hematuria, and lower abdominal pain. *Escherichia coli* is the most common causative agent of UTI.

Renal disease in the form of acute pyelonephritis may be characterized by the previously described manifestations of UTI plus pain in the lumbar area (usually right side), tenderness, malaise, high fever, and gastrointestinal disturbances. Uterine irritability is an important complication of pyelonephritis. It is wise to look for renal disease in any client with premature labor.

Women with chronic renal disease and renal transplants are now living long enough to bear children. During pregnancy they may be treated with corticosteroids such as prednisone. The prognosis for pregnancy after transplantation is good if the woman's general health is optimum, blood pressure is normal, and there are no signs of graft reaction. Hemodialysis may be performed for failing renal function during pregnancy.

One of the major complications of chronic renal disease is hypertension; the two conditions in combination may be associated with fetal growth retardation and increased perinatal mortality. Infants born to mothers who have been taking steroids are prone to hyperglycemia at birth owing to suppression of fetal insulin activity by corticosteroids.

As part of the prenatal education, the nurse should provide instruction on personal hygiene practices, since most UTIs result from bacteria ascending through the urethra. Screening for renal disease during pregnancy is performed by carefully collecting a midstream clean-catch urine specimen. To ensure an adequate specimen the nurse should instruct the client as to the proper method of collecting the sample. An examination of the urinary sediment as well as a culture and antibiotic sensitivity studies should be carried out.

Hospitalization is recommended for treatment of acute pyelonephritis, since intravenous therapy and bed rest in the left lateral position are prescribed. Temperature elevation is controlled by antipyretics, analgesics, and cool sponge baths.

Women with diagnosed UTIs or pyelonephritis are treated with appropriate antibiotics (tetracycline, kanamycin, and gentamicin are contraindicated). The nurse should carefully review the actions, side-effects, and administration of the prescribed drug, as well as stress the importance of maintaining good fluid intake (3 to 4 liters/24 hr) orally or parenterally, if necessary. It is also necessary to reculture urine 1 week after completion of the 7- to 10-day antimicrobial therapy. Recurrences are common, causing some authorities to recommend long-term suppressive antimicrobial therapy.

Chorioamnionitis

Chorioamnionitis is an intrauterine infection involving mononuclear and polymorphonuclear leukocytic infiltration of the fetal membranes and amniotic fluid. Symptoms of the disease are maternal fever and fetal tachycardia. Premature rupture of the membranes (PROM) is believed to be the most common cause of the disease; however, some studies have suggested that chorioamnionitis may be the precursor to PROM.

The danger of this disease is increased by repeated vaginal examinations and intrauterine manipulation. In many hospitals it has become common practice to give antibiotics prophylactically to women with PROM. When membranes are ruptured more than 24 hours the incidence of chorioamnionitis rises dramatically.

Interventions include culturing of the amniotic fluid and maternal blood for causative organisms (most often *E. coli*, anaerobic and aerobic streptococci and staphylococci), administering appropriate intravenous antibiotic therapy, and carefully monitoring the fetus.

Labor is induced in cases of mild infection if delivery may be accomplished within 6 to 8 hours. In severe cases or when the fetus is distressed, cesarean delivery is elected.

Thyroid Disease

Hyperthyroidism

Hyperthyroidism is probably the second most significant endocrinopathy in pregnancy, second only to diabetes mellitus. Approximately 2 of 1000 pregnancies are complicated by hyperthyroid disease. Although a woman with uncontrolled hyperthyroidism is likely to be anovulatory and thus unable to conceive, many with milder disease do conceive, and in some cases the hyperthyroidism is first diagnosed during pregnancy. If the condition is not detected and treated properly, spontaneous abortion and premature labor are common. There is a greater risk for delivering SGA infants. Diagnosis may be somewhat of a problem in milder cases, since some thyroid enlargement and confusing hyperdynamic symptoms occur in normal pregnancy.

Helpful signs for identifying hyperthyroidism during pregnancy are tachycardia that exceeds the increase caused by normal pregnancy, a high pulse rate while sleeping, an enlarged thyroid gland, exophthalmos, and failure to gain weight normally.[7]

Laboratory studies may be confusing, since there is increased protein binding of thyroid hormone in pregnancy, resulting in higher values for studies such as the protein-bound iodine and total thyroxine (T_4), with lower triiodothyronine (T_3) uptake. Multiple studies and newer methods, however, can overcome the confusion.

Once-popular surgical treatment (subtotal thyroidectomy) has been replaced by medical approaches, except in special cases (*e.g.*, reaction to the antithyroid drugs, unusually large dosage requirements). The problem with medical therapy is that the antithyroid drug (propylthiouracil) crosses the placenta and if doses are excessive the fetal thyroid can be suppressed, leading to fetal goiter or even cretinism. This is best avoided if the level of control is maintained at slightly hyperthyroid levels.

Women with exophthalmic goiter produce a long-acting thyroid stimulator (LATS), which is an immunoglobulin G (IgG). This crosses the placenta and if present can cause hyperthyroidism in the newborn.

A major complication of hyperthyroidism is the rare occurrence of *thyroid storm* during pregnancy and the puerperium. This condition is manifest by high fever, tachycardia, sweating, severe dehydration, and occasional cardiac decompensation. Treatment consists of early recognition followed by in-hospital intense therapy with large doses of propylthiouracil and potassium iodide and possibly intravenous administration of steroids.

Severe Hypothyroidism

Severe hypothyroidism is rare during pregnancy because the condition is usually associated with amenorrhea and anovulation. Women with mild hypothyroidism may conceive, but are at greater risk for spontaneous abortion. Infants of hypothyroid mothers with mild disease generally appear healthy; however, there is an increased risk of congenital goiter or cretinism in infants of more severely hypothyroid mothers.

Infectious Diseases

Although most infectious diseases have no established specific ill effects on mother or baby, there are those that produce profound effects. Diseases with particular fetal effects such as the TORCH syndrome are discussed in Chapter 42. For purposes of this discussion, infectious diseases complicating pregnancy are subdivided into two classifications, sexually transmitted diseases and other diseases that are not sexually related but that cause unique problems.

Common Cold

Susceptibility to acute upper respiratory tract infections is apparently slightly greater during pregnancy. The common cold often precedes more serious conditions affecting the upper respiratory tract. Therefore, the nurse should advise pregnant women to make every effort to avoid contact with these infections. The administration of aspirin or acetaminophen (Tylenol) is unnecessary for symptomatic treatment of mild respiratory congestion during pregnancy and should be reserved for febrile episodes. There is some evidence associating maternal aspirin ingestion within the last 2 weeks of pregnancy with coagulation problems in neonates.

Influenza

The occurrence of influenza infection during pregnancy poses serious risks of maternal and fetal morbidity and has been correlated with higher premature labor and abortion rates. Symptoms of influenza include high fever, muscle aches and back pain, sore throat, and prostration.

Although the pregnant woman is not more likely to contract influenza, she is more prone to the development of complicating pneumonia, especially if she is in the third trimester, during which time the diaphragm is elevated and respiration is compromised. The development of pneumonia represents a serious threat to the gravida, since maternal mortality increases significantly when this complication occurs.

In the face of an epidemic involving a specific strain of influenza virus, immunization with a killed or attenuated virus vaccine is indicated. Nonspecific polyvalent vaccines are probably ineffectual.

Measles (Rubeola)

Ill effects are not commonly noted in pregnancy, but pregnant women who contract measles are said to be more likely to have spontaneous abortions and pre-mature labor. No other definite effects are reported, although eruptions have been noted on infants at birth and premature infants are particularly prone to adverse sequelae from measles infection.

Chickenpox (Varicella)

Varicella during pregnancy is rare; however, when it does occur, it is likely to be severe. If varicella pneumonia develops as a complication, it is often fatal. Treatment includes maintaining adequate oxygenation, controlling bacterial superinfection, and administering acyclovir.

Some studies suggest that maternal chickenpox during the first trimester may be associated with congenital malformations,[20] and exposure of the fetus to the virus just prior to delivery poses serious risk for disseminated visceral and central nervous system disease.

Typhoid Fever

Typhoid fever, which is now relatively rare in the United States, in former years caused serious complications in pregnancy, resulting in abortion, prematurity, and infant mortality. Treatment with chloramphenicol or ampicillin is usually quite effective in arresting the disease. Immunization is not contraindicated during pregnancy, and antityphoid vaccine should be administered when necessary.

Tuberculosis

In recent years the incidence of tuberculosis is actually rising, especially among Southeast Asian refugees and Mexicans who have experienced substantial preexisting nutritional deprivation associated with low socioeconomic status.[21]

The average case of tuberculosis in itself has only a slight effect on the course of pregnancy, since it rarely predisposes to abortion, premature labor, or even stillbirth. Fortunately, the disease is seldom acquired congenitally, although a small number of authentic cases have been reported in which, in addition to a tuberculous condition of the placenta, tubercle bacilli were found in the cord blood, together with tuberculous lesions in the infant.

Medical opinions differ, but the consensus is that pregnancy does not exert an adverse effect on tuberculosis when properly managed. It is generally agreed, however, that only a woman in an arrested state should consider becoming pregnant. Pregnancy is undertaken with some risk, for although a tuberculosis lesion may remain latent for an indefinite time, provided that the natural resistance is not overtaxed, it must be noted that pregnancy is one of the factors responsible for overtaxing the resistance sufficiently to convert a latent, inactive lesion into an active one. Maintenance of proper nutrition does much to prevent activity in a latent focus.

Treatment with modern antituberculosis drugs, streptomycin, isoniazid (INH), ethambutol hydrochloride, and para-amino-salicylic acid (PAS), has completely altered management in general, as well as during pregnancy. New advanced cases are rare, and a majority of women are managed as outpatients. No deleterious effects on the fetus have been reported. Mothers may exhibit nausea, vomiting, malaise, and fever while on isoniazid. Optic nerve disturbances have been related to ethambutol administration in the mother. When isoniazid is given during pregnancy, supplemental pyridoxine should be administered to minimize the potential for neurotoxic fetal effects.

Some authorities recommend isoniazid therapy in the third trimester and puerperium for the inactive client who has had active disease within 2 years of pregnancy.

Labor and delivery are conducted in a normal fashion, avoiding inhalation anesthesia, and mother and baby are separated if disease is active. Breast-feeding may be permitted when the disease is inactive.

Poliomyelitis

Poliomyelitis generally does not complicate pregnancy or delivery, except in the very unusual cases in which respiratory paralysis develops; in these rare cases cesarean birth has given satisfactory results. Fortunately, as a result of immunization, the disease has virtually disappeared.

Viral Hepatitis

The hepatitis viruses are the most common causes of liver disease in pregnancy. Refugees from Southeast Asia and Africa, as well as drug abusers, are at particular risk for developing hepatitis B virus (HBV). Clinical symptoms range from mild to severe, with anorexia, nausea, and vomiting being the most characteristic symptoms of hepatitis. Since 75% of affected women do not exhibit clinical jaundice, the diagnosis may be missed or delayed in women exhibiting the nausea and vomiting characteristic of pregnancy, or cases may be misdiagnosed as hyperemesis gravidarum. In contrast to the latter, in hepatitis the liver is characteristically enlarged and tender and bilirubin levels rise as high as 25 mg/dl. When nausea and vomiting persist unabated in pregnancy, hepatitis should be considered and ruled out.

The diagnosis of hepatitis A is usually established by the detection of antibody to hepatitis A virus (anti-HAV) of the IgM class, whereas the serologic diagnosis of hepatitis B is established most often by the detection of circulating hepatitis B surface antigen (HB_sAg).

Untreated hepatitis is associated with an increased incidence of abortion, premature labor, and stillbirth. There is no evidence that HAV or HBV is teratogenic. Maternal mortality rates from viral hepatitis vary and have been reported at from 1% to 17%. Its course is substantially influenced by the nutritional status of the client, and hence maternal mortality is higher in the less developed regions of the world. Prompt diagnosis and treatment with hospitalization, bed rest, good nutrition, and intravenous therapy generally result in favorable outcome. The pregnant woman who has been recently exposed to hepatitis should receive γ-globulin prophylactically. Since there is now some evidence suggesting that hepatitis B is sexually transmitted, all pregnant women should be cautioned against intimate contact with infected individuals. In addition, women at risk for hepatitis A should be advised that the virus is shed in the stools of infected persons and that fecal–oral transmission is the predominant mode of spread.

The fetus may acquire the virus *in utero* or during delivery, and the newborn may develop active hepatitis or a carrier state. It has been shown that about 90% of the infants born to carrier mothers positive for hepatitis B_e antigen are infected with HBV.[22]

Prompt treatment of the newborn with hepatitis B immune γ-globulin is recommended. Since HB_sAg has been detected in breast milk and the virus is present in maternal serum, which could be transmitted from excoriations around the nipple, breast-feeding should be avoided.

Sexually Transmitted Infectious Disease (STD)

The sexually transmitted diseases include a variety of conditions that range from very mild and easily treated (*e.g.,* vaginitis) to potentially very harmful to maternal–fetal health (*e.g.,* acquired immune deficiency syndrome (AIDS), syphilis). Because all of these diseases are spread through coitus, they are classified as sexually transmitted. It should be noted that initial infection with any of these diseases does not produce immunity. Some diseases are incurable, while others may cause repetitive episodes of outbreaks. Each condition is presented individually, followed by a general discussion on the nursing care of a pregnant woman with a STD.

Syphilis

The most serious form of syphilis is congenital infection caused by *Treponema pallidum*. Until recently, it appeared that public-health controls were effectively decreasing the incidence of intrauterine infection and late abortion or stillbirth. However, the number of cases of congenital disease has risen by 38%.[23] Syphilis selectively affects socioeconomically disadvantaged populations, especially blacks and foreign-born Hispanics.

An antenatal blood test for syphilis (VDRL) is required by law, and, except for the instances in which prenatal care is nonexistent, maternal syphilis can be detected and adequately treated, thereby protecting the fetus.

Syphilis can occur at any stage during pregnancy. The primary stage is usually apparent because of the classic lesions (chancres), which are deep and painless ulcers often found on the genitalia, lips, or rectal area. In the secondary stage of syphilis a macular rash appears on the entire body. In latent syphilis the diagnosis is based upon a positive serology; the most difficult problem occurs when the serology is repeatedly positive and the client denies a history. Biologic false-positives occur in a number of circumstances, but, fortunately, new, more specific tests (FTA-ABS is a specific antibody test for syphilis) are now available that can be used in the questionable case.

A pregnant woman is contagious during the primary, secondary, and latent stages. The disease can be transmitted through the placenta after the 18th week of pregnancy. The final or third stage of syphilis involves the appearance of neurologic symptoms, including slurred speech, mental confusion, and ataxia.

Treatment is indicated in the following circumstances:

- When a diagnosis of early syphilis is made, regardless of stage
- When late symptomatic syphilis is discovered
- When latent syphilis is diagnosed by repeated positive serologic tests and the woman's history corroborates the diagnosis, and when there has been either inadequate or no treatment
- When the diagnosis is made by repeated positive tests, even though the history does not confirm, and when either the more specific tests are not available or there is not time for adequate therapy. Re-treatment in subsequent pregnancies is necessary if there is any doubt about the adequacy of previous therapy.

The aim of therapy is to prevent the spread of congenital syphilis, which can cause congenital anomalies. The treatment consists of a course of penicillin (benzathine penicillin G or procaine penicillin G) or erythromycin if penicillin allergy exists. The mother who has been treated successfully may become reinfected during pregnancy; therefore, it is important to treat her sexual partner as well. Both mother and baby should be carefully followed by serologic tests postpartum. It is significant to note that even the unaffected baby will have a positive test because the mother's test is positive;

however, the titer in the baby will be lower than that of the mother and will become negative within 3 months. Infants born of mothers treated with erythromycin for syphilis during pregnancy should be managed as though they have congenital syphilis.[7]

Gonorrhea

Gonorrhea is of special concern in maternity care because of the consequences to the mother at the time of labor and during the puerperium, as well as the risk of permanent injury to the baby's eyes at the time of birth.

The disease is caused by the gram-negative coccus *Neisseria gonorrhoeae*, an organism that may attack the mucous membrane, but most commonly affects the mucosa of the lower genital tract. The endocervical glands and urethra are common foci, but for complete detection, the anus and oropharynx should be cultured.

Gonorrhea is spread by sexual contact and in the majority of women remains asymptomatic except for a nonspecific vaginal discharge. This is particularly the case in pregnancy, in which the normal route of spread through the endometrial cavity to the tubes is occluded by the pregnancy. The rate of symptomatic carriers in pregnancy is reported to be as high as 5% to 10% in many clinics.

Although gonorrhea causes few problems for the client during pregnancy, it can produce serious puerperal infection if present in the cervix at the time of delivery. Routine gonorrhea cultures or blood drawn for gonorrheal antibodies are recommended in early pregnancy. Gram-stained smears are suggestive but not conclusive in women.

The treatment of asymptomatic gonorrhea involves a single injection of 4.8 million units of aqueous procaine penicillin intramuscularly, preceded by 1 g of probenecid orally to produce the high level of penicillin needed to eradicate the increasingly resistant gonococcus. Cure should be proven by reculture, although reinfection is possible and should be watched for. Sexual partners should be evaluated and treated appropriately.

The organism can infect the infant's eyes at birth, and if prophylactic treatment of the eyes is not adequate, blindness may result from *ophthalmia neonatorum*.

Genital Herpes

Two types of herpesviruses that are immunologically and clinically distinct may involve the genital tract. Type I herpes hominis is mainly associated with nongenital lesions, but may also involve the genital tract. Type II herpes hominis is almost entirely genital and is generally sexually transmitted. Herpes type II is one of the most rapidly spreading STDs, with between 5 and 20 million American adults infected.

Approximately 1% to 2% of pregnancies are complicated by herpesvirus infection. The incubation period is 3 to 14 days for the primary infection and 7 to 10 days for the secondary infection. The lesions are characterized by painful vesicles in the vulva and perineal areas that commonly rupture and become secondarily infected (Fig. 37-1). The cervix and vagina are also commonly infected with lesions that are asymptomatic and may shed for several months. The infected woman may experience flulike symptoms. Inguinal adenopathy may be severe. Cytologic smears reveal large multinucleate cells with eosinophilic inclusion bodies, and unsuspected herpes is frequently diagnosed as an incidental finding by Pap smear. The initial herpes symptoms usually disappear within 3 weeks; however, recurrences are frequent and associated with stress or illness.

The maternal infection is only rarely transmitted transplacentally to the fetus, but when this occurs in the first trimester, spontaneous abortion or severe fetal abnormalities may result. After the 20th week of gestation, infection increases the risk for premature birth but not for fetal abnormalities. The fetus is most likely to be infected following rupture of the membranes or during the course of delivery, since the virus can be transmitted through lesions in the genital tract. Detection of active herpes infections prior to delivery is most important, since congenital and neonatal herpes is often lethal and ocular and central nervous system damage occurs in nearly half of the survivors (see Chap. 42 for further discussion).

Since there is at present no effective treatment for genital herpes, when viral cultures are positive cesarean birth is recommended to avoid exposure to the lower genital tract.

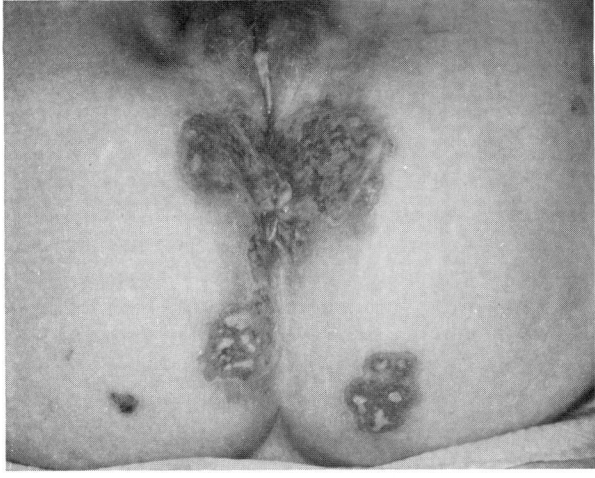

FIGURE 37-1

Herpes genitalis lesions are characterized by painful vesicles in the vulva and perineal areas.

Topical application of acyclovir (Zovirax) may be given to modify the symptomatology and shorten healing time of lesions, if the benefits of its use during pregnancy justify the potential risk to the fetus. Broad-spectrum antibiotic therapy is often prescribed to treat secondary infection. Perineal comfort may be promoted by taking sitz baths two to three times per day and keeping the infected region clean and dry.

When an uninfected pregnant woman has a sexual partner with a history of genital herpes, condoms should be used to reduce the possibility of transmission, even in asymptomatic phases of the disease. In addition, women with a history of genital herpes should be advised to have Pap smears performed annually, since there is now evidence suggesting that herpes type II may have a causal role in cervical carcinoma.[24]

Chlamydial Infections

Infections caused by *Chlamydia trachomatis* are becoming the most prevalent of the STDs in the United States. During pregnancy the organism has been associated with an increased risk of premature birth, stillbirth, ophthalmia neonatorum, and newborn chlamydial pneumonia. Endometritis is a maternal complication that may occur in the postpartum period.

Chlamydial infection may be difficult to diagnose, since culture techniques are not yet available in many clinics. Pregnant women whose sexual partners have nongonococcal urethritis should be treated. Erythromycin is administered on an empty stomach in oral doses of 500 mg four times a day for at least 7 days. The male partner should be simultaneously treated with tetracycline. The infected infant is given tetracycline ophthalmic ointment for several weeks following birth or until negative eye cultures are obtained.

Trichomonas vaginalis

Trichomonas vaginalis is found in as many as 20% of pregnant women; a large number of these women remain asymptomatic. The disease is characterized by a white to gray green discharge, which is foamy. Pruritus and irritation may also be present.

Diagnosis of *Trichomonas vaginalis* is made based upon microscopic examination of vaginal discharge (saline wet smear). During the first half of pregnancy, the woman is treated symptomatically. Metronidazole (Flagyl) is prescribed in the last half of pregnancy when the possibility of teratogenic effects may be avoided. In combination with alcohol, Flagyl causes acute nausea and vomiting. Therefore, women should be advised about this potential drug interaction. Other medications that may be administered as a vaginal suppository include Tricofuron and Vagisec. The pregnant woman's sexual partner also requires treatment to prevent reinfection of the couple. *Trichomonas vaginalis* usually does not affect the infant.

Listeria monocytogenes

Listeria monocytogenes is a rather uncommon gram-positive bacillus that causes a sexually transmitted perinatal infection. It can be transmitted by an asymptomatic carrier and may invade the fetoplacental unit and the newborn. In the United States, the Centers for Disease Control reports that 17% of the cases of listeriosis occur in neonates.[25] The onset of newborn listeriosis may be immediate at birth, with clinical symptoms including respiratory distress, cyanosis, skin lesions, and hypothermia, or may be delayed 1 to 6 weeks following birth and manifested in the form of meningitis. Mortality rates may be above 50% for infected neonates. The organism is easily cultured with routine blood and urine culture techniques.

Pregnant women who clinically manifest a fever of unknown origin should be screened for *Listeria monocytogenes*. Treatment of infected women consists of a combination of ampicillin or penicillin with gentamicin.

Candida albicans

Candida albicans (*Monilia*) is present in the vagina of about 25% of women approaching term. The causative organism is a fungus that uses glycogen for survival. Symptoms of the disease include intense burning and itching. A thick, white vaginal discharge, resembling cottage cheese, may be present. The vaginal walls are often covered with white patches. In some women the symptoms are absent and the condition is asymptomatic, requiring no treatment.

When therapy for *Candida albicans* is indicated, a vaginal cream or tablet of miconazole (Monistat), chlordantoin (Sporostacin), or nystatin (Mycostatin) may be inserted twice daily for 7 to 10 days. A single tablet of clotrimazole (Gyne-Lotrimin) may be inserted at bedtime for 7 days.

Candidiasis may be transmitted to the newborn through the birth canal, leading to an oral infection known as *thrush* (see Chap. 46).

Acquired Immune Deficiency Syndrome

AIDS, a recently recognized major health problem primarily among homosexual men, also poses a serious threat to women. Several cases of AIDS have been reported among infants of women with diagnosed AIDS or epidemiologic risk factors for its development, suggesting *in utero* or perinatal transmission.[26] The finding of multiple affected siblings with different fathers suggests that the mother is the main determinant of the AIDS infection of her offspring and that she may remain continuously infected herself.[27,28] Certain precautions

are encouraged to prevent and limit the transmission of AIDS, including management of single-partner lifestyles and sexual discretion.

Nursing Process Applied to Pregnant Women with (at Risk for) STDs

Assessment. At the time of the first prenatal visit all pregnant women should be screened for evidence of STD. Risk factors often include unmarried status, multiple sex partners, age under 20 years, past history of STD, lack of prenatal care, and a sexual partner with STD. Serologic testing for syphilis is performed on *all* pregnant women, using either the VDRL test or the rapid plasma reagin (RPR) test. For most of the other STDs, diagnosis may be verified by a positive culture or blood test. Testing may not be routinely ordered unless a particular STD is suspected. Women with negative VDRL or gonorrhea results are often reassessed in the eighth or ninth month of pregnancy if risk factors continue to exist. It is also common for women with a history of herpes type II to receive periodic culturing during pregnancy.

A physical examination is also performed during the initial evaluation. The labia, vulva, perineum, and rectal areas are carefully observed for lesions or other skin eruptions. Vaginal discharge is assessed for color, odor, and quantity. Internal vaginal examination is necessary for inspection of the cervix and collection of a cervical smear. The client should be questioned about the presence of painful urination or systemic symptoms (fever, chills, headache, malaise) urinary incontinence, and pain or itching of the vulva.

Nursing Diagnosis. The nursing diagnoses include knowledge deficit related to STD and risks; risk of increased perinatal morbidity related to STD and its complications; anxiety and disturbance in self-concept related to acquisition of STD; and alteration in comfort related to the inflammatory process.

Nursing Intervention. Client education is an essential component of nursing intervention for pregnant women with a potential or actual STD. The exact information given will depend upon the nature of the STD. Basic components of any educational program include signs and symptoms of infection, incubation period, transmission and methods for prevention, treatment and basic comfort measures, follow-up appraisal, perinatal implications—method of delivery, and neonatal concerns.

Several teaching sessions are needed to review and reinforce the extensive information presented. Opportunities should be provided for expressing emotions and anxieties and for questioning. If possible the client's

(text continued on page 803)

The Pregnant Woman with a Sexually Transmitted Disease

Nursing Objectives

1. Identify early the woman with STD during pregnancy.
2. Provide appropriate prenatal care and treatment of the woman with an STD.
3. Implement a comprehensive client education program on the STD (*e.g.*, epidemiology, perinatal considerations, treatment).
4. Accept the woman's psychosocial response(s) to the STD.
5. Prevent complications of the STD during pregnancy.

Assessment	Potential Nursing Diagnosis	Planning/Intervention	Evaluation

Risk factors
  Unmarried
  Adolescent
  No prenatal care
  Previous STD
  Multiple sex partners
History
  Known or suspicious lesion during pregnancy
  Sexual partner with a known or suspected past STD
  Urinary retention
Physical examination
  Lesions on cervix, vulva, rectum
  Edema of perineal area
  Inguinal adenopathy
  Discharge (odor, color, amount)
  Vital signs
Laboratory studies
  Blood for VDRL, RPR (syphilis) on first prenatal visit and repeat as necessary
  Vaginal smear for gonorrhea and repeat as necessary
  Other tissue cultures as necessary
  Pap smear
Reculture for STD on a frequent basis
Educational needs: knowledge of STD
	Knowledge deficit related to STD and risks	Appropriately screen for STD (routine cultures for syphilis and gonorrhea)
		
		Question pregnant woman about her past history of STD or infected sexual partner
		
		Refer sexual partner for treatment as indicated by diagnosis
		
		Provide basic client education about STD
		  Characteristics and epidemiologic considerations
		  Signs and symptoms
		  Incubation period
		  Transmission
		  Treatment
		  Basic comfort measures
		Explain importance of regular follow-up (*e.g.*, cultures for herpes, VDRL, Pap smears)
			Woman submits positive (negative) culture for STD
			
			Woman freely discusses sexual history and past STD
			
			Sexual partner seeks treatment for STD
			
			Woman discusses basic facts about STD and treatments
			
			Woman returns for follow-up as recommended

Fetal well-being evaluated as necessary Fetal heart tones	Risk of increased perinatal morbidity related to STD and its complications	Provide instructions on perinatal risk factors and fetal effects	Woman freely discusses perinatal risk factors and fetal effects

(continued)

Assessment	Potential Nursing Diagnosis	Planning/Intervention	Evaluation
Sonography Nonstress tests Fetal movement		Explain appropriate therapy	
		Administer medications as prescribed (*e.g.*, penicillin for syphilis; topical ointments for lesions)	Woman receives prescribed medications
		Employ appropriate skin isolation techniques when caring for client with active disease (*e.g.*, herpes type II)	
		Gown and glove	
		Double-bag linen	
		Promote comfort of infected sites by	Woman states she has only minimal discomfort
		Keeping lesions clean and dry	
		Sitz baths 2–3 times per day	
		Exposure to heat lamp	
		Instruct mother on techniques of hand washing and personal hygiene	Woman performs a repeat demonstration of hygiene techniques
		Monitor fetal well-being	
		Fetal heart tones, nonstress testing	
		Ultrasonography	
		Prepare for cesarean section, if indicated	
Expressions of fear, guilt, shame Verbalizations about sexual partner's role in transmission Expectations of how disease will impact on lifestyle	Anxiety and disturbance in self-concept related to acquisition of the STD	Allow opportunities to express fear that disease has been transmitted to sexual partner	Woman expresses fear, anger, or other emotions concerning the disease and possible transmission
		or	
		Allow opportunities to express anger that sexual partner may have been transmission source of disease	
		Demonstrate acceptance of emotions displayed regarding body image, self-concept, guilt about impact of disease upon fetus	Woman shows ease and confidence in expressing her emotions to nurse
		Invite client's sexual partner to attend counseling session (if agreeable to client)	Woman's sexual partner attends counseling sessions
		Counsel regarding sexual modification in life-style necessitated by disease (*e.g.*, abstinence during acute episodes)	Woman clarifies questions she has concerning her lifestyle

(text continued from page 800)

sexual partner should be invited to attend the teaching sessions so that his questions may be presented and answered by the nurse. In responding to the emotional responses of the client and her sexual partner, it is essential that the nurse demonstrate a nonjudgmental and accepting attitude, as well as an empathetic manner.

Modifications in sexual behavior and alternative methods of expressing sexuality need to be discussed with the pregnant woman and her partner. The nature of information presented will vary with the specific STD. Abstinence is recommended during periods when the active disease may be transmitted (both primary and recurrent infections). Sexual activity should not be resumed until a negative culture or blood test is obtained *or* symptoms have resolved for a minimum of 7 to 10 days (herpes).

To relieve any local discomfort, the client with STD may be advised to take sitz baths two to three times per day, expose the infected area to a heat lamp, or apply wet compresses. It is essential that all lesions be kept clean and dry and good personal hygiene be maintained. Douching should be avoided for most diseases. Topical antibiotics or steroid creams are applied as prescribed by the physician. Intramuscular antibiotics such as penicillin are administered for selected STDs.

Substance Abuse During Pregnancy

The effects of substance abuse on fetal growth and development have been a focus of increasing scientific inquiry. The results of a variety of clinical studies have demonstrated an association between maternal substance abuse and adverse perinatal outcome. The use of common household substances, such as alcohol, caffeine, and nicotine, has been correlated with higher rates of abortion, premature birth, and stillbirth. A full discussion of the influence of these substances on perinatal outcome is provided in Chapters 8 and 22.

"With rare exception, any drug that exerts a systemic effect in the mother will cross the placenta to reach the embryo and fetus."[7] The effects on the fetus cannot be accurately determined by observing maternal behavior; they are related to the chemical constituents of the drug, the dosage administered, and the interaction of the drug with other substances. It should be noted that most drug abusers take more than one drug during pregnancy and generally do not seek prenatal care until late in pregnancy or during the intrapartum period.

The use of hard drugs such as heroin during pregnancy produces direct maternal–fetal effects, as well as increases the risk of coincidental infections. Malnutrition, a frequent condition accompanying drug addiction,

increases the pregnant woman's susceptibility to anemia and infections such as hepatitis, STD, UTI, and vaginitis. Acute maternal withdrawal may result in premature labor secondary to uterine hyperirritability. Accompanying violent fetal movements often occur owing to fetal withdrawal.

Marijuana

Marijuana is perhaps the most frequently abused illegal drug of women during the childbearing years. It is estimated that about 43 million Americans have used marijuana and about 16 million are currently using it.[29] Use of this substance is especially high for adolescents and young adults. Marijuana consists of a complex of about 400 chemical substances contained in *cannabis sativa;* its major psychoactive component is tetrahydrocannabinol (THC).

Since it is unethical and illegal to administer marijuana for research purposes to childbearing women, much of the information obtained on marijuana effects is based upon animal research. Depressed testosterone levels, decreased follicle-stimulating hormone and luteinizing hormone, inhibited ovulation, menstrual cycle disruptions, and decreased sperm concentrations are among the reported actions of marijuana on the reproductive system. In mice, THC increases the incidence of intrauterine deaths and reduces fetal birth weight. Teratogenic effects do not appear to be of major significance in humans; however, effects on placental function and fetal endocrine physiology may be potentially harmful. In a prospective study examining women who reported use of marijuana before or during pregnancy, or both, babies born to heavy users showed significantly more symptoms associated with nervous system abnormalities, interpreted as suggesting immaturity.[30] Other studies have found similar behavioral alterations in the offspring of marijuana users.

In addition, laboratory analysis of maternal and neonatal blood indicates that THC is transferred to the newborn and may lead to depressed activity. Based upon these clinical findings, the Surgeon General has warned that use of marijuana during pregnancy may harm the infant's health.

Heroin

The pharmacologic actions of heroin are largely attributable to morphine, which produces major effects on the central nervous system and bowels. Heroin crosses the placenta rapidly, and fetal blood levels are in proportion to those of the mother. Abuse of heroin during pregnancy increases the risks for delivery of a low-birthweight infant, prematurity, late-pregnancy bleeding, pregnancy-induced hypertension, and malpresentation.

Approximately one half of the infants born to heroin addicts will develop withdrawal symptoms, usually within 24 to 48 hours of birth. The longer the maternal addiction, the larger her habit, and the closer to delivery the last dose, the higher is the probability of neonatal withdrawal symptoms. Management of the heroin-addicted newborn is further discussed in Chapter 46.

Methadone

Methadone is often used as a substitute drug in treatment programs for pregnant addicts. The effects of this drug are believed to be less harmful to the fetus/newborn than heroin. Withdrawal symptoms commonly manifest about 1 week following birth in infants of methadone-maintained mothers.

The incidence of complications of pregnancy is less in methadone-addicted women than in heroin addicts, probably due to their more frequent involvement in prenatal care.

Phencyclidine

Phencyclidine (PCP, angel dust) is an increasingly popular synthetic street drug with effects that sometimes mimic uppers and other times mimic downers. Individuals taking PCP experience distortions in reality. The gross psychological changes that occur as a consequence of PCP abuse have been attributed to decreased ability to process stimuli from the environment. The possible teratogenic effects of PCP have been described in several case studies of infants born to PCP abusers. Reportedly, the affected infants had congenital dysmorphic facial features, poor head control, nystagmus, central nervous system irritability, and coarse flapping movements of the extremities.[31] Numerous animal studies clearly demonstrate that PCP readily crosses the placenta and influences postnatal behavior.

Diagnosis of PCP use is made through toxicologic screening of maternal and newborn urine. There are six signs that are useful in identifying the suspected PCP user: unusual, bizarre, or inappropriate behavior; combined vertical and horizontal nystagmus; incoordinated gait or gait ataxia; a blank stare; muscle rigidity, and blood pressure elevation.[32]

Other Drugs

Nonnarcotic substances known to cause addiction with resulting maternal and newborn withdrawal include *stimulants* (uppers or speed), such as amphetamines, which cause a feeling of "high" or increased produc-

tivity, and *depressants* (downers), such as barbiturates, tranquilizers, and alcohol, which create feelings of calmness and passivity. The symptoms of abstinence from these drugs are similar to those of narcotic withdrawal and affect the central nervous system, gastrointestinal system, and sleep patterns.

Cocaine and lysergic acid diethylamide (*LSD*) may have potent effects on neurotransmission; any use during late pregnancy is likely to be associated with behavioral and functional disabilities in the newborn. Fetotoxicity is believed to be mediated by biotransformation.[33] LSD is suspected of causing chromosomal breakage with resulting congenital malformations. Results of recent studies suggest a strong association between cocaine abuse during pregnancy and later learning disabilities in offspring.

Nursing Process Applied to the Substance Abuser

Nursing Assessment

Efforts toward managing drug-addicted pregnant women should ideally begin with prevention and early identification of abusers. Nurses employed in hospital and community settings play a key role in recognizing the signs and symptoms of substance abuse. As educators, nurses should caution all women in the childbearing age-group about the potential dangers that substance abuse places on reproductive capacity and maternal–child health. Detailed drug histories including use of household, prescribed, and illegal substances should be obtained at the time of the first prenatal visit. Specific information should be collected about the woman's drug habit, including names of drugs used, dosage, frequency of use, and time of last administration.

Prenatal care is of prime importance for improving perinatal outcome of substance abusers. Nutritional assessment and counseling should be provided on an ongoing basis, since many addicts have inadequate dietary intake to maintain maternal and fetal health. A comprehensive assessment of the client is performed with special attention to skin lesions and infections, central nervous system disturbances, and evidence of STD. Gestational age is carefully determined by a variety of methods, since menstrual history is often unreliable.

Nursing Diagnosis

Assessment of the client for signs and symptoms of substance abuse during pregnancy may lead the nurse to some of the following nursing diagnoses: alteration in nutrition: less than body requirements secondary to loss of appetite; potential for self-injury related to impaired mental processes associated with drug abuse; ineffective individual coping: dependence or denial related to inability to effectively manage life stressors without drugs/alcohol; alteration in family and other social relations; potential for neonatal withdrawal/addiction secondary to maternal substance abuse.

Nursing Intervention

The professional services of an expert interdisciplinary health team are critically important for helping the pregnant addict reduce the stresses that often have contributed to her addiction. It is sometimes necessary to initiate a referral program for withdrawal or reduction of the addict's maintenance dose to the lowest level possible. Financial assistance, adequate housing, and psychological support are often essential elements for the woman to continue treatment and prenatal care. It is also particularly desirable to involve other members of the client's family in her rehabilitation program.

Perhaps the most significant key to success in providing nursing care to pregnant substance abusers is establishing a positive and trusting nurse–client relationship. Many addicts are distrustful of professionals and fear legal actions against themselves. The nurse should explain that information will be kept confidential and used to plan appropriate intervention. The importance of full disclosure of drug habits in relation to predicting the onset of withdrawal symptoms in the fetus/newborn should be stressed. The nurse should also consider the possibility of multiple-drug use and the serious problems it poses as she counsels the addicted pregnant woman or new mother.

References

1. Brown ZA: Diabetes in pregnancy. FCH/Perinatal Health Promotion 1:43–46, 1978
2. O'Sullivan JB, Mahan CM: Criteria for the oral glucose tolerance test in pregnancy. Diabetes 13:278–285, 1964
3. Hollander P, Maeder EC: Diabetes in pregnancy, no longer a barrier to successful outcome. Postgrad Med 77:132–146, 1985
4. Leveno KJ, Whalley EJ: Dilemmas in the management of pregnancy complicated by diabetes, in symposium on diabetes mellitus. Med Clin North Am 66:1325–1341, 1982
5. National Diabetes Data Group: Classification of diabetes mellitus and other categories of glucose intolerance. Diabetes 28:1039, 1979
6. White P: Classification of obstetric diabetes. Am J Obstet Gynecol 130:229, 1978
7. Pritchard JA, MacDonald PC, Gant NF: Williams' Obstetrics, 17th ed. Norwalk, CT, Appleton-Century-Crofts, 1985
8. Good-Anderson B: Home blood glucose monitoring in the pregnant diabetic. JOGNN 12:89–92, 1983
9. Ueland K: Pregnancy and cardiovascular disease. Med Clin North Am 61:17–41, 1977
10. de Sweit M: Pregnancy and heart valve replacement. Int J Cardiol 5:741–743, 1984
11. Chyun DA: Pregnancy and cardiac valvular prostheses. JOGNN 14:38–44, 1985
12. Burwell CS, Metcalfe J: Heart Disease and Pregnancy. Boston, Little, Brown & Co, 1958
13. Shaul WL, Hall JG: Multiple congenital abnormalities associated with oral anticoagulants. Am J Obstet Gynecol 127:191–198, 1977
14. Carson M, Reed M: Warfarin and fetal abnormality. Lancet 1:1127, 1976
15. Sherman S, Hall BD: Warfarin and fetal abnormality. Lancet 1:692, 1976
16. Kneut C: Sickle-cell anemia. Issue Compr Pediatr Nurse 4:19–27, 1980
17. Ship-Horowitz T: Nursing care of the sickle cell anemic patient in labor. JOGN Nurs 12:381–386, 1983
18. Anionwu E: Sickle cell disease. Health Visitor 55:336–341, 1982
19. Richardson EA, Milne RS: Sickle cell disease and the childbearing family: An update. MCN 8:417–422, 1983
20. De Nichola LK, Hanshaw JB: Congenital and neonatal varicella. J Pediatr 94:175, 1979
21. Davis JM, Goldenring J, McChesney M et al: Pregnancy outcomes of Indochinese refugees, Santa Clara County, California. Am J Public Health 72:742–744, 1982
22. Kanai K et al: Prevention of perinatal transmission of hepatitis B virus to children of e antigen-positive HBV carrier mothers by hepatitis B immune globulin and HBV vaccine. J Infect Dis 151:287–290, 1985
23. Handsfield HH, Lukehart SA: Editorial: Prevention of congenital syphilis. JAMA 252:1750–1751, 1984
24. Olds SB, London ML, Ladwig PA: Maternal-Newborn Nursing: A Family-centered Approach, 2nd ed. Menlo Park, CA, Addison-Wesley Publishing, 1984
25. Osborne NG, Pratson L: Sexually transmitted diseases and pregnancy. JOGNN 13:9–12, 1984
26. Rubinstein A et al: Acquired immunodeficiency with reversed T4/T8 ratios in infants born to promiscuous and drug-addicted mothers. JAMA 249:2350–2356, 1983
27. Wykoff RF et al: Immunologic dysfunction in infants infected through transfusion with HTLV-III. N Engl J Med 312:294–296, 1985
28. Scott GB et al: Mothers of infants with acquired immunodeficiency syndrome. JAMA 252:363–366, 1985
29. Asch RH, Smith CG: Effects of marijuana on reproduction. Contemp OB/GYN 22:217–225, 1983
30. Fried PA, Watkinson B, Gant A et al: Changing patterns of soft drug use prior to and during pregnancy: A prospective study. Drug Alcohol Depend 6:323, 1980
31. Nicholas JM, Lipshitz J, Schreiber EC: Phencyclidine: Its transfer across the placenta as well as into breast milk. Am J Obstet Gynecol 143:143–146, 1982

32. Linder RL, Lerner SE, Burns RS: PCP: The Devil's Dust. Belmont, CA, Wadsworth, 1980
33. Butnarescu GF, Tillotson DM, Villarreal PP: Perinatal Nursing. New York, John Wiley & Sons, 1980

Suggested Reading

Chyun DA: Pregnancy and cardiac valvular prostheses. JOGNN 14:38–44, 1985

Higgins SD, Gavite TJ: Late abruptio placentae in trauma patients: Implications for monitoring. Obstet Gynecol 63 (Suppl 3):10, 1984

Mocarski V: Asymptomatic bacteria: A silent problem of pregnant women. MCN 5:238–241, July/August 1980

Perley NZ, Bills BJ: Herpes genitalis and the childbearing cycle. MCN 8:213–217, 1983

Quilligan EJ, Kretchmer N: Fetal and Maternal Medicine. New York, John Wiley & Sons, 1980

Richardson EAW, Milne LS: Sickle-cell disease and the childbearing family: An update. MCN 8:417–422, 1983

Schuler K: When a pregnant woman is diabetic: Antepartal care. Am J Nurs 79:448–450, 1979

Tilden VP: The relation of life stress and social support to emotional disequilibrium during pregnancy. Res Nurs Health 6:167–174, 1983

Ueland K: Cardiovascular diseases complicating pregnancy. Clin Obstet Gynecol 21:429, 1978

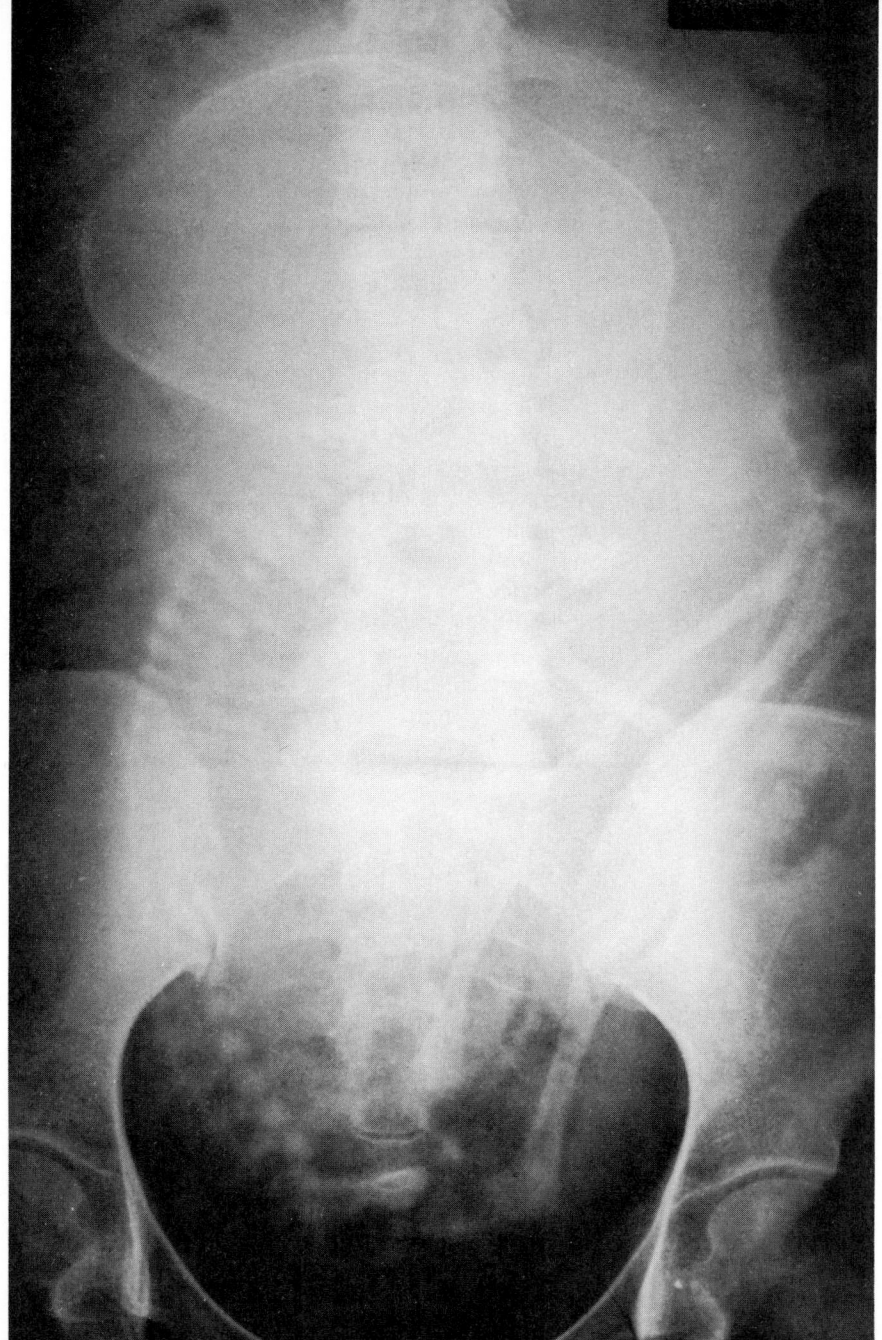

CHAPTER 38

Complications of Labor

A complicated labor requires sensitive and astute nursing care, for it represents a period of great stress for the laboring woman, her partner, nurses, and physicians. The principles of nursing care during normal labor (see Chap. 25) also apply when the labor is complicated, with certain modifications depending upon the nature of the problems. The nurse's ability to use clinical judgment is crucial, as the nursing diagnoses and care deriving from such judgments may be of lifesaving significance for both the mother and the infant. Assessment skills including observation, interviewing, and physical examination provide important data on the nature and extent of the problem. Reporting, recording, and professional intercommunication promote accurate decision making and implementation of appropriate treatment. Physical and emotional supportive measures assist the mother and father to understand and cope with the unusual events in the labor experience, which is often prolonged and painful.

Dystocia

Dystocia, or difficult labor, is a term usually used to refer to a labor that is made longer or more painful by problems with the mechanics of the labor, involving the "3 P's," the powers, passageway, and passenger, (which were discussed in Chapters 23 and 24). A fourth "P," the person or psyche, is often added to the list because certain aspects of maternal response to labor can also affect the length of labor. These problems in mechanics of labor may include any or a combination of the following:

Powers. The uterine contractions may not be sufficiently strong or appropriately coordinated during the first stage of labor to effect cervical dilatation and effacement, or during the second stage, voluntary pushing combined with uterine contractions may not be sufficient to effect descent and expulsion of the fetus.

Passageway. There may be variations in the size and shape of the bony pelvis or other abnormalities of the reproductive tract that interfere with engagement, descent, or expulsion of the fetus.

Passenger. There may be faulty presentation or position, unusual size, or abnormal development of the fetus that prevents entrance into or passage through the birth canal.

Psyche. Maternal factors such as anxiety, lack of preparation, and fear can interact with the other factors, or sometimes operate alone, to cause prolongation of the labor.

Therefore, for progress in labor to be made, and the birth to occur, the forces or *powers,* including uterine contractions and maternal "bearing down" in second stage, must be coordinated and of adequate strength to propel an irregular object, the fetus, or *passenger*, through the birth canal, or *passageway*. The passenger must be of appropriate size and shape and able to undergo the necessary maneuvers to pass through the different dimensions of the birth canal. The passageway must also be of normal size and configuration and not present undue obstacles to the descent, rotation, and expulsion of the baby.

Problems with the Powers— Uterine Dysfunction

Classification and Research

Many attempts have been made to classify labors that do not follow the usual pattern, so that the problems may be more easily identified and managed. One method is classification according to the *quality* of uterine contractions. Ineffectual contractions can be described as hypotonic, hypertonic, or incoordinate.[1] A second classification is by *time of onset*. Primary inertia (dysfunction) occurs at the beginning of labor. Secondary inertia develops after labor is established.

Dysfunctional labor may also be classified by the *pattern and timing* of the disruption of progress. Friedman has plotted cervical dilatation and degree of descent against lapsed time on a graph, demonstrating the normal labor pattern as an S-shaped curve (see Fig. 24-1). Categories of delayed progression according to Friedman are prolonged latent phase, protraction disorders, and arrest disorders (Fig. 38-1).[2]

There is some overlapping between these classifications. Hypertonic uterine dysfunction, primary inertia, and prolonged latent phase all occur in early labor and are most common in the nullipara. Hypotonic uterine dysfunction, secondary inertia, and protraction or arrest of the active phase all occur later in labor and tend to be more common in the multipara.

A number of researchers have contributed to the understanding and measurement of uterine contractions. Larks described the stimulus of a contraction as starting in one cornu and developing several milliseconds later in the other cornu, then joining and descending down over the fundus and upper uterine segment, resulting in a pulling up of the isthmus and cervix.[3] Caldeyro-Barcia and associates in Montevideo determined that the pressure of a contraction necessary to dilate the cervix is at least 15 mm Hg. Measurement of contractions in terms of Montevideo units, the average intensity of the uterine contractions multiplied by the number of contractions in a 10-minute period, also comes from the work of this group.[1] In normal labor the intensity or amplitude of the contractions is usually

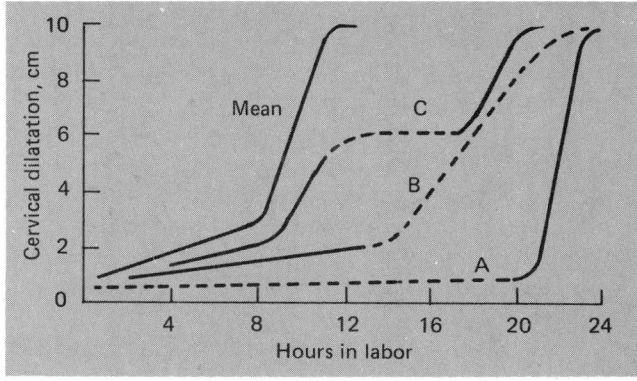

FIGURE 38-1

The major labor aberrations shown in comparison with the mean cervical dilatation time curve for nulliparas. A = prolonged latent phase, B = protracted active phase dilation, and C = secondary arrest of dilation. (Friedman E: Greenhill Obstetrics, 13th ed. Philadelphia, WB Saunders)

between 30 and 50 mm Hg and the frequency is usually two to five contractions in 10 minutes.[4]

Friedman's division of the first *stage* of labor into two *phases*, the latent phase and the active phase, and his use of curves to plot both dilatation and descent have been found to be very useful in detecting and estimating the severity of dysfunctional labor.[5] There are those who feel, however, that the latent phase is the end of several weeks of "prelabor," which is a preparatory period for labor.

As defined by Friedman, the *latent phase* is a period of effacement and beginning dilatation of the cervix, lasting an average of 8½ hours in a nullipara and a somewhat shorter time in the multipara. During this phase, 3 to 4 cm of dilation is accomplished. The *active phase*, or clinically apparent labor, is briefer and consists of an acceleration phase, a phase of maximum slope, and a deceleration phase before full dilatation is accomplished. This phase of labor lasts approximately 3½ to 4 hours in the primigravid patient.

Friedman classifies dysfunction by the length of the phases of labor rather than by the quality of the contractions. However, his prolonged latent phase occurs during the onset and first phase of labor and hence can be associated with hypertonic dysfunction. By definition, the latent phase is prolonged if it lasts longer than 20 hours in the primigravida or 14 hours in the multigravida. In practice, however, the diagnosis should be suspected and treatment instituted many hours before these time intervals have elapsed.[1]

Friedman describes two types of dysfunction that can occur during the active phase of the first stage of labor: protraction disorders and arrest disorders.[2] Protraction disorders are characterized by a slower than normal rate of cervical dilation and by delayed descent of the fetal head in the active phase of labor. The expected rate of cervical dilation is 1.2 cm or more per hour for nulliparas and 1.5 cm or more for multiparas. The rate of descent for the fetal head should be approximately 1.0 cm/hr for nulliparas and 2.0 cm/hr for multiparas.[6] Although a slowing of progress can be an indication of cephalopelvic disproportion, especially in a nullipara, most of the patients with protraction disorders, given supportive fluids, reassurance, and minimum sedation, go on to dilate fully, although more slowly than usual.[7]

Arrest disorders are diagnosed when cervical dilation or descent of the fetal head has ceased for more than 2 hours in the active phase of labor. These disorders may follow protraction disorders, or a normally progressing labor may suddenly stop. Arrest disorders are frequently associated with cephalopelvic disproportion.[6]

Hendricks and associates have described slightly different curves for normal labor (Fig. 38-2).[8] They found in normal active labor that there is a rather constant active acceleration phase without the deceleration described by Friedman. Also, although it is often assumed that the nullipara will progress more slowly than the multipara, these investigators found that cervical dilation progressed at about the same rate in both after 4-cm dilation was reached.[8] Despite variations in the description of normal labor, any significant prolongation of any of the phases described by Friedman or any significant variation from the curves presented by Hendricks and associates constitutes uterine dysfunction.[1,2,8]

When there is failure to progress in early labor despite the presence of uterine contractions, one of the first factors to consider is whether or not the patient is actually in labor. It is not unusual for a woman in late pregnancy to experience Braxton Hicks contractions that are so strong and regular that they can easily be mistaken for true labor. Progressive cervical changes must take place to signify true labor, since true labor contractions do accomplish at least some cervical effacement

and dilatation. Appearance of bloody show assists in the diagnosis of labor, particularly when it accompanies cervical changes. Without signs of progress to confirm labor, uncomfortable uterine contractions signify false labor. For the diagnosis of dystocia, cervical changes must have occurred and progressed, only to have the progression slowed or halted at some point.

Etiologic Factors

The chief factors associated with uterine dysfunction are injudicious use of analgesia (*i.e.,* excessive or too early administration of the drugs), minor degrees of pelvic contraction, and fetal malposition of even a small degree, such as a slight extension of the head as seen in some occiput posterior positions. Postmaturity and large infants have also been found to be significantly related to dysfunctional labor. These conditions may occur singly or in combination in cases of dysfunction.

Other factors that are associated with this condition include overdistention of the uterus, grand multiparity, excessive cervical rigidity, and maternal age. Although the latter group of factors has been shown to play some etiologic role, this is less important than was once believed. In over 50% of the cases, the cause is unknown. Considering the possible role of corticosteroids in the initiation of labor, and their relation to stress states, the effects of emotional factors in dystocia cannot be overlooked when no other cause is apparent. More research at the cellular level will have to be done to obtain increased definitive knowledge concerning the etiologic factors in this condition.

Complications

Uterine dysfunction can result in complications for both mother and fetus. Fetal injury and death are the most serious potential outcomes. For the mother, exhaustion and dehydration may occur if labor is allowed to become

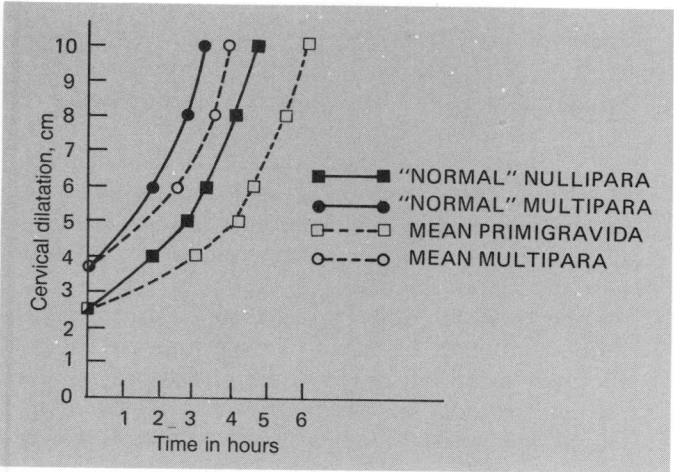

F I G U R E   3 8 - 2

Cervical dilatation in normal nulliparous and multiparous women after the onset of true labor. (Hendricks, Brenner, Kraus: The normal cervical dilatation patterns in late pregnancy and labor. Am J Obstet Gynecol 106:1065, 1970)

too prolonged. Intrauterine infection is a common maternal complication, especially if the membranes are ruptured, even if the mother is placed on antibiotics.

Fortunately, there have been several significant advances in the treatment of uterine dysfunction in the past few decades. First, there is a better understanding of the role of prolonged labor as a contributor to perinatal mortality and morbidity. Second, the judicious use of dilute intravenous oxytocin has been found to facilitate the progress of some types of dysfunctional labor. Third, cesarean deliveries are used more frequently in place of difficult high forceps or midforceps procedures when oxytocin fails or is inappropriate for use.[1]

Hypotonic Dysfunction

When the uterine contractions decrease in strength and uterine tone is less than usual after the onset of true labor the patient is considered to have hypotonic dysfunction. Minimum uterine tension during the resting stage is about 8 mm Hg to 12 mm Hg in the normally functioning uterus, while normal labor contractions reach an intrauterine pressure of 50 mm Hg to 60 mm Hg at the acme. These values are reduced in hypotonic dysfunction, and contractions are not strong enough to dilate the cervix. Contractions may also become farther apart and irregular (Fig. 38-3). This condition usually occurs in the acceleration or active phase, but contractions may become hypotonic during the second stage of labor also (Table 38-1).

Management. Possible courses of action for the management of hypotonic uterine dysfunction include simple corrective measures, amniotomy or oxytocin administration, and cesarean delivery. The decision is usually made on the basis of the general condition of the mother and fetus and on the presence or absence of mechanical obstruction. If the mother is becoming fatigued or dehydrated, rest and fluids may be tried first. If a marked degree of disproportion is found to exist or there is an uncorrectable malposition or marked fetal distress, a cesarean section is employed to effect delivery. If these conditions are not present, stimulation of labor is generally the treatment of choice, rather than "watchful waiting" for more effective labor to resume spontaneously.

If membranes are intact and the head is engaged, initial treatment may be to rupture the membranes artificially (amniotomy). (See Chapter 39 for further discussion.) This procedure alone may stimulate effective contractions, but it must be used judiciously, since it is a commitment to deliver the baby within a reasonable time.[5] Augmentation of labor by the use of intravenous oxytocin is usually the treatment of choice when strong, regular contractions with progressive effacement and dilation, or fetal descent, fail to occur or when membranes are already ruptured.

Oxytocin Stimulation.
Oxytocin acts on the myometrium, causing it to contract. Natural oxytocin is produced in the body by the hypothalamus and stored in the posterior pituitary gland. Maternal levels of oxytocin increase as gestation progresses, although the exact role of this increase in human labor is not known. Animal extracts of oxytocin were once used to stimulate uterine contractions. Synthetic oxytocin is as effective as the natural substance, is chemically pure, and eliminates the danger of reaction to animal protein. Therefore,

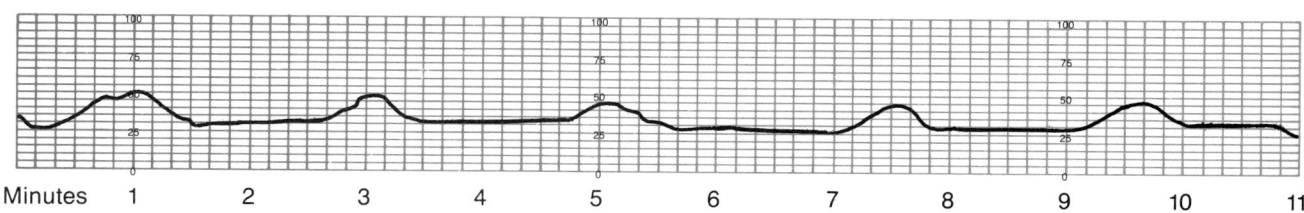

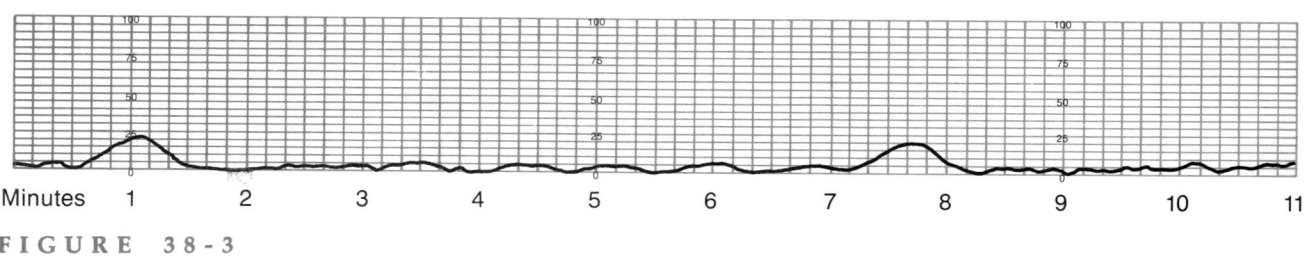

FIGURE 38-3

Hypotonic bottom and hypertonic top uterine motility.

synthetic oxytocin is the product used in modern ob-stetrics.[4] In relation to stimulation of labor, oxytocin may be used to initiate (induce) labor contractions or to augment contractions that are weak and ineffective, as in cases of hypotonic dysfunction. The role of oxytocin in the postpartum period, to contract the uterus and control bleeding, is discussed in Chapter 25.

Contraindications to Use of Oxytocin. The fol-lowing are usually considered to be contraindications to the use of oxytocin for either augmentation or in-duction:[1,4]

- Any obstruction that would interfere with descent of the fetus, such as cephalopelvic disproportion or anomaly of the birth canal
- Conditions that would increase the danger of uterine rupture, such as high parity (greater than four), previous uterine incision (cesarean section or extensive myomectomy), or overdistention of the uterus (twins, polyhydramnios)
- Hypertonic or incoordinate uterus, because oxyto-cin makes the condition worse and may lead to formation of a constriction ring
- Fetal distress, because the change in the contrac-tions brought about by the oxytocin may add to the distress
- Placenta previa

Method of Oxytocin Administration. The amount and rate of oxytocin administration must be carefully controlled, and this can be done effectively only by use of the intravenous route. Optimally, an infusion pump is used to administer the intravenous oxytocin, to help provide a consistent and precise rate. Types of solution, amount of oxytocin added, and rate of infusion vary according to agency protocols or physician preference (see Nursing Guidelines for Oxytocin (Pitocin) Induction and Augmentation, pages 814–815). The usual choice of solution is 5% dextrose in water, normal saline, or lactated Ringer's solution; 10 units (10,000 mU) of oxy-tocin is added to 1000 ml of solution and started at a rate of 0.5 mU to 2 mU/min.

A piggyback system, using two bottles of the same solution, one containing oxytocin and the other without, is recommended because this makes it possible to dis-continue the oxytocin if necessary and still keep the intravenous line open. Contractions and fetal heart rate are carefully evaluated, and if no problems develop, the infusion is gradually increased. The usual maximum is 20 mU/min, but levels above 10 mU/min are seldom needed for augmentation of labor and levels of 30 mU to 40 mU/min may be needed for some inductions.[1] Ideally the contractions stimulated by the oxytocin will mimic natural labor as closely as possible, with uterine contractions of moderate to strong intensity occurring every 2 to 3 minutes, lasting no more than 45 to 60 seconds, and with at least a 30-second rest between

contractions. Signs of fetal distress must be carefully watched for and the infusion slowed or stopped if any signs are detected. Use of external or internal electronic monitors is mandatory when oxytocin stimulation of labor is employed. Internal monitoring of uterine activity has the advantage of providing a more accurate picture of the intensity of the contractions than external mon-itoring.

Extreme caution is necessary, especially at the be-ginning of the oxytocin infusion, because of the unpre-dictability of individual response. Sensitivity of the in-dividual client should be carefully assessed by beginning with very small amounts. Sensitivity to oxytocin varies widely from client to client and from time to time in the same client depending on a variety of influencing factors. Increased sensitivity is associated with ruptured membranes, term gestation, high parity, favorable cervix (soft, effacing, dilating, and anterior), and irritable uterus.[9]

Dangers of Oxytocin Use. When oxytocin is ad-ministered to the pregnant woman it is potentially dan-gerous to both mother and fetus. These dangers can be minimized by careful monitoring of the administration of the drug, the character of the contractions, and the condition of the fetus. When the contractions increase in frequency, strength, and length above normal levels, the fetal and placental circulation may be impaired and fetal distress may result. Another potential danger to the fetus is possible birth injuries from being propelled too rapidly through the birth canal or being forced through a pelvis that is too small for it. Tetanic and tumultuous contractions can result in abruptio placentae or rupture of the uterus, resulting in adverse effects on both mother and fetus. Cervical lacerations from too rapid passage of the fetus through the pelvis and am-niotic fluid embolism are additional dangers for the mother when this type of contraction occurs.[4,10]

Side-Effects. Oxytocin infusion may also have some maternal side-effects. Hypertension may develop, with frontal headache. Both of these effects disappear when the drug is discontinued. Oxytocin has antidiuretic properties that can lead to water intoxication when used in large amounts. The prevalence of this problem can be decreased by using an electrolyte solution for the infusion rather than dextrose in water and by avoiding infusion of a large volume of fluid.[10]

Complications of Hypotonic Dysfunction. Un-treated hypotonic uterine dysfunction exposes the mother to the dangers of exhaustion, dehydration, and intrapartum infection. Signs of fetal distress often do not appear until intrapartum infection has developed. While treatment of intrauterine infection with antibiotics offers protection to the mother, it appears to be of little value in protecting the fetus (Table 38-1).

Hypertonic Dysfunction

Hypertonic dysfunction, the least common type of uterine dysfunction, generally occurs at the onset of labor.[1] The gradient of the contraction is distorted either by the midsegment contracting with more force than the fundus or by complete asynchronism of the electrical impulses originating in each cornu. There is an elevation of the resting tone of the uterus, but the contractions are of poor quality (see Fig. 38-3).

Although the contractions in this type of dysfunction are ineffectual in accomplishing dilatation, the increased uterine tone usually results in maternal discomfort. These contractions are often described as "colicky" and extremely painful. The uterus may be tender to palpation, even between contractions (see Table 38-1).

Management. Treatment for this type of dysfunction usually consists of rest and administration of fluids. When medication is indicated to produce the needed rest and relaxation, an injection of 10 mg to 15 mg of morphine may be prescribed because it usually stops the abnormal contractions. A short-acting barbiturate may also be administered to help promote rest. Intravenous fluids are used to maintain hydration and electrolyte balance, and in most instances normal labor resumes when the client awakens. Tocolytic agents such as ritodrine have been used with some stated success, especially in other countries.[1]

Oxytocin is usually contraindicated in treating this type of dysfunction, although there is some disagreement on this point.[5,6] With the uterus in a constant state of increased muscle tone, oxytocin presents the danger of causing an even greater resting tension, which might interfere with fetal oxygenation. Also, it may not correct the uncoordinated action of the two segments, which underlies this problem.

Occasionally the contractions remain uncoordinated and ineffective even after the client has been rested. In these cases cesarean delivery is usually the choice, especially if any signs of fetal distress are evident.[1]

Complications. Fetal distress tends to appear quite early in labor when there is hypertonic dysfunction. The constant increase in uterine tone predisposes to fetal hypoxia. Occasionally prolonged rupture of membranes may accompany this condition and can lead to intrapartum infection.

Assessment in Dysfunctional Labor

Ongoing nursing assessment is an essential component of the care of the client with uterine dysfunction, to aid in detecting the condition, to assist in decisions about the course of treatment, and to monitor maternal and fetal well-being during attempts to promote more ef-

TABLE 38-1

Criteria for Differentiating Dysfunctional Labor

Criteria	Hypertonic	Hypotonic
Phase of labor	Latent	Active
Symptoms	Painful	Painless
Fetal distress	Early	Late
Medication		
Oxytocin	Unfavorable reaction	Favorable reaction
Sedation	Helpful	Little value

(Modified from Pritchard JA, McDonald PC: Williams Obstetrics, 16th ed, p 660. New York, Appleton-Century-Crofts, 1980)

fective contractions. The labor room nurse is often the one to detect the first deviations from the normal labor pattern. Either an internal or an external electronic fetal monitor is helpful to the nurse in assessing the length and frequency of contractions, but the external monitor does not accurately portray the strength of the contraction. It is important for the nurse to be able to evaluate the intensity of labor contractions by palpation, without relying exclusively on the electronic monitor. (See Chap. 25 for evaluation of uterine contractions.) Subjective statements of pain and related behavior, such as crying and moaning, are often not reliable indicators of the strength of contractions and should be evaluated in light of objective data from tactile examination and the electronic monitor, rather than be taken at face value.

Assessing the condition of the fetus is also important. The nurse needs to watch the monitor for changes in the fetal heart rate and baseline variability. She should also be alert for other signs of fetal distress, such as meconium-stained amniotic fluid and increased fetal activity.

Maternal vital signs should be checked frequently. Elevation of maternal temperature and increased pulse rate are clinical signs that may alert the nurse to the onset of secondary complications such as infection. Urine should be checked for acetone. Acetonuria is a sign of exhaustion and dehydration. A record of intake and output is also helpful in assessing hydration.

Nursing Diagnosis

From her assessment the nurse assists with recognizing the medical diagnosis of dysfunctional labor. She will also make a number of potential nursing diagnoses, which could become actual depending on the progress of the situation. Some of the nursing diagnoses might be potential fluid volume deficit related to prolonged labor and restricted fluid intake; potential for infection related to prolonged rupture of membranes; alteration in comfort related to ineffective uterine contractions; and anxiety or fear related to unexpected length of labor.

Nursing Guidelines for Oxytocin (Pitocin) Induction and Augmentation*

Physician Responsibilities

1. The physician evaluates the patient and determines if the client is to be started on intravenous oxytocin.
2. The physician obtains at least a 10-minute baseline monitor strip of uterine contractions and fetal heart rate, using an external system if membranes are intact.
3. The physician writes on the client's order sheet that oxytocin is to be started at 1.0 mU/min or at a level to be determined by the physician and may progress to 10 mU/min by increasing the oxytocin infusion by 1 mU/min every 15 to 20 minutes.
4. The physician evaluates the client when the dosage of oxytocin reaches 10 mU/min. If continuation is needed, the physician writes on the client's order sheet that the oxytocin infusion is to be increased every 15 to 20 minutes until a dose of 20 mU/min is reached. The following dose schedule should be used:

Oxytocin infusion continues at	12 mU/min
	16 mU/min
hold at	20 mU/min

5. The resident physician consults with the Chief Resident when oxytocin infusion has reached 20 mU/min.
6. The physician must be present on the Labor and Delivery Floor while oxytocin is being infused. (At least one physician is present at all times.)
7. The physician frequently observes the client's progress, at least hourly or more often if indicated.

Nursing Responsibilities

1. Prepare the oxytocin solution as follows:
   10 units of oxytocin are added to 500 ml of normal saline. This yields a solution with a concentration of oxytocin of 20 mU/ml to be used with an infusion pump.
2. Take infusion pump to bedside.
3. Assemble infusion pump with oxytocin solution.
4. Set infusion pump to correspond to the oxytocin dosage that was ordered.
5. Start oxytocin infusion (secondary line) by inserting needle into the connector most proximal to the primary line. Be sure to keep primary line running at a slow rate.
6. Turn on oxytocin infusion pump at set rate.
7. Observe contraction pattern and fetal heart rate on the monitor. If no abnormalities are noted in 15 to 20 minutes, increase the oxytocin infusion so that the uterine contractions are observed every 2 to 3 minutes and last approximately 60 seconds.
8. Once a regular contraction pattern is established, hold the oxytocin infusion at that rate or decrease the infusion rate and determine if a regular contraction pattern will still be sustained.
9. If at any time a question arises as to the possibility of hyperstimulation (less than 2 minutes between contractions or contractions lasting longer than 60 seconds) or an abnormal fetal heart rate pattern, the nurse immediately does the following:
   a. Turns off oxytocin infusion.
   b. Turns client on left side.
   c. Starts oxygen by mask at 6 to 8 liters/min.
   d. Notifies physician.
10. Notify the physician if the contraction pattern slows and labor is not well established.
11. Check the oxytocin infusion bottle as to the amount being absorbed and the rate of infusion, at least every ½ hour.
12. Remember that all clients receiving intravenous oxytocin must be continuously observed by a qualified member of the nursing staff who is under the direct supervision of a registered nurse.
13. Continuously assess the client's progress both physically and emotionally as well as by the monitor tracings. Remember that the client, and not the monitor, is being treated.
14. Notify the physician when 10 mU/min of oxytocin is reached so that an evaluation of the client may be made by the physician.
15. Carry out the written prescription for oxytocin infusion, if it is to be continued to 20 mU/min, according to number 4 under Physician Responsibilities.
16. Take vital signs and fetal heart rate every 15 minutes and record these on the intrapartum flow sheet as well as on the monitor strip.

(continued)

(continued)

17. Record the characteristics of the contraction pattern every 15 minutes on the intrapartum flow sheet. These observations include palpation of the intensity of the uterine contraction and their frequency at least every ½ hour.
18. Accurately record intake and output every 2 hours.

Note. If in doubt at any time about the response of the mother or fetus to oxytocin, turn the oxytocin infusion off and notify the physician immediately.

Chart Notations

Intrapartum Flow Sheet

1. Dosage of oxytocin, the name, and amount of the solution
2. Rate of the flow of oxytocin increased, held, or decreased
3. Contraction pattern every 15 minutes
4. Vital signs and fetal heart rate every 15 minutes
5. Vaginal exams and results done by the physician
6. Adjustment to the monitor

Nurse's Record

1. Intake
   a. Oral
   b. Intravenous
2. Output
   a. Urine
   b. Vomitus
   c. Other
3. 8-hour summary of intake and output
4. Vaginal exams and results done by the physician
5. Treatments
6. Nursing care
   a. Physical
   b. Emotional
   c. Teaching

Monitor Tracings

1. Dosage of oxytocin and time started
2. Time and the dosage of oxytocin when increased, held, or decreased
3. Vital signs every 15 minutes and the time
4. Exams and procedures by physician and the time
5. Any movement or changes to the client or monitor that may interfere with recording of the tracing

(After Hospital of the University of Pennsylvania, Department of Nursing, Department of Obstetrics and Gynecology)

Planning/Intervention

The nurse plans interventions based on the nursing diagnoses and on the medical plan of treatment. Care will include comfort measures, emotional support, and explanations of what is happening, as well as administering and monitoring effects of ordered medications.

Emotional Support. Labors of this type are extremely discouraging for the mother and the father. The diagnostic procedures as well as the therapy take a certain amount of time, and carrying out these measures requires patience and waiting on the part of everyone concerned. It is essential that the couple know and understand this fact. The physician and nurse need to spend sufficient time with the parents to explain what is happening in depth and in terms that are appropriate for them. It is very possible that repeated reinforcement of the explanations, progress, and so on will be needed. In stressful situations, people often do not hear all that is said. Feedback from the parents should be encouraged, so that their level of understanding and acceptance can be ascertained. The normal tension and anxiety found in any labor certainly is intensified in a dysfunctional labor, and it is important that it not be compounded by fantasy or misunderstanding.

Since dysfunctional labor is so variable, it is often impossible (and unwise) to give the parents any definite reassurances as to when effective labor will commence or when the birth will occur. Yet some kind of boundaries must be placed on when this ineffective phase will end and progress will begin, so that the mother will have some goal to look forward to and to work for. Therefore, it is important to reassure the client, reminding her that her case is not unique (after many hours clients think that theirs is the longest labor in obstetric history), that certain specific measures are known and can be taken to help effective labor to begin, and that competent medical and nursing care will be given throughout labor.

An explanation of the plan for treatment enables the parents to anticipate more realistically what is in store and therefore reassures them that certain definite measures are available and are being employed.

Comfort Measures. In addition, all the comfort measures that promote relaxation should be used. Sponge baths, various changes in position, soothing back rubs, quiet conversation, reading or other diversionary activities, and clean, dry linen, as well as a quiet, restful environment, are all appropriate. However, isolating the client in a dark room on the premise that she needs sleep or rest only contributes to her fear unless she is actually sleeping and then frequent observations are needed to see when she awakens. Human contact is one of the most important items of "treatment" in cases of complicated labor and should never be neglected. The presence of the same person, nurse, or physician is very helpful for the reasons already mentioned in Chapter 25. Allowing the client to have with her a familiar person of her choice, such as husband or mother, is also important. Coaching the client in breathing patterns and relaxation techniques also can be comforting and helps to conserve her strength.

Certain comfort measures can actually aid in correction of some dysfunctional labor patterns. For example, an overdistended bladder may not be noticed by the client, but may add to her discomfort. Encouraging emptying of the bladder often speeds cervical dilatation, possibly by allowing the fetal head to descend further with better proximity to the cervix. Similarly, emptying the rectum by means of an enema has also been found to enhance uterine contractions.[5]

Position changes may also improve uterine contractions. In general, uterine contractions come less frequently but tend to be better coordinated and more intense when the mother is in the side-lying position, as compared with the supine position.[5] She may need some encouragement to assume the side-lying position at first, but usually will try it willingly when told that it may improve her contractions. Walking in the hall or sitting in a comfortable chair may also assist in the resumption of effective contractions in some cases. However, the client should not be allowed out of bed if the membranes have ruptured and the head is not well engaged.

Oxytocin Monitoring. If oxytocin stimulation of labor is used, the mother must have someone in attendance at all times during the infusion. The physician is usually required to be present in the labor and delivery suite, but the nurse may be the one who is actually in the client's room. The dosage and rate of oxytocin are specified by the physician, and the nurse ascertains that the infusion is running at the prescribed rate and also reports any changes in maternal or fetal condition immediately.

In setting up a piggyback system for the infusion, the nurse should make sure that the bottle containing the oxytocin is clearly labeled as such, that the piggyback line is inserted in the port closest to the client, and that contamination is avoided during the insertion.[10] If an infusion pump is not used the drip rate must be counted frequently to be sure that it has not changed with changes in the client's position. Even with the use of an infusion pump, observation is necessary, since there is always the possibility of a pump malfunction.

Although uterine contractions and fetal heart tones are being continuously monitored electronically, they need to be assessed by the nurse at least every 15 minutes. If there is any doubt about the accuracy of the monitor, especially if external monitors are being used, the contractions should be evaluated by palpation and the heart tones checked by Doppler. Any contraction lasting over 90 seconds indicates that the uterus is being overstimulated, and the rate of flow should be either decreased or temporarily discontinued. The fetal heart rate pattern should be observed for changes. Late decelerations or severe variable decelerations are an indication for discontinuation of the oxytocin infusion. With any signs of fetal distress the oxytocin should be turned off, the mother turned on her left side, oxygen started by mask, and the physician notified.

Maternal blood pressure and pulse are to be checked every half hour. Owing to oxytocin's antidiuretic properties, intake and output should also be monitored carefully and decreased urinary output reported. Another concern is the monitoring of labor progress. With the stimulation of more effective uterine contractions, cervical dilation may occur much more rapidly, and this needs to be detected soon enough for preparations to be made for the birth.

It is important to have a method for recording the times, amount, and rate of oxytocin infused, the fetal heart tones, the maternal blood pressure and pulse, the frequency, intensity, and length of contractions, and other relevant comments. The client's labor record may be used, or there may be a specific "oxytocin record" or flow sheet that provides an easily accessible record of the client's progress during the infusion. Significant information is also written at the appropriate times on the electronic monitor strip.

Recording and reporting the physiological signs and symptoms cannot be stressed enough during these infusions. However, supportive care continues to be important, and the nurse must avoid the pitfall of "monitoring the monitor" instead of caring for the client. Since the nurse will be with the client continuously over a period of time, this time can be used to establish rapport and provide adequate explanations and reassurance. Before the oxytocin infusion is started the nurse can help prepare the client by explaining the procedure and expected changes in the uterine contractions. The often rapid change from mild to strong uterine contractions can be difficult for the client to adjust to, but anticipatory guidance and assistance with breathing and relaxation can make the adjustment easier. Although the infusion stimulates contractions, and therefore discomfort, the mother and her partner often look upon this treatment optimistically, since it marks the end of a desultory, ineffective period in labor and brings with it promise of termination of a difficult time. The nurse's explanations and reassurance can reinforce this positive attitude.

Other Problems with the Expulsive Forces

Inadequate Voluntary Expulsive Force. When the cervix is fully dilated, most women cannot resist the urge to push or bear down during a uterine contraction. The combined force of the maternal use of abdominal musculature and the contraction of the uterus helps propel the fetus down the vagina and through the vaginal outlet. The urge and ability to push can be interfered with by such factors as anesthesia and heavy sedation. Fatigue or intensification of pain during pushing can also cause the woman to push with less effectiveness. In rare instances a physical problem such as a spinal cord injury may be the reason for insufficient expulsive efforts.[1]

Management is usually related to the cause. Careful selection and timing of analgesia and anesthesia can be helpful in preventing the problem. If continuous epidural anesthesia is used, it may be necessary to allow the effects to wear off sufficiently for the woman to be able to push. For the woman who is "holding back" because of pain, analgesia may be needed. In any event, appropriate encouragement, support, instruction, and positioning can be very helpful.

Precipitate Labor and Delivery. Labor that lasts less than 3 hours is called precipitate labor. It is most often due to lack of resistance of maternal tissues allowing the fetus to pass easily through the pelvis. It can also be due to contractions with an amplitude over 50 mm Hg, or occasionally to the mother's lack of awareness of the sensations of vigorous labor.[1] Precipitate delivery may, but does not necessarily, follow precipitate labor and may occur after a labor of normal length. Although rapid labor is sometimes associated with increased danger of maternal lacerations or fetal asphyxia from interference with the placental circulation, some recent studies have shown that the risk to mother and child is not necessarily increased greatly over that of the average labor.[4] If labor is progressing rapidly because of tetanic contractions caused by infusion of an oxytocic agent, the infusion should be stopped immediately. Spontaneous forceful contractions are difficult to modify, but tocolytic agents may be effective.[1]

Pathologic Retraction and Constriction Rings. Localized rings or constrictions of the uterus sometimes occur in association with prolonged rupture of the membranes or long labors (Fig. 38-4). The *pathologic retraction ring* (Bandl's ring) is the most common. It is an exaggeration of the normal physiologic retraction ring, which occurs at the junction of the upper and lower uterine segments (see Chap. 24). The uterus above the ring becomes thicker, while the lower uterine segment thins out and will rupture unless the obstruction is relieved or delivery is accomplished by cesarean section.[5] *Constriction rings* are rare and not well understood. They usually conform to a depression in the baby, such as the neck or abdomen, and do not go all the way around. The area of spasm is thick, but the lower uterine segment does not become stretched or thinned out.[4] Cesarean birth, using an anesthetic that relaxes the uterus, is usually the treatment of choice.

Problems with the Passageway

The second major category of factors causing dystocia is that related to variations or abnormalities of the maternal reproductive tract, especially the pelvis, that interfere with engagement, descent, or expulsion of the fetus.

Contracted Pelvis

Disproportion between the size of the infant and the size of the birth canal is caused most frequently by a contracted pelvis. The pelvis may be contracted, or reduced in size, at the inlet, the midpelvis, or the outlet.

In the case of *inlet contraction*, the anteroposterior diameter of the inlet is decreased to 10 cm or less or the greatest transverse diameter is 12 cm or less. Either of

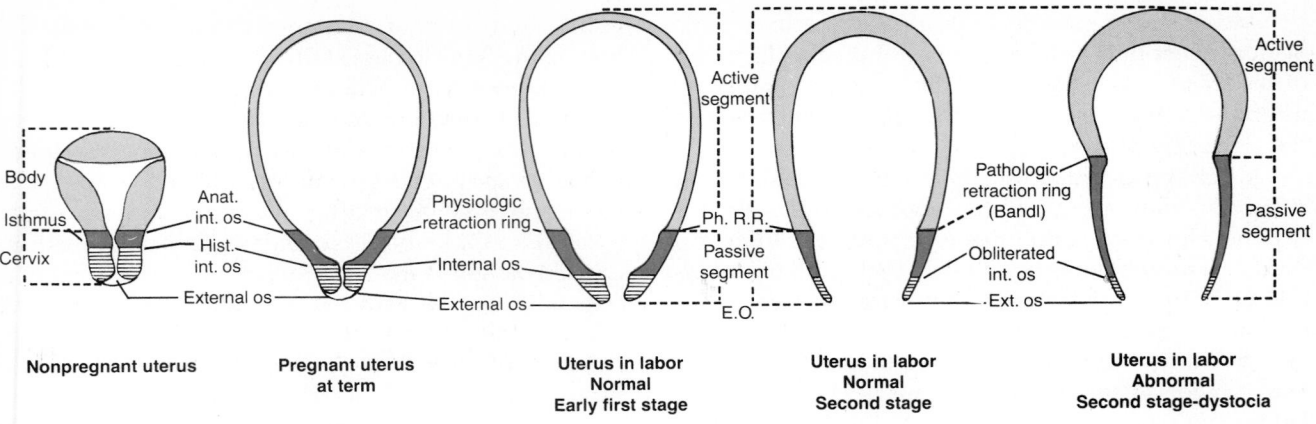

Nonpregnant uterus   Pregnant uterus at term   Uterus in labor Normal Early first stage   Uterus in labor Normal Second stage   Uterus in labor Abnormal Second stage-dystocia

FIGURE 38-4

Sequence of development of the segments and rings in the uterus in pregnant women at term and in labor. Note comparison between the uterus of a nonpregnant woman, the uterus at term, and the uterus during labor. The passive lower segment of the uterine body is derived from the isthmus; the physiologic retraction ring develops at the junction of the upper and lower uterine segments. The pathologic retraction ring develops from the physiologic ring. (*Anat. Int. Os*, anatomical internal os; *Hist. Int. Os*, histologic internal os; *Ph. R. R.*, physiologic retraction ring; *E.O.*, external os) (After Pritchard JA, MacDonald PC, Gant NF: Williams Obstetrics, 17th ed, Chap 15, p 308. New York, Appleton-Century-Crofts, 1985)

these contractions results in an increase in obstetric difficulties. The incidence of difficult labors is increased even more when both diameters are contracted.[1] Contraction of the inlet may be the result of rickets or generally poor development. A small woman is more likely to have a pelvis that is small in all dimensions, but she is also more likely to have a small baby. Effects of a contracted pelvic inlet on the fetus include failure of the presenting part to engage, increased incidence of malpositions and deflexed attitudes, and extreme molding of the presenting part. Since the presenting part does not fit the inlet well, prolapsed umbilical cord is also more likely.

Midpelvic contraction is less well defined than contraction of the inlet or outlet; however, the midpelvis is considered contracted when the distance between the ischial spines is less than 9.0 cm (normal is 10.5) or when the sum of the interspinous and the posterior sagittal distance is less than 13.5 cm (normal is 15.0 cm–15.5 cm). Contraction of the midpelvis is a fairly frequent cause of dystocia. Management can be more difficult than in inlet contraction because the condition is more difficult to recognize, since the presenting part is able to engage in the pelvis. As labor progresses, molding and caput formation may give the impression that the head is lower than it actually is, and a difficult forceps delivery may result. Transverse arrest of the head may also occur.

Contraction of the pelvic outlet is identified when the distance between the ischial tuberosities is less than 8 cm. Other dimensions of the outlet are also important in determining the degree of difficulty caused by the outlet contraction. The incidence of perineal tears and the need for forceps are increased, but cesarean section is rarely necessary. Severe dystocia is usually the result of an association with a midpelvic contraction.

Variations in Pelvic Shape

The shape of the pelvis may be equally important or more important than its size, although these factors may complement each other. For example, large size may compensate for a shape that is not optimal. The normal female or *gynecoid* pelvis has the best dimensions in all planes for the passage of the fetus. The other three pelvic variations adversely influence the prognosis for a vaginal delivery (see Chap. 9 for discussion of pelvic types).

Cephalopelvic Disproportion

The term *cephalopelvic disproportion* (CPD) implies a relationship between the size of the fetal head and the size of the pelvis. This of course indicates that the problem could originate with either the passageway or the passenger, or a combination of the two. It involves an interplay between the factors in the preceding section and those in the following section. Cephalopelvic (or fetopelvic if the head is not the presenting part) disproportion can be either absolute or relative. When the fetus cannot pass safely through the birth canal under any circumstances, it is considered absolute. In many cases, however, whether or not the fetus can be delivered vaginally will depend on the efficiency of the uterine contractions, the stretchability of the maternal soft tissues, the attitude, presentation, and position of the fetus, and the moldability of the fetal head.[4]

Extreme degrees of pelvic contraction or problems with the fetus can often be detected during antepartal care and a decision made about the advisability of cesarean delivery. In doubtful cases, the client may be given a "trial labor" of 4 to 6 hours to determine whether or not with adequate contractions the head will pass through the pelvis. For these mothers labor may be even more anxiety provoking than usual, depending partly on the support and information they have received. If cesarean delivery is the eventual outcome, there may be a great deal of disappointment and perhaps even a feeling of failure. The warm empathic attitude of the nurse is particularly needed for these clients. Frequent reports on the progress of labor should not be overlooked, whether or not the progress is favorable. The perinatal team does the client a disservice in avoiding the subject if progress is not made in labor.

Problems with the Passenger

The position and presentation of the fetus at the beginning of labor can greatly influence the progress of the labor. Even slight deviations can affect the uterine contractions adversely or prevent the fetus from passing through the birth canal.

Persistent Occiput Posterior and Transverse Arrest

The fetal head usually enters the pelvic inlet transversely and therefore must traverse an arc of 90° in the process of internal rotation to the direct occiput anterior position (see Fig. 23-2). In about a quarter of all labors, however, the head enters the pelvis with the occiput directed diagonally posterior, that is, in either the R.O.P. or the L.O.P. position. Under these circumstances the head must rotate through an arc of 135° in the process of internal rotation.

With good contractions, adequate flexion, and a baby of average size, the great majority of these cases of occiput posterior position undergo spontaneous rotation through the 135° arc as soon as the head reaches the pelvic floor. This is a normal mechanism of labor. It must be remembered, however, that labor is usually prolonged, and the mother has a great deal of discomfort

in her back as the baby's head impinges against the sacrum in the course of rotating (Fig. 38-5).

Nursing intervention is aimed at relieving the back pain as much as possible. Sacral pressure, back rubs, and frequent change of position from side to side can be helpful, and they should be employed to the degree that seems to be well tolerated by the client.

In a minority of cases, however (perhaps 10% or less), these favorable circumstances do not exist, and rotation may be incomplete or may not take place at all. If rotation is incomplete, the head becomes arrested in the transverse position, a condition known as *transverse arrest*. If anterior rotation does not take place at all, the occiput usually rotates to the direct occiput posterior position, a condition known as *persistent occiput posterior*. Both transverse arrest and persistent occiput posterior position represent deviations from the normal mechanisms of labor. It is thought that narrowing of the midpelvis plays a role in the etiology. These conditions appear to have, in some cases, an adverse effect on uterine behavior. Here the malposition is the cause rather than the effect of uterine inefficiency. This conclusion can be verified by the following findings. (1) When the fetal head is rotated or rotates spontaneously, uterine action improves. (2) Oxytocin therapy for dysfunction associated with an occipitoposterior position does not cause the infant's head to rotate.[11]

Some controversy persists in the management of persistent occiput posterior. When labor progresses, although first and second stages tend to be prolonged in primigravidas, management is the same as for occiput anterior positions and results in no increased risk to the fetus. Premature operative intervention, particularly if the station is high, seems contraindicated. Forceps rotation on the perineum is appropriate to reduce lacerations if this can be easily accomplished.[1]

Breech Presentation

The breech is the presenting part in 3% to 4% of singleton deliveries and is more common when the baby is premature or there is multiple gestation. The reasons for breech presentation are not always apparent, although associated factors include great parity, twinning, hydramnios, hydrocephalus, placenta previa, and implantation of the placenta in the cornual fundal regions of the uterus. Studies have not indicated a positive correlation between breech presentation and contracted pelvis.[1]

Classification. Breech presentations are classified as follows:

Complete. The buttocks present with the feet and legs flexed on the thighs and the thighs flexed on the abdomen (Fig. 38-6A).

Woman with Dysfunctional Labor

Nursing Objectives

1. Identify presence of dysfunctional labor patterns.
2. Maintain fluid and electrolyte balance.
3. Provide information to client and family about labor pattern, progress of labor, and planned interventions.
4. Minimize pain and discomfort.

Assessment	Potential Nursing Diagnosis	Planning/Intervention	Evaluation
Uterine contractions for dysfunctional patterns		Monitor frequency, duration, and intensity of contractions	
Level of fatigue and ability to cope with pain	Alteration in comfort related to ineffective uterine contractions	Stay with client or have partner stay continuously; coach in breathing and relaxation techniques; record and report behavior; assist as needed with position changes, effleurage, concentration or distraction for pain management; keep linen clean and dry; provide quiet environment	Client avoids exhaustion Client attains as much comfort as possible
Emotional status	Anxiety or fear related to unexpected character or length of labor	Explain labor progress, plan of treatment, and what can be expected; reassure as appropriate	Client avoids panic and discouragement
Hydration	Potential fluid volume deficit related to prolonged labor and restricted fluid intake	Give oral or intravenous fluids as ordered Check for dryness of lips and for decreased skin turgor	Client retains normal fluid volume
Bladder		Encourage client to void frequently; catheterize as necessary	Client avoids bladder distention

(continued)

Frank. The buttocks present with the hips flexed and the legs extended against the abdomen and chest (Fig. 38-6B); this is the most common type of breech presentation.

Incomplete. One or both feet or the knees extend below the buttocks (Fig. 38-6C); this type of presentation is also known as a single or double footling breech.

Compound. The buttocks present together with another part such as a hand (very rare).

Delivery Methods for Breech Presentation.

Choosing the route of delivery for an infant in the breech presentation is the subject of much debate. Many studies have shown that neonatal morbidity and mortality are considerably higher when infants with breech presentations are delivered vaginally as compared to the outcome of cesarean deliveries. Therefore, the incidence of cesarean delivery for breech presentation has increased substantially in the last decade. Several studies have found that, even with delivery by cesarean section, the infant in breech presentation is at increased risk for morbidity and mortality.[1]

There is no significantly increased danger for the life of the mother in breech presentations, although there is increased incidence of lacerations of the birth canal, episiotomy extensions, cesarean deliveries, and postpartum infections. Labor is not prolonged, contrary to previous belief.[1] For the infant, however, there is considerably increased risk of both death and injury in comparison to vertex presentations. Factors related to breech presentation, such as prematurity and congenital

Assessment	Potential Nursing Diagnosis	Planning/Intervention	Evaluation
Vital signs Signs of infection	Potential for infection related to prolonged rupture of membranes	Check temperature-pulse-respiration and blood pressure every 2 hours or more frequently if indicated	Client remains free of infection
		Report and record temperature increase or other changes in vital signs	
		Use clean technique in client care with good hand washing	
Response to oxytocin (if given)		Monitor oxytocin infusion; maintain rate as ordered	Client progresses in labor
		Monitor uterine contractions and fetal heart rate carefully; report and record	Client remains free of complications
Fetal well-being	Potential fetal distress related to prolonged labor	Monitor fetal heart rate tracing for changes in variability, reactivity, rate, or pattern or auscultate fetal heart tones frequently if fetal monitor not in use	Fetus remains in good condition
		Check for meconium staining of amniotic fluid or sudden increase in fetal activity	
		If signs of fetal distress are detected, position client on left side, start oxygen, turn off oxytocin (if in use), notify physician	

malformations, account for a good number of the deaths and long-term sequelae. Mortality from vaginal delivery for all preterm and term infants in breech presentation is about 5.5 times that of infants in vertex presentation. Even with preterm infants excluded, the perinatal mortality in many studies is still 3.5 times higher than for vertex.[12] In term breech births, the majority of perinatal deaths are related to cord prolapse and other cord complications or to tentorial tears and cerebral hemorrhage, which occur during delivery of the aftercoming head.

Other factors related to death or damage of the baby include asphyxia from aspiration of amniotic fluid due to breathing before the head is born, injury due to trapping of the head by the incompletely dilated cervix and injury, such as fractures, resulting from manipulation and possible rough handling during the delivery.[4]

Although increasing the cesarean delivery rate may decrease the perinatal morbidity and mortality, it increases the maternal morbidity related to major surgery.[1,10] The question, then, is how to select those cases in which the infant can be delivered vaginally with minimum risk, so that the cesarean delivery rate can be kept as low as possible.

Several scoring systems have been developed to evaluate the feasibility of vaginal delivery in breech presentations. The Zatuchni-Andros Prognostic Index (Table 38-2) is an example. These systems are designed to serve as a guide in deciding on the route of delivery. The effectiveness of low scores in predicting patients at risk for infant morbidity and mortality, prolonged labors, and eventual cesarean delivery has been reported. The recommendation is that a score of three or less is

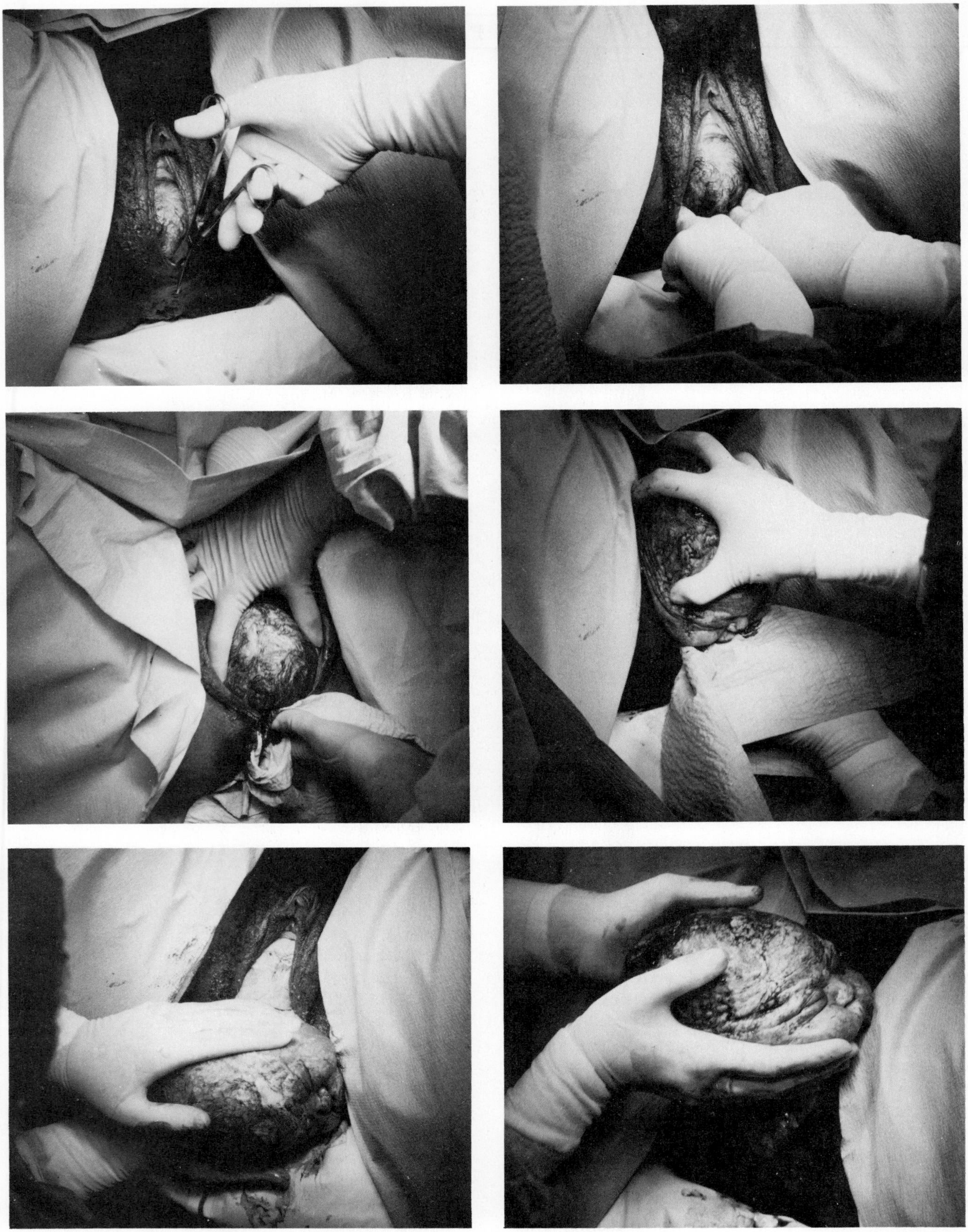

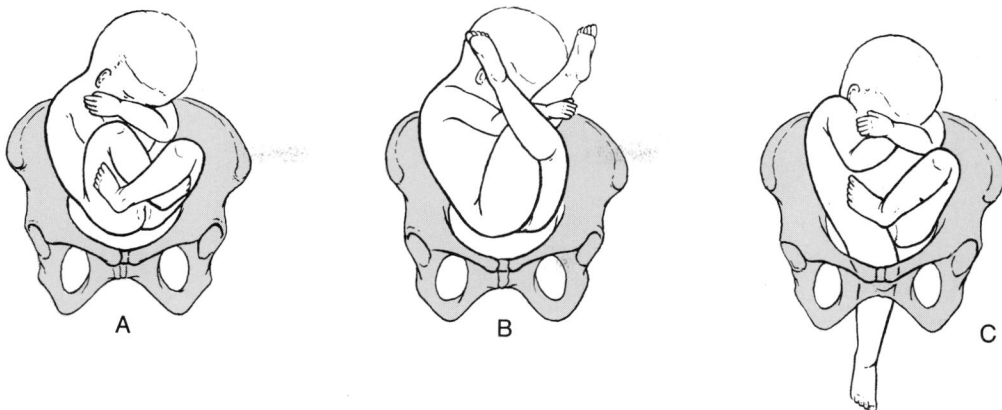

FIGURE 38-6

Breech presentation may be (*A*) complete breech, (*B*) frank breech, and (*C*) an incomplete or footling breech.

a good indication for a cesarean birth, a score of four requires further observation and subsequent evaluation, and a score of five or more will hopefully result in a successful vaginal delivery. Some investigators have found that low scores are of great prognostic value, but that high scores are less significant and may still be associated with high morbidity and mortality.[12]

One problem with the scoring system is that it does not take into account all of the important factors that must be considered; therefore, it should not take the place of the obstetrician's clinical judgement for each individual woman.

Circumstances in association with breech presentation that are usually considered to be indications for cesarean delivery and those generally considered favorable for vaginal delivery are listed on page 824.[1,12]

Of the breech presentations, frank breech is usually considered most favorable for vaginal delivery because the buttocks fits into the pelvis more evenly, helping to prevent cord prolapse and acting as a better cervical dilator than other breech presentations. The splinting effect of the baby's extended legs, however, may impede delivery by preventing lateral flexion.[12]

It would seem that the small preterm infant might be easy to deliver vaginally. In reality, these infants are apt to have proportionately larger heads. The cervix dilates sufficiently for the breech to pass, but the head may become trapped by the cervix. The deflexed head represents another situation in which a baby's head may become trapped, but this time by the bony pelvis.

FIGURE 38-5

First several steps in spontaneous vaginal delivery of a baby in occiput posterior presentation. (Courtesy of Dr. Mastroianni)

A most important consideration in the delivery decision is the obstetrician's knowledge of and skill in vaginal breech deliveries. This can be a problem, since the current trend toward cesarean delivery for breech presentation does not allow opportunity for much practice in breech vaginal delivery.

External Version. With the increasing use of cesarean birth for breech presentation, many obstetricians are taking a new look at external version as a way to prevent breech deliveries. This is most likely to be attempted if the breech presentation is recognized during the third trimester. Some fetuses do return to the breech position after version, but studies have shown a significant decrease in breech deliveries when external version is used. There is a difference of opinion among obstetricians concerning the degree of risk with this procedure, and whether the results are worth the risk. Researchers have reported antepartal hemorrhage, premature labor, premature rupture of membranes, and fetal death as complications. Fetal-maternal bleeds have also been reported and led to the recommendation of giving anti-*D* globulin to Rh negative women prior to attempting external version.[1]

Vaginal Delivery. The *mechanism of labor* in breech delivery, except for the reversal of polarity, is comparable to that for vertex presentations. The steps are shown in Figure 38-7. Descent is slower initially in the case of a breech but among women of similar parity, dilatation and effacement are approximately the same for breech and vertex presentations.

Spontaneous breech deliveries sometimes occur, but usually some degree of assistance is necessary. Assistance is most often needed for delivery of the aftercoming head. This may be accomplished by the application

---

Factors Used in Clinical Decisions Related to Delivery Method for Breech Presentations

Circumstances Considered Indications for Cesarean Delivery

A large fetus

Any degree of contraction or unfavorable shape of the pelvis

A hyperextended head

Either maternal or fetal indications for delivery, but not in labor

Complications of labor, such as acute fetal distress, placenta previa, abruptio placentae, prolapsed cord, or uterine dysfunction

An apparently healthy preterm fetus of 26 or more weeks gestation; mother in active labor or in need of delivery

Severe fetal growth retardation

Previous pregnancies resulting in perinatal death or birth trauma

A firm request for sterilization

Footling presentation

Circumstances Usually Favorable for Vaginal Delivery

Gestational age between 36 and 38 weeks

Estimated fetal weight between 6 and 7 pounds

Presenting part at the beginning of labor at 0 station or below

Soft, effaced cervix, dilated to 3 cm or more

Ample pelvis with expectation of head entering in direct occiput anterior position

Prior obstetrical history of breech delivery of infant weighing greater than 7 lb, or vertex delivery of infant weighing greater than 8 lb

Frank breech presentation

---

of Piper forceps (see Chap. 39) or by one of several maneuvers, such as the Mariceau-Smellie-Veit maneuver (Fig. 38-8). Maintenance of flexion of the head is important, and suprapubic pressure by the obstetrician or an assistant is usually needed.[12]

Many physicians prefer local or pudendal anesthesia for vaginal breech deliveries because it does not interfere with labor and allows the mother to participate actively. Epidural anesthesia is also preferred for the same reasons and, additionally, it permits more comfortable intravaginal manipulation and extractions. For difficult breech deliveries a general anesthetic such as halothane might be used since these agents inhibit uterine contractions and make intravaginal manipulation easier.

Assessment in Breech Presentation. As with all complicated labors, nursing assessment is an important

---

T A B L E   3 8 - 2

Zatuchni–Andros Prognostic Index*

	Points		
	0	**1**	**2**
Parity	Primigravida	Multipara	
Gestational age	39 weeks or more	38 weeks	37 weeks or less
Estimated fetal weight	8 lb (3630 g)	7 lb–7$^{15}/_{16}$ lb (3629 g–3176 g)	<7 lb (3173 g)
Previous breech†	0	1	2 or more
Dilation‡	2 cm	3 cm	4 cm or more
Station‡	−3 or higher	−2	−1 or lower

* Zatuchni GI, Andros GJ: Prognostic index for vaginal delivery in breech presentation. Am J Obstet Gynecol 98:854, 1967.
† Greater than 2500 g.
‡ Determined by vaginal examination on admission.

Woman with Breech Presentation

Nursing Objectives

1. Identify abnormal presentation.
2. Provide client and family with information about presentation and possible interventions.
3. Monitor fetal and maternal condition.
4. Provide comfort measures.

Assessment	Potential Nursing Diagnosis	Planning/Intervention	Evaluation
Signs of breech presentation Leopold's maneuver: head in fundus; breech in pelvis Vaginal examination: breech presenting Passage of meconium		Check for fetal presentation and position; report and record findings	
Progress of labor	Potential alteration in labor progress related to abnormal fetal presentation	Monitor uterine contractions Monitor changes in cervical dilatation and effacement and in fetal presentation and position	Client progresses in labor
Condition of fetus Fetal heart rate and pattern Fetal movement	Potential for fetal distress related to increased risk of prolapsed cord	Monitor fetal heart rate tracing for changes, particularly variable decelerations; check for increased fetal movement; (passage of meconium not indication of fetal distress in breech presentation)	Fetus remains free of distress
Indications for cesarean delivery Fetal distress Position other than frank breech (complete or footling breech position) Evidence of CPD	Knowledge deficit related to breech birth Anxiety/fear related to concern about possible cesarean section	Gather data to assist in decision concerning route of delivery Keep client and family informed of progress of labor and plan of treatment Reassure as appropriate Prepare for surgery, if decision made for cesarean section: have lab work done, shave abdomen, insert Foley, do preoperative and postoperative teaching	Client verbalizes understanding of breech birth and cesarean delivery Client verbalizes relief from anxiety and fear Infant is born in good condition

part of the care of the woman in labor with a breech presentation. This will include, but not be limited to, use of the electronic monitors. Initial assessment might include being the one to detect a possible breech presentation. In breech presentation the infant often passes meconium during the course of labor. After the membranes have ruptured, the black, tarry substance may be found coming from the patient's vagina. The nurse needs to ascertain that the presentation is, in fact, a breech, for if the fetus is in the vertex presentation, passage of meconium would be an indication of probable fetal distress.

When breech presentation is confirmed, continuing knowledge of the condition of both the mother and the

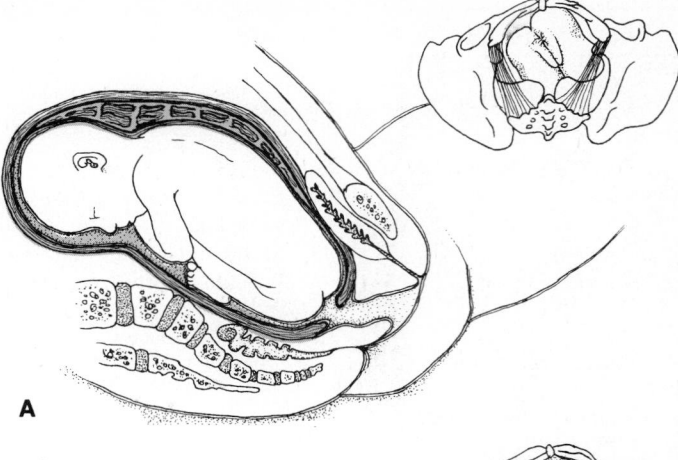

A

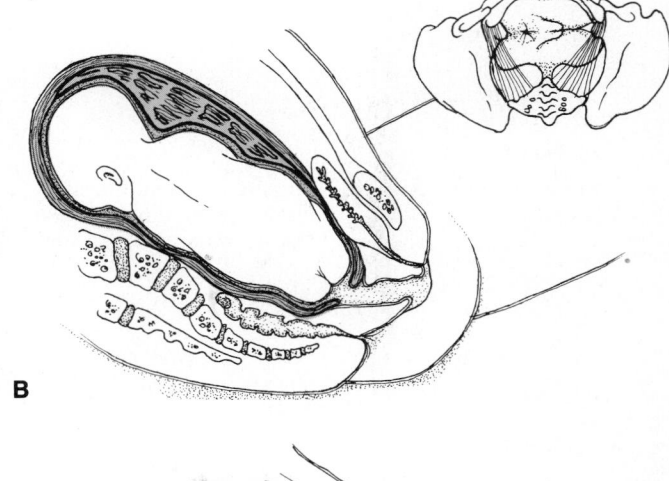

B

FIGURE 38-7

(*A*) Engagement, R.S.A. The bitrochanteric diameter has passed through the inlet of the maternal pelvis (side view). (*B*) Internal rotation of the breech, R.S.A. to R.S.T. With further descent, the anterior hip of the fetus meets the resistance of the pelvic floor of the mother and rotates 45° so that the bitrochanteric diameter of the fetus lies in the anteroposterior diameter of the maternal pelvis (side view). (*C*) Birth of the buttocks by lateral flexion. Birth of the posterior buttock over the perineum (side view). (*D*) Birth of the anterior buttock under the pubic arch (side view). (*E*) Birth of the baby up to the umbilicus. Loop of cord is being brought down. (*F*) Engagement of the shoulders. The bisacromial diameter is in the right oblique diameter of the maternal pelvis (perineal view). (*G*) Delivery of the anterior shoulder under the pubic arch (side view). (*H*) Delivery of the posterior shoulder over the perineum (side view). (*I*) Mauriceau-Smellie-Veit maneuver (with an assistant). The occiput is directly under the symphysis pubis. The assistant applies suprapubic pressure (side view). (*J*) Delivery of the head is attempted after the hairline is visible at the introitus (perineal view). (*K*) Mauriceau-Smellie-Veit maneuver continuing. Delivery of the head by flexion upward over the perineum with continuous suprapubic pressure (side view).

C

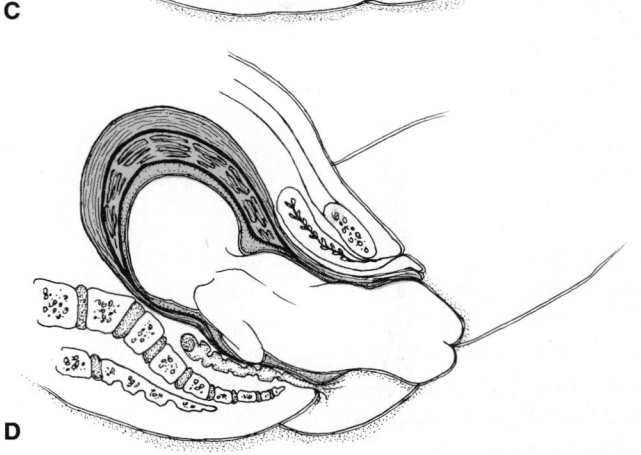

D

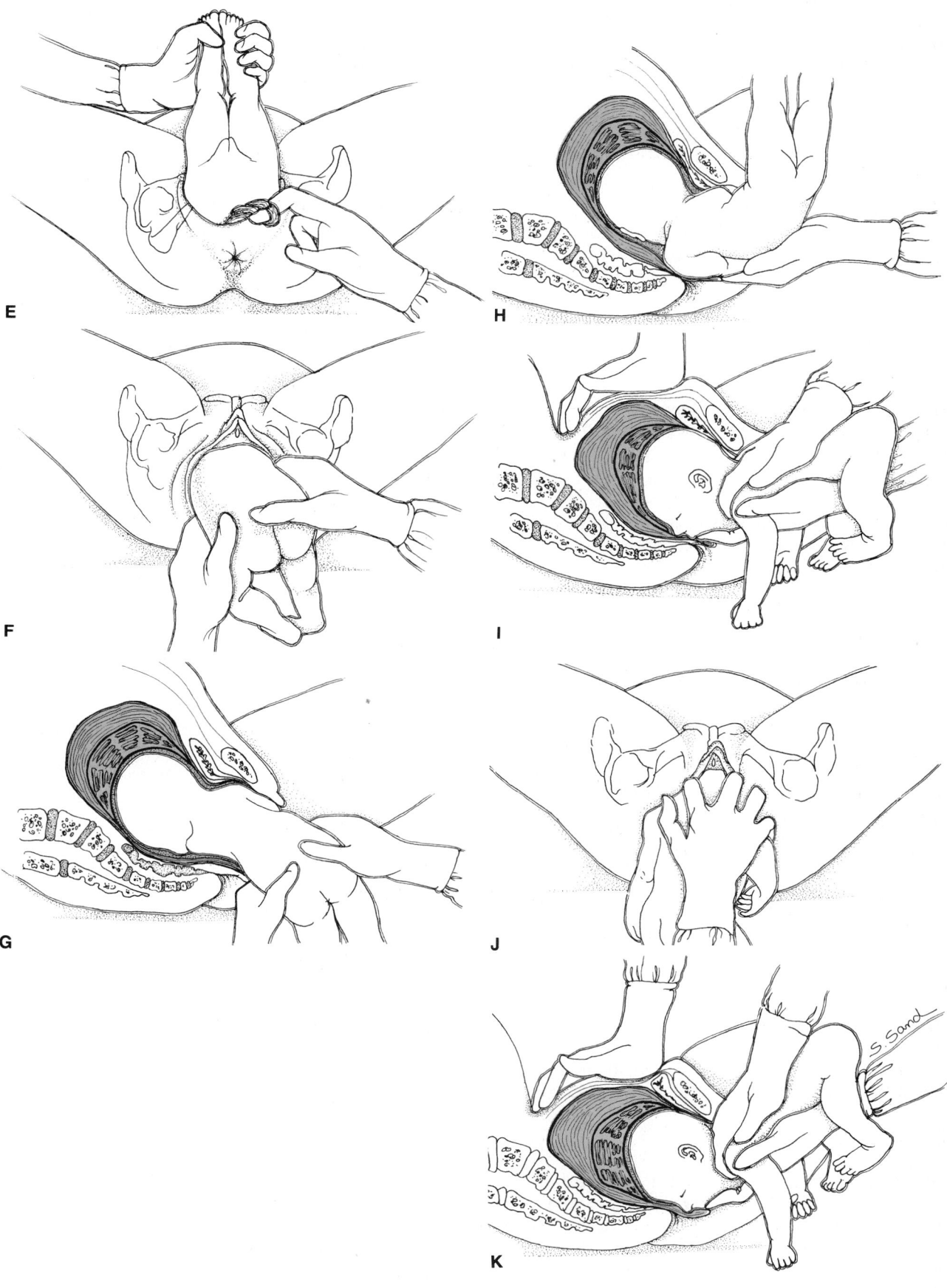

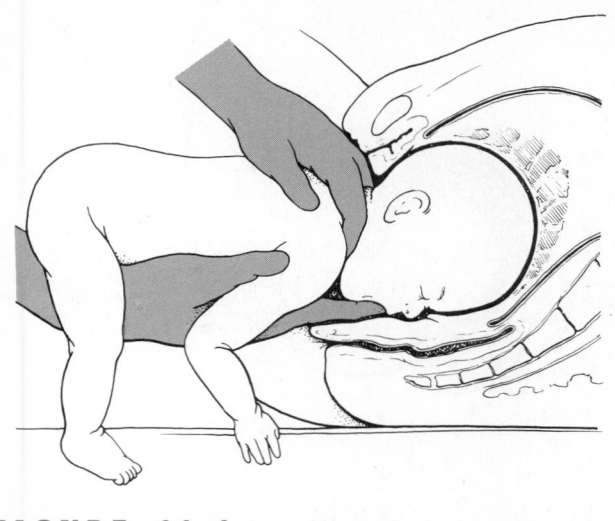

FIGURE   38-8

Mauriceau-Smellie-Veit maneuver for extracting the head in breech delivery.

fetus plays an important part in the decision making and the nurse is often the one to provide this information for the obstetrician.

Nursing Diagnoses.   The following nursing diagnoses might be used: potential for fetal distress related to increased risk of prolapsed cord, anxiety/fear related to concern about possible cesarean section, potential for postpartum hemorrhage related to interventions necessary for delivery, or knowledge deficit related to breech birth.

Planning and Implementation.   Planning and implementation of care should include comfort measures and explanations to the parents of what is happening. Explanation and appropriate reassurance are important for mothers who have breech presentations because many have heard frightening stories of what may happen if the baby is ''breech.'' The anxiety and fear may interfere with the woman's ability to work effectively with her labor. With modern obstetric techniques and knowledge, labor need not be prolonged or exceptionally painful, and cesarean section is now a safer viable alternative to vaginal delivery. If a cesarean delivery is to be done, teaching should be implemented to prepare the client for her preoperative and postoperative care.

Abnormal Presentations

Shoulder Presentation.   Shoulder presentation, or ''transverse lie,'' occurs when the infant lies crosswise in the uterus instead of longitudinally. The shoulder is usually the fetal part in the brim of the inlet, but sometimes it is the back, abdomen, ribs, or flank, depending on how the infant is positioned. Studies have shown

this complication to occur once in 300 to 500 cases, and it is seen most often in multiparas, owing to relaxation of the abdominal wall. Other common etiologic factors are prematurity, placenta previa, and contracted pelvis.[1]

This is a serious complication that increases the hazards of delivery for the mother and even more so for the fetus. Frequently an arm prolapses into the vagina, making the problem of delivery even more difficult. If neglected, this presentation results in rupture of the uterus and death of both mother and fetus.

External version in late pregnancy or early labor is occasionally successful, especially in the multipara, in converting the shoulder to a longitudinal lie. A transverse lie with the woman in active labor is generally an indication for cesarean delivery. Internal podalic version and extraction is a very hazardous procedure frequently associated with rupture of the uterus (see Chap. 39). It is rarely justified except in the case of a second twin.

Face Presentation.   Face presentations are seen in about 1 of 600 patients. Factors that favor extension of the head and prevent flexion are implicated in these presentations, a contracted pelvis being paramount among these. These infants may deliver spontaneously if labor is effective and the pelvis is adequate. The face comes through the vulva with the chin anterior (Fig. 38-9). However, if there is indication that the pelvis is contracted or that there is fetal distress, a cesarean delivery is indicated. As edema of the scalp is common in vertex presentations, facial edema is often present to the extent that the landmarks resemble a breech presentation. The edema and purplish discoloration disappear within a few days, but the infant's appearance gives the parents a great deal of concern. The nurse can be very helpful in reassuring the parents that the condition is temporary and will resolve without sequelae.

Brow Presentation.   Brow presentations are somewhat more rare than the other malpresentations. They are impossible to deliver as long as the brow presentation persists, since the largest diameter of the fetal head, the occipitomental, presents. They are, however, an unstable presentation, and often spontaneously convert to an occiput or face presentation. The same etiologic factors that underlie a face presentation pertain here. The principles of treatment are the same as for face presentations. If the labor is progressing and it is not unduly vigorous and there is no fetal distress in the closely monitored infant, no intervention is necessary. If labor does become tumultuous or, more likely, desultory, then prompt cesarean section is indicated.[1]

Compound Presentations.   Compound presentations are found when an extremity prolapses alongside, and enters the pelvis at the same time as, the presenting part. The most common combination is for an upper extremity to prolapse alongside the head. Prolapse of a

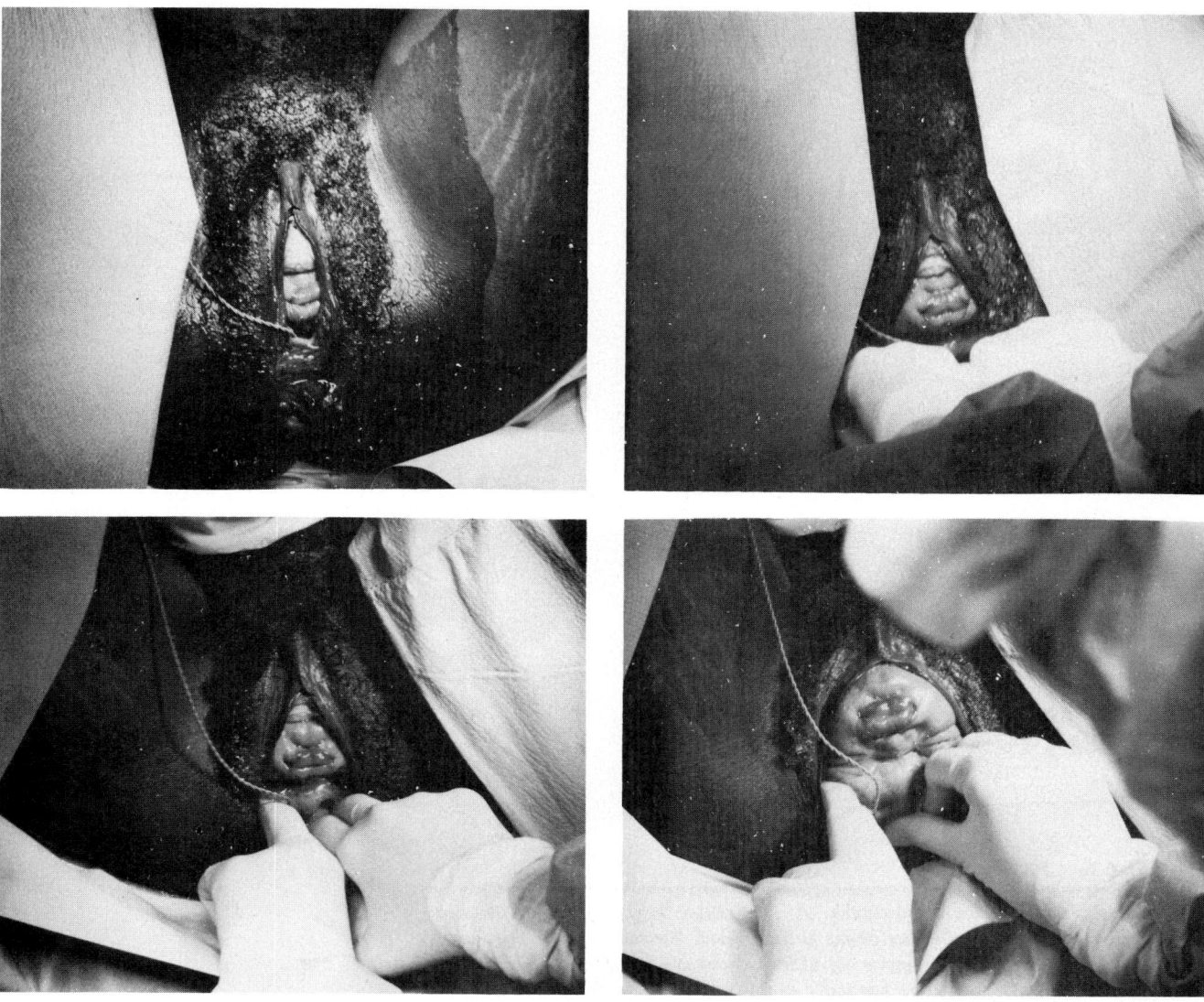

FIGURE 38-9

Face presentation. (Courtesy of Dr. Mastroianni)

leg in cephalic presentations or an arm in breech presentations does occur, but it is uncommon. The major problem with any of these presentations is increased incidence of prolapse of the umbilical cord. If left alone, the situation often is corrected spontaneously. When progress is arrested an attempt may be made to reposition the prolapsed part. If this is unsuccessful, or if there are indications that vaginal delivery should not be attempted, the baby should be delivered by cesarean section.

Oversized Baby

Excessive size of the infant (4000 g or more) may be a cause of serious dystocia, especially when the fetus weighs over 4500 g (10 lb). About 1 infant in 138 falls into this class. The trauma associated with the passage of such huge infants through the birth canal causes a decided increase in fetal mortality; this has been estimated as 13% (almost 1 in 7), in contrast with the usual death rate of 4% for infants of normal size. Uterine dysfunction is frequent in labors with excessive-size infants because the head becomes not only larger but harder and less malleable with increasing weight. Even though these infants are born alive, they often do poorly in the first few days because of a variety of conditions.

Excessive size of the fetus is usually due to maternal diabetes, large size of one or both parents, or multiparity. Postmaturity due to prolonged gestation is thought to be a cause of excessive-size infants in some instances. Tremendously large infants weighing over 13 lb are extremely rare, and almost all are born dead. Most oversized babies are boys. Although studies have shown a relationship between maternal diet and growth and

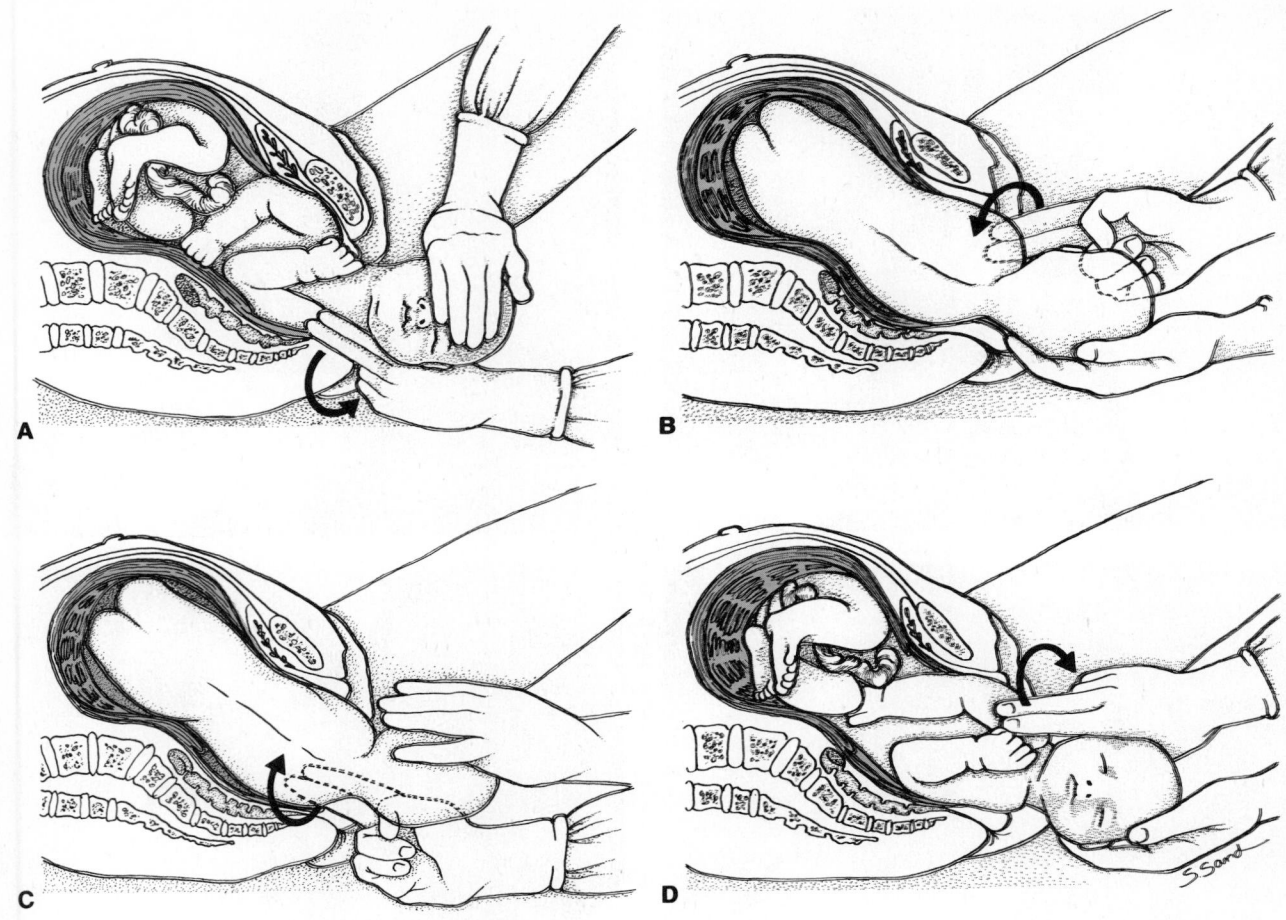

FIGURE 38-10

Maneuvers to relieve shoulder dystocia. (*A*) First phase beginning. The posterior shoulder is rotated 180°. (*B*) First phase is completed. Former anterior shoulder is now posterior, and former posterior shoulder is now anterior. There will be an attempt to deliver the shoulders normally at this time. If the attempt fails, the physician proceeds to the second phase. (*C*) Second phase beginning. The newly posterior shoulder is rotated 180°. (*D*) Second phase is completed. Original anterior shoulder is now anterior once again, and the original posterior shoulder is now posterior once again. The remainder of the delivery is performed in the usual way.

survival of the fetus, it is doubtful that strict regulation of diet during pregnancy can significantly reduce excessive growth of the infant. However, large women who are heavy may tend to have larger babies.

Shoulder Dystocia

One serious complication of an oversized infant is shoulder dystocia. After the head has passed through the pelvic canal, the infant's unusually large shoulders may arrest at either the pelvic brim or the outlet. The incidence of shoulder dystocia is 1.7% in infants over 4000 g, and the mortality rate is about 16%. The time between delivery of the head and delivery of the body must be short to ensure an uncompromised fetus. A large mediolateral episiotomy and adequate anesthesia

are mandatory. The infant's nose and mouth are cleared. Then, without using force, the physician sweeps the posterior arm across the chest and delivers it. The shoulder girdle is then rotated into one of the oblique pelvis diameters (Fig. 38-10). At this time the anterior shoulder can usually be delivered. Care must be taken not to apply vigorous traction on the head or neck or to excessively rotate the body. Occasionally deliberate fracture of the clavicle is necessary to save the infant's life.[1]

Fetal Anomalies

Any fetal anomaly that increases the size of a fetal part or parts can be a cause of dystocia. This occasionally occurs owing to a large fetal abdomen from a greatly distended bladder or enlargement of the kidneys or liver. Another rare cause of problems is incomplete twinning, resulting in double monsters or conjoined ("Siamese") twins.

Hydrocephalus. The most common fetal anomaly causing dystocia is hydrocephalus, or an excessive accumulation of cerebrospinal fluid in the ventricles of the brain with consequent enlargement of the cranium. This condition is encountered in approximately 1 fetus in 2000 and accounts for some 12% of all malformations at birth. Associated defects are common, spina bifida being present in about one third of the cases. Varying degrees of cranial enlargement are produced, and frequently the circumference of the head exceeds 50 cm, sometimes reaching 80 cm. The amount of fluid present is usually between 500 and 1500 ml, but as much as 5 liters has been reported. Since the distended cranium is too large to fit into the pelvic inlet, breech presentations are exceedingly common, being observed in about one third of such cases.

Whatever the presentation, gross disproportion between the size of the head and that of the pelvis is the rule, and serious dystocia is the usual consequence (Fig. 38-11). The mother is in danger of an obstructed labor resulting in rupture of the uterus, especially when the condition is undetected. Hydrocephalus may be suspected when the enlarged fetal head is palpated as a large symmetrical mass in the fundus or above the symphysis pubis. The condition is often accompanied by polyhydramnios, however, which makes abdominal palpation of the enlarged head more difficult. Ultrasound is a useful tool in making this diagnosis, since the width of the ventricles can be assessed, the thickness of the cerebral cortex evaluated, and the size of the head compared to that of the thorax and abdomen. By vaginal examination, large fontanels, wide suture lines, and an indentable, thin cranium may be palpated.

Except in mild cases, the obstetrician most often finds it necessary to puncture the cranial vault and aspirate some of the cerebrospinal fluid in order to reduce the head to a size that can pass through the birth canal. With a cephalic presentation the ventricle is tapped transvaginally after the cervix is dilated to about 3 cm; for a breech presentation it is done at the base of the skull after the breech and trunk are delivered.[1] When this type of aspiration is necessary, fetal mortality is the usual outcome.

When hydrocephalus is diagnosed early through the use of ultrasound, shunts are attempted *in utero* to minimize fetal brain damage and to delay delivery until the fetus is more mature. Although this treatment has not been very successful to date, there is hope for the future.

Labor and birth with a hydrocephalic fetus are very difficult for all concerned—The mother must undergo a difficult labor with increased danger to herself and

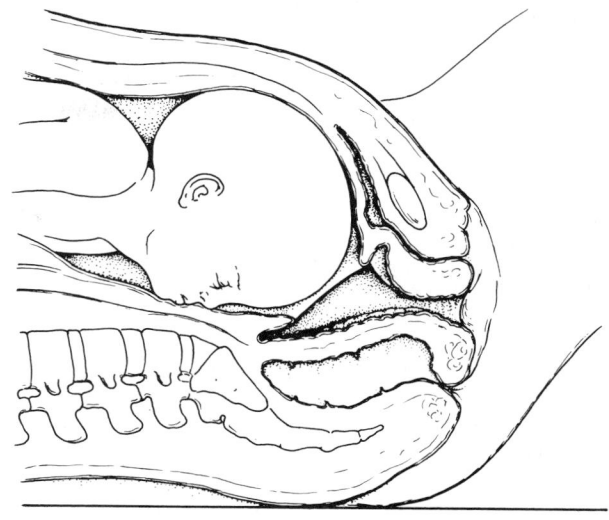

FIGURE 38-11

Severe dystocia from hydrocephalus, cephalic presentation. Note the disparity between the small size of the face and the rest of the cranium.

high probability of death for the fetus; the father is stressed by the high risk situation; and the physician and nurse must cope with a grave crisis and a poor prognosis. This is a situation in which the nurse is called on to exercise all of her nursing skill, both during the labor and after the delivery. The components of care that are useful in helping the parents in such a crisis are discussed in Chapter 45.

Problems with the Psyche

The client's psyche may influence the duration and character of labor considerably.[5] The woman who is fearful, anxious, or even extremely excited may become tense and have difficulty working with her contractions. These women often have longer, more uncomfortable labors. The release of catecholamines in response to stress is thought to interfere with the activity of the myometrium, and the woman's increased tension leads to fatigue. Childbirth preparation classes in many instances help to prevent these problems. Supportive nursing care during labor can also aid the woman in relaxation.

Hemorrhagic Complications

Hemorrhage is probably a more important cause of maternal death in the United States than statistics indicate, because national vital statistics are based only on the *immediate* cause of death. The death of a woman who hemorrhaged after labor, contracted postpartum infection, and died would be classified as due to infection, although hemorrhage was the real underlying cause. The major causes of hemorrhage associated with childbearing are placenta previa, abruptio placentae (see Chap. 36), and uterine atony.

Postpartum Hemorrhage

Hemorrhage during the postpartum period is the most common cause of serious blood loss associated with pregnancy, and it causes about one fourth of all maternal deaths from hemorrhagic complications. The debilitation and lowered resistance that often accompany it are related to postpartum infections, another leading cause of maternal death. To a large extent, death from postpartum hemorrhage is preventable if the condition is diagnosed early and treated aggressively.

Definition and Incidence

Postpartum hemorrhage is commonly defined as loss of more than 500 ml of blood during the first 24 hours after giving birth. However, ordinary blood loss following vaginal delivery frequently is more than 500 ml by accurate measurement. Most obstetricians estimate the amount of bleeding at delivery, and studies show that estimated blood loss is usually only about one half of actual loss. Therefore, an *estimated* blood loss over 500 ml serves to alert the nurse and physician that the client has bled excessively and is in danger of postpartum hemorrhage.

Bleeding of this degree occurs once in every 20 or 30 cases despite the most skilled care. Hemorrhages of 1000 ml and over are encountered once in about every 75 cases, whereas blood losses of 1500 and 2000 ml are encountered less frequently. Postpartum hemorrhage is a fairly common complication of labor, and one with which the nurse should be intimately familiar, since nurses are expected to assume an important role in its prevention, detection, and treatment.

Causes

In order of frequency, the three immediate causes of postpartum hemorrhage are uterine atony, lacerations of the birth canal (perineum, vagina, and cervix), and retained placental fragments. Clotting defects, uterine tumors, and infections as well as obstetric accidents such as inversion of the uterus, can also be classified as causes of postpartum hemorrhage, but they are less common and of a more indirect nature.

Uterine Atony.   Uterine atony is by far the most common cause of postpartum hemorrhage. The uterus contains huge blood vessels within the interstices of its muscle fibers, and those at the placental site are open and gaping. It is essential that the muscle fibers contract down tightly on these arteries and veins if bleeding is to be controlled. They must *stay* contracted down, because relaxation for only a few seconds gives rise to sudden, profuse hemorrhage. They must stay *tightly* contracted down, because continuous, slight relaxation gives rise to continuous oozing of blood, one of the most treacherous forms of postpartum hemorrhage.

In a study of 56 maternal deaths from pregnancy-related hemorrhage over a 9-year period in California, 19 were due to uterine atony. The majority of these women died within 4 hours of delivery, possibly before the seriousness of their bleeding was recognized. Generally, these patients were older multiparas with spontaneous term deliveries; most of the deaths were avoidable had the hemorrhage been diagnosed earlier and adequate treatment instituted in time.[1]

Lacerations.   Lacerations of the perineum, the vagina, and the cervix are naturally more common after operative delivery. Tears of the cervix are particularly likely to cause serious hemorrhage. Bright red arterial bleeding in the presence of a hard, firmly contracted uterus (no uterine atony) suggests hemorrhage from a cervical laceration. The physician establishes the diagnosis by actual inspection of the cervix (retractors are necessary) and, after locating the source of bleeding, repairs the laceration.

Perineal and vaginal tears also contribute to postpartum blood loss. In addition, perineal tears may do great damage in destroying the integrity of the perineum and in weakening the supports of the uterus, the bladder, and the rectum. Unless these lacerations are repaired properly, the resultant weakness, as the years go by, may cause prolapse of the uterus, cystocele (a pouching downward of the bladder), or rectocele (a pouching forward of the rectum). These conditions, which often originate from perineal lacerations at childbirth, give rise to many discomforts and often necessitate operative treatment.

Lacerations of the birth canal sometimes occur during the process of normal delivery and may be unavoidable even in the most skilled hands.

Retained Placental Fragments.   Small, partially separated fragments of placenta may cause postpartum hemorrhage by interfering with proper uterine contraction (Fig. 38-12). Careful inspection of the placenta to determine whether a piece is missing should be routinely carried out at delivery. If a portion is missing, exploration of the uterus is indicated to remove the placental

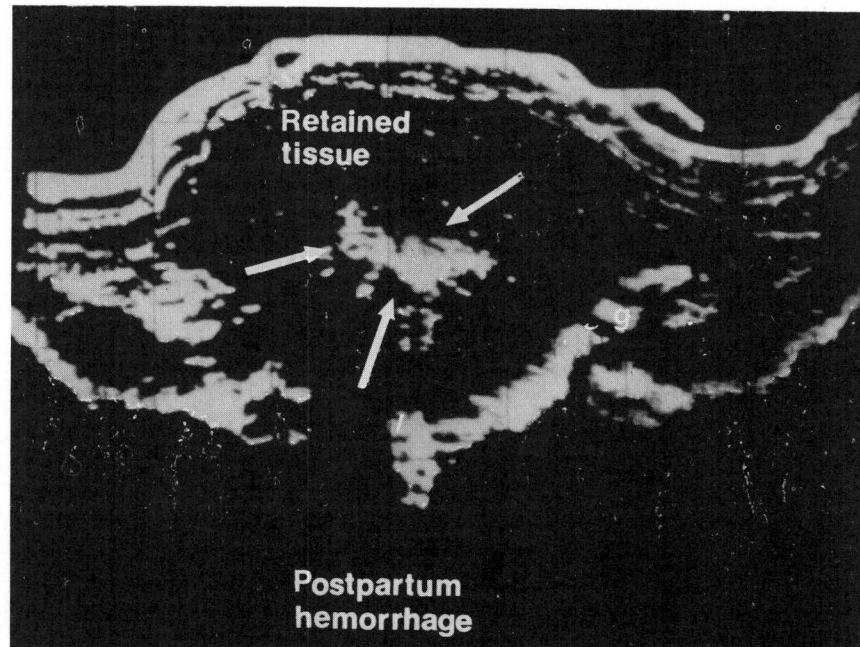

FIGURE 38-12

Postpartum hemorrhage. Retained tissue demonstrated on sonogram. This requires surgical evacuation. (Cavanagh D, Woods RE, O'Connor TCF, Knuppel RA: Obstetric Emergencies, 3rd ed. Philadelphia, Harper & Row, 1982)

fragment. In the case of continued postpartum bleeding, retention of placental fragments is generally ruled out by manual exploration. However, this is rarely a cause of immediate postpartum hemorrhage and is more commonly implicated in late hemorrhage in which profuse bleeding occurs suddenly a week or more after delivery.

Predisposing Factors

There are certain factors that predispose to postpartum hemorrhage, so in a majority of cases it may be anticipated in advance. Hemorrhage due to uterine atony can be anticipated following labors with overdistention of the uterus (large baby, twins, polyhydramnios), labors in which deep anesthesia was used, and labors in which there were either very vigorous contractions or hypotonic contractions. High parity or previous postpartum hemorrhage also puts the woman at increased risk for hemorrhage due to uterine atony.

Delivery of a large baby, midforceps or forceps rotation, intrauterine manipulation, and delivery after cesarean section are examples of situations in which trauma is likely to lead to postpartum hemorrhage, probably from lacerations of the uterus or birth canal. Attempts to hasten the delivery of the placenta in the third stage of labor may also lead to hemorrhage.

It should be noted that a small woman withstands blood loss less well than a woman of average size or larger. An average-sized, relatively healthy mother can lose up to 1% of her blood volume without immediate crises. It is not difficult to relate body weight to blood volume, since 1 ml of blood equals 1 g. Therefore, if a woman loses 1% of her body weight through blood loss, she is considered to have a hemorrhage.[13]

Clinical Picture

Excessive bleeding may occur prior to the birth of the placenta, but is seen more commonly following the third stage. Although it is occasionally torrential, the most common type is a continuous trickle, minute by minute. These small constant trickles are not alarming in appearance and are therefore more treacherous, since no one may become concerned and no action may be taken.

The condition and size of the client determine the amount of blood loss that can be tolerated, with exhaustion from prolonged labor or antecedent anemia or chronic disease reducing the ability of the body to compensate. When hemorrhage has been profuse enough, the pulse becomes rapid and thready, the skin becomes pallid and clammy, and chills and disturbed vision occur. As shock deepens, air hunger develops, with restlessness and sweating; unconsciousness and death may follow. The pulse and blood pressure may not change significantly until large amounts of blood have been lost; then the vascular mechanism fails and shock ensues. Vascular collapse may lead to death when intravenous infusion cannot be maintained for blood replacement. Cardiac arrest may also occur at this point.

Shock

During any stage of pregnancy, hemorrhage poses a severe threat to the mother. This is especially true of postpartum hemorrhage because the shock that accompanies the blood loss is often out of proportion to the amount lost.

When hemorrhaging occurs, the body activates certain compensatory mechanisms. The adrenals release catecholamines, which cause the arterioles and venules of the skin, liver, gastrointestinal tract, lungs, and kidneys to constrict. This diverts blood to the brain and heart. When shock persists, cellular oxygenation continues to be reduced, which results in accumulation of lactic acid and consequent acidosis. Serum acidosis in turn causes arteriole vasodilatation, but venule vasoconstriction persists. Thus, a downward spiral is established in which the decreased perfusion, increased tissue acidosis and anoxia, edema, and blood pooling further decrease perfusion of the tissues. Eventually, cellular death occurs and the patient dies.[14] Acceptable ranges in various systems while managing shock are given in Table 38-3.

Management. Medical interventions for the woman experiencing a postpartum hemorrhage will depend on the cause of the hemorrhage and the stage at which it is detected. If the bleeding occurs prior to delivery of the placenta, the physician may find it necessary to remove the placenta manually. Early postpartum hemorrhage due to uterine atony will usually be treated with fundal massage and oxytocics. If the hemorrhage is the result of lacerations or retained placental fragments, the

TABLE 38-3

Goals of Shock Management

Variables	Acceptable Adult Ranges
Cardiovascular	
Pulse rate	<90 beats/min
Arterial pulse pressure	>30 mm Hg
Central venous pressure	5 cm–12 cm H_2O
Pulmonary arterial pressure	
Systolic	25 mm Hg–30 mm Hg
Diastolic	8 mm Hg–10 mm Hg
Pulmonary wedge pressure	8 mm Hg–15 mm Hg
Hematocrit	35%–45%
Hemoglobin	>11 g/dl
Respiratory-metabolic	
Respiratory rate	12–15 breaths/min
Arterial PO_2	80 mm Hg–100 mm Hg
Arterial PCO_2	37 mm Hg–45 mm Hg
Arteriovenous O_2 extraction	40 ml/liter
Arterial pH	7.35–7.45
Renal	
Urinary output	30 ml–50 ml/hr

(Court D: Maternal cardiovascular and renal disorders: Maternal shock in pregnancy. In Creasy RK, Resnik R (eds.): Maternal-Fetal Medicine. Philadelphia, WB Saunders, 1984)

client may be returned to the delivery room for repair or uterine evacuation.

It is necessary that there be *fluid replacement* for serious hemorrhage to combat hypovolemia. Pritchard recommends two general guidelines. First, lactated Ringer's solution and whole blood are given in amount and proportion to maintain a urine flow of at least 30 ml/hr and preferably 60 ml/hr (1 ml/min). In addition, the hematocrit is maintained at 30% or slightly higher. Second, if initial vigorous fluid replacement therapy does not maintain or restore the urine flow, then the central venous pressure (CVP) is monitored and fluids are adjusted accordingly.

CVP readings provide important information regarding fluid needs and can aid in preventing circulatory overload. The normal range is between 5 and 8 cm H_2O. Values below 5 cm H_2O are indicative of significant hemorrhage and the need for transfusion of whole blood. Elevation of the CVP above 15 cm H_2O occurs with fluid overload, pulmonary embolus, and left heart failure.[15] To institute this type of monitoring, a catheter is inserted into the subclavian vein, between the clavicle and the first rib (Fig. 38-13).

A more accurate assessment of cardiopulmonary status and problems can be supplied through measurement of *pulmonary wedge pressure* by means of a Swan-Ganz catheter. This double lumen catheter, tipped with an inflatable balloon, is introduced into the external jugular, subclavian, or femoral vein, and its progress is followed by continuous pressure monitoring, with electronic transducers and an oscilloscope, while it is threaded into the right atrium. The balloon is inflated and is carried by blood flow through the right ventricle and into the pulmonary artery. The balloon is then deflated and the catheter secured.[15–17]

Since *blood transfusion* plays an important role in preventing serious shock, the blood groups of *all* maternity clients should be known before labor, and cross-matched blood should be available for those in whom hemorrhage is anticipated or appears imminent. Seeing that the blood typing is carried out, ordering and calling for the cross match, and making sure that the blood is sent to the unit are usually responsibilities of the nurse. Time is of the essence for these clients; therefore, the nurse must preplan and establish priorities with rapidity.

If oxytocin therapy fails to stop the bleeding, the physician probably will carry out bimanual compression of the uterus. This provides the most efficient means of compressing the site of bleeding. Packing the uterus with gauze, a procedure once considered valuable to promote hemostasis in such cases, is seldom used today. It is considered by many to be inadequate treatment and conducive to infection.

Immediate treatment of hemorrhagic shock suggested by Danforth[15] includes elevation of the legs to a 30° angle, oxygen by mask, rapid infusion of lactated

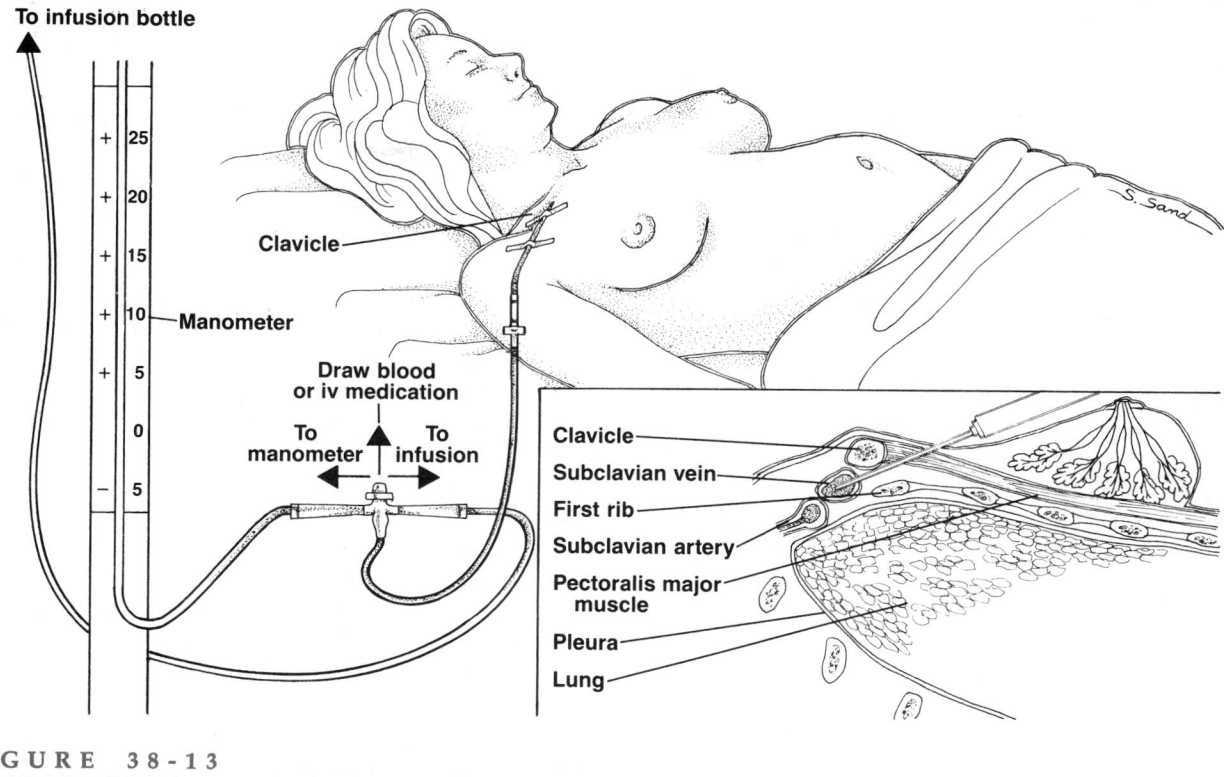

FIGURE 38-13

(*A*) Insertion of CVP catheter into subclavian vein. (*B*) Plastic catheter and CVP setup in place. (Modified from Malinak et al: Am J Obstet Gynecol 92:447, 1965)

Ringer's solution, and drawing blood for type and cross matching. This would be followed by close monitoring of vital signs, including CVP monitoring, insertion of a Foley catheter to monitor urine output, and blood transfusion, if indicated. The Trendelenburg position is avoided because it may interfere with cerebral circulation and respiratory exchange.

Assessment in Hemorrhagic Complications

The nurse plays a primary role in the prevention, detection, and treatment of postpartum hemorrhage, especially that caused by uterine atony. Routine nursing assessment of vital signs, condition of the uterus, and amount of bleeding in the early postpartum period is directed toward detecting uterine atony and subsequent increased bleeding (see Chaps. 25 and 31). Assessment should include review of the chart to identify any factors that would place the client at risk for hemorrhage. For the client at risk, or any client with increased bleeding, the vital signs, fundus, and amount of bleeding should be checked more frequently than routine. The client should also be monitored for other signs of impending shock, such as changes in skin color and temperature, decreased urinary output, or changes in level of consciousness (Fig. 38-14 and Table 38-4).

Nursing Diagnosis

Assessment of the client for signs and symptoms of postpartum hemorrhage may lead the nurse to some of the following nursing diagnoses: fluid volume deficit related to excessive blood loss and manifested by increased pulse rate, decreased blood pressure, and decreased urinary output; potential for infection related to decreased resistance secondary to excessive blood loss; fear/anxiety related to concern about bleeding as a life-threatening situation.

Planning/Intervention

If one suspects that a woman may be hemorrhaging, it is important that the nurse remain with her constantly. The fundus should be checked immediately. The physician needs to be notified, and the emergency equipment must be easily accessible, including intravenous tray with large-bore (#18) needles, retention catheter, and oxygen, suction, blood pressure, and CVP apparatus.

Massaging the Fundus. The uterus should be grasped immediately and massaged gently but firmly. The lower uterine segment is supported with the edge

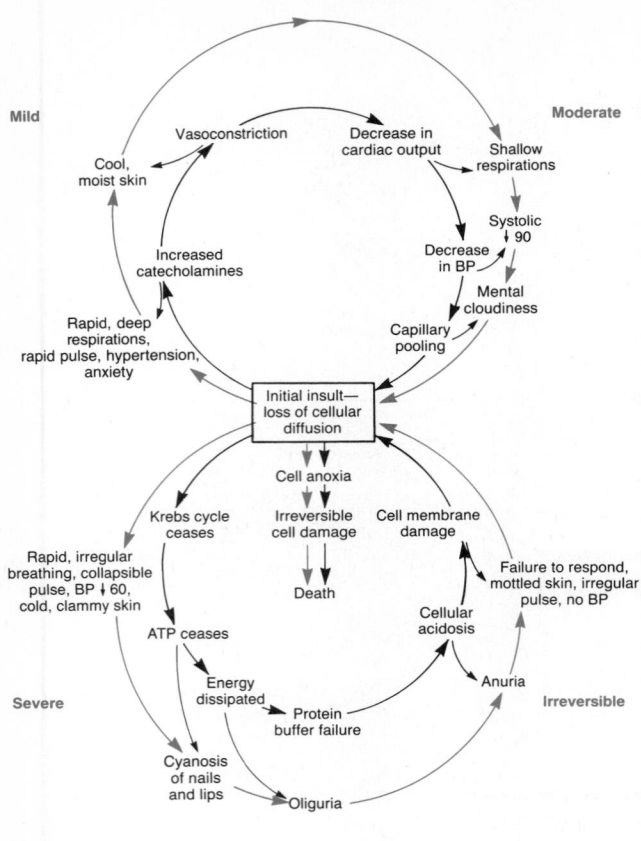

Mild

Moderate

Severe

Irreversible

FIGURE   38-14

Diagram of physiological alterations in shock in relation to symptoms. (Royce JA: Shock: Emergency nursing implications. Nurs Clin North Am 8:377, 1973)

of the hand a little above the mother's symphysis, while the fundus is massaged with the other hand (see Fig. 25-19). Thus, the uterus is cupped between the two hands and is supported as it is massaged. Massage is to be continued until the uterus assumes a woody hardness; if the slightest relaxation occurs, the massage must be reinstituted. In many cases the uterus stays contracted most of the time, but occasionally it relaxes; it is therefore obligatory to keep a hand on the fundus constantly for a full hour after bleeding has subsided. When the uterus is well contracted, care should be taken to *avoid overmassage*, because such practice contributes to muscle fatigue, which in turn further encourages uterine relaxation and excessive bleeding.

It must be remembered that relaxation sometimes occurs 2 or more hours after delivery; in these cases the uterus may balloon with blood, with very little escaping externally. Accordingly, the consistency, size, and height of the uterus should be checked frequently until several hours have elapsed. Ordinarily, the height of the fundus after delivery is about at the level of the umbilicus. If the uterus becomes distended with blood, or if the

bladder becomes full and presses upward against the uterus, causing it to rise in the abdomen, then the fundus can be palpated several centimeters above the umbilicus. The nurse must make absolutely certain that the uterus is in fact being massaged, and not a roll of abdominal fat or a distended bladder. When properly contracted, the uterus should feel about the size and consistency of a small, firm grapefruit.

Frequently, a big, boggy, relaxed uterus is difficult to outline through the abdominal wall, and it may be necessary to push the hand well posteriorly toward the region of the sacral promontory to reach it. The very fact that the uterus is hard to identify usually means that it is relaxed, but palpation and massage will often cause it to become firm.

Allaying Anxiety.   The frequent massage and deep palpation are often painful to the mother; at best, they are disturbing, since they come at a time when she wants nothing more than to rest and sleep after her great effort. If she is awake and alert, then the continued attention and scrutiny may increase her anxiety. It must be remembered that apprehension is a natural concomitant of hemorrhage and shock. Quick and efficient nursing observations and appropriate explanation and reassurance help allay the concerns of both the mother and her partner.

This aspect of nursing care may be difficult to implement. If the mother or the father expresses concern and questions the activity by asking "What's wrong?", then the nurse can simply say, "The uterus has a tendency to relax and must be massaged so that it will contract down as it should." Usually, such a statement suffices. This indicates the reason for the continued activity without associating hemorrhage and its fearsome consequences with the actions of the attendants. If the mother drifts off to sleep between the nurse's observations, then the nurse can gently rouse her by speaking her name before commencing massage, so that the mother is not awakened abruptly to the painful sensation of someone squeezing her abdomen.

Other Aspects of Care.   Vital signs must be checked every 5 to 15 minutes, and any variation, however slight, is to be reported immediately. Skin condition, level of consciousness, and urinary output are also monitored.

One way that the nurse can keep a more accurate account of the blood loss is by keeping a perineal pad count. A record is kept of the number of pads saturated, how fully they are saturated, and the time it took for the saturation to occur. Thus, the nurse's notes might read: "Two pads ¾ saturated in 20 minutes." This type of report is more helpful to the physician than a more general, vague statement like, "Saturating perineal pads quickly."

TABLE 38-4

Symptoms of Shock

	Mild	Moderate	Severe	Irreversible
Respirations	Rapid, deep	Rapid, becoming shallow	Rapid, shallow, may be irregular	Irregular, or barely perceptible
Pulse	Rapid, tone normal	Rapid, tone may be normal but is becoming weaker	Very rapid, easily collapsible, may be irregular	Irregular apical pulse
Blood pressure	Normal or hypertensive	60 mm Hg–90 mm Hg systolic	Below 60 mm Hg systolic	None palpable
Skin	Cool and pale	Cool, pale, moist, knees cyanotic	Cold, clammy, cyanosis of lips and fingernails	Cold, clammy, cyanotic
Urine output	No change	Decreasing to 10 ml/hr–22 ml/hr (adult)	Oliguric (less than 10 ml) to anuria	Anuric
Level of consciousness	Alert, oriented, diffuse anxiety	Oriented, mental cloudiness or increasing restlessness	Lethargy, reacts to noxious stimuli, comatose	Does not respond to noxious stimuli
CVP	May be normal	3 cm H$_2$O	0 cm H$_2$O–3 cm H$_2$O	

(Royce JA: Shock: Emergency nursing implications. Nurs Clin North Am 8:377, 1973; Wagner MM: Clinical Nursing Specialist, University of Iowa Hospitals and Clinics)

Rupture of the Uterus

Rupture of the uterus is fortunately a rare complication, occurring about once in every 2000 pregnancies. It constitutes one of the gravest accidents in obstetrics, however, since the mortality rate for the infant is 50% to 75% and virtually all untreated mothers die of hypovolemia from hemorrhage or, less often, of infection. In this condition, the uterus simply bursts because the strain placed upon its musculature is more than it can withstand. Uterine rupture may occur in pregnancy but is far more frequent in labor.[1]

While the incidence has not changed to any degree in the past several decades, the etiology has changed, and the outcome has improved significantly. Today, the most common cause is attributed to rupture of the scar from a previous cesarean section, especially from a classical incision. Women in labor after a cesarean are observed closely for any signs of uterine rupture. The second most common etiologic agent is felt to be injudicious stimulation of labor with oxytocin. Other contributing factors include previous surgery involving the myometrium, prolonged or obstructed labor, certain faulty positions or fetal abnormalities, multiparity, excessive fetal size, and traumatic delivery, such as version and extraction, or injudicious use of forceps.[13]

When rupture occurs, the patient complains of a severe, sudden, lancinating pain during a strong labor contraction. The rupture may be complete or incomplete; pain and abdominal tenderness are usually present in both cases. If there is complete rupture, regular contractions cease because the torn muscle can no longer contract. There is an outpouring of blood into the abdominal cavity and sometimes into the vagina. The uterus may be palpated abdominally as a hard mass lying alongside the fetus. The patient soon exhibits signs of shock.

If the rupture is incomplete, the contractions may continue, and the signs of shock may be delayed, since the blood loss is slower. As soon as the diagnosis of rupture of the uterus is made, rapid preparations for an abdominal operation should ensue, since hysterectomy is the usual treatment. In addition, antibiotics are administered to combat infection, and blood transfusions and fluids are given to replace lost blood and to alleviate shock.

Since this accident gravely compromises the lives of both the infant and the mother, prevention, early diagnosis, prompt treatment, blood transfusions, and antibiotics are essential components in improving the prognosis.

The nursing care is essentially that for any complicated delivery with potential hemorrhage and shock. Whenever possible it is advisable to have the nurse who has been attending the mother during labor remain with her until the anesthetic for the cesarean section is given. This provides some measure of continuity of care and help in reassurance and comfort of the parents.

Inversion of the Uterus

Inversion of the uterus is a highly fatal accident of labor in which, after the birth of the infant, the uterus turns inside out. Shock is profound, and hemorrhage may occur, which if not treated quickly will cause the death of the mother.

There are two common causes of this accident, both of which are preventable: (1) pulling on the umbilical cord and (2) trying to express the placenta when the uterus is relaxed. In the former case, the traction on the attached placenta simply pulls the uterus inside out, while in the latter, the hand pushes the relaxed muscular sac inside out. Thus, the umbilical cord should never have strenuous traction applied nor should the uterus be pushed downward unless it is firmly contracted.

It is imperative that several steps in treatment be taken promptly and simultaneously. (1) Two intravenous infusion systems are instituted, one with lactated Ringer's solution and one with whole blood. These are given promptly to refill the intravascular compartment and support cardiac output. (2) An anesthesiologist gives a general anesthetic, usually halothane, to relax the uterus. The placenta is left in place until the infusions are operational and uterine relaxation has been accomplished. If the placenta is removed prematurely, hemorrhage is increased. Attempts are then made to replace the uterus in the vagina by placing the palm of the hand on the center of the fundus with the fingers extended to identify the cervical margins. The fundus is then pushed up through the cervix. When the uterus is returned to its normal shape, anesthesia is discontinued and oxytocin is begun to help the uterus remain contracted. Bimanual compression also aids in this. The uterus is then monitored transvaginally until normal tone is assured.

If the uterus cannot be placed from below because of a constriction ring, a laparotomy is performed so that the uterus can be pulled up simultaneously from above and pushed up from below. The constriction ring may be incised. A traction suture in the fundus aids in repositioning. Treatment continues as previously described. Subsequent inversion is unlikely.[1]

Disorders of Placental Attachment

Other important causes of bleeding associated with labor are those related to the placenta. Placenta previa and abruptio placentae have been discussed previously as complications of pregnancy (see Chapter 36). At times, however, the first signs of these problems become evident during labor, and the nurse in the labor and delivery area should be familiar with their diagnosis and management.

Placenta Previa

The cardinal sign of placenta previa is painless, bright-red vaginal bleeding. If bleeding from this condition has not been identified until after labor begins, contractions and bloody show may confuse the situation.

Identification depends on accurately assessing the extent of vaginal bleeding. Overt hemorrhage with huge blood loss is not difficult to diagnose, but it requires fine judgment to decide when bloody vaginal discharge ceases to be heavy "show" and becomes potential hemorrhage. Any vaginal bleeding that the nurse believes is excessive should be reported to the physician, and vaginal examination of these patients should be avoided.

Abruptio Placentae

Abruptio placentae can be a true obstetric emergency if the area of separation is extensive. The signs that alert the labor and delivery room nurse to this complication include a hypertonic uterus that does not relax well between contractions, an area of extreme sensitivity when the uterus is palpated, sudden sharp and persistent uterine pain, and symptoms and signs of shock that seem greater than the observable blood loss would indicate. An extremely hard, boardlike uterus that cannot be indented and does not relax indicates a severe degree of placental separation and bleeding.

Marginal sinus rupture was formerly treated as a separate clinical entity, but now is felt to be a mild type of abruptio placentae in which slight separation occurs at the edge of the placenta. The marginal sinus is located under the edge of the placenta and is one of the large maternal sinuses bathing the placental villi. If the placenta separates at a point along its margin, this maternal sinus is disrupted and bleeding occurs. There is usually no increased pain or uterine tension, and the amount of vaginal bleeding may vary considerably. If the area of separation is small, as it usually is in marginal sinus rupture, there is no danger of hypoxia to the fetus and generally are no changes in fetal heart rate. When there is excessive vaginal bleeding during labor and placenta previa and abruptio placentae have been ruled out, the most probable cause is a small marginal separation of the placenta. Nursing care is the same as for other hemorrhagic conditions.

Placenta Accreta

At times the attachment of the placenta to the uterus is so firm that the placenta does not separate spontaneously from its site of implantation during the third stage of labor. The term *placenta accreta* is used to describe any implantation of the placenta in which this abnormally firm adherence to the uterine wall exists. This condition is usually the result of partial or total absence of the decidua basalis, which allows the placental villi to attach to the myometrium. Other terms may be used to denote deeper penetration of the villi: *placenta increta* when the villi *invade* the myometrium and *placenta percreta* when they *penetrate* the myometrium. The abnormal adherence may be total, partial,

Woman with Postpartum Hemorrhage

Nursing Objectives

1. Identify client at risk for early postpartum hemorrhage.
2. Detect excessive vaginal bleeding as early as possible.
3. Control bleeding through early and continued intervention.
4. Maintain stable vital signs.

Assessment	Potential Nursing Diagnosis	Planning/Intervention	Evaluation
Risk factors for postpartum hemorrhage:		Review chart for risk factors	
Overdistention of uterus (large baby, twins, polyhydramnios)	Potential for excessive vaginal bleeding related to relaxation of uterine muscle secondary to twin pregnancy	Identify client at risk, and monitor uterus, lochia, and vital signs closely	
Abnormal uterine contractions (hypotonic, tetanic)			
Oxytocin induction or augmentation of labor			
Grandmultiparity			
Previous postpartum hemorrhage			
Difficult (traumatic) delivery			
Condition of uterus		Check uterus every 15 minutes times 4 or until it remains firm without excessive bleeding	Client has a firm fundus with return to normal lochia
Firmness			
Size			
Height of fundus		Massage fundus until firm, express blood and clots as necessary	
Lochia			
Amount		Estimate amount of bleeding	
Color		Initiate pad count	
Presence of clots		Observe for continuous trickle of blood in presence of contracted uterus	
		Start IV line if not in place	
		Maintain IV with oxytocin at ordered rate	
		Administer other medications as ordered	
Vital Signs	Fluid volume deficit related to excessive blood loss and manifested by increased pulse rate, decreased blood pressure, and decreased urinary output	Check every 15 minutes or as ordered	Client avoids hypovolemic shock
Temperature-pulse-respiration		Report and record	Client's vital signs stabilize
Blood pressure			
CVP (if used)			
Urinary output		Keep accurate intake and output record; insert Foley catheter for more accurate output, if indicated	Client voids as planned
		Encourage emptying of bladder	

(continued)

Assessment	Potential Nursing Diagnosis	Planning/Intervention	Evaluation
Skin: color and temperature		Observe for pallor; cool, moist skin	
Level of consciousness		Check orientation of client by speaking to her frequently	
Emotional status	Fear/anxiety related to concern about excessive bleeding as life-threatening situation	Keep client and family members informed about what is happening and what is being done	Client verbalizes her confidence in recovery
		Reassure as indicated	
Lab values		Make sure that type and cross match are done if indicated	
		Make sure that hemoglobin, hematocrit, other lab work are done, as ordered	
Need for surgical intervention		Make sure client is informed about procedure	Client repeats information she understands about procedures
		Complete surgical checklist	
	Potential for infection related to decreased resistance to pathogenic organisms secondary to excessive blood loss	Maintain aseptic technique	Client remains free of infection

or focal, depending on the number of cotyledons involved.[1]

Predisposing factors to placenta accreta are implantations where decidual formation may be defective, such as in the lower uterine segment (placenta previa), over a previous cesarean section scar, or after uterine curettage. The reported incidence varies, but was stated as 1 per 2562 deliveries in a 1980 study.[1] The condition is usually not recognized until the third stage of labor when the placenta does not separate. Maternal hemorrhage may be profuse, and hysterectomy is often necessary.

Preterm Labor

Preterm labor is defined as labor that begins before 37 completed weeks of pregnancy. The lower limit is not well established. Twenty-eight weeks was most frequently used in the past, but with the increasing ability to care for the infant born prior to 28 weeks, 20 weeks

is now more frequently used as the lower limit. The infants resulting from these preterm labors account for a significant proportion of perinatal morbidity and mortality. Preterm labor occurs in approximately 5% to 7% of pregnancies.[18] Prevention of preterm delivery is now considered to be the most important problem to be dealt with in improving the outcome of pregnancies in which there are no congenital anomalies.[19]

The problem of preterm labor is currently the focus of many studies. These studies are directed toward several different aspects of the problem, including prediction, prevention, early detection, diagnosis, and management. In the absence of conclusive data in any of these areas, interventions and protocols in different institutions or geographic areas are varied.

Prediction

Certain maternal factors have been shown to be related to increased risk for preterm labor and delivery. Most of these are the same risk factors that place the expectant mother at increased risk for other pregnancy problems. Those factors suggested by Hobel to be most clearly related to preterm labor are stress from interrelated factors, including age under 18, poor nutrition, poor hygiene, employment, smoking; obstetric-gynecologic history such as previous second-trimester abortion or previous preterm birth; and such current pregnancy factors as multiple pregnancy or hydramnios.[20]

Creasy and associates have developed a risk assessment tool (Table 38-5) that successfully identified 64% of the women in their study population who subsequently delivered prior to term.[19] However, approximately two thirds of the women with high-risk scores did not go into labor prematurely. The development of biochemical and biophysical measurements to be used with the tool could improve the accuracy of predicting the woman at risk. The women in the study who were identified as being at high risk were started on a treatment protocol when beginning signs of preterm labor were identified. These interventions resulted in lowering the preterm birth rate in the experimental group compared with the control group. The tool and protocols are now being used in other areas with the hope of replicating these results. In some studies it has proved to be less successful. Main and co-workers suggest that the tool may need modification for use with different populations.[21]

Prevention

Efforts to prevent preterm labor are directed toward prevention or detection of risk factors and treatment of these factors as appropriate. Interventions to prevent the onset of labor in women found to be at risk have not proved to be very effective in most cases. Good dietary counseling and encouragement to reduce or preferably eliminate maternal cigarette smoking or use of unnecessary drugs are appropriate interventions for pregnant women in general, but may be particularly helpful for the woman at risk for preterm labor. Bed rest has proved useful in preventing preterm labor with multiple gestations, but its usefulness in single gestation is not known. Bacterial infection of the lower genital tract is suspected by some researchers to contribute to the onset of preterm labor. Prevention of infection might help prevent some preterm labors. Avoiding intercourse has also been suggested as a preventive measure, both for reducing the risk of infection and because the prostaglandins in seminal fluid are thought possibly to stimulate uterine contractions.[20]

Cervical cerclage has been found to be effective in preventing preterm labor related to incompetent cervix, but its use in preventing preterm births from other causes is in doubt. To the contrary, there is some evidence that placement of a cerclage after 20 weeks may promote uterine contractions.[19]

There have been some efforts to use pharmacologic methods prophylactically. Use of progesterone in preventing preterm labor has shown mixed results. Suggestions of possible teratogenic effects have resulted in a ban on the use of progestins during pregnancy by the United States Food and Drug Administration (FDA). The usefulness of prophylactic β-adrenergic therapy is also unclear after several studies.[19]

Early Detection and Diagnosis

Prevention of preterm birth through early detection and treatment of preterm labor has become more possible since the discovery of new, more effective tocolytic agents to arrest labor. Preterm labor must be detected early if tocolytic agents are to be used, since their effectiveness decreases with the advance of labor. Client education and frequent evaluation of the cervix for high-risk patients have proved effective in early identification of preterm labor in some studies.[19]

Diagnosis of preterm labor in time to prevent preterm birth is often difficult. The presence of regular uterine contractions does not always mean true labor has begun. Rupture of the membranes accompanied by regular uterine contractions establishes the diagnosis, but attempting to stop the labor at this point may not be wise. Progressive cervical effacement and dilatation can also establish the diagnosis, but, again, advanced dilatation is a contraindication to tocolysis.

The following criteria are usually used in the diagnosis of preterm labor when membranes are intact: (1) uterine contractions at least once every 10 minutes and lasting at least 30 seconds and (2) documented cervical change or cervical effacement of 80% or dilatation of 2 cm.[19]

Management

Until fairly recently measures available to arrest the progress of preterm labor were limited to conservative treatment such as bed rest. Today there are a number of drugs that are used to try to inhibit preterm labor. These are referred to as *tocolytic agents*. If preterm labor begins, the question becomes whether or not to use these agents in an attempt to prevent preterm birth. Indications for use of a tocolytic drug to inhibit labor are a client suspected of being in preterm labor, gestational age greater than 20 weeks but less than 36 weeks, estimated fetal weight less than 2500 g, and no contraindications to continuing the pregnancy.[22]

Contraindications to attempting to inhibit labor are ruptured membranes, active uterine bleeding, maternal medical complications such as diabetes or severe preeclampsia, chronic fetal distress such as intrauterine growth retardation, acute fetal distress, intrauterine infection, cervical dilatation greater than 3 cm, major fetal anomalies incompatible with life, and intrauterine fetal death.[22,23]

TABLE 38-5

System for Determining Risk of Spontaneous Preterm Delivery*

Points Assigned	Socioeconomic Factors	Previous Medical History	Daily Habits	Aspects of Current Pregnancy
1	Two children at home Low socioeconomic status	Abortion ×1 Less than 1 year since last birth	Works outside home	Unusual fatigue
2	Maternal age <20 years or >40 years Single parent	Abortion ×2	Smokes more than 10 cigarettes per day	Gain of less than 5 kg by 32 weeks
3	Very low socioeconomic status Height <150 cm Weight <45 kg	Abortion ×3	Heavy or stressful work Long, tiring trip	Breech at 32 weeks Weight loss of 2 kg Head engaged at 32 weeks Febrile illness
4	Maternal age <18 years	Pyelonephritis		Bleeding after 12 weeks Effacement Dilation Uterine irritability
5		Uterine anomaly Second-trimester abortion Diethylstilbestrol exposure Cone biopsy		Placenta previa Hydramnios
10		Preterm delivery Repeated second-trimester abortion		Twins Abdominal surgery

* Score is computed by adding the number of points given any item. The score is computed at the first visit and again at 22 to 26 weeks' gestation. A total score of 10 or more places client at high risk of spontaneous preterm delivery.
Creasy RK: Disorders of parturition: Preterm labor and delivery. In Creasy RK, Resnik R (eds) Maternal-Fetal Medicine: Principles and Practice. Philadelphia, WB Saunders, 1984

If the decision is made to attempt to halt the labor, a combination of supportive and pharmacologic interventions will probably be implemented.

General Measures.   Bed rest in the left lateral position is sometimes effective in reducing the frequency and intensity of uterine contractions. Hydration, usually by intravenous infusion, is also used. It is thought to decrease release of antidiuretic hormone and oxytocin from the posterior pituitary gland.[23] Unnecessary vaginal manipulation should be avoided.

Use of Tocolytic Agents.   *Ethyl alcohol (ethanol)*, administered intravenously to the mother, was the first tocolytic agent used with success and was a popular intervention in the 1960s and 1970s. However, the high levels needed to suppress uterine contractions caused intoxication in the mother and fetus; ethanol has also been found to cause metabolic problems, and with the growing concern over the effects of alcohol on the fetus, it has mostly been abandoned for use in arresting preterm labor.[1]

β-adrenergic agonists are currently in use as tocolytic agents. This group of drugs includes ritodrine (Yutopar), terbutaline (Brethine), isoxsuprine (Vasodilan), and others. Only ritodrine is currently approved by the FDA for use in inhibiting preterm labor, but the others are used in other countries and have been used in the United States on an experimental basis. These drugs are primarily β_2 stimulators and lead to relaxation of bronchial, vascular, and uterine smooth muscle, but they also exhibit some β_1 effects, stimulating myocardial contractility and heart rate. Common side-effects of these agents are maternal and fetal tachycardia, hypotension, and nervousness, with occasional more severe side-effects such as cardiac arrhythmias, hypokalemia, or pulmonary edema.[24] These drugs are usually given intravenously, but some may be given orally, and this route is used for maintenance after contractions have stopped (Table 38-6).

Magnesium sulfate has been used with some success in arresting preterm labor, although it is not yet approved for this purpose by the FDA. The mode of action is thought to be reduction of myometrial activity by lowering the intracellular concentration of calcium.[4] Complications are rare, but may include hypotension and respiratory depression in the mother and hypotonia in the infant.

Prostaglandin synthetase inhibitors are another class of drugs that have been shown to reduce uterine activity. Indomethacin and aspirin are two of the drugs in this group. Because of potential dangers to the fetus, they are not advocated for use in inhibiting preterm labor at this time.[4]

Use of Steroids.   Although the ideal objective of the treatment of preterm labor is to prevent delivery until term, when the fetus will be mature, realistically this is possible only about 20% of the time with our current methods.[20] A short-term objective that is more attainable is to temporarily stop labor for 24 to 48 hours to allow time for maturation of the fetal lungs. Respiratory distress syndrome (RDS) is the most common cause of morbidity and mortality in preterm infants. This condition is related to a deficiency of surfactant in the immature lungs. Some studies have shown a decrease in RDS when betamethasone or dexamethasone is administered to the mother prior to delivery. Few side-effects have been demonstrated, but long-term effects are not known, so the drugs are not used indiscriminately. The treatment seems to be most effective for gestations of less than 33 weeks.[4]

Assessment in Preterm Labor

Initial assessment of the woman who is thought to be in labor prior to 37 weeks' gestation includes basic information about her health and obstetric history plus evaluation of her current condition. The nurse can assist in determining the presence of true labor by monitoring the frequency, intensity, and duration of contractions, checking for cervical effacement and dilatation, and observing for other signs of labor, such as rupture of membranes and bloody show. Assessment of the fetus for approximate size, maturity, and signs of fetal distress is also important. Prenatal history, fetal monitoring, ultrasound, and determination of the lecithin/sphingomyelin ratio are all methods that might be used in the assessment.

Once treatment is begun, the nurse continues to assess the signs of labor and also assesses for side-effects of the treatment on both mother and fetus. Continuous electronic fetal and contraction monitoring is used, and the nurse assesses the monitor strip for any changes.

Nursing Diagnosis

Preterm labor is an alteration in the childbearing process. The nurse is an active participant, with the physician, in making and interpreting the assessment data to make the diagnosis of preterm labor and arrive at decisions for interventions. There are also specific nursing diagnoses that might be made during this time to guide the nurse in providing appropriate nursing care. Possible nursing diagnoses would include anxiety/fear related to unpredictable prognosis for the continuation of the pregnancy; alteration in comfort related to uterine contractions; alteration in comfort related to prolonged bed rest in the side-lying position; and alteration in family processes related to the effect of the mother's extended hospital stay on the family.

Planning/Intervention

The woman who is admitted in preterm labor, and her family, can be expected to have a high level of anxiety. This is understandable, since they are usually not prepared for the labor physically or emotionally and may be fearful that the baby will not survive. Support from a primary nurse who can be with them through the admission process and provide information about what is and will be happening can be very helpful in allaying their anxiety.

Bed rest in the side-lying position and adequate hydration, either oral or intravenous, are interventions that are usually instituted while the decision on further treatment is being made. An intake and output record should be kept. Comfort measures should be employed as with any labor (see Chap. 25), and analgesic medications should be avoided or kept to a minimum.

Care of the Woman Receiving Tocolytic Treatment.   The nurse's role is an important one in the care of the woman receiving a tocolytic agent by intravenous infusion. She can help determine whether the mother understands the nature of the treatment and the possible side-effects. The mother should be helped to maintain the left lateral position in bed to minimize the risk of supine hypotension. Baseline data should be obtained before the infusion is started. This includes fetal heart rate, uterine activity, and maternal vital signs. The physician also usually orders baseline laboratory studies, including complete blood count with differential, blood glucose, and serum electrolytes; urinalysis and urine culture to check for latent urinary tract infection; and a baseline electrocardiogram.[25]

The nurse may be responsible for starting the intravenous line and mixing the medication. The protocol will vary according to the hospital, the doctor's orders, and the drug to be used. A large-gauge intravenous catheter is usually used, and the solution should be administered with the use of an infusion pump so the dosage can be carefully titrated. The usual initial dosage of ritodrine is 0.1 mg/min, with the infusion rate being increased by increments of 0.05 mg/min every 10 minutes until uterine activity ceases, the maximum of 0.35 mg/min is reached, or significant side-effects develop.[26]

Although the side-effects for the different β-adrenergic agonists vary somewhat, ritodrine is fairly typical and will be used in this example. While the infusion

(text continued on page 849)

TABLE 38-6

Drugs Used for Preterm Labor

Tocolytic Agents

General indications for use: Signs of preterm labor
Gestational age >20 wks but <36 wks
Estimated fetal weight >500 g but <2500 g
No contraindications to continuation of pregnancy

General contraindications: Pregnancy <20 wks
Ruptured membranes, especially with signs of infection
Active uterine bleeding
Maternal medical complications such as diabetes mellitus or severe preeclampsia
Acute or chronic fetal distress
Major fetal anomalies
Intrauterine fetal death
Any maternal or fetal condition contraindicating the continuation of pregnancy
Advanced labor with cervical dilatation beyond 3 cm

Drug	Action	Additional Contraindications	Side-effects/Complications	Dosage and Route	Remarks
Beta Adrenergic Agonists					
Ritodrine (Yutopar)	Exerts preferential effect on beta$_2$ receptors in smooth muscle of uterus inhibiting contractility; in blood vessels causing vasodilation	Maternal cardiac disease, renal disease, or hyperthyroidism Known hypersensitivity to drug	Maternal: Cardiovascular: Increased heart rate Widening pulse pressure: Slightly increased systolic BP Decreased diastolic BP Increased cardiac output Hyperglycemia Hypokalemia Fluid retention Pulmonary edema Subjective reactions Palpitations Tremors Nausea and vomiting Headache Nervousness Restlessness Anxiety Chest tightness or pain	Intravenous infusion: 150 mg ritodrine to 500 ml of solution = 0.3 mg/ml Begin at 0.05 mg to 0.1 mg/min; increase by 0.05 mg/min every 10 min until UCs stop or side-effects are unacceptable to maximum recommended dose of 0.35 mg/min; continue IV 12 hrs after labor ceases; 30 min prior to discontinuing IV, start ritodrine PO Oral: Ritodrine 10 mg every 2 hrs for 24 hrs, then 10–20 mg every 4–6 hrs for maintenance	Risk of pulmonary edema increased when given concurrently with corticosteroids Nurse should be alert for signs of pulmonary edema

Drug	Action	Contraindications	Side Effects	Dosage	Comments
			Dyspnea Fetal: tachycardia Neonatal: hypoglycemia		
Isoxsuprine hydrochloride (Vasodilan)	Similar to ritodrine		Higher rates of cardiovascular side-effects, hypotension, fetal distress. Others similar to ritodrine	Intravenous infusion: 80 mg in 500 ml solution Begin at 0.25 to 0.5 mg/min; increase to maximum of 0.75 to 1.0 mg/min; continue with: Intramuscular maintenance doses: 10 mg every 6 hrs for 12 to 24 hrs; continue with: Oral maintenance: 10–20 mg 4 times/day	Not approved by FDA for tocolytic use
Terbutaline (Brethine, Bricanyl)	Similar to ritodrine	Client taking terbutaline for asthma Others same as ritodrine	Similar to ritodrine	Intravenous infusion: 0.01 mg/min, increase to 0.085 mg/min maximum Oral maintenance dose: 2.5 mg every 4 to 6 hrs	Not approved by FDA for tocolytic use
Magnesium Sulfate	Exact mode of action unknown—depresses uterine activity when maternal serum magnesium levels 6–8 mEq/L	CNS depression Cardiac dysfunction Renal pathology	Maternal: Related to increasing serum magnesium levels hypotension, respiratory depression, hypotonus Magnesium toxicity: Respiratory arrest Circulatory collapse Cardiac arrest Fetal: distress in response to mother's symptoms Neonatal: respiratory depression, hypotonus	Intravenous infusion: Loading dose: 4 g by slow IV push or over 30 min by infusion Maintenance: 2 g/hr until UCs stop or signs of toxicity appear	Not approved by FDA for tocolytic use Nursing responsibilities: Monitor VS q 5 min during loading dose and q 15 min during maintenance Stop infusion and report if: BP is 90/60, respiration is 12/min; there is no patellar reflex; urine output is 30 cc/hr Keep calcium gluconate at bedside

TABLE 38-6 (continued)

Drug	Action	Additional Contraindications	Side-effects/Complications	Dosage and Route	Remarks
Prostaglandin synthetase inhibitors					
Indomethacin Naproxen Aspirin	Interfere with synthesis of prostaglandins	Gastrointestinal lesions Coagulation defects Allergy to specific drug Epilepsy Psychiatric disturbance	Maternal: Nausea and vomiting GI bleeding Headache Drowsiness, dizziness, and vertigo Allergic reactions Postpartum hemorrhage Fetal/neonatal: Premature closure of ductus arteriosus Other cardiac and pulmonary changes Hyperbilirubinemia Hemorrhagic disorders	Route: Oral Dose: No routine dose established	Advantage: Tocolysis without hypotension Disadvantages: Potential danger to mother and fetus/infant which currently outweigh advantage—not recommended for use with preterm labor at this time in United States

Corticosteroids

Drug	Action	Indications	Contraindications	Side-effects/Complications	Dosage and Route	Remarks
Betamethasone (Celestone) Dexamethasone	Increased production of surfactant in fetal lungs	Preterm labor at gestational age of 28 to 32 wks L/S ratio not known or <2:1 Fetal membranes intact Possibility of delaying delivery for 48 hrs after initiation of therapy without undue risk to mother or fetus	Inability or contraindications to delaying delivery Gestational age 34 wks L/S ratio ≥2	Maternal: May increase adverse effects of diabetes or preeclampsia Increased risk of infection Delayed wound healing if cesarean birth Fetal/neonatal: No reports of serious side-effects, but long-term effects not known	12 mg IM, repeat in 12–24 hrs. × 1; 6 mg IM, repeat in 12–24 hrs × 1; then weekly until L/S ratio 2:1 Effects seem to be transitory, peak at 48 hrs and last approximately 1 wk	Not approved by FDA for this use; controversy exists about effectiveness and potential dangers Use with tocolytic agent appears to increase risk of pulmonary edema

The Patient at Risk for Preterm Labor

Nursing Objectives:

1. Identify woman at risk for preterm labor.
2. Identify early signs of preterm labor.
3. Provide nursing care to promote maternal and fetal well-being during:
   Attempts to inhibit or delay labor
   Labor and birth of preterm infant
4. Identify adverse responses to tocolytic treatment.

Assessment	Potential Nursing Diagnosis	Planning/Intervention	Evaluation
Risk factors associated with preterm labor: Maternal age <18 or >40 Low socioeconomic status Poor nutritional status Employment outside of home Heavy cigarette smoking Alcohol or drug abuse Previous reproductive loss Previous low birthweight or preterm infant Maternal disease or infection Present pregnancy: Bleeding, over distention of uterus, premature rupture of membranes	Knowledge deficit regarding factors related to risk of preterm labor	Take history at first antepartum visit to determine presence of risk factors; reassess at each antepartum visit Teach client to identify risk factors Teach methods of possible risk reduction: Improve nutrition Decrease or stop smoking Avoid alcohol and drugs Reduce stress	Clients at risk are identified Client identifies risk factors Client takes steps to reduce risks
Signs of labor Contractions q 10 min lasting 30 sec or more Cervical change, Effacement = 80% Dilatation = 2 cm	Knowledge deficit regarding signs of preterm labor	Provide information about signs of preterm labor to clients at risk: menstrual-type cramps, lower abdominal tightening or pressure, intermittent back ache, bloody show, watery vaginal discharge Provide information about when and how to contact health care provider and/or come to hospital	Client describes signs of preterm labor Client seeks medical care appropriately
Labor progress Continued cervical changes Frequency, intensity, and duration of uterine contractions Rupture of membranes or leaking amniotic fluid Bloody show	Anxiety/fear related to unexpected early labor	On admission to labor unit: observe for signs of labor and progressive changes; obtain lab values—CBC, urinalysis; test vaginal discharge with nitrazine paper for presence of amniotic fluid Encourage left side-lying position	Client responds positively to care aspects

(continued)

847

Assessment	Potential Nursing Diagnosis	Planning/Intervention	Evaluation
		Provide oral or intravenous fluids to maintain hydration—initial 200 ml to 500 ml bolus as ordered	
		Monitor and record intake and output	
Maternal emotional status		Provide appropriate, factual information to client and family about progress of labor and plan of care	Family understands client's condition and plan of care
		Allow husband or other person of client's choice to be present as desired	Client acknowledges reduction of fear

Gestational age
  EDC
  Height of fundus
  Ultrasound
		Assist in estimation of gestational age to help determine choice of treatment	

Fetal well-being Fetal heart rate, baseline, periodic changes, variability		Apply external fetal monitor and observe for fetal status	Fetal distress is detected early and appropriate measures instituted
Fetal movement		Prepare client for ultrasound or amniocentesis if ordered	
Tests of fetal maturity, L/S ratio, ultrasound		Explain all procedures and their purposes	
Response to tocolytic treatment		Explain procedures to client	Client understands procedure
Uterine contractions		Follow agency protocol for starting and monitoring infusion	
Side-effects (depending on agent used): Maternal vital signs: changes in heart or respiratory rate, blood pressure, or temperature		Monitor vital signs, fetal heart rate, uterine activity, maternal subjective reactions	
Fetal heart rate		Report side-effects or complications	
		Provide physical and emotional support	
Maternal subjective reactions: tremors, palpitations, nausea and vomiting, restlessness, chest tightness or pain, dyspnea	Alteration in comfort related to unpleasant side-effects and prolonged bedrest	Provide comfort measures, additional pillows for positioning, back rub, assistance with personal hygiene, restful atmosphere	Client responds to comfort measures
Boredom, discouragement	Ineffective individual coping related to prolonged hospitalization	Provide for appropriate diversions or companionship as desired	Client copes effectively
Family concerns	Alteration in family process related to the effect of extended hospital stay on family functioning	Provide opportunity to discuss concerns about family	Client verbalizes concerns for family

(continued)

Assessment	Potential Nursing Diagnosis	Planning/Intervention	Evaluation
		Allow visits of other children when hospitalization is long-term	Children visit mother as appropriate
		Make referrals to public health nurse or social service as needed for assistance	
		Provide information about possible continuation of preterm labor; teach about labor and delivery, cesarean delivery, facilities, and care available for preterm infant	
Contraindications to tocolytic treatment: Pregnancy <20 weeks >36 weeks Active uterine bleeding Maternal illness Fetal distress or intra-uterine death Advanced labor—cervical dilatation >3 cm Ruptured membranes	Fear for self and fetus related to imminent preterm delivery	Keep client and family informed concerning progress of labor, plan of treatment, status of fetus Provide physical and emotional support, avoid leaving her alone Monitor signs of progress of labor and fetal well-being Prepare for preterm delivery or cesarean delivery—alert surgical team and neonatal intensive care team	Client and family are knowledgeable about situation Client affirms that her fear has been minimized Infant receives prompt and efficient resuscitation as needed

(text continued from page 843)

rate of the ritodrine is being increased, the pulse and blood pressure are taken at least every 15 minutes, and after that every 30 minutes until the infusion is stopped. Significant side-effects to be reported are maternal pulse rate greater than 120 beats per minute, chest pain, dyspnea, blood pressure less than 90/60 or a significant decrease from the mother's baseline, or fetal tachycardia greater than 180 beats per minute.[25,26] These symptoms may require discontinuation of the therapy and the administration of propranolol as an antidote. Milder symptoms, such as headache, restlessness, or nausea, may respond to a slight decrease in the dosage.[25]

If uterine contractions are successfully inhibited, the woman may be put on oral maintenance therapy. The initial oral dose should be given 30 minutes before the intravenous ritodrine is discontinued. Vital signs should be taken every 2 hours for the first 24 hours, then every 4 hours. Uterine activity and side-effects should also be monitored. The side-effects of the oral drug can sometimes be minimized by taking it with food.

Women on tocolytic therapy need lots of emotional and physical support. Not only are they concerned about the outcome for themselves and their baby, but they may be uncomfortable from the side-effects of the drug and from the enforced bed rest. Helpful hints from a nurse who was also a patient on long-term intravenous tocolytic therapy include the following:

- Suggesting use of a mattress pad or "egg-crate" mattress to help alleviate the hip discomfort from the side-lying position
- Encouraging use of pillows from home for comfort and to brighten up the room
- Assisting with personal hygiene such as brushing teeth and washing hair
- Providing passive range of motion or isometric exercises to assist in maintaining muscle tone
- Assisting with finding activities that can be accomplished while lying in bed
- Providing comfort measures such as back rubs[27]

Prolapse of Umbilical Cord

In the course of labor, the cord prolapses in front of the presenting part about once in every 400 cases. It is a grave complication for the fetus, since the cord is then compressed between the presenting part and the bony pelvis, and the fetal circulation is shut off (Fig. 38-15). Any factor that prevents proper adaptation of the presenting part to the maternal pelvis predisposes to prolapse of the cord. The accident occurs most commonly in shoulder and footling breech presentations and less often with frank breeches and multiple pregnancy. In cephalic presentations, it rarely occurs unless there is pelvic contraction or excessive development of the fetus. There is an increased incidence with prematurity, probably because the small fetus is poorly fitted to the pelvic inlet.

Prolapse frequently occurs following rupture of the membranes when the head, the breech, or the shoulder is not sufficiently down in the pelvis to prevent the cord from being washed past it in the sudden gush of amniotic fluid. After the membranes rupture, the cord comes down, and it may be either a concealed or an apparent prolapse. In the latter instance, the diagnosis is made when the cord is seen; when the cord is not visible, the correct diagnosis is made when the mother is examined and the cord is felt or when examination of the fetal heart reveals distress due to pressure on the cord. This is why it *must* be a routine practice to listen to and to record the fetal heart sounds immediately after the membranes rupture and again in about 5 to 10 minutes. When fetal heart tones are electronically monitored, moderate to severe variable decelerations may be seen with the cord compression resulting from a cord prolapse.

The immediate treatment of cord prolapse is to minimize the pressure of the presenting part upon the cord and the resultant impaired umbilical circulation. The head of the bed or table should be lowered, the hips should be elevated with a pillow, or the woman should be placed in a knee–chest position to raise the level of the hips above the shoulders and allow the presenting part to gravitate away from the pelvis (Fig. 38-16). Additionally, the presenting part may be pushed upward by pressure from a sterile gloved hand in the vagina.

The physician and other staff must be notified at once so emergency procedures can be instituted. No attempt should be made to reposition the cord, and with a live baby near term, the goal of therapy is to effect delivery as soon as possible. If dilatation is incomplete, immediate cesarean section yields the best results for fetal salvage. In occasional carefully selected cases, prolapsed cord in vertex presentations with nearly complete dilatation can be delivered with minimal trauma to mother and infant using vacuum extraction.

Perinatal mortality with cord prolapse, which is usually about 26%, can be reduced to 5% to 10% when delivery is accomplished within one half hour after diagnosis. More frequent vaginal examinations, checking the fetal heart after rupture of membranes, and active rapid treatment combine to reduce mortality.

This particular complication is not painful for the mother; however, it can be very frightening, since many mothers realize it can result in their infant's death. Also, whether they realize the grave implications or not, the increased activity, various position changes, and quickened responses of the attendants give them an indication that all is not well. Therefore, again, the calmness, warmth, and efficiency of the nurse are needed to reassure the mother that all possible measures are being taken to bring the situation under control.

It goes without saying that these women never should be left unattended, and their partners, if they are present, should be treated with consideration. It is difficult, when any crises occur, to deal with the relatives of the mother with appropriate thoughtfulness, since most of the energy is directed toward meeting the pressing (and often lifesaving) demands of the situation.

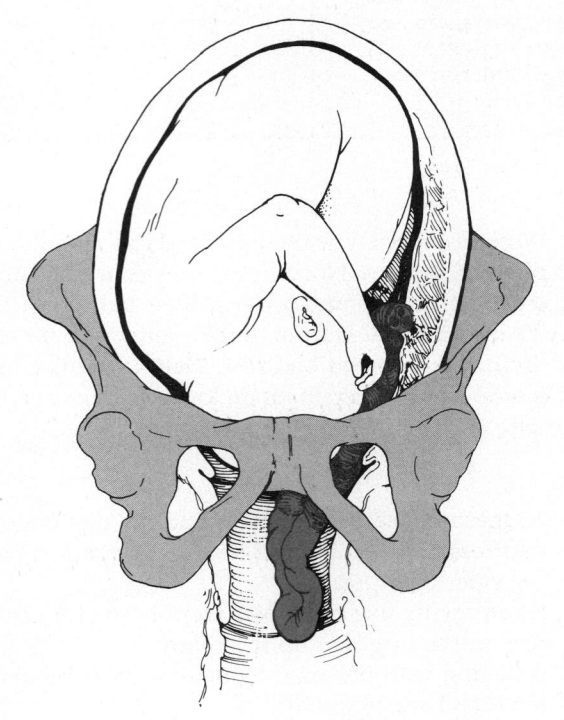

F I G U R E   3 8 - 1 5

Prolapse of the cord. As the head comes down, the compression of the cord between the fetal skull and the pelvic brim will shut off its circulation completely.

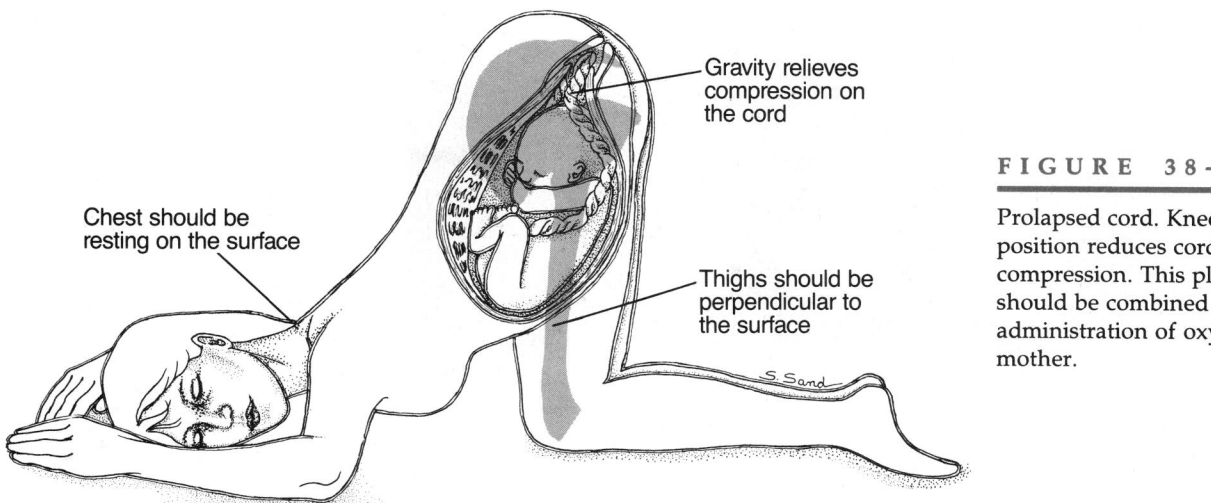

Chest should be resting on the surface

Gravity relieves compression on the cord

Thighs should be perpendicular to the surface

S. Sand

FIGURE 38-16

Prolapsed cord. Knee–chest position reduces cord compression. This placement should be combined with administration of oxygen to the mother.

However, it must be remembered that the mother and her family are considered as a unit, and a few moments usually can be found to provide essential information.

Amniotic Fluid Embolism

When amniotic fluid enters into the maternal circulation, it may reach the pulmonary capillaries, resulting in amniotic fluid embolism. For this to occur, there must be a tear through the amnion and chorion, an opening into the maternal circulation, and increased intrauterine pressure to force the fluid into the venous circulation. The most likely sites of entry are the endocervical veins and the uteroplacental area, and it usually follows a tumultuous labor.[1]

Amniotic fluid invariably contains small particles of matter, such as vernix caseosa, lanugo, and sometimes meconium, and these form multiple tiny emboli, which reach the lungs and cause occlusion of the pulmonary capillaries. This complication, amniotic fluid embolism, is almost invariably fatal and, as a rule, causes the death of the mother within 1 or 2 hours. Fortunately, this tragic condition is rare, occurring only once in many thousand labors.

The clinical characteristics of the condition are sudden dyspnea, cyanosis, pulmonary edema, profound shock, and uterine relaxation with hemorrhage. A highly important feature of amniotic fluid embolism is a diminution in the fibrinogen content of the blood, or hypofibrinogenemia. The mechanism is similar to, if not identical with, that which occurs in abruptio placentae and missed abortion, as described in Chapter 36.

The treatment consists of oxygen therapy, blood transfusion and the intravenous administration of fibrinogen, but, as indicated, this is usually futile.

Multiple Pregnancy

When two or more embryos develop in the uterus at the same time, the condition is known as multiple pregnancy. These are considered complicated pregnancies since there is an appreciable increase in morbidity and mortality. Multiple pregnancies account for about 2% to 3% of all viable births. The frequency of identical (monozygotic or one-egg) twins is apparently relatively constant throughout the world at about 1 set in every 250 pregnancies. Moreover, their appearance is largely independent of race, heredity, maternal age, parity, infertility drugs, and environmental factors. On the other hand, fraternal (dizygotic, two-egg) twins are influenced by these factors. Their incidence in the white race is about 1 set in 95 and in the black race 1 set in 78. Twinning among Orientals is less common. Women who were themselves a dizygotic twin tend to have more multiple pregnancies. Similarly, increased age, parity, endogenous gonadotropin, and taking infertility drugs also increase the probability of multiple pregnancy.[28]

Types of Twins

Multiple fetuses result from two basic processes. Twin fetuses more commonly result from the fertilization of two different ova. This type of twinning is known as dizygotic, or fraternal twins. About one third as often, twins arise from the fertilization of a single ovum, monozygotic or identical twins. Either or both processes may be at work in the production of larger numbers of fetuses in one birth. Quadruplets, for instance, may arise from one to four ova.[1] An interesting feature of twinning is that although dizygotic twins are not in the strict sense true twins because they result from the union of two

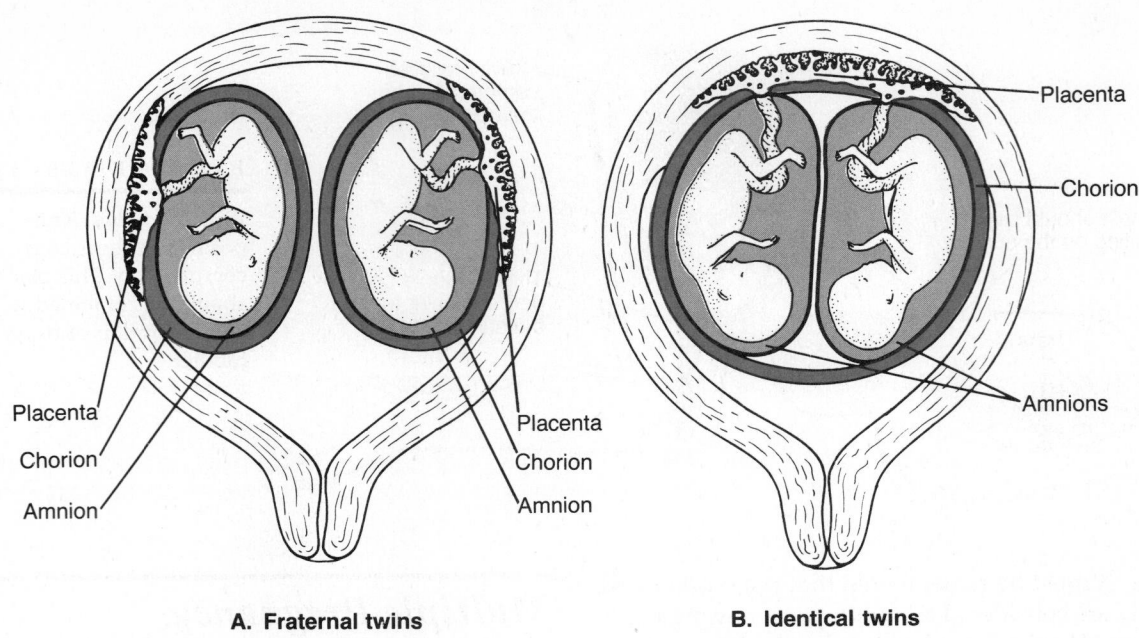

A. Fraternal twins

B. Identical twins

FIGURE 38-17

Twin pregnancy. (*A*) Fraternal twins with two placentas, two amnions, and two chorions. (*B*) Identical twins with one placenta, one chorion, and two amnions.

separate ova and sperm, if they are of the same sex, they often resemble each other as closely at birth as a pair of monozygotic twins. The process of the division of one fertilized zygote into two does not always result in an equal sharing of the protoplasm; thus, the growth of monozygotic twins is often dramatically discordant.[1]

Basically, two types of placentas exist in twins, those with monochorial (one chorion) and those with dichorial (two chorions) membranes (Fig. 38-17). Also, the placentas may be fused, separate, or a single disk, and there may be one or two amnions. However, each fetus usually has its own umbilical cord. The possible combinations thus include the following:

1. Monozygotic (identical)
   a. Diamniotic dichorionic (two amnions, two chorions), 30%
   b. Diamniotic monochorionic (two amnions, one chorion), most common
   c. Monoamniotic monochorionic (one amnion, one chorion), very rare
2. Dizygotic (fraternal or nonidentical)
   a. Diamniotic dichorionic (two amnions, two chorions)

Examination of the fetal membranes is used to assist in diagnosing the zygosity of twins but is not always accurate. Only monozygotic twins can have a single chorion, which establishes identical twinning. Two chorions are always present in dizygotic twins, but are also the placentation of about 30% of monozygotic

twins. If the sexes are different, the twins are obviously fraternal, but if twins are the same sex and dichorionic, the diagnosis is uncertain.[1,28] The usual twin placentations are shown in Figure 38-18. In the United States, 33% of twins are identical.

Diagnosis

Early diagnosis of multiple pregnancy is an important factor in improving the perinatal outcome. Detection late in pregnancy or at delivery correlates with increased risk for perinatal morbidity and mortality. One of the advantages of early diagnosis is that it allows time for the mother and her family to be informed of the differences involved in multiple pregnancy and what can be done to improve the outcome.[29] Referral to a perinatal center can also be made at a more optimum time.

Twins are suspected whenever uterine size is greater than ordinarily expected for any point in the pregnancy. In addition, the palpation of three or four large parts in the uterus, the auscultation of two fetal heart tones of differing frequencies, or the history of twins "running in the family" all serve to alert the obstetrician or nurse to the possibility of a multiple pregnancy.

Ultrasound can aid in the diagnosis of multiple pregnancy, and the use of routine ultrasound screening of all pregnancies before the 20th week is practiced in some areas. At present there is no biochemical test that clearly differentiates between multiple and single preg-

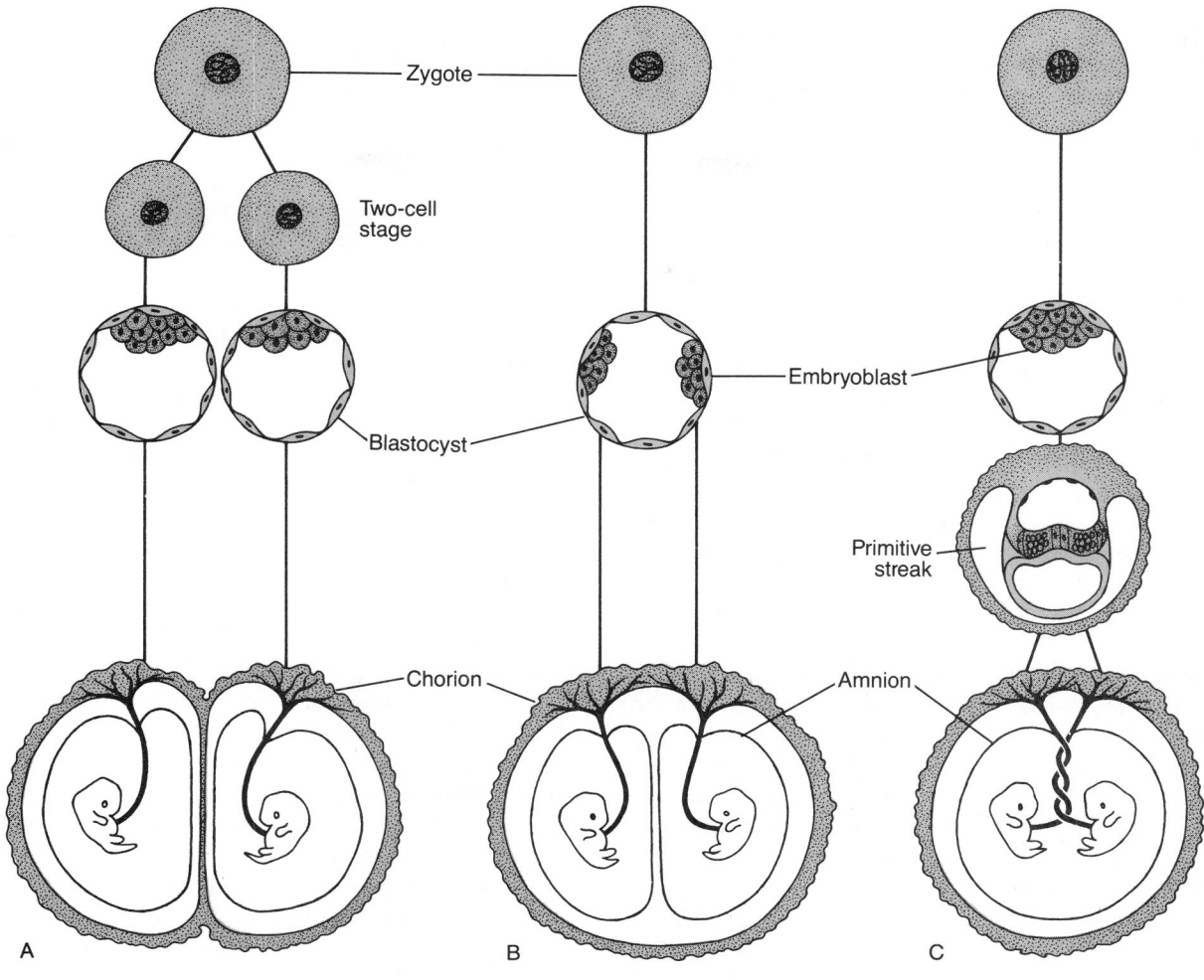

FIGURE 38-18

Membranes and placenta in twin pregnancies. (*A*) Two placentas, two amnions, two chorions (from either dizygotic twins or monozygotic twins with early cleavage of the zygote. (*B* and *C*) Single ovum twins. (*B*) One chorion and two amnions and one placenta. (*C*) One chorion and one amnion (note entanglement of cords, a danger when there is only one amnion)

nancies, but assay of one of the hormones, such as chorionic gonadotropin or placental lactogen, that are usually elevated during multiple pregnancy has been suggested.[29]

Pathophysiology

Several high-risk conditions are associated with multiple pregnancy. These include premature delivery (50%), hemorrhage (20%), hypertensive disorders, preeclampsia and eclampsia (25%), abnormal presentation and position (10%), hydramnios (7%), and uterine dysfunction (10%). Cord compression and entanglement, intrauterine growth retardation, and operative delivery also contribute to morbidity and mortality. In addition, monozygotic twins are less hardy than dizygotic twins. Weight differences are more pronounced, and they have a higher incidence of congenital anomalies and neonatal mortality.

Some of these problems may be due to the monochorionic placenta, which is thought to be less competent than the dichorionic variety. The problems center on placental vascular disorders. The most serious of these is the shunting of blood due to vascular anastomosis, which results in a twin-to-twin transfusion syndrome (intrauterine parabiosis). The anastomosis may be artery-to-artery, artery-to-vein, or vein-to-vein. An artery-to-vein anastomosis is the most serious and accounts for the disparity in size and appearance seen in these supposedly identical infants. The *donor* twin is pallid, anemic, dehydrated, growth retarded, and hypovolemic. Hydrops and cardiac decompensation may be present, as well as polyhydramnios. In contrast, the *recipient* twin appears healthy, large by contrast, and ruddy. However, this appearance is due to edema, plethora, and hypertension. Kernicterus, ascites, glomerular-tubal hypertrophy, enlarged heart and liver, or congenital heart anomalies may be accompaniments. Fetal polyuria and hydramnios may also be present. These infants are at great risk for death in the first 24 hours of life.[1,29]

Management

Because of the antepartal and perinatal risk, the mother needs to be monitored carefully during the antepartal period. She is asked to see the obstetrician more frequently, at least every 2 weeks in the second trimester and at least weekly in the third trimester if there are no complications. Diet is regulated to allow for adequate weight gain. An increase of 300 Kcal or more per day in energy sources in the diet is not too much. Protein intake is supervised, and iron, folic acid, and vitamin supplements are increased. Rest periods on the side may be prescribed, although the efficacy of complete bed rest even in the last trimester for higher socioeconomic status women seems equivocal.[1] Pritchard and associates, however, have found that women who are socioeconomically deprived seem to benefit from hospitalization with some ambulation privileges during the last trimester. In their opinion there are better outcomes in the incidence of premature labor and preeclapsia and a generally lowered perinatal mortality.[1]

The latter weeks of a twin pregnancy are likely to be associated with heaviness of the lower abdomen, back pains, and swelling of the feet and the ankles. Abdominal distention makes sleeping difficult, and therefore the physician may prescribe a hypnotic. A well-fitting maternity girdle makes daytime more comfortable. Because of the excessive abdominal size, the mother may find that frequent small feedings are more suitable than the usual three larger meals a day. The nurse can be very helpful in giving the mother anticipatory guidance regarding these matters during the antepartal period.

Travel is curtailed because labor may begin at any time without warning, and delivery in strange surroundings may be hazardous.

Labor and Delivery

If not already hospitalized, the mother is requested to come to the hospital at the first sign of labor. When labor is confirmed, a decision must be made on route of delivery, taking into account the presentation of the twins, the presence of any maternal or fetal complications, the gestational age, and the availability of anesthesia, an experienced obstetrician, and neonatal intensive care.[29] During the labor, steps are taken to ensure a successful outcome for mother and fetuses.

First, the mother is attended at all times by a qualified perinatal team member. Here the nurse can be invaluable. Fetal heart rates must be monitored continuously and maternal vital signs recorded. A combination of external and internal fetal monitoring after the membranes have ruptured proves satisfactory. A liter of cross-matched blood or its equivalent is to be available and in the area. In addition, an intravenous infusion system capable of delivering the blood is to be instituted. Lactated Ringer's solution alternated with a 5% dextrose solution at 60 ml to 120 ml/hr has been found to be satisfactory in the absence of hemorrhage or metabolic disturbance during labor.[1]

It is recommended that two obstetricians be available and scrubbed for the delivery and an anesthesiologist be in attendance, especially for the contingency of a cesarean delivery. Moreover, *two* individuals, with at least one being skilled in resuscitation, are needed for *each* fetus at the time of delivery.

A local or pudendal block is preferred to minimize the effect of anesthetic on the infants. However, a combination of thiopental, nitrous oxide plus oxygen, and succinylcholine given in timed, appropriate doses has been found to be effective when cesarean section is indicated. The general anesthetic halothane also may be used when operative intervention is needed.[1]

The first twin is delivered either by vertex or assisted breech delivery. If the first infant is transverse, an external version is used to bring about a deliverable presentation.

If the twins are monozygotic, the first infant's cord must be clamped to prevent the second twin from bleeding through it. The cords should be labeled. The position of the second twin is ascertained and it is brought into position by a combination of vaginal and abdominal manipulation. If there is a second sac, it is carefully ruptured to allow a slow loss of fluid and to guard against cord prolapse. A spontaneous or a prophylactic forceps vertex delivery is preferred. If the breech presents, then the physician may have to assist in the extraction. If descent does not come about, then a version and extraction may be required. These require astute management on the part of both the obstetrician and the anesthesiologist.[1]

Routine use of oxytocin is delayed until after the delivery of the second twin, when 1 ml is given intravenously. The uterus is not massaged until after the placenta(s) are expelled, then massage is continued until the uterus remains hard and contracted (15–30 min). One ml of ergonovine is given after expulsion of the placenta(s), if the mother is not hypertensive.

As with any delivery, the nurse has the responsibility of supportive care for the mother as well as assisting the physician in whatever activities are indicated.

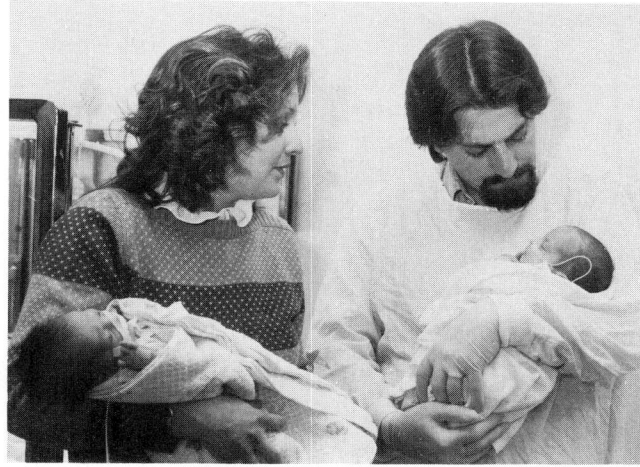

FIGURE 38-19

Parents of twins need support from the nursing staff, even if twins were expected. (Courtesy of The Children's Hospital of Philadelphia)

Since these infants are apt to be small, oxygen or resuscitative measures may be necessary. The care is similar to that for any premature baby (see Chap. 44). The supplies or equipment that may be needed (*e.g.*, resuscitator, oxygen apparatus) should be procured early in the delivery and kept in readiness (but out of the mother's sight, if possible). Maternal vital signs as well as the fetal heart rate should be checked frequently.

Postpartum

Physically, the care required by the mother will depend on her general condition and the type of delivery. Complications are the same as those following single births, but the frequency of complications such as uterine atony may be increased.

The birth of more than one infant can be a psychological shock to the parents, even if expected (Fig. 38-19). One additional child may be desired and acceptable; two may impose an emotional or financial burden. The parents may wonder if they can manage the care of two newborns simultaneously. Problems may be compounded in feeding, especially if the mother plans to breast-feed, and in providing two of everything.

Parents need anticipatory guidance and support during the initial adjustment period. Some may need referral to a social worker or public-health nurse to assist with plans for the unexpected new baby. Many also appreciate information about special clubs for mothers of twins, or introduction to other mothers who have successfully coped with the first few months after the birth of twins. If the infants are very small the parents will need the same type of extra support given to other parents of preterm infants (see Chap. 44).

References

1. Pritchard JA, MacDonald PC, Gant NF: Williams Obstetrics, 17th ed, Chap 29. New York, Appleton-Century-Crofts, 1985
2. Friedman EA: Labor, Evaluation and Management. New York, Appleton-Century-Crofts, 1978
3. Larks SD: Electrohysterography. Springfield, IL, Charles C Thomas, 1960
4. Oxorn H: Human Labor and Birth. Norwalk, CT, Appleton-Century-Crofts, 1985
5. Hendricks CH: Dystocia due to abnormal uterine action. In Danforth D (ed): Obstetrics and Gynecology, 4th ed. Philadelphia, Harper & Row, 1982
6. Bowes WA Jr: Clinical aspects of normal and abnormal labor. In Creasy RK, Resnik R (eds): Maternal-Fetal Medicine: Principles and Practice. Philadelphia, WB Saunders Co, 1984
7. Friedman EA: Dysfunctional labor. In Cohen W, Friedman EA (eds): Management of Labor. Baltimore, University Park Press, 1983
8. Hendricks CH et al: The normal cervical dilatation patterns in late pregnancy and labor. Am J Obstet Gynecol 106:1065, 1970
9. Beischer NA, Mackay EV: Obstetrics and the Newborn, 2nd ed. Sydney, WB Saunders, 1986
10. Malinowski JS: Nursing Care of the Labor Patient, 2nd ed. Philadelphia, FA Davis, 1983
11. Phillips RD, Freeman M: The management of the persistent occiput posterior position. Am J Obstet Gynecol 43:171, February 1974
12. Danforth DN: Dystocia due to abnormal fetopelvic relations. In Danforth DN (ed): Obstetrics and Gynecology, 4th ed. Philadelphia, Harper & Row, 1982
13. Douglas RG, Stromme WB: Operative Obstetrics, 3rd ed. New York, Appleton-Century-Crofts, 1976
14. Royce JA: Shock: Emergency nursing implications. Nurs Clin North Am 8:377, 1973
15. Danforth DN: Shock. In Danforth DN (ed): Obstetrics and Gynecology, 4th ed. Philadelphia, Harper & Row, 1982
16. Court D: Maternal shock in pregnancy. In Creasy RK, Resnik R (eds): Maternal-Fetal Medicine: Principles and Practice. Philadelphia, WB Saunders, 1984
17. Berkowitz RL: The Swan-Ganz catheter and colloid-osmotic pressure determinations. In Berkowitz RL (ed): Critical Care of the Obstetric Patient. New York, Churchill Livingstone, 1983
18. Stubblefield PG: Causes and prevention of preterm birth. In Fuchs F, Stubblefield PG (eds): Preterm Birth—Causes, Prevention and Management. New York, Macmillan, 1984
19. Creasy RK: Preterm labor and delivery. In Creasy RK, Resnik R (eds): Maternal-Fetal Medicine: Principles and Practice. Philadelphia, WB Saunders, 1984
20. Hobel CJ: Prevention of preterm delivery. In Beard RW, Nathanielsz PW (eds): Fetal Physiology and Medicine, 2nd ed. New York, Marcel Decker, 1984
21. Main DM, Gabbe SG, Richardson D et al: Can preterm deliveries be prevented? Am J Obstet Gynecol 151:892–898, 1985

22. Bowes WA Jr: Delivery of the very low birth weight infant. Clin Perinatol 8:173–195, 1981
23. Whitley N: A Manual of Clinical Obstetrics. Philadelphia, JB Lippincott, 1985
24. Clewell WH, Makowski EL: Management of premature labor and breech delivery. In Warshaw JB, Hobbins JC (eds): Principles and Practice of Perinatal Medicine. Menlo Park, Addison-Wesley, 1983
25. Aumann GM, Blake GD: Ritodrine hydrochloride in the control of premature labor. JOGN Nurs 11:75–79, March/April 1982
26. Shortridge LA: Using ritodrine hydrochloride to inhibit preterm labor. MCN 8:58–61, January/February 1983
27. Cagney EN: Nursing care during the treatment of preterm labor. In Fuchs F, Stubblefield PG (eds): Preterm Birth: Causes, Prevention and Management. New York, Macmillan, 1984
28. Benirschke K, Chung KK: Multiple pregnancy, Pt 1. N Engl J Med 288:1276–1284, June 14, 1973
29. Mac Lennan AH: Multiple gestation: Clinical characteristics and management. In Creasy RK, Resnik R (eds): Maternal-Fetal Medicine: Principles and Practice. Philadelphia, WB Saunders, 1984

Suggested Reading

Barden TP: Premature labor. In Fanaroff AA, Martin RJ (eds): Behrman's Neonatal-Perinatal Medicine, 3rd ed. St. Louis, CV Mosby, 1983
Bills BJ: Nursing considerations: Administering labor-suppressing medications. MCN 5:252–256, July/August 1980
Cohen WR, Friedman EA (eds): Management of Labor. Baltimore, University Park Press, 1983
Frederiksen MC: Tocolytic therapy with β-adrenergic agonists. Ration Drug Ther 17:1–4, June 1983

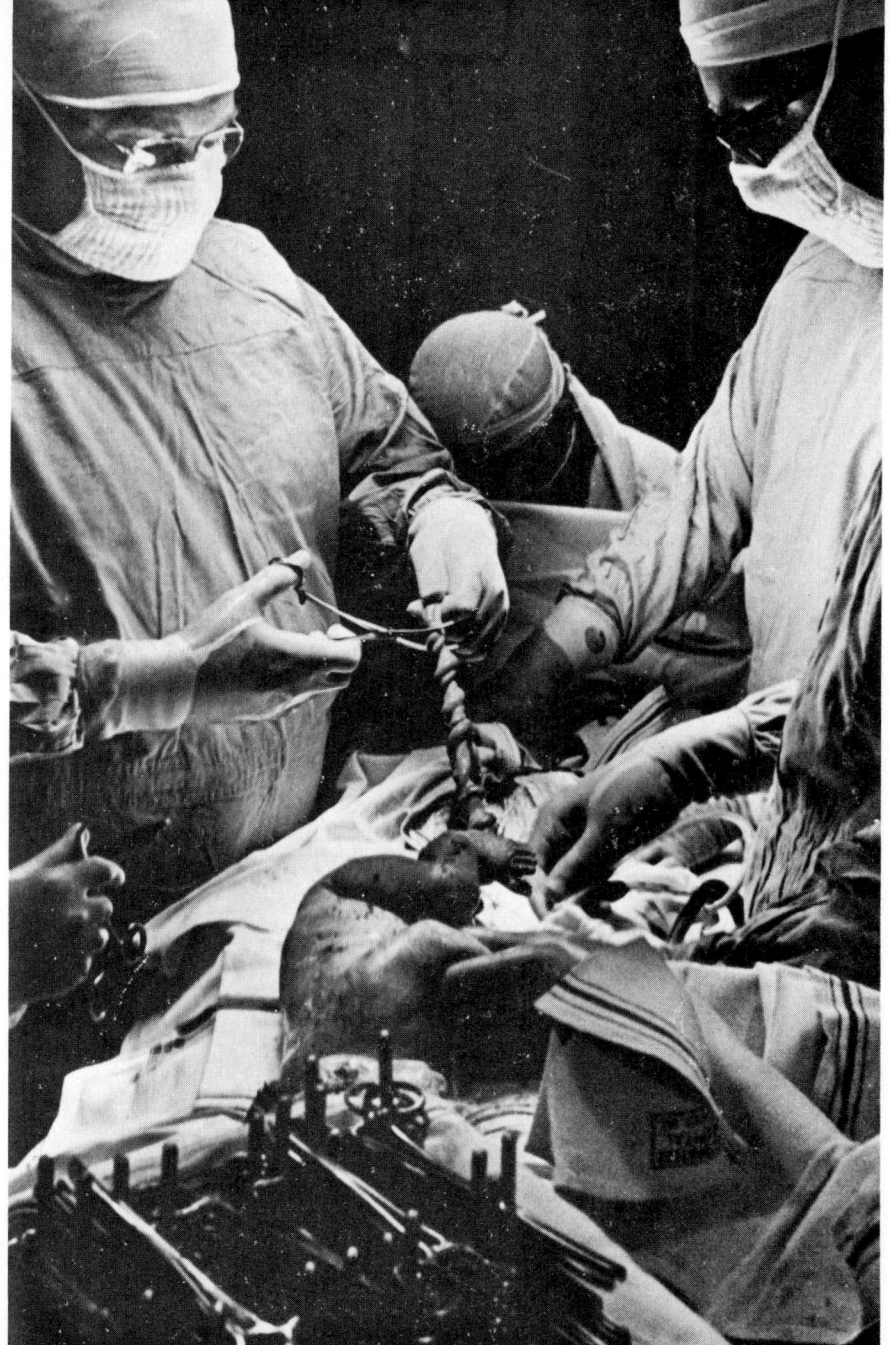

CHAPTER 39

Operative Obstetrics

There are several special procedures that the physician may use to assist the mother in labor and delivery. They come under the heading of operative obstetrics. These include version, induction of labor, the application of forceps or a vacuum extractor, repair of lacerations, and cesarean birth.

Version

Version consists of turning the baby in the uterus from an undesirable position to a desirable position. There are two types of version, external and internal.

External Version

External version is an operation designed to change a breech presentation into a vertex presentation by external manipulation of the fetus through the abdominal and the uterine walls. It is attempted in the hope of averting the difficulties of a subsequent breech delivery. Obstetricians find the procedure most successful when done about a month before full term; it often fails, however, either because it proves to be impossible to turn the fetus around or because the fetus returns to its original position within a few hours. Some obstetricians disapprove of it altogether.

Internal Version

Internal version is sometimes called internal podalic version, which is a maneuver designed to change whatever presentation may exist by converting it into a breech presentation (Fig. 39-1).

When cervical dilatation is complete, the whole hand of the operator is introduced high into the uterus and one or both of the baby's feet are grasped and pulled downward in the direction of the birth canal. With the external hand, the obstetrician may expedite the turning by pushing the head upward. The version is followed by breech extraction.

Internal version is most useful in cases of multiple pregnancy in which the birth of the second twin is delayed or when the second twin is in a transverse lie. It is now almost never used in other circumstances.

Induction of Labor

Induction of labor means the artificial initiation of labor after the period of viability. Induction of labor is indicated when continuation of pregnancy would adversely affect maternal health or when there are conditions in the mother that would affect fetal well-being. Compli-

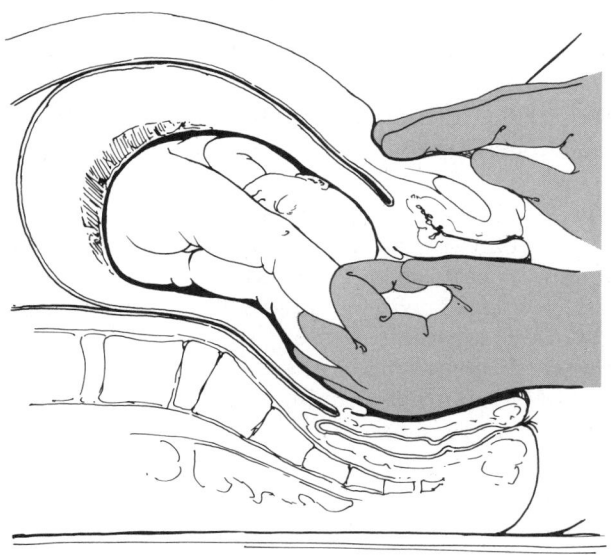

FIGURE 39-1

Internal podalic version.

cations of pregnancy that may require induction include hypertensive disease of pregnancy, diabetes, hemolytic disease, and postmaturity (see Chap. 36, Complications of Pregnancy, and Chap. 37, Concurrent Diseases in Pregnancy).

Before induction is attempted the physiologic readiness of both the mother and the fetus should be evaluated. Tests of fetal maturity and fetal well-being are usually done before the decision is made to induce labor. (See Chapter 42 for information about these tests.) Maternal readiness refers to the condition of the cervix and the likelihood that induction will be successful.

Several numerical scoring systems to assess readiness of the cervix have been developed based on the physical characteristics of the cervix as determined by vaginal examination. The characteristics to be assessed include dilatation, effacement, consistency and position of the cervix in the vagina, plus station of the presenting part. Each of these criteria is assigned a specified number of points, with conditions most favorable for successful induction being assigned the most points. The Bishop Score, which is one of the earlier scoring systems, is still used today. With this system, a score of 9 or more is very favorable for induction, while a score of 4 or less indicates the likelihood of a failed induction.[1] A more recent scoring system by Lange and associates[2] deletes the position of the cervix as a criteria and gives double weight to cervical dilatation.

When the cervix is found to be unfavorable for induction (unripe) and prompt delivery of the fetus is deemed necessary, an attempt may be made to prime the cervix by one of several methods.

Laminaria tents. Laminaria tents are used to ripen the unfavorable cervix prior to induced abortion or induction of labor. *Laminaria digitata* is a specific type of seaweed that is dried and sterilized. When inserted in the cervical os, the smooth, rounded stem absorbs moisture and swells to three to five times its original diameter. Insertion of the laminaria the night before induction is planned usually causes gradual softening and dilatation of the cervix begins by morning. Induction by amniotomy or intravenous oxytocin infusion can then be instituted with an increased chance of success.

Prostaglandins. Prostaglandin E_2 (PGE_2) in the form of vaginal suppositories, tablets, or cervical gel has been shown to be effective in ripening the cervix.[1] The two physiologic actions thought to be involved are biochemical changes in the cervix, resulting in softening and stimulation of uterine contractions. This method is approved only for experimental use in the United States, but it is more widely used in other countries.

Oxytocin. Oxytocin may be given as an intravenous infusion for a number of hours daily over a period of

ASSESSMENT TOOL

Bishop Score to Assess Readiness of Cervix for Delivery

Factor	Points			
	0	*1*	*2*	*3*
Dilatation of cervix (cm)	0	1–2	3–4	≥5
Effacement of cervix (%)	0–30	40–50	60–70	≥80
Consistency of cervix	Firm	Medium	Soft	
Position of cervix	Posterior	Mid	Anterior	
Station of presenting part	−3	−2	−1, 0	≥+1

Bishop EH: Pelvic scoring for elective induction. Obstet Gynecol 24:266, 1964

several days. This is sometimes referred to as serial induction. The oxytocin induced contractions often bring the fetal head down into the pelvis and assist in ripening the cervix.[1] The infusion is usually stopped at night so the client can eat and rest.

Methods of Induction

Since it was believed that the intestinal peristalsis produced by a cathartic is somehow transferred to the uterus, with the consequent initiation of uterine contractions, castor oil has long been employed to induce labor. It was often followed by the administration of a hot soapsuds enema. While this is a harmless approach, it is at the very least uncomfortable and it usually fails.

Oxytocin Administration

An efficient and safe method for the induction of labor is the administration of oxytocin by intravenous drip. The properties of this oxytocic agent and its use in the third stage of labor are discussed in Chapter 24; its use in induction and augmentation of labor is considered in detail in Chapter 38.

Artificial Rupture of the Membranes

Amniotomy, or artificial rupture of the membranes, is a common method of enhancing labor, and has been used to induce labor. When the client is near term and the cervix is favorable, amniotomy is almost always followed by labor within a few hours.

The intact membranes serve as a barrier against bacterial invasion. For this reason, delivery should be accomplished expeditiously once this barrier has been eliminated by amniotomy. Many obstetricians now feel that the procedure should be delayed until after the initiation of good contractions with intravenous oxytocin. Besides the danger of infection, amniotomy also increases the risk of cord prolapse and fetal head compression. Amniotomy is contraindicated when the presenting part is high or there is an abnormal presentation such as breech or transverse lie.

To perform an amniotomy the obstetrician inserts the first two fingers of one hand into the cervix until the membranes are encountered. A long hook, usually an Allis clamp or a plastic Amnihook, is inserted into the vagina and the membranes are simply hooked and torn by the tip of the sharp instrument. The fluid may initially come out with a gush or leak out slowly. Leaking of amniotic fluid from the vagina usually continues throughout labor. The color, odor, and consistency of the amniotic fluid should be noted. It is usually clear and almost odorless and deviations can indicate problems. For example, brownish or greenish discoloration is a sign that the infant has passed meconium *in utero* and a foul odor is a sign of infection.

Nursing Process in Amniotomy. Assessment is an ongoing part of the nurse's responsibility when an amniotomy is performed. The condition of mother and fetus are assessed before, during, and after the procedure, and any changes are reported to the physician. Possible nursing diagnoses might include potential for infection related to rupture of membranes, alteration in comfort related to increasing strength of uterine contractions, or anxiety or fear related to an unfamiliar procedure.

Nursing planning and intervention involves preparing the client for the procedure and carrying out the necessary assessments. The nurse should explain the procedure to the client, reassure her that it is no more uncomfortable than a vaginal examination, and describe the warm, wet sensations that she will probably experience. Expectations for increased strength of uterine contractions should also be explained.

Prior to the procedure the nurse can assist the client in assuming a position on her back with her knees flexed and separated. Antiseptic preparation of the vulva is carried out according to hospital policy. Fetal heart tones should be checked before and immediately after the amniotomy for possible changes indicating prolapse of the cord. They should continue to be checked frequently because of the increased possibility of cord prolapse. The time of the amniotomy and the color, amount, and odor of the fluid should be recorded on the chart. If an electronic fetal monitor is in use, the time of the amniotomy should also be recorded on the graph. The bed linens should be changed as often as necessary to keep the client comfortable.

Forceps Deliveries

There are occasions when it becomes necessary to mechanically help in the delivery of the fetus. Forceps are instruments that may be used in maternal care for holding and extracting the fetal head.

Reasons for Forceps Delivery

It may become necessary to deliver the baby by forceps for the mother's welfare (maternal indications) or because of conditions associated with the baby's condition (fetal indications). Maternal indications include inability of the mother to push after full dilatation of the cervix because of conduction anesthesia, exhaustion, or heart disease, or any condition affecting the mother that is likely to be improved by delivery.

The chief fetal indications for forceps delivery are fetal distress, as suggested by a slow, irregular fetal heart, and, in general, conditions that would potentially cause fetal distress, such as placental abruption or prolapsed umbilical cord.

Many obstetricians, however, deem it desirable to deliver almost all primigravidas with forceps electively, in the belief that the operation spares the mother many minutes of bearing-down efforts and relieves pressure on the baby's head. This is usually referred to as "elective forceps."

Forceps delivery is never attempted unless the cervix is completely dilated and the vertex is engaged (*i.e.,* the greatest biparietal diameter of the fetal head is at, or has already traversed, the pelvic inlet). Usually, but not always, when engagement has occurred, the vertex is at or below the ischial spines.

Types of Forceps

Some of the common types of obstetric forceps are illustrated in Figure 39-2. The instrument consists of two steel parts that cross each other like a pair of scissors and lock at the intersection. The lock may be of a sliding type, as in the first three types shown, or a screw type, as in the Tarnier instrument.

Each part consists of a handle, a lock, a shank, and a blade; the blade is the curved portion designed for application to the sides of the fetal head. The blades of most forceps (the Tucker–McLean is an exception) have a large opening or window (fenestrum) to give a better grip on the head and usually consist of two curves, a cephalic curve, which conforms to the shape of the head, and a pelvic curve, to follow the curve of the birth canal. Axis-traction forceps, such as the Tarnier, have a mechanism attached below that permits the pulling to be done more directly in the axis of the birth canal. An axis-traction handle is also available for use on standard forceps.

The two blades of the forceps are designated as right and left. The left blade is the one that is introduced into the vagina on the client's left side; the right blade goes in on the right side.

Types of Forceps Delivery

In the vast majority of instances today, the forceps delivery is carried out at a time when the fetal head is on the perineal floor (visible or almost so) and internal ro-

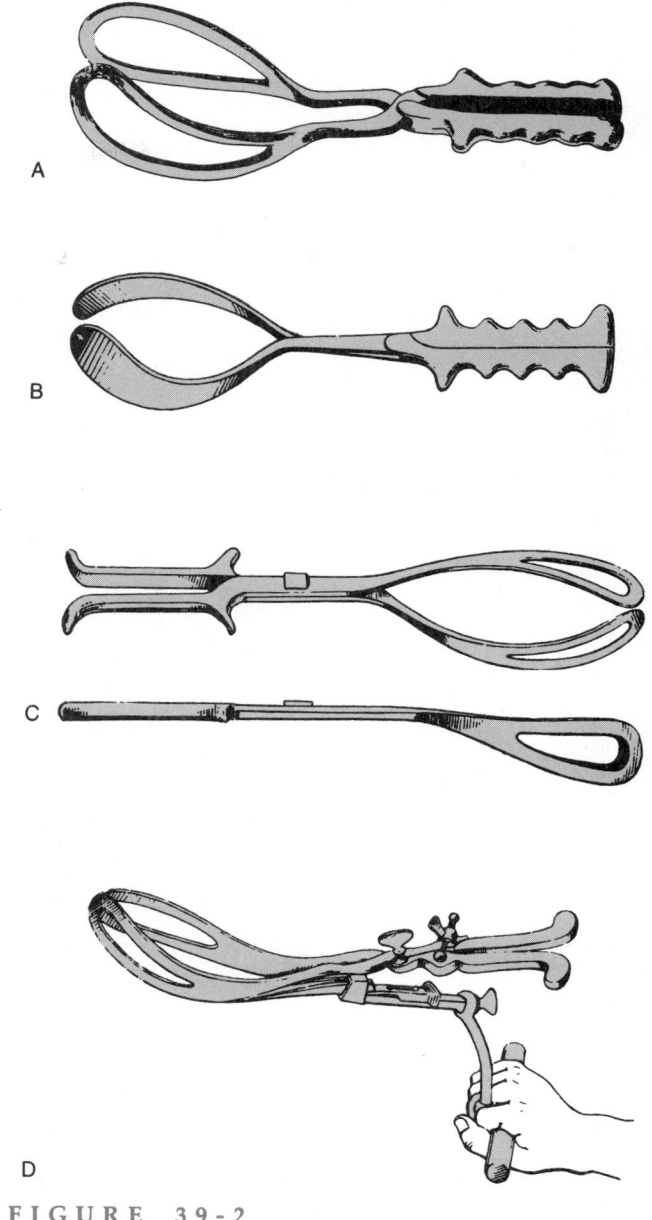

FIGURE 39-2

Types of forceps. (*A*) Simpson forceps. (*B*) Tucker–McLean forceps. (*C, top*) Kielland forceps, front view. (*C, bottom*) Kielland forceps, side view. (*D*) Tarnier axis-traction forceps.

tation may have already occurred, so that the fetal head lies in a direct anteroposterior position. This is called *low forceps,* or "outlet forceps." When the head is higher in the pelvis but engaged and its greatest diameter has passed the inlet, the operation is called *midforceps.* If the head has not yet engaged, the procedure is known as *high forceps.* High-forceps delivery is an exceedingly difficult and dangerous operation for both mother and baby and is rarely done. Increasingly, cesarean birth is preferred to a potentially difficult midforceps delivery.

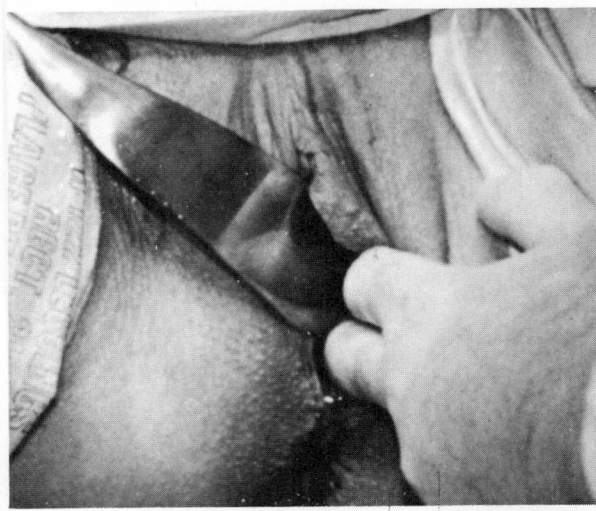

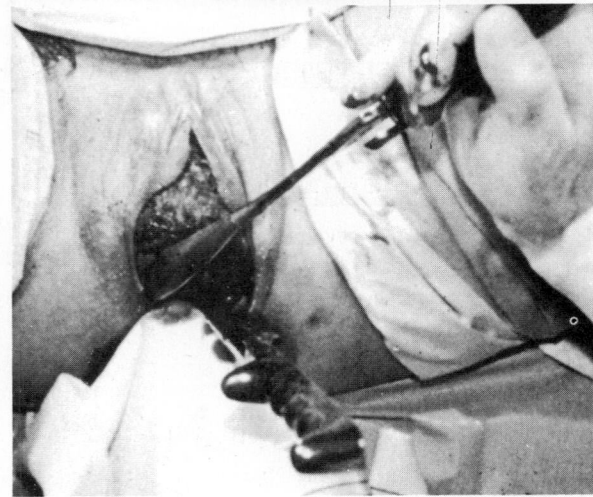

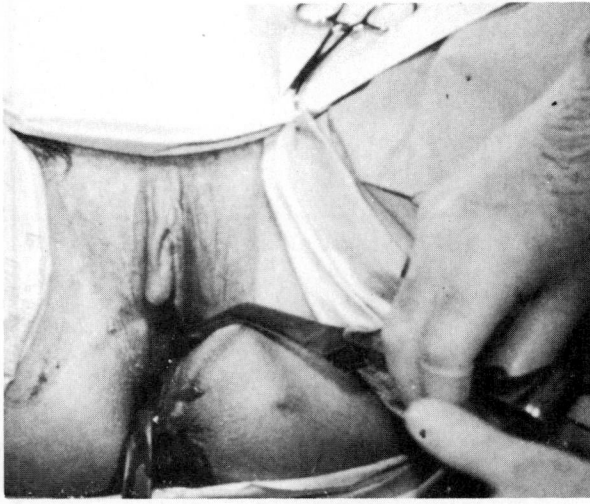

Procedure

After a decision is made to use forceps, the obstetrician selects the type of instrument to be used. Several pairs of the generally approved forceps, each encased in suitable wrappings, are autoclaved and kept in the delivery room for immediate use. The other instruments needed for a forceps delivery are the same as those required for a spontaneous delivery.

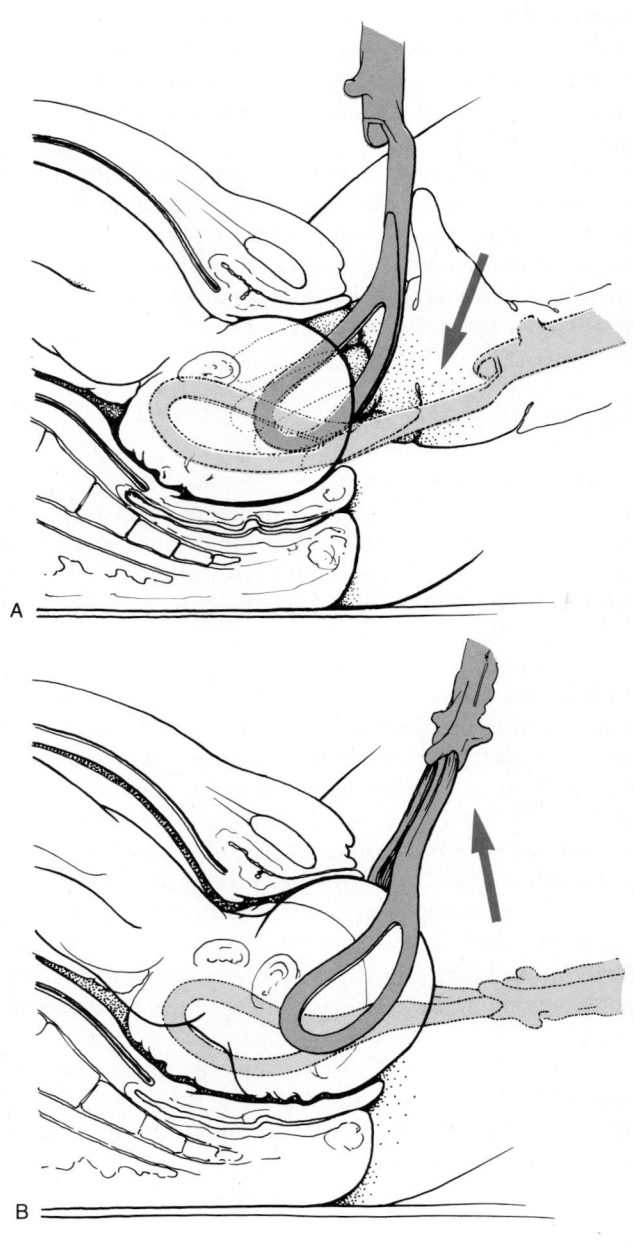

FIGURE   39-3

Insertion of the two blades of the forceps. (From the film *Human Birth*, published by JB Lippincott, Philadelphia)

FIGURE   39-4

(*A*) Insertion of forceps blade and (*B*) applied forceps and direction of traction.

Anesthesia is recommended, but in low-forceps deliveries it may be light, and in most institutions this type of operation is performed in association with conduction anesthesia or under pudendal block anesthesia. The client is placed in the lithotomy position and prepared and draped in the usual fashion. For a midforceps delivery the bladder should be emptied by catheterization.

After checking the exact position of the fetal head by vaginal examination, the physician introduces two or more fingers of one hand into the left side of the vagina; these fingers guide the left blade into place and at the same time protect the maternal soft parts (vagina and cervix) from injury. The other hand is used to introduce the left blade of the forceps into the left side of the vagina, gently insinuating it between the baby's head and the fingers of the hand (Fig. 39-3). The same procedure is carried out on the right side, and then the blades are articulated. Traction is not continuous but intermittent (Fig. 39-4), and between traction, the blades are partially disarticulated to release pressure on the fetal head. Episiotomy is now routine in these cases.

Nursing Care

When forceps delivery is anticipated, the nurse can briefly explain the procedure and its necessity to the mother and father. The mother will feel pressure and pulling, but will not feel pain with adequate regional or spinal anesthesia. Breathing techniques to prevent muscle tensing and pushing during application of the forceps should be encouraged, as well as other techniques used by the mother/couple to cope with labor.

The nurse provides the physician with the required type of forceps. This often can be determined in advance, and the forceps put on the delivery table. Once the forceps are applied, the nurse monitors contractions and advises the physician, so traction with the forceps can be coordinated with contractions. The mother is also encouraged to continue pushing as the physician applies traction. Continuous fetal heart rate monitoring is a nursing responsibility. Bradycardia from head compression is common when forceps traction occurs.

Appropriate infant resuscitation equipment should be available, and a pediatrician should be called if the infant is depressed or the forceps delivery is difficult. Bruises from forceps on the infant's head are not uncommon, and the parents should be informed that these will disappear in a few days.

Piper Forceps for Breech Delivery

The Piper forceps have been designed to assist in the delivery of the aftercoming head in breech presentations (Fig. 39-5). They are applied after the shoulders have been delivered and the head has been brought into the pelvis by gentle traction combined with suprapubic pressure. Suspension of the body and arms with a towel facilitates application of the blades. The left blade is

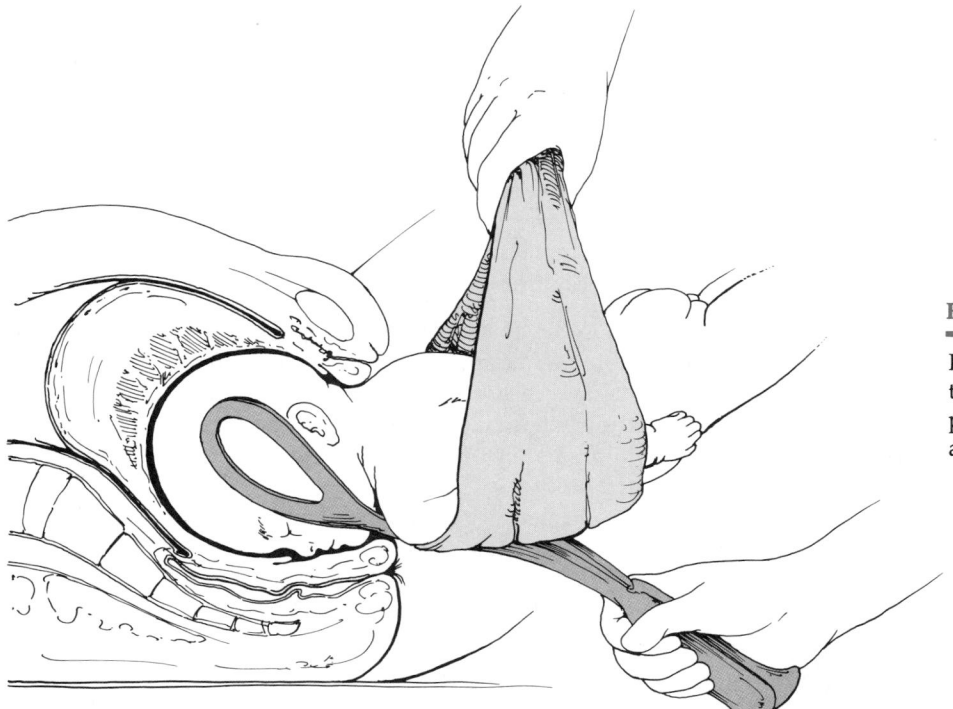

FIGURE 39-5

Piper forceps are used to deliver the aftercoming head in breech presentations, while the body and arms are suspended in a towel.

introduced in an upward direction along the fetal head on the left side, and the right blade is then applied in a similar fashion. The forceps are locked in place, and their position on the head is confirmed by palpation. An episiotomy is made and, as traction is applied, the chin, mouth, and nose emerge over the perineum. The Piper forceps are often used electively as a substitute for the Mauriceau-Smellie-Veit maneuver, or when the Mauriceau-Smellie-Veit maneuver for delivery of the fetal head has failed (see Chap. 38).

Vacuum Extraction

Occasionally, an instrument known as the vacuum extractor is used in place of the forceps. The vacuum extractor consists of a cup that is applied to the fetal head and tightly affixed there by creating a vacuum in the cup through withdrawal of the air by a pump. Cups are supplied in various sizes. The largest cup that can be applied with ease is selected for use. Vacuum is built up slowly, and the suction creates an artificial caput within the cup, providing a firm attachment to the fetal scalp. Traction can then be exerted by means of a short chain attached to the cup, with a handle at its far end.

Nursing Care

The nurse should briefly explain the procedure and its necessity to the mother and father. The mother will feel pressure and pulling sensations, but will not feel pain with adequate regional or spinal anesthesia. Breathing techniques to prevent tensing and pushing are encouraged during application of the vacuum extraction cup. The mother is kept informed by the nurse during the procedure.

The nurse provides the physician with the vacuum extraction equipment, including the size cup requested and sterile tubing. After the physician assembles the cup and tubing, the nurse attaches the distal end to suction. With the cup applied to the fetal head, the nurse activates the suction. To avoid damaging vaginal tissues, suction must be released if the cup slips off the fetal head. The nurse encourages the mother to push during contractions to aid birth, while traction is applied by the physician (Fig. 39-6).

The fetal heart rate should be monitored frequently by the nurse during the procedure. Infant resuscitation equipment should be available, and the pediatrician should be called if complications are expected with the infant. Parents are informed that the baby's head will have a caput (chignon) where the cup was applied, but that this will disappear in a few hours.

Repair of Lacerations

Except for clamping and cutting the umbilical cord, episiotomy is the most common operative procedure performed in obstetrics. In view of the fact that this incision of the perineum, made to facilitate delivery, is employed almost routinely in primigravidas, the procedure has been discussed in the section on the conduct of normal labor (see Chap. 25).

Lacerations of the perineum and the vagina that occur in the process of delivery have also been discussed previously, because some tears are unavoidable, even in the most skilled hands. The suturing of spontaneous perineal lacerations is similar to that employed for the repair of an episiotomy incision, but may be more difficult because such tears often are irregular in shape with ragged, bruised edges.

Cesarean Delivery

Cesarean delivery is the removal of the fetus from the uterus through an incision made in the abdominal wall and the uterus.

The main indications for cesarean delivery fall into the following groups:

- Disproportion between the size of the fetus and that of the bony birth canal—that is, contracted pelvis, tumor blocking birth canal, and so on
- In certain cases in which the client has had a previous cesarean section, myomectomy, or uterine reconstruction, the operation is done because of the fear that the uterus will rupture in labor
- Certain cases of severe preeclampsia or eclampsia
- Certain cases of placenta previa and premature separation of the normally implanted placenta
- Actual or pending fetal distress
- Malpresentation (breech or transverse)

When a cesarean delivery is done prior to the onset of labor, as the result of a prearranged plan, it is called *elective* cesarean delivery (as with elective low forceps, the obstetrician is not forced to perform the operation immediately, but elects to do it as the best procedure for mother and baby).

Prematurity is the most common fetal complication of elective cesarean delivery, occurring because the duration of gestation is misjudged. This can now be avoided by evaluating fetal maturity preoperatively through determination of the amniotic fluid lecithin/sphingomyelin (L/S) ratio (see Chap. 41).

The incidence of cesarean birth has increased dramatically in the past several years, from about 4.5%

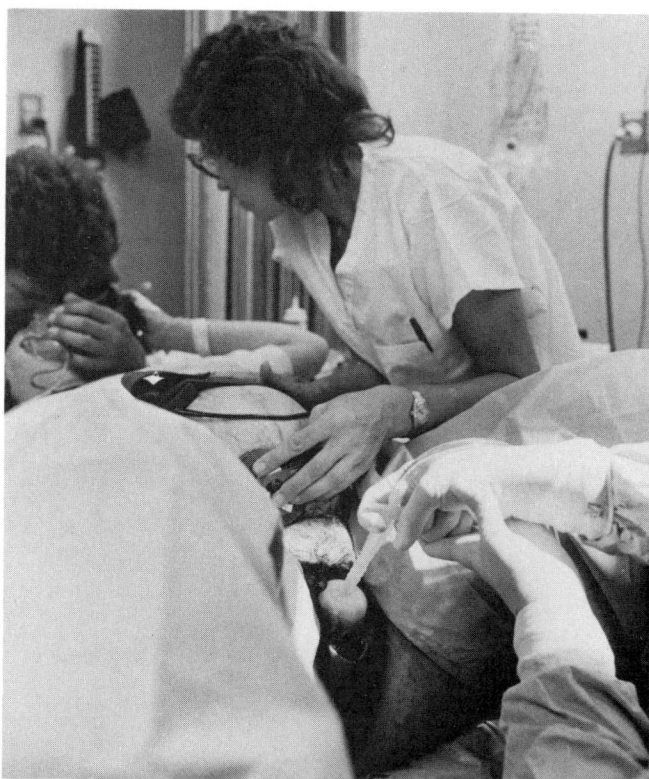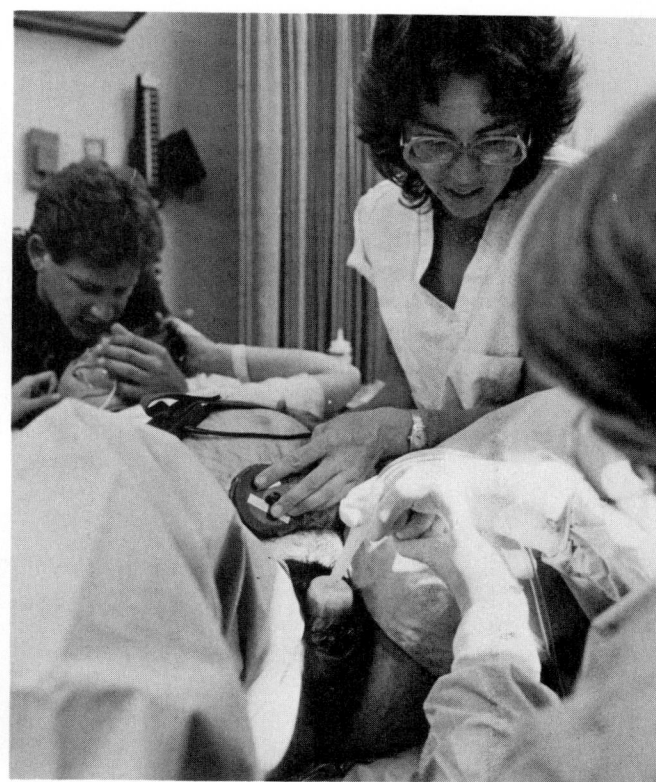

FIGURE 39-6

The nurse keeps the couple informed during the procedure and encourages the mother to push during the contractions, and monitors the fetus as traction continues. (Photos by Kathy Sloane)

prior to 1965 to 20% to 22% in certain types of hospitals.[3] This substantial increase has engendered a great deal of controversy, and the necessity for the large numbers of operative deliveries has come under public scrutiny. This controversy is discussed later in the chapter.

Main Types of Cesarean Delivery

Although there are four types of cesarean delivery, the lower-segment section is usually the operation of choice. In this operation, the uterus is entered through an incision in the lower segment. Other types of cesarean delivery include the classical cesarean section, in which the incision is made directly into the wall of the body of the uterus; the extraperitoneal cesarean section, in which the operation is arranged anatomically, such that the incision is made into the uterus without entering the peritoneal cavity; and cesarean section–hysterectomy, which involves a cesarean section of any variety followed by removal of the uterus.

Low-Segment Cesarean Delivery

Low-segment cesarean delivery is usually the operation of choice for a number of important reasons. Since the incision is made in the lower segment of the uterus, which is its thinnest portion, there is minimal blood loss, and the incision is easy to repair. The lower segment is also the area of least uterine activity, and thus the possibility of rupture of the scar in a subsequent pregnancy is lessened. Since the incision can be properly peritonealized, the operation is associated with a lower incidence of postoperative infection.

The initial incision (the abdominal cavity having been opened) is made transversely across the uterine peritoneum, where it is attached loosely just above the bladder. The lower peritoneal flap and the bladder are now dissected from the uterus, and the uterine muscle is incised either vertically or transversely (Fig. 39-7A through D). The membranes are ruptured, and the baby is delivered (Fig. 39-7E through L). The placenta is extracted (Figs. 39-8 and 39-9), and intravenous Pitocin

(text continued on page 868)

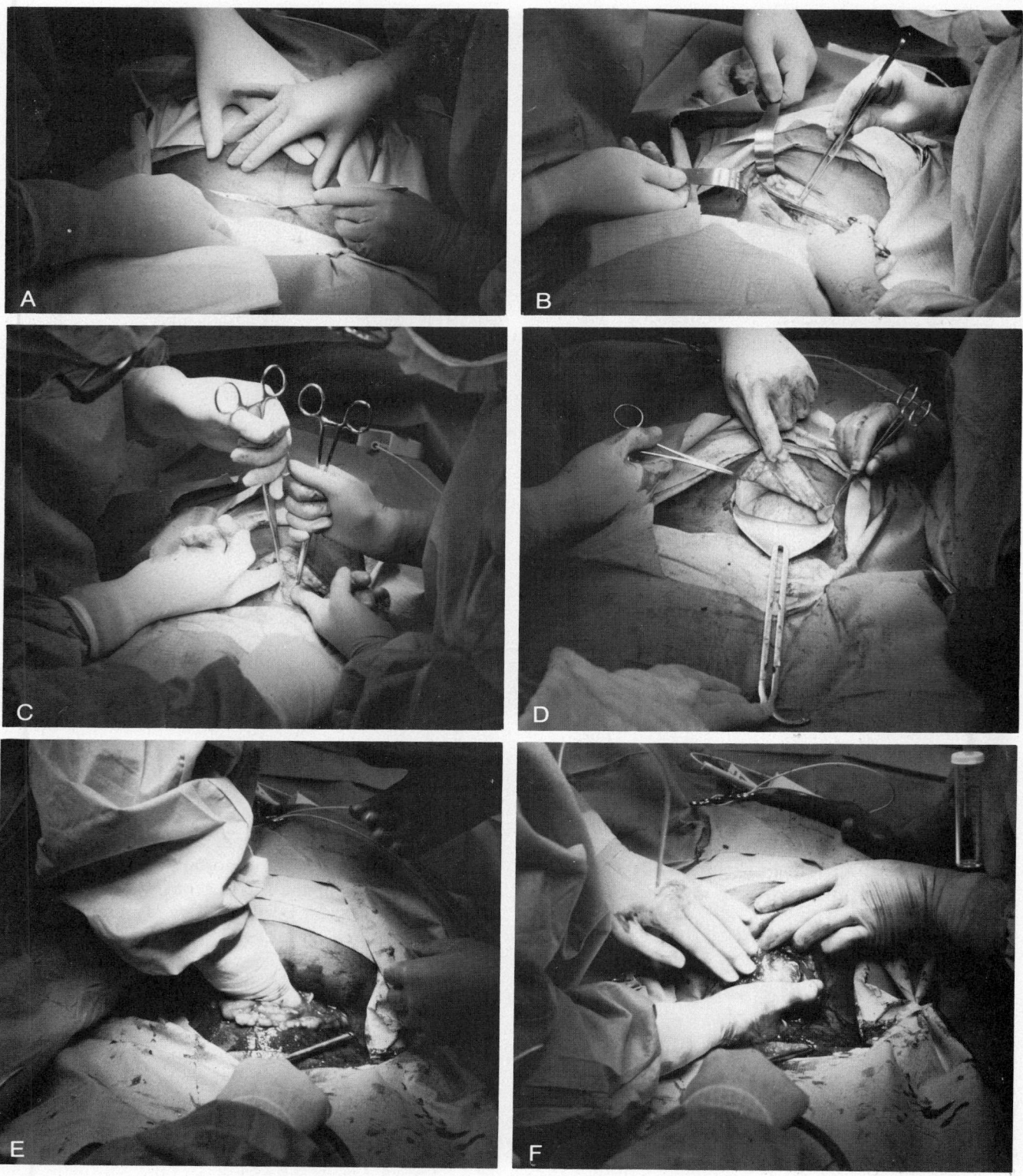

FIGURE 39-7

Cesarean birth. (*A*) Pfannenstiel's incision through the skin at the start of the operation. (*B*) The fascia has been nicked at the midline and is being opened in a smiling fashion with heavy scissors. (*C*) The fascia is separated from the underlying rectus muscle in a combination of blunt (shown in picture) and sharp dissection. (*D*) The peritoneum has been opened (hemostats on the edges), and the bladder blade has been positioned. The lower uterine segment is visible through the incision.

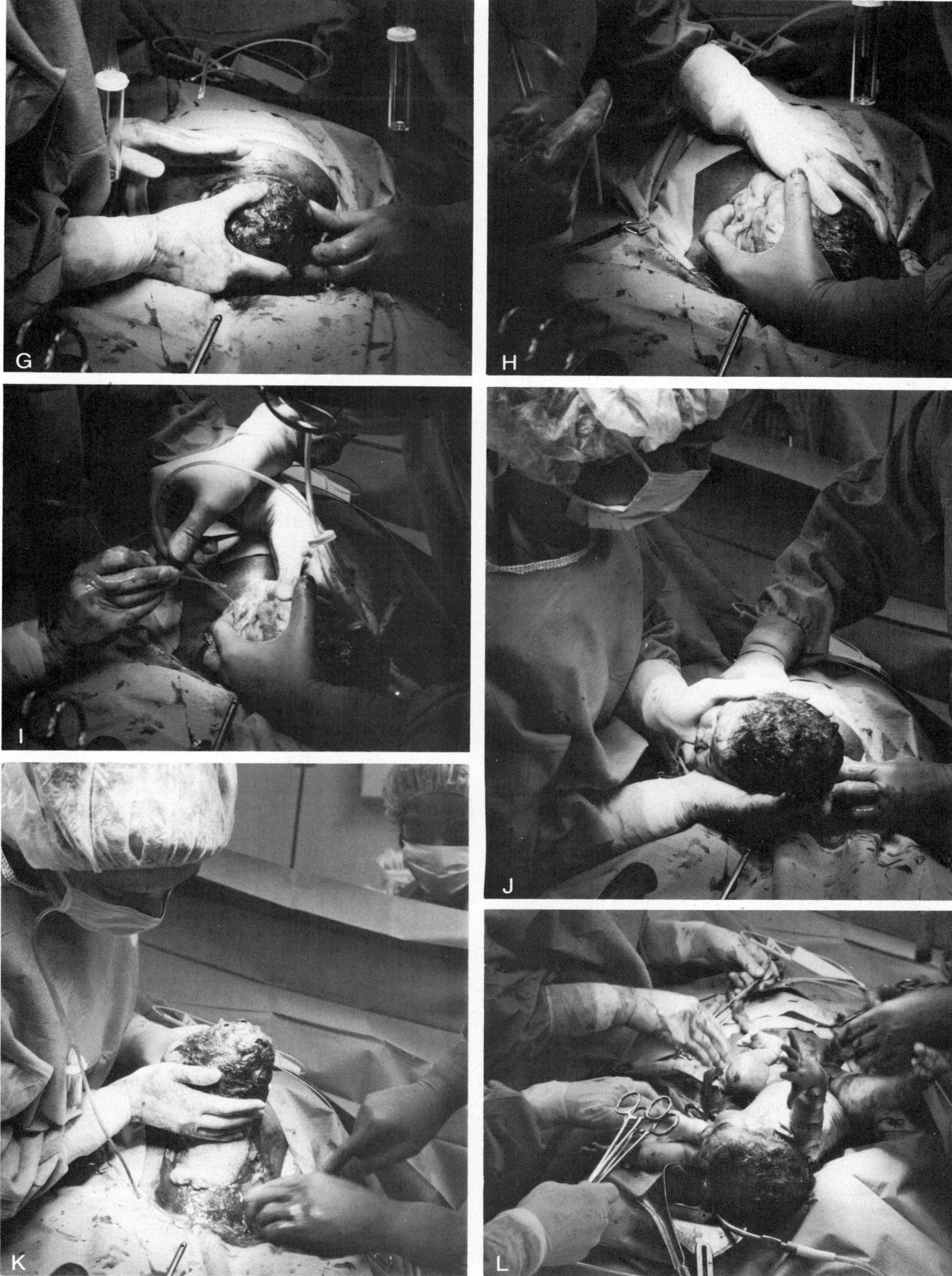

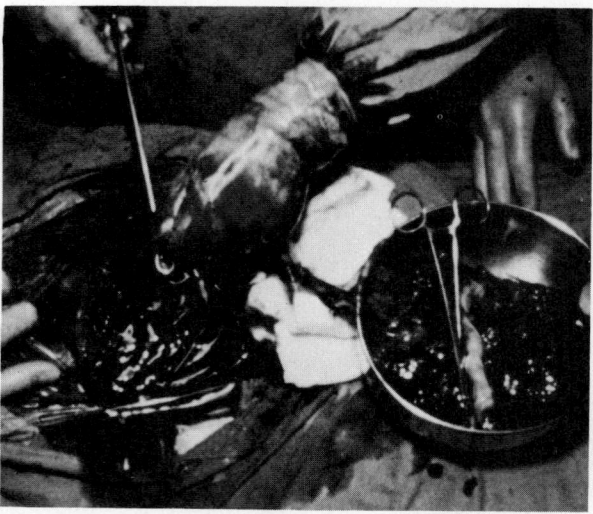 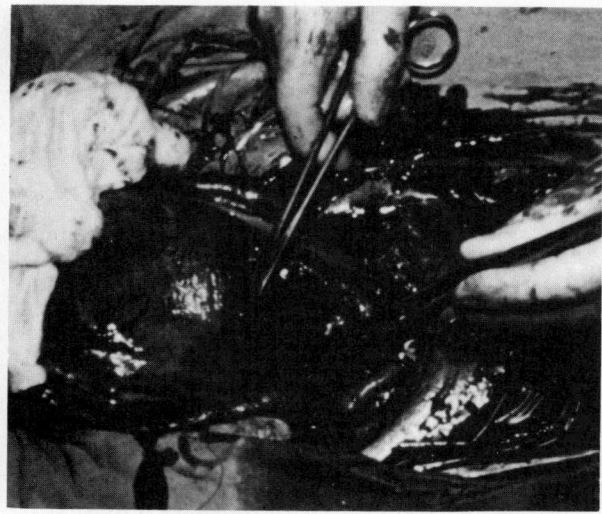

FIGURE 39-8

The placenta is extracted through the abdominal incision. (From the film Human Birth, published by JB Lippincott, Philadelphia)

(text continued from page 865)

is administered to contract the uterus. The uterine incision is sutured, and the lower flap is imbricated over the uterine incision. This two-flap arrangement seals off the uterine incision and is believed to prevent the egress of infectious lochia into the peritoneal cavity.

Classical Cesarean Delivery

A vertical incision is made directly into the wall of the body of the uterus; the baby and the placenta are extracted, and the incision is closed by three layers of absorbable sutures. Thus, this approach requires tra-

versing the full thickness of the uterine corpus. It is still recommended in certain circumstances. It is particularly useful when the bladder and lower segment are involved in extensive adhesions resulting from a previous cesarean section and occasionally is selected when the fetus is in a transverse lie or when there is an anterior placenta previa.

Extraperitoneal Cesarean Delivery

By appropriate dissection of the tissues around the bladder, access to the lower uterine segment is secured without entering the peritoneal cavity. The baby is de-

FIGURE 39-7 *(continued)*

(*E*) The bladder flap has been created; a low transverse uterine incision has been made, and the operator's hand is introduced in the lower uterine segment to facilitate the delivery of the fetal head. (*F*) The vertex has been brought to the site of the uterine incision, and the operator's right hand is guiding the delivery of the head. Fundal pressure from the right hand of the surgical assistant is facilitating the process. (*G*) The fetal head is gently being delivered through the uterine and abdominal incisions. (*H*) The fetal head has been delivered; the index finger of the assistant is being introduced into the baby's mouth to facilitate oropharyngeal suctioning of the amniotic fluid and secretions prior to the baby's first breath. (*I*) Nasopharyngeal and oropharyngeal suctioning are being performed by both the operator and the assistant using DeLee catheters. (*J*) Delivery *first* of the posterior shoulder through the uterine and abdominal incisions by gentle upward traction. (*K*) Delivery of the anterior shoulder by gentle downward traction. (*L*) The baby has been delivered, and the umbilical cord has been clamped with Kelly clamps and cut.

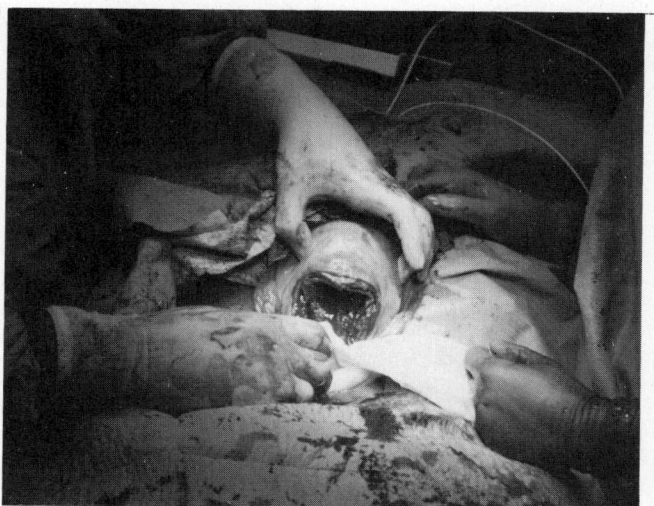

FIGURE 39-9

Following delivery of the baby and placenta, the low transverse incision is clearly visible.

livered through an incision in the lower uterine segment. Since the entire operation is done outside the peritoneal cavity, neither spill of infected amniotic fluid nor subsequent seepage of pus from the uterus can reach the peritoneal surfaces. This approach was used extensively in the preantibiotic era, but is rarely if ever employed today.

Cesarean Delivery–Hysterectomy

Cesarean delivery–hysterectomy is also known as Porro's operation. This operation comprises cesarean birth followed by removal of the uterus. It may be necessary in certain cases of *premature separation of the placenta* and placenta accreta and in women with multiple *fibroid tumors of the uterus;* in rare circumstances it is done electively for sterilization purposes.

Increasing Cesarean Delivery Rates

Despite recommendations of the National Consensus Development Conference (1980), cesarean delivery rates are still rising. Few hospitals except teaching institutions provide peer review for the dystocia diagnosis. Trials of labor in women with low-segment transverse cesarean births are not universally accepted. Vaginal deliveries of breech presentations have not found much support. More accurate diagnosis of fetal distress using fetal *p*H scalp monitoring is practiced only in a minority of hospitals. Despite costs to the health-care system and risks to the mother from unnecessary cesarean delivery, powerful incentives for both physicians and hospitals fueled by an unhealthy medicolegal climate, will probably keep the rate above 15% no matter what educational and administrative efforts are made.[4]

Factors Contributing to Increased Cesarean Births

Numerous factors are involved in the rising cesarean rate, and understanding their interrelations and relative importance is a complex task. Standards of obstetric practice in managing certain labor complications contribute significantly to the increased cesarean birth rate. Four diagnostic categories account for about 80% of all cesareans and for 80% to 90% of the rise in the rate: repeat cesareans, dystocia, breech presentation, and fetal distress.

By and large, the increase in the incidence of cesarean birth is attributable to fetal indications. Fetal monitoring has permitted earlier diagnosis of fetal distress, and modern methods for assessment of fetal well-being during the course of pregnancy also provide a basis for early delivery. In the latter circumstances, cesarean delivery is a justifiable substitute for prolonged and difficult medical induction. Cesarean birth is a less traumatic substitute for some previously preferred operative procedures, such as difficult midforceps and vaginal breech delivery in the primigravida or mother in preterm labor, to avoid trauma to the aftercoming head.

Those who support this trend point to reduced perinatal mortality and morbidity, but others suggest that complex medicolegal factors underlie the rise. The decision to carry out a cesarean delivery cannot be taken lightly. Maternal morbidity and mortality are more frequent than with vaginal delivery. For this reason, cesarean delivery should not be performed unless there is obstetrically sound justification.

Childbirth Complications. The purpose of operative intervention in cases of maternal disease or labor complications is to improve the fetal outcome. A virtual explosion of obstetric technology has occurred to assist physicians in monitoring the condition of the fetus and diagnosing the presence of a dangerous situation. Included are such procedures and equipment as amniotomy, prenatal stress testing, chemical induction and stimulation of labor, amniocentesis, electronic fetal monitoring (EFM), internal pressure transducers for measuring the strength of uterine contractions, assessment of fetal scalp blood *p*H, and various other blood and chemical studies. In nearly all cases, the technology itself has inherent risks, both direct and indirect, to the well-being of mother and infant. The following are the most common indications for cesarean birth.

Previous Cesarean Birth. About 98% of women in the United States with a previous cesarean birth had, until recently, operative deliveries with subsequent births. Almost one third of all cesarean births are done for this indication, and it accounts for 25% to 30% of the rise in the cesarean rate. Because of the increasing rate of primary cesareans, this category multiplies the overall rate increase. Increasingly, the client is offered the option of attempting labor and vaginal delivery, especially when the previous cesarean birth occurred for reasons other than cephalopelvic disproportion (CPD).

Dystocia. Dystocia includes such diagnoses as cephalopelvic disproportion (CPD), prolonged labor, uterine dysfunction, and failure to progress in labor. It accounts for 30% of the rise in the cesarean rate, the largest single category for primary operations. Several factors are involved in the increased rate for dystocia. Absolute CPD is rare. Much of the increase stems from a change in obstetric management from less anatomical emphasis to a functional definition of the progress of labor. Labor graphs are used that set parameters for normal progress in terms of time, centimeters dilatation, and effectiveness of contractions. When women in labor deviate from graphic definitions of normal progress, indications arise for cesarean delivery. Suggestions have been made to reduce the incidence of cesareans in this category. Approaches include managing prolonged labor with rest, hydration, sedation, ambulation, and, if effective labor does not ensue, use of oxytocin stimulation with discretion. The amount of time allowed for response to treatment of dysfunctional labor needs to be evaluated; the implication is that intervention comes too soon. Childbirth preparation, a supportive labor environment, more freedom of maternal movement and choices, and avoidance of technological intervention are associated with decreases in cesarean births for dystocia.[5]

Breech Presentation. Changes in the medical philosophy of breech management have led to an increase in cesareans for breech presentation. About 10% to 15% of the rise in cesarean rate is due to breech presentation. Many studies have indicated increased morbidity and mortality among breech-born infants, but there is other evidence that overall perinatal mortality is not significantly lessened with cesarean deliveries. When mothers of equal parity with infants in equal weight groups are compared, there is no significant decrease in perinatal mortality in infants delivered by cesarean in the great majority of groups.[6] The National Institutes of Health (NIH) Consensus Development Task Force on Cesarean Childbirth recommended that vaginal breech delivery continue to be an accepted practice with a full-term baby not over 8 lb, a normal pelvis, frank breech presentation without hyperextended head, and an experienced obstetrician. This last requirement is becoming more and more difficult to fulfill, however, because of the diminishing experience of resident physicians in delivering breech infants vaginally. Because of policies tending toward cesarean delivery as standard for all breech presentations, residents have less and less experience with vaginal breech deliveries. They become reluctant to do this when in practice later and are also concerned with possible lawsuits for not doing cesareans if the infant is injured by vaginal birth.

Fetal Distress. Over the past 10 years the most rapidly increasing indication for cesarean delivery has been fetal distress. This category has had an eightfold increase and now accounts for 10% to 15% of all cesareans. The association of fetal distress, cesarean birth, and EFM is complex and controversial. Although the increased cesarean rate and introduction of widespread EFM occurred about the same time, there is no proof of causality, and this may only reflect a greater reliance on technology and intervention in obstetrics generally. The key question is whether EFM permits more accurate identification of fetal distress than auscultation, or whether fetal distress is being overdiagnosed. It is recognized that the monitors malfunction, that physicians and nurses misread the tracings, and that abnormal tracings do not always correlate with low Apgar scores or low scalp *p*H. In addition, EFM appears involved indirectly in increasing cesarean rates for indications other than fetal distress. Some studies have found a higher incidence of dystocia in women who are monitored during labor. The stress produced by procedures used to insert monitors, by tension in the environment, and by fear of the implications of EFM could contribute to reduced uteroplacental perfusion and general muscular tension in the woman. Having to lie stationary on her back to accommodate the equipment's needs is detrimental to effective labor and the woman's ability to cope with contractions. Monitors might also lead to premature diagnosis of failure to progress, with physicians allowing less time to determine effective labor.

Medicolegal Factors. Obstetricians are more willing to perform operative deliveries now than in the past, for a number of reasons.

Safety. Cesarean birth is relatively safe for the mother, with maternal mortality reported between 20 and 70 per 100,000 operations. Maternal mortality has continued to decline despite sharply rising cesarean birth rates. Perinatal mortality has also decreased and is less than one third that of 30 years ago. It has continued to decline even with the increase in cesarean deliveries. Improved diagnosis of fetal maturity has helped to prevent premature delivery by the physician. EFM and functional (graphic) definitions of labor have provided more scientific rationales for operative deliveries. Although overall perinatal mortality is higher for abdominal than vaginal delivery, the selective use of cesarean deliveries can improve the fetal prognosis in a number of conditions.

Medical Training. Changes in medical training are also important. Obstetric residents receive less preparation and experience in the use of forceps, especially midforceps. They deliver fewer breech presentations vaginally and are taught to rely more on cesarean deliveries. Obstetric residents learn values that support more active physician intervention in the childbirth process and are less inclined to wait and encourage natural processes to take place. Extreme adherents of such values hold that normal birth is dangerous for infants, owing to forces and pressures on the fetal head that lead to risk of brain damage, and suggest that the majority of women will eventually be delivered by surgery.[7]

Providers of Maternal Care. Certain changes in characteristics of the obstetric population may also lead to greater inclination by physicians to perform cesareans. The proportion of nulliparous mothers has increased, and the average age of the obstetric population has risen recently. Both of these groups have higher incidences of cesarean births. A greater proportion of maternity care is being provided by obstetricians (rather than family or general practice physicians), who perform cesarean sections more frequently than nonobstetricians.

Economics and Malpractice. Economic factors may be involved; cesareans are about three times more costly than vaginal deliveries, but the evidence concerning cesarean births in prepaid, military, and governmental facilities (where there should be no fee incentive) is mixed. The threat of malpractice suits appears to be an enormous concern for many physicians, who fear loss of community trust and goodwill even in unsuccessful suits. However, suits involving cesareans are related more to events occurring during the operation than to failure to perform the cesarean.

Hospitals. The characteristics of hospitals affect cesarean delivery rates. Hospitals with neonatal intensive care units are most likely to provide cesareans.

Public hospitals have slightly lower, and proprietary hospitals slightly higher, cesarean rates than voluntary hospitals. Cesarean rates rise with hospital bed size. The age mix and complications of clients in various types of hospitals play important roles in the indications for surgical delivery. However, hospitals with medical school affiliations and neonatal intensive care units (NICU) have the most serious case mixes, but are least likely to do cesareans for several types of complications.[3] The teaching function in hospitals appears to provide some control over appropriate use of technology.

Disadvantages in Cesarean Delivery

There are, of course, disadvantages to delivering by cesarean. Maternal mortality and morbidity are involved along with the discomforts occurring following any surgery. Maternal–infant bonding may be affected, including development of mothering skills and breast-feeding. These drawbacks are spelled out in Maternal Risks in Cesarean Birth.

Maternal Risks in Cesarean Birth

Maternal mortality, although rare, is 4 times higher with cesarean delivery than with vaginal delivery. Half of this increase is due to complications leading to the cesarean or to maternal disease. The other half is due to the surgery itself.

Maternal mortality in repeat cesarean is about twice that in vaginal deliveries.

Maternal morbidity is much greater after cesarean; the major risks are from:
  Infection of uterus and other genital tract structures
  Infection of respiratory or urinary tract
  Hemorrhage

Postoperative discomforts occur frequently, including incisional pain, gas, weakness, and difficulty in movement.

Maternal–infant bonding is interfered with through common hospital practices such as:
  General anesthesia during surgery
  Separation of mother and infant during recovery and first day
  Analgesics given the mother for pain relief
  Isolation necessary for infections

Development of mothering skills is interfered with because of:
  Disorientation following anesthesia and surgery
  Pain limiting activities and requiring sedation
  Weakness, which limits the energy the mother can give to infant caretaking
  Postoperative complications further reducing mother–infant contact
  Emotional turmoil and the need to process feelings (anger, loss, confusion, fear, inadequacy, etc.) associated with undergoing cesarean birth and operative procedures
  Delay and increased difficulty gaining a sense of mastery over the mother's body

Breast-feeding is more difficult or impossible because of:
  Pain, weakness, limited activities
  Infections or other serious complications
  Medications that may be excreted in breast milk
  Sense of inadequacy related to childbearing capabilities

Education to Avoid Cesarean Delivery

Women and their partners can benefit from understanding how they can help avoid unnecessary cesarean birth. Often a series of occurrences from early pregnancy through the labor process leads to the decision for surgical delivery. Different choices by parents, or different actions in relation to health providers, might lead to a different outcome. Choice of birth attendant, locale for delivery, health practices, level of knowledge about childbearing, and participation in childbirth preparation can all affect the type of delivery[8] (see Avoiding Unnecessary Cesarean Birth).

Vaginal Birth After Cesarean

The practice of "once a cesarean always a cesarean" has been standard in American obstetrics since 1916, although in Europe vaginal delivery after cesarean birth is not uncommon. Fear of uterine rupture deterred physicians from allowing a woman to deliver vaginally after a cesarean in what is called trial of labor/vaginal birth after cesarean (VBAC).

Several studies have documented the safety of allowing selected women to deliver vaginally after a cesarean birth. These studies also found that between 60% and 65% deliver successfully, involving the same or fewer risks than repeat cesareans.[9] The NIH Consensus Development Task Force on Cesarean Childbirth recommended in its 1980 report that labor and vaginal delivery is a safe, relatively low-risk choice following a previous low-segment transverse uterine incision. It also recommended that trials of labor take place in facilities with capability of an immediate emergency cesarean delivery if necessary.[10] See Report of the NIH Consensus Development Task Force on Cesarean Childbirth for further information.

Nursing Care for Cesarean Birth

The woman undergoing a cesarean birth is in need of the same sensitive and supportive care recommended for vaginal births by the Interprofessional Task Force on Health Care of Women and Children.

With the increased incidence of cesarean birth, nursing care that assists the mother and family to have a satisfying childbirth experience is extremely important. Having an operative delivery increases anxiety, adds numerous factors that must be understood and accepted, makes postdelivery recovery more difficult, places an additional strain on the developing mother–infant relationship, and creates a need for processing and integrating the altered birth experience.

Women facing a repeat or elective cesarean birth, who know in advance that their birth will be operative, have time to prepare psychologically for the experience. Other women do not know in advance and must contend with the decision for a cesarean delivery while

CLIENT EDUCATION

Avoiding Unnecessary Cesarean Birth

Cesarean births are necessary for a small proportion of women with serious conditions threatening fetal or maternal life. For many other women, a series of events takes place that, in their combined effects, leads to an inevitable decision for cesarean birth, which is usually necessary at that time, but which might have been prevented had different choices been made. Some approaches to minimizing the risk of cesarean birth follow:

- Carefully choose a birth attendant who will be most supportive of your needs and desires for the birth experience. A nurse–midwife, if available, might be more compatible with your chosen style of birth.
- Select a birth environment that provides the type of setting compatible with your objectives for the birth experience. This may be an alternate birth center, or a hospital with policies permitting many choices.
- Become informed about childbearing, its potential risks, choices available at various decision points, and legal rights and responsibilities.
- Participate in childbirth-preparation classes, which increase knowledge and reduce fear, provide tools for positive management of labor and delivery, and help the mother attain optimal physical and emotional condition for undergoing labor and birth.
- Maintain your general health through appropriate nutrition, exercise, weight, and activities; avoid habits or practices that increase risk such as smoking, alcohol or drug use.
- When the birth attendant is an obstetrician, discuss his or her beliefs and practices related to cesareans, such as indications for surgery, induction, or labor stimulation and the percentage of deliveries done by cesarean section (above 10% increases risk).
- Determine the hospital's policies regarding cesarean operations and fetal monitoring and what percentage of deliveries are by cesarean section (above 30% increases risk).

Report of the NIH Consensus Development Task Force on Cesarean Childbirth

In 1979 the National Institutes of Health convened a Consensus Development Task Force to examine cesarean childbirth. A group of experts from medicine, research, law, social sciences, and the public examined all available evidence about cesareans and arrived at consensus recommendations for practice. In 1980, their report was published with these recommendations for lowering the cesarean birth rate:

1. Labor and vaginal delivery is a safe, relatively low-risk choice following a previous low-segment transverse uterine incision.
2. Trials of labor after previous cesareans should take place in facilities with the capability of a prompt emergency cesarean if necessary. Hospitals that lack such facilities should inform clients in advance and refer them to the nearest fully equipped hospital.
3. Prolonged labor (dystocia) should be treated with such measures as rest, hydration, sedation, ambulation, and oxytocin stimulation before resorting to cesarean.
4. Research should continue into means for evaluating the progress of labor, the effects of conservative treatment of dystocia, and the effects of emotional support and regional anesthesia.
5. Vaginal breech delivery should continue to be an accepted practice with a full-term baby not expected to be over 8 lb, normal pelvis, frank breech presentation without hyperextended head, and an experienced obstetrician.
6. All clients should have the choice of regional anesthesia.
7. Fathers should be allowed to be present at cesarean births.
8. Parents and infants should not be routinely separated after birth, unless indicated by the mother's or infant's condition.
9. Parent education and information about cesareans should be provided during pregnancy by childbirth educators and health professionals.

---

undergoing labor. Each situation presents its particular stresses and coping demands.

Prenatal Preparation

Childbirth classes in preparation for cesarean birth are increasing in number. Some educators feel all childbirth classes should present information about cesareans, even when vaginal delivery is anticipated. Considering that in some medical centers the cesarean rate is nearly one in four deliveries, this approach has merit.

Cesarean prenatal classes usually cover content common to all prenatal classes, including onset of labor and contact person should labor begin at home. Special emphasis is given to prenatal testing (*i.e.,* tests of fetal condition, preoperative tests), surgical procedures, analgesia and anesthesia, technologies (sonography, intravenous fluids, urinary retention catheter), the operating room experience, and postoperative recovery.

Techniques for increasing comfort and relaxation are taught. Although labor is not anticipated, the woman will find these techniques useful during tests and examinations and to alleviate pain after surgery. Hospital policies are reviewed, including the father's presence in the operating room and following surgery. The delivery and care of the infant are detailed, including procedures in the operating and recovery rooms and normal vari-

ations in early mother–infant relations. The course of postoperative recovery, both in the hospital and at home, is related to the pacing of caretaking responsibilities and needs for assistance at home.

Psychoemotional factors are very important for couples experiencing cesarean birth. Many describe feelings of fear, disappointment, frustration over loss of control, grief over losing their ideal birth experience, anger or victimization, or confusion over the necessity for the procedure. Mothers are particularly susceptible to decreased self-esteem. They may have disturbed body image and role expectations and may feel they have failed in reproductive functions. Worry about the scar affecting their attractiveness and the effects of the surgery on sexual processes is often present.

The nurse must be prepared to deal with these feelings, fears, and uncertainties. Opportunity for exploration and expression of feelings and clarification of uncertainties and misunderstandings must be provided either in group or individual discussions. Working within a crisis framework, the nurse can assist women and their partners to progress through appropriate stages to achieve acceptance and a sense of readiness.

Emphasizing that cesarean birth can be a satisfying and fulfilling experience creates a positive context. Both parents can mature, expand their self-concepts, and grow in self-esteem by effectively handling this expe-

CLIENT EDUCATION

Some Alternatives Available to Women Undergoing Cesarean Birth

- Regional (epidural) anesthesia so you can be awake during the birth
- Partner or other support person present during surgery and birth
- Hands freed from restraints for touch contact with father and baby
- Dropping the screen (which prevents view of the surgery) at the time of delivery
- Having an advocate (usually a nurse) who describes to parents what is going on during the operation and delivery
- Touching or holding the baby immediately after birth
- Delaying instillation of silver nitrate drops into the baby's eyes for the first hour after birth
- Continual contact between mother, father, and baby during first hour of life if the baby is stable
- Breast-feeding the infant immediately after birth in delivery or recovery room
- Initiation of rooming-in as soon as you desire
- Extended or unlimited visiting privileges for the father (or support person) during the postpartum period
- Utilization of medications (when necessary) that are not secreted in significant amounts in the breast-milk[11,12]

rience. They can develop a nurturing relationship with the baby and increase their mutuality as a couple. Being well-prepared for physical and emotional events can be key in the couple's success.

Preoperative Preparation

Cesarean birth involves preparation both for surgery and for the infant. The usual preparations of laboratory tests, physical examination, typing and cross matching blood, abdominal shaving, and other customary procedures are carried out. The physician discusses the type of operation and anesthesia with the woman and family, and informed consent is obtained.

When the client is admitted for an elective cesarean section, nursing care includes checking fetal heart tones and being alert to prodromal signs of labor. Oral intake should be discontinued for at least 8 hours prior to surgery. A short time before the operation the abdomen is shaved, beginning at the level of the xiphoid cartilage and extending out to the far sides and down to the pubic area. A retention catheter is inserted and attached to a constant drainage system to ensure that the bladder remains empty during the operation. The nurse should make certain that the catheter is draining properly before the procedure.

An intravenous infusion (commonly Ringer's lactate solution or 5% dextrose in water, 1000 ml) is started. Valuables are taken for safekeeping, and routine preoperative precautions are taken, such as removing fingernail polish, dentures, glasses, and contact lenses. Preoperative medications are administered, usually including atropine and an analgesic.

Unanticipated Cesarean Delivery. Emergency cesareans are performed when fetal or maternal complications pose serious risks. Complications may arise at any stage of labor, but often the decision for surgery is made after hours of nonprogressive labor or as a result of abnormal tracings on the fetal monitor. The woman is often discouraged, exhausted, very worried about her own or the baby's condition, and possibly dehydrated with low glycogen reserves. Preoperative preparations usually must be done rapidly, leaving little time for explanations.

The nurse should provide short, simple, and very concise explanations of reasons for the surgery and procedures that must be done. It is important that the nurse offer as much reassurance about the mother's and baby's conditions as can reasonably be given. However, the client's and her partner's anxiety level will be high, and they may not recall much or may misunderstand. After the operation, the nurse should spend time reviewing events leading up to the surgery, what occurred in the operating room, and the baby's status to allow the parents to understand and integrate their experiences.

Care During Surgery

Nurses assist during cesarean birth by either scrubbing or circulating in the operating room. The surgical team consists of obstetrician, surgical assistant, anesthesiologist, pediatrician, and nurses. Many cesareans are done under conduction anesthesia, so the woman is aware of events. The father, gowned appropriately, may also be in the room, sitting close to the mother's head. The surgical team must take the above into consideration in their communications with each other. The nurse has a special role in keeping parents informed, providing calm reassurance, and interpreting events.

The birth can be exciting, as parents hear the baby's first cries and are able to see him shortly after delivery. Special procedures to allow parents closer contact with the baby immediately after birth are discussed later.

Care of the Infant

In addition to the preparation of the operating room for the surgical procedure, preparation for the care of the infant must be accomplished. There must be a warm crib and equipment for the resuscitation of the infant. An infant resuscitator, equipped with heat, suction, oxygen (open mask and positive pressure), and an adjustable frame to permit the proper positioning of the infant is most useful. A competent person should be present at cesarean birth to give the infant initial care and to resuscitate if necessary. This person may be an experienced nurse. In many hospitals it is customary to have a pediatrician at hand to take over the care of the infant as soon as it is born and thus free the obstetrician to devote full attention to the mother.

The nurse can encourage and foster the parent–infant bonding process by providing the mother (when she is awake) and the father the opportunity to touch and hold the newborn. When it is difficult for the mother to actually hold the infant herself, the nurse can hold the infant in an *en face* (face-to-face) position to facilitate the maternal–infant bonding process.

Immediate transport to the NICU must be available, in case the infant is compromised at birth. Depending on the infant's condition and hospital policies, newborn care and evaluation may be done in the operating room. The father may be given the baby to hold and show to the mother, or they may be united in the recovery room.

Postoperative Postpartum Care

The woman who has had a cesarean delivery has undergone both abdominal surgery and a birth. Postoperative care includes the same procedures as for any abdominal surgery with the added dimension of postpartum care.

Assessment

Blood Loss. Bleeding is assessed the same as in any delivery. The woman must be watched for hemorrhage by frequently inspecting the perineal pad and checking the fundus. Usually the abdominal dressings are not bulky, and the nurse can palpate the fundus to see if the uterus is well contracted. Skin and uterine sutures are secure, and gentle but firm pressure can be used to assess uterine consistency. This may cause some discomfort, but will not disturb the sutures. Oxytocics are usually ordered to contract the uterus and control bleeding.

The amount and character of lochia are noted, using the same guidelines as with vaginal deliveries. Some women have less lochia following cesarean birth because of operative techniques used in placenta removal and hemostasis. The skin incision is examined regularly for signs of hematoma, bleeding, or infection. Vital signs are taken every 4 hours for the first few postoperative days, or until stable. It is particularly important to watch for signs of shock or infection.

Input and Output. If the retention catheter is to remain in place until the following morning, it should

remain attached to "constant drainage" and should be watched to see that it drains freely. Intravenous fluids are usually administered during the first 24 hours, although small amounts of fluids may be given by mouth after nausea has subsided. A record of the mother's intake and elimination is kept for the first several days or until the need is no longer indicated.

Intervention

Comfort and Respiratory Function. Analgesic drugs should be used to keep the mother comfortable and encourage her to rest. Her position in bed during the early postoperative hours may be dictated by the type of anesthesia that she received. She should be encouraged to turn from side to side every hour. Deep breathing and coughing should also be encouraged to promote good ventilation. Most mothers who deliver cesarean are allowed early ambulation. This contributes considerably to maintaining good bladder and intestinal function.

Pain following cesarean birth most often involves the incisional site, gas pain as bowel function is restored, flank pain from stretching of abdominal muscles during surgery, muscle aches from immobility, afterpains, and sometimes discomfort from bladder distention. Analgesic medication should be timed to provide maximum relief during the times the mother will spend feeding and caring for the baby. Then she can devote her energy to the infant and avoid the distraction of postoperative pain.

General Postpartum Care

After the immediate postoperative period, the mother receives routine postpartum care and continued post-surgery observations. Postpartum care includes vital signs, lochia observation, fundal assessment, breast and perineal care, attention to bladder and bowel elimination, ambulation, and hygiene.

Assessment. Care related to the surgery includes observation of the skin incision, pain control, respiratory function, and increased needs for rest and restoration. Showers may be taken by the second day after surgery, if a spray dressing or other protection of the incision is used.

Assessment and intervention in the development of mothering skills, and family adaptations to cesarean birth are of central importance. The woman's and family's response to the birth process must be carefully observed. Especially in unanticipated cesareans, the levels of anxiety, anger, disappointment, and confusion may be high. Many women feel overwhelmed by an unexpected cesarean birth and are completely unprepared for their physical and emotional responses. They express feelings of anxiety for themselves or the baby. They

(text continued on page 878)

The Woman Experiencing Cesarean Delivery

Nursing Objectives
1. Prepare mother and family for cesarean birth experience.
2. Guide mother and father in maximal preparation in the birth process and appropriate decision making.
3. Prevent complications or detect them early.
4. Promote comfort and recovery of body functions.
5. Support mothering activities and development of maternal–child bonding.
6. Assist parents in understanding and integration of the cesarean birth into a positive self-concept and satisfying childbearing.

Assessment	Potential Nursing Diagnosis	Intervention	Evaluation
Preparation for cesarean birth (unanticipated, elective)	Knowledge deficit related to reasons for cesarean, procedures, relaxation, pain relief.	Include cesarean birth in childbirth preparation classes	Parents recognize the potential for cesarean birth and feel prepared
	Fear related to condition of self or baby, pain, procedures, outcomes, aftermath	Provide information and explanation of reasons for cesarean, preparations for surgery, and processes to anticipate	Parents verbalize understanding, accept need and processes, cooperate in preparations
		Assist parents to express their feelings of fear, disappointment, grief, powerlessness, etc.	Parents express feelings freely and begin to accept and prepare for cesarean delivery
		Provide information and reassurance (as much as possible) about condition of mother and baby	Parents feel reasonably reassured or able to cope with risks
Postoperative condition: Fundal contraction Bleeding Vital signs Input and output Incision Respiratory function Comfort	Potential complications: hemorrhage, uterine atony, hematomas, shock, depressed respiratory function	Monitor postoperative progress, report early signs of problems, take emergency actions as needed	
	Alteration in comfort: pain related to incision, afterpains, stretched abdominal muscles	Administer analgesics, change position, adjust bedding	Mother reports increased comfort or sleeps or rests
Early bonding with infant Mother Father	Potential alteration in parenting related to lack of early contact, complications, pain, anesthesia, disappointment over birth, powerlessness	Provide opportunity for parents to see, hold, and explore infant in recovery area (if possible); or report on infant's condition and characteristics (sex, weight, normalcy, progress)	Parents have satisfying early contact or have their questions about the baby answered and feel well-informed
	Potential alteration in parenting related to lack of early contact due to exclusion, condition of mother or infant, powerlessness, disappointment	Discuss parents' feelings and reactions to cesarean birth; provide information and explanations	Mother is awake and reasonably comfortable; can hold/interact with baby
			Parents express feelings freely, fit missing pieces together, begin to integrate the experience
Postpartum observations: Incision healing Pain Fluids and nutrition	For general postpartum care, see Nursing Care in the Postpartum Period, Chapter 31. Observations specific to cesarean sections are included here.	Monitor condition of incision, input and output, bowel and bladder function, respiratory function	Mother takes fluids and food, moves bowels as expected, voids well after removal of catheter, and aerates lungs adequately

(continued)

Assessment	Potential Nursing Diagnosis	Intervention	Evaluation
Bowel function Bladder function Respiratory function	Potential complications: infection, hematoma, incisional bleeding, wound dehiscence	Identify signs of complications early; report and take action	Mother feels comfortable
	Alteration in comfort related to incision, afterpains, stretched abdominal muscles, gas	Administer analgesics, assist in positioning, teach splinting and movement to minimize pain	Mother reports increased comfort, holds and cares for infant, and interacts with partner satisfactorily
	Potential complications: persistent nausea and vomiting, continued intravenous therapy, lack of appetite, decreased gastrointestinal functioning		
	Alteration in bowel elimination: decreased functioning related to anesthesia and surgery (decreased peristalsis and activity), gas, constipation		
	Alteration in patterns of urinary elimination related to surgery, anesthesia, indwelling catheter; potential for urinary retention		
	Potential complications: decreased oxygenation due to limited ventilation, pneumonia, pulmonary embolus		
Mothering skills	Potential alteration in parenting related to discomfort following surgery, disappointment with birth, feeling incomplete or powerless, anger, inexperience	Provide pain relief, explanations and information about cesarean, opportunity to explore events surrounding cesarean birth	Mother is comfortable, expresses feelings freely, gains understanding and acceptance of cesarean birth
	Knowledge deficit of special needs following cesarean birth, effect of postsurgical recovery on strength and emotions, managing discomforts	Teach parents about special needs of mother for rest, recovery, and emotional processes	Parents understand and accept special needs, make provisions for these
Adjustment to cesarean birth	Potential disturbance in self-concept related to body changes (incision), failure to have "normal" birth, insufficient "control" over childbearing, time required for recovery	Encourage mother to express feelings, support positive interpretations, reinforce normal aspects	Mother expresses feelings and identifies positive aspects of cesarean birth
	Anxiety/fear related to effects of surgery on self or infant		

(continued)

Assessment	Potential Nursing Diagnosis	Intervention	Evaluation
Family adjustment	Potential alteration in family processes related to disappointment, anger, powerlessness, blame seeking, coping inexperience, or lack of understanding	Encourage parents to express feelings, clear misunderstandings, process their experience, relate it to needs for home management	Parents express feelings, integrate the experiences surrounding cesarean birth, make plans for managing at home
	Impaired home maintenance management related to increased needs of mother for rest and recovery time following cesarean	Discuss sexuality after cesarean birth; correct misunderstandings	Parents understand effects of cesarean birth on sexual functioning, feel prepared to accept limits, are supportive of each other
	Potential sexual dysfunction related to misunderstandings or fears of surgery effects on sexual functioning		

(text continued from page 875)

experience anger or depression because they expected a normal birth. They tend to feel a sense of loss over not experiencing vaginal delivery, not witnessing the birth, and not having their partner's or family's participation. There are often altered body perceptions as well as many concerns surrounding mothering the infant during their recovery from surgery.[13]

The physical discomfort of the mother after the surgery, combined with her feelings of disappointment or guilt, can interfere with her ability to bond to her infant. The long-term consequences of inadequate or delayed maternal–infant bonding can range from poor growth and development of the infant to blatant child abuse.

However, mothers who were allowed early and continuous contact with their infants following cesarean birth (with spinal anesthesia and delivery of a healthy, normal infant) were found to have significantly more positive perceptions of their infants in the early postpartum period. They also displayed more maternal behavior in caretaking at this time and when the infant was 1 month old than cesarean mothers who only had brief contact in the first 12 hours after birth.[14]

At this time, the woman finds herself burdened with an abdominal operative procedure. Her needs for physical and emotional recovery may dominate her mothering interests initially. She may need to deal with her reduced ability to care for the infant, separation from the infant (especially with maternal or neonatal complications), discomfort in holding and feeding, and concern about the infant's well-being. The father likewise may have needs to review and integrate the experience and to learn the new processes involved in recovery and procedures following cesarean birth.

Intervention. The nurse has a large responsibility in providing explanations of events and decisions, and in giving support through physical contact, calmness, comfort measures, verbal reassurances, and assisting the mother to gain mastery of her body and infant-care tasks.

Nursing care must provide opportunity to review events, seek understandings of what happened and why, remember responses and work these through, clear up questions and misunderstandings, and alter self-concept and expectations to be congruent with reality.

One or 2 days after the birth, a visit from the labor and delivery nurse who assisted the couple during the childbirth is often beneficial for the integration of the event into their lives. The filling in of missing pieces is important for all women who experience gaps in their memories of the labor and births of their infants.[15] This may be more important when the woman is attempting to understand the reasons for surgical intervention in what is often expected to be a natural process. Visits such as this also provide the couple with the opportunity to discuss any feelings of failure, guilt, or anger they may be experiencing. A sensitive and responsive nurse can effectively help the couple work through such feelings by remaining open to their comments and honestly addressing their concerns. If the family unit is to be strengthened through the childbearing process, and if childbirth is to be a family-centered event, then every attempt should be made by the obstetric staff to help families incorporate this experience into their lives.

Discharge Planning

Hospitalization after cesarean birth usually lasts 4 to 6 days. Discharge preparation includes that for any postpartum patient (Chap. 31) and also teaching specific to postoperative considerations. Mothers may be prescribed analgesics for use at home and should be reminded of their increased need for rest. Exercises may begin when abdominal pain has decreased, but lifting heavy objects should be avoided for 2 to 3 weeks. Most mothers are able to lift their infants without problem.

Instruction about complications is important, including signs of infection (fever, dysuria, flank pain), hemorrhage, thrombosis (severe chest or leg pain, leg swelling), and wound dehiscence. Guidelines for contacting physician or clinic are given. Intercourse may be resumed when lochia has ceased and there is no undue abdominal or perineal discomfort. Contraceptive information is provided as for other postpartum patients. A return visit is usually scheduled for 3 weeks following delivery, and another at 6 weeks.

Destructive Operations

Destructive operations (designed for the most part to reduce the size of the baby's head and thus to expedite delivery) are rarely done in modern obstetrics. Even in large maternity hospitals many years may pass without a single destructive operation. This salutary state of affairs is attributable in part to the widespread extension of prenatal care, in part to better management of women in labor, and in part to the availability of cesarean section, which makes it safe to effect abdominal delivery even in neglected cases.

References

1. Oxorn H: Human Labor and Birth. Norwalk, CT, Appleton-Century-Crofts, 1986
2. Lange AP, Secher NJ, Westergaard JG et al: Prelabor evaluation of inducibility. Obstet Gynecol 60:137, 1982
3. Goldfarb MG: Who receives cesareans: Patient and hospital characteristics. National Center for Health Services Research, Hospital Cost and Utilization Project Research Note. Rockville, MD, DHHS Publication No. (PHS) 84-3345, September 1984
4. Gleicher N: Cesarean section rates in the United States: The short-term failure of the National Consensus Development Conference in 1980. JAMA 252:3273, 1984
5. Beck NC, Hall D: Natural childbirth: A review and analysis. Obstet Gynecol 52:371–379, 1978
6. Minkoff HL, Schwarz RH: The rising cesarean section rate: Can it safely be reversed? Obstet Gynecol 56(2):135–143, August 1980
7. Corea G: The cesarean epidemic. Mother Jones V, VI:28–35, July 1980
8. Young D: Unnecessary cesareans: Ways to avoid them. Birth Fam J 8(1):47+, Spring 1981
9. Shy K, LoGerfo J, Karp L: Evaluation of elective repeat cesarean section as a standard of care: An application of decision analysis. Am J Obstet Gynecol 139(2):123, 1981
10. Final Report of the NIH Consensus Task Force on Cesarean Childbirth, Office of Research Reporting, Bldg. 31, NICHD, 9000 Rockville Pike, Bethesda, MD, 1980
11. Enkin MW: Having a section is having a baby. Birth Fam J 4(3):99–102, Fall 1977
12. Hedahi KJ: Cesarean birth: A real family affair. Am J Nurs 80(3):471–472, March 1980
13. Affonse DA, Stichler JF: Cesarean birth: Women's reactions. Am J Nurs 80(3):468–470, March 1980
14. McClellan MS, Cabianca WA: Effects of early mother–infant contact following cesarean birth. Obstet Gynecol 56(1):52–55, July 1980
15. Affonso D: 'Missing pieces'—a study of postpartum feelings. Birth Fam J 4(4):159–164, Winter 1977

Suggested Reading

Boyd ST, Mahon P: The Family-Centered Cesarean Delivery. MCN 5:May/June 1980

Cain RL, Pedersen FA, Zaslow MJ et al: Effects of the father's presence or absence during a cesarean delivery. Birth 11(1):10–15, Spring 1984

Chi IC, Su-Wen Z, Balogh S et al: Post-cesarean section insertion of intrauterine devices. Am J Public Health 74(11):1281–1282, November 1984

Danforth DN: Cesarean section. JAMA 253:811, 1985

Digest: Avoiding unnecessary repeat cesarean deliveries may help stem overall rise in C-section rates. Fam Plann Perspect 17(3):125–127, May/June 1985

Marieskind HI: An evaluation of cesarean section in the United States. Final report to the US Dept. of Health, Education, and Welfare, Office of the Assistant Secretary for Planning and Evaluation/Health, June 1979

Paul RH, Phelan P, Yeh S: Trial of labor in a patient with a prior cesarean birth. Am J Obstet Gynecol 151:297, 1985

Placek PJ, Taffel S, Moien M: Cesarean section delivery rates: United States, 1981. Am J Public Health 73:861, 1983

Porreco RD: High cesarean section rate: A new perspective. Obstet Gynecol 65:307, 1985

Prichard JA, Macdonald PC, Gant MF: William's Obstetrics, 17th ed. New York, Appleton-Century-Crofts, 1985

Shearer E: NIH Consensus Development Task Force on Cesarean Childbirth: The process and the result. Birth Fam J 8(1):25–30, Spring 1981

White E, Shy KK, Daling JR: An investigation of the relationship between cesarean section birth and respiratory distress syndrome of the newborn. Am J Epidemiol 121:651, 1985

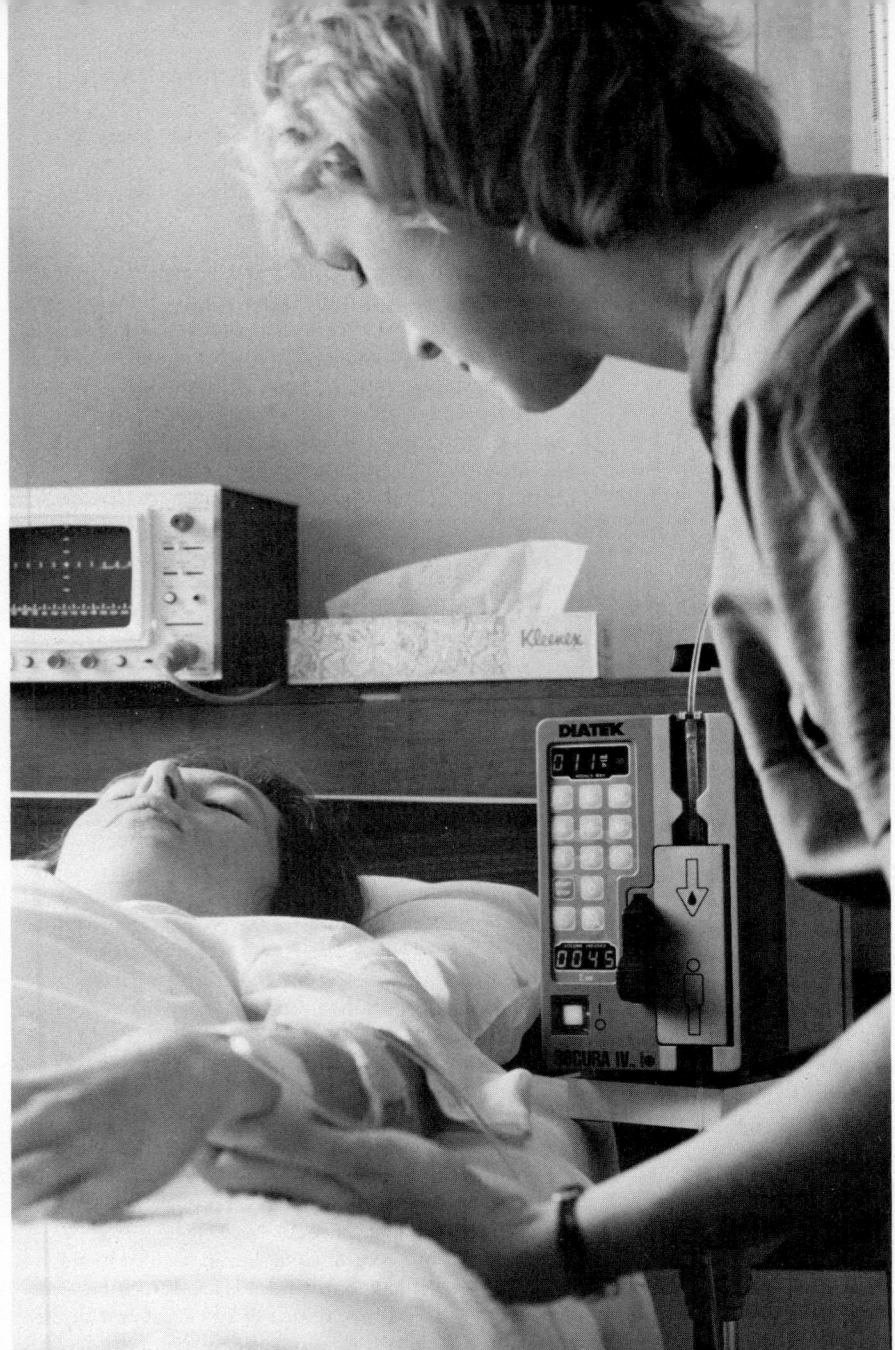

CHAPTER 40

Postpartum Complications

The postpartum period is a time of increased physiological stress, as well as a phase of major psychological transition. During this time the woman's body is more vulnerable because of the energy depletion and fatigue of late pregnancy and labor, the tissue trauma of delivery, and the blood loss and propensity for anemia that frequently occur. Most women recover from the stresses of pregnancy and childbirth without significant complications. When postpartum complications do occur, the most common are *infection* involving the genital tract, urinary system, and breasts; *hemorrhage,* immediate or delayed; *embolic and thrombotic clotting disorders;* and *uterine subinvolution.* The potentially critical nature of many postpartum complications, the associated pain and procedures, medications, frequent need to be isolated or removed from the maternity unit, and emotionally disruptive effects of the physiological malfunction can interfere with the maternal–infant bonding process (see Common Postpartum Complications).

Applying the Nursing Process in Postpartum Complications

Assessment

Postpartum nursing assessment focuses upon identifying complications early, monitoring progress and physiological functions, noting needs for comfort promotion and education, identifying psychoemotional reactions and needs, and monitoring postpartum involution. (General biophysical aspects and psychosocial aspects of the postpartum period were discussed in Chaps. 29 and 30. General care for the postpartum woman, including assessment, was discussed in Chap. 31.)

    The signs and symptoms of each specific complication are noted, as well as vital signs, condition of perineum and uterus, character of lochia, condition of extremities and breasts, and status of bladder and bowel function. The mother's needs for physical comfort are assessed, including rest and sleep, nutrition and hydration, and pain relief. Psychosocial assessment covers relationship with the infant, patient and family responses to the complication, and relationship with the husband or partner.

Nursing Diagnosis

The nursing diagnosis may involve a potential complication, such as hemorrhage, uterine atony and subinvolution, lacerations, hematomas, retained placental fragments, or urinary retention. Another set of diagnoses includes potential for infection involving the vagina, perineum, uterus, breasts, or abdominal incision related

881

Common Postpartum Complications

Genital tract infections
    Infection of episiotomy or lacerations
    Endometritis
    Parametritis (pelvic cellulitis)
    Pelvic abscess
    Peritonitis
    Salpingitis
    Early or late postpartum hemorrhage
Pelvic or femoral thrombophlebitis
Cesarean section wound infection
Pulmonary embolism
Subinvolution of the uterus
Vulvar hematomas
Mastitis, breast abscess
Urinary tract infection
    Cystitis
    Pyelonephritis

---

to bacterial invasion secondary to trauma during labor and delivery. Alteration in comfort may result from pain associated with infectious or hemorrhagic complications. Urinary tract infections may produce an alteration in patterns of urinary elimination.

Knowledge deficits may be associated with lack of information about specific complications, their progression and treatment, and implications for self and mothering. Mothers may not know how to attain greater comfort when suffering from postpartum complications. They may need to learn signs and symptoms of complications and progression. The presence of complications may be related to alterations in parenting, because they may require separation of mother and infant, may cause pain and anxiety, and may lead to feelings of incompetency and powerlessness.

Planning/Intervention

Nursing care assures prompt diagnosis and treatment of postpartum complications to reduce their dysfunctional effects. Treatment regimens are carried out and their effects monitored (*e.g.*, vital signs, disease progression, symptoms, specimen collection). Comfort measures for pain are provided and nutrition and fluid intake are enhanced to promote healing and well-being.

It is important to encourage maximum mother–infant contact, given the requirements of the specific complication. Attachment can be enhanced by providing information about the infant, discussing the baby's behavior and characteristics, providing pictures of the baby, and supporting visits to the nursery. When the complication allows, the mother can be assisted to hold and care for her infant as much as possible.

Explanations can be provided about the complication and its expected course and treatment. The partner should be involved in these discussions when possible and helped to understand and provide support for the mother's emotional needs. The nurse also can respond to the mother's or family's needs for emotional support and encouragement and can assist them to work through fears of the consequences or grief about the effects of complications on the postpartum experience. The nursing-care plan at the end of the chapter further develops the care given for various complications.

Evaluation and Reassessment

A return to normal adaptation to the postpartum period marks recovery from a postpartum complication. Vital signs have become stable, and appetite has returned. The woman is able to void normally, and she is afebrile and free of pain. Her uterus and lochia are normal for the stage of involution. She is able to rest and sleep well. She assumes self-care and infant caretaking. Her partner provides support, and she continues breast-feeding if she had been breast-feeding previously.

Postpartum Infections of the Genital Tract

When inflammatory processes develop in the birth canal postpartally, as a result of bacterial invasion of these highly vulnerable areas, the condition is known as puerperal infection. It is really a postpartum wound infection of the birth canal, usually of the endometrium. As is true of other wound infections, the condition often remains localized but may extend along various pathways to produce diverse clinical pictures. Febrile reactions of more or less severity are the rule, and the outcome varies according to the portal of entry; the type, the number, and the virulence of the invading organisms; the reaction of the tissues; and the general resistance of the client. Puerperal infection is one of the most common causes of death in childbearing.

Febrile morbidity in the postpartum period is defined by the Joint Committee on Maternal Welfare as a temperature elevation of 38°C (100.4°F) or more occurring after the first 24 hours postpartum on two or more occasions that are not within the same 24 hours.[1] Low-grade temperature elevations postpartally are not uncommon and have been attributed to such factors as dehydration, infusion of fetal protein, breast engorgement, and respiratory infection. However, the endometrial cavity is the site of significant anaerobic bacterial growth in the immediate postpartum period, and probably most women with temperature elevations in the first 24 hours do have genital tract infections. When delivery has occurred vaginally, the spontaneous clearance of necrotic decidua and blood from the uterine cavity is adequate to remove bacteria in most cases. The transient temperature elevation seen in the first 24 hours after delivery represents this process. When the delivery has been by cesarean section, there is a much higher risk of postpartum infection. The maternal mortality rate is two to four times higher than for vaginal delivery,[2] with febrile morbidity ranging from 29% to 85%.[3] Figures 40-1 and 40-2 show febrile patterns of transient temperature elevation in the first 24 hours and clinically significant postpartum infection.

Prevention of Infection

The prevention of infection throughout the maternity cycle is an important factor in the maintenance of health and the prevention of disease. During pregnancy, complete blood counts or hematocrit and hemoglobin tests are done routinely and iron is prescribed as necessary, not only for the immediate value but also because anemia predisposes to puerperal infection. Health teaching is emphasized at this time, particularly in regard to diet, rest, exercise, and general hygiene. The client is advised to avoid possible sources of infection, especially upper respiratory tract infections.

During labor, care should be exercised to limit bacteria from extraneous sources. In the hospital, cleanli-

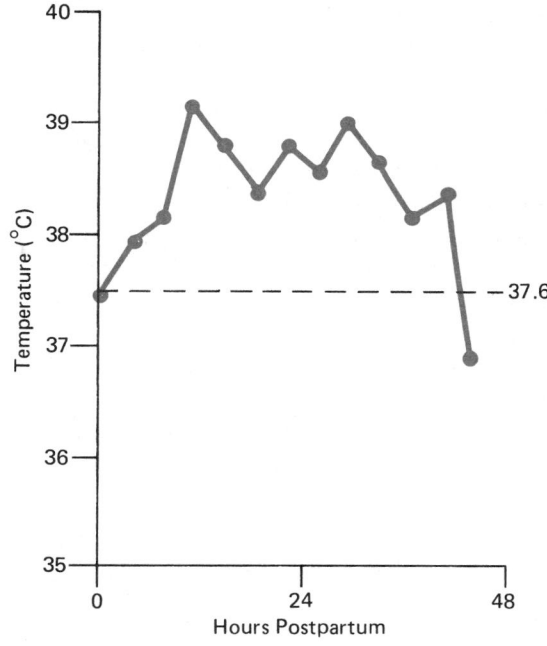

FIGURE 40-2

The pattern of fever (>38.4°C) in the first 24 hours post partum following either spontaneous vaginal delivery or cesarean section. (Filker R, Monif GRG: The significance of temperature during the first 24 hours postpartum. Obstet Gynecol 53(3):358–361, 1979)

ness and good housekeeping are imperative, but, nevertheless, individual care technique reduces the chance of contamination from other clients. Each client should have her own equipment, which includes her own bedpan. This bedpan should be cleansed after each use and sterilized once a day. Careful hand washing on the part of all personnel after contacts with each client helps to prevent the transfer of infection from one client to another.

The strictest rules should be enforced for surgical cleanliness during labor and delivery. No one with an infection of the skin or the respiratory tract should work in the maternity department. The nasopharynx of attendants is the most common exogenous source of contamination of the birth canal. Regular nasopharyngeal cultures of maternity personnel are often required. To be effective, masks worn during delivery must cover the nose and the mouth and be clean and dry; thus, they must be changed frequently and should not hang around the neck when not in use.

During the puerperium the same precautions should be carried out. For many days following the delivery, the surface of the birth canal is a vulnerable area for pathogenic bacteria. The birth canal is well protected against the invasion of extraneous bacteria by the closed vulva, unless this barrier is invaded. Clients, therefore, are to be taught the principles of perineal hygiene and how to care for themselves without using the fingers to

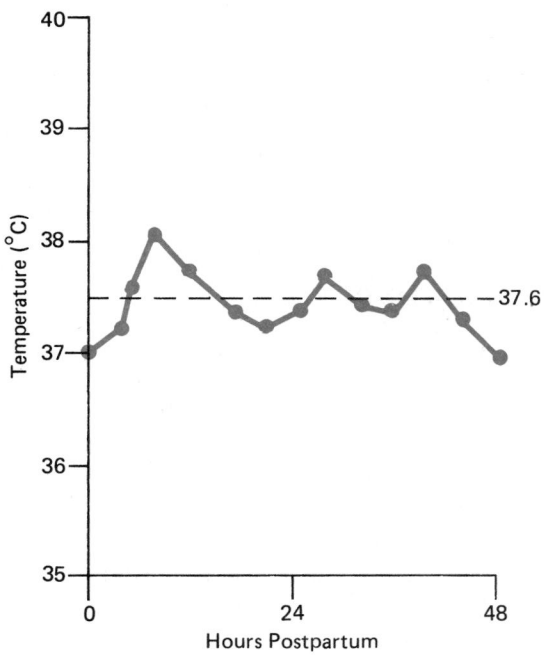

FIGURE 40-1

The pattern of resolving postpartum fever (single spike) following spontaneous vaginal delivery. (Filker R, Monif GRG: The significance of temperature during the first 24 hours postpartum. Obstet Gynecol 53(3):358–361, 1979)

Prevention of Postpartum Infection

Well-balanced diet, good nutrition before and during pregnancy

Prompt recognition and treatment of anemia

Early and regular prenatal care

Healthful activities during pregnancy (*e.g.*, adequate rest, exercise, general hygiene, maintaining normal weight)

Accurate diagnosis and early treatment of urinary tract infections during pregnancy

Infection control and monitoring in the hospital

Conscientious aseptic technique by hospital personnel

Regular nasopharyngeal cultures of maternity personnel

Minimization of pelvic examinations during labor

Avoidance of early rupture of membranes

Intrauterine fetal monitoring only when absolutely necessary

Prevention of cesarean section

Avoidance of general anesthesia

Avoidance of manual removal of placenta

Prevention of hemorrhage

Minimization of delivery trauma (*e.g.*, forceps, episiotomy, lacerations)

---

separate the labia, because this permits the cleansing solution to enter the vagina.

Causative Factors

The most common organisms causing postpartum infections are anaerobic nonhemolytic streptococci, coliform bacteria, bacteroides, and staphylococci. Most infections are caused by mixed anaerobic bacteria. There is reduced incidence of beta-hemolytic streptococcal infection owing to improvements in obstetric care and aseptic technique. Multiple bacterial pathogens are present in the cervix and lower uterine segment during pregnancy and for a short time after delivery. Generally, such organisms harbored in the female genital tract do not cause infections, but the trauma of birth and the alteration of immunologic function and resistance caused by fatigue and stress make the postpartum woman more susceptible. Hemorrhage and anemia also predispose to postpartum infection.

Endogenous infections are caused by bacteria in the genital tract that enter and colonize wounds in the perineum, vagina, cervix, or endometrium at the site of placental attachment. Existing infections in other organs

or septicemia may also be a cause. Exogenous infections are caused by introduction of organisms into the genital tract. Nurses, physicians, and other personnel are the most frequent source of exogenous (nosocomial) infections.

Although attending personnel wear gloves, the hands and the instruments used may become contaminated by pathogenic bacteria as the result of droplet infection from the nasopharynx or improper sterilization. Even in modern obstetrics, this is a very common mode of infection, and unless the utmost vigilance is used in masking all attendants in the delivery room (both nose and mouth) and in excluding all persons suffering or recovering from an upper respiratory tract infection, it is a constant source of danger.

Although a less common means of transfer today than a few decades ago, careless physicians and nurses have been known to carry bacteria to the parturient from countless extraneous contacts: from other cases of puerperal infection, from suppurative postoperative wounds, from cases of sloughing carcinoma, from patients with scarlet fever, from infants with impetigo neonatorum, and from umbilical infections of the newborn. The physician and nurse, themselves, may have an infection such as an infected hangnail or furuncle.

Coitus late in pregnancy may introduce extraneous organisms to the birth canal or carry upward bacteria already present on the vulva or in the lower vagina. However, there is little risk unless the membranes are ruptured, in which case coitus should be avoided.

During the second stage of labor, the chances of fecal matter being transferred to the vagina are great, another source of introducing coliform bacteria.

In addition to traumatic labor and postpartum hemorrhage, other factors are prolonged labor, prolonged rupture of the membranes, retention of placental tissue, and retained blood clots.

Pathophysiology

Uterine–peritoneal puerperal infection is most commonly a result of colonization of these tissues by bacteria present in the cervix or vagina. Cervicovaginal organisms enter the uterine cavity during labor, which explains the high correlation between duration of labor and postpartum endometritis. Although in most cases the organisms enter the amniotic fluid when the membranes are ruptured, the presence of organisms within amniotic fluid with intact membranes has recently been demonstrated. Amniotic fluid colonization during labor (with intact membranes) may be a common occurrence, but without clinically significant infection resulting. Amniotic fluid has an antibacterial effect, related to a polypeptide linked with zinc and other lysozyme and immunoglobulin systems.[4]

The upper endometrial cavity is probably sterile in most women without postpartum infection. However, it is known that the postpartum cervix and vagina contain numerous potentially pathogenic bacteria, and these increase during the postparum period. The lower uterus is probably colonized by such bacteria, but at some point colonization ceases and the uterine cavity becomes sterile. The exact location in the cavity at which colonization ceases is unknown, but is presumed to be close to the cervical–endometrial junction.

When large numbers of virulent bacteria enter the uterine cavity during labor (by mechanisms such as discussed in the preceding section), they can attach to the uterine decidua following delivery and cause endometritis. In some cases, the bacteria gain entrance into the large venous vascular channels to produce parametritis, or bacteria enter the fallopian tubes to cause salpingitis. It is often difficult to accurately identify the causative organism in such infections because of the lack of sensitivity and specificity in sampling and diagnostic techniques. For example, transcervical sampling of the uterine cavity almost always is contaminated by cervical organisms, blood cultures may identify only one organism in a mixed infection, and fundal aspiration is infrequently done because of difficulty in obtaining the sample and being certain that it is from the uterine cavity.

Types of Genital Tract Infection

Genital tract (puerperal) infection can be divided into two main types, *local lesion processes* and *extensions of the original lesion process*. When a lesion of the vulva, the perineum, the vagina, the cervix, or the endometrium becomes infected, the infection may remain localized in these wounds. However, the original inflammatory process may extend along the veins (the most common way) and cause thrombophlebitis and pyemia, or through the lymph vessels to cause peritonitis and pelvic cellulitis.

Lesions of the Perineum, Vulva, and Vagina

These lesions are highly vulnerable areas for bacterial invasion in the early puerperium. The most common is a localized infection of a repaired perineal laceration or episiotomy wound.

The usual symptoms are elevation of temperature, pain and sensation of heat in the affected area, and burning on urination. The area involved becomes red and edematous, and there is profuse seropurulent discharge. If a wound of the vulva becomes infected, the entire vulva may become edematous and ulcerated. Infections involving the perineum, the vulva, and the vagina cause the patient considerable discomfort and alarm.

These local inflammatory processes seldom cause severe physical reactions, provided that good drainage is established and the patient's temperature remains below 38.4°C (101°F). To promote good drainage, all stitches may be removed to lay open the surface. Because the drainage itself is a source of irritation and contamination, the wound must be kept clean and the perineal pads changed frequently. Care must be exercised in cleansing the wound to see that none of the solution runs into the vagina.

Treatments by such means as sitz baths or the perineal heat lamp are generally used for the relief of pain. Antibiotics are prescribed to combat the infection. If drainage is impaired, the patient not only has more pain but also may have a chill, followed by a sudden elevation of temperature.

Endometritis

Endometritis is a localized infection of the lining membrane of the uterus. Bacteria invade the lesion, usually the placental site, and may spread to involve the entire endometrium (Fig. 40-3).

When endometritis develops, it is usually manifest about 48 to 72 hours after delivery. In the milder forms the patient may have no complaints or symptoms other than a rise in temperature to about 38.4°C (101°F), which persists for several days and then subsides. On the other hand, the more virulent infections are often ushered in by chills and high fever, with a comparable rise in pulse rate (Fig. 40-4). In the majority of severe cases the patient experiences a chilly sensation or actual chills at the onset and often complains of malaise, loss of appetite, headache, backache, and general discomfort.

It is not unusual for the patient to have severe and prolonged afterpains. The uterus is usually large and is extremely tender when palpated abdominally. The lochial discharge may be decreased in amount and distinguished from normal lochia by its red brown appearance and foul odor. In some cases, particularly those caused by the hemolytic streptococcus, the lochia may be odorless.

If the infection remains localized in the endometrium, it is usually over in about a week or 10 days. When extension of the infection occurs to cause peritonitis, pelvic thrombophlebitis, or cellulitis, the disease may persist for many weeks, often with dramatic temperature curves and repeated chills.

Treatment depends on the severity of the condition. Mild cases with temperature under 37.8°C (100°F) and no chills are best handled by simple measures. Fowler's position facilitates lochial drainage. Ergonovine four times daily for 2 days promotes uterine tone, and forced fluids provide additional support. The lochia is cultured and the patient is treated with the appropriate antibiotic

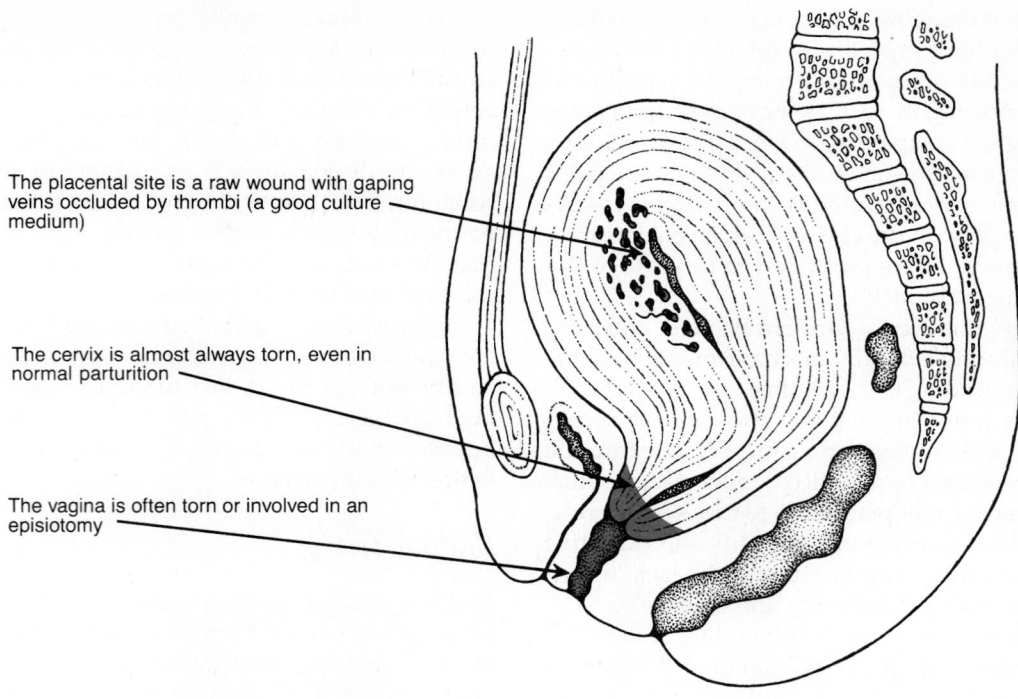

The placental site is a raw wound with gaping veins occluded by thrombi (a good culture medium)

The cervix is almost always torn, even in normal parturition

The vagina is often torn or involved in an episiotomy

FIGURE 40-3

Sites of common postpartum infection.

(Table 40-1). Isolation is desirable to protect other patients and to afford the mother greater rest. In this group it is unnecessary to discontinue breast-feeding.

In severe cases, breast-feeding is discontinued not only because it exhausts the mother but also because it is usually futile in the presence of high fever.

Pelvic Cellulitis or Parametritis

Pelvic cellulitis is an infection that extends along the lymphatics to reach the loose connective tissue surrounding the uterus. It may follow an infected cervical laceration, endometritis, or pelvic thrombophlebitis. The

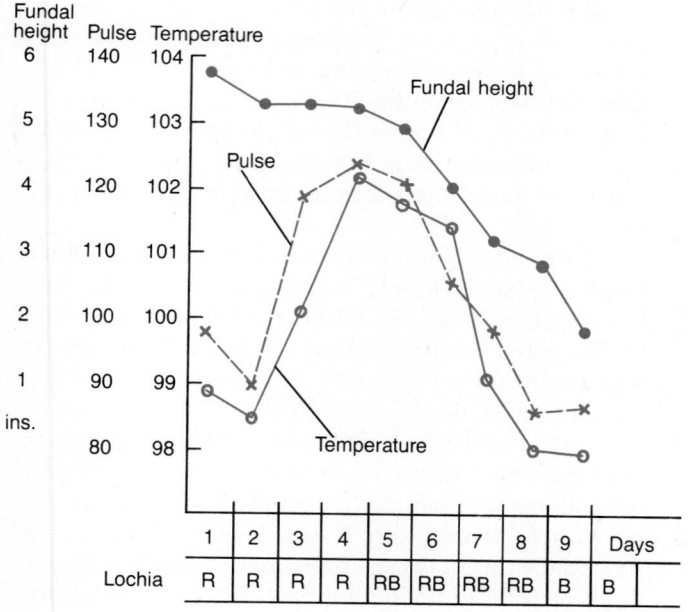

FIGURE 40-4

Febrile pattern in endometritis. The four classic signs of postpartum endometritis are temperature elevation to 101°F (38.4°C), increase in pulse rate (100–120), delayed involution with fundal height not decreasing, and lochia remaining red with foul odor. (*R*, red; *B*, brown)

TABLE 40-1

Antibiotic Activity Against Common Endometrial Infections

	Penicillin	Penicillin & Aminoglycoside	Ampicillin	Cephalosporin	Aminoglycoside & Clindamycin	Penicillin & Chloramphenicol
Aerobic organism						
Streptococci	+	+	+	+	+	+
Enterococci	−	+	+	−	−	±
Escherichia coli	±	+	±	+	+	+
Gardnerella vaginalis	+	+	+	+	+	+
Staphylococcus aureus	−	+	−	+	+	±
Anaerobic organism						
Peptostreptococci	+	+	+	+	+	+
Peptococci	+	+	+	+	+	+
Bacteroides sp.	+	+	+	+	+	+
B. fragilis or *B. bivius*	−	−	−	−	+	+

+, 95% of organisms susceptible; ±, more than 50% of organisms susceptible; −, less than 50% of organisms susceptible. (Eschenbach DA, Wager GP: Puerperal Infections. Clin Obstet Gynecol 23(4):1020, December 1980).

patient has a persistent fever and marked pain and tenderness over the affected area. The problem is usually unilateral but may involve both sides of the abdomen. As the process develops, the swelling becomes very hard and finally either undergoes resolution or results in the formation of a pelvic abscess. If the latter occurs, as the abscess comes to a point, the skin above becomes red, edematous, and tender. Recovery is usually prompt after the abscess is opened (Figs. 40-5 and 40-6).

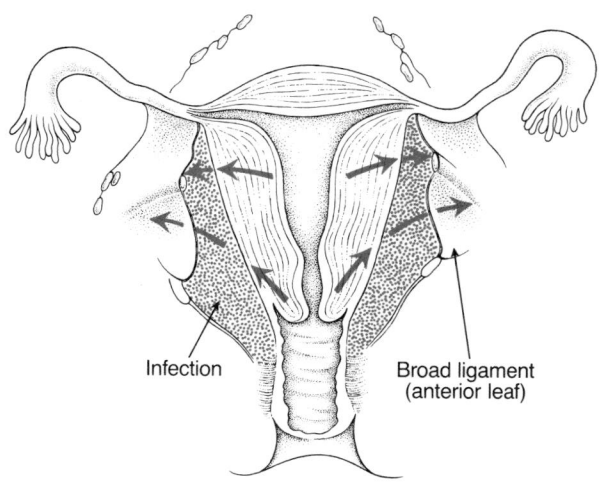

FIGURE 40-5

Parametritis or pelvic cellulitis. Infection may spread from the uterus, a cervical laceration, or thrombophlebitis into the loose connective tissue. It may extend retroperitoneally in any direction, commonly between leaves of the broad ligament, and around the vagina or rectum. Pelvic examination reveals a large, hard mass representing a pelvic abscess in some instances.

Parametritis usually occurs later than endometritis, during the second postpartum week. Fever and malaise are the typical presentation, and lochia usually remains red and is heavy. There is less pain than might be expected. This condition is treated with antibiotics.

Peritonitis

Peritonitis is an infection, either generalized or local, of the peritoneum. Usually the infection reaches the peritoneum from the endometrium by traveling through the lymphatic vessels, but peritonitis may result also from the extension of thrombophlebitis or parametritis (Fig. 40-7).

The clinical course of pelvic peritonitis resembles that of surgical peritonitis. The patient has a high fever

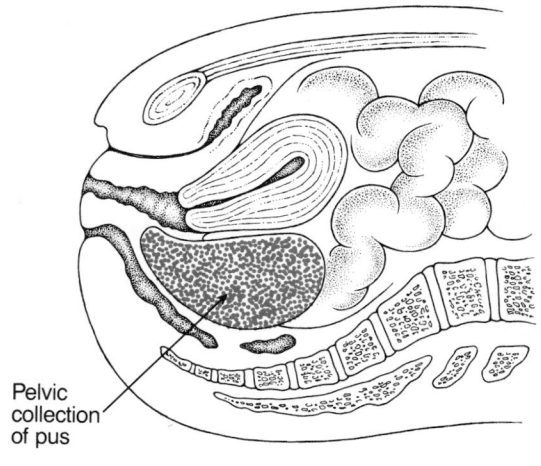

FIGURE 40-6

Pelvic abscess.

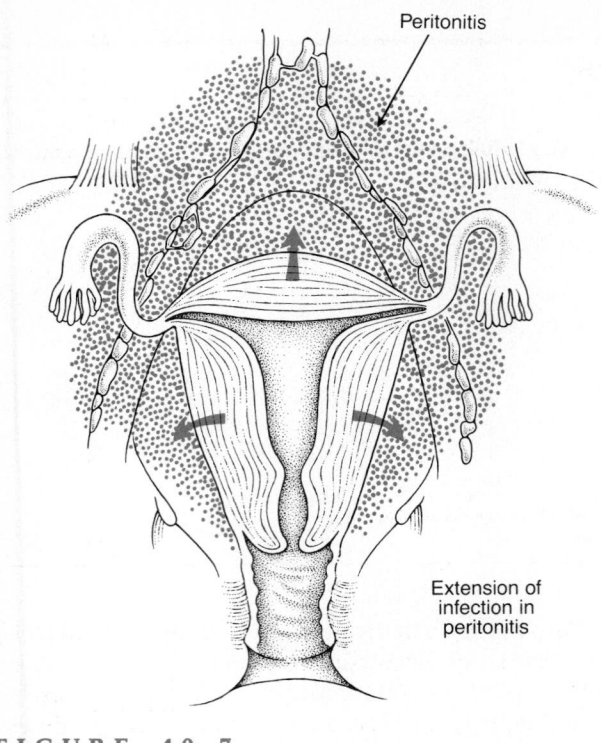

F I G U R E 4 0 - 7

Postpartum peritonitis. The pelvic peritoneum may become involved in an infection in the same ways as the parametrium. Generalized peritonitis may occur with development of paralytic ileus. Although uncommon, peritonitis can be severe and life threatening.

and rapid pulse and, in general, has the appearance of being profoundly ill. She is usually restless and sleepless and has constant and severe abdominal pain. Hiccups, nausea, and vomiting, which is sometimes fecal and projectile, may be present.

Antimicrobial therapy is given to combat the infection, analgesic drugs are prescribed for discomfort, and mild sedative drugs are given to relieve the restlessness and apprehension. If there is intestinal involvement, oral feedings are withheld until normal intestinal function is restored; meanwhile, fluids are administered intravenously. Blood transfusions and oxygen therapy may be indicated for supportive treatment. A record of intake and output must be kept.

Salpingitis

Acute salpingitis is infection of the fallopian tubes following childbirth. Bacteria may ascend from the uterine cavity or travel by the venous route to cause salpingitis. The symptoms resemble peritonitis, and the two are difficult to distinguish diagnostically. High fever, rapid pulse, nausea and vomiting, abdominal pain, and rigidity are common findings. Although usually bilateral, unilateral salpingitis may be impossible to distinguish from appendicitis when it occurs on the right side. An exploratory laparotomy or laparoscopy may be necessary to establish the correct diagnosis.

Treatment is with antibiotics, analgesics, and sedatives as with peritonitis. Tubal patency and subsequent fertility is always a concern with salpingitis (Fig. 40-8).

Thrombophlebitis

Thrombophlebitis is an infection of the vascular endothelium with clot formation attached to the vessel wall. It may be of two types: pelvic thrombophlebitis, an inflammatory process involving the ovarian and the uterine veins, or femoral thrombophlebitis, in which the femoral, the popliteal, or the saphenous vein is involved (Fig. 40-9). Early ambulation may be a factor in preventing this complication.

Femoral Thrombophlebitis. Femoral thrombophlebitis presents a special group of signs and symptoms. It is a disease of the puerperium characterized by pain, fever, and swelling in the affected leg. These symptoms are due to the formation of a clot in the veins of the leg itself, which interferes with the return circulation of the blood. When this condition develops, it usually appears about 10 days after labor, although it may manifest itself as late as the 20th day. As in all acute febrile diseases occurring after labor, the secretion of milk may cease.

The disease is ushered in with malaise, chilliness, and fever, which are soon followed by stiffness and pain in the affected part. If it is in the leg, the pain may

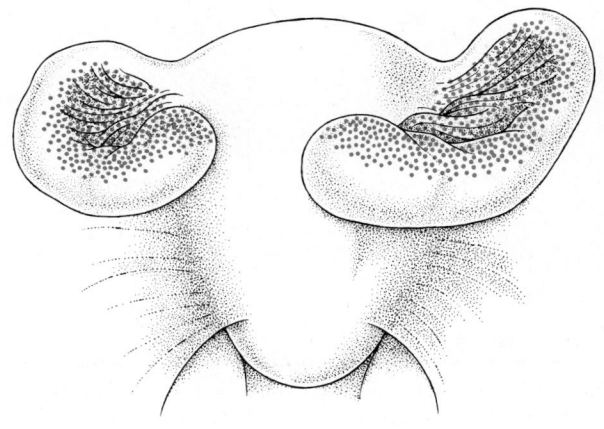

F I G U R E 4 0 - 8

Postpartum salpingitis. Infection of the fallopian tubes leads to hyperemia, edema, and purulent discharge into the tubal lumina. The tubes are enlarged, swollen, and tender. Tubal abscesses may occur, creating tender adnexal masses.

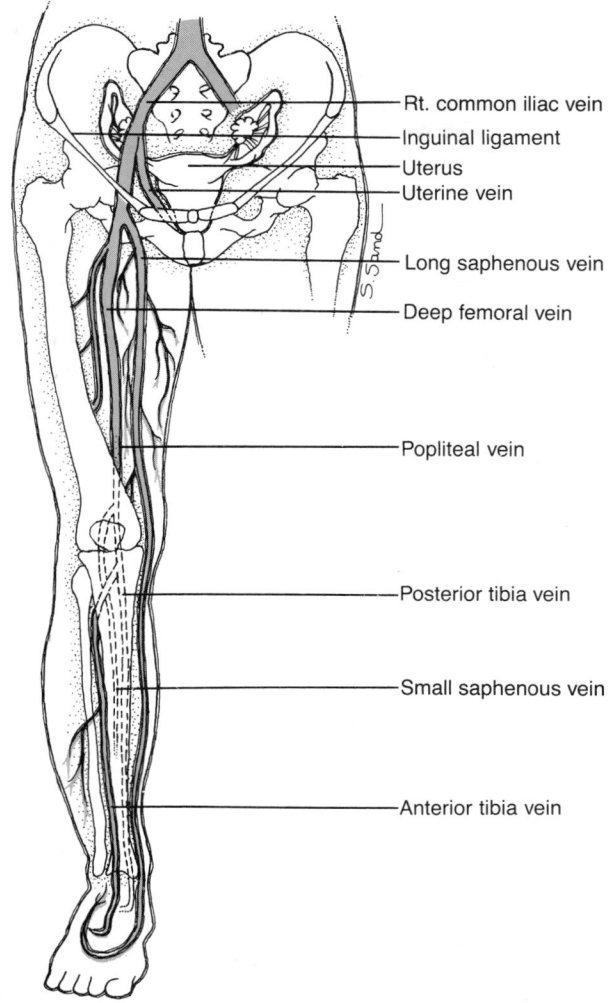

- Rt. common iliac vein
- Inguinal ligament
- Uterus
- Uterine vein
- Long saphenous vein
- Deep femoral vein
- Popliteal vein
- Posterior tibia vein
- Small saphenous vein
- Anterior tibia vein

FIGURE 40-9

Sites of postpartum thrombophlebitis. Pelvic thrombophlebitis involves the uterine and ovarian veins. Femoral thrombophlebitis involves the femoral, popliteal, and long saphenous veins. When the small saphenous vein is involved, the term is *phlebothrombosis*, because the thrombus is caused more by stasis than infection, although deep calf thrombi do become infected.

begin in the groin or the hip and extend downward, or it may commence in the calf of the leg and extend upward. In about 24 hours the leg begins to swell, and although the pain then lessens slightly, it is always present and may be severe enough to prevent sleep. The skin over the swollen area is shiny white.

The acute symptoms last from a few days to a week, after which the pain gradually subsides and the patient slowly improves.

The disease lasts 4 to 6 weeks. The affected leg is slow to return to its normal size and may remain permanently enlarged and troublesome.

The prognosis is usually favorable. However, in some of the very severe cases, abscesses may form and the disease may become critical and produce fatality. Since the clot tends to be attached to the vessel wall somewhat loosely, there is a tendency for the clot to dislodge and produce a pulmonary embolism, which is also fatal in the majority of cases.

Treatment of femoral thrombophlebitis consists in rest, elevation of the affected leg, and analgesics as indicated for pain. Anticoagulants, such as heparin and dicumarol, may be prescribed to prevent further formation of thrombi. Antimicrobial drugs may be used in cases in which more generalized infection is known or suspected. A "cradle" is used to keep the pressure of the bedclothes off the affected part. Heat or icebags may be used along the course of the affected vessels.

Surgical treatment may be indicated in some severe or nonresponding cases and consists in incision of the affected vessel, removal of the clot, and repair of the vessel. Ligation of the major vessels is sometimes resorted to as a preventive measure for pulmonary embolism.

Under no circumstances should anyone rub or massage the affected part. The leg should be handled with the utmost care when one is changing dressings, applying a bandage, making the bed, or giving a bath.

Pelvic Thrombophlebitis.

Pelvic thrombophlebitis is a severe complication in the puerperium. The onset usually occurs about the second week following delivery with severe repeated chills and dramatic swings in temperature. The infection is usually caused by anaerobic streptococci, and although it is difficult to obtain a positive blood culture, bacteria are present in the bloodstream during chills. Antimicrobial therapy is used and is effective in treating most strains of this organism; as long as the chills and the fever persist, blood transfusions may be given. Heparin and dicumarol may be prescribed to prevent the formation of more thrombi. A further problem is likely to arise with metastatic pulmonary complications, such as lung abscesses or pneumonia.

These patients are often depressed and discouraged and feel physically unwell. Breast-feeding may have been interrupted and the significant emotional and physiological changes following childbirth may be compounded by the illness.

Astute nursing care at this time is particularly essential. Accurate observing, recording, and reporting and paying particular attention to details of the physical care aspects are extremely important in helping to resolve the disorder and to prevent further complications. Supportive care to help the mother (and family) work through the depression and discouragement is another crucial aspect of care. The principles outlined in the discussion of grief are appropriate here (see Chap. 45).

Management of Genital Tract Infection

The use of antimicrobial therapy has vastly improved the prognosis of puerperal infection. Antibiotic drugs are effective in combating most of these infections, but, nevertheless, the management and the care of patients with puerperal infections are highly important and demand the utmost skill. Penicillin is effective against the hemolytic streptococcus, the clostridium bacillus, and certain staphylococci. Since penicillin is not effective against the colon bacillus and certain strains of staphylococci, a broad-spectrum antibiotic such as ampicillin, tetracylcine, or cephalosporin may be prescribed for infections caused by these organisms. Many types of antimicrobials are available, some specifically for the gram-positive or gram-negative organisms and the penicillin-resistant organisms (see Table 40-1). The se-

lection and dosage of these drugs depend upon the severity of the disease and the type of offending organism. Sensitivity series are often done to help determine the appropriate antibiotic.

Assessment

In its typical form each of the clinical types of puerperal infection presents a very characteristic set of signs and symptoms, although occasionally one form of the disease is combined with another. The distinctions between these different types of infections are important because the clinical course, the treatment, and the prognosis depend on the particular form of infection (Table 40-2).

It is very important that the nurse recognizes and reports early signs and symptoms of postpartum genital tract infection so that proper treatment may be instituted without delay. When such puerperal infection develops,

T A B L E 4 0 - 2

Types of Postpartum Genital Tract Infections

Type of Infection	Etiology	Signs and Symptoms	Treatment
Perineal and vulvar lesions	Bacterial invasion of episiotomy, laceration, traumatized tissue	Fever, localized pain Edema, erythema, seropurulent discharge from lesion	Antibiotics Removal of stitches and promotion of drainage, sitz baths, perineal heat lamp, analgesics
Endometritis	Bacterial invasion of placental site or entire endometrium	Fever about 38.4°C (101°F), chills, rapid pulse Malaise, headache, backache, loss of appetite, cramps Relaxed, tender uterus with foul-smelling discharge, dark or profuse lochia	Antibiotics, ergonovine Fowler's position to promote drainage, hydration
Pelvic cellulitis or parametritis	Bacterial invasion by way of lymphatics to tissue surrounding uterus (often following endometritis)	Fever, chills Pain and tenderness of lower abdomen, edema Signs of endometritis may be present also	Antibiotics Hydration, blood transfusion for dropping hemoglobin Bed rest, analgesics
Femoral thrombophlebitis	Infection of thrombi and vascular endothelium	Fever, chills, malaise Stiffness, pain, swelling of affected area	Rest, elevation of leg, heat or ice to leg Anticoagulants, antibiotics, analgesics
Pelvic thrombophlebitis	Infection of thrombi and pelvic veins	Severe repeated chills and dramatic temperature swings	Anticoagulants, antibiotics, blood transfusion, bed rest
Peritonitis	Spread of infection to peritoneum, local or generalized	High fever, rapid pulse Severe abdominal pain Vomiting, restlessness Distention	Antibiotics, analgesics, sedatives Bed rest, hydration, blood transfusion, oxygen, IV infusions

one of the first symptoms usually seen is a rise in temperature. Although temperature elevations in the puerperium may be caused by upper respiratory tract infections, urinary tract infections, and the like, the majority are due to genital tract infection.

The symptoms may vary, depending on the location and the extent of the infectious process, the type and the virulence of the invading organisms, and the general resistance of the patient. The affected area is usually painful, reddened, and edematous and the source of profuse discharge. The patient may complain of malaise, headache, and general discomfort. The temperature is elevated, and in the more severe infections, chills and fever may occur.

The nurse can maintain particular alertness for symptoms and signs of puerperal infection in providing care for women with increased risk factors. The risk factors that increase the probability of developing postpartum uterine and pelvic infections fall into three major categories: factors related to general risk of infection, factors related to events during labor, and factors related to operative procedures. Table 40-3 lists these risk factors by each category.

Women are at increased risk for thrombophlebitis during the postpartum period if they cannot ambulate soon after delivery and if they have a previous history of embolic disorders.

Uterine cultures are taken to gain information about the organism; in severe cases blood cultures may be taken, but if they are to be of real diagnostic value, they must be taken at the time of the chill.

Nursing Diagnosis

Among potential nursing diagnoses in genital tract infections are knowledge deficit related to the cause and care of the particular infection; alteration in comfort (pain) related to fever and progress of infection may be evident.

Planning/Intervention

The curative treatment is antibiotic therapy, but good nursing care is also essential. The patient should be kept as comfortable and quiet as possible; sleep and rest are important. Conserving the patient's strength in every way, along with giving her nourishing food and appropriate amounts of fluids, helps to increase her powers of resistance. The head of the bed should be kept elevated to promote drainage and to keep the patient comfortable.

The infected lesions are treated the same as those of any surgical wound. Drainage must be established, and since this discharge is of a highly infectious nature, care must be taken to see that it is not spread and that all contaminated pads and dressings are wrapped and burned.

Care must be exercised to prevent the spread of the infection from one patient to another. Isolation of infected patients from others is desirable to protect the healthy maternity clients. Ideally, the patient with puerperal infection should be away from the maternity divisions. If it is impossible to arrange for such complete segregation, the nurse must consider every patient with puerperal infection as "in isolation" and follow scrupulous technique accordingly.

Regardless of the situation, the nurse who is caring for a patient with puerperal infection (or any infection, for that matter) should not attend other maternity clients. The hands of all attendants need special attention and should be scrubbed thoroughly after caring for a mother who has an infection. In certain cases strict isolation technique, with special gowns, masks, and rubber gloves, is essential. Clean isolation gowns, masks,

T A B L E   4 0 - 3

Risk Factors for Developing Postpartum Infections

Related to General Infection Risk	*Related to Labor Events*	*Related to Operative Risk Factors*
Anemia	Prolonged rupture of membranes	Cesarean section
Poor nutrition	Chorioamnionitis	General anesthesia
Lack of prenatal care	Intrauterine fetal monitoring	Urgency of operation
Obesity	Number of exams during labor	Breaks in operative technique
Low socioeconomic status		Manual placental removal
Sexual intercourse after rupture of membranes		Hemorrhage
		Forceps delivery
		Episiotomy
		Lacerations

(Eschenbach DA, Wager GP: Puerperal Infections. Clin Obstet Gynecol 23(4):1004, December 1980)

and gloves should be available for all persons who attend the isolated patient, and after being used these should be left in the room and disposed of in special hampers or containers. This apparel should not be worn outside the patient's room. Nurses who care for these patients must be fully acquainted with principles of good isolation technique.

Evaluation

The goal is to have infections resolved and wounds healing normally. The patient's temperature has returned to normal, her lochia is normal, and there is an appropriate fundal size. She is able to manage her own self-care and to care for her infant.

Genital Tract Infection Following Cesarean Delivery

The incidence of genital tract infection is significantly increased when delivery is cesarean. This is frequently related to several factors, such as duration of ruptured membranes, number of vaginal examinations, length of labor, various complications, and the need for invasive procedures. However, the operative trauma itself increases infectious morbidity, generally caused by a mixed anaerobic/aerobic infection by organisms present in the genital tract at the time of labor and delivery. Surgical trauma, with devitalization of tissue and collection of blood and serum in the myometrium or endometrium, which have become infected with organisms that have ascended from the lower genital tract to the amniotic fluid, plays a key role in the development of postpartum endometritis, myometritis, incisional wound abscesses, and pelvic abscesses.[5]

The incidence of wound infection following cesarean section is between 6% and 11%. Risk factors for development of wound infections include obesity, diabetes, number of vaginal examinations, length of time in the hospital prior to delivery, emergency cesarean section, duration of operation, use of electrocautery, and placement of wound drains. The bacteria causing wound infections usually originate from the patient's own flora, either bacteria from the skin or coliforms or anaerobes from the uterine cavity. However, some particularly virulent infections are due to hospital-acquired organisms.

The initial signs of wound infection usually begin on or after the second postoperative day, with unexplained temperature elevation often occurring before other physical findings. Pain, induration, and erythema of the incision are the classic signs and symptoms. Areas of fluctuance often develop, and these, as well as abscesses, need to be drained.

Management

Treatment is by antimicrobial therapy and drainage of abscesses; the antibiotics commonly used include penicillin, tetracycline, kanamycin, and clindamycin. The organisms most frequently causing infections following cesarean section are anaerobic streptococci, aerobic streptococci, *Bacteroides* species, *E. coli*, and less often *Clostridium* species and staphylococci. A particularly strong relationship has been found between membranes ruptured for longer than 6 hours and post-cesarean-section infection (myometritis).[5] Early treatment of endometritis with agents having both gram-negative aerobic and anaerobic spectra can be very effective.[3]

Treatment also consists of debridement of necrotic tissue and packing the wound to keep it open and draining several times daily with saline sponges, as well as antibiotics. Suggested preventive measures include wound irrigation with topical antimicrobials instead of saline during surgery, prophylactic systemic antibiotics, and delayed primary closure in cases complicated by obesity or established infection.

The complications of abdominal wound infection may be most serious. Synergistic bacterial gangrene widens the wound and must be treated by wide surgical excision and systemic antibiotics. Necrotizing fasciitis may be difficult to diagnose initially, requires debridement of the entire necrotic area, and is associated with high mortality. Wound dehiscence has mortality rates as high as 35%, with predisposing factors including obesity, ileus with vomiting and coughing, intestinal obstruction, fluid and electrolyte imbalance or hypoproteinemia, and wound infection. This surgical emergency needs immediate exploration of the wound, debridement, and secondary fascial closure with retention sutures. Postoperatively, nasogastric decompression and systemic antibiotics are usually needed.[4]

Subinvolution of the Uterus

Subinvolution occurs when normal involution of the puerperal uterus is retarded and there is a delay in return to normal size and function. The causes of subinvolution include retained placental tissue and membranes, endometritis, and presence of uterine fibroids.

Subinvolution is characterized by a large and flabby uterus, lochial discharge prolonged beyond the usual period, sometimes with profuse bleeding, backache, and dragging sensation in the pelvis. When infection is present there may also be leukorrhea and uterine tenderness.

The fundus is higher in the abdomen than expected with subinvolution. Lochia does not follow normal progression from rubra to serosa to alba, but may remain rubra longer than expected. In another pattern, lochia returns to rubra after it has been serosa or alba. Women may experience irregular or prolonged bleeding or delayed hemorrhage as a result. This must be reported immediately.

Treatment is aimed at correcting the cause of subinvolution. Oxytocic medication, such as methylergonovine maleate (Methergine) or ergonovine, may be administered to maintain uterine tone and prevent the accumulation of clots in the uterine cavity. Curettage is employed to remove any retained placental tissues or secundines. Endometritis requires antimicrobial therapy.

Early ambulation appears to decrease the incidence of subinvolution. Breast-feeding, which stimulates uterine contractions, may contribute to preventing subinvolution.

Late Postpartum Hemorrhage

Late postpartum hemorrhage occurs when blood loss is greater than 500 ml after the first 24 hours following delivery. These late postpartum hemorrhages may take place any time between the seond day and the sixth week. They are usually sudden in onset and may be so massive as to produce shock. Late postpartum hemorrhage is uncommon, occurring perhaps once in 1000 cases.

The most frequent causes of late postpartum hemorrhage are subinvolution of the placental site, retained placental tissue, and infection. Regeneration of the placental site takes longer (about 42 days) than the rest of the endometrium (about 21 days). Regeneration of the placental site begins from the remains of the epithelial glands; if these are not functional, regeneration must occur from the spread of the surrounding epithelial tissue in the rest of the endometrium. Until the site is firmly epithelialized, sloughing of clots may cause bleeding. Certain factors are associated with clot sloughing and hemorrhage, including low-grade fever, a history of abortion or uterine bleeding during pregnancy, hormonal influences, and non-breast-feeding.

When placental fragments have been retained, these may become necrosed. As fibrin is deposited and builds up, a pseudopolyp can form.[6] When such pseudopolyps become detached, brisk bleeding may occur from the placental site, which has not accomplished adequate hemostasis. This leads to late postpartum hemorrhage.

Treatment of late postpartum hemorrhage is to identify and correct the cause of bleeding. Oxytocics are often administered, with curettage if necessary to remove retained placental tissue. Antibiotics are administered if infection is present. Fluids and blood are replaced as necessary.

Nursing Care

During the acute phase of bleeding, the nurse assesses vital signs, blood loss, and cardiovascular function, administers medications, and assists with operative procedures such as curettage. Informing the family of the client's condition and progress is important. The nurse assists with arrangements for care of the infant, especially if hospitalization will involve several days. Measures to support breast-feeding (if appropriate), such as emptying the mother's breasts and providing the breast milk to family members for infant feeding, can be instituted.

Intervention includes allaying anxiety that may affect parenting by allowing expression of concerns, providing accurate information about condition and progress, correcting misconceptions, giving reasonable encouragement, and assisting the client and family to put the experience in perspective. Knowledge deficits about the complications and their causes, consequences, and treatment can be alleviated by client teaching.

If the mother must return to the hospital, this undoubtedly upsets the beginning relationship with the newborn to some degree. Much of the mother's anxiety or desire to return home as quickly as possible may arise from the often abrupt and temporary arrangements that she has had to make. Understanding and counseling the mother about these concerns and helping with planning can relieve much anxiety. Arrangements for the mother to get adequate rest upon her return home are helpful.

Early postpartum hemorrhage, occurring within the first 24 hours of delivery, is discussed in Chapter 38.

Pulmonary Embolism

Pulmonary embolism is usually caused by a thrombus fragment (embolus) carried by venous circulation to the right heart. The thrombus usually originates in a uterine or a pelvic vein. When the embolus occludes the pulmonary artery, it obstructs the passage of blood into the lungs, either wholly or in part, and the patient may die of asphyxia within a few minutes. If the clot is small, the initial episode may not be fatal, but recurrent emboli increase the mortality risk. Emboli may follow infection, thrombosis, severe hemorrhage, or shock.

Nursing Care

The symptoms of pulmonary embolism are sudden intense pain in the chest; severe dyspnea; unusual apprehension; syncope; feeble, irregular, or imperceptible pulse; pallor in some cases, cyanosis in others; and eventually air hunger. Death may occur at any time from within a few minutes to a few hours, according to the amount or degree of obstruction to the pulmonary circulation. If the patient survives for a few hours, it is likely that she may recover.

When embolism occurs, rapid emergency measures to combat anoxia and shock must be carried out promptly. Oxygen is administered without delay, and anticoagulants are given. Morphine or Demerol may be given to help relieve the patient's apprehension and pain. To prevent recurrent emboli, dicumarol and heparin therapy is continued for as long as 6 weeks to 6 months, depending on clinical response. During hospitalization the patient must be kept warm, quiet, comfortable, and as free from worry as possible. She may be given a light, nourishing diet during early convalescence.

Preventive measures include careful aseptic technique during labor and delivery to prevent infection. Early ambulation is important, since circulatory stasis is a causative factor in thrombus formation. Prompt identification and treatment of thrombophlebitis can assist in preventing emboli.

Whether emboli occur before discharge or at home, the mother–infant relationship is severely disrupted because of the mother's acute, life-threatening complication. Nursing measures to provide information and reduce knowledge deficits, to allay anxiety, and to minimize alterations in parenting are indicated. See suggestions for nursing measures in the section on Late Postpartum Hemorrhage.

Vulvar Hematomas

Blood may escape into the connective tissue beneath the skin covering the external genitalia or beneath the vaginal mucosa to form vulvar and vaginal hematomas. The condition occurs about once in every 500 to 1000 deliveries.

Vulvar hematomas cause severe perineal pain and the sudden appearance of a tense, fluctuant, and sensitive tumor of varying size covered by discolored skin. When a hematoma develops in the vagina, it may temporarily escape detection, but the pain and the patient's inability to void should alert the nurse to this complication.

Small hematomas are usually treated supportively and allowed to resolve of their own accord. However, if the pain is severe or the hematoma enlarges, incision and evacuation of the blood, with ligation of bleeding points, is required. Large genital hematomas nearly always result in a blood loss that is more than the clinical estimate. Hypovolemia and anemia should be prevented by blood replacement as necessary.

Vulvar or vaginal hematomas may become infected, particularly those that must be opened and drained. Therefore, attention must be given to prevention of contamination both through careful aseptic technique of attendants and by teaching the patient perineal and bowel hygiene. Dressings or perineal pads must be changed frequently and early signs of infection such as foul-smelling discharge or temperature elevation reported at once. Broad-spectrum antibiotics may be instituted.

Mastitis

Mastitis, or inflammation of the breast, may vary from a "simple" inflammation of the tissues around the nipple to a suppurative process that results in abscess formation in the glandular tissue. Mastitis is the result of an infection, usually caused by *Staphylococcus aureus* or hemolytic streptococcus organisms. The disease in most instances is preceded by fissures or erosions of the nipple or the areola, which provide a portal of entry to the subcutaneous lymphatics, although under conducive conditions organisms present in the lactiferous ducts can invade the tissues and cause mastitis.

The usual route for transmission of organisms to the mother's breasts is from the nasopharynx of her infant, who has become colonized by *S. aureus* in the hospital nursery. Although organisms usually enter through fissures, there need be no break in continuity of the skin of the breast or nipple. Once these organisms are introduced into the mother's breast, milk provides a superb culture medium for them. Efforts to prevent puerperal mastitis cannot be limited to the care of the mother's breasts but must extend to the hospital nursery, where the infant may acquire penicillin-resistant strains. In the nursery such equipment as soap-solution containers, cribs, mattresses, blankets, and linens, as well as floors, can harbor the organisms.

The nasopharynx of newborns tends to become readily infected with *S. aureus*, and the infection may persist for some weeks after the infant leaves the hospital. Studies of puerperal mastitis or breast abscess after discharge from the hospital did not show evidence of the resistant strain of the organism in cultures of the mothers' nares on admission to the hospital. In these cases the infants were the source of infection, because the offending organism was cultured from the nose, the throat, or the skin of the infants.

The patient's hands can be a source of infection, particularly when mastitis is caused by organisms other than *S. aureus*. On occasion, epidemics of mastitis occur when organisms are transmitted by nursery personnel to many infants, and by infants to mothers. Any hospital personnel having direct physical contact with infant or mother can be a source of infectious organisms.

Nursing Care

Assessment

Puerperal mastitis may occur any time during lactation but usually occurs about the third or fourth week of the puerperium. There is usually marked engorgement of the breast preceding mastitis, although engorgement *per se* does not cause the infection. When the infection occurs, the patient complains of acute pain and tenderness in the breast and often experiences general malaise, a chilly sensation, or a chill followed by a marked rise of temperature (40.5°C or 105°F) and an increased pulse rate. On inspection the breast appears hard and reddened. The inflammation may be generalized or confined to a lobe or local area of the breast, with induration, tenderness, and erythema of the involved area. Mastitis is usually unilateral. In advanced cases there may be local abscess formation (Fig. 40-10). The obstetrician should be notified at once and treatment instituted promptly before the infection becomes localized as an abscess.

Nursing Diagnosis

Many of the mother's problems may stem from knowledge deficit related to care of the breasts. But present problems involve pain related to spread of infection;

alteration in parenting related to the mother's inability to continue breast-feeding; and anxiety related to infection and her inability to breast-feed.

Planning/Intervention

Mastitis usually is preventable by prophylactic measures. Prevention is initiated when the expectant mother learns about breast hygiene and begins to take special care of her breasts during the later months of pregnancy (see Chaps. 21 and 22).

After delivery, breast care helps prevent the development of fissures, but if they do occur, proper treatment must be given promptly. Any time the mother complains of sore, tender nipples, they should be inspected immediately. There may be no break in the surface, but if the condition is neglected, the nipple may become raw and cracked. The nurse may detect a very small crack in the surface of the nipple when inspected carefully. Fissures can be treated with tincture of benzoin, lanolin, and use of a nipple shield. Once a break in the skin occurs, the chances of infection mount.

With early treatment with antibiotics, the inflammatory process may be brought under control before suppuration occurs. The choice of antibiotics depends upon results of a culture taken from the milk. The antibiotic-resistant behavior of the organism (usually *S. aureus*) determines drug selection. Penicillin is still ef-

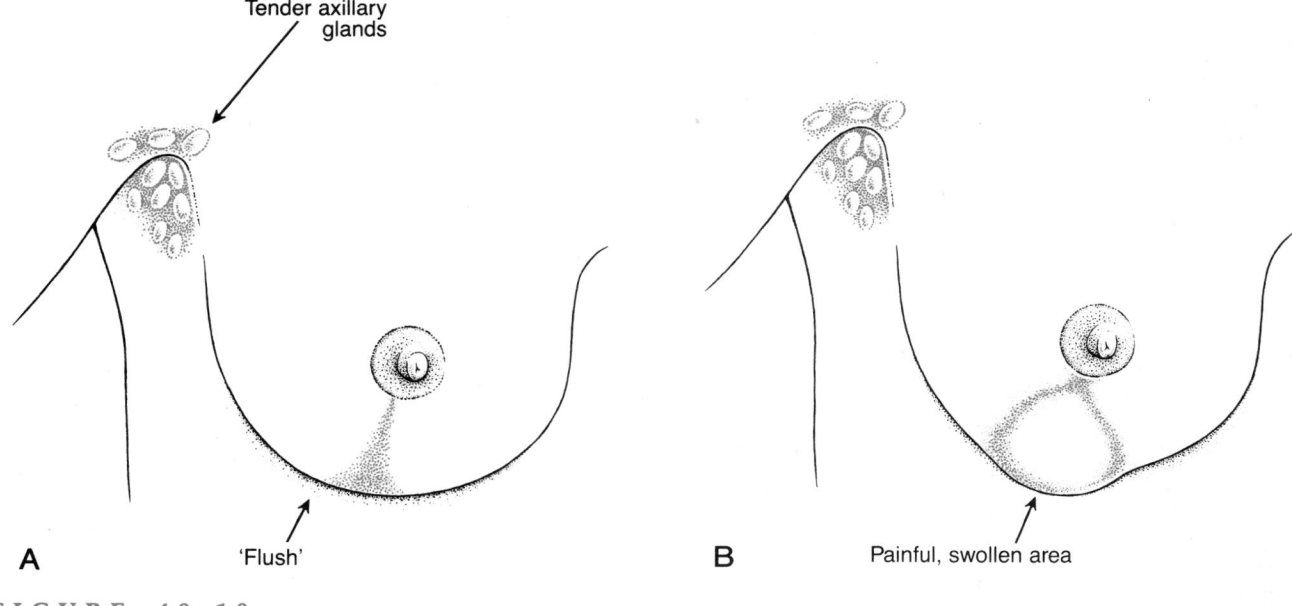

FIGURE 40-10

Mastitis. (*A*) Early mastitis. Fever is followed by a painful area on the breast and a "flush" that is red and tender but not fluctuant or swollen. (*B*) Overt inflammation in mastitis. A swollen, painful, red-to-brawny area develops. The purulent drainage gradually localizes into an abscess; when fluctuant, it must be incised and drained.

fective in some cases, but the prevalence of penicillin-resistant organisms favors use of other antibiotics, such as erythromycin or kanamycin.[7] Depending upon virulence and resistance, intensive therapy may be needed with cephalosporin or vancomycin, drugs that are particularly effective against staphylococcal infections.

The breasts should be well supported with a firm breast binder or well-fitted brassiere. While the breasts are very painful, small side pillows used for support may increase the mother's comfort. Icecaps may be applied over the affected part. When suppuration is inevitable, heat applications may be ordered to hasten the localization of the abscess. Breast-feeding may be discontinued in cases of mastitis.

When abscess formation occurs measures have to be taken to remove the pus. During incision and drainage the incision is made radially, extending from near the areolar margin toward the periphery of the breast, to avoid injury to the lactiferous ducts. After the pus is evacuated, a gauze drain is inserted (Fig. 40-11). Following the operation the care of the patient is essentially the same as for a surgical patient. Complete recovery is usually prompt. Nursing measures are taken to reduce knowledge deficits, to allay anxiety, and to minimize alterations in parenting related to the impact of mastitis.

Prevention is especially important and is a major nursing responsibility. Some methods to help control the spread of infection at its source include careful nursery aseptic technique on the part of all personnel, measures to prevent the spread of organisms from infant to infant, such as proper spacing of cribs, and the ex-clusion of carriers from the maternity divisions as soon as they are identified. The nurse, in her care of the mother, should emphasize health teaching, not only concerning hygienic measures for the prevention of skin infections but also the urgency for prompt treatment of any member of the family if carbuncles, boils, burns, or other skin lesions develop.

Evaluation and Reassessment

When care has been successful, evaluation of the patient should indicate a normal temperature and pain-free breasts. The mother has continued nursing, has indicated she has knowledge about breast-feeding, and has demonstrated her ability to nurse accurately and well. The mother is relaxed in her infant care. The family has returned to or adapted to appropriate parenting behaviors.

If a decision has been made to discontinue breast-feeding, assessment should be made of the woman's acceptance of this fact and adjustment to the role.

Urinary Tract Infection

Postpartum urinary retention is a common occurrence owing to increased bladder capacity, decreased tonus, and decreased perception of the urge to void due to perineal trauma. If the patient is unable to fully empty the bladder, the urine that is retained serves as a culture medium for bacterial growth, often leading to cystitis or pyelonephritis. Urinary tract infections occur in about 5% of postpartum patients and are usually caused by coliform bacteria. This incidence increases to 15% in women who receive intrapartum catheterization.[4]

The increased circulatory volume of the mother that was necessary for the growth and development of the fetus during pregnancy diminishes rapidly after delivery. The two main avenues for the diminution of the circulating blood volume are the skin and the kidneys. Consequently, the newly delivered mother perspires copiously and excretes large quantities of urine within 24 to 48 hours of delivery. As much as *500 ml to 1000 ml* may be voided at *each* urination; that is two to three times what is usual in the nonparturient.

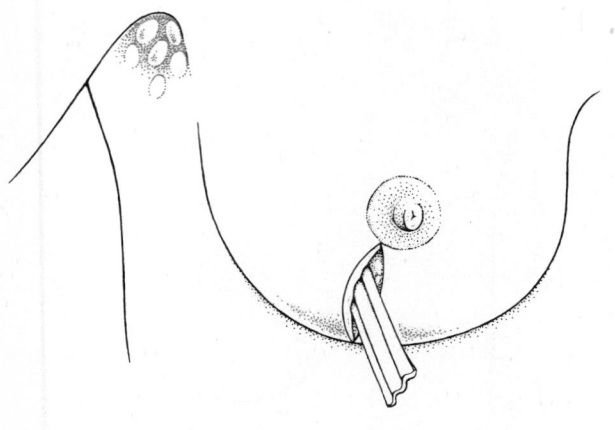

F I G U R E   4 0 - 1 1

Drainage of breast abscess. A radial incision is made in the breast, to avoid injuring the lactiferous ducts, that extends from near the areolar margin toward the periphery. All pus pockets must be broken down and evacuated. A gauze drain is left in for about 3 days. The wound is closed when clean. Antibiotic therapy is given.

Retention and Residual Urine

Because of the trauma of labor or operative delivery, the bladder is not as sensitive to distention as usual. Overdistention and incomplete emptying may occur, resulting in residual urine. Retention of urine due to the inability to void is more frequently seen after operative delivery. It often lasts 5 or 6 days, but may persist longer. The main cause is probably edema of the trigone muscle, which may be so pronounced that it obstructs the urethra. Very temporary urinary retention may be due to the effects of analgesia and anesthesia received in labor.

Nursing Care

The patient should void within 6 hours after delivery (see Chap. 29). If the patient has not done so within 8 hours, or depending upon the degree of distention, catheterization is necessary.

When the mother continues to void small amounts of urine at frequent intervals, this may indicate an overflow of a distended bladder with residual urine. In many cases of residual urine the patient's only symptoms are frequent, scanty urination, but others may experience suprapubic or perineal discomfort. The treatment is usually catheterization after each voiding until the residual urine becomes less than 30 ml; in persistent cases constant drainage by an indwelling catheter may be indicated.

Catheterization for residual urine, to be completely accurate, must be done with 5 minutes after the patient voids. If 60 ml or more of urine still remains in the bladder, voiding is considered incomplete. It is not uncommon for the catheterization to yield 800 ml or more of residual urine. Large amounts of urine (from 60 ml–1500 ml, as shown by catheterization) may remain in the bladder, even though the patient may feel she has completely emptied the bladder when she voided. Such lack of tone in the bladder wall is more likely to occur when the mother's bladder has become overdistended during labor. A distended bladder requires prompt attention because of the resultant trauma; moreover, it may be a predisposing cause of postpartum hemorrhage.

Repeated catheterization may be necessary for several days.

Cystitis and Pyelonephritis

The normal bladder is very resistant to infection, but when stagnant urine remains in a traumatized bladder and infectious organisms are present, there is danger of cystitis. When cystitis occurs, the patient often has a low-grade fever, frequent and painful urination, and marked tenderness and discomfort over the bladder. A catheterized specimen of urine for microscopic examination is collected, and with significant leukocytosis in association with residual urine, the diagnosis of cystitis is confirmed. To avoid urinary stasis, an indwelling bladder catheter may be inserted. In addition, antibiotics are prescribed and fluids should be forced.

If the infection spreads and involves the ureters and kidneys (pyelonephritis), the patient often has a high fever and chills and flank pain over the affected kidney(s).

Nursing Care

Nursing care includes assisting in the diagnosis of urinary tract infections by collecting urine samples. The technique of catheterization is discussed in Chapter 31. It may be preferable to avoid catheterization, especially if the mother is not having difficulties in voiding. Catheterization increases the risk of infection. Therefore a "clean catch" specimen may be indicated.

One method for this type of collection is as follows:

1. The patient is requested not to void for at least 2 hours and to drink as much fluid as she can in the meantime.
2. Then she is taken to the bathroom (or placed in a sitting position on a bedpan if she cannot ambulate) and the vulva and introitus are cleansed.
3. A large sterile cotton ball is placed over the introitus.
4. The mother is then requested to void a little urine forcefully into the toilet or bedpan, but *not to empty her bladder.*
5. Next, a sterile urine specimen bottle or sterile basin is placed under the stream and a specimen of urine is caught. It is sent to the laboratory for examination.

This method yields very good results in obtaining uncontaminated specimens, if done carefully under the continued supervision of the nurse. It also avoids the possibility of introducing bacteria into the bladder at the time of catheterization.

Diagnosis of urinary tract infection is confirmed by urine culture. Sensitivity studies are usually performed to identify the appropriate antibiotic for the causative organism. Medication is usually administered orally, except in acute febrile pyelonephritis, in which intravenous antibiotics are often used. Symptoms are usually relieved within 24 to 48 hours, and treatment is continued for 10 days to 2 weeks. Repeat urine cultures are performed following the course of therapy to be certain the urine is free of organisms.

When indwelling catheters are necessary because of inability to void and persistent residual urine, it has been found that patients with catheters in place for longer than 4 days have a significantly higher incidence of bacteriuria than those whose catheters are removed before this time. Almost all such infections are caused by *Escherichia coli.* Therefore, it is recommended that patients with indwelling catheters for longer than 24 hours be treated with suppressive antimicrobial therapy,

(text continued on page 900)

The Woman with Postpartum Complications

Nursing Objectives

1. Provide prompt diagnosis and treatment of postpartum complications to minimize risk of morbidity, mortality, and dysfunctional effects.
2. Promote comfort and recovery through physical-care measures, nutrition, and pain-relief therapies.
3. Provide client and family teaching to assist their understanding and integration of the experience.
4. Minimize separation of mother and infant and assist developing the mother–infant relationship through information, support, and encouragement of mother–infant attachment.
5. Assist client and family to deal with anxiety, anger, grief, and fear through self-expression and acceptance.

Assessment (For All Complications:)	Potential Nursing Diagnosis	Intervention	Evaluation
Physiological assessment			
Vital signs	Potential for infection (complications such as hemorrhage, urinary tract infection, urinary retention, infection of the genital tract, embolism, subinvolution, vulvar hematoma, mastitis) related to abnormal conditions of the puerperium	Record and report signs and symptoms	Mother's vital signs are stabilized
Patterns of temperature elevation		Administer medications and treatments	Mother voids completely
Condition of perineum and uterus		Monitor vital signs	Mother remains symptom free
Character of lochia		Monitor fluids and hydration	
Tenderness and pain		Collect specimens	
Condition of legs			
Condition of breasts			
Status of bladder and voiding			
Physical comfort			
Rest and sleep	Alteration in comfort: pain related to spread of the infection	Provide physical care to promote comfort (*e.g.*, bath, backrub, clean and dry linens, positioning)	Mother rests and sleeps well
Appetite, nutrition, and hydration		Enhance fluid and food intake (relaxed atmosphere, preferences)	Mother takes adequate fluids and food
Pain or discomfort		Carry out treatments promptly and efficiently (*e.g.*, sitz baths, medications, dressings)	Mother reports relief of pain and discomfort
Psychosocial assessment			
Relation to infant	Knowledge deficit related to cause, progress, and care of complication	Encourage maximum mother–infant contact, provide continuous information on infant	Mother assumes as much caretaking of infant as condition permits
Response to complication	Alteration in parenting related to physical or emotional effects of complication	Explain and discuss complication, expected course and treatment	Mother maintains interest in infant
Response of partner			Mother understands treatment and expected course of complication

(continued)

Assessment	Potential Nursing Diagnosis	Intervention	Evaluation
		Involve partner in education about complication, relating to infant, understanding mother's emotional needs, providing support	Partner understands above and provides support
			Mother expresses grief and fear
		Respond to needs for support and encouragement, working through grief and fear	
Genital Tract Infection			
Fundal size, consistency, tenderness; lochia odor, character; temperature; condition of perineum, wound, legs	Alteration in comfort: pain related to progress of infection	Obtain specimens, report findings, administer antibiotics/medications, note response, isolate as needed, monitor	Mother is pain free
	Knowledge deficit of self-care related to particular infection		Mother performs self-care
Subinvolution and Hemorrhage			
Fundal size, consistency, tenderness; amount of lochia, clots, character; pulse and blood pressure; blood loss	Potential for injury: complications such as hemorrhage related to subinvolution	Massage uterus, facilitate voiding, report blood loss, prepare for IVs and transfusion, monitor for shock, administer medications and oxygen, keep family informed	Mother returns to stable condition
			Mother and family understand events and treatment
Pulmonary Embolism			
Respiratory distress and pain, hypotension, cyanosis, hemoptysis	Potential for injury: pulmonary embolism	Evaluate respiratory status, report signs/symptoms and frequent vital signs, administer medications and oxygen, note response to treatment, obtain specimens, institute emergency CPR/therapy if needed	Mother breathes normally
			Mother returns to symptom-free condition
			Mother's vital signs and cardiopulmonary condition stabilize
Mastitis			
Temperature and pulse; swelling, pain, redness of breasts; nipple soreness, fissures; axillary nodes, tenderness	Alteration in comfort: pain related to infection	Obtain specimens for milk culture, report findings, assist at procedures (incision and drainage), change dressings, administer antibiotics/medicines, provide ice packs or hot compresses and comfort measures (support brassiere), monitor vital signs and progress of healing	Mother's vital signs are stable
	Knowledge deficit related to care of breasts		Mother returns to symptom-free condition
			Mother continues nursing

(continued)

Assessment	Potential Nursing Diagnosis	Intervention	Evaluation
Urinary Retention/Infections			
Frequency and amount of voiding, dysuria, hematuria, suprapubic or flank pain, temperature and pulse, height and consistency of uterine fundus	Potential for injury: complications (urinary retention, cystitis, pyelonephritis) related to trauma or decreased tonus Alteration in comfort: pain or discomfort related to infection	Obtain specimens, report findings, administer antibiotics/medications, insert intermittent or indwelling catheter as needed, note response to treatment, isolate as needed, monitor signs/symptoms	Mother voids normally Mother is pain free Mother's vital signs are stabilized

(text continued from page 897)

usually with such antimicrobial drugs as nitrofurantoin, sulfamethoxazole, or ampicillin.[9]

Other Complications

Sheehan's Syndrome

Sheehan's syndrome, an uncommon complication, is also called postpartum anterior pituitary necrosis; it occurs in about 15% of women who survive severe hypovolemic shock associated with postpartum hemorrhage. There is loss of function of the pituitary gland, resulting in deficiency in thyroid, adrenocortical, and ovarian functions. Symptoms include failure of lactation, decreased breast size, loss of pubic and axillary hair, genital atrophy, and myxedema in severe cases. Most women never menstruate again, although in less severe cases, there may be occasional ovulation and scanty menses.

Treatment consists of hormone replacement, usually thyroid, cortisone, and estrogen. A high-protein diet with ample carbohydrates is prescribed to counteract the typical cachexia. The prognosis depends on the degree of pituitary deficiency, and infertility is usual. Reasonable health can often be maintained with proper hormone replacement, but premature aging frequently results.

Chiari–Frommel Syndrome

The Chiari–Frommel syndrome is a rare condition characterized by prolonged lactation (galactorrhea), which can occur following normal delivery, whether or not the mother is breast-feeding. There is profuse leakage of fluid from the breasts, with headaches, hearing or visual loss, and genital atrophy. The cause is often unknown, but it may be due to pituitary tumor or prolonged phenothiazine therapy. Gonadotropin and urinary estrogen excretion are reduced or absent. There is no effective treatment, although clomiphene citrate may induce ovulation and menstruation, and abnormal lactation can be suppressed by 2-bromocriptine. Estrogen therapy or oral contraceptives may also control galactorrhea, but symptoms usually recur following discontinuation of medication.

Postpartum Vulvar Edema

Vulvar edema in the postpartum period is an unusual syndrome that is frequently fatal and involves massive perineal edema. In the instances reported, following normal pregnancy, labor, and delivery, in which local or regional anesthesia and episiotomy were used, unilateral perineal edema and induration developed beginning about the second postpartum day. This progressed to generalized vulvar, vaginal, perineal, and gluteal edema and induration. Over 2 or 3 days, the edema gradually spread to the other side and into the inner pelvis. Fever and marked leukocytosis also occurred, and in those patients who died, there was also vascular collapse. No definite etiology has been found, and while infections were present in some cases, this was not always true. Treatment consisted of various antibiotics, local heat, heparin, steroids, and crystalloids, but none was particularly effective. Early recognition of asymmetrical vulvar edema, associated with low-grade fever and an elevated white blood cell count, is recommended as possibly preventing maternal death by aggressive treatment with antibiotics and steroids.[8]

References

1. Pritchard JA, MacDonald PC, Gant NF: Williams' Obstetrics, 17th ed. Norwalk, CT, Appleton-Century-Crofts, 1985
2. Gleicher N: Cesarean section rates in the United States: The short-term failure of the National Consensus Development Conference in 1980. JAMA 252:3273, 1984
3. McNellis D: The role of antibiotics in the management of infections associated with pregnancy. Fam Comm Health 6(3):13–21, November 1983
4. Eschenbach DA, Wager GP: Puerperal infections. Clin Obstet Gynecol 23(4):1003–1037, December 1980
5. Gilstrap LC, Cunningham FG: The bacterial pathogenesis of infection following cesarean section. Obstet Gynecol 53(5):545–549, May 1979
6. Danforth DN (ed): Obstetrics and Gynecology, 4th ed. Philadelphia, Harper & Row, 1982
7. Romney SL, Gray MJ, Little AB et al: Gynecology and Obstetrics: The Health Care of Women, 2nd ed. New York, McGraw-Hill, 1981
8. Ewing TL, Smale LE, Elliott FA: Maternal deaths associated with postpartum vulvar edema. Am J Obstet Gynecol 134(2):173–179, May 15, 1979
9. Harris RE: Postpartum urinary retention: Role of antimicrobial therapy. Am J Obstet Gynecol 133(2):174–175, January 1979

Suggested Reading

Axnick KJ, Yarbrough M (eds): Infection Control: An Integrated Approach. St Louis, CV Mosby, 1984

Clarke-Pearson DL, Creasman WT: Diagnosis of deep venous thrombosis in obstetrics and gynecology by impedance phlebography. Obstet Gynecol 58:52, July 1981

Dilts CL: Nursing management of mastitis due to breastfeeding. J Obstet Gynecol Neonatal Nurs, July/August 1985, pp 286–288

Eschenbach D, Wager G: Puerperal infections. Clin Obstet Gynecol 23(4):1003, 1980

Faro S: Group B beta hemolytic streptococci and puerperal infections. Am J Obstet Gynecol 139(6):686, 1981

Friedman C: Maternal infections: Problems and prevention. Nurs Clin North Am 15(4):817, 1980

Ott WJ: Primary cesarean section: Factors related to postpartum infection. Obstet Gynecol 57(2):171, 1981

Visscher HC, Visscher RD: Early and late postpartum hemorrhage. In Sciarra JJ (ed): Gynecology and Obstetrics, vol. 2. Philadelphia, Harper & Row, 1982

Watson, Besch H, Bowes WA: Management of acute and subacute puerperal inversion of the uterus. Obstet Gynecol 55:1222–1226, 1980

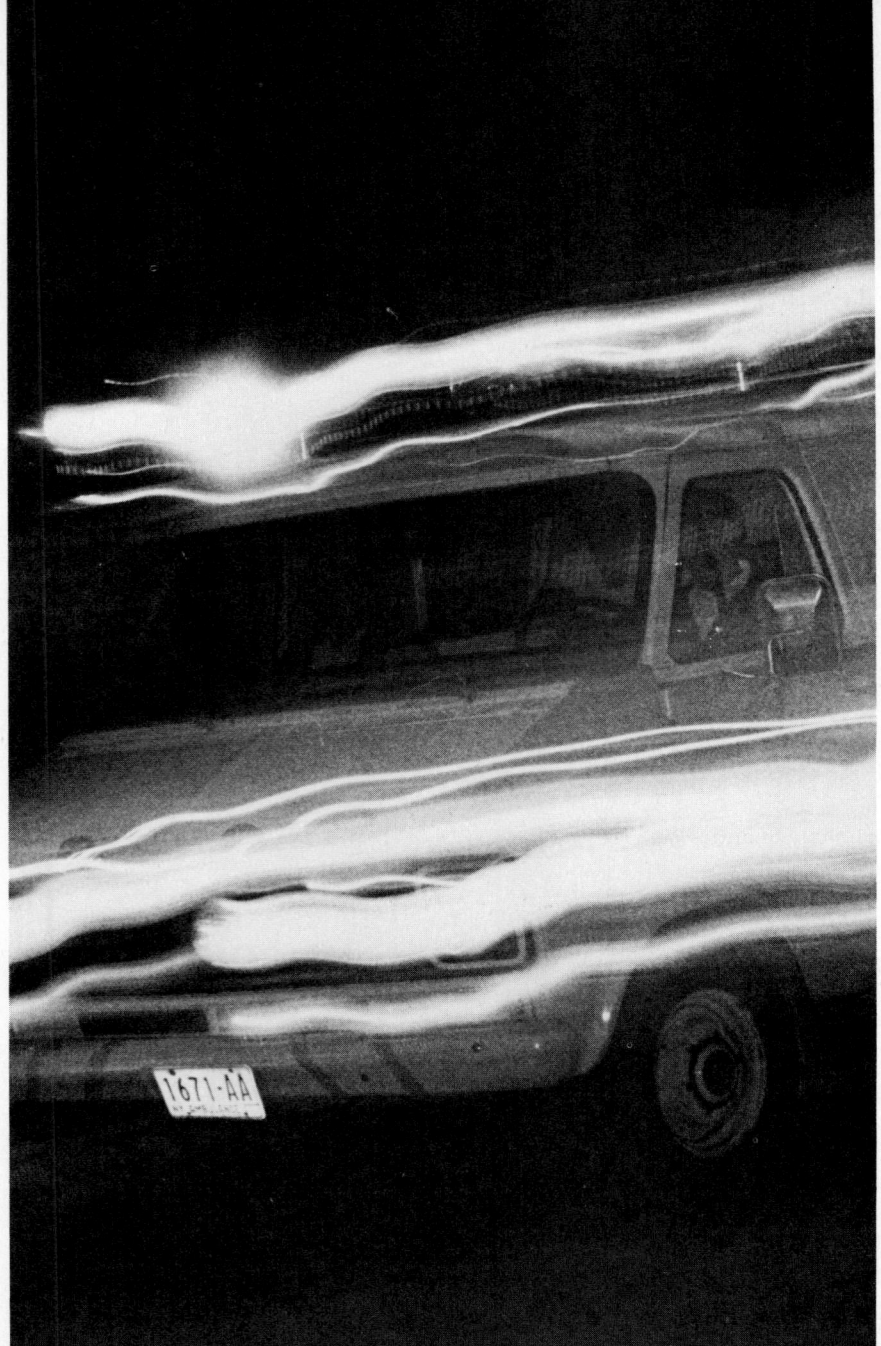

CHAPTER 41

Emergencies in Maternity Practice

Precipitate and Emergency Deliveries

Labor occasionally progresses so rapidly that the maternity nurse must deliver the infant. These precipitous deliveries tend to occur in multiparas with a history of rapid labors, in certain adolescent primiparas, in women who experience little pain during labor and have inadequate warning that delivery is approaching, and in unanticipated premature labors.

At other times the labor may not be precipitate, but the laboring woman is far from a hospital or labor is brought on unexpectedly by an unforeseen emergency. Her only attendant may be a member of the family or a nurse. Common circumstances that often surround emergency deliveries are illustrated in Figure 41-1.

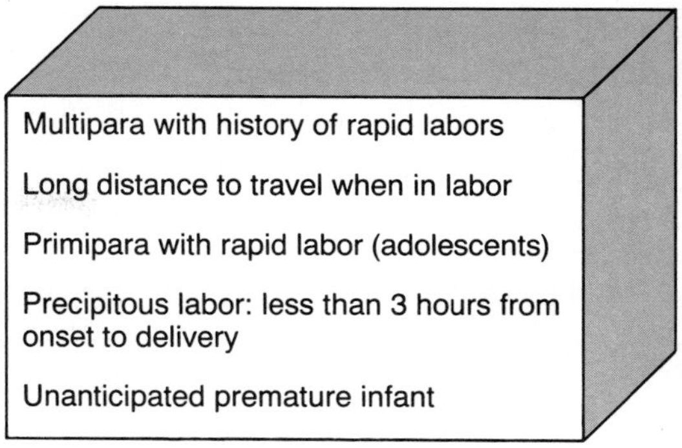

Nurses who practice in the area of maternity nursing need a basic working knowledge for providing a safe birth without benefit of the usual institutional supports. A knowledgeable maternity nurse can help to ensure a safe birth and an emotionally satisfying experience for the mother, father, and others involved.

The nurse's composure and ability to convey calm is one of the cornerstones in a successful delivery. Whenever possible, the mother should be told what to anticipate and what she can do to cooperate effectively. Teamwork with the mother is essential and can be accomplished if confidence is instilled by competence in both physical and emotional aspects of care. If the father is present, he can help care for the mother and infant in whatever capacity seems most appropriate and in accord with his ability. He might be involved directly in some aspect of the delivery, or he might help best by taking care of the other children or by calling the physician.

General Considerations for Delivery

Location for Delivery. If the mother is on a delivery table, it is wise *not to break* the table because it takes practice to handle the infant over a dropped table while accomplishing the following three critical objectives:

- Holding the baby close to the introitus to prevent tension and pulling on the cord
- Holding the baby's head down to promote drainage of secretions
- Holding the infant at or above the level of the introitus to prevent transfusion of the baby by gravity flow[1]

If the mother is laboring in a bed or stretcher, there may not be sufficient space to deliver the shoulders.

Multipara with history of rapid labors

Long distance to travel when in labor

Primipara with rapid labor (adolescents)

Precipitous labor: less than 3 hours from onset to delivery

Unanticipated premature infant

FIGURE 41-1

Common circumstances surrounding emergency deliveries.

Also, the perineum may not be readily visible and it may be difficult to keep the infant's nose and mouth free from the blood and amniotic pool, especially when it comes time for suctioning the infant.

These problems can be overcome by placing an upside down padded bedpan (or similar object) under the mother's hips. This gives about five extra inches of space between the perineum and the bed. If there is no bedpan or similar object available, the nurse can ask the mother to raise her hips by placing her feet firmly on the bed. If this is not feasible, then one or two persons can raise her buttocks a few inches off the bed until the necessary procedures are performed.[1]

Positioning the Mother. The mothers' head needs to be elevated about 45° by any means available. If the mother is in the supine position during delivery her vena cava and aorta are compressed and the uteroplacental blood flow is compromised. This is likely to result in a hypoxic baby, and in an emergency situation the nurse wants to avoid this circumstance at all costs.

Elevating the head also helps the mother to maintain eye contact with her attendants. This can help allay any fears she might have and help her to see and hear instructions.

Many authorities recommend the lateral Sims position for emergency deliveries because it places the least strain on the perineum and affords the best possible visualization of the birth. It also allows for necessary space for delivering the shoulders.[1,2]

Maintaining Clean Technique. Sterility and asepsis are not priorities, since surgery, vaginal intrusion, or the use of instruments is not involved in these deliveries. Normally the vagina has a high bacterial count and few women have sterile uterine cavities during the postpartum period. Repeated vaginal examinations are the primary cause of puerperal infection. The infant also does not need to be in a sterile environment after birth.

Priorities in Clean Technique

1. Cleanse attendant's hands
2. Cleanse mother's perineum and thighs
3. Have attendant put on gloves if available
4. Drape mother if drapes available
5. Prevent fecal contamination of birth canal and baby

The priorities for clean technique are as follows: (1) cleansing the attendant's hands, (2) cleansing the mother's skin, (3) putting on gloves if they are available, (4) placing clean or sterile drapes on the mother if they are available, and (5) preventing fecal contamination of the birth canal and baby.[2]

Protecting the Perineum.   It is important that the nurse not perform an episiotomy unless she is legally and professionally qualified to do so. The nurse's greatest contribution is assisting a slow birth of the infant's head (Fig. 41-2*A*). Massaging and supporting the perineum may be helpful as described below. The inexperienced nurse should give priority to safe delivery of the infant.

Delivery

Delivery of the Head.   As the head distends the perineum at the acme of a contraction, gentle, even pressure is exerted against the head to control its progress and prevent perineal lacerations. This kind of *control* applied during each contraction prevents the head from suddenly pushing through the vulva and causing subsequent complications. *The head must never be held back.* The mother should be encouraged to pant through the contraction to prevent bearing down, particularly as the head, which is supported by the nurse, is being delivered. Preferably, the head is delivered between contractions.

The nurse can place the index finger inside the lower vagina and the thumb opposite on the perineum and gently massage the area to stretch perineal tissues and prevent lacerations. This is "ironing the perineum." The nurse supports the perineum with one hand and controls the delivery of the head with the other hand. The head should be allowed to emerge slowly. Rapid delivery of the head can cause perineal tears, and the sudden change of pressure within the fetal skull may cause subdural or dural tears.

Rupture of the Membranes.   If the membranes have not ruptured previously, they may remain intact until they appear as a smooth, glistening object at the vulva.

If they protrude, they may rupture with the next contraction. If the membranes have not ruptured before the head is delivered, they must be broken immediately (by nipping them at the nape of the infant's neck) to prevent aspiration of fluid when the infant takes its first breath.

Precautions Concerning the Cord.   As soon as the head is delivered, the nurse should feel for a loop or loops of cord around the neck by inserting one or two fingers along the back of the fetal neck (Fig. 41-2*B*). If the cord is found, it is gently slipped over the baby's head, if this can be done easily, or pulled on gently to slacken it. If the cord is coiled too tightly to permit this, it must be doubly clamped and cut (between the clamps) before the rest of the body is delivered. One or more loops of cord around the fetal neck occur in about a quarter of all deliveries.

Suctioning.   As the head extends upward, the infant's mouth and nose are wiped gently to remove mucus, blood, and fluid. The mouth, nasal passages, and throat are suctioned with a bulb syringe. Lacking these, the nurse can use a finger to wipe the throat and squeeze fluid from the nares.

Delivery of the Infant's Body.   After external rotation of the head, which is usually spontaneous, there is no occasion for haste in the delivery of the body. Gentle downward pressure with the hands on either side of the head, over the ears, may be exerted to direct the anterior shoulder under the symphysis pubis, then reversed upward to deliver the posterior shoulder over the perineum (Fig. 41-2*C*). The *posterior* shoulder should be controlled by the nurse's hand. When the axilla of the *anterior* shoulder is seen, the hand is slid along the posterior shoulder to hold the arm close to the infant's body to prevent its flapping with delivery and tearing the mother's perineum. The infant's body now follows easily and quickly and should be supported as it is born.

As the body emerges, the nurse can slide her hand down the baby's back, cradling the buttocks in one hand and the head and back in the other. The head is held lower than the trunk (Fig. 41-2*D*). The newborn is kept close to the introitus to prevent tension on the cord and held at the level of the uterus for placental blood flow. The nose and mouth can be suctioned again, and the newborn is dried, including the head, to prevent heat loss.

Immediate Care of the Infant

Gentle stimulation by rubbing the back as the infant is dried is helpful to stimulate crying and respiration after the airway is clear. A clear airway is essential, since the

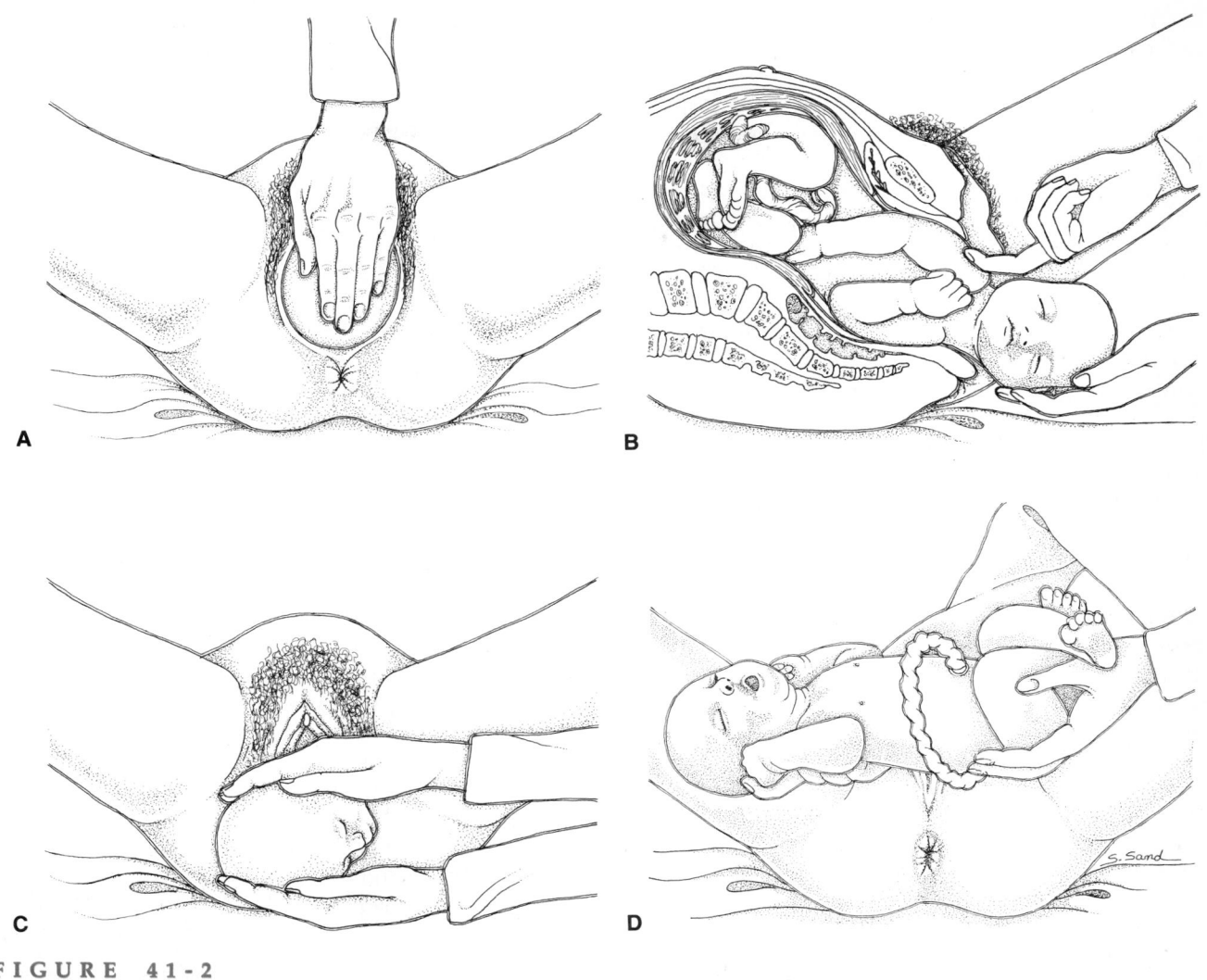

FIGURE 41-2

Assisting an emergency birth. (*A*) Apply gentle, even pressure with the flat of your hand, fingers and thumb close together, on the emerging head to slow the baby's progress and protect the mother's perineum. (*B*) While gently supporting the head, during restitution and external rotation, feel around the neck for the umbilical cord, pulling gently to slacken it if necessary. (*C*) Placing palms over baby's ears, apply gentle traction downward until the anterior shoulder appears fully at the introitus, then upward to lift out the other shoulder. (*D*) As the body emerges, slide your hand down the baby's back, cradling the buttocks in one hand, the head and the upper back in the other. Hold the head lower than the trunk.

newborn only aspirates material into the lungs if encouraged to cry with an occluded airway.

The infant can then be placed on the mother's abdomen and steadied until she can hold him. She should be helped to keep the head lower than the rest of the body.

The infant must be kept warm. This is most easily done by having the mother hold the baby skin-to-skin. The pair can then be covered by warmed, dry blankets or several layers of whatever cloth is available. The ba-

by's head should be covered. The mother's body serves as a reliable heat source, and the layers of cloth prevent heat loss through evaporation.[1]

If necessary, the airway can continue to be cleared and the Apgar can be done. After the airway is cleared, the mother is encouraged to put the baby to breast. Even if the infant only nuzzles or licks rather than sucks, oxytocin is released from the mother's pituitary, which stimulates uterine contractions and aids in the separation of the placenta and prevention of hemorrhage.

Delivery of the Placenta and Cutting the Cord

Shortly after the Wharton's jelly in the cord is exposed to cool air, and the infant cries, the umbilical vessels stop pulsating and blood flow ceases. The baby on the mother's abdomen stimulates release of oxytocins that stimulate uterine contractions and aid placental separation. There is no rush to cut the cord; the nurse can wait until after delivery of the placenta. However, the cord should not be milked, since this can cause hypervolemia, leading to respiratory distress or hyperbilirubinemia (and additional antibodies in cases of isoimmunization). It is important to *wait* for the placenta to separate before attempting to deliver it. More harm is done by injudicious "assistance" than by letting nature take its course. The signs of placental separation are a slight gush of dark blood from the vagina, lengthening of the cord, and change in uterine contour from discoid to globular.

The mother usually feels another urge to push, has a contraction, or feels pressure in her vagina. The nurse instructs the mother to push and can then lift the placenta from the vagina by holding onto the umbilical cord. Uterine inversion can be guarded against by placing the flat of one hand gently but firmly on the lower abdomen just above the symphysis pubis. Force is not to be used, and the placenta can be guided along the curve of Carus (the curved angle from the cervix to the introitus that forms almost the lower fourth of a circle). If the umbilical cord is held near the introitus, it is less likely to break or tear than if held further back.[1]

The membranes may trail behind the placenta and can be teased out with a gentle up, down, and out motion. The nurse inspects the placenta to see if it is intact. The uterus can be massaged gently to maintain firmness and to help the uterine vessels constrict down. Vigorous or continuous massage is to be avoided to prevent muscle fatigue or prolapse or inversion of the uterus (see Chap. 25).

The umbilical cord is clamped placing two sterile clamps about 2 to 4 inches from the newborn's abdomen. The cord is cut between the clamps with sterile scissors. A sterile cord clamp or sterile cord ties are placed adjacent to the clamp on the newborn's umbilical cord. Only sterile equipment is to be used to clamp and cut the cord. Materials can be boiled in water if no sterile packs are available and can include a Kelly clamp, an umbilical clamp, or tape or boiled shoelaces. If the cord is clamped with unsterile materials, neonatal tetanus can result, which is a highly fatal but preventable condition.[1] The placement of tapes and scissors for cutting the cord is illustrated in Figure 41-3. Double loops of tape or laces need to be placed around the cord and secured with at least two square knots. The cord should then be observed frequently for any bleeding.

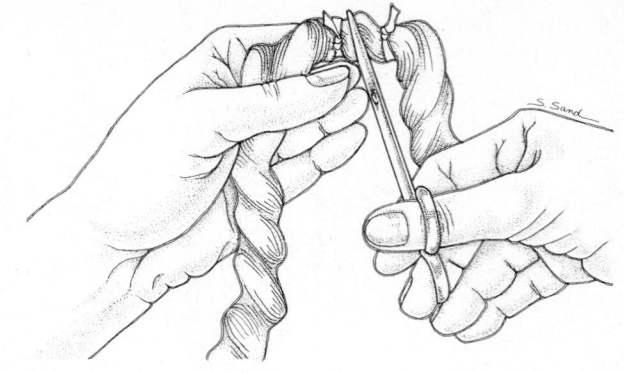

FIGURE 41-3

Placement of tapes and scissors for cutting the cord. To prevent the possibility of neonatal tetanus, it is important to use sterile materials.

Continuing Care for Mother and Infant

When the infant is breathing satisfactorily, he can remain skin-to-skin with the mother and the pair is covered with warmed dry, clean covers if they are available. It is important to be sure the infant's head is covered because that is his largest body area and heat dissipates very readily with no covering. Later, if clean clothes are available for the infant, he can be dressed after the vernix and birth secretions are *wiped* away. There is no need under emergency conditions to attempt to bathe the infant. The infant can also be allowed to nurse at will.

The mother is cleansed under the buttocks and made comfortable. Her perineum is inspected for lacerations. Bleeding from lacerations can be controlled by pressing a clean perineal pad against the area and having the mother keep her thighs pressed together. Fundal firmness is checked, and the uterus is gently massaged as needed to stimulate contraction. To prevent or minimize hemorrhage, the uterus is kept contracted by gentle massage, expulsion of clots, avoiding bladder distention, and putting the infant to breast or manually stimulating the mother's breasts.

The mother, father, and others present should be complimented on their courage, persistence, and helpfulness. Explanations and reassurance, as is possible, should be provided about the situation and the condition of mother and infant. The mother and father should be encouraged to touch and look at the baby to support bonding.

If the physician arrives soon after delivery, the nurse can assist with examination of the mother, newborn, and placenta. If the newborn is premature or is having respiratory distress, the baby should be transported immediately to the nursery. The newborn must be properly identified before he leaves the delivery area.

Record Keeping. The nurse should record the following information on the delivery record: fetal presentation and position, presence of the cord around the neck, time of delivery, Apgar at 1 and 5 minutes, sex, character of amniotic fluid, time of placental expulsion, intactness of placenta, condition of mother and infant, and any medications given or unusual occurrences.

Out of Hospital Births

Emergency deliveries may occur in various locations outside of the hospital. Births at home are considered emergencies when they are unplanned and unexpected. Women in labor need to be transported to the nearest hospital or care facility whenever possible. When birth is imminent, however, transport should not be attempted and the delivery should be attended to by the most skilled person present. Important considerations for these deliveries include privacy, a clean place for the birth, and measures to protect the mother from infection and hemorrhage and the newborn from infection, chilling, and respiratory distress.

The nurse (if present) needs to provide a calm, competent image and to reassure the mother that all will be done to make the birth a safe and satisfying experience. The mother should not be separated from her partner or other support people, but does need to be screened from bystanders, both for privacy and asepsis. A clean surface for the birth should be provided using whatever clean material is available (newspapers, towels, blankets, garment bags turned inside out, coats or slacks turned inside out, etc.)

A warm environment is important, if it can be provided. If clean water is available, the nurse or attendant should wash the hands (soap is even better, if possible).

Emergency Delivery Pack

Drape for mother's buttocks to provide sterile field

4 × 4 gauze pads for wiping the newborn's face and removing secretions from mouth

Bulb syringe to suction newborn's nose and mouth

2 sterile clamps for umbilical cord (Kelly, Rochester)

Sterile scissors to cut umbilical cord

Sterile umbilical cord clamp (Hesseltine, Hollister)

Package of sterile gloves

Baby blanket for wrapping newborn

Record Keeping for Emergency Delivery

Fetal presentation and position

Presence of cord around neck

Time of delivery

Apgar at 1 and 5 minutes

Sex of infant

Character of amniotic fluid

Time of placental expulsion

Intactness of placenta

Condition of mother after birth

Condition of infant after birth, anomalies

Medications given to mother or newborn

Unusual occurrences during the delivery

The nurse should gather equipment and have it handy. If delivery occurs in a shelter or other facility with a delivery pack, these items should be present: bulb syringe, cord clamp, scissors, basin, blankets, sheets, towels, pillows, baby shirts, a dozen diapers, ophthalmic silver nitrate solution, sterile water and eyedropper (to rinse baby's eyes), peripads, and a sanitary belt. Substitutions must be made as needed. A clean, soft cloth can be used to wipe the newborn's face and mouth and dry the hair. New shoestrings can be used to tie the umbilical cord, and a new razor or scissors (clean or boiled) can be used to cut it. If these are not available, the cord may be left intact and the placenta wrapped in a blanket with the baby, making sure there is no traction on the cord.

The delivery is conducted as described for a hospital precipitous birth. Usually emergency deliveries proceed rapidly with few complications. The newborn must be protected from heat loss, infection, and overstimulation. Drying the newborn thoroughly and placing it skin-to-skin with the mother as they are both wrapped warmly prevent heat loss. Coats, garment bags turned inside out, blankets, towels, or even newspapers can be used to cover the mother and infant. Overstimulation is prevented by reducing the noise level and having dim lighting. People should be kept away (except the father and other close persons) to reduce stimulation and the risk of infection.

If the newborn is having mild respiratory depression, the nurse must ascertain a clear airway, wipe mucus from the mouth and nares, facilitate mucus drainage by gravity, stimulate the newborn by rubbing the back and stroking the bottoms of the feet, and ensure the baby is dry and warm. If additional measures are needed, the nurse can give mouth-to-mouth resuscitation to encourage respiratory effort.

Parent–infant bonding can be encouraged, even in the most unusual circumstances for birth. The parents need praise for coping with a difficult situation and reassurance that mother and newborn are in good condition (as possible). The parents can be encouraged to hold, touch, and look at their newborn. Its normal behavior and appearance can be described. The mother can put the baby to breast when it nuzzles or sucks its fingers. Being able to care for the baby and assure themselves of its normalcy helps alleviate the parents' fear of adverse effects from a delivery under unusual circumstances.

Large-Scale Disasters

When any large-scale emergency arises, it is usually sudden and calls for immediate action, whether it is caused by earthquake, hurricane, flood, fire, or war. In the event of such a catastrophe, babies are likely to be born rapidly, and many woman may abort. When organized rescue work is hampered, it may fall to those who are in the immediate area to manage as best they can. The nurses in the area need to be able to assist with measures for the safety and the welfare of maternity clients and their newborns.

All nurses who have completed the basic course in maternity nursing are familiar with antepartal care, the conduct of labor, and the immediate care of the newborn, but their preparation has been carried out, for the most part, in an organized environment, such as a hospital, where supplies, equipment, and medical direction are available. It requires considerable imagination to cope with an emergency situation in which facilities are not available. Yet in any large-scale disaster, whole communities may be isolated and left to their own resources when telephone and radio communications are wrecked; roads may become impassable if they are inundated by water and blocked by debris, and an area may be without safe water, means of power and light, and medical supplies.

Characteristics of Disasters

It has been established that all disaster emergencies have certain similarities and differ only in scope, intensity, and effect.[3] There are usually two kinds of people remaining, those who *need* help and those who *are able* to help. In any extreme, large-scale emergency, the medical-health requirements of the surviving population create a great need for hospital space (improvised if necessary) and for skilled professionals to care for the ill and injured and to keep the well as healthy as possible.

In extreme disaster conditions nursing care is usually administered on an austere basis, but in accordance with established principles designed to save life, prevent the spread of disease, alleviate suffering, and promote recovery. If the emergency is confined to an area, the resources and manpower of the unaffected regions can be used.

Every responsible practitioner will want to be familiar with basic emergency and disaster nursing techniques (see Suggested Reading). It is important to remember, however, that the required knowledge and skills for nursing under these conditions are essentially the same as those required in daily client care; *only the priorities change.* Thus, treatment will be based on available personnel, drugs, supplies, and equipment.

Nursing Services During Disasters

Disasters strike with little if any warning, and a hospital's emergency department must be prepared to face almost any situation. Definitions of disaster vary. Some disaster authorities define a major accident as having occurred when there are 50 or more living casualties. From a hospital's point of view, a disaster or emergency occurs when, with no warning, more casualties of varying severity arrive than the hospital is prepared or staffed to handle at that particular time.

With all the attendant noise, confusions, horror, and tragedy of a disaster, there is no time to begin planning the management of mass casualties. Thus, planning must have been carried out beforehand so that the hospital is in readiness.

The following paragraphs provide an outline of one suggested plan that has proven successful.

Alert

When such facilities are available, the emergency or accident service usually has the responsibility of alerting the rest of the hospital; the message can be conveyed to the hospital telephone operator by some person designated as the alerting or casualty officer. Hospitals that do not have specific emergency room facilities *per se* can set aside some room that might serve this purpose. If the physical plant is such that this is impossible, these hospitals might act as "overflow" facilities for those casualties who are not so badly injured.

When the various wards of the hospital are alerted, the following information about the disaster needs to be given: the type of disaster, where and when it took place, the number of casualties involved, and the nature of the injuries. The hospital's preparation for multiple injury cases from a plane crash, for instance, differs from that required for a large number of burned patients or casualties suffering from smoke inhalation or exposure to cold.

Phased Response

The casualty officer (person designated to give the alert) is responsible for deciding the level of response initially required by the hospital to cope with the disaster. For instance, a Phase 1 response might be designed to cope with an internal disaster affecting the hospital itself, such as fire, explosion, or bomb threat. A Phase 2 response might cope with a small number of casualties involving just the emergency room facilities. Finally, a Phase 3 response alerts and mobilizes the entire hospital to deal with a classic disaster.[3]

Disaster Chest

Once a disaster has been declared, the nurse or other member of the staff in charge (and there should be a special person so designated) goes to the "disaster chest," which is easily identifiable and contains all the necessary documents and equipment for organizing the emergency service. Some item of identification, an arm band, badge, and the like, must be available for the disaster officer to wear. This is also appropriate for any of her deputies, as many bottlenecks and disorganization are created by not being able to identify appropriate personnel in charge of activities. In addition to the identifying material, each box ought to contain a number of "action" cards, which incorporate written informa-

---

Basic Contents of a Disaster Chest

Applicator sticks
Arm bands (medical)
Baking soda
Bandages (adhesive, gauze roller, head, muslin roller, triangular)
Basins (emesis)
Bedpans
Blankets (disposable, fireproof, and waterproof)
Cotton (absorbent)
Cups (paper)
Dressings (tubular gauze, 4 × 4s and other sizes)
Eyepads (adult and child sizes)
Instrument sets (4 hemostats, 1 tissue forceps, 1 scissors)
Matches (safety)

Muslin (uncut)
Paper toweling
Pencils (indelible, red and white skin-marking)
Pitchers (2-quart)
Safety pins
Salt (table)
Sanitary pads, binders, or belts
Scissors
Soaps (hand, tincture of green soap)
Splints (basswood)
Swabs (alcohol)
Tags (medical)
Tape (adhesive)
Tongue depressors
Tourniquets
Twine

---

tion, advice, and instruction for members of the nursing staff. Standard 5 × 8-inch cards can be used for basic instructions; for more complicated diagrams, larger cards may be necessary. These instructions need to be clear, short, and unambiguous.

The contents of the disaster chest are described above.[4] These chests and their contents are also suitable for transfer to the scene of a disaster (with suitable action cards) if it is advisable to give emergency treatment at the scene. Hospital and civil disaster officials caution against including drugs, particularly narcotics, in the disaster chest, even when it is to be used exclusively in the hospital, because they are subject to theft and deterioration. Arrangements can be made to assure that local physicians, hospitals, police, and ambulance and rescue teams provide drugs at the disaster scene if the chest is to be transported there.

Triage or Casualty Sorting

The process of casualty sorting in the saving of lives bears repeating here. The aim of this endeavor is to identify those casualties whose lives can be saved by the early application of medical skills and resuscitation procedures and to concentrate available medical and nursing resources on these people. An experienced physician is appointed as triage officer, and as each casualty is brought in he is rapidly assessed and assigned one of the following priorities:

Priority 1—these individuals can easily die and may need blood transfusions, plasma infusions for burns, or surgery soon to close cavity wounds. Laboring women, especially if wounded, are assigned to this category, and the delivery as well as treatment of injuries is given first priority.

Priority 2—these casualties are unlikely to die immediately or soon from the injuries sustained. Pregnant women who are not in labor may be given this priority unless they are wounded or some complication is anticipated.

Priority 3—these persons are obviously dying from the injuries sustained.

It has been suggested that Priority 2 patients be given first aid, and then be left in the care of first aiders until more help can be given. After Priority 1 casualties have been attended to and when resources permit, attention can then be redirected to Priority 2 casualties. Those who are dying need to be offered comfort and compassion by auxiliary personnel but not by medical and nursing personnel, whose efforts need to be directed toward saving the lives of those who can be helped.[5]

Primary Treatment Areas

Several kinds of facilities are needed; they may have to be improvised. The *resuscitation rooms* must be close to the ambulance entrance and suitably equipped so that hemorrhage can be controlled, airways established by tracheostomy if necessary, and fractures supported and stabilized. Once the patient has been resuscitated he can be reassessed and moved to another treatment area as quickly as possible.

In the *urgent treatment area*, wounds are covered, splints are applied, shock is treated, and patients are prepared for later care. Operation priorities are made before the patients leave this area. In the *nonurgent treatment area*, which may include the *ambulatory casualty area*, patients are received for care of minor wounds, burns, and simple fractures. Special provision is made for those with minimal or no injuries who are suffering from the effects of emotional shock. If a woman is near term or is having any cramping, she may be held in the ambulatory area until further assessment can be made.

It is recommended that two registered nurses staff each of these areas, one of whom has some experience with disaster nursing. In addition, two nurses need to help the triage officer, while the casualty officer supervises the total operation. Nursing auxiliary personnel or volunteers can escort patients to other parts of the hospital.[3,5]

Some communities have instituted a mobile Disaster Nurse Corps whose members go to the scene of a disaster and carry out most of the procedures described above. Working with physicians and other paramedical personnel, they are able to render life-saving care to many victims whose injuries would have been compounded by improper handling.[5]

Disaster Protection for Mothers and Infants

Ensuring the lives and health of pregnant women and their newborn during national or extensive local disasters requires planning that is predicated on the belief that detailed plans and preparations prior to these events are essential and imperative.

In planning for the safeguarding of mothers and newborns prior to a disaster, certain assumptions can be made and specific factors considered. Pregnant women will be subject to all of the risks and injuries to which men and nonpregnant women will be exposed. Their general care should be in accordance with provisions made for the population at large. However, their obstetric care does require additional planning and facilities; it should be separate from hospital and emergency facilities for casualties if possible. Two lives are at stake, lives of particular importance to the future of the country. The need for care of the pregnant woman is predictable, since sooner or later she must inevitably be delivered and in the process will need medical attention to a greater or lesser extent. In the vast majority of instances, probably in 90% of all cases, the birth process, whether it results in a viable infant or abortion, will be essentially uncomplicated. The most formidable complications to be encountered with any frequency will be hemorrhage, obstructed or prolonged labor, infection, and mild and severe toxemias of pregnancy and miscellaneous medical and surgical conditions accompanying pregnancy.

It is estimated that at any given time approximately 2% of the total population will consist of women in various stages of pregnancy. In applying this prevalence rate to a given geographic area, allowance must be made for the character of the area because the rate will, of course, be affected by the presence of large industrial plants and offices employing large numbers of women and younger men establishing families.

Adequate preparation for the care of mothers and babies during a disaster, particularly a large-scale one, requires that plans be made for the training of families for their own protection and survival. This is especially true for the pregnant woman and her family. Thus, a large percentage of the population needs to be trained to carry out minimal essentials of care (buddy system) to save the lives of other people.

In any major disaster, physicians, nurses, and other specially trained professional personnel will be almost completely absorbed in the task of caring for casualties. Normal women in labor at such times may have to rely largely on nonprofessional personnel for their needs, such as other women who have received instruction in the procedures described. Each community should contain a corps of laywomen who understand the basic concepts of attending normal childbirth and have been given at least minimal training in providing this type of care. Preparation for disaster is a family and community effort. Those responsible for planning and implementing disaster plans have the unique responsibility for making this information available to individuals in communities in a way that they can understand and accept.

Every expectant mother needs to know her physician's expectation of the kind of delivery she will have, so that if she needs any special facilities, she will be able to go where these are available. She needs to understand the care she and her baby will need during delivery and immediately afterward.

Essential Equipment

Essential equipment for childbirth is quite minimal and is available to almost every woman in her own home. A package should be made up and kept accessible with other emergency supplies if the area is disaster prone. Contents include a clean sheet, towels, washcloth, and soap; blankets, clothing, a nipple and a bottle for the baby; a pair of blunt scissors; two pieces of clean linen tape, 6 inches long and ¼ inch wide, separately wrapped from the other articles; and a package of powdered milk for the mother. A 72-hour supply of bottled drinking water is also imperative. A can of powdered infant formula is also good insurance in the event that the establishment of lactation is delayed.

Meeting the Pregnant Disaster Victim's Needs

Those who are giving care to pregnant women need to understand that the pregnant woman's normal dependent needs may be greatly enhanced by separation from and concern for her husband and family and by increased fear for herself and her baby. Providing understanding and a warm accepting environment increases the confidence of the pregnant woman in her ability to go through labor, comforts her, and relieves some of her fear and apprehension. Someone should be with the patient throughout labor. The emotional support that patients in labor (who have had some preparation) derive from each other should be used.

Preparations for Impending Labor and Delivery

There are certain preparations for impending labor or abortion that can be made in the immediate period of evacuation. As quickly as possible after a shelter, Field Aid Point, or First Aid Station is occupied, all pregnant women should be registered and the expected date of birth recorded.

The pregnant women of special concern are those who are in labor or expecting at any time, those who are expecting within a week or two, and those who

have had difficulty with previous confinements or who have reason to expect difficulty by reason of disease or abnormalities. *They should be apprised of these facts by their physicians.*

A delivery area can be selected away from the general living or gathering area if space permits. It should be prepared with respect to quiet, warmth or coolness, cleanliness, available supplies, and equipment. The mother will need a clean surface to lie on for the delivery. Clean plastic material or paper can be used for padding the delivery bed. The mother will need clean towels or a clean garment or sheet. A warmer covering such as a sweater, jacket, or blanket is also desirable. Hopefully, she will have brought these articles for the baby with her. The infant's crib can be improvised from a carton and lined with any suitable material (*e.g.,* paper or a blanket) available. The mother's confidence may be temporarily shattered, but the nurse can encourage her that labor and delivery can progress normally. The mother may be able to better mobilize her resources to proceed through labor. The nurse will instruct the mother or attendant to report the first evidence of the onset of labor. This will usually give enough time to make the immediate preparations for delivery.

Essentials of care during labor and delivery do not differ significantly from those described early in the chapter.

Continuing Care

Mother and baby can be considered an inseparable unit. If a mother cannot take care of her baby, full-time mothering care must be provided to enhance the baby's chances of survival and to promote his well-being. Frequent observations of the baby are made for irregularities in breathing, mucus in air passages, weak sucking reflex, skin irritation, and unstable temperature-regulating mechanism.

Breast-feeding is preferable. The infant may be put to breast immediately after birth and as necessary thereafter until the milk supply is established. Once the milk supply is sufficient to satisfy the baby, feedings are given as often as necessary to meet the need. Artificial feedings may be necessary in instances in which the mother is unable to nurse. Formula may be prepared from powdered infant formula or dried skim milk immediately prior to feeding, as there will be no refrigeration facilities. If a bottle and nipple are unavailable, the baby can suck on a teaspoon placed on his lower lip, or milk can be dropped on the inside of the cheek with a medicine dropper. The formula does not have to be heated. Disposable diapers are preferred, but sheets substitute nicely. Of course, any absorbent material can be used if these are not available.

The newborn is particularly susceptible to infection. Anyone with any evidence of infection, such as rash, diarrhea, or upper respiratory tract infection, should not give infant care.

When the infant is found to be premature and in need of special care, or to have congenital malformations, the emergency facilities that have been developed for such conditions can be used.

When the mother and infant are ready to leave the place where care has been given during labor and delivery, arrangements must be made with the family and others for the mother to be relieved of responsibilities, except the care of her baby and herself, if possible. The mother, the family, and the attendant should know where and whom to call if she or the baby have any conditions or symptoms that need medical care.

Psychological Reactions to Emergency Situations

Human behavior during disasters falls into fairly predictable patterns. The nurse needs to know these reactions because coping with large numbers of persons suffering massive emotional shock is equally important as rendering help for physical trauma and illness. This will also help the nurse understand her own responses to the catastrophe.

Periods of a Disaster

Disaster can be divided into various periods. These may include a prodromal or warning period, an impact period, an immediate-reaction period, and, finally, a delayed-response period. During these segments there are characteristic modes of behavior that people may exhibit.

In the *prodromal or warning period* certain persons tend to demonstrate disorganized or destructive behavior. They mill around, disobey instructions, break things, or lash out at anyone getting in their way. Others, however, are able to function in the face of even grave personal danger incredibly effectively; still others become immobilized and, for all practical purposes, helpless.

Some of the above individuals may respond to the warning signals as if catastrophe had already occurred and demonstrate a penchant for ineffective action. These persons fall into two general groups. The first are those who have been through a similar experience before in which they were helpless and have developed a subsequent fear or helpless response to disaster or its warnings. The second are those who always become helpless in any dangerous or frightening situation. These persons often present a difficult problem for helping personnel because if left to themselves, they often precipitate wild panic in others owing to their own panicky behavior. They need to be taken aside and given definite tasks to

do, no matter how simple. Clear, brief instructions and frequent reassurance help these people to regain control of their emotions.[6]

At the *impact period*, almost everyone will experience many frightening feelings, no matter how adequate the training or drilling; thus, there will be at least some period of confusion. This is especially true in the case of an emergency in which there is no warning, such as a dam breaking, a sudden explosion, or an electrical storm. Many respond with physical signs and symptoms. They may exhibit shortness of breath, rapid pulse and respiration, trembling, sweating, and so on. Adequate anticipatory training and drilling have been found to shorten the period of this uncontrolled activity, thus reducing the confusion period.

The *immediate reaction period* after impact is most crucial. Noneffective behavior at this point exacts a heavy toll in terms of the lives and well-being of the survivors. On the other hand, effective action will save lives, diminish disability, reduce abnormal behavior, and decrease the confusion immeasurably. It is imperative that normal behavior be resumed as quickly as possible, not only for each individual's personal safety but also to assure help for those unable to act because of an injury.

Immediately following impact, especially in a disaster of any magnitude, almost all persons will be unable to think, move, or express concern, although given a reasonable length of time, most will make a tremendous effort to adjust. Some will manage this more quickly than others, and they will have to help their slower brethren in their adjustments. Help will usually be available from the relatively uninjured, since professionals are often not available. The less able should team with those who appear more able; the buddy system is more effective and often invaluable.[6]

The *delayed response period* begins when the immediate danger has passed. Groups often unite for mutual protection, and it is at this period that the less acutely affected psychological casualties can be salvaged. It is important to remember that minimal attention may be all that is needed, but it *must be given* and *given early* in this period. Those afflicted are often highly suggestible and will follow almost any advice or take cues for action from the behavior of others. This can be a double-edged sword, for while they respond well to instructions and reassurances, they also tend to become infected easily with anxiety and panic and will, in turn, precipitate panic reactions in others if they are not carefully watched. It is important at this time for all to realize that the menace has passed; thus, verbal reinforcement and reiteration are important. Valuable information can also be conveyed by signs and facial expressions to aid individuals in achieving some measure of security.[6]

Types of Behavior

Various types of behavior may be demonstrated in response to danger or threat in general. A summary of these behavioral reactions follows.

Normal Reactions.
Apparent calmness, at least for a time, is a normal reaction during disaster. More usually seen, however, are physical or body manifestations such as sweating, trembling, weakness, or rapid pulse. Included here also are nausea, vomiting, and diarrhea of a temporary nature. Confusion, crying, and immobilization of a short duration are not uncommon and can still be classified as "normal." The ability and the length of time required to collect oneself with or without help seem to be the most likely criteria for classification in the "normal" category.[6]

Abnormal Reactions.
When the above reactions become prolonged or incapacitating, the individual condition is thought of as more serious. "Conversion hysteria" can occur in which the person unconsciously converts his massive fear into a belief that some part of his body has ceased to function. And in fact, the organ does not function in spite of the fact that no organic damage can be demonstrated. These people cannot be treated as malingerers or "fakers." Since the disability is at the level of the unconscious, the person is as truly disabled as if he had had physical injury to the limb or organ. Nausea and vomiting arising from emotional origins are also seen in prolonged and incapacitating cases. Difficulty arises in diagnosis because these symptoms are indicative of radiation sickness also. Moreover, the person may interpret his symptoms as due to radiation exposure. Problems of isolation and decontamination multiply. These cases tax both the diagnostic astuteness and the emotional reserve of those dealing with them.

Panic and Depression.
Somewhere between the normal reactions and the gross abnormal reactions fall panic and depressed and overactive responses. Panic is not expressed as frequently as one might expect, but its danger lies in its contagiousness. It can spread and cause a mass headlong flight of a crowd. Persons in the grip of this phenomenon often crush and trample one another as they are driven by a compulsion to flee. Purposeless uncontrolled motor behavior is indicative of a panic stage; it is evidenced by such behavior as uncontrolled weeping and running around. Sheer horror, such as the sight of maimed family, and the belief that avenues of escape are being blocked are the two most frequent precipitating conditions. Helping to move individuals and a crowd away from the presenting danger *in an orderly fashion* is the best preventive for this phenomenon.

Depressed reactions are characterized by a general slowing down of motor and mental processes. Persons sit and stare; they seem numb and confused. They do not respond when spoken to, or if they do, it is with monosyllables. These individuals cannot initiate action even to escape threat. Fortunately, they can be salvaged if help can be given to get them moving before too long a period. Other victims respond with a flurry of overactive responses. They will chatter ceaselessly about inappropriate topics, they run back and forth and are avid rumor spreaders. If given a task, they are soon off doing something else, although to their minds, they have completed it to perfection. An unreal confidence in their abilities is their hallmark. This causes them to assume more responsibility than they can possibly discharge and to become very intolerant of other ideas or plans. They are especially troublesome to those who are demonstrating effective leadership.[6]

Principles of Behavior for Nurses Helping in Disasters

It is not possible to present a blueprint for dealing with these situations and behavior. There are some principles of behavior that the nurse can use and that can be easily conveyed to those who will help. First of all the nurse must accept *each person's right to his own feelings*. A quick appraisal of one's own feelings at this time makes one realize how difficult it is to make a conscious choice of one's deeper feelings. An ability to make a conscious choice depends upon what we do about our feelings to relieve the tensions they create within us. Nothing is gained by trying to deny the existence of the distressed feelings in ourselves or others, simply because they appear different from what we would ordinarily expect or experience in everyday life. If we can help someone to take appropriate action, the distressed feelings may change, either quickly or gradually. Each person brings to the disaster a varied experiential background that contributes to or detracts from coping with the effects of the disaster. Letting a person know that you understand *how he feels at the moment* will be the first step toward helping him. Pity will overwhelm him. When the nurse tries to see the events through his eyes and can convey this by gesture or short conversation, it helps him to find constructive outlets for his feelings.

A second principle involves *accepting a person's limitations*. If a person is obviously physically injured, one does not expect him to carry on as usual. Yet, when the nurse is tired, frustrated, and trying to maintain emotional equilibrium, it is easy to resent the vague "unseen" disabilities of others. The feeling of irritability will be enhanced because others will seem to have "pulled themselves together" considering the circumstances. Again, these people need understanding and patience, not resentment, because they too are laboring under a great load.

A third principle involves the *ability to accurately and quickly assess the capabilities of others.* A very upset person can easily cause the nurse to forget that he can be of real assistance; therefore, it is wise to be on the lookout for skills and other assets that might be revived and used. The nurse can begin to help the patient reorganize his world by inquiring into what has happened to him and letting him reply in his own way. Allowing him to talk of his experiences, without letting him ramble on or become more upset, will greatly relieve some of his feelings of despair and helplessness. The nurse can briefly explore his concern about his family and friends, giving him an honest estimate regarding the possibility of his reestablishing contact with his dear ones. If he is too depressed to talk freely, the nurse can talk to him about what may have happened to him and to them. This may increase his confidence in the nurse to the point where he can make conversation. Brief questions regarding his occupation will give clues to his interests and basic capabilities. The nurse can then draw conclusions as to how he can best be used. While this may sound exploitive, keeping someone gainfully occupied is a genuine therapeutic coup. Treating someone as a potentially valued member of the disaster team will increase his effectiveness immeasurably.[6]

Finally, the last but perhaps the most important principle, try to *accept your own limitations in the relief role.* The nurse will want to do a great deal in a disaster; some things, however, will be beyond the nurse's strength and skill. The nurse will need to establish a set of priorities with respect to client care in the realm of responsibility generally. The first priority is to whatever emergency job has been assigned or volunteered for. In practice this job may well be more than full time; therefore, the nurse must select those activities that will be worth trying and those that would be a waste of time. While pushing to the limits of capacity, it is imperative that the nurse not extend beyond those limits because illness may result. If pushing beyond endurance is a personality characteristic, then it is wise to acknowledge it early and set a pace accordingly. A reasonable candid self-appraisal is an important prereq-

uisite for anyone attempting psychological first aid. If one is to deal effectively with others, then one's own concerns must be dealt with *first and promptly.* If they are, the nurse will be less likely to become bogged down when trying to aid others. No matter how thorough the nurse's training has been, it is important to recognize that personal disturbance is likely when the community experiences a terrible tragedy. The first psychological job then is to understand oneself reasonably well. Only then may the nurse justifiably hope to endure and control personal anxieties in the midst of a communitywide disaster and render excellent assistance to those in need.

Reactions of Nurses to Disaster Situations

Research has indicated that while nurses may experience a great deal of anxiety and stress in a disaster while ministering to patients, this does not apparently interfere with effective performance.[7] Causes of greatest stress for the nurse appear to be excessive physical demands and concern for one's own safety. Next most stressful is concern about supplies, either because supplies are inadequate or because they cannot be replenished. Other concerns include worry about one's own family, disorganization, and concern for those who have lost their home and all their possessions.

Excerpts from the following interviews with nurses who have encountered disasters are instructive.

"We had to walk up several flights of stairs, back and forth, up and down, for anything we needed (no elevators because of power loss). We carried water up the stairs. We helped carry trays up. The hardest thing was having to move all the patients into the halls. It was hard physical work because we had all the windows shut and there was no air-conditioning and it was very hot."

"I think, trying to safeguard the patients during the worst part of the hurricane, when it just looked like the walls were going to come down. I heard that all the windows had blown in and I tried so desperately to get over there. Some men forced open the hall door so I could go down the stairwell and I was kind of sorry after I got in the stairwell, because I was in there by myself and I have never felt such pressure in my life. I felt as though my ears would burst."

"I didn't know what was happening to my family; that was the most stressful thing. I didn't know until three o'clock the next day, except I knew they weren't dead because there weren't that many people killed. I felt like they weren't."

Nursing Guidelines: Principles of Behavior for Helping in Disasters

1. Accept each person's right to his own feelings.
2. Accept the person's limitations.
3. Assess others' capabilities quickly and accurately.
4. Accept your own limitations.

"I think what really got me most was the people with large families that had small children. Small children that didn't even have a place to lie down or rest, and not a change of clothes, and no food. One lady with six or eight children came in and I asked her what I could do for her. She said, 'Oh, I'm not too concerned about myself right now; I am more concerned about my children, and if I could just get a bottle of water for my children and for my baby.' "[7]

Trauma in the Pregnant Woman

The leading cause of death in women under the age of 35 is trauma, principally that related to automobile accidents. Since most pregnant women are under the age of 35, they are at risk for accidental trauma. The use of seat belts during pregnancy should be reviewed with every pregnant woman and the maternity nurse must be familiar with the issues. As term approaches, seat belts are increasingly uncomfortable and the woman is disinclined to use them. In a collision the sudden deceleration that occurs upon impact delivers substantially more force to the lower abdomen when a seat belt is used than when it is not, with a high potential for fetal injury by compression. In pregnancies beyond 20 weeks the sudden increase in intrauterine pressure directed upward through the amniotic fluid is associated with a high incidence of premature separation of the placenta. On the other hand, the leading cause of fetal death associated with trauma is death of the mother; when the effect of the seat belt on the fetus is evaluated statistically, there is no significant difference in fetal loss between surviving pregnant women who are belted and those who are not. Among unrestrained pregnant victims the causes of maternal death include head trauma and internal injuries.

The use of a shoulder harness offers a substantial advantage to the pregnant woman in that it redistributes the points of pressure. A study of these issues concludes, "Our study provides no evidence that lap belt restraint increases the mortality of either mother or fetus when pregnant women are victims of severe collisions. In addition, severe mortality of unbelted victims is statistically related to ejection from the car. Seat belts which usually prevent such ejection should be recommended for pregnant travelers."[8]

Management

The management of the injured pregnant woman usually occurs initially in the emergency room. The maternity nurse and obstetrician should be involved in treatment at an early point.

Immediate priorities are the same as those for the nonpregnant victim. These include control of bleeding, assuring airway patency, immobilization of fractured extremities, vertebrae, and pelvis in an effort to reduce blood loss in the surrounding tissues, and blood replacement. The pregnant woman is different from her nonpregnant counterpart in the following ways:

- Because blood volume is normally increased during pregnancy, blood replacement should be generous. If blood is not immediately available, fluid replacement should be substituted until it is.
- The pregnant woman maintains her vital signs for a longer period of time in the face of excessive hemorrhage than does the nonpregnant woman. Pulse and blood pressure may be sustained at virtually normal levels until almost immediately before vascular collapse. Failure to recognize and treat the difference in pregnancy can lead to sudden collapse and irreversible shock.
- When the victim is supine, in late pregnancy the weight of the uterus and its contents creates pressure on the vena cava. The resulting reduction in the return of venous blood to the heart reduces cardiac output and maternal blood pressure and reduces placental blood flow. It may also increase venous pressure in the lower half of the body, producing more bleeding in injured extremities. Pregnant women, therefore, should be placed on their left side in virtually all cases. This allows the uterus to fall forward and relieves vena cava pressure.
- The fetus must also be considered. The maternity nurse usually is responsible for appropriate monitoring (including, if possible, application of the fetal monitor). In this way early signs of fetal distress can be detected and the appropriate action taken.

One of the principal issues in the management of the traumatized pregnant woman is the use of x-ray. Obviously, unnecessary x-rays should be avoided. The decision not to get a radiograph must be weighed against the damage that could occur if a maternal skull fracture or pelvic fracture is missed. Radiographs should be taken as indicated regardless of the pregnant state.

Assessment of fetal viability, and therefore salvageability, is an important part of the management of the pregnant trauma victim. In the event of premature labor, preparation should be made to care for the premature infant on delivery. In some circumstances, a cesarean section should be given serious consideration. In the severely injured woman this decision must be carefully weighed, since it could very easily increase the hazard to the mother. The presence of the fetus should never delay or compromise maternal therapy but rather highlight the need for prompt action. In general, the tests and immediate management that are indicated for the mother are also likely to foster the best interest of the fetus.

References

1. Jennings B: Emergency delivery and how to attend to one safely. MCN 4:148–153, May/June 1979
2. Fowler S, Butler–Manuel R: Modern Obstetrics for Student Medicine, p 360. Chicago, Year Book Medical Publishers, 1974
3. Hirst W, Savage P: Disaster planning. Nurs Times 70: 186–189, February 1974
4. Zanotelli P: Civil disasters? These nurses are ready. RN 34:50–52, September 1971
5. Zanotelli P: Major disasters and plans to deal with them. Nurs Mirror 130:40–41, June 28, 1974
6. Isler C: The psychology of disaster. Nurs Clin North Am 2:349–368, June 1967
7. Laub J: Psychological reactions of nurses in disaster. Nurs Res 22:343–347, July/August 1973
8. Crosby WM: Traumatic injuries during pregnancy. Clin Obstet Gynecol 26:902, 1983

Suggested Reading

Antonetti M: Staff training for fire emergencies. J Am Health Care Assoc 1:49–50, July 1975

Cain HD: Flint's Emergency Treatment and Management, 17th ed. Philadelphia, WB Saunders, 1985

Ellenbogen C: Treatment priorities for septic shock. Am Fam Physician 25(2):163–167, February 1982

Higgins SD, Gavite TJ: Late abruptio placentae in trauma patients: Implications for monitoring. Obstet Gynecol 63(suppl 3):10, 1984

Miller M: Emergency management of the unconscious patient. Nurs Clin North Am 16(1):59–73, March 1981

Rosenblum EH, Jones AL: What would you do in a disaster? Nursing 76:72–73, September 1976

Swedberg J, Driggers D, Johnson R: Hemorrhagic shock. Am Fam Physician 28(1):173–177, July 1983

Wert BJ: Stress due to nuclear accident: A survey of an employee population. Occupational Health Nursing, pp 16–24, September 1979

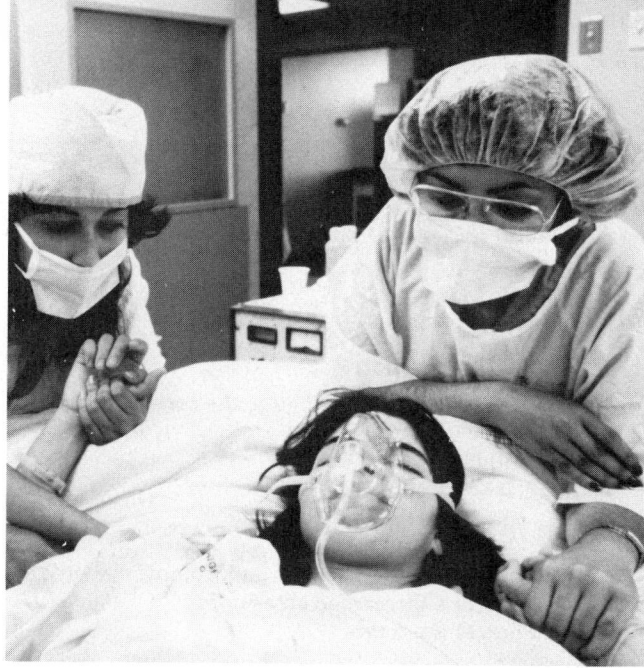

S T U D Y   A I D S

Unit VII:
Assessment and Management of Maternal Disorders

Conference Material

1. A mother, Para 2, is admitted to the hospital at 42 weeks' gestation for induction of labor. Her membranes have been artificially ruptured and intravenous oxytocin has been started. Discuss the nursing care of this mother from this time until she is in active labor.

2. What specific nursing care would you give to a mother who sustained a third-degree perineal laceration as the result of a maximal breech delivery?

3. A 38-year-old gravida 5 had an uneventful pregnancy until the last trimester, when she developed preeclampsia. Now, at term, she is admitted to the hospital because of suspected abruptio placentae and, after consultation, is to have an emergency cesarean section. Discuss the nursing care of this mother from time of admission until she is taken to the operating room for surgery.

4. A primigravida, who has 3-year-old adopted twins, is delivered by low cervical cesarean section because of pelvic injuries received in an auto accident 6 years earlier. Discuss the nursing care of this mother following cesarean section.

5. J.W. is a 25-year-old multipara whose labor was prolonged with early rupture of membranes. There were no complications of delivery. On her second postpartum day, her temperature spiked to 39°C with a pulse rate of 118. She also reported increased afterpains and headache. On examination, you note fundal tenderness and a foul odor to the lochia, which is decreased and red-brown in color. After the physician's examination, the diagnosis of endometritis is established, cultures are taken, and antibiotic therapy is begun. J.W. is breast-feeding her infant and planning to leave the hospital early tomorrow. How will you counsel her regarding (a) the infectious process and treatment, (b) breast-feeding, and (c) hospital discharge? What physical care activities will be added to the care plan as part of the management of her endometritis?

6. Three common infectious processes during the postpartum period are mastitis, urinary tract infection, and thrombophlebitis. For each of these conditions, discuss the following:
   A. Measures that may be taken prenatally, intrapartally, and postpartally to prevent their development
   B. The mechanisms by which these infections develop
   C. Their clinical manifestations (signs and symptoms)
   D. Their medical management and delegated nursing functions
   E. The nursing care plan that you would institute, including the areas of patient education, maternal–infant bonding, postpartal psychological processes, infant care and feeding, discharge planning, and follow-up care after hospitalization.

7. One of the responsibilities of the nurse in an antepartal clinic is to provide childbirth education classes to parents. In preparing material for these classes, you have decided to include a class on cesarean birth, even though the women are having normal pregnancies and are generally low-risk patients. Part of your reason for doing this is the knowledge of the rising cesarean rate, which in some medical centers is one of every four deliveries. Discuss in detail (a) how you decide which areas of content related to cesarean births you include in this 1-hour class, and (b) write a brief content outline of these topics and the specific points you plan to make in each area.

8. You are caring for a mother having her fourth child who is in very active labor. Suddenly, the membranes rupture, and she begins to bear down. As you observe the perineum, you see the infant's head crowning. Since you are alone with this mother at the time, what will you do?

9. Your community has been devastated by a sudden tornado. What types of behavior would you expect from some of the survivors? What interventions would you plan to help them?

10. How would you go about finding out what preparations your community has taken for disaster protection?

Multiple Choice

Read through the entire question and place your answer on the line to the right.

1. Which of the following signs and symptoms should the nurse anticipate when a pregnant patient has a history of heart disease?
   A. Dyspnea
   B. Slow pulse rate
   C. Decrease in blood pressure
   D. Hemorrhage
   Select the number corresponding to the correct letter or letters.
   1. A only
   2. B only
   3. A, C, and D
   4. All of the above _____

2. Which of the following factors influence the answer that you have given in Question No. 1?
   A. Increased need for oxygen intake
   B. Increase blood volume
   C. Toxic damage to the heart
   D. Failure of kidneys to excrete
   Select the number corresponding to the correct letters.
   1. A and B
   2. A and C
   3. B, C, and D
   4. All of the above _____

3. Which of the following signs and symptoms would the patient with a ruptured fallopian tube manifest?
   A. Hegar's sign
   B. Intense pain
   C. Profound shock
   D. Irregular fetal heart tones
   E. Vaginal bleeding
   Select the number corresponding to the correct letters.
   1. A and B
   2. A, C, and D
   3. B, C, and E
   4. B, D, and E _____

4. In the management of hypertensive disorders of pregnancy, which of the following symptoms during labor should be reported to the physician promptly?
   A. Regular uterine contractions
   B. Epigastric pain
   C. Dimness of vision
   D. Headache
   E. Decrease in urinary excretion
   Select the number corresponding to the correct letters.
   1. A, C, and D
   2. B, D, and E
   3. B, C, and D
   4. B, C, D, and E _____

5. Which of the following are causes of bleeding in the first trimester of pregnancy?
   A. Abortion
   B. Abruptio placentae
   C. Placenta previa
   D. Ectopic pregnancy
   Select the number corresponding to the correct letters.
   1. A and B
   2. A and D

3. A, B, and C
4. B, C, and D _____

6. Which of the following are common causes of bleeding in the third trimester of pregnancy?
   A. Menstruation
   B. Abortion
   C. Abruptio placentae
   D. Placenta previa
   E. Ectopic pregnancy
   Select the number corresponding to the correct letters.
   1. A and B
   2. A, B, and C
   3. C and D
   4. A, C, and D _____

7. By what criterion or criteria is an incomplete abortion distinguished from a threatened abortion?
   A. Dilatation of the cervix
   B. Bleeding
   C. Passage of placental tissue
   D. Pain
   Select the number corresponding to the correct letter or letters.
   1. A only
   2. A and B
   3. C only
   4. A, C, and D _____

8. A patient in the third trimester of pregnancy reports to the nurse by phone that she has experienced vaginal bleeding. This is unassociated with pain and she feels otherwise well. She should be advised
   A. To report to the hospital immediately for evaluation
   B. To go to bed and call again if bleeding persists
   C. That this is commonly seen just prior to labor and not to worry
   D. To report this to the physician at the time of the next prenatal visit _____

9. The patient described above continues to bleed vaginally. The most serious condition that must be ruled out is
   A. Placental abruption
   B. Bloody show
   C. Chronic cervicitis
   D. Hydatidiform mole _____

10. The warning signals of preeclampsia that should be watched for during the course of routine prenatal care include
   A. Sudden excessive weight gain (greater than 2lb/week–3 lb/week)
   B. Generalized skin rash
   C. An elevation of blood pressure greater than 15 mm Hg in diastolic pressure over previously observed levels
   D. An elevation of more than 30 mm Hg in systolic pressure above previously observed levels.
   Select the number corresponding to the correct letters.
   1. A, B, and C
   2. A, C, and D

3. A and D
4. B and C   ____

11. Match the statements below with the hemoglobinopathy they most accurately describe.
   A. No increased fetal morbidity or maternal morbidity, but an increased incidence of urinary tract infection in pregnancy   ____
   B. Only slight increased perinatal mortality but greatly increased maternal morbidity and mortality   ____
   C. 50% of pregnancies end in spontaneous abortion, neonatal death, or stillbirth   ____
      1. Sickle cell trait
      2. Sickle cell hemoglobin C disease
      3. Sickle cell anemia   ____

12. Diabetes may have a deleterious effect in pregnancy in the following ways:
   A. Increased fetal size with a greater risk of difficult vaginal delivery
   B. A 4-fold increase in the incidence of preeclampsia
   C. An increased incidence of hydramnios
   D. Increased incidence of urinary tract infection
   Select the number corresponding to the correct letters.
   1. A and B
   2. A and C
   3. B and C
   4. All of the above   ____

13. Match the following statements with the condition listed below.
   A. Potentially lethal infection of the newborn that may occur during delivery   ____
   B. Eyes may be affected at birth and, unless promptly treated, blindness may result   ____
   C. Characterized by anorexia, nausea, vomiting, and elevated serum bilirubin levels   ____
      1. Gonorrhea
      2. Herpes genitalis
      3. Viral hepatitis   ____

14. Breech presentations
   A. Should never be delivered vaginally
   B. Considerably increase the risk of mortality and morbidity for the infant
   C. Cause an increased risk of morbidity for the mother
   D. Generally result in prolonged labor
   E. Always require cesarean section
   Select the number corresponding to the correct letters.
   1. All of the above
   2. A, B, and C
   3. C, D, and E
   4. B and C
   5. C and D   ____

15. The three most frequent causes of postpartum hemorrhage are
   A. Retained placental fragments
   B. Full bladder

C. Uterine atony
D. Lacerations of the perineum, cervix, and vagina
E. Clotting defects
F. Uterine infections
Select the number corresponding to the correct letters.
1. A, B, and C
2. A, C, and D
3. B, C, and D
4. C, E, and F
5. B, C, and F   ____

16. What is the effect of tetanic contractions on the pregnant uterus?
   A. Descent and rotation are hastened.
   B. Ruptured uterus is a great risk.
   C. Fetal head may be compressed and ruptured.
   D. Uterine inertia may follow
   E. Perineal lacerations may occur.
   Select the number corresponding to the correct letter or letters.
   1. A only
   2. B only
   3. A, C, and D
   4. B, C, and E   ____

17. A patient in the first stage of labor develops hypertonic dysfunction. Which of the following are important in the treatment of this condition?
   A. Pitocin
   B. Sedation
   C. Fluids
   D. Bed rest
   E. Ambulation
   Select the number corresponding to the correct letters.
   1. A, B, and D
   2. A, C, and E
   3. B, C, and D
   4. B, C, and E   ____

18. Which of the following principles should be observed in the use of intravenous oxytocin to stimulate labor?
   A. The condition of the fetus must be satisfactory.
   B. It should be used only in cases of primary uterine inertia.
   C. It should not be given to a multipara who has had five or more full-term pregnancies.
   D. It should be used in cases of borderline pelvis.
   E. A responsible person should be in constant attendance while the mother is receiving intravenous oxytocin.
   Select the number corresponding to the correct letters.
   1. A and B
   2. A, C, and E
   3. B, D, and E
   4. All of the above   ____

19. What specific treatment should be included in the care given a mother who has had a repair of a third-degree laceration of the perineum?
   A. Give daily routine perineal care.
   B. Begin stool softeners early.
   C. Omit enemas until the fifth postpartal day.

D. Limit activities in regard to early ambulation.

E. Encourage the mother not to sit erect until wound has healed.

Select the number corresponding to the correct letter or letters.

1. A only
2. A and B
3. A, C, and D
4. All of the above _____

20. Which of the following structures are involved when an episiotomy is performed?

A. The vaginal mucosa
B. The levator ani muscle
C. The glans clitoris
D. The cardinal ligament
E. The fourchette

Select the number corresponding to the correct letter or letters.

1. A only
2. A and B
3. A, B, and E
4. All of the above _____

21. Obstetrical forceps are frequently used to facilitate delivery. In which of the following conditions could it be indicated to delivery the infant by forceps?

A. The cervix fails to dilate completely.
B. The mother has heart disease.
C. The mother has a contracted pelvis.
D. Prolapse of the umbilical cord.
E. Passage of meconium-stained amniotic fluid in vertex presentation at full dilatation

Select the number corresponding to the correct letters.

1. A and B
2. B, D, and E
3. C and E
4. All of the above _____

22. A. What type of fetal heart rate pattern would be most likely to appear if the cord prolapses?

1. Combined acceleration waveform
2. Isolated acceleration waveform
3. Severe variable deceleration waveform
4. Late deceleration waveform
5. Early deceleration waveform _____

B. If the nurse suspects a prolapsed cord, in what position should she place the mother, with the hope of relieving pressure on the cord?

1. Knee-chest or head-down position
2. Fowler's position
3. Sims's position
4. A prone position _____

C. In addition to changing the mother's position to relieve pressure on the cord, what other measures may the nurse employ if she observes the umbilical cord prolapsed out of the vagina?

1. Immediately wash the cord with warm antiseptic solution and replace in vagina.

2. Push the presenting part up with a sterile gloved hand in the vagina
3. Apply a clamp to the exposed cord and cover with a sterile towel.
4. Keep the cord warm and moist by continuous applications of sterile saline compresses. _____

D. What is the main objective of emergency care when prolapsed cord occurs?

1. To prevent cold air from prematurely stimulating respiration
2. To prevent drying of the cord while it is still pulsating
3. To stimulate and restore circulation in the cord by vasodilatation
4. To prevent or relieve pressure on the cord _____

23. A major nursing goal in caring for the pregnant substance abuser is

A. Immediate withdrawal from the drug(s)
B. Initiation of childbirth instruction
C. Provision of nutritional counseling
D. Psychiatric referral _____

24. *Candida albicans* is caused by which of the following agents?

A. Virus
B. Bacteria
C. Parasite
D. Fungus _____

25. Nurses providing antepartum counseling to women with cardiac disease should emphasize the importance of

A. Avoiding all sexual activity during pregnancy
B. Avoiding contact with individuals suffering from infectious disease
C. Participating in a natural childbirth
D. Restricting all physical activity _____

26. Mrs. Alvarez is diagnosed as having pregnancy-induced hypertension (PIH). The nurse would suspect this condition if she found which of the following data in her assessment?

A. Ankle edema and glucosuria
B. Glucosuria and proteinuria
C. Proteinuria and hypertension
D. Hypertension and hyporeflexia _____

27. All of the following physiologic changes may be present in Mrs. Alvarez except

A. Increase in arterial blood pressure
B. Decrease in peripheral vascular resistance
C. Decrease of plasma renin activity
D. Increase in pressor responsiveness to angiotensin II _____

28. Magnesium sulfate is ordered for Mrs. Alvarez. The nurse should withhold the medication if

A. Respirations are 16 per minute
B. Reflexes are 2+

C. Irritability and nervousness are evident
D. Urinary output is <20 ml per hour   ____

29. The organisms that most often cause postpartal infections of the genital tract include
A. Anaerobic nonhemolytic streptococci
B. Beta-hemolytic streptococci
C. Coliform bacteria and bacteroides
D. Staphylococci
E. Pseudomonas
Select the number corresponding to the correct letters.
1. A, B, and C
2. B, C, and D
3. A, C, and D
4. B, C, and E
5. All of the above   ____

30. By which routes do bacteria usually colonize genital tissues?
A. Cervicovaginal organisms entering the uterine cavity during labor
B. Amniotic fluid colonization prior to or during labor
C. Colorectal organisms introduced vaginally by examinations
D. Urinary colonization with vaginal contamination   ____

31. Risk factors that increase the probability of developing postpartal infection include
A. Anemia
B. Prolonged rupture of membranes
C. Intrauterine fetal monitoring
D. Manual removal of placenta
E. Hemorrhage
Select the number corresponding to the correct letters.
1. A, B, and C
2. B, C, and D
3. C, D, and E
4. All of the above   ____

32. Risk factors for developing wound infection after cesarean section include
A. Obesity
B. Diabetes
C. Longer time in hospital prior to delivery
D. Multiple vaginal examinations
E. Longer duration of surgery
Select the number corresponding to the correct letters.
1. A, B, and C
2. B, C, and D
3. C, D, and E
4. All of the above.   ____

33. Signs and symptoms of pulmonary embolism include
A. Sudden intense chest pain
B. Severe dyspnea
C. Flushing
D. Irregular or feeble pulse
E. Cyanosis

Select the number corresponding to the correct letters.
1. A, B, and C
2. A, B, C, and D
3. A, B, D, and E
4. All of the above   ____

34. What is the treatment of puerperal mastitis before suppuration occurs?
A. Antibiotics, breast support, ice application
B. Antibiotics, breast support, heat application
C. Antibiotics, aspiration, breast support
D. Antibiotics, incision and drainage, breast support   ____

35. Measures to prevent puerperal mastitis include
A. Keeping skin of nipples intact
B. Careful asepsis in the nursery
C. Conscientious handwashing by nursing personnel
D. Regular nasopharyngeal cultures of nursery staff
E. Prophylactic antibiotics to nursing mothers
Select the number corresponding to the correct letters.
1. A, B, and C
2. A, B, C, and D
3. A, B, C, and E
4. All of the above   ____

36. Urinary tract infections during the postpartum period are common because of which of these contributing factors?
A. Bladder trauma leading to decreased sensitivity to distention
B. Distention leading to incomplete emptying of the bladder
C. Urinary stasis due to residual urine
D. Colonization of residual urine by recto-genital organisms
E. Dehydration due to restriction of fluids during labor
F. Diuresis due to rapid decrease in blood volume after delivery
Select the number corresponding to the correct letters.
1. A, B, C, and D
2. A, B, C, D, and E
3. A, B, C, E, and F
4. All of the above   ____

Discussion

37. List the four classical signs of endometritis.

38. How does peritonitis differ from parametritis?

39. List the signs and symptoms of femoral thrombophlebitis.

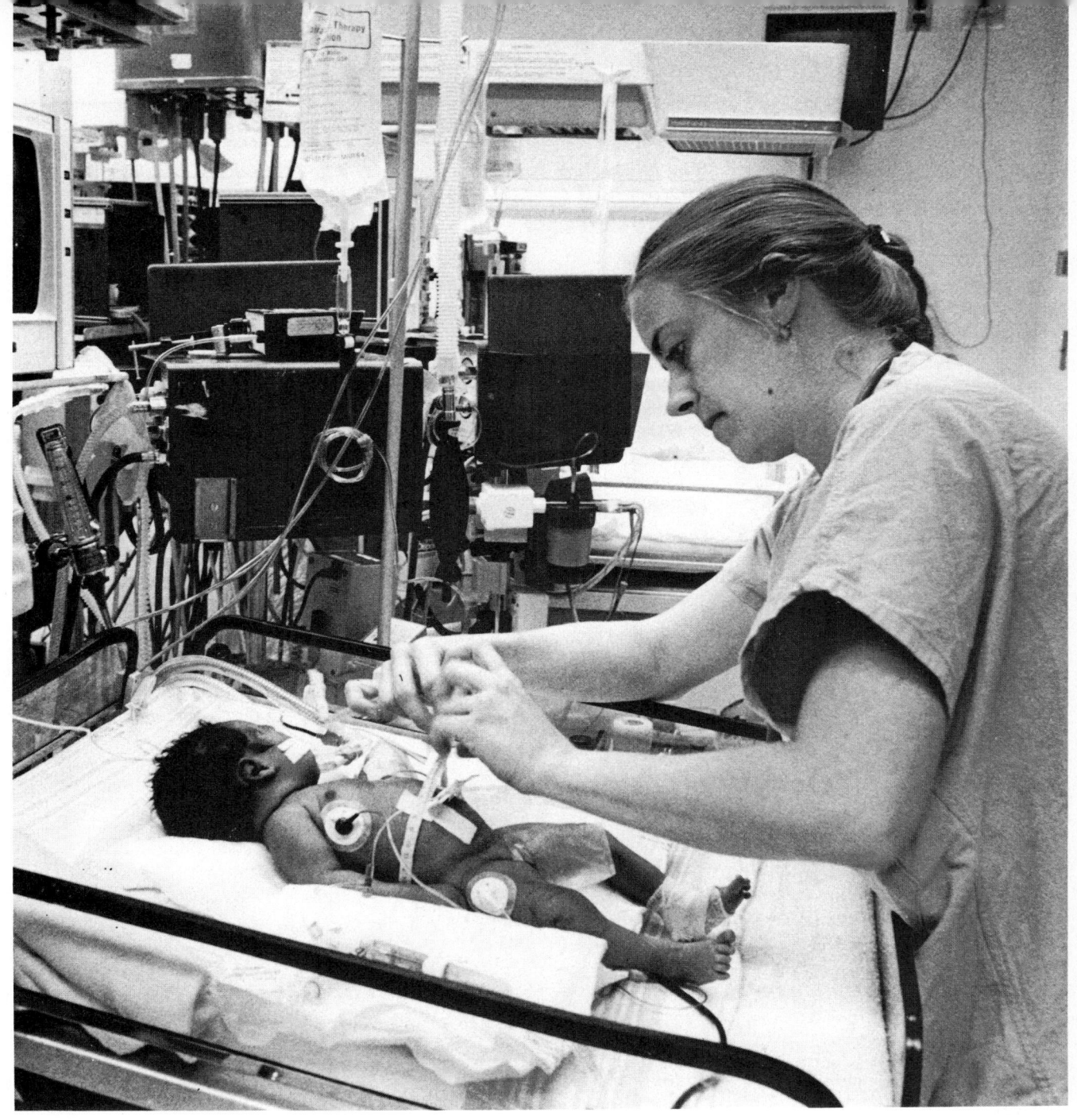

UNIT VIII

Assessment and Management of Perinatal Disorders

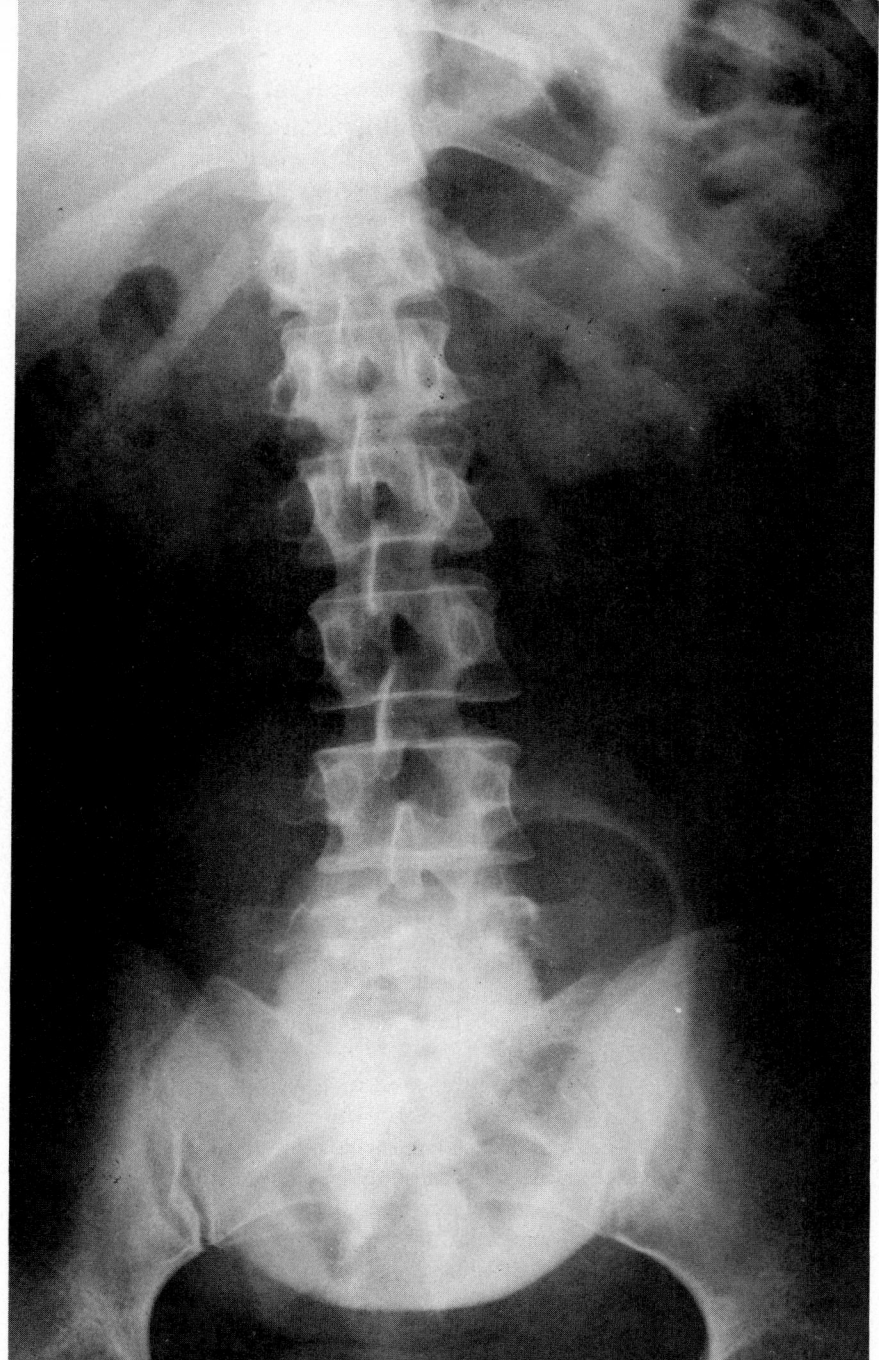

CHAPTER 42

Fetal Diagnosis and Treatment

Prior to the middle of the 20th century the fetus was generally regarded as a passive participant in the entire reproductive process. Fetal evaluation was limited to gross observation of growth and auscultation of the fetal heart. X-ray films were used to assess fetal position and major bony abnormalities, but these methods clearly fell short of precisely determining fetal age and well-being. In the last few decades, however, a series of rapidly evolving developments have opened the way to increasingly accurate approaches. These developments include safer use of amniocentesis (which has allowed greater access to amniotic fluid, for cytogenetic and biochemical assessment of the fluid), ultrasound techniques, and electronic and biochemical fetal monitoring.

In addition to these technical advances, which permit evaluation of the fetus, there have been advances in understanding that permit significant, albeit limited, treatment of the fetus beyond simply converting the fetus to a newborn. The proliferation of this technology has been accompanied by a parallel proliferation in professional and supportive personnel in the broad area of perinatology. Subspecialties have evolved for both maternal/fetal medical specialists and neonatologists. Obstetric anesthesia has emerged as a growing and well-defined area of study. Training programs have been developed for perinatal nurse clinicians, and the concept of the perinatal team has become well established. Such a team includes the obstetrician, neonatologist, anesthesiologist, nurse specialist, nutritionists, genetics counselor, social worker, and other supporting consultants.

In the general area of fetal evaluation, two broad areas of concern are the determination of fetal age and the evaluation of fetal well-being. In the latter category are included assessment in early pregnancy for congenital disorders, later evaluation of well-being in pregnancy complications, and intrapartal monitoring by electronic means.

Regionalization of Perinatal Care

It is impractical for every hospital regardless of size and population served to have all the personnel and equipment necessary to deliver the most sophisticated levels of care. The concept of regionalization or centralization of perinatal care, in which three levels of care are identified, has evolved.

The goals of this system are to make complex care available to entire populations within the constraints of geography, costs, population distribution, and availability of specialists and subspecialists. To make such a regionalized structure effective, it is necessary for health providers to develop and maintain a network through communication, consultation, transportation, and outreach education. A review of the various levels is given in Table 42-1.

The regionalized structure consists basically of four types of facilities: physicians' offices and clinics, local facilities for uncomplicated deliveries, larger urban facilities providing a fairly full range of obstetric and neonatal services, and perinatal centers and specialized units offering the full range of services for maternal and neonatal complications.

Primary-care units for mothers during pregnancy, and for mothers and infants following delivery, are generally physicians' offices and maternal–child health clinics. These provide primary perinatal care, including promotion of good health, screening for complications of pregnancy, and treatment of intercurrent diseases and problems.

Level I facilities are generally community hospitals that are designed to provide care for mothers and neonates without major complications. These are local facilities that relate closely to the community. Because all complications cannot be identified in advance, level I units must be able to provide emergency services of a more complex nature until the mother or infant can be transferred to a facility with greater capacity.

Level II facilities are hospitals in larger, usually urban, communities that offer a wider range of maternal and neonatal services. These serve as referral sources to local hospitals and physicians for high-risk pregnancies or neonatal care. They provide an intermediate level of complex services and can manage the more common complications of childbearing and the newborn.

Level III facilities are the regional perinatal centers that provide the full range of services for perinatal complications of both mother and infant. These units can generally meet most maternal or neonatal needs related to high-risk conditions and may contain specialized units such as children's cardiac centers, units for management of pregnant diabetics, or units for intrauterine exchange transfusions in the cases of severe Rh sensitization.

Implicit in this concept is the identification of the high-risk mother or newborn and the transfer of that patient as required to a hospital with the appropriate level of care. Scoring systems and computerized and problem-oriented record systems have been developed to aid in identifying these patients. The key is early recognition of problems by the health-care provider in order that transport may be carried out at the earliest and most optimal time. Whenever possible, infant transport is best accomplished *in utero* rather than after birth, when the newborn is already in a compromised state. There is considerable evidence that the outcome is far superior when intensive neonatal care begins at the moment of delivery. This is not always possible because occasionally high-risk babies are born to low-risk mothers, and even when the mother at risk is identified, delivery may occur before transfer can be arranged. Despite the obvious value of this concept of regionalization and mother and infant transport, there are significant problems relating to the social and emotional aspects

T A B L E   4 2 - 1

Regionalized Perinatal Health Care

Primary Care	*Level I Facilities*	*Level II Facilities*	*Level III Facilities*
Physicians' offices Prenatal clinics Well-child clinics	Community hospitals (local facilities)	Larger, urban hospitals	Regional perinatal centers
Provide primary perinatal care, including health promotion, identification of complications, treatment of intercurrent diseases and problems	Provide maternal and neonatal care of uncomplicated patients, with emergency services of more complex nature until transfer to another facility with greater capacity can occur	Provide wider range of maternal and neonatal services, serve as referral source for local hospitals and physicians for high-risk pregnancies and neonatal care; intermediate level of complexity, manage the more common complications of childbearing and the newborn	Provide full range of services for perinatal complications of mother and infant, can care for most high-risk conditions, may contain specialized units for neonatal problems or pregnancy complications
Relate through a network involving communication, consultation, transportation, and outreach education			

of patient care. Separation of patients from their families, familiar surroundings, and physicians can create tremendous anxiety and require special sensitivity on the part of all involved in their care.

Determination of Fetal Age

Although it is customary to use Nägele's rule to determine the period of gestation and estimated date of confinement from the first day of the last menstrual period, this method is fraught with error for various reasons. These include failure to remember exact dates, irregular cycles, bleeding in the first trimester, and late registration for prenatal care. In the case of an uncomplicated pregnancy, not knowing the exact length of gestation may not represent a serious problem. However, in the high-risk mother for whom timing of the delivery is critical, the information is vital. Thus, the degree to which the determination should be pursued depends upon the clinical situation.

Means for Determining Fetal Age

Physical Measurements

Estimation of uterine size by pelvic examination in the first trimester is a helpful indicator of gestational growth, whereas determination of uterine size in the second trimester is less valid. Measuring the fundal height above the pubic symphysis at each visit can give useful information about growth or lack of growth. Between 20 and 31 weeks the fundal height in centimeters reasonably accurately corresponds to the gestational age in weeks. Estimation of fetal weight is notoriously inaccurate, with the greatest errors at the higher and lower weights.

Radiographic Studies

Radiographic studies can be helpful in determining maturity. If both the distal femoral and the proximal tibial epiphyses are calcified, one can be assured of a mature fetus (Fig. 42-1). However, if the epiphyses are not calcified one cannot assume immaturity, since there is considerable variation based on sex, race, and fetal weight, along with technical problems related to the position of the fetal knee relative to the maternal skeleton. Because of these inaccuracies, as well as concerns about radiation and the fetus, radiographs are only very rarely performed for the purpose of determining fetal age.

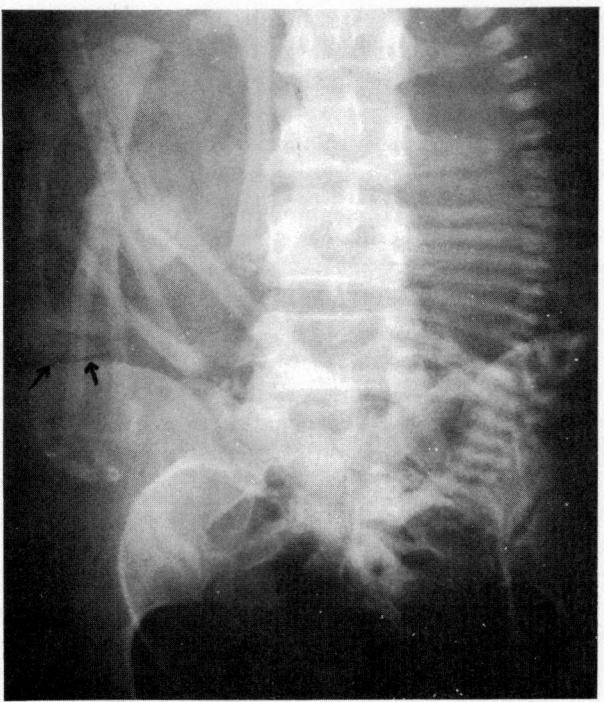

FIGURE   42-1

Abdominal roentgenogram showing a fetus with calcification of both distal femoral and proximal tibial epiphyses (*arrows*).

Ultrasound

Diagnostic ultrasound is now widely used in obstetrics for a variety of purposes, including early diagnosis of pregnancy, confirmation of fetal viability, placental localization, confirmation of fetal death, and estimation of fetal age. The most useful techniques are the B-mode scan and the real-time scan. The *B scan* provides a visual cross-sectional picture that allows identification of the size, shape, and location of structures. *Real time* uses a generator that produces multiple pulses and echoes. Since these are activated in sequence, they detect movement, including vessel pulsations, cardiac action, and breathing. The diagnosis of early pregnancy and estimation of the period of gestation can be made by either technique, but real time offers the advantage of documenting viability as well, since cardiac activity as well as fetal movement can be seen by that technique from early on (uniformly by 8 weeks).

The most common approach to the determination of gestational age is to measure the biparietal diameter of the fetal head. This is especially useful if done between 16 and 24 weeks, and is further enhanced by making two measurements, 3 to 4 weeks apart, which will not only better fix the gestational age, but also confirm a normal rate of growth.

Fetal head growth generally proceeds at a normal rate despite late pregnancy problems that might retard overall fetal growth. This occurs because the brain is spared under such circumstances and brain growth is the major determinant of head size. To detect this type of growth retardation with head sparing, additional measurements must be made, including the femur length, abdominal circumference, and head circumference. These measurements can be used to calculate fetal weight within an error of 10%. It must be emphasized that, although it is commonly done, a single measurement of the biparietal diameter late in the third trimester is of very little value in establishing the period of gestation.

Concerning the safety of diagnostic ultrasound, there is no conclusive evidence of harm to mother or fetus from ultrasound. However, there is a hypothetical risk because high sound intensities over a long time can result in thermal changes within cells, cavitation (small gas bubbles that can rupture cell membranes), and viscous stresses. Benefits must be weighed against potential risks and mothers informed of these as well as clinical indications and alternatives.

Endocrine Studies

Of all the assays available, estriol (or total estrogens) and human placental lactogen (hPL)—also known as human chorionic somatomammotropin (hCS)—are the most commonly used. Both have normal curves that rise progressively during pregnancy. Serum and 24-hour urine samples are assayed. The range of normal is wide, however, making these techniques less valid in determining fetal age than fetal well-being. It is possible for a given value to be in the normal range for both 35 and 40 weeks, and therefore the age differentiation cannot be made. These assays are not often used in clinical practice today.

Amniotic Fluid Studies

Transabdominal amniocentesis has become a standard technique in modern obstetric practice (see Fig. 17-2). It must not be regarded as a totally innocuous procedure and should be undertaken only on the basis of well-founded indications. Potential complications include fetal bleeding, placental disruption, Rh sensitization, and fetal puncture. The frequency of these complications is poorly recorded and is greatly influenced by such factors as the experience of the person carrying out the procedure and the use of ultrasound to localize the placenta. The incidence of complications is probably in the 1% range. Given a sample of amniotic fluid, the following determinations are useful in evaluating fetal age.

Gross Appearance. The presence of large amounts of vernix caseosa generally indicates maturity. Meconium is often present in the significantly postdate pregnancy. Neither, however, is sufficiently consistent for precise age estimation because the meconium may be present as a sign of fetal distress in the less than mature pregnancy.

Cytology. The cells in amniotic fluid come from the fetus and the membranes. The bulk of fetal cells are desquamated squamous cells from the skin. Cells from the respiratory, urinary, and gastrointestinal tracts are also present. If amniotic fluid is mixed with a vital stain for fat (Nile blue sulfate) and a smear is made, a varying number of the squamous cells take up the stain and appear orange on the smear. These cells originate from the sebaceous glands; normally they first appear at 34 to 35 weeks of gestation and increase in number as term is approached. Generally 15% to 20% indicates a mature fetus, while at term the presence of 50% fat-containing cells and free-fat droplets is the rule. This technique has the distinct advantage of being easily done and the information can be immediately available. With more accurate methods available, this technique is rarely used.

Creatinine. The concentration of creatinine in amniotic fluid gradually rises as the fetus's kidneys mature, increasing their ability to excrete creatinine, and also as the fetus's muscle mass increases, which causes an increase in creatine to creatinine metabolism. Values of 2 mg/dl are indicative of fetal maturity. Increased maternal plasma creatinine causes increased amniotic fluid levels. Hence, if creatinine is to be used to evaluate fetal maturity, it is important to be sure that the mother's levels are not elevated.

Bilirubin. Although the determination of bilirubin in amniotic fluid by spectrophotometry has its greatest application in evaluating the fetus in Rh sensitization, it can also be applied in evaluating the age of the fetus in nonsensitized clients. Because of the maturation of the fetal liver and the placenta, the concentration of bilirubin in amniotic fluid is progressively decreased toward term and disappears at about 37 to 38 weeks, strongly suggesting fetal maturity. This evaluation is not sufficiently valid to be used as the sole standard but does complement the other assays.

Osmolality. Although amniotic fluid in early pregnancy is isotonic with maternal plasma, as pregnancy progresses the fluid becomes more hypotonic, presumably because of the increasing contribution of fetal urine. Values of 250 mOsm/liter/kg or less are generally associated with maturity, but variation is considerable.

Phospholipids. The most important and germane studies of fetal maturity have evolved through extensive investigation of fetal pulmonary fluids and the genesis of respiratory distress syndrome. Because there are respiratory movements *in utero*, the composition of amniotic fluid does reflect the content of pulmonary fluids. Consequently, several techniques measuring surfactant activity in amniotic fluid have been devised to determine fetal pulmonary maturity.

Surfactant is synthesized by the type II pneumocytes in the lung, and although present in small quantities from midpregnancy, the mature pathway for surfactant synthesis (choline incorporation) is activated at 35 weeks in the normal pregnancy. In certain stressful circumstances such as preeclampsia, Class D and F diabetes, and premature rupture of the membranes, the process is accelerated. In others, such as Class A, B, and C diabetes, it may be delayed. As will be discussed subsequently, the administration of corticosteroids may, under certain conditions, accelerate pulmonary maturity.

There are several techniques for measuring this activity, including the "Shake" test, lecithin/sphingomyelin (L/S) ratio, and Felma measurement. The Shake test determines the stability of foam on the surface of mixtures of ethyl alcohol and various dilutions of amniotic fluid (Fig. 42-2); maturity is indicated when the foam is stable in the presence of a 2:1 dilution. A kit (Lumadex-FSI Test) that uses these principles is commercially available.

The most widely used technique is the L/S ratio. Lecithin is a major constituent of surfactant. Since the concentration of sphingomyelin remains relatively constant, a rising L/S ratio indicates increasing surfactant production. The separation of lecithin and sphingomyelin is achieved by thin-layer chromatography. The ratio is determined either by visual inspection or by densitometry. Pulmonary maturity is established when the L/S ratio exceeds 2:1.

More recent studies of specific phospholipids in amniotic fluid, phosphatidylglycerol (PG), and phosphatidylinositol (PI) have proved to be valuable in borderline cases and especially in women with Class A, B, and C diabetes in whom fetal pulmonary maturity is often delayed to 37 weeks or later. An accurate 15-minute immunologic agglutination test for PG is available commercially.

Antepartal Assessment of Fetal Well-Being

There are several circumstances in which the fetus might be in jeopardy; it is therefore desirable to evaluate the fetal status. Such instances range from the first-trimester client with a threatened abortion, with whom there is the need to determine the viability of the pregnancy, to midtrimester pregnancy studies to determine congenital disorders (see Chap. 17). In the third trimester, serial evaluations are necessary in chronic disorders such as diabetes and hypertension as well as in more acute problems such as preeclampsia and the postdate pregnancy. At the present time the application of sophisticated tests to determine fetal well-being is limited to clients with a determined fetal risk, while normal pregnancies are evaluated largely by clinical means. It is entirely possible that some or all of these techniques may soon be routinely applied as a form of antenatal screening.

The action to be taken when the fetus at risk is in fact in jeopardy is limited and determined by the period of gestation. If in the first trimester it is determined that the pregnancy is nonviable, the uterus can be evacuated. This is basically an all-or-none evaluation, and qualitative assessment of the first-trimester pregnancy is not currently possible. As one deals with the midtrimester and a previable fetus, assessment of well-being is of

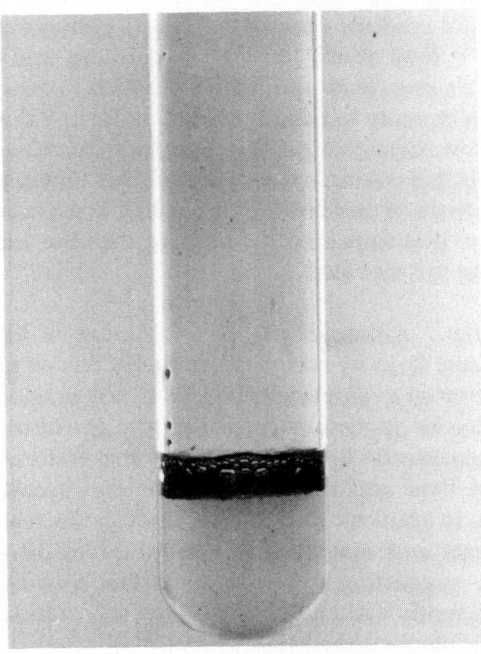

FIGURE   42-2

Shake test. Note bubbles on the surface maintained by surfactant in the amniotic fluid.

little moment because there is generally no recourse if serious fetal problems are uncovered, given the fact that delivery is unacceptable. There are some exceptions to this in which therapy can be directed toward the fetus while allowing the pregnancy to continue. The classic example of this situation is intrauterine transfusion in the severely affected fetus with Rh hemolytic disease. In the vast majority of cases, however, these evaluations are done in the third trimester and the choice is between delivery of a potentially viable premature infant or prolongation of intrauterine life with the risk of fetal death. When the indications of *in utero* jeopardy are severe, the decision to deliver often results in the birth of a seriously ill newborn and a potential neonatal death. More commonly, however, the studies are reassuring and permit prolongation of the pregnancy.

Assessment in Early Pregnancy: Threatened Abortion

A common problem in the first trimester is assessing the significance of bleeding and deciding whether a pregnancy is viable and should be allowed to continue despite the persistent symptoms. Standard immunologic pregnancy tests may remain positive for some time following the point at which viability is lost. Several β-subunit titers are particularly reassuring if their values display progressively higher levels that are appropriate for the gestational period. B-mode ultrasound scans can define a gestational sac as early as 5 weeks following the last menstrual period. The integrity of the sac and its appropriate dimensions are reassuring up to 10 weeks. The fetus is generally visible within the sac by 8 weeks, and fetal activity and heartbeat can be discerned by 10 weeks with real-time equipment. These techniques have considerably more precision in assessing progress than clinical examinations evaluating uterine growth. They can therefore provide reassurance in a situation involving considerable anxiety and offer a definitive answer in situations of nonviability, thereby permitting uterine evacuation.

Assessment in Late Pregnancy

Estrogens

Estrogen levels in maternal serum and urine rise progressively during the course of normal pregnancy, following a sigmoid curve as seen in Figure 42-3. Although estrone and estradiol also increase during pregnancy, it is estriol that is the predominant estrogen, increasing 1000-fold and accounting for 90% of the total estrogen. This makes it feasible in the case of 24-hour urinary

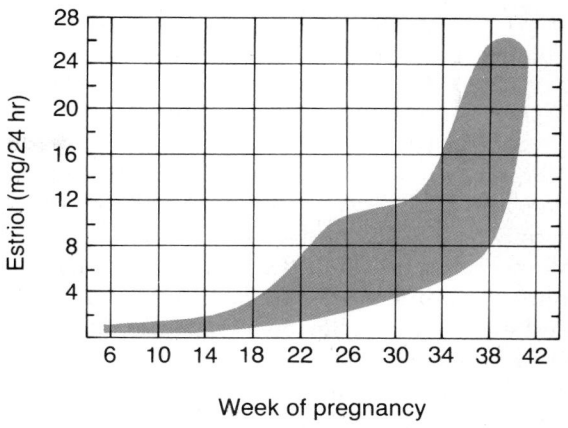

FIGURE 42-3

Pattern of urinary estriol excretion in normal pregnancy.

determinations to measure either estriol or total estrogens. Even more important in the clinical application of estriol measurements for problem pregnancies is the fact that at least 90% of the estrogen precursors are produced by the fetal zone of the fetal adrenal cortex, largely as sulfates of dehydroepiandrosterone (DHEAS) and 16αOH DHEAS. Much of the DHEAS is converted to 16αOH DHEAS by the fetal liver. The conversion of these androgen precursors to estriol is a function of the placenta by processes involving the splitting off of the sulfate and conjugation. Finally, estriol is excreted by the maternal kidney mostly in the conjugated form. Thus it becomes clear that in order for there to be a normal quantity of estriol in a 24-hour urine specimen, the several parts of the cycle must be intact, including the live healthy fetus with intact adrenals producing normal amounts of androgen precursors, a normally functioning placenta capable of making the conversion to estriol, and healthy maternal liver and kidneys competent to conjugate and then excrete the estriol. Consequently, estriol values that are normal for the gestational age are quite reassuring. Most commonly, measurements are made in 24-hour urine collections. Although there may be some day-to-day variation, a fall of more than 30% to 40% must be considered significant and the impression of fetal jeopardy pursued. Serial measurements must be done, and the frequency of determination is dependent upon the seriousness and the stability of the clinical situation. In a hospitalized unstable diabetic, daily estriols may be needed, while less frequent studies are sufficient in a less critical situation.

Because urinary estriols require a 24-hour collection, with the possibility that it may be incomplete as well as inconvenient for the mother, and because this, in effect, brings about a lag in the assessment process, a number of alternatives have been suggested. Simultaneous measurement of urinary creatinine can provide a constant that then enables the clinician to use shorter collection periods, of 4 or 8 hours, for example, and still get meaningful information by calculating the estriol/creatinine ratio. It should also be noted that there are a number of factors that can interfere with urinary estriol determinations. Obviously, in the presence of impaired maternal renal function, the test loses its validity and cannot be used to assess the fetal status. Maternal administration of ampicillin, methenamine mandelate, and corticosteroids all interfere with the measurement, as does a large quantity of glucose in the urine. The latter can be dealt with by diluting the specimen for the assay.

Because of these problems, a number of workers have turned to the use of plasma estriol measurements. The normal curve is similarly shaped to that for urinary measurements, although the quantities are measured in micrograms rather than milligrams. The use of plasma values does not eliminate all problems because levels vary during the day. Therefore, samples must be obtained at the same time each day for proper comparison. Abnormal renal function can result in false elevations of plasma levels. Furthermore, this technique is somewhat more difficult than urinary assays. The methodology has been improved, however, by the use of radioimmunoassay, and currently this technique, applied to unconjugated estriol, is gaining in favor.

Estetrol (15αhydroxyestriol) measurements have been proposed by some as a better means of fetal evaluation. This estrogen is derived from placental estradiol and estrone, with the final synthesis taking place in the fetal liver. Both serum and urinary assays have been suggested, but the current consensus, after an initial surge of enthusiasm, is that estetrol measurements offer no advantage over estriol.

Progesterone

This steroid hormone is produced by the placenta in progressively increasing quantities during pregnancy. It can be measured as serum progesterone or urinary pregnanediol, but has little value in evaluating fetal well-being, since progesterone does not require fetal precursors and can, in fact, persist in significant quantities even after an intrauterine fetal death has occurred.

Human Chorionic Gonadotropin

Human chorionic gonadotropin (hCG), produced by the trophoblast, normally peaks in early pregnancy and falls off to relatively low levels in the second and third trimesters. It is the basis for most pregnancy tests, as well as for the follow-up of hydatid moles and choriocarcinoma, but is of limited value in problem pregnancies. An exception occurs in the case of severely affected erythroblastotic infants. Because of placental hypertrophy, hCG values may be quite high; however, by the time these values are reached, the fetus is usually beyond saving.

Human Placental Lactogen

Also known as human chorionic somatomammotropin, human placental lactogen (hPL) is synthesized by the syncytiotrophoblast of the placenta in progressively increasing quantities throughout pregnancy. Human placental lactogen shows an incomplete immunologic cross-reaction with human pituitary growth hormone. The value of this assay in monitoring fetal well-being has been a rather controversial subject, and one can probably conclude that hPL is a valuable adjunct but should not be regarded as the sole end point for testing fetal jeopardy. It is generally concluded that those clinical situations in which fetal compromise is the direct result of impaired placental function will be heralded by falling hPL values approaching a danger zone (below 4 mg/ml after 30 weeks of gestation). Thus, hPL assay is most useful with hypertension disorders of pregnancy, placental insufficiency with fetal growth retardation, and especially postdate pregnancies. Because placental function is not impaired in such conditions as Class A and B diabetes without hypertension, congenital malformation, and hemolytic disease, the study has no predictive value for such women.

Maternal Blood Enzyme Measurement

A number of enzymes increase in concentration in maternal serum during pregnancy, including heat-stable alkaline phosphatase (HSAP), diamine oxidase (DAO), and oxytocinase.

Heat-Stable Alkaline Phosphatase. An isoenzyme of alkaline phosphatase, HSAP originates in the placenta and rises in concentration progressively throughout pregnancy. A sudden rapid rise in late pregnancy seems to indicate placental damage and potential fetal death. In some studies this has been shown to take place prior to a drop in estriol. As with hPL, most feel this easy-to-do study is a good adjunct but not an end in itself.

Plasma Diamine Oxidase. DAO is probably produced by retroplacental decidua, perhaps to protect the pregnant woman against histamine produced by the fetus. It rises at a rapid linear rate in early pregnancy, but, unfortunately, it tends to plateau in the third trimester, making it less useful for fetal evaluation.

Oxytocinase. Cystine aminopeptidase enzyme (oxytocinase) inactivates oxytocin during pregnancy and is synthesized by the placenta. As with hPL and HSAP, it seems to be a rather pure indicator of placental function, does not reflect distress, which is primarily fetal, and is therefore useful as an adjunct but not for primary evaluation of well-being.

Amniotic Fluid Studies

Most amniotic fluid studies are directed toward the determination of fetal maturity or genetic diagnosis, which is discussed in Chapter 17. A major exception is the measurement of bilirubin in amniotic fluid as a means of judging the severity of hemolytic disease.

When chorioamnionitis is suspected, but the diagnosis is not clear, examination of amniotic fluid for the presence of polymorphonuclear leukocytes and Gram-stained bacteria may be helpful. Although there are some conflicting reports concerning the importance of the white blood cells, the presence of bacteria is clearly significant.

The presence of meconium in amniotic fluid is an indication that there may have been an episode of fetal stress at some time prior to the observation, but not necessarily as an ongoing situation. Indeed, the presence of meconium does not indicate a fetus in distress unless there are other indicators, such as a significant alteration in the fetal heart rate (FHR). The mechanism of passage of meconium is presumably hyperperistalsis secondary to the hypoxic insult. In most cases, the observation of meconium-stained fluid is made intrapartally after rupture of the membranes, although transabdominal amniocentesis or transvaginal amnioscopy may also be used. The latter procedure is limited to late pregnancy when the cervix is open enough to admit the lighted speculum. An advantage is that the procedure can be done repeatedly to monitor well-being in certain cases, such as the postdate pregnancy. Disadvantages of the technique are that fluid samples cannot be obtained for analysis and that occasionally the membranes may be inadvertently ruptured.

Physiological Studies

Because it is not feasible to measure directly the critical respiratory and nutritional function of the placenta, a number of indirect approaches have been developed. Fetal movements and especially a change in the pattern of fetal movement are felt to be indicators of well-being. Some have suggested that mothers be instructed to count the number of fetal movements in a given time period each day and record the information. Even without this formal quantifying of fetal movement, when a mother reports a reduction in fetal movements, it must be evaluated further, especially if there is an underlying reason to suspect fetal jeopardy.

With the advent of real-time ultrasound, which enables one to observe fetal activity, it is possible to observe cardiac activity and respiratory movements. The latter, it has been suggested, is a good index of fetal well-being.

Antepartum Fetal Heart Rate Monitoring

Periodic electronic fetal monitoring during the third trimester has become a common method for evaluating the fetus in a high-risk pregnancy. As with many other forms of fetal assessment, a normal result is highly accurate in indicating fetal well-being. On the other hand, false-positive results occur with a relatively high frequency. This has required that two or more different tests of fetal well-being be carried out before premature delivery or other remedial measures are instituted.

The observation of changes in FHR associated with spontaneous or evoked fetal movement has become known as the *nonstress test* (NST). Evaluation of FHR in the presence of spontaneous or oxytocin-induced contractions is termed the *contraction stress test* (CST) or *oxytocin challenge test* (OCT). The CST was widely applied clinically prior to the more recent development of the NST. The ease of performing the NST and its apparent reliability as a screening tool have greatly reduced the number of CSTs performed. An example of a clinical protocol for applying these tests is given in the nursing guidelines for these tests.

Contraction Stress Testing

The CST requires administration of oxytocin by intravenous infusion. Continuous external fetal monitoring is applied, and oxytocin is administered in increasing dosages until uterine contractions (UCs) occur. The occurrence of repeated late decelerations with contractions is classified as a positive or abnormal test. The lack of late decelerations with each of three contractions during a 10-minute interval is classified as a negative result or a passed test.

Other terms used for classification of tests include *unsatisfactory, suspicious,* and *equivocal.* Unsatisfactory tests occur when interpretable tracings cannot be obtained, or the criterion of three contractions in a 10-minute interval is not met. Unsatisfactory tests are repeated within a short time interval (usually 24 hours). It has been suggested that the interpretation of the test should be based on a 10-minute testing segment known as a "testing window." The classification of *equivocal* and elimination of the term *suspicious tests* (occasional decelerations) have been proposed in conjunction with the concept of a 10-minute testing window. Equivocal tests are those in which nonrepetitive late decelerations are observed (*i.e.,* no positive or negative testing win-

---

Nursing Guidelines for Performing The Contraction Stress Test

A. Procedure for the CST:

1. Take client to a labor room or antepartal testing unit.
2. Explain to client the testing procedure and the time involved. (The test itself requires an average of about 90 minutes, but it is not uncommon for the procedure to take 3 hours.)
3. Have client change into a gown.
4. Place client in a semi-Fowler's position at a 30° to 45° angle with a slight left tilt.
5. Place client on an external monitor. A phonotransducer or ultrasound transducer is used to record the FHR and a tocodynamometer to measure UC.
6. Record client's blood pressure initially and at 5- to 10-minute intervals.
7. Obtain at least a 10-minute baseline recording of FHR and observe for spontaneous UC.

    If spontaneous UCs without late decelerations are noted at a frequency of less than three (3) in 10 minutes or no spontaneous uterine activity is observed, proceed with oxytocin infusion.
8. Prepare and begin an oxytocin infusion according to the institutional protocol or as indicated by the physician.

   a. Start the oxytocin infusion (secondary line) by inserting the needle into the connector of the primary line at the connector most proximal to the primary line. Be sure to keep primary line running at a slow rate.
   b. Client is evaluated by the physician when the dosage of oxytocin reaches 10 mU/min. If the oxytocin infusion is to be continued, the physician must write an order to increase the dosage.

B. Interpretation of the CST

1. Test is read as:
   a. Negative—no late deceleration of the FHR when an adequate frequency of three contractions in 10 minutes has been established, a "negative window"
   b. Positive—late decelerations occurring with three contractions in 10 minutes, a "positive window"
   c. Equivocal—no positive or negative window
   d. Hyperstimulation—excessive uterine activity is present in association with a deceleration of the FHR
   e. Unsatisfactory—inadequate UC or FHR record

(*Courtesy of Patricia M. Graef, BSNEd.)

---

dow) or in which decelerations are associated with maternal hypotension or uterine hyperstimulation. Since external methods of pressure monitoring are used, uterine hyperstimulation cannot be defined on the basis of true intrauterine pressure (mmHg) but rather is defined on the basis of the frequency of contractions (more than three contractions in 10 minutes) or a tetanic contraction. It is suggested that equivocal tests be repeated in 24 hours. In some areas of the country, the CST is interpreted without the use of the testing window. If the test shows any late decelerations, it is considered equivocal and is repeated within 24 hours.

Early investigators found that positive CSTs were associated with a relatively high frequency of poor outcome, such as intrauterine fetal death, fetal distress, or poor condition of the infant at birth. A normal CST gave a high degree of confidence for continued fetal survival *in utero* during an arbitrarily set limit of 1 week. Further experience has confirmed this observation. Instances of fetal death within 1 week of a negative CST are very infrequent. When this has occurred, the fetal deaths have often been attributed to factors other than the primary indication for testing (*e.g.,* abruptio placentae or fetal malformation). Some have suggested performing CSTs more frequently when there is deterio-

ration of the maternal condition (*e.g.,* increasing severity of pregnancy-induced hypertension) or in certain very high-risk disorders (*e.g.,* diabetes with vascular disease).

Clinical studies in which clients were induced to labor and electronically monitored following a positive CST have demonstrated a high false-positive rate (25%–40%), that is, late decelerations did not recur in labor. Because of this experience, it has been suggested that more than one test of fetal well-being should be carried out before a *preterm* delivery for fetal compromise is indicated. Clearly the greatest benefit of the CST lies in the reassurance that allows continuation of a high-risk pregnancy when the test result is normal.

Nipple Stimulation Test. Another noninvasive technique has been developed in antepartal testing for the achievement of a CST. It is called the nipple stimulation test. This technique is based on the principle that nipple stimulation causes oxytocin to be released from the neurohypophysis, and, if successful, the need for intravenous infusion of Pitocin is eliminated. With this method, the nurse applies warm, moist towels over the woman's breasts and instructs her to twist her nipples gently. This technique is similar to the nipple-rolling breast preparation that is recommended antepartally.

If, after a reasonable time, sufficient contractions do not result, the nurse proceeds with the CST procedure.

Nonstress Testing

Observation of accelerated FHR associated with fetal movements led to the development of the NST. This form of testing does not require intravenous administration of drugs and thus can be safely and more quickly performed in an outpatient area. These features, coupled with the apparent reliability of the NST as a screening test, have resulted in a marked reduction in the number of CSTs performed.

Various criteria have been applied for interpreting the NST. The occurrence of five accelerations of greater than 15 beats per minute for more than 15 seconds in 20 minutes was initially required as a normal or reactive test. More recent studies have suggested that fewer accelerations of the same magnitude may be adequate. Because the fetus has cyclic periods of rest, external stimulation by manipulation has been used to elicit movement for the testing. Failure to demonstrate a reactive pattern owing either to lack of accelerations with movement or to lack of fetal movement is taken as an indication for further evaluation of the fetus by a CST (Fig. 42-4).

Nursing Care. The NST and CST have been almost exclusively performed by nurses. Along with this function, nurses have assumed the role of educating the clients about the tests and screening the test results. A notable secondary benefit of these functions has been the opportunity for nurses working in both the antepartal and labor and delivery areas to establish a nurse-client relationship with high-risk clients during the antepartal period. The benefits of this relationship in the delivery of nursing care during labor, delivery, and the puerperium should be obvious.

Specific Fetal Problems

Acute fetal distress is covered in Chapter 43 in relation to intrapartum fetal monitoring, although many of the chronic fetal problems that are discussed here can produce acute distress as well. In addition, some of these problems, such as preeclampsia, have significant maternal implications that are covered elsewhere.

Hemolytic Disease—Rh Factor

Hemolytic disease is one of the complications of pregnancy in which there may be devastating fetal effects with virtually no maternal risk. Although the fetal pathology of severe hemolytic disease had been described before the turn of the century, the exact nature of the problem was not known until after the discovery of the Rh factor in 1940. The disease is most unusual in that within 30 years the cause, treatment, and methods for prevention have been worked out. Most of the attention has been focused on the Rh factor as a cause, but the ABO blood groups may also cause a form of hemolytic disease, as do other lesser blood groups.

The incidence of hemolytic disease is related to the occurrence of blood groups. In the white population, 15% are Rh negative. In blacks, Orientals, and American

---

Nursing Guidelines for Performing The Nonstress Test

A. Procedure for the NST

1. Take client to the antepartal testing unit.
2. Explain the procedure to the client, including the time involved. The test requires an average of 30 minutes.
3. Have client change into a gown.
4. Place client in a semi-Fowler's position at a 30° to 45° angle with a slight left tilt.
5. Place client on an external monitor using ultrasound transducer or phonotransducer to record the FHR. A tocodynamometer is used to document fetal activity and spontaneous uterine activity.
6. Record client's blood pressure initially and at 5- to 10-minute intervals.

7. The client is asked to indicate each time fetal movement occurs by pressing the record button on the monitor. A 10- to 20-minute strip is obtained.

B. Interpretation of the NST

1. Test is read as:
   a. Reactive—2 FHR accelerations greater than 15 bpm above the baseline and lasting 15 seconds or more with fetal movement in 10-minute period
   b. Nonreactive—no or one FHR acceleration greater than 15 bpm and lasting 15 seconds or more with fetal movement in a 10-minute period or accelerations less than 15 bpm or lasting less than 15 seconds

(*Courtesy of Patricia M. Graef, BSNEd.)

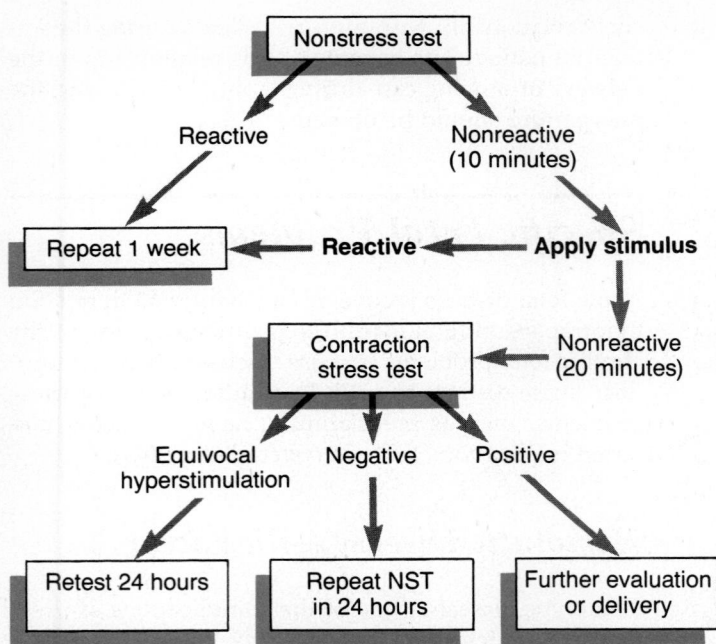

FIGURE 42-4

An example of a protocol for antepartal fetal heart rate testing (NST and CST).

Indians this figure is only 5%. The frequency of Rh hemolytic disease is therefore much less in these groups. Approximately 13% of American marriages have the setup of Rh problems (Rh-negative wife, Rh-positive husband), and 22% have the combinations for ABO disease. Ninety-eight percent of all hemolytic disease is related to either Rh or ABO incompatibilties. Fetal involvement with hemolytic disease formerly occurred with a frequency of approximately 1 in 100 deliveries; however, this incidence has been markedly reduced by the introduction of prevention by Rh immunoglobulin.

Anti-D Globulin

The ability to prevent Rh sensitization has been an established fact since Rh (anti-D) globulin became commercially available in 1969. This substance, which was initially obtained from the plasma of sensitized women, is now obtained by deliberately sensitizing Rh-negative male volunteers. It prevents sensitization by clearing the fetal cells from the material circulating and perhaps also by depressing the client's immune response. A single dose (300 mcg) is capable of clearing up to 15 ml of fetal erythrocytes. Lower doses (50 mcg) have been made available for use in situations in which only small fetomaternal transfusions are likely, such as first-trimester abortion and ectopic pregnancy.

Candidates for Rh immunoglobulin are unsensitized Rh-negative clients who (1) have delivered Rh-positive babies, (2) have had untypeable pregnancies such as stillborns, ectopic pregnancies, or spontaneous or induced abortions, (3) have received ABO-compatible Rh-positive blood, or (4) have had amniocentesis. It is

of no value in the client who is already sensitized, and although the recommendation is that it should be administered within 3 days of delivery this should not preclude administration at a later time if for some reason the 72-hour deadline has been missed.

Although most failures to prevent sensitization are due to failure to administer Rh immunoglobulin or inadequacy of the dose to cover the size of the fetomaternal bleed, there is a small risk (1%–2%) of sensitization even when proper technique is followed. The inadequate dose problem can be dealt with by doing appropriate follow-up studies 48 hours after the anti-D globulin. This involves doing either a Kleihauer Betke smear to demonstrate that fetal cells are no longer present or, even more simply, an indirect Coombs' test to show that there is excess antibody present. If the indirect Coombs' test is negative at 48 hours, an additional dose of immunoglobulin should be given. The remainder of the failures are probably related to fetomaternal bleeding episodes that occurred long enough prior to delivery that the postpartum administration of anti-D globulin will not protect. Several projects are underway to reduce this problem by evaluating the administration of immunoglobulin antepartally in the third trimester either routinely or when there are predisposing occurrences such as third-trimester bleeding.

With all of these developments, Rh hemolytic disease is becoming increasingly uncommon, but there does seem to be an irreducible group of clients who are sensitized for the reasons mentioned above. Because the problem is becoming more rare, it is important that the care of the severely sensitized client be delegated to a perinatal center.

Pathophysiology

The pathogenesis of Rh hemolytic disease is based on the fact that even though the maternal and fetal circulations are normally completely separated, breaks in this barrier permit the entry of fetal red blood cells into the maternal circulation during the second and third trimesters and at delivery in up to 50% of pregnancies. Such breaks also occur with abortions beyond 6 to 8 weeks of pregnancy. If these cells are Rh positive (*e.g.*, containing the Rh+ or D antigen), the mother may react to this mismatched "minitransfusion" by forming protective antibodies. Since the formation of antibodies takes time, and since the unsensitized woman probably does not react until after she delivers, there is rarely a problem in the first pregnancy unless the woman has received a mismatched transfusion in the past. Antibodies formed as the result of the first exposure persist for life. When the woman becomes pregnant again, and the fetus is Rh positive, she will respond with rapid antibody formation as soon as she is exposed to Rh-positive cells. Thus, once antibodies have been formed, all subsequent pregnancies with Rh-positive infants will be a problem.

There are two types of Rh antibodies. The larger type (gamma M, or 19S) does not cross the placenta as readily as the smaller (gamma G, or 7S). In the case of ABO disease in which the mother who lacks the antigen has the antibody (*e.g.*, type O has neither A nor B antigen, but has both anti-A and anti-B antibodies, type A has A antigen and anti-B antibody, and so on), these naturally occurring antibodies are the large 19S variety. Also, because these antibodies require a break in the placental barrier to get into the fetal circulation, and because this is most likely to occur at the time of delivery of the placenta, ABO disease is almost always milder than Rh disease, and rarely is the child stillborn or severely affected at birth. In addition, because the AB antigens are present in all body cells, this tends to absorb excess antibody and reduce the effect on the red cells.

However, in Rh disease, there are both 19S and 7S antibodies (the result of sensitization). The 7S antibodies cross readily into the fetal circulation by a facilitated transport mechanism and are responsible for the destruction of the fetal red blood cells. This produces anemia, and if it is severe enough, heart failure results in an edematous hydropic infant and possibly a stillbirth.

While the fetus is *in utero*, the mother is able to remove the breakdown products of the red cells (bilirubin) and handle them in her own liver; thus, the baby is not born jaundiced.

Genetic Determination

The inheritance of Rh blood type follows the simple dominant–recessive rules, with Rh+ being a dominant. Each person receives two genes (one from each parent) to determine Rh blood type. It is necessary to receive two Rh-negative genes to be negative, whereas one can be Rh positive with one Rh-positive and one Rh-negative gene (heterozygous) or two Rh-positive genes (homozygous). Thus, if the husband is heterozygous, there is a fifty–fifty chance of having an Rh-negative, unaffected child (Fig. 42-5). If the father is homozygous, all offspring will be Rh positive and subject to hemolytic disease.

In the ABO system, a person may have genes for A, B, AB, or no antigens. Thus, the contribution to the offspring may be A or B or none. For example, type O individuals receive neither A nor B from the parents; a type A individual may receive an A gene from each (AA) or an A from one and none from the other (AO). The same is true for the type B individual (BB or BO). The AB individual receives an A from one parent and a B from the other.

All pregnant women should have a blood group determination, at least with the first pregnancy. If adequate records are available, this need not be repeated with subsequent pregnancies. If the woman is Rh negative or type O (the most common maternal type for ABO disease), the husband's blood should also be typed.

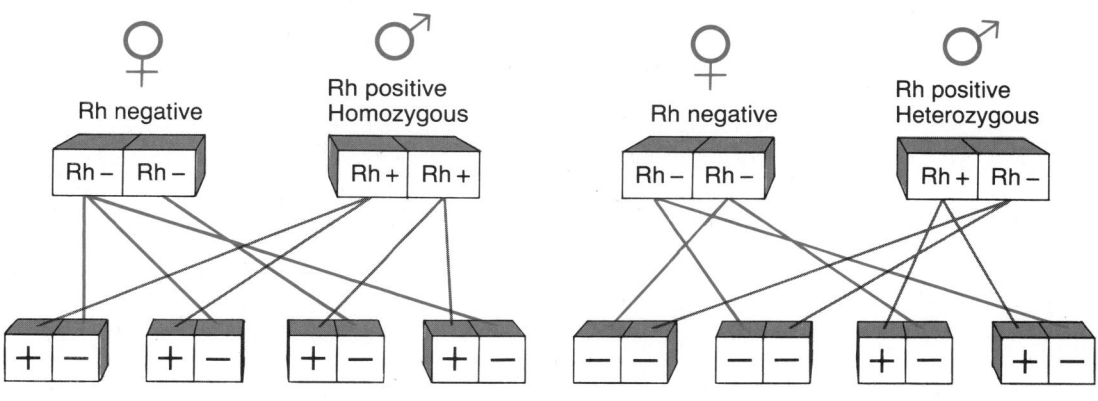

FIGURE 42-5

Inheritance patterns for the Rh factor.

If he is Rh positive, a genotype may be done to determine whether he is homozygous or heterozygous. Also, the Rh-negative woman's blood should be examined for the presence of antibodies to the Rh factor (D). This is accomplished by the indirect Coombs' test and is reported in dilutions (*e.g.*, positive 1:2, 1:4, 1:8, and so on). If the initial screening or titer is negative (*i.e.*, shows no antibodies), this should be repeated at approximately 30 and 36 weeks of pregnancy. If both of those titers are negative, it is safe to assume that there will be no significant problem and to permit the pregnancy to run its normal course. If the titer is positive, it becomes necessary to decide how seriously the fetus is affected (*i.e.*, how anemic it is). Because it is not possible to approach the fetus directly and do a hemoglobin or hematocrit, less direct means must be used. In the past, the physician merely repeated the antibody titer, watching for a rise, and combining with this the woman's past history arrived at a plan of management.

Bilirubin Levels in Fetal Diagnosis

It has now been well established that the severity of the hemolytic anemia in the fetus can best be determined by the quantity of *bilirubin* in the amniotic fluid (*i.e.*, the higher the bilirubin level, the lower the fetal hemoglobin). Thus, amniocentesis with analysis of the bilirubin in the fluid is the best basis for making therapeutic decisions in the sensitized woman. Because the quantity of bilirubin is small in the mildly sensitized or unsensitized woman, standard techniques for measuring bilirubin cannot be used, and therefore a spectrophotometric approach is used. Bilirubin produces an optical density peak at 450, and it is the height of this peak (or the ΔOD_{450}) that is used to evaluate fetal involvement (Fig. 42-6). Amniocentesis is used to evaluate the fetus in all women with significant sensitization. In most laboratories, a significant antibody titer below which fetal morbidity is unlikely can be determined. Although this varies from institution to institution, titers above 1:8 to 1:16 are generally considered significant. Amniocentesis is usually instituted at 24 to 25 weeks, since intrauterine transfusion is impractical before that, although in instances with previous early stillbirths the procedure may be instituted as early as 20 weeks. The frequency of repeated amniocentesis is determined by the level of the ΔOD_{450}, weekly taps being indicated if values are high.

The common method for evaluating the ΔOD_{450} is the Liley chart illustrated in Figure 42-6. Values in the

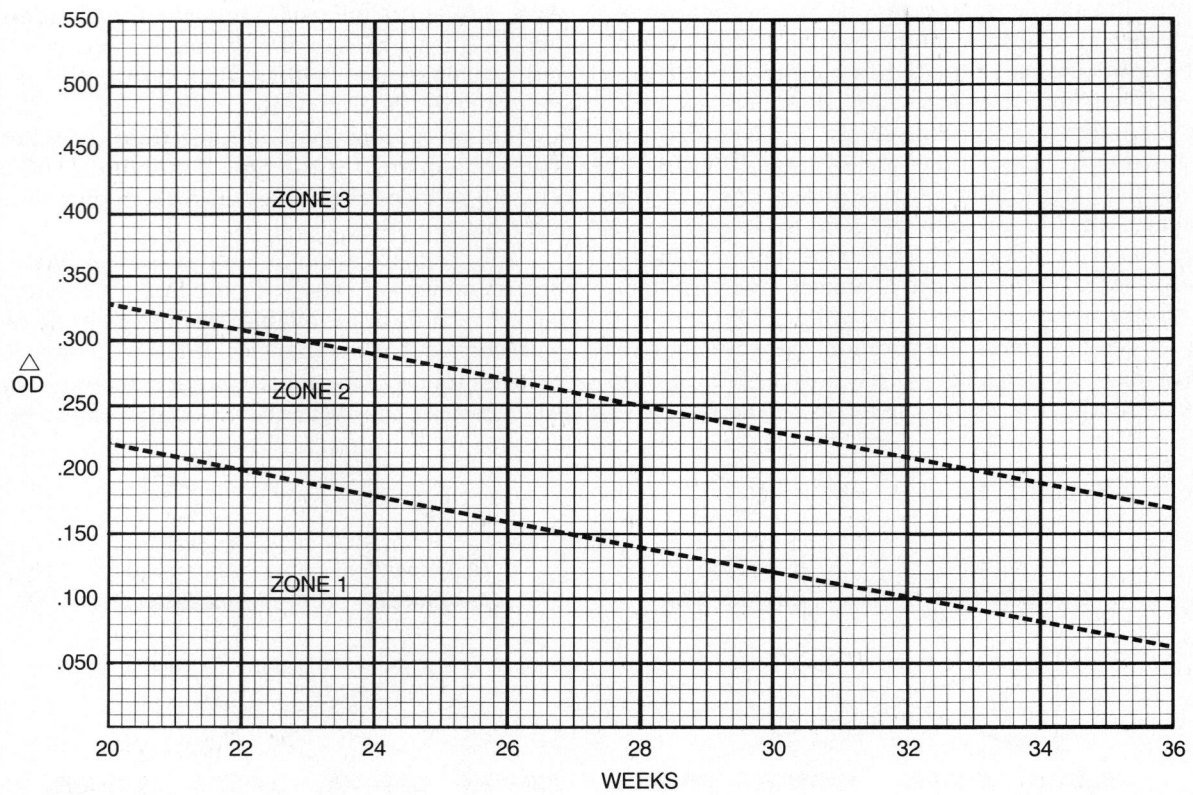

FIGURE   4 2 - 6

Modified Liley graph for relating ΔOD_{450} to weeks of gestation in determining severity of hemolytic disease. (Management of Erythroblastosis [Technical Bulletin, No. 17]. ACOG, Chicago, July 1972)

lower zone for the particular gestation indicate a mildly affected or even unaffected fetus, whereas those in the middle zone indicate an affected fetus, but one not in immediate danger of death. Values in the upper zone suggest the fetus will not survive 10 to 14 days without intervention. Management decisions are not based on single values but rather on the trend. If the ΔOD_{450} remains in the lower zone, no interference is indicated and the pregnancy can be allowed to proceed to term. If the values remain in the middle zone, the fetus is best delivered as soon as there is evidence of maturity, especially of the lung, by using the L/S ratio. Upper zone values indicate immediate intervention by delivery if beyond 33 to 34 weeks or by intrauterine transfusion if before that gestational age.

This dramatic procedure was first described in 1963 by Liley and involves the instillation of Rh-negative red blood cells into the peritoneal cavity of the fetus under ultrasound control. The fetus is able to absorb these intact cells. If the procedure is repeated successfully every 10 to 14 days until the point of maturity (approximately 34–35 wk), a stillbirth may be avoided.

The overall survival rate is in the 50% range, although in some centers a 75% survival rate of hydropic fetuses has been attained. This increased success is largely the result of improved fetal evaluation using real-time sonography. Often the fetus is very sick when the procedure is initiated, and these results are dramatic when compared with no survivors, which was often the case without the procedure.

Fetus of the Diabetic Mother

The problem of diabetes and pregnancy is discussed in Chapter 37, and the management of the newborn is discussed in Chapter 45. Here we discuss impact of the disease on the fetus.

Perinatal Mortality.
The specific impact of diabetes mellitus on the fetus is best indicated by the increase in perinatal mortality. Despite marked improvements in neonatal care and in the management of pregnancies complicated by diabetes mellitus, the overall perinatal mortality remains greater than that observed in the normal population. The rate is a direct function of the degree of maternal glycemic control achieved during gestation. The severity (White classification) of the diabetes also has been correlated with perinatal outcome. Stillbirths are rarely seen with Class A clients. Class F/R diabetics, however, may have not more than a fifty–fifty chance of having a surviving infant, depending on the severity of renal and ophthalmologic involvement. It has long been known that there is a small but significant risk of stillbirth in diabetic pregnancy. This may result from the effect of diabetes on the blood vessels of the uterus and placenta, producing premature aging. Hyperglycemia and subsequent fetal acidosis have also been proposed as mechanisms for fetal death. To avoid these stillbirths, routine early delivery has been a popular plan of management. This has unfortunately resulted in an increase in neonatal deaths because of the propensity of diabetic offspring to respiratory distress syndrome. Current improved survival is related to selective early delivery and antepartal testing for fetal pulmonary maturity.

Respiratory Distress Syndrome.
Controversy exists as to whether there is increased susceptibility of the diabetic offspring to the respiratory distress syndrome. Hyperinsulinism, however, has been associated with a delay in the onset of surfactant production by the type II cells of the fetal lung. This seems to occur more commonly in Class A, B, and C diabetics, whereas in class D and F diabetics, in whom vascular disease predominates, pulmonary maturity may be accelerated.

Metabolic Problems.
In addition to pulmonary problems, there are several metabolic problems that are more commonly observed in the fetus of the diabetic mother. Glucose crosses the placenta readily by carrier-mediated facilitated diffusion. Fetal glucose levels reflect the level in the mother. Insulin, on the other hand, does not cross, and consequently the fetus may respond to hyperglycemia by hypertrophy of pancreatic islet cells and the overproduction of insulin. The combination of high levels of insulin and glucose and other growth factors is at least partially responsible for the increased size of fetuses in diabetic pregnancies. Fetal overgrowth is a result of increased subcutaneous fat deposition and is more commonly observed with inadequate control of maternal blood glucose levels. Macrosomia increases the likelihood of mechanical problems at delivery, including shoulder dystocia and traumatic injury. Excessive fetal size also contributes to the high rate of cesarean delivery among diabetics.

Birth Defects.
Congenital malformations are increased three times in infants born to diabetic women, and lethal defects are six times as likely. Although defects of every organ system are observed, skeletal defects involving the caudal portion of the skeleton (caudal regression) and ventricular septal defects are the most characteristic. There is now overwhelming evidence that poor control around the time of fetal organogenesis is responsible for these malformations. It follows that preconception counseling and careful assessment of maternal glycemic control may enable the woman to plan the optimal time for attempting a pregnancy.

Prolonged Pregnancy

The average duration of pregnancy is roughly 280 days from the first day of the last menstrual period, or 267 days from the time of conception if the menstrual cycle is of average length. Only 5% of women deliver on the actual due date, although most deliver within 10 to 14 days in either direction from the date. Since the placenta has a normal life span equal to the duration of pregnancy, one may be justifiably concerned that if the due date is exceeded by more than 2 weeks, the aging placenta may no longer be able to support the fetus adequately. Fortunately, in most instances the placenta is capable of such support. In fact, in a great number of women who are postdates, the date has been miscalculated or based on faulty memory. In addition to those postmature pregnancies in which there is placental insufficiency, there is another group of late pregnancies in which the placenta functions well and the fetus becomes oversized, creating potential mechanical problems in labor and delivery.

If the circumstances including the status of the cervix, the size and position of the baby, and the size of the maternal pelvis are all favorable, induction of labor should be carried out when a pregnancy exceeds the due date by 10 to 14 days. If there is any question about the dates, efforts should be made to verify the gestational age by techniques already discussed. It is important to recognize, however, that a single determination in late pregnancy has a rather significant inherent error. This is especially true of ultrasound measurements of the biparietal diameter, since linear growth stops after 30 weeks. When a pregnancy is 10 to 14 days postdate and conditions are not favorable for induction of labor, the well-being of the fetus must be established to permit the continuation of the pregnancy. Urinary or serum estriols may be used. Because the adequacy of placental function is not necessarily static under such circumstances, these studies can provide only limited assurance and must be repeated two or three times weekly. They are rarely used today.

The OCT and NST are especially valuable in evaluating the postdate pregnancy. Because of the possibility of a rapid progressive decline in placental function, the OCT cannot provide the usually accepted promise of 7 days of well-being for the fetus.

In addition to establishing maturity in the case of uncertain gestational age, the examination of amniotic fluid for meconium may be helpful in such cases. Clear fluid is reassuring, although it does not rule out fetal jeopardy. Meconium staining and scant fluid suggest an affected fetus, and, although not sufficient alone to indicate aggressive action, they are confirmatory in the presence of other signs of fetal compromise. Aspiration and severe pulmonary consequences for the newborn are possible when meconium is present. However, prevention is a dilemma. Even prompt cesarean delivery does not necessarily obviate aspiration, since respiratory movements can occur *in utero*.

On the surface, it would seem simple to determine the due date and the probability that the pregnancy has gone beyond that point, but there are a number of pitfalls. Many women do not record or cannot recall when they had their last period. Others have long cycles, with ovulation and conception occuring later than the 14th day. This is especially true in women discontinuing oral contraceptive therapy, in whom the first ovulation may not occur until 4 to 6 weeks after the last withdrawal flow. One must assess these factors carefully before overtreating a mother for supposed postmaturity.

Preeclampsia-Eclampsia

Although the manifestations of preeclampsia (hypertension, edema, and proteinuria) and eclampsia (convulsions in addition) are primarily maternal (see Chap. 36), the fetal impact cannot be ignored. Progressive placental insufficiency is an inherent part of the syndrome, and intrauterine fetal growth is frequently retarded prior to the development of maternal manifestations. With the appearance of clinically evident preeclampsia, placental function continues to decline and fetal death may result if the pregnancy is allowed to continue. Occasionally, a woman with moderate or severe preeclampsia may appear to respond so favorably to therapy that there is the temptation to allow the pregnancy to continue, to permit further fetal maturity. Such a decision is fraught with risk of failure of the fetus to prosper and the possibility of a stillbirth. In most cases it is unwise. Should such a course be considered, amniocentesis for detection of pulmonary maturity (L/S ratio) should be done first because pulmonary maturity is often markedly accelerated in such circumstances. To attempt to prolong a pregnancy in the face of significant preeclampsia is not appropriate if the fetal lungs are already mature. If the L/S ratio is at immature levels, and a conservative course is to be followed, fetal well-being must be carefully assessed frequently. This is not a simple matter, since urinary estriol excretion may be reduced by impaired renal function, whereas serum levels may be falsely elevated. Interpretation of OCTs and NSTs is also difficult in the immature fetus.

The perinatal wastage in preeclampsia is largely a function of the stage of pregnancy at which the process develops and therefore the degree of maturity of the infant delivered. If preeclampsia does not develop until after the 36th week of gestation, the perinatal loss should be quite low. Perinatal mortality is high when convulsions (eclampsia) occur. Recent reviews indicate a mortality rate of approximately 20%.

Chronic Hypertension

Approximately 75% of women with benign essential hypertension go through pregnancy with no maternal or fetal problems. Unfortunately, some 15% develop preeclampsia. When this happens, the fetal prognosis is less favorable, especially if preeclampsia occurs at a time when the fetus is significantly premature. The perinatal mortality rate in this group is approximately 20%.

In the case of the hypertensive mother without superimposed preeclampsia, the fetal risk is not great, but it is greater than that for women with normal blood pressure. Because of this, it is recommended that fetal evaluation be initiated for all hypertensive women in the third trimester to identify the occasional benign hypertensive woman whose fetus is in jeopardy and for whom preterm delivery is indicated. There is, in addition, an increased frequency of abruptio placentae in these hypertensive women, with the added perinatal wastage characteristic of that problem.

TORCH Infections Affecting the Fetus

As diagnostic skills and technology improve, more infections are being discovered that are detrimental to fetal development and well-being. The effects these infections have on the fetus are related to the gestational age at which infection occurs. Early infections might precipitate spontaneous abortion. Others may cause deafness or cataracts. Infections during the birth process can cause neonatal sepsis. Some problem infections are indicated in Figure 42-7.

When only a few of these infections were classified, the term *TORCH* was applied to perinatal infections (*T*, toxoplasmosis; *O*, other; *R*, rubella; *C*, cytomegalovirus; *H*, herpes). The term is still meaningful, but the "*O*, other" is rapidly becoming the most frequent cause of perinatal infection.

Toxoplasmosis. Toxoplasmosis is caused by the protozoan organism *Toxoplasma gondii*, which is contracted from oocytes in cat feces or by eating uncooked meat. Only cats that are unconfined and eat infected rodents are a hazard. When primary infection, which is generally asymptomatic, occurs just before or during early pregnancy, congenital infection may result. This can lead to the birth of a child who is mentally and physically retarded, and who suffers from chorioretinitis and microcephaly. Approximately 10% to 15% of these babies die, and most of the survivors are severely compromised. If the disease is recognized clinically or by seroconversion in early pregnancy, abortion is recommended. If abortion is not accepted or the infection occurs later in pregnancy, treatment with triple sulfa may reduce the fetal impact.

Other. Other infections make up a growing category that includes syphilis, varicella, acquired immunodeficiency syndrome (AIDS), hepatitis, and group B β-hemolytic streptococcus (GBBS).

GBBS is found in the vagina of 20% of asymptomatic normal women. It can, however, cause a severe

Transplacental
Toxoplasmosis
Rubella
Cytomegalovirus
Herpes simplex
Group B coxsackievirus
Varicella
Malaria
L. Monocytogenes
Group B β-hemolytic
   streptococcus
Gonococcus (?)
Tuberculosis (rare)
AIDS (HTLV-III)

Ascending infection and infections acquired by direct contact with birth canal
E. coli and other
   gram-negative bacilli
L. monocytogenes
Vibrio
C. albicans
M. hominis
Varicella
Herpes simplex
Gonococcus
Group B β-hemolytic
   streptococcus

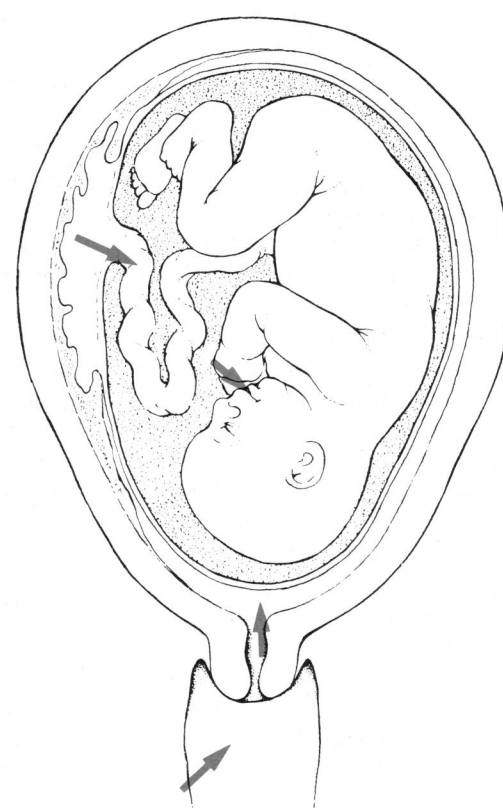

FIGURE 42-7

Arrows indicate probable routes of fetomaternal infection. (Adapted from Evans ME, Glass L: Perinatal Medicine. Hagerstown, Harper & Row, 1976)

sepsis and pneumonia in the newborn. Factors that place the fetus at particular risk of contracting GBBS are prematurity, premature rupture of the membranes, and prolonged labor. The infection is usually controlled in the birth process, but it has been seen in infants born by cesarean section to mothers with intact membranes.

Universal screening of pregnant women would be fruitless, since many women are chronic carriers of GBBS. Screening should focus on women at risk of delivering premature infants. Also, whenever premature rupture of the membranes occurs and conservative therapy is being contemplated, a culture for GBBS should be obtained.

AIDS has become a major public-health concern. This syndrome is caused by the HTLV-III virus. It is spread through sexual and blood-borne contact. AIDS causes the immune system to function abnormally, and patients develop fulminant infections. The incubation period is variable and may be longer than 5 years.

AIDS can be transmitted from mother to fetus. AIDS is seen frequently in intravenous drug abusers and hemophiliacs who have received multiple transfusions. These women should possibly be screened for AIDS. The national blood supply is now being tested for anti-HTLV-III, and clients should be reassured that our blood supply is safe from AIDS. Clients suspected of having AIDS should undergo blood and secretion precautions.

Rubella. Although most concerns are for infection in the first trimester, serious problems are known to occur when the infection develops as late as the fifth month of gestation, and later infections may be responsible for more subtle problems. Infections in the first trimester may result in abortion in more than 33% of cases. Congenital rubella (*i.e.,* the expanded rubella syndrome) may be difficult to differentiate clinically from the other TORCH infections, although cultures of the virus or specific IgM measurements are diagnostic. These babies and their placentas are highly infectious, and contact with nonimmune pregnant personnel should be avoided.

When the pregnant woman is exposed to rubella, she should have immediate serologic testing for rubella antibody. If this indicates immunity she is protected (85%–90% of adults in the United States are immune). If she is not immune she should be carefully followed for development of clinical rubella or development of antibodies. If either of these developments occurs, abortion should be recommended in view of the high rate of fetal involvement. Gamma globulin is not recommended in rubella exposure unless abortion is unacceptable, and then it is important for the client to realize that, although the disease may be modified, fetal effects are not necessarily obviated.

Special care must be taken to avoid immunizing the pregnant woman. Although the exact risk is not known, the vaccine virus is known to have access to the fetus.

Cytomegalovirus. Cytomegalovirus is the most common of the congenital infections. It occurs in about 1% of births, and approximately 10% of infected newborns exhibit permanent damage. The diagnosis can be established by viral culture or serology. There is no specific therapy unless the diagnosis can be established sufficiently early to provide an abortion option.

Herpes Simplex. There are two strains of this virus: type I, which is primarily responsible for oral lesions, and type II, which is primarily responsible for genital lesions. These distinctions are not absolute, but hold in the majority of cases. Type II herpes infection can be sexually transmitted and is discussed further in Chapters 37 and 46.

Two problems are evident in pregnancy. More commonly, neonatal infection can be contracted during delivery by exposure to the virus in genital lesions or in the asymptomatic carrier state. Congenital infection, which is extremely rare, can occur when a primary infection (absent antibodies, viremia) occurs in pregnancy. Like other TORCH infections, the impact is greatest when this occurs in early pregnancy, and the result is similar (*i.e.,* mental retardation, microcephaly, cerebral calcification, chorioretinitis).

Infections due to Premature Rupture of Membranes

Intrauterine infection as a result of premature rupture of the membranes is probably the most common infectious threat to the fetus. It is well recognized that the frequency of such infection parallels the length of time from the rupture of the membranes to the onset of labor. Infection of the fetus occurs by way of the amniotic fluid to the fetal tracheobronchial tree, as well as from the membranes and placenta through the cord vessels, producing fetal sepsis. The organisms most commonly involved are anaerobic streptococci and gram-negative bacilli.

Since it is difficult to achieve therapeutic levels of antibiotics in the amniotic fluid once the patient becomes febrile, the treatment is delivery by either induction or cesarean. More important, however, is the prevention of infection. This is accomplished by delivery (most often by induction, but by cesarean if necessary) of any woman with premature rupture of the membranes whose fetus is larger than 1500 g to 1800 g. This weight range is selected because in most clinics the survival data for babies of that size are such that the risk of delivery and prematurity appears to be less than the risk of intrauterine infection. Recent data have suggested, however, that with premature rupture of the membranes, the fetal lung may mature within 24 to 48 hours, and therefore a delay may be indicated. This

The Fetus and Family at Risk

Nursing Objectives

1. Give appropriate prenatal care to assess and maintain a state of well being.
2. Ensure that the baby is born as close to term as possible in a hospital that is equipped to care for the high-risk infant.
3. Provide appropriate care for the mother and support person(s).

Assessment	Potential Nursing Diagnosis	Planning/Intervention	Evaluation
Care of the Fetus			

Gestational age
  Nägele's rule
  Fundal height
  Ultrasound
	Potential for injury (asphyxia, meconium aspiration, hypoglycemia, polycythemia, specific health problems) related to early delivery or complications	Review prenatal record
		Obtain history from mother
		Calculate gestational age
		Perform fundal height measurement
		Prepare mother for ultrasound
			The fetus' age is determined and documented
			The fetus is delivered as close to term as possible
			The fetus survives birth with no or few complications

Nutrition Growth and development of the fetus	Potential alteration in nutritional status: less than body requirements related to disease process (*i.e.*, chronic hypertension, prolonged pregnancy	Do serial fundal heights with prenatal care Provide nutritional counseling for the mother Take maternal weight at each prenatal visit Ultrasound examination Fetal activity determination Results reported to physician Initiate antepartal testing if appropriate	Fetal well-being is determined and maintained Fetus is delivered at appropriate time if it is in jeopardy
Need for delivery of the high-risk infant Level of care the hospital provides		Monitor FHR and report findings to physician Facilitate transfer if needed Prepare for high-risk delivery Have appropriate neonatal resuscitation equipment available and in working condition Have qualified personnel present to care for the infant at the delivery	High-risk infant is born in a hospital that can provide appropriate care
Care of Mother and her Support System			
Communication Coping behaviors	Fear of injury to, or death of, infant related to high risk factors Ineffective individual coping (depression, guilt) related to perceived parental role failure	Allow communication by utilizing open-ended questions Allow time for the parents to ask questions and voice fears Assist and promote effective coping behavior Explain procedures Facilitate the parents' meeting with the neonatal staff prior to the birth	Client/family communicates freely with each other and staff Client/family voices fears Client/family indicate understanding of procedures by repeating and discussing information Client/family develop coping behaviors indicated by their words and actions
Learning capabilities Determine factors or situations causing learning deficit Assess readiness to learn	Knowledge deficit of etiological factors and care related to the high-risk condition	Develop a teaching plan Provide teaching that is client/family specific	Client/family achieves learning goals Client/family participate actively in health management plan

effect has yet to be clearly established in maturing the fetal lung.

Fetal Growth Retardation

Fetal growth retardation is one term applied to the clinical syndrome in which the fetus fails to prosper *in utero*. The terms *dysmaturity, placental insufficiency, small-for-date babies, uteroplacental insufficiency,* and *stunted fetus* have also been applied. The syndrome may occur with maternal diseases such as diabetes with severe vascular involvement, chronic renal disease, and chronic hypertension with renal involvement. Intrauterine infection with rubella, toxoplasmosis, and cytomegalovirus are causes. The most severe growth retardation is produced by multiple congenital malformations. In some cases the syndrome may be idiopathic and recurrent. In general, the earlier in gestation that retardation is apparent, the poorer the outlook.

At birth these babies appear to have lost subcutaneous fat, their skin is often wrinkled, and the fingernails and toenails are long. The amniotic fluid, cord, and nails are heavily stained with meconium. The stillbirth rate is high, and the frequency of respiratory problems in the newborn is increased. The most significant management problem from the obstetric viewpoint is differentiating (antepartally) the growth-retarded fetus from a premature fetus of appropriate size. After delivery, this differentiation is less difficult and can be based on weight (particularly weight gain patterns), certain developmental criteria such as ear cartilage development and plantar skin creases, and behavior patterns.

The question of erroneous menstrual dates often arises, and this necessitates the use of the method described in Determination of Fetal Age. Once the diagnosis is suspected, some search for an etiology is indicated. Heroic approaches to the fetus are certainly not indicated if a diagnosis of congenital rubella or cytomegalovirus infection has been established. However, this may not be simple to do if, on the other hand, the diagnosis is not ominous. The fetus must be evaluated and followed with an index of well-being (such as urinary estriol). Delivery must be timed appropriately. In the presence of uteroplacental insufficiency, fetal tolerance to labor may be reduced and the need for cesarean delivery increased.

Disproportionate Twin Development

Twins with disparity in size may be accounted for by the possibility of a connection between the placental circulations. This is especially true in single-ovum twins. When this happens in early pregnancy and one heart pumps more strongly than the other, there may be monopolization of a larger area of the placenta by one twin and thus a disparity in size. Such twins are not only greatly different in size at birth, but the smaller one is often anemic and may require transfusion. The larger twin may be hypervolemic and require a phlebotomy to prevent heart failure and jaundice. This type of placental anastomosis, when it occurs in double-ovum twins, accounts for those rare situations known as "chimerism," in which an individual may have two populations of cells, as evidenced by blood groups or sex chromatin. The other important clinical significance of disparity in twin sizes is that difficulties may be encountered in delivery if the smaller of the twins is delivered first through a cervix that is not completely dilated.

Fetal Treatment

The art of fetal treatment is at this time far less developed than that of fetal diagnosis. The most common approach to the fetus by the obstetrician is to select an appropriate time for delivery, convert the fetus to a newborn, and thus allow active treatment by the neonatologist. Perhaps the most important approach to the fetus is to provide appropriate support throughout the pregnancy. This includes adequate prenatal diet, as well as glucose and oxygen during labor, especially if there is fetal distress.

Treatment in the case of a positive prenatal diagnosis of congenital disease is generally limited to therapeutic abortion. However, in some instances of metabolic errors, maternal dietary modification may be effective in protecting the fetus with an enzyme defect.

Drug Therapy

Many drugs administered to the mother cross the placenta into the fetal circulation. Transplacental passage is generally a function of the molecular size of the drug. Substances with molecular weights less than 500 cross readily by simple diffusion. Although there should always be concern over the possible deleterious effects of drugs, one can sometimes achieve a desirable therapeutic effect in the fetus by treating the mother. One example of this is the administration of digitalis to the mother when the fetus is found to suffer from supraventricular tachycardia. This cardiac arrhythmia is suspected when there is an elevated fetal heart rate and is confirmed by fetal echocardiography. Administering digitalis through the mother to the fetus is the treatment of choice.

Another example of fetal drug therapy is the administration of glucocorticoids to the mother to induce the production of surfactant by the type II cells of the fetal lung and thereby reduce the risk of respiratory distress syndrome. The evidence is that if this is done between 26 to 28 and 32 to 34 weeks of gestation, and if delivery can be delayed for 24 to 48 hours, there will be a significant reduction in respiratory distress. The effect appears to be transient; the frequency of respiratory distress increases when delivery is delayed for more than 7 days following treatment. The effectiveness of this approach is still under investigation. Those who do not favor its use point out that the long-term effects on the child of exposure to glucocorticoids *in utero* are not known and that glucocorticoids may increase the risk of *in utero* infection. This treatment is still under review.

Transfusion

Intrauterine fetal transfusion in Rh disease is the most publicized form of treatment. It is hoped that the use of Rh immune globulin prophylaxis will ultimately eliminate the need for this procedure.

Surgery and Needle Aspiration

Refinements in sonography have resulted in earlier and more accurate diagnosis of fetal abnormalities. Efforts to treat these have received substantial press coverage, captured public attention, and engendered substantial public and professional debate. Successful intrauterine treatment of obstruction of the lower urinary tract that would otherwise result in extensive kidney damage has been reported. Particularly noteworthy is the intrauterine treatment of hydrocephalus. Efforts have been made to relieve the hydrocephalus by intermittent sonographically directed needle aspiration through the mother's abdomen or even by the surgical insertion of a shunt to provide continuous drainage into the amniotic sac. The risk/benefit ratio of these procedures is not established, and they must still be looked upon as experimental. Clearly, there are substantial ethical issues, as such treatment could allow the survival of a severely retarded child who might otherwise have died *in utero*.

Future Therapy

The future undoubtedly holds many advances—from the prenatal correction of congenital defects to the unscrambling of genetic mishaps. There may well be treatments of maladies that are presently unknown in this rapidly developing area of fetal medicine.

Suggested Reading

Bourgeois F, Thiagarajah S, Harbert G: The significance of fetal heart rate decelerations during nonstress testing. Am J Obstet Gynecol 150:213, 1984

Chamberlain P, Manning F, Morrison I et al: Ultrasound evaluation of amniotic fluid volume: I. The relationship of marginal and decreased amniotic fluid volumes to perinatal outcome. Am J Obstet Gynecol 150:245, 1984

Creasy R: Biophysical aspects of management of the growth retarded fetus. Semin Perinatol 8:56, 1984

Depp R: Postmaturity. In Queenan JT (ed): Management of the High Risk Pregnancy. Oradell, NJ, Medical Economics Book Division, 1980

Devoe L, McKenzie J, Searle N et al: Clinical sequelae of the extended nonstress test. Am J Obstet Gynecol 151:1074, 1985

Diagnostic ultrasound in pregnancy. US Department of Health and Human Services, Public Health Service, National Institutes of Health, NIH Publication No. 84-667, 1984

Druzin M, Gratacos J, Paul R et al: Antepartum fetal heart rate testing: XII. The effect of manual manipulation of the fetus on the nonstress test. Am J Obstet Gynecol 151:61, 1985

Freeman R, Anderson G, Dorchester W: A prospective multi-institutional study of antepartum fetal heart rate monitoring: I. Risk of perinatal mortality and morbidity according to antepartum fetal heart rate test results. Am J Obstet Gynecol 143:771, 1982

Freeman RK, Garite TJ: Fetal Heart Monitoring. Baltimore, Williams & Wilkins, 1981

Friede A, Rochat R: Maternal mortality and perinatal mortality: Definitions, data, and epidemiology. In Sachs B (ed): Obstetric Epidemiology. Littleton, MA, PSG Publishing, 1985

Harman CR, Manning FA, Bowman JR et al: Severe Rh disease: Poor outcome is not inevitable. Am J Obstet Gynecol 145:823, 1983

Huddleston J, Sudiff G, Robinson D: Contraction stress test by intermittent nipple stimulation. Obstet Gynecol 63:669, 1984

Keegan K, Paul R, Broussard P et al: Antepartum fetal heart rate testing: V. The nonstress test: An outpatient approach. Am J Obstet Gynecol 136:81, 1980

Khouzami V, Johnson J, Hernandez E et al: Urinary estrogens in postterm pregnancy. Am J Obstet Gynecol 141:205, 1981

Liston R, Cohen A, Mennuti M et al: Antepartum fetal evaluation by maternal perception of fetal movement. Obstet Gynecol 60:424, 1982

Manning F: Ultrasound in perinatal medicine, p 203. In Casey RK, Resnik R (eds): Maternal-Fetal Medicine. Philadelphia, WB Saunders, 1984

Scott JR (guest ed): Isoimmunization in pregnancy. Clin Obstet Gynecol 25:241–456, 1982

Seeds AE (guest ed): Diabetes in pregnancy. Clin Obstet Gynecol 24:1–324, 1981

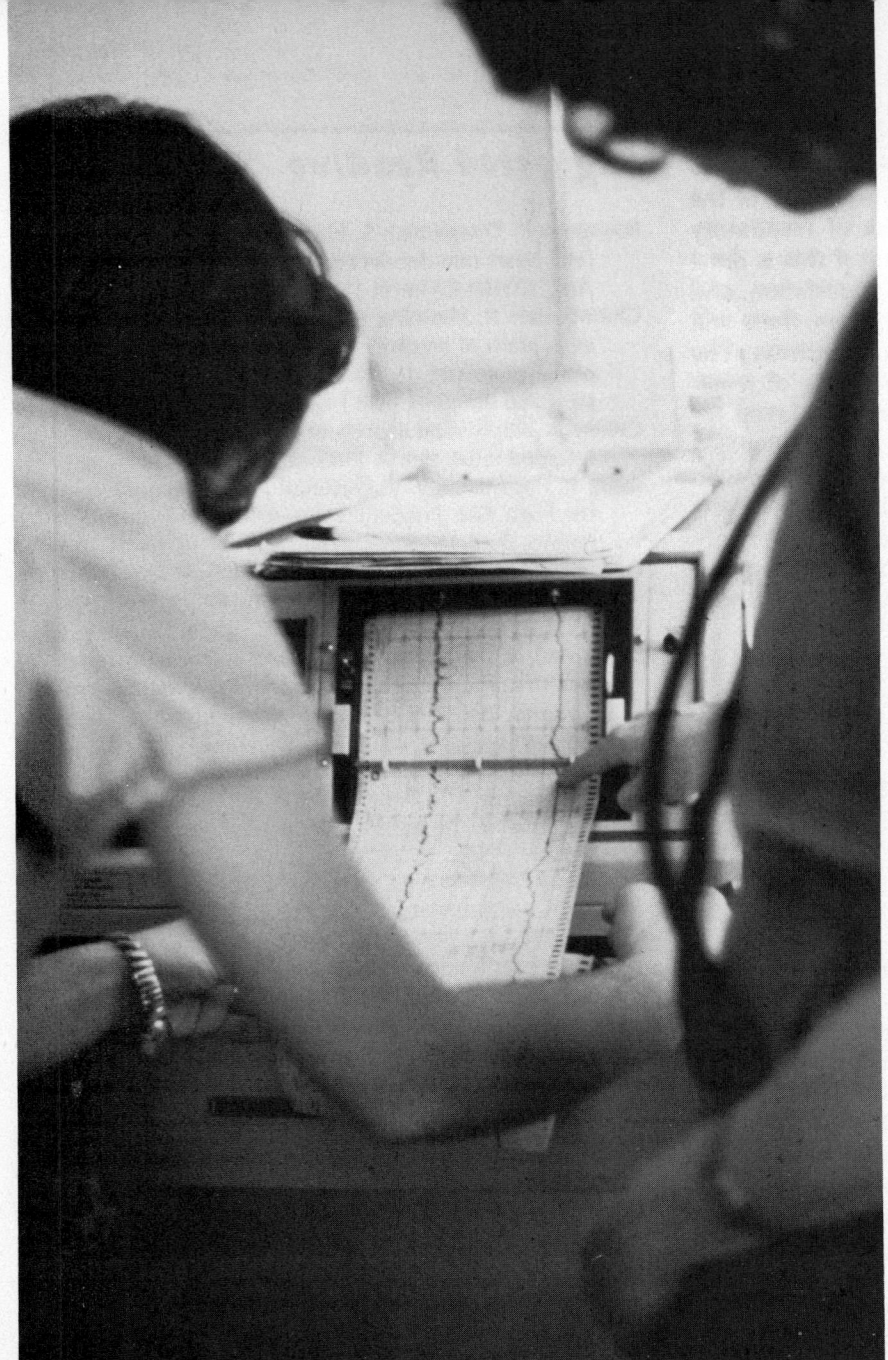

CHAPTER 43

Intrapartum Fetal Monitoring and Care

The fetus, as a "patient," has always been relatively inaccessible to the nurse and the physician. For many years, the forces of labor and the well-being of the fetus could be evaluated only by palpation of the maternal abdomen and by periodic sampling of the fetal heart rate (FHR) through auscultation. A greater understanding of fetal cardiorespiratory physiology and methods to measure certain maternal and fetal functions have developed over the past three decades. Among these methods, continuous electronic monitoring of FHR and uterine activity (UA) have had the widest clinical application. Experience with intrapartum fetal monitoring has resulted in an improved understanding and clinical interpretation of intrapartum events.

The development and application of continuous fetal monitoring has dramatically expanded the role of the nurse in caring for the family during labor and delivery. With this expanded role have come additional responsibilities in parent education, counseling, client care, and surveillance.

Fetal Monitoring

Pros and Cons

Several nonrandomized studies suggest that the majority of intrapartum fetal deaths are avoidable when the FHR is monitored continuously. It is also generally accepted that continuous fetal monitoring enables early detection of intrapartum fetal hypoxia (distress) and, when accompanied by appropriate therapy, results in lower neonatal morbidity and mortality, as well as improved neurologic development following birth. Most obstetricians believe that continuous fetal monitoring offers substantial benefit in this regard. Clinical studies of its value, however, have produced conflicting results, especially concerning its use in low-risk clients during normal labor. Although the observation of normal fetal monitoring data is predictive of a good fetal outcome, the interpretation of abnormal patterns has been fraught with difficulty and with considerable false-positive diagnosis (*i.e.*, an apparently abnormal finding when the fetus is well). All of this has led the medical community, governmental agencies, and the consumer to question the value of routine fetal monitoring. It is apparent that valid "cost-benefit" and "risk-benefit" analyses will require more data from long-term prospective studies.

The application of internal fetal monitoring devices presents severe potential risks to the mother and fetus. Complications such as uterine perforations with hemorrhage are fortunately rare. Neonatal scalp infection, which generally resolves with local antibiotic therapy, is observed in fewer than 1% of cases. The relationship of internal fetal monitoring to maternal infectious morbidity remains a concern, although several studies indicate that other contributing factors, such as prolonged rupture of membranes, the need for cesarean delivery, and an excessive number of vaginal examinations, more significantly increase the incidence of postpartum endometritis in internally monitored clients. Finally, there is concern regarding the contributions of electronic fetal monitoring to the increasing rate of cesarean sections. Although this is difficult to evaluate, a number of investigators have suggested that the effect is not substantial. In fact, some have claimed that experience with appropriate use of monitoring can reduce the frequency of cesarean sections that are performed for fetal distress.

Selection of Patients

In spite of these controversies, the use of electronic fetal monitoring has become commonplace. Because not every high-risk fetus can be identified prior to labor, some physicians advocate electronic monitoring of all patients during labor. However, uncertainty of the benefit in normal pregnancy and limited availability of equipment frequently result in selective monitoring of high-risk patients and those receiving oxytocics or conduction anesthetics.

Because labor may be a stressful event to the fetus in a certain number of uncomplicated pregnancies, it is important to screen expectant mothers for the potential use of continuous monitoring techniques. Careful auscultation of FHR by nursing personnel may detect decelerations and prompt the initiation of electronic monitoring.

Nurse's Involvement

The role of the nurse during labor has therefore expanded to caring for the fetus as well as for the mother. As with other diagnostic procedures, it is the nurse's responsibility to inform the client about the purpose and the procedure of the monitoring and to screen and interpret the data initially.

With consumerism becoming an increasingly important factor in the delivery of obstetric care, the need for fetal monitoring by those intent on natural, nonintervention childbirth has been questioned. The principles of fetal monitoring and the scientific basis for interpreting the data have become well understood. Although it seems logical to presume that the detection and alleviation of fetal stress or the detection of fetal distress should be of benefit to all, the long-term benefits of clinically applied fetal monitoring are not as yet well substantiated. In counseling parents, the nurse should state the intended benefits of fetal monitoring without

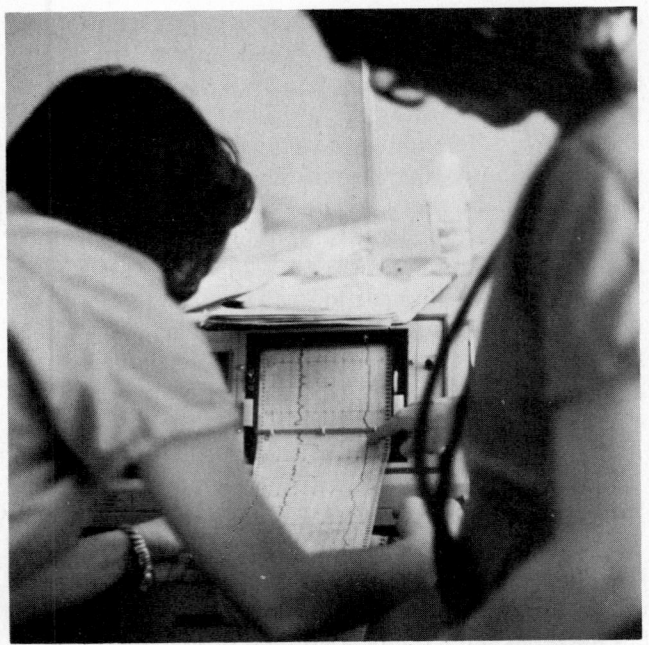

FIGURE 43-1

Professional labor nurses are trained to apply and read monitor equipment. (Photo by Kathy Sloane)

ignoring the infrequent complications. The nurse should never tell the family that intrapartum monitoring guarantees a healthy neonate.

Continuing interpretation of data and the use of new equipment or tests are imperative. In many institutions, nursing guidelines have been established concerning the application of fetal monitors, the interpretation of data, and the institution of remedial change when abnormalities are detected. Thus, to use the fetal monitor, the nurse must be familiar with the equipment, have an understanding of the fundamental principles involved, and have access to updated information concerning interpretation and management of the data.

When fetal monitoring first became widely used, concerns were raised that there would be a tendency to nurse the monitor rather than the client. On the contrary, fetal monitoring has had the beneficial result of freeing the nurse from repetitive tasks and providing an opportunity for more and better quality care for the mother and the fetus. In applying monitoring, the nurse makes independent assessments of maternal and fetal pathophysiology and initiates action to correct abnormalities as they develop. These tasks have led to the concept of the nurse caring for a high-risk mother and fetus as an "intensivist." As a result, greater appreciation of the need for primary personal continuous nursing care during labor and delivery has developed. Thus, monitoring is an important factor in enhancing the quality of nursing care during labor and delivery (Fig. 43-1).

Assessment by Fetal Monitoring

Methods of Monitoring

Uterine Activity

UA may be monitored by either external or internal methods. External monitoring provides a recording of the frequency and duration of uterine contractions (UC), while internal monitoring provides an accurate measurement of intrauterine pressure for assessing both baseline tone and the intensity of the contractions.

The use of an internal pressure catheter permits the most accurate assessment of UA, both quantitatively and temporally. Thus, the internal method is particularly useful in evaluating clients receiving oxytocic drugs or in instances when the temporal relationship of changes in FHR to UC is unclear. Internal uterine monitoring is also helpful in documenting the adequacy of labor in clients who experience an arrest of cervical dilatation. Often a labor pattern of frequent contractions of low intensity will appear impressively strong when using the external technique. The clinical impression of weak contractions perceived by an experienced nurse may be confirmed with internal pressure monitoring. In such cases, Pitocin augmentation may be necessary. Nevertheless, the majority of labors that are monitored can be adequately assessed by the external method. The method used, and any change of method, should be noted directly on the fetal monitoring record as well as in the nursing note or nursing flow sheet.

External Pressure Monitoring. UA is monitored by a pressure transducer called a *tocodynamometer* (Fig. 43-2). A transducer converts one form of energy to an-

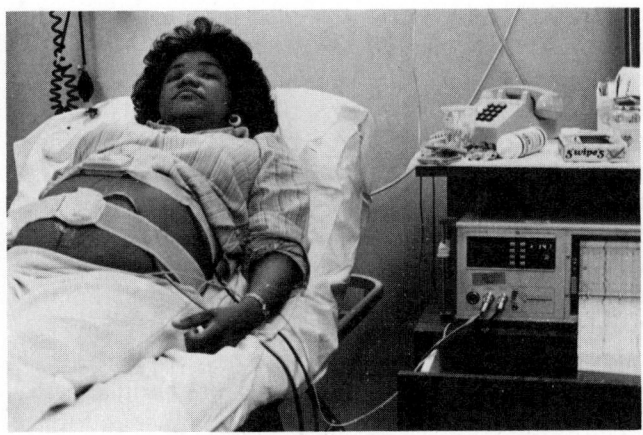

FIGURE 43-2

A tocodynamometer is used to monitor uterine activity. The disk is secured to the mother's abdomen with an elastic belt. (Photo by Kathy Sloane)

other; this transducer converts pressure to electrical signals. The tocodynamometer is a flat disk with either a protruding or a flush plunger. It is secured to the mother's abdomen with an elastic belt. As the uterus contracts, the abdominal wall rises and presses against the transducer. The subsequent movement of the plunger is converted into an electrical signal and is recorded on the paper, giving a continuous record of the frequency and duration of contractions.

Correct placement of the tocodynamometer is necessary if interpretable data are to be gathered (see the Nursing Guidelines for detailed nursing procedure). The transducer is placed over the area where the greatest displacement of the uterus occurs during a contraction (*i.e.,* the uterine fundus). Displacement of the abdominal wall by the uterus may not be adequate to record UC in a client with a small uterus (*i.e.,* less than 20 weeks' gestation) or in one who is extremely overweight. Movement of the maternal abdominal wall caused by respirations, coughing, or position changes may be reflected on the fetal monitoring record. Any such interfering factors should be noted as such on the monitor tracing. It may not be possible to obtain consistent data with this method from clients who are extremely restless. Occasionally, clients who are experiencing pain find that the firm elastic straps become uncomfortable

---

Nursing Guidelines for Application of the External Fetal Monitor

Equipment needed

Fetal monitor

Monitor paper

Ultrasound transducer

Tocodynamometer

2 straps and buttons

Conductive jelly

Preparation of equipment

Plug ultrasound transducer into outlet on front of monitor.

Plug tocodynamometer into outlet on front of monitor.

Turn monitor on.

Test monitor by pushing FHR button.

Procedure

Nursing Intervention	*Rationale*
1. Explain procedure to mother and support person.	• Allays fears and gains cooperation; promotes compliance
2. Elevate head of bed 15°–30° degrees.	• Decreases aorta and vena caval compression
3. Powder 2 straps and place under client.	• Promotes comfort
4. Apply conductive jelly to ultrasound.	• Aids in transmission of ultrasound wave
5. Place ultrasound on client's abdomen and move around until strong FHR is heard and consistent waveform appears on oscilloscope.	• Locates the point of maximum FHR; verifies clarity of input
6. Attach straps to ultrasound using buttons to fasten.	• Should be firmly attached but not tight
7. Push recorder button if haven't done so already.	• Will not record otherwise
8. Place tocodynamometer on the fundal portion of uterus.	• Location of greatest uterine displacement
9. Attach straps to tocodynamometer using buttons to fasten.	• Should be firmly attached but not tight
10. Adjust sound and equipment as needed, particularly when a procedure is performed or client's position is changed.	• Monitor sensitive to change or disturbance to equipment

or interfere with breathing techniques and effleurage. When this occurs, repositioning the tocodynamometer and straps may be useful.

Internal Method. A soft plastic catheter filled with sterile water is passed, usually by a physician, into the uterus beyond the presenting fetal part by means of a firmer plastic introducer (Fig. 43-3). This, of course, requires that the cervix be partially dilated. Although a catheter or balloon may be placed extra-amniotically, for clinical use, the placement is intra-amniotic and requires that the membranes be previously ruptured. The catheter is connected to a pressure transducer (strain gauge). The intrauterine pressure is transmitted from the amniotic fluid through the sterile water in the catheter to the pressure transducer. The transducer produces an electrical signal that is amplified by the recorder. Changes in the intrauterine pressure that occur with contractions or increased intra-abdominal pressure from, for example, the Valsalva maneuver or coughing are recorded on the monitor (see the Nursing Guidelines for procedure).

The internal pressure catheter provides a means of sampling amniotic fluid for meconium or bacteria during labor if this becomes clinically useful. If the catheter becomes plugged by vernix, meconium, or blood, intrauterine pressure will not be transmitted to the transducer. Flushing with small amounts of sterile water

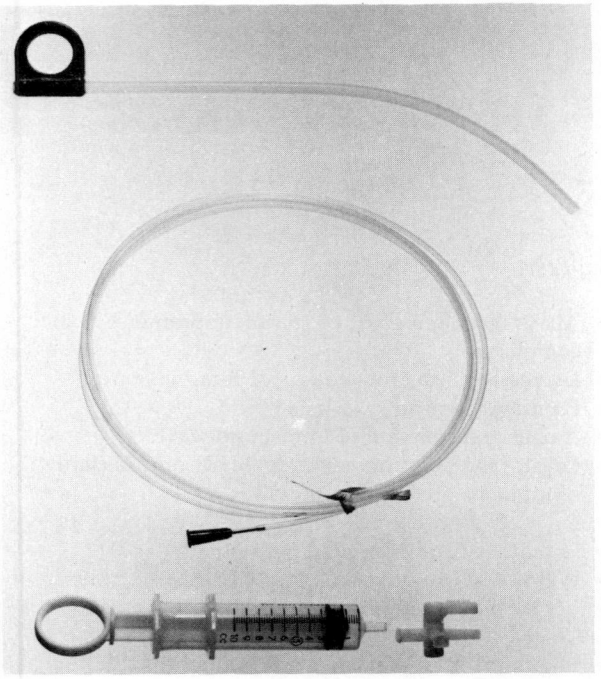

F I G U R E   4 3 - 3

Equipment for internal pressure monitoring includes plastic introducer, catheter, stopcock, and syringe.

usually corrects the problem. When this fails, the catheter should be withdrawn slightly and repositioned. This may relieve kinking of the catheter or entrapment between the lower uterine segment and fetus. The portion of the catheter in the vagina or outside the client should not be advanced into the uterus. Not only may this result in bacterial contamination, but it is generally ineffective because the flexibility of the catheter will cause it to coil alongside the presenting fetal part. Perforation of the uterus and injury to the placenta should be considered when excessive vaginal bleeding occurs after placement of the catheter and when UC fail to be recorded. Perforation into the broad ligament has been reported, in which case hemorrhage was concealed. The presence of maternal hypotension and tachycardia following catheter insertion might suggest this rare complication.

Fetal Heart Rate

Prior to the development of fetal monitoring, evaluation of FHR was restricted to periodic auscultation during the interval between contractions. FHR changes occurring with the contractions or during the first 30 seconds following the contraction were usually not detected. The ability to diagnose fetal distress was limited to sustained and extreme variation in FHR, such as severe bradycardia. With auscultation, the evaluation of periodic changes, that is, those occurring over short time intervals (decelerations or accelerations), remains somewhat subjective, especially when they occur at a rate that is within the normal range.

With continuous FHR monitoring, the time interval between two successive heartbeats is calculated at a rate and is recorded graphically. For example, a lapse of 375 milliseconds between beats would constitute a rate of 160 beats per minute (bpm). For this calculation to be made, the fetal signal obtained with a transducer is amplified and then counted by a cardiotachometer. This is converted to a rate between successive beats and recorded continuously during, and in the interval between, contractions.

External Method. Several methods for monitoring the FHR through the maternal abdomen are available.

Phonocardiography. Phonocardiography uses a transducer, which is essentially a microphone. With this technique, the heart sounds of the fetus constitute the signal. Extraneous sounds or "noise" from within the uterus, maternal abdomen, or abdominal wall may also be detected as a signal. Thus, electronic filtering is required.

Fetal Electrocardiogram. Fetal electrocardiogram (FECG) is a method for obtaining the electrical signal

Nursing Guidelines for Application of the Intrauterine Pressure Catheter

Equipment needed

Fetal monitor

Monitor paper

Disposable catheter pack

Transducer

Transducer dome

2 three-way stopcocks

2-ml syringe

18-gauge needle

2 sterile towels

Procedure

1. Explain the purpose, rationale, and procedure for using the intrauterine catheter to client and support person.
2. Prepare transducer by placing 1 drop of sterile water directly on the strain gauge and covering with a sterile dome. Connect two three-way stopcocks to the openings on the dome.
3. Fix the transducer at miduterine level by the bed.
4. Position client for vaginal examination.
5. Open the sterile towel packs while physician is sterile gloving, so that he may place sterile drape around the perineal area.
6. Open sterile catheter pack and a 18-gauge needle pack for physician.
7. Hold a 30-ml vial of sterile water while the physician draws up 20 ml for priming the intrauterine catheter.
8. After proper placement of the catheter by the physician, tape it securely to the client's inner thigh and connect the catheter and the 20-ml syringe to the portholes on one of the three-way stopcocks. Turn the stopcock valve off to the dome and flush the catheter with 10 ml of sterile water.
9. Turn the stopcock valve off to the catheter. Open the other three-way stopcock to air, filling the dome with the sterile water from the 20-ml syringe. Allow a small amount of sterile water to flow out of a porthole on the empty stopcock to ensure there are no trapped air bubbles within the dome that can alter the pressure measurement.
10. To calibrate the strain gauge to atmospheric pressure, allow the empty stopcock to stay open to air and remove the syringe on the other stopcock, making sure that the valve is turned off to the catheter. Adjust the penset on the monitor to zero. Turn the valve on the catheter stopcock off to the syringe.
11. Turn the other three-way stopcock off to air and test the system by asking the client to cough. Proper functioning of the catheter is assured if there is an inflection on the chart paper when the client coughs.
12. Palpate the uterus lightly to determine when relaxation occurs, and observe the pressure reading. The uterine resting tone should be 5 mm Hg to 15 mm Hg, with an average of 8 mm Hg to 12 mm Hg during normal labor.
13. Make certain the transducer is placed at the height that approximates that of the catheter tip. If the level of the catheter is above the transducer, a falsely elevated pressure recording results. If the catheter tip is below the transducer, a falsely low or negative pressure may be recorded.

of the fetal heart from the maternal abdominal wall. When the abdominal wall FECG is used as the signal, the larger maternal ECG complex is censored or edited out by the machine. When the maternal signal coincides with the fetal signal, the machine may edit the maternal signal and insert a fetal beat automatically. This is known as *compensation*. Monitoring of the FECG through the maternal abdominal wall will result in clin-ically useful tracings in only a portion of cases in which it is attempted.

Doppler/Ultrasound. The Doppler or ultrasound method is the most commonly used method of external monitoring (Fig. 43-4). With this technique, high-frequency sound waves are transmitted from a crystal and are reflected from the moving fetal heart to a re-

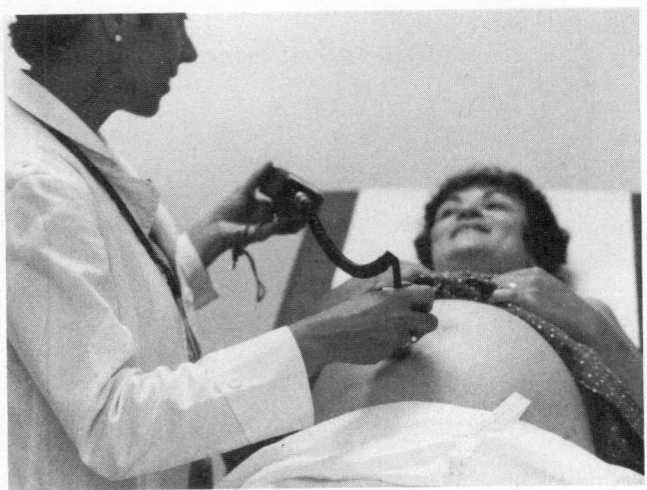

FIGURE   43-4

In the Doppler or ultrasound method of monitoring, high-frequency sound waves are transmitted, giving a signal that is amplified. (Courtesy of Booth Maternity Center, Philadelphia)

ceiving crystal. The difference in frequencies of the transmitted and the reflected sound waves constitutes the signal, which can be amplified for counting by the cardiotachometer and is also heard as an audible signal from the machine. Filtering is needed for other intra-abdominal motion, which constitutes noise. More recently, a bidirectional Doppler has been employed in fetal monitoring that permits selection of motion either toward or away from the transducer. With this technique, whichever constitutes the better signal is selected for recording. To obtain clinically useful tracings with the Doppler, "averaging" over two or three successive beats is performed. Some machines are also equipped with logic circuitry such that rates above a certain level (*e.g.,* 180) will be halved on the recorder, whereas rates below a preset level (*e.g.,* 90) will be doubled. Variations in equipment function such as this illustrate the importance of being familiar with the particular equipment in use.

When the Doppler transducer is used, the transducer is applied to an area that is directly over the fetal heart. This site is selected by auscultation and by palpating the fetus. By trial and error, the position from which the sharpest (not necessarily the loudest) audible fetal signal can be heard is determined before securing the transducer with an elastic belt. Periodic changes of fetal or maternal position may require readjustment of the transducer to maintain high-quality data (see Nursing Guidelines for Application of the External Fetal Monitor, given earlier).

Internal Method.   In most centers, direct FECG is the most widely used method for FHR monitoring dur-

ing labor. Following rupture of the membranes, the transducer, which is a small electrode, is attached to the skin of the presenting part of the fetus, usually the scalp. This small, silver silver-chloride electrode is commonly referred to as a *clip* because the first electrodes available were attached by two prongs to the fetal scalp. At present, the most commonly used electrode is a small spiral wire that is advanced into the fetal skin by clockwise rotation while gentle pressure is applied (Fig. 43-5). Application of the electrode requires that the membranes be ruptured and that the cervix be dilated at least 1 cm to 2 cm or more. The presenting part must be known and fixed in the pelvis. Attempts to apply the scalp electrode when the fetus is floating are hazardous and may dislodge the fetus to an abnormal lie, increasing

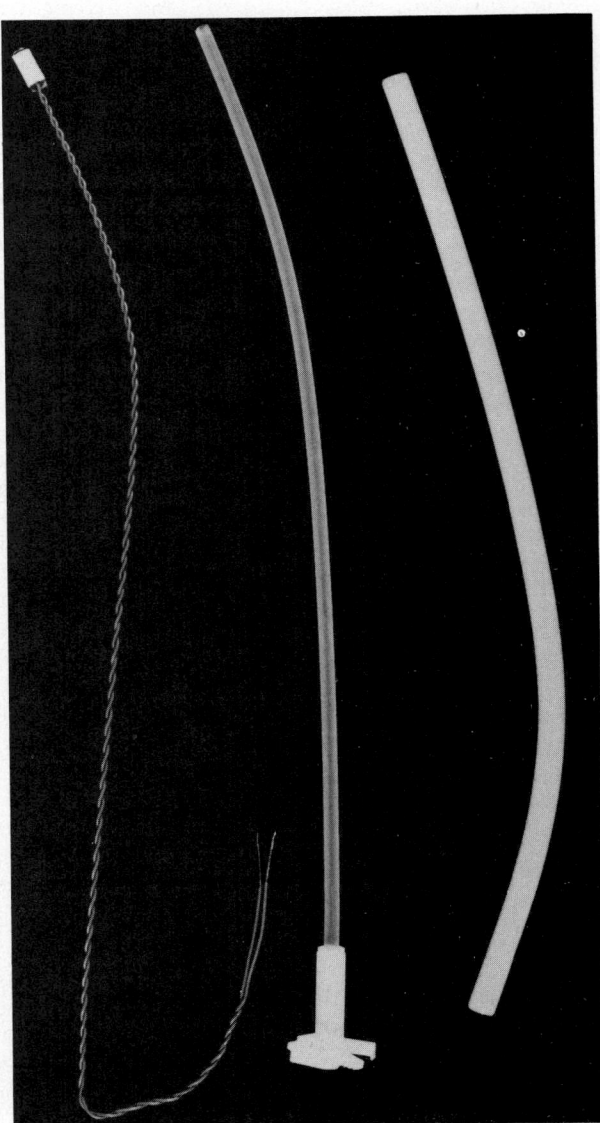

FIGURE   43-5

Scalp electrode and introducer for fetal heart monitoring.

Nursing Guidelines for Application of a Fetal Scalp Electrode (Clip)

Equipment needed

Fetal monitor

Monitor paper

Leg plate

Leg strap

Fetal scalp electrode

Procedure

1. Explain purpose, indications, and procedure for internal FHR monitoring to the client and the support person.
2. Test leg plate before beginning the procedure by plugging into monitor where indicated. It should read out a test rate of 120 bpm.
3. Position client for a vaginal examination.
4. Open spiral electrode pack with sterile technique.
5. Remove applicator and attach color-coded wires to appropriate push post on the leg plate following application of spiral electrode to baby's scalp by physician or certified nurse.
6. Apply electrode paste to leg plate and secure firmly with leg strap to mid-inner or anterior thigh.
7. Observe oscilloscope for FECG waveform, making sure it correlates simultaneously with an audible signal and a clear interpretable tracing.

the risk for umbilical cord prolapse (see Nursing Guidelines for Application of a Fetal Scalp Electrode [Clip]).

The FECG serves as the fetal signal for counting. On occasion, the maternal signal obtained by this method may produce an artifactual tracing (*e.g.*, the maternal ECG may be conducted through a dead fetus). The use of real-time ultrasonography to evaluate fetal heart motion can usually resolve this question and avoid unnecessary cesarean delivery. Editing of the direct FECG may result in failure to detect fetal cardiac arrhythmias. With direct FECG there is no need for averaging, and the true beat-to-beat variation in FHR can be evaluated. Spiral electrodes are easily removed before or after delivery by gentle counter-clockwise rotation of the attached wires.

pH of Fetal Blood Scalp Samples

Determination of *p*H of fetal scalp blood is clinically useful for the diagnosis of fetal distress. For this measurement, a small volume of fetal blood may be obtained by puncturing the fetal scalp and collecting the blood samples in fine glass capillary tubes. To perform this procedure, the membranes must be ruptured, the cervix

must be dilated 3 cm to 4 cm, and the fetal presenting part must be fixed in the pelvis. The procedure requires the client to be in the lithotomy position. It may be performed in bed or in the delivery room. Serial determinations are often obtained 20 to 30 minutes apart. Regardless of where the procedure is carried out, the obstetric team must be prepared to act immediately should the *p*H determination reveal severe fetal acidosis ($pH \leq 7.20$).

A conical vaginal endoscope is used to visualize the vertex of the fetus during fetal blood sampling (Fig. 43-6). Because of the invasive nature of the procedure, sterile technique is used throughout. The perineum is covered with sterile drapes and prepared with a

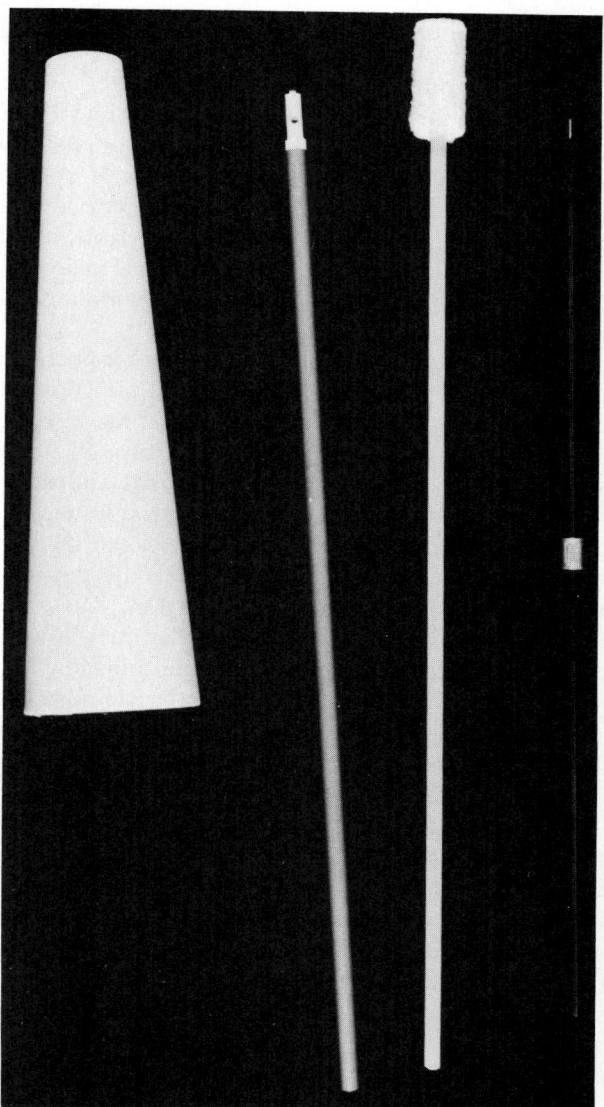

FIGURE 4 3 - 6

Scalp sampling equipment includes plastic amnioscope, scalpel, cotton sponge, and heparinized capillary tube.

povidone-iodine solution. The amnioscope is inserted into the vagina and the dilated cervix. A light source is then attached to the amnioscope. A light film of silicone jelly is applied to the scalp. This causes droplets of fetal blood to bead and aggregate, making it easier to collect the blood samples in the capillary tubes. A small metal blade attached to a long handle is used to puncture the scalp. The narrow 2×2-mm detachable blades are mounted in plastic to control the depth of the puncture. A single brisk motion is used to penetrate the skin in a manner similar to that used to obtain a "finger stick." The scalp sampling should not be performed overlying a suture line or fontanel. The beaded drops of fetal blood are allowed to aggregate and are collected in the long, heparinized capillary tubes. Heparinized capillary tubes hold 250 μl of fetal blood when full. Modern instruments require only 25 μl to 40 μl of fetal blood to obtain a determination of blood gases. The tube is then passed to the waiting nurse, who inserts a fine metal bead or short wire into the capillary tube prior to sealing it with wax. A magnet passed along the outside of the tube moves the metal wire and stirs the sample to prevent clotting. Exposing the sample to atmospheric air can cause an exchange of oxygen and carbon dioxide, which will alter the hydrogen ion concentration. Placing the capillary tube on ice will retard cellular respiration and thus retards a change in pH.

After an adequate sample of scalp blood is obtained, the physician applies firm pressure to the puncture site through the next two contractions to guarantee adequate hemostasis. The site should be observed through a third contraction, and if there is no bleeding, the endoscope may be removed. Repeated scalp blood sampling may be safely performed if necessary. The risks of the procedure include continued bleeding from the puncture site, ecchymosis, hematoma, and infection.

Following scalp blood sampling, the nurse should observe the client for excessive vaginal bleeding that may be fetal in origin. In addition, sustained fetal tachycardia may be observed on the monitor tracing when fetal blood loss occurs externally or a massive hematoma forms.

The partial pressure of oxygen and carbon dioxide, as well as bicarbonate ion concentration, can be measured on these samples. The pH, however, has proven to be the simplest, most rapid, and most clinically useful measurement that can be performed on a small sample of blood. The pH of the fetal scalp blood normally ranges between 7.25 and 7.35 during labor. This correlates well with the acid–base status of the blood in the umbilical vessels. A mild progressive decline of pH within the normal range has been noted with contractions and as labor progresses. When the fetus becomes hypoxic, anaerobic glycolysis occurs, resulting in an excess production of lactic acid and an increase in hydrogen ion concentration. The increased hydrogen ion concentration is measured as a decrease in pH (acidosis). Thus,

the development of acidosis reflects the effects of hypoxia on cellular metabolism, or respiration.

Generally, cord compression with resultant variable decelerations results in a rapid increase in fetal pCO_2, resulting in a mild respiratory acidosis that quickly subsides. Persistent variable decelerations and late decelerations are strongly suggestive of fetal metabolic acidosis.

Clinical studies have demonstrated a correlation between the pH of fetal scalp blood and abnormalities in FHR, Apgar scores, and umbilical cord pH. As a result of these observations, the measurement of the pH of fetal scalp blood has become an increasingly important method for diagnosing and confirming fetal distress. This measurement helps when the interpretation of fetal monitoring data is unclear and reduces the chances of false-positive diagnoses of fetal distress using fetal monitoring. Traditionally, a scalp blood pH of 7.20 or less is considered to be indicative of fetal acidosis or fetal distress; pH values between 7.20 and 7.25 are borderline and warrant repeat sampling. Generally, one does not act on a single pH determination. Equivocal and low values should be repeated while the physician is preparing for a possible rapid delivery.

As is true of other antepartal and intrapartum methods of fetal evaluation, measurement of scalp blood pH may produce false-negative results (normal values when the fetus is hypoxic). Events that occur following fetal blood sampling, but before delivery (*e.g.*, continued cord compression), may account for many of the false-negative results observed. Abnormal maternal acid–base status may be transmitted passively to the fetus through the placenta and account for a portion of the false-positive cases (abnormal values when the fetus is well). This is possible in the diabetic client who is prone to develop ketoacidosis. For this reason, obtaining a simultaneous blood sample from the mother to determine the pH of her blood is occasionally of value in interpreting the fetal pH and will reduce the frequency of false-positive results. Because these problems occur in only a small proportion of cases, they do not detract substantially from the clinical value of fetal pH measurement. In fact, it has been suggested by some physicians that the diagnosis of fetal distress should *always* be based on the finding of fetal acidosis. However, rapid fetal deterioration, inability to obtain samples, or suspicion of false-negative results makes this test impractical as an absolute criterion in all cases.

Care of the Newborn.

Following delivery of an infant in whom fetal blood sampling has been performed, umbilical venous and arterial blood samples should be obtained from a doubly clamped segment of cord. Measurement of blood gases and pH on these samples makes it easier to correlate the fetal monitor tracing, the scalp blood pH measurements, and the neonatal condition.

When assessing the newborn, the nurse should

closely inspect the scalp of the infant to identify the puncture site(s). In many institutions, cleansing with an antiseptic solution and applying an antibiotic ointment are routine. Personnel in the nursery should be alerted to the number and the status of scalp puncture sites at the time the infant is transferred to the nursery. In this way, any complications resulting from the procedure can be detected immediately and treated.

Other Intrapartum Methods of Fetal Evaluation

A number of other techniques for intrapartum fetal evaluation are under investigation in the laboratory or have reached the stage of clinical trials. These include percutaneous monitoring of oxygen tension, continuous scalp *p*H measurement, electroencephalography, and observation of fetal movements, particularly respirations, using real-time ultrasound.

Application of the Fetal Monitor

The decision to apply the fetal monitor should be based on institutional policy and requires the consent of the client. In some institutions, fetal monitoring is employed in all laboring clients. The responsibility for selection of clients to be monitored rests with the physician and with the nurse. The nurse's role in selection is particularly important when the number of clients who are in labor exceeds the number of available monitors, and priorities for monitoring must be established. In general, the decision to monitor is made on the basis of one of three primary indications:

1. Antepartum risk factors, including maternal complications such as diabetes, hypertension, and cardiac, renal, and hematologic diseases. Fetal problems such as suspected intrauterine growth retardation or post-dates pregnancy are included.
2. Intrapartum risk factors, such as third-trimester bleeding, passage of meconium, or abnormalities of FHR determined by auscultation
3. Other obstetric factors (*e.g.*, to evaluate abnormal progress of labor or the effects of drugs such as oxytocics and some anesthetic agents)

After the decision has been made to monitor a client, the method of monitoring is selected. This is contingent upon four factors: (1) status of the cervix and membranes, (2) the indication for monitoring, (3) client acceptance, and (4) availability. When the membranes are intact or the cervix is not dilated, external methods of monitoring must be used. If adequate data cannot be obtained with the available external systems, internal monitoring should be considered. In cases in which the most accurate data are required (*e.g.*, true beat-to-beat variation, temporal relationship of decelerations to con-

---

Nursing Guidelines for Care During Fetal Heart Rate Monitoring

1. Continue to perform nursing care that is given to all laboring mothers.
2. Explain to mother and support person what fetal monitoring consists of.
   - Allow mother to express herself and to participate in decision making.
   - Obtain a signed consent form if institution requires.
   - If FHR monitoring is routine for all clients and this mother refuses, follow institution guidelines for releasing institution and personnel from liability.
3. Explain steps involved for FHR monitoring before or while applying either external or internal monitoring.
4. Recognize mother's fears and concerns and that she needs reinforcement and support. Common fears include the following:
   - Harm to baby from ultrasound
   - Harm to baby from scalp clip to head
   - Something wrong with baby
5. The following procedures can be done to maximize client comfort:
   - Noisy machine volume can be adjusted so that mother can relax and be comfortable.
   - The mother will have to stay in bed but may change her position frequently to feel less confined.
   - If available, monitoring by telemetry would further allow client mobility.
   - Powdering and reapplying the monitor straps every 2 hours may minimize discomfort from tight straps.
6. Remember to always greet and speak to the client before evaluating the monitor tracing. The laboring mother and fetus are our main focus. The monitor assists with their care.

---

tractions, or true intrauterine pressures), internal monitoring must be used.

See the Nursing Guidelines for nursing care during FHR monitoring.

Fetal Monitor Tracing and Nursing Documentation

Fetal monitors are equipped to provide a continuous recording of FHR and UA. This information is recorded on perforated paper that folds "accordion style" (Fig. 43-7). The UA is generally recorded on the lower channel. The recording paper provides a vertical scale for measuring the intrauterine pressure, usually in millimeters of mercury (mm Hg). Most monitors are

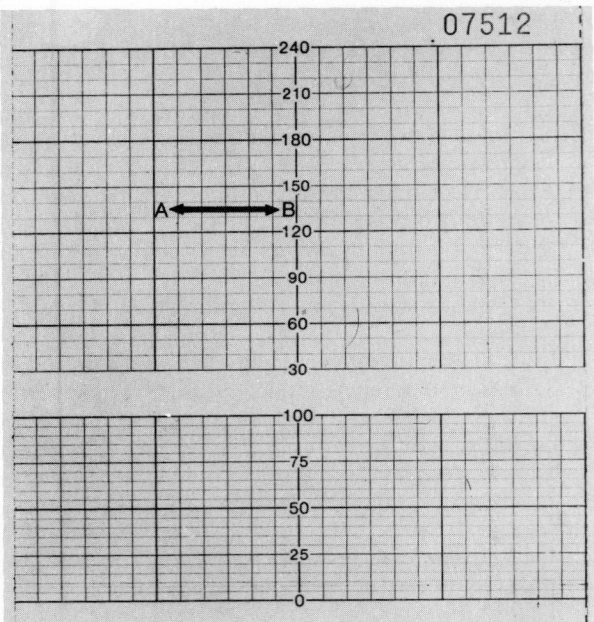

07512

F I G U R E   4 3 - 7

Recording paper for fetal monitor. Note FHR (bpm) recorded on upper channel, UA (mm Hg) recorded on lower channel, and panel number at top of sheet. Distance from A to B equals 1 minute when paper speed is 3 cm/min.

equipped with a zeroing and calibration device to ensure that the record accurately reflects the true intrauterine pressure. The FHR in beats per minute is displayed on the upper channel. Some monitors are also equipped with a digital display of the FHR and a small oscilloscope screen for viewing the FECG.

The paper speed is usually set at 3 cm/min. Divisions on the horizontal scale provide a measurement of the time elapsed and are useful as markers to correlate events on both channels. Numbering on the individual sheets of the record provides a reference for rapid calculation of elapsed time for longer intervals.

Because the data obtained become a part of the client's permanent record, it is important that a systematic method of identification be used at the beginning of each new fetal monitor tracing paper and following delivery. A sample format for identification is shown in Figure 43-8. In addition, it has become common practice to record the clock-time and important clinical data, such as vital signs, vaginal examinations, rupture of membranes, physician review of the tracing, medications (dose and route of administration), and client activity, directly on the monitor record. This information is important for interpreting the record and is invaluable when reviewed retrospectively for teaching purposes.

In addition to recording events on the tracing itself, nursing documentation is necessary either on a flow sheet or in a nurse's note. The flow sheet is usually self-explanatory. The nurse's note should include descriptive rather than diagnostic information, as follows:

9:30 AM. Continuous fetal external monitoring, FHR ranges between 130 and 142 bpm with variability ranging between 6 and 8 bpm since 8:00 AM. Refer to flow sheet.

10:00 AM. Uterine contractions occurring every 3 minutes with intensity to 75 mm Hg. FHR dropped to 120 from 146 for 45 seconds recovering thereafter—Variability ranging between 3 and 5 bpm, Dr. Smith notified @ 9:52 AM. Client turned on left side, discontinued oxytocin infusion, applied oxygen by mask at 101/min, peripheral IV infusion at 125 ml/min. Dr. Smith in to see client and review tracing @ 9:55 AM.

It is critical to remember that these notes are an integral part of the client record. An attempt should be made to legitimately correct any discrepancies concerning nursing and physician notes at the time of labor and delivery. If an error is made, it should be so stated. Crossing out information is not acceptable. In summary, the careful nursing documentation of all important events may prove helpful if a case is later reviewed in a court of law.

Interpretation of Data

To properly interpret the data obtained from electronic fetal monitoring, a systematic approach should be used to examine the tracings and correlate them with clinical events. The interpretation of monitor tracings can be learned from annotated atlases of monitor tracings (see Selected Reading) and of course clinical experience. It is important to bear in mind that expertise in this area often takes several years to acquire. To provide teaching in monitoring interpretation, many institutions have periodic in-service programs and, more important, conferences in which tracings are reviewed by members of the team caring for the clients.

Evaluation of Uterine Activity or Uterine Contractions

External Methods

Only the frequency and duration of UC may be determined with external monitoring. The onset of the contraction is determined by the upswing of the pen and is followed by the *increment*. The peak of the contraction or highest level recorded is called the *acme*. The progressive relaxation of the uterus following the acme is referred to as the *decrement*. When the baseline is reached, the contraction is completed. The total duration of the contraction and the interval from the onset of

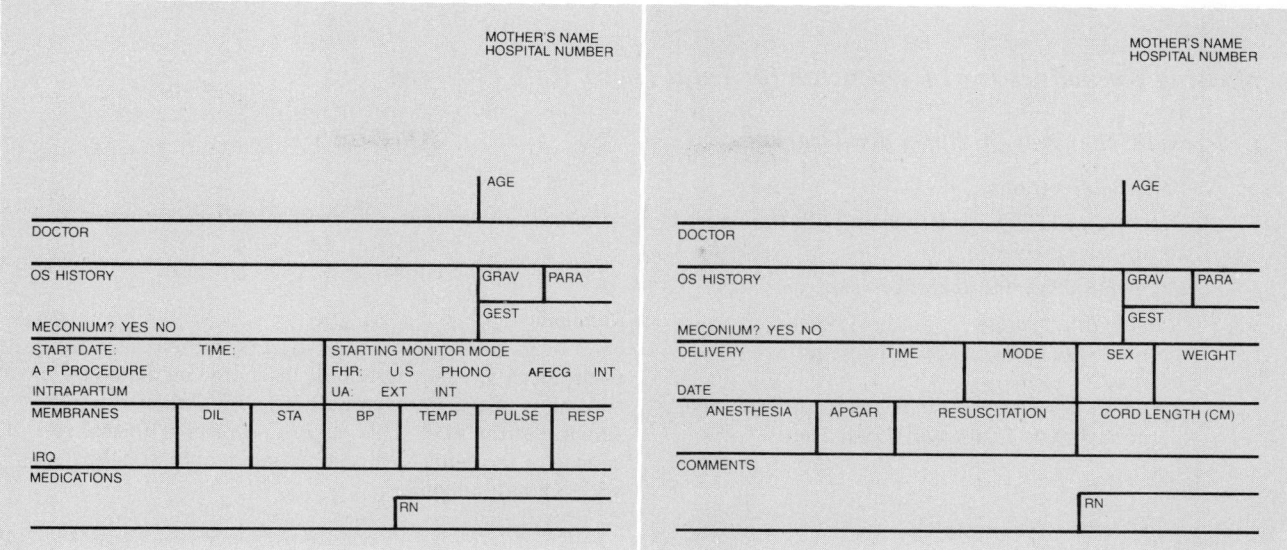

FIGURE 43-8

(*Left*) Label provides identification and clinical information for interpretation of tracing and is applied when monitoring is initiated and at the start of each new monitor strip. (*Right*) Label provides identification and clinical information for correlation of monitor data with neonatal condition and is applied following delivery.

one contraction to the onset of the next contraction may be calculated when the paper speed is known (3 cm/min). Maternal respiratory movement may be noted as fine "saw-tooth" deflections confirmed by comparing the rate with that observed clinically. Coughing, sneezing, and so on appear as large spiking deflections. Bearing-down efforts, or pushing, cause multiple sharp spikes superimposed on the contractions. Changes of position cause sudden sharp changes of the baseline.

Internal Method

Intrauterine pressure can be quantitated (following proper zeroing and calibration) only when internal monitoring is used. The baseline uterine tone is measured as the height of the baseline during the interval between contractions and is usually in a range of 5 mm Hg to 15 mm Hg.

An elevated baseline pressure may indicate any of the following:

- Misplacement of the pressure transducer in relationship to the catheter tip
- Excessive oxytocin administration
- Abruptio placentae
- Hypertonic uterine dysfunction

The contraction amplitude may range from 30 mm Hg to 60 mm Hg or more. Although contraction amplitudes of less than 25 mm Hg to 30 mm Hg may occur in normal active-phase labor, they are most frequently associated with early labor or hypotonic uterine dysfunction.

Hypertonic labor occurs when UC amplitudes exceed normal, the frequency between onset of contractions is less than 2 minutes, or the resting interval between contractions is less than 1 minute. Coalescence of UC or a contraction of 2 minutes' or greater duration is a tetanic contraction. Hypertonic labor or uterine tetany is observed with administration of an excessive amount of oxytocic drugs, abruptio placentae, or hypertonic uterine dysfunction. Hypertonic uterine activity may have a deleterious effect upon the fetus. Sustained increases in intramyometrial pressure will retard blood flow and, consequently, delivery of oxygen to the fetus. The effects of hypertonicity are most immediately reflected in FHR including late or prolonged decelerations. Efforts to abolish hypertonia include cessation of oxytocin administration and occasionally the administration of uterine relaxants.

Evaluation of the FHR

FHR Baseline

During very early fetal development, cardiac activity is initiated by the intrinsic rhythmicity of the myocardial cells. Soon after, the sinoatrial node (SA node) assumes the function of initiating the impulses, which are trans-

(text continued on page 960)

Nursing Guidelines for Intervention for Fetal Heart Rate Patterns

I. *Periodic changes—uniform decelerations*

A. Early decelerations

Description: FHR begins to slow with the onset of the uterine contractions and returns to baseline when the contraction is over.

Pathophysiology: Head compression

Nursing Intervention	*Rationale*
1. Be aware that the FHR slows with a contraction. 2. Chart descriptive note or chart on flow sheet according to institutional practice.	Fetal head compression associated with the contraction, resulting in a parasympathetic discharge mediated by the vagus nerve. Parasympathetic stimulation results in slowing of the FHR. This pattern represents normal response of the fetus to this stimulus and is associated with a good outcome.

B. Late decelerations

Description: FHR begins to fall at height of contraction and returns to baseline after the contraction has ceased. Usually the FHR remains within the normal range. Decelerations may be subtle but still ominous.

Pathophysiology: Uteroplacental insufficiency

Nursing Intervention	*Rationale*
1. Recognize the pattern on the tracing as well as be alert for audible changes in the rhythm of the FHR.	Nursing personnel must have knowledge and experience in FHR monitoring.
2. Follow institution policy: do you assess and wait for next deceleration to occur before notifying physician or proceed to intervention #3?	Effective nursing and physician management to provide for safe labor and delivery for mother with an uncompromised infant; compliance with institution policies is important.
3. Turn client to her left side and give oxygen by mask @ 10 liters/min.	Changing position relieves aorta or vena cava pressure. Hypotension, hyperstimulation or conduction anesthesia may also be the cause and need to be addressed by nurse and physician.
4. Chart a descriptive note or chart on flow sheet.	Nursing management is dictated by institution policies.

II. *Nonuniform Decelerations*

A. Variable decelerations

Description: A slowing of the FHR either with a contraction or between contractions. The pattern of the deceleration is often either a U or V shape that drops suddenly from the baseline and returns abruptly to the baseline.

Pathophysiology: Cord compression

Nursing Intervention	*Rationale*
1. Recognize the pattern and assess the frequency, depth, and duration of the deceleration.	There is correlation between the severity of the variable deceleration and fetal condition.
2. Follow institution policy: do you assess before notifying the physician and carrying out the interventions of #3?	Some institutions have 24-hour physician coverage on the unit; in other institutions the nurse must inform the physician by phone, since they have standing orders.
3. Turn client to her left side or to knee–chest position and give oxygen by mask @ 10 liters/min.	Changing position may help to remove the pressure on the cord. If this is not effective, physician may attempt upward displacement of presenting part.

(continued)

(continued)

III. *Baseline changes*

A. Tachycardia

Description: A baseline FHR of more than 160 bpm persisting 10 to 15 minutes
   Mild: 160–179 bpm
   Marked: 180 or more bpm

Pathophysiology: Fetal hypoxia, maternal fever, idiopathic maternal anxiety, prematurity, drug related, fetal arrhythmia

Nursing Intervention	Rationale
1. Confirm by auscultating FHR.	Confirm that monitor is operating properly and FHR has increased. Tachycardia may be in response to fetal movement.
2. Monitor maternal vital signs.	Tachycardia may be due to maternal fever.
3. Monitor contractions.	FHR may increase in response to excessive contractions.
4. Change maternal position.	Aortoiliac compression is alleviated.
5. Continue to watch closely by reviewing tracings for changing patterns.	Etiologic factors might be identified. Tachycardia may be a sign of fetal distress; arrhythmias may be identified by fetal EKG.
6. Chart descriptive note or chart on flow sheet.	Nursing management is dictated by institution policies.

B. Bradycardia

Description: An FHR of less than 120 bpm persisting 10 to 15 minutes
   Mild: 100–119
   Marked: Less than 100

Nursing Intervention	Rationale
1. Change maternal position.	Changing position alleviates uterine pressure on the aorta and vena cava.
2. Give oxygen by mask @ 10 liters/min.	Baby may have congenital heart abnormality.
3. Continue to watch closely for:	Ominous signs indicate fetal distress, even impending death.
Marked bradycardia with loss of variability and late decelerations	This is a sign of fetal distress.
Mild bradycardia with good FHR variability and absence of late decelerations	This is generally not a sign of fetal distress.
Bradycardia due to heart block	This is not a sign of acute fetal distress.
4. Chart descriptive note or chart on flow sheet.	Nursing management is dictated by institution policies.

C. Variability

Description: A variation of the resting FHR
   Average: 6–10 bpm
   Minimal: 3–5 bpm
   None: 0–2 bpm

Pathophysiology: Maternal medication, fetal acidosis, fetal neurologic immaturity.

Nursing Intervention	Rationale
1. Observe variability of the FHR.	Variability is an indication of normal neurologic control of heart rate and a measure of fetal reserve.
2. Increased variability requires no nursing intervention.	This may be due to external uterine palpitation, UC, fetal activity, or maternal activity.
3. Decreased variability: follow physician's order based on cause.	Possible causes include prematurity, drugs, hypoxia and acidosis, fetal sleep, fetal cardiac arrhythmias.
4. Chart descriptive note or chart on flow sheet.	Nursing management is dictated by institution policies.

(text continued from page 957)

mitted throughout the conduction system of the heart, resulting in the mechanical events known as the heartbeat. Nursing interventions applied to various rhythms are presented in the Nursing Guidelines on pages 958 and 959.

Tachycardia and Bradycardia

The FHR decreases slightly as pregnancy advances and normally ranges between 120 and 160 bpm. Elevation of the FHR baseline above 160 bpm for periods greater than 10 minutes is referred to as *baseline tachycardia.* Rates between 161 and 180 bpm are classified as *mild tachycardia* and those greater than 180 bpm as *marked tachycardia.* Rates below 120 bpm are referred to as *bradycardia.* Those between 100 and 119 bpm are classified as *mild bradycardia* and those less than 100 bpm as *marked bradycardia.* Either fetal tachycardia or bradycardia may be related to fetal hypoxia (low oxygen content of the fetal blood or inadequate delivery of oxygen to the fetal tissues). Fetal tachycardia may be an early warning sign of fetal hypoxia, whereas fetal bradycardia occurs somewhat later in the sequence of events. Abnormalities in baseline FHR may also be due to arrhythmias (abnormal discharge or transmission of impulses through the conduction system of the heart). These are usually benign and transient, but may at times be associated with congenital heart defects or heart failure. Fetal tachycardia may also be associated with maternal

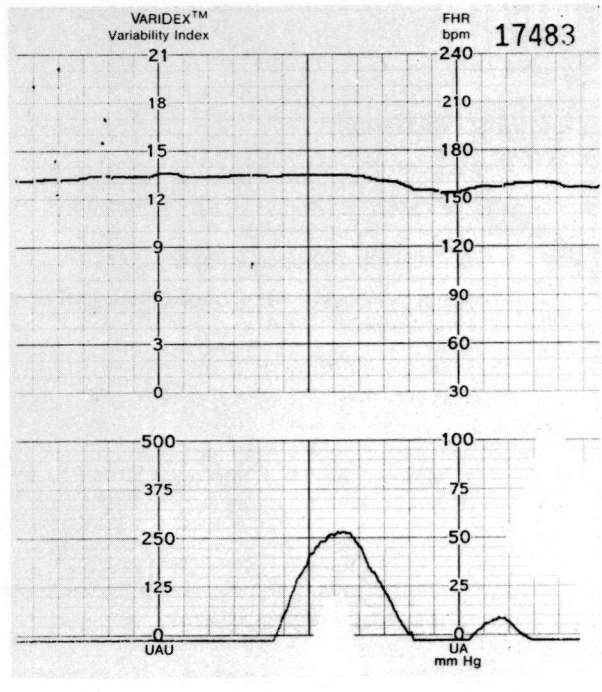

FIGURE 43-10

Fetal heart rate tracing with absent beat-to-beat variability. Note subtle late deceleration.

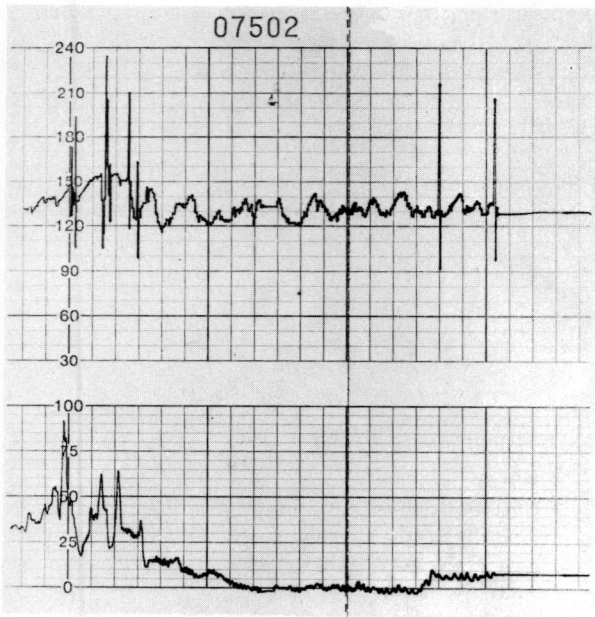

FIGURE 43-9

Fetal heart rate tracing. Note fine irregularity or beat-to-beat variability.

fever, fetal infection, maternal thyrotoxicosis, fetal anemia, and fetal tachyarrhythmias. Because core temperature (internal body temperature) rises earlier and is higher than that measured either orally or rectally, fetal tachycardia may precede maternal fever by a short time. Likewise, fetal bradycardia may be associated with maternal hypothermia, but this is an unusual event clinically. Fetal bradycardia may also be caused by drugs administered to the mother, such as β-blockers. Fetal congenital heart block may produce a baseline bradycardia. This phenomenon has been observed in infants of mothers with systemic lupus erythematosus, who produce an antibody that crosses the placenta and destroys the fetal conducting system.

Variability

As fetal development advances, the autonomic nervous system assumes an increasingly important role in modulating FHR. Discharge of sympathetic nerves causes an increase in rate, whereas discharge of parasympathetic nerves causes a slowing of the heart rate. The normal continuous opposition of these two stimuli results in the beat-to-beat variability noted in the heart rate of the normal fetus. It is reflected by the fine irregularity seen on the normal FHR tracing (Fig. 43-9). A fetus of at least 28 weeks' gestational age should demonstrate normal beat-to-beat variability which usually ranges from 2 bpm to 10 bpm around the average heart rate.

It is important to note that true beat-to-beat variability can be assessed only by direct fetal electrography (*i.e.*, internal monitoring using the spiral electrode). In the past, variability of the FHR baseline was often overlooked as an indicator of fetal status. However, it is now apparent that normal beat-to-beat variability is probably the most reliable indication of fetal well-being. When beat-to-beat variability is normal (*i.e.*, ≥6 bpm) it is thought to indicate an intact nervous system with normal regulatory influence over the FHR. Whereas several factors may be responsible for the loss of heart rate variability, a flat FHR baseline in the absence of explainable causes is considered ominous and potentially indicative of hypoxia (Fig. 43-10).

Nowhere in FHR monitoring is the influence of drugs more obvious than in the assessment of FHR variability. It has become increasingly apparent that a large proportion of drugs administered to the mother will cause diminished or absent FHR variability. Specific drugs that decrease variability include narcotics, barbiturates, phenothiazines, atropine, and tranquilizers. For this reason, it is often useful to evaluate FHR variability by internal monitoring before these drugs are administered.

Periodic Changes

When changes in the FHR occur in association with uterine contractions, they are described as being periodic. The fetus is equipped with cardiovascular reflexes that may cause periodic or transient changes in the FHR from its normal baseline. Some of these responses (*e.g.*, accelerations with fetal movement) are indicative of normal fetal status, whereas others (*e.g.*, variable deceleration with cord compression) are designed to compensate for alterations in cardiovascular dynamics. Both periodic and nonperiodic changes require careful evaluation for the diagnosis of fetal stress and distress.

Accelerations. Transient increases of the FHR (>15 bpm for >15 sec) have been noted during labor since fetal monitoring was first used (Fig. 43-11). They are at times associated with contractions, but often are unrelated to UA. The outcome of fetuses demonstrating accelerations in labor has been uniformly good. It is believed that the increased FHR is due to transient discharges of the sympathetic nervous system. It has also been suggested that accelerations associated with contractions might be caused by partial compression of the cord, which results in selective occlusion of the umbilical vein and causes fetal hypotension and a transient increase in the FHR. The observation that accelerations are associated with fetal movement in the healthy fetus is the basis of the nonstress test (NST) for antepartal evaluation of the high-risk fetus.

Early Decelerations. Transient slowing of the FHR in a pattern that is almost a mirror image of the contractions is known as an *early deceleration*. These decelerations are believed to be related to the fetal head compression associated with the contraction, resulting in a parasympathetic discharge mediated by the vagus nerve. Parasympathetic stimulation results in slowing of the FHR. This pattern represents a normal response of the fetus to this stimulus and, in the absence of other periodic FHR changes, is associated with a uniformly good outcome.

Characteristically, these decelerations have a waveform that coincides with and resembles an inverted UC (Fig. 43-12). They are uniform in shape, of short duration, and of low amplitude. The FHR at the *nadir* (lowest point) of the deceleration is usually 100 bpm or greater. When slower FHRs are observed with contractions, the decelerations are usually of the variable type (see below). Early decelerations do not respond to oxygen administered to the mother or to position change.

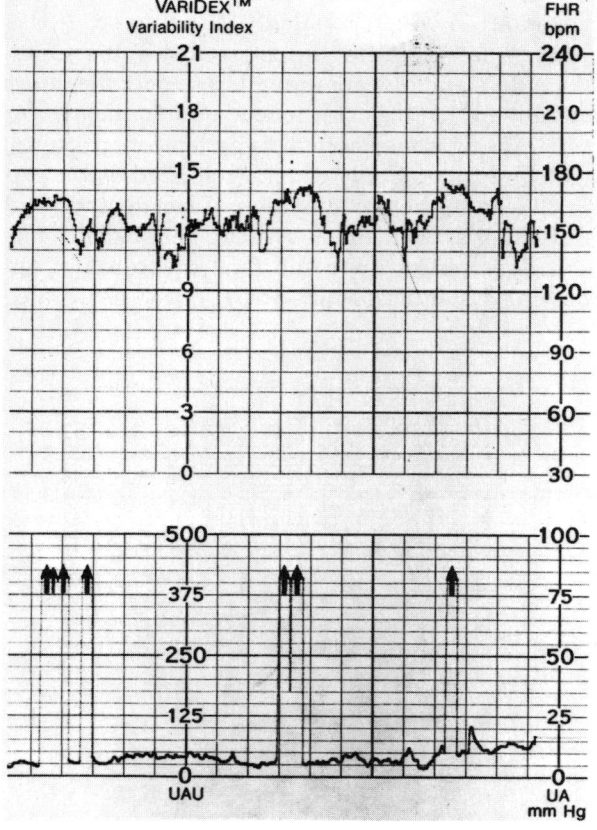

FIGURE 43-11

Transient accelerations of fetal heart rate noted during NST. Arrows were made by the client to indicate when fetal movements were perceived.

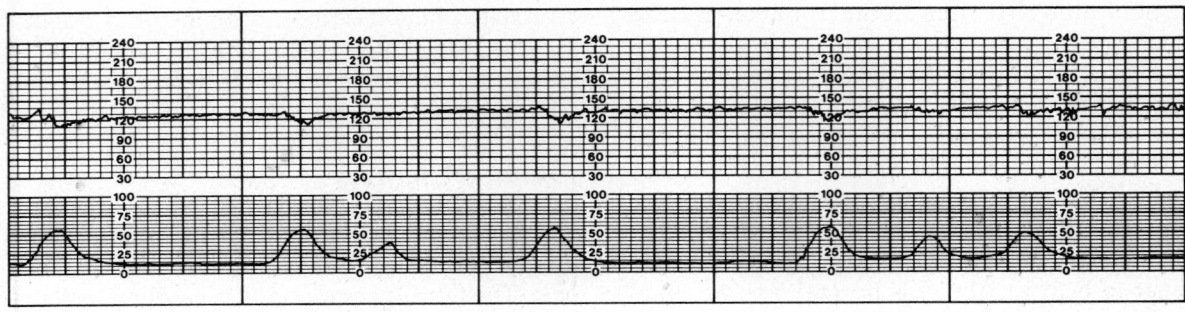

FIGURE 43-12

Early deceleration. The FHR baseline is in the normal range, with diminished variability. Uterine activity is normal with oxytocin augmentation. Early deceleration patterns are evident, approximating a mirror image of the uterine pressure curve. The nadir of the early deceleration occurs at the same time as the peak of the uterine contraction. (Parer JT, Puttler OL Jr, Freeman RK: In Freeman RK (ed): A Clinical Approach to Fetal Monitoring. San Leandro, CA, Berkeley Bio-Engineering, 1974)

They may be abolished when atropine (a vagolytic agent) is administered. However, because of the benign nature of this pattern, remedial action is not necessary.

Late Decelerations. Like the term *early decelerations,* the designation *late decelerations* indicates a uniform shape and a consistent relationship of the deceleration to contractions. In contrast to early decelerations, the onset of the late deceleration, its nadir, and its recovery do not coincide with the onset, amplitude, and recovery of the UC but rather are delayed (Fig. 43-13). Unlike variable decelerations, late decelerations may be quite subtle, entirely within the normal FHR range, and yet ominous. This is particularly true if FHR variability is absent or diminished. Several studies have demonstrated that subtle late decelerations accompanied by reduced heart rate variability are more likely to be associated with fetal acidosis than are more obvious late decelerations in which variability is preserved. A classification of late decelerations is given in Table 43-1.

Late decelerations are thought to reflect the effects of intermittent hypoxia on the fetal autonomic nervous system, causing transient fetal hypertension, triggering a vagally mediated bradycardia. Prolonged tissue hypoxia will lead to the accumulation of lactate and result in fetal acidosis. Such effects on acid–base balance may have a direct effect upon the fetal myocardium and conducting system, causing slowing of the heart rate.

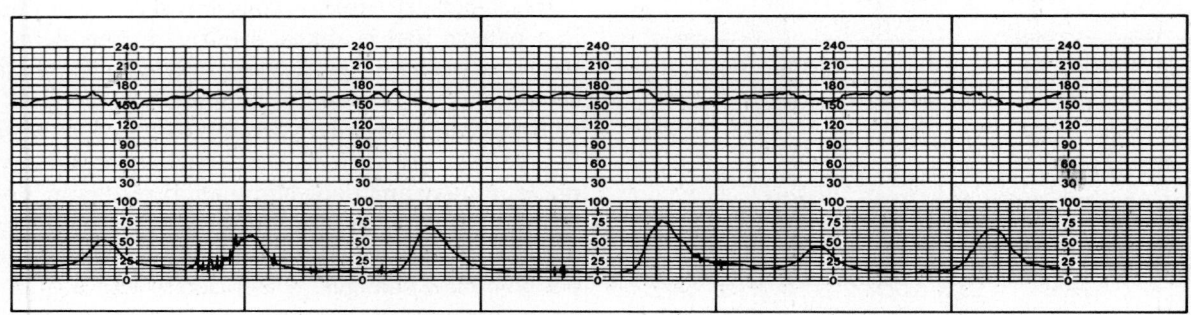

FIGURE 43-13

Moderate late deceleration. There is a mild fetal tachycardia, ranging between 160 and 170 beats per minute, with decreased variability. Uterine activity is normal. The nadir of late deceleration occurs when the uterine contraction is nearly over. A scalp capillary blood sample had been taken just prior to the first portion of this panel, and mild fetal acidosis was demonstrated, with scalp blood pH 7.21. (Parer JT, Puttler OL Jr, Freeman RK: In Freeman RK (ed): A Clinical Approach to Fetal Monitoring. San Leandro, CA, Berkeley Bio-Engineering, 1974)

TABLE 43-1

Principles of Grading Variable and Late Decelerations

	Criteria of Grading		
	Mild	*Moderate*	*Severe*
Variable deceleration			
Level to which FHR drops and duration of deceleration	<30-sec duration irrespective of level >80 bpm irrespective of duration 70–80 bpm <60 sec	<70 bpm >30 <60 sec 70–80 bpm >60 sec	<70 bpm >60 sec
Late deceleration			
Amplitude of drop in FHR	<15 bpm	15–45 bpm	>45 bpm

The hypoxia reflected in late decelerations results from the reduced oxygen delivered by the placenta due to diminished intervillous blood flow that occurs with the UC. A direct and specific relationship between hypoxia and late decelerations has been demonstrated experimentally in monkeys. Hypoxia causing late decelerations may be elicited when less oxygen is delivered to the uterus (*e.g.*, with maternal hypoxia or hypotension), when abnormally strong UC occur (hypertonus), or when relative placental insufficiency exists (*e.g.*, intrauterine growth retardation or hypertensive disorders of pregnancy).

Transient late decelerations associated with maternal hypotension or uterine hypertonus that responds to remedial action are thought to signal fetal stress. Removing or correcting the stress often results in fetal recovery. On the other hand, a pattern of consistent and persistent late decelerations that do not respond to remedial measures suggests fetal distress and is often associated with hypoxia, acidosis, and low Apgar scores at birth. This latter group of findings, of course, indicates prompt delivery.

Variable Decelerations. Variable deceleration is the most commonly observed FHR change during labor. The nomenclature of this pattern is based on the fact that the relationships of these decelerations to the contractions and the waveform are both variable (Fig. 43-14). These decelerations represent a reflex response to umbilical cord compression. They are often observed in association with UC, a situation in which cord compression is more likely to occur; the cord can be wrapped around the fetal trunk, the neck, or an extremity. They may also represent compression of the cord against the uterine wall during a contraction. Variable decelerations are often seen when oligohydramnios is present. This is a circumstance during which the cord is particularly vulnerable. When the umbilical cord is compressed, fetal peripheral resistance rises. The fetal

(text continued on page 966)

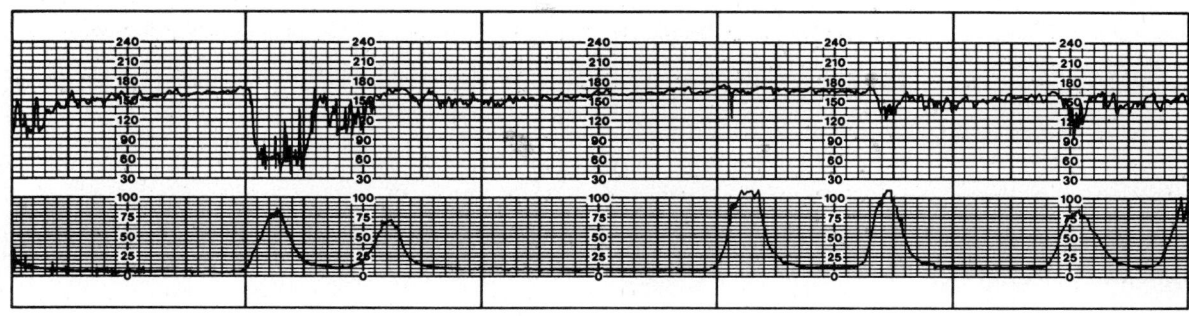

FIGURE 43-14

Severe variable deceleration. There is a mild fetal tachycardia with normal baseline variability. Uterine activity is normal. The deceleration is corrected by changing the client's position. Subsequent deceleration patterns are much less severe. (Parer JT, Puttler OL Jr, Freeman RK: In Freeman RK (ed): A Clinical Approach to Fetal Monitoring. San Leandro, CA, Berkeley Bio-Engineering, 1974)

The Woman Participating in Intrapartum Fetal Monitoring

Nursing Objectives
1. Determine if fetal monitoring is needed during labor.
2. Use careful monitoring to determine status of fetus.
3. Assist in delivering a healthy baby in the best possible way.
4. Provide supportive care to mother and father.

Assessment	Potential Nursing Diagnosis	Planning/Intervention	Evaluation
Determination of need for electronic fetal monitoring (EFM)			
Assess current maternal physical status	Potential for injury (fetal distress) related to unexpected factors	Review maternal records and fetal data if available Check maternal vital signs and question regarding maternal subjective impressions and observations regarding physical status	Mother's data is within normal limits; EFM may not be needed Mother's data shows prenatal factors associated with possible fetal distress; monitor is indicated
Assess labor progress		Review chart and question mother regarding onset and quality of contractions, condition of the membranes and other pertinent data Observe for behavioral manifestation of normal/abnormal labor progress Report and record as necessary (this to be done as indicated throughout)	Mother's assessment indicates abnormal labor pattern; monitor is indicated
Assess FHR Assess amniotic fluid at time of rupture of membranes		Auscultate FHR Observe or review records as to quality and quantity	FHR abnormalities; apply monitor Scant, excessive, or meconium-stained fluid may indicate fetal disease, abnormality, or distress; monitor indicated
Assess couple's knowledge of EFM	Knowledge deficit of fetal monitoring related to purpose	Review records for evidence of prenatal preparation classes Question couple, allowing time for feedback	Couple exhibits satisfactory knowledge

Assessment indicates application of EFM	Knowledge deficit of fetal monitoring procedures related to lack of interest or opportunity to discuss prior to this time	Apply EFM—external or internal as indicated
		  Explain (or reexplain) rationale for use
		  Explain methods to be used
			Parents understand rationale for use, procedure for monitoring, and interpretation of EFM data
			
			Parents participate in decision making

(continued)

Assessment	Potential Nursing Diagnosis	Planning/Intervention	Evaluation
		Apply monitor so that mother is comfortable; explain about position changes	Mother is comfortable and understands need for position changes
		Place monitor in mother's view; review initial tracings	Mother understands timing for breathing and relaxation techniques
		Review tracings with parents periodically; answer *all* questions	Parents understand labor course
			Parents observe labor progress with data
Problem Assessment			
Determine baseline bradycardia by strip review and observations of mother's verbal and behavioral input	Fear of possible loss of fetus related to unknown outcome	Evaluate FECG; identify arrhythmia	Client appreciates support of nurse
	Powerlessness related to outcome	Review tracing for periodic deceleration and baseline variability	Client discusses fears
	Alteration in comfort: pain related to immobility	Review record for drugs	Client understands and asks for comfort measures
		Institute remedial measures for fetal distress	Client understands possible outcomes and verbalizes
		Turn to left lateral recumbent position	Client asks questions concerning procedures
		Discontinue oxytocin if applicable	Support person is a comfort to the woman
		Administer O_2 by mask	
		Report and record verbally and in writing	
		Remain with client; institute primary nursing (one-to-one); answer questions	
		Comfort measures as necessary	
		Be alert for possible deterioration	
		Review strips frequently and regularly	
		Confirm by auscultation	
		Evaluate FECG; identify arrhythmias	
		Take maternal temperature	
		Review drugs administered to mother	
		Review tracings for periodic decelerations and baseline variability	
		Institute remedial measures for fetal distress as outlined above	

(text continued from page 963)

pO_2 falls and pCO_2 rises. This triggers baroreceptors, which stimulate the vagus nerve and cause a fall in the FHR. The firing of the vagus nerve is erratic, resulting in the variable onset, shape, severity, and duration of the contraction. The sudden hypoxia from cord compression may trigger aortic arch chemoreceptors also playing a role in the pathogenesis of these decelerations.

Variable decelerations may be classified as mild, moderate, or severe (see Table 43-1). Because there is a correlation between the severity of variable decelerations and fetal condition, it is important that the nurse evaluate the frequency, depth, and duration of these decelerations.

The variable decelerations must be judged in context with the entire fetal tracing. What is the baseline FHR? Has it shifted upward or downward during the course of labor? Is the baseline variability acceptable? The answers to these questions will help the nurse and physician decide whether these variable decelerations are the harbinger of poor fetal outcome or whether they represent a period of transient cord compression. Anytime a fetus experiences repetitive variable decelerations, the nurse should take initiative and institute maternal position change in an attempt to relieve the cord compression. The usual first move is to roll the client in the left lateral recumbent position. If this is ineffective, other position changes should be attempted to relieve the decelerations. If the client is receiving oxytocin and persistent, severe variable decelerations are present, oxytocin infusion should be stopped until the physician has the opportunity to evaluate the tracing.

Mild variable decelerations are usually of little clinical significance. Moderate and severe variable decelerations can cause a significant reduction in umbilical blood flow, resulting in an increase in fetal pCO_2 and a transient respiratory acidosis. Repetitive severe variable decelerations can result in fetal metabolic acidosis.

This requires early intervention by the physician. Therefore, with repetitive moderate and severe variable decelerations, fetal scalp sampling or delivery should be performed.

Sinusoidal Pattern.   An unusual abnormality in FHR in which there is a repetitive undulation of the baseline resembling a "sine wave" has been called a *sinusoidal pattern* (Fig. 43-15). Occasionally, tracings of a normal fetus appear to have a transient sinusoidal pattern. This has not been correlated with any particular fetal abnormality. On occasion, a persistent sinusoidal pattern is indicative of fetal hypoxia or severe fetal anemia. The latter is most frequently observed in fetuses suffering from hydrops fetalis due to Rh isoimmunization.

Severe fetal anemia can also be seen in cases of fetal–maternal hemorrhage. This can occur spontaneously from a chronic placental abruption or following transplacental amniocentesis.

The pathophysiology of the development of a sinusoidal pattern is not understood. It has been hypothesized that this pattern may reflect an absence of autonomic nervous control over the FHR due to severe hypoxia. This pattern has been observed, and is considered ominous in the hydropic fetus.

Nursing Diagnosis

A variety of nursing diagnoses may be made through the various stages of intrapartum fetal monitoring. Examples are anxiety related to perceived loss of fetus; alterations in comfort; pain related to position or equipment used in monitoring; ineffective individual coping related to an unsatisfactory support system; knowledge deficit of monitoring procedures related to inability to concentrate/understand nurses' instructions; power-

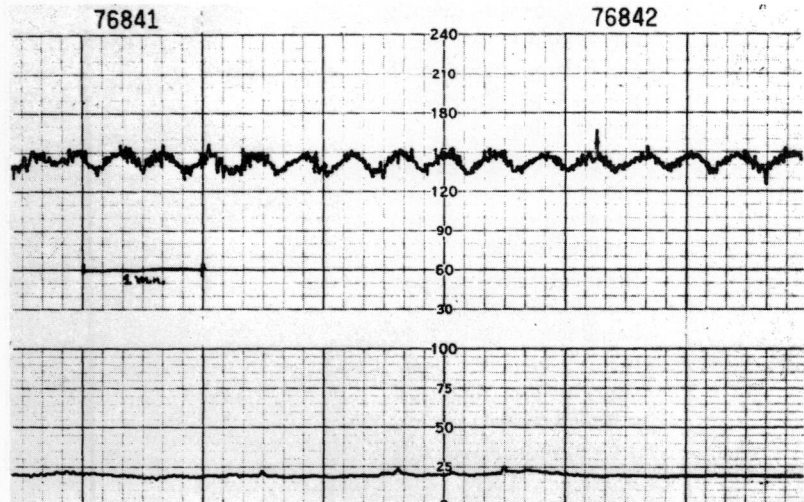

F I G U R E   4 3 - 1 5

Fetal heart rate tracing demonstrating sinusoidal pattern prior to labor. The fetus was severely anemic owing to Rhesus isoimmunization.

lessness related to being confined to bed by monitoring equipment.

Nursing Intervention: Remedial Measures for Fetal Distress

Abnormalities in FHR Tracing

The keys to excellent nursing care in the client with abnormalities in the FHR tracing are careful attention to detail and fast, calm action. Early decelerations do not usually require intervention.

In the event of repetitive late decelerations, oxytocin should be discontinued if it is being used. Oxygen should be delivered by face mask at 5 to 6 liters/min. Maternal blood pressure should be ascertained. If the client is hypotensive, an attempt should be made to physiologically raise the blood pressure. This can be accomplished by maternal position change and increasing the rate of intravenous crystalloid infusion. If the client has received regional anesthesia and this has caused hypotension, an anesthesiologist should be summoned so that an appropriate vasopressor agent can be administered.

In the event of repetitive late decelerations that do not correct with the above measures, fetal scalp sampling should be performed quickly or delivery should be effected.

If severe variable decelerations occur, the same steps should be taken as in the case of late decelerations. Also, an immediate vaginal examination should be done to rule out an occult prolapse of the umbilical cord. If cord prolapse is found, the fetal head should be elevated vaginally and the client placed in the Trendelenburg or knee–chest position and taken to the delivery room immediately.

Impaired Maternal Oxygen Delivery

Impaired delivery of maternal oxygen may result from a number of maternal disorders. Maternal pulmonary dysfunction, associated with an acute severe asthmatic attack, amniotic fluid embolism, thromboembolism, tonic–clonic seizure, or general anesthesia, may result in maternal hypoxia delivering less oxygen to the placenta and fetus. Heart failure and hypotension can keep normally oxygenated blood from reaching the uterus. Hypotension may be caused by maternal blood loss, compression of the vena cava by the gravid uterus, or autonomic blockade associated with conduction anesthesia.

When maternal oxygen uptake or delivery of oxygen to the uterus is impaired, oxygen should be administered by mask and the mother turned to the left lateral recumbent position. This position displaces the gravid uterus off of the inferior vena cava, thus promoting venous return to the heart and improved cardiovascular function. Then, if necessary, pharmacologic correction of the respiratory, cardiac, or autonomic disorder can be initiated.

Impaired Placental Exchange of Oxygen

The cause of impaired placental oxygen exchange may be placental insufficiency. This may be caused by excessively strong contractions that either occur spontaneously or are caused by hyperstimulation with oxytocin. Such contractions result in transient interruption of blood flow in the intervillous space and thus diminish oxygen exchange. When this occurs, administration of oxytocin should be discontinued if it is being used. Improving maternal oxygenation and oxygen delivery by administration of oxygen and use of the left lateral position are also helpful. Uteroplacental insufficiency may also be seen in intrauterine growth retardation, placental abruption, and post-dates pregnancy.

Impaired Fetal Circulation or Oxygen Transport

Cord compression is the most common example. In this situation, prolapse of the cord should be determined rapidly by perineal inspection and vaginal examination. This complication requires prompt delivery, usually by cesarean section. When there is evidence of cord compression, the previously mentioned measures should be initiated (*i.e.,* maternal oxygen administration, left lateral position, and discontinuation of oxytocics). Positions other than left lateral (*e.g.,* right lateral or knee–chest) may also be useful in alleviating variable decelerations and should be tried when the pattern does not respond to the initial remedial measures. Fetal oxygen transport to the tissues may also be impaired when there is severe fetal anemia, as is seen in Rh isoimmunization and fetal–maternal hemorrhage. When the fetal tracing does not respond to appropriate nursing measures, the physician may elect to obtain a fetal scalp pH determination or proceed with immediate delivery.

Psychological Aspects of Fetal Monitoring

Fetal monitoring can occasionally have important psychological impact on the clients. It is hoped that the need for fetal monitoring has been discussed with the client before the onset of labor. If it has not, this task may fall upon the labor room nurse. It is important to

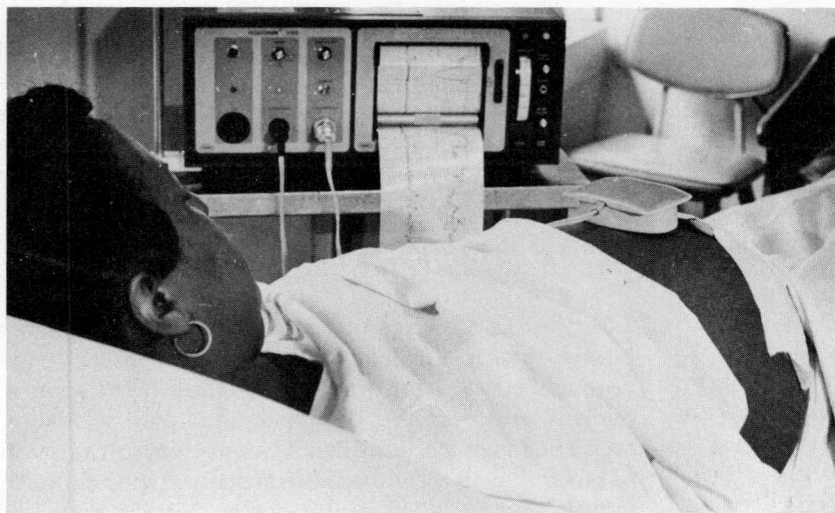

FIGURE 43-16

Client with external fetal monitor applied. Note that the monitor function can be observed by the client.

stress to the parents that the purpose of monitoring is to detect any evidence of fetal distress before the fetus is damaged, *not* because the physician feels that the fetus is already in danger. This will usually alleviate much of the client's fear. The nurse must make the client aware that the FHR is consistently changing and that there is a wide range of normal variation. The nurse must also assure the client that with external FHR tracing, movement by the mother or fetus can cause a temporary loss of the FHR on the monitor. The client must know that this is a mechanical phenomenon and does not reflect a real loss of the FHR. Often the nurse is also called upon to explain to the client that internal monitoring is safe for the fetus.

Because most clients desire to observe the monitor tracing, the equipment should be placed in view of the mother, father, and nurse (Fig. 43-16). Couples often find that observing the onset and decrement (downslope) of the contractions is useful in applying breathing techniques. This is particularly true for the father. The reassurance obtained from observing or listening to the fetal heartbeat during labor is often a secondary benefit to the couple.

Fetal monitoring requires a nurse who is professional, composed, and diplomatic. The nurse must be ready to take initiative. If an abnormal FHR pattern is noted, the nurse must take immediate action and at the same time allay the client's anxiety and notify the physician. Also, should scalp pH sampling or cesarean delivery become necessary, the nurse must exert a calming influence on the client while helping prepare her and equipment for the appropriate procedure.

Indeed, the responsibility of helping the mother cope with the psychological aspects of fetal monitoring usually rests with the labor nurse. This individual must be a competent, compassionate, secure individual who can help the client understand the purpose of and pro-

cedures involved in fetal monitoring. This individual should also be able to act swiftly in the event of an emergency and still maintain the client's confidence and allay her fears.

Suggested Reading

Freeman RK, Garite TJ: Fetal Heart Rate Monitoring. Baltimore, William & Wilkins, 1981

Goodlin RC: History of fetal monitoring. Am J Obstet Gynecol 133:323, 1979

Hess OW: Impact of electronic fetal monitoring on obstetric management. JAMA 244:682, 1982

MacDonald D, Grant A, Sheridan-Pereitra M et al: The Dublin randomized controlled trial of intrapartum fetal heart rate monitoring. Am J Obstet Gynecol 152:524, 1985

Perkins R: Evidence of fetal jeopardy in the intrapartum period. In Bishop EH, Cefalo RC (eds): Signs and Symptoms in Disorders of Pregnancy, pp 159–174. Philadelphia, JB Lippincott, 1983

Westgren M, Holmquist P, Svenningsen NW et al: Intrapartum fetal monitoring in preterm deliveries: Prospective study. Obstet Gynecol 60:99, 1982

Yeh SY, Diaz F, Paul RH: Ten-year experience at intrapartum fetal monitoring in Los Angeles County/University of Southern California Medical Center. Am J Obstet Gynecol 143:496, 1982

Young DC, Gray JH, Luther EK et al: Fetal scalp blood pH sampling: Its value in an active obstetric unit. Am J Obstet Gynecol 136:276, 1980

Zanini B, Paul RH, Huey JR: Intrapartum fetal heart rate: Correlation of scalp pH in the preterm fetus. Am J Obstet Gynecol 136:43, 1980

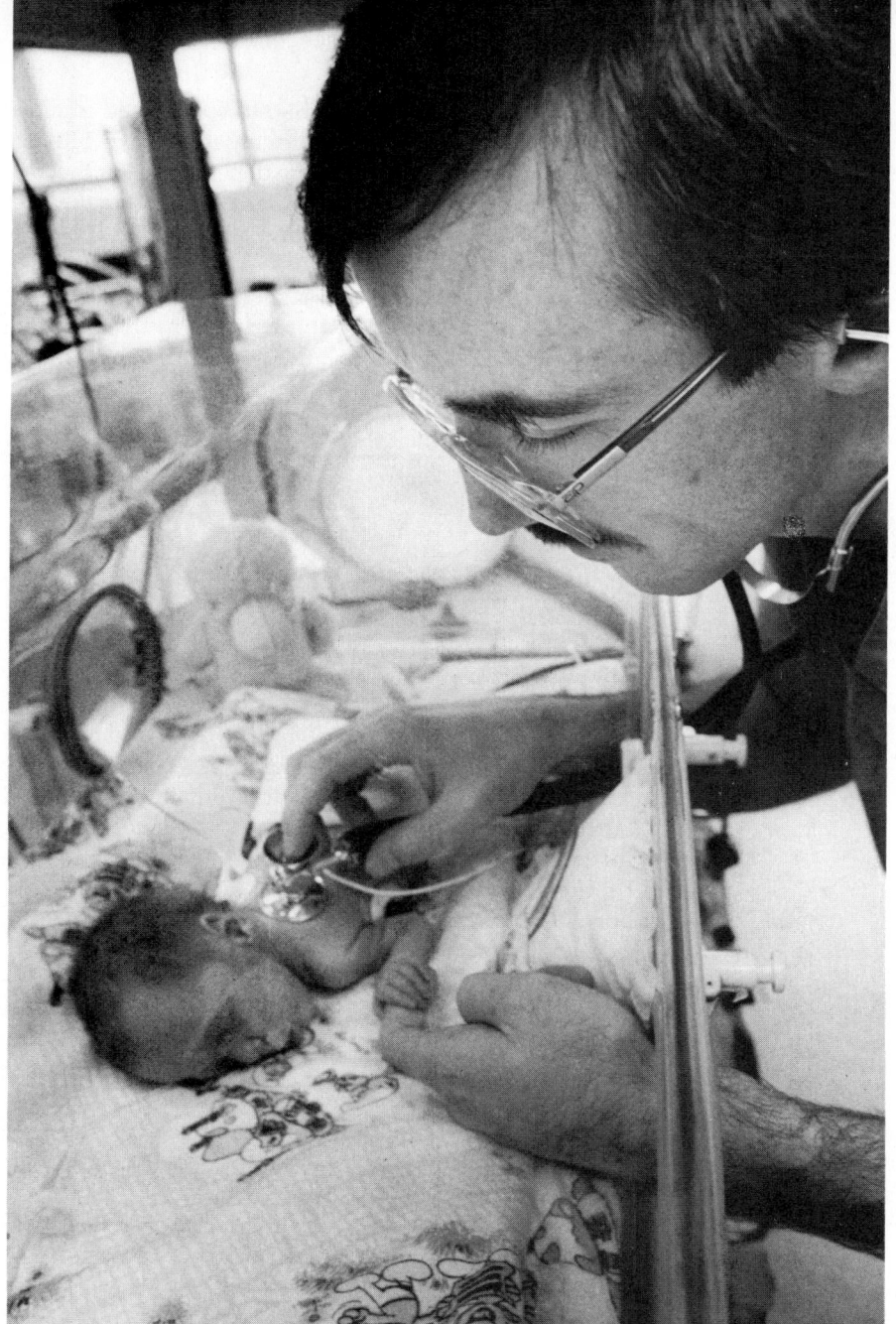

CHAPTER 44

The High-Risk Infant: Disorders of Gestational Age and Birth Weight

The particular, precise, and highly specialized practice of neonatal nursing could cover an entire text. The neonate and the family's complete dependence on the skill of the primary caretaker, the neonatal nurse, makes her task that much more demanding, challenging, rewarding, stressful, and draining.

From the time of birth, resuscitation, stabilization, possible transport, and continued care in the neonatal intensive care unit (NICU), the neonate is cared for by an ever-vigilant specialized team.

Overview

Disorders of Gestational Age and Birth Weight

The size of an infant at birth is influenced by many factors that affect the maternal and fetal environments. The relationship between low birth weight and perinatal morbidity and mortality has long been recognized. Only recently, however, have the different implications of birth weight relative to gestational age been established. Infants of low birth weight may be of appropriate size for their gestational age but immature because they are born before pregnancy has progressed to full term. These infants are classically "premature"—born before their organ systems have matured to the point of physiological functioning. Other low-birth-weight infants may be undersized for the length of their gestation, whether delivered before or at term. These infants are called *small for gestational age*. Often they are physiologically mature but have not attained the size and weight appropriate for gestational age for numerous reasons.

Infants experiencing disorders of gestational age and birth weight also include those who are large for gestational age and who are postmature—born after pregnancy has progressed beyond full term. The associated problems and potential causes are different among these various types of altered fetal growth, requiring individualized assessment and approaches to management. The particular causes of alterations in fetal growth also determine the newborn's immediate and long-term prognosis. The challenge to effective assessment and management of fetal growth disorders begins with an understanding of the intricate and complex mechanisms that control normal fetal growth.

Classification of Infants by Birth Weight and Gestational Age

In the past, all newborns weighing 2500 g or less were termed premature and those weighing more were designated full term. This approach assumed that intra-

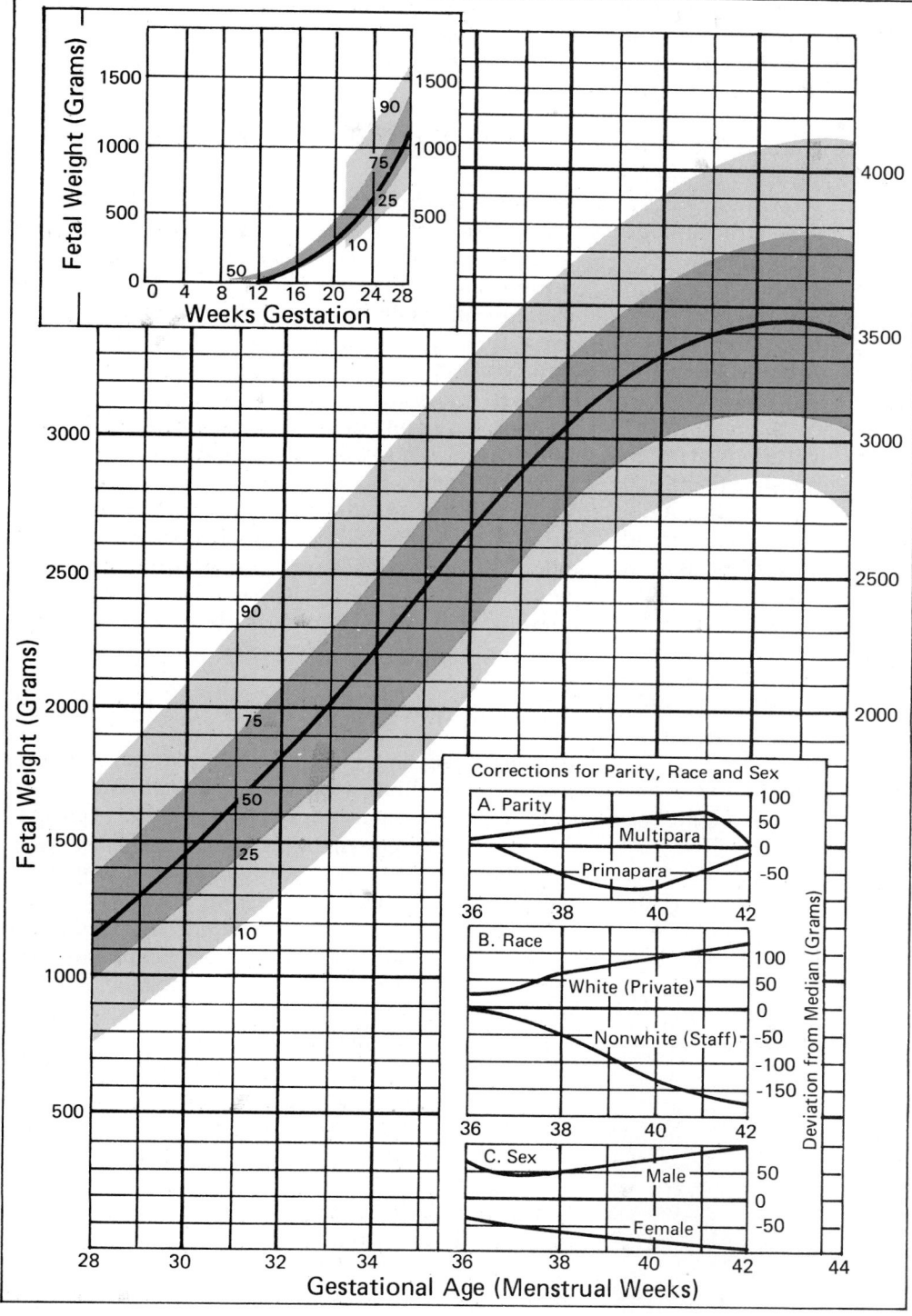

FIGURE 44-1

Fetal weight. The 10th, 25th, 50th, 75th, and 90th percentiles of fetal weight in grams throughout pregnancy and correction factors for parity, race (socioeconomic status), and sex are graphed. Data obtained from 31,202 prostaglandin-induced abortions and spontaneous deliveries. (Courtesy of Brenner WE, Edelman DA, Hendricks CH: A standard of fetal growth for the United States of America. Am J Obstet Gynecol 126: 555–564, 1976)

uterine growth rates were essentially the same for all fetuses and that birth weight corresponded to gestational age. A considerable amount of data has now accumulated to demonstrate the inaccuracy of this assumption, and the two dimensions of *birth weight* and *gestational age* are now considered separately.

The World Health Organization (WHO) has designated a *term birth* as one occurring between 38 weeks' and 42 weeks' gestation, with age calculated from the date of the onset of the mother's last menstrual period. WHO advises that newborns not be classified as *premature* on the basis of weight alone. Gestational age must be used to assign categories of preterm, term, and post-term births. Also, it must be recognized that an infant weighing less than 2500 g is not necessarily premature.

Intrauterine growth standards are used to compare an infant's weight and gestational age with population averages. Although these have shortcomings in application to particular situations (*e.g.,* differences in weight due to race, parity, sex, altitude), they are useful as guides in the assessment of high-risk infants. The most widely used growth chart was developed in Colorado and gives percentiles of intrauterine growth for weight, length, and head circumference. However, the altitude effects made this estimate low for the rest of the country. A more recent fetal growth chart includes correction factors for parity, race, and sex and presents average fetal weights for the 10th, 25th, 50th, 75th, and 90th percentiles (Fig. 44-1). Infants may be classified in any one of nine groups (Fig. 44-2).

Weight serves in the assessment of growth, and gestational age in the assessment of maturity. An infant born at 40 weeks' gestation and weighing less than 2500 g (below the 10th percentile for weight or length) would be mature but undergrown. This disorder is called *intrauterine growth retardation*, with the infant classified as *small for gestational age* (SGA). An infant born at 36 weeks' gestation and weighing 3500 g (above the 90th percentile for weight) would be immature but overgrown. Such *large for gestational age* (LGA) infants are typical for diabetic mothers. Although this infant has attained average term weight, it is actually premature, with incomplete maturation of organ systems.

The term *premature* seems appropriate for the *preterm*, immature infant, regardless of birth weight. Preterm infants are those infants born before 37 weeks' gestation. Preterm infants may also be SGA, implying that at least two factors are involved, that causing the early delivery and that retarding the growth rate *in utero*.

The term *low-birth-weight infant* defines any live-born infant weighing 2500 g or less. A *very-low-birth-weight infant* weighs 1500 g or less (Figs. 44-3 and 44-4).

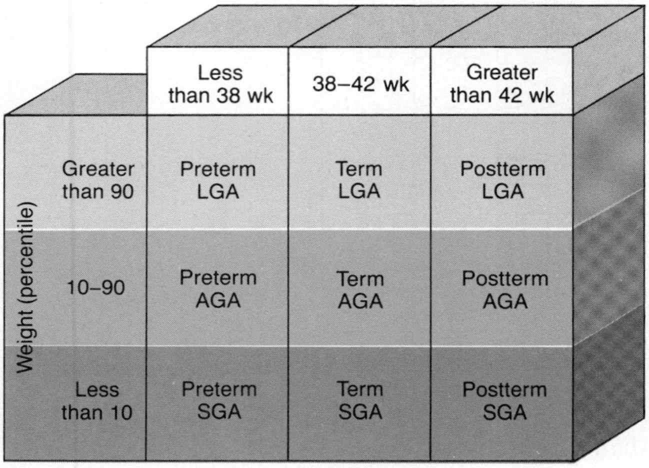

Factors That Affect Fetal Growth

Fetal growth is influenced by a variety of factors of maternal, placental, and fetal origin. Genetic predispositions, the mother's nutritional and health status, fetal nutrition, fetal and maternal endocrine functions, developmental insults, environmental stressors, and placental function are variably involved in this process. Maturation is affected by biochemical determinants, enzymes, genes, and hormones, particularly adrenal and thyroid. Development of the various organs follows a different time sequence, with hormonal action triggering a certain organ to grow and mature at a particular time during gestation. As different organs mature at different times, there are critical periods when stressors can significantly alter normal development. After these critical periods, the organ is less susceptible to damage and more capable of functioning in the extrauterine environment.

Maternal Factors

Although genetic factors certainly play an important role in determining fetal measurements and weight, other environmental influences have also been associated with fetal growth. Maternal nutritional status, as measured by prepregnancy weight and the slow steady weight gain experienced during pregnancy, is a definitive influencing factor. (See Chap. 21 for further discussion on adequate maternal nutrition to promote fetal growth.) Adjunct risk factors in this area include those women who are experiencing malnutrition for various reasons, pregnant adolescents, women of low socioeconomic status, women with low pregnancy weight or inadequate weight gain during pregnancy, women having frequent pregnancies, and women who have delivered other infants of low birth weight.[1]

Pregnancy-induced hypertension poses a threat to fetal growth since it promotes a decrease in uterine blood flow. (See Chap. 36 for more discussion of this maternal syndrome.) Advanced maternal diabetes mellitus and its accompanying vascular insufficiency promote intrauterine growth retardation.

Substance abuse of alcohol and heroin has been correlated with decreased fetal growth. The use of prescribed drugs such as propranolol, warfarin, and steroids has also been correlated with SGA infants. Cigarette smoking is directly related to SGA births, with the number of cigarettes smoked and the duration of smoking implicated in the fetal weight result. Birth weight is decreased on the average of 170 g as a result of 10

FIGURE 44-2

Birth weight–gestational age groups as defined by Lubchenko and co-workers. (Clewell WH: Prematurity. J Reprod Med 23(5):237–244, 1979)

Weight (percentile)	Less than 38 wk	38–42 wk	Greater than 42 wk
Greater than 90	Preterm LGA	Term LGA	Postterm LGA
10–90	Preterm AGA	Term AGA	Postterm AGA
Less than 10	Preterm SGA	Term SGA	Postterm SGA

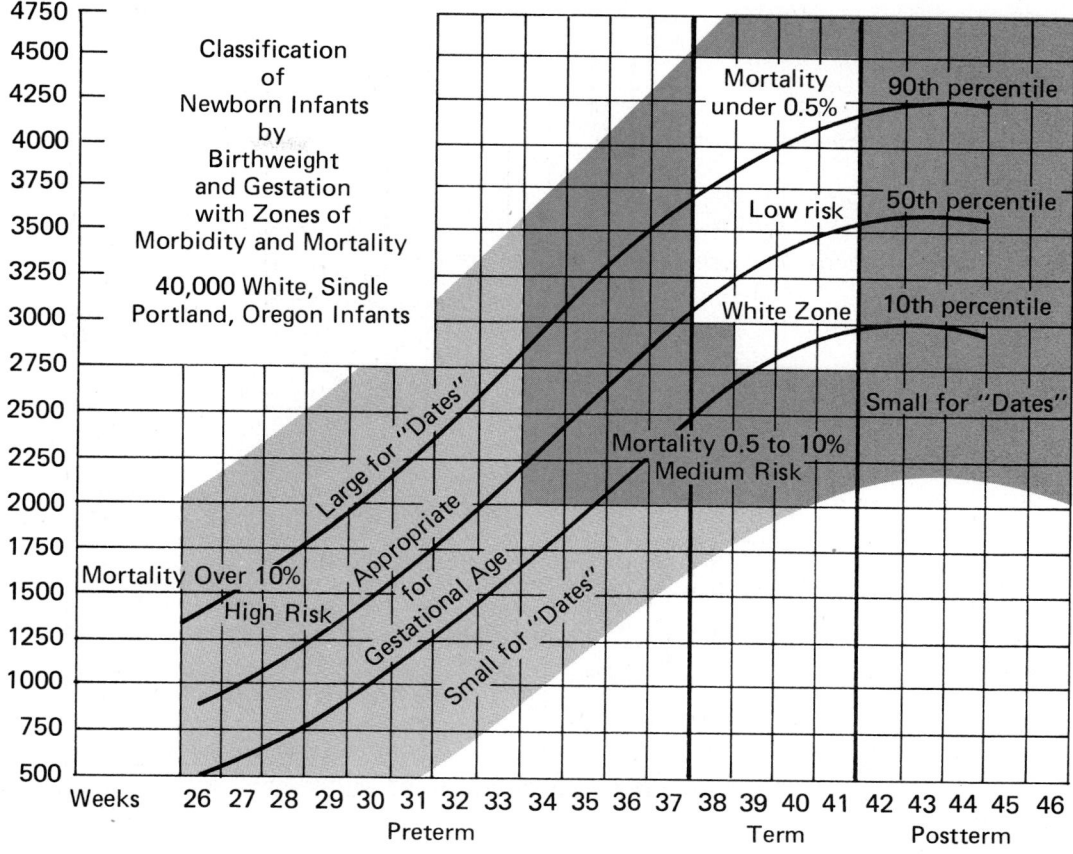

Weeks — Preterm — Term — Postterm

FIGURE 44-3

Classification of newborn by birth weight and gestation with areas of morbidity and mortality. (Babson SG, Benson RC, Pernoll ML, Benda GI: Management of High-Risk Pregnancy and Intensive Care of the Neonate. St Louis, CV Mosby, 1975)

cigarettes smoked a day and 300 g as a result of 15 cigarettes smoked a day.[1]

It has been demonstrated that infants born at higher altitudes experience decreased birth weight as a result of the decrease in oxygen tension.

Placental Influences

Under normal conditions, the size of the placenta is a major determinant of fetal size. When there is severe maternal nutritional deprivation, it appears that the maintenance needs of the placenta are met first, leading to reduction of fetal growth. In a fetus with growth retardation, however, the placenta is relatively smaller than with a normally growing fetus of the same gestational age. This is associated with higher levels of asphyxia at birth and perinatal morbidity seen among SGA infants. Placental mechanisms for maintaining optimal transfer of nutrients and gases between maternal and fetal blood are necessary for an adequate supply of growth-promoting substances to the fetus. The dif-

fusion capacity of the placenta increases proportionately with fetal weight during pregnancy. Any impairment of oxygen transfer has a deleterious effect on fetal growth. Transfers of minerals, electrolytes, and trace metals, which are necessary in an adequate supply for proper fetal growth, are also related to placental function.[2]

There appears to be no single placental abnormality common to infants who are SGA, and placental and cord defects are present in only a small number of cases. When lesions are present, the most common are infarction, villous avascularity, fibrinosis, premature aging, and nonspecific chronic villous inflammation.

Fetal Endocrine Influences

The hypothalamic-pituitary axis acts through the pancreas to modify fetal growth. This is an interactional situation between mother and fetus. In the normal-birth-weight fetus of a normal mother, the pancreas has 2% endocrine tissue with 40% beta cells. In infants

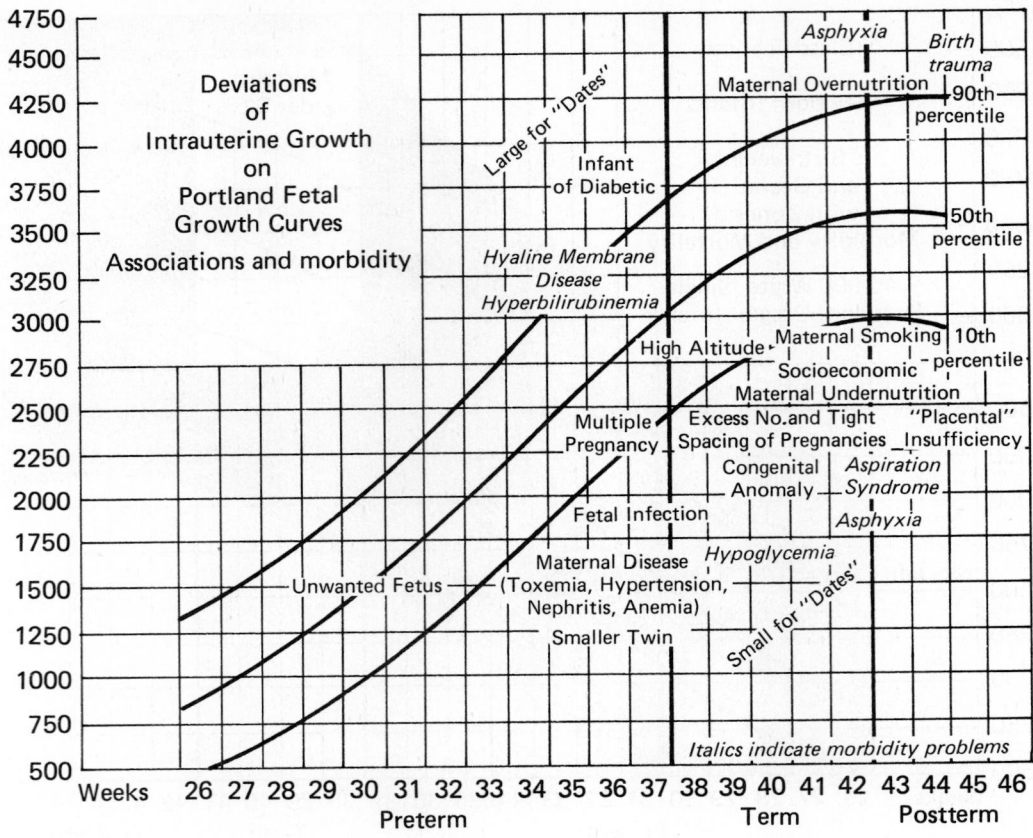

FIGURE   44-4

Intrauterine growth curves and associations with perinatal mortality and morbidity. (Babson SG, Benson RC, Pernoll ML, Benda GI: Management of High-Risk Pregnancy and Intensive Care of the Neonate. St Louis, CV Mosby, 1975)

of gestational diabetic mothers, endocrine tissue is 10% with 60% beta cells, leading to significantly higher fetal insulin levels. The percentages of endocrine tissue and insulin levels are directly proportional to the excess fetal weight observed in infants of diabetic mothers. There appears to be a competitive effect between adrenal cortical hormones and insulin. This relates to lung maturation and the formation of surfactant. Cortisol slows cell growth but enhances antagonist to glucocorticoids. This effect seems related to the higher incidence of respiratory distress syndrome (RDS) in infants of diabetic mothers. A similar relationship between insulin levels and glucocorticoids occurs with enzyme and glucose metabolism in the liver. Insulin, acting unopposed in the fetus, directly influences cytoplasmic growth and increases triglyceride concentrations in the brain, liver, and lung.[2]

Thyroid and adrenal hormones are important to fetal maturation. Inadequate levels of thyroid hormone are associated with decreased fetal size, delayed skeletal ossification, delayed maturation, and mental retardation. Infants of hyperthyroid mothers may have advanced neurologic development for gestational age, greater body weight, greater placental weight, and advanced skeletal development. They appear several weeks older than their gestational age. Corticosteroids are used to induce organ maturation, for instance, to promote lung maturation. They also affect maturation of the foregut (absorption of antibodies), pancreas, liver, and small bowel. Liver glycogen depends on the presence of corticosteroids. It is possible that growth hormone may play a role in brain growth. Somatomedins (growth hormone ancillary factors) may be important in cell multiplication in the fetus, as high levels are found in large infants at birth and low levels are found in SGA infants. Through an endocrine chain, hormonal regulation of fetal growth may be finely regulated by the central nervous system.[2]

Other Fetal Factors

Infants of multiple gestation have a more pronounced decrease in growth late in the third trimester. Certain congenital malformations, chromosomal disorders, and congenital infections promote intrauterine growth retardation. Examples of such disorders are trisomies 8, 13, 18, and 21, congenital heart disease, and rubella.

Assessment (Identification) of the High-Risk Neonate

Although the causes of prematurity and altered fetal growth are not completely understood, several associated factors have been identified that alert nurses and physicians to the possibility of these problems. Early recognition of mothers with high-risk pregnancies and careful prenatal care can often contribute to a better outcome for the infant and the mother.

Many of the factors contributing to the birth of a high-risk infant are not specific for a particular problem or condition, but are generally related to increased morbidity and mortality. Others have specific associations with neonatal disorders or fetal abnormalities. Those related to prematurity include diabetes, placental insufficiency, multiple pregnancy, preeclampsia and hypertensive disorders, and infection. Several overlap with increased incidence of SGA infants, including preeclampsia and hypertensive disorders, placental insufficiency, infections, discordant twin, and altitude. Congenital anomalies are more highly correlated to term SGA infants.

Chapter 32 covers assessment of gestational age. Assessment considerations related to SGA and LGA neonates may be found in those sections of this chapter. Factors associated with high-risk infants are listed in Table 44-1.

Small-for-Gestational-Age Infants (Intrauterine Growth Retardation)

Significance of Gestational Age

Infants whose weights fall below the 10th percentile for their gestational age have experienced impairment of the normal growth process during the prenatal period. Some physicians use the limiting criterion of birth weight of two standard deviations below the mean of gestational age. This condition may occur at any gestational age, but the majority of SGA infants are born at, or close to, term and weigh less than 2500 g. Under the old classification, these would have been called *premature*, although their period of intrauterine life was not significantly shortened. Though small, these infants are mature in comparison with infants of similar weight but lower gestational age.

Growth-retarded infants have an increased risk of perinatal morbidity and mortality and are estimated to account for about 25% of the entire perinatal mortality.[3] The infant's condition is a product of a process of intrauterine deprivation that begins many weeks before birth. It is often related to abnormalities of the pregnancy or of the fetus.

There are two types of intrauterine growth retardation, which may occur separately or simultaneously. Fetal growth involves both an increase in the number of cells (hyperplasia) and an increase in the size of cells (hypertrophy). Embryonic growth involves a rapid increase in the number of cells as the organs and body structures are formed. These cells increase in size later in pregnancy. If an insult to the fetus occurs early in gestation, mitosis is impaired and fewer new cells are formed. This results in small organs of subnormal weight. The cells, however, are of normal size. If interference with growth occurs later, the cells are normal in number but smaller in size, again resulting in smaller organs, but in this instance due to reduced amounts of cytoplasm. An intrauterine insult throughout both phases of growth results in cells that are fewer in number and smaller in size. The classic example of the latter condition is the infant with the rubella syndrome.

Maternal preeclampsia, which tends to be more prominent during later pregnancy, creates the second type of growth retardation in which cell numbers are normal, but cell size is reduced.[4]

Assessment

Common physical characteristics of the SGA infant are listed below. However, assessment of gestational age according to physical characteristics may be altered or misleading for several reasons. Vernix is often decreased or absent. Consequently, the skin is more exposed to amniotic fluid. As a result, sole creases appear more mature than is actually true. Breast tissue formation is reduced in SGA infants. In females the adipose tissue covering the labia is decreased; thus, external genitalia appear less mature. In the SGA infant neurologic criteria tend to be more accurate than physical criteria.[1]

Physiological Problems

In adaptation to extrauterine life, the problems encountered by the SGA infant are different from those of the appropriate-for-gestational age, preterm infant. If the problem of poor growth *in utero* has been detected during pregnancy, nurses and physicians skilled in resuscitation should be present at delivery.

Certain disorders tend to occur more frequently in

TABLE 44-1

Identification of High-Risk Infant: Associated Factors

Antepartal Factors

Maternal Characteristics

Age under 15 or over 35
Low socioeconomic status
Unmarried
Family or marital conflicts
Emotional illness or family history of
   mental illness
Persistent ambivalence or conflicts
   about the pregnancy
Stature under 5 feet
20% underweight or overweight
Malnutrition

Reproductive History

Parity greater than 8
Two or more previous abortions
Previous stillborn or neonatal death
Previous premature labor or low-
   birth-weight infant (<2500 g)
Previous excessively large infant
   (>4000 g)
Infant with isoimmunization or ABO
   incompatibility
Infant with congenital anomaly,
   genetic disorder, or birth damage
Preeclampsia or eclampsia
Uterine fibroids >5 cm or submucous
Abnormal Pap smear
Infertility
Prior cesarean section
Prior fetal malpresentations
Contracted pelvis
Ovarian masses
Genital tract abnormalities
   (incompetent cervix, subseptate or
   bicornate uterus)
Pregnancy occurring 3 months or less
   after last delivery
Previous prolonged labor or significant
   dystocia

Substance Abuse

Drugs
Alcohol
Heavy smoking (>2 packs/day)

Medical Problems

Chronic hypertension
Renal disease (pyelonephritis,
   glomerulonephritis, polycystic
   kidney)
Diabetes mellitus (Classes B to F)
Heart disease (aortic insufficiency,
   pulmonary hypertension, diastolic
   murmur, cardiac enlargement, heart
   failure, arrhythmia)
Sickle cell trait or disease

Anemias with hemoglobin <9 g and
   hematocrit <32%
Pulmonary disease (tuberculosis,
   chronic obstructive pulmonary
   disease)
Endocrine disorders (hypothyroidism
   or hyperthyroidism, family history
   of cretinism, adrenal or pituitary
   problems)
Gastrointestional or liver disease
Epilepsy
Malignancy (including leukemia and
   Hodgkin's disease)

Complications of Present Pregnancy

Low or excessive weight gain
Hypertension (mean arterial pressure
   >90, blood pressure 140/90,
   increase >30 mmHg systolic or >20
   mm Hg diastolic)
Recurrent glycosuria and abnormal
   fasting blood sugar or glucose
   tolerance test
Uterine size inappropriate for
   gestational age (either too large or
   too small)
Recurrent urinary tract infections
Severe varicosities or thrombophlebitis
Recurrent vaginal bleeding
Premature rupture of membranes
Multiple pregnancy
Hydramnios with a single fetus
Rh negative with a rising titer
Late or no prenatal care
Exposure to teratogens (medications,
   x-ray, radioactive isotopes)
Viral infections (rubella,
   cytomegalovirus, herpes, mumps,
   rubeola, chickenpox, shingles,
   smallpox, vaccinia, influenza,
   poliomyelitis, hepatitis, Western
   equine encephalitis, coxsackie virus
   B)
Syphilis, especially late pregnancy
Bacterial infections (gonorrhea,
   tuberculosis, listeriosis, severe acute
   infection)
Protozoan infections (toxoplasmosis,
   malaria)
Postmaturity
Anemia with hemoglobin of 9 g or
   less
Severe preeclampsia, eclampsia
Abnormal contraction stress test
Falling urinary estriol levels

Intrapartum Factors

Complications of Labor and Delivery

Labor longer than 24 hours in
   primigravida

Labor longer than 12 hours in
   multigravida
Second stage longer than 1 hour
Ruptured membranes more than 24
   hours
Abnormal presentation or position
Heavy sedation or injudicious
   anesthesia
Maternal fever or infection
Placenta previa or abruptio placentae
Cesarean section
Meconium-stained amniotic fluid
Fetal distress caused by monitoring or
   scalp blood sampling
Prolapsed cord
High forceps or midforceps delivery,
   difficult or operative delivery
Premature labor
Severe preeclampsia, eclampsia
Precipitous labor less than 3 hours
Elective induction
Oxytocin (Pitocin) augmentation

Immediate Problems of Infant

Malformation or other significant
   abnormality
Birth injury
Asphyxia (Apgar <6 at 5 minutes)

Neonatal Factors

Characteristics of Infant

Preterm or premature
SGA or LGA
Birth weight under 5½ pounds or over
   9 pounds
Low-set ears
Enlargement of one or both kidneys
Single palmar crease
Single umbilical artery
Small head size

Clinical Problems

Feeding problems
Anemia
Hyperbilirubinemia
Temperature instability
Respiratory distress
Hypoglycemia
Polycythemia
Sepsis
Rh or ABO incompatibilities
Hypocalcemia
Persistent cyanosis
Shock
Seizures
Heart murmur

Common Physical Characteristics of SGA Infant

- Decrease in subcutaneous tissue
- Loose, dry skin
- Decrease in normal chest and abdominal circumference
- Sunken abdomen
- Thin, slightly yellow, dull, dry umbilical cord
- Sparse scalp hair
- Wide-eyed look[4]

---

the SGA infant and therefore should be anticipated by the caregiver.

Asphyxia

Any neonate may be a victim of asphyxia during the labor and delivery process or immediately after birth. Moreover, SGA infants appear to be particularly vulnerable to this immediate neonatal complication.

The process of asphyxia may be a result of one of the following three mechanisms:

1. Fetal asphyxia from lack of umbilical circulation
2. Fetal asphyxia due to lack of placental exchange, as in abruptio placentae, or the SGA infant's chronic hypoxia *in utero*
3. Fetal asphyxia from inadequate perfusion of the maternal side of the placenta

Furthermore, neonatal asphyxia may be the result of excess fluid in the lungs, airway obstruction, or ineffective respiratory effort.[5]

The failure to initiate or maintain normal respirations at birth is a severe life-threatening emergency requiring immediate intervention to prevent anoxic cellular damage and to save the infant's life.

Nursing personnel need to be able to predict when an asphyxiated infant may be born and require a resuscitative effort. Fetal monitoring during labor and delivery plays a significant role in that process. Indications of fetal distress on the monitor assist the staff and prepare them for a depressed infant. (See Chap. 43 for more details on monitoring and indications of fetal distress.) Other maternal indices are prolapsed cord, uterine rupture, abruptio placentae, placenta previa, and maternal seizures. These occurrences compromise fetal oxygenation status and thus promote fetal asphyxia.

The Apgar score is the most universally known indicator of neonatal well-being at 1 and 5 minutes of life. Usually, normal respiratory patterns are established almost immediately, and by 1 minute the infant is pink, crying, and active, with a heart rate of 120 to 160 beats per minute, normal reflexes and muscle tone, and an Apgar score of 8 to 10. If asphyxia has occurred, the infant is apneic.

Primary apnea occurs when asphyxia has been prolonged over 1 minute to 2 minutes, with mild bradycardia and hypotension. The newborn is cyanotic, with diminished reflexes, bradycardia of 60 to 100/minute, and an Apgar score of 3 to 5. Following gentle suctioning and the administration of oxygen, gasping respirations usually begin after about 2 minutes. Rapid improvement often follows, with the 5-minute Apgar score reaching 8 to 10. Without other complicating conditions, these infants have an excellent immediate and long-term prognosis.

Secondary apnea occurs when there is severe bradycardia and hypotension, and death follows shortly if there is not immediate resuscitation. The newborn is ashen, heart sounds are distant, with weak pulses and bradycardia between 20 and 60 beats per minute, reflexes are absent, and the Apgar score is 1 to 3. No gasping movements are initiated with stimulation, and the infant must be resuscitated (see further discussion in this chapter). Spontaneous respiration may not begin for 5 to 15 minutes after resuscitation is started. There is danger of irreversible effects of anoxia, with long-term disabilities.[6]

The three causes of intrauterine injury of the central nervous system, narcosis, hypoxia, and brain hemorrhage, all produce a similar clinical syndrome of asphyxia, characterized by apnea. The course and prognosis of this syndrome vary with the degree of hypoxia, the location and extent of the hemorrhage, and the degree of hypercapnia and acidosis. This acidotic asphyxial state is more injurious and difficult to correct than hypoxia alone.

The normal oxygen saturation of the arterial blood of the fetus at birth is approximately 60%, but in severe cases it may drop as low as 12%. In addition, the blood of these infants has a high concentration of lactic acid and a very low *p*H.

Management is aimed at correcting metabolic acidosis as well as maintaining tissue oxygenation. Any underlying disorder (hypoglycemia, anemia) must also be identified and corrected.

Meconium Aspiration Syndrome

Aspiration of meconium into the alveoli, occurring *in utero* or after birth, results from fetal hypoxia. The fetal response to hypoxia includes reflex relaxation of the anal sphincter and accelerated intestinal peristalsis, in addition to reflex gasping, which draws the meconium into the tracheobronchial system.[7]

Meconium in the respiratory tract acts like a foreign body and blocks the flow of air into the alveoli. Increasing inflation of the alveoli distal to the obstruction can lead to their rupture and the leakage of air into the interstitial tissue (Fig. 44-5). This initiates a series of complications such as pulmonary interstitial emphysema, pneumomediastinum, and pneumothorax. The asphyxia that results from these meconium effects on the lungs leads to the involvement of the central nervous system, kidney, erythropoietic system, and metabolism, which is associated with the meconium aspiration syndrome. The syndrome may be prevented or minimized through appropriate obstetric management of the mother in whom there is evidence of meconium-stained amniotic fluid and prompt removal of meconium from the infant's upper respiratory tract immediately after birth.[4] Direct visualization and suctioning are essential preventive measures.

Hypoglycemia

Neonatal hypoglycemia is a frequent occurrence in SGA infants. Hypoglycemia is defined as a blood glucose level of 20 mg to 25 mg/dl in the low-birth-weight infant and 30 mg to 35 mg/dl in the term infant during the first 3 days of life. After 72 hours of life, glucose should be at 40 mg/dl.[4]

Although hypoglycemia usually occurs during the first 12 hours of life, it may appear as late as 48 hours. Blood sugars may be monitored by Dextrostix and verified by routine laboratory tests if abnormalities are suspected. Blood sugars must be carefully monitored and early feeding instituted as necessary. Intravenous glucose supplement may be necessary if the infant does not tolerate oral feedings.

Infants are at increased risk of hypoglycemia if their growth retardation is due to maternal undernutrition or placental insufficiency. When the placental–fetal transfer of substrates is markedly reduced, the reserve for substrates (in this case, glycogen) is also reduced. At birth, increased amounts of glucose are used to supply the energy required for various physiological adaptations. Increased glucose utilization, lack of substrate reserve, inefficient gluconeogenic mechanism, and insufficient intake of glucose then result in a fall in blood glucose with consequent hypoglycemia.

Symptoms such as tremors, cyanosis, convulsions, apnea, abnormal cry, cardiac arrest, hypotonia, hypothermia, and tachypnea are often nonspecific. Continuous low blood sugar may result in increased risk of cerebral damage.

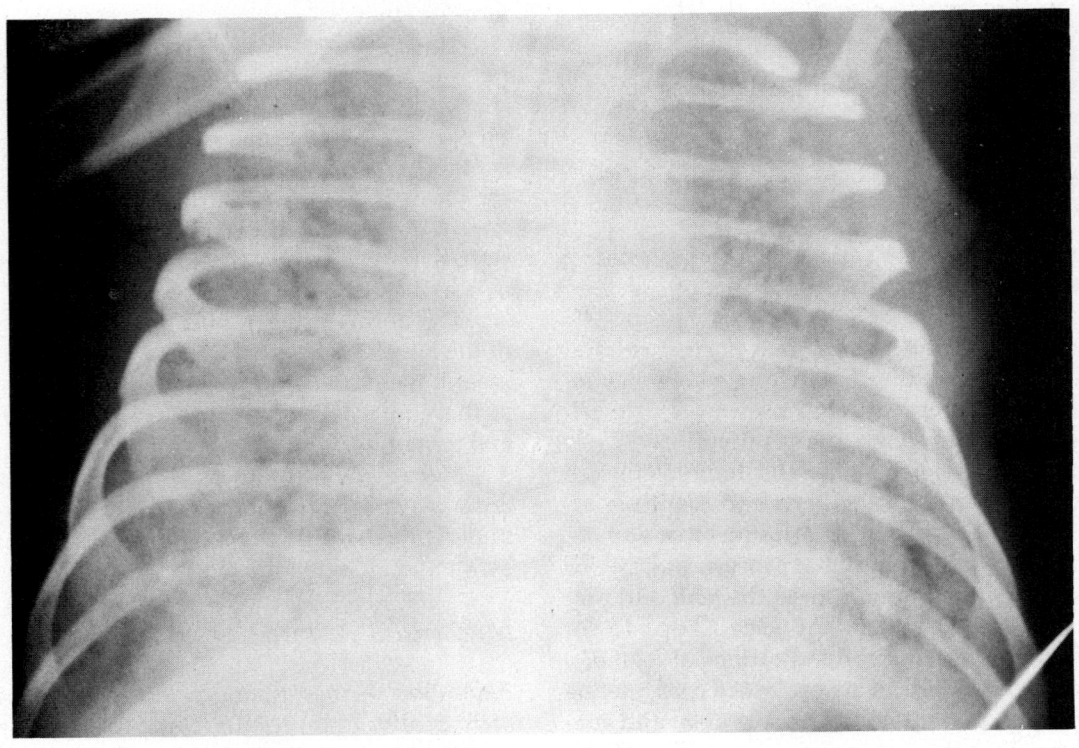

FIGURE 44-5

Severe meconium aspiration syndrome, showing shaggy heart border and irregular densities throughout both lungs, and having a wooly quality in this patient. (Avery GB: Neonatology: Pathophysiology and Management of the Newborn. Philadelphia, JB Lippincott, 1981)

Small-for-Gestational-Age Infant

Nursing Objectives

1. Perform gestational-age assessment soon after birth.
2. Identify infants who are SGA soon after birth.
3. Diagnose and treat promptly typical complications of the SGA infant.

Assessment	Potential Nursing Diagnosis	Planning/Intervention	Evaluation
Observation of infant for SGA characteristics: Decrease in subcutaneous tissue Loose, dry skin Decrease in normal chest and abdominal circumference Sunken abdomen Thin, slightly yellow, dull, dry umbilical cord Sparse scalp hair Wide-eyed look Gestational-age assessment and weight Risks: maternal nutrition problems, pregnancy-induced hypertension, advanced maternal diabetes, maternal smoker, maternal abuse of drugs/alcohol, multiple gestation, congenital infections, chromosomal disorders, congenital malformations, meconium-stained amniotic fluid	Potential for injury (asphyxia, meconium aspiration, hypoglycemia, temperature instability, polycythemia) related to intrauterine growth retardation	Prepare for possible resuscitation of asphyxiated infant at delivery Perform direct visualization and suctioning when meconium is present in amniotic fluid Frequently monitor Dextrostix Provide thermoneutral environment Check hematocrit for abnormal increases Treat complications	Infant maintains normal respirations Infant is pink, crying, and active Infant accepts early feedings Infant maintains normal temperature Infant responds to treatment for complications

Thermal Regulation

Lacking subcutaneous tissue and fat, SGA infants have difficulty maintaining body temperature. In addition to body composition, basal metabolic rates differ from normal. Effects of asphyxia are aggravated by cold stress.

Polycythemia

On the average, SGA infants have a higher plasma volume than appropriate for gestational-age infants. This polycythemia/hyperviscosity state may be due to intrauterine hypoxia, which stimulates erythropoiesis. Furthermore, a placental–fetal blood shift may occur during labor or as a result of fetal asphyxia. The alteration in blood viscosity leads to hypoxia and hypoglycemia. With a hematocrit greater than 65 and symptoms of hypoxia and hypoglycemia present, treatment is required. A partial exchange transfusion may be necessary.[1]

Nursing Intervention

In addition to the nursing care discussed above, further intervention is discussed at the end of the chapter. The steps of the nursing process are followed in the accompanying nursing-care plan.

Post-term Infants

Considering an accurate gestational age of greater than 42 weeks, the post-term infant may experience the effects of the placental insufficiency due to aging. Since this infant is usually larger than the term infant, cephalopelvic disproportion may be a problem during the birth process. Resultant birth trauma may also present significant problems as a result of vaginal deliveries. With placental insufficiency occurring in the latter part of the gestation, physical characteristics resemble those of the SGA infant.

Physical characteristics of postmature infants include decreased or absent vernix caseosa/lanugo; abundant scalp hair; dry, cracked, thin skin; little subcutaneous fat; yellow staining of skin, nails, and cord; and an alert, wide-eyed look.

Clinical problems of post-term infants include hypoxia/perinatal asphyxia, meconium aspiration, hypoglycemia, polycythemia, and thermal regulation problems.

Nursing care is delineated in the nursing-care plan.

Large-for-Gestational-Age Infants

The best example of an LGA infant is the infant of a diabetic mother. For an extended discussion of this type of infant, see Chapter 46.

Preterm or Premature Infants

Factors That Affect Prematurity

Premature or preterm infants are born before the 37th week of gestation, regardless of birth weight. Most babies who weigh less than 2500 g at birth are premature, as are almost all those weighing less than 1500 g. However, as previously stated, not all infants weighing less than 2500 g are necessarily premature. The main criterion is gestational age. The majority of these preterm infants are of appropriate weight for gestational age, but some are small-for-dates. The causes of early delivery in the cases of those infants who are appropriately sized remain obscure.

The majority of instances of premature labor have an unknown etiology. Conditions that have been clearly related to premature labor can be divided into categories of maternal, fetal, or placental etiology. *Maternal factors* include preeclampsia, eclampsia, uterine anomalies or tumors, sepsis, cervical incompetence, cardiovascular or renal disorders, diabetes, abdominal surgery, and trauma. *Fetal factors* include multiple pregnancy, hydramnios, rubella, toxoplasmosis, syphilis, and premature rupture of membranes. *Placental factors* include placenta previa and abruptio placentae. Mortality rates are inversely proportional to gestational age and birth weight.

Assessment

The length of gestational age greatly affects the preterm infant's chances for survival. Survival is unlikely in the 24- to 27-week gestational age range. Current neonatal technology offers a better chance for the 28- to 30-week-old infants. Older infants, from 31 to 36 weeks, have a good chance for survival with appropriate therapy. Those preterms of 36 to 38 weeks' gestation will need minimal therapy.

Assessment was discussed in Chapter 32 and is also presented in the nursing-care plan at the end of this section.

Physiological Problems

Cardiovascular System

Changes in fetal circulation that occur at birth are covered in Chapter 12. The most common cardiovascular defect occurring in the preterm infant is the patent ductus arteriosus. The ductus, being the fetal structure acting as a pathway for blood between the pulmonary artery and aorta, remains open owing to the preterm birth. The preterm infant has a lower pulmonary vascular resistance as a consequence of decrease in the muscular development of the pulmonary arterioles. Vasoconstrictive efforts are not as responsive to increases in oxygen levels. While the ductus remains open there is an increase in the amount of blood shunted to the pulmonary circuit, leading ultimately to pulmonary edema, increase in respiratory effort, and oxygen consumption.

Respiratory System

The preterm infant is at risk for respiratory problems. The lungs are not fully mature until 37 to 38 weeks' gestation. Surfactant, acting as an agent to decrease surface tension in the lung, is deficient in the preterm infant. In addition, it is not until 34 to 36 weeks that mature alveoli are present in the fetal lung. (For more discussion of the problem of respiratory distress syndrome, see the section "Special Health Problems of the Preterm Infant," in this chapter.)

Post-term Infant

Nursing Objectives

1. Identify the post-term infant promptly.
2. Prevent or treat potential complications early.

Assessment	Potential Nursing Diagnosis	Planning/Intervention	Evaluation
Gestational-age assessment	Potential for injury (birth trauma) related to vaginal delivery of large infant	Observe, record and report typical characteristics:	Infant breathes normally
Birth weight		Decreased or absent vernix caseosa/lungs	Infant maintains normal temperature
Maternal diabetes	Potential for injury (asphyxia, meconium aspiration, hypoglycemia, polycythemia) related to aging of the placenta	Abundant scalp hair	Infant responds to treatment for complications
Genetic influences		Dry, cracked, thin skin	
Gestation of 42 weeks or more	Potential for injury (temperature problems) related to size	Yellow staining of skin, nails, cord	
		Alert, wide-eyed look	
		Prepare for possible resuscitation of asphyxiated infant at delivery	
		Perform direct visualization and suctioning when meconium is present in amniotic fluid	
		Frequently monitor Dextrostix	
		Provide thermoneutral environment	
		Check hematocrit for abnormal increases	
		Observe for potential birth injuries—limpness, abnormal movement of extremities	

Generally speaking, the preterm infant's respiratory patterns may be regular or may exhibit increasing and frequent periods of apnea. It has been presumed that infants of less than 33 weeks' gestation have immature responses to lowered carbon dioxide levels. However, a direct relationship between decreased carbon dioxide responsiveness and the apnea of prematurity has not been clearly delineated. Neonates also do not consistently respond to hypoxic states as adults do, with a steady increase in ventilation. Rather, neonates have transient increases in ventilation in response to a decrease in inspired oxygen concentration, followed by a steady depression of ventilation.

Patterns of periodic breathing in the preterm (pauses of 5 to 10 seconds) have been reported quite commonly. True apneic episodes, however, last for 10 to 15 seconds, accompanied by pallor, cyanosis, hypotonia, and bradycardia. Repeated apneic episodes occur most often in preterm infants weighing less than 1500 g. This disorder represents the immaturity of the respiratory control systems in the brain. Many disorders may precipitate apneic episodes in the neonate, which must be treated promptly, if possible.

1. Temperature instability
2. Central nervous system problems
3. Drugs (maternal/fetal)
4. Infection
5. Metabolic disorders
6. Neonatal asphyxia

The use of tactile stimulation, water beds, low nasal continuous positive airway pressure (CPAP) at 3 cm to 5 cm H_2O, and xanthine drugs have all been helpful in managing apneic episodes.[8]

Gastrointestinal System

Maturity of the gastrointestinal tract is established by 36 to 38 weeks' gestation. Therefore, the preterm infant's gastrointestinal tract is not as functional as its mature potential. The preterm infant is subject to the following factors, which may interfere with mature gastrointestinal functioning:

1. Uncoordinated sucking and swallowing
2. Incompetent cardiac sphincter
3. Delayed gastric emptying time
4. Decreased absorption of fat
5. Incomplete digestion of protein
6. Decreased or uncoordinated motility[9]

Central Nervous System

Sleep/wake cycles are difficult to evaluate in the preterm infant. Preterm infants experience more quiet sleep, less active sleep, and higher pO_2 levels in the prone position. More quiet sleep is experienced in a neutral thermal environment.

Very little facial expression is noted before 30 to 32 weeks' gestation. Little spontaneous crying occurs before 30 to 32 weeks. From this time on, hunger is expressed by crying. Rhythmic nonnutritive sucking is noted only after 33 weeks' gestation. The auditory system functions from 26 weeks' gestation. Consistent auditory responses are noted at 32 to 34 weeks.

A gradual increase in muscle tone is noted with increasing gestational age. As muscle tone increases, the extremities gradually assume a flexed position. This posturing and flexible nature of the extremities represent a part of the gestational age assessment scoring. By 36 weeks muscle movements become more coordinated.

The stage of development of the nervous system at birth is dependent upon the degree of maturity. The fetus has a majority of neurons by 18 to 20 weeks' gestational age. The basement membrane of brain capillaries is of minimum thickness compared with the adult brain. This phenomenon may be one factor predisposing the preterm infant to subependymal and intraventricular hemorrhage. Reflexes, such as Moro and tonic neck, are present in the preterm infant.[10]

Renal System

In the preterm infant the kidneys and related urinary structures have immature properties. The kidneys do not concentrate urine well or excrete large amounts of fluid. Further, drug excretion takes longer. Glomerular filtration rate efficiency parallels gestational age. The buffering capacity of the kidneys is low, predisposing the neonate to acidosis with decreased excretion of bicarbonate and acid.[11]

Hepatic System

The preterm's immature liver presents serious problems during the immediate neonatal period. Bilirubin levels rise more rapidly than in the term infant, owing to inability of the liver to process bilirubin. Infants weighing less than 1500 g may be placed on prophylactic phototherapy.[12]

Hypoglycemia of the neonate may be due to low liver glycogen stores. Lower serum protein levels, deficiency of blood-clotting factors, and deficient conjugation and detoxification of certain drugs are all attributed to liver immaturity.

Immunologic Problems

The preterm infant lacks the immunity of IgG, which largely is acquired during the last trimester. IgA, present in breast milk, may not be received by the neonate who is given nothing by mouth (NPO) due to illness.

Skin

The skin of the preterm is thin, transparent, and covered with abundant vernix. There is a high rate of insensible water loss, especially with infants of less than 30 weeks' gestational age. Further, the preterm infant's skin absorbs chemicals readily, so precautions must be taken with topical ointments and solutions covering the skin. Finally, the skin is very vulnerable to damage from adhesive materials, so care must be taken with the amount and kind of adhesive used with monitors and other items placed on the skin.[13]

Thermal Regulation

The following factors foster temperature regulation problems in the preterm infant.

1. High surface/mass ratio
2. Lack of subcutaneous fat
3. Increase in insensible water loss
4. Respiratory distress fostering insensible water loss with work of breathing
5. Extended posture of extremities[4]

Special Health Problems of the Preterm Infant

Respiratory Distress Syndrome

Also known as hyaline membrane disease (HMD), RDS type I is a developmental disease of preterm infants appropriate for gestational age (AGA).[14] By estimate 40,000 infants develop HMD each year in the United

Preterm Infant and Family

Nursing Objectives

1. Make an accurate determination of gestational age by physical characteristics and neurologic behaviors.
2. Minimize loss of birth weight and establish weight gain pattern.
3. Maintain temperature within normal limits and prevent cold stress.
4. Maintain skin integrity without breakdown or abrasions.
5. Maintain hydration without evidence of any fluid loss.
6. Prevent infection by taking strict precautions.
7. Anticipate and prevent common complications.

Assessment	Potential Nursing Diagnosis	Planning/Intervention	Evaluation
Maternal Factors			
Placenta previa	Impaired gas exchange related to lack of surfactant	Observe, record, and report signs and symptoms of respiratory distress:	Infant breathes normally or at ease with ventilator
Abruptio placentae			
Hypertensive disease of pregnancy			
Cervical incompetence		Tachypnea	
Premature rupture of membranes		Cyanosis	
		Retractions	
Uterine anomalies		Grunting	
Infections		Nasal flaring	
Previous preterm delivery	Fluid volume deficit related to insensible water loss and inadequate fluid intake	Diminished breath sounds	
		Keep airway open by suctioning as needed	
		Administer oxygen along with appropriate monitoring of blood gases	
		Monitor ventilator function and settings	
		Change position frequently. Use chest physical therapy	
		Maintain intravenous lines and monitor closely for any infiltration	Infant maintains normal fluid/electrolyte balance
Fetal Factors			
Multiple gestation		Administer correct fluid and correct amount per hour	Infant loses minimal birth weight and gains steadily
Infections		Total intake per shift and daily	
		Observe for signs of dehydration:	
		Check skin turgor	
		Check urine output	
		Check mucous membranes	
		Check character of fontanel	

(continued)

Assessment	Potential Nursing Diagnosis	Planning/Intervention	Evaluation
		Monitor color, odor, specific gravity, clinitest, and amount of urine	
		Weigh daily at approximately the same time	
		Use heat shields or plastic sheeting with radiant warmers	

	Alteration in nutrition: less than body requirements related to actual intake less than caloric requirements	Provide adequate calorie intake with most efficient method according to individual needs:
		  Nipple
		  Gavage
		  Nasojejunal
		  Gastrostomy
			Infant adjusts to method of feeding
			
			Infant maintains normal bowel movements

		Measure abdominal girth as needed	
		Measure residuals and replace	
		Allow parents to participate in feeding plan	
		Observe stool patterns closely and report any abnormalities	
	Impairment in skin integrity related to tapes and other abrasive materials used with monitoring devices	Place as little tape as possible on skin	Infant maintains healthy skin
		Use OpSite for other skin devices	

(continued)

States. Due to improvements in management, incidence and mortality appear to be on the decrease.[15]

Pathophysiology. In RDS, the alveoli and the alveolar ducts are filled with a sticky exudate, a hyaline material, that prevents aeration. Although it is known that the hyaline material is a protein, the cause of hyaline membrane formation is not definitely known.

Three main theories have been postulated. The first proposes an alteration in the fibrinolytic enzyme system in the lung or blood that leads to the proliferation of the protein (fibrin) exudate. The second suggests alterations in or lack of the pulmonary surfactant that reduces alveolar ventilation and promotes atelectasis. The third indicates pulmonary hypoperfusion rather than surfactant deficiency. This hypoperfusion begins with intrauterine asphyxia and results in reduced alveolar ventilation and atelectasis. Whatever the exact causes and mechanisms, surfactant activity is indeed deficient, and, as a result, there is incomplete expansion of the lung and failure to establish normal, functional residual capacity (lack of alveolar stability). Thus, the lungs are atelectatic, and this is a hallmark of the disease.

Several factors may result in a deficiency of surfactant, including the following:

1. Immature cells lining alveoli
2. Decreased rate of production of surfactant as a result of transient fetal or early neonatal stress
3. Inadequate release mechanism for surfactant from the lining of type II alveolar cells (usually functioning at 35 weeks)
4. Death of cells that produce surfactant[16]

Assessment	Potential Nursing Diagnosis	Planning/Intervention	Evaluation
		Keep any lotions having direct skin contact to a minimum	
		Place infant on water bed or sheepskin	
		Turn and reposition frequently	
	Potential for injury (cold stress) related to immature temperature-regulating mechanism	Maintain neutral thermal environment	Infant does not experience cold stress
		Monitor skin temperature by probe method	Infant maintains stable temperature
		Frequently check temperature of heating unit	
		Avoid subjecting infant to heat losses by evaporation, convection, conduction, and radiation	
	Potential risk of infection related to immature immune system	See Care Plan for infection, Chap. 46	Infant remains or becomes infection free
	Anticipatory grief of parents related to loss of perfect infant	See Care Plan for grieving family, Chap. 45	
	Parental knowledge deficit related to care of the preterm infant	Give parents adequate and realistic information regarding infant's condition	Parents indicate knowledge and skill by performing caretaking tasks
		Encourage parents to perform many caretaking tasks	Parents voice confidence in caring for the infant
		Refer to public-health nurse, social services, parental support group	Parents follow through on referrals

Lecithin is thought to be the surface-active (surfactant) phospholipid responsible for maintaining alveolar stability. The production of lecithin normally begins around the 32nd to 36th week of gestation, with the initial functioning of enzyme systems producing this phospholipid. The high glucocorticoid levels found in the fetus after the 34th week of gestation accelerate production and synthesis of surfactant and lead to lung maturation. It has been found that chronic stress conditions that increase cortisol levels, such as intrauterine infections, premature rupture of the membranes, maternal hypertensive disorders, and partial abruptio placentae, are associated with a lower incidence of RDS because these stressors lead to stimulation of earlier lung maturation. The use of the synthetic steroidal hormone betamethasone a few days prior to anticipated premature delivery stimulates maturation of the fetal lungs and holds promise of improving the outlook of RDS in the small premature infant.

Clinical Manifestations. Pulmonary compliance, or the capacity of the lung to increase in volume in response to a given amount of applied pressure during inspiration, is diminished in RDS. The stiffness of the lungs and their limited distensibility contribute significantly to the work of breathing in these sick babies (Fig. 44-6). Pulmonary vasoconstriction is another injurious factor of major importance. This vasoconstriction results in increased resistance within the pulmonary circuit and causes hypoperfusion of alveolar capillaries; hence, the lungs are ischemic as well as atelectatic. The fetal circulatory state persists in varying degrees, and

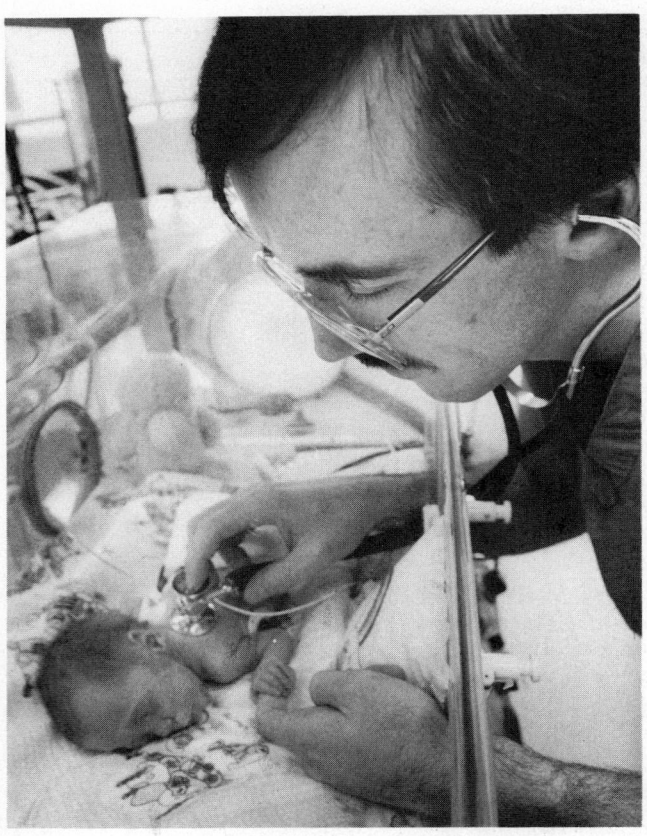

FIGURE 44-6

The nurse performs a respiration assessment. (Courtesy of The Children's Hospital of Philadelphia)

this becomes life-threatening to the neonate. After a few breaths, continued impairment of gas exchange enhances hypoxia, hypercapnia, and acidosis. This, in turn, increases the pulmonary vasoconstriction and ischemia; surfactant activity is further diminished, and atelectasis becomes more extensive. Pulmonary compliance decreases and the energy required for the simple act of breathing increases intolerably. This leads to further impairment of gas exchange and a vicious cycle that soon becomes incompatible with life. Intensive treatment is necessary to remedy this situation.[16]

The Silverman score (Fig. 44-7) is a standard index of measuring behaviors indicating respiratory distress. Symptoms usually occur within 6 hours of life. Nasal flaring, grunting, tachypnea, seesaw respirations, and cyanosis may be observed (Fig. 44-8). The infant becomes flaccid and hypotonic. Diminished breath sounds are auscultated. The typical x-ray picture is demonstrated in Figure 44-9.

Renal Changes. Neonates with RDS demonstrate decreases in urine volume, glomerular filtration rate, and renal plasma flow. Diuresis usually occurs at 24 hours of age and peaks at 60 hours.

Gastrointestinal Problems. Infants with HMD may be stricken with necrotizing enterocolitis as a result of bowel ischemia secondary to hypoxia.

The prevention of atelectasis is vital in the treatment plan. Oxygen therapy is instituted; ventilatory measures such as continuous positive airway pressure or positive-

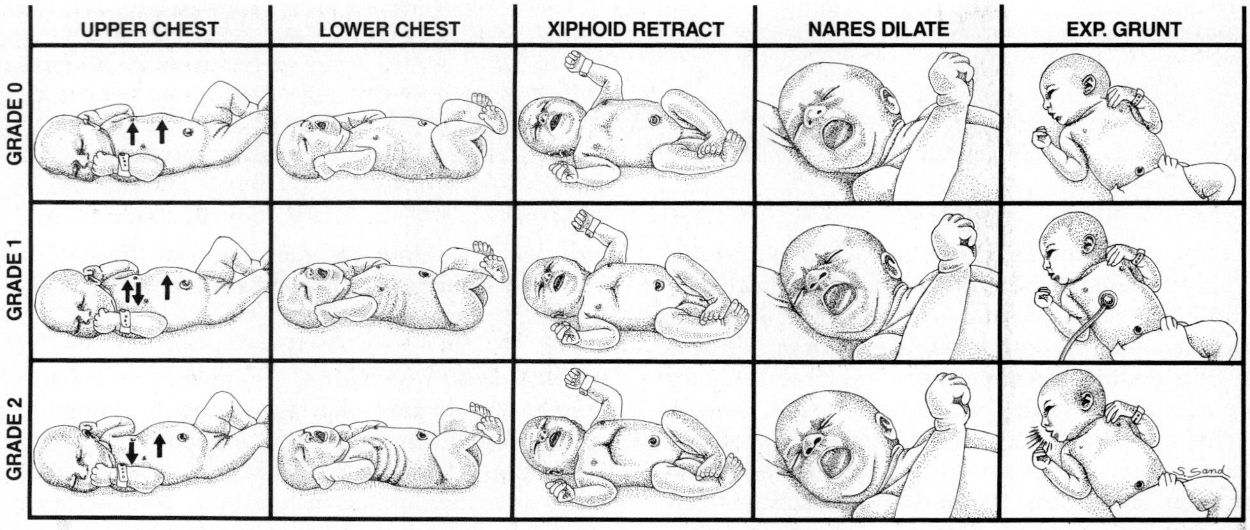

	UPPER CHEST	LOWER CHEST	XIPHOID RETRACT	NARES DILATE	EXP. GRUNT
GRADE 0					
GRADE 1					
GRADE 2					

FIGURE 44-7

Observation of retractions using the Silverman score. An index of respiratory distress is determined by grading each of five arbitrary criteria. Grade 0 indicates no difficulty; grade 1 indicates moderate difficulty; and grade 2 indicates maximum respiratory difficulty. The retraction score is the sum of these values; a total score of 0 indicates no dyspnea, whereas a total score of ten denotes maximal respiratory distress.

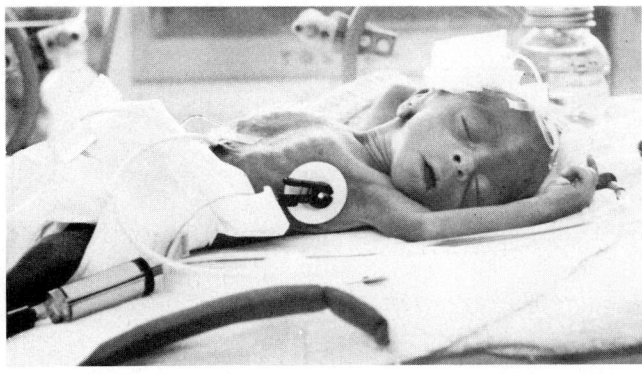

FIGURE 44-8

Respiratory distress syndrome. This infant exhibits marked substernal and intercostal retractions, "seesaw" respirations, and nasal flaring.

pressure ventilation are used. A thermoneutral environment is maintained. Continuing fluid balance and correction of acidosis are ongoing. For related nursing care, see later sections of this chapter and nursing care plans.

Prognosis. Usually symptoms begin to lessen as surfactant production is established at about 48 to 72 hours of life. The following complications may occur as a result of RDS:

- *Respiratory:* Pneumothorax, pneumomediastinum, bronchopulmonary dysplasia
- *Cardiovascular:* Hypotension, hypovolemia, hypoxemia, myocardial failure, patent ductus arteriosus
- *Central nervous system:* Cerebral edema, intracranial hemorrhage
- *Sepsis*
- *Renal failure*[15]

Bronchopulmonary Dysplasia

Bronchopulmonary dysplasia (BPD) is a chronic lung disorder estimated to occur in approximately 5% of all infants admitted to neonatal intensive care and requiring intermittent positive-pressure ventilation. The disease process ranges from a broad spectrum of mild pulmonary infiltrates to severe cystic emphysema. It is difficult to wean these infants from ventilator therapy and oxygen therapy.[8]

Risk Factors. The following factors have been linked to the development of BPD. Inspired oxygen concentrations greater than 50% given over a period of many days present a higher risk to the patient. It is not precisely clear what numbers are most damaging; this depends on many factors. The use of positive-pressure assisted ventilation and endotracheal tubes also appear to contribute to the patient's risk. Oxygen alone cannot be implicated, since infants placed in negative-pressure ventilators with high oxygen concentration are not affected by BPD.[8]

The use of nasal CPAP with oxygen is not implicated either. The disease affects not only the preterm infant but also term infants requiring ventilatory support.

Pathophysiology. There are destructive inflammatory changes occurring in the lung tissue as scarring and emphysema. Clinical characteristics include airway obstruction, abnormal alveoli, hypoxemia, hypercarbia, and compensatory respiratory acidosis.[17]

Prognosis. Infants may experience respiratory difficulties due to BPD for as long as 2 years. During the first year of life the mortality rate with severe BPD is

(text continued on page 990)

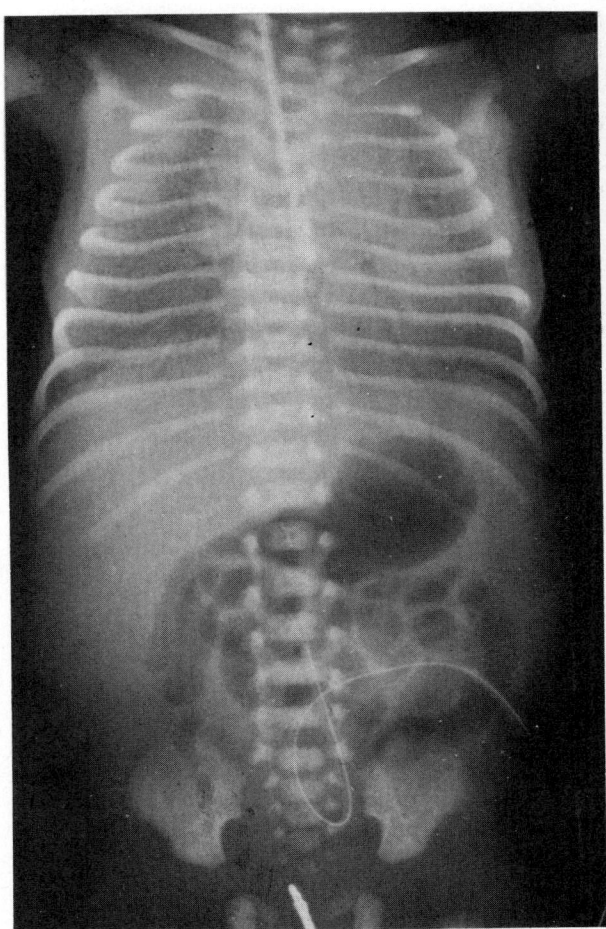

FIGURE 44-9

Severe hyaline membrane disease (HMD). Note diffuse density of the lung fields compared with intestinal gas, with well-defined air bronchograms. Both lungs are uniformly involved. An umbilical artery catheter lies at the aortic bifurcation (third lumbar vertebra). (Avery GB: Neonatology: Pathophysiology and Management of the Newborn. Philadelphia, JB Lippincott, 1981)

Family and Neonate With Respiratory Distress Syndrome

Nursing Objectives

1. Assess and quickly correct acid–base imbalances.
2. Recognize and provide early treatment for complications.
3. Recognize and treat concurrent common complications of the preterm infant.

Assessment	Potential Nursing Diagnosis	Planning/Intervention	Evaluation
Preterm delivery	Impaired gas exchange related to lack of lung surfactant	Deliver oxygen according to needs displayed by transcutaneous readings or arterial blood gas samples	Infant breathes with assistance
Evidence of fetal hypoxic episode		Use appropriate delivery method:	Infant returns to normal acid–base balance
Previous family history		Oxygen hood	
		Flooding of isolette	
		Check oxygen concentration every hour	
		Calibrate oxygen sensors as per protocol	
		Manage ventilatory assistance	
		CPAP	
		Monitor pressure readings	
		Check nasal prongs for patency	
		Lubricate nasal prongs	
		Check nares for pressure areas	
		Ventilator	
		Maintain ordered settings	
		Keep bag and mask nearby in case of ventilator failure or extubation	
		Monitor blood gases soon after ventilator or oxygen changes made	
		Observe color	
		Observe respiratory effort	
		Auscultate and assess breath sounds, heart rate	
		Observe general activity	
		Recognize and promptly correct alterations in acid–base balances by:	
		Changes in ventilator settings	
		Bagging	
		Administration of drugs	
		Volume replacement	
	Ineffective airway clearance related to an increase in secretion production	Use suction for brief periods using intermittent pressures	Infant responds to treatment

(continued)

Assessment	Potential Nursing Diagnosis	Planning/Intervention	Evaluation
	and inability to clear airway by coughing	Use sterile procedure with saline instillation with endotracheal tube	
		Bag before and after suctioning with 100% oxygen to prevent atelectasis	
		Suction only as needed	
		Observe and describe infant's tolerance to the procedure as well as the amount, color, and character of secretions	
		Turn frequently and use chest postural drainage to mobilize secretions	
		Keep well hydrated to promote secretion liquefaction	
	Fluid volume and electrolyte imbalances related to disease, sensible and insensible water losses, and use of parenteral fluids	Record daily weights	Infant establishes balanced input and output
		Monitor laboratory values as ordered	Infant reaches and maintains fluid and electrolyte balance
		Observe for signs and symptoms of electrolyte imbalances, fluid overload, and dehydration	Infant steadily gains weight
		Deliver correct type and amount of IV fluid	Infant maintains skin integrity
		Monitor output. Check specific gravity, Clinitest, color, odor	
		Maintain positioning of peripheral IV site	
		Observe site for infiltration	
		Restrain infant as needed	
		Secure umbilical catheter as needed to prevent any dislodgment from tubing	
		Observe extremities for blanching or discoloration of hands and feet	
		If discoloration or blanching occurs, contralateral foot may be wrapped briefly—if adverse reaction of vasospasm not relieved, removal of catheter is required	
		For subclavian catheter, change dressing as per protocol using sterile technique	

(continued)

Assessment	Potential Nursing Diagnosis	Planning/Intervention	Evaluation
		For all intravenous lines, change tubing every 24 hours	
	Alteration in nutrition, less than body requirements, related to larger caloric expenditure than intake	Provide adequate calories per kilogram of body weight	Infant adapts to type of feeding used
		Minimize volume by using special higher caloric preterm formulas	Infant maintains stable temperature
		Minimize caloric expenditure with heat loss by maintaining thermoneutral environment	Infant gains weight
		Use hats when out of isolette	
		Conserve energy by minimizing bottle feedings	
		Gavage feed as necessary	
		Place head of bed up after feedings	
		Measure residuals and abdominal girth	
	Parental knowledge deficit related to disease process	Provide informative, realistic explanations to parents regarding short-term and long-term prognosis	Parents visit NICU regularly
		Encourage parents to visit and provide caretaking tasks for infant	Parents provide caretaking
			Parents demonstrate understanding of prognoses by discussing problems freely
	Potential complications related to RDS and preterm	Observe for and record signs and symptoms of:	Infant responds to treatment of complications
		Bronchopulmonary dysplasia	
		Pneumothorax	
		Retrolental fibroplasia	
		Necrotizing enterocolitis	
		Intraventricular hemorrhage	
		Patent ductus arteriosus	
		Treat for complications	

(text continued from page 987)
high (30%–40%), usually as a result of respiratory failure or infection.[8]

Nursing Care. These infants need to be observed closely for signs of infection and treated with antibiotics as necessary. Infants who experience episodes of bronchospasm may benefit from bronchodilator therapy.

Transient Tachypnea of the Newborn (RDS Type II)

Transient tachypnea of the newborn may occur in preterm or term infants. The major clinical sign is delayed reabsorption of fetal lung fluid.[14]

Some mild degree of pulmonary immaturity may be associated with this disease, as demonstrated by a study suggesting that a 1-minute Apgar score of less than 7, negative amniotic fluid phosphatidylglycerol, and less than 33 weeks' gestation were characteristics of these infants.[18] Other contributing factors are a diabetic mother and cesarean delivery. Cesarean delivery babies do not experience the thoracic compression, which assists in clearing the lungs, of infants born by vaginal delivery.

Clinical signs are similar to those of RDS, such as tachypnea, nasal flaring, grunting, and retraction. There is a degree of mild hypoxia and hypercapnia. Diagnosis is made by chest radiographic findings. Recovery usually occurs by 72 hours of life. Nursing management involves administration of oxygen as needed and other maintenance measures.

Pneumothorax

Frequency of pneumothorax is about 1% of all live births. In cases of assisted ventilation and PEEP (positive end-expiratory pressure), incidences rise to over 40%.[8]

Clinical signs indicate a sudden rapid deterioration in condition, especially in an infant with respiratory disease. Tachypnea, grunting, pallor, or cyanosis may occur. Breath sounds may be decreased. Cardiac apex may shift away from the affected side. Bradycardia and hypotension may occur.

Diagnosis may be ascertained by transillumination of the chest followed by definitive chest films. The air leak is then decompressed by needle aspiration and subsequent placement of a chest tube with water-seal drainage and suction of 10 cm to 20 cm H_2O. Oxygen administration may be necessary. When air movement in the tube and bubbling cease, the tube is clamped and removed in 24 hours if the infant's condition remains stable.

Retrolental Fibroplasia

Retrolental fibroplasia is an acquired disease, associated with prematurity, in which retinal pathology occurs in those infants receiving continuous oxygen therapy in high concentration. The incidence of the condition depends on the concentration of oxygen given and the degree of immaturity of the eyes at the time when oxygen is given. Incidence is inversely proportional to birth weight. Other risk factors are preterm twin or other multiple pregancies, preterms receiving exchange transfusions, and preterms weighing less than 1500 g or less than 37 weeks.

The preterm infant is susceptible owing to the immaturity of retinal development. The active stage of the disease usually begins during the first month after birth. Reese divides the progression of the disease into stages prior to complete retinal detachment.

> ### Active Stages in Progression of Retrolental Fibroplasia
>
> Stage I: Dilation and tortuosity of retinal vessels
>
> Stage II: Stage I plus neovascularization and some peripheral retinal clouding
>
> Stage III: Stage II plus retinal detachment in the periphery of the fundus
>
> Stage IV: Hemispheric or circumferential retinal detachment
>
> Stage V: Complete retinal detachment[19]

Management. When detected early and proper measures are instituted promptly (*i.e.*, reduction in concentration of oxygen administered), the condition in the infant may regress at any stage of the disease; on the other hand, partial or complete blindness may result.

Extensive research, carried on during the years since retrolental fibroplasia was first described, has established the cause and the means of prevention of the disease. It is now a fact that almost all cases of retrolental fibroplasia in the premature infant are the result of intensive oxygen therapy. Today, oxygen is administered to an infant in the lowest concentration compatible with life and is discontinued as soon as feasible. Blood gases are monitored frequently to keep arterial oxygen pressure at acceptable levels.

High doses of vitamin E may reduce the incidence and severity of retrolental fibroplasia.[19] It is recommended that all infants at risk be examined by an ophthalmologist, ideally at 3 to 4 weeks of age.

Intraventricular Hemorrhage

Intraventricular hemorrhage (IVH) occurs in the preterm infant and is being recognized as a major disorder in this group with increasing frequency. Incidence increases with decreasing gestational age. IVH is a leading cause of death. Survivors may experience moderate or severe neurologic handicap.

Risk Factors. Obstetric and neonatal factors that may serve as stimuli for bleeding include birth asphyxia, hypotension, assisted ventilation, HMD, pneumothorax, hypercarbia, thrombocytopenia, fluid and electrolyte imbalances, and volume expanders.

Pathophysiology. A highly vascular area, the subependymal germinal matrix, is very evident between 28 and 32 weeks. Very little of this structure is present at term. The subependymal germinal matrix is located at the level of the foramen of Monro and the head of the

---

Classification of Severity of Intraventricular Hemorrhage

Grade I: Isolated subependymal hemorrhage

Grade II: Intraventricular hemorrhage without ventricular dilation

Grade III: Intraventricular hemorrhage with ventricular dilation

Grade IV: Intraventricular hemorrhage with ventricular hemorrhage and hemorrhage into the parenchyma of the brain[21]

---

caudate nucleus. Bleeding is thought to originate from the capillaries of the germinal matrix.

As a stimulus to increased cerebral blood flow and resultant venous congestion, hypoxia and hypercarbia dilate cerebral vessels. Furthermore, hypoxia and acidosis injure the endothelium of the vessels, making them rupture easily.

In preterm infants the mechanism for keeping cerebral blood flow constant may be impaired. Arterioles dilate as stimulated by hypoxia or hypercarbia. A rise in blood pressure at this point may result in capillary rupture and hemorrhage. Bleeding may be isolated in the subependymal germinal matrix or extend into the neighboring ventricles.[20] The classification system can be used to isolate the severity of the hemorrhage.

Clinical Manifestations.   Clinical signs may range from none to a dramatic change in condition. Observations of a deterioration may come about very quickly. The nurse may notice apnea, bradycardia, hypotension, seizures, or decerebrate posturing. The anterior fontanel bulges, and the temperature becomes unstable, indicative of increasing intracranial pressure.

Diagnosis.   Spinal fluid shows increased number of red blood cells, elevated protein, and low glucose. Computed tomography (CT) and ultrasound techniques can pinpoint the location and size of the hemorrhage.

Prevention.   Studies are ongoing to determine the usefulness of drugs in preventing hemorrhage (*i.e.*, phenobarbital and ethamsylate).[20] Nurses can prevent intracranial insult by identifying the infant who is at risk for IVH and providing as safe an environment as possible given the many factors involved.

Careful monitoring of intake and output and its subsequent effects on blood pressure is advised. Avoidance of the head-down position as used frequently in chest physiotherapy is essential. Administration of sodium bicarbonate slowly and well diluted is recommended. Avoidance of stress for the infant, which can

raise the blood pressure, may be accomplished by grouping nursing activities and providing rest periods. Activities that lead to hypoxia, such as suctioning and intubation, should be time-limited. Administration of preoxygenation and postoxygenation by bag and mask is essential.

Treatment.   The activity of hemorrhages can be monitored by CT scan and ultrasound. Small hemorrhages will not require any treatment and resolve spontaneously. Others will require removal of the blood by spinal tap, direct ventricular puncture, or ventricular reservoir.

If posthemorrhagic hydrocephalus occurs, surgery is required to place a ventriculoperitoneal shunt. This shunt drains the accumulated cerebrospinal fluid into the peritoneal cavity where it is reabsorbed.

Nursing Care.   Continuing observation of the neonate at risk can alert the nurse to those subtle cues indicative of a change in status. Status of the fontanels (*i.e.*, flat, full, tense, or bulging) should be noted regularly. Seizure activity may be very subtle (*i.e.*, brief apnea) and may be very difficult to pick up.

In an infant diagnosed with IVH, the nurse must continue to be alert for signs of increasing intracranial pressure, such as apnea, bradycardia, hypotension, and temperature instability. Repeat measurements of head circumferences and observation of fontanels are required. Assistance with treatment procedures and care of drains may be essential.

Patent Ductus Arteriosus

The process of the patent ductus arteriosus is more likely in the preterm infant than in the term. Incidence overall in the preterm infant is 20.2%, with a 12% incidence of significant patent ductus arteriosus.[22]

Physiology.   The ductus arteriosus in the fetus serves as a connection between the pulmonary artery and the aorta. It functions as a bypass for the lungs and, possibly, as a volume recipient from the left ventricle.

In the term infant the ductus arteriosus closes in stages. Early or functional closure occurs in the first 24 hours. Later or anatomical closure of the tissue occurs in a few days. In the preterm infant these events occur also, but at a later time, when age and weight approach that of a term infant.

The appearance of clinical signs of a patent ductus arteriosus depends on the balance between the pulmonary and systemic vascular beds. If the pulmonary vascular resistance is low, there may be a left-to-right shunt, increasing the work of breathing for the neonate. If there is severe RDS, pulmonary vascular resistance is high, resulting in a right-to-left shunt.

Clinical Manifestations. Signs are more evident on the third or fourth day, when RDS would be resolving. Murmurs can be auscultated. Wide pulse pressures, tachycardia, and bounding pulses are noted. Signs and symptoms of pulmonary edema occur, such as tachypnea, grunting, retractions, and rales.[22]

Diagnosis. Diagnostic studies confirm clinical findings. A chest film is frequently used, along with echocardiography.

Treatment. Fluid restriction is necessary to decrease the work load of the heart. Adjustments are necessary in the case of the use of overhead warmers to combat insensible water loss. Diuretics such as furosemide (Lasix) may be used to control volume on board. Controversy exists as to whether the use of digoxin in the preterm infant is really therapeutic. Preterm infants exhibit a high incidence of arrhythmias. Since anemia can increase the heart's work load, the hematocrit needs to be kept as close to 45 as possible.[22]

The role of prostaglandins and indomethacin's inhibitory effort are fairly recent medical advances in the treatment of patent ductus arteriosus. Overall, indomethacin has been successful, although in some neonates the ductus has reopened; since it affects the kidney, it should not be administered if the blood urea nitrogen is above 25 or the creatinine is above 1.8.[22] Renal function will be affected, with a decrease in urine output, decrease in serum sodium, and increase in potassium. These effects last only 72 hours. A total of three doses is given every 12 hours intravenously, orally, or rectally. If there is not subsequent improvement in status, surgical intervention may be necessary. The timing of medical or surgical intervention and the choice of candidates remain open to debate and the individual situation.

Nursing Care. Frequent assessment is necessary to assist in the diagnosis, and treatment can prevent further complications. Ongoing electrocardiographic monitoring and skilled interpretation are essential. Precise monitoring of vital signs and intake and output and correct administration of drugs ordered are additional nursing interventions.

Necrotizing Enterocolitis

Necrotizing enterocolitis (NEC), a disease of the neonate characterized by necrosis of the bowel, occurs in 1% to 7.5% of neonates admitted to the NICU.[23] Mortality figures range widely from 15% to 75%. NEC is the most frequent preoperative diagnosis for infants going to surgery. The average age at onset of the disease is 4 days. The majority of infants with NEC are low-birth-weight preterm infants.[24] Seventy-five to 90% of these infants weigh less than 2500 g; 80% to 90% are less than 38 weeks' gestation. Other factors that seem to be predisposing include a history of resuscitation at birth due to a low Apgar score, RDS, apneic spells, and cyanosis.[23,24]

Etiology and Pathophysiology. Factors that have been cited in the literature that lead to an episode of NEC are feeding, mucosal injury in the bowel, and bacterial colonization.[23]

Most infants developing NEC were fed a cow's milk formula; few were fed only breast milk. Intestinal ischemia may be a result of vasospasm in response to asphyxia as blood is shunted to vital organs of the heart and brain. Bacterial colonization of the gut normally begins at delivery and progresses to 10 days in a healthy neonate. However, infants in the NICU experience a more sterile environment, and colonization is delayed. Bacteria most commonly tied to NEC are normal flora: *Escherichia coli*, *Klebsiella*, and clostridia.

Diagnosis. Signs indicative of NEC are abdominal distention along with gastric retention and vomiting. Others mentioned are lethargy, irritability, apnea, diarrhea, unstable temperature, and gastrointestinal bleeding. X-ray films of the abdomen indicate multiple dilated loops of bowel and pneumatosis.

Treatment

Medical. If the diagnosis is made early, surgery may be avoided. Cultures of blood, urine, and stool are obtained. The neonate is place on NPO status to rest the bowel. Intravenous fluids are given, a nasogastric tube is placed to low suction, and intravenous or gastric antibiotics are given. Serial abdominal films are obtained to monitor any changes in the gut.

Surgical. Resection of necrotic segments of bowel and enterostomy are performed if the disease progresses to intestinal perforation and peritonitis.

Nursing Care. Nurses must identify early those infants at risk. Preventive nursing care of infants receiving early feedings include abdominal evaluation for distention by measurement of abdominal girth and measurement of gastric residual prior to feedings.

Following diagnosis of NEC, the infant is observed closely for changes in abdominal status. This can be accomplished most effectively by exposing the infant's entire abdomen. The abdomen is observed for distention by measurement of abdominal girth and visual inspection for tight, shiny skin. Any changes in vital signs may be indicative of shock secondary to intestinal perforation. Careful intake and output measurements are essential, especially measurement and description of gastric contents. All stools must be hematested. Postoperative care is similar to that of other abdominal surgeries, with special attention to stoma care. Infants with NEC usually are placed on long-term total parenteral nutrition (TPN) therapy until the bowel is reanastomosed.

Parents of infants with NEC require simple explanations of the baby's condition, opportunity for frequent contact, and increasing caretaking of the infant over the long course of therapy.

Nursing Diagnosis in High-Risk Neonatal Care

To intervene most successfully, the nurse needs to formulate appropriate nursing diagnoses. The following are examples of nursing diagnoses pertaining to the preterm neonate: potential fluid volume deficit related to insensible water loss and inadequate fluid intake; potential impairment of gas exchange related to lack of surfactant; potential for cold stress related to immature temperature-regulating mechanism, and potential risk of infection related to immature immune system.

The SGA infant is at potential risk of asphyxia, hypoglycemia, and temperature instability related to intrauterine growth retardation. The post-term infant is at risk of potential birth trauma related to vaginal delivery of a large infant. The infant experiencing RDS is at risk for potential complications of this disease.

Planning/Intervention in High-Risk Neonatal Care

Resuscitation

An NICU nurse, neonatologist, and respiratory therapist should attend all high-risk deliveries. These personnel should also be on rotating call in the event that unanticipated problems occur with the newly born infant. A cart containing all necessary resuscitation equipment should be readily available near the labor rooms and delivery areas. Equipment needs to be replaced as it is used, and the cart should be checked for inventory, expiration dates, and drugs every shift (see Neonatal Resuscitation Equipment).

Resuscitation technique encompasses the skills of maintaining an open airway, assistance with breathing, and maintaining circulation, the ABCs of cardiopulmonary resuscitation (Fig. 44-10). All procedures should be carried out under the open warmer to allow easy access along with continuous temperature monitoring of the neonate. The neonate should be dried thoroughly and wrapped to avoid evaporative heat loss.

Airway

As the head emerges at the time of birth, the nose and mouth are cleared of mucus with a bulb syringe or Delee trap.

If further suctioning is required, the infant should be placed in the radiant warmer. The mouth is again suctioned first, followed by the nose to avoid reflex aspiration if the nose is stimulated first. Intermittent suction with a suction catheter for brief periods (10–15 seconds) is recommended. Continuous heart rate monitoring should be maintained, since suctioning can stimulate the vagus, resulting in bradycardia. Oxygen should be administered under intermittent positive-pressure ventilation at 3 to 4 liters/min. The neonate should be mechanically ventilated between suctioning if he is apneic.[25]

Breathing

Bag and Mask. The infant is placed in the so-called sniffing position, without hypertension of the neck; some neonates may require a towel roll under the shoulders to maintain this position. The mask is placed over the nose and mouth to create a seal. Various mask sizes should be available, since mask size must be appropriate for each particular infant. The bag should have a one-way valve on the neck piece to allow for expiration. The bag should also have a collar and reservoir to permit 100% oxygen to be administered. Some bags have a pop-off valve to control maximum peak pressures, although others have attached gauges to give this information.[26] One type of bag is shown in Figure 44-11.

Oxygen Concentration. Most infants require 100% oxygen during a resuscitation effort. Some infants already receiving oxygen therapy may require only the percentage they are receiving.

Rate. The usual rate for hand bagging is from 40 to 60 breaths per minute, to simulate the usual respiratory rate (Table 44-2).

Amounts of Pressure. Peak pressure is the highest pressure in the lungs during normal inspiration. It is recommended to use 40 cm to 60 cm H_2O pressure from the first breath of assisted hand ventilation, and 16 cm to 20 cm H_2O pressure for subsequent ventilation in neonates with normal lungs. In neonates with diagnosed lung disease, 20 cm to 25 cm H_2O pressure may be necessary. Excess pressure could cause pneumothorax.

Positive end-expiratory pressure (PEEP) is the lowest positive pressure measured during expiration. If the pressure is not allowed to drop to zero, then PEEP is given. Infants with diseased lungs may require some

Neonatal Resuscitation Equipment

1. Oxygen and air tanks with oxygen diluter, corrugated tubing
2. Infant warmer with suction machine, thermometer, 2 bottles of sterile water for suctioning, and stethoscope
3. Cardiac monitor with leads, strain gauge (to be brought to room when delivery expected)

Shelf supplies

IV instrument tray

Catheter-assist tray (see next section)

Blood-culture tube, culturettes

Blood-collecting tubes

Dextrostix with heel-stick equipment

Hematocrit tubes with sealing material

Extra syringes—8 each of tuberculin, 3 ml, 5 ml, and 10 ml

Safety pins

Feeding tubes—2 No. 8

Suction supplies—1 connecting tube; 2 each of numbers 5, 8, and 10 DeLee

Endotracheal suction tubes (2) and adapter

Sterile gloves—4 of each size

Sterile drapes (2 packs)

Sterile towels (4)

Ice basins for blood gases

Infant hood

2 continuous positive airway pressure (CPAP) set-ups—1 always set up and 1 extra

Face masks—1 each of 3 different infant sizes

Chart and pens on clipboard

Oxygen analyzer—brought in before delivery

Lab slips and white tape for identification labels

Stop watch

Stockinet and safety pins for restraints

1 hemoset

1 metriset

1 250-ml $D_{10}W$

1 150-ml $D_5/2$ NS

Betadine

Needle electrodes

Catheter-assist tray:

1 20-ml syringe

2 10-ml syringes

2 5-ml syringes

5 3-ml syringes

5 tuberculin syringes

4 packages 4-0 silk suture

4 No. 20 knife blades

4 disposable No. 16 blunt needles (Luer stub adapters)

4 disposable Tomac stopcocks

4 No. 5 arterial catheters

4 No. 3½ arterial catheters

1 roll of 1-in pink tape

Cord clamp and cord tie

Disposable scalpels

Alcohol sponges

Corks

Extra 2 × 2 gauzes

4 steri-drapes

2 intraflo

Medicine tray:

4 Heparin, 1000 units/ml

1 20-ml vial of 1% Xylocaine and 1% Xylocaine for IV use

2 calcium gluceptate, 200 mg/ml

2 sodium bicarbonate

2 each normal saline and sterile water vials

1 KCl vial; 1 NaCl vial

1 salt-poor 25% albumin

2 adrenalin 1:1000 (dilute 0.1 ml to total volume of 1 ml)

Neosporin ointment

Narcan 0.4 mg/ml, 1 vial

50% dextrose, 50-ml bottle

Intubation tray:

Laryngoscope with regular and premature size blades and batteries

Forregger tubes—1 each of sizes 2.5, 3.0, 3.5, 4.0, 8, 10, 12, 14, 16

Portex tubes—2 each of sizes 2.5, 3.0, 3.5, and 4.0

Benzoin and cotton swabs

Elastoplast, pink tape, precut tapes (preemie and regular)

Pneumothorax equipment

Needle holder, tweezers, and scissors

4-0 sutures and stylette

(Waechter EH, Phillips J, Holaday B: Nursing Care of Children, 10th ed. Philadelphia, JB Lippincott, 1985; adapted from the *Nursing Manual*, Nursery, Mt. Zion Hospital and Medical Center, San Francisco, CA)

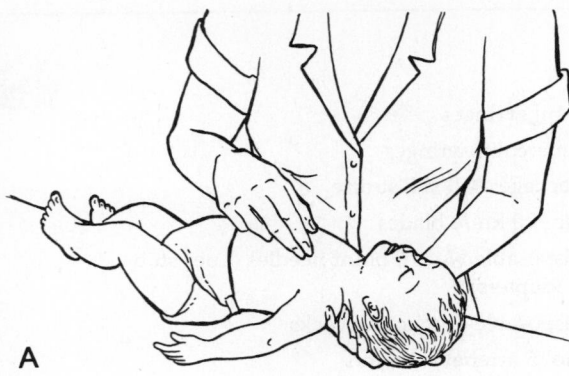

Airway
Clear the airway of mucus, if present.
   Use your finger in a sweeping
   motion.
Tilt the infant's head backward
   slightly. Forceful extension of the
   neck may obstruct the infant's
   pliable breathing passages.

A

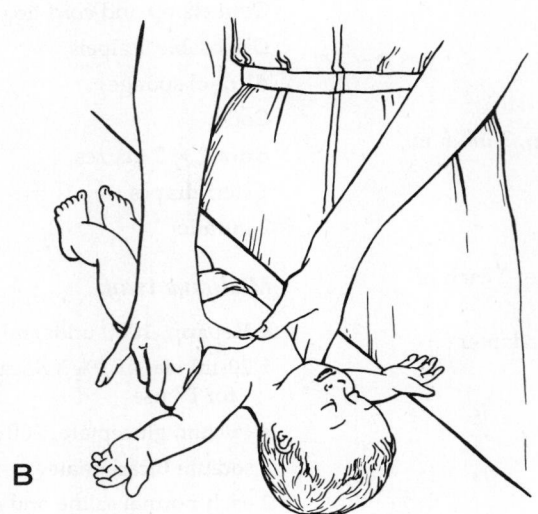

Circulation
Circle chest with hands and
   compress sternum with both
   thumbs.
Maintain a rate of 80 to 100
   compressions per minute.
Ventilate quickly, once after each five
   compressions.
Do not interrupt compression during
   ventilation.

B

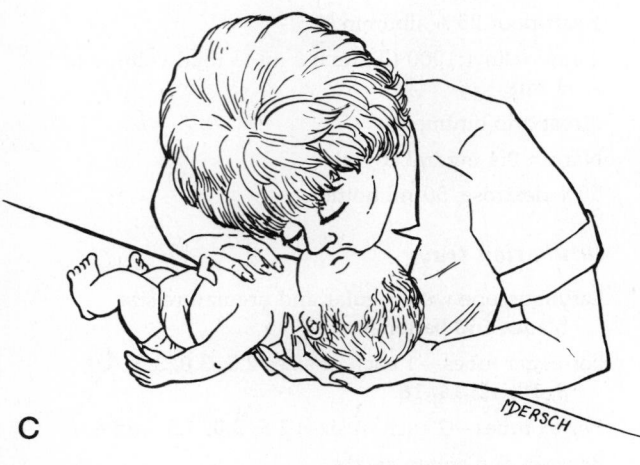

Breathing
Support infant's back and head with
   your hand.
Cover the infant's nose *and* mouth
   with your mouth.
Use small breaths or puffs from
   cheeks to inflate the lungs once
   every three seconds.

C

FIGURE   44-10

Techniques of cardiopulmonary resuscitation in an infant. (*A*) Airway.
(*B*) Circulation. (*C*) Breathing.

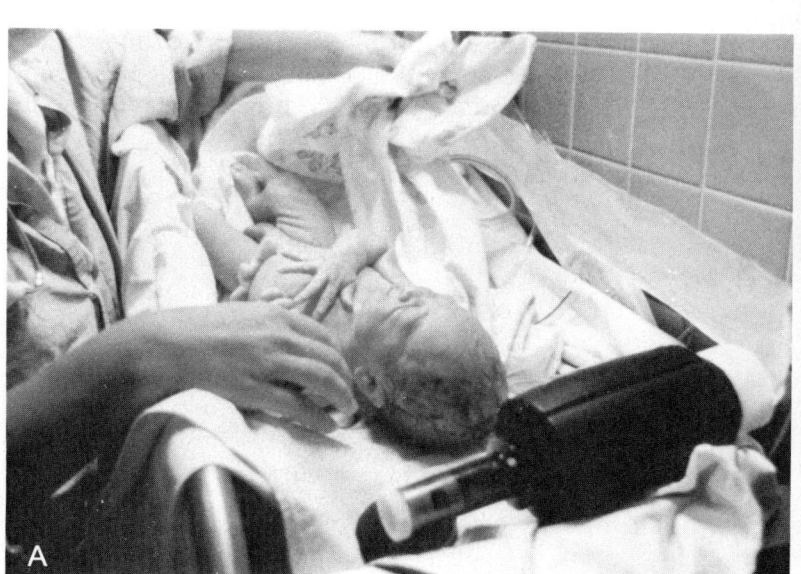
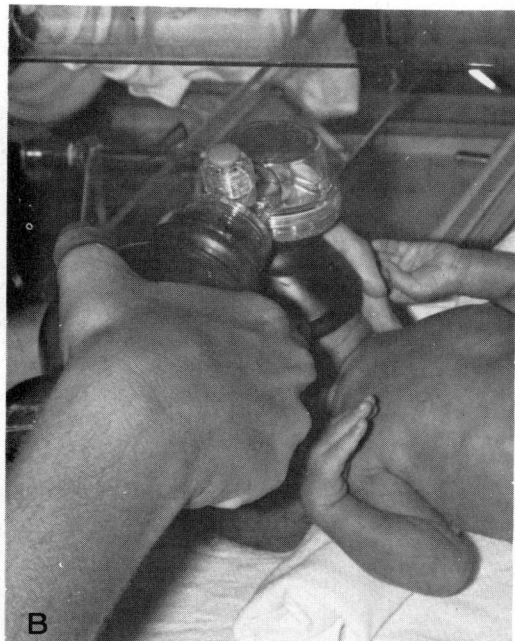

FIGURE 44-11

Bagging in resuscitation. (*A*) An Ambu resuscitation bag stands ready in case it is needed. (*B*) Appropriate technique for bagging. A towel is placed under the newborn's shoulders to maintain the sniffing position. (*A*, courtesy of Booth Maternity Center, Philadelphia)

small PEEP pressures, while infants with normal lungs do not require any PEEP.[26]

Chest movement should be observed with each mechanical breath. Some respiratory effort and improvement of color should ensue.

If spontaneous respirations do not quickly occur, endotracheal intubation should be quickly accomplished by an experienced resuscitator.

Endotracheal Intubation. The infant is again placed in the proper position to straighten the airway. Once positioning is accomplished, the laryngoscope is

TABLE 44-2

*Suggested Methods of Emergency Hand Ventilation**

Condition of Neonate	Rate in Breaths per Minute (BPM)	Concentration of Inspired Oxygen (FiO₂)	Peak Pressure (cm H₂O pressure)	Positive End Expiratory Pressure–PEEP (cm H₂O pressure)
Depressed neonate in delivery room (state of lungs unknown)	40–60	100%	Very first breath: 40–60 Other breaths: 16–25	0
Neonate with normal lungs (acute distress)	40–60	If witnessed deterioration, may try less than 100% If unwitnessed, 100%	16–20	0
Neonate with known diseased lungs (as initial stabilization before transport)	40–60	100%	16–25	Up to +5

* If efforts do not result in improvement of neonate's condition, other appropriate measures to be taken include (1) reassessment of airway (that is, need for suctioning and intubation); (2) emergency medicines including correction of hypovolemia; and (3) use of other bagging techniques such as increasing the FiO₂, increasing the rate, using a PEEP or increasing the PEEP, and carefully increasing peak pressure (these techniques create increased risk of complications).
(Reprinted with permission from Mason TN: A hand ventilation technique for infants. MCN 7(6):367, November/December 1982. Copyright © 1982, American Journal of Nursing Company)

inserted and the endotracheal tube of correct size is inserted on the right side of the mouth and advanced into the trachea. If is helpful to measure the distance from mouth to suprasternal notch before placing the tube (Fig. 44-12). The pressure of bilateral breath sounds when bagged with 100% oxygen means that placement is accurate. If one side has diminished breath sounds, the tube is probably placed too far. An x-ray film will confirm placement, which really cannot be done during a delivery area resuscitation. After insertion is accomplished, the infant is mechanically ventilated by rapid bagging with 100% oxygen. It is important to secure

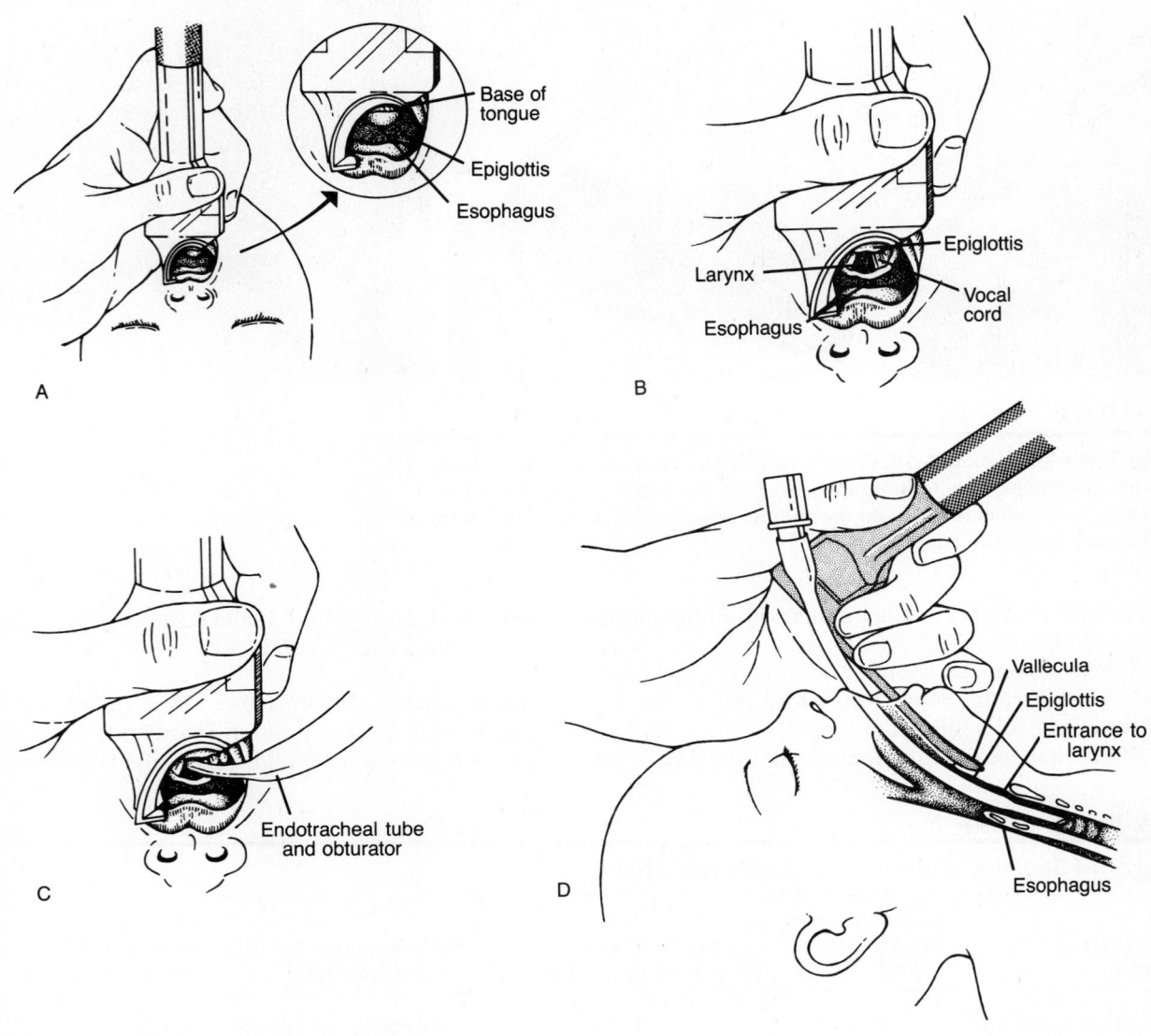

FIGURE 44-12

Technique of endotracheal intubation. The Miller blade should be inserted near the midline and moved to the left side of the mouth, gently deflecting the tongue. As it is advanced, the base of the tongue and epiglottis are visualized. The blade should be advanced in the same plane of movement into the vallecula (see *D*); as the blade is gently raised, the epiglottis swings anteriorly, revealing the opening of the larynx. If secretions or meconium is noted, gentle suctioning should be done before insertion of the endotracheal tube. On certain occasions when the epiglottis is not adequately raised, the blade tip may be placed posterior to the epiglottis, which can then be gently raised to expose the vocal cords. The endotracheal tube is advanced from the right corner of the mouth and inserted while maintaining direct visualization. The laryngoscope blade is then carefully withdrawn while the position of the tube is maintained by the right hand on the infant's face. Note the tip of the blade in the vallecula.

the tube somewhat before transporting the infant from the delivery area. Application of tincture of benzoin to the upper lip and cheeks followed by adhesive strips helps stabilize the tube until it can be more permanently secured for long-term care (Fig. 44-13).[25]

Circulation

While other resuscitative measures are being accomplished, the pulse should be monitored and cardiac compression performed in the event of cardiac arrest. Two fingers should be placed in the middle of the sternum and compressed halfway to the spine at a rate of about 80 to 100 per minute (see Fig. 44-10*B*).

It is imperative to maintain the cardiac massage and the ventilation. This can be accomplished by alternating the two maneuvers. A 5:1 ratio of cardiac massage to assisted ventilation of 100% oxygen should be used. The two procedures must not be performed simultaneously because the pressure applied during cardiac massage may rupture a lung that has just been inflated by the ventilation. If the procedure is effective, the femoral or temporal artery pulses are palpable in synchrony with depression of the sternum. The procedure is to be discontinued periodically to determine the presence of spontaneous cardiac activity. When this occurs, cardiac compression may be discontinued.

Drugs

Drugs may be required in a resuscitative effort (Table 44-3). Drugs are not the primary emphasis in a resuscitative effort, but their indications and usual dosages should be reviewed.

Environment

Infants who are at risk for cold stress are low birth weight, SGA, preterm, or asphyxiated. These infants are at risk owing to the lack of fat deposits and less brown fat available for generation of heat. Less subcutaneous fat is available for heat conservation. Brown fat thermogenesis is decreased in the asphyxiated infant who has been hypoxic. Precautions must be taken to observe these infants closely to prevent any further environmental insult. Once other resuscitative measures have been accomplished—airway, breathing, circulation, and drugs—the infant's axillary temperature should be taken. Controlled heat and slow rewarming are recommended, with continuous temperature monitoring by temperature probe taped to the abdomen. The infant with cold stress may exhibit RDS symptoms of tachypnea, flaring, grunting, and retractions. These symptoms disappear as the temperature returns to normal.[25]

Once the infant is supported and stabilized, immediate transport to the NICU is recommended, whether in-house or to a regional center. Parents should be informed of all events and permitted to see their infant as soon as possible.

Transport of the Infant at Risk

Recent advances and specialization in the care of the neonate have resulted in the regionalization of services for the high-risk neonate. (See Chapter 47 for a discussion of the structure of various regional centers.)

Transport is accomplished when sick infants are identified and admitted to a tertiary-care center. In some cases, *in utero* transport can be carried out when the birth of a critically ill neonate is anticipated. Unfortunately, it is not always possible to transport the mother, so most centers have a transport team available to accompany the neonate from the referral hospital to the center. Transportation is accomplished by ground or air ambulance. The transport team usually consists of a registered nurse or physician and a registered respiratory therapist. General indications for neonatal transport and the equipment required are listed.

It is essential that the parents have the opportunity to see the infant before the transport team departs. It is helpful for the parents to have a picture of the infant to keep with them.

Neonatal Intensive Care Unit

NICUs, developed to provide highly skilled nursing and medical care to the high-risk neonate, require extensive sophisticated equipment (Fig. 44-14). The first of such types of nurseries emerged in the mid-1960s in the United States. Nurses provide 24-hour care, with one nurse for every one or two critically ill neonates. With the emphasis now on the development of the whole infant and family, sole physical care is obsolete. Nurseries are designed with infant stimulation in mind as well as a comfortable setting for the families involved.

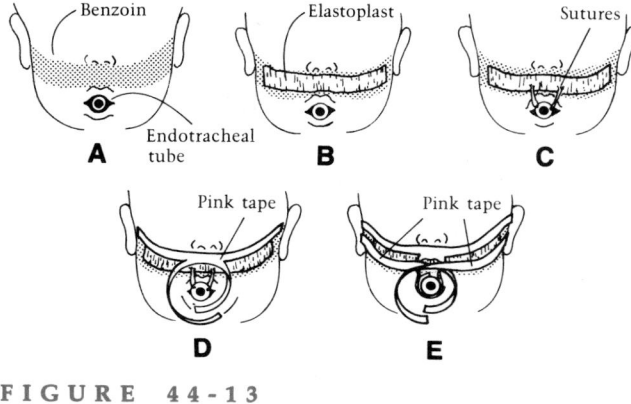

FIGURE 44-13

Technique for securing an orotracheal tube. (Redrawn from Gregory GA: Respiratory care of newborn infants. Pediatr Clin North Am 19:317, 1972)

TABLE 44-3

Drugs Used in the Resuscitation of Infants and Children

Agent*	How Supplied	Recommended Dose†	Uses
Atropine sulfate	0.4 mg/ml ampule	IV 0.01 mg–0.05 mg/kg/dose	To reverse or prevent the effects of the vagus nerve on the heart, tracheobronchial tree, and mucous membranes
Calcium	Calcium gluconate, a 10% solution containing 100 mg Ca gluconate/ml (9.7 mg elemental calcium/ml)	100 mg/kg day (1 ml–2 ml/kg/day) or 0.1 ml–0.2 ml/kg 1 dose IV slowly, with heart rate monitored for bradycardia	Calcium is a potent stimulant of cardiac contractile force, used to increase cardiac output
	Calcium chloride, a 10% solution containing 100 mg Ca chloride/ml (27.2 mg elemental calcium/ml)	10 mg/kg (0.1 ml/kg) IV slowly, with the same precautions as for gluconate. May repeat every 3–5 min to maximum dose of 2 ml/kg	
Dextrose (50%)	50-ml ampules, vials	1 ml/kg initially. May be repeated	Used to correct hypoglycemia; stimulates cardiac contractile force
Dopamine	200 mg in 5 ml	Dilute 100 mg in 100 ml normal saline to produce solution of 1 mg/ml. Give 5 μg–10 μg/kg/min initially, titrate up to 50 μg/kg/min	Used as a support for failing circulation
Epinephrine (Adrenalin)	1:1000 solution	Dilute to 1 mg/10 ml by adding 1 ml of 1:1000 epinephrine to 9 ml of normal saline. Give 0.1 ml of this solution/kg body weight (0.01 mg/kg)	A potent stimulant of cardiac contractile force and excitation; valuable for initiating contraction in the arrested heart
Isoproterenol	0.2 mg/ml 1.0 mg/5 ml	Dilute 1 mg in 100 ml normal saline to produce solution of 10 μg/ml, or 1 mg in 250 ml normal saline to produce solution of 4 μg/ml. Give 0.05 μg–0.5 μg/kg/min, IV	Cardiac stimulant that increases cardiac output; used to maintain blood pressure in shock; smooth muscle relaxant used for severe bronchospasm
Lidocaine	1% solution (10 mg/ml)	0.5 mg–1 mg/kg slowly IV every 20 min‡	Used to decrease ventricular irritability, maintain a normal rhythm following defibrillation, and increase the chances of successful defibrillation
Sodium bicarbonate	Ampules of 50 mEq/50 ml or 10 mEq/10 ml	2 mEq–5 mEq/kg slowly IV. May repeat at 5- to 10-min intervals, if needed	Used to correct acidosis, which is always associated with inadequate circulation and reduced peripheral perfusion occurring during an arrest

Defibrillation: 2 to 5 watt-sec/kg initially

* Most emergency drugs are toxic. Review the package insert for complete information about dosage and side-effects, toxicities, contraindications, and need for special monitoring.
† Consult package insert for information about administration and maximum doses.
‡ Doses not definitely established for infants and children.
(Waechter EH, Phillips J, Holaday B: Nursing Care of Children, 16th ed. Philadelphia, JB Lippincott, 1985)

Neonatal Transport

General neonatal indications for transport:
- Low birth weight or preterm
- Respiratory assistance needed
- High acuity level
- Life-threatening surgery
- Seizures
- Persistent fetal circulation

Equipment required:

Battery-operated monitors for vital signs, blood pressure

Transcutaneous oxygen monitor

Suction equipment

Intravenous pump, equipment

Respirator

Blood-drawing equipment

Resuscitation equipment

Transport equipment should be checked every shift*

* For details see OGN Nursing Practice Resource, Maternal-Neonatal Transport, No. 8, June 1983.

Continuing Management

Providing a Thermoneutral Environment

A thermoneutral environment keeps the infant's metabolic rate and oxygen consumption at a minimum and temperature within normal range. Skin temperature should be maintained between 36.1°C and 36.7°C (96.8°F to 97.8°F). Axillary temperature should be kept at or about 36.7°C (97.8°F). Infants of low birth weight have more difficulty maintaining a normal temperature owing to a decrease in subcutaneous fat, a small body mass to larger surface area, thin fragile skin, and an extended limbs posture.[27]

Temperature of the neonate may be assessed by one or several of the following means:

- Probe taped to skin
- Axillary temperature
- Anal (core) temperature

Environmental temperature should be assessed frequently in conjunction with the infant's temperature.

Several types of equipment may be used for the provision of heat in the neonate. The standard isolette does not provide as much accessibility as the overhead warmer. Isolettes can provide humidity and isolation (Fig. 44-15). The isolette can be flooded with oxygen but only to a maximum of about 40%. The temperature of the isolette can be adapted by a servocontrol mechanism and Thermistor probe taped to the skin. Double-walled units or heat shields can help reduce heat loss incurred upon entering the isolette.

The radiant overhead warmer provides improved visibility and accessibility to the neonate (Fig. 44-16). A temperature probe unit adjusts the heat flow in accordance with the infant's skin temperature. One significant disadvantage of the radiant warmer is insensible water loss. Insensible water loss represents that water lost from the lungs and skin through the mechanism of convection and evaporation. The use of plastic sheeting has been found most effective in reducing insensible water loss. The use of heat shields may interfere with radiant heat transfer and impede the servocontrol function.[27]

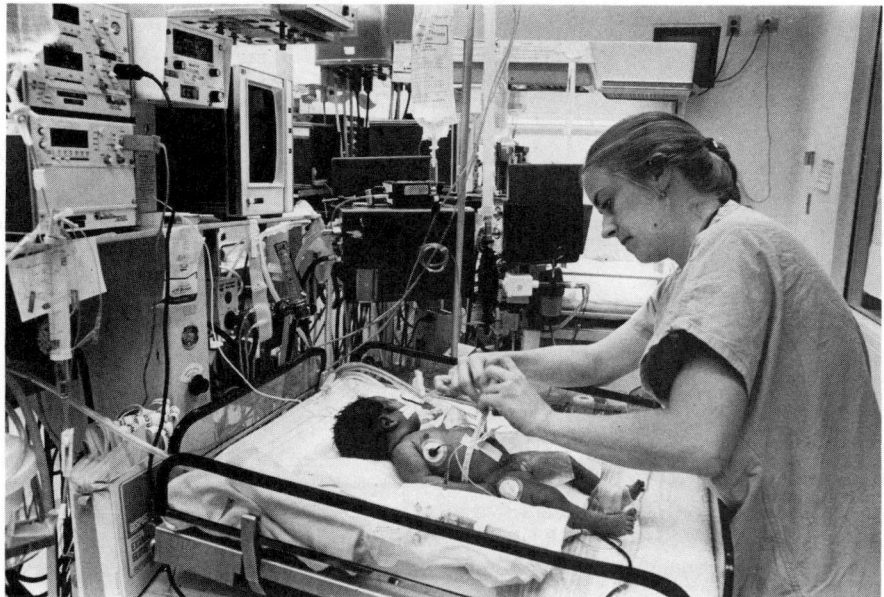

FIGURE 44-14

Sophisticated equipment and highly skilled nursing and medical care are the hallmark of the NICU. (Courtesy of The Children's Hospital of Philadelphia)

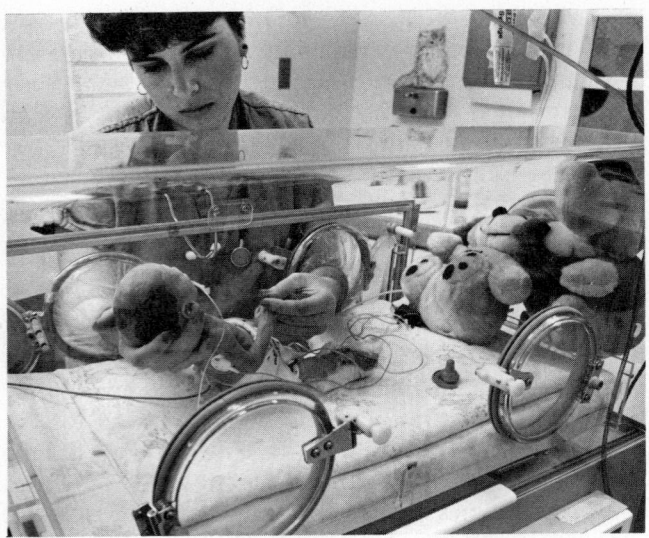

Isolette. Access to the neonate is provided through hand holes so that the carefully controlled environment will not be disturbed. (Courtesy of The Children's Hospital of Philadelphia)

All equipment used must be checked thoroughly and frequently for correct functioning. Temperature probes used must be kept taped on the skin. Units housing infants should be kept away from drafts.

All those caring for infants should always use warm hands, warm surfaces, warmed oxygen. All procedures should be carried out in a warm area or under a radiant heat source.

Nurses should observe infants for signs of cold stress, such as tachypnea, apneic spells, and color changes.

If infants do become chilled they should be warmed slowly over a period of hours to avoid apnea. The heating unit's desired temperature should be increased very gradually until the infant's temperature is stable.

As the infant's condition stabilizes, he can be weaned slowly from an isolette. Initially he is dressed in a shirt and diaper as the isolette's temperature is gradually lowered. If this is successful, the portholes are opened, the heat is turned off, and the infant eventually is transferred to an open crib.

Maintaining Skin Integrity

The skin functions as a barrier against infection, helps regulate body temperature, stores fats, discharges electrolytes and water, and protects organs.

The preterm's skin is particularly fragile and susceptible to trauma and irritation. The outside layer of the epidermis, the stratum corneum, becomes thicker as maturation occurs. Skin permeability decreases with increasing gestational age. Finally, bonds between the layers of epidermis and dermis strengthen with increasing gestational age.[28]

The use of tape is necessary to secure monitor leads and other pieces of equipment used in the NICU. The choice of tape deserves due consideration, as well as the amount and placement. Skin blankets with porous adhesive backing, such a Hollihesive and Stomahesive, have been used with success in some neonatal units. This material is pliable, is easy to remove, and can be cut into various shapes. Tape can then be placed on top of the "skin blanket" without directly touching the skin.[28] Problems are encountered with electrodes, which must be in direct skin contact. Electrodes can be wrapped on with kling. The use of limb electrodes is a possibility.

Op-Site, when used for a dressing for burns and other skin problems, is very useful owing to its transparent and waterproof nature.

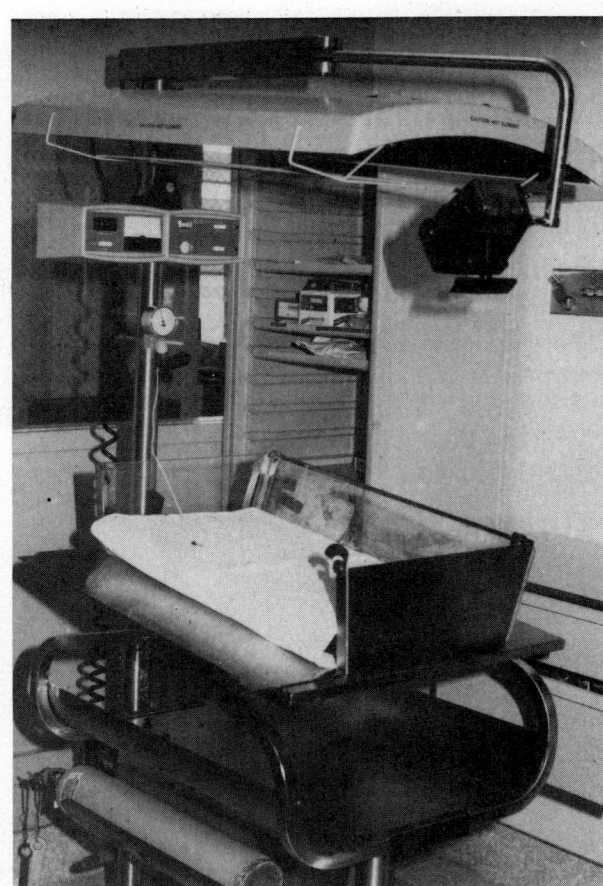

The radiant overhead warmer. Although visibility and accessibility are provided with the radiant warmer, a problem is insensible water loss.

The preterm infant's skin is extremely permeable to topical ointments, so great care should be taken with their application.

Preventing Infection

The nurse should observe the preterm infant carefully for signs of sepsis. Every item that comes into contact with the infant must be kept scrupulously clean. Each infant should have his own stockpile of equipment for his own use. Frequent cultures should be taken of items in the environment. Personnel should adhere to the hand-washing routines and dress codes of their particular unit. Any personnel with contagious illnesses should not contact the susceptible neonate.

Some nurseries place all infants weighing less than 1000 g on reverse isolation: incubator, sterile linens, and gloves.[27]

Respiratory Care

Assessment.   Observation of the preterm infant provides numerous clues as to respiratory status.

Respirations should be counted for a full minute, since irregularity is common (Fig. 44-17). Instances of periodic breathing are to be expected; however, apnea may be of a more pathologic nature. The usual respiratory rate ranges from 40 to 60 breaths per minute.

The infant's color should be generally pink. In the first few hours after birth, acrocyanosis may occur owing to vasomotor instability.

Respiratory movements should be symmetrical. The abdomen can be seen rising and falling as breaths are inspired and expired.

Respiratory distress is indicated by tachypnea, retractions, grunting, nasal flaring, cyanosis, pallor, hypotonia, and bradycardia.

Additional data regarding respiratory status are provided by auscultation to ascertain abnormal breath sounds and indications of airway obstructions. Accurate identification of abnormal breath sounds requires considerable practice and skill on the part of the nurse. The infant's chest size requires the use of a stethoscope with a small diaphragm so that it picks up more local sounds than those transmitted across the small chest. Breath sounds should be auscultated bilaterally, moving the stethoscope down the chest along the midaxillary line both laterally and anteriorly.[14] Abnormal or diminished breath sounds should be noted. Infants may present with rales, rhonchi, or decreased breath sounds in various disease states. Breath sounds should be equal bilaterally.

Upon auscultation of the chest the heart sounds are assessed by counting the rate, describing the quality and location of the point of maximal impulse (PMI).

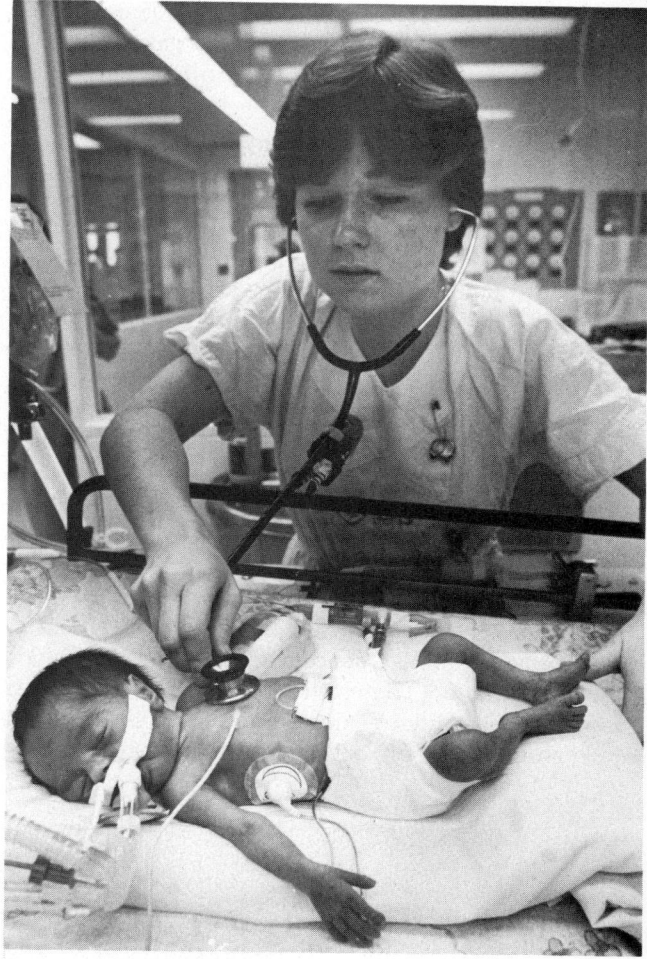

FIGURE 44-17

Respirations are assessed by the nurse for a full minute. The usual rate ranges from 40 to 60 breaths per minute. (Courtesy of The Children's Hospital of Philadelphia)

Murmurs may be noted as well as displacement of the PMI. The PMI is usually located in the fourth intercostal space to the left of the sternum in the midclavicular line. A displacement of the PMI may be indicative of pneumothorax.

Monitoring of Blood Gas Status.   Those infants experiencing respiratory distress and thus requiring additional oxygen or ventilatory support must have frequent blood gas samples taken to titrate oxygen requirements and ventilatory settings.

Blood gases may be monitored by several techniques: indwelling catheter, intermittent punctures, capillary sampling, and transcutaneous monitoring.

The use of an indwelling catheter is by far the most accurate of methods for measuring blood gases; however, it can subject the neonate to complications of emboli and arterial spasm. Indwelling catheters provide easy access to obtaining periodic blood gas samples.

Intermittent arterial punctures require great skill on the part of the technician. Crying by the infant may alter the PO_2 reading.

Heel-stick capillary samples are much easier to obtain but are not reliable for PO_2 readings.

Transcutaneous oxygen tension ($TcPO_2$) monitoring has been developed recently and is being used increasingly in the neonatal intensive care settings. This device is noninvasive and provides continuous monitoring of PO_2 readings. The monitoring of continuous status is helpful to observe the neonate's response to nursing interventions such as weighing, nasogastric feedings, suctioning, and postural drainage. One nursing research study demonstrated significant decrease in $TcPO_2$ during suctioning and repositioning but not during heel-stick procedures.[29] Another study showed a modest increase in $TcPO_2$ and heart rate during nonnutritive sucking in preterm infants of less than 33 weeks' gestation and weighing less than 1500 g.[30] Placement of the electrode requires a space with good capillary blood flow and little fat. The electrode should not be placed on a bony prominence. Commonly used sites are the upper chest, abdomen, and inner thigh. The site should be changed and the electrode recalibrated minimally every 4 hours.[14] Some reports of skin erosion beneath the electrode make diligent assessment of skin a vital task.

Administration of Oxygen and Ventilatory Support.

Flooding of the isolette with oxygen presents problems since the maximum concentration able to be maintained is probably no more than 30% to 40%. Frequent opening of the portholes makes maintaining a constant flow impossible.

When other ventilator support is not necessary, administration of oxygen by hood is an option (Fig. 44-18). An oxygen analyzer must be kept in the hood to measure the percent of oxygen administered. Oxygen should be warm and kept at a stable temperature. The neonate should be suctioned periodically to maintain the open airway. Blood gases should be monitored every 4 hours and 10 to 20 minutes following each change in FIO_2.

Continuous positive airway pressure results from a machine applying pressure throughout the lungs of the neonate. This type of pressure helps to keep the alveoli open, thus decreasing the work of breathing and oxygen requirements. Infants with RDS benefit the most from

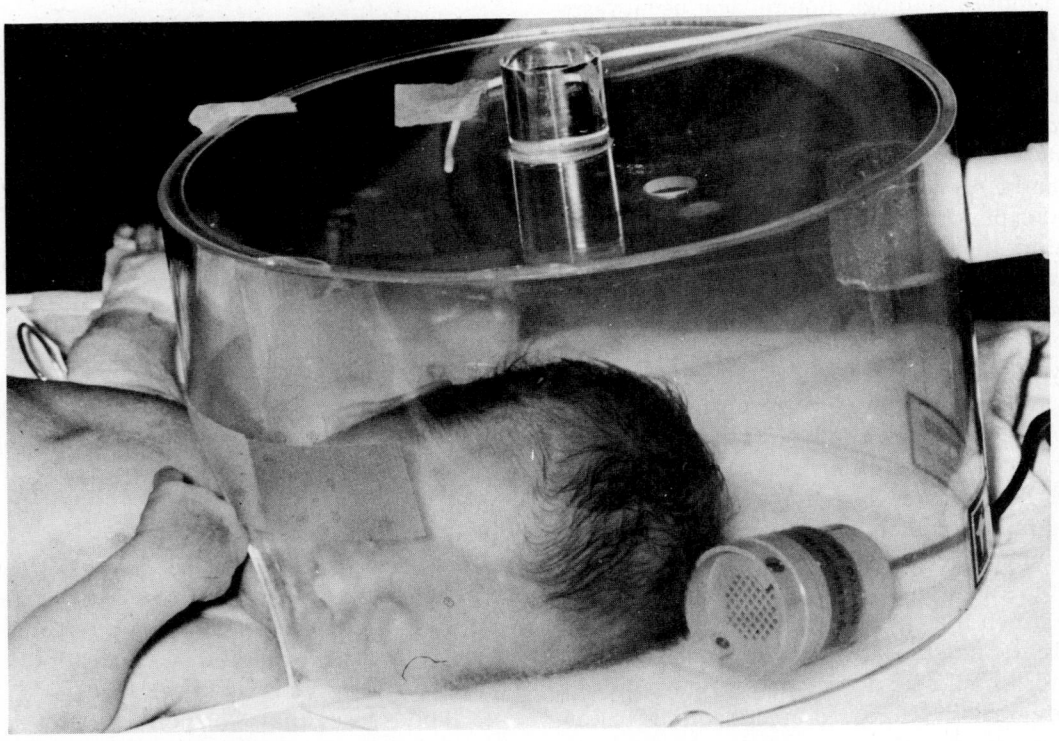

FIGURE 44-18

Oxygen hood for administration of controlled oxygen concentration. Note the temperature probe passing through the lid and the sensor of oxygen analyzer next to infant's face. (Avery GB: Neonatology, 3rd ed. Philadelphia, JB Lippincott, 1987)

CPAP, since atelectasis is a common complication. The use of CPAP is indicated for a PaO_2 of less than 50 mm Hg in the presence of 60% oxygen.[14]

CPAP pressure is measured in centimeters of H_2O. Initial amount delivered is usually 4 cm to 6 cm. This pressure is slowly increased until oxygenation is sufficient as measured by blood gas readings. CPAP is usually delivered by nasal prongs or endotracheal intubation (Fig. 44-19). The nurse must observe for complications of pneumothorax.

Mechanical Ventilation.

In the event of apnea or inability to maintain adequate oxygenation with CPAP, endotracheal intubation and positive-pressure ventilation may be essential for respiratory assistance. PaO_2 of less than 50 mm Hg, $PaCO_2$ of greater than 60, and pH of less than 7.25 in 100% oxygen with CPAP indicate that respiratory assistance is required. Other indicators are apnea, severe retractions, respiratory rate over 80, and cyanosis.[31]

In the preterm infant with RDS the ideal PaO_2 should be maintained between 50 and 75 mm Hg to avoid complications of retrolental fibroplasia and BPD.[31]

Several kinds of positive-pressure ventilators are available (Table 44-4). The nurse must become intimately familiar with the particular machine used in her unit as well as the implications of the various settings. Various parameters that may be altered to provide maximal assistance for each individual patient are peak inspiratory pressure (PIP), respiratory rate, inspiratory/expiratory ratio (I/E), PEEP, and oxygen flow rate delivered (FiO_2). It is important once the endotracheal tube is placed for the infant to be bagged to estimate ventilator settings before placing the infant on the ventilator itself. Securing of the tube is essential for anticipated long-term therapy.

Once the infant is placed on the respirator, ventilator settings and alarms must be checked frequently. Blood gases must be checked at least every 4 hours and 10 to 20 minutes past a change in ventilator settings.

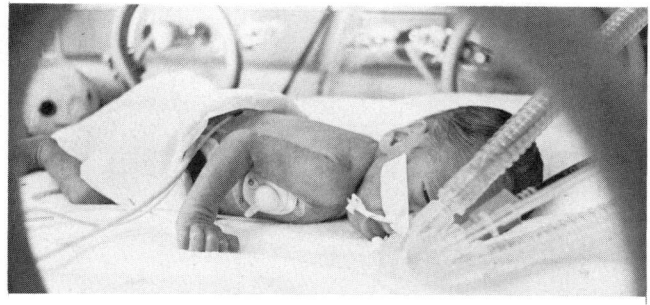

TABLE 44-4

Commonly Used Positive-Pressure Ventilators

Volume Type

Bournes LS 104–150 (Bournes Medical Systems, Riverside, California)

Servo 900B (Siemens Corporation, Union, New Jersey)

Pressure Type

Time Cycled

Bournes BP 200 (Bournes Medical Systems, Riverside, California)

Bear BP 2001 (Bear Intermed, Riverside, California)

Healthdyne 100 (Healthdyne, Inc., Marietta, Georgia)

Sechrist IV-100 (Sechrist Industries, Inc., Anaheim, California)

Pressure Cycled

Baby Bird II (Bird Corporation, Palm Springs, California)

Cavitron PV-10 (Healthdyne, Inc., Marietta, Georgia)

(Spitzer AR, Fox WW: Use and abuse of mechanical ventilators. In Stern L (ed): Hyaline Membrane Disease: Pathogenesis and Pathophysiology. Orlando, Grune & Stratton, 1984. By permission)

Suctioning is essential to keep the airway open. Suctioning should be carried out as a sterile procedure, following the instillation of a small amount of normal saline. The neonate should be oxygenated by bagging before and after the procedure. Chest physical therapy may be necessary to assist in the mobilization of secretions (Fig. 44-20). Various devices such as padded nipples and electric toothbrushes may be used for percussion and vibration techniques.[32] The head-down position must be used with caution, since it may be implicated in the development of intracranial bleeding.

Muscle relaxant drugs may need to be administered to enhance respiratory assistance put forth by the ventilator. Pancuronium bromide (Pavulon) is the drug most commonly used in the neonate. One additional drug used to correct metabolic acidosis is sodium bicarbonate, which must be administered at a very slow rate.

Blood Pressure

It is essential for nurses to be able to measure intraarterial blood pressure in the critically ill neonate. Owing to decrease in peripheral perfusion, the indirect Doppler method is less reliable. Some changes in neonatal clinical status may become evident in blood pressure prior to observation of other behavioral changes. Thus, the ability to monitor blood pressure intra-arterially is a critical nursing function. Although the most common route is the umbilical artery, peripheral arteries may also be used (Fig. 44-21).

In addition to monitoring and recording the blood pressure, the nurse must care for the system (*i.e.,* cali-

(text continued on page 1008)

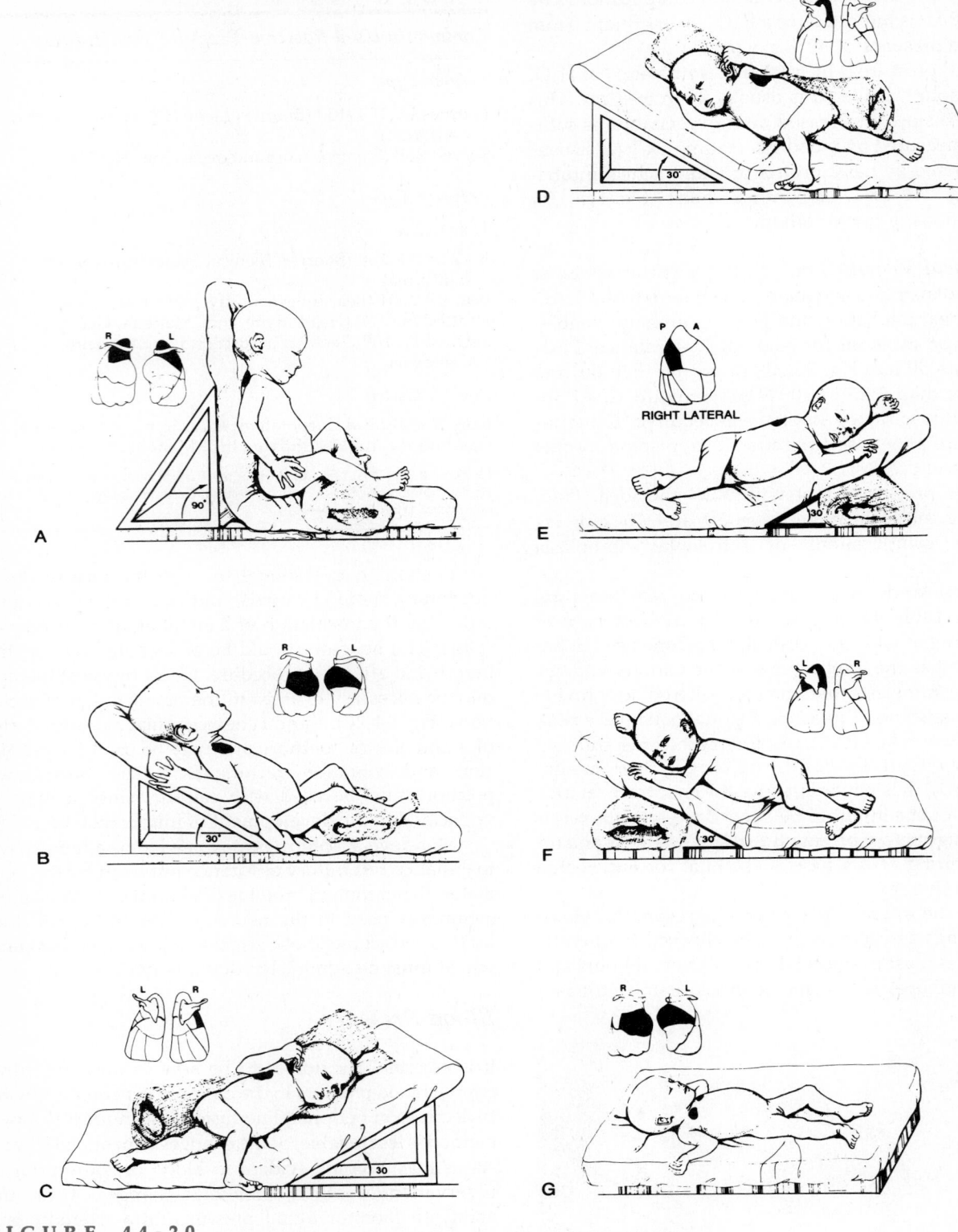

FIGURE 44-20

Postural drainage positions. Insets indicate the segments drained for each position. Shading on the infant indicates the area for chest percussion and vibrations. (Fletcher MA, MacDonald M, Avery G: Atlas of Procedures in Neonatology. Philadelphia, JB Lippincott, 1983)

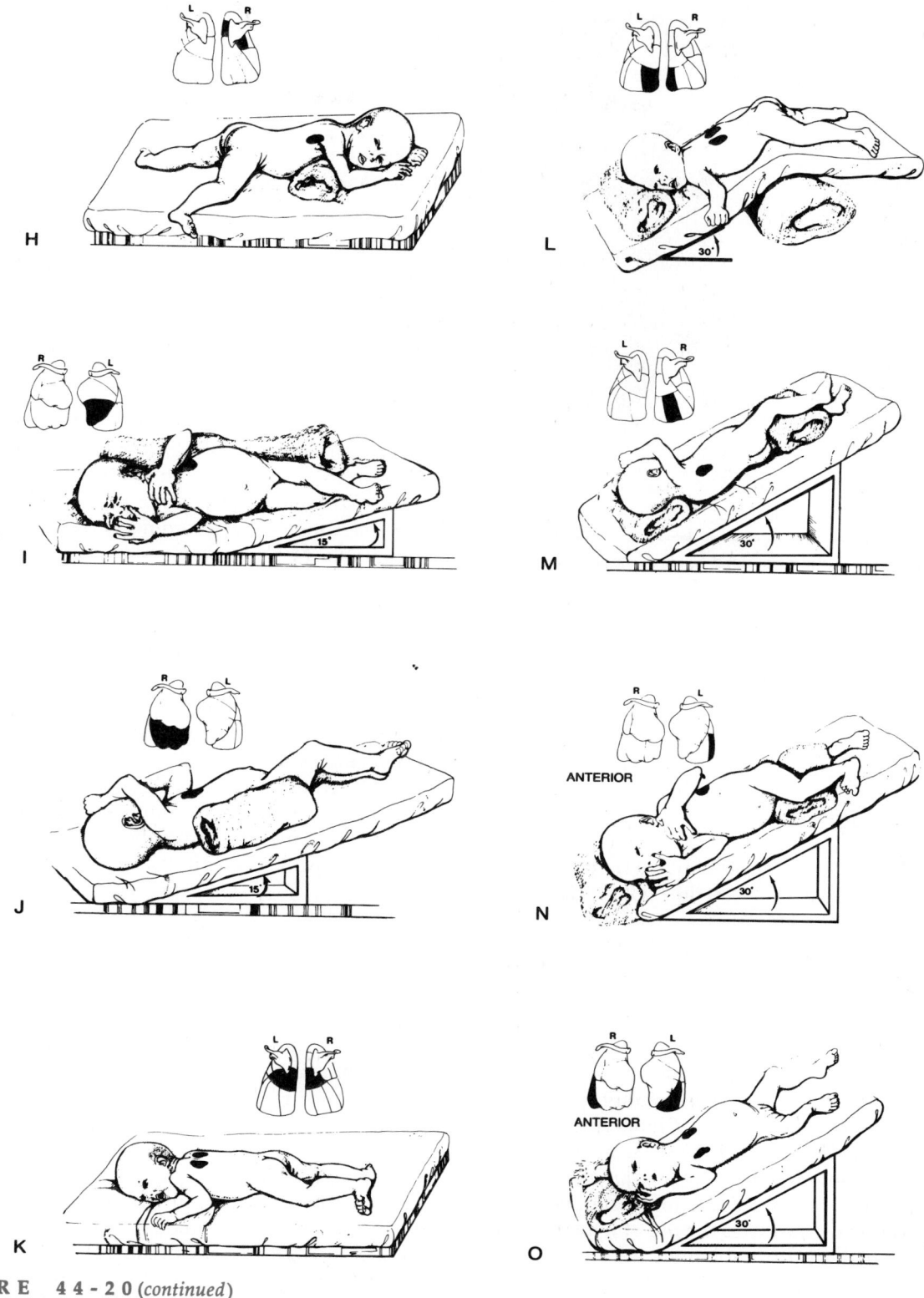

FIGURE 44-20 (continued)

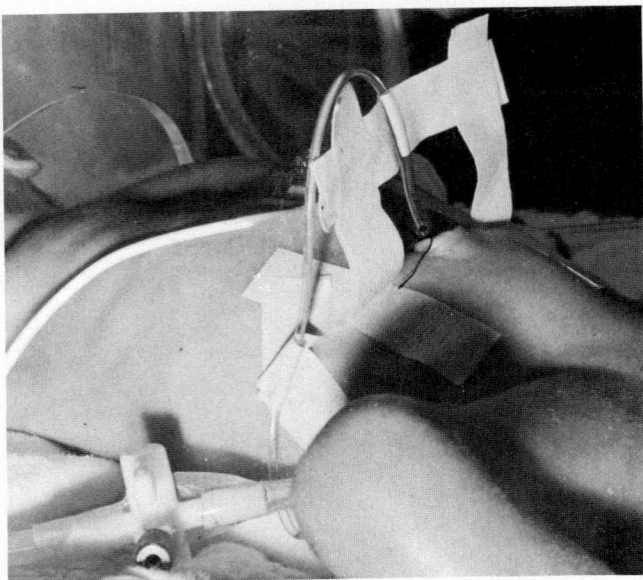

FIGURE 44-21

An umbilical artery catheter is used to monitor blood pressure. This is a sterile procedure. A bridge is taped over the catheter to secure it. (Symansky MR, Fox HA: Umbilical vessel catheterization: Indications, management, and evaluation of the technique. J Pediatr 80:820, 1972)

(text continued from page 1005)
bration, expelling of air bubbles, changing of tubing, and checking alarms).

Nutritional Support

Fluid Therapy.　Since preterm infants are particularly susceptible to water losses due to the high surface/body mass ratio, permeable skin, and use of radiant warmers, they require adequate fluid intake at all times. Further, most preterm infants initially are too critically ill to tolerate enteral feedings. Several routes of parenteral fluid administration may be used.

Peripheral or central catheters may be used for the administration of fluids. When administration of fluids is supplemented or considered temporary, peripheral lines may be the optimum route. If long-term therapy is anticipated, especially with TPN, placement of a central line into the internal and external jugular is warranted. The catheter is threaded into the superior vena cava. This placement facilitates the use of hyperosmolar solutions and high dextrose solutions such as TPN.

Fluid volume requirements range from an initial 80 ml to 120 ml/kg/day to 120 ml to 180 ml/kg/day by the first week. Due to their immature gastrointestinal systems, even small changes in fluid intake may adversely affect the preterm infant, such as fluid overload precipitating congestive heart failure or patent ductus arteriosus.

Certain criteria may be measured by the nurse to ensure adequate nutritional intake.

1. Continued weight gain of 20 g to 30 g/day
2. Adequate urine output of 1 ml to 3 ml/kg/hr
3. Specific gravity of urine 1.006 to 1.013, negative glucose
4. Normal Dextrostix

Accurate assessment of intake and output is essential. All gains and losses must be accounted for, such as catheter flushes. The prescribed amount of intravenous fluid must be administered per hour. Skin turgor and the state of the fontanel are other measures of hydration. Infants should be weighed at the same time every day.[7]

Specific Nutritional Requirements.　Not all is known regarding specific nutritional requirements for the low-birth-weight and preterm infants.

Caloric requirements on the average are 120 mg/kg/day, but may vary according to the individual situation (Table 44-5).

Protein requirements range from approximately 2.25 g/kg/day to 5 g/kg/day. Some higher-calorie, higher-protein formulas have been developed to meet these requirements. Human milk contains specific immunologic properties. Milk of mothers who deliver prematurely may have a 20% higher protein content, and such milk promotes growth. However, human milk is ordinarily relatively low in protein.[33]

Fats should account for 40% to 50% of the total caloric intake. The introduction of medium-chain triglycerides results in better fat absorption. It is not clear whether or not this actually leads to improved weight gain.

Carbohydrate requirements have not been determined.

Iron needs to be supplemented at about 8 weeks when stores are depleted; 2 mg/kg/day is the recommended dosage.[34]

Vitamins can be provided in the form of a multivitamin supplement. Folic acid and B_{12} need to be supplemented separately. Vitamin E needs to be supplemented, with a dose range of 5 IU to 25 IU.

Feeding Schedule.　In planning the feeding schedule for the premature and low-birth-weight infant, it is important to establish a food tolerance, since the intestinal tract (as well as other organs) is underdeveloped. The caloric needs of the low-birth-weight baby are estimated according to the body weight. At first, the feeding should be in small amounts, increasing gradually to the amount that will produce a consistent gain. Vomiting and consequent aspiration, distention, and diarrhea may be due to overfeeding. Early and more nearly optimal feeding, in the case of the larger infant, will contribute

TABLE 44-5

Daily Feeding Requirements of Low-Birth-Weight and Premature Infants

Premature, appropriate for gestational age		Low birth weight		
Item	Calories/kg/24 hr	Nutrient requirements	First week of life	Active growth period
Resting	40–50 (depending on age)	Water (ml)	80–200	130–200
Activity	10–15	Calories	50–100	110–150*
Cold stress	5–10 (depending on environmental temperature)	Protein	1–2	3–4
		Glucose (g)	7–12	12–15
		Fat	3–4	5–8
Specific dynamic action	8–8	Sodium	1–2	2–3
		Potassium	1–2	2–4
Fecal loss	2*–12	Chloride	1–2	2–3
Growth	25–25	Calcium (mEq)	1–2	3–5
Total	90–120	Phosphorus	1–2	2–4
		Magnesium		0.5–1
		Iron (mg)		1.5–2

* Above 120 calories/kg applies to infants with perinatal undergrowth.
(Babson SG, Benson RC, Pernoll MI et al: Management of High-Risk Pregnancy and Intensive Care of the Neonate. St Louis, CV Mosby, 1975)

to lessening mortality and morbidity by preventing nutritive depletion and maintaining biochemical homeostasis.

Those infants in good condition (these are usually but not always the larger infants) with active peristalsis may be started on oral 5% to 10% glucose or sterile water. Studies have shown that sterile water, if aspirated, is less damaging to the lung than dextrose water or milk.[35]

For the infant in poor condition, no matter what the cause, oral feedings are usually withheld for several days if necessary. Parenteral fluids are instituted instead. If the infant is fed orally, some physicians begin the infant on a trial of plain water; if it is retained, then glucose water or dilute modified cow's milk formula is instituted at 2-hour intervals. Thus, there is a gradual replacement of water feedings by milk feedings. A gradual increase in the amounts of milk and water at each feeding should continue until caloric and fluid requirements are met. If an infant is taking about 180 ml of full-strength modified cow's milk formula per kilogram of body weight per day, he is getting about 120 calories per kilogram per day, which ensures an adequate weight gain (see Table 44-5).

Premature infants who weigh 1.4 kg (approximately 3 lb) or less may be fed every 2 or 3 hours. Infants who weigh over 1.4 kg (approximately 3 lb) may be placed on a 3- to 4-hour feeding schedule. The stomach of the premature baby needs rest between feedings as much as that of the full-term baby; therefore, the interval should be regulated accordingly. The schedule should be as near that of a normal infant as is compatible with its progress.

Gavage Feeding. Feeding by gavage, whether intermittent or continuous, is a common means of feeding infants who cannot tolerate oral feedings for a period of time and whose gastrointestinal tract is intact. Infants who may require this feeding assistance include those of less than 32 weeks' gestation and those with central nervous system depression and poor sucking reflexes. Appropriate-for-gestational-age infants who become very tired may require gavage to avoid needless energy expenditure and loss of calories.

For intermittent gavage feeding, a 5 F or 8 F feeding tube is chosen according to the infant's size and tolerance. Vagal stimulation with subsequent bradycardia may be a problem as the tube is introduced. The tube is measured from the tip of the nose or mouth to the tip of the earlobe, ending at the tip of the xiphoid process (Fig. 44-22). The tube may also be measured from the bridge of the nose to the umbilicus. The tube is then marked at the point of measurement, ensuring that it will be inserted only to that point.

The infant is positioned either on his back or on his side with his head elevated. The infant may need to be restrained in a mummy restraint or held during the procedure.

After the tube is lubricated with sterile water, the infant's head is held still with one hand and the tube is inserted up to the mark with the other hand. Tubes may be inserted through the mouth or the nares. Nose insertion may obstruct the passage of a nose breather and irritate the nasal mucosa (Fig. 44-23).

Correct placement of the feeding tube may be checked by aspiration of the gastric residuum and injection of 3 cc of air while listening with the stethoscope.

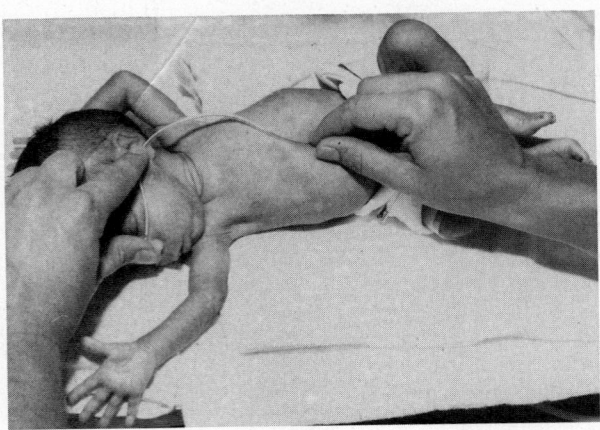

FIGURE 44-22

Measurement for gavage feeding.

Gastric residual should be measured and returned to the stomach unless otherwise ordered. If cyanosis, severe gagging, or coughing ensues, the tube may be misplaced and should be removed and reinserted properly.

Upon ascertaining correct placement, the syringe is separated from the tube. The plunger is then removed from the barrel, and the barrel is reconnected to the tube. The desired amount of formula is poured into the syringe. The syringe is elevated 6 to 8 inches over the infant's head, and the feeding is allowed to flow in by gravity.

When the formula is absorbed, the tube is rinsed with 2 ml to 3 ml of sterile water. The tube is folded over onto itself and removed with one smooth motion.

If the infant could not be held during the feeding, this is an appropriate time to hold him. Some infants enjoy sucking on a pacifier during the feeding. Sucking

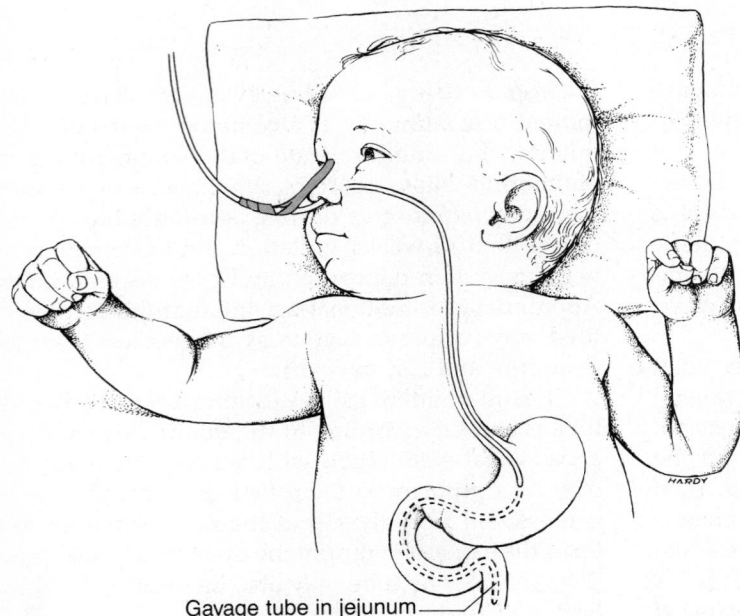

Gavage tube in jejunum

FIGURE 44-23

Gavage feeding.

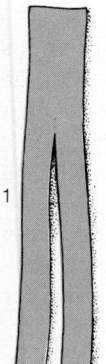
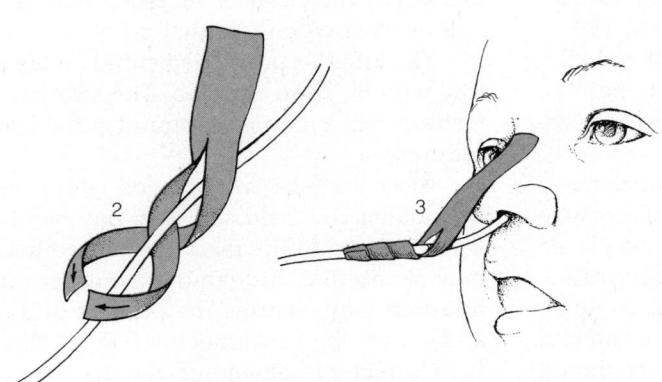

Steps in preparing adhesive tape to retain gavage tube

helps the infant to practice the reflex and associate it with a full stomach.

After feeding the infant should be positioned on his right side or his abdomen with the head slightly elevated to facilitate digestion.

Continuous gavage feedings by nasogastric tube may minimize problems of distention and aspiration. While a nasogastric tube is left securely taped in place, formula is pumped in by continuous drip. The tube may be clamped or removed when each feeding is complete. Residual as well as abdominal circumferences are checked frequently.

Nasojejunal and Nasoduodenal Feedings.

Continuous infusions by the nasojejunal and nasoduodenal routes represent alternative methods of nutritional support. The tube is passed into the stomach, and placement is checked by x-ray film when a gastric residual *p*H of 5 to 7 is obtained. Continuous infusion, advancing from glucose water to the infant's full fluid and caloric requirement, may be given. Hypertonic formulas should not be introduced directly into the small intestine. Perforations have been reported, because polyvinyl or polyethylene catheters become stiff after a week or so of continuous use. Oral feedings should be begun as soon as the infant's condition permits.[35]

The nurse needs to assess the infant for signs of abdominal distention by inspection and measurement of abdominal girth. Tubing is changed routinely to prevent bacterial growth. Residual is also checked and reported as per agency policy. Stool guaiac test needs to be performed to see that the infant is tolerating the feedings. Infants may need some form of restraint so that the tube will not be pulled out. Nonnutritive sucking may be enjoyed by the infant.[36]

Gastrostomy.

Gastrostomy tubes may be inserted, usually in surgical patients, to allow feedings to drip slowly into the stomach. Residual is checked prior to feeding. The tubing is left open between feedings about 10 cm to 12 cm above the abdominal wall.[35]

Bottle-Feeding.

Behaviors indicating that the infant may be ready to advance to bottle-feeding include a strong, vigorous suck, coordination of sucking and swallowing, sucking in response to the gavage tube, and wakefulness before feedings. The infant may be challenged with feedings slowly. Bottle-feedings could begin with once a day, then once a shift, then every other feeding, and so on, as tolerated. If the infant requires more than 30 minutes to finish the feeding, the next feeding should be a gavage feeding.[37]

A soft, average-sized nipple with an adequate opening is used. The infant may be helped to open his mouth to accept the nipple by applying gentle pressure

on his chin and touching his lips with the nipple. The infant is held in the semierect position to facilitate "burping" and nursing. After the feeding, the infant is positioned as described under gavage feeding.

There are several precautions to be aware of. The infant is not to be urged to accept more formula than is easily taken. Moreover, the bottle should be removed if the infant appears to be getting the milk too fast, in which case the infant usually gasps, chokes, or swallows so quickly as to interfere with respiration. Any infant who has been feeding well and shows reluctance to eat on two successive occasions needs critical reassessment.

Feedings are to be discontinued if the baby vomits, becomes cyanotic, overdistends, or develops frequent or diarrheal stools. Feedings should also be reevaluated if residual is increasing.

Total Parenteral Nutrition.

TPN, also known as *hyperalimentation*, is an aseptically prepared hypertonic solution composed of protein, carbohydrates, electrolytes, vitamins, and minerals (Table 44-6).

In cases in which oral feedings must be delayed for a long time, TPN has been able to provide adequate nutrition to the neonate. Indications for the use of TPN include low-birth-weight infants, surgical infants in whom the gut needs to be rested, NEC, and prolonged diarrhea.[35]

Central catheters for TPN infusion may be inserted in various sites: external or internal jugular, or internal jugular into superior vena cava (Fig. 44-24). Peripheral lines may also be used. TPN is infused at a carefully calculated rate by way of an infusion pump. A filter is placed close to the insertion site to help prevent infection. A sterile dressing is placed securely over the in-

TABLE 44-6

Daily Requirements of Total Parenteral Nutrition

Protein	2.5–3.5 g/kg
Fat Emulsion	2–4 g/kg
Calories	90–110 kcal/kg
H_2O	125–150 ml/kg or as needed
Na	3–4 meq/kg
K	2–3 meq/kg
Ca	50–100 mg/kg depending on size of infant
P	1–1.5 mmol/kg
Mg	1 meq/kg
Multivitamins* (MVI® Pediatric)	10 ml (65% of dosage to infants less than 3 kg; 30% to infants less than 1 kg)

* Multivitamin preparations are undergoing scrutiny because of the preservatives in them. Practitioners must keep abreast of current recommendations.
(From Avery GB, Fletcher AB: Nutrition. In Avery GB (ed): Neonatology, 3rd ed. Philadelphia, JB Lippincott, 1987)

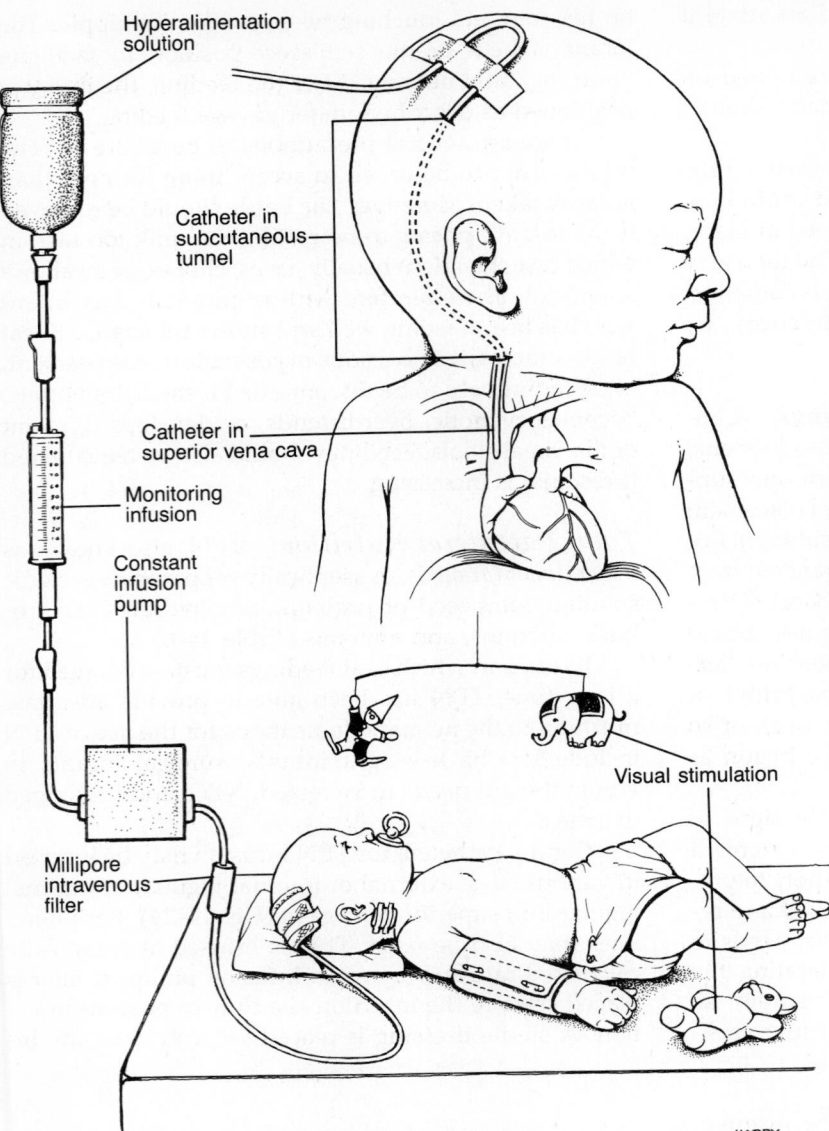

Hyperalimentation solution

Catheter in subcutaneous tunnel

Catheter in superior vena cava

Monitoring infusion

Constant infusion pump

Millipore intravenous filter

Visual stimulation

HARDY

FIGURE 44-24

Hyperalimentation (total parenteral nutrition) aseptically feeds the infant through, in this case, the superior vena cava. The solution is infused at a carefully calculated rate by way of an infusion pump.

sertion site. Neither medications nor blood should be given through the line.

Nursing care for the infant receiving TPN involves monitoring the equipment, the infusion, and the infant.

The solution is prepared aseptically in the pharmacy and refrigerated until used. The solution container, tubing, and filter must be changed minimally every 24 hours and labeled. The container label is carefully checked against the physician's order for correct ingredients and amounts.

Peripheral lines must be watched very carefully for any signs of infiltration. Severe tissue necrosis and sloughing can occur owing to the hyperosmolar solution. The insertion site dressing is changed at least three times a week using strict aseptic technique and following agency procedure. The infusion itself is maintained at the desired rate.

Various parameters are measured, such as Dextrostix, urine specific gravity, sugar and acetone, intake and output, and daily weights. Blood studies are done frequently to check electrolyte requirements (*i.e.*, hemoglobin, hematocrit, electrolytes, and serum osmolarity). The infant's sucking needs may be satisfied by a pacifier.

Intralipid. Intralipid is a Swedish soybean oil–egg emulsion designed to deliver extra calories and lower glucose concentration in addition to TPN. Infants on TPN alone develop fatty-acid deficiencies quite rapidly.

Intralipid should be infused slowly (preferably for 24 hours) in a line separate from other intravenous solutions, but may be run in the same line through a Y connector or close to the insertion site. Serum is checked for turbidity daily to ensure fat clearance. Serum fatty acids and triglyceride levels should be monitored weekly. The American Association of Pediatrics recommends that amount of lipids not exceed 3 g/kg/day, or 33 calories.[38]

Care of the Parents

The parents of high-risk newborns often have adaptational needs or problems that necessitate sensitive and thoughtful nursing care. Not only are they making the transition to new parenthood, with all its requirements, but they must cope with the unusual situation of a small, different, and often sick baby. The importance of the early postpartum period for the establishment of bonds between the parents and the newborn and the laying of the groundwork for healthy attitudes toward future relationships with the child must not be underestimated (Fig. 44-25).

Interactional Deprivation

Prolonged mother–infant separation has been studied for its effects on attachment. As soon as possible after the infant's birth, the mothers in the early-contact group were admitted into the nursery and encouraged to touch

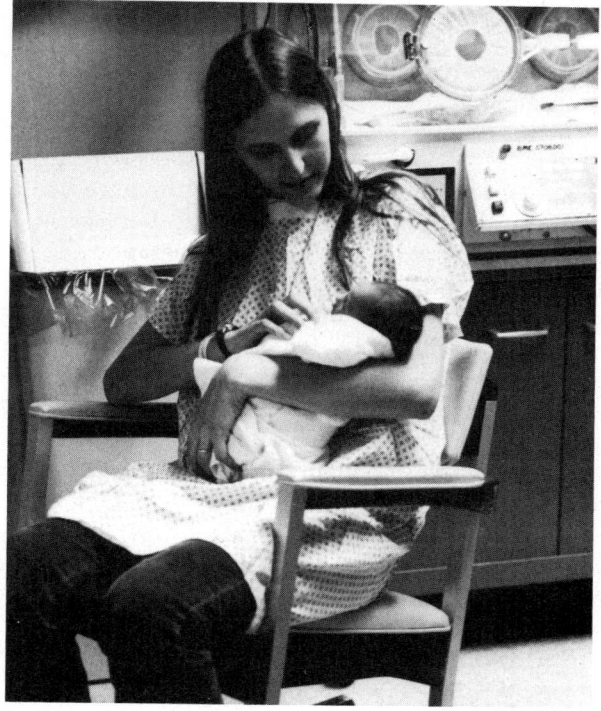

FIGURE 44-25

En face contact between mother and infant should be encouraged when the infant is removed briefly from the incubator.

their babies and to perform such caretaking duties as the infant's condition allowed. Mothers in the late-contact group were not permitted into the nursery until after their infants reach almost 1 month of age. Results revealed detectable differences in mothering performance between these two groups. In one study, high-contact mothers had higher scores on an attachment interview, on maternal performance, on *en face* feeding, and on the amount of fondling of infants when tested 1 month after delivery.[39] In another study comparing late- and early-contact mothers 1 month after discharge of the infants, and after 200 feedings at home, the late-contact mothers held their babies differently and changed their positions less, bubbled their infants less frequently, and were not as skillful in feeding.[40] Some mothers who were barred from interaction with their babies in the nursery resumed prior interests when they returned home. The babies then had to compete with these interests when they were discharged.

Such studies suggest that prolonged separation may adversely affect commitment or attachment between mother and infant, may reduce confidence in mothering abilities, and may interfere with the mother's ability to develop an efficient routine of care. When mothers were allowed into the high-risk nursery for early and frequent contact and caretaking of their infants, there was no increase in nursery infections or disruption of nursery routine.[41]

Modifying hospital routine to allow mothers early contact with their high-risk infants appears to have a positive effect on later maternal behavior. This lends support to the concept of a sensitive time for bonding to occur between the mother and her infant. This time is probably within the first several hours of delivery. Greater maternal attentiveness and better caretaking seem related to later exploratory behavior in infants; thus, removing barriers to maternal attachment during the sensitive period may have a potent influence on the later development of these babies.

Parental Reactions and Psychological Tasks

The birth of a premature or high-risk infant is often experienced as an acute emotional crisis by the family (Fig. 44-26). This causes a certain amount of disorganization in the parents before they are able to master their feelings and come to accept the event. Since the baby may be born before term, parents are often deprived of the last 6 to 8 weeks in which the final psychological (and sometimes material) preparation for the birth is made. Few of the physical and emotional signs of approaching labor (enumerated in Chap. 24) may happen. These are helpful to the mother in alerting her to the approach of another new phase in the childbearing process, and this awareness in turn assists her in achieving psychological preparation. The result may

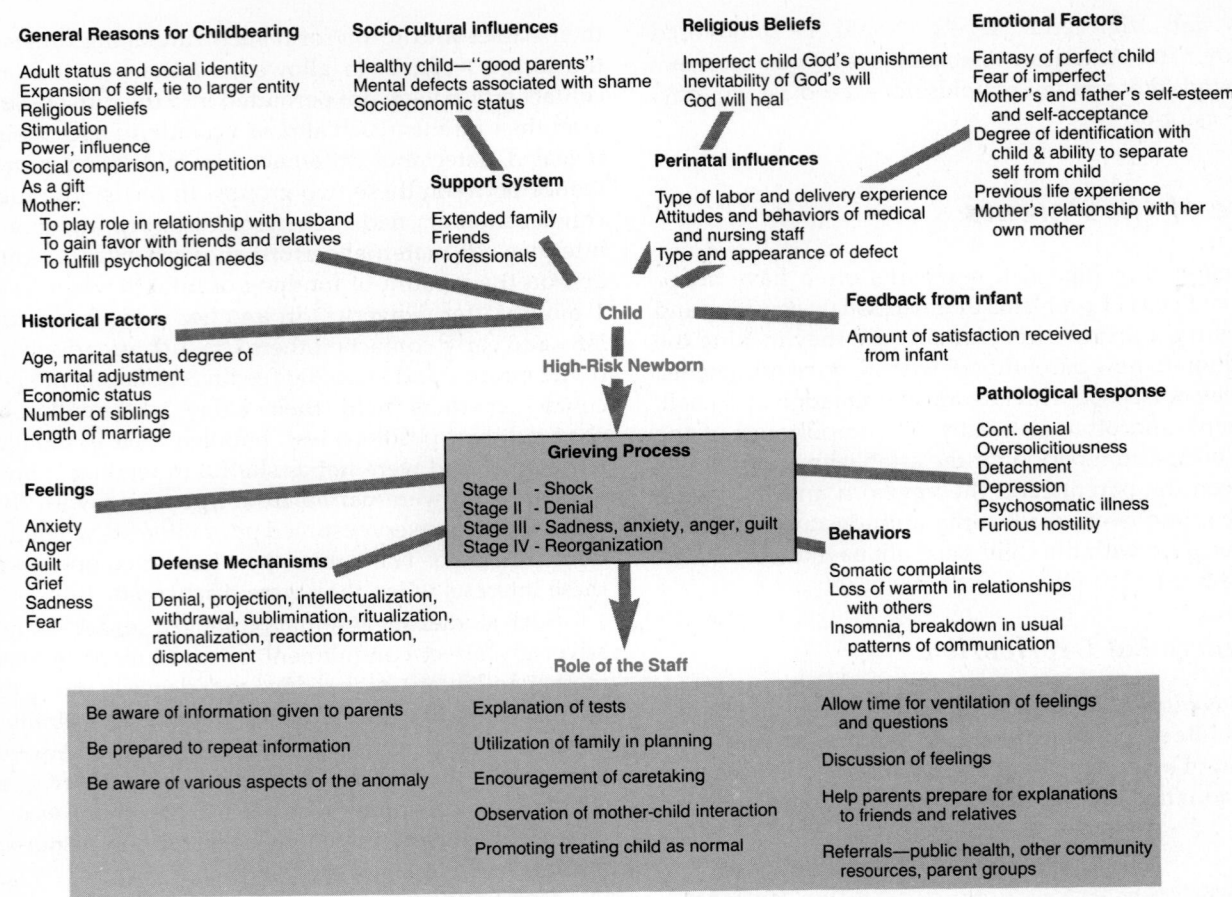

General Reasons for Childbearing

Adult status and social identity
Expansion of self, tie to larger entity
Religious beliefs
Stimulation
Power, influence
Social comparison, competition
As a gift
Mother:
  To play role in relationship with husband
  To gain favor with friends and relatives
  To fulfill psychological needs

Socio-cultural influences

Healthy child—"good parents"
Mental defects associated with shame
Socioeconomic status

Support System

Extended family
Friends
Professionals

Religious Beliefs

Imperfect child God's punishment
Inevitability of God's will
God will heal

Perinatal influences

Type of labor and delivery experience
Attitudes and behaviors of medical
  and nursing staff
Type and appearance of defect

Emotional Factors

Fantasy of perfect child
Fear of imperfect
Mother's and father's self-esteem
  and self-acceptance
Degree of identification with
  child & ability to separate
  self from child
Previous life experience
Mother's relationship with her
  own mother

Historical Factors

Age, marital status, degree of
  marital adjustment
Economic status
Number of siblings
Length of marriage

Child

High-Risk Newborn

Feedback from infant

Amount of satisfaction received
  from infant

Pathological Response

Cont. denial
Oversolicitiousness
Detachment
Depression
Psychosomatic illness
Furious hostility

Feelings

Anxiety
Anger
Guilt
Grief
Sadness
Fear

Defense Mechanisms

Denial, projection, intellectualization,
  withdrawal, sublimation, ritualization,
  rationalization, reaction formation,
  displacement

Grieving Process

Stage I - Shock
Stage II - Denial
Stage III - Sadness, anxiety, anger, guilt
Stage IV - Reorganization

Behaviors

Somatic complaints
Loss of warmth in relationships
  with others
Insomnia, breakdown in usual
  patterns of communication

Role of the Staff

Be aware of information given to parents

Be prepared to repeat information

Be aware of various aspects of the anomaly

Explanation of tests

Utilization of family in planning

Encouragement of caretaking

Observation of mother-child interaction

Promoting treating child as normal

Allow time for ventilation of feelings
  and questions

Discussion of feelings

Help parents prepare for explanations
  to friends and relatives

Referrals—public health, other community
  resources, parent groups

FIGURE 44-26

Parental response to the high-risk newborn.

then be a rather abrupt arrival of the infant. The event may be surrounded by several anxiety-provoking features, such as an unattended delivery, a longer hospital stay for her baby and perhaps herself, separation from her infant, and, most heartrending of all, a delicate infant who may be in danger of death.

Guilt feelings and a certain amount of grieving in both parents are an invariable accompaniment. The parents ask themselves time and again such questions as, "What went wrong? What did we do? What made it happen? Can I really carry babies?" These guilt feelings and grief may be manifested in a variety of ways, including general anger with the whole situation, self-deprecation, numerous complaints, blaming the spouse or attendants, insistent bids for reassurance and attention, profuse crying, or extreme quiet and immobilization.

Loneliness is also a problem because the mother may have no opportunity to see, hold, feed, and examine her child as the other mothers have. We are all familiar with the wistful figure at the nursery window, gazing longingly through the glass, while the other mothers are occupied with feeding, changing, and cud-

dling their infants. The loneliness continues when the parents go home without their infant. Because of the continued separation, the task of integrating the new member into the household is delayed.

In addition, most mothers are concerned about whether they will be able to take adequate care of their babies when they do bring them home. The mother may still carry a picture of the frail infant surrounded by all the nursery paraphernalia and not realize that her baby will be reasonably mature when discharged from the hospital.

To cope with this concern, she may ask many questions while she is in the hospital and may demand reassurance about the baby's condition; on the other hand, she may be quiet and uncommunicative, quite overwhelmed with the anticipated enormous responsibility.

Supportive Care

Although there is much that is specialized in the physical care activities for the premature infant, the mother's physical care remains generally the same as that for any normal postpartum course. Thus, the emphasis on care

---

Psychological Processes Parents Go Through After Birth of a High-Risk Infant

Shock, disbelief, and denial

Anger and searching self and others for causes

Grieving over loss of fantasized perfect infant

Grieving over own inability to produce perfect infant

Anticipatory worrying over loss of infant

Initiation of contact with infant

Belief and desire that infant will live

Readiness to establish caretaking relationship (see Fig. 44-27).

---

for these mothers is twofold: (1) they need help to facilitate their emotional adjustment (this holds true for the father as well) and (2) they need help in preparing for the care of the infant when they bring it home.

The nurse can do much to strengthen the mother's ego by helping her work through her guilt feelings and grief and thus reinforcing her concept of herself as an adequate, worthy person. To do this, the nurse must provide opportunities for the mother to ventilate her feelings and to question the situation. It is often difficult for the nurse to answer all the questions the mother and father ask, especially if the prognosis for the baby is guarded. Yet, to avoid the questions or problems is to deprive the parents of a valuable avenue of coping with the problem. The fears and fantasies engendered by not knowing are often worse than the facts, even though the facts are unpleasant.

As the nurse listens to the mother and the father and reflects their concerns, they are helped to arrive at a clearer notion of the reality of the situation. Thus they are able to separate fact and fancy and to work through to a more positive acceptance of their situation. The nurse can expect some negative feelings to be expressed, and the patient may go through a period of self-pity. An accepting, nonjudgmental attitude will help the patient move to a more positive frame of mind.

Keeping the lines of communication open between the nursery staff and the patient is another useful supportive measure. The nurse on the postpartum unit can be prepared with the latest reports regarding the baby's condition so that this information can be given to the parents. Especially when the mother cannot be taken to see her baby in the premature nursery, it is very helpful if the nurse in the premature unit can inform her of her infant's progress. If circumstances within the unit prevent this, contact with the mother by telephone may be substituted. This two-way communication between the floor and the nursery helps the patient to feel that everyone is "tuned in" to her situation and concerned about her. It also gives her the opportunity to know the personnel who are responsible for the care of her baby, and this is reassuring in itself.

In the event that the infant is transported to a level III center, the parents need to be informed of the circumstances and encouraged to see and touch the infant before transport occurs. It is helpful for the parents to be given a snapshot of the infant. Some nurseries have developed a pamphlet describing the unit. The nurse should explain to the parents that they are permitted to visit and telephone at any time and should encourage them to do so.

Visiting the Nursery. The father may often be the first parent to visit the neonatal unit and assume the role of communicator to the mother. Either the mother is not housed at the transport hospital or her physical condition may not permit her to visit immediately.

The father's first visit may be overwhelming at first, though the nurse may have tried to prepare him in advance. It is best to simply explain the equipment and its functions and then allow the father to ask questions. The nurse may encourage him to touch the baby and begin the attachment process at a tolerable pace.

The mother's first visit can be handled in a similar fashion. If she plans to breast-feed she should be taught how to express and save her milk. This is a positive act that can definitely enhance the mother–child relationship.

As visits continue parents may be encouraged to bring small objects from home such as toys and clothes. Siblings and other relatives may be allowed to visit, depending on the unit policy.

As time goes by, specific caretaking tasks may be assumed by the parents under the nurse's supervision (Fig. 44-27). This will prepare the parents gradually for the time of discharge, greatly enhance their self-confidence, and promote attachment. Any pamphlets that will help stress important information are always appreciated.

In the event that the level III center is far from the parents' home, a return transport may be offered and be acceptable to the parents.[42]

Other Sources of Support

All avenues of support are to be explored with the parents. If the mother seems to benefit from visitors or visiting with the other patients, then there need be no restriction on visiting privileges. There is no reason to isolate a mother in a room by herself (even if there has been a fetal death) without ascertaining whether the mother needs to be alone for a time. If possible, the same nurse should be assigned to her care. If the mother is to work through her feelings, she must have time to build trust, and this takes at least several encounters.

Other personnel, such as the social worker, may be helpful if aid is needed financially or strict budgeting is

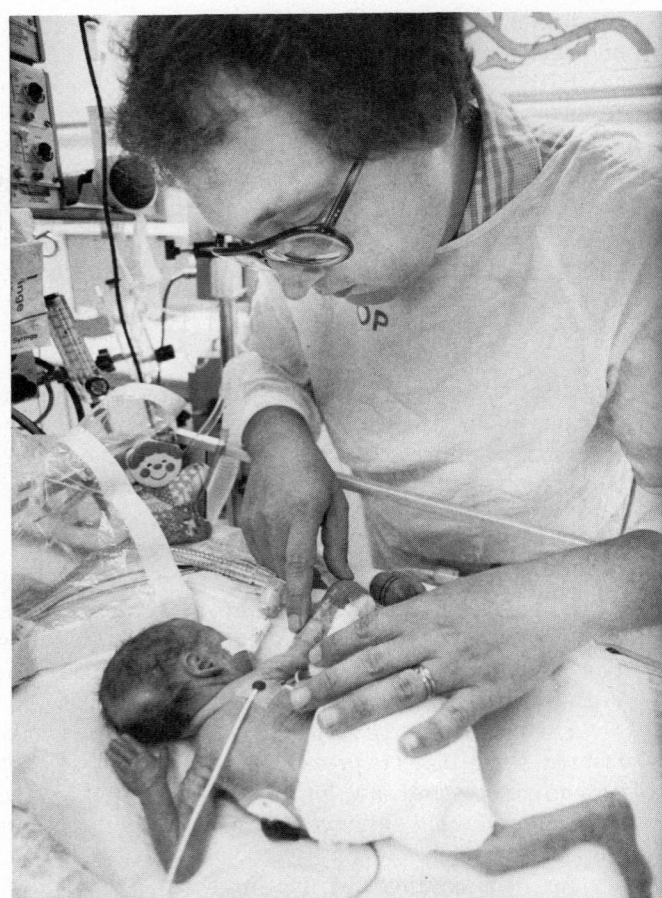

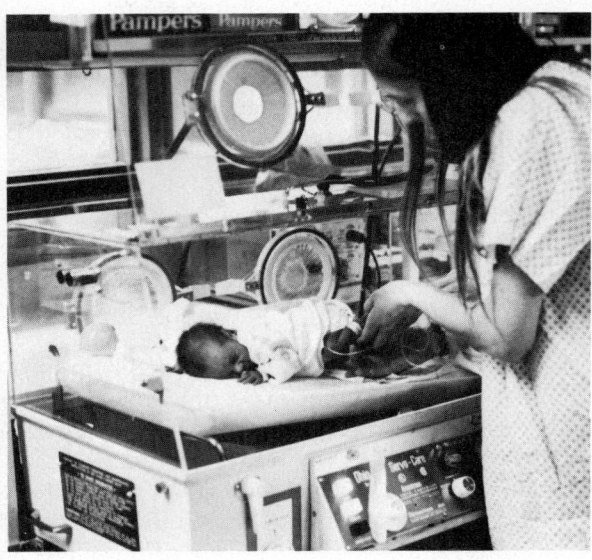

FIGURE 44-27

Allowing parents to stroke their infant or to perform caretaking tasks enhances bonding. (Left photo courtesy of The Children's Hospital of Philadelphia)

necessary. Another source of help that can prove invaluable is the public-health or visiting nurse. The need for a referral for these patients and their infants should never be overlooked. Most patients are delighted to have someone to rely on during the first difficult days when they bring the baby home. Furthermore, some patients cannot make much progress in expressing their feelings or in working the problem through during their short hospital stay. Thus, they are helped in this, as well as in making necessary arrangements in preparation for the baby's homecoming. Finally, parent support groups led by neonatal nurses can prove to be of great assistance in terms of emotional support.

Crisis Management

In implementing care, the nurse should remember that the advent of a high-risk birth is a crisis in itself; however, the parents may have to adjust to various related crises (*e.g.*, a sudden, downward turn in the baby's condition, financial embarrassment, unexpected developments regarding other children and relatives). Nurses must be prepared to help the parents deal with these as they arise and to seek appropriate resources for them if the matter lies beyond their competence. Knowledge

of the principles of communication and supportive care will be used here as they would be in any other crisis. Willingness and ability to allow the parents to work through and vent their feelings about the situation are of prime importance. The nurse is one of the key persons in the care of high-risk infants and their parents.

Preparation for the Future

Studies of high-risk infants born since the introduction of perinatal intensive care in the past 2 decades indicate that mortality and morbidity have significantly decreased. Contributing to this improvement have been early identification of high-risk pregnancies, maintenance of an appropriate thermal environment for the neonate, and early correction of neonatal acidosis, hypoglycemia, and hyperbilirubinemia.

Refinement and widespread use of continuous positive pressure and ventilators have also been contributing factors.

In terms of developmental outlook, 90.5% of those infants weighing over 1500 g exhibit no residual handicap. Those infants weighing less than 1500 g exhibit a low incidence of cerebral palsy, which is rising slightly. In the less than 1000-g range there is an increasing in-

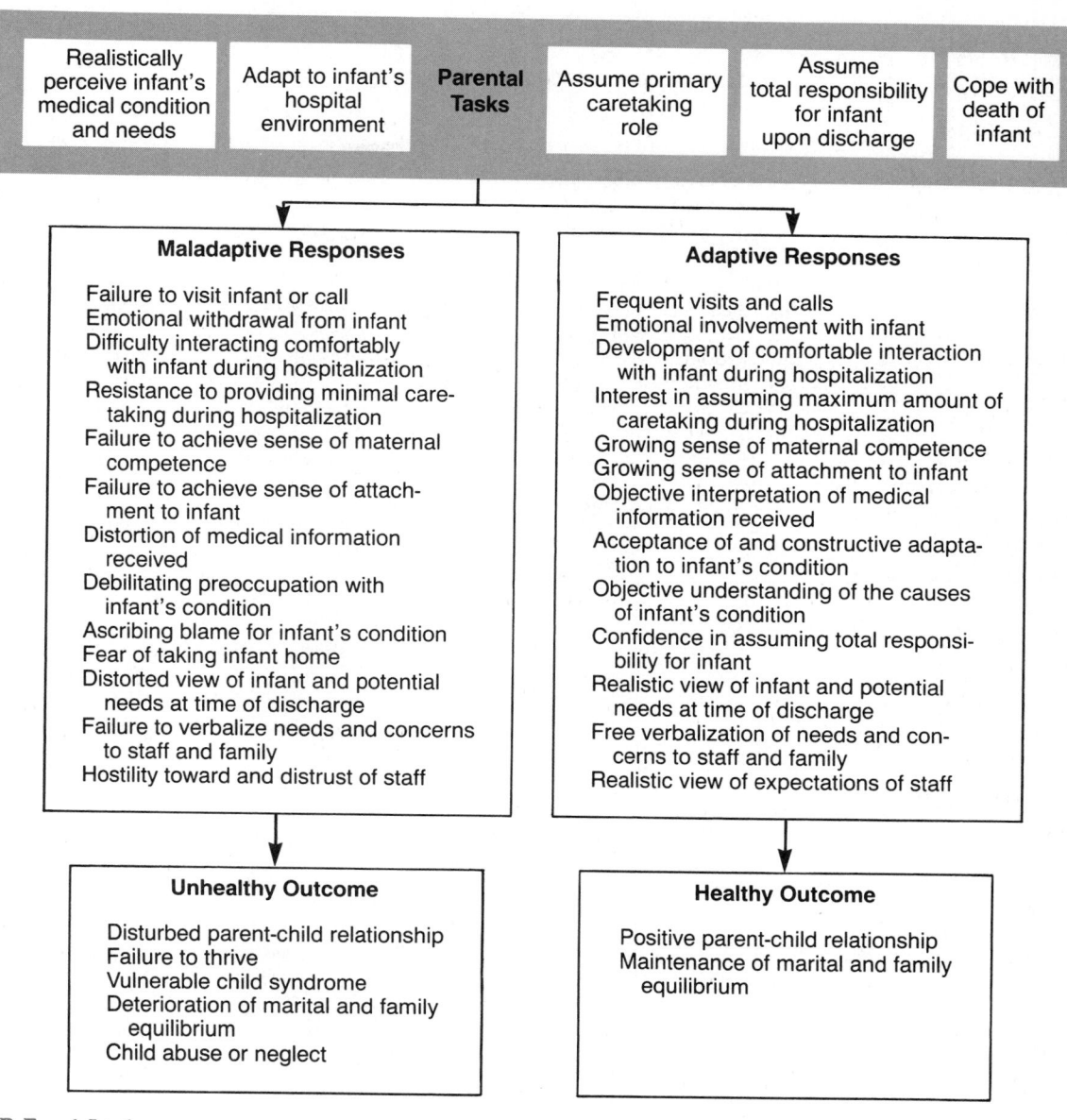

Realistically perceive infant's medical condition and needs	Adapt to infant's hospital environment	**Parental Tasks**	Assume primary caretaking role	Assume total responsibility for infant upon discharge	Cope with death of infant

Maladaptive Responses

Failure to visit infant or call
Emotional withdrawal from infant
Difficulty interacting comfortably with infant during hospitalization
Resistance to providing minimal caretaking during hospitalization
Failure to achieve sense of maternal competence
Failure to achieve sense of attachment to infant
Distortion of medical information received
Debilitating preoccupation with infant's condition
Ascribing blame for infant's condition
Fear of taking infant home
Distorted view of infant and potential needs at time of discharge
Failure to verbalize needs and concerns to staff and family
Hostility toward and distrust of staff

Adaptive Responses

Frequent visits and calls
Emotional involvement with infant
Development of comfortable interaction with infant during hospitalization
Interest in assuming maximum amount of caretaking during hospitalization
Growing sense of maternal competence
Growing sense of attachment to infant
Objective interpretation of medical information received
Acceptance of and constructive adaptation to infant's condition
Objective understanding of the causes of infant's condition
Confidence in assuming total responsibility for infant
Realistic view of infant and potential needs at time of discharge
Free verbalization of needs and concerns to staff and family
Realistic view of expectations of staff

Unhealthy Outcome

Disturbed parent-child relationship
Failure to thrive
Vulnerable child syndrome
Deterioration of marital and family equilibrium
Child abuse or neglect

Healthy Outcome

Positive parent-child relationship
Maintenance of marital and family equilibrium

FIGURE 45-1

Parental response during crisis period. (Grant P: Psychosocial needs of families of high-risk infants. Fam Community Health 1(3):93, November 1978. An Aspen Publication. Article code 0160-6379/78/0013-0091)

perience a feeling of numbness. Physiological reactions are loss of appetite, palpitations, fatigue, shortness of breath, and so on. A tendency to withdraw from the situation may be observed in the case of a defective or critically ill neonate. This coping mechanism allows the potential loss to be less painful if attachment has not occurred.

Searching. The second stage involves seeking of an answer or reason for the event by the parents. Behaviors of anger, guilt, hostility, and emptiness are commonly seen. Parents may feel that their actions are to blame

for the loss. Health-care professionals may be the target of their anger.

Disorientation. Disorientation is a bridge stage to reorganization. During this time gradual change to normal activities will occur. Parents may still be experiencing depression and may have little emotional energy to deal with setbacks (*e.g.*, a complication in the health course of the preterm infant).

Reorganization. Over a considerable period of time, parents accommodate to the loss. Minimal energy is de-

The Grieving Family

Nursing Objectives

1. Identify the family experiencing grief.
2. Assess the impact of the experience on the family structure.
3. Determine if the family is appropriately working through its grief.

Assessment	Potential Nursing Diagnosis	Planning/Intervention	Evaluation
Perinatal loss 　Abortion 　Stillbirth 　Neonatal death Intrauterine fetal death Infant of low birth weight or preterm Infant with a congenital anomaly Infant with a life-threatening illness Family support systems available Past grief experiences Religious beliefs Age and maturity level of parents	Anticipatory or dysfunctional grieving related to a perinatal loss	Anticipate various stages of the grief process Allow family time to ventilate feelings Provide facts sought by family Allow family time to see and hold baby—describe how baby will look, and wrap as a normal newborn Ask if parents wish to name baby Provide photographs or other remembrances of baby if family wishes Seek parents' permission for an autopsy Ask if parents wish baby baptized Notify clergy Provide information on hospital policy regarding funeral options Refer to a community support group, social worker, counselor Provide follow-up care as needed In case of ill baby encourage parents to visit nursery as much as possible Assist in mobilization of resources Be realistic regarding prognosis and any long-term ramifications	Family is supportive of one another Family applies its energy to working through grief Family applies healthy coping mechanisms Family adapts to crisis Parents verbally repeat understanding of prognosis and resources Parents of ill children visit nursery

voted to the grief process and most energy is directed toward normal living.[1]

Working Through a Crisis

During pregnancy, all women wish for and fantasize about a perfect child. They also fear that their babies might be abnormal. Their fantasies of the expected child are a composite of the images of the people who are important to or admired by them. When the infant deviates drastically from the anticipated child, the simultaneous occurrence of the sudden loss of the idealized child and the necessity of accepting a deviant child can be overwhelming. The greater the deviation from normal, the greater the impact of the experience can be.

Becoming a parent is a turning point in life, and it is particularly so for the parents of a child who has a disorder. They can emerge from this crisis less mentally and emotionally healthy than they were, or they can move on to increased maturity. If they use maladaptive coping mechanisms to deal with the crisis, the former no doubt will occur; if they can be helped to work through the problems positively, this experience will stand them in good stead for future stressful situations.

Nursing Care During Crisis

It is the responsibility of the nurse and other members of the health team to help the parents cope with this situation. However, nurses are only human and at times are hampered by their own anxieties, feelings, and fantasies. Thus, it is especially important for them to understand the psychodynamics occurring in both the parents and themselves so that they may choose a therapeutic course of action to help the parents.

Variables. It is important to remember that the parents have to grieve for the lost perfect child before they can form an attachment to the imperfect one. The process of grief involves anger, which can be directed toward anyone involved in the situation, including the infant. Mourning also impairs the capacity to recognize, evaluate, and adapt to reality appropriately. Thus, whenever possible, long-range planning for the infant should be delayed until the parents, particularly the mother, can participate in them; otherwise, the mourning and depression may persist for an undue length of time.

Anxiety is another dominant reaction. It is thought that the sources of the most serious anxiety are the threats to the parents' sense of adequacy, self-esteem, and social status. One of the earliest questions expressed, "What caused this?" is charged with feelings of biologic inadequacy. Indeed, what the parents are really asking is, "What's the matter with us as progenitors of children?" Particularly for the mother, her failure to produce what she has so long prepared herself to create may well be a threat not only to her femininity but to her whole unique personhood as well. Moreover, these feelings hold true even for those who have not consciously planned the child or who have had several children. Procreating a defective child strikes at the very core of the woman's being. This is very understandable; the child just born is still, in effect, an extension of the mother, and a defect in him is tantamount to a defect in herself. The degree of the mother's anxiety is also related to a deep narcissistic wound, since the psychological work during pregnancy includes an increase in narcissism. Feelings of shame and embarrassment are the general accompaniment of personal feelings of inadequacy.[2]

Some of the variables affecting the parents' coping behaviors include past experiences the parents have had in their own growing-up period. If their childhood ex-

periences have fulfilled their needs for mastery, they will have gained trust, security in human relationships, feelings of optimism and the ability to cope, and freedom from crippling guilt and fear. They will also have learned tolerance for frustration. All of these will be of great help to them in their present crisis. Positive experiences with other handicapped or developmentally disabled adults and children can also affect the degree of concern and attitude the parents have. On the other hand, if they remember hostility directed toward a defective person, or if they (or others) responded to that person with guilt, pity, repugnance, or overprotectiveness, these feelings may become reactivated as they confront the abnormality of their child.

Another variable that may influence the response of the parents to their stress is the degree of energy they have at their disposal at the time of the crisis. The mother who has had a long, physically exhausting labor has less energy for coping with stress than the mother who has had a rapid, nonexhausting one. The father who has been at the mother's side coaching her during labor and delivery has less reserve than one who has not performed the physical and emotional effort that accompanies coaching. In addition, having to attend to other-related life situations, such as making emergency preparations for the care of other children or making arrangements for job-related problems and the like, also takes away valuable energy needed for coping.[3]

Many other variables, such as differences in class, economic background, the physical and emotional maturity of the parents, the birth order of the child, and its sex, appearance, and prognosis, also influence the responses of the parents. All of these variables may have important bearing on the immediate significance the event will have for them.

Applying the Nursing Process to Grief

The nursing-care plan that follows delineates the steps of the nursing process in caring for the family that is grieving in the loss of their newborn.

Congenital and Genetic Abnormalities

The etiology of birth defects is not completely understood, but a multifactor etiology is generally accepted. It is recognized that most of these defects have an environmental component in their causes.

Malformations may arise from (1) genetic factors, such as change in the chromosome number, mutation, or structural abnormalities, or (2) environmental factors, such as irradiation, infection, and drugs.

The most frequent of the generally influenced malformations are multifactorial. These defects result from interactions among multiple genetic and environmental factors.

There are approximately 250,000 babies born each year with abnormalities that cause a significant alteration in the structure or function of their bodies. The incidence of these disorders has not changed greatly over the decades; however, the techniques of prenatal diagnosis, repair, and correction have improved immensely, thus offering a great deal of hope and consolation to the parents and children who are afflicted with these conditions. Indeed, there is increasing specialization in *teratology*, the study of the relationship of genetic and environmental factors in the production of congenital abnormalities.

Congenital deformities may range from minor abnormalities, such as supernumerary digits, to grave malformations incompatible with life, which include anencephaly (absence of the brain), hydrocephalus (excessive amount of fluid in the cerebral ventricles with tremendous enlargement of the head), and various heart abnormalities. These grave defects are second only to accidents as a cause of death in childhood. Moreover, these youngsters represent a serious community-health problem when one considers the numerous sequential surgical procedures and the attendant expense these families must undergo. In addition, the special rehabilitation and education that many require, plus the drain on the parents' time and emotional and physical reserves, can have a grave social impact.

Because these conditions are so numerous and varied, this section presents selected disorders, those more commonly seen that are apparent at birth or soon thereafter or those with which the maternity nurse will have to deal. The care of these infants and their parents presents a great challenge to the nurse, who must give competent and, at times, complex nursing care to the babies as well as help the parents to convert their feelings of disappointment and despair into constructive efforts at rehabilitation of the infant.

Congenital Heart Disease

At the time of birth and for weeks thereafter, there are great changes in the circulatory system of the newborn. When the cord is clamped and expansion of the lungs occurs, the pulmonary circulation increases in volume. The foramen ovale, the ductus arteriosus, and the ductus venosus are no longer needed and therefore close gradually over a period of several months. Usually the foramen ovale is closed by the third month of life and the ductus by the second; during the period of closure, signs or symptoms of patency rarely occur. When they do, they may be an indication of defects in these structures or other parts of the heart.

Congenital heart disease has an incidence of about 8 per 1000 at birth. Cardiovascular malformations account for approximately 1.2 deaths in 1000 births during infancy.

The role of heredity as an etiologic agent is not yet well understood. Congenital lesions may be recorded in as many as three generations, and siblings seem to manifest the disease more often than in the preceding or succeeding generations. *Maternal disease* during pregnancy, such as rubella or diabetes, influences the bodily structures of the developing fetus. Yet the etiology and dynamics of cardiovascular lesion are not known definitely. However, there is a higher incidence of other congenital defects such as Down's syndrome among infants with congenital heart disease. Thus, the infant may suffer from multiple disorders.

Types of Congenital Cardiac Anomalies

Major types of congenital cardiac anomalies are illustrated in Figure 45-2.

Transposition of the Great Vessels. The aorta originates in the right ventricle rather than the left, and the pulmonary artery originates in the left ventricle rather than the right. Survival depends on other intercirculatory lesions such as atrial septal defect (ASD), patent ductus arteriosus (PDA), or ventricular septal defect (VSD).[4]

Atrial Septal Defect. An abnormal opening between the right and left atria persists after birth, with left-to-right shunting of blood. This may result from failure of the foramen ovale to close properly, or there may be other defects high in the ostium secundum or basally in the ostium primum.[4]

Patent Ductus Arteriosus. The vascular connection between the pulmonary artery and the aorta, which is functional during fetal life, persists after birth, rather than closing as it normally does. When the duct remains patent after birth, the direction of blood flow through it is reversed because of the higher pressure in the aorta, thus shunting oxygenated aortic blood into the pulmonary vasculature. During fetal life, the shunt is from the pulmonary artery to the aorta.[4]

Ventricular Septal Defect. There is an abnormal opening between the right and left ventricles. This varies in size and may occur in the muscular or membranous portion of the septum. Shunting of blood from left to right ventricles occurs during systole because of higher left ventricular pressure. If, however, pulmonary vascular resistance produces pulmonary hypertension, the shunt is reversed and occurs right to left with resultant cyanosis.[4]

Transposition of the great arteries

This anomaly is an embryologic defect caused by a straight division of the bulbar trunk without normal spiraling. As a result, the aorta originates from the right ventricle, and the pulmonary artery from the left ventricle. An abnormal communication between the two circulations must be present to sustain life.

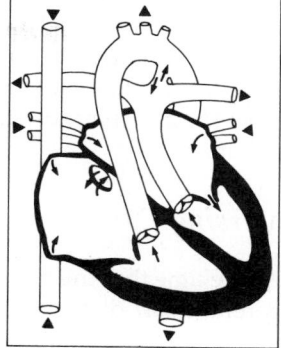

Atrial septal defect

An atrial septal defect is an abnormal opening between the right and left atria. Basically, three types of abnormalities result from incorrect development of the atrial septum. An incompetent foramen ovale is the most common defect. The high ostium secundum defect results from abnormal development of the septum secundum. Improper development of the septum primum produces a basal opening known as an ostium primum defect, frequently involving the atrioventricular valves. In general, left to right shunting of blood occurs in all atrial septal defects.

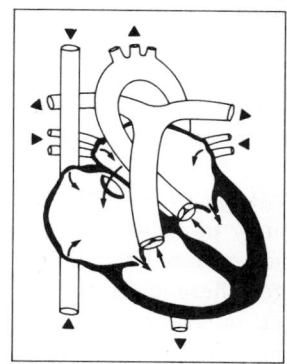

Patent ductus arteriosus

The patent ductus arteriosus is a vascular connection that, during fetal life, short circuits the pulmonary vascular bed and directs blood from the pulmonary artery to the aorta. Functional closure of the ductus normally occurs soon after birth. If the ductus remains patent after birth, the direction of blood flow in the ductus is reversed by the higher pressure in the aorta.

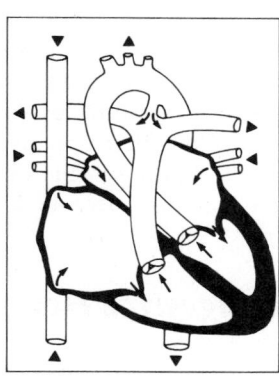

Ventricular septal defect

A ventricular septal defect is an abnormal opening between the right and left ventricle. Ventricular septal defects vary in size and may occur in either the membranous or muscular portion of the ventricular septum. Due to higher pressure in the left ventricle, a shunting of blood from the left to right ventricle occurs during systole. If pulmonary vascular resistance produces pulmonary hypertension, the shunt of blood is then reversed from the right to the left ventricle resulting in cyanosis.

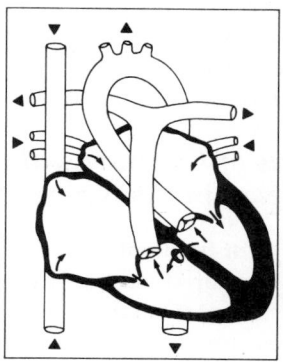

Coarctation of the aorta

Coarctation of the aorta is characterized by a narrowed aortic lumen. It exists as a preductal or postductal obstruction, depending on the position of the obstruction in relation to the ductus arteriosus. Coarctations exist with great variation in anatomical features. The lesion produces an obstruction to the flow of blood through the aorta causing an increased left ventricular pressure and work load.

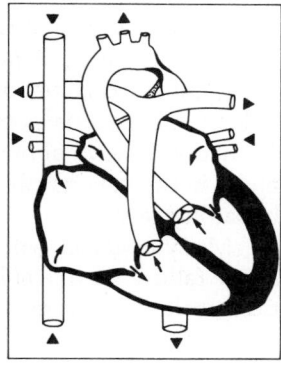

Tetralogy of Fallot

Tetralogy of Fallot is characterized by the combination of four defects—(1) pulmonary stenosis, (2) ventricular septal defect, (3) overriding aorta, and (4) hypertrophy of right ventricle. It is the most common defect causing cyanosis in patients surviving beyond two years of age. The severity of symptoms depends on the degree of pulmonary stenosis, the size of the ventricular septal defect, and the degree to which the aorta overrides the septal defect.

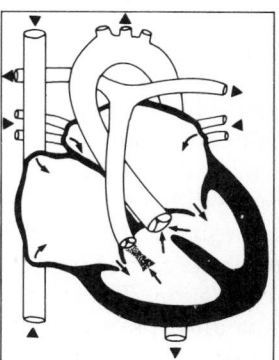

FIGURE 45-2

Six types of congenital anomalies. (Courtesy of Ross Laboratories)

Coarctation of the Aorta. There is a constriction of the aorta, causing narrowing of the lumen; this partially obstructs blood flow, creating increased left ventricular pressure and work load. The coarctation may occur before or after the ductus arteriosus, and there are great variations in anatomical features of coarctations.[4]

Tetralogy of Fallot. Four defects are combined in tetralogy of Fallot, which is the most common defect causing cyanosis in children who survive beyond 2 years of age. There is pulmonary stenosis, ventricular septal defect, overriding aorta, and hypertrophy of the right ventricle. The severity of symptoms depends on the size of the ventricular septal defect, the degree of pulmonary stenosis, and the degree to which the aorta overrides the septal defect.[4]

Other Cardiac Defects. There are other types of cardiac anomalies, including tricuspid atresia, pulmonary and aortic stenosis, overriding aorta and truncus arteriosus, and anomalous venous return. Surgery can repair some of these defects and in some instances restore the infant to normal cardiac functioning. Others cannot be repaired and often are incompatible with life.

Signs of Cardiovascular Disease in the Neonate

The *most* frequent reason for suspicion of neonatal cardiovascular disease is the observation of cyanosis or signs of heart failure. Other signs of cardiovascular heart disease are tachypnea, retractions, grunting, nasal flaring, decreased response to stimuli, shallow respirations, absent or unequal pulses, enlarged liver, peripheral edema, arrhythmias, murmurs, cardiomegaly, abnormal electrocardiogram (ECG), and changes noted on echocardiography.

Medical Management

A more specific diagnostic tool used to pinpoint the specific congenital defect is the use of cardiac catheterization. In the cardiac catheterization procedure, a radiopaque catheter is inserted through a peripheral blood vessel, usually the femoral vein, into the heart. Angiography is carried out by the injection of dye through the circulation. The data obtained indicate defects in the anatomy, pressure changes and oxygen saturation of blood in the chambers of the heart and great vessels, and changes in cardiac output or stroke volume. Complications of this procedure are hemorrhage, arrhythmias, infection, reactions to dye, and obstruction in the vessels.[5] The data obtained from this procedure greatly assist the surgical team if surgery is warranted. Once the lesion is definitely identified, the decision can be made whether medical or surgical intervention is the best approach. Further medical interventions used to stabilize the neonate are monitoring, maintenance of fluid and electrolyte status, use of supplementary oxygen, thermoneutral environment, and use of medication. Most often used medications are digoxin, furosemide (Lasix), spironolactone (Aldactone), and morphine sulfate.

Nursing Care

At the time that the neonate is suspected of having congenital heart disease the nurse is very much involved in gathering observational data, assisting, and preparing the infant for various diagnostic procedures. Small, frequent oral feedings should be tried to avoid overtiring the infant. Strict intake and output records are kept, as well as daily weight. Parenteral nutrition may be necessary if oral feedings are not tolerated. Oxygen is administered safely as needed while monitoring blood gas status. Digoxin is administered safely by checking the dosage and route with another nurse. The apical pulse is counted prior to administration, and the drug is held if the pulse is less than 90 to 100. If diuretics are being given, potassium levels are monitored frequently and adjusted with supplements in intravenous fluid or given orally. Cardiovascular drugs and nursing considerations are listed in Table 45-1.

Congestive Heart Failure

Neonates with left-to-right shunts and obstructive lesions may demonstrate signs of pump failure. When this complication occurs, the heart is unable to pump blood in accordance with the body's needs.

Those infants with left-sided failure, with resultant backup of blood into the pulmonary system, are often those who have coarctation of the aorta, hypoplastic left heart, or aortic stenosis.

Right-sided failure often occurs in infants diagnosed as having large atrial septal defects, pulmonary stenosis, or tricuspid valve abnormalities. There is a backup of blood in the venous circulation, resulting in edema and hepatomegaly.

Many neonates will have both left-sided and right-sided failure as a result of patent ductus arteriosus, transposition of the great vessels, and ventricular septal defects.[6]

Applying the Nursing Process to Congestive Heart Failure

Assessment. The nurse carefully observes the neonate for signs of congestive heart failure (see Physical Assessment Criteria for Heart Failure).

TABLE 45-1

Cardiovascular Drugs/Diuretics

Drug	Dosage/Route	Nursing Considerations
Digoxin	Premature: 0.02 mg–0.04 mg/kg IV (total digitalizing dose) 0.01 mg/kg/day divided every 12 hr (maintenance) Full term: 0.04 mg/kg IV (total digitalizing dose) 0.01 mg/kg/day divided every 12 hr PO (maintenance)	*Cardiotonic* Monitor apical pulse for bradycardia Monitor serum potassium Watch for nausea, vomiting Check dosage carefully Observe for ECG changes
Hydralazine	0.2 mg/kg/dose or 1.7 mg–3.5 mg/kg/day divided every 4–6 hr IV, IM 1 mg/kg/day divided every 6 hr to increase as needed up to 7.5 mg/kg/day	*Antihypertensive* Monitor blood pressure and apical pulse Watch for nausea, vomiting, diarrhea
Lidocaine	0.5 mg–1.5 mg/kg/dose by slow IV push; may be repeated every 5–10 min as needed 20 μ–50 μ/kg/min continuous IV infusion	*Antiarrhythmic* Use infusion pump for accurate IV administration Use cardiac monitor
Procainamide	2 mg/kg/dose given over 5 min IV 40 mg–60 mg/kg/day divided every 6 hr PO	*Antiarrhythmic* Use with caution in congestive heart failure Monitor blood pressure, ECG
Propranolol	0.01 mg–0.15 mg/kg/dose by slow IV push; then 0.5–1.0 mg/kg/day divided every 6 hr PO Starting dose: 1 mg/kg/day divided every 6 hr PO 0.15 mg–0.25 mg/kg/dose IV	*Antiarrhythmic* Check apical pulse rate Monitor blood pressure, ECG, pulse
Chlorothiazide	20 mg–30 mg/kg/day divided every 12 hr PO	Monitor intake/output, serum electrolytes Monitor serum creatinine and blood urea nitrogen levels
Ethacrynic acid	2 mg–3 mg/kg/day divided every 12 hr PO 0.5 mg–2.0 mg/kg/dose IV	Very potent diuretic Monitor potassium levels Oral solutions should be stored in refrigerator
Furosemide	1 mg–2 mg/kg/dose every 6–8 hr PO 0.5 mg–2.0 mg/kg/dose every 12 hr IM or IV	Potent loop diuretic Monitor serum potassium
Spironolactone	1.7 mg–3.3 mg/kg/dose divided every 6–8 hr	When used alone diuretic effect may take 2–3 days. May be used in addition to another diuretic Potassium-sparing diuretic Monitor potassium, electrolytes, intake/output, weight

Nursing Intervention. Oxygen administration by various methods is used in cyanotic infants. Digoxin and furosemide may be used to promote cardiac efficiency and diuretic effect. Potassium supplements may be necessary. Strict records of intake and output, monitoring of daily weights, and monitoring of electrolytes are essential. When oral feedings are tolerated, a low-sodium formula may be used, such as Lonalac or Similac PM 60/40. Parents need experience and teaching for planned home interventions.

Postoperative and Postcatheterization Nursing Care. Areas of particular importance to note following cardiac catheterization are the equality of peripheral pulses and the temperature and color of the affected extremity.

Postoperatively, the neonate requires close observation in the intensive care unit. Monitors are attached to constantly record vital signs, blood pressure, and temperature. All readings should be compared with the baseline. Environmental and anesthetic influences may decrease the temperature initially. In addition, some temperature elevation due to the inflammatory process may be noted in the first 24 to 48 hours postoperatively. Any elevation after this may be indicative of infection.

All lines and dressings are observed and changed

Infant with a Congenital Heart Defect

Nursing Objectives

1. Make early identification of the infant with congenital cardiac defects.
2. Plan intervention to place minimal stress on the cardiovascular system.

Assessment	Potential Nursing Diagnosis	Planning/Intervention	Evaluation

Familial history of congenital heart defects	Ineffective breathing patterns related to congestive heart failure	Observe infant for:
		  Cyanosis
		  Murmurs, arrhythmias
			Infant breathes normally

Presence of:
  Cyanosis
  Murmur
  Congestive heart failure
  Respiratory distress
	Impaired gas exchange related to congenital cardiac defect	Absent or unequal pulses
		Tachypnea
		Retractions
		Grunting
		Nasal flaring
		Edema
			Infant returns to normal feedings
			Infant's respiratory and heart rates stabilize
			Infant gains weight

Other congenital anomaly present	Alteration in nutrition, less than body requirements related to difficulty breathing, sucking, and swallowing	Decrease in urine output Difficulty in coordination of breathing, sucking, swallowing	
	Fluid volume excess related to congestive heart failure	Provide continuous monitoring	
	Decreased cardiac output related to congestive heart failure, congenital heart defect	Monitor vital signs frequently	
		Provide assistance with diagnostic procedures: chest film, echocardiogram, cardiac catheterization	
		Give small frequent feedings with rest periods	
		Put up head of bed after feeding	
		Record strict intake and output	
		Monitor daily weights	
		Administer drugs as ordered	
		Administer oxygen	

as needed. An intra-arterial line is suggested with heparinized saline. Central venous pressure readings are taken frequently.

Respiratory status is monitored carefully by turning, postural drainage, and assessment of breath sounds. Suctioning accompanied by prebagging and postbagging with oxygen may be necessary to remove secretions. Chest tubes are present postoperatively. The Pleurevac system is checked for adequate functioning and color and amount of drainage.

Fluid and electrolyte requirements are calculated according to the infant's weight and electrolyte reports. Initial fluids are parenteral, since feedings are gradually resumed. Blood replacement may be necessary: frequent monitoring of hematocrit, hemoglobin, and blood levels is essential.

All nursing activities are designed to allow maximum rest periods for the neonate.[5] Other steps in the nursing process are given in the nursing-care plan Infant with a Congenital Heart Defect.

---

*Physical Assessment Criteria
for Heart Failure*

Tachypnea (respiratory rate greater than 50)

Tachycardia (140–180 heart rate)

Liver enlargement

Cardiomegaly

Rales, rhonchi

Feeding difficulties

Peripheral edema

Inappropriate sweating

Gallop rhythm

Various ECG and echocardiogram changes[7]

Cleft Lip and Cleft Palate

The cleft lip and the cleft palate, which may occur separately or in combination, result from the failure of the soft or bony tissues of the palate and the upper jaw to unite during the fifth to tenth weeks of gestation. The defect may be unilateral or bilateral (Fig. 45-3). Only the lip may be involved, or the disunion may extend into the upper jaw or the nasal cavity.

Each year about 1 in 700 white infants and 1 in 2000 black infants are born with a cleft lip or cleft palate; thus, this condition is one of the most common birth defects. More males than females appear to be affected by the combination cleft lip and cleft palate disorder. Cleft palate alone has an increased incidence in females.

A clear-cut etiologic pattern for these deformities remains obscure. Variables found to be associated with them include genetic factors, drugs (particularly corticosteroids), radiation, hypoxia *in utero*, maternal viral illness during pregnancy, and dietary influences. The hypothesis has been put forward that palatolabial defects may be due to sex-modified multifactorial inheritance.[8]

Surgical Treatment

The plan of treatment and the outcome depend on the severity of the condition. If only the lip is involved, surgery may take place within the first few days, although some physicians prefer to wait until the child weighs 10 lb or more because they feel that there is more tissue available at that time to facilitate operative precision. When the palate is involved, the repair is usually postponed until the infant is 16 to 24 months old or weighs 20 lb or more. Time is not the only salient

variable; it is even more important that the child be free of infection and nutritionally sound.

When surgery is performed later, a prosthetic speech device usually is fitted so that speech development may not be hindered. Cleft palates usually involve other difficulties, such as frequent respiratory tract infections and orthodontia and speech problems. Therefore, the care of these children involves the coordinated activities of the pediatrician, plastic surgeon, orthodontist, hospital and community-health nurses, speech therapists, and, very often, the social worker. Fortunately, modern treatment is so effective that these defects become a relatively minor handicap.

Nursing Care

Support. The parents require a great deal of supportive help initially, especially since this disorder is so disfiguring. When this condition occurs, particularly if the baby is a girl, it may come as a tremendous shock and burden to the parents. However, repair is generally successful, and it is very helpful if the parents know and understand this. Members of the team involved in the reconstruction process can visit the parents after a comprehensive assessment of the infant has been made. To assure them that the defect is correctable, color transparencies are shown of an infant with a similar defect and the results of the surgery. Such visual reassurance has been found to be more effective than any verbal explanation.

The pattern of treatment is explained so parents can understand and begin to participate in the feeding and care of the child. Parents may be informed of support groups such as the Cleft Palate Club.

Feeding. Feeding is usually one of the most immediate and difficult problems in the daily care of the infant with a cleft lip or cleft palate. It can best be accomplished by placing the infant in an upright position and directing the flow of milk against the side of the mouth. This will decrease the possibility of aspiration as well as the amount of air swallowed during feeding.

Since sucking strengthens and develops the muscles needed for speech, a nipple is used for feeding whenever possible. A variety of nipples may be tried, including a regular nipple with enlarged holes, a soft rubber nipple, a presoftened "preemie" nipple, a Beniflex Nurser, a lamb's nipple, or a duck-bill nipple (Fig. 45-4). The last two are more expensive, and specific instructions are necessary for their use. If the infant cannot use any of the nipples, then a spoon or a rubber-tipped asepto syringe may be tried. The flow of milk must be adjusted to the infant's swallowing and should not be stopped until the infant attempts to suck.

The feedings are given at a pace that neither causes

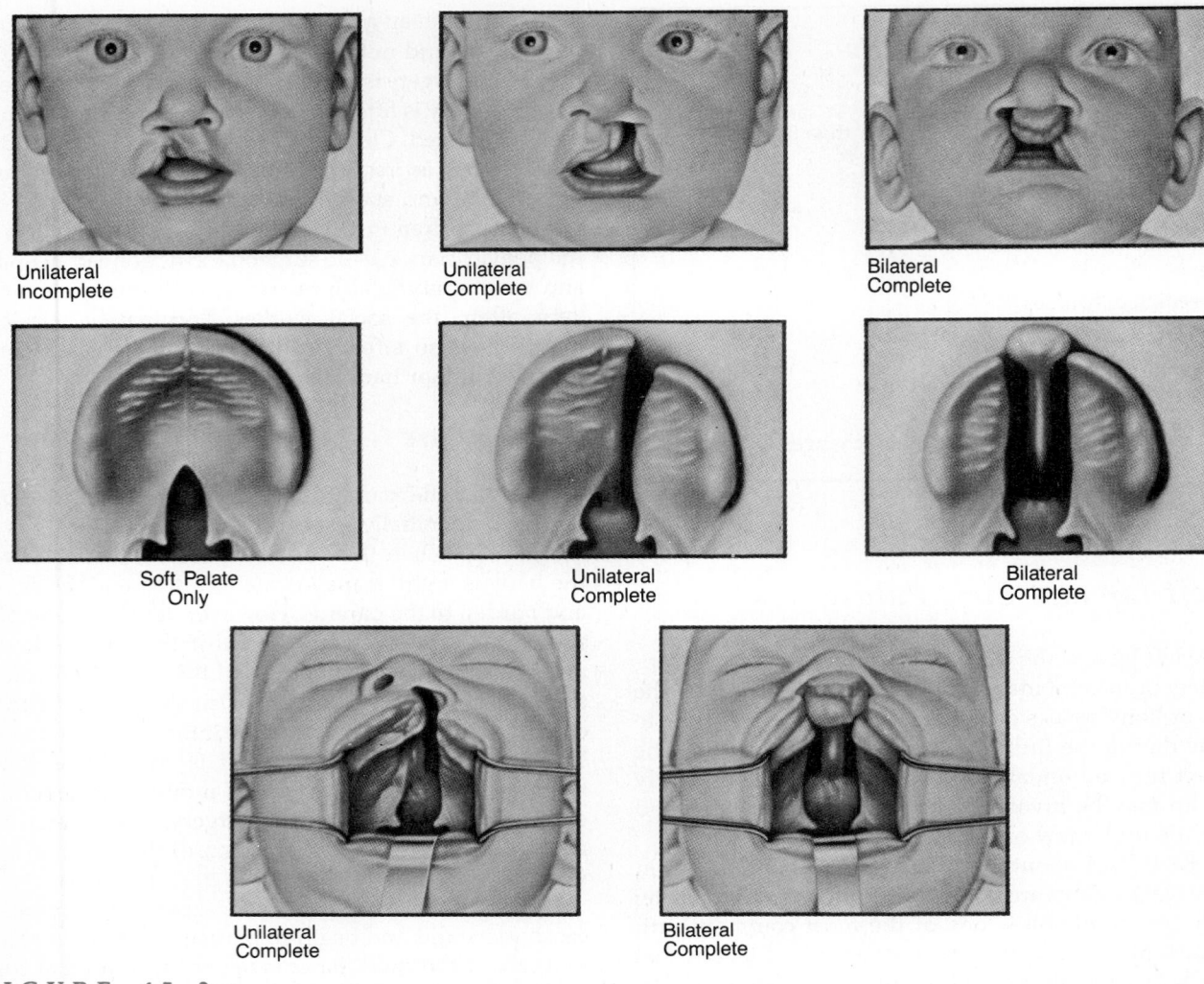

Unilateral
Incomplete

Unilateral
Complete

Bilateral
Complete

Soft Palate
Only

Unilateral
Complete

Bilateral
Complete

Unilateral
Complete

Bilateral
Complete

FIGURE 45-3

Illustrations of cleft lip and cleft palate. (Redrawn from drawing provided by Ross Laboratories)

the infant to become unduly tired nor results in aspiration of the liquid. Thickened formulas are often used. Since these infants tend to swallow large amounts of air, they should be bubbled at frequent intervals. The mother needs to be instructed in this technique.[5]

The nurse should help the mother to attain ease in feeding her baby and should arrange to stay with her during several of the sessions. This is one way of assessing how well the mother is progressing.

Gavage usually is unnecessary and should be used only when the other methods fail, since it does not stimulate the sucking and swallowing reflexes and it promotes aspiration.

The mother may want to breast-feed her infant, and there is no contraindication as long as the milk can be given in a way that the baby can take it. This may mean that the mother may have to express her milk and offer it in a bottle.

Hypospadias and Epispadias

In *male hyposadias,* the urethra opens on the undersurface of the penis proximal to the usual site. Minor degrees of this condition are quite common, and no surgical intervention is necessary. If the opening is at the base of the penis or far back on the shaft, plastic surgical repair is necessary. In *male epispadias,* the urethral opening is on the dorsal surface of the penis. There is a congenital absence of the upper urethral wall. If the defect is pronounced, it also will require repair. Surgical correction is usually made by 3 to 5 years of age. Definitive urethroplasty should be performed before the boy enters school so that it will be possible for him to urinate in the standing position. Since the foreskin is used in the repair, boys with hypospadias are not to be circumcised (Fig. 45-5).[9]

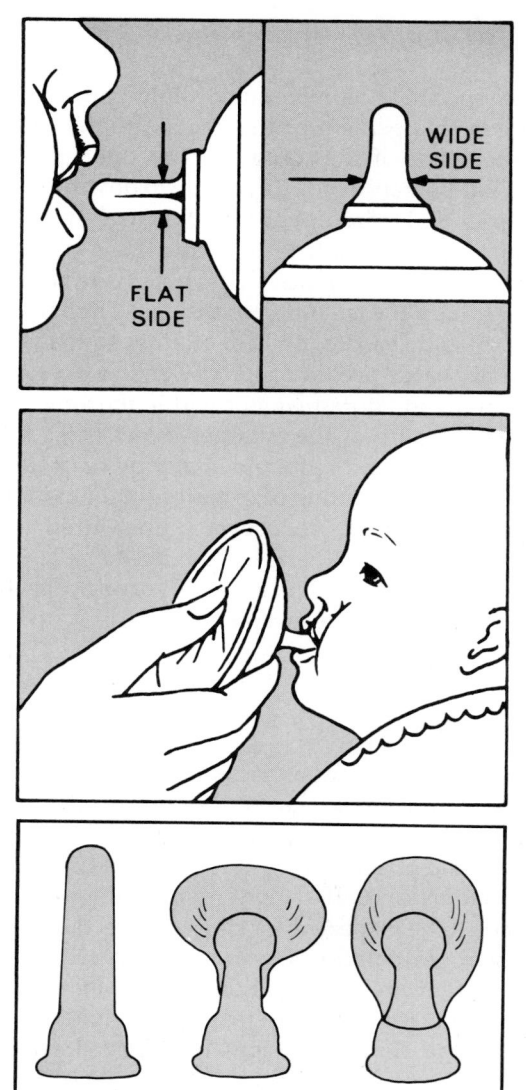

FIGURE 45-4

Nipples used for feeding babies with cleft lip and palate. (*A*) Beniflex Nurser. (*B*) Other types of nipples. (Beniflex Nurser courtesy of Mead Johnson)

In *female hypospadias,* the urethral meatus opens into the vagina, whereas in *female epispadias,* the upper urethral wall is absent, with possible exstrophy of the bladder. Serious types of genitourinary abnormalities often occur with numerous anomalies.

Ambiguous Genitalia

Infants may be born with ambiguous or uncertain genitalia or with characteristics of both male and female genitals (Fig. 45-6). Abnormal sexual differentiation in

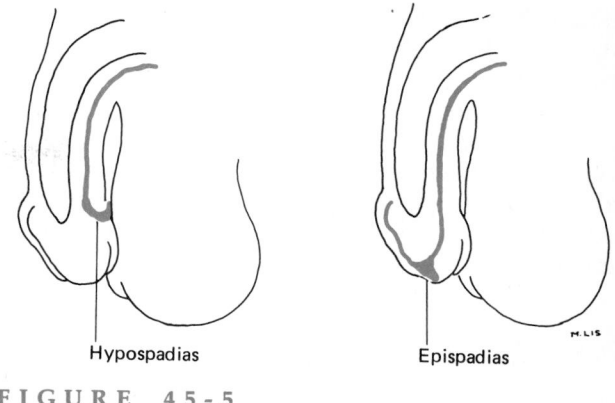

FIGURE 45-5

Illustration of hypospadias and epispadias.

fetal development can be due to genetic defects (adrenogenital syndrome, Klinefelter's syndrome, Turner's syndrome) or to the intrauterine hormonal environment (steroid sex hormone therapy given to the mother to prevent abortion). It is important for the nurse to report any instances of questionable genitalia because establishment of genetic sex and sexual rearing are critical to later compatible psychosexual development. Chromosomal sex, as well as the morphologic characteristics of internal and external sex organs, is taken into consid-

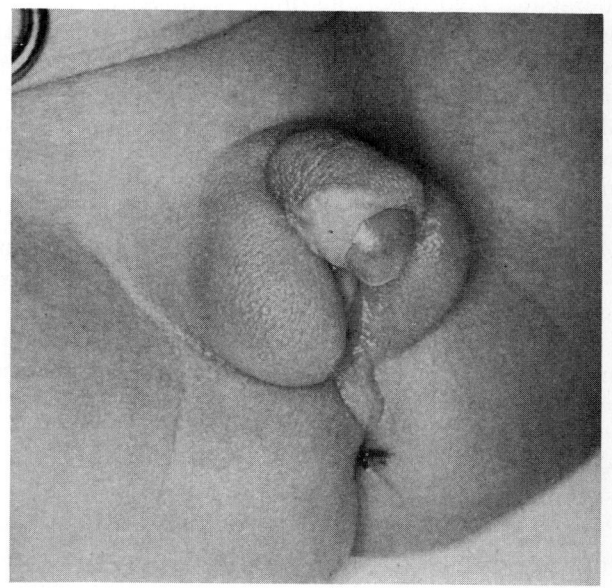

FIGURE 45-6

Infant born with ambiguous genitalia. From this photograph it is difficult to tell whether this patient has an atypical penis with penoscrotal hypospadias or whether there is extreme masculinization of the clitoris and scrotal changes of the labia majora. (Avery GB: Neonatology: Pathophysiology and Management of the Newborn, 2nd ed. Philadelphia, JB Lippincott, 1981)

eration in sex assignment. The diagnostic evaluation takes only 2 or 3 days, at which time sex assignment can be made.[9]

Often surgery to convert genitalia to one or the other sex is necessary, as well as later hormonal therapy to promote the development of secondary sex characteristics. Intersex problems represent an area of specialty, and appropriate referrals to experts in this field are indicated.

Spina Bifida

Spina bifida is a rather common malformation (1 in 500 live births) and is due to the congenital lack of one or more vertebral arches, usually at the lower part of the spine (Fig. 45-7A). When the membranes covering the spinal cord bulge through the opening, the condition is known as *meningocele* (Fig. 45-7A). It forms a soft, fluctuating tumor filled with cerebrospinal fluid. The tumor can be diminished by pressure. It enlarges when the baby cries. The extrusion of the cord along with the coverings is known as *meningomyelocele* (Fig. 45-7A and B). Most surgeons advocate early surgical closure, in the first 12 to 18 hours after birth. Surgical closure should take place within 24 hours to prevent further deterioration of the spinal cord and roots.[10]

When the repair is massive, the outlook can be discouraging. Hydrocephalus may occur if not already present. The situation and prognosis for the infant may be guarded, and the parents need a good deal of support and instruction about the continuing care of their infant. Many infants with neural tube defects die or suffer from neuromuscular impairments if they survive. Permanent impairment depends upon the level of the defect and the extent of central nervous system tissue involvement. Major urologic and orthopedic defects are usually involved. Prenatal diagnosis can identify neural tube defects through the use of ultrasound, amniography, or increased levels of α-fetoprotein in the amniotic fluid or maternal serum. Anencephaly can also be diagnosed prenatally by these techniques.

Nursing Care

Prevention of infection at the defect site is an essential part of nursing care. Until any surgical correction is performed the infant must be maintained in the prone position. Sterile dressings or other solutions may be ordered for protection of the sac. The site should be kept clean, without contamination by urine or feces.

Range of motion of extremities is important. Frequent change of position following surgery is important. The bladder may need to be emptied periodically by the Credé method, since dribbling often occurs.

Parents require much support as well as long-term medical, social, and parent-group referrals.

Hydrocephalus

An abnormal accumulation of fluid in the cranial vault causes enlargement of the head, atrophy of the brain, prominence of the forehead, and the typical "setting sun" appearance of the eyes due to downward pressure (Fig. 45-8). Hydrocephalic infants frequently have other anomalies, are subject to perinatal complications, and have a high incidence of mental retardation, neuromuscular defects, and convulsions. The incidence is 1 per 2000 deliveries, or 12% of all birth malformations. The abnormal accumulation of fluid may occur between the brain and dura mater or within the ventricles of the brain. Because of the enlarged head, these infants are often breech and require delivery by cesarean section.

Surgical shunting of cerebrospinal fluid is the treatment indicated to reduce pressure within the cranial vault; otherwise, there will be irreversible neurologic damage and death. Not all cases are operable, however, and observations over time are necessary to determine therapy.[10]

Nursing Care

Nursing interventions include prevention of complications and assessment of disease process by frequent measuring of head circumference, palpation of the fontanel, and observation of behaviors of increasing intracranial pressure. If a shunt is surgically placed, the site needs to be inspected for signs of infection and inflammation. Antibiotics may be ordered prophylactically. The infant must be positioned carefully depending on the shunt location. Parents need to be taught how to pump the shunt and signs of obstruction. Long-term referrals are essential for multidisciplinary services.

Anencephaly

In anencephaly, there is complete or partial absence of the infant's brain and of the skull overlying the brain. The cause is not known. Although there is a familial tendency in occurrences, multiple environmental factors seem to be involved. About 70% of anencephalic infants are female. Often the pregnancy involves polyhydramnios. If infants survive labor and delivery, their life expectancy is quite short. Supportive care is provided the infant; it seldom lives more than a few days. The parents also need much support in grieving and integrating this traumatic situation.

Microcephaly

The microcephalic infant has a head that is considerably smaller than normal and a smaller brain with accompanying mental retardation. Several causes of micro-

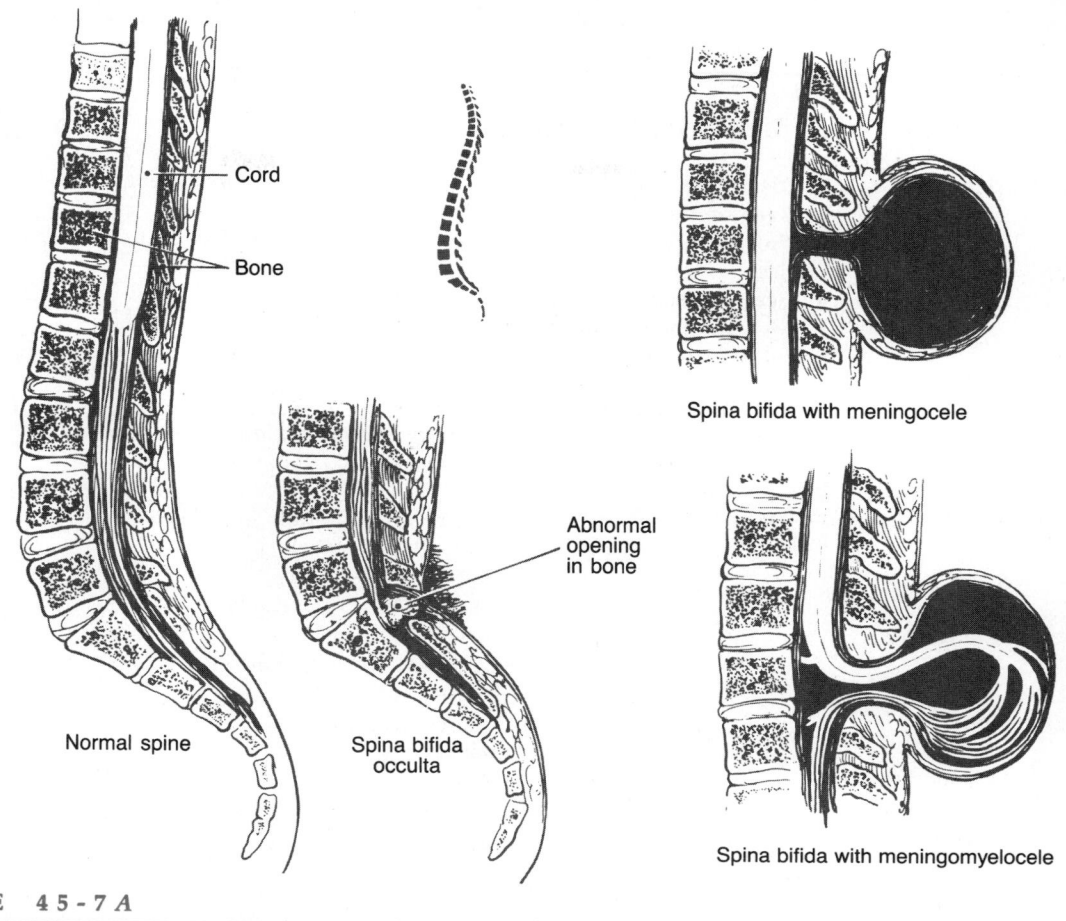

Cord

Bone

Normal spine

Spina bifida
occulta

Abnormal
opening
in bone

Spina bifida with meningocele

Spina bifida with meningomyelocele

FIGURE 45-7A

Spina bifida. (Spina Bifida: Hope Through Research. PHS Publication No. 1023, Health Information Series No. 103, 1970)

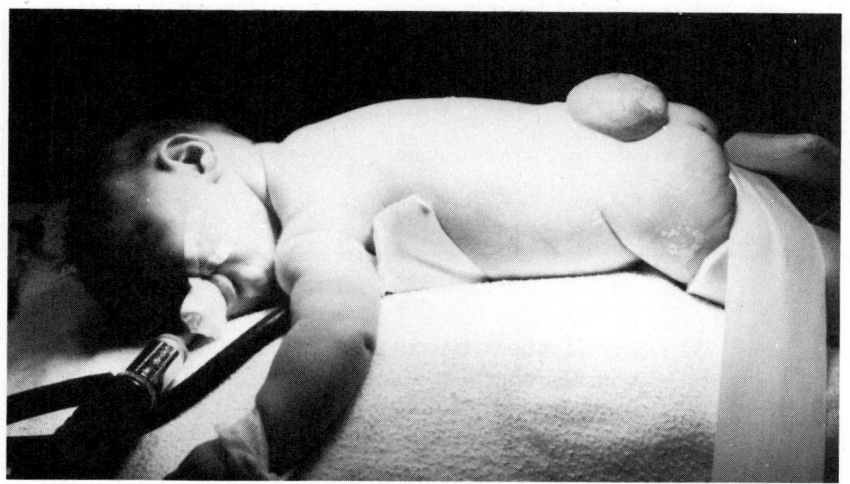

FIGURE 45-7B

Meningomyelocele in the lumbosacral area. The patient is in a prone position with supporting blanket rolls beneath a heating blanket. (The heating blanket is not shown.) (Mayer BW: Pediatric Anesthesia: A Guide to Its Administration. Philadelphia, JB Lippincott, 1981)

cephaly have been identified, including exposure of the pregnant woman to x-rays or viruses. Congenital microcephaly is also part of many chromosomal abnormalities and other syndromes.[10]

Many of these infants survive and need varying amounts of custodial care depending upon the extent of retardation. As with Down's syndrome, parents need assistance with decisions involving caring for the infant or child at home or seeking placement for institutional care.

Family of Neonate with Meningomyelocele

Nursing Objectives

1. Identify early the neonate's lesion site and related involvement.
2. Keep rupture site free of infection.
3. Provide care so that the neonate does not experience trauma to the lower extremities.
4. Reassess regularly for developing hydrocephalus.
5. Maintain the neonate's bowel and bladder functions.
6. Inform parents regarding long-term care and prognosis.

Assessment	Potential Nursing Diagnosis	Planning/Intervention	Evaluation
Neural tube dysfunction ascertained during pregnancy testing	Infection related to neural tube defect and occasional leakage of fluid	*Preoperatively* Protect sac by carefully positioning neonate on abdomen or side	Neonate's vital signs are stable
Herniated sac noted at delivery		Cover defect with dressing as ordered	
Complications of disease process:		Use doughnut-shaped device for support	
Decrease in sensation and movement below lesion		Observe sac for fluid drainage	
Bowel and bladder dysfunction		*Postoperatively* Protect incisional site from contamination by urine or feces	
Potential for hydrocephalus		Position on side or abdomen	
		Take temperature frequently	
		Inspect incisional site for redness or swelling	
	Potential for injury: trauma to lower extremities related to level of defect and lack of motion and sensation	Provide passive exercises to lower extremities frequently	Neonate responds to passive exercise
		Change position frequently	Neonate is comfortable
		Refer to physical therapy	

(continued)

Diaphragmatic Hernia

Diaphragmatic hernia is caused by a defect in the development of the diaphragm that allows abdominal organs to herniate into the thoracic cavity (Fig. 45-9). The majority of cases involve the left leaf of the diaphragm. Neonates present with cyanosis, severe respiratory distress, absent breath sounds on the involved side, and a scaphoid abdomen.

The mortality rate is high. Stabilization of the infant prior to a surgical repair requires placement of a naso-gastric tube to decompress the abdomen, correction of acidosis, administration of oxygen, and ventilatory assistance.[11]

If the defect is small, it can be easily repaired. This must be done soon after birth because the herniated abdominal organs interfere with adequate respiration. Large defects in the diaphragm allow extensive herniation, which can prevent normal intrauterine development of pulmonary tissue, and can be incompatible with life. The outcome depends upon the size of the defect, the amount of normal pulmonary development, and the success of surgery to close the hernia.

Assessment	Potential Nursing Diagnosis	Planning/Intervention	Evaluation
	Alteration in bowel and bladder function related to level of nerve involvement	Note urine function—if stream or frequent dribbling	Neonate empties bladder
		Use Credé's method of emptying bladder	
		Observe anal sphincter functioning by stimulation	Neonate responds to stimulation of anal sphincter
	Potential for injury: hydrocephalus related to meningomyelocele	Measure head circumference daily	Neonate's head stops growing
		Observe for signs of increasing intracranial pressure	Neonate has stable signs
		Note bulging or tenseness of fontanel	
		Observe for irritability, change in behavior	Neonate behaves normally
	Impaired physical mobility related to loss of nerve innervation below lesion	Provide frequent range of motion exercises	Neonate responds to exercises
		Change position	Neonate is comfortable
		Support extremities	
		Consider long-term referral	
	Parental anxiety related to uncertainty of long-term diagnosis	Allow parents to discuss situation at length	Parents freely discuss the situation and prognosis
		Provide realistic information regarding long-term care and prognosis	Parents acknowledge understanding of long-term care
		Teach parents signs of increasing intracranial pressure, how to Credé bladder, how to provide range of motion exercises	Parents identify signs of increasing intracranial pressure
			Parents perform return demonstration on teaching
			Parents care for infant under supervision in the nursery setting
		Refer to multidisciplinary agencies, parental support group, spina bifida clinic	Parents follow through on support groups

Obstructions of the Alimentary Tract

Esophageal Atresia and Tracheoesophageal Fistula

The incidence of esophageal atresia and tracheoesophageal fistula is 1 per 3000 live births.

Atresia of the esophagus, although less common than some that have been mentioned, is quite serious, and immediate steps must be taken to prevent aspiration. The defect occurs during embryonic development and results in the esophagus ending in a blind pouch rather than a stomach. A fistula usually occurs into the trachea near the bifurcation of the esophagus and the trachea. When the infant attempts to swallow liquids or even normal secretions, there is an overflow into the trachea from the blind pouch (Fig. 45-10).

This malformation should be suspected whenever the infant demonstrates excessive drooling, coughing, gagging, or respiratory distress during feeding. Abdominal distention may occur as air travels through the fistula to the esophagus and into the stomach. Rales, rhonchi, or decreased breath sounds may be auscultated. Diagnosis is made by insertion of a radiopaque catheter

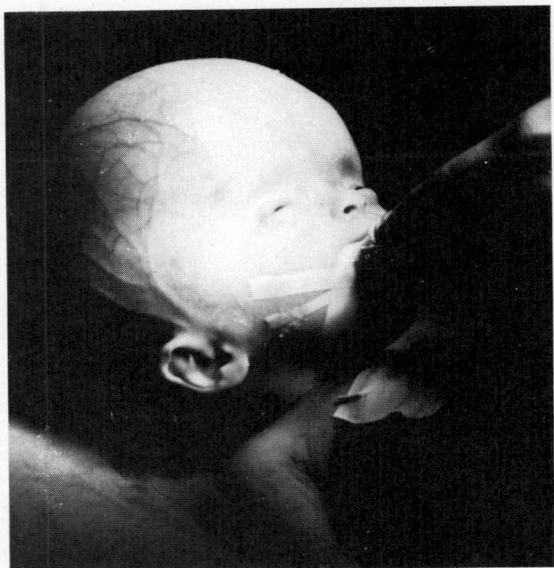

FIGURE 45-8

Hydrocephalus. Note the enlargement of the head, the prominent veins in the skin, and the "setting sun" appearance of the eyes. (Mayer BW: Pediatric Anesthesia: A Guide to Its Administration. Philadelphia, JB Lippincott, 1981)

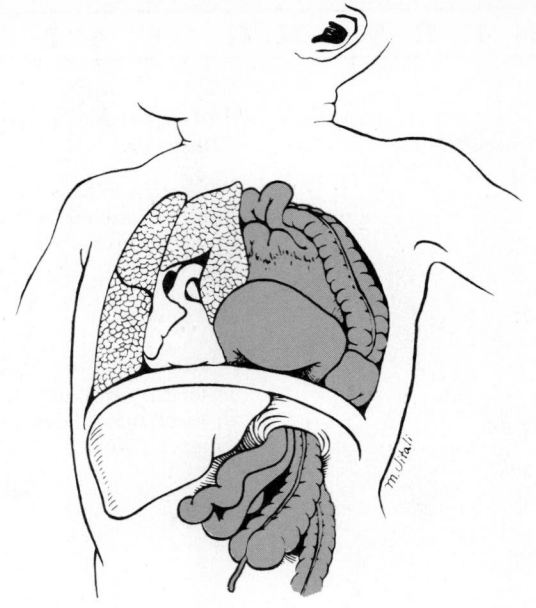

FIGURE 45-9

Diaphragmatic hernia showing abdominal contents within the thoracic cavity. This is considered a true pediatric emergency. (Mayer BW: Pediatric Anesthesia: A Guide to Its Administration. Philadelphia, JB Lippincott, 1981)

into the blind pouch to encounter resistance. Subsequent x-rays will reveal its path.[11]

Unless necessary surgery to correct the defect is prompt, the infant will contract bronchitis or pneumonia from repeated aspiration of milk and secretions.

The infant is placed in the supine position, with his head elevated 30° or more to prevent any gastric secretions from rising into the trachea through the fistula. The infant usually is placed in a heated, humidified incubator after surgery. This atmosphere is needed to liquefy the tenacious mucus that collects. A sump suction catheter (Replogle tube) is placed in the upper pouch to eliminate mucus. The nurse should watch carefully for any cyanosis or labored respiration that indicates the need for this measure. Blood, plasma, parenteral fluids, and antibiotics are also given. The extent of the repair and the condition of the infant determine when oral feeding should begin.

Pyloric Stenosis

Pyloric stenosis is a congenital anomaly with an incidence of 2 to 5 per 1000 live births. It usually manifests its symptoms between the second and sixth week by the onset of vomiting that becomes projectile and occurs within 30 minutes after every feeding. The infant loses

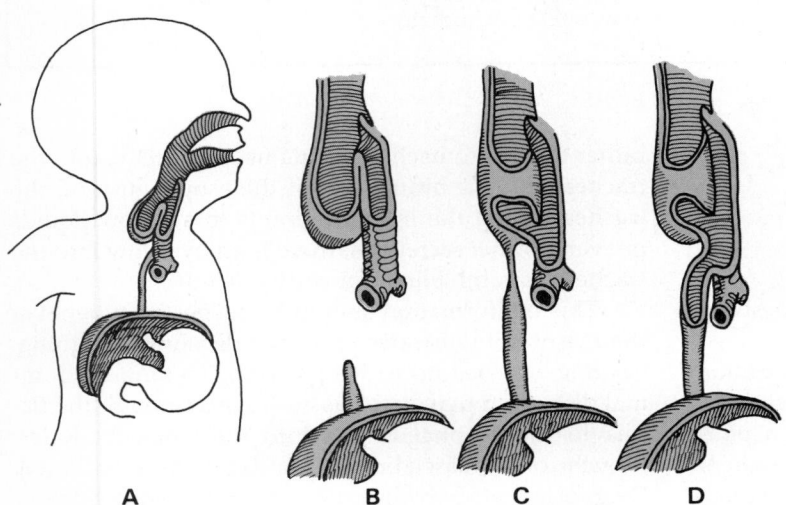

FIGURE 45-10

Esophageal atresia. (A) The most common form of esophageal atresia. (B) Both segments of the esophagus are blind pouches. (C) The esophagus is continuous, but with a narrowed segment. (D) The upper segment of the esophagus opens into the trachea.

A   B   C   D

NURSING CARE PLAN

Infant with a Tracheoesophageal Fistula

Nursing Objectives:
1. Prevent aspiration pneumonia by early diagnosis and treatment.
2. Carry out surgical correction when infant is stabilized.
3. Prevent potential complications.

Assessment	Potential Nursing Diagnosis	Planning/Intervention	Evaluation
Maternal history of hydramnios	Ineffective airway clearance related to structural defect	*Preoperatively*	Neonate remains free of aspiration pneumonia
Neonatal regurgitation and cyanosis with first feeding	Impaired gas exchange related to aspiration	If suspected anomaly due to large amounts of secretions and respiratory distress, do not feed	
Inability to pass nasogastric tube		Use sterile water for first feedings if necessary	
Respiratory distress		Assist with diagnostic tests	
		Manage double-lumen indwelling suction tubing	
		Raise head of bed slightly	
		Postoperatively	Neonate's nutrition is adequate to prevent dehydration and promote weight gain
		Chest tube maintenance:	
		Keep tube secure	Neonate remains free of postoperative complications
		Keep clamp nearby in case of dislodgement; clamp close to chest wall	
		Record and describe drainage from chest tube	
		Position with head of bed raised	
	Alteration in nutrition: less than body requirements related to surgical procedure (inability to feed immediately postoperatively)	Administer oxygen as ordered	
		Monitor intake/output	
		Administer gastrostomy feedings as tolerated and as ordered	
		Suction gently—mark suction catheter to minimize vigorous suctioning and any damage to suture lines	

weight, bowel elimination lessens, highly colored urine becomes scanty, and the symptoms of dehydration appear. Upon examination, gastric peristalsis is found, and the pyloric "acornlike" tumor may be palpated. Surgery is the treatment of choice.

The operation is not usually an emergency, leaving sufficient time for supportive treatment to correct any dehydration or electrolyte imbalance beforehand. Fluids, electrolytes, and blood replacement may be necessary, depending on the condition of the infant. Gastric lavage, from 1 to 2 hours before operation, may be done until returns are clear. Maintaining body heat before and after surgery is essential.

Postoperative feedings are resumed gradually, beginning with glucose water, in limited amounts, at about 6 hours. Feedings are advanced slowly to full-strength formula with close observation and recording of the infant's tolerance.

As soon as the infant is tolerating feedings, breast-feeding may be resumed. With an uncomplicated course, the infant should be discharged within 4 to 6 days postoperatively.[12]

Obstruction of the Duodenum and Small Intestine

Obstruction of the duodenum or small intestine is relatively easy to diagnose. Vomiting occurs following the first feeding, as no meconium is passed. The emesis may be bile stained or fecal stained, depending on whether the obstruction is high or low in the intestinal tract. If the obstruction is low, usually there is marked distention. An x-ray film, indicating a dilated small bowel without gas in the colon, confirms the diagnosis, and immediate surgery is indicated.[11]

The surgery (duodenoduodenostomy or duodenojejunostomy) is accompanied by continuous parenteral fluids, blood replacement as needed, and nasogastric suction. Postoperative care includes maintaining body temperature and providing intravenous fluids until peristalsis is established (about a week). This is followed by feedings as given in pyloric stenosis. If distention occurs, nasoduodenal suction may be necessary.

Imperforate Anus

Imperforate anus consists of atresia of the anus, with the rectum ending in a blind pouch. Careful examination of the infant in the delivery room usually reveals the condition. Surgical treatment is, of course, imperative. Later continence depends upon the nature of the anorectal abnormalities and the effectiveness of surgery. The incidence is 1 in 5000 births.

More males are affected by imperforate anus than females. Most females who are affected have a small fistula. This is uncommon in males (Fig. 45-11). The fistulous connection may be into the vagina, bladder, or urethra or through the perineum. Male fistulas may lead into the bladder or urethra or through the perineum

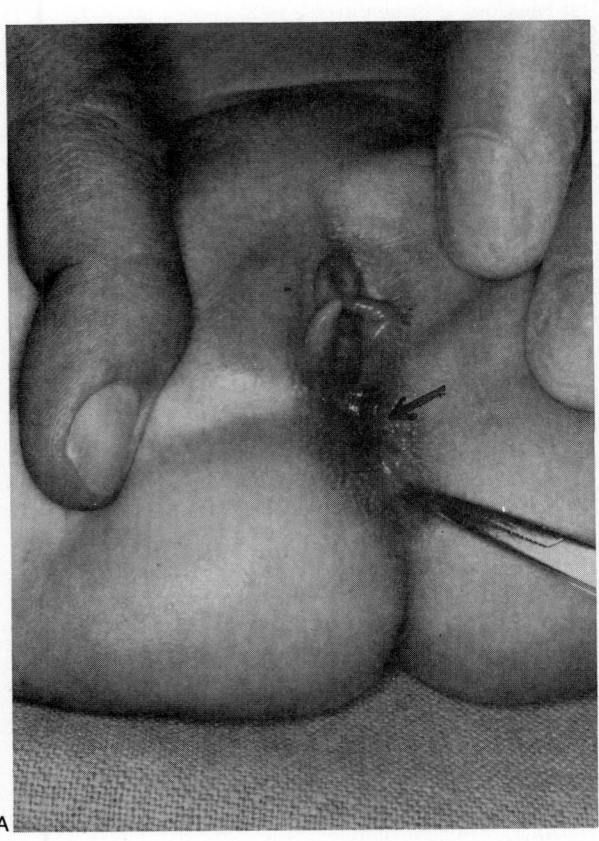
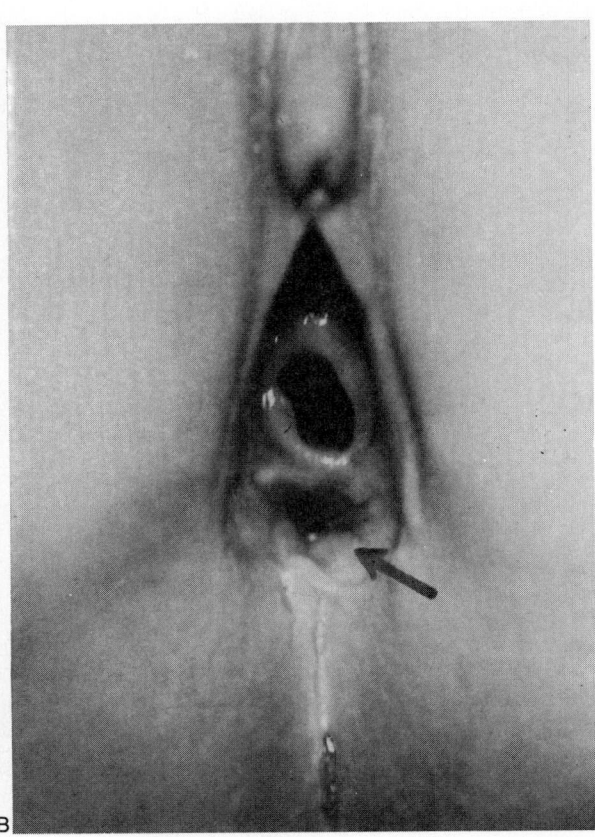

FIGURE 45-11

(A) Female with imperforate anus. The arrow demonstrates perineal fistula opening. The clamp is at the point where a normal anus would open. (B) Closeup of female with imperforate anus and an introital fistula just inside the labia minora and immediately beneath the hymenal ring. This is the most common form of fistulous opening in female imperforate anus. (Avery GB: Neonatology: Pathophysiology and Management of the Newborn, 2nd ed. Philadelphia, JB Lippincott, 1981)

(Fig. 45-12). If there appears to be an anal opening, the nurse can check for patency by inserting a well-lubricated probe (thermometer, tubing, small finger) and can observe physiological functioning by stroking the anus and watching for the normal "wink" response of the sphincter. X-ray examination confirms definitive diagnosis.

Abdominal Wall Defects

Omphalocele

Omphalocéle is a congenital abdominal wall defect, occurring in 1 in 5000 births, in which an amount of abdominal contents protrudes at the base of the umbilicus (Fig. 45-13). Omphaloceles develop between the eighth and tenth week of fetal life. The mass is covered with a layer of peritoneum and amnion and may rupture at delivery. Omphaloceles are often seen in conjunction with other cardiac, genitourinary, and extraintestinal anomalies.[11] Treatment requires covering of the mass

with sterile gauze soaked in saline, nasogastric tube placement, and immediate total or staged surgical repair. Sepsis is a serious and potential complication.[13]

Gastroschisis

Gastroschisis is a similar defect that occurs less frequently than omphalocele, with an incidence of about 1 in 50,000 births or less. The lesion is not covered with membrane, and the umbilical cord protrudes lateral to the defect in the abdominal wall (Fig. 45-14). Treatment is similar to that for omphalocele.

Chromosomal Anomalies

When a particular chromosome is in triplicate rather than the usual duplicate (pair), it is called *trisomy*. Three such trisomies, trisomy 13 (D trisomy), trisomy 18 (E trisomy), and trisomy 21,22 (Down's syndrome), have typical clinical pictures and can be recognized at birth.

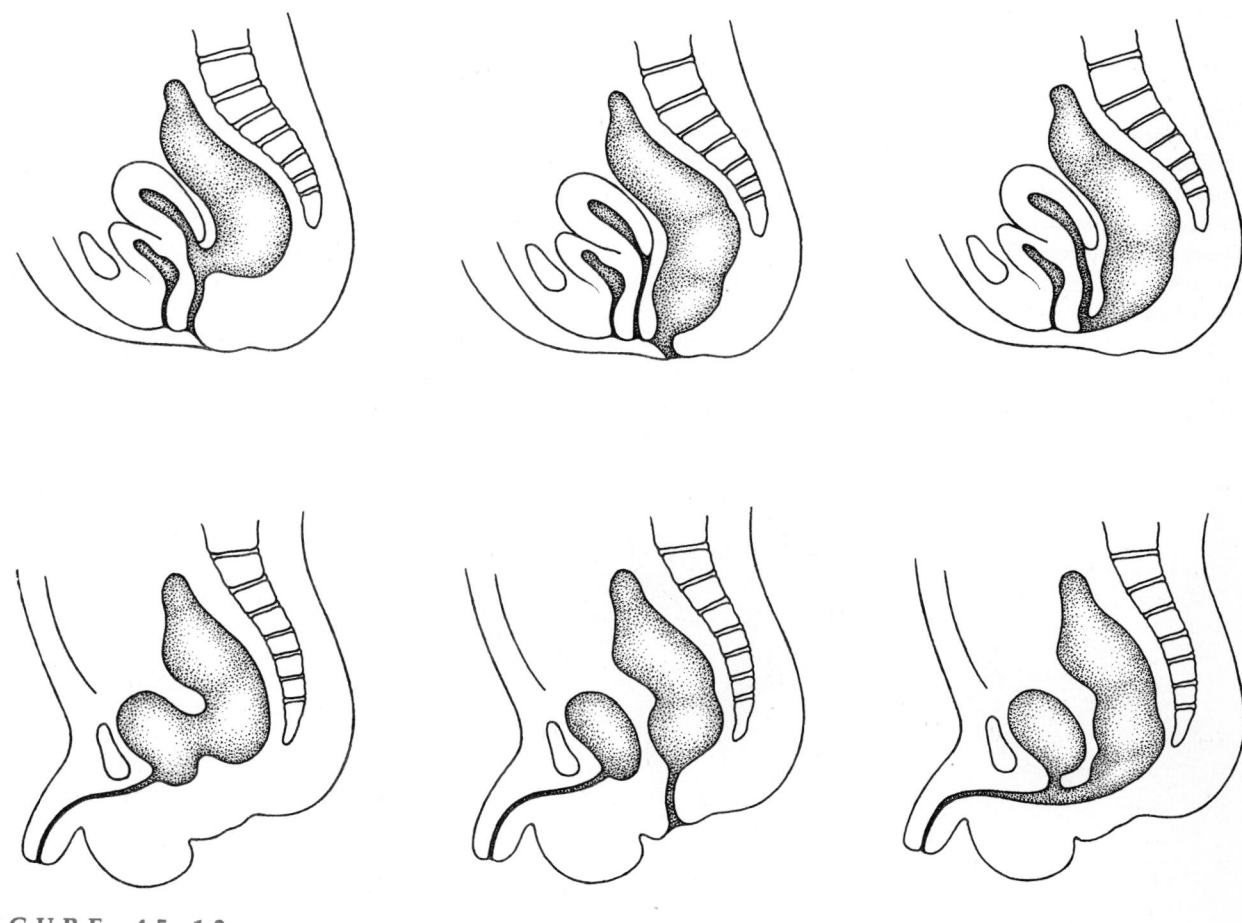

FIGURE 45-12

Types of imperforate anus.

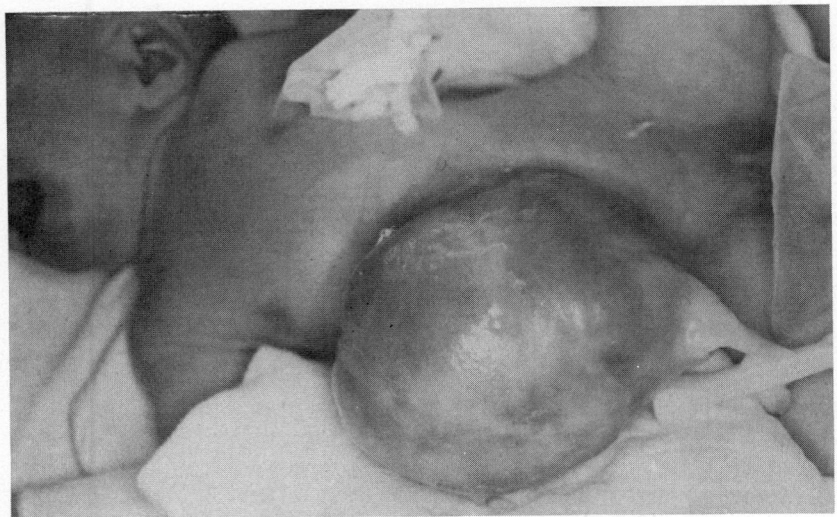

FIGURE 45-13

Large omphalocele. Note covering of the sac and its relationship to the umbilicus, which protrudes from the lower portion. (Avery GB: Neonatology: Pathophysiology and Management of the Newborn, 2nd ed. Philadelphia, JB Lippincott, 1981)

As discussed in Chapter 11, in the normal person, there are 46 chromosomes in 23 pairs, one pair of sex-determining chromosomes, and 22 pairs of autosomes. The extra chromosome found in trisomy results from nondisjunction (see Chap. 17), which can occur at any time in a cell's lifetime, during either meiosis or mitosis. Two different cytologic pictures emerge in trisomic cells. In the first, there is a free extra chromosome, giving 47 chromosomes, or a chromosome is lacking, giving only 45. This is called nondisjunction. In the second, the extra chromosome is translocated, that is, attached to another chromosome. The total number is 46, but one of the chromosomes is the size of two chromosomes combined.

There is an increased incidence of all three types of trisomy with advanced maternal age. This phenomenon is thought to be related to the long storage of oocytes in the mother. These germ cells are laid down during the mother's own fetal life; they wait, however, until the time of their individual ovulation to complete their meiotic divisions. Thus, it appears that nondisjunction tends to occur in older oocytes.

Trisomy 13, or D

Trisomy 13 is characterized by an extra chromosome in the D group, which includes pairs 13 through 15 (see Chap. 17). Infants with this abnormality frequently have difficulty establishing and maintaining respiration. One of the most striking features is the abnormal cranial development. The cranium is usually small, with a sloping forehead. The ears may be malformed and low set, and the eyes usually have some defect (cataracts, iris defects, unusual smallness), often bilaterally. Cleft palate and lip are commonly present. In addition, the hands and feet are often grossly deformed. Extra digits are common on both hands and feet. The thumbs may be retroflexible (double-jointed). The foot frequently has

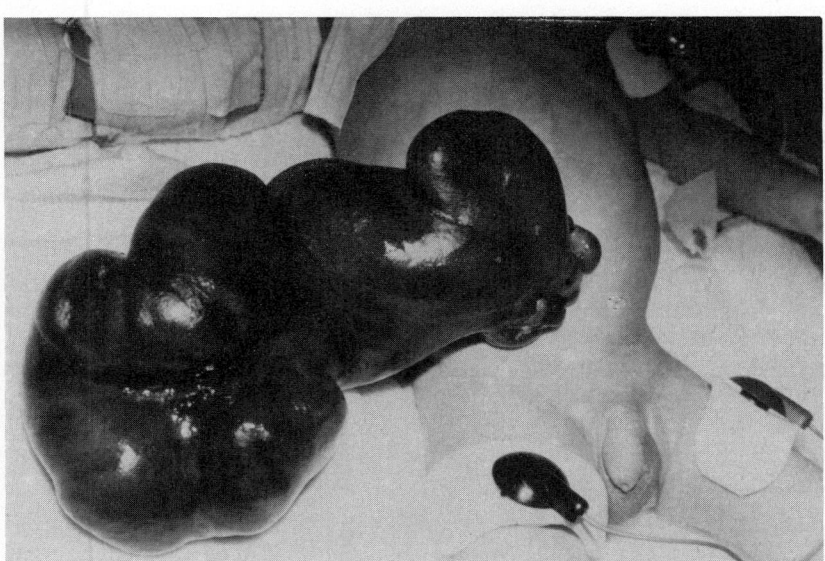

FIGURE 45-14

Patient with gastroschisis. Note edematous, matted bowel, the result of the intestines floating freely in the amniotic fluid. Remarkably, these distorted viscera will ultimately fit back into the abdominal cavity and will finally assume a normal appearance and function. (Avery GB: Neonatology: Pathophysiology and Management of the Newborn, 2nd ed. Philadelphia, JB Lippincott, 1981)

a posterior prominence of the heel sometimes accompanied by a convex sole, known as "rocker-bottom" foot. Other defects may include a bulbous nose, umbilical and diaphragmatic hernias, abnormal genitalia, scalp defects, and extensive capillary hemangiomatas far in excess of what is usually found in the normal newborn.

Neurologic examination reveals these infants to have a weak or absent Moro reflex and little or no response to loud noises; hence, they appear to be deaf. They are prone to develop myoclonic seizures. All suffer from apneic spells of unknown origin. Autopsy often reveals the complete lack of olfactory nerves and tracts. All of these infants are mentally retarded, and the majority have severe cardiac defects (dextroposition of the heart, ventricular septal defect), which are the major contributors to death. The average life span is less than a year, although several have lived to the age of 5 years.[14]

Trisomy 18, or E

Trisomy 18 is characterized by an extra chromosome in the E group, which includes pairs 17 and 18 (see Chap. 17). These babies are usually born at term, but are small, averaging about 2 kg (5 lb). Their placentas are often very small. The head is small with a prominent occiput, but is in proportion to the body size. The eyes are usually normal, but the ears are generally malformed and low set. The mouth appears small because of the short upper lip, and the mandible is small, giving a receding chin.

The hands of these babies are always malformed, but in a different way from those in trisomy 13 infants. They give the best diagnostic clue to the condition. These babies keep their fists clenched most of the time, with the index finger overlying the third finger.

Profuse lanugo covers the forehead, back, and extremities, and the skin usually has a mottled appearance. The sternum is very short; thus, the abdomen appears long. The pelvis is small, with limited abduction of the hips. There also may be abnormal genitalia. Inguinal and umbilical hernias are frequent; diaphragmatic eventration (elevation of a thinned portion of the diaphragm) occurs more often than frank hernia in these patients.

Neurologic examination reveals abnormal muscle tone. These babies progress from a hypertonic state to frank opisthotonus. Since the sucking reflex is poor, gavage feeding is often instituted. Unlike trisomy 13, trisomy 18 babies demonstrate no gross brain abnormalities. Cardiac abnormalities are common, and either these or aspiration accounts for the death of these babies.

The life span of these infants is less than 6 months on the average. During this time they become progressively undernourished and present a failure-to-thrive syndrome. As with trisomy 13, some infants have survived to childhood, so that death in infancy cannot be predicted.[14]

Trisomy 21, or Down's Syndrome

In Down's syndrome, an extra chromosome belonging to pair 21 or pair 22 or a translocation of 15/21 is found (see Chap. 17). Although these babies are apt to have congenital defects and are more susceptible to infection, they can be expected to live much longer and have less severe mental retardation (although it can be very severe) than the other trisomy infants.

The eyes are set close together and are slanting, have narrow palpebral fissures, and contain Brushfield's spots. The nose is flat. The tongue is large and fissured and usually is very obvious because it protrudes from the open mouth. The head is small, and posteriorly the occiput appears flat above the broad, pudgy neck (Fig. 45-15). The hands are short and thick, especially the fingers (the little finger is curved), with simian creases apparent on the palmar surfaces. In addition to having defective mentality and the deformities mentioned above, these infants have underdeveloped muscles, loose joints, and heart and alimentary tract abnormalities.[14]

Incidence and Etiology. The incidence of Down's syndrome has been estimated at 1 in 500 births. However, this ratio has dropped with the lowering of maternal age. For statistics on incidence with increasing maternal age, see Chapter 17.

Types. The most common chromosomal defect of the ovum in Down's syndrome is trisomy of chromosome 21 or 22. This results in a total chromosomal count of 47 instead of the normal number of 46. This type, commonly referred to as standard trisomy, usually occurs in infants born to older women and is rarely familial. The incidence of standard trisomy is 1 in 600 births.

The second type of abnormality results from a 15/21 translocation; in this type the actual chromosomal count is 46. The translocation type of Down's syndrome usually occurs in infants born to younger parents, is of the familial type, and is rare.

The third type of the disorder, mosaicism, is very rare. A unique factor in mosaicism is that one person may have cells with different chromosomal counts. Laboratory tests may demonstrate that the affected person's blood cells, for example, have 47 chromosomes, whereas his skin cells may show 46 chromosomes. This is not a familial type of Down's syndrome, and, moreover, the abnormalities may be less severe.

Prognosis. The usual causes of death in these babies are heart defects and infectious illnesses. The survival

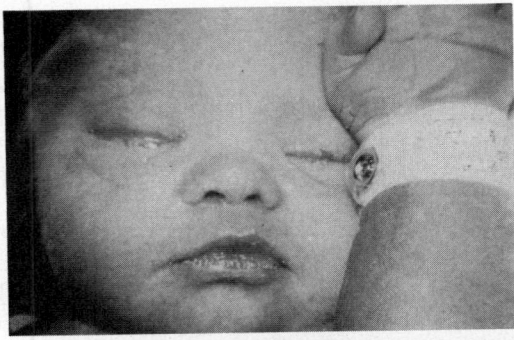

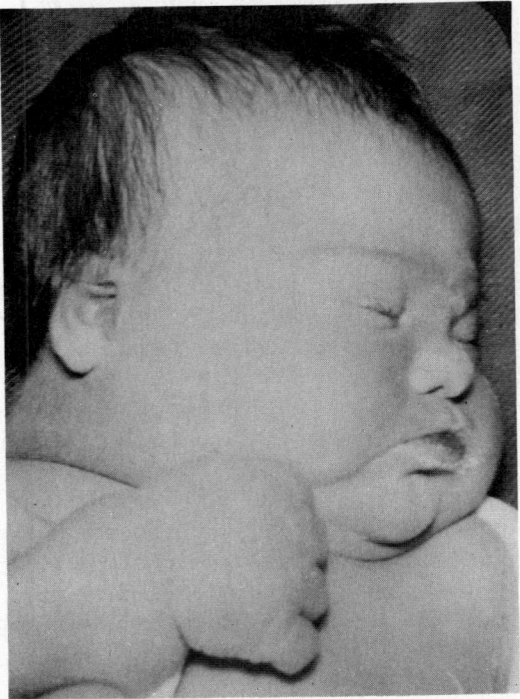

FIGURE 45-15

Patient with Down's syndrome. (Avery GB: Neonatology: Pathophysiology and Management of the Newborn, 2nd ed. Philadelphia, JB Lippincott, 1981)

rate is variable. Children with Down's syndrome are essentially retarded but have been found to be far more educable than was previously thought.

Prevention

The key approach to trisomy conditions lies in prevention because treatment does not alter the long-range prognosis. Education of the public regarding the effect of maternal age is the key issue in prevention. The incidence of all three trisomies goes up with increased maternal age. The later thirties and the forties are less safe for childbearing (from many points of view). Childbearing is less risky when the mother is younger. Genetic counseling is another aspect of public education

(see Chap. 17). Parents who have had a trisomic child (or if trisomy has appeared among their siblings) would benefit from counseling concerning the risk of having another affected child. In some families, trisomies are not the result of nondisjunction and therefore have an appreciable chance of recurring. This depends on the interaction of the variables of family history, maternal age, and chromosomal arrangement.

Nursing Care

Immediate care is supportive for the infant. Warmth, prevention of infection, maintenance of fluid and electrolyte balance, and, often, oxygen therapy are provided. Nursing therapy is aimed primarily at supporting the parents in helping them to work through their grief. The latter aspect is particularly important because of the grave prognosis for these babies. It is often helpful to institute community-health or visiting nurse referrals because the parents may need technical help upon arriving home with the infant. If a fetal death occurs, supportive help from a public-health nurse is also beneficial.

Phocomelia

Phocomelia (seal limbs) is a defect in one or several limbs. Thalidomide has caused the lack of an intermediate part or a deformity of a distal part. Since the early 1960s, the United States Food and Drug Administration has tightened the regulation of drugs. Often, the etiology of stunting or amputation of limbs is unknown. Nurses need to be supportive of parents while they attempt to cope with this crisis. Multiprofessional referrals are needed to begin the complicated rehabilitative process.

Inborn Errors of Metabolism

Numerous metabolic disorders, so-called inborn errors of metabolism, are now known to originate from mutations in the genes that alter the genetic constitution of a person to the extent that normal function is disrupted. These biochemical disorders arise because of the disturbance (mutation) in a molecule of the gene itself. They *do not* stem from some mishap or alteration during the embryonic development of tissue or organs. The mode of transmission of these inborn errors usually is recessive (*i.e.*, to be affected, an infant must receive a pair of defective genes, one from the mother and one from the father). The mother and father in these cases would be carriers of the defective genes but would not be affected by the resulting disorder *per se*. Fortunately, defective genes are found rather infrequently in the general population, and the chance of their joining is rare; hence, the diseases they produce are rare.

It is important to remember that these inborn errors of metabolism do not usually produce symptoms that are apparent at birth. Therefore, the maternity nurse will rarely see evidence of these disorders although she is involved in neonatal screening tests.

Neonatal Screening Test

Many states require screening for neonatal disorders, the most common being phenylketonuria. Others that may be tested are galactosemia, hypothyroidism, maple syrup urine disease, and homocystinuria. The same blood sample collected on filter paper can detect all of these diseases.

Phenylketonuria

Phenylketonuria, the result of an inborn error of metabolism, reflects the absence of the liver enzyme phenylalanine hydroxylase. Without this enzyme, phenylalanine cannot be converted to tyrosine. As a result, toxic levels of phenylalanine and its metabolites phenylpyruvic acid and phenylacetic acid accumulate in blood, urine, and the central nervous system. The affected child has a musty odor, decreased pigmentation of skin and hair, and progressive mental retardation. The incidence is about 1 in 1500 live births. Minimal central nervous system damage will be done if early diagnosis is made and treatment is begun before 3 months of age.

The most commonly used screening method is the Guthrie method, which uses small amounts of blood placed on filter paper. Accuracy of the test is dependent upon adequate ingestion of protein for 24 to 48 hours. With current short hospital stays, a repeat test may be necessary in a few weeks. Phenylalanine levels of about 4 mg to 8 mg/dl are considered a presumptive positive. Parents can also check the infant's urine against a test strip at about 6 weeks of age. A green color reaction is positive. Treatment must begin before 3 months of age to prevent mental retardation.

The only treatment is dietary restriction to keep phenylalanine levels between 3 and 10 mg/dl. Allowances of phenylalanine consumption average about 500 mg to 600 mg daily. The average adult consumes several thousand milligrams of phenylalanine daily. Products containing Nutrasweet (aspartame) are labeled with a warning that it contains phenylalanine. Lofenalac is a formula low in phenylalanine that may be given to the neonate. There is no agreed upon time at which to discontinue the restricted diet.[15]

Parents need support from resources such as dietitian, social services, pediatrician, and public-health nurse to fully understand the disease and strict dietary regimen.

Galactosemia

Galactosemia is an autosomal recessive disease and an inborn error of carbohydrate metabolism. The body is unable to metabolize galactose and lactose owing to lack of complex enzyme structures. Levels of galactose in the blood lead to cataract formation, renal disease, liver dysfunction, and some degree of mental retardation. Formulas such as Nutramigen or ProSobee may be used as treatment since they are lactose free. Other treatment may be necessary for concomitant clinical problems.[16]

Congenital Hypothyroidism

Thyroid deficiency is believed to have been present at or before birth. Factors that may be responsible are inborn error of metabolism, maternal iodine deficiency, or maternal ingestion of antithyroid drugs.

Early signs include hypotonia, lethargy, large fontanels, respiratory distress, feeding problems, hypothermia, constipation, pallor, and poor cry.

Other features that appear at about 6 months of age include depressed nasal bridge; relatively narrow forehead; puffy eyelids; coarse hair; large tongue; thick, dry, cold skin; abdominal distention; bradycardia; hypotension; and hyporeflexia.

Treatment of thyroid replacement should be initiated immediately. Although physical recovery is usually good, it is uncertain how complete the mental recovery will be.[16]

Maple Syrup Urine Disorder

In maple syrup urine disease, three branched-chain amino acids are unable to be metabolized. The result is a rapidly progressing disease characterized by severe depression of the central nervous system and ultimately death from respiratory failure. Treatment is the use of a diet low in leucine, isoleucine, and valine.[16]

Homocystinuria

Homocystinuria is an automosomal recessive disease with progressive clinical symptoms. There is a reduction in the activity of cystathionine synthetase, which leads

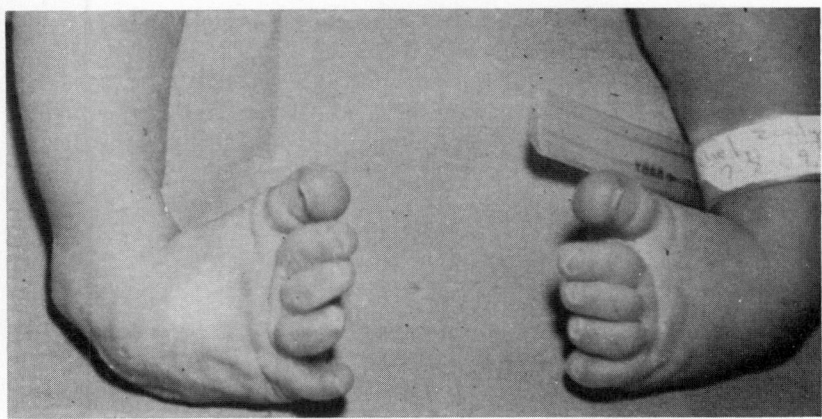

F I G U R E   4 5 - 1 6

Talipes equinovarus (clubfoot). (Avery GB: Neonatology: Pathophysiology and Management of the Newborn, 2nd ed. Philadelphia, JB Lippincott, 1981)

to the building of homocystine in the blood and urine and methionine in the blood. A gradual buildup of metabolites does not clinically present until 2½ to 3⅓ years. Signs are dislocation of lenses, skeletal deformities, thrombotic episodes, and mental retardation. Treatment is the administration of pyridoxine or a diet low in methionine and high in cystine.[17]

Care should be taken so that the parents of an affected child are not led to believe that all babies treated will have the usual pattern of growth and development (intellectual development may be slow, for instance). This cannot be guaranteed. *Early detection* and *prompt treatment* prevent mental retardation. The control of this condition demands consistent and disciplined supervision and follow-through on the part of the parents.

Musculoskeletal Disorders

Talipes Equinovarus (Clubfoot)

Clubfoot occurs twice as often in males as in females, with an overall incidence of 1 in 1000 births.[18] The three elements of this deformity are equinus or plantar flexion of the foot at the ankle, varus or inversion deformity of the heel, and forefoot adduction (Fig. 45-16). All three are present in classic talipes equinovarus. Infants with this deformity should be examined for associated anomalies, especially those of the spine. There is a hereditary pattern in some families. Clubfoot may also be part of a generalized neuromuscular syndrome. Therapy begins early. If the foot can be manipulated to the other direction, simple exercise may correct the abnormality. Plaster casts may be applied after the affected foot structures have been stretched and manipulated. Casts are applied sequentially, correcting first the forefoot adduction, then inversion of the heel, and lastly the equinus flexion at the ankle. Serial casting is needed as the infant grows. After correction is obtained, braces

are usually needed for months to years to prevent recurrences of the deformities. Surgery is rarely required.[18]

Congenital Hip Dysplasia

Congenital hip dysplasia refers to malformations of the hip involving various degrees of deformity that are present at birth. Congenital hip dysplasia occurs in 1 in 50 to 1000 births. It occurs more frequently in females than in males. One fourth of the cases are bilateral; if unilateral, it more often involves the left hip than the right.

There is an association between congenital hip disorders and breech deliveries owing to the abnormal position *in utero.*

Three categories of congenital hip can be noted. The first is *acetabular dysplasia* (or preluxation). In this instance, there is bony hypoplasia of the acetabular roof. The femoral head remains in the acetabulum. The second is *subluxation,* involving a majority of dysplasias. There is incomplete dislocation, in which the femoral head remains in contact with the acetabulum but is slightly displaced. In *dislocation,* the femoral head loses contact with the acetabulum and is displaced posteriorly and superiorly over the fibrocartilaginous rim.[5]

Prognosis is best if diagnosis is established while the newborn is still in the nursery. Ortolani's sign demonstrates that the femoral head can be lifted into the acetabulum as the thigh is abducted in flexion and that it dislocates as the hip is adducted (Fig. 45-17).[19]

Treatment should begin promptly for best outcome. The longer that treatment is delayed, the poorer the prognosis.

In infants under 1 year of age, treatment may be any method designed to keep the hip in full abduction. Methods range from triple diapering to a device made of plastic, metal, or leather or a soft Frejka pillow splint (Fig. 45-18). If these methods are ineffective, a hip spica cast may be applied followed by a brace. Successful treatment is usually accomplished in 3 to 4 months.[18]

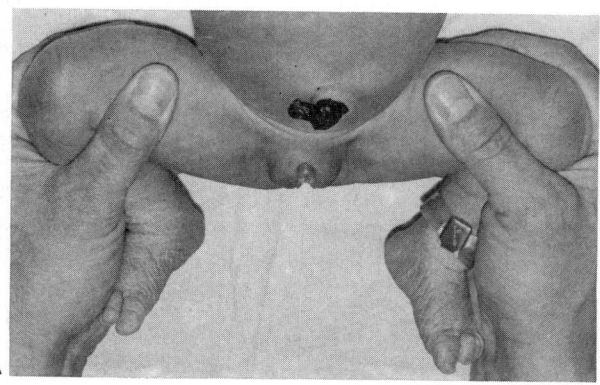
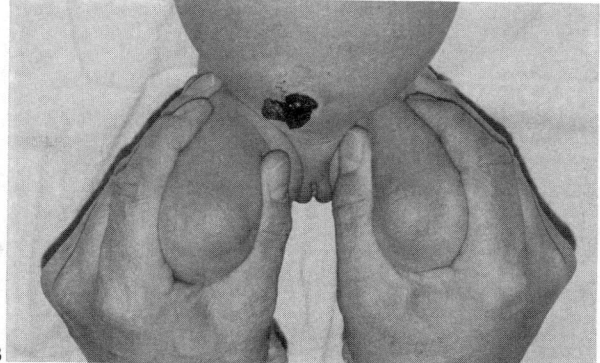

FIGURE 45-17

(*A*) Ortolani's sign. The fingers are on the trochanter and the thumb grips the femur as shown. The femur is lifted forward as the thighs are abducted. If the head was dislocated it can be felt to reduce. (*B*) The thighs are adducted and if the head dislocates it will be both felt and seen as it suddenly jerks over the acetabulum. (Avery GB: Neonatology: Pathophysiology and Management of the Newborn, 2nd ed. Philadelphia, JB Lippincott, 1981)

Parents need education and support in applying corrective measures or appliances, using adaptive feeding and holding techniques, and understanding the course of treatment and expected results. If the patient is identified and treated early, the long-term prognosis for correction is good.

Polydactyly

A hereditary condition, polydactyly consists of extra digits on the hands and feet. If the digits do not include bones, ligation with a silk suture during the neonatal period is often adequate to cause sloughing of the tissue,

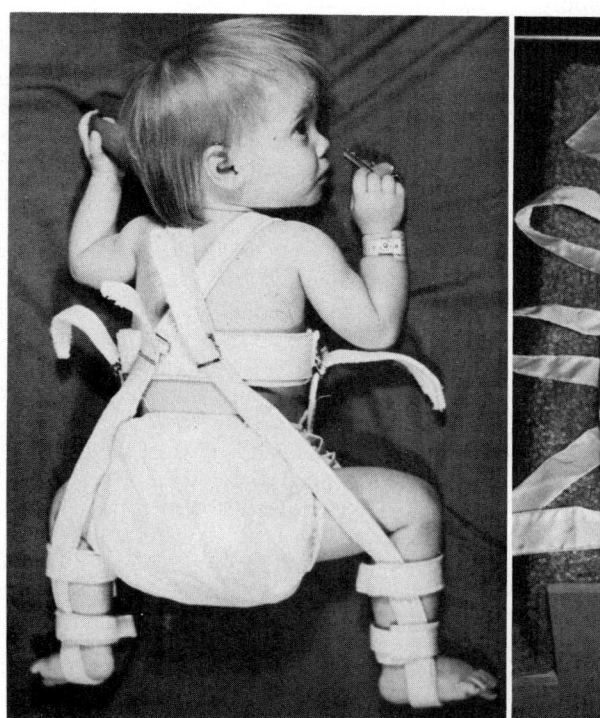
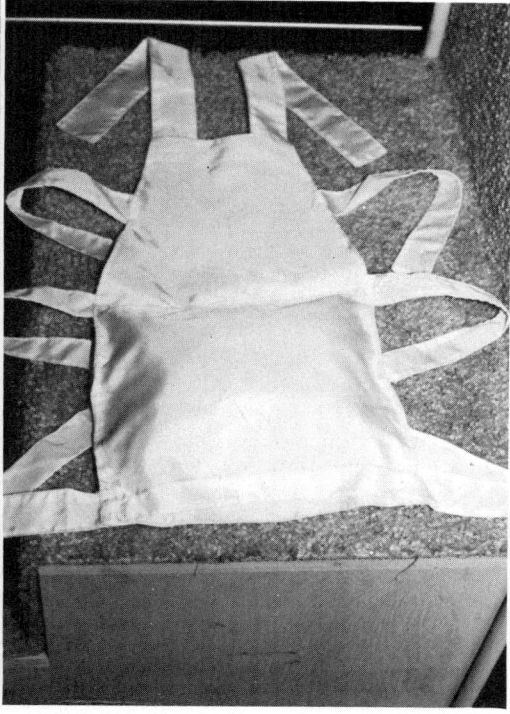

FIGURE 45-18

Nonrigid Frejka apron, an abduction device used to correct a dislocated hip. (Coleman S: Congenital Dysplasia and Dislocation of the Hip. St Louis, CV Mosby, 1978)

leaving only a small scar after a few days. Surgery is required if bones are present in the extra digits. Surgery should wait until the function of each of the duplicated digits is certain.

References

1. NAACOG OGN Nursing Practice Resource: Grief Related to Perinatal Death, 13:2–3, June 1985
2. Grant P: Psychosocial needs of families of high-risk infants. Fam Community Health 1(3):91–102, November 1978
3. Waechter EA: Bonding problems of infants with congenital anomalies. Nurs Forum 16(3 and 4):298–318, 1977
4. Waechter EA, Phillips J, Holaday B: Nursing Care of Children, pp 823–829. Philadelphia, JB Lippincott, 1985
5. Whaley LF, Wong DL: Nursing Care of Infants and Children, pp 383, 1283–1286. St Louis, CV Mosby, 1983
6. Olds SB, London ML, Ladewig PA: Maternal-Newborn Nursing, p 893. Menlo Park, CA, Addison-Wesley, 1984
7. Lees MH, Sunderland CO: The cardiovascular system. In Fanaroff AB, Martin RJ (eds): Behrman's Neonatal-Perinatal Medicine, pp 539–542. St Louis, CV Mosby, 1983
8. Kurcynski TW: Congenital malformations. In Fanaroff AB, Martin RJ (eds): Behrman's Neonatal-Perinatal Medicine, p 1035. St Louis, CV Mosby, 1983
9. Danish RK: Metabolic and endocrine disorders. In Fanaroff AB, Martin RJ (eds): Behrman's Neonatal-Perinatal Medicine, pp 923–926. St Louis, CV Mosby, 1983
10. Brann AW, Schwartz J: Central nervous system disorders. In Fanaroff AB, Martin RJ (eds): Behrman's Neonatal-Perinatal Medicine, pp 380–386. St Louis, CV Mosby, 1983
11. Sunshine P, Sinatra F, Mitchell CH et al: The gastrointestinal system. In Fanaroff AB, Martin RJ (eds): Behrman's Neonatal-Perinatal Medicine, pp 483–530. St Louis, CV Mosby, 1983
12. Randolph JG, Altman RP, Anderson KD: Surgery of the neonate. In Avery GB (ed): Neonatology: Pathophysiology and Management of the Newborn, pp 790–831. Philadelphia, JB Lippincott, 1981
13. Babson SG, Pernoll ML, Benda GI: Diagnosis and Management of the Fetus and Neonate at Risk, pp 284–285. St Louis, CV Mosby, 1980
14. Polin RA, Mennuti MT: Genetic disease and chromosomal abnormalities. In Fanaroff AB, Martin RJ (eds): Behrman's Neonatal-Perinatal Medicine, p 1019. St Louis, CV Mosby, 1983
15. Wyatt DS: Phenylketonuria: The problems vary during different developmental stages. MCN 3(5):296, 1978
16. Nicholson JF: Inborn errors of metabolism. In Fanaroff AB, Martin RJ (eds): Behrman's Neonatal-Perinatal Medicine, pp 831–892. St Louis, CV Mosby, 1983
17. Morishima A: Metabolic and endocrine disorders. In Fanaroff AB, Martin RJ (eds): Behrman's Neonatal-Perinatal Medicine, p 820. St Louis, CV Mosby, 1983
18. Dick HM: Orthopedic disorders. In Fanaroff AB, Martin RJ (eds): Behrman's Neonatal-Perinatal Medicine, pp 1011, 1012. St Louis, CV Mosby, 1983
19. Griffin PP: Orthopedics in the newborn. In Avery GB (ed): Neonatology: Pathophysiology and Management of the Newborn, pp 890–909. Philadelphia, JB Lippincott, 1981

Suggested Reading

Avery GB (ed): Neonatology. Philadelphia, JB Lippincott, 1985

Berman W Jr: Management of congestive heart failure in the neonate. Perinatology and Neonatology 8(4):16–17, 20, 22, July–August 1984

Berry HK: Screening newborns for genetic disease: The PKU model. Diagn Med 7(1):50–59, January 1984

Cassani VL: Tracheoesophageal anomalies. Neonatal Network 3(2):20–27, October 1984

Colten JM: A comprehensive nursing approach to the neonate with myelomeningocele. Neonatal Network 2(4): 7–16, February 1984

Grosfeld JL et al: Congenital abdominal wall defects: Current management and survival. Surg Clin North Am 61(5):1037, 1981

Harrell-Bean HA et al: Neonatal ostomies. JOGN 12(3):695–735, May–June 1983

Hazinski MF: Congenital heart disease in the neonate: Acyanotic defects producing an increase in pulmonary blood flow. Neonatal Network 2(5):12–25, April 1984

Hazinski MF: Congenital heart disease in the neonate: Common congenital heart defects producing hypoxemia and cyanosis. Neonatal Network 2(6):36–51, June 1984

Hazinski MF: Congenital heart disease in the neonate. Neonatal Network 3(2):7–19, October 1984

Hazinski MF: Congenital heart disease in the neonate: Admission of the neonate with heart disease. Neonatal Network 2(3):7–19, December 1983

Johnson DL: Postop low caloric output in infancy. Heart Lung 12(6):603–611, November 1983

Klaus MH, Fanaroff AA: Care of the High Risk Neonate. Philadelphia, WB Saunders, 1983

Korones SB: High-Risk Newborn Infant. St Louis, CV Mosby, 1983

Smith EJ: Galactosemia: An inborn error of metabolism. Nurse Pract 5(2):8, March/April 1980

Waechter EA et al: Nursing Care of Children. Philadelphia, JB Lippincott, 1985

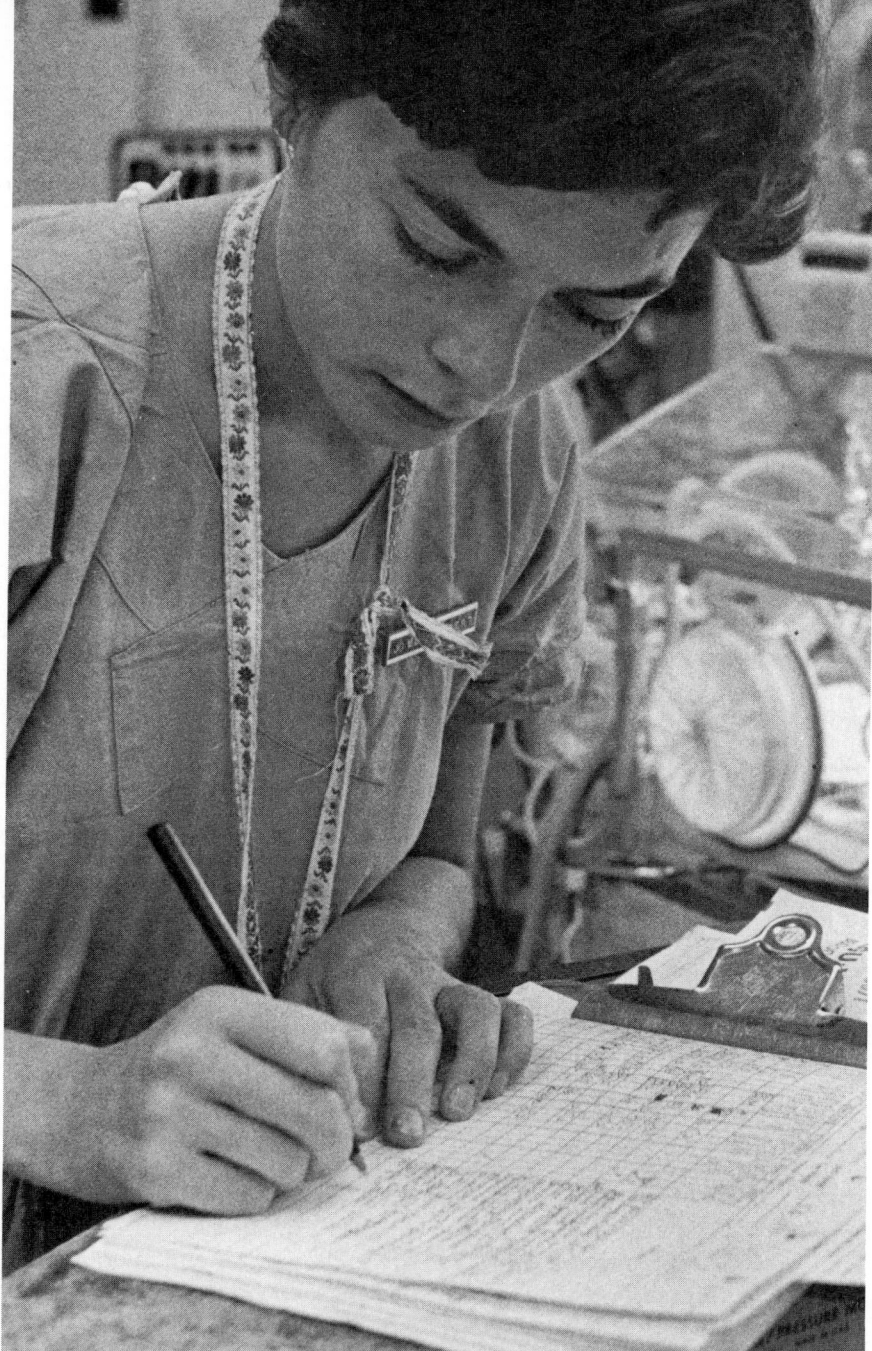

CHAPTER 46

The High-Risk Infant: Acquired Disorders

Certain factors have an impact upon the neonate's transition to extrauterine life. These include maternal disorders, birth trauma, and postnatal infections and physiological processes as affected by the newborn's environmental systems. Most neonates make the transition to extrauterine life smoothly. For those neonates that do not, the professional's skills in the delivery room and the nursery are important to their future development.

Infants with acquired disorders may be only mildly affected, or they may be confined to intensive care for months. Parents of these infants need teaching from nurses to be able to cope with any unexpected illness of the infant. Parents also need assistance in dealing with guilt associated with this traumatic experience.

Birth Trauma

Assessment

Immediate observation of the newborn in the delivery room usually permits the nurse to identify injuries or anoxia resulting from the birth process. A thorough neonatal assessment (discussed in Chap. 32), alertness to subtle changes in the newborn's behavior and condition, and careful recording of observations are important in the ongoing care.

Nursing Diagnosis

Nursing diagnoses will help to determine intervention in physical problems of the neonate and psychological problems concerning the family. Diagnoses for the newborn may include such items as alteration in comfort, pain related to the specific injury; impairment of skin integrity related to immobility (in casting of fractures); potential for injury, shock related to intracranial hemorrhage.

Knowledge deficit related to the type of disorder, its prognosis, and home care may be an important diagnosis concerning the family.

Planning/Intervention

Some kinds of birth trauma require emergency intervention to save the infant's life; others can be treated later or resolve spontaneously in several days. Facility with emergency techniques enables the nurse to promote the well-being of the high-risk infant with an acquired disorder.

After managing the emergency situation, the major responsibility of the nurse is to minimize the pain. Medication usually is not given to the newborn, and the nurse must use judgment in using procedures that will alleviate pain or lessen it as much as possible. Gentle handling of the infant is important. Positioning will also aid in pain relief. The newborn's vital functions must be supported.

In some cases immobilization of a fracture will be necessary, and the nurse must take steps to avoid skin breakdown. Observations and management used in general cast care are adapted to the newborn.

Communicating with parents by providing information and support is a major nursing responsibility (see Chap. 44). The nurse should not hide the facts but share with the parents the description of the condition and possible outcomes. They should be shown how to handle the baby and given time for touching and stroking if the newborn's movements must be kept to a minimum. Training in home care will give the family confidence in its ability to care for the newborn when he is released. Follow-up appointments should be made and a telephone number provided that the parents may call for additional help.

Specific interventions are included with each condition.

Evaluation

As mentioned earlier, some injuries will resolve spontaneously. Other newborns may be moved to a neonatal intensive care unit, and still others will go home with their parents. Evaluations will differ in each case. Major concerns will be that the newborn has little pain or is pain free; that the newborn has stable vital signs; and that the parents are knowledgeable about their newborn's condition and confident about their ability to care for the infant at home.

Head Trauma

Caput Succedaneum

Soft edematous swelling of the scalp frequently occurs over a portion of the presenting part. Pressure from the uterus or birth canal can precipitate the accumulation of serum or blood above the periosteum. Swelling may cross suture lines. No treatment is indicated. A caput succedaneum usually resolves spontaneously in a few days (Fig. 46-1).[1]

Cephalhematoma

Cephalhematoma is not as common as caput succedaneum. The incidence is 0.4% to 2.5% of all live births. It is due to a collection of blood between the bone and periosteum. The suture lines are not crossed by this hematoma. Usually it is unilateral, but it may be bilateral. Cephalhematoma occurs during labor and delivery owing to the rupture of blood vessels crossing the skull to the periosteum. It may be precipitated by prolonged labor or the use of forceps. Since the bleeding is a slow process, it may take hours or days for the swelling to be obvious. The swelling may be obvious by the second or third day. Most cephalhematomas resolve in 2 weeks to 3 months, with the majority resolving by 6 weeks of life (Figs. 46-2 and 46-3).[1] Rare complications accompanying cephalhematoma are skull fracture and intracranial hemorrhage.

The nurse's role in caring for infants with caput succedaneum and cephalhematoma is the reassurance of parents that both conditions will resolve without treatment.

Intracranial Hemorrhage

The following categories of intracranial hemorrhage in the newborn can be associated with birth trauma.

Subarachnoid Hemorrhage. Subarachnoid hemorrhage may be discovered only by bloody spinal fluid, may be asymptomatic, and may be of no clinical significance. Seizures may develop later when the infant had initially appeared normal.

Subdural Hemorrhage. Subdural hemorrhage is rare today. The history is usually that of a primipara with precipitate labor or difficult delivery of a large-for-

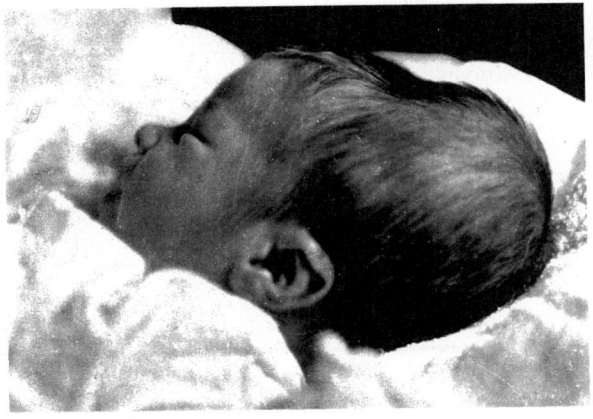

FIGURE 46-1

Caput succedaneum. (MacDonald House, University Hospitals of Cleveland)

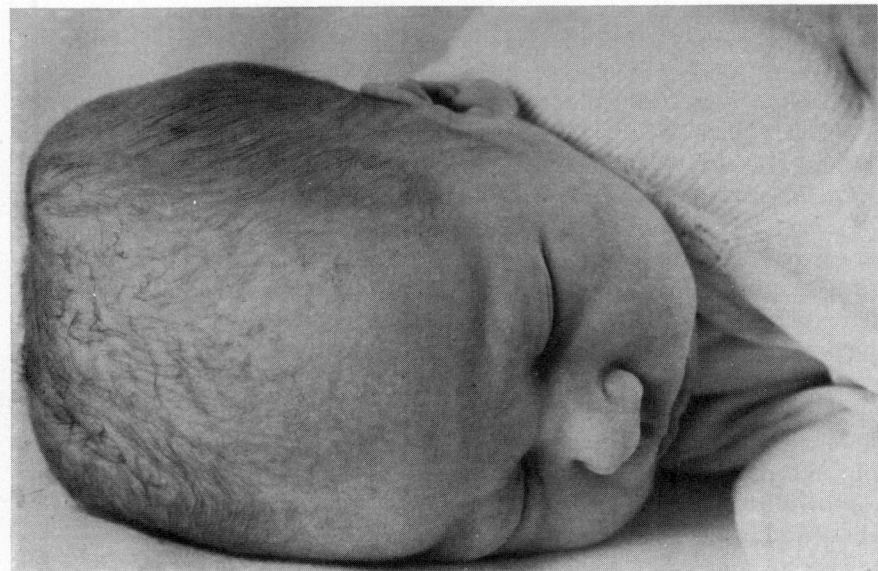

FIGURE 46-2

Cephalhematoma. (Courtesy of Mead Johnson Laboratories)

gestational-age infant. The infant may exhibit signs of increasing intracranial pressure: increasing head circumference, poor feeding or vomiting, and occasional seizures. Management consists of observation of reabsorption of fluid and occasional subdural taps.[2]

Perinatal Hemorrhage and Shock

Blood loss from hemorrhage can occur at any time in the perinatal period: prenatal, intranatal, or neonatal. If there are significant amounts of blood loss, the end result may be shock. Anemia occurring early in neonatal life may also be due to some form of perinatal hemorrhage.

Perinatal Influences

Fetomaternal transfusion is common but not usually severe enough to cause anemia in the newborn. Fetal-to-fetal transfusion occurs only in identical twins. Sig-

nificant anemia occurs in only 15% of the cases. Major blood loss can occur from various obstetric problems (Table 46-1).

Management of shock due to blood loss requires resuscitative measures as well as instillation of volume expanders, blood, and fluids. Milder anemias may require only transfusions and iron replacements.

Nursing staff must be knowledgeable concerning the infant's history to be prepared for early transfusions. Observation for signs of hemorrhage and shock must be frequent and accurate (Table 46-2).

The sites at which laboratory work is obtained are important to note. Capillary values for hematocrit and hemoglobin are higher than central methods (Table 46-3). As replacement transfusions are administered slowly, over several hours, nurses should observe the neonate for tachycardia and apnea. Transfusion reactions may be exhibited by respiratory distress, increase in temperature, vomiting, hematuria, flushing, tachypnea, cyanosis, pulmonary edema, hypotension, and seizures.[3]

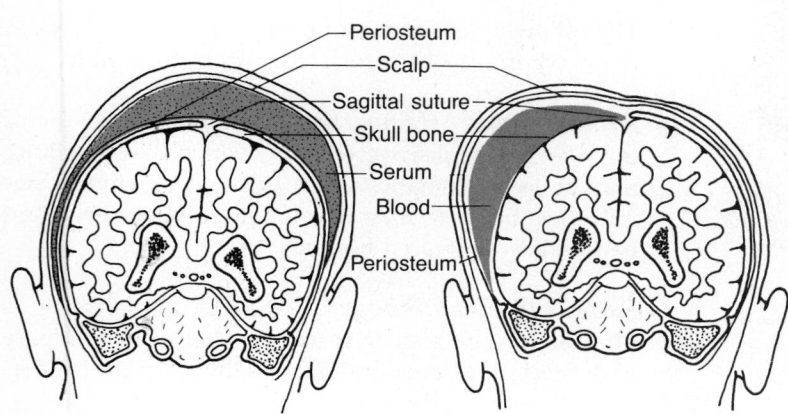

Periosteum
Scalp
Sagittal suture
Skull bone
Serum
Blood
Periosteum

FIGURE 46-3

Comparative diagram of the underlying pathophysiology in caput succedaneum *(Left)* and cephalhematoma *(Right)*.

T A B L E   4 6 - 1

Types of Blood Loss Experienced by the Neonate

Perinatal	Neonatal
Fetomaternal transfusion	Intracranial hemorrhage
Fetal-to-fetal transfusion	Intraventricular hemorrhage
Rupture of umbilical cord	Organ hemorrhages
Rupture of placental vessels	Cephalhematomas
Placenta previa	Iatrogenic loss due to blood
Abruptio placentae	sampling[3]

Nervous System Problems

Facial Paralysis

Facial paralysis due to pressure on cranial nerve VII may occur as a result of a difficult vaginal delivery or pressure of forceps on the facial nerve, which may cause temporary paralysis of the muscles of one side of the face so that the mouth is drawn to the other side. This will be particularly noticeable when the infant cries. Other signs noted are inability to close the eye on the affected side and absence of wrinkling of the forehead.[4] The condition is usually transitory and disappears in a few days, often in a few hours. No medical treatment is necessary. Because the infant can look grotesque, the parents will need an explanation concerning the temporary nature of this affliction (Fig. 46-4).

If the mother is allowed to feed the baby, the nurse should be with her consistently during the first feedings to help her as necessary. Sucking may be difficult for the infant, and the mother needs to develop patience and skill in the feeding of her baby.

If one eye remains open because of the affected muscles, the physician prescribes such treatment as is appropriate. Artificial tears may need to be instilled daily to prevent drying, or a protective eye patch may be used. Any necessary instruction regarding continuing care after discharge should be given the mother before she leaves the hospital.

Very often when disorders occur parents are afraid to handle their infant for fear of hurting him. This may happen even if the condition is short-term and fairly innocuous. Thus, parents should be encouraged to hold and cuddle their infants whenever the condition permits.

Arm Paralysis

Brachial plexus injury is the most common nerve injury of the newborn. Damage to the upper plexus (Erb's palsy) is more common than damage to the lower plexus (Klumpke's palsy).

Erb's palsy usually occurs as a result of pulling or stretching the shoulder away from the head, a result of vertex or breech delivery.

Symptoms are a limp arm with elbow extended, wrist pronated, and arms internally rotated. The grasp reflex is present, but the deep tendon reflex is absent. Moro is lessened or absent on the affected side (Fig. 46-5).

Treatment includes maintaining the correct alignment by proper positioning, intermittent immobilization, and frequent full range of motion exercises to prevent

T A B L E   4 6 - 2

Differential Characteristics of Acute and Chronic Blood Loss in the Newborn

Blood Loss	Clinical Characteristics	Venous Pressure	Hemoglobin	Course	Treatment
Acute	May have acute distress with pallor and shallow, rapid, and often irregular respirations; increased heart rate; weak or absent peripheral pulses; low or absent blood pressure; hepatosplenomegaly is not present	Low	Usually is normal initially, then quickly drops during the next 24 hours of postnatal age.	Must treat the anemia and shock promptly to prevent death.	IV fluid therapy and transfusion of whole blood. May need iron therapy later.
Chronic	May have marked pallor with evidence of distress. Occasionally signs of congestive heart failure may be present with hepatosplenomegaly	Normal to increased	Initially low	Usually uneventful	Transfusion of packed red blood cells may be necessary. Iron replacement therapy usually is indicated.

(Baune KW, Lacey L: Common Hematologic Problems of the Immediate Newborn Period. JOGN May/June 1983; Adapted from Oski F, Naiman J: Hematologic Problems in the Newborn, 2nd ed. Philadelphia, WB Saunders, 1972)

TABLE 46-3

Normal Hematologic Values During the First Week of Postnatal Life in the Preterm and Term Infant

Value	Cord Blood	1 Week (PNA)
Preterm (≤1500 g)		
Hemoglobin (grams per deciliter)	13.0–18.5	14.8
Hematocrit (volume percentage)	49.0	45.0
Reticulocytes (percentage of erythrocytes)	10	3
Platelets		150,000–350,000
Term		
Hemoglobin (grams per deciliter)	14–20	17.0
Hematocrit (volume percentage)	53.0	54.0
Reticulocytes (percentage of erythrocytes)	3–7	0–1
Platelets		200,000–400,000

(Baune KW, Lacey L: Common Hematologic Problems of the Immediate Newborn Period. JOGN May/June 1983; Adapted from Oski F, Naiman J: Hematologic Problems in the Newborn, 2nd ed. Philadelphia, WB Saunders, 1972)

contractures. Immobilization may be completed by a splint or pinning the shirt sleeve to the mattress.

Symptoms of lower plexus injury are limited to the forearm and hand. There may be edema and cyanosis of the part. The wrist and hand are limp and the deep tendon reflex is present but the grasp is absent. Treatment is similar to that for Erb's palsy.[1]

Phrenic Nerve Injury

Phrenic nerve injuries occur most often in conjunction with brachial palsy, most often being due to difficult breech delivery. Since the phrenic nerve is the only nerve innervating the diaphragm, paralysis of the diaphragm occurs, usually unilaterally. Symptoms are those of respiratory distress. The infant should be positioned on the affected side and given intravenous fluids and oxygen if necessary. More severe respiratory distress may require mechanical ventilation. Surgical intervention to move the diaphragm down may be necessary if spontaneous recovery does not occur over a period of time. Most infants recover spontaneously over a period of weeks or months with supportive treatment. A potential complication is the occurrence of pneumonia in the atelectatic lung.[1]

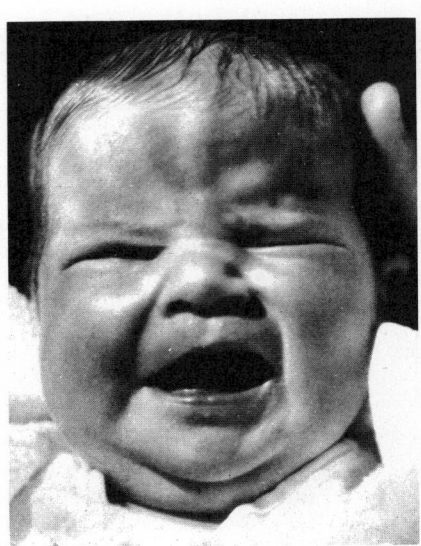

FIGURE 46-4

Facial nerve paralysis. Note the asymmetry of the mouth during crying.

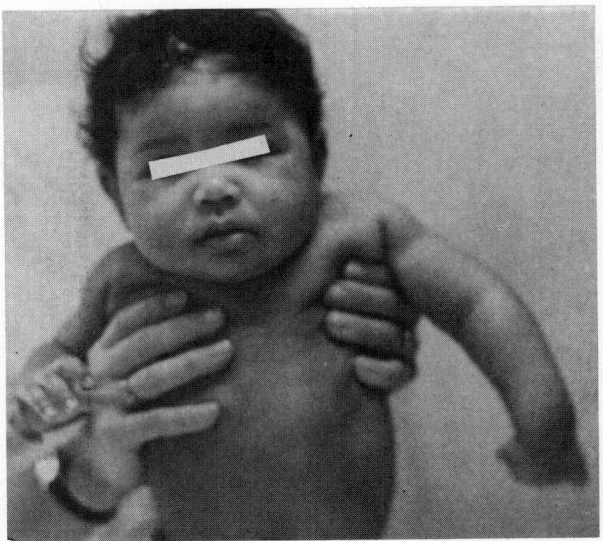

FIGURE 46-5

A 2-month-old baby girl with a left Erb's palsy. (Avery GB: Neonatology: Pathophysiology and Management of the Newborn, 3rd ed. Philadelphia, JB Lippincott, 1987)

Fractures

Clavicle

The clavicle is the bone most commonly fractured during delivery, usually as a result of dystocia (*i.e.*, shoulder delivery in vertex or extended arms in breech). The infant may be asymptomatic. Symptoms that might be observed are decreased or absent mobility of the affected arm, discoloration of the site, crepitus along the clavicle, and absence of the Moro reflex on the affected side. No treatment or interventions are necessary other than gentle handling to minimize pain and proper alignment.[1]

Long Bones

The humerus is the bone most often fractured following the clavicle. Fracture of the femur is the most common fracture of the lower extremities.

Fracture of the humerus occurs with difficult delivery of the arms or shoulders in a vertex delivery. The sign noted is immobility of the affected arm. The Moro reflex is absent on the affected side. The affected arm must be immobilized in the adducted position for 2 to 4 weeks to allow healing to occur. Immobilization may be carried out by splints or a cast.

Fracture of the femur may occur during a breech delivery. Deformity of the thigh, swelling, or immobility may be noted. Treatment is traction, suspension, and casting for about 3 to 4 weeks.[1]

Skull

Due to the flexibility and molding of the infant's head, skull fractures are uncommon. They occur as a result of prolonged, difficult labor or forceps delivery. Fractures may be linear or depressed; the majority are linear. The infant will be asymptomatic with a linear fracture unless blood vessels become involved leading to a subdural hematoma. Depressed fractures may require surgery if brain tissue is involved.[5]

Neonatal Infections

Infectious diseases during pregnancy are discussed in Chapter 37. The following is a continuation of those diseases as found in the neonate. The neonate is particularly vulnerable to infection for two reasons: the protective environment of the uterus is no longer available, and the neonate has not acquired defenses against disease. The fetus may have become infected *in utero*, or the neonate may become infected during passage through the birth canal or when exposed to the environment of the hospital and caregivers (including the mother). Overall incidence for bacterial infections is 1% to 2% of live births, and viral infections account for 6% to 8% of live births.

Assessment

Nurses are the chief observers of the neonate. They are in the presence of the neonate for longer periods of time than other caregivers, are experienced in recognizing signs and symptoms of sepsis, and can be aware of very slight changes in the newborn's condition. The behaviors, signs, and symptoms of sepsis in the neonate are often subtle and are noticed only by experienced caregivers. Clinical signs of sepsis are listed in the chart.

Neonatal nurses have the responsibility to note such behaviors so that diagnosis and treatment may be begun early. Their observations may also prevent an epidemic of infection within the newborn nursery.

Clinical Signs of Sepsis in the Neonate

Central Nervous System

Full fontanel
Lethargy
Jitteriness
Temperature instability
Irritability
Hypotonia
Tremors/seizures

Gastrointestinal

Feeding problems
Vomiting
Diarrhea

Skin

Rashes
Jaundice

Respiratory

Apnea
Cyanosis
Grunting

Laboratory

Positive blood cultures
WBC over 35,000, less than 25,000
Sedimentation rate greater than 5 mm/hr

Neonates at Risk

Maternal factors influencing neonatal sepsis include symptomatic bacteriuria during pregnancy, smoking (indirectly promotes low birth weight), low socioeconomic status, and minority race.

At delivery, mothers with bacterial or viral infections of the urinary tract, vagina, or cervix may infect their infant during the birth process. Rupture of the membranes for longer than a 24-hour period has been associated with increased incidence of neonatal infection. Other factors associated with neonatal infection are bleeding secondary to placenta previa or abruptio placentae, fetal distress, and prolonged second stage.[6] Scalp abscesses have been observed following internal fetal monitoring. Cephalhematomas occasionally lead to complications of osteomyelitis of the skull.

Male infants are more often infected than females. The neonate is more vulnerable to infection than even older children. Antibody levels are low, particularly IgA and IgM, since IgG is the only immunoglobin acquired transplacentally. Decrease in the bacterial capacity, deficient leukocyte response, and deficient phagocytosis have been documented in the neonate. Serum complement components of Cl_Q, C3, and C5 and low levels of serum properdin have been demonstrated. Colostrum has been demonstrated to be effective protection against infection.[6]

Nursing Diagnosis

Nursing diagnoses involving the newborn may include the following: alteration in bowel elimination, diarrhea related to the infection; fluid volume deficit related to vomiting, diarrhea, or feeding problems; alteration in respiratory functions, ineffective airway clearance related to specific infection; and alteration in comfort, pain related to the infection.

The family may be diagnosed for the following: knowledge deficit of care related to specific infection and alteration in family processes related to stress of involvement and care.

Planning/Intervention

An important aspect of infection control is prevention. Prevention of infection is discussed in Chapter 33, Nursing Care of the Normal Newborn. Once an infection is found in a neonate, steps must be taken to prevent further spread. Antibiotics used in infection management are listed in Table 46-4. Further interventions are discussed with each condition and in the nursing-care plan at the end of this section.

Bacterial Infections

Gastroenteritis

Agents most commonly associated with infant diarrhea are *Escherichia coli, Salmonella, Shigella, Yersinia, Campylobacter,* and, rarely, *Pseudomonas, Klebsiella, Enterobacter,* and *Candida albicans.* Classic symptoms are fever, vomiting, abdominal distention, and severe diarrhea.[6]

Management and Prevention. Any infant suspected of harboring an infection should be isolated, following agency procedure. In the case of diarrhea, rectal swabs for culture should be taken from the suspect infant, as well as from others in the nursery. Prior to receiving culture reports, therapy for the primary infant and prophylactic therapy for other infants may be instituted. Medications of choice are *neomycin* or *colistin sulfate.*[7] Other therapy includes fluid and electrolyte maintenance through parenteral or oral routes.

An outbreak of diarrhea in the nursery may necessitate closure of the nursery to any new admissions and a thorough cleaning of the physical environment. All personnel who come in contact with newborns should review infection-control techniques as a preventive measure against future outbreaks.

Infections of the Skin

Skin infections are common and may be due to bacteria, viruses, or fungi. Infections due to *Staphylococcus aureus* are on the increase since the cessation of the practice of bathing all newborns with hexachlorophene. *Staphylococcus aureus* is characterized by abscesses, pustules, or bullous lesions. Diagnosis is made by a smear or culture of the lesions. Skin infections are treated with systemic antibiotics.[6]

Congenital Syphilis

Transmission of syphilis to the fetus occurs by transplacental passage or contact with active genital lesions at birth.[7] The extent of the disease in the newborn depends on the time during gestation that the diagnosis was made, the extent of the disease in the mother, and the success of maternal treatment. If the mother is treated before the 18th gestational week, disease in the fetus is almost always prevented. Langhans' layer of the chorion, which provides a protective barrier, deteriorates between 16 and 18 weeks. Treatment after the 18th week may cure fetal spirochetemia in organ systems, but late changes of congenital syphilis may still occur. All organ systems are involved. The characteristic skin rash, usually appearing at 7 days of age, is copper colored and noted around the mouth, nose, and diaper

TABLE 46-4

Antibacterial Drugs

Drug	Dosage/Route	Nursing Considerations
Ampicillin	0–7 days: 50 mg–100 mg/kg/day divided every 12 hr IV, IM >7 days: 100 mg–200 mg/kg/day divided every 6–8 hr IV, IM	Initial vial dilution is stable for 1 hr only. Check package insert for IV use.
Carbenicillin	0–7 days: 200 mg–300 mg/kg/day divided every 8 hr IV, IM >7 days: 300 mg–400 mg/kg/day divided every 6–8 hr IV, IM	Usually used with another antibiotic such as gentamicin. Chemically incompatible with aminoglycosides. Do not mix in IV. Give 1 hr apart.
Cefazolin	0–7 days: 25 mg–50 mg/kg/day divided every 12 hr >7 days: 25 mg–100 mg/kg/day divided every 8 hr	Use large muscle for IM. Change sites every 3 days. Clinitest may produce false-positive. Clinistix, Tes-Tape not affected.
Gentamicin	0–7 days: 5 mg/kg/day divided every 8–12 hr, IV, IM >7 days: 7.5 mg/kg/day divided every 12 hr IV, IM	Monitor renal function—output, specific gravity, urinalysis, blood urea nitrogen, and creatinine.
Kanamycin	0–7 days: 15 mg–20 mg/kg/day divided every 12 hr >7 days: 20 mg–30 mg/kg/day divided every 8 hr	Antagonist to parenteral penicillins: do not mix together in IV. Monitor renal function.
Methicillin	0–7 days: 50 mg–100 mg/kg/day divided every 12 hr IV, IM >7 days: 100 mg–200 mg/kg/day divided every 6–8 hr IV, IM	Mix with normal saline for IV use. Anemia may develop with long-term use.
Nafcillin	0–7 days: 50 mg–100 mg/kg/day divided every 12 hr IV >7 days: 100 mg–200 mg/kg/day divided every 6–8 hr IV	Mix with dextrose 5% in water or normal saline for IV use.
Penicillin G	0–7 days: 100,000–150,000 units/kg/day divided every 12 hr IV, IM 0–7 days: 50,000–100,000 units/kg/day divided every 12 hr IV, IM >7 days: 150,000–400,000 units/kg/day divided every 6–8 hr IV, IM >7 days: 75,000–100,000 units/kg/day divided every 8 hr IV, IM	Meningitis dose Other Indications Meningitis dose Other indications
Tobramycin	0–7 days: 5 mg/kg/day divided every 12 hr IV, IM >7 days: 7.5 mg/kg/day divided every 8 hr IV, IM	Tobramycin is less nephrotoxic than gentamicin. Continue to monitor renal function.

area and on palms and soles. The rash may extend to the trunk and extremities. There may be poor feeding, fever, and a characteristic syphilitic rhinitis or serosanguineous drainage from the nose. Condylomata in the perianal area may develop, which are raised hairs resembling warts. Lips are cracked and tough and may exhibit rhagades (radiating scars). Loss of hair and nails

may occur. Other complications are hepatitis, lymphadenopathy, pneumonia, anemia, and hepatosplenomegaly. X-ray films of bone may show skeletal lesions in a majority of infants by 3 months.

Diagnosis is most commonly suggested by the signs, symptoms, and radiographic findings and is confirmed by serum antibody testing.

Symptomatic congenital syphilis should be treated with penicillin in two intramuscular or daily intravenous doses for 10 days.

Late congenital syphilis may still appear with more complications of interstitial keratitis, deafness, bone, joint, and skin involvement.[6]

Ophthalmitis

Chemical conjunctivitis usually is observed soon after birth, lessening considerably after 2 days of age. Bacterial conjunctivitis is usually noted during the first week of life. Organisms most likely responsible are *Neisseria gonorrhoeae* and *Chlamydia trachomatis*. Purulent discharge of the eyes and redness and edema of the lids are noted. With *Neisseria gonorrhoeae*, corneal involvement may occur as lesions develop and progress to corneal perforations. With *Chlamydia* there may be little or great inflammation, swelling, and a yellow discharge. The cornea is rarely affected with *Chlamydia*.

Treatment of gonococcal infection is parenteral administration of aqueous penicillin G and irrigation of the conjunctival sacs. Inclusion conjunctivitis should be treated with 10% sulfacetamide ophthalmic drops or ointment or 1% tetracycline ointment.[6]

Prevention includes the instillation of 1% solution of silver nitrate, erythromycin, or tetracycline ointments. Silver nitrate is not effective against *Chlamydia*.

Thrush

Thrush is an infection of the mouth caused by the organism *Candida albicans*, the organism that causes monilial vaginitis in the mother. The infant may acquire the infection as it passes through the birth canal of a mother so infected. However, the infection may be transferred from infant to infant on the hands of attendants and is favored by lack of cleanliness in feeding, in the care of the mother's nipples, or in the care of the bottles and the nipples. It is most likely to occur in weak, undernourished babies and in those receiving antibiotic therapy, because the use of certain antibiotics alters the oral flora, making it more susceptible to this opportunistic organism.

The condition appears as small white patches (due to the fungus growth) on the tongue and in the mouth. These white patches may be mistaken at first for small curds of milk. The infant's mouth must be kept clean, but great gentleness is required to avoid further injury to the delicate epithelium. Any attempt to wipe away the plaques usually causes bleeding.

Management. Nystatin (Mycostatin) is the drug of choice in treating oral monilial infections. It is applied directly to the mucosa with a cotton-tipped applicator or is given as an oral instillation (100,000 units/ml), 1

ml four times a day at intervals of 6 hours. The solution is slowly and gently instilled so that there is an opportunity for it to be widely distributed throughout the oral cavity before it is swallowed. It is important to keep equipment used for this baby, such as linen, clothing, diapers, and feeding equipment, especially clean. Breastfeeding mothers may be instructed to treat their nipples with topical nystatin.

Pneumonia

Pneumonia is a significant factor in 10% of neonatal deaths. Three types of pneumonia exist, depending on the time of presentation and the route of acquisition.

Transplacental pneumonitis is a congenital infection acquired *in utero*. Symptoms are manifest early and may be connected with infections such as cytomegalovirus, herpes, rubella, toxoplasmosis, and *Listeria monocytogenes*.

Aspiration pneumonia, acquired as part of the birth process, is manifest in the first few days of life. Organisms most often involved are group B β-hemolytic streptococci, group D streptococci, pneumococci, and coliform organisms.

Acquired pneumonia at delivery or in the postpartum period is the third type. *Staphylococcus aureus* and coliform organisms are commonly implicated in postnatally acquired pneumonia. Symptoms of respiratory distress may vary, but include nasal flaring, tachypnea, retractions, diminished breath sounds, and rales.

Diagnosis is based on blood cultures and chest roentgenogram.

Treatment consists of appropriate antibiotic therapy, oxygen, and supportive measures. Many newborns with aspiration pneumonia do not require antibiotic therapy.[8]

Group B Streptococci

Group B streptococci are now the leading cause of early neonatal sepsis. Previously, coliform organisms retained this distinction. Five types of group B streptococci have been isolated. Sites of culture of the organisms are the throat, stools, and genital tract.[9] The maternal carrier rate is about 30%, remaining relatively the same regardless of trimester. Incidence is about 1 to 3 in 1000 live births, with a mortality rate of 40% to 75%.

Two separate clinical syndromes have been identified. Early onset has a higher mortality than late onset. Early-onset disease usually is manifest within 3 to 5 days of life and most often within 12 to 24 hours. Early-onset symptoms closely resemble those of respiratory distress syndrome (RDS).[9,10] It produces a fulminant pneumonia with a very high mortality (greater than 40%). The organism is sexually transmitted and is carried asymptomatically in the cervix and vagina in a significant number (over 20%) of pregnant women. The infection is thought to be contracted by contact during the birth process and is especially likely to occur when predisposing factors such as prematurity, prolonged labor, and premature rupture of the membranes exist. The rate of newborn colonization is high; however, the attack (infection) rate is low (1%–2% of colonized babies become infected). Screening of all gravidas and treatment of carriers had been recommended, but the practicality of the approach is open to serious question.

The late-onset syndrome, occurring between 10 and 50 days of age, presents as nonspecific signs of irritability, lethargy, apnea, failure to nurse, and fever. Meningitis often is the consequence of late-onset disease. The source is not necessarily the cervix or vagina or even the mother. Mortality in late-onset infection is considerably less.

Diagnosis is presumed based on isolation of the organism from the neonate's gastric contents and confirmed by positive blood or cerebrospinal fluid cultures. Treatment is supportive in addition to appropriate therapy following laboratory studies.[10] Penicillin or ampicillin is the drug of choice.[11]

Chlamydia

Chlamydia trachomatis is a parasite primarily inhabiting the genital tract and commonly transmitted during sexual activity. It is transmitted to the neonate during birth. Pneumonia may develop in approximately 40% of infants who develop chlamydial conjunctivitis. This conjunctivitis begins 5 to 12 days after birth. Incidence of pneumonia due to *Chlamydia* is 3 to 8 per 1000 live births. Infants are treated with erythromycin as the drug of choice. Silver nitrate is not effective against *Chlamydia*.[11]

Listeria monocytogenes

Listeria monocytogenes is a gram-positive bacillus, sexually transmitted, which may infect the fetus *in utero* or the neonate. Like group B streptococci, *Listeria* has both an early-onset and a late-onset component. The early-onset component is manifest at birth with symptoms of respiratory distress, cyanosis, and hypothermia. If the infant is not treated at this point, meningitis and death may ensue. A late form of the disease may be manifest at 1 to 6 weeks of life owing to postnatal acquisition. Mortality rate is high for *Listeria*.[11] Treatment of choice is ampicillin.[6]

TORCH Viruses

There are over a dozen viral infections that the newborn may contract during the prenatal, intrapartum, and postpartum periods. They are categorized in the acronym TORCH.

Toxoplasmosis

Congenital toxoplasmosis results from transplacental transfer of the parasite *Toxoplasma gondii* to the fetus. The neonatal incidence is 0.3 to 6 per 1000 live births. Not all infants born to a mother infected with toxoplasmosis during the pregnancy are affected by this disease. Most infants are without symptoms at birth (60%–75%).

Classic congenital defects are chorioretinitis, microcephaly, hydrocephalus, and cerebral calcifications.[12] Other indications of the disease include prematurity, intrauterine growth retardation, seizure disorders, and hepatosplenomegaly.

Laboratory diagnosis isolates anti-*Toxoplasma* IgM fluorescent antibodies in cord or neonatal blood. Drugs of choice are pyrimethamine (1 mg/kg/day orally) and sulfadiazine (25 mg/kg/day). Both drugs should be administered over a 21- to 30-day period. Folinic acid, 2 mg to 6 mg, should also be given three times a week to prevent anemia. These drugs may not reverse neurologic damage already incurred, but may prevent further adverse effects.[13]

Other

Hepatitis B Virus. The incidence of hepatitis B virus (HBV) infecting the newborn is 0 to 7 per 1000 live births. Routes of transmission are varied. Most infants are affected primarily during the last trimester of gestation, or at the time of delivery from contaminated secretions in the birth canal.[14] Other potential routes in the postpartum period are contact with infected maternal saliva, urine, feces, serum, or breast milk.

Acquisition of the virus *in utero* may lead to low birth weight of the newborn. A small number of infants infected with HBV around the time of delivery may present with acute hepatitis accompanied by liver changes. Most remain asymptomatic. HBV may be cultured from amniotic fluid as a diagnostic measure. The presence of IgM may be noted in cord blood or neonatal serum. It is recommended that hepatitis B immune globulin (HBIG) be given to infants of infected mothers.[13]

Rubella

The incidence of congenital rubella has been noted as 0.5 to 0.7 per 1000 or 3 to 5 per 1000 during epidemics.[13] Although rubella is generally considered to be a relatively mild illness, for the fetus whose mother has been exposed with subsequent transplacental transmission, the consequences may be disastrous. Damage to the fetus may occur without obvious illness in the mother. Consequences in the fetus depend upon the virulence of the virus and the gestational age of the fetus. The fetus is at a critical developmental stage during the first 4 weeks of pregnancy, when there is a 50% chance of a resulting anomaly. From the fifth to eighth week chances decrease to 25%. From the 9th to 12th week an 8% to 17% chance exists. There is a low percentage of 10% resulting in defects when maternal rubella occurs between 13 and 24 weeks.[15]

Major defects identified with infection occurring up to 4 weeks prior to pregnancy or during the first trimester are cardiac defects, cataracts, and deafness. There is a higher rate of spontaneous abortions and stillbirths.[16] Some additional problems of infants infected in the first trimester are intrauterine growth retardation, glaucoma, hepatosplenomegaly, hepatitis, lesions in long bones, meningitis, and pneumonia.[10] Psychomotor retardation, microcephaly, and deafness result from second-trimester infection. Infection during the last trimester of pregnancy may also result in problems.[10] Approximately two thirds of neonates are asymptomatic.[13]

In addition, the effects of the disease may be evident later, usually by age 5. Some may even exhibit neurologic deficits after age 10.

Diagnosis is established by hemagglutination inhibition (HI) or complement fixation (CF) antibodies in blood or rubella-specific IgM from cord or neonatal serum. Finally, rubella virus can be cultured from amniotic fluid, the placenta, and the neonate's throat, urine, or spinal fluid.

Treatment of the neonate consists in supportive management, surgical correction of defects as feasible, and multidisciplinary referral.

Cytomegalovirus

Cytomegalovirus (CMV) is the most common of perinatal infections. In addition to transplacental transmission, contact with contaminated vaginal or nasopharyngeal secretions, urine, or feces can transmit the virus. Finally, less frequently viral transmission occurs from blood transfusion or breast milk. CMV has been noted in preterm infants receiving multiple transfusions. The incidence of congenital occurrence in the neonate is 6 to 34 per 1000 live births. The rate of perinatal infection has been estimated at 20 per 1000 live births. As with other congenital viruses, many neonates are asymptomatic. Congenital defects include bone lesions, anemia, low birth weight, hepatomegaly, splenomegaly, jaundice, petechiae, heart disease, pneumonia, cataracts, chorioretinitis, microcephaly, obstructive hydrocephaly, intracranial calcifications, and encephalitis.[12] The most common findings are hepatosplenomegaly and jaundice.[13]

Diagnostic tools are positive viral cultures of amniotic fluid or neonatal serum, anti-CMV IgM antibodies in cord or neonatal serum, or the presence of CMV inclusion cells in urine or cerebrospinal fluid.

Treatment is supportive. Long-term follow-up is essential to monitor growth and development. Immunization to prevent infection is in the experimental stages. Drug therapy with antimetabolites and antiviral agents is also experimental.

Herpes Simplex Virus (HSV)

Most neonates are affected by herpes simplex, type 2, the genital version. Other neonates are infected by type 1, the oral virus. Herpes is the most common virus in pregnant women following CMV.

The majority of neonates come in contact with the virus at delivery when the infant passes through the infected maternal birth canal. However, the virus also can ascend during pregnancy or following rupture of the membranes. Some cases of transplacental infection have been reported. Finally, sites other than the genital area in the mother and other nonmaternal sources have been demonstrated.[13]

The incidence in the neonate is 0.03 to 0.05 per 1000 live births. The greatest risk to the neonate at delivery occurs when the mother has had a primary herpetic lesion during the last 3 weeks of pregnancy. Thirty to 50% of neonates delivered through the infected birth canal are affected. Cesarean delivery should be performed when active lesions or positive herpes cultures are noted during the previous 2 weeks and when the membranes have been ruptured less than 6 hours or are intact. There has been demonstrated a significant decrease in neonatal infection if cesarean delivery is performed within 4 hours of membrane rupture.[12]

The incubation period for neonatal herpes is *usually* 6 to 11 days from birth to onset of disease. Some infants may be asymptomatic. Lesions may be seen in the eyes, throat, mouth, and skin. Disseminated disease is indicated by jaundice, purpura, respiratory distress, shock, and central nervous system involvement. Diagnosis is established by viral cultures of eyes, nose, throat, blood, urine, or cerebrospinal fluid. In addition, identification of herpes-specific IgM antibodies in cord or neonatal serum can be made. The use of systemic antimetabolites (vidarabine or 5-iodo-2-deoxyuridine), γ-globulins, and interferon stimulants (poly IC) has been documented as potential treatment.[12] The success or failure of these various drugs is unclear at this point.

Acquired Immune Deficiency Syndrome (AIDS).

Various types of immunodeficiencies and infections have been noted in infants born to women at risk for AIDS. Some infants may have been the recipients of contaminated blood transfusions or blood products.

Nursing Care: Prevention

Primarily, nursing management of infants suspected of harboring viruses is focused on prevention of infection in other infants and health-care providers in the im-

Neonates with Infections (Prevention and Management)

Nursing Objectives

1. Identify infants infected *in utero* or at delivery.
2. Begin early treatment for infected infants.
3. Identify infants at risk for infection.
4. Institute preventive measures in the newborn nursery.

Assessment	Potential Nursing Diagnosis	Planning/Intervention	Evaluation
Maternal Factors Smoking Low socioeconomic status Bacterial or viral infections of the urinary tract, vagina, or cervix Rupture of membranes more than 24 hours Amnionitis Maternal bleeding **Neonatal Factors** Male sex Preterm Invasive procedures (surgery, diagnostic) Certain congenital malformations (*i.e.*, meningomyelocele, gastroschisis)	Potential infection related to immature immune system, environmental factors, maternal exposure or actual infectious disease process, sharing of nursery Alteration in bowel elimination, diarrhea related to infection Fluid volume deficit related to vomiting, diarrhea, or feeding problems Alteration in respiratory functions, inefficient airway clearance related to specific infection	Continue to observe newborn for signs and symptoms: Skin: rashes, lesions, jaundice CNS: hypotonia, temperature instability, irritability, lethargy, full or bulging fontanel Respiratory: tachypnea, apnea, cyanosis, grunting, retractions, nasal flaring Gastrointestinal: vomiting/diarrhea, feeding problems Circulatory: hypotension; cool skin, mottling Provide assistance in performing diagnostic tests Obtain various lab specimens as orderd Frequently monitor vital signs and intake and output Pay careful attention to environmental temperature Administer antibiotics as ordered Use infection protocol as per agency procedure—strict hand washing and any required isolation	Newborn passes normal bowel movements Newborn is free from vomiting Newborn voids properly Newborn takes adequate feedings Newborn breathes normally without assistance Newborn's vital signs are stabilized Newborn is comfortable Other newborns in the nursery remain symptom free

mediate environment. All of the TORCH viruses except toxoplasmosis can be spread easily by direct contact. Isolation procedures should be followed scrupulously. Infants may be isolated with their mothers in a private room. The nurse or primary caregiver should use gowns and gloves for direct contact, disposing carefully of contaminated linen and disposable items. Good handwashing techniques must be used.

The Centers for Disease Control recommends strict isolation for congenital rubella or disseminated neonatal herpes, respiratory isolation for rubella, secretion precautions for herpes, and enteric, blood, and secretion precautions for hepatitis.[12]

Pregnant women with inadequate antibody titers should not care for infected mothers or babies. Staff members with herpetic lesions on exposed body areas should not be assigned to care for neonates.

Caring for parents includes disseminating information on each disease entity, including its mode of transmission, and preventing further spread of illness.

For example, HBV and CMV may be transmitted through breast milk. CMV is often found in the infant's urine for a number of years, so parents should take appropriate precautions. The nursing staff needs to support those mothers who express guilt feelings in regard to their affected infants.

Infant of a Diabetic Mother

The successful control of diabetes with insulin has led to survival and fertility of an increasing number of women. Better control of the diabetic state during pregnancy has increased the infant's chances for a healthy state at birth. However, the infant of a diabetic mother (IDM) still presents with a number of clinical problems that are best dealt with in the intensive care nursery setting.

IDMs may be large for gestational age, but most are appropriate for gestational age. Typically the infant has a round face, soft skin, an abundance of subcutaneous fat tissue (Fig. 46-6), and a plethoric appearance.

Clinical Problems and Related Management

Hypoglycemia.   The most common metabolic problem is hypoglycemia. Maternal hyperglycemia is accompanied by fetal hyperglycemia. The fetal pancreas is thus stimulated, leading to hypertrophy of islet cells and hyperplasia of beta cells with subsequent increase in insulin content. Upon delivery, the neonate is no longer dependent on maternal glucose; thus, a hypoglycemic state ensues. Since insulin acts to stimulate fetal organ growth, a hyperinsulin state produces an increase in organ size and macrosomia (large for gestational age). There is an impetus for increased deposition of fat in the third trimester.[12] Potential birth injuries may occur with attempted vaginal delivery of very large neonates. These potential birth injuries include cephalhematoma, subdural hemorrhage, facial palsy, ocular hemorrhage, clavicular fracture, and brachial plexus injury.[17] Hypoglycemia is defined as a blood glucose value below 30 mg/dl in the term infant and below 20 mg/dl in the preterm infant. Blood glucose levels usually drop within the first 30 to 60 minutes of life. Most IDMs are asymptomatic. Signs or symptoms that do occur are lethargy, irritability, coarse tremors, apnea, and convulsions.[17] Treatment is the administration of intravenous glucose, either by high-concentration bolus, 25% to 50% glucose, or by constant infusion, 10% to 15%, calculated according to the weight of the neonate. In lieu of intravenous administration, early feedings may be begun within the first 30 minutes after delivery.

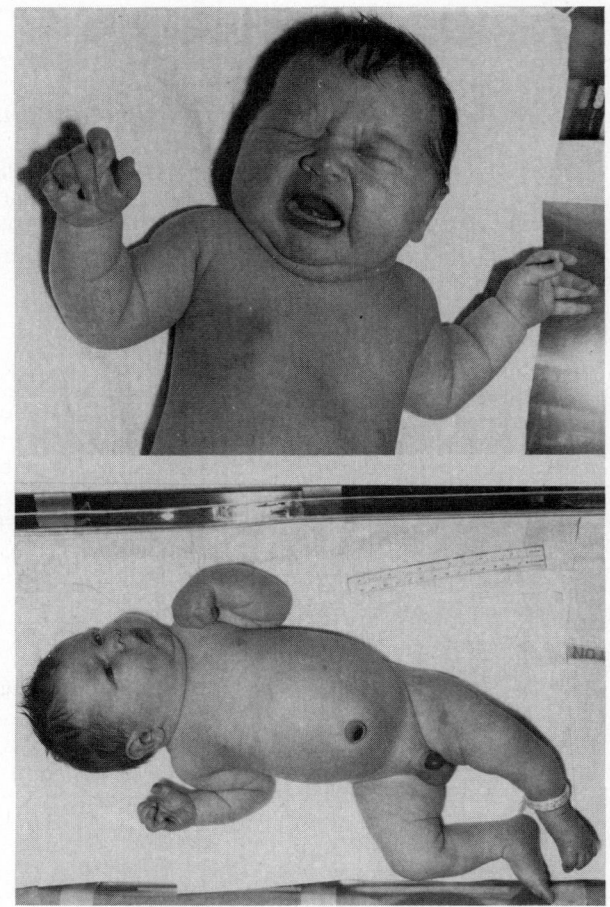

F I G U R E   4 6 - 6

The infant of a diabetic mother showing typical features. (Avery GB: Neonatology: Pathophysiology and Management of the Newborn, 3rd ed. Philadelphia, JB Lippincott, 1987)

Hypocalcemia.   Hypocalcemia is defined as a calcium level below 7 mg/dl and is one of the most common clinical problems for the IDM. About 50% of infants born to insulin-dependent women experience hypocalcemia during the first 3 days of life. During pregnancy there exists a maternal hyperparathyroid state that seeks to increase maternal calcium that has been diverted to the fetus. After delivery, serum calcium falls owing to the levels of parathyroid hormone (PTH), vitamin D, and calcitonin. Subsequently, PTH and vitamin D levels rise to correct this deficiency. Symptoms of hypocalcemia are jitteriness, convulsions, and twitching. Calcium in oral form may be administered with feedings with calcium levels are stabilized.

Hyperbilirubinemia.   The etiology of hyperbilirubinemia in IDMs is not clear, although several theories have been postulated. Of these, polycythemia commonly seen in IDMs emerges as a significant factor as-

Infant of a Diabetic Mother

Nursing Objectives
1. Identify and screen infants of diabetic mothers for common metabolic complications.
2. Initiate early treatment for pertinent problems.

Assessment	Potential Nursing Diagnosis	Planning/Intervention	Evaluation
History Maternal diabetic classification/method of control during pregnancy **Neonatal** Weight Apgar score Gestational age	Potential for birth injury (cephalhematoma, subdural hemorrhage, facial palsy, ocular hemorrhage, clavicular fracture, brachial plexus injury) related to macrosomia Fluid volume deficit related to maternal diabetes	Identify the infant of a diabetic mother from history and neonatal physical characteristics Document characteristics: Plethoric Round face Soft skin Abundance of subcutaneous tissue Observe for metabolic problems *Hypoglycemia* Jitteriness Irritability Apnea Dextrostix less than 45 Continue to monitor frequent Dextrostix Check with blood glucose as needed. Must be above 30 mg/dl in term infant and 20 mg/dl in the preterm Carry out treatment orders if required: Frequent early feedings Intravenous fluids *Hypocalcemia* Tremors, convulsions, twitching Prolonged QT interval Calcium levels below 7 mg/dl Carry out orders for calcium replacement (either intravenous or oral) *Hyperbilirubinemia, RDS* See related care plans	Newborn is free of birth injury Newborn is comfortable despite birth injury Newborn retains skin integrity Newborn voids and has normal bowel movements Newborn achieves fluid and electrolyte balance

sociated with hyperbilirubinemia. Treatment is the same as for jaundice due to other factors.

Respiratory Disease. The IDM appears to develop hyaline membrane disease later than other neonates.[17]

Some also note problems due to transient tachypnea of the newborn. The fetus's hyperinsulinic state may interfere with the ability of the lungs to use phospholipids. There appears to be an increased number of "false-positive" lecithin/sphingomyelin (L/S) ratios among all diabetic classes. RDS has been noted with an L/S ratio of greater than 2.0 in the IDM.[18] Since diligent pregnancy monitoring has become so commonplace, the trend to deliver diabetic patients early is diminishing. Treatment for IDMs with RDS is frequent monitoring of blood gases and accordingly providing respiratory support of oxygen, ventilators, fluids, and appropriate nutrition. See nursing-care plan for detailed nursing information.

Pathologic Jaundice in the Neonate

Hyperbilirubinemia in the neonate may occur due to numerous causes. Physiologic jaundice, evident after 24 hours of age, is a common phenomenon (see Chap. 32).

Pathologic forms of jaundice may be the result of a variety of factors. Hemolytic disease of the newborn (*e.g.*, Rh or ABO incompatibility) is significant but decreasing in severity owing to preventive measures. The administration of anti-D globulin (RhoGAM) to eligible women has been an important intervention combating Rh incompatibility and erythroblastosis fetalis. ABO incompatibility has always been less of a threat to the newborn than the Rh problem. For extensive discussion of the pathophysiology of these entities see Chapter 42.

Other factors that may produce hyperbilirubinemia by the overproduction of unconjugated bilirubin are the following:

- Enclosed hemorrhage (*e.g.*, cephalhematoma)
- Ecchymosis from bruising, as in a breech delivery
- Congenital enzyme deficiency, as in glucose-6-phosphate-dehydrogenase deficiency (G6PD)
- Drug-induced hemolytic anemia, such as that produced by excessive amounts of vitamin K

The following factors delay or alter bilirubin conjugation into the water-soluble form:

- Immaturity of glucuronyl transferase enzyme system
- Asphyxia, hypoglycemia, hypothermia
- Liver cell damage due to sepsis or medications[10]

Finally, hepatitis, biliary duct obstruction, and galactosemia can lead to impaired excretion of bilirubin.

Pathologic forms of jaundice pose a serious threat to the neonate owing to the possibility of the complication of kernicterus. Kernicterus results from the accumulation of unconjugated and unbound bilirubin in brain cells. Neurologic signs occur, and ultimately intellectual function is impaired. The exact bilirubin level at which kernicterus occurs varies with each individual infant, occurring sooner in the preterm infant.

Assessment

Pathologic disease may be suspected if jaundice is evident within the first 24 hours of life and lasts more than 7 days in the term infant or 10 days in the preterm infant or if serum bilirubin increases by greater than 5 mg/dl every 24 hours. Further investigation is also needed if bilirubin levels are greater than 12 mg/dl in the term infant and 15 mg/dl in the preterm infant during the first 48 hours.[19] Finally, infants with erythroblastosis fetalis (severe isoimmunization) present with generalized edema, pallor, hepatosplenomegaly, hydrothorax, and severe anemia.

Diagnostic tests that may be used are direct and total serum bilirubin, blood typing of mother and baby, complete blood count, total serum protein, and direct Coombs' test. The direct Coombs' test is performed on neonatal cord blood, measuring whether neonatal red blood cells are coated with maternal antibodies.

A noninvasive screening tool that may be used to correlate skin color with a total serum bilirubin value is transcutaneous bilirubinometry. A hand-held fiberoptic instrument illuminates the skin and measures the intensity of the yellow color. This method should be accompanied by a total serum bilirubin test and should not be relied upon solely to institute treatment.

Nursing Diagnosis

Potential for injury is high in the list of possible nursing diagnoses. These potential injuries might include kernicterus related to elevated bilirubin levels; dehydration or hyperthermia related to phototherapy; and hyperbilirubinemia, electrolyte imbalances, hypoglycemia, and hypothermia related to exchange transfusion rebound. There may also be an alteration in bowel elimination (diarrhea) related to phototherapy. Alteration in family processes is another potential problem related to the infant's eyes being covered during phototherapy and even the confinement during phototherapy.

Planning/Intervention

In the event of a positive Coombs' test or very low birth weight infant, phototherapy may often be initiated without waiting for bilirubin results. Treatment could involve immediate exchange transfusion, as in the event of a hydropic infant. More often than not, however, the more conservative treatment of phototherapy is used.

Phototherapy

The use of intense fluorescent light to reduce serum bilirubin has gained acceptance in the treatment of hyperbilirubinemia (Fig. 46-7). Blue light decomposes bil-

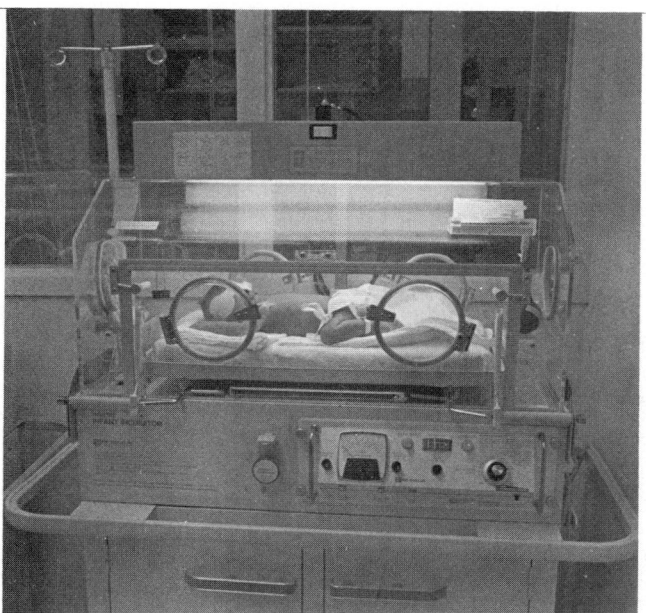

FIGURE 46-7

Phototherapy, using fluorescent lights, is considered conservative treatment for jaundice.

irubin by photo-oxidation, which appears to take place in the skin. The chemical nature of the products formed in the breakdown of bilirubin has not been precisely determined, nor have long-term outcomes been evaluated, as well as the theoretic effects of intense light upon a wide spectrum of biologic processes. For these reasons, there are some reservations about the unqualified use of this treatment for all jaundiced babies.

Phototherapy is applied by exposing the nude infant to fluorescent daylight bulbs that supply 200 to 400 foot-candles on the skin surface. Success is measured by serial bilirubin level.

To avoid retinal damage, the infant's eyes are shielded from the light by means of patches (Fig. 46-8). The nurse should make sure that the lids are closed when the patches are applied. The nurse must check frequently for correct positioning of the eye patches, that the eyes are indeed covered, and that the nares are not occluded. The eye patches are to be removed at least once each shift to inspect the eyes for conjunctivitis and to allow eye contact with parents and visual stimulation.

Some centers cover the genital areas with a face mask as a "bikini diaper," while others do not. Effects of exposure to light, particularly with male genitalia, are unknown. Monitoring of temperature is important because additional heat from the light necessitates adjustments in environmental temperature. Infants in open cribs may exhibit heat loss. Fluids need to be increased to compensate for insensible water loss. Expected changes in elimination patterns are loose green stools

and green urine. Evaluation of skin color with the light turned off is necessary. The newborn needs frequent repositioning to expose all skin surfaces to light. Finally, the neonate needs to have tactile stimulation as often as possible, whether with parents or the nursing staff. Parental contact will provide reassurance to the family of the infant's progress.

Exchange Transfusion

Exchange transfusions are performed in those infants subjected to hemolytic disease (*i.e.*, Rh incompatibility or ABO incompatibility) (Table 46-5). The exchange transfusion will decrease levels of bilirubin and correct any anemia. The donor blood used must be compatible with both infant's and mother's serum.[20]

Procedure. An exchange transfusion alternately removes a small amount of blood from the infant and replaces it with the same amount of donor blood. An umbilical catheter is used to perform the exchange, usually a double-volume type. In a double-volume exchange, the amount of donor blood is twice that of the newborn volume. Small amounts up to 20 ml are exchanged at a time. An infusion of albumin can be given several hours prior to the procedure to increase the number of bilirubin binding sites. This would make the exchange more efficient.

Pre-Exchange. The nurse is the primary caregiver who assesses the infant's color as becoming more jaun-

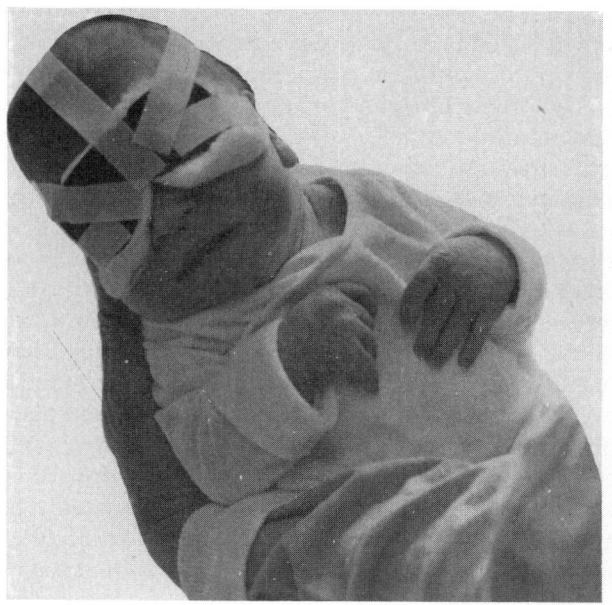

FIGURE 46-8

Infant prepared with eye shield in place for phototherapy treatment.

TABLE 46-5

Indications and Blood Products for Exchange Transfusions in Hemolytic Disease of the Newborn

Indications for Exchange Transfusions	Type of Donor Blood Used for Exchange Transfusions
Rh Incompatibility Anemia (hematocrit < 45%) Positive Coombs' test and rate of rise in serum bilirubin > 0.5 mg/hr	Rh Incompatibility 1. Rh-negative blood of infant's type that cross matches with mother's serum 2. Type O, Rh-negative red blood cells, Rh-negative plasma 3. Type O, Rh-negative "low titer" whole blood
ABO Incompatibility Rate of rise in serum bilirubin > 1.0 mg/hr	ABO Incompatibility 1. Type O, Rh-specific with low titers of anti-A antibody and anti-B antibody 2. Type O, Rh-negative red blood cells resuspended in type AB, Rh-negative plasma

(Baune KW, Lacey L: Common Hematologic Problems of the Immediate Newborn Period. JOGN May/June 1983; Adapted from Klaus M, Fanaroff A: Care of the High-Risk Neonate. Philadelphia, WB Saunders, 1979 and Katlwinkel J, Cook LJ, Ivey HH et al: Book II, Newborn Care: Concepts and Procedures. Charlottesville, University of Virginia Medical Center, Unit 16, 1979)

diced and behavior as increasingly lethargic, necessitating more diagnostic work-up. The nurse checks to see that all pre-exchange blood samples have been collected. An informed consent must be signed by the parents. Donor blood ordered must be checked for the type, unit number, and expiration date. Usually a hematocrit of donor blood is obtained. The desirable donor hematocrit is between 45 and 55. Blood must be warmed slowly. Blood-warming units keep blood at an even temperature during the procedure. The infant must be placed on monitors and restrained. The nurse prepares the infant for umbilical artery catheterization if needed by restraining the infant and setting up the sterile tray, solutions, and surgical gloves.

Procedural Tasks. The infant's temperature and other vital signs are taken and recorded at frequent intervals during the procedure. Vital signs are recorded on the infant's flow sheet as well as the exchange record itself. An exchange record is provided in the standard exchange transfusion tray. The amount of blood placed in and out is recorded on the exchange transfer sheet as well as any drugs given. For example, a dose of calcium may be given for every 100 ml exchanged. Total amounts of blood infused and withdrawn are recorded. Postexchange blood samples are withdrawn at the end of the procedure.

Post-transfusion. Frequent vital signs continue following the procedure. Some complications to anticipate and keep in mind are rebound hyperbilirubinemia, electrolyte imbalances, hypoglycemia, and hypothermia.

Evaluation

Evaluation and reassessment indicate that the newborn retains healthy eyes during phototherapy. Time is allowed for eye contact with the parents and visual stimulation. Tactile stimulation is given as often as possible. Despite the use of monitors and restraints during exchange transfusions, the neonate receives as much tactile stimulation and care as possible.

Fluid and electrolyte balance and temperature must be maintained, and the infant's temperature and vital signs are stabilized.

Breast Milk Jaundice

The incidence of increased bilirubin at about the fourth to seventh day with a peak at 2 weeks has been reported in 1% to 2% of breast-fed babies.[20]

The exact etiology of breast milk jaundice is unknown. Theories have focused on the roles of pregnanediol, increased enzyme activity, and increased free fatty acids in breast milk. Current investigation appears to be focused on the high levels of lipase activity and increased levels of free fatty acids in breast milk. The

Neonate with Pathologic Jaundice

Nursing Objectives

1. Identify infants at risk for hemolytic disease of the newborn.
2. Begin prompt and appropriate treatment of infants affected by hemolytic disease of the newborn.

Assessment	Potential Nursing Diagnosis	Planning/Intervention	Evaluation
Jaundice noted within first 24 hours	Potential for injury, kernicterus related to elevated bilirubin levels	Observe for levels of jaundice, note any progression	Newborn is free of kernicterus
Positive direct Coombs' test	Potential for injury, dehydration, hyperthermia related to phototherapy treatment	Use transcutaneous bilirubinometry as a screening tool	Newborn's vital signs and temperature are stabilized
Maternal/neonatal blood typing indicative of Rh or ABO incompatibility	Alteration in bowel elimination, diarrhea related to phototherapy	Obtain bilirubin specimens, monitor lab results	Newborn maintains fluid and electrolyte balance
	Potential for injury, (hyperbilirubinemia, electrolyte imbalances, hypoglycemia, hypothermia) related to exchange transfusion rebound	Give frequent feedings and monitor intake and output, skin turgor	Newborn is free of diaper rash
		Initiate phototherapy as ordered	Newborn participates in visual stimulation
		Remove infant's clothing	Newborn interacts with parents
		Place eye shield securely on infant. Remove at least every 4 hours to observe for conjunctivitis and allow for visual stimulation	
		Monitor temperature of infant and of isolette or warmer frequently	
		Observe diaper area for loose stools	
		Keep skin as clean as possible	
		Change position frequently	
		Remove from phototherapy for interaction/feeding with parents PRN	
		Prepare infant for exchange transfusion—restraints, monitors	
		Assist with insertion of catheter	
		Assist with collection of all blood samples	
		Check blood for correct typing	
		Use blood-warming equipment for procedure	

lipases found in breast milk are able to completely break down triglycerides to glycerol plus free fatty acids. Additionally, free fatty acids may interfere with the conjugation of bilirubin by inhibiting glucuronyl transferase. Evidence to support this theory has not really been forthcoming. Theories about the exact etiology of breast milk jaundice remain as indefinite conclusions.[20]

Treatment for elevated bilirubin levels due to breast milk jaundice may vary. Whether or not the temporary termination of breast-feeding is appropriate is debatable. Some physicians may simply monitor bilirubin levels closely and use phototherapy as deemed appropriate. Others may have the mother discontinue breast-feeding and substitute formula during the few days of peak bilirubin level.

Nurses need to give information to the parents, assuring them that this condition is only temporary. The mother may need help in learning to pump her breasts, if cessation of breast-feeding is recommended.

Infants of Drug-Addicted Mothers

The life-style of addicted women during the childbearing years promotes other health problems affecting the fetus and subsequently the neonate. There is a typical pattern of sporadic or no prenatal care. There may be a history of malnutrition, anemia, syphilis, and hepatitis.

Heroin Abuse

Heroin abusers' infants are often of low birth weight (50%); of those, 50% are small for gestational age. The incidence of anomalies is no higher than that of the general population. Fifty to 75% of infants born to heroin-addicted women will exhibit signs of withdrawal in the first day or two. The incidence of symptoms depends upon the duration of the addiction and the dosage and time of last dose. These infants demonstrate behaviors of a lack of quiet sleep and nonnutritive sucking patterns. Other signs are tremors, jitteriness, irritability, high-pitched cry, fist sucking, regurgitation, vomiting, diarrhea, hypertonia, hyperthermia or hypothermia, and, rarely, seizures. There exists a low incidence of RDS, which may be attributed to the action of heroin speeding up the production of surfactant.[21]

Methadone Maintenance

Infants born to mothers on methadone maintenance have a lower incidence of growth retardation than those of heroin-addicted mothers. There is no increase in congenital anomalies. The appearance of withdrawal behaviors depends upon the timing of the last maternal dose. Behaviors are similar but more intense than those of heroin withdrawal. The average onset is 24 to 52 hours postpartum. There is some occurrence of a late 2- to 4-week withdrawal period.

Diagnosis can be made by various types of urine screening.

Treatment

Treatment consists in providing of a quiet environment and adequate intake and administering medications to temper withdrawal behaviors. Phenobarbital is the drug of choice, followed by paregoric, diazepam, and thorazine.[21]

Addicted babies are harder to hold, less cuddly, and more difficult to console, and they show depressed visual response and exaggerated auditory response. They appear to be less alert, are more irritable, have increased muscle tone, and are more labile in alternating between hyperactivity and lethargy. These characteristics make addicted infants harder to mother in a situation in which every support is needed to enhance mother–infant bonding. Minimizing separation of infant and mother and assisting the mother in experiencing satisfying caretaking episodes are critical in promoting the relationship. An honest and open approach in discussing the effects of addiction on the baby and his needs may help the mother feel more confident in her mothering ability. She may experience guilt and anxiety, and the question of care for the infant after discharge must be discussed. A multidisciplinary approach involving drug counselors, social workers, and community-health nurses is useful in providing follow-up care for both mother and baby.

Fetal Alcohol Syndrome

Fetal alcohol syndrome, discussed earlier regarding the mother's intake of alcohol while pregnant, has become the third most commonly recognized cause of mental retardation in the United States, exceeded only by Down's syndrome and an incompletely enclosed spinal cord. It is estimated that the incidence is 2 to 3 per 1000 live births.

The risk of congenital anomalies to the fetus from maternal alcohol intake increases with increasing amounts of intake. The risk is 10% if a mother's intake is more than 1 or 2 oz of absolute alcohol a day, 19% if 2 oz or more, and 40% if more than 5 oz.[21] Infants affected exhibit typical craniofacial and limb defects, cardiovascular defects, intrauterine growth retardation, and developmental delay. It is not certain whether alcohol or its breakdown, acetaldehyde, is responsible for

Infants Born to Drug Abusers

Nursing Objectives

1. Test and diagnose suspected infants.
2. Minimize withdrawal symptoms in the neonate.
3. Discharge infants to a safe home environment.

Assessment	Potential Nursing Diagnosis	Planning/Intervention	Evaluation
Known history of maternal drug abuse	Sleep/rest disturbance related to hyperirritability	Observe for withdrawal symptoms:	Infant is diagnosed as infant of drug-addicted mother
Amount, type of drug, and time of last dosage	Potential for injury, blisters related to frantic sucking of fists	Lack of quiet sleep	Infant adjusts and quiets down to quiet environment
	Alteration in nutrition, potential for less than body requirements related to uncoordinated and ineffective sucking and swallowing reflexes	Nonnutritive sucking patterns	Infant accepts adequate nutrition
		Tremors	
		Jitteriness	
		Irritability	
		High-pitched cry	
		Fist sucking	
		Regurgitation	
		Vomiting	
		Diarrhea	
		Hypertonia	
		Hyperthermia or hypothermia	
		Assist with diagnostic testing—collection of urine specimen	
		Provide a quiet environment	
		Carefully compute intake/output	
		Administer drugs as ordered	
	Potential for alteration in parenting related to continuing maternal drug abuse	Refer to community services for home assessment and long-term follow-up	Infant leaves hospital for safe environment
			Infant receives follow-up care

the fetal damage. Alcohol interferes with protein synthesis and the absorption of numerous nutrients, and heavy consumption is most likely to affect fetal development during the first trimester when organogenesis is occurring. Spontaneous abortion is common among alcoholics, but improved nutrition and vitamin fortification now allow many of these pregnancies to continue. If excessive alcohol consumption occurs during the second trimester, infant weight is most affected, which leads to growth retardation.

One study found that daily consumption of 1 oz of absolute alcohol before pregnancy is associated with a decrease in birth weight of 91 g. The same amount in late pregnancy is associated with a decrease in birth weight of 160 g.[22]

Characteristic anomalies seen in the fetal alcohol syndrome include microcephaly, short palpebral fissures, epicanthal folds, cleft palate, maxillary hypoplasia, altered palmar creases, joint defects, cardiac defects, anomalous genitalia, fine motor dysfunction, and capillary hemangiomas (Fig. 46-9). Postnatally, there often is developmental delay and growth deficiency. There may be severe mental retardation with depressed sucking and swallowing reflexes or slight retardation that is not detected until later when developmental problems occur. The extent of immediate fetal depression at birth

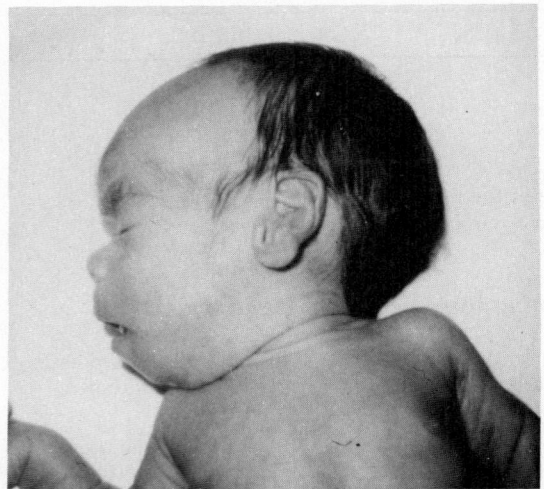

FIGURE 46-9

Infants born with fetal alcohol syndrome exhibit an altered pattern of growth and development, low birth weight, short stature, small heads, and a variety of joint and heart defects, as well as mental retardation and fine motor dysfunctions.

depends upon the time and amount of the mother's last intake of alcohol, as well as such problems as anoxia or aspiration perinatally. Difficulties in feeding and disturbances of sleep are common in the newborn with this syndrome. Prenatal detection of excessive alcohol consumption and counseling to stop or reduce drinking are the most important preventive measures.[23]

References

1. Mangurten HC: Birth injuries. In Fanaroff AB, Martin RJ (eds): Behrman's Neonatal-Perinatal Medicine. St Louis, CV Mosby, 1983
2. Brann AW, Schwartz JF: Central nervous system disturbances. In Fanaroff AB, Martin RJ (eds): Behrman's Neonatal-Perinatal Medicine. St Louis, CV Mosby, 1983
3. Braune KW, Lacey L: Common hematologic problems of the immediate newborn period. JOGN 12(Suppl)(3): 21s–24s, 1983
4. Jensen MD, Bobak IM: Maternity & Gynecologic Care, p 1080. St Louis, CV Mosby, 1985
5. Korones SB: High-Risk Newborn Infants, p 58. St Louis, CV Mosby, 1981
6. Feigin RD, Callanan DL: Postnatally acquired infections. In Fanaroff AB, Martin RJ (eds): Behrman's Neonatal-Perinatal Medicine. St Louis, CV Mosby, 1983
7. Reynolds DW, Stagno S, Alford CA: Chronic congenital and perinatal infections. In Avery GB (ed): Neonatology: Pathology and Management of the Newborn, pp 748–789. Philadelphia, JB Lippincott, 1981
8. McCracken GH: Bacterial and viral infections in the newborn. In Avery GB (ed): Neonatology: Pathology and Management of the Newborn, pp 723–747. Philadelphia, JB Lippincott, 1981
9. Daum RS, Smith AL: Bacterial sepsis in the newborn. Clin Obstet Gynecol 22:391–395, June 1979
10. Babson SG, Pernoll ML, Benda GI: Diagnosis and Management of the Fetus and Neonate at Risk, pp 211–274. St Louis, CV Mosby, 1980
11. Osborne NG, Pratson L: Sexually transmitted disease and pregnancy. JOGN 13(1):9–12, January-February 1984
12. Devore N, Jackson V, Piening SL: Torch infections. Am J Nurs 83(12):1660–1665, December 1983
13. Glasgow LA, Overall JC: Viral and protozoal perinatal infections. In Fanaroff AM, Martin RJ (eds): Behrman's Perinatal-Neonatal Medicine, pp 690–707. St Louis, CV Mosby, 1983
14. Ogra PL: Neonatal Infections, Nutritional and Immunologic Interactions, p 133. San Diego, Grune & Stratton, 1984
15. Haggerty L: TORCH: A literature review and implications for practice. JOGN 14(2):124–129, 1985
16. Brown SG: The devastating effects of congenital rubella. Am J Maternal Child Nurs 3(1):16–21, January/February 1978
17. Epstein MF: Medical and parental expectations in the care of the infant of a diabetic mother. Diabetes Educator 9(2):44s–46s, Summer 1983
18. Cowett RM, Schwartz R: The infant of the diabetic mother. Pediatr Clin North Am 29(5):1213–1231, October 1982
19. Maisels MJ: Neonatal jaundice. In Avery GB (ed): Neonatology: Pathophysiology and Management of the Newborn, pp 473–544. Philadelphia, JB Lippincott, 1981
20. Brooten D, Brown L, Hollingsworth A et al: Breast-milk jaundice. JOGN 14(3):220–223, 1985
21. Rosen TS: Infants of addicted mothers. In Fanaroff AB, Martin RJ (eds): Behrman's Neonatal-Perinatal Medicine, pp 934–937. St Louis, CV Mosby, 1983
22. Lindor E, McCarthy AM, McRae MG: Fetal alcohol syndrome. JOGN 9(4):222–228, 1980
23. Luke B: Maternal alcoholism and fetal alcohol syndrome. Am J Nurs 77(12):1924–1926, December 1977

Suggested Reading

Avery GB (ed): Neonatology. Philadelphia, JB Lippincott Co, 1985

Gennaro S: Listeria infection: Nursing care of mother and infant. MCN 5(6):390–392, November/December 1980

Greene JW et al: Integrative Clinicopathological Conference:

A neonate and her diabetic mother. Hosp Pract 19(9): 29, 33–34, September 1984

Klaus MH, Fanaroff AA: Care of the High-Risk Neonate. Philadelphia, WB Saunders, 1983

Korones SB: High Risk Newborn Infants. St Louis, CV Mosby, 1983

Leland D et al: Use of TORCH titers. Pediatrics 72(1):41–43, July 1983

Mangione RA et al: Neonatal complications associated with maternal diabetics. Neonatal Network 2(3):36–41, December 1983

Mogan-Capner P et al: Fetal and neonatal infection. Nurs Times 8(4):49, 52–54, July/August 1984

Ogata ES: Diabetes-related problems of the newborn. Perinatology and Neonatology 8(1):48–53, January/February 1984

Waechter EA, Phillips J, Holaday B: Nursing Care of Children. Philadelphia, JB Lippincott, 1985

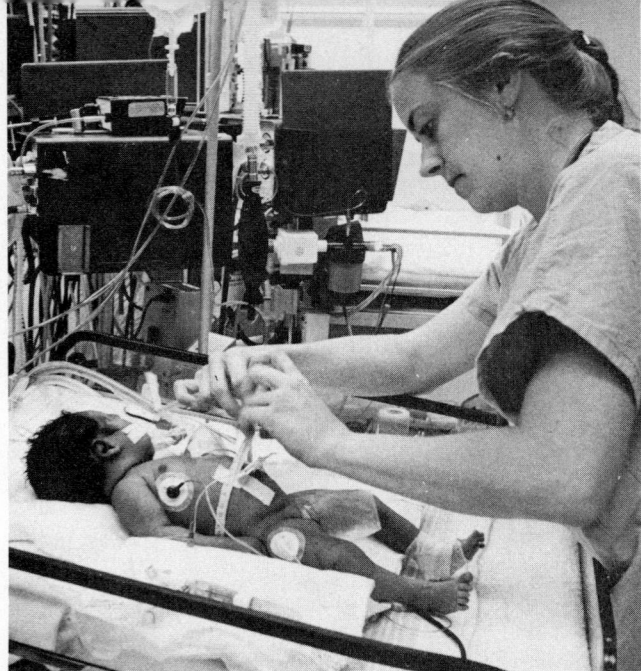

S T U D Y   A I D S

Unit VIII:
Assessment and Management of Perinatal Disorders

Conference Material

1. In your own hospital setting, evaluate the facilities for and the care of the newborn infants in relation to the prevention of infection.

2. A mother's firstborn infant has a cleft lip and cleft palate. The infant is apparently normal otherwise. The distraught mother can see only "my poor deformed baby girl" and blames herself for this "tragedy," because she did not follow her physician's instructions during pregnancy, particularly in relation to good nutrition. How might the nurse handle the nursing problems in this situation?

3. How do you account for the high infant mortality during the neonatal period?

4. What community agencies in your city render services for handicapped children? What is the procedure for making the referral to such agencies? How can the public health nurse function most effectively in such cases?

5. What legislation in your city or state has contributed to reducing the incidence of congenital syphilis?

6. What methods are used by your hospital, well-baby clinics, or other community agencies for the detection of phenylketonuria?

Multiple Choice

Read through the entire question and place your answer on the line to the right.

1. Which of the following factors may predispose to the production of an erythroblastotic infant?
   A. Rh-negative mother
   B. Rh-positive father
   C. Rh-positive fetus
   D. Rh-positive substance from the fetus finds its way into the mother's bloodstream to build up antibodies
   E. Mother has had a previous Rh-positive pregnancy or transfusion.
   Select the number corresponding to the correct letters.
   1. A and D
   2. A, C, and D
   3. B, C, and E
   4. All of the above   ————

2. Which of the following statements concerning diabetes complicated by pregnancy are correct?
   A. The size of the placenta tends to be in direct relationship to the size of the infant.
   B. Toxemia occurs more frequently than in nondiabetic pregnancies.
   C. Deliveries are always performed by cesarean section, usually 2 weeks prior to term
   D. The fetus tends to be large.
   E. Hypoglycemia occurs in the infant following delivery.
   Select the number corresponding to the correct letters.
   1. A and B
   2. B, D, and E
   3. B, C, D, and E
   4. All of the above   ————

3. The most effective treatment of erythroblastosis is accomplished by blood transfusion. Which of the following is the best method to use?
   A. Exchange transfusion with Rh-negative blood
   B. Exchange transfusion with Rh-positive blood
   C. Exchange transfusion with blood plasma
   D. Repeated small transfusions with Rh-negative blood
   E. Repeated small transfusions with Rh-positive blood
   F. Repeated small transfusions with blood plasma   ————

4. Hemolytic disease of the newborn may be produced by the union of parents with which of the following blood types?
   A. Rh-positive mother with Rh-negative father
   B. Rh-negative mother with Rh-negative father
   C. Rh-negative mother with Rh-positive father
   D. Type O mother with type A father
   E. Type A mother with type B father
   Select the number corresponding to the correct letters.

1070

1. A and C
2. B and D
3. C and D
4. All of the above   ————

5. Which one of the following infectious diseases, when contracted by the mother during the first trimester of pregnancy, will most often produce congenital anomalies in the infant?
   A. Scarlet fever
   B. Rubella
   C. Diphtheria
   D. Rubeola
   E. Typhoid fever   ————

6. Some disorders that affect the infant in the neonatal period are manifestations of inborn errors of metabolism. Which of the following conditions would this include?
   A. Phenylketonuria
   B. Icterus neonatorum
   C. Galactosemia
   D. Down's syndrome
   E. Erythroblastosis fetalis
Select the number corresponding to the correct letter or letters.
   1. A only
   2. A and C
   3. B, C, and D
   4. B, D, and E   ————

7. What has recently become the best method to prevent erythroblastosis fetalis?
   A. Injection of the mother soon after delivery with Rh-immune globulin to prevent maternal sensitization
   B. Transfusing the mother during pregnancy
   C. Transfusing all Rh-negative fathers
   D. Transfusing all Rh-negative babies
   E. Repeated small transfusions of Rh-positive blood to the mother
Select the number corresponding to the correct letter or letters.
   1. A only
   2. A and B
   3. B, C, and D
   4. C, D, and E   ————

8. Sampling of amniotic fluid can be useful in determining fetal lung maturity. The determination that is carried out for this purpose is
   A. Bilirubin
   B. Cytology
   C. Creatinine
   D. Lecithin-sphingomyelin (L/S) ratio   ————

9. Certain behaviors indicate that a preterm infant may be ready to advance from gavage feedings to nipple feedings. Which of the following are these behaviors?

   A. Strong, vigorous suck
   B. Sucking and swallowing coordinated
   C. Competent gag reflex
   D. Sucking on gavage tube
   E. Wakefulness before feeding time
Select the number corresponding to the correct letters.
   1. B, C, and E
   2. C and D
   3. A and C
   4. All of the above   ————

10. Nursing care of an infant receiving TPN includes which of the following interventions?
   A. Changing tubing every 48 hours
   B. Changing the insertion site dressing once a week
   C. Frequent checking of Dextrostix
   D. Measuring head circumference
   E. Offering pacifier to infant
Select the number corresponding to the correct letters.
   1. A, B, and E
   2. B and C
   3. A and D
   4. All of the above   ————

11. Small-for-gestational-age infants exhibit which of the following clinical problems?
   A. Hyperglycemia
   B. Anemia
   C. Congenital disorders
   D. Hypercalcemia
   E. Temperature instability
Select the number corresponding to the correct letter or letters.
   1. A and B
   2. B, C, and E
   3. C and E
   4. All of the above   ————

12. When the mother learned that her preterm infant was receiving gavage feedings, she asked the nurse why this was being done. Which of the following reasons may be correct for the nurse to reply?
   A. "This method of feeding your baby was indicated because he became exhausted when he tried to swallow."
   B. "Feeding your baby this way prevents him from vomiting and thus eliminates the danger of his aspirating formula into his lungs."
   C. "Feeding your baby this way conserves his strength and permits him to receive food into his stomach when sucking or swallowing may be difficult."
   D. "Your baby can be given his formula quickly this way and thus he does not have to be handled as much."
   E. "A tiny baby's resistance to infection is poor, so gavage feeding is really a protective measure

against such infections as thrush, which he
might acquire if he were bottle-fed."
Select the number corresponding to the correct letter or
letters.
1. A only
2. C only
3. B, C, and D
4. B, D, and E   ____

13. Signs of neonatal congestive heart failure include
A. Tachypnea
B. Bradycardia
C. Hepatomegaly
D. Edema
E. Sternal retractions
Select the number corresponding to the correct letters.
1. A, C, D, and E
2. B, C, and E
3. A and D
4. B and E   ____

14. Which of the following conditions are congenital
disorders?
A. Patent ductus arteriosus
B. Brachial palsy
C. Hydrocephalus
D. Retrolental fibroplasia
E. Caput succedaneum
Select the number corresponding to the correct letter or
letters.
1. A and C
2. B, C, and D
3. B, D, and E
4. All of the above   ____

15. Factors that may produce hyperbilirubinemia by the
overproduction of unconjugated bilirubin are
A. Rh incompatibility
B. Asphyxia
C. Ecchymosis from bruising
D. Liver cell damage due to sepsis
E. Hepatitis
Select the number corresponding to the correct letters.
1. B, C, and D
2. A, D, and E
3. A and C
4. All of the above   ____

16. The following are examples of viral infections in the
neonate:
A. Herpes simplex type II
B. Rubella
C. Syphilis
D. Toxoplasmosis
E. Cytomegalovirus
Select the number corresponding to the correct letters.
1. A, B, C, and E
2. B, C, D, and E
3. A and C
4. All of the above   ____

17. Which of the following clinical problems are possible
in the infant of a diabetic mother?
A. Small-for-gestational age
B. Respiratory distress syndrome
C. Hyperglycemia
D. Hyperbilirubinemia
E. Hypercalcemia
Select the number corresponding to the correct letters.
1. A, C, and E
2. B and D
3. B, C, and E
4. All of the above   ____

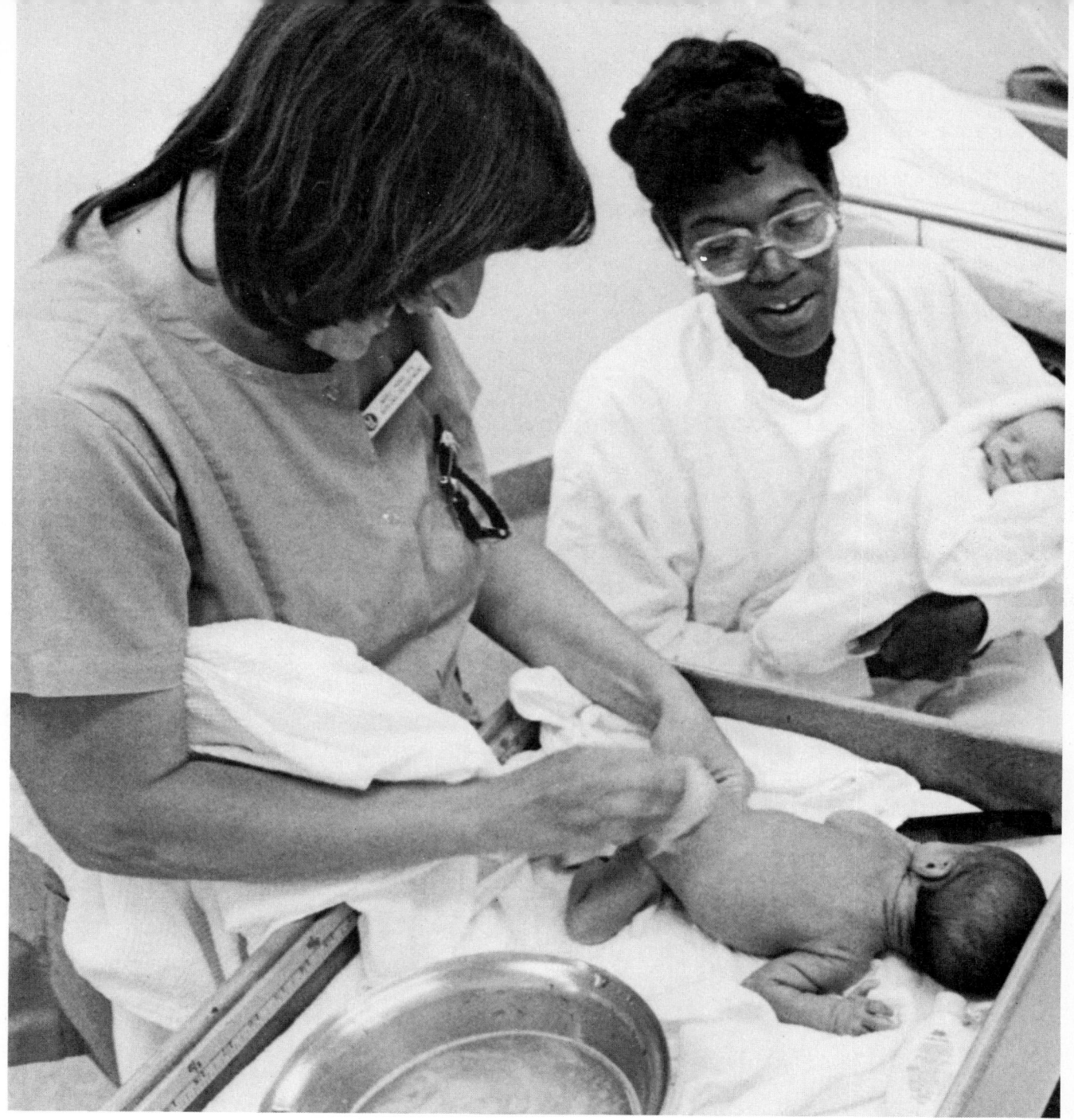

UNIT IX

*Special Considerations
in Maternity Nursing*

Evolution of Maternity Nursing

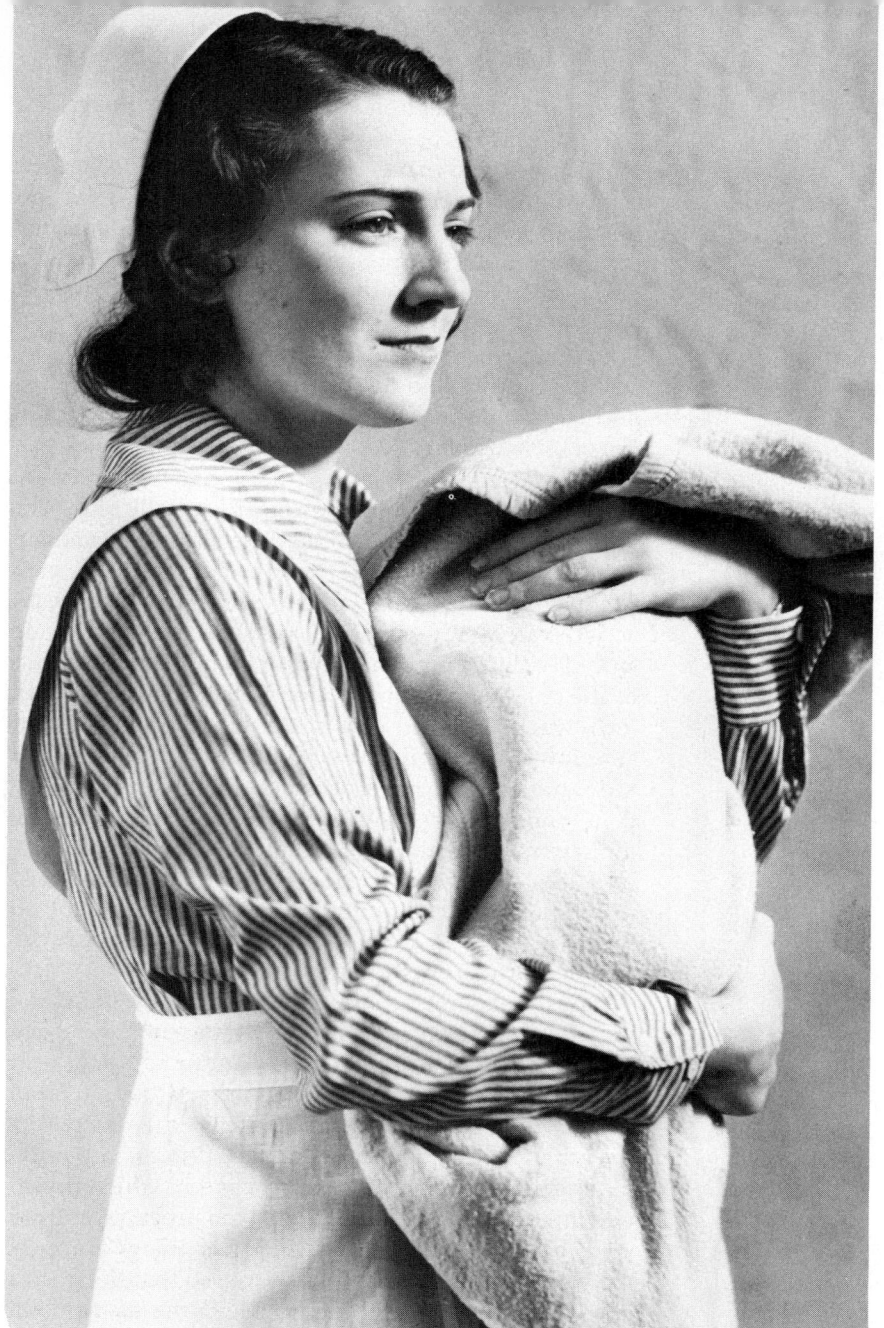

CHAPTER 47

Evolution of Maternity Nursing

The bearing of children is an event of enormous social significance that has certain symbolic meanings. Traditions, rites, and practices have been developed around this event in all societies to encourage positive outcomes for the individual and society. Roles for attendants during the reproductive process have been formalized and differ greatly among cultures. Involvement of the sciences in childbearing grew gradually through the ages, but continued to be interwoven with folk beliefs and customs. In the less-developed countries, ancient folk practices continue to prevail in the care provided during pregnancy, delivery, and the postpartum period.

The birth of a baby was traditionally a family and community event. Labor and delivery usually took place in the home, with the mother attended by a midwife and with the support of family members and close friends. Children were familiar with birth and death, as were all family members, because these events occurred within their living environment. The acceptance of the childbearing process, with its inherent risks and joys, was a common part of the fabric of life. The institution of prenatal care and hospital deliveries, and the entrance of the medical profession into the maternity field, undoubtedly contributed to the marked decrease in maternal and neonatal mortality that has characterized the 20th century. However, improved maternal nutrition, improved sanitation, and the declining birth rate may be even more significant factors in reducing the mortality of mothers and neonates.

As knowledge continues to advance, there is a growing appreciation of the fine balance of natural ecosystems and the wisdom of restraint in applying technology to the reproductive process. Although recent developments in reproductive care include increasing scientific intervention in the natural process, a point of diminishing returns has been reached in which continued interventions frequently lead to iatrogenic morbidity. A balance is required, in which technology is applied more discriminately in childbearing, so that the normal reproductive process can proceed with the least amount of interference.

Early Childbirth Practices

Prehistory

Study of customs and practices of primitive peoples gives some insight into prehistoric and ancient societies.[1] Primitive cultures usually have healers skilled in use of medicinal herbs and knowledgeable about physiological processes and diseases. Often there is overlap between spiritual and healing roles, particularly as primitive cultures usually have holistic views of life.

Traditional healers knew many uses of herbs for women's health needs and problems. Goldenseal was used as a douche for vaginal infections and was combined with squawvine as a female genitourinary tract tonic. It was used in small doses with cloves in spearmint tea for morning sickness. Large doses contract the uterus and may have contraceptive effects. False unicorn root (chamailirium) was used to treat female sterility and prevent miscarriage, when taken daily for several months. It was also useful for amenorrhea, painful menses, irregular menses, and leukorrhea. Uva ursi (bearberry) has traditionally helped to reduce postpartum hemorrhage and aid involution. Rehmania is an important Chinese herb formula to treat menstrual irregularities and stop postpartum hemorrhage.[2] Many other herbs have been used and continue as part of contemporary traditional herbalists' treatments.

Childbirth among ancient peoples was usually a process of social importance to the entire tribe. Rituals surrounded birthing, and female healers or other childbirth attendants were present. Appeals by the priests for the gods' assistance were common. Customs varied; some tribes had special places for childbirth, while others used customary sleeping places. Many tribes used kneeling, squatting, or sitting positions for delivery. Fathers participated in some cultures and were excluded in others. In one culture, the father held the mother on his lap, reclining against his chest, while he and the midwife applied pressure to the uterus during contractions.[3] Even without the benefit of science, childbearing was a complex process among ancients to which a substantial repertoire of naturalistic knowledge, traditional skills, and important social customs were applied.

Egyptian, Hindu, and Chinese Societies

In ancient Egypt, a highly organized society existed, with complex childbearing practices. The priesthood in Egypt was concerned with all the activities of society. Priests had supervisory interest in normal childbirth and took an active part in the care of abnormal or operative cases. Ancient Egyptians are known to have had obstetric forceps, to have performed cesarean sections on dead mothers, and to have carried out podalic version.

There were special rooms in temples for giving birth to a pharoah or divinity, and reliefs on temple walls give a visual idea of the Egyptian method of delivery. Parturient women are shown kneeling, sitting on their heels, or sitting on two bricks with a space between them. One midwife supported the woman from behind, and another received the infant. Ancient papyrus documents contained remedies for assisting labor, including vaginal suppositories, manual massage, and oral potions. There seems to have been a large body of gynecological and obstetric knowledge in Egyptian society, with many approaches to assisting women in conception, pregnancy, and childbirth, as well as with gynecologic problems.

Surata, an early and prolific Hindu writer, lived sometime between 600 BC and 500 AD. His knowledge of menstruation and gestation was quite modern. He knew and described intelligently the management of normal and abnormal labor. He described the use of forceps and cesarean section upon dead mothers to remove living children and gave excellent antepartal and pospartum advice. He advised cleanliness on the part of the attendant, such as cutting the beard, the hair, and the nails closely, wearing clean gowns, and disinfecting the operating rooms prior to operation or delivery. His surgical antiseptic technique includes many modern principles.

The Chinese have a long and ancient tradition of care based on holistic, energetic models. Eastern healing arts have traditionally included herbal remedies, energy flow balancing through acupuncture and pulse diagnostics, and life-style analysis and change. Many monographs have been written on childbearing, advising various techniques and remedies and counseling patience in attending labor and avoiding unnecessary interference. In China and Japan, only midwives were permitted to care for women having normal births. Physicians assisted only difficult births in many early societies.

Ancient Greece

Normal childbearing was generally the domain of midwives, while physicians attended complicated births. Some midwives were of high social standing, such as the mother of Socrates and the wife of Pericles. Aristotle remarked on the wisdom and intelligence of midwives. Men attending births were called "man-wives," and at one point these male physicians attempted to have laws passed preventing nonphysician midwives from practicing. Agnodice, a high-ranking Athenian woman, trained as a midwife in Alexandria and practiced in men's clothing. When found out and brought to court, she won her case with support from other powerful Athenian women. Athens subsequently licensed midwives to perform deliveries and treat women's diseases.[4]

Hippocrates, the "Father of Medicine," wrote many advanced medical books. His books have few references to childbirth, probably because men (physicians) rarely attended birth and nursing care was carried out by women, who were kept distinctly separate from men in many activities.[1] One book does discuss a case of puerperal sepsis. Physicians attended very difficult births and performed destructive operations (Fig. 47-1).

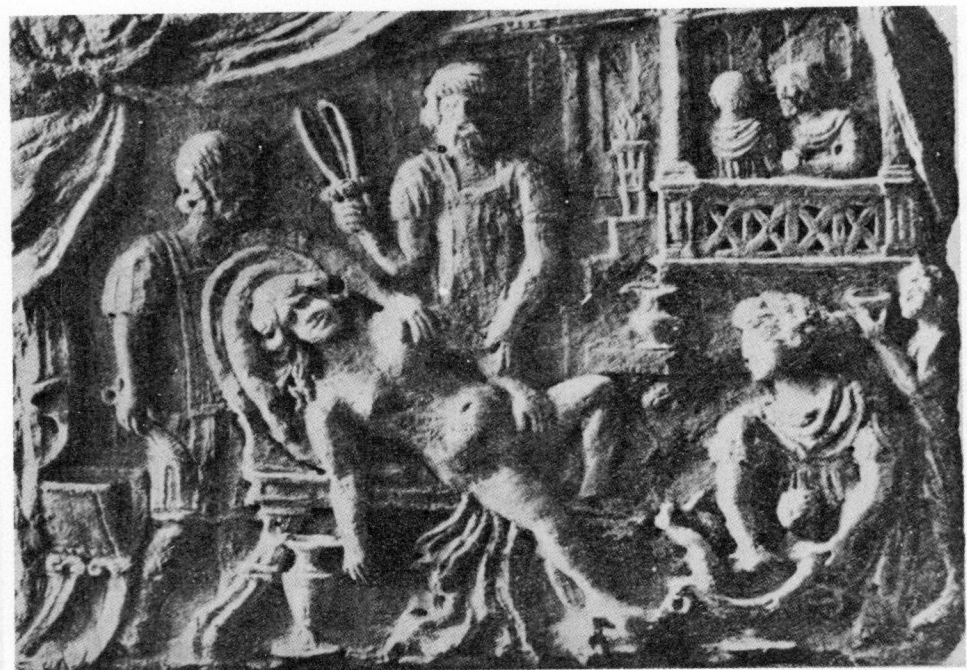

FIGURE 47-1

Bas-relief (second or third century AD near Rome) depicting birth scene. Note that the physician (center) holds a pair of obstetric forceps aloft in his right hand. (Danforth DN (ed): Obstetrics and Gynecology. Philadelphia, Harper & Row, 1982)

Soranus, the "Father of Obstetrics," studied in Alexandria and practiced in Rome. He wrote books about obstetrics that included descriptions of podalic version, care during pregnancy, use of birthing chairs, and abortion. He instructed midwives and advocated trimmed nails and warm hands, as well as supporting the perineum with a linen cloth as the head advanced, to prevent perineal lacerations. For contraception, he advised use of cedar or rancid oil, honey, thin strips of lint, or pessaries.

Early Judeo–Christian Era

Although the ancient Jews specified little assistance to the woman during labor and delivery, they were interested in the hygiene of pregnancy and cleanliness at the time of childbirth. Hygiene and sanitation were practices integrated into religious law. In instances of difficult deliveries, the women "were comforted until they died." The stool or obstetric chair was used at this time and continued to be used until about the 19th century AD. Reference is made to this chair in the Bible, in the first chapter of Exodus, "when you do the office of the midwife to the Hebrew women, and see them upon the stools. . . ."

The teachings of Christianity promoted compassion for the sick and suffering and upheld the equality of women (although not all Christians accepted this). Several examples of the nursing role appear in the New Testament. The deaconess Phebe was "a succourer of many," and widows were noted to provide relief to the afflicted (Romans 16:1–2; 1 Timothy 5:9–10). Organized nursing services were provided by early Christian religious orders. The Sisters of Hôtel Dieu were the first order of nuns with nursing care as their sole mission. This order formed in AD 660.[5]

Middle Ages

Much of the knowledge of medicine and nursing care developed during Greek and Roman times was lost during the Middle Ages. Religious institutions, particularly the early Catholic church, taught that women were sources of sin and evil. Literal, narrow interpretations of biblical passages led to the idea that women deserved to suffer, especially in childbirth, because Eve was condemned to bring forth children in sorrow after causing the Fall from Eden. Practices related to childbearing were often cruel and barbarous.

Disease was rampant during these Dark Ages. Syphilis, smallpox, bubonic plague, and leprosy were widespread. Women were in great danger of puerperal sepsis, especially if they delivered in hospitals. In the Moslem world, however, the knowledge of scientific medicine was sustained. During the eighth to tenth centuries, many great hospitals were built in Arabia.[6] Some of this knowledge was brought back to Europe by returning Crusaders.

Renaissance Period

The Renaissance was characterized by advances in medicine and maternity care commensurate with those in other fields. During this time the first English text on obstetrics, the *Byrthe of Mankynde* (1545), was published by Raynalde. Both it and its German counterpart by Roesslin, the *Rosegarden of Pregnant Women and Midwives* (1513), are copies of Soranus, and with their publication podalic version was reintroduced to obstetric practice. Many famous men were responsible for the progress in obstetrics, among them Leonardo da Vinci (who made the first accurate sketches of the fetus *in utero*) and Vesalius (who first accurately described the pelvis).

Cesarean delivery had been practiced upon dead mothers since antiquity, but the first authentic cesarean delivery performed upon a living mother is credited to Trautman, of Wittenberg, in 1610. According to the records, the woman had a large ventral hernia that contained the uterus. Prior to this, Nufer, a sow gelder, is reputed to have performed the operation on his wife after obstetricians and midwives had failed to deliver her. Reportedly, Jane Seymour was delivered by a cesarean section done by Frere, a noted surgeon of the time, at the request of Henry VIII. That she died a few days after the birth of Edward VI adds credence to the story. Due to the frightful mortality from hemorrhage and sepsis, cesarean birth did not become popular in spite of the advocacy of the Church. Through the following centuries it was done occasionally, but not until the advent of uterine sutures and aseptic technique did it become a practical procedure.

Ambrose Paré (1510–1590), the dean of French surgeons and obstetricians, made podalic version a practicable procedure to be used in preference to cesarean delivery in difficult labor. His work helped establish obstetrics as an independent branch of medicine. Schools were established during this period to train midwives, and laws passed to regulate their practice.

Francois Mauriceau, a famous French obstetrician, wrote an advanced treatise on midwifery (1668). Many well-known obstetricians taught midwives and shared new knowledge with them. Louise Bourgeois (1563–1637) was a French midwife who used and advocated podalic version. A school for midwives was established at Hôtel Dieu in Paris, which became known for improving midwifery skills (late 16th century).

VanDeventer, of Holland, has been called the father of modern obstetrics and is credited with the first accurate description of the pelvis, its deformities and their effect on parturition. He also shares with Ould, of Dublin, the first description of the mechanism of labor.

Obstetric forceps have been used in Greek, Roman, Hindu, and Arabic cultures for many centuries. Peter Chamberlen, son of a Huguenot who left France for England to escape religious persecution, is credited with inventing a modern version of forceps, in about 1580. Five generations of Chamberlen obstetricians guarded forceps as a family secret. By the time their forceps was revealed in 1813, other types had been developed.

Although most maternity care was provided by midwives, a gradual shift in attitude began during the 15th and 16th centuries. Prominent people and nobility increasingly sought male physicians and birth attendants, probably because of perceptions that they possessed new scientific knowledge. The French dauphine and the mistress of Louis XIV of France were delivered by physicians (male midwives). The French term *accoucheur* replaced *midman* and *man-midwife*. Similar events in other countries led to greater use of physician birth attendants.

The 16th century witnessed severe population losses due to plagues, wars, and natural disasters. In England, William Pelty realized that controlling communicable diseases and saving infant lives would prevent continued diminution of the population. To this end he recommended isolation of plague patients and maternity hospitals for unmarried pregnant women. Such ideas were too far in advance of the time, however, and had no immediate consequences.

Eighteenth Century

Population continued to be a great general concern to the governments of the world. Those who were concerned with general matters of health felt that governments ought to take a more active role in overseeing health matters. Between 1779 and 1817, Johan Peter Frank in Germany wrote several volumes entitled *System einer vollstandigen medicinischen Polezey*. This work is even today considered a landmark in the history of thought on the social relations of health and disease. His recommendations concerning childbirth were many and, as with Pelty, farsighted for his time. He insisted that all childbirth be attended by trained persons and further urged that a midwife be consulted prior to the expected date of confinement. In addition, he proposed legislation to enforce a reasonable period of bed rest during the puerperium and to free the mother for several weeks from any work in or outside the house that might prevent her from giving the necessary attention to her infant. When necessary, he felt that the state should support parturients for the first 6 weeks after delivery. He then expanded upon the above and outlined a detailed child welfare program. Acceptance of his work and ideas spread to all countries in close cultural contact with Germany.

William Smellie (England, 1697–1763) taught obstetrics with a manikin and made improvements on the obstetric forceps in use at the time, adding a steel lock and curved blades. He also laid down the first principles for their use and differentiated by measurement between contracted and normal pelves.

William Hunter, though a pupil of Smellie, was opposed to the use of forceps and frequently exhibited his rusted blades as evidence of their uselessness. In conjunction with his brother he laid the foundation of modern knowledge of placental anatomy.

Charles White published a thesis on obstetrics advocating the scrubbing of the hands and general cleanliness on the part of the accoucheur; he was the pioneer in aseptic midwifery. John Harvie, 90 years before Credé, advocated external manual expression of the placenta. It is known that a similar procedure was in use in Dublin at that time.

There were many famous obstetricians on the Continent during this period. Chief among them was Baudelocque, who invented the pelvimeter and named and described various positions and presentations.

Events in America

The physician Fuller and his highly esteemed midwife spouse came to the new world on the Mayflower in 1620. Anne Hutchinson was an early American midwife who practiced in Boston and Rhode Island (circa 1640). She faced religious persecution as a witch and heretic, but escaped the stake.

An 18th century New York City ordinance regulated midwives, requiring an oath that included the promise to help any woman in labor, rich or poor; to identify the newborn's true parents; to prevent harm or murder of newborns; to consult with other midwives as needed; to not give medicines to cause abortions; to not conceal a bastard's birth; and to be of good behavior.[7]

William Shippen, a famous American physician who was a student of Smellie and Hunter, opened a school for midwifery in Philadelphia in 1762. Because he provided convenient lodgings for the accommodation of poor women during confinement, he may be said to have established the first lying-in hospital in America. With Morgan, he founded the School of Medicine of the University of Pennsylvania, becoming its first Professor of Anatomy, Surgery, and Midwifery.

In America, prejudices against men in midwifery were carried over from Europe; as late as 1857 a demonstration before the graduating class at Buffalo roused such a storm of criticism that the American Medical Association had to intervene. Their judgment was that any physician who could not conduct labor by touch alone should not undertake midwifery.

Growth of Science and Modern Maternity Care

Nineteenth Century Scientific Progress

The increased knowledge and ability that trained midwives and physicians brought to maternity care were largely offset by the increased mortality due to puerperal fever. During the 17th, 18th, and 19th centuries it became a pestilence, at times wiping out whole communities of puerperal women. The mortality rates varied in the best European clinics at Paris and Vienna from 10% to 20%. The origin and the spread of the disease were little understood or studied. Obstetricians spent futile hours on a study of minor alterations in instruments or technique and ignored the vast loss of life from puerperal fever. Oliver Wendell Holmes, of Harvard, first presented his views on the contagiousness of puerperal fever in 1843. In 1855 he reiterated them in a monograph on *Puerperal Fever as a Private Pestilence*. This was, and still remains, a medical classic on the subject. His statements aroused great controversy in America, and he received considerable abuse and criticism from Meigs and Hodge, two of the foremost American obstetricians of the day. One of them stated that it was ridiculous to conceive of any gentleman carrying contamination on his hands from patient to patient.

Whereas Holmes first conceived the correct idea of the nature of the disease, Ignaz Philipp Semmelweiss finally recognized and proved without question the nature of its source and transmission. He was an assistant in the Viennese clinic for women. While his associates were fussing with details of technique, he was studying and mourning the tremendous death rate among puerperal women in the clinic. He observed that the death rate in Clinic I, where women were delivered by medical students or physicians, was always higher than in Clinic II, where midwives officiated and received instruction. After fruitless study and manifold changes in technique to follow more closely that of Clinic II, the cause of the disease was brought home to him in a desperate and startling fashion. His friend, Kalletschka, an assistant in pathology, died after performing an autopsy upon a victim of puerperal fever, during which Kalletschka had sustained a slight cut on his finger.

Postmortem findings were identical with those of puerperal sepsis, and Semmelweiss concluded that the disease was transmitted from the dead by contact from the physicians and the students, who often went directly from the postmortem room to deliveries. Accordingly, he immediately instituted and enforced a ruling that made it obligatory that all physicians and students wash their hands in a solution of chloride of lime after attending autopsies and before examining patients or delivering babies. In 7 months he had reduced the mortality in Clinic I from 12% to 2%. In the subsequent year Clinic I had a mortality lower than Clinic II, a hitherto unheard-of feat. Subsequently, he observed that puerperal sepsis could be transmitted from patient to patient, or from attendants to patient, by contact of contaminated material, as well as from the postmortem room. In 1861 he published his immortal work on *The Aetiology, Concept, and Prophylaxis of Puerperal Fever*.

The history of medicine provides pitiful figures in profusion, but none, it seems, met such a cruel reception and ultimate fate as Semmelweiss. His colleagues (for the most part, but with a few notable and loyal exceptions) distorted and criticized his teachings.

Semmelweiss apparently was not a skilled writer, and this, combined with his poor interpersonal relations, hampered acceptance of his work. He was known to call another physician a murderer and a Nero, and he personally blamed his superior for the terrible conditions on the hospital wards. Medical colleagues carried their distaste for his views to the point of persecution. Semmelweiss was forced to leave Vienna and go to Budapest, where a similar attitude—if possible a more malignant one—awaited him. A disappointed man, he died in 1865 from a brain abscess that may have originated in an infection similar to that of his friend Kalletschka.

Further scientific developments eventually supported Semmelweiss's work and led to changes in medical practices that resulted in reduction and eventual prevention of puerperal fever. Louis Pasteur (1822–1895) and Sir Joseph Lister (1827–1912) demonstrated the presence and actions of microorganisms in causing infection. This paved the way to acceptance of the "germ theory" and promotion of antiseptic techniques in surgical procedures and wound care.

The 19th century initiated the use of drugs to alleviate the pains of childbirth. The use of ether as an anesthetic was first discovered in America, but it was first used for childbirth by Simpson in Great Britain. He brought back the lost art of podalic version by making it a safer procedure. Eventually he substituted chloroform for ether. As with almost every advance in medicine, it was opposed bitterly. The opposition was loudest and most vehement from the clergy, but, in 1853, Queen Victoria accepted it for delivery and by her action silenced most of the criticism. Nitrous oxide had been used in 1880 and has continued to be popular since that time.

Nursing and Maternal–Infant Care in America

Early efforts to organize and train nurses in America were spearheaded by wealthy laywomen inspired by "social feminism," which promoted use of maternal instinct and women's special sensitivity to human needs to make communities more homelike, warm, kind, and harmonious. Nurses, mainly working-class women, were not social feminists, but shared the "sanitary ideal" with the leisure-class women. This grew out of Florence Nightingale's work advocating order, discipline, and efficiency to attain cleanliness, health, and productivity and avoid waste. Early nurse training programs were instituted owing to pressure by upper-class women on hospital boards of directors, and often over the objections of physicians.[8]

During the 19th century, a laissez-faire ideology in the United States worked against physicians' efforts to organize and obtain licensure. There were many competing forms of health practitioners, including botanists, bonesetters, herbalists, nostrum vendors, homeopaths, and osteopaths. Medical schools proliferated without regulation, with many women students and some schools devoted to women or minorities (mainly blacks).[9]

Elizabeth Blackwell, the first woman to graduate from a "regular" US medical school (Geneva, New York, Medical College, 1849), founded the New York Infirmary for Women in 1857 and established the first recognized school of nursing in the United States at the New England Hospital for Women and Children (1872).[10] Women physicians of this period promoted educating the public (primarily women as gatekeepers to family health) about physiology, nutrition, exercise, cleanliness, and fresh air.[11]

Hospitals did not employ graduate nurses because nursing care was provided much more cheaply by students. Graduate nurses sought work in public-health and private-duty practice. At the turn of the century, this situation provided a perfect solution for several interrelated social and economic problems in American society. Nurses could serve a socializing and communicable-disease-control function by caring for the sick poor at home, providing health care to working-class families, including education into the sanitary ideal. As many such families were immigrants, this was an important way to socialize them into American values as well as to control infectious disease. Public-health nursing and visiting nurses' associations grew rapidly after 1900. However, the nursing profession had little control over this, with multitudes of agencies and companies operating their own nursing services.

Medical reformers at this time sought to reduce rates of disease and death by widespread application of scientific medicine and technology. Effective state licensing of medical schools began requiring longer training, standards for laboratories and basic science instruction, higher tuitions, and more rigorous licensing examinations. These raised the cost of medical education and decreased the student pool.

The Goldmark Report (1923), sponsored by the Rockefeller Foundation, investigated the problems in nursing and offered solutions. Several Goldmark recommendations encouraged upgrading educational standards, lengthening nurses' training to 2 years, starting nursing schools in universities, and recruiting women with high capacity.[12] However, by 1922, the supply of public-health nurses was large and their salaries were quite low. Decreasing immigration and improved economic status reduced the need for indigent home care and immigrant socialization. Infectious diseases were coming under control, urban death rates were dropping, and fewer sick were receiving home care as hospitals became more widely accepted and accessible. The separation between sick care and prevention was made wider by federal legislation and or-

Milestones in Maternal–Infant Health: United States

1876. The beginning of child-welfare legislation in the United States was the act passed by the New York State Legislature, granting to the *Society for the Prevention of Cruelty to Children* a charter that gave it wide power in the protection of child life.

1900. The *United States Census Bureau* was made a permanent organization. Up to this time, vital statistics were considered to be of so little importance in the United States that as soon as the population was tabulated and classified, the bureau was disbanded, to be reestablished and reorganized every 10 years.

1908. The *Division of Child Hygiene* was established in New York City, the first in the United States, and it was important enough to be recognized nationally. Josephine Baker, M.D., was appointed chief. This was a pioneer achievement, and the methods that evolved had no precedent.

1909. The *American Association for the Study and Prevention of Infant Mortality* was organized and held its first meeting in New Haven, Connecticut. This committee was composed of both professional and lay members and devoted itself entirely to problems connected with child life, particularly to studying and trying to correct the high mortality. At this time there were no records of births or deaths, and the causes of deaths were unknown.

The work of this organization was of profound significance. In 1918, its expanding activities caused it to change its name to the *American Child Hygiene Association,* and in 1923 the name was changed to the *American Child Health Association.* In 1935, after having contributed to every angle of this pioneer work, the association was disbanded.

1915. The *Birth Registration Area* was established by a federal act. The information is compiled in a uniform manner, giving the birth and the death statistics on which our information on mortality rates is based.

1919. The *American Committee on Maternal Welfare* was founded to stimulate medical cooperation with public and private agencies to protect the lives and health of mothers and infants and to teach principles and practice of personal hygiene and health to parents, physicians, nurses, and others dealing with the problems of maternity. The Committee was incorporated as a nonprofit organization in 1934 for the purpose of studying the maternal mortality rate in the United States and to publishing the *Bulletin of Maternal and Child Health.*

1921. The *Sheppard–Towner Bill* was passed by Congress, an act for the promotion of the welfare and hygiene of mothers and infants to be administered by the United States Children's Bureau. This bill was introduced in the 65th Congress by Congresswoman Jeanette Rankin of New Jersey. It was reported out of committee favorably but failed to pass.

In the 67th Congress the bill was again introduced by Senator Sheppard and Congressman Towner and, after much agitation, finally passed—an epoch in child-welfare legislation.

Because of this legislation there was created at once, in the states that did not already have them, departments that now are quite uniformly labeled Divisions or Bureaus of Maternal and Child Health.

1944. The *Public Health Service Act* brought together all existing laws affecting the public-health service. In addition, the act revised existing laws, provided authority for grants, and authorized expansion of the federal–state cooperative public-health programs that had bearing on maternal and child health programs. This act was to have a great indirect influence on the care of mothers and infants because of its provisions funding research and education of personnel needed in these areas.

1946. The *World Health Organization,* an agency of the United Nations, became a reality. The object of the organization is "the attainment of the highest possible level of health of all the peoples."

1962. The *National Institute of Child Health and Human Development* was authorized. The goal of this Institute was support of research and training in special health problems and needs of mothers and children. This Institute also conducts and supports research in the basic sciences relating to the processes of human growth and development, including prenatal development.

1964. The *Nurse Training Act,* one of the amendments of the Public Health Act, was an indirect aid to maternal and infant care. This act authorized grants for the expansion and improvement of nurse training, assistance to nursing students, scholarship grants to schools of nursing, and the establishment of a National Advisory Council on Nurse Training.

1965. *Amendments to the Social Security Act* provided for a new 5-year program of special project grants for comprehensive health care and services for school and preschool children, particularly in low-income family areas. These amendments also increased the authorization for money to support maternal and child health service programs.

PKU testing became mandatory for all infants in the states of Illinois and Michigan, thus setting a precedent for other states.

1966. The *Department of Health, Education, and Welfare,* (DHEW) issued a policy statement on birth control that stated that the Department would support, on request, health programs making family-planning information and services available. Due to this unique statement, federally supported family-planning programs have since slowly begun to evolve.

The *Federal Food, Drug and Cosmetic Act* was instituted on June 14, 1966. This legislation required label-

(continued)

(continued)

ing of ingredients of food represented for special dietary use. Infant foods, particularly, were specified.

The *Child Protection Act of 1966* banned the sale of toys and children's articles containing hazardous substances, regardless of labeling.

1967. *Medicaid* programs were increasing among the states to provide health care for low-income families. Care during pregnancy and child care were included.

1968. *Head Start* programs provided educational opportunities for underprivileged children of preschool age. These programs are often associated with nutritional and health screening programs.

1969. The *National Center for Family Planning* was established under the Health Services and Mental Health Administration, DHEW, to serve as a clearinghouse for information about contraception.

1973. The *United States Supreme Court* struck down almost all state statutes prohibiting or restricting abortion, leaving the abortion decision to the woman and her physician during the first 3 months of pregnancy; after this time the state could regulate abortion procedures only in the interest of maternal health. Essentially, the decision to abort became the right of the individual woman, with the state unable to interfere in her choice except to ensure that the abortion be performed under safe conditions.

National Center on Child Abuse and Neglect was established in DHEW's Office of Child Development to act as clearinghouse on information about child abuse. A *National Commission* was formed to study the role of the federal government in this area and the adequacy of state laws. Funds were made available to regional child-abuse prevention and treatment demonstration programs.

1975. The *National Advisory Council on Maternal, Infant and Fetal Nutrition* was established. Annual reports submitted to the President and Congress make continuing recommendations for administrative and legislative changes in programs aimed at low-income individuals at nutritional risk (PL 94–105).

The *WIC* program (Special Supplemental Food Program for Women, Infants and Children) was intended to provide low-income families with supplemental foods and nutrition education through local agencies, as an adjunct to good health during critical times of growth and development.

1976. The *Early and Periodic Screening, Diagnostic and Treatment* program (EPSDT) provided Medicaid-eligible children with regular health screening and treatment through federal funding.

1977. The *Child Health Assessment Act* (CHAP) extended the early and periodic screening program (EPSDT) to broaden eligibility and to require that treatment be given for conditions discovered during assessment, with exceptions of mental retardation, mental health, developmental problems, and dental care. This legislation also expanded and improved community-health centers.

1979. By this year *all 50 states had enacted laws* requiring every child to be immunized as a condition of entry into school.

1980. The *Children's Bureau* was disbanded after 68 years of significant contributions to the welfare of United States children. This is viewed by many as evidence of weakening of child advocacy in America.

1981. Congress authorized *Medicaid payments for services of nurse–midwives,* making this alternate care available to many women who previously lacked access.

---

ganized medicine's campaign to limit government involvement in health care.

The Sheppard-Towner Act (1921) was passed over medical opposition. It provided federal funds to states for educational programs promoting maternal and infant welfare, which public-health nurses would carry out through health-department programs. The nursing role became largely confined to infectious disease control and prevention and health education for the poor, in addition to specifically mandated maternal–child programs. By about 1930, voluntary nursing agencies declined as the demand for home care fell off. The major arena for public-health nursing became government health departments. As nurses gradually won mandatory licensure struggles, largely by making compromises that protected interests of their powerful adversaries (organized medicine and hospital associations), the labor

market shifted toward hospital employment. Efforts to limit entry into nursing or to increase the cost and length of education were compromised so hospitals would have an abundant labor supply. Medical dominance over policy-making groups and nursing education was also a legacy of the sexism and economic and social forces operating at the time nursing emerged as a profession.[13]

Nursing Contributions to Maternal–Child Health

Even within the confines of sociopolitical oppression, nurses made significant contributions to promoting the health of mothers and children in this country. In 1873, the New York Diet Kitchen Association organized a soup kitchen to take nourishing food to the sick at home. In

The Infant Milk Saga in New York

1873. The *New York Diet Kitchen Association,* the oldest public-health organization in America, was opened at the request of doctors from "de Milt Dispensary" on the lower East Side of New York City. It was first organized as a soup kitchen, and milk, gruel, beef tea, and cooked rice were taken to the sick in their homes, with the idea of restoring health. In 1892, they began to make formulas for sick babies and still later dispensed free milk, or sold it at 3 cents a quart.

1893. The first *Infant Milk Station* in the United States was established in New York City by Nathan Strauss. Through his persistence, milk was finally made safe through pasteurization, and many such stations were set up.

1907. The *New York Milk Committee* was organized. Its object was the reduction of infant mortality through the improvement of the city's milk supply. It established milk depots that proved beyond question their great value in the reduction of infant mortality by dispensing clean, pasteurized milk and by educating mothers.

1911. In New York City *the first strictly municipal baby-health stations* were organized under the jurisdiction of the Department of Health. The full cost of the work was borne by the municipality. Soon the dispensing of milk came to be of minor importance, and emphasis was placed on prevention. They are now called *Child-Health Stations.*

The *New York Milk Committee* (1907) made an investigation at the baby-health stations and found that 40% of all infant deaths (112 in 1000) occurred within the first month of life before the mothers registered their babies at the health stations. This indicated the necessity for care *before* birth. The committee then decided to carry out an experiment in antepartal work. They were convinced that much could be hoped for as a result of organized antepartal care.

1912. The *Babies' Welfare Association* (formerly the *Association of Infant Milk Stations* [1893]) represents the first comprehensive and successful attempt to coordinate the various child-welfare agencies in any community. All of the organizations of this type agreed to coordinate their activities by preventing duplication and overlapping without interfering with the organizations. In 1922, the name was changed to the *Children's Welfare Federation* of New York City. It continued to act as a clearinghouse and, among its other activites, managed the *Mother's Milk Bureau.*

1892 they began making formulas for sick babies and later dispensed free milk. Maria L. Daniels was the first nurse director and contributed a great deal to public and indigent health care (see chart above).

In 1926, this group was organized as the *Children's Health Service of New York.* The organization grew with the times, changing its program from curing the sick to preventive work—keeping well babies well. Although the organization devoted its major effort to work with babies and preschool children, it also included antepartal care in its program.

Clara Barton, a nurse in the American Civil War, was an early leader of the American Red Cross (organized in 1881). The Red Cross later recruited, taught, and certified nurses to teach prenatal classes, having an important early influence on childbirth education in the United States. In 1907 Mr. George H. F. Schrader gave money to the *Association for Improving Conditions of the Poor* (now the *Community Service Society*) for the salaries of two nurses to do antepartal work. This was the first consistent effort to prevent deaths of babies by caring for the mothers *before* the babies were born. The main reason given why antepartal care would be of value was that nurses in convalescent homes for postpartum mothers thought that if clients had better care during pregnancy, the health of mothers would be improved.

Between 1909 and 1914 Mrs. William Lowell Putnam, of Boston, promoted a demonstration of organized antepartal care. It was called the *Prenatal Care Committee* of the Women's Municipal League. The members of this committee worked in cooperation with the Boston Lying-In Hospital through Robert L. DeNormandie, M.D., of Harvard Medical School, Dr. Ruggles, of the then Homeopathic Hospital, and the Instructive District Nurses Association. The committee functioned long enough to establish the fact that good obstetric care was not possible without antepartal care.

Margaret Sanger, famous for her landmark work in promoting and making available birth control in the United States, was a public-health nurse when she opened the first birth control clinic in America (Brooklyn, 1916). She recognized the plight of many families overburdened with more children than they could feed or clothe. Poverty and ignorance compounded their problems. Since there was virtually no contraceptive information in the United States, Sanger went to France and learned about methods used for generations to prevent large families. She returned to the United States and published periodicals and other literature about limiting births. Because she used the mails, the Justice Department indicted her for violation of the Comstock Law (which classified birth control information as obscene and pornographic and prohibited contraception and abortion). She left the country to prepare her defense, traveling in Canada, England, and the Netherlands (where birth control was accepted and maternal mortality was one third that in the United States). Influential friends convinced President Wilson to drop the case against Sanger that time, but when she opened the first birth control clinic in 1916, she and her sister (Ethel Byrne, also a nurse) were arrested and spent 30 days in a workhouse. Sanger continued her work by teaching, holding conferences, founding organizations, and writing publications. Sanger founded the *National Committee on Federal Legislation for Birth Control,* which later became the *Planned Parenthood Federation of America* (1928) and the *International Planned Parenthood Federation* (1952).

Between 1910 and 1930, the birth rate in women ages 15 to 44 dropped 38%.[14] Sanger probably influenced the New York Academy of Medicine's milestone resolution to support birth control in 1931. The American Medical Association announced its support in 1937. Sanger testified before Congress in 1932 as an authority on birth control. She was inducted into the Nursing Hall of Fame, American Nurses' Association, in 1976.

Lillian Wald, a nurse, has been credited with suggesting the formation of a federal children's bureau. She is also a member of the Nursing Hall of Fame (1983). In 1906 the United States Census Bureau published mortality statistics that drew attention to the appalling loss of life among babies and children. Up to this time, very little thought had been given to maternal and infant protection.

Although the first legislative efforts to form a children's bureau in 1906 failed, President Roosevelt convened the First White House Conference on Children in 1910. The group of professional and lay people at the conference recommended a bureau be formed, and in 1912 the *United States Children's Bureau* was established. The bureau was to set up special machinery to study and protect the child and to study all matters pertaining to the welfare of children and child life among all classes of people, to assemble and accumulate factual information, and to disseminate this information throughout the country.

The *National Society for the Prevention of Blindness* was created in 1916 after much pioneer work and investigation, locally and throughout the states, by Carolyn Van Blarcom, R.N. Through these investigations it was learned that by far the greatest cause of blindness was ophthalmia of the newborn. This finding led to the passing of a law compelling all physicians and midwives to use prophylaxis in newborn babies' eyes. Also, as a direct result of Miss Van Blarcom's surveys, a school for lay midwives, Belleview School for Midwives (no longer in existence), was started. Miss Van Blarcom took out a midwife's license and was the first nurse in the United States so to register. The first obstetric nursing textbook to be written by a nurse is credited to Miss

Van Blarcom. Her later contribution to the better care of mothers and babies was to secure for Johns Hopkins Hospital the E. Bayard Halsted Fund for medical research.

In 1917 the Women's City Club of New York organized an antepartal clinic that became the *Maternity Service Association.* Francis Perkins was the first executive secretary, and Miss Mabel Choate, as president, provided stimulating leadership. Dr. Ralph W. Lobenstine, a famous obstetrician, gave much time, labor, authority, and direction as chairman of the medical board. In 1918, this organization was incorporated as the *Maternity Center Association* and carried out the first extensive piece of organized antepartal work in the United States. Miss Anne Stevens was director. Miss Annie W. Goodrich's wise counsel, as a member of the nursing committee, gave impetus to the organization's accomplishments. Louis I. Dublin, Ph.D., associated with this movement from the beginning, made an analysis of the first 4000 records collected by the association. This revealed the startling fact that, through antepartal care, 50% of the lives of mothers might be saved and 60% of the lives of babies. Antepartal training and experience were extended to nurses throughout the world. This piece of intensive antepartal work fired increased interest in the care of mothers and babies. In 1929, the Maternity Center Association opened a school for the training of nurse–midwives.

Emergence of Professional Maternity Nursing

A variety of factors, cultural, social, and technological, have had important roles in shaping the growth and development of maternity nursing. One of the most important and most direct of these factors was the shift from home to hospital delivery. At the turn of the century, almost all women were delivered at home by a midwife or a physician. At the present time, more than 90% of mothers deliver in the hospital. Two other factors, in turn, brought about this change to hospital delivery and helped shape the kind of care received there. An increase in the understanding of asepsis made physicians much more attentive to this aspect of care, particularly for maternity clients. A growing conviction developed that delivery in a hospital was mandatory.

As more women began delivering in hospitals, provision had to be made for quick, efficient, aseptic care. Certain timesaving devices and work-simplification procedures were borrowed from industry. "Assembly-line care" soon flourished. Compliance with timesaving techniques, performance of the somewhat ritualistic procedures called for to maintain asepsis, and the increasingly bureaucratic structure generated by the complex, modernizing hospital all went into defining and shaping the very essence of maternity care. Hence, there arose the ritualistic, rigid adherence to rules and procedures (with rather little thought to the mother) that characterizes so much of maternity care even today. It was during these early times that antepartal care was conceived and developed as an aspect of preventive medicine. Thus, women increasingly had longer contact with their physicians during the childbearing time and this, together with the still prevalent Victorian notion of dependency, served to cement the obstetric relationship. To justify this relationship, physicians began to insist even more strongly on hospital deliveries.

Maternity nursing developed as obstetrics developed and, not surprisingly, was based on the medical model of obstetrics in which pathology was the main focus. Thus, the nursing student's experiences were oriented to the physical care of her clients, with emphasis on technical competence. Much of the student's clinical experience was in reality service to the hospital. This type of service-to-the-institution, technical competence orientation produced a nurse who was efficient in organizing care for many clients. However, because of the great number of clients, no in-depth nursing therapy was either attempted or possible. Little or no public-health experience was offered, and the nurse gradually became more institution (*i.e.,* hospital) oriented. The nurse became the physician's veritable right arm.

Compartmentalization and Routinization

In the third and fourth decades of this century, hospitals became larger and more complex and the nurse gradually had to assume more and more administrative and organizational duties. Similarly, medical science enlarged and, with the new knowledge and progress, more functions, formerly in the province of the physician, were delegated to the nurse. These factors, together with the acute hospital personnel shortage precipitated by World War II, combined to develop and promote impersonal routinized care for the mother and her infant.

As more became known about the transmission and control of pathogenic organisms, various subunits were designated for the use of the mother, the well newborn, the sick newborn, and the premature infant. Thus, restrictions and compartmentalization of nursing function (nursery nurse, postpartum nurse, and so on) proliferated in the name of better technique but at the expense of unity in the mother–infant relationship. Perhaps even worse was the compartmentalization of thinking and communication that also evolved. The postpartum nurse knew and cared about the progress of the particular mothers in her charge while they were on the ward. She rarely knew how they responded to their pregnancy in general. She might know something about how they had withstood their labors, but only in the physical

sense, and then only in relation to their immediate postpartum course. The nursery nurse knew about the babies in her nursery, but very little about the parents who would take them home or the environment into which they would go.

The experience of childbearing, once common to all members of the social group and centered in the home, with involvement of most family members, had now become a disjointed, technical, and alien process about which parents were generally ignorant. Complex and mystical, childbirth had become the province of physicians and specialized nurses, to be enacted in a strange, threatening institution in which the parents were the most powerless members.

Impact on the Woman and Family

As a result of these practices, a woman felt generally in the dark regarding her pregnancy, labor, and delivery. There was usually little or no exchange of educational information between the physician and the pregnant woman, and most of the decisions made about the pregnancy were made by the physician. Much of the information that a woman might obtain about childbearing and childbirth was provided by family members and friends who would share their experiences with the woman. Often these stories would emphasize the pain and suffering women had to endure to give birth—information that only increased the pregnant woman's feelings of anxiety and apprehension about her forthcoming labor and delivery.

When a woman's labor started, she usually was taken to the hospital. Once the woman was admitted to the hospital, she usually was separated from the father. The labor and delivery rooms were off-limits to the father, relatives, and friends of the woman for the duration of the intrapartum period. With little knowledge about the usual course of labor and birth, and having been isolated from all support persons, the laboring woman relied heavily on the advice of the obstetric staff to help her cope with the discomfort and apprehension she was experiencing. Analgesics and anesthetics that were administered by the well-meaning obstetric staff to relieve the woman's pain also relieved her of her sense of control and self-esteem. More often than not, a woman would awaken after childbirth unaware that she had, in fact, given birth. It was not uncommon for the father, not the mother, to be the first to become acquainted with the newborn, though usually only through the nursery room window.

During the postpartum period the mother would feed her infant according to the hospital schedule. When this task was completed, the infant usually was returned to the nursery where the father, mother, and other children could gather to view the newborn. In some hospitals, fathers were not allowed to touch their infants until the infant was discharged. The importance of efficiency and competency at specific medical tasks was often emphasized in the nurse's role during this period, and client advocacy and education had little or nothing to do with maternity nursing. It is not difficult to understand why consumers became dissatisfied with this kind of maternity care. They began to question healthcare professionals about the rationales for some of these practices; gradually their demands for more involvement in pregnancy and childbirth began to have a significant impact on maternity care in this country (Table 47-1).

Family-Centered Care

The concept of *family-centered maternity care* began to gain support among nursing circles during the 1960s. This approach advocated consideration of other members of the family, particularly the father, during predelivery and postdelivery care. The pregnant woman, who had been viewed largely in isolation as a medical problem, was recognized as having social and emotional needs that deserved the nurse's attention as did her physical needs. It seems strange now that nurses had to be reminded that pregnant women had families with psychological needs for some involvement in this most

TABLE 47-1

Characteristics of Maternity Care and Emergence of Maternity Nursing

Maternity Care	Maternity Nursing
Birth a family and community event, integrated into everyday life	Midwives usual birth attendants, precursors to maternity nurse
Development of scientific medicine and physician participation in childbirth	Gradual replacement of midwives by physicians as birth attendants
Increasing understanding of asepsis and increased technology in obstetrics	Nursing emerged as women's occupation, paralleling growth of scientific medicine
Growing emphasis on hospital deliveries rather than home births	Nurses in obstetrics taught by medical (pathological) model
Increasing numbers of women delivering in the hospital	Nursing students focused upon technical competence and physical care of clients in hospitals
Necessity for efficient, organized aseptic care in hospitals, due to organizational structure	Nursing students provided service to hospitals where trained
Borrowing of timesaving approaches and work-efficient procedures from industry	Nursing orientation was toward efficient care of a number of clients, without in-depth nursing therapy (as there was no theoretical foundation)
"Assembly-line care" in hospitals	Institution-oriented nurses became the physician's "right arm"
Ritualistic practices, rigid adherence to rules and procedures	Development of the humanistic-supportive nursing model as distinct from the pathological-intervention medical model
Impersonal, routine care	
Resurgence of family and participant focus in childbearing, through natural childbirth and consumer movements	Expansion of the maternity nurse's role to include personalized care, parent education, counseling and psychosocial support, advocacy, alternative-care services to childbearing families
Pressure for change in hospital routines and procedures, alternative birth approaches	
Development of family-centered maternity care, participant childbirth, rooming-in, alternate birth centers	Emergence of new roles (nurse practitioner, clinical specialist) and resurgence of nurse–midwifery

momentous event, as well as very real practical problems and social concerns that often could be helped by nursing attention. But this had been the outcome of years of emphasis on efficiency and routinization on the one hand and influence of the medical model on the other.

Prepared Childbirth

Contributing to family-centered maternity care was the *participant childbirth movement*, which brought about significant changes in the practice of obstetrics through consumer pressure. Its purposes closely paralleled the family-centered approach, but even greater involvement of the father was advocated. As the ideas and techniques of Dick-Read, Lamaze, and Bradley caught on in the United States, childbearing women and their partners began to seek knowledge and demand a right to make choices in the conduct of their own pregnancies, labors, and deliveries. Women wanted to be aware and awake, to feel a central part of the process, to become equipped to cope with the stress of labor without heavy medication, and to have their partners by their side to share the experience. Prepared childbirth usually involved education about the processes of parturition and instruction in techniques to reduce pain perception and enhance the sense of control over the process (see Chaps. 20 and 26).

Fathers frequently served as labor coaches, and through this type of involvement pressure was brought to bear on hospitals to allow their presence in the labor room. It seemed ludicrous to allow fathers to assist their partners during labor, only to dismiss them at the climax of the entire process. This gain was not achieved easily, and it took some years before reluctant physicians and nurses accepted the fact that prepared fathers were not going to faint or become irate over necessary procedures or during unexpected complications (Fig. 47-2).

Mother–Baby Couple Care

Following increased concern about family involvement in the childbearing process, *mother–baby couple care* was instituted in many postpartum units to facilitate development of the early mother–infant relationship. The forerunner of this practice was *rooming-in*, when mothers who elected to do so (and who could afford a private room or could be placed with a roommate who also wanted rooming-in) would have their babies placed in the room with them during the hospitalization period. Rooming-in had a varying course over the years, with persistent professional resistance that mothers had to overcome, often only to be left largely on their own with their new babies.

Mother–baby couple care represents a commitment on the part of the postpartum and nursery staff to re-

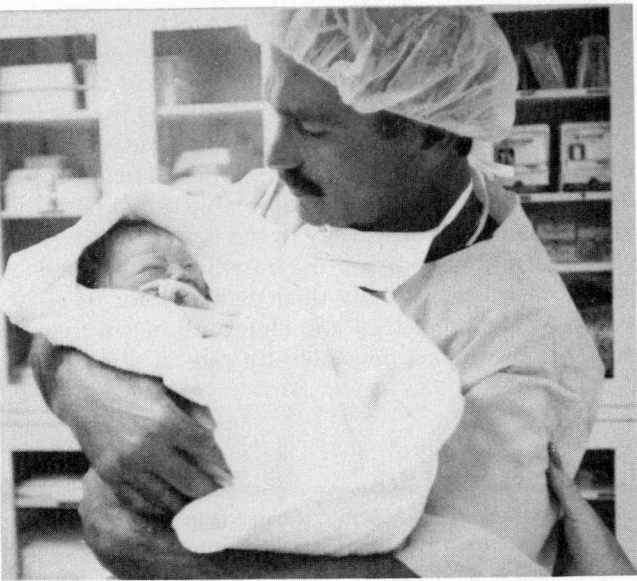

FIGURE 47-2

A father who has participated in the labor and delivery proudly holds his newborn minutes after the birth. (Courtesy of Memorial Medical Center of Long Beach, Long Beach, CA)

structure the hospital units so mothers and babies may be together the greater part of the day and night. Usually satellite nurseries are developed to serve each wing of the maternity unit, and postpartum and nursery nurses move back and forth within the wing or area. Babies are with their mothers except for specified times when they are in the nursery for physical examinations, tests, or procedures, or if the mother or baby is temporarily sick.

Although the logistics of mother–baby couple care require some working out, and although nurses need some retraining in the area of their lesser experience, the benefits of each mother–baby couple having the same nurse responsible for their care are enormous. In this way, the same nurse knows the condition and needs of both mother and baby, enhancing the development of the mother–infant relationship through intimacy and close contact, immediate response to needs or problems, and elimination of the communication gap.

Breast-Feeding

The back-to-nature movement that was an expected reaction to the increasing use of artificial substances and chemical additives in a wide variety of materials and products served as an impetus to the rediscovery of *breast-feeding*. Organizations such as the LaLeche League were formed to help mothers relearn the art of breast-feeding and to encourage success through information and support. In response to maternal need, postpartum nurses began to learn how to help mothers initiate satisfactory breast-feeding patterns during their first days of nursing their babies in the hospital.

Expanding Roles in Maternity Nursing

In the mid-1960s experiments began to expand nursing roles to include greater responsibility for primary-care treatment of common problems and health needs. Early programs were started by physician–nurse teams (Ford, R.N. and Silver, M.D. in Denver; Resnick, R.N. and Lewis, M.D. in Los Angeles) to expand nursing roles in pediatrics[15] and adult health.[16] In 1971 the *National Commission for the Study of Nursing and Nursing Education*, Jerome Lysaught, director, reported a study of nursing roles and recommended that nursing roles be expanded, educational systems repatterned, and nursing input into health care increased. Also that year the American Nurses Association (ANA) and American Academy of Pediatrics jointly developed guidelines for *training pediatric nurse associates* and held a national conference to implement these. The ANA and American College of Obstetricians and Gynecologists also met to draw up guidelines for training clinical nurse specialists in obstetrics–gynecology.

In 1972 the *Committee to Study Extended Roles for Nurses* reported to the secretary of DHEW that functions of nurses "need to be broadened [so they can] assume broader responsibility in primary care, acute care, and long-term care." The new nurse practitioner was functioning in expanded nursing roles in many areas, including obstetrics, pediatrics, psychiatry, and medical–surgical nursing.

In 1973 the *National Commission for the Study of Nursing and Nursing Education*, directed by Jerome Lysaught, reported on the implementation phase of its study. To encourage the expansion of nursing practice, it conducted educational and informational activities aimed at nursing professionals and the public, developed a national joint practice commission between medicine and nursing with state counterparts, and developed statewide planning committees to generate changes in patterns of education and practice.

These expanded nursing roles developed in two general directions. The nurse practitioner role focused mainly on primary, ambulatory care and the nurse clinical specialist role focused on secondary–tertiary, hospital care.

Nurse Practitioner

As the nurse practitioner role evolved, it encompassed additional skills in the techniques of physical diagnosis that were formerly in the realm of medicine, as well as the knowledge base to diagnose and treat common problems and minor illness. Health prevention and maintenance, including examination, testing, and education, as well as management of stabilized chronic illness, are also included in nurse practitioner functions. The nurse practitioner combines the nurse's sensitivity to emotional needs and focus on adaptation and social aspects of client care with the techniques and knowledge of medicine to diagnose and treat pathophysiological problems. These nurses usually practice in a primary-care setting, defined as the first contact with the health-care system in any given episode of illness, and are responsible for continuance of care, including maintenance of health, evaluation and management of symptoms, and appropriate referrals.[17,18]

Maternity Nurse Practitioner. The maternity nurse practitioner, or ob-gyn nurse practitioner, provides prenatal care for uncomplicated pregnancies in conjunction with a physician consultant. The nurse takes a health and pregnancy history, performs the physical and obstetric examination, orders and interprets laboratory and other diagnostic studies, plans for necessary treatments and medications in conjunction with the physician, and assesses family relationships and psychosocial needs.

Throughout the pregnancy, the maternity nurse practitioner sees the woman on antepartal visits, sometimes alternating with the physician, evaluates the progress of the pregnancy, and manages minor physical problems. Information and counseling related to pregnancy and childbirth and assessment of the couple's adjustments and family problems are also part of the nurse practitioner's role. Referrals to community agencies, prepared childbirth classes, and other medical specialties may also be made. Most maternity nurse practitioners are skilled in provision of contraception and can select appropriate methods for the client, including oral contraceptives, intrauterine devices, and diaphragms, and teach about their use and about other methods.

Family Nurse Practitioner. Family nurse practitioners also provide care during pregnancy. They are generalists who care for all family members similarly to family-practice physicians. In addition to the functions described above for maternity nurse practitioners, family nurse practitioners provide postdelivery care for the baby as it grows, thus providing continuity throughout the reproductive process except during the intrapartum phase.

Maternity Clinical Specialist

Maternity clinical specialists undergo advanced study of maternity nursing at the graduate level and are able to provide in-depth intervention for many of the ad-

The Pregnant Patient's Bill of Rights

American parents are becoming increasingly aware that health professionals do not always have scientific data to support common American obstetrical practices and that many of these practices are carried out primarily because they are part of medical and hospital tradition. In the last forty years many artificial practices have been introduced which have changed childbirth from a physiological event to a very complicated medical procedure in which all kinds of drugs are used and procedures carried out, sometimes unnecessarily, and many of them potentially damaging for the baby and even for the mother. A growing body of research makes it alarmingly clear that every aspect of traditional American hospital care during labor and delivery must now be questioned as to its possible effect on the future well-being of both the obstetric patient and her unborn child.

One in every 35 children born in the United States today will eventually be diagnosed as retarded; one in every 10 to 17 children has been found to have some form of brain dysfunction or learning disability requiring special treatment. Such statistics are not confined to the lower socioeconomic group but cut across all segments of American society.

New concerns are being raised by childbearing women because no one knows what degree of oxygen depletion, head compression, or traction by forceps the unborn or newborn infant can tolerate before that child sustains permanent brain damage or dysfunction. The recent findings regarding the cancer-related drug diethylstilbestrol have alerted the public to the fact that neither the approval of a drug by the U.S. Food and Drug Administration nor the fact that a drug is prescribed by a physician serves as a guarantee that a drug or medication is safe for the mother or her unborn child. In fact, the American Academy of Pediatrics Committee on Drugs has recently stated that there is no drug, whether prescription or over-the-counter remedy, which has been proven safe for the unborn child.

The Pregnant Patient has the right to participate in decisions involving her well-being and that of her unborn child, unless there is a clear-cut medical emergency that prevents her participation. In addition to the rights set forth in the American Hospital Association's "Patient's Bill of Rights" (which has also been adopted by the New York City Department of Health) the Pregnant Patient, because she represents TWO patients rather than one, should be recognized as having the additional rights listed below.

1. *The Pregnant Patient has the right*, prior to the administration of any drug or procedure, to be informed by the health professional caring for her of any potential direct or indirect effects, risks or hazards to herself or her unborn or newborn infant which may result from the use of a drug or procedure prescribed for or administered to her during pregnancy, labor, birth, or lactation.
2. *The Pregnant Patient has the right*, prior to the proposed therapy, to be informed, not only of the benefits, risks, and hazards of the proposed therapy but also of known alternative therapy, such as available childbirth education classes which could help to prepare the Pregnant Patient physically and mentally to cope with the discomfort or stress of pregnancy and the experience of childbirth, thereby reducing or eliminating her need for drugs and obstetric intervention. She should be offered such information early in her pregnancy in order that she may make a reasoned decision.
3. *The Pregnant Patient has the right*, prior to the administration of any drug, to be informed by the health professional who is prescribing or administering the drug to her that any drug which she receives during pregnancy, labor and birth, no matter how or when the drug is taken or administered, may adversely affect her unborn baby, directly or indirectly, and that there is no drug or chemical which has been proven safe for the unborn child.
4. *The Pregnant Patient has the right*, if cesarean section is anticipated, to be informed prior to the administration of any drug, and preferably prior to the hospitalization, that minimizing her and, in turn, her baby's intake of nonessential preoperative medicine will benefit her baby.
5. *The Pregnant Patient has the right*, prior to the administration of a drug or procedure, to be informed if there is NO properly controlled follow-up research which has established the safety of the drug or procedure with regard to its direct and/or indirect effects on the physiological, mental and neurological development of the child exposed, via the mother, to the drug or procedure during pregnancy, labor, birth, or lactation (this would apply to virtually all drugs and the vast majority of obstetric procedures).
6. *The Pregnant Patient has the right*, prior to the administration of any drug, to be informed of the brand name and generic name of the drug in order that she may advise the health professional of any past adverse reaction to the drug.
7. *The Pregnant Patient has the right* to determine for herself, without pressure from her attendant, whether she will accept the risks inherent in the proposed therapy or refuse a drug or procedure.

(continued)

(continued)

8. *The Pregnant Patient has the right* to know the name and qualifications of the individual administering a medication or procedure to her during labor or birth.
9. *The Pregnant Patient has the right* to be informed, prior to the administration of any procedure, whether that procedure is being administered to her for her or her baby's benefit (medically indicated) or as an elective procedure (for convenience or teaching purposes).
10. *The Pregnant Patient has the right* to be accompanied during the stress of labor and birth by someone she cares for, and to whom she looks for emotional comfort and encouragement.
11. *The Pregnant Patient has the right* after appropriate medical consultation to choose a position for labor and for birth which is least stressful to her baby and to herself.
12. *The Obstetric Patient has the right* to have her baby cared for at her bedside if her baby is normal, and to feed her baby according to her baby's needs rather than according to the hospital regimen.
13. *The Obstetric Patient has the right* to be informed in writing of the name of the person who actually delivered her baby and the professional qualifications of that person. This information should also be on the birth certificate.
14. *The Obstetric Patient has the right* to be informed if there is any known or indicated aspect of her or her baby's care or condition which may cause her or her baby later difficulty or problems.
15. *The Obstetric Patient has the right* to have her and her baby's hospital medical records complete, accurate, and legible and to have their records, including Nurses' Notes, retained by the hospital until the child reaches at least the age of majority, or, alternatively, to have the records offered to her before they are destroyed.
16. *The Obstetric Patient*, both during and after her hospital stay, *has the right* to have access to her complete hospital medical records, including Nurses' Notes, and to receive a copy upon payment of a reasonable fee and without incurring the expense of retaining an attorney.

It is the obstetric patient and her baby, not the health professional, who must sustain any trauma or injury resulting from the use of a drug or obstetric procedure. The observation of the rights listed above will not only permit the obstetric patient to participate in the decisions involving her and her baby's health care, but will help to protect the health professional and the hospital against litigation arising from resentment or misunderstanding on the part of the mother.

(Reprinted by permission of the Committee on Patient's Rights, Box 1900, New York, N.Y. 10001)

aptational and physiological problems encountered in maternity care. Frequently, clinical specialists have an area of expertise within the specialty field, such as a maternity clinical specialist with special expertise in the care of pregnant diabetics, breast-feeding mothers, parents experiencing neonatal death or abnormalities, Rh-sensitized mothers, and so on. These nurses with master's degrees also serve as consultants to other maternity nursing staff, assisting them to plan care for difficult problems or special situations encountered in the unit. Although clinical specialists also may be involved in staff education, their primary function is direct client services using a high degree of knowledge, skill, and competence in their area of specialty.[19]

Directions for Maternity Nursing

To remain congruent with changes in the health-care delivery system, maternity nursing also must adapt and grow in new and diverse directions. The desires of the consumers of maternity care also signify a growing need for changes. This is because the routinized and standardized care organized in settings more convenient for the providers than for the consumers of care are less and less acceptable. Parents are asking for full participation in all phases of childbearing, the right to be involved in decisions affecting their bodies and health, and the right to institute practices that they believe are important for the happiness and well-being of parents and baby (see The Pregnant Patient's Bill of Rights).

A growing body of literature and research is reaffirming the importance of early and continued close contact between mother and baby. The importance of natural practices, such as breast-feeding and avoidance of highly processed and chemically preserved foods, suggests that health professionals support rather than discourage parents who wish to follow these practices.

The appropriateness of routine delivery of normal, uncomplicated maternity clients in the hospital with its focus on disease and illness is being questioned. However, new data about the importance of immediate, active intervention in delivery of high-risk pregnancies and the postdelivery care of depressed, sick, or anoxic infants reinforce the need for highly trained personnel and well-equipped delivery rooms and intensive care nurseries. The situation appears paradoxical, and answers will not be easy.

Whatever the future portends, its hallmark will be change. Health care, medical care, and nursing care are all undergoing major upheavals. The issues of national health insurance, Diagnostic Related Groups (DRGs), the role of third-party payers, problems with malpractice insurance, federal controls, and peer review organizations, changing practice laws of nursing and medicine, the exorbitant costs of health care and the increasingly vociferous consumer advocacy movement, and the development of health-maintenance organizations and community-health networks, all signify that health care in this country is experiencing radical changes. Maternity nursing must ride the winds of change, and nursing leaders must take the initiative in shaping the new form this specialty will take in the years to come to serve the best interests and needs of families during all phases of childbearing.

Nursing Roles and the Women's Movement

Part of the reason why nursing was so subjugated by medicine was the powerless status of women when nursing emerged as a profession. Working women were viewed with suspicion and distaste in the early 1900s.

Nurses have conducted, with more or less vigor, the long struggle toward more responsibility and autonomy that parallels the women's movement for full and equal status. Nursing leaders during the first part of the 20th century kept their focus on improving nurse training and obtaining licensure and failed to see the significance of more pervasive feminist issues such as the right to vote, independent legal status, and comparable professional status.[20] When hospital nursing responsibilities expanded after World War II, assuming greater technical skills once medicine's domain, with strategic positions in the institution and middle-management duties, cultural prescriptions for a domestic woman's role were threatened. The authority vested in nursing positions was viewed as anomalous and unnatural, and there were fears that women with power would abuse it and insinuations that competent nurses were questionable women. The perceived conflict between work and femininity was resolved by reverting to the old argument that women, by their nature, had a special fitness for nursing care.[21]

The women's movement that exploded during the 1960s rejected this feminine mystique and all the supporting social structures and ideologies based on concepts of female inferiority, submissiveness, frailty, and limited abilities. It upheld women's rights to equal status and economic rewards and questioned sex-based oc-

cupational roles. Through years of struggle in the courts, classrooms, lecture halls, media, and political arenas, women have made enormous strides in attaining greater independence, work opportunities, educational opportunities, and recognition in society. In nursing, the attitudes, values, and strategies used by feminists have influenced economic gains (increased wages and benefits), power and status (recognized structures for nursing input in workplace decision making), political gains (expanded practice through legislation and regulation, reimbursement, consultative powers), and the nurse–physician relationship (less gaming, more honest and equitable interactions).

The women's health movement has had profound effects on the care of women and children. Its work falls into three main categories: changing established health institutions, changing consumer and provider consciousness, and providing health-related services. Some results have been expanding health-insurance benefits to include contraception and abortion, developing guidelines to prevent sterilization abuse, client information and labeling for drugs, greater availability of nondrug and non-invasive contraceptives, growth of self-help groups, more emphasis on self-examination and knowledge of one's body, greater availability of abortion and changes in laws, and many other educational and women's health-clinic services.[22] Women's health groups also have supported childbirth preparation, alternative birthing, greater parental control over the processes of pregnancy, labor, and delivery, early discharge after normal delivery, and prevention of cesarean delivery. Natural approaches to treating many common women's problems are advocated and published in the growing body of literature fostered by the women's health movement.[23] Many nurses are involved in writing feminist health literature and providing services.

Alternatives in Maternity Care

Resurgence of Home Births

Routine maternity care in many areas of the country includes expensive, sophisticated tests and procedures that many women, and their partners, regard as invasive and interfering manuevers on the part of health-care professionals. The increasing reliance of obstetricians on such procedures as routine fetal monitoring, amniotomy, administration of intravenous fluids, and administration of oxytocic drugs during the course of uncomplicated labors and births illustrates the still prevalent belief that pregnancy and childbirth are pathological, not normal, processes.[24,25] Furthermore, the increasing cost of maternity and obstetric services, especially when unnecessary tests and procedures are used routinely, is a very real concern of expectant families. As a result, there has been a gradual increase in the number of home births occurring in this country during the past decade.[26,27]

This current trend concerns both the consumers and providers of maternity care. The primary concern of both these groups is the potential complications that can occur during any normal birth but that can be even more life-threatening to either the mother or the fetus when the birth occurs at home without adequate medical backup or quick access to emergency equipment. Although some physicians and nurses are proponents of home births that use good medical and emergency backup systems, most health-care professionals regard this practice as exposing the mother and the fetus to unnecessary danger.[28]

For a small but increasing number of women, however, home birth remains the birth alternative of choice. Although there are many different types of women choosing to deliver at home, the general profile has been found to be a white, married, 25-year-old woman who has attended college. The five most important reasons given by women for electing a home birth are the following:

- Desire to have the baby close to the mother after birth
- Desire to have the father present during birth
- Viewing pregnancy as a normal process and hence out of place in a hospital
- Having more control over the childbirth experience at home
- Wanting to give birth in familiar surroundings[29]

Mistrust of the hospital and negative feelings about the hospital environment are important factors in the decision to give birth at home. The main issues involved are fear of medical intervention, loss of control over the labor process, the delivery and postdelivery environment, and dislike of hospital routines and professional attitudes. Many women view their labor as a vulnerable time and want their energies free to focus on this demanding process. They do not want a confrontation over such practices as using drugs for pain relief, stimulation of labor with oxytocins, use of monitoring devices, use of amniotomies, or such medical interventions as forceps or episiotomies at delivery. Many women also feel that they cannot maintain as much control over their environment at the hospital, even in birthing centers. There is an inherent tension in the hospital atmosphere that is perceived as increasing a woman's pain and complications. Hospital routines are seen as more in the interest of the institution and its staff than in the interest of the childbearing family. Women are concerned about early and continued physical contact with

the infant, early cutting of the umbilical cord, use of silver nitrate in the infant's eyes, and giving babies sugar water to supplement breast-feedings. They also want to be able to use the delivery position of their choice and to avoid being moved just before delivery.

Birth to such women is a natural, normal phenomenon, and home is the natural setting when there are no medical problems. The hospital is seen as a place for the ill, not the healthy undergoing a normal physiological process. The hospital poses additional dangers in some women's views. Medical intervention during labor and delivery is associated with increased risks for the mother and infant, and women fear unnecessary intervention when in an atmosphere supportive of it. The risk of infection is seen as greater in the hospital because of virulent germ strains (as has often been seen in nosocomial infections) and staff errors and oversights leading to breaks in technique or exposure to contamination. Alternative birth centers are unattractive to some women for many of these same reasons. The hospital atmosphere still prevails, and if there are any complications (even minor ones) the woman is transferred to the regular labor unit. One woman expressed her concerns as follows:

> They charge a lot of money to pretend you're having the birth at home. People there are still trained in complications. I was afraid they'd think, since the machinery's here, why not use it?[29]

Women who give birth at home generally find that the experience surpasses their expectations. It is a powerful reinforcement of their ability to undergo childbirth and to maintain control without much pain. The bonding between mother, father, and infant has been described as "unbelievable." Siblings observing the birth also undergo remarkable bonding. It is described as a very strengthening experience for the family.

Because the home offers many qualities not available in hospitals, women continue to choose to deliver at home. Health practitioners who oppose home births deny this alternative to their clients and eliminate a practice option for themselves; their expertise cannot be brought to bear in assisting women to have optimal birth experiences. Greater responsibility for providing emergency obstetric equipment and transportation in the event of complications has been suggested as an appropriate response by health professionals.

Alternative Birth Centers

In 1978, a joint statement entitled "The Development of Family-Centered Maternity/Newborn Care in Hospitals" was issued by the Interprofessional Task Force on Health Care of Women and Children.[30] This task force was composed of representatives from the American College of Nurse–Midwives, the American Nurses' Association, the Nurses' Association of the American College of Obstetricians and Gynecologists, the American College of Obstetricians, and the American Academy of Pediatrics. The representatives from these groups collaborated and agreed upon the following definition of family-centered maternity/newborn care:

> Family-centered maternity/newborn care can be defined as the delivery of safe, quality health care while recognizing, focusing on, and adapting to both the physical and psychological needs of the client-patient, the family, and the newly born. The emphasis is on the provision of maternity/ newborn health care which fosters family unity while maintaining physical safety.[30]

The joint statement prepared and issued by this group of professionals also provided guidelines for implementing family-centered maternity/newborn care in hospitals interested in incorporating such programs into their obstetric units. The statement advocated the establishment of such services as the following:

- Childbirth classes for the entire family
- Continuing education for maternity staff, including information on current childbirth trends and techniques
- A more liberal definition of family to include other supportive persons important to the mother
- Development of birthing rooms as options in addition to standard labor and delivery rooms
- Development of the option of early discharge of mother and infant with appropriate follow-up visits to assess early postpartum progress

This professional statement in 1978 reflects increased awareness of consumer demands and changing client values related to maternity care. As a result of a number of forces, childbearing couples are more knowledgeable and concerned consumers. The prepared childbirth movement, the women's health movement, and the rise of consumer consciousness are among these forces.[31] Two common themes are the emphasis on client control and decision-making power, and the desire for highly personalized health care. The unmet needs of a large group of uncomplicated, low-risk pregnant women within the traditional hospital obstetric service led to demands for alternatives; the concept of a *birth center* was one alternative that emerged recently. For many expectant families, the alternative birth center (ABC) provides an acceptable option to the traditional medical delivery of an infant in the hospital, as well as a safe alternative to giving birth at home.

Physical Setup and Procedures

An ABC usually consists of one or more private birthing rooms where a woman labors and gives birth to her infant. The woman can be accompanied by the father and, in some ABCs, by her children and other family members or friends. The physical setup of the birthing room is quite different from the standard labor and delivery rooms used in traditional obstetric units. Usually there is a bed that is large enough for the mother, father, and their newborn to recline comfortably. Chairs and a dresser are included in the furnishings, as are plants and pictures. In some ABCs parents are encouraged to bring their own pictures and wall hangings to decorate the room so that the room is similar to their own home environment. Often a stereo is provided in the room for the laboring woman to listen to her favorite music as a means of relaxing and maintaining inner calm during the labor and birth. Private bathroom facilities are incorporated into each birthing room for the convenience and comfort of the mother. The standard equipment used during childbirth is usually stored in cabinets in the room until it is needed. Emergency equipment that might be needed during the intrapartum period is readily available to the staff and is similarly stored.

ABCs are subject to the organizational demands of their hospital; therefore, considerable variation occurs in appearance as well as policies and procedures. The room decor ranges from unmodified labor rooms to very homelike bedrooms. Policies and procedures vary less and usually include options for the presence of family and friends, minimal medical intervention, no separation of parents and infant, and early discharge (usually 6 hr–24 hr after birth). The choice of attendant for the birth varies with hospital policy and professional availability, but may include nurse–midwives, family-practice physicians, obstetricians, and specially trained nurse practitioners or physician's assistants.

Client Selection

Most ABCs are located within hospitals and are designed for use by women who have had normal pregnancies and who are experiencing uncomplicated intrapartum periods. Strict criteria are used by physicians, nurse–midwives, and nurse practitioners during the prenatal and intrapartum periods to evaluate women who desire to give birth in an ABC. If a woman is considered to be in a high-risk category during her pregnancy, she is usually not eligible for an ABC. When a woman with a normal prenatal course is initially admitted to an ABC but develops a complication during labor, she is usually transferred to the regular obstetric unit of the hospital.

There is considerable variation in policies for determining risk factors that exclude a client from the ABC

Patient Selection in ABC Programs

High-Risk Factors Excluding Admission to ABC Programs

Preeclampsia or chronic hypertension

Premature labor (occurring prior to 37 weeks' gestation)

Abnormal presentations (other than vertex) or multiple births

Third-trimester bleeding

Prolonged rupture of membranes (more than 24 hours before onset of labor)

Previous cesarean section

History of postpartum hemorrhage

Genital herpes (at the time of labor)

Postdatism (41 wk–43 wk gestation)

Maternal history of heart disease, kidney disease, psychiatric disorder or severe emotional problems, previous stillbirths, Rh sensitization, diabetes, tuberculosis, chronic or acute pulmonary problems

Estimated fetal weight less than 5 lb or greater than 9 lb

Anemia (hemoglobin less than 9.5 g–10 g)

Primiparas over 35 years old or multiparas over 45 years old

Polyhydramnios or oligohydramnios

Treatment during pregnancy with any drugs that could adversely affect the infant

Criteria Requiring Transfer Out of ABC After Labor Admission

Anemia (hemoglobin less than 9.5 g–10 g)

Temperature elevation (greater than 38°C)

Significant variation in maternal blood pressure from prenatal values

Signs of preeclampsia (hypertension, proteinuria, edema, visual disturbances)

Meconium-stained amniotic fluid

Abnormal fetal heart rate or pattern—development of need for continuous fetal heart rate monitoring

Prolonged labor (more than 24 hours)

Second-stage arrest (longer than 2 hours for primigravidas or longer than 1 hour for multiparas)

Significant vaginal bleeding

Mother's desire for repeated medication or regional anesthesia

Any condition of mother or infant that birth attendant feels requires greater management than ABC provides

or complications that require a transfer out of the ABC. In some hospitals, a woman will be transferred if she requires any or more than a small amount of analgesia (*e.g.*, 25 mg of nisentil or Demerol), whereas in others any procedure short of forceps delivery can be done in the ABC.[32] Examples of factors excluding clients from an ABC and criteria requiring transfer out of the ABC after labor admission are given below.

Supportive Atmosphere

In an ABC, a woman is free to move about during her labor. She is allowed to drink fluids and often is encouraged to bring beverages to the ABC from her home so she will have the type of fluids she desires. Analgesics are available in some ABCs; however, most couples are required to attend childbirth classes during the pregnancy so that the women will learn some breathing techniques to decrease or eliminate her need for analgesics during labor. Although one-to-one nursing care is provided for the woman, active participation of the father (or coach) is encouraged and supported by the nurse. In some ABCs, children are allowed to be present during the birth, but a responsible adult (other than the parents or nursing staff) must accompany the child or children to observe them and attend to their needs throughout this event.

The atmosphere in an ABC is usually relaxing and congenial as a woman labors and gives birth. Because nursing care is provided on a one-to-one basis, the opportunity for establishing rapport between the expectant family and the nurse is excellent. Often a nurse meets the family during the prenatal period and contracts with that family to be their obstetric nurse throughout the labor and birth of their child. The nurse becomes familiar with the members of the family prior to the birth and is better able to assess their special needs and intervene appropriately to meet these needs during the intrapartum period.

Labor and Delivery Practices

In an ABC, the goal of the staff is to meet the individual desires and needs of the woman during a safe, normal childbirth while they carefully monitor the progress of her labor and the birth of her child. Enemas, pubic shaving, and stirrups are not routine in the majority of ABCs. Similarly, episiotomies are not routinely done; rather, attempts are made to stretch the woman's perineum naturally through gentle massaging of the vaginal introitus during the second stage of labor. The actual birth of the infant can occur in any position that is safe and comfortable for the mother. Since much of the amniotic fluid contained in the infant's lungs, trachea, and nasal passages is squeezed out as the infant passes through the birth canal, suctioning of the newborn's mouth and nose is not standard after the birth, but is performed only when necessary.

With the safe emergence of the infant's head and shoulders (Fig. 47-3), many birth attendants encourage the mother (or the father) to actually complete the birth by lifting the newborn onto the mother's abdomen. While the mother, father, and children become acquainted with the newborn through sight and touch, the nurse observes and assesses the newborn's transition to extauterine life without interfering in the parent–infant bonding process (Fig. 47-4). In some ABCs, the instillation of silver nitrate in the newborn's eyes is de-

layed for 30 minutes to 1 hour so that the infant can have eye-to-eye contact with the mother and father—an important factor in the bonding process. Breast-feeding soon after the birth is encouraged because it enhances maternal attachment and increases uterine contractions, which facilitates placental separation. After the umbilical cord pulsations cease, the birth attendant clamps and cuts the umbilical cord (or allows the father to do this) and then delivers the placenta.

During the postpartum period, the mother and her newborn are carefully observed for several hours. If there are no complications, the mother and her infant may be discharged after the infant has been examined

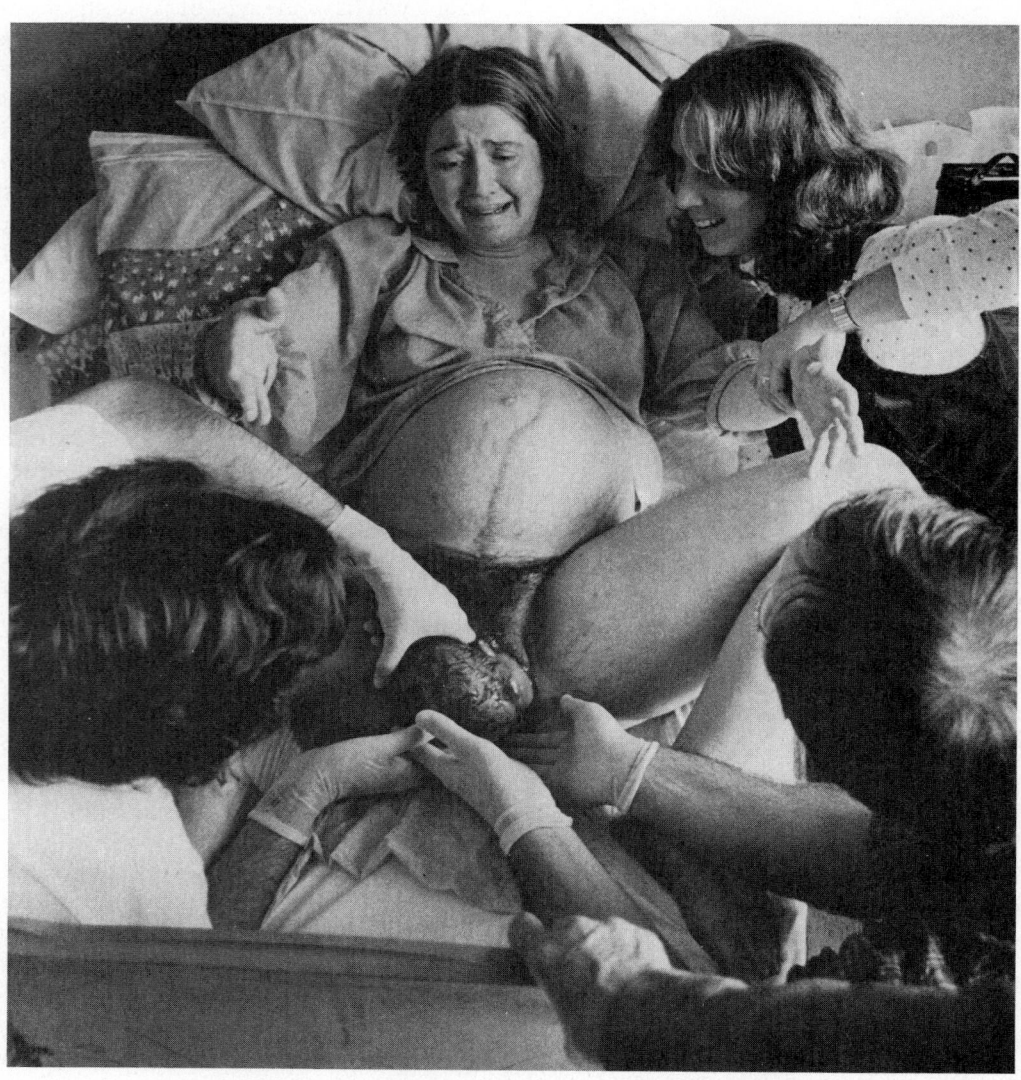

F I G U R E   4 7 - 3

Delivery in the alternative birth center usually is conducted in the labor bed. The father assists the obstetrician in the delivery while the mother watches the birth of her baby in the mirror being held in the foreground. The nurse, who is supporting the mother, does not wear a traditional uniform at this particular alternative birth center. (Photo by Michael Alexander)

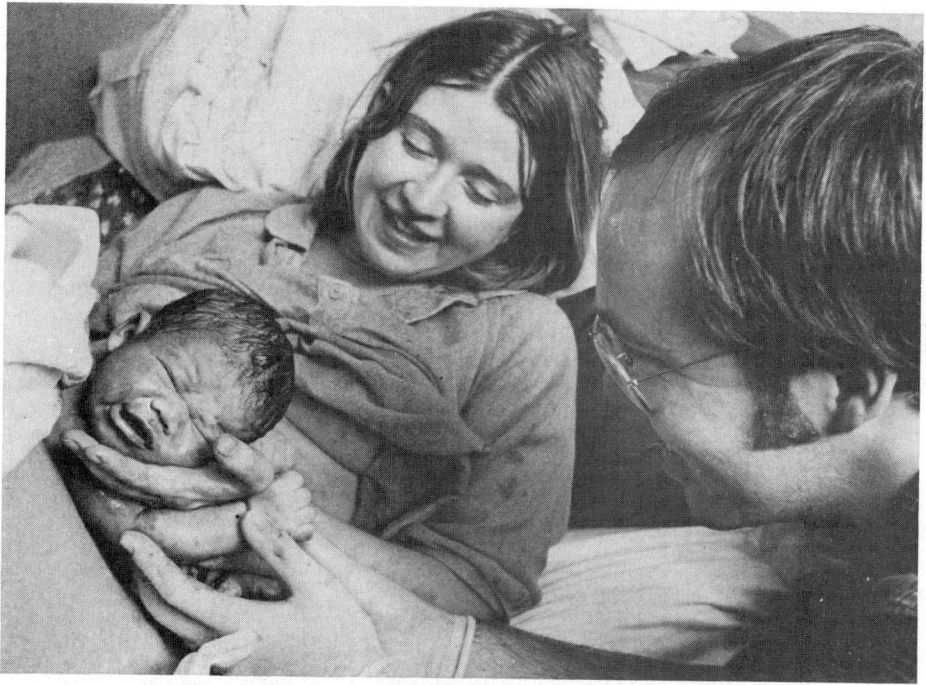

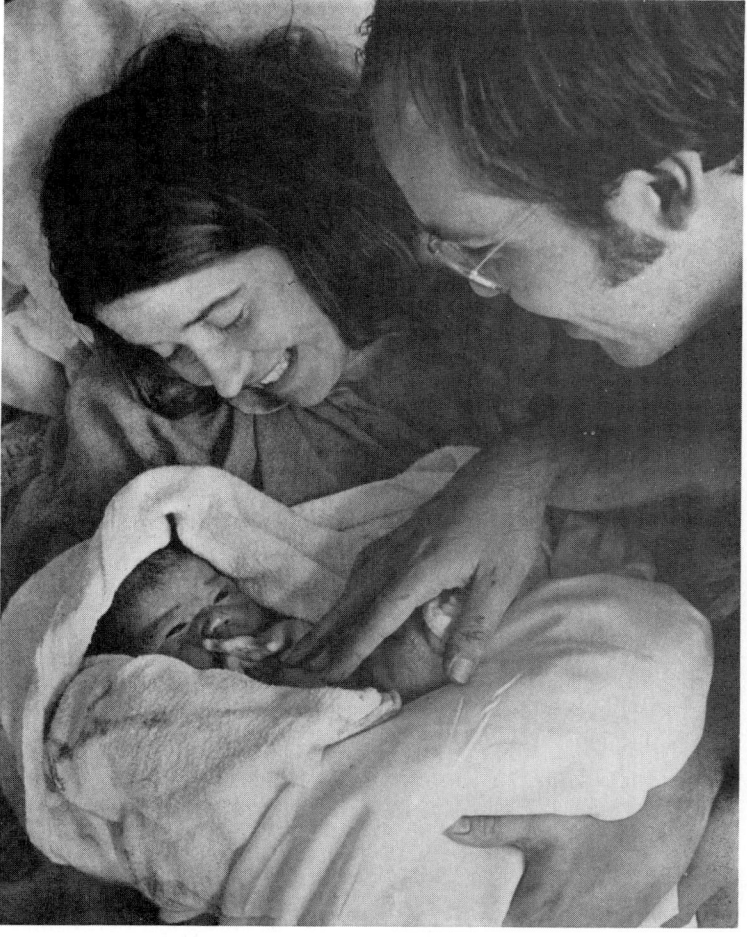

FIGURE 47-4

The parents have the opportunity to become acquainted with their new baby immediately after delivery. (Photos by Michael Alexander)

by a pediatrician or the family physician. Many ABC programs employ nurses who make follow-up home visits during the first postpartum week to assess the health of the mother and the infant. Samples for such tests as the phenylketonuria (PKU) and thyroxine (T_4) can be obtained during one of these home visits.

Growth of ABCs

The positive responses of families that have used ABCs, combined with the economic advantages of the lower cost for obstetric care in this type of facility, have contributed to the feasibility of establishing such programs within the traditional setting of the hospital and in out-of-hospital settings (Fig. 47-5).[33-35]

Women are very interested in options in childbearing, as demonstrated by a study in which there was an increase from 33% to 66% of women preferring nontraditional facilities after reading a brief description of the characteristics of a birth center or birthing suite. There was no significant difference in age, education, religion, annual income, and parity among women preferring traditional services and women preferring various nontraditional options. There is a variety of interested, potential ABC clients. A market was demonstrated for the ABC. Emphasis was placed on the need to educate women regarding its availability and characteristics.[36]

Nurse–Midwifery

Another alternative in maternity care that is returning in many parts of the country is the nurse–midwife as childbearing attendant. Throughout most of the world, nurse–midwives or lay midwives provide the preponderance of maternity care. In the United States, nurse–midwives are registered nurses who have completed a recognized program of study and clinical experience leading to a certificate in nurse–midwifery. They are prepared to give comprehensive care to childbearing couples, including physical management and educational-counseling aspects. Nurse–midwives are prepared to assume primary responsibility for prenatal, intrapartum, and postpartum care of women having normal pregnancies (Fig. 47-6).

Midwifery: Historical Perspectives

In every primitive society, there seems to have been someone present to care for the mother and the infant. Usually this task fell to women who, in essence, were the ancient forerunners of maternity nurses. Midwives no doubt have existed for centuries untold; Homer made reference to a nurse–midwife in the *Iliad*. They continued to attend the majority of deliveries in Roman and medieval times, although the role of physicians was enlarging. During the 18th century maternity cases began to receive more attention, since many lying-in

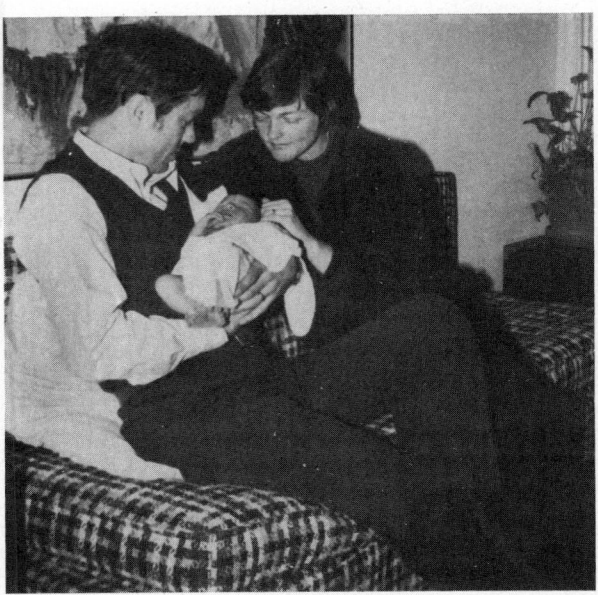
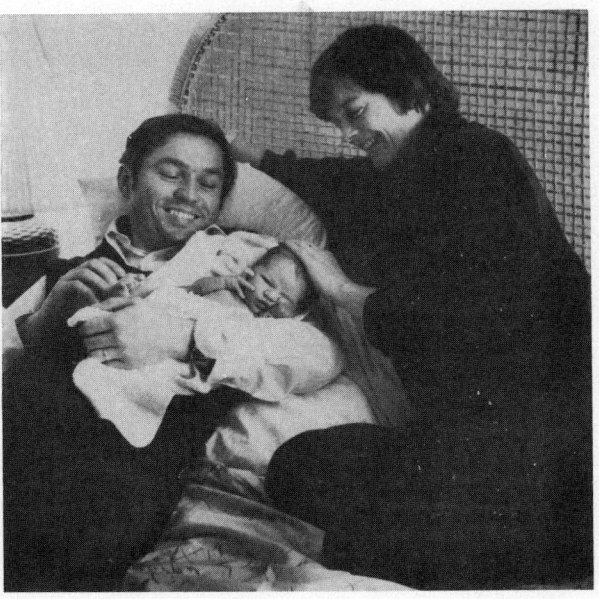

FIGURE 47-5

Parents enjoy their new baby in the homelike setting of the Alternative Birth Center, Alta Bates Hospital, Berkeley, California. (Photos by Jeff Weissman. By permission of Alta Bates Hospital, Berkeley, California)

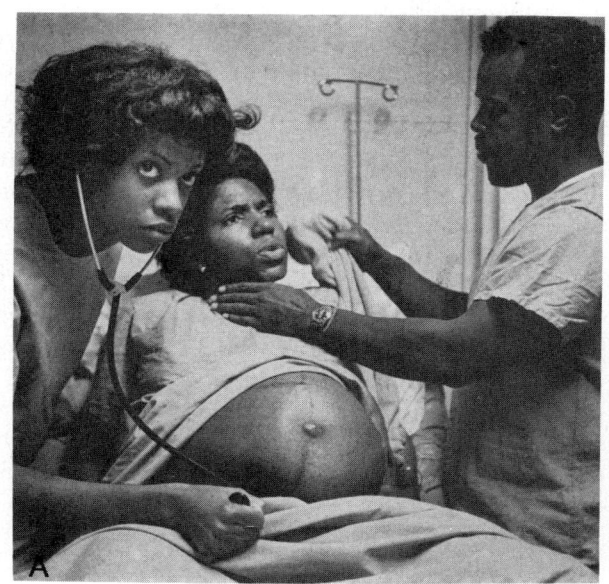

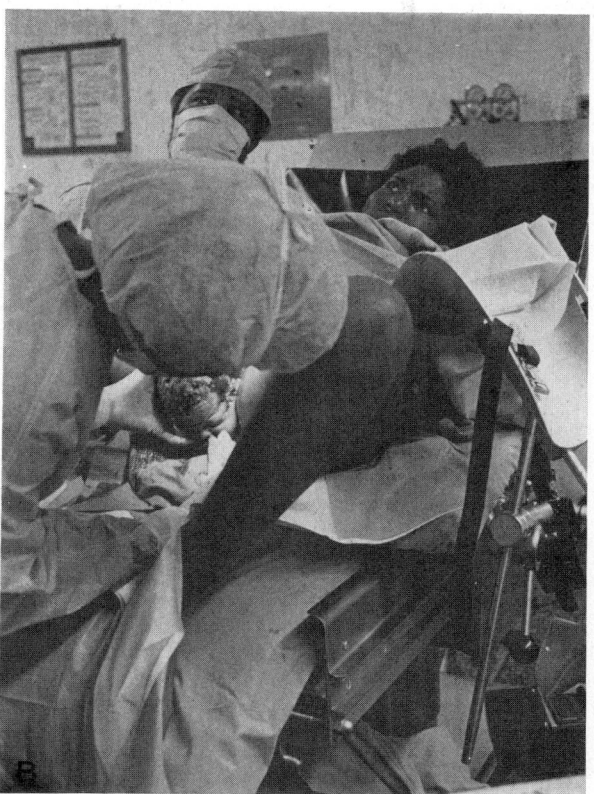

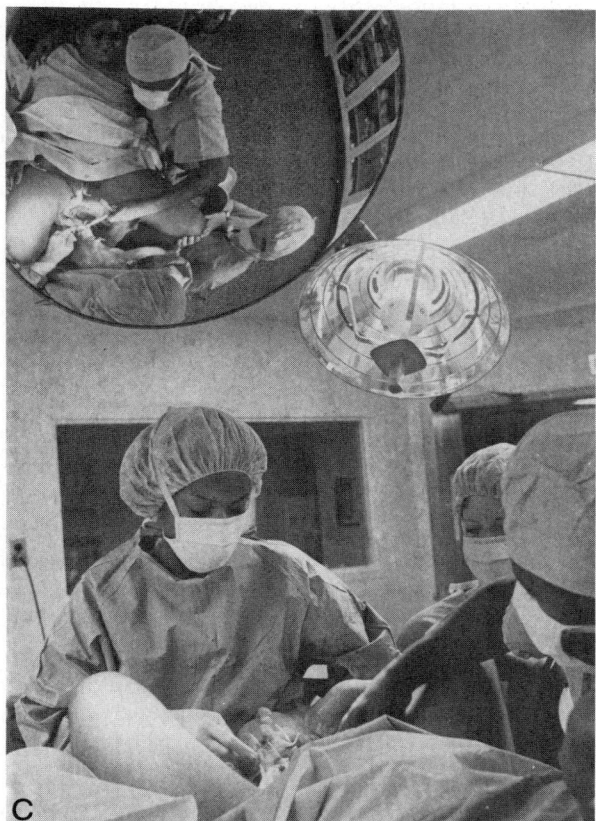

FIGURE 47-6

Labor conducted by a nurse–midwife. (*A*) The nurse–midwife monitors the fetal heart, while the father coaches the mother to keep her Lamaze breathing light and high in the chest. (*B*) The nurse–midwife delivers the baby with the mother out of stirrups in the semi-upright position. The parents watch the birth in the overhead mirror. (*C*) The nurse–midwife supervises the father as he cuts the umbilical cord. (Photos by Allison Wachstein)

charities were formed and midwives were included in training programs in London and Paris.

As midwifery assumed a more scientific status, special lying-in hospitals increased, and the last 50 years of the 18th century saw a remarkable decrease in maternal and infant deaths in these hospitals owing to better techniques of nursing management. The male physicians remained mostly uninvolved in parturient care unless needed for special procedures in difficult labors. It was not until the 19th century that physicians participated extensively in obstetrics.

History of Nurse–Midwifery in the United States.

In the United States there was a gradual transition from maternity care by trained midwives to care by medical doctors (allopathic medicine).

In early colonial times, midwives were important to the continued growth of the newly settled territories. Midwife services were guaranteed by several charter companies to induce women to travel to the colonies. Midwives were given first transportation on ferry boats (along with physicians) as an indication of their status and the importance of their services.

In the 17th and 18th centuries, midwives were held in equal esteem as "physicians and chirurgeons."[37] In the late 19th century, the use of physicians as childbirth attendants started as a new vogue, leading to the use of forceps and a trend toward selection of the hospital as the location for delivery and for physician training in obstetrics. At the beginning of the 20th century, several pivotal changes in American society and medical care set the stage for the subsequent virtual elimination of midwives as birth attendants. The medical profession, plagued by sectarian divisions throughout the 19th century, began to coalesce just as turn-of-the-century waves of European immigration brought increased demand for midwifery. Immigrants were accustomed to relying on midwives for childbirth and shunned the hospital, which tended to be remote and alien. Many midwives with excellent European training accompanied the new settlers and flourished in their communities. Rather than giving the midwife a distinct place in the US system and assuring proper training and supervision, the obstetricians elected to eliminate their competitor, no doubt with significant economic concerns involved.[37]

Obstetric specialists sought to educate the public about the nature of the obstetrician's skills and the science and art of obstetrics. They also warned of dangers from an "untrained" birth attendant (believing no amount of training short of medical would produce a competent birth attendant). Although a few municipalities tried to establish regulatory schemes for midwives and public-health officials urged regulation, mid-

wives remained "declassed persons" who never fit into reformers' constructs of scientific technicians bringing order to the chaos of urban industrial society. Midwives were tolerated in public-health prenatal centers (a concession to immigrants), but only as a stopgap measure until they could be replaced by physicians.

Public-health activists had statistical proof of the midwife's capabilities, showing decreased maternal mortality and infant blindness (from gonococcal ophthalmia) when midwives provided care. However, they did not crusade on the midwives' behalf or challenge medical resistance. To legitimate the midwife's work would threaten the economic and social status of medicine and undermine the "germ theory" paradigm. Midwives, as independent practitioners, were never subjugated to physicians as were hospital nurses. The midwife's naturalistic approach demystified childbirth and reduced the scientific content of obstetrics, compared with medicine and surgery. It was essential for obstetricians to argue that their unique services (*e.g.* anesthesia, forceps, and cesarean deliveries) were critical to modern, scientific (and thus quality) childbirth care.[37]

Another important factor in the decline of midwives was the choice women themselves made. Following earlier trends, wealthy women had abandoned the midwife in favor of the physician as a birth attendant by the early 20th century. As daughters of immigrant families matured into womanhood, they were eager to adopt American ways. They began turning to obstetricians and hospitals for delivery, because midwives carried the stigma of outdated, Old World cultures to which their parents clung. As families' economic conditions improved, the midwife was abandoned. A final blow was dealt when Congress restricted immigration in the 1920s. Demand for midwife services fell sharply.

However, midwifery continued in rural and inner-city areas with development of the nurse–midwife and institution of training programs.

The first nurse–midwifery service in the United States was founded by Mary Breckenridge as the Frontier Nursing Service. Its purpose was to provide primary health care and maternity services in the mountain counties of Kentucky. Begun in 1925, this rural health service has a medical center and outpost clinics that are staffed by nurse–midwives and nurse practitioners. Traveling rough country roads, usually by jeep, nurse–midwives at times need to travel by horseback to reach families in the more remote areas. This organization has demonstrated that nurse–midwives can help lower mortality in a large population in rural and isolated areas. The Frontier Nursing Service also operates a graduate school of midwifery and a family nurse practitioner program.

The Maternity Center Association was founded in New York in 1918 and in 1932 established a school of nurse–midwifery for graduate nurses in association with the Lobenstine Midwifery Clinic. Consolidated as the Maternity Center Association 3 years later, this organization graduated and certified over 400 nurse-midwives over the next 30 years. The school was transferred to the Kings County Hospital in affiliation with Downstate University of New York in Brooklyn in 1958. This move initiated hospital-based formal midwifery education. Other midwifery schools were developed at Yale, Johns Hopkins, Columbia, Catholic University, several state universities, Loma Linda, Emory, Meharry Medical College, and New Jersey College of Medicine, and by the US Air Force.

The American College of Nurse–Midwifery was established in 1955 as an organization of nurse–midwives to study and evaluate midwifery activities, plan and develop educational programs, and respond to professional needs. The college is a member of the International Confederation of Midwives. In 1969, the name was changed to the American College of Nurse–Midwives, with objectives including improving services to mothers and newborn babies in cooperation with other groups, establishing qualifications for midwifery activities, developing educational programs, establishing communications channels with other groups, and sponsoring research and literature.

Although physicians had long opposed widespread use of nurse–midwives, and many barriers to practice through restrictive legislation and denial of hospital privileges had been created, the American College of Obstetricians and Gynecologists took a positive stance in 1970. Together with the Nurses Association of the American College of Obstetricians and Gynecologists (NAACOG) and the American College of Nurse–Midwives, the physicians' organization issued a "Joint Statement of Maternity Care," published in 1971, which allowed midwifery to reenter the mainstream of American health care. The statement provided that, as part of a medically directed health team, "qualified nurse-midwives may assume responsibility for the complete care and management of uncomplicated maternity patients."[38] Also in 1971, the American College of Nurse–Midwives initiated a National Certification Examination to standardize the level of basic competency among nurse–midwives.

Nurse–Midwifery Practice

Nurse–midwifery practice encompasses the care of essentially normal women and emphasizes the promotion and maintenance of health. Most midwives offer a comprehensive approach to maternity care, functioning

---

Nurse–Midwifery

What is a Certified Nurse-Midwife?

A certified nurse–midwife (CNM) is an individual educated in the two disciplines of nursing and midwifery, who possesses evidence of certification according to the requirements of the American College of Nurse–Midwives.

What is Nurse-Midwifery Practice?

Nurse–midwifery is the independent management of care of essentially normal newborns and women, antepartally, intrapartally, postpartally, and/or gynecologically, occurring within a health-care system that provides for medical consultation, collaborative management, or referral and is in accord with the *Functions, Standards, and Qualifications for Nurse–Midwifery Practice* as defined by the American College of Nurse–Midwives.

The nurse–midwife provides care for the normal mother during pregnancy and stays with her during labor, providing continuous physical and emotional support. She evaluates progress and manages the labor and delivery. She evaluates and provides immediate care for the normal newborn. She helps the mother to care for herself and for her infant, to adjust the home situation to the new child, and to lay a healthful foundation for future pregnancies through family planning and gynecologic services. The nurse–midwife is prepared to teach, interpret, and provide support as an integral part of her services.

(J Nurse–Midwifery 26(2):42, March/April 1981)

---

as a member of a health-care team. In addition to managing the complete care for mothers with normal pregnancies, the certified nurse–midwife (CNM) is prepared to function in all areas of women's health maintenance, including family planning and childbirth, and also provides perinatal care and newborn management. The CNM in the United States usually delivers in the hospital setting, where most American births take place. The CNM is an employee of a hospital or medical center, or works for a community-based maternal and child health service, or is in private practice with an obstetrician or family physician.

A recent examination of the content and process (methods) used by nurse–midwives in providing prenatal care found that the clinical practice of CNMs reflected their philosophy of comprehensive, personalized maternity care. The nurse–midwives had longer visits with clients than most physicians and varied the content according to the client's needs. They discussed topics

Content of Topics Discussed by Nurse–Midwives in Prenatal Visits

Health Status

Pregnancy progress interim history
Danger signs
Exercise/rest
Explain illness
Signs/symptoms of labor
Discomforts of pregnancy
Laboratory tests/results
Nutrition/diet history
Breast care
Weight gain/weight loss
BP/vital signs
Emotions of pregnancy
Other

Preventive Health Care

Accident prevention
Dental care
Family planning
Community-health resources
Smoking
Ultrasound
Other

Treatments

Vitamins or iron
Other medications
Other

Preparation for Labor

Conduct of labor and delivery
Alternate birth options/orientation
Prenatal education classes
Reading by client
Cesarean section
Job/employment
Explain CNM role
Other

Preparation for Parenthood

Breast-feeding
Infant care
Rooming-in
Pediatrician
Circumcision
Attitudes toward pregnancy/parenting
Other

Miscellaneous

Charting/paperwork
Hospital admission procedures
Other

(After Lehrman EJ: Lehrman Nurse–Midwifery Practice: Descriptive Study of Prenatal Care, Nurse Midwifery 26(3):33, 1981)

including health status and pregnancy, preventive health care, preparation for labor and parenthood, and treatments prescribed for the client (see list of topics). Some type of physical examination was included in every visit and used as participative care. The nurse–midwife would have the woman or partner palpate fetal parts or listen to the fetal heartbeat and would often use this as a departure point for parent education. A significant other (usually husband or partner) was present in about one third of the visits. Client and family education was a dominant focus in most visits, with the midwives showing openness to working with the woman and family in meeting their wishes for alternatives for hospital birth.[39]

Many nurse–midwives have assumed nonclinical positions because of the restriction on or prohibition of their practice that was common until recently. In a 1977 survey of graduates of the Yale nurse–midwifery program, it was found that 32% of the graduates were clinicians, 32% were teachers, 14% were administrators, 10% had both clinical and teaching positions, 2.3% were other, and 13% were not working. Those who were clinicians provided primary care for groups of clients, which included health checks and screening, health supervision and maintenance, maternity care, family planning, and diagnosis and management of acute illness.[40] Another study of midwives in the 11 Western states who were in practices that included provision of prenatal care revealed the following areas of employment.[41]

Hospital	39.1%
Nurse–midwifery maternity service	30.4%
Private nurse–midwifery practice	30.4%
Private practice with a physician	21.7%
Nurse–midwifery educational program	17.4%
Public-health agency	8.6%
Prepaid health plan	4.3%
Military	4.3%*

Nurse–Midwives and Pregnancy Outcome

The aggressive management of human parturition that is characteristic of obstetrics in the 1970s and 1980s is not generally in the best interests of the great majority of mothers and infants. In developed countries that have a significantly lower incidence of infant mortality than that of the United States, highly trained nurse–midwives provide most of the family-planning and obstetric services. Nurse–midwives who are well trained practice nonintervention obstetrics that integrates updated scientific research, while respecting and supporting the delicately balanced natural mechanisms of the labor process. The medical expertise of the physician is used only when the pregnant woman develops a significant illness or when labor and birth is anticipated to be, or found to be, abnormal.

Many obstetric practices are known to be or are suspected of being potentially injurious to the mother, infant, or their developing relationship. Electronic or ultrasonic devices used to ascertain and monitor fetal status may pose dangers to the fetus. Animal studies have revealed delayed neuromuscular development, electroencephalographic changes, altered emotional behavior, and anomalies when such devices are used. Amniotomy has been associated with increased risk of umbilical cord compression and prolapse and increased pressure on the fetal brain. Confining a woman to bed during labor tends to prolong labor by 2.5 hours; increases the woman's need for analgesics, uterine stimulants, and forceps deliveries; and increases the incidence of abnormal fetal heart rates and poor infant Apgar scores. Drugs that are potentially teratogenic or carcinogenic may depress the infant's cardiovascular, respiratory, and thermoregulatory mechanisms and may have subtle permanent effects on the infant's brain circuitry.[41]

* Total is more than 100% because of part-time work in more than one type of position. Figures indicate a significant amount of dual positions or holding of more than one job in this nurse–midwife population.

Data from the North Central Bronx Hospital in New York indicate that the outcome of pregnancy may be significantly improved, even among higher-risk clients, with the use of nurse–midwives. The maternity service is essentially run by nurse–midwives, with appropriate physician consultation. About 30% of the clients are clearly medically high risk, and their care is much the same as for low-risk clients. If there is a medical indication for intervention, care is provided by a board-certified obstetrician or chief pediatric resident. Only severely Rh-sensitized expectant mothers were transferred to another hospital. A review of 2608 birth records during 1979 showed an outstanding maternal and infant outcome, including the high-risk clients. Of the total population of mothers, 83% were successfully delivered by midwives; these were spontaneous vaginal deliveries without fundal pressure. Fewer than 30% of all labors required analgesia or anesthesia. Of infants above 1000 g, 93% had Apgar scores of 7 or above at 1 minute and 98.3% had such scores at 5 minutes. The neonatal mortality rate among infants 1000 g or heavier was 4.2 in 1000. The incidence of instrumental deliveries (forceps, vacuum extraction) was 2.34%, and the cesarean section rate was 9% (7% primary and 2% repeat). All mothers who had delivered previously by cesarean section were allowed to labor spontaneously; of these, 37% gave birth vaginally. Fewer than 50% of clients were monitored electronically, including the 30% who were high risk. Episiotomy was done in only 26% of births; 45% of clients gave birth over an intact perineum, and 26% had first- or second-degree tears. Uterine stimulants (oxytocin) were used in only 3% of labors, and only when there was a medical indication.[41]

The skilled and supportive care provided by nurse–midwives made possible these low-intervention and positive-outcome rates. Childbirth education was a key component of the program, and the presence of loved ones for support during labor was important. Other practices during labor and delivery included allowing low-risk mothers to eat and drink during labor, avoiding enemas, not prepping or shaving the perineum, minimizing vaginal examinations (three to five times per labor), taking great care not to rupture membranes, having most mothers give birth in their labor beds in the labor room, allowing mothers to give birth in the semisitting position without stirrups, and delivering low-birth-weight infants over an intact perineum unless there was insufficient stretch. On this service, there were no elective inductions of labor.

Although the highly trained obstetrician's skills are critical in medically complicated childbirth, and although the neonatologist contributes significantly to saving very premature, ill, and defective infants, care during pregnancy and childbirth that is noninterventionist and supportive of health and well-being remains the most important factor in most normal pregnancies. Nurse–midwives are particularly suited by training and philosophy to provide such care.

References

1. Bullough B, Bullough VL: The Care of the Sick: The Emergence of Modern Nursing. New York, Prodist Publishers, 1978
2. Tierra M: The Way of Herbs: Simple Remedies for Health and Healing. Santa Cruz, CA, Unity Press, 1980
3. Graham H: Eternal Eve. Garden City, NY, Doubleday & Co, 1951
4. Findley P: Priests of Lucina. Boston, Little, Brown & Co, 1939
5. Stewart IM, Austin AL: A History of Nursing, 5th ed. New York, GP Putnam's Sons, 1962
6. Griffin GL, Griffin JK: History and Trends in Professional Nursing. St Louis, CV Mosby, 1973
7. Bookmiller MM, Bowen GL: Textbook of Obstetrics and Obstetric Nursing, 2nd ed. Philadelphia, WB Saunders, 1954
8. Armeny S: Organized nurses, women philanthropists, and the intellectual bases for cooperation among women, 1898–1920. In Lagemann HC (ed): Nursing History: New Perspectives, New Possibilities, pp 1–12. New York, Teachers' College Press, 1983
9. Starr P: The Social Transformation of American Medicine, pp 40–43; 56–58; 120–121. New York, Harper & Row, 1982
10. DeYoung L: The Foundations of Nursing. St Louis, CV Mosby, 1972
11. Morantz RM: Self-healing in the nineteenth century: A women's movement. In Weiss K (ed): Women's Health Care: A Guide to Alternatives, pp 147–155. Reston, VA, Reston Publishing, 1984
12. Clemen SA, Eigsti DG, McGuire SL: Comprehensive Family and Community Health Nursing, pp 16–17. New York, McGraw-Hill, 1981
13. Tomes N: The silent battle: Nurse registration in New York State, 1903–1920. In Weiss K (ed): Women's Health Care: A Guide to Alternatives, pp 107–132. Reston, VA, Reston Publishing, 1984
14. Kalisch PA, Kalisch BJ: The Advance of American Nursing. Boston, Little, Brown & Co, 1978
15. Silver HK, Ford L et al: The pediatric nurse practitioner program: Expanding the role of the nurse to provide increased health care for children. JAMA 204(4):298–302, April 22, 1968
16. Lewis CE, Resnick BA: Nurse clinics and progressive ambulatory patient care. N Engl J Med 227:1236–1241, December 7, 1967
17. National Commission for the Study of Nursing and Nursing Education, Jerome Lysaught, Director: An Abstract for Action. New York, McGraw-Hill, 1970
18. Extending the Scope of Nursing Practice. A Report of the Secretary's Committee to Study Extended Roles for Nurses. Washington, DC, Department of Health, Education and Welfare, November 1971
19. Riehl JP, McVay JW: The Clinical Nurse Specialist: Interpretations. New York, Appleton-Century-Crofts, 1973
20. Ashley JA: Hospitals, Paternalism and the Role of the Nurse, pp 98–117. New York, Teachers' College Press, 1977
21. Melosh B: Doctors, patients and 'big nurse': Work and gender in the postwar hospital. In Lagemann HC (ed): Nursing History: New Perspectives, New Possibilities, pp 157–179. New York, Teachers' College Press, 1983
22. Marieskind HI: Women in the Health System, pp 289–295. St Louis, CV Mosby, 1980
23. Downer C: Self-healing in the twentieth century: Self-help and vaginal disease. In Weiss K (ed): Women's Health Care: A Guide to Alternatives, pp 379–386. Reston, VA, Reston Publishing, 1984
24. Anderson SF: Childbirth as a pathological process: An American perspective. MCN—Am J Maternal Child Nurs 2(4):240–244, July/August, 1977
25. Arms S: Immaculate Deception. Boston, Houghton-Mifflin, 1975
26. Hazell LD: A study of 300 elective home births. Birth Fam J 2(1):11–15, Winter 1974/1975
27. Birthing alternatives: A matter of choice and turf, pp 42–48. Medical World News, May 28, 1984
28. Estes MN: A home obstetric service with expert consultation and back-up. Birth Fam J 5(3):151–157, Fall 1978
29. Searles C: The impetus toward home birth. J Nurse-Midwifery 26(3):51–56, May/June 1981
30. The development of family-centered maternity/newborn care in hospitals. A joint position statement prepared by the Interprofessional Task Force on Health Care of Women and Children. New York, The National Foundation/March of Dimes, June 1978
31. Patterson KA, Peterson VL: The Alternative Birth Center Movement in the San Francisco and Bay Area. J Nurse-Midwifery 25(2):23–27, March/April 1980
32. DeVries R: The development and future of the hospital-based alternative birth center. J Nurse-Midwifery 24(6):37–38, November/December 1979
33. Ernst EKM, Forde MP: Maternity care: An attempt at an alternative. Nurs Clin North Am 10(2):241–249, June 1975
34. Kerner J, Ferris CB: An alternative birth center in a community teaching hospital. Obstet Gynecol 51(3):371–373, March 1978
35. Lubic RW: The childbearing center. J Nurse-Midwifery 21(3):24–25, Fall 1976
36. Mather S: Women's interests in alternative maternity facilities. J Nurse-Midwifery 25(3):3–8, May/June 1980
37. Brickman JB: Public health, midwives and nurses, 1880–1930. In Lagemann HC (ed): Nursing History: New Perspectives, New Possibilities, pp 65–75. New York, Teachers' College Press, 1983

38. American College of Obstetricians and Gynecologists; the Nurses Association of the American College of Obstetricians and Gynecologists; and the American College of Nurse-Midwives: Joint statement on maternity care. ACOG Newsletter, February 1971
39. Lehrman EJ: Nurse-Midwifery practice: Descriptive study of prenatal care. J Nurse-Midwifery 26(3):27–40, May/June 1981
40. Burgess HA: Nurse-midwives from Yale—what are they doing now? J Nurse-Midwifery 25(5):43–45, September/October 1980
41. Haire D: Improving the outcome of pregnancy through increased utilization of midwives. J Nurse-Midwifery 26(1):5–8, January/February 1981

Suggested Reading

Adams CJ: Management of delivery by United States certified nurse-midwives. J Nurse-Midwifery 30(1):3–8, January/February 1985

Anderson EM, Leonard BJ, Yates JA: Epigenesis of the nurse practitioner role. Am J Nurs 74:1812–1816, October 1974

Formato LS: Routine prophylactic episiotomy: Is it always necessary? J Nurse-Midwifery 30(3):144–147, May/June 1985

Koehler NU, Solomon DA, Murphy M: Outcomes of a rural Sonoma County home birth practice: 1976–1982. Birth 11(3):156–169, Fall 1984

Perry DS: The early midwives of Missouri. J Nurse-Midwifery 28(6):15–21, November/December 1983

Piechnick SL, Corbett MA: Reducing low birth weight among socioeconomically high-risk adolescent pregnancies. J Nurse-Midwifery 30(2):88–98, March/April 1985

Shannahan MD, Cottrell BH: Effect of the birth chair on duration of second stage labor, fetal outcome, and maternal blood loss. Nurs Res 34(2):89–92, March/April 1985

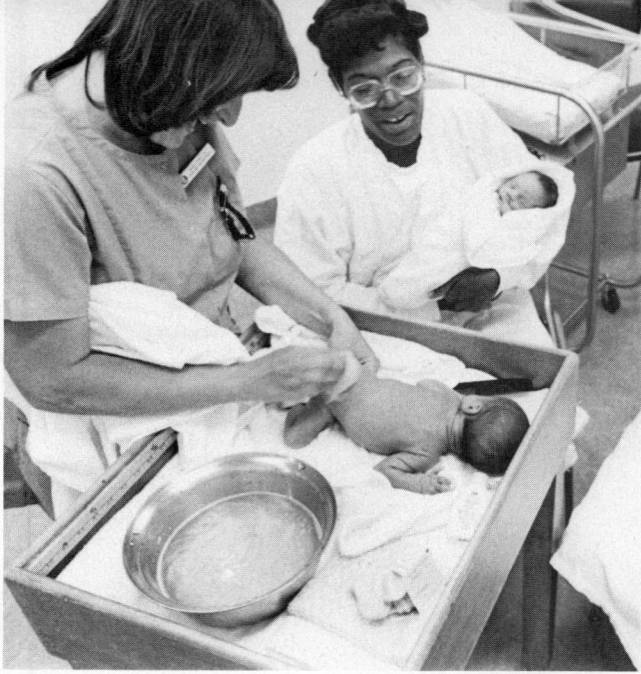

Unit IX:
Special Considerations
in Maternity Nursing

Conference Material

1. Alisa K. is a 22-year-old primigravida in the first trimester, who is in excellent health with no apparent risk factors. She and her husband Ron have sought your advice as a community health nurse regarding childbirth options. They believe strongly in natural birth with full family participation in a supportive and comfortable setting. The couple has been considering a home birth and is seeking information about this as well as other options and about having a nurse-midwife as a birth attendant. How do you counsel Alisa and Ron about (a) advantages and risks of various childbirth options, and (b) advantages and disadvantages of various childbirth attendants?

2. Discuss the changing emphasis of practice that occurred in nursing from the late 1800s to the present, taking into consideration social and cultural conditions, the status of women, the growth of scientific medicine, the development of the hospital as an institution, and the evolution of nursing as a profession. Give specific examples relevant to maternity nursing and the care of childbearing families.

3. Discuss future directions for maternity nursing practice based upon recent developments in the maternal–infant care field and the nursing profession. Take into consideration population and demographic changes, consumer preferences, economic considerations, trends in health-care system organization, and other relevant factors you may identify. Create a scenario of what the nurse's practice

might be like (*e.g.*, setting, types of clients, services provided, compensation, interprofessional relations, etc.) if a particular future direction is realized.

4. What do you see as the coming trends in maternity nursing in the next 10 years? What past social trends and technologies are shaping the evolution of maternity nursing?

Multiple Choice

1. Manual massage of the uterus was first used in
   A. Egypt
   B. Assyria
   C. Greece
   D. Sumatra   ____

2. A very early recorded description of podalic version was written by
   A. Surata
   B. Hippocrates
   C. Soranus
   D. Aristotle   ____

3. The first order of nuns with nursing care as their sole mission was
   A. Sisters of Mercy
   B. Sisters of Hotel Dieu
   C. Sisters of St. Lazarus
   D. Sisters of St. Claire   ____

4. Though practiced upon dead mothers since antiquity, the first authentic cesarean section performed upon a living mother occurred in the
   A. 1200s
   B. 1400s
   C. 1600s
   D. 1800s   ____

5. The invention of modern forceps is credited to
   A. Mauriceau
   B. Pare
   C. Van Deventer
   D. Chamberlen   ____

6. External manual expression of the placenta was advocated first in the 18th century by
   A. Harvie
   B. Credé
   C. Hunter
   D. Smellie   ____

7. The first lying-in hospital and school for midwives in North America was established in the mid 1700s by
   A. Fuller
   B. Hunter
   C. Shippen
   D. Hutchinson   ____

8. Semmelweis became convinced that puerperal sepsis was transmitted by contact with blood of infected patients by
A. Observations that there were fewer deaths from puerperal sepsis in wards where midwives performed deliveries
B. Identifying the microorganism in an infected blood sample using an early microscope
C. Postmortum findings on his pathology assistant who died after cutting his finger doing an autopsy on a victim of puerperal sepsis that were identical with those of women who died of puerperal sepsis ____

9. The first recognized school of nursing in the United States, at the New England Hospital for Women and Children, was established by
A. Elizabeth Blackwell
B. Lavinia Dock
C. Lillian Wald
D. Margaret Sanger ____

10. The Goldmark Report (1923) made recommendations to improve nursing that resembled those made by Flexner (1910) to improve medicine, including
A. Upgrading educational standards (longer programs, more scientific content)
B. Placing nursing schools in universities
C. Recruiting women with high capacity (high school graduates)
D. All of the above ____

11. The first birth-control clinic in America was established in Brooklyn (1916) by
A. Clara Barton
B. Margaret Sanger
C. Maria Daniels
D. Lillian Wald ____

12. The importance of antepartal care in saving lives of mothers and infants was demonstrated in the 1920s through an analysis of records by
A. The Children's Bureau
B. The Belleview School for Midwives
C. The Maternity Center Association
D. The U.S. Census Bureau ____

13. The main concepts in family-centered maternity care include
A. Consideration of other family members, especially the father
B. Attention to social and psychological needs of pregnant women
C. Participant childbirth
D. Rooming in and early mother-child contact
Select the number corresponding to the correct letters.
1. A and B
2. A, B, and C
3. A, B, C, and D ____

14. The expanded role of the nurse practitioner was first introduced in
A. The 1950s
B. The 1960s
C. The 1970s ____

15. Some results of activities of the Women's Health Movement have included an impact on
A. Expanding health insurance benefits to include contraception and abortion
B. Patient information inserts and drug labeling
C. Growth of self-help groups
D. Changes in abortion laws to increase availability
E. Increased alternatives in childbearing
Select the number corresponding to the correct letters.
1. A, B, and C
2. B, C, and D
3. A, B, C, and D
4. All of the above ____

16. The major reasons why women elect home births include
A. Desire to have the baby close to the mother after birth
B. Desire to have the father present during birth
C. Viewing pregnancy as normal and out of place in a hospital
D. Wanting more control over the childbirth experience
E. Wanting to give birth in familiar surroundings
Select the number corresponding to the correct letters.
1. A, B, and C
2. B, C, and D
3. A, B, C, and D
4. All of the above ____

17. Factors that would exclude a woman from labor and delivery in an alternative birth center include
A. Estimated fetal weight below 5 lb or above 9 lb
B. Anemia
C. Membranes ruptured longer than 24 hours before onset of labor
D. Breech presentation
E. Primiparas over 35 years old or multiparas over 45 years old
Select the number corresponding to the correct letters.
1. A, B, and C
2. A, C, and E
3. A, B, C, and E
4. All of the above ____

18. Factors requiring transfer out of an alternative birth center after admitted include
A. Temperature elevation (>38°C)
B. Meconium-stained amniotic fluid
C. Prolonged labor (>24 hours)
D. Abnormal fetal heart rate
E. Second stage arrest (>4 hours for primigravidas; >2 hours for multiparas)

Select the number corresponding to the correct letters.
1. A, B, and C
2. A, B, C, and D
3. A, B, D, and E
4. All of the above   ____

19. Significant factors in the decline of midwives in the early 20th century include
   A. Lack of support by public health authorities
   B. Medical profession opposition and discrediting of midwives
   C. Trends toward physician birth attendants among wealthy women
   D. Desire of immigrant second-generation women to adopt American ways
   E. Congressional restriction of immigration

Select the number corresponding to the correct letters.
1. A, B, and C
2. B, C, and D
3. A, B, C, and D
4. All of the above   ____

20. Professional standards for nurse-midwife education have been established since the mid 1950s by
   A. The American College of Obstetricians and Gynecologists
   B. The American College of Nurse-Midwives
   C. The American Nurses' Association
   D. The Nurses' Association of the American College of Obstetricians and Gynecologists   ____

21. The three areas that employ the greatest number of nurse-midwives include
   A. Public health agency, physician practice, nurse-midwife practice
   B. Prepaid health plan, nurse-midwife maternity service, physician practice
   C. Hospital, nurse-midwife maternity service, nurse-midwife practice
   D. Hospital, public health agency, nurse-midwife maternity service   ____

22. Low-intervention and positive-outcome rates in nurse-midwife-run maternity services (even with a proportion of high-risk mothers) have been attributed to
   A. Childbirth education
   B. Presence of supportive persons
   C. Encouraging hydration and nutrition
   D. Avoiding enemas, prepping, and shaving
   E. Minimizing vaginal examinations
   F. Not rupturing membranes
   G. Birth in labor beds in semiupright position

Select the number corresponding to the correct letters.
1. A, B, C, and D
2. A, B, C, E, and F
3. B, C, E, F, and G
4. All of the above   ____

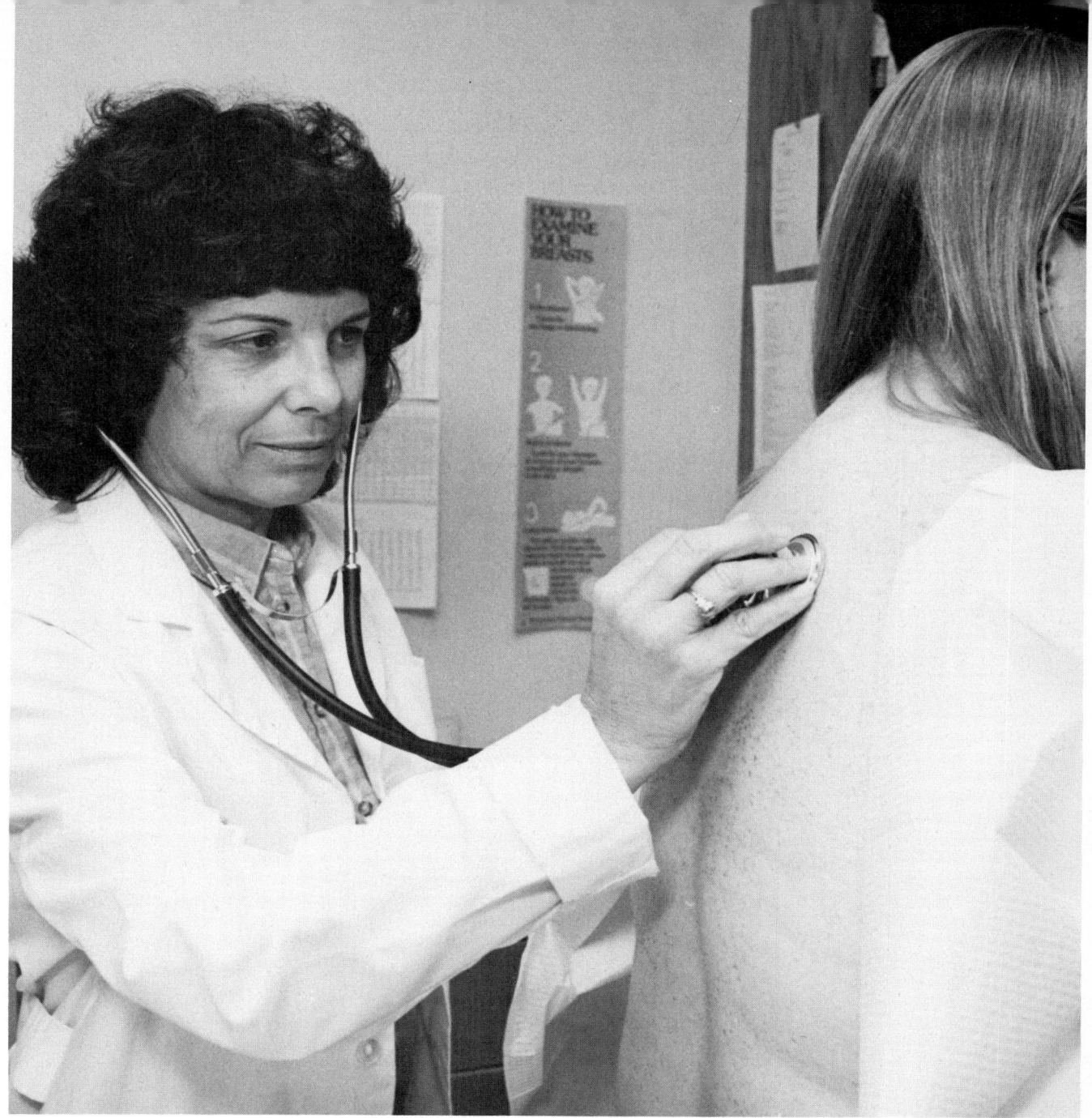

UNIT X

Assessment and Management in Women's Health Promotion

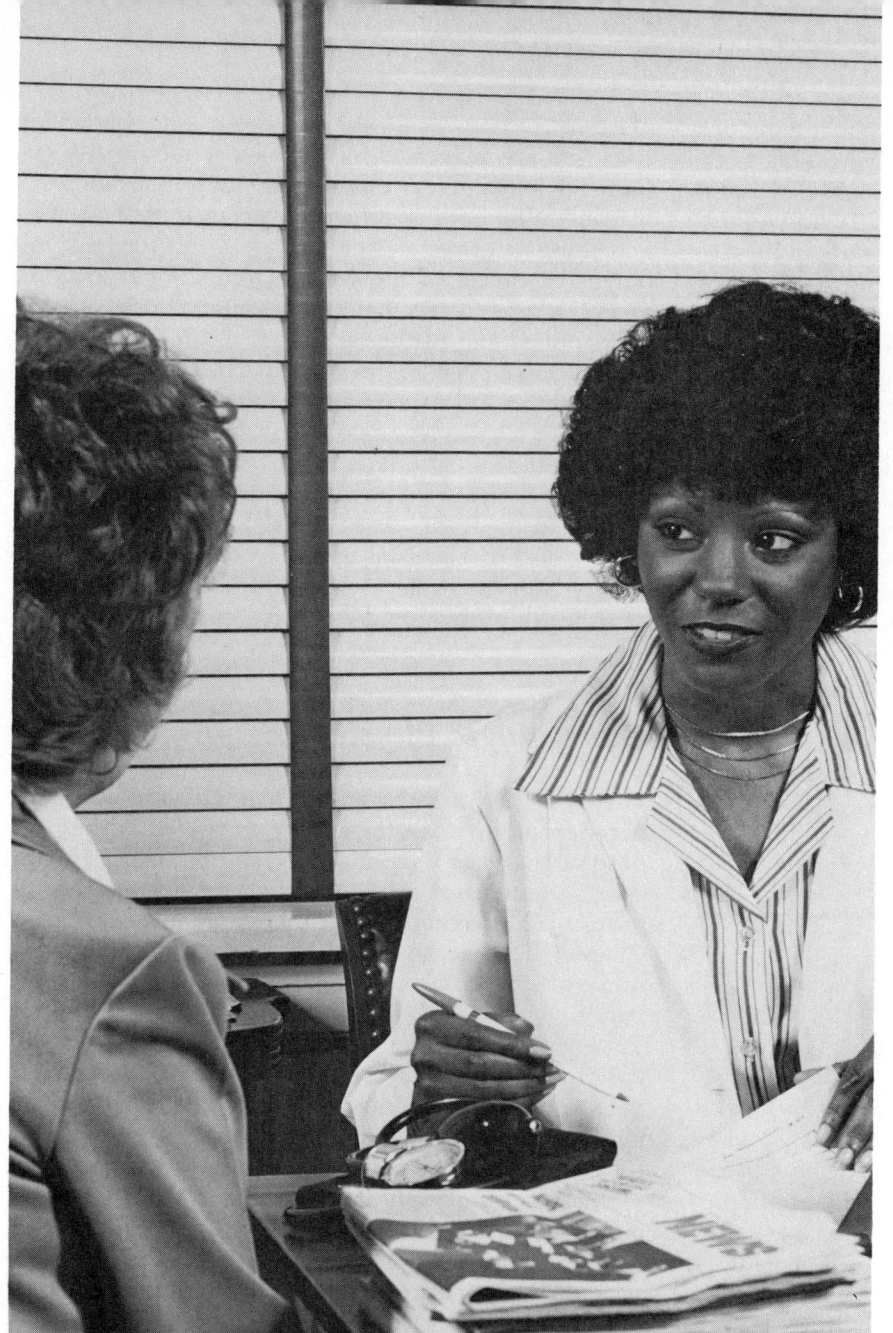

CHAPTER 48

Promoting Gynecologic Health

Nurses who provide care to women have many opportunities to promote individual and family health and to help reduce the risk of illness in their clients. The roles of nurses in maternity care have blended into various areas of women's health care, depending upon the setting and client needs. The nurse working on the maternity unit, in the Ob-gyn clinic, or in the physician's office may respond to health-care needs that encompass both reproductive care and gynecologic care. Health promotion and the prevention or early detection of illness are important responsibilities.

The areas of gynecology most often encountered by the nurse who is primarily in the maternity role include health promotion in numerous forms; growth and development needs, including such life stages as adolescence and menopause; and common gynecologic disorders such as menstrual problems and genital infections. Nurses are particularly sensitive to women's problems because of mutual perceptions and common experiences. Nursing care is often highly acceptable to the female client, since nurse and client often share perspectives and the nurse represents a care provider who is understanding, is attuned to women's concerns, and keeps communications open.

Assessment

Gynecologic Health History

The assessment process may include a general health history, or it may be focused upon particular systems or areas of concern. The nurse must decide how broad or focused the assessment will be, depending upon the clinical setting, the major purpose of the client encounter, and the health needs or problems of the client. A postpartum nurse may need to assess the new mother's concern about possible exposure to diethylstilbestrol (DES) with a focused health history. The clinic nurse may do a thorough health history at an intake visit for a gynecologic problem.

A more thorough history usually includes identifying data, occupation, family structure, menstrual history, obstetric history, significant illnesses (with emphasis on gynecologic problems), immunizations, life-style and behaviors history, sexual history, and family health history. A review of systems often is included to assess their current status.

An important component of the history is a review of periodic screening procedures that are recommended for early detection of gynecologic problems, such as breast and cervical cancer. The woman is asked about her performance of breast self-examination and about her most recent Pap smear and the results. Particular risks that are suggested by the history are further explored. For example, women with multiple sexual partners are at higher risk for sexually transmitted disease, and those with rectal bleeding are at greater risk for polyps or cancer of the colon. Occupational hazards and high stress levels that place women at risk can also be identified and further explored.

The health history described in Chapter 22 (Nursing Care During the Antepartal Period) can be used as a guide. For a complete health history, additional questions should be asked about current health practices, life-style, occupational and environmental conditions, and health concepts (see Special Emphases in Gynecologic Health History). Specific points in the health history relevant to developmental needs and gynecologic health promotion are covered in the sections that follow.

Gynecologic Physical Examination

The nurse performs an appropriate physical examination depending upon the systems involved or the purpose of the visit. Examinations may be focused upon specific systems or may be general, as with the health history. The format closely follows that described in Chapter 22. Age and risk status of clients direct the nurse to emphasize certain components of the examination.

For the adolescent, particular attention is paid to the progress of sexual development by noting stage of the secondary sex characteristics (see Sex Maturity Ratings in Girls). Examination for scoliosis also is important for adolescents. The pelvic examination is often critical, as the most common health problems of adolescent girls include dysmenorrhea, irregular menses, vaginitis, and contraception. The first pelvic examination is a rite of passage into American womanhood and must be conducted gently and with great sensitivity. Special techniques for the first pelvic examination have been described.[1] The nurse's attitudes and actions at this time may affect the adolescent's emerging sexual identity either positively or negatively, an influence that could remain for many years.

Women in young and middle adulthood generally have health needs or problems centering around contraception, pregnancy, menstrual problems, vaginal and urinary infections, and neoplasms of the breasts or reproductive organs. Examinations focus upon these areas, especially the breast and reproductive systems. In older adulthood, menopausal concerns become important and the physical examination can focus upon physiological changes expected with declining hormonal function. Cancer of the breast, reproductive organs, and colon

ASSESSMENT TOOL

Special Emphases in Gynecologic Health History

Personal Data
Age, marital/relationship status
Education and occupation
Cultural/ethnic group
Children/persons living in home
Religion
Support systems

Menstrual History
Menarche or menopause
Menstrual cycle characteristics
    Length of cycle
    Days of flow
    Character of flow
    Premenstrual symptoms
    Degree of discomfort
    Medications or remedies used
Date and results of last Pap smear
If menopausal, any vaginal bleeding or other
    symptoms
If menstruating, any irregular bleeding

Pregnancy History
Age at first pregnancy
Total number of pregnancies and outcomes
Pregnancy complications

Contraceptive History
Current contraceptive (if any)
Other contraceptives used
Satisfaction and problems with contraceptive
    methods
Future fertility plans

Major Illnesses or Health Problem
Date and type of illness/health problem
Date and type of operations/hospitalizations
Current medical treatment and medications

Family Health History
Type of illness/health problems of relatives
    Heart attack   High blood pressure
    Stroke   Blood clots (lungs, legs)
    Cancer   Mental illness
    Diabetes   Obesity

Current Health Status
Client's definition of state of health
Concerns about symptoms or possible problems
Self-care activities
Last physical, gynecological, and dental examination

Life-Style and Habits
Nutrition and eating patterns
Sleep and rest
Exercise and recreation
Elimination (bladder, bowel, skin)
Sexual patterns
Stress and stress management
Leisure activities
Environment at home and work (hazards, satisfactions,
    concerns)
Smoking
Alcohol use
Drug use (prescription, over-the-counter, recreational)

becomes a greater risk, which must be carefully assessed during examination.

Periodic Screening

Women at different ages are particularly susceptible to certain diseases. Periodic screening tests or examinations have been recommended according to an age-related schedule. The most critical screening procedures for women include breast examination, mammography, pelvic examination, Pap smear, hematocrit or hemoglobin, rectal examination, stool guaiac, and height, weight, and blood pressure. The nurse can perform many of these procedures both in the hospital and in the clinic or office. A schedule for screening tests and examinations is suggested in Table 48-1.

Nursing Diagnosis

Data from the assessment process provide the foundation for making the nursing diagnosis. A common diagnosis might be alterations in health maintenance, in which the woman experiences or is at risk of experiencing a disruption in her state of wellness. These disruptions are often caused by inadequate preventive measures or an unhealthy life-style.[2a] Many factors may contribute to alterations in health maintenance, including lack of knowledge, poor learning skills, crisis or changing support systems, health or religious beliefs, financial changes, and poor self-esteem.

Depending upon assessment data, the nursing diagnosis might also be noncompliance; potential for injury; alterations in nutrition; diversional activity deficit;

Sex Maturity Ratings in Girls: Breasts

Stage 1

Preadolescent. Elevation of nipple only

Stage 2

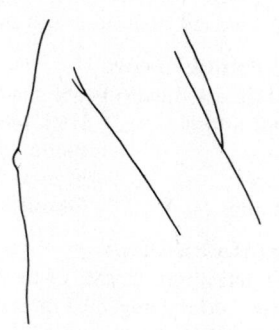

Breast bud stage. Elevation of breast and nipple as a small mound; enlargement of areolar diameter

Stage 3

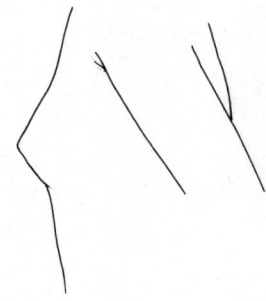

Further enlargement and elevation of breast and areola, with no separation of their contours

Stage 4

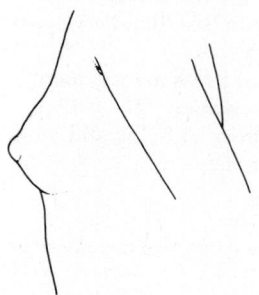

Projection of areola and nipple to form a secondary mound above the level of breast

Stage 5

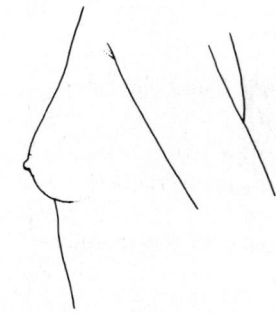

Mature stage; projection of nipple only. Areola has receded to general contour of the breast (although in some normal individuals the areola continues to form a secondary mound)

(Illustrations courtesy of W. A. Daniel, Jr, Division of Adolescent Medicine, University of Alabama, Birmingham)

---

ineffective coping; or powerlessness. Women who do not follow health-related advice given by the nurse may have a nonsupportive family, may lack autonomy in health-seeking behavior, or may not have an effective therapeutic relationship with the nurse. When nutrition is in excess of body requirements, the weight gain may be associated with anxiety or depression, stress, sedentary life-style, or lack of nutritional knowledge. Powerlessness can be a problem in carrying out health-promoting behaviors when the woman experiences social displacement, insufficient finances, adolescent dependence on peer groups, or (in the elderly) sensorimotor deficits.

Planning/Intervention

The nursing-care plan and nursing actions follow directly from the assessment and diagnosis. Key points in assessment, diagnosis, and nursing care are discussed for several common gynecological health conditions.

Breast Conditions

Every nurse should be well versed in teaching breast self-examination (BSE). This is a professional service nurses are in unique positions to offer clients in a variety

Sex Maturity Ratings in Girls: Pubic Hair

Stage 1
Preadolescent. No pubic hair except for the fine body hair (vellus hair) similar to that on the abdomen

Stage 2

Stage 3

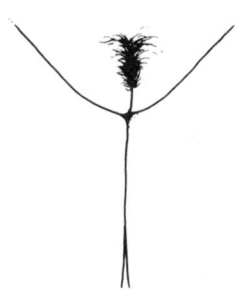

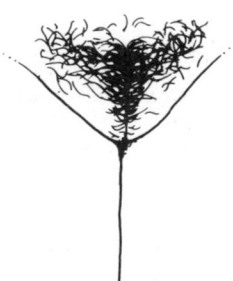

Sparse growth of long, slightly pigmented, downy hair, straight or only slightly curled, chiefly along the labia

Darker, coarser, curlier hair, spreading sparsely over the pubic symphysis

Stage 4

Stage 5

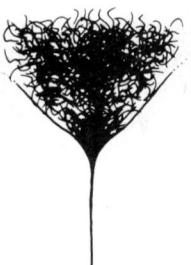

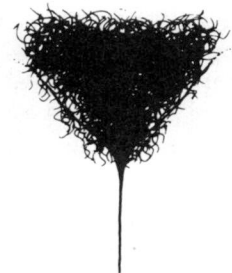

Coarse and curly hair as in adults; area covered greater than in stage 3 but not as great as in the adult and not yet including the thighs

Hair adult in quantity and quality, spread on the medial surfaces of the thighs but not up over the abdomen

(Illustrations courtesy of W. A. Daniel, Jr, Division of Adolescent Medicine, University of Alabama, Birmingham)

of settings. Its importance for early detection of minimal breast lesions has been clearly demonstrated.[3a] BSE is usually taught initially at an adolescent health examination and should be reviewed and reinforced by the nurse every 2 to 3 years. It is recommended that women perform BSE every month about 1 week after their menses. The American Cancer Society's approach to teaching BSE is shown on page 1117.

Clients with problems involving the breasts may present with various symptoms and signs, such as pain, lumps, nipple discharge, skin rashes or discolorations, and changes in size or shape. Any of these could be benign or could signal a malignant neoplasm. Differentiating breast problems is often complex and difficult. Any sign or symptom that cannot be identified readily as a benign problem should be referred to the physician for further evaluation. The nurse can obtain additional data by asking questions about the following:

How long the lump, thickening, or other symptom has been present, and whether or not it has changed
Character of breast pain, if present
Presence of nipple discharge, and characteristics of this
Presence of rash or eczema on the nipple
History of breast trauma, family history of cancer risk

T A B L E   4 8 - 1

Schedule for Periodic Screening for Women

Screening Test or Examination	Age of Woman			
	12–20	20–40	40–60	60–80
Breast exam	Annual	Annual	Annual	Annual
Mammogram	*	Baseline	Every 1–2 years depending on risk	Every 1–2 years depending on risk
Pelvic exam/Pap smear	Annual if sexually active	Annual	Annual	Annual or every 2 years
Hematocrit/hemoglobin	Every 2 years	Every 2 years	Every 5 years	Every 5 years
Rectal exam	*	*	Annual	Annual
Stool guaiac	*	*	Annual	Annual
Height/weight	Annual	Annual	Annual	Annual
Blood pressure	Every 2 years	Every 2 years	Annual	Annual
Urinalysis	*	Every 5 years	Every 5 years	Annual

* Not indicated unless increased risks or symptoms are present.

In the physical examination, the nurse particularly assesses any skin changes (dimpling, erythema, rash), nipple discharge, and thickenings or lumps felt. It is important to perform the examination with the client in both sitting and supine positions. Characteristics of lumps help differentiate among various types of lesions. Combining examination data with information from the history and data on incidence, conclusions can be drawn about the probable nature of the breast lesion (Table 48-2).

Benign Breast Disease

Fibrocystic disease is the most common benign breast problem among women aged 25 to mid-40s; it usually subsides with menopause. This condition is also called *chronic cystic mastitis* and *cystic hyperplasia* and is thought to be estrogen related because its symptoms follow menstrual cycles and decrease after menopause. Fibrocystic disease is characterized by multiple, usually bilateral breast lumps that become more tender prior to menses. The lumps are usually firm, mobile, well defined, and tender to palpation. They increase in size premenstrually, can fluctuate rapidly in size, and regress after menses. The most common location is the upper outer breast quadrants, although the lumps may occur in any area of breast tissue. Nipple discharge is rare.

Diagnosis is often based upon history and physical examination that reveal the above patterns. Any lumps that are unusual in size, shape, consistency, or behavior should be referred for aspiration or biopsy. A baseline mammogram is strongly recommended, because it is difficult to distinguish cystic lumps from early breast cancer. Alteration in comfort: pain is a common nursing diagnosis, since many women experience quite severe discomfort of a cyclic nature. Knowledge deficit related to the medical condition, diagnostic procedures, and treatments is usually present. The woman also may have little knowledge of breast physiology and cyclic changes. Disturbance in self-concept related to pain or potential loss of body part or function also can occur. Women often fear cancer when they experience breast lumps and pain, so a nursing diagnosis of fear related to potential surgery, life-threatening disease, loss of body part or function, and other factors may be indicated.

Nursing care focuses on pain relief, education, and emotional support. The woman is advised to wear a good supportive brassiere both day and night and to avoid trauma to the breasts. Dietary factors may affect the extent of breast pain, and the nurse can recommend avoiding chocolate, coffee, and black tea and restricting sodium intake. When pain is acute, ice packs to the tender areas may help, and pain relievers such as salicylates or anti-inflammatory medications may be used. The hormone inhibitor danazol (Danocrine) may be ordered when these therapies are not effective. Up to 70% to 80% of women using danazol report relief of pain and nodularity; however, the side-effects include menstrual pattern changes and weight gain.[4]

Health teaching is an important intervention. Women must learn BSE thoroughly and feel confident in identifying unusual lumps or changes in their breasts. By explaining the relationship of fibrocystic disease to the monthly cycle, the nurse can help alleviate fears of cancer while reinforcing the need for further evaluation of suspected abnormalities. Providing support for discussion of the client's emotional responses to the threat of cancer can dissipate fears and develop effective coping strategies. Women with fibrocystic disease are encouraged to have regular breast examinations by a phy-

CLIENT EDUCATION

Breast Self-Examination Technique

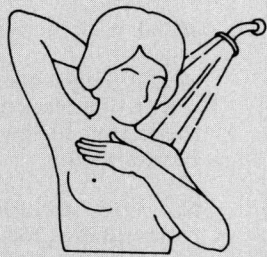

1. *In the shower.*

Examine your breasts during bath or shower; hands glide easily over wet skin. With fingers flat, move them gently over every part of each breast. Check for any lump, hard knot, or thickening.

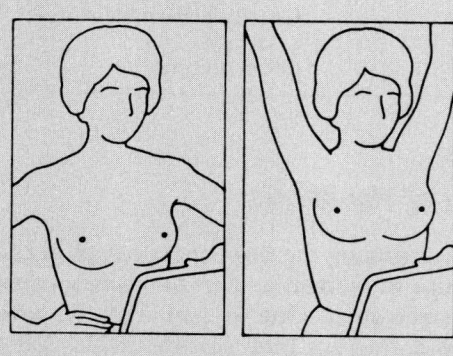

2. *Before a mirror.*

Inspect your breasts with arms at your sides. Next, raise your arms high overhead. Look for any changes in contour of each breast—a swelling, dimpling of skin, or changes in the nipple. Then rest palms on hips and press down firmly to flex your chest muscles. Left and right breast will not match exactly—few women's breasts do. Regular inspection shows what is normal for you and will give you confidence in your examination.

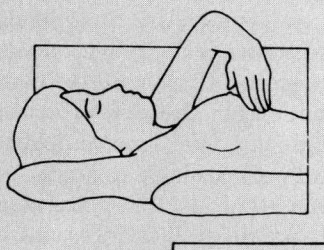

3. *Lying down.*

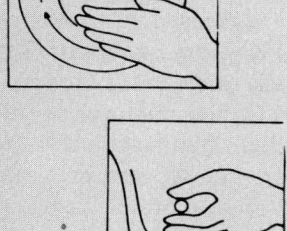

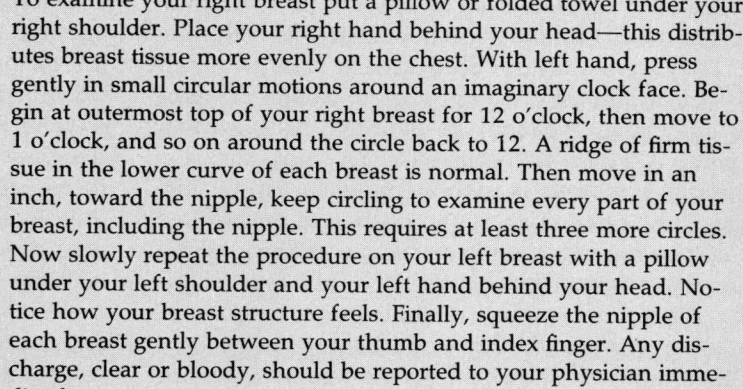

To examine your right breast put a pillow or folded towel under your right shoulder. Place your right hand behind your head—this distributes breast tissue more evenly on the chest. With left hand, press gently in small circular motions around an imaginary clock face. Begin at outermost top of your right breast for 12 o'clock, then move to 1 o'clock, and so on around the circle back to 12. A ridge of firm tissue in the lower curve of each breast is normal. Then move in an inch, toward the nipple, keep circling to examine every part of your breast, including the nipple. This requires at least three more circles. Now slowly repeat the procedure on your left breast with a pillow under your left shoulder and your left hand behind your head. Notice how your breast structure feels. Finally, squeeze the nipple of each breast gently between your thumb and index finger. Any discharge, clear or bloody, should be reported to your physician immediately.

sician or nurse practitioner, and periodic mammography as indicated.

Fibroadenoma is the third most common breast tumor (following fibrocystic disease and carcinoma) and occurs primarily in women in their teens and early 20s.

In adolescents, the cause is associated with breast hypertrophy during the pubertal growth spurt. The lump is typically well defined, firm and rubbery, freely movable, rounded, and nontender. A solitary nodule ranging from 1 cm to 5 cm is common, but multiple tumors

TABLE 48-2

Differentiating Among Breast Masses

	Fibrocystic Disease	Fibroadenoma	Cancer
Usual age	30–55, regresses after menopause	15–20+, occurs up to 55	30–80, peak incidence 42–48
Number	Usually multiple, may be single	Usually single, may be multiple	Usually single, but may coexist with other lesions
Shape	Round	Round, discoid, or lobular	Irregular or stellate
Consistency	Soft to firm, bumpy nodular breasts	Usually firm, may be soft	Firm or hard
Delimitation	Usually well delineated	Well-delineated, clear margins	Not clearly delineated from surrounding tissue
Mobility	Mobile	Very mobile, slippery	May be fixed to skin or underlying tissue
Tenderness	Often tender	Usually nontender	Usually nontender, but not always
Retraction signs	Absent	Absent	Often present

occur in about 15% of cases. These tumors are responsive to hormones and can increase rapidly in size. There is no significant association with malignancy.

Diagnosis is based upon tumor characteristics identified during examination. If there are unusual characteristics, a biopsy or mammogram may be necessary. Watchful observation with eventual surgical excision is the usual course of treatment. Although cancer is unlikely, it cannot be completely ruled out in any discrete lump. Nursing diagnoses could include knowledge deficit, disturbance in self-concept, and fear. Nursing care includes education and support similar to that described for fibrocystic disease, with explanations appropriate for fibroadenoma.

Intraductal papillomas are tiny tumors (2 mm–3 mm) most commonly located in a major subareolar collection duct. They have a central fibrovascular stalk with delicate papillae and are often too small to palpate. Tumors are usually single but may be multiple. No particular age-group is typical for occurrence. The most common presenting symptom is serosanguineous nipple discharge. During examination, the location of the affected duct may be found by gently pressing with the fingertip at successive points around the circumference of the areola. A point may be found where pressure produces the discharge. A small lump or thickening also may be felt. If no lump is palpable and the lesion cannot be localized, mammography is used to locate the papilloma.

Although papillomas are usually benign, low-grade malignancy may exist. The lesion must be excised and examined histologically. Excision is the definitive treatment for papillomas, with follow-up because they may recur. Multiple lesions are more difficult to manage, requiring several excisions. Nursing diagnoses can include knowledge deficit, disturbance in self-concept, and fear, with nursing care as described above.

Carcinoma of the Breast

Breast cancer is among the three most common causes of breast lumps in women and is the leading cause of cancer deaths in women. One woman in 11 will develop breast cancer during her lifetime. About 119,000 new cases are diagnosed and 38,000 deaths reported annually from breast cancer. Women are most likely to develop breast cancer after the age of 35, with the peak incidence between the ages of 40 and 60. Individual risk increases steadily with age. Theories of causality include hormonal mechanisms involving endogenous steroids, viral agents, and immunologic deficiencies.

Risk factors have been identified that place women at increased risk for breast cancer. Risk increases with age, and 75% of breast cancers occur after age 40. Race is a factor, with white women at higher risk than nonwhite. Hereditary factors may be important, since women have increased risk with mothers, sisters, or daughters having breast cancer. Reproductive factors increasing risk include nulliparity, early menarche (before age 12), late menopause (more than 30 years after menarche), first pregnancy after age 35, oophorectomy before age 40, and breast cancer in the other breast. Nutritional patterns associated with increased risk include diets high in fat and protein and low in selenium. Other possible factors include exposure to radiation, having other malignancies, being under chronic psychological stress, and being of higher socioeconomic status (See Risk Factors for Gynecologic Cancer).

Assessment. A breast mass is the most common sign of breast cancer. It is usually discovered by the woman or her sexual partner. In early stages, the lump is usually single, firm, and dense, may be movable or fixed to skin or underlying tissue, and may be circumscribed or ir-

ASSESSMENT TOOL

Risk Factors for Gynecologic Cancer

Breast Cancer

Over 40 years of age

White

Living in cold climate, Western hemisphere

Unmarried

Higher socioeconomic status

Nulliparous or first pregnancy after age 35

Family history of breast cancer (grandmother, mother, sister, daughter)

Previous breast cancer or fibrocystic breast disease

Early menarche (before age 12)

Late menopause (more than 30 years after menarche or after age 50)

Diet high in fat and protein, low in selenium

Other malignancies, lowered immunocompetency

Cervical Cancer

Multiple sexual partners

Beginning sexual contact before age 20

First pregnancy at an early age

High parity

Intercourse with men who have had venereal disease or prostatic cancer

History of sexually transmitted disease (herpes, trichomoniasis, chlamydia, genital warts, syphilis)

Ovarian Cancer

Delayed onset of childbearing

Low parity

Infertility

Nulliparity

Several spontaneous abortions

Family history of ovarian cancer

Caucasian of European or North American origin

Endometrial Cancer

White, middle class

Irregular menses

Infertility

Late menopause

Obesity, hypertension, and diabetes mellitus

Personal or family history of other cancers

History of atypical endometrial hyperplasia

Postmenopausal bleeding

---

regular. The most frequent location is the upper outer quadrant. Other signs that usually appear later may include nipple discharge or retraction, skin edema or dimpling, and enlarged axillary lymph nodes. Breast cancer is usually nontender, but tenderness may occur and the woman may report pain or tingling sensations.

There are several types of breast cancer with differing rates of growth and severity. The two most common types are adenocarcinomas and ductal carcinomas (comprising about 65% of all breast cancers). Breast cancers tend to be spatially and temporally multicentric. Over half of the carcinomas have been found with multiple sites of apparently primary lesion, often microscopic in size and only identifiable by pathologic examination. Metastasis occurs early, and by the time a breast cancer is palpable (about 1 cm) micrometastases are almost certainly present. The length of time required for cancers to grow to 1 cm in size has been estimated at between 3 months and 2½ years.[3b] However, some speculate that as long as 30 years may be required for malignancies to progress from a single cell to a palpable

mass. Metastasis first occurs in surrounding tissue, then through the ductal system, lymph channels, and circulatory system to distant metastatic sites such as bones, liver, and lungs.

Diagnosis. Diagnostic tests most often used for evaluation of suspected breast cancer are mammography and biopsy. Mammography is very accurate when typical findings of cancer are present, such as microcalcifications or increased density with stippling. However, at least 50% of breast cancers discovered by palpation in asymptomatic women may have negative mammograms.[3c] With a suspicious breast mass, biopsy must be performed. Needle or aspiration biopsy withdraws a core of tumor cells or cystic fluid for microscopic examination. Incisional biopsy, which can be done under local anesthesia, removes a portion of tumor for cytologic examination. Careful examination of a permanent tissue specimen generally takes several days.

If biopsy confirms malignancy, staging is done to determine if the disease is local (confined to the breast)

The Woman with Breast Problems

Nursing Objectives

1. Ensure accurate identification of type of breast problem.
2. Identify early the woman with breast cancer.
3. Provide thorough education on breast problem and BSE.
4. Prevent breast problems by reducing risk whenever possible.
5. Implement effective nursing care to minimize risk, reduce complications, promote adjustment of client and family, and enhance health status.

Assessment	Potential Nursing Diagnosis	Planning/Intervention	Evaluation

Risk factors
  Age, race
  Family history
  Menstrual patterns
  Pregnancy history
  Dietary patterns
  Life-style patterns
	Knowledge deficit related to risk factors for various breast problems	Teach BSE
		Teach risk factors for cancer
		Teach characteristics of women with benign breast diseases
			Client performs BSE correctly and verbalizes confidence in evaluating breast tissue
			Client can describe risk factors
			Client can describe characteristics of women with benign breast disease

History of problem and physical examination/laboratory tests	Anxiety or fear related to potentially serious breast mass	Explain procedures and possible outcomes; provide support	Client less anxious, able to cope with waiting for results, understands rationales
Benign breast disease Fibrocystic disease	Knowledge deficit related to the medical condition	Teach client about type of breast disease	Client relates understanding of her type of breast problem
Fibroadenoma Intraductal papilloma	Alterations in comfort: pain	Provide pain relief measures (medications); teach client self-care methods of pain relief	Client obtains relief of pain through self-care methods or medications
	Disturbance in self-concept related to pain or potential loss of body part or function	Encourage client to express her concerns; clarify misconceptions	Client verbalizes concerns, understands risk, and accepts self-concept

(continued)

or if metastasis has occurred. Chest x-ray films, lung scans, blood tests (primarily for alkaline phosphatase), and liver and bone scans are usually done. Node biopsies may also be indicated. This information permits staging or classification of the tumor in order to decide on the most appropriate treatment. Two approaches to classifying (staging) tumors are used: the Columbia Clinical Classification and the TNM System of the American Joint Committee for Cancer Staging.

Nursing Diagnoses. Several nursing diagnoses may be appropriate for clients with breast cancer. Knowledge deficit related to medical condition, tests, and surgical procedures is likely to be present. Ineffective coping

patterns due to anxiety may affect cognitive abilities. Disturbance in self-concept related to potential loss of body part or function is probable, since therapy often involves some degree of breast removal. Fear related to anticipated pain, surgery, life-threatening disease, loss of body part or function, or change in relationship with partner may be present. During hospitalization and recovery, numerous other nursing diagnoses could be relevant, such as alterations in bowel elimination; alterations in comfort; ineffective individual coping; alterations in family processes; and powerlessness.

Treatment. Surgical treatment for breast cancer ranges from local excision of the tumor to total resection

Assessment	Potential Nursing Diagnosis	Planning/Intervention	Evaluation
	Fear related to potential life-threatening disease, surgery, or loss of body part or function	Encourage client to express fears and clarify her misconceptions	Client verbalizes fears, has realistic view of risk, carries out prevention and early detection measures
Breast cancer	Anxiety or fear related to effects of cancer, such as surgery, pain, death, loss of body part or function, change in relationships	Encourage client to express fears and clarify her misconceptions	Client verbalizes fears, finds ways of coping, is able to accept loss of breast
	Knowledge deficit related to medical condition, tests, hospitalization and surgical procedures, recovery	Teach client about procedures and routine related to treatment	Client describes procedures and routine, understands treatment and recovery process
	Disturbance in self-concept related to loss of body part or function	Encourage client to express her concerns and feelings	Client verbalizes feelings and concerns, is able to accept altered self-concept
	Ineffective individual coping related to anxiety, interpersonal conflicts, disfigurement, altered appearance, inadequate resources	Assist client to identify ineffective coping and find more effective approaches	Client voices problems affecting coping, can describe other approaches, is able to carry out normal daily activities and interests
	Sexual dysfunction related to loss of body part, disrupted relationship with partner	Encourage expression of feelings and involve sexual partner, promote comfort with body changes, refer to sexual counseling	Client and partner express feelings about body changes and sexuality, accept breast loss, resume satisfying sexual relationship, or seek sexual counseling
	During hospitalization: numerous physiological disruptions (circulatory, respiratory, infection, elimination, fluids) as well as above	Monitor vital signs, dressings, wound; promote respiratory and eliminative functions; promote hydration and nutrition; provide pain relief; minimize side-effects of surgery or other therapy	Stable physiological function, wound heals, client recovers strength, discomfort is managed, side-effects of therapy do not interfere significantly with daily activities and interests

of the breast, chest wall muscles, and axilla. The extent of surgery depends upon the clinical staging of the disease, the histologic characteristics of the tumor, and other considerations, such as age and health status. Recent data indicate that conservative breast surgery combined with radiotherapy yields survival rates similar to those with modified radical mastectomy.[5] Radiation therapy is often used as an adjunct to local excision or simple mastectomy, to shrink large tumors to operable dimensions, and as primary treatment for inflammatory breast cancer or inoperable tumors (see chart on page 1123).

Medical oncology uses antineoplastic drugs and endocrine therapy to affect tumor growth. Chemother-apy is often used as preferred adjuvant therapy to surgery when there is axillary node involvement. The systemic effects of drugs halt microscopic metastatic disease and can lengthen the period before relapse. For advanced breast cancer, chemotherapy is primarily palliative. When breast tumors are hormone sensitive, their growth can be retarded by using estrogen, androgen, or progestin, depending upon tumor receptors.

Planning/Intervention. Major problems with chemotherapy and hormone therapy are caused by side-effects, making alterations in comfort a common nursing diagnosis.

Nursing care is related to the stage of the disease,

the point in medical or surgical therapy, and the nursing diagnoses identified. Interventions commonly used include client teaching, support during procedures, emotional support and counseling, physiological monitoring and technical procedures, comfort measures, family counseling, and coordination of resources for family support and recovery (see Nursing Care Plan).

Cervical Conditions

Maternity nurses need to be conversant with Pap smears and the management of cervical intraepithelial neoplasia. Women of all ages are concerned about cervical cancer, and the widespread use of Pap smears for screening has increased awareness over the past several decades. Some controversy exists over the frequency of screening intervals. The American Cancer Society and the National Cancer Institute recommend Pap smears every 3 years after two annual negative tests. The Canadian Task Force recommends tests every year between the ages of 18 and 35, then every 5 years after two negative annual tests after age 35. The American College of Obstetricians and Gynecologists continues to recommend annual Pap smears from beginning of sexual activity.[6]

Cancer of the cervix is the second most frequent cancer in women (after breast cancer), and about 2% of women will develop it before the age of 80. The death rate from cervical cancer has fallen steadily over the past 40 years, with most cases diagnosed as carcinoma in situ because of Pap smear screening. The average age at diagnosis of carcinoma in situ is 35 years and at diagnosis of invasive disease, 45 years. However, increasing numbers of women in their teens and early 20s are being diagnosed in both stages of disease. Cervical cancer is progressive, with most untreated clients developing invasive disease in 5 to 9 years after carcinoma in situ.[3d]

Women are at increased risk for cervical cancer when they have multiple sexual partners, begin sexual contact before age 20, have their first pregnancy at an early age, have high parity, have intercourse with men who have had venereal disease or prostatic cancer, and have had sexually transmitted diseases themselves (such as herpes, trichomoniasis, chlamydial disease, genital warts, or syphilis).

It is proposed that all types of cervical dysplasia, from moderate through actual carcinoma in situ, be considered part of the same process called cervical intraepithelial neoplasia (CIN). Histologically, the changes in tissue involve the same processes but are a matter of degree. When normal squamous metaplasia proceeds to atypical changes, these cells over many years can result in a cervical epithelium having varying degrees of dysplasia.[7]

Assessment. Nurses must be able to identify women at increased risk for cervical cancer, and must have the skills to perform vaginal examinations and Pap smears. Women often have no symptoms associated with CIN, and the condition usually is detected on routine Pap smear. Associated conditions, such as vaginal infections or cervicitis, may cause symptoms and signs of increased or odorous vaginal discharge, itching or burning of the perineum, urinary frequency or burning, dyspareunia, or lower abdominal discomfort. A history of sexual, menstrual, and pregnancy patterns is critical in evaluating cervical conditions.

Staging (Classification) of Breast Cancer

Columbia Clinical Classification

A1 No clinically involved axillary nodes
 2 No grave signs as in clinical stage C
B1 Clinically involved axillary nodes less than 2.5 cm transverse diameter
 2 No grave signs as in clinical stage C
C Any of the five grave signs
 1 Edema of skin, limited extent (less than one third of skin involved)
 2 Ulceration of skin
 3 Solid fixation primary tumor to chest wall
 4 Axillary nodes 2.5 cm or more transverse diameter
 5 Fixation axillary nodes to overlying or surrounding tissue
D All more advanced cases

TNM* System of the American Joint Committee for Cancer Staging

Stage I
(T) Tumor less than 2 cm diameter
(N) Nodes in axilla, if present, not felt to contain metastasis
(M) No distant metastases

Stage II
(T) Tumor less than 5 cm diameter
(N) Nodes in axilla, if present, not fixed
(M) No distant metastases

Stage III
(T) Tumor greater than 5 cm or tumor of any size with skin invasion or attachment
(N) Nodes in supraclavicular area
(M) No distant metastases

Stage IV
(T) Tumor of any size with extension to chest wall and skin
(N) Any amount of nodal involvement
(M) Distant metastases are present

* (T, tumor; N, nodes; M, metastases)

Types of Surgery for Breast Lesions

Radical mastectomy (Classical, Halsted). Through a vertical incision the entire breast is removed with a significant margin of skin around nipple and areola and tumor. The pectoralis major and minor muscles are removed, the axillary vein is dissected, and the axillary lymph nodes are dissected. A skin-thin surgical flap is left, but, depending upon the amount of skin removed, skin grafting may be necessary.

Extended radical mastectomy. Includes the above procedure plus excision of the internal mammary lymph nodes. Some sections of the ribs must be removed to reach the internal mammary nodes. The supraclavicular nodes may also be removed. This operation is rarely done today.

Modified radical mastectomy. The entire breast and most of the axillary lymph nodes are removed, but the pectoralis muscles are preserved. Some surgeons dissect the entire axillary chain, while others leave the upper third intact. The axillary vein is stripped.

Simple (or total) mastectomy. The entire breast is removed, but the axillary nodes and pectoralis muscles are not. Some surgeons biopsy the last lymph node in the tail of the breast. If it has been invaded, either the axilla is irradiated or a radical mastectomy is done.

Partial mastectomy (segmental resection, wedge resection). The tumor and a wide segment of surrounding breast tissue, underlying fascia, and overlying skin are removed, usually about one-third of the breast. Some surgeons also dissect the axillary nodes.

Lumpectomy, tylectomy, or local excision. The tumor and 3 cm to 5 cm of tissue on either side are removed, retaining other breast tissue and skin.

Subcutaneous mastectomy. Breast tissue, including the axillary tail, is removed through an incision beneath the breast. All breast skin including the nipple and areola and a small button of tissue under the nipple remains. A silicone implant is inserted, either during the initial surgery or several months later.

A complete pelvic examination is done, including speculum examination, bimanual examination, and collection of specimens. Before taking the Pap smear, the cervix is inspected and its condition noted. Findings may include nabothian cysts, ectropion, erosion, cervicitis, polyps, or other lesions, such as leukoplakia, herpes, or frank carcinoma (Fig. 48-1).

Nurses have increasing responsibility for Pap smear screening, particularly those in extended roles such as nurse practitioners and clinical specialists. The Pap smear is taken using a cotton-tipped applicator and a spatula (wooden or plastic). The cervix is wiped gently only if there is excessive mucus. Lubricating jelly should not be used because it distorts the cell sample; water is permissible to aid speculum insertion. Samples are taken from the endocervical canal with the cotton-tipped applicator, which may be wetted with saline. The applicator is placed high in the cervix, rotated a few times, then withdrawn and applied to a slide in the opposite direction. The spatula, with the long tip placed into the cervical os, is used to scrape the ectocervix. The material is spread thinly on a slide. Slides are sprayed or immersed immediately in a fixative; air drying can distort cells. Vaginal pool specimens are recommended for women over the age of 50, when they can be helpful in detecting endometrial cancer.[6] Pap smears generally are reported descriptively and identify the degree of cervical epithelial changes that have occurred. The presence of inflammation or infection is also noted on the Pap report.

Depending upon symptoms and vaginal or cervical signs, other specimens may be taken for microscopic examination, such as wet mounts prepared with saline or potassium hydroxide, or gonorrhea cultures. With a history of exposure to DES, samples are obtained with a spatula by scraping the vaginal walls, placing on a slide, and fixing as above.

Diagnosis. The Pap smear report describes the condition of the cervix. If the report is abnormal, further evaluation is necessary. Women with an atypical Pap smear that also identifies presence of a microorganism (with or without inflammation) are treated with the appropriate medication, such as antifungal, antitrichomonal, or antibiotic drugs. The Pap is then repeated in 3 to 6 months. If significant atypia still is present, the woman is referred for colposcopy or biopsy.

Women with Pap smears showing dysplasia require prompt management because this can be a precursor to cancer. Initial treatment consists in colposcopy and biopsy. Colposcopy uses a binocular stereoscopic microscope of low magnification to view the cervix through a vaginal speculum. The cervix is swabbed to remove mucus, and 2% acetic acid is applied to enhance cellular patterns. A green filter and Schiller's iodine solution may also be used to accentuate vascular patterns and

Normal nulliparous cervix

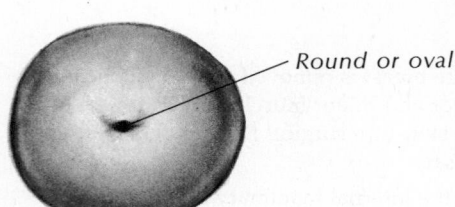

Round or oval

The nulliparous cervical os is small and either round or oval. The cervix is covered by smooth pink epithelium.

Normal parous cervix

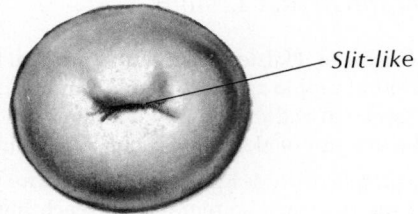

Slit-like

After childbirth, the cervical os presents a slit-like appearance.

Cervical polyp

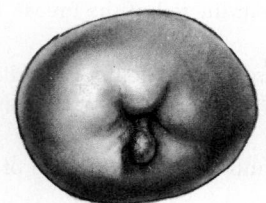

Cervical polyps usually arise from the endocervical canal, becoming visible when they protrude through the cervical os. They are bright red, soft and rather fragile. When only the tips are seen they cannot be clinically differentiated from polyps originating in the endometrium.

Nabothian or retention cysts

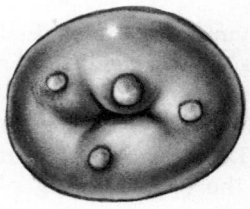

Retention or Nabothian cysts are another accompaniment of chronic cervicitis. Variable in size, single or multiple, they appear as translucent nodules on the cervical surface.

Ectropion & erosion

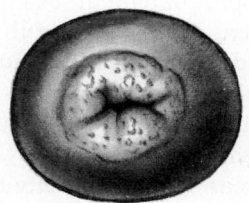

Ectropion is extension of endocervical columnar epithelium (reddish, bumpy) onto the ectocervix. This physiologic condition often occurs with increased estrogen activity (eg, pregnancy). If inflammation or infection occurs, the tissue becomes friable and bleeds easily. This is referred to as erosion.

F I G U R E   4 8 - 1

Common cervical conditions.

identify suspicious cells. The transformation zone of the cervix (area of change from squamous to columnar epithelium) is carefully examined for vascular patterns, intercapillary distance, surface pattern, color tone and opacity, clarity, and demarcation. Typical findings include white epithelium, mosaic structure, punctation, and leukoplakia.

Biopsy specimens are taken from suspicious areas of the cervix. This is usually adequate if the upper margin of the transformation zone can be seen on the ec-

tocervix. If the upper margin is not visible, endocervical curettage is necessary to sample the transformation zone adequately. Based upon cytologic examination of these specimens, medical treatment can be planned.

Nursing Diagnoses. Nursing diagnoses related to CIN are similar to those for breast tumors. Both conditions potentially involve cancer, which is life-threatening and may require loss of body parts. Common nursing diagnoses might be knowledge deficit; ineffec-

Descriptive Pap Smear Reports

Findings inadequate for diagnosis
Findings essentially normal
Atypical cells present and suggestive of cytologic findings consistent with:

CIN grade I (mild dysplasia): isolated abnormal nuclei within framework of a reasonably orderly epithelium

CIN grade II (moderate dysplasia): substantial proportion (50%) of abnormal cells, although retaining the basic makeup of the epithelium

CIN grade III (severe dysplasia with carcinoma in situ): intraepithelial lesion composed of cancer cells, which may be classified as keratinizing type, large cell type, or small cell type

Invasive squamous cell carcinoma

Inflammation (mild, moderate, severe) present
Microorganisms present (fungi, *Trichomonas*, bacteria)
Estrogen level: adequate, increased, decreased, absent

---

tive coping patterns; disturbance in self-concept; anxiety; fear; sexual dysfunction; and powerlessness.

Treatment. Medical treatment depends upon the extensiveness of the CIN. If cells from the endocervical canal have been found free of disease, and the abnormal cells from the cervix range from mild/moderate dysplasia to carcinoma in situ, techniques are used that completely destroy the surface of the transformation zone and penetrate at least 4 mm to 5 mm to destroy any dysplastic extensions into the gland crypts. Cryosurgery, carbon dioxide laser therapy, and radical electrocautery are all effective techniques that can be performed on an outpatient basis or in surgical centers. Local or general anesthesia can be used, and pain during the healing process is usually minimal.[7]

When CIN has progressed to the microinvasive stage, conization is the initial treatment. It is used when colposcopy and biopsy fail to reveal the source of abnormal cells and when the upper margin of the transformation zone cannot be visualized. Surgical conization removes a cone-shaped wedge from the cervical canal with a knife. Depending on the extent of invasion, hysterectomy may follow conization.

Invasive cervical cancer is staged according to extent of stromal involvement and whether vaginal or pelvic wall extension, rectal or bladder extension, kidney involvement, and distant metastases have occurred. Treatment consists in hysterectomy (simple or radical), irradiation, or chemotherapy, depending upon the extensiveness of disease, the woman's age and general health, and the presence of other abnormalities. Some

controversy exists over use of surgery or radiotherapy, but in general all women with stages beyond stage I and stage IIA are treated with radiotherapy. Surgery for stages I and IIA disease is reserved for young women in whom preservation of ovarian function is desired.[3e]

Planning/Intervention. Nursing care is similar to that for breast problems and breast cancer (see Nursing-Care Plan). Of particular consideration is the meaning of reproductive ability to the woman and her partner. Some women suffer severe alterations in self-concept when they can no longer have babies, and their spouses often hold similar attitudes that devalue nonprocreative women. Interventions in these cases focus upon the process of accepting physical and psychoemotional changes and finding other qualities for which the woman can be valued. In other instances, loss of the uterus and reproductive capacity does not significantly diminish self-concept. The woman may have other valued roles or may be at a point in life when childbearing is no longer desired. For some women who have been experiencing considerable pain with menses and disruption in routines, hysterectomy may be viewed with relief. If cancer is diagnosed, many women find the

Staging of Cervical Cancer

Stage 0	Carcinoma in situ, intraepithelial carcinoma
Stage I	Carcinoma strictly confined to the cervix
IA	Microinvasive carcinoma (early stromal invasion)
IB	All other cases of Stage I (occult cancer = occ)
Stage II	Carcinoma extends beyond the cervix but has not extended to the pelvic wall. The carcinoma involves the vagina, but not as far as the lower third.
IIA	No obvious parametrial involvement
IIB	Obvious parametrial involvement
Stage III	Carcinoma has extended to the pelvic wall. On rectal examination, there is no cancer-free space between the tumor and the pelvic wall. The tumor involves the lower third of the vagina.
IIIA	No extension to the pelvic wall
IIIB	Extension to the pelvic wall or hydronephrosis or nonfunctioning kidney
Stage IV	Carcinoma has extended beyond the true pelvis or has clinically involved the mucosa of the bladder or rectum.
IVA	Spread of carcinoma to adjacent organs
IVB	Spread to distant organs

Nomenclature of the International Federation of Gynecology and Obstetrics (FIGO).

threat to life vastly more important than the loss of reproductive capacity. Nursing interventions then focus upon expressing fear, placing realistic parameters on expectations, values clarification and spiritual supports, enhancing family and community resources, and finding personal strengths for coping.

Pelvic Masses

Conditions involving pelvic organs and producing varying degrees of pain are common among women of reproductive age. Maternity nurses may be consulted about pelvic symptoms and need a working knowledge of the kinds of conditions that might be involved. Menstrual and bleeding problems are covered in Chapter 49. Common pelvic masses are discussed here, particularly ovarian tumors and uterine masses. Among younger women, these conditions tend to be benign; the risk of cancer increases with age. However, cancer must be considered in every type of pelvic mass until diagnosed otherwise.

Ovarian masses common among women between the ages of 20 and 40 include functional ovarian cysts, cystadenomas, cystic teratomas, fibromas, endometriomas (chocolate cysts), and tubal/ovarian pregnancies. Unless quite large, these masses usually cause no symptoms and are discovered incidentally during an examination. When symptoms are present, they are usually vague and may include lower abdominal discomfort, aching, feelings of fullness, pressure, dyspareunia, or discomfort with menstruation or defecation. Tubal/ovarian pregnancies cause acute abdominal pain prior to and during rupture and are discussed in Chapter 36.

Ovarian cancer also is generally silent, making its diagnosis in early stages difficult. The most common types are cystadenocarcinomas and adenocarcinomas, which may be either solid or cystic. Ovarian metastasis from other primary cancers may occur. In early stages, ovarian cancer may feel no different from benign cystic or solid ovarian masses. Later, cancers may become fixed, heavy, and hard and have ill-defined margins. Malignant tumors frequently are nontender and cause few symptoms except vague pelvic fullness or aching. Infectious ovarian or pelvic masses are usually readily identifiable because of associated findings of fever, leukocytosis, tenderness, nausea, and vomiting.

Ovarian cancer is infrequent under age 35; the greatest incidence is among women aged 50 to 59. Risk rises steadily to age 75, after which it declines. Ovarian cancers constitute about 4% of all female cancers and are the fifth leading cause of death for women in the 35- to 54-year-old age-group. Factors that increase risk include delayed onset of childbearing, low parity, in-

fertility, nulliparity, several spontaneous abortions, and family history of ovarian cancer. White women of European and North American origin are more likely to contract ovarian cancer than black women of African origin or Oriental women of Asian origin. There is some evidence that women with irregular menses and premenstrual tension may be at increased risk.[8]

Assessment. The health history focuses upon age, menstrual history, present menstrual status, parturition history, family history—especially of cancers, and race. Symptoms involving the lower abdomen and reproductive organs are explored. Weight gain must be carefully evaluated; it may be related to ascites or ovarian enlargement. Some women may notice increased abdominal girth, but may interpret this as midriff bulge or middle age. As the tumor enlarges, it progressively compresses surrounding pelvic structures and blood vessels, leading to urinary frequency, edema of lower extremities, constipation, and pelvic discomfort. Gastrointestinal symptoms may include heartburn, bloating, anorexia, and food intolerance. Unusual vaginal bleeding is a common symptom during reproductive years, including amenorrhea and irregular or excessive menses. Many types of ovarian tumors can affect menstrual patterns. Late signs of cancer are pelvic pain, cachexia, and anemia; unfortunately, much ovarian cancer is not discovered until an advanced stage with such signs, and prognosis is poor.

Physical examination usually reveals an ovarian enlargement; specific characteristics depend upon the type of tumor (Table 48-3). An experienced examiner can often make a reliable assessment based upon tumor characteristics and associated history of symptoms, taking risk characteristics into consideration. Functional ovarian cysts that fail to resolve with conservative management must be further evaluated, as are solid masses, using such techniques as ultrasonography, laparoscopic examination, and biopsy.

Diagnosis. Medical diagnosis is based upon tumor characteristics and results of diagnostic tests. In some instances, surgical removal of the tumor with pathologic examination establishes the diagnosis. When ovarian cancer is diagnosed, it must be staged so appropriate therapy can be planned. An international system for staging ovarian cancer has been developed. Pap tests of vaginal, pleural, or peritoneal fluids; lung and bone scans; blood tests; and radiographic studies of chest, kidneys, and gastrointestinal system complete the diagnostic work-up.

Nursing Diagnosis. Nursing diagnoses may include knowledge deficit; disturbance in self-concept; ineffec-

Staging of Ovarian Cancer

Stage I	Growth limited to the ovaries
IA	Growth limited to one ovary, no ascites
IB	Growth limited to both ovaries, no ascites
IC	Growth limited to one or both ovaries, ascitic fluid containing malignant cells is present
Stage II	Growth involves one or both ovaries with pelvic extension
IIA	Extension or metastases to uterus or tubes only
IIB	Extension to other pelvic tissues
Stage III	Growth involves one or both ovaries with widespread intraperitoneal metastases (omentum, bowel, peritoneum, etc.)
Stage IV	Distant metastases outside the peritoneal cavity

International system for staging cancer of the ovary.

tive coping; fear; anxiety; powerlessness; alterations in comfort; sexual dysfunction; and spiritual distress.

Treatment. Functional ovarian cysts may be managed conservatively, since these usually resolve spontaneously within several weeks. The client is reexamined during different phases of the menstrual cycle after an interval of 1 to 3 months. Failure of the mass to resolve by 12 weeks requires further diagnostic procedures. Solid benign tumors are generally removed surgically, with ovarian resection or removal depending upon extent of tumor involvement. Ovarian cancer is treated according to stage of the disease. Surgical removal of as much of the tumor as possible is usually done first and can range from simple removal of one ovary to radical hysterectomy and bilateral salpingo-oophorectomy. Chemotherapy or radiotherapy often follow, the combinations and extent dependent upon the stage of cancer and aggressiveness of the malignancy.

Planning/Intervention. Nursing care is related to the type of ovarian tumor, medical treatment, and client and family's responses. For simple benign problems, interventions emphasize client teaching, support during procedures, and emotional support to cope with fear and anxiety. When ovarian cancer is present, interventions include the above as well as physiological monitoring and technical procedures, comfort measures, support for family coping and adjustment, expressing and dealing with fear, coordination of resources for family support and recovery, values clarification and spiritual supports, and finding personal strengths for coping.

Uterine Masses

Uterine masses often present as an enlarged or irregularly shaped uterus, although a pedunculated fibroid can be felt as an apparently separate pelvic mass. Evaluation of an enlarged uterus is to some extent related to age; certainly among women in the childbearing age pregnancy must always be considered. Infections, adenomyosis, polyps, fibroids, hyperplasia, and malignancy are among the more common causes of uterine enlargement. Endometrical carcinoma is the third most frequent malignancy in women; 90% of these are adenocarcinomas. The peak incidence is between ages 50 and 70, and it is more common in postmenopausal women. The etiology of endometrial cancer is unclear; it is possibly triggered by metabolic abnormalities involving pituitary hyperactivity and impaired glucose metabolism. Prolonged exogenous estrogen use, especially in postmenopausal women, has been associated with increased incidence of endometrial cancer.

Assessment. Risk for endometrial cancer is greater in white, middle-class women who experience irregular menses, infertility, or late menopause. An association has long been observed between obesity, hypertension, and diabetes mellitus and endometrial cancer, but the causal connections are not well understood. Other risk factors include personal or family history of cancers, atypical endometrial hyperplasia, and postmenopausal bleeding.

The history includes exploration of the above risk factors and questions about related symptoms. Fever, abdominal pain, nausea, and anorexia are indicative of an infection. Urinary frequency, nausea and vomiting, breast tenderness, and amenorrhea suggest possible pregnancy. Bleeding patterns are extremely important; irregular menses and abnormal bleeding are the most common symptoms of endometrial cancer. Postmenopausal bleeding requires immediate investigation because cancer is more frequent in this age-group and this is a hallmark symptom. Hormone use must be carefully assessed.

Pelvic examination is done to determine size, shape, and consistency of the uterus and to evaluate the ovaries and adnexa. Depending upon symptoms and risk factors, endometrial biopsy or fractional curettage of the endocervix and endometrium often is done. Over 80% of endometrial cancers will be diagnosed with these methods.[3f] The Gravlee Jet Washer is another diagnostic aid used in women over the age of 35. This method obtains endometrial cells by washing the uterine cavity with normal saline in a collecting system.[9]

Diagnosis. Clinical findings may be used for initial diagnosis of uterine masses thought to be benign, such

T A B L E   4 8 - 3

Characteristics of Pelvic Tumors

Condition	Location	Size	Consistency	Mobility
Ovary				
Functional cyst (follicular, corpus luteum)	Adnexa, usually unilateral	5 cm–6 cm	Cystic	Mobile
Benign neoplastic (cystadenoma, cystic teratoma)	Adnexa, usually unilateral	6 cm–12 cm	Cystic	Mobile unless large
Malignant (cystadenocarcinoma, adenocarcinoma)	Adnexa, usually unilateral	5 cm–25 cm	Cystic or solid	Mobile early, fixed or frozen late
Endometrioma (chocolate cyst)	Adnexa, usually unilateral; cul-de-sac	>10 cm	Cystic	Usually fixed
Fallopian tubes				
Tubo-ovarian abscess	Adnexa, bilateral; cul-de-sac	Varies	Solid	Fixed
Parovarian cyst	Adnexa, usually unilateral	5 cm–8 cm	Cystic	Mobile
Ectopic pregnancy	Adnexa, unilateral; cul-de-sac	5 cm–6 cm	Solid	Mobile
Uterus				
Fibroid pedunculated	Midline; adnexa or cul-de-sac	Varies	Firm and rubbery	Mobile
Adenomyosis	Midline	8–12 cm	Firm to hard	Mobile uterus
Endometrial carcinoma	Midline	Often normal	Firm	Mobile uterus
Endometritis	Midline	Often normal	Firm	Mobile uterus

as fibroids or adenomyosis. Diagnostic tests help establish other causes, such as pregnancy test for pregnancy and biopsy or curettage for hyperplasia or cancer. Blood tests such as white blood cell count with differential and erythrocyte sedimentation rate aid diagnosis of infections.

Nursing Diagnosis. Nursing diagnoses are related to the type of medical problem, the stage of disease if cancer is diagnosed, and the responses of the client and her family. Refer to discussion under ovarian tumors.

Treatment. Benign conditions such as uterine fibroids are often managed conservatively if the tumors are not increasing in size significantly. Management includes regular evaluation by pelvic examination and diagnostic tests. If the fibroids enlarge or other signs or symptoms cause concern, abdominal surgery may be required, with possible tumor resection or hysterectomy. The management of adenomyosis and hyperplasia is discussed in Chapter 49. Endometrial cancer is treated according to its stage and the age and health status of the client. For early stages of adenocarcinoma, total abdominal

Shape	Tenderness	Pain	Fever	N/V/D	Other Associated Factors
Round to ovoid	None to slight	None to dull, aching	No	No	Delayed menses; spontaneous resorption in 6–12 weeks
Round to ovoid	None	None or vague fullness, aching	No	No	Disturbed menses ±
Varies	None	None or vague fullness, aching	No	No	Disturbed menses ±
Irregular	±	±	No	No	Nodules on uterosacral ligaments; fixed retroflexed uterus; cul-de-sac nodules
Poorly defined	++++	Severe constant	Yes	N/V	Elevated white blood cells, erythrocyte sedimentation rate; history of venereal disease or pelvic inflammatory disease ±; movement of cervix painful
Round to ovoid	None	None or vague, aching	No	No	Ovary separately palpable
Ovoid	++ to ++++	Mild to severe	No	N/V	Menstrual irregularities; signs, symptoms of pregnancy; peritonitis if ruptured
Irregular	No	None or vague aching	No	No	Uterus enlarged, nodular, irregular contour; pressure; irregular menses
Uterus globular	+++	Cramps	No	No	Abnormal bleeding, dysmenorrhea; multipara age 40–50
Usual	None	None usually	No	No	Abnormal bleeding
Usual	+++	Cramps, aching	±	±	History of venereal disease, vaginal discharge; menstrual changes

hysterectomy with bilateral salpingo-oophorectomy is the usual treatment. For more extensive disease, radiotherapy, chemotherapy, and hormone therapy in various combinations are used.

Planning/Intervention.
Nursing care for uterine masses follows the general approaches previously described for benign and malignant ovarian and breast conditions. Care for clients who are pregnant has been presented earlier; care for infectious conditions and bleeding-related problems is discussed in Chapters 49 and 50.

Evaluation.
Nursing intervention is evaluated by observing for changes in the client's behavior, level of knowledge, and attitudes. The client is able to express a clear understanding of the health problem, its cause, treatment, and outcomes. She understands measures that can be taken to prevent illness or complications and expresses willingness to undertake these. Behavioral changes might be observed that indicate therapeutic

Staging for Endometrial Cancer

Stage I   The carcinoma is confined to the uterine corpus.

IA   The length of the uterine cavity is 8 cm or less.

IB   The length of the uterine cavity is more than 8 cm.

Stage II   The carcinoma involves the corpus and the cervix.

Stage III   The carcinoma has extended outside the uterus but not outside the true pelvis.

Stage IV   The carcinoma has extended outside the true pelvis or has involved the mucosa of the bladder or rectum.

The Stage I cases are subgrouped by histologic type of adenocarcinoma as follows:

G1   Highly differentiated adenomatous carcinomas

G2   Differentiated adenomatous carcinomas with partly solid areas

G3   Predominantly solid or undifferentiated carcinomas

Classification system developed by the International Federation of Gynecology and Obstetrics (FIGO).

progress, such as weight loss, normal physiologic tests, medication compliance, general appearance, and affect. A positive attitude and seeking family support indicate effective emotional responses to health problems. Following through on referrals for psychological counseling or social support agencies indicates effective intervention. Regular breast self-examination and having regular Pap smears are evidence that preventive measures are being carried out. Rapport with the nurse is shown when the client openly discusses concerns and asks questions.

Women and Stress

Stress is an integral component of life, and nurses providing care to gynecologic and maternity clients will encounter numerous opportunities to intervene in stress-related problems. Stress is conceptualized as a person–environment relationship that taxes or exceeds the resources of the individual to deal with the resulting demands.[10] The body's response to stress includes physical, mental, emotional, and chemical reactions. Factors that contribute to stress can be those that frighten, excite, confuse, endanger, or irritate the person. A certain amount of stress is natural and probably necessary for life, but continuous stress at a sufficiently high level can often have adverse effects on health.

Most of the studies of stress have been based upon men's experiences. Common stress inventories include events more pertinent to a man's life and perceptions, and often leave out stresses related to social and sex-role changes that impact women. Another shortcoming is failure to consider that the same life events may impact women differently than men. A mother of young children starting a new job not only faces the usual stressors of learning new tasks, relating to a new social group, and adjusting to the work environment, but also may need to cope with attitudes that she should not be working at all. Her own feelings about working when her children are small may be another stressor. Women's historic oppression is often not considered in studies of stress and life events. Research indicates that higher levels of symptoms are experienced by those with oppressive life conditions, such as financial insecurity, abusive families, unemployment, and social isolation. Women, minorities, and the poor with such oppressive conditions have more physical and emotional health problems.[11]

Various factors contribute to the stressors women encounter as well as to women's reactions to stress. These factors are, to varying degrees, inherent and universal among women, whether socially based or individual. There are biologic differences between women and men that lead to characteristic patterns and rates of illness, longevity, and causes of death. While women are more resistant to infectious and degenerative disease and to major illness (*e.g.*, cancer, heart disease), they do have more acute, limited conditions than men. Women seek care earlier and more often than do men, and for less serious problems. Physical or physiological factors affect women's stress at work, and often stress is increased when work environments do not accommodate women's unique characteristics.

Such factors as changing family patterns, divorce, employment and unemployment, inequities in earnings and promotions, sexual discrimination, discounting the female experience, and learned helplessness influence women's experiences of and responses to stress.

Stress and Work. The number of women in the work force has increased dramatically to 43% of all workers, or 46 million women, in 1985.[12] This proportion has increased from 35% in 1954 and 41% in 1980. Over 90% of all women work for at least some period during their lives. Some reasons for this increase include feminism, a decreasing birth rate, more service jobs, more female heads of households, antidiscrimination legislation, increased education, economic pressures, and changing family patterns and values. Although about half of women workers are responsible for financially maintaining their families, they continue to earn less than men with the same or less education.[13]

Work outside the home often produces role conflict and other stress as women face expanded demands from obligations both at home and at work. The International Labor Office calculates that the average woman worldwide works 80 hours each week at home and at work, while the average man works 50 hours each week at home and at work.[13] This dual employment of women results from continued major responsibility for home activities, such as cooking, cleaning, and child care. Women in effect have two full-time jobs, and trying to do both well leads to considerable stress. Interestingly, women performing multiple roles of wife, mother, and career woman reported that they were coping with more stressful life events than single working women or married women at home, but tended to be least vulnerable to both illness and depression. It is hypothesized that emotional support by the family and personal control and success at work interacted for women in multiple roles and provided resources for coping.[14]

Physical Hazards. Physical hazards are workplace stressors, and women's biologic differences in body structure and strength can be risks if the work environment does not make accommodations. Because women have about 60% as much muscle mass as men of the same height and weight, their work capacity for carrying weight and gripping is less. When tools, equipment, and work environments are designed for men, women experience a higher incidence of repeated traumas and have more risk for back strain and other musculoskeletal disorders.[13,15] Noise exposure and hot and cold environments are sources of stress. Women have less heat tolerance because of a greater proportion of body fat and reduced sweating.

Chemical Hazards. Chemical hazards have great risk for women in reproductive years, especially during pregnancy. Although toxic substances have received much attention as threats to women's health, the majority of threshold limit values set by the National Institute of Occupational Safety and Health (NIOSH) for toxic substances are based on levels determined by research conducted only on men. In addition, there is very little research on the response of women to toxic substances in the workplace. Most of the protective equipment used is designed to fit the average male, so may offer reduced protection to women.

Work Characteristics Hazards. Work characteristics hazards may impact women differentially than men. In the past decade, movement of women into male-dominated jobs has decreased, and increasingly women are holding traditionally female jobs. These types of jobs have certain characteristics that are associated with high stress levels. Jobs in food service, health

care, manufacturing, and clerical work are characterized by the predictors of job dissatisfaction: lack of control over work and environment, powerlessness, less recognition, excessive hours of work, low pay, underutilization of skills, and demanding requirements.[16] This job dissatisfaction is a significant risk factor for coronary artery disease, hypertension, and ulcers. Clerical workers participating in the Framingham Heart Study had twice as much risk for coronary artery disease as other working women. Their limited job mobility, a nonsupportive boss, and suppressed hostility at work were more strongly predictive of coronary artery disease than were serum cholesterol, blood pressure, smoking history, and glucose intolerance.[17]

Some traditionally female jobs are being restructured by technology. Widespread use of computers not only requires retraining, but health effects are beginning to be recognized. Clerical workers using video display terminals full-time for information processing were found to have the highest rate of stress ever recorded, even more than that of air traffic controllers.[18]

Nurses face significant work-related stress because of work characteristics as well as chemical and physical hazards. Most nurses have a dual role as wage earner and homemaker, perceive their pay as inequitable when their education and levels of responsibility are considered, face limited opportunities for advancement within the hospital structure, and often find their work task oriented and repetitive. In addition, the hospital setting is based upon authoritarian power models, and many nurses feel the lack of independent decision-making opportunities and the subtle discrimination of operating in a male-dominated organization. However, nurses do not seem to have any greater stress than other working women. When nurses and other female hospital employees were compared on a stress scale with other employed women, their mean scores were in the average or below average ranges. The scale included stressful life events, frustration level, time pressure, boredom, nutritional habits, self-perception, type A behavior, and anxiety level. The nurses had experienced more recent stressful life events, but had better scores for nutritional habits and self-concept than other working women.[19]

Substance Abuse. Substance abuse among women in the workplace is a significant stressor of increasing dimensions. Current estimates are that 50% of all alcoholics are women, but a lower proportion of clients in workplace alcoholism programs are females. Data on drug use are limited, showing age correlations (more illicit drugs for persons aged 21 to 29) and indicating that women use more prescription and over-the-counter drugs than men. Multiple drug use and abuse are increasing, including combining drugs and alcohol. Women are not being reached effectively by traditional identification and referral mechanisms. Research on patterns of abuse behaviors looking at the relationship of family and job stressors to drug and alcohol use has focused on male behavioral models rather than female. There is speculation that work characteristics of traditional women's occupations contribute to substance abuse.

Stress levels have been tied generally to substance abuse. Being both a woman and a parent increases stress symptoms, and working exacerbates these problems. The origins, context, and control of employed women's substance abuse differ from those of men and seem related to issues of familial responsibilities, low self-esteem, job and pay discrimination, sex-role conflicts, and stress and conflict management.[20]

Tobacco.   Tobacco is another substance with great health risks that is used by many women. Although smoking rates have dropped substantially for men, they continue to increase for women, with the greatest increase among female adolescents. Heavy smoking by women (25 or more cigarettes each day) rose sharply from 1970 to 1980, especially in the 17- to 44-year-old age range. Nurses continue to smoke at higher rates than other professional women and than physicians. About 39% of female nurses were smokers in 1975, compared with 19% of other professional women and 14% of physicians. By 1981, 25% of nurses were still smokers. Psychiatric and mental-health nurses tend to smoke more than those in other specialties, reported variously as 52% and 48%. Smoking among women has been related to work characteristics, stress and concerns about weight. Many women see smoking as the lesser of two evils (*e.g.*, stress, obesity). Cigarette smoking has been called a feminist issue, especially among younger women.[21]

The health consequences of smoking can be severe, including such diseases as emphysema, hypertension, coronary artery disease, and lung cancer. Smoking is reported to be responsible for 43% of cases of lung cancer in women.[22] The incidence of lung cancer among women is increasing. Women smokers using oral contraceptives are at greatly increased risk for heart attack, especially after the age of 35 to 40. Smoking during pregnancy retards fetal growth and increases the rates of spontaneous abortion and perinatal mortality. Women who smoke have a three to four times greater risk for severe cervical abnormalities.[23] Nonsmokers also are harmed by "sidestream smoke," because this smoke coming directly from the burning tip of the cigarette contains higher concentrations of toxic chemicals than smoke inhaled into the lungs through a filter. Cigarette smoke is a mixture of particles and gases that contain at least 3800 chemicals, of which over 50 are known

carcinogens.[20] Estimates are that about 5000 people die annually in the United States from lung cancer that results from sidestream smoke, with the total number of deaths including those from diseases in the range of 10,000 to 50,000.[24]

Assessment.   Stress in women may be assessed by observation and by history taking. A person under severe stress usually manifests it in appearance and behavior, looking drawn, haggard, or poorly groomed and exhibiting a number of behavioral symptoms such as irritation, fatigue, anxiety, nervousness, confusion, distraction, or depression. Many people express stress through physical symptoms such as headaches, back pain, constipation or diarrhea, gastric distress, anorexia or overeating, palpitations, hyperventilation, insomnia, and increased susceptibility to infections. When the nurse suspects that stress is related to the client's symptoms or problems, further assessment can be done using a stress assessment tool. Involving the client in self-assessment is integral to using such tools for assessing stress levels. Coping strategies are usually included in the assessment process.

Substance abuse may require a somewhat different focus in assessment, because indicators are often subtle. Early indicators may include depression, dependency, low self-esteem, and learning problems. These are often followed by insomnia, anxiety, worry, inadequacy either felt or expressed through poor role performance, few leisure activities, missing appointments, and evasiveness. Late indicators include disrupted social relations, severe depression, inability to work, gastritis, fractures and injuries from falls, suicidal tendencies, isolation, and other substance abuse. Other clues the nurse might observe are changes in appearance, heavy perfume or mouthwash, emphasis on somatic complaints (especially menstrually related), and concealing parts of the body (arms, legs). On physical examination, alcoholics may have spider angiomas, tender or enlarged liver, tachycardia, hypertension, and gastric tenderness. Depending upon route of administration, drug users may have tracks on arms or legs.

Smokers usually do no attempt to conceal their cigarette use. Signs that indicate heavy smoking, however, include the smell of smoke on clothing or hair, brown discoloration of index and middle finger, discolored teeth, and thickened or ridged fingernails. Most smokers have changes in lung sounds, such as scattered rhonchi that clear with coughing, or wheezing.

Nursing Diagnosis.   Ineffective individual coping is the most direct nursing diagnosis related to stress. It is defined as the individual's inability to manage internal or environmental stressors adequately due to inadequate

ASSESSMENT TOOL

Stress Assessment

I. Personal Information

Age
Children
Living arrangements
Health state
Financial state

Marital status
Relatives/friends
Work
Limitations/disabilities

II. Stressors

Life events

Events that have been experienced in the last 12 months. How important (rank: little to great)

	Check if happened	How important
Relationship change	___	___
Career change	___	___
Illness/death	___	___
Personal illness	___	___
Work problems	___	___
Financial problems	___	___
Family problems	___	___
Legal problems	___	___
Health/body changes	___	___
Psychological stress	___	___

Life conditions

Reasonably consistent patterns in life: Describe usual situation related to each of these that is important.

Living space
Family relations
Employment/career
Financial state
Health state
Recreation/activities
Spiritual values

Coping strategies

Usual ways used to cope with stress. Describe how well these work.

Eat/drink more/less
Use alcohol or drugs
Sleep more/less
Exercise more/less
Use relaxation technique
Smoke more
Avoid problem/pretend not there
Clarify/set goals
Time management/efficiency
Make changes in job, relations
Pray, meditate, seek spiritual help
Analyze/understand conflicts
Talk with spouse, friends
More recreation/activities
Block out feelings
Desensitize fears, aversions
Seek new relations
Enter therapy/support group
Other

resources (physical, psychological, or behavioral).[25] Some maturational factors contributing to ineffective coping include career choices and pressures, child-rearing and marital problems, retirement, and aging. Situational factors may include sensory overload (work environment, effects of urban living) and inadequate psychological resources (poor self-esteem, helplessness, lack of motivation).

Other nursing diagnoses potentially related to stress include sleep pattern disturbance; alterations in thought processes; anxiety; fear; powerlessness; disturbance in self-concept; impaired communication; and alterations in parenting.

Planning/Intervention. Nursing care focuses on assisting the woman to identify and interpret her stressors and responses to them. Once this is done, the goal is to reduce or reinterpret stress so it becomes feasible for the woman to cope effectively. Using counseling and teaching skills, the nurse may assist the client in any of these areas: problem solving, decision making, exploration of alternative behaviors and strategies, drawing upon other internal and external resources, analyzing usual ways of coping, assessing what works and what does not, and learning specific stress reduction techniques.

In the work setting, nurses can identify and evaluate stressors affecting women and develop recommendations or programs for stress management. Some approaches could be flexible time, child-care programs, educational campaigns, stress reduction workshops, health screening and promotion, time management, conflict management, family problem solving, personal growth groups, fitness programs, stop-smoking programs, assertiveness training, and support groups. When serious problems are identified, such as alcohol or drug abuse, referrals to substance abuse programs are indicated. Psychotherapy or other emotional counseling can be recommended for severe emotional problems.

Many approaches to stress reduction are available (see Suggested Reading). To obtain maximum benefit, all these techniques should be used regularly for a certain period. Three common approaches are briefly described here.

Progressive relaxation uses tensing and relaxing of muscle groups progressively throughout the body to attain a state of deep relaxation. Beginning in a sitting or lying position, the woman takes a few deep breaths, then progressively tenses and relaxes toes, feet, calves, knees, thighs, buttocks, stomach, lower back, chest, upper back, shoulders, arms and hands, neck, face, eyes, and forehead. Next, the entire body is tensed and relaxed, followed by a few deep breaths and a period of stillness.

Guided imagery has the client focus on images that create a relaxed state. Sitting or lying in a comfortable position, the women closes her eyes and takes several deep breaths. Then she creates a mental image of a scene that she finds satisfying and peaceful, such as a beach, stream, meadow, mountain, or forest. She imagines smells, sounds, textures, colors, and any other aspects of the situation that produce a good feeling. Some advise this image be written, polished, and put on audiotape. It is then played back for relaxation.

Meditation is an approach to quiet the mind and focus on the deep inner silence or peace. A quiet place is needed, and the woman sits comfortably. She may select a word or sound to chant, a symbol or object to gaze at, or music to focus the mind. Meditation is continued for 15 to 20 minutes, with a passive attitude that accepts thoughts and distractions, then gently refocuses attention on the meditation object.

Evaluation. The first indication of positive action occurs when the woman identifies stressors and her responses to them. She then chooses an approach and follows the techniques to reduce her stress. She reports better sleep and the ability to think more clearly. Depending on her situation, her enhancement of parenting abilities is manifest in both her speech and her actions, or she takes definite steps to overcome her feelings of powerlessness in the workplace and faces her anxieties and fears.

Family Violence Against Women

Family violence is an area of growing national concern. Spouse abuse and battering is a social problem affecting every stratum of society and is one of the most common but least reported forms of violence in the United States. An estimated 3 to 4 million women are battered annually,[26] and 30% of couples reported at least one episode of violence in their marriage, although estimates are that closer to 50% to 60% of marriages experience abuse, much of which is unreported or concealed in divorce statistics.[27] There are serious immediate effects of battering, including severe injury or death. About one fourth of all murders are domestic, and of these 50% are spouse killings. Domestic violence falls disproportionately upon women; about 40% of all female but only 10% of all male homicide victims are killed by spouses.[28] Longer-term effects include neglect or abuse of children, perpetuation of patterns of family violence, serious psychopathology, family disruption, and criminal and civil proceedings.

No coherent theoretical foundation has yet been

developed about the causation of spouse abuse, although many correlates have been identified. While myths persist, no stereotypic abuser and abused have been established. Some common characteristics borne out in various studies describe abused women as having low self-esteem, believing myths about battering relationships, being traditionalists, believing in the stereotypical feminine role in the home, accepting responsibility for the batterer's actions, feeling guilt, denying their terror and anger, and voicing severe psychophysiological complaints. Characteristics of battering men include having low self-esteem, believing myths about battering relationships, believing in male dominance and the stereotypical masculine role in the family, blaming others for their actions, not believing violent behavior should have negative consequences, and using drinking, sex, and battering to cope with stresses and enhance self-esteem. Several characteristics are the same for abused and abuser, suggesting a basis for their symbiotic relationship.[29]

Family violence generally follows cycles, which occur over weeks or months. Tension builds over minor conflicts or disagreements, with the woman becoming compliant, passive, or withdrawn to avoid or deflect the man's anger. The man senses her anger and interprets lack of action as weakness, which further exacerbates his aggressiveness. Tension continues to build over incidents, eventually exploding into acute battering that often is triggered by an unrelated event. Common precipitants are arguments over spending money, jealousy by the husband over slights, sexual problems, drinking or drug use, conflicts over childrearing, the husband's unemployment, or pregnancy. The battering phase

usually lasts 2 to 24 hours, though it could be a week or more. After severe beating, the woman usually does not seek care at once, experiencing a state of shock or disbelief and minimizing the injuries. Fear and helplessness may prevent the woman from seeking help. In the final phase, relief is felt by both, and the man often expresses extreme love and kindness and is contrite over his behavior. He may promise it will never happen again and may give her gifts. The woman wants to believe him and to think that this is his real nature and that he will change his abusive behavior.[30]

The cycle repeats itself over the years. Violence usually begins early in marriage, and many women remain for 6 to 7 years in a violent home situation, especially if they have small children. Most women leave the man two to four times and return before they permanently end the relationship. The longer the woman waits to take action, the more entrenched the family dynamics become. Unhealthy interaction patterns are reinforced, with each partner knowing how to hurt the other emotionally. As months and years pass, the woman withdraws from other relatives, friends, and neighbors. She is reluctant to be seen with injuries and is fearful or embarrassed to talk about the beatings, and the husband is possessive and jealous of all outside relations. Social isolation increases with growing helplessness and powerlessness. Accepting abuse and pain as a part of life, the women often develops serious psychoemotional and somatic problems, such as paralyzing anxiety, nightmares, depression, tremors, sweating, alcohol and drug abuse, hypertension, ulcers, and paranoia.

Assessment. Women experiencing family violence are often difficult to identify because they wish to conceal their problems. Risk for battering is increased in women with a history of alcohol or drug abuse, child abuse, or prior spouse abuse in another marriage. Other signs that could indicate a violent family situation include neglected grooming and appearance; depression manifest by fatigue, somatic complaints, or feelings of hopelessness; expressions of helplessness and powerlessness; and an unequal decision-making structure typified by the authoritarian male and submissive, passive female. Women who do not have a network of relatives and friends whom they see regularly, and from whom they receive support, may be at increased risk for abuse.

When a woman is seen in the clinic or office and reports an injury, or the nurse notices bruising or other injuries, certain cues of abuse can be sought. The woman may have an inappropriate explanation for the injury (fell down stairs, ran into the door). The site and types of injuries tend to be typical, including bruises, abra-

---

Myths About Battering Relationships

Battering is uncommon and occurs only in a small percent of marriages or long-term relationships.

Lower socioeconomic class families experience the great preponderance of battering and abuse.

Battered women were themselves almost always abused as children.

Battered women have masochistic personalities.

Battered women invite physical violence by provoking their mates.

Battering is caused by alcohol and drug abuse.

Battering men and battered women can rarely ever change their behaviors.

Battered women can leave the abusive relationship easily if they would only choose to do so.

sions, or contusions of the head, eyes, back of neck, throat, chest, breasts, abdomen or genitals. Usually the injuries are multiple, in contrast to single or dual sites on extremities (ankles, wrists, feet, hands) in nonabusive injuries. A period of time (days to weeks) may have elapsed before injuries are reported, while nonabusive injuries usually are reported promptly. The abused woman is often hesitant or evasive in providing details on how the injury occurred, and her affect may be inappropriate (avoiding eye contact, embarrassment, fright, disorientation, depression). If her husband is present, she may appear anxious and glance at him or seek approval to answer questions. He may be reluctant to leave her alone with the nurse, may interject answers to questions, or may demand to be present.

Often the nurse must build a trusting relationship with the woman before abuse can be disclosed. The nurse needs to convey unconditional acceptance, understanding, sensitivity, and positive regard for the woman. A conditional statement may open the door for discussing abuse, with the nurse saying, "Many women are physically hurt by their husbands (partners). Has this ever happened to you?" If the woman reveals abuse, this may be accompanied by a flood of emotion with crying and pouring out details of years of abuse. The nurse must listen empathetically and convey emotional support without judgment.

Nursing Diagnosis. Abuse trauma related to family violence would be an appropriate nursing diagnosis that would most directly identify the problem. Several other nursing diagnoses might also be appropriate, such as ineffective family coping in which the family demonstrates destructive behavior in response to an inability to manage stressors due to inadequate psychological or behavioral resources. Fear related to threat of injury or death, powerlessness related to personal and interpersonal characteristics, disturbance in self-concept related to abusive dynamics, and social isolation related to extreme anxiety, depression, or paranoia could be diagnoses. Rape trauma syndrome also could apply, even within the context of marriage or a continued relationship. This is defined as forced, violent sexual assault against the woman's will and without her consent and includes an acute phase of disorganization of the victim's and family's life-style.[2b] Other nursing diagnoses are related to the physical trauma and medical treatment of injuries.

Planning/Intervention. Counseling, support, reassurance, and education are used by nurses throughout the care of battered women. Empathetic listening and acceptance provide the environment in which the woman can express, examine, and work through her

situation. She will be facing choices among "unacceptable" alternatives, none of which seems a perfect solution. The nurse must be understanding of her ambivalence toward the batterer; the woman would not remain in a cycle of violence unless there were powerful ties to her spouse. During this process, the nurse identifies and clarifies myths and misunderstandings. The woman's capacity to change, to make and follow through with decisions, and to clarify her values and beliefs is constantly supported. This helps the woman increase self-esteem and explore self-beliefs that keep her caught in the cycle of violence, such as guilt, powerlessness, and self-blame.

The battered woman has three basic alternatives: leave the relationship (with threat of homicide, child custody battles, loss of material support); stay and hope that the man will change through counseling, therapy, or legal intervention (data show change is unlikely, and risk of abuse or death continues); or stay and resign herself to no change (risk of abuse or death continues). No alternative seems perfect, yet the woman must choose and make her own decision. Nurses can become frustrated at indecision or the choice to remain in the relationship, but rescuing the battered woman is impossible and the cycle will not stop until she takes the initiative. The woman needs to reestablish a sense of control over her life and feel safe enough to function. The nurse assists this process by building a trusting relationship, allowing expression of fear, providing empathy no matter how terrible the story becomes, and extending dignity by regard for the woman's worth.

The nurse informs battered women of services available in the community, especially women's shelters and safe houses. Physical safety is a central concern. The woman also needs to learn of her legal rights and the processes of law enforcement that can protect her from battering. If she decides to leave, she should be advised to take the children (if any) to protect them from abuse and to make obtaining custody easier, and to bring extra clothing, important documents, money, and emergency supplies. If the woman decides not to leave, she needs to know that resources are available and that the nurse continues to view her with respect and to offer a supportive relationship.

Breaking the symbiosis with the battering spouse is often very difficult. The nurse works toward increased autonomy through use of "I am" statements, values clarification, grief therapy, and support for independent decisions. The woman is aided to identify her strengths and resources and to build upon these. Support groups, individual counseling, and psychotherapy can be recommended. The nurse must remember that leaving a violent family situation is a long process, taking on average about 4 to 7 years. Most women who enter a shelter return home. Abused women often need rehabilitation that takes years, as they slowly gain ego strength and self-esteem. The nurse contributes to this process by effective counseling and support at every contact with a battered woman.

Evaluation. Recovery from the trauma of abuse is a long process. Even though the client may make progress in her steps toward autonomy, there may be periods of backsliding. These are part of the process.

When the woman seeks safety or acknowledges she needs help, she has made a first step. Another sign of progress is that she trusts the nurse enough to express her fears. She identifies her strengths and resources and builds on them; she explores and clarifies her values and beliefs as part of her acknowledgment of who she is. She indicates she has attained knowledge and understands her legal rights by acting on them. She makes choices from "unacceptable" alternatives and follows through with her decisions. As she progresses through these steps, she establishes a sense of control over her life and feels safe enough to function.

Menopause

Although menopause is defined as the age of the last menstrual period, it commonly refers to the 1 to 2 years of most marked decline in ovarian function. The average age at which menopause occurs is 50 years, with a range from 48 to 52 years. Most women have experienced menopause by age 55. Nurses working in hospitals, offices, and clinics often encounter perimenopausal women, most often during the course of other care, since many women do not seek care specifically for menopausal symptoms. Maternity nurses are likely to be asked questions about menopause by older mothers, as well as by friends and neighbors. The most common symptoms of menopause are hot flashes with associated vasomotor changes (sweating, faintness) and atrophic vaginal and vulvar changes. The physiology of menopause is discussed in Chapter 9.

Menopause has traditionally been associated with emotional instability, although evidence fails to support a direct relationship between menopause and emotional symptoms. It is a developmental transition as the woman's childbearing years come to an end and a new phase of life is entered. In cultures that glorify youth, menopause can signify aging and cause stress related to body changes. Women of higher socioeconomic status with careers have been found with no emotional distress and few symptoms related to decreased estrogen, when

compared with women of lower socioeconomic status who did not work or had low-status and low-paying jobs.[31]

Osteoporosis

Osteoporosis, demineralization of the bones and general reduction in skeletal bone mass, has been estimated as occurring in up to 85% of the female population in the United States.[32] About 25% to 30% of white women will have a fracture related to osteoporosis. Decreasing levels of estrogen are associated with loss of bone calcium, which is evidenced by high levels of circulating calcium in the plasma that is then excreted by the kidneys. At menopause, women may begin losing bone at a rate of 1% to 3% each year until death. In most women, no symptoms are present until a fracture occurs. Unfortunately, fractures represent a late stage of osteoporosis. Clinical signs include reduced height, back pain, and the "dowager's hump," as vertebral fractures cause wedging and collapse of the vertebrae. When the vertebral column is altered, the rib cage size is decreased, which impairs breathing. Bending and exertion become difficult, and pain may result from compression of nerve roots. Wrist fractures also are common, typically resulting from a fall. Hip fractures usually result from falls, most commonly in women over age 70. Fewer than half of these women ever regain mobility; 15% die within 6 months of the fracture, and nearly 30% are dead within a year, usually from emboli, pneumonia, thrombosis, or heart failure.[33]

Assessment. Risk factors for osteoporosis include white women with small body structure, poor nutrition, inadequate dietary calcium, diet rich in meat, decreased physical activity, heavy cigarette smoking, and excessive alcohol use. Family history of relatives with osteoporotic symptoms (*e.g.*, dowager's hump, wrist and hip fractures) also increases risk. The physical examination should include periodic measurements of height and weight, particularly measurement of the distance from pelvis (symphysis pubis) to head and pelvis (symphysis pubis) to heel. These two measures should be about equal; if the pelvis-to-head measurement is less, it could indicate vertebral collapse.

Blood tests are not useful, because women with osteoporosis can have normal levels of serum calcium, phosphorus, and alkaline phosphatase. Radiographic photodensitometry can detect finger bone density, and single photon absorptiometry can measure mineral content in the radius and ulna. The computed tomographic scanner gives the most accurate measurement of early bone loss in the spine.

Nursing Diagnosis. Nursing diagnoses may include activity intolerance; alterations in comfort (pain); potential for injury; impaired physical mobility; alterations in nutrition (less than body requirements for calcium); and knowledge deficit related to cause, prevention, and treatment of osteoporosis.

Treatment. Menopausal women absorb only about 25% of their calcium intake. Hence, it is especially important to emphasize proper dietary intake of calcium and give serious consideration to calcium supplementation. On average, women in the United States who are in the menopausal age-group take in only about 500 mg of elemental calcium daily. They need about 1.5 g, and when intake is maintained at that level it may have a protective effect on bone loss.

The use of estrogen to treat menopausal symptoms and osteoporosis is controversial. Estrogen is capable of inhibiting osteoporosis and relieving vasomotor symptoms, but other complex factors also are involved. The serious complications of estrogen therapy include endometrial carcinoma, thromboembolic disease, hypertension, gallbladder disease, and possibly breast cancer. If estrogen therapy is to be used, it must be started shortly after menopause; therapy after 6 years following menopause has marginal, if any, effect on reducing bone loss. Other issues surround the dosage, length of administration, and combination of estrogen with cyclic progestin to protect the endometrium. Withdrawal bleeding is often a consequence of this combination, cyclic approach.

One must weigh the severity of the symptoms against the potential hazards of estrogen treatment and the quality of life. Signs and symptoms that interfere with working outside or inside of the home or with a good sex life are clear indications for treatment. Prevention of osteoporosis is also a major concern. Absolute contraindications to estrogen treatment include liver disease, cerebrovascular disease, venous thrombosis and embolism, and an estrogen-dependent malignancy of the breast or uterus.

The nurse can play a pivotal role in prevention of postmenopausal osteoporosis through client education. It is helpful to have on hand a list of calcium-containing foods that can be used as a basis for discussion. Calcium supplementation (Table 48-4) is especially important when dietary calcium intake is marginal, which more often than not is the case.

Client education about nutrition is important. In addition to dietary sources of calcium and calcium supplements, protein intake should be discussed. There is evidence that doubling of protein intake can result in a 50% increase in calcium excreted in the urine. The recommended 44 g of protein per day for adult women should not be exceeded, and red meat should be minimized. Menopausal women also need to limit their salt intake, because women with high sodium excretion also lose more calcium in the urine. A moderate salt diet would include from 500 mg to 1500 mg sodium daily. Adequate vitamin D (100 IU–500 IU) is necessary because it increases calcium absorption in the intestines and also increases resorption of calcium through the

TABLE 48-4

Calcium Supplements

Type	Selected Brands	Elementary Calcium Per Tablet (mg)	Approx. Price per 1200 mg*
Calcium carbonate	Caltrate 600 (Lederle)	600	19¢
	BioCal chewable (Miles)	250	44¢
	BioCal swallowable (Miles)	500	26¢
	Tums (Nordoff Thayer)	200	15¢
	Cal-Sup 300 (3M)	300	25¢
	Suplical chewable (Warner Lambert)	600	20¢
	Generic	600	7¢
Oyster shell (calcium carbonate)	Oscal (Marion)	500	23¢
	Generic	500	12¢
Calcium phosphate	Posture (Ayerst)	600	21¢
Calcium lactate	(Lilly)	47	$1.05
Calcium gluconate	(Lilly, Thompson)	45	$2.00
Bone meal, dolomite	NOT RECOMMENDED BECAUSE OF POSSIBLE CONTAMINATION		

* Prices may vary around the country. Different formulations of the same brand may vary in price.
(University of California, Berkeley Wellness Letter 2(9):3, June 1986)

kidneys. The use of fluoride to treat osteoporosis is experimental; although it increases bone density, the bone formed may be abnormal.

Women must be advised about the effects of cigarette smoking and alcohol upon bone demineralization. Physical activity on a regular basis is strongly advised both to prevent and to treat osteoporosis. Exercise that combines movement, pulling, and stress on the long bones is best, such as walking, jogging, hiking, jumping rope, bicycling, or rowing.

Nurses serve as an important resource to women about menopause and osteoporosis. Through community efforts at increasing women's awareness, osteoporosis can largely be prevented.

Evaluation. The goal is prevention, and outcomes will signify the menopausal or postmenopausal woman's comprehension of this. The woman conveys her grasp of knowledge about osteoporosis and its prevention and treatment by taking active steps in self-care. Perhaps she stops smoking or cuts her alcohol intake. She develops an exercise program that is convenient to her life-style and time limits. She limits salt and protein in her diet. She makes decisions about estrogen or calcium replacement and takes her medication faithfully.

References

1. Hein K: The first pelvic examination and common gynecological problems in adolescent girls. Women Health 9(2–3):47–63, Summer/Fall 1984
2. Carpenito LJ: Handbook of Nursing Diagnosis. a, p 28; b, p 53. Philadelphia, JB Lippincott, 1985
3. Romney SL et al: Gynecology and Obstetrics: The Health Care of Women, 2nd ed. a, p 1198; b, pp 1196–1197; c, p 1188; d, p 1030–1031; e, p 1043; f, p 1074. New York, McGraw-Hill, 1981
4. Humphrey LJ: Medical management of the fibrocystic breast. In The Fibrocystic Breast. Boston, Tufts University Press, 1983
5. Fisher B et al: Five-year results of a random clinical trial in the management of primary breast cancer. N Engl J Med 292:117–122, 1975
6. Baldwin KA, Goodwin K: The Papanicolaou smear. J Nurs Midwifery 30(6):327–332, November/December 1985
7. Berman RL: Current perspectives in gynecology. Ciba Clin Symp 37(1):2–29, 1985
8. Sargis N: Detecting ovarian cancer: A challenge for nursing assessment. Oncology Nurs Forum 10(2):48–52, Spring 1983
9. Austin JM et al: The Gravlee method: An alternative to the Pap smear? Am J Nurs 83(7):1057–1058, July 1983
10. Lazarus R, Launier R: Stress-related transactions between person and environment. In Pervin LA, Lewis M (eds): Perspectives in Interactional Psychology. New York, Plenum Press, 1978
11. Bowles C, Dam-Rabolt M: Stress response and coping patterns. In Griffith-Kennedy J (ed): Contemporary Women's Health: A Nursing Advocacy Approach, pp 126–154. Menlo Park, CA, Addison-Wesley, Health Sciences Division, 1986
12. Statistical abstract of the United States, 1986. US Department of Commerce, Bureau of the Census, 106th ed, p 390, 1986
13. Wysocki LM, Ossler C: Women, work and health: Issues of importance to the occupational health nurse. Occup Health Nurs 31(11):18–23, 56–61, November 1983
14. Married or single. University of California, Berkeley Wellness Letter, 2(9):1, June 1986
15. Randolph SA: Stress, working women, and an occupational stress model. Occup Health Nurs 32(12):622–625, December 1984
16. Moore EC (ed): Women and health. Public Health Rep V:95(suppl):35, 1980
17. Haynes S, Feinlieb M: Women, work and coronary heart disease. Am J Public Health 70(2):133–141, 1980
18. Tabor M: Workers health in the automated office. Occup Health Saf, pp 22–26, April 1983
19. Posner I, Lester D, Leitner L: Stress in nurses and other working females. Psychol Rep 54(1):210, February 1984
20. Vicary JR et al: Substance use among women in the workplace. Occup Health Nurs 33(10):491–495, 527–530, October 1985
21. Charbonneau L: Smoking or health: How long can nurses ignore the facts? The Can Nurse 81(7):27–32, August 1985
22. Doyle NC: Smoking among women—an equal opportunity tragedy. American Lung Association Bulletin 66:10–13, July/August 1980
23. Mayberry RM: Cigarette smoking, herpes simplex virus type 2 infection, and cervical abnormalities. Am J Public Health 75(6):676–678, June 1985
24. Collishaw NE et al: Tobacco smoke in the workplace: An occupational health hazard. Can Med Assoc J 131:1199–1204, November 15, 1984
25. Carpenito LJ: Handbook of Nursing Diagnosis, pp 15–17. Philadelphia, JB Lippincott, 1985
26. Stark E et al: Wife Abuse in the Medical Setting. National Clearinghouse on Domestic Violence, Rockville, MD, 1981
27. Straus MA: Wife beating: How common and why. Victimology: An International Journal 2:443–458, 1978
28. Dobash RE, Dobash RP: Wives, the "appropriate" victims of marital violence. Victimology: An International Journal 2:426–442, Fall 1977–1978
29. Reeder S: Ethical Dilemmas for Health Providers in Cases of Spousal Abuse. Unpublished paper presented at conference on Bridging the Gaps in Women's Health Care, October 1983, San Antonio, Texas. Mimeographed

30. Griffith-Kennedy J: Abuse and battering. In Griffith-Kennedy J (ed): Contemporary Women's Health: A Nursing Advocacy Approach, pp 198–220. Menlo Park, CA, Addison-Wesley, Health Sciences Division, 1986

31. Severne L: Psychosocial aspects of menopause. In Voda A et al (eds): Changing Perspectives on the Menopause. Austin, University of Texas Press, 1982

32. Gregory CA: Possible influences of physical activity on musculoskeletal symptoms of menopausal and post-menopausal women. J Obstet Gynecol Nurs 11(2):103–107, March/April 1982

33. Graham BA, Gleit CJ: Osteoporosis: A major health problem in postmenopausal women. Orthop Nurs 3(6):19–26, November 1984

Stern PN, Harris CC: Women's health and the self-care paradox: A model to guide self-care readiness. Health Care Women Int 6(1–3):151–163, 1985

Suzuki S: Zen Mind, Beginner's Mind. New York, Weatherhill, 1980

Wabrek AJ, Gunn JL: Sexual and psychological implications of gynecologic malignancy. JOGN Nurs 13(6):371–376, November/December 1984

Woodard D: Treatment of osteoporosis. N Engl J Med 312(10):617, March 1985

Suggested Reading

Burgess S: DES daughters: Fighting fear with facts. Am J Nurs 85(6):639–640, June 1985

Butnarescu G: Women's health: An investment in the future. Issues Health Care Women 4(2–3):93–105, March/June 1983

Dean A: Our own worst enemy—the female profile. Nurs Success Today 2(11):39–C3, November 1985

Golas V: The Lazy Man's Guide to Enlightenment. New York, Bantam Books, 1980

Haughey BP et al: Nurses' ability to detect nodules in silicone breast models. Oncology Nurs Forum 11(1):37–42, January/February 1984

Jacobson E: Progressive Relaxation. Chicago, University of Chicago Press, 1974

Keyes K: Handbook to Higher Consciousness. Marina Del Rey, CA, DeVorss & Co, 1975

Krouse HJ: A psychological model of adjustment in gynecologic cancer patients. Oncol Nurs Forum 12(6):45–49, November/December 1985

Kutzner SK, Toussie-Weingarten C: Working parents: The dilemma of child rearing and career. Top Clin Nurs 6(3):30–37, October 1984

LeShan L: How to Meditate. New York, Bantam Books, 1974

MacPherson KI: Osteoporosis and menopause: A feminist analysis of the social construction of a syndrome. Adv Nurs Sci 7(4):11–22, July 1985

Mamon JA, Zapka JG: Improving frequency and proficiency of breast self-examination: Effectiveness of an education program. Am J Public Health 75(6):618–624, June 1985

Mulligan JE: Some effects of the women's health movement. Top Clin Nurs 4(4):1–9, January 1983

Rimer B, Glassman B: The fitness revolution: Will nurses sit this one out? Nurs Econ 1(2):84–89, 144, September/October 1983

Sinnott JP: Stress, health and mental health symptoms of older women and men. Int J Aging Hum Dev 20(2):123–132, 1984–1985

Spreads C: Breathing—The ABC's. Hagerstown, MD, Harper & Row, 1978

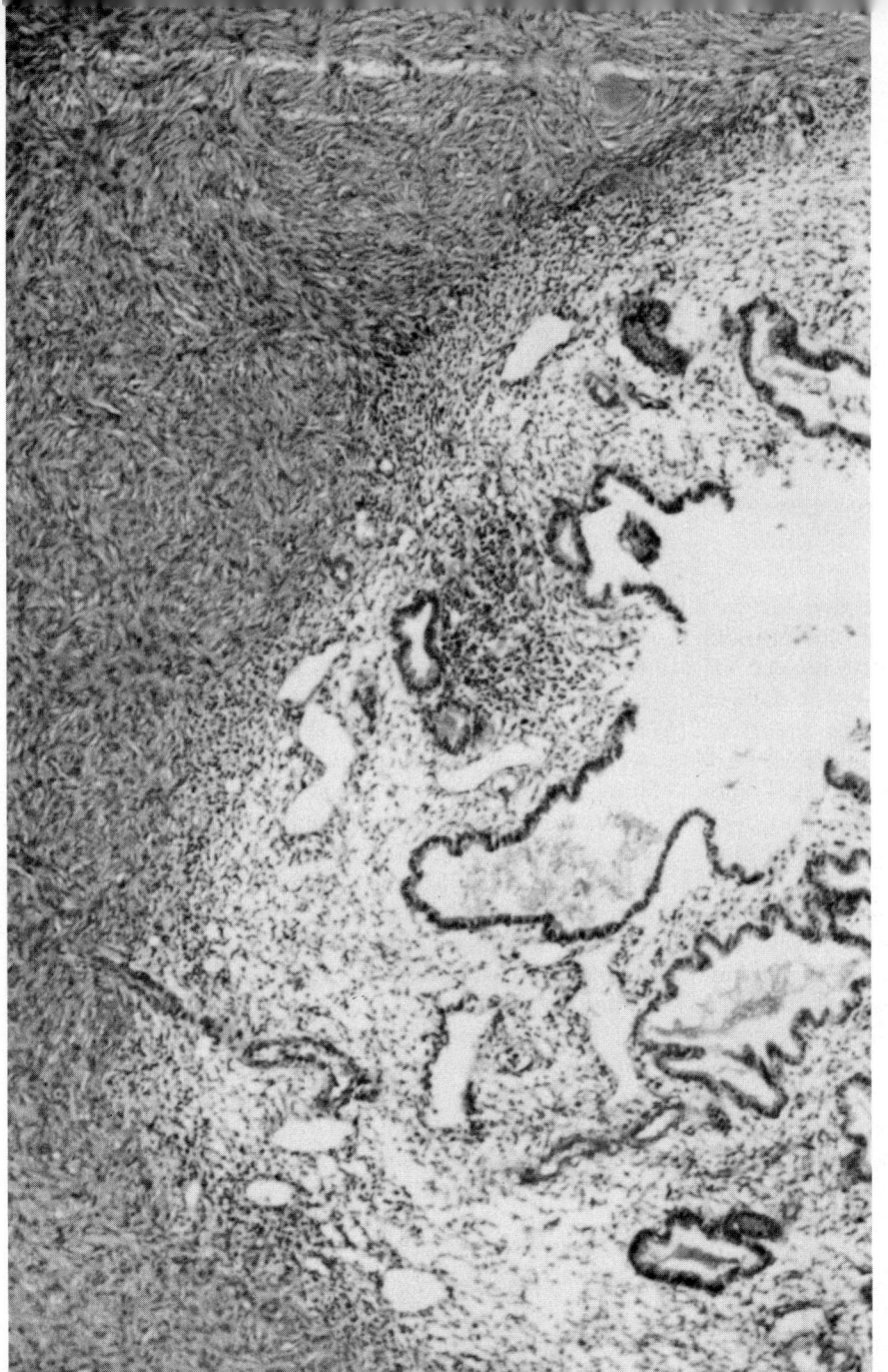

CHAPTER 49

Nursing Care in Menstrual and Bleeding Disorders

Women may experience problems with menstruation or irregular bleeding throughout the reproductive years. Less commonly, prepubertal girls and postmenopausal women have bleeding disorders. Maternity nurses will find many occasions when clients in the hospital and in clinics express concerns about menstruation or irregular bleeding not associated with pregnancy. It is important that nurses providing care to women be familiar with common disorders and be able to undertake appropriate assessment and nursing care.

Assessment

Clients reporting bleeding disorders are assessed by a careful menstrual history, a history of the bleeding problem, and a personal and family health history. Often the history provides the most significant data for determining the diagnosis, especially for menstrual problems such as premenstrual syndrome (PMS) and dysmenorrhea. The physical examination focuses upon a speculum and bimanual pelvic examination, with specimens and diagnostic tests as indicated (see Menstrual History).

The menstrual history establishes the woman's usual patterns associated with the menstrual cycle. This provides a baseline from which to evaluate her current symptoms. The nurse must determine what the client means by "bleeding," including the onset, duration, frequency, and intervals between the usual bleeding episodes. The amount of bleeding must be assessed, and this may be difficult. The nurse asks if the bleeding is enough to use a pad or tampon, how often the pad/tampon is changed, and how saturated it is when changed. The number and degree of saturation of pads/tampons used over a set time period, such as 4 hours, can give some idea of the extent of bleeding. Women vary in patterns of changing pads/tampons, of course, and in their estimations of time and saturation.

Associated symptoms provide additional diagnostic cues. The patterns of pain or discomfort in relation to bleeding are important: Does pain occur before or after onset of bleeding? Does it continue or cease when bleeding begins? The nurse can assess the severity of pain by asking how much it affects life-style and daily activities. With severe pain, the client may lie down or go to bed and be unable to continue activities. Less severe pain affects activities to varying degrees. The client is asked to describe the character of the pain; such descriptors as aching, cramping, sharp, shooting, burning, or piercing may be used.

The presence of foul-smelling vaginal discharge or a foul smell to blood may indicate infection, especially when fever also occurs. If the client experiences urinary discomfort or burning, the nurse must carefully assess whether the blood comes from the vagina or the urinary meatus. Other areas to check include sudden changes in weight, recent major stress or life changes, severe dieting, drug use, signs of pregnancy, other illness, and contraceptive use. To gain perspective, the client should be asked if she has ever experienced these symptoms before and, if so, when and what was done. Factors that relieve the symptoms, or make them worse, can help in assessment.

The pelvic examination provides data on the condition of the perineum, vagina, cervix, uterus and adnexa, urethra, and rectum. Some women may mistake bleeding from hemorrhoids or the urinary meatus as coming from the vagina. If vaginal bleeding does occur, it may originate from vaginal, cervical, or uterine structures. Careful inspection may reveal vaginal lacerations or inflammation, or cervical polyps, infection, or lesions. Bimanual examination may reveal uterine enlargement, tenderness, or masses; nodules on the rectovaginal septum, ligaments, or cul-de-sac; or adnexal masses, fullness, or tenderness. Combined with data from the history, pelvic findings can affirm the diagnosis. Specimens of vaginal or cervical discharge should be taken for culture or microscopic examination, and Pap smears should be done if indicated. The nurse may perform or assist in the pelvic examination, depending upon skills and expertise (see Chap. 22).

Other diagnostic tests that might be indicated include hematocrit and hemoglobin, complete blood count and differential, stool guaiac, serum iron and iron-binding capacity, pregnancy test, gonorrhea culture, *Chlamydia* culture, serology, and sonogram.

Nursing Diagnosis

The nursing diagnosis is generally related to the medical (pathophysiological) diagnosis and the client's responses to her condition and symptoms. Potential complications can be a nursing diagnosis for almost all conditions, and a prime concern of nursing care is to detect and prevent such complications. For many menstrual and bleeding problems, alterations in comfort (pain) is an appropriate diagnosis because of the cramping that is a common symptom. Sexual dysfunction related to painful intercourse or infertility could occur. Anxiety/fear related to the unpredictable nature of the disease or uncertainty of outcomes is possible. Knowledge deficits are common nursing diagnoses, related to the pathophysiological condition, myths and misunderstandings, signs and symptoms of complications, medical treatment, needs for nutrition and rest, and non-pharmaceutical therapies. In chronic conditions that affect life-style or daily activities significantly, there is the potential for ineffective individual and family coping.

Nursing diagnoses for specific menstrual and bleeding problems are included in the following section.

Planning/Intervention

The key points in assessment, diagnosis, and nursing care are discussed for several common menstrual and bleeding disorders. Age-specific causes of bleeding are listed in Table 49-1.

Bleeding Problems

Increased Cyclic Bleeding

Heavy menstrual flow (hypermenorrhea, menorrhagia) may be normal for some women, although anemia must be ruled out. If heavy bleeding is a change from the woman's usual pattern, a good menstrual and symptom history must be taken and the amount of bleeding carefully evaluated. Heavy bleeding commonly occurs in association with the use of contraceptives. There is a 10% incidence of significant increase in menstrual flow with an intrauterine device (IUD).[1] After discontinuing oral contraceptives, women may experience increased flow. Women occasionally have an episode of very

heavy bleeding while taking oral contraceptives. Pelvic examination in these cases is normal. Knowledge deficits are the usual nursing diagnoses, and nursing care includes education and reassurance, or referral for further evaluation of potential complications.

Endometrial infections can cause heavy menstrual bleeding because of disturbance of clotting mechanisms. Menses are usually painful, and the blood may be foul smelling. The woman may have fever, uterine tenderness and enlargement, and mucopurulent cervical discharge. When the tubes or ovaries are involved in pelvic infections, there may be adnexal fullness, masses, or tenderness. When pelvic inflammatory disease (PID) is suspected, cultures are taken for *Neisseria gonorrhoeae* and *Chlamydia* organisms, and a white blood cell count with differential is ordered. PID is treated with antibiotics and, if severe, may require hospitalization. Nursing diagnoses include alterations in comfort (pain); knowledge deficits; and potential complications. Nursing care includes education about the condition and medical treatment, information about comfort measures and analgesic medications, and evaluation for complications, as well as teaching the client about identifying and preventing complications.

Recurrent heavy menses over months and years in the woman aged 30 to 45 can be due to *endometriosis* (adenomyosis) or uterine *myomas* (fibroids) (Fig. 49-1). The typical history includes "flooding," in which the woman bleeds through super tampons and peripads in a short time. She may have pain or cramping with menstrual flow, particularly with adenomyosis, in which there is usually increasing pain over time. Pelvic examination is critical in identifying causes of the heavy

TABLE 49-1

Common Causes of Gynecologic Bleeding

Age 5–13	Age 14–25	Age 25–35	Age 35–45	Age 45+ (postmenopausal)
Foreign bodies	Pregnancy	Pregnancy	Pregnancy	Estrogen therapy
Self-inflicted lacerations	Oral contraceptives or IUD	Oral contraceptives or IUD	Anovulation	Endometrial hyperplasia or polyps
Vaginitis (nonspecific)	Cervical eversion or cervicitis	Cervical eversion or cervicitis	Endometrial hyperplasia	Endometrial carcinoma
Rule out urinary tract infection and rectal bleeding	Anovulation	Cervical polyps	Uterine fibroids	Uterine fibroids
	Vaginal lacerations or infections	Anovulation	Adenomyosis	Coital injuries
	Foreign bodies	Vaginal lacerations or infections	Endometriosis	
	Adenosis	Foreign bodies	Endometrial carcinoma	
	Cervical polyps	Uterine fibroids	Oral contraceptives or IUD	
		Endometrial hyperplasia	Cervical polyps	
			Other cervical and vaginal causes	

ASSESSMENT TOOL

Menstrual History

Menarche
   Age menses began_____
   Menstrual patterns first few years:
      Regularity of cycles_____
      Cramping or pain_____
      Length and character of flow_____
   Preparation for menses (extent, who informed her, circumstances)

_____
_____

   Reaction to menarche (feelings, attitudes)

_____
_____
_____

Menstrual cycle characteristics
   Length of cycles (regular, irregular)

_____
_____

   Length and character of flow (how many days, amount of blood, clots)

_____
_____

   Discomfort or pain with menses:
      When pain begins (days, hours before flow; with onset of flow)

_____
_____

      How long pain lasts (hours, days)_____
      Severity of pain (extent of interference with activities, debility)

_____
_____

   Medications or remedies used, effectiveness

_____
_____

   Use of tampons, pads, sponges, etc.

_____
_____

(continued)

bleeding. If fibroids are present, the uterus may feel irregular in shape or nodular, or it may be enlarged with submucous fibroids. In adenomyosis, there are endometrial implants, which bleed monthly into the uterine muscle. The uterus feels slightly enlarged, boggy, and tender. Endometrial nodules also may be felt on the ligaments, rectovaginal septum, or tubal structures. Medical treatment may include dilatation and curettage (D&C) to control endometrial hyperplasia, hormone therapy to resolve or control endometriosis, surgery to remove myoma, or hysterectomy. Continued surveillance is necessary to rule out cancer, as uterine masses could be malignant.

Nursing diagnoses include knowledge deficits; alterations in comfort (pain); anxiety/fear; potential complications (anemia, surgery); ineffective individual or family coping; and disturbance in self-concept. Education, counseling, and support are nursing interventions for most diagnoses. Fear and self-concept disturbances may be related to the threat of cancer, because uterine enlargements and masses might be malignant. The nurse provides support through the medical diagnostic process, education, and reassurance as indicated. Continued pain and flooding with menses disrupt the woman's life-style and that of her family, affecting their coping and the woman's self-concept. The nurse can

A S S E S S M E N T   T O O L   *(continued)*

Premenstrual symptoms
    Onset of symptoms (days or hours preceding menstrual flow)_____
    Progression of symptoms (worse, better, when they end)_____
    Types of symptoms and relative severity

    _____

    Factors associated with symptoms (food, rest, activity)

    _____

    Medical treatment or self-treatment, results

    _____

    Interference with work or daily activities

    _____

    Effects on spouse, family

    _____

Attitudes toward menstruation
    Feelings about menstruation (positive, negative)_____
    Feelings about menstrual symptoms_____
    Perception of relation between menstrual symptoms and woman's status

    Feelings about important others' responses to menstrual behaviors

    _____

    Beliefs about effects of menstrual symptoms on women's cognitive or functional abilities

    _____

Knowledge about menstruation
    Physiology of menstrual cycle_____
    Psychology of menstruation_____
    Social constructs related to menstruation_____
    Dysmenorrhea (cause, symptoms, treatment)_____
    PMS (cause, symptoms, treatment)_____

---

assist with developing effective ways of coping, improving communications, and supporting a more positive self-concept.

There may be *systemic causes* of heavy cyclic bleeding. Several drugs are known to increase menses, including thiazide diuretics, anticoagulants, anticholinergics, hypothalamic depressants (morphine, reserpine), and phenothiazines. When other causes have been ruled out by history, physical examination, and diagnostic tests, and the drug appears to be the cause of heavy bleeding, the client is counseled about the benefits and risks of continuing the drug. Anemia must be evaluated and treated, if present. Knowledge deficits are corrected

and anxiety/fears allayed. The client is assisted to decide whether to continue the drug, and alternatives are explored.

Decreased Cyclic Bleeding

Short, scant menstrual flow occurring at regular intervals can be a normal pattern for some women. Menstrual flow may be very light, or the woman may have spotting for 1 to 2 days. It is important to determine the length of time between bleeding episodes, because very short cycles (17–20 days) may indicate *anovulation*. Women under 30 years old with consistent anovulatory cycles

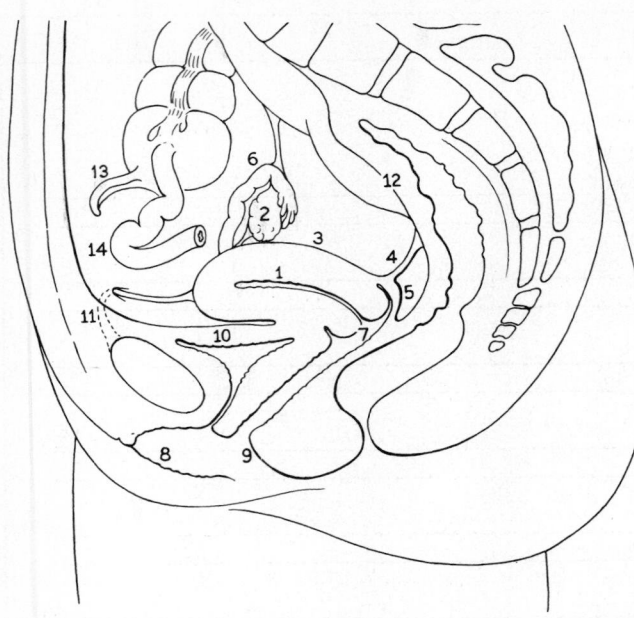

FIGURE 49-1

Schematic drawing of sites of endometriosis (numbered, beginning with the ovary, in approximate order of frequency). (*1*) Adenomyosis site, (*2*) ovary, (*3*) serous surface of uterus, (*4*) uterosacral ligament, (*5*) cul-de-sac, (*6*) tube, (*7*) cervix, (*8*) vulva, (*9*) peritoneum, (*10*) bladder, (*11*) extraperitoneal portion of round ligament, (*12*) rectosigmoid, (*13*) appendix, (*14*) ileum. (Mattingly RF, Thompson JD: Te Linde's Operative Gynecology, 6th ed. Philadelphia, JB Lippincott, 1985)

are more prone to infertility and are at increased risk for endometrial carcinoma. If the physical examination is normal, the woman is instructed in keeping a menstrual calendar, basal body temperature chart, and cervical mucus observations to document presence or absence of ovulation. If she is ovulating, she may need reassurance that her pattern is normal. If she is anovulatory, further work-up is needed depending upon her concerns and childbearing goals (Chap. 16 discusses managing infertility).

Oral contraceptives often cause light menses because they create a relative estrogen deficiency or have an androgenic influence on the endometrium. If other symptoms of estrogen deficiency are not present, the woman may be reassured that there is no cause for concern. Knowledge deficits are corrected by education and explanations. If the woman is not comfortable with very light flow, another contraceptive pill may be used with more estrogenic or less androgenic effects.

Cervical stenosis may cause light menses with dark brown spotting and cramping. The cervical os may appear occluded on pelvic examination, or it may not admit a sound. Referral is indicated for medical treatment,

which often includes progressive cervical dilatation. Knowledge deficits and alterations in comfort are common nursing diagnoses.

Decreased menstrual flow also may be due to *severe weight loss* diets and inadequate protein. Eating disorders may underlie this problem (anorexia, bulimia). Heavy use of *marijuana* can decrease menstrual flow by inhibiting normal estrogen function.[2] Such problems are suspected when physical examination is normal and history does not indicate other causes. Nursing diagnoses include alterations in nutrition; ineffective individual coping; disturbance in self-concept; and alterations in thought processes. Interventions are complex and long-term.

Intermenstrual Bleeding or Spotting

Bleeding or spotting between menses is often a sign of an organic problem, although there may be functional causes. Thorough menstrual and symptom histories are needed, with particular attention to the amount, character, and duration of bleeding and any associated symptoms. Pelvic examination helps to confirm the diagnosis and guide treatment.

Midcycle spotting (mittelstaining) is light pink spotting that lasts a few hours to a day and is associated with ovulation. This functional condition is caused by a relative estrogen dip at midcycle just prior to ovulation. Some women may experience occasional and periodic midcycle spotting. When the history and physical examination are negative for other conditions, the woman may identify other signs of ovulation to help confirm the diagnosis (*e.g.*, drop then sustained rise in basal body temperature, ovulation pain, ferning, and characteristic ovulatory changes in cervical mucus). Usually no medical treatment is needed, although small doses of estrogen around the time of ovulation can prevent the spotting.[3] Knowledge deficit related to ovulatory physiology is the nursing diagnosis, and treatment includes education and reassurance.

Vaginitis or *cervicitis* may cause intermenstrual spotting or light bleeding. Often vaginitis is associated with increased discharge, itching, dysuria, spotting after intercourse, or discomfort with intercourse. Pelvic examination may reveal increased vaginal discharge, erythema, cervical discharge, polyp, or inflammation. A Pap smear is indicated for cervical evaluation, and saline or potassium hydroxide slides are taken for examination of vaginal discharge. When vaginitis is diagnosed, treatment is specific for the organism (see Chap. 50). Abnormal Pap smears lead to further diagnostic evaluation (see Chap. 48). Nonpatterned bleeding may be an early sign of cytologic changes caused by diethylstilbestrol (*DES*), especially when this occurs in adolescents and young adults. Pap smears and colposcopy are needed for thorough evaluation.

Foreign bodies are another cause of intermenstrual spotting that does not follow a pattern. These are more frequent in young girls and adolescents, although it is not uncommon for women to forget a tampon or diaphragm in the vagina for several days. Associated symptoms include lower abdominal cramping, increased foul smelling vaginal discharge, and pressure. The foreign body can usually be seen on speculum examination, when it can be removed. The nursing diagnosis is commonly knowledge deficit, and care includes an explanation of the situation and resultant symptoms. If indicated from other observations, alterations in thought processes may be related to inserting or forgetting the foreign body.

When the cause of unpatterned genital bleeding is not evident from the history or examination, *trauma* must be considered. Sexual abuse is a common problem in both female children and adult women and is one of the most frequent causes of genital trauma. Sensitive questioning in a supportive, accepting atmosphere may be necessary to obtain a history of abuse. Nursing diagnoses and nursing care are discussed in Chapter 48. Other causes of trauma may be scratching, falls, and lacerations from using tampon or diaphragm inserters.

Oral contraceptives cause a type of breakthrough bleeding that may occur at any time in the menstrual cycle, is usually not cyclic and regular, but can be recurrent. The amount of bleeding ranges from light spotting to frank, heavy bleeding and may last from a few hours to several days. Ordinarily there is little or no pain or cramping. Breakthrough bleeding occurs when endometrial sloughing is incomplete during withdrawal menses, and areas build up with varying thickness until the estrogen levels provided by the oral contraceptive are not enough to maintain the endometrium. When other data from history and examination are normal, and breakthrough bleeding is the most likely medical diagnosis, the nursing diagnosis usually is knowledge deficit. Intervention consists of educating the woman about oral contraceptive effects and the physiology of breakthrough bleeding. Usually she is advised to continue the same pill, unless bleeding occurs frequently and higher-dose estrogen or a different combination is indicated. Depending upon the woman's response to contraceptives and bleeding, other nursing diagnoses could be disturbance in self-concept; anxiety/fear; noncompliance; or ineffective individual coping.

Pregnancy must always be considered as a possible cause of intermenstrual bleeding in women of childbearing age. Even those using contraceptives must be evaluated for pregnancy due to contraceptive failure and misuse. The typical symptoms of pregnancy are explored during the history, and the pelvic examination provides information about whether characteristic changes of pregnancy have occurred (Chadwick's sign, Hegar's sign—softened uterine isthmus, uterine enlargement). Some women continue to have light bleeding at the time their menses would be due, even though they are pregnant.

Endometrial hyperplasia related to hormone imbalances is a frequent cause of sudden, heavy bleeding without a cyclic pattern, particularly in women approaching the cessation of ovarian function. The aging ovary fails to produce estrogen and progesterone with smooth cyclic release in sufficient quantities, and ovulation becomes erratic. Adequate progesterone is necessary to regulate endometrial breakdown during the menstrual phase. When estrogen influences the endometrium in the absence of sufficient progesterone, the endometrium continues to proliferate and grow in thickness. During menses, the endometrium is incompletely sloughed, leading to irregular areas of thick buildup. When the hormone levels no longer support this hyperplastic endometrium, sudden bleeding occurs that can be extremely heavy, with large clots, and can last up to 2 weeks.

A good history is necessary to identify the character of the bleeding and associated factors. The pelvic examination serves to rule out other causes of bleeding, such as fibroids, endometriosis, or pregnancy. As the woman becomes older, endometrial carcinoma is an increasing concern. Diagnostic tests are usually done, including a Pap smear and endometrial biopsy or jet wash. Some physicians prefer to perform a D&C instead of an endometrial biopsy if the woman is about 40 years old or older, because the entire endometrium is available for cytologic examination. Biopsies and jet washes only sample a portion of the endometrium, and malignancies can be missed (see Chap. 48).

When diagnostic tests show endometrial hyperplasia, treatment may be surgery (D&C) or hormone therapy. Frequently, a progestational drug is used, such as medroxyprogesterone acetate (Provera), during the last part of the menstrual cycle to regulate endometrial breakdown and control bleeding. Acute bleeding episodes can be stopped by administering progesterone or estrogen in high doses, followed by an oral contraceptive or estrogen–progesterone combination to control subsequent menstrual bleeding. Careful monitoring of response to treatment is necessary for irregular bleeding in premenopausal women, because of the risk of cancer. This type of intermenstrual bleeding also is called *dysfunctional uterine bleeding.*[4]

Nursing diagnoses may include knowledge deficits related to pathophysiological conditions and medical treatments; anxiety/fear, especially if cancer risk is high;

potential complications such as anemia and infections; disturbance in self-concept related to altered body functions; alteration in comfort (pain); and sexual dysfunction. Nursing care could include education and information about the condition, its causes and medical treatments, and support during procedures. Counseling is indicated when anxiety/fear is present, including clarification of misconceptions, setting boundaries on fears, and finding ways of handling anxiety. Women approaching menopause may need assistance dealing with body and functional changes through active listening, support, reassurance, and acceptance. Measures to alleviate pain, such as medications, relaxation, or thermal applications, can be provided. Sexual dysfunctions must be identified and appropriate counseling or referral provided.

Amenorrhea

The absence of menses, or skipping periods, is a common problem among women during the reproductive years. Primary amenorrhea occurs when a girl reaches 18 years of age and has never menstruated. The most frequent causes are structural, congenital, and endocrine abnormalities, such as gonadal dysgenesis, imperforate hymen, absent vagina or uterus, androgen insensitivity syndrome, prepubertal ovarian failure, congenital adrenal hyperplasia, and hypopituitarism. Secondary amenorrhea occurs when a previously menstruating woman ceases to menstruate; the causes may be pathologic (organic) or functional. A careful menstrual history usually suggests the most likely cause of amenorrhea, and further data are provided by the physical examination and diagnostic tests.

Pregnancy is probably the most common cause of secondary amenorrhea in women aged 16 to 45. Typical symptoms of pregnancy are elicited in the history, and the pelvic examination may reveal typical physiological changes of pregnancy. A pregnancy test confirms the diagnosis, and counseling with referral is offered for interruption or continuation of pregnancy. *Oral contraceptives* frequently cause women to skip one or more menses, particularly low-dose estrogen and progestin-only pills, and patterns of use must be carefully explored. If the woman is taking the pills properly, she is advised to continue for a few more cycles. Withdrawal menses will likely occur in subsequent cycles. If amenorrhea continues, and the woman is disturbed by lack of menses, a higher-dose or different estrogen pill can be prescribed. Usually nursing diagnoses are knowledge deficits; anxiety; or alterations in self-concept. Nursing care includes education, counseling, reassurance, and increasing options or coping strategies.

Ovarian cysts may cause amenorrhea, the most common types including follicular and corpus luteum cysts. When the graafian follicle fails to rupture, it may continue to increase in size and secrete estrogen. The ovary may be enlarged to 6 cm to 8 cm. Since ovulation does not occur, the luteal phase is not entered and the endometrium continues to proliferate under estrogen influence. Usually these cysts resolve spontaneously in several weeks, and menstruation is restored. Oral contraceptives may be used for one to two cycles to cause involution of the cyst. In corpus luteum dysfunction, progesterone continues to be secreted and the secretory endometrium is maintained, similar to early pregnancy. These cysts also tend to regress spontaneously, and regular cycles are restored in a few weeks. Nursing diagnoses include knowledge deficits and anxiety, and nursing care focuses on education and reassurance.

Organic causes of secondary amenorrhea include pituitary necrosis (Sheehan's syndrome), hyperthyroidism, galactorrhea, adrenal or ovarian virilization (Stein-Leventhal syndrome), and Cushing's syndrome.

Discomfort

Dysmenorrhea

Discomfort associated with menstruation is a common experience among women. Two clinical syndromes have been identified: dysmenorrhea and PMS. PMS is discussed in the following section. Although definitions vary, dysmenorrhea largely is regarded as pain that occurs shortly before onset or during menstrual flow. *Primary dysmenorrhea* occurs without pelvic pathology and is the largest category of menstrual pain. *Secondary dysmenorrhea* results from organic or pathologic causes, such as endometriosis, adenomyosis, PID, cervical stenosis, IUD, or trauma. The focus of this section is on primary dysmenorrhea.

Characteristic symptoms are experienced to varying degrees by women with primary dysmenorrhea. Painful menses is the hallmark symptom. The pain is located in the suprapubic region and can be sharp, gripping, cramping, or dull aching. It often is accompanied by pelvic fullness or bearing down sensations that may radiate to the inner thighs and lumbosacral area. Some women experience nausea/vomiting, headache, fatigue, dizziness, faintness, diarrhea, or emotional instability during this time.

Incoordinate, spasmodic uterine contractions are thought to cause the menstrual pain. These are possibly related to prostaglandins present during the luteal phase of the menstrual cycle. Women with dysmenorrhea have been found to have higher intrauterine pressure during the menstrual period and to have more prostaglandins in their menstrual flow than women without pain. Pain relief is often obtained with oral contraceptives, which cause atrophy of the endometrium and consequent reduction of prostaglandin synthesis. Women with dysmenorrhea also have decreased uterine blood flow during menses, which has been relieved by β-sympathomimetic drugs with vasodilating properties. This suggests that ischemia plays a role in causing dysmenorrhea.[5]

The onset of dysmenorrhea is typically shortly after menarche, once ovulatory cycles are established. Anovulatory bleeding is usually painless. The highest incidence is between the ages of 14 and 25, and pregnancy often markedly improves subsequent menstrual discomfort. Oral contraceptives tend to provide relief. There is a family tendency toward primary dysmenorrhea; women whose mothers had dysmenorrhea are more likely to have the same problem.

There is conflicting information about the impact of the woman's social environment on dysmenorrhea. Female patients in mental hospitals indicated more menstrual pain when they had less acceptance of the female role, and more pain was reported among college students scoring higher on a masculinity scale. In contrast, femininity scores on a personality inventory were positively correlated with menstrual symptoms in college women and women at a family-planning clinic. Traditionally feminine women (homemakers with no personal career ambitions) were found to have more menstrual symptoms, and another study found no associations between perimenstrual discomfort and traditional or feminist orientations. Demographic and social characteristics (race, employment status, marital status) have been described as weak correlates of dysmenorrhea, with a negative correlation between dysmenorrhea and income, education, and age. Both negative and positive attitudes associated with menses were correlated with dysmenorrhea; women who felt menstruation should not affect a woman's behavior had less pain, and those who experienced degrees of debilitation during menstruation had more pain.[6]

Assessment. Assessment of dysmenorrhea includes a thorough menstrual history and careful exploration of pain and other associated symptoms (see Important Causes of Pelvic Pain). It is important to distinguish dysmenorrhea from PMS, because the treatments are quite different. The amount of disruption in daily activities caused by dysmenorrhea helps assess the severity of pain and debilitating effects of symptoms. The role of stress and anxiety in menstrual pain is complex. While tension could certainly contribute to increased pain, recurrent painful menses and debilitation also could create anxiety and stress surrounding menstruation. A life-style and stress history is taken to evaluate the role tension and anxiety may play. The physical examination assists in eliminating significant pathology as the cause of

---

Important Causes of Pelvic Pain

Cyclic, Recurrent Menstrual Pain

Dysmenorrhea (primary, secondary)
Endometriosis
Adenomyosis
IUDs
Endometritis or PID

Recurrent Pain Not During Menses

Midcycle ovulation pain (mittelschmerz)
Ovarian cysts (follicular, corpus luteum)
Ovarian or uterine malignancies
Psychogenic pain

Acute, Severe Nonmenstrual Pain

Ectopic pregnancy, actual or pending rupture
Twisted fallopian tube, ovary, or ovarian cyst
Ruptured ovarian cyst
Appendicitis
Acute PID
Acute lower bowel lesions

---

menstrual pain, and the pelvic examination should be normal in primary dysmenorrhea. Diagnostic tests to rule out pathology might include a complete blood cell count, urinalysis, sedimentation rate, and pelvic ultrasonography.

Diagnosis and Treatment. In the absence of pelvic pathology, and with a symptom history typical for dysmenorrhea (see Characteristic Symptoms of Dysmenorrhea), the diagnosis is made. Initial medical treatment may consist of mild analgesics such as aspirin and acetaminophen; aspirin has a slight anti-prostaglandin effect that provides significant relief for some women. If these analgesics are not effective, nonsteroidal anti-inflammatory drugs are often used, which have a stronger antiprostaglandin effect. Popular prescription drugs are naproxen (Anaprox), mefenamic acid (Ponstel), and ibuprofen (Motrin); these are reported to have a 70% chance of significantly reducing pain.[7] Common side-effects of these medications include gastric irritation and gastritis; less frequently they may cause headaches, nausea, allergic reactions, and asthma. Oral contraceptives may be used to relieve dysmenorrhea unless contraindicated or unacceptable to the client. Most often, low-dose combination pills with 50 mcg estrogen or less are prescribed.

Nursing Diagnosis. Nursing diagnoses related to dysmenorrhea may include alterations in comfort (pain);

Characteristic Symptoms of Dysmenorrhea

Onset of pain a few hours before or with menstrual flow

Pain located in suprapubic region, may radiate to inner thighs and lumbosacral area

Character of pain is sharp, gripping, cramping, or dull aching

Pain often accompanied by pelvic fullness or bearing-down sensations

Duration of pain is several hours to about 2 days

Associated symptoms may include:

  Nausea/vomiting

  Headache

  Fatigue

  Dizziness

  Diarrhea

  Emotional instability

knowledge deficits; ineffective individual coping; alterations in nutrition; and disturbance in self-concept.

Planning/Intervention.   Nursing care is based upon diagnoses for individual clients. Nursing care for pain can include a number of nonpharmacologic approaches. Heat has pain-relieving properties because it causes vasodilation and increased blood flow to the affected area and decreases hypertonic muscle contractions, thus affecting both causes of dysmenorrhea (ischemia, hypertonia). Either dry heat with a heating pad or wet heat in a tub or shower may be effective. Massage or effleurage of the lower abdomen is often therapeutic, because it increases the pain threshold by providing a secondary stimulus. Relaxation techniques such as biofeedback, autogenic training, yoga, progressive relaxation, and meditation have been used effectively to relieve menstrual pain.[8]

Knowledge deficits related to the pathophysiology of dysmenorrhea and psychosocial factors can be alleviated by education and counseling. Many women have heard that dysmenorrhea is a psychosomatic problem and may have had negative experiences in the health-care system. Nurses can explain how attitudes and beliefs about dysmenorrhea have developed and can correct misinformation and misconceptions by discussing current research and understandings of the problem. Women can be assisted to find ways to prevent or minimize menstrual discomfort. Exercise that tones muscles and increases circulation can allay ischemia. Swimming is excellent for building muscle tone, and other aerobic exercises also can be helpful. Getting adequate rest seems to reduce menstrual pain for some women. Sleep

needs often are increased during menstruation, and increased sleep time can relieve tension.

Alterations in nutrition with less intake of B vitamins than needed may contribute to dysmenorrhea. The B vitamins increase protein utilization and help relieve fatigue, tension, and depression. Premenstrually, carbohydrate metabolism may be altered, with mild glucose intolerance and hypoglycemia. A diet high in protein and complex carbohydrates, taken in small frequent amounts, should provide relief for hypoglycemia symptoms.

Women experiencing disturbance in self-concept have negative feelings about or views of themselves related to menstrual pain. They may have 1 or more days of significant debility, which contributes to lower self-esteem and less effective role performance. Women may have internalized social myths and prejudices surrounding menstrual discomfort, and may feel less worthy in comparison to men. Nursing care focuses on helping these clients to formulate more positive attitudes toward menstruation and toward themselves as normal, healthy women. They need reassurance that their attitudes toward femininity and women's roles are not the cause of dysmenorrhea. Explanations of menstrual physiology and psychology can help correct misconceptions. Planning to anticipate and prepare for days when functioning is decreased can help the woman feel more in control. Finding effective methods of pain relief, if possible, can help improve self-concept disturbances.

Ineffective individual coping may result when menstrual pain causes additional stress and the woman has inadequate resources to handle her stressors. The woman may feel overwhelmed, may withdraw and become noncommunicative, may become irritable and defensive, and may be prone to accidents. Usually other factors in the woman's life help create a situation in which she is unable to respond effectively; dysmenorrhea is one of many difficulties. Nursing care seeks to identify sources of stress and assist the woman to find ways to remove, reduce, or alleviate causes of stress. Any measures to reduce menstrual pain will be very helpful. In addition, there may be a need for individual or family therapy, social agency referrals, motivational and values-clarification techniques, and increasing the woman's social and family networks. This problem may be anticipated at important transition points in maturation, such as leaving home, making career choices, getting married, having children, and launching children.

Premenstrual Syndrome

An estimated 20% to 40% of menstruating women in the United States experience premenstrual symptoms severe enough to cause some degree of temporary men-

---

Characteristic Symptoms of PMS

Onset of symptoms 4 to 10 days before menstrual flow

Recurrent, cyclic symptoms affecting all or many menstrual cycles

Multiple somatic, behavioral, and emotional symptoms that tend to be a typical complex for each individual woman

Symptoms improve after onset of menstrual flow

More common PMS symptoms include:

Fluid retention and peripheral edema

Anxiety, nervousness

Irritability, frustration

Agitation, argumentativeness

Depression, lowered self-esteem

Impaired concentration, being accident prone

Food or sweet/salt craving, hunger, eating binges

Fatigue, lethargy

Headaches, dizziness

Painful breasts, abdominal bloating, pelvic cramping

Crying, emotional instability

Feelings of panic or loss of control

---

tal or physical incapacitation.[9] About 5% to 15% have very severe symptoms.[10] Up to 90% have recurrent premenstrual symptoms, but most experience no debilitation with these. PMS has emerged as a complex of physical and emotional symptoms that occur on a cyclic basis prior to onset of menstruation. It is caused by different mechanisms than dysmenorrhea and often responds to different therapeutic approaches. Although PMS has been studied since as early as 1930, and the term was coined by Dalton in 1953, much is still unknown about etiology.

PMS is characterized by a complex of behavioral, physical, and emotional symptoms that begin to appear about 4 to 10 days before menses. As many as 74 to 150 different recurrent symptoms have been associated with PMS.[11,12] Fluid retention produces edema, possibly due to increased estrogen, progesterone, and aldosterone. Increased prolactin levels may affect water excretion, leading to bloating and edema. Edema produces symptoms of depression, anxiety, irritability, and mood changes. Progesterone acts to elevate monoamine oxidase (MAO) levels, which may cause depression. Vitamin B₆ (pyridoxine) regulates MAO production, and deficiencies may contribute to mood fluctuations. Pyridoxine acts as a coenzyme in the conversion of tryptophan to dopamine and serotonin, and reductions are associated with depression.

Altered glucose metabolism, particularly hypoglycemia, is thought to be responsible for PMS symptoms of hunger and food cravings, fatigue, nervousness, sweating, headaches, and gastrointestinal distress. Premenstrual women have a flattening of the glucose tolerance curve, with possible increases in insulin receptor concentration or endorphin effects on glucose metabolism. Endorphins (endogenous opiate peptides) may contribute to PMS through their neurotransmitter functions, which regulate release of pituitary hormones and other neuroendocrine changes, leading to both physical and psychological symptoms.[9] Prostaglandins and vasopressin may be involved in PMS symptomatology. Opiates are known to inhibit the actions of prostaglandins, and they may affect the release of prolactin and vasopressin.[13] These substances affect water excretion and uterine tone and contractility.

The most frequently reported PMS symptoms are tension states such as anxiety, nervousness, irritability, frustration, agitation, and argumentativeness. Edema and fluid retention and depression or lowered self-esteem are experienced by many women with PMS.

PMS Resources

Premenstrual Assessment Form

Self-administered form to assess premenstrual symptoms; includes 95 items and instructions. Send request and self-addressed stamped envelope to:

Jean Endicott, PhD
Director, Premenstrual Evaluation Unit
Columbia Presbyterian Medical Center
722 West 168 Street
New York, NY 10032

PMS Access

Several types of resources are available, including diet logs, symptom charts, PMS training for health personnel, PMS newsletter, a mail-order service, and a toll-free hotline. Contact:

PMS Access
Madison Pharmacy Associates, Inc.
1603 Monroe Street
Madison, WI 53711

Toll-free hotline (800) 222-4PMS

Premenstrual Symptom Calendar

Calendar for charting premenstrual symptoms. Send written request and self-addressed stamped envelope to:

Candice Telis, RN
2 Main Street
Flemington, NJ 08822

Less frequent are food cravings, fatigue, headache, painful breasts, and crying. Feelings of panic and loss of control or violent acts and child battering have been reported by a small number of women. Increased accidents and injuries and suicidal ideation are infrequent symptoms.[11] With increasing numbers of women in the work force, concern has surfaced about the impact of PMS on absenteeism, decreased work performance, and increased error and accident rates. While women do report subjective changes in work performance, various studies have not found objective alterations in cognition and motor performance during the premenstrual phase.[14] Absenteeism due to PMS has been estimated to lose as much as 5 billion dollars yearly to industry.[15]

The relationships between PMS and psychological symptoms such as depression, anxiety, and other tension states is not clear. While edema no doubt plays a role in these symptoms, the causal paths and networks among factors are complex and mediated by multiple variables. The anticipation of symptoms that are unpleasant and disruptive may cause women to become anxious and depressed, rather than these resulting from a direct physiological effect of PMS. Negative attitudes toward menstruation have been correlated with menstrual symptoms. For some women, such attitudes and life stresses may exacerbate physiological mechanisms to increase symptomatology. Further research into psychophysiological factors in the premenstrual phase is needed.[14]

Assessment.   Assessment includes a menstrual history focused upon the onset and progression of menstrual symptoms, as well as the woman's attitudes and responses over time. A nutritional history is taken with particular attention to salt intake, protein and carbohydrate balance, and use of caffeine and alcohol. A general health history provides information about other problems that could contribute to or be confused with PMS. As part of the assessment, the client can fill out a symptom calendar for 1 to 3 months, noting carefully the timing, type, and severity of each premenstrual symptom. Because there are so many different PMS symptoms, assessment is very individualized and self-assessment is particularly important. The client needs to identify which symptoms are most frequent and most troublesome, so therapies can be focused on these. The physical examination seeks evidence of pathology or abnormalities that might be related to symptoms, with particular attention in the pelvic examination to uterine or ovarian enlargement, signs of endometriosis or adenomyosis, and structural abnormalities (see PMS Resources).

Nursing Diagnosis.   Diagnosis of PMS is made when physical examination and diagnostic tests indicate nor-

mal pelvic conditions, and the woman's symptoms in the premenstrual and menstrual phases follow the typical patterns. Nursing diagnoses related to PMS could include alterations in comfort (pain); anxiety/fear; ineffective individual or family coping; fluid volume excess; knowledge deficit; alterations in nutrition; disturbance in self-concept; and sexual dysfunction.

Treatment.   Treatment for PMS varies according to which symptoms are most disturbing to the client. There are no entirely effective drugs, although medical treatment has included diuretics and hormones, primarily progesterone. The most effective therapies include dietary, life-style, and behavioral adjustments; between 36% and 75% of women with PMS have obtained significant symptomatic relief from these.[15] These types of therapies are particularly suitable for nurses to implement and are entirely within the domain of nursing. The definitive treatment of PMS is a nursing, not medical, responsibility.

Planning/Intervention.   Pain and discomfort associated with PMS can be treated with mild analgesics such as aspirin or acetaminophen and with application of dry or moist heat. However, cramping is not as much of a problem with PMS as it is with dysmenorrhea. Relaxation techniques are very useful, because they also affect PMS symptoms of irritability, depression, and anxiety (nursing diagnosis of anxiety/fear). Knowledge deficit is treated by teaching clients about the physiology and psychology of PMS and by clarifying myths or misconceptions about its social and psychological origins and impacts. Public education could be another nursing intervention, especially in schools, so young girls can gain accurate information about the menstrual cycle and such problems as dysmenorrhea and PMS. Classes in community clinics, family associations, and women's groups can further educate the public.

Alterations in nutrition, either by deficits or excesses, are important factors in PMS symptomatology, and considerable therapy is aimed at correcting these. Caffeine, chocolate, and other xanthine derivatives should be eliminated because of their tendency to increase irritability, insomnia, mood changes, and depression. Salt and other forms of sodium should be reduced, especially 7 to 9 days before menstruation, because of fluid retention properties. Women need to be reminded to drink at least 1 quart of water daily and to use such natural diuretics as cranberry or grapefruit juice. They are advised to cook without salt or avoid salting cooked foods and to eliminate foods high in sodium, such as pickles, potato chips, pork, catsup, sauces, prepared soups, and so forth. Fresh or frozen foods are preferable to canned ones, which contain sodium. Hypoglycemia-type symptoms (fatigue, headache, dizziness, food cravings) are relieved by avoiding sweets and refined carbohydrates and by eating a diet high in protein and complex carbohydrates. Frequent small meals keep blood glucose levels more stable.

Vitamin B_6 is often recommended to reduce irritability and depression. Some nurses use calcium, magnesium, and chromium supplements because of their hypothesized role in neurotransmitter functioning. Vitamin E has been recommended for breast tenderness. A multivitamin/multimineral supplement may be sufficient for some women, but at least 100 mg of vitamin B_6 are needed, which may require taking additional B_6 tablets.[15-17]

Exercise on a regular basis can reduce stress and cramping and helps relieve depression and moodiness. Various relaxation techniques such as biofeedback, autogenic training, progressive relaxation, meditation, and breathing exercises are effective for reducing stress and depression. When these therapies improve PMS symptoms, alterations in self-concept related to the effects of PMS on ability to work and undertake daily activities are remedied. If a problematic self-concept derives in part from negative attitudes toward menstruation based on social stereotypes, education and counseling to change these attitudes are indicated. Women's group therapy has been effective in correcting these stereotypes, because women with PMS are able to recognize that other women with desirable personality and behavioral characteristics have the same symptoms. The supportive relationships developed in groups, and the sharing of experiences and techniques to alleviate symptoms, help improve the self-concept.[14]

Ineffective individual coping may result when women with PMS feel they cannot handle their environmental stressors adequately. A substantial proportion of women with PMS are married, highly educated, and working outside the home. These woman may suffer from the "superwoman syndrome" and expect to excel in all areas of their lives nearly all the time.[15] They need counseling to make life-style adjustments that recognize their own needs and to accept their limitations without feelings of unworthiness. Setting aside time for themselves to relax or pursue hobbies or interests is important. Some of these women may need to learn limit setting and more effective sharing of responsibilities with family and co-workers. They also may be taught self-management practices that enable them to put off decisions or prepare ahead for important events that will fall in the premenstrual phase. Women who experience a great deal of anxiety, depression, moodiness, and irritability may particularly want to use such self-management. However, it is important to view this approach as a self-selected technique, not a societal dictum that women cannot be trusted to make important decisions premenstrually.

CLIENT EDUCATION

Self-Care for PMS

Women with PMS often can reduce symptoms through self-care measures appropriate to their symptom complex:

Fluid retention (breast tenderness, abdominal bloating, peripheral edema):

   Cook without salt or avoid salting cooked foods

   Use fresh or frozen vegetables instead of canned

   Eliminate foods high in sodium (pickles, potato chips, pork, catsup, sauces, prepared soups and other foods, soy sauce)

   Drink 1 quart of water daily

   Use natural diuretics (teas, cranberry and grapefruit juice)

Depression, irritability, mood swings

   Get adequate sleep (at least 7–8 hours per night; more may be needed)

   Get regular exercise (walk about 2 miles/day, swim, bicycle)

   Use multivitamin and multimineral supplements daily

   Be sure to take at least 100 mg of vitamin B_6 per day or eat foods high in B_6 (corn, whole wheat, yeast, tomatoes, sunflower seeds, peanuts)

   Increase calcium, magnesium, and chromium

   Develop support systems (friends, spouse, women's group) for expressing feelings

   Use relaxation techniques (yoga, autogenic training, progressive relaxation, biofeedback, visualization, imagery, meditation)

Headaches and hypoglycemia-type symptoms

   Avoid sweets and refined carbohydrates

   Eat diet high in protein and complex carbohydrates

   Eat several small meals per day

   Avoid caffeine, chocolate, xanthine derivatives

   Do not skip meals

   Snack on fresh fruit or vegetables

The family may be coping ineffectively when PMS causes significant debility to the mother/wife. Providing relief for severe PMS symptoms is a first step in nursing care for this problem, because the woman will have better ability to meet responsibilities and carry out daily activities. When patterns of family interaction have developed that are disruptive or negative, family therapy may be necessary to restore communications and func-

The Woman with Premenstrual Syndrome (PMS)

Nursing Objectives
1. Accurately identify women with PMS.
2. Involve the woman in thorough assessment of symptoms and associated factors.
3. Provide education on PMS to clients, families, and the public.
4. Implement effective nursing care to reduce symptoms and debility from PMS.
5. Encourage and support self-care to prevent and minimize effects of PMS.

Assessment	Potential Nursing Diagnosis	Planning/Intervention	Evaluation

Menstrual history
  Menarche, menstrual patterns, reactions, preparation
  Menstrual cycle character and symptoms
  Attitudes toward menstruation
	Knowledge deficit related to menstrual physiology and psychology	Teach menstrual physiology and psychology
		Clarify myths, misconceptions
		Provide information and data on social and psychological factors
			Client describes correct understanding of menstrual physiology and psychology; myths and misunderstandings are cleared

Knowledge about menstruation Physical/pelvic examination negative for pathology	Alteration in self-concept related to negative attitudes and perceptions toward menstruation	Provide education and counseling about menstruation as normal female functioning Reduce PMS symptoms Suggest group therapy to build positive attitudes and correct social stereotypes	Client accepts normality of menstruation and symptoms Client states positive attitudes and corrects former stereotypes
Specific PMS symptoms Pain, cramping	Alteration in comfort: pain	Prescribe mild analgesics (acetylsalicylic acid, acetaminophen) Apply dry or moist heat Teach relaxation techniques Stress regular exercise	Client says pain and cramping are decreased

Fluid retention:
  Breast tenderness
  Abdominal bloating
  Peripheral edema
  Weight gain
	Fluid volume excess
	Alteration in nutrition: more sodium than body requirements
		Reduce or avoid sodium in foods
		Drink 1 quart of water daily
		Use natural diuretics (teas, cranberry and grapefruit juice)
			Client states she has less bloating and her symptoms are improved

(continued)

tions. Education can be an important nursing contribution. Family members who understand the psychology and physiology of the menstrual cycle are better equipped to accept and be supportive of the mother/wife. The family can become involved in care related to diet, exercise, relaxation, and rest, which facilitates positive coping behaviors and reduces family stress. Sexual dysfunction related to PMS may be simple discomfort and avoidance of intercourse premenstrually, which is treatable by reducing PMS symptoms. More complex sexual problems may be augmented by PMS and need referral to sexual therapy.

Assessment	Potential Nursing Diagnosis	Planning/Intervention	Evaluation
Depression, irritability, mood swings, frustration, impaired concentration, nervousness, anxiety, emotional instability	Alteration in nutrition: more xanthines than body requirements	Eliminate or reduce caffeine, chocolate, other xanthines; increase vitamin B$_6$, calcium, magnesium	Client adopts nutritional patterns and feels better
	Ineffective individual coping related to PMS symptoms and stress	Stress regular exercise	Client develops coping strategies and performs daily activities more effectively
		Teach relaxation techniques	
		Counsel on life-style adjustments, limit setting, self-management practices	
Headaches	Alteration in nutrition: less than body requirements for protein and complex carbohydrates; more for simple carbohydrates	Avoid sweets and simple or refined carbohydrates	Client adopts new nutritional patterns and feels better
Hypoglycemia-like symptoms: fatigue, dizziness, food cravings, hunger		Eat diet high in protein and complex carbohydrates	
		Eat several small meals each day	
		Do not skip meals	
		Snack on fresh fruit or vegetables	
Family conflicts or sexual problems	Ineffective family coping related to effects of PMS symptoms on communications and functions	Provide relief of PMS symptoms	Family communicates well, copes more effectively, and redistributes functions
		Provide education and counseling of family about menstrual physiology and psychology; PMS causes and symptoms	
		Teach effective communication techniques to family	
		Involve family in care (diet, exercise, relaxation, rest)	
		Refer for family therapy	
	Sexual dysfunction	Provide relief of PMS symptoms	Couple establishes a satisfying sexual relationship
		Provide education and counseling on sexual response/patterns	Couple makes accommodations to premenstrual problems
		Teach appropriate sexual techniques	
		Refer for sexual counseling for more complex sexual problems	

Evaluation. The effectiveness of nursing care is evaluated by observing for desired changes in client attitudes and behaviors. With PMS, the client can report whether or not particular symptoms have improved, and to what extent. For specific therapies related to a nursing diagnosis, the nurse must reassess by questioning the client or by physical examination and observations. For example, a diet record kept for a week before and a week after nutritional education and counseling can document changes in nutritional patterns. Discussions with the client about attitudes toward menstruation and PMS or administration of attitude scales provides data about change in these areas. The client's ability to perform work and family roles and her perceived levels of stress in doing these premenstrually give an overall indication of how effective the therapeutic program has been.

In a larger context, nursing research is needed to improve the quality of care provided to clients with PMS. Many research questions about the causes and manifestations of PMS, its impact upon the individual and the family, and the effectiveness of specific therapies remain to be answered. Development and testing of assessment tools, monitoring instruments, and therapeutic protocols are all fruitful areas for nursing research. Since nursing provides the definitive therapies for PMS, the nursing profession has major responsibility for extending knowledge in this area through research.

References

1. Romney SL et al: Gynecology and Obstetrics: The Health Care of Women, 2nd ed, p 438. New York, McGraw-Hill, 1981
2. Anderson PO, McGuire GG: Delta-9-tetrahydrocannabinol as an antiemetic. Am J Hosp Pharm 38:641, May 1981
3. Martin LL: Health Care of Women, pp 109–110. Philadelphia, JB Lippincott, 1978
4. Lauver D: Irregular bleeding in women: Causes and nursing intervention. Am J Nurs 83(3):396–401, March 1983
5. Lichter ED, Warfield CA: The pain clinic: Pelvic pain syndrome. Hosp Pract 20(3):32E, H, K, March 15, 1985
6. Brown MA, Woods NF: Correlates of dysmenorrhea: A challenge to past stereotypes. JOGN Nurs 13(4):256–265, July/August 1984
7. Nichols DH, Evrard JR: Ambulatory Gynecology, pp 58–59. Philadelphia, Harper & Row, 1985
8. Fogel CI, Woods NF: Health Care of Women: A Nursing Perspective, pp 242–243. St Louis, CV Mosby, 1981
9. Reid R, Yen SSC: Premenstrual syndrome. Am J Obstet Gynecol 139(1):85–104, 1981
10. Chakmakjian ZH, Zaven H: A critical assessment of therapy for the premenstrual tension syndrome. J Reprod Med 28(3):530–537, August 1983
11. Brown MA, Zimmer PA: Personal and family impact of premenstrual symptoms. JOGN Nurs 15(1):31–38, January/February 1986
12. Rupp SL: Premenstrual syndrome. NAACOG Update Series, Lesson 15, Vol 2, p 3. Princeton, NJ, Continuing Professional Education Center, 1985
13. Craig GM: Prostaglandins in reproductive physiology. Postgrad Med J 51(592):74–84, 1975
14. Coyne CM, Woods NF, Mitchell ES: Premenstrual tension syndrome. JOGN Nurs 14(6):446–454, November/December 1985
15. Frank EP: What are nurses doing to help PMS patients? Am J Nurs 86(2):136–140, February 1986
16. Zwack B: Premenstrual syndrome. Can Nurs 81(1):51–53, January 1985
17. Kirkpatrick MD, Grady TR: Premenstrual syndrome: A self-help checklist. Occup Health Nurs 33(2):90–92, February 1985

Suggested Reading

Abraham GE: Nutritional factors in the etiology of the premenstrual tension syndromes. J Reprod Med 28(7):446–464, 1983
Brooks-Gunn J, Ruble D: The menstrual attitude questionnaire. Psychosom Med 42:503–512, 1980
Brown MA: Primary dysmenorrhea. Nurs Clin North Am 17(1):145–153, 1982
Edelin KC: Evaluation of female pelvic pain, part 2. Hosp Med 19(2):37–39, 42–44, 46, February 1983
Garner CH: Endometriosis. JOGN Nurs (suppl) 14(6):10s–20s, November/December 1985
Harrison M: Self Help for Premenstrual Syndrome. New York, Random House, 1982
Lark SM: Premenstrual Syndrome Self Help Book. Los Angeles, Forman Publishers, 1984
Lauersen NH, Stukane E: Premenstrual Syndrome and You. New York, Simon and Schuster, 1983
Norris RV, Sullivan C: PMS: Premenstrual Syndrome. New York, Rawson Associates, 1983
Woods NF: Women's roles and illness episodes. Res Nurs Health 3(4):137–145, 1980
Woods NF, Most A, Dery G: Prevalence of perimenstrual symptoms. Am J Public Health 72:1257–1264, 1982

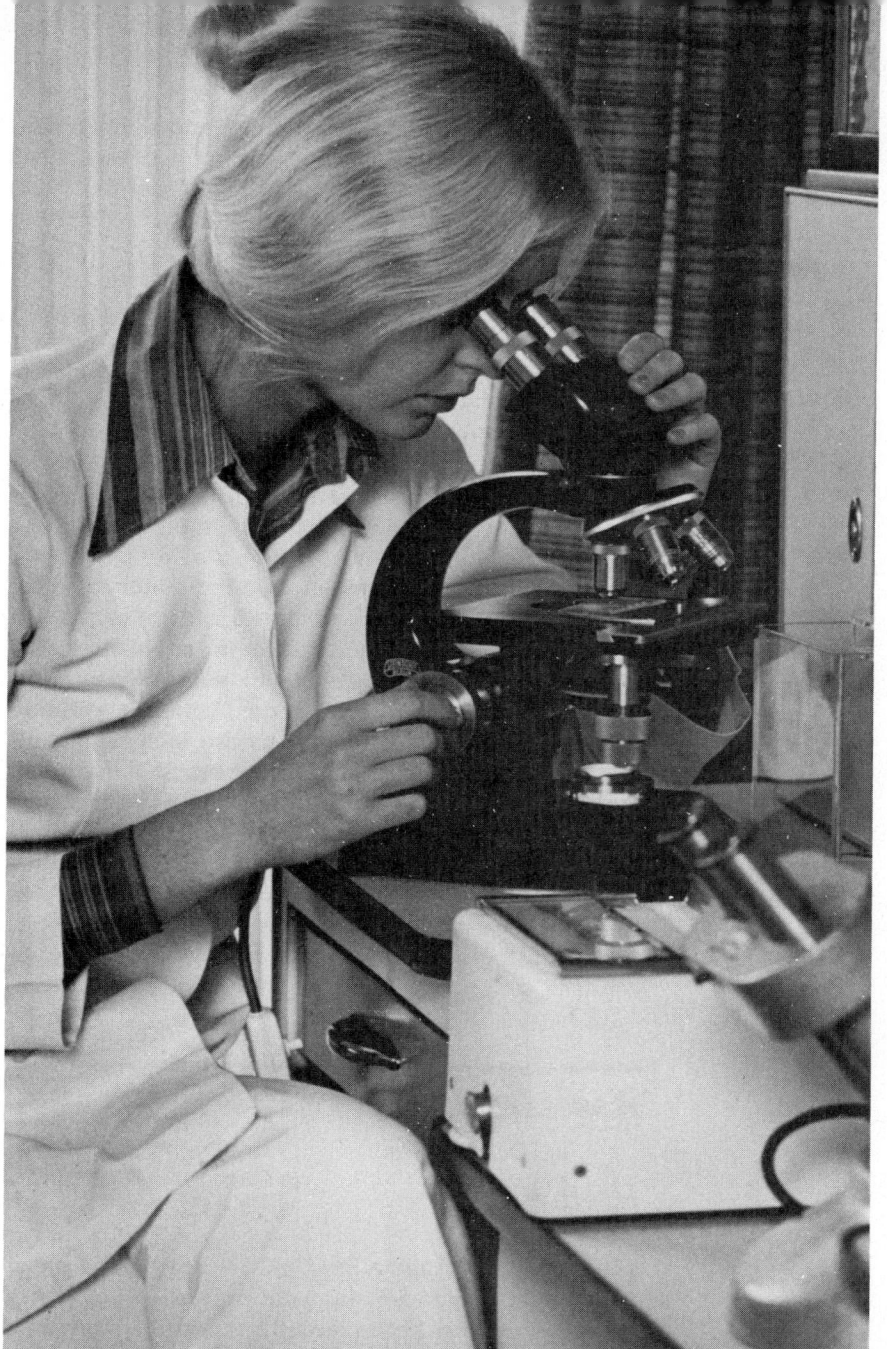

CHAPTER 50

Nursing Care in Vaginal and Pelvic Infections

Vaginal secretions of varying amount and character are normal for women during the years of active gonadal function, from about ages 11 to 50. Menstrual cycle stages with associated hormonal patterns affect vaginal physiology. Discharge may be related to other factors, such as contraceptive use, emotional state, sexual activity, and pathologic conditions. Vaginal discharge and itching are among the most frequent reasons women seek gynecological care. Nurses who practice in maternity units or clinics commonly will encounter problems related to vaginal discharge and lower abdominal discomfort, many of which are due to vaginal or pelvic infections. These nurses need skill in assessing common gynecologic infections and providing indicated nursing care and referral.

Vaginitis is an infectious or inflammatory process involving the vagina or vulva and can be caused by several microorganisms. Less commonly, allergic or traumatic processes contribute to vaginal infections. Cervicitis is infection of the cervix, commonly due to microorganisms. Pelvic infections can include the endometrium, tubes, and ovaries, or some combination of these, and are often referred to by the more inclusive term *pelvic inflammatory disease* (PID). Vaginal and pelvic infections are frequently, but not always, transmitted sexually. Infections that are sexually transmitted diseases (STDs) can be spread by various types of heterosexual and homosexual contact, both genital and nongenital.

Assessment

History

The history for vaginal and pelvic infections focuses on the onset, characteristics, and progression of symptoms. If symptoms began recently, this signifies an acute (new) infection in contrast to a chronic condition with long-standing symptoms. The duration of symptoms is important as an indication of potential damage to reproductive structures. The character of the discharge provides clues about the involved microorganism (Table 50-1). Serous or blood-tinged discharge suggests a foreign object or possible cervical lesion. The amount of discharge is ascertained, using the woman's estimate of slight, moderate, or copious. If the woman wears a pad or tampon, this usually indicates heavier discharge. A foul-smelling odor to the discharge might indicate a particular pathogen or presence of a foreign body. Some women can identify changes in odor, even if not foul. Others may perceive discharge as malodorous even when the nurse finds it inoffensive.

Associated symptoms are explored during the history. The nurse should ask specifically about itching,

TABLE 50-1

Common Types of Vaginitis: Characteristics and Treatment

Type of Vaginitis	Erythema/ Itching	Discharge	Saline Mount	Potassium Hydroxide Mount	Culture/ Other	Medication/Other Treatment
Candida albicans (Monilia)	Vulva, labia, perineum, thighs Mild to severe	Mild to moderate Curdy white	Hyphae or spores Many lactobacilli	Hyphae or spores	Nickerson's grows brown or black colonies	Vaginal tablets or cream: Mycostatin, miconazole, chlordantoin
Trichomonas vaginalis	Severe vulval itching, ±erythema Petechiae of cervix and vagina	Copious Yellow-green frothy	Trichomonads Few lactobacilli Many WBCs	Negative	None	Metronidazole (Flagyl) orally or clotrimazole vaginal tablets (treat sexual partner)
Gardnerella vaginalis	Mild to moderate	Mild to moderate Homogeneous Gray, foul	Clue cells Small rods Many WBCs Few lactobacilli	Negative	Blood agar ± colonies	Metronidazole (Flagyl) orally or ampicillin orally (treat sexual partner)
Chlamydia trachomatis	None to mild	Slight to moderate, varies	Many WBCs Few lactobacilli	Negative	Pap smear with inclusion bodies *Chlamydia* culture	Erythromycin, tetracycline, or doxycycline orally (treat sexual partner)
Allergic or irritative	Mild to severe	Varied	Unremarkable	Negative	No growth	Remove source of allergy or irritation Topical steroid if severe inflammation
Foreign body	Mild or absent	Serous, purulent, fetid	Many WBCs	Negative	+specific organism if 2° infection	Remove foreign body Treat 2° infection with specific antibiotic

because it is characteristic of *Candida* (*monilia*) and *Trichomonas* infections. Vulvar irritation can be caused by any discharge that creates persistent drainage, although *Candida* is particularly implicated in severe vulvar irritation and inflammation. Abdominal or pelvic discomfort may be reported in association with endometritis and PID. The severity of pain is assessed by asking how much it interferes with daily activities, what measures are used to relieve pain, and whether the client must lie down. Patterns of pain are important; does it occur with intercourse, urination, menstruation, movement, certain foods, and so forth? Other important symptoms might include fever, nausea/vomiting, decreased appetite, constipation, and stress.

Menstrual history and current patterns are important in assessing possible pelvic infections. Recent changes in amount of flow, painful menstruation, or presence of clots could indicate endometritis or PID. Certain vaginal infections seem to become more intense following menstruation, such as *Candida* (*monilia*) vaginitis, because of increased vaginal glycogen during the premenstrual and menstrual phases of the cycle. The

last menstrual period is determined as an indication of possible pregnancy. The woman is asked when she had her last Pap smear and whether the results were normal.

A focused general health history provides useful data. The client is asked whether she has ever had a similar problem before, and if so, what was the diagnosis and treatment. The results of treatment are important; did she receive symptomatic relief and did the problem resolve? A history of recurrent vaginitis could indicate an STD that is being passed back and forth between sexual partners. Chronic illnesses or current health problems may make the client more susceptible to infections, especially diabetes, eating disorders with poor nutrition, conditions under treatment with antibiotics, and immunosuppressed conditions.

Contraceptive use can affect susceptibility to certain vaginal or pelvic infections. The intrauterine device (IUD) has been associated with increased incidence of PID, especially in women who have never been pregnant.[1] Oral contraceptives that have a strong androgenic effect and cause a relatively thin endometrium may predispose women to chlamydial infections.[2] Estrogenic

A S S E S S M E N T   T O O L

History for Vaginal and Pelvic Infections

Onset and progression of symptoms

Characteristics of symptoms
  Discharge (color, amount, odor, consistency, timing)
  Itching (severity, location, timing)
  Burning or stinging
  Dysuria
  Pain or discomfort (location, type, duration, severity)
  Fever, flulike symptoms
  Skin rash
  Nausea/vomiting
  Constipation
  Dyspareunia
  Decreased appetite

Personal habits and hygienic practices (use of perfumes, sprays, deodorants, powders, antiseptic soaps, or ointments in perineal or vaginal areas)

Self-care remedies used (douches, vaginal instillations, topical creams, teas, over-the-counter drugs)

Menstrual history
  Menarche
  Menstrual patterns
  Last menstrual period (length of flow, amount of flow, character, discomfort, usual pattern or different)
  Relation of symptoms to menstrual flow
  Use of tampons or pads; type of tampons used

Contraceptive history
  Type of current contraceptive (especially note IUD and type, if known—and diaphragm use)
  Side-effects or problems with method
  Use of condom by sexual partner(s)

Sexual history
  Number of sexual partners
  Recent change in sexual partner or new sexual contact
  Sexual patterns of sexual partner(s)
  Sexual practices (oral–genital, anal–vaginal, other)
  Known exposure to STD
  Partner with history of genital tract infection

Personal health history
  General state of health
  History of significant illness or hospitalization
  Current illness or disease, chronic disease
  Under medical treatment or taking regular medication(s)
  Health habits (smoking, alcohol and drug use, exercise, stress reduction, nutrition)
  Current stress level and ways of dealing with stress

effects of oral contraceptives may make women more prone to monilial infections and possibly more susceptible to gonorrhea if exposed. Contraceptive foams, creams, or sponges can cause irritative or allergic vaginitis in sensitive women. Some women are allergic to the rubber used in diaphragms and condoms and may develop vaginitis. Tampon use can be the cause of toxic shock syndrome (TSS), which also may be caused by a cervical cap or diaphragm left in place too long.

Personal habits and hygienic practices may be associated with vaginitis. A variety of perfumes, deodorant sprays, powders, antiseptic soaps, or ointments applied to perineal or vaginal tissue can lead to irritations and allergic reactions. Resultant inflammation or tissue damage can provide access for pathogens to establish infections. Excessive douching can upset the normal vaginal flora and reduce resistance to pathogenic organisms. Some believe that nylon panties or pantyhose or tight-fitting jeans contribute to infections by retaining perineal moisture or causing mechanical irritation.

A focused sexual history is clearly indicated for vaginal and pelvic infections. Having multiple sexual partners is one of the greatest risk factors for STD. In a sensitive and nonjudgmental way, the nurse must explore whether or not the woman has more than one sexual partner. Of course, a woman may have a single male partner, but he may have several sexual contacts unknown to her. The diagnosis of an STD in a woman who reports an exclusive sexual relationship can be quite traumatic and needs supportive nursing intervention. It is important to ascertain if the woman's male partner has a history of prior STD, because this increases the risk of PID. Sexual practices may be implicated, especially anal–vaginal penetration. Herpes infections are transmitted by oral–genital contact as well as intercourse.

The woman's level of stress is explored in the history, because sustained significant stress can alter immune responses and resistance. Sources of stress are elicited, including those at work and home, and intrapersonal conflicts or issues related to self-esteem, goals, personal growth, and others. The relationship with the woman's sexual partner may be a source of stress, especially in cases involving STD.

Physical Examination

The physical examination includes a thorough speculum and bimanual pelvic examination and examination of the abdomen to assess extrapelvic sources of symptoms. The client is instructed to void before the examination, and a clean-catch urine specimen is obtained in case urinalysis is indicated. The external genitalia and perineum are examined for erythema, swelling, lesions, and discharge. The appearance of the urethra and Skene's and Bartholin's glands is noted, and signs of inflammation include swelling and redness. The urethra is milked for discharge, and if cysts of the glands are present, they are palpated for size, tenderness, and discharge. All discharge should be cultured for gonorrhea.

The speculum examination includes inspection of the vagina and cervix for discharge, inflammation, and lesions. The characteristics of any discharge are noted, and specimens are taken for saline or potassium hydroxide (KOH) slides, as indicated (Fig. 50-1). If there is suspicious cervical discharge (yellow, purulent) or if the history indicates exposure to gonorrhea, a gonorrhea culture is taken from the cervical os. In some clinics or offices, appropriate culture media are available for *Chlamydia trachomatis* and herpes simplex type 2. Specimens for culture are taken as history and examination findings indicate. If cervical lesions are present, or the condition of the cervix is questionable, a Pap smear is

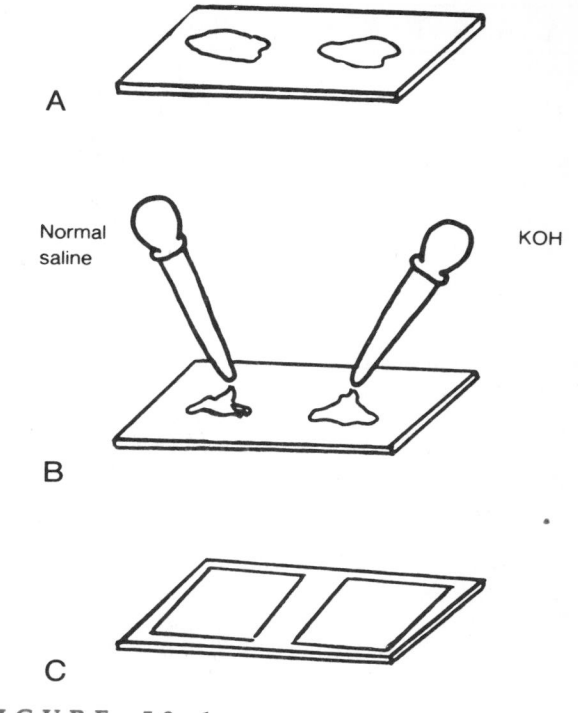

FIGURE 50-1

Preparation of wet mount of vaginal discharge for microscopic examination. *A.* Using a cotton-tipped applicator or Pap stick, place two separate drops of the vaginal discharge on a glass slide and spread thinly. *B.* Add one drop of normal saline to one specimen for microscopic examination for *Trichomonas vaginalis.* Add one drop of 10% to 20% potassium hydroxide (KOH) to the other specimen for microscopic examination for *Candida albicans.* *C.* Place separate coverslips over each specimen and blot excess moisture with a paper towel. Examine slides under high- and low-power lenses of microscope. (Nursing Services Manual, Newton, MA, Preterm Institute, 1976)

taken for cytologic evaluation. The bimanual examination follows, in which the condition of cervix, uterus, tubes, and ovaries is evaluated. A very tender cervix may indicate cervicitis or PID; tenderness of the uterus, tubes, or ovaries may indicate local infections or PID. An enlarged uterus needs further evaluation if the cause is not evident. Ovarian enlargements or adnexal fullness or masses may indicate PID or tumors, and further evaluation is required (see Chap. 48 for pelvic masses and tumors). A rectovaginal examination is usually done to rule out rectal lesions and better evaluate the rectovaginal septum and posterior vaginal wall. An abdominal examination, with superficial and deep palpation of organs and auscultation of bowel sounds if needed, should be included.

Specific findings from the physical examination and results of diagnostic tests are discussed under the appropriate type of vaginal or pelvic infection in the following sections.

ASSESSMENT TOOL

Physical Examination for Vaginal and Pelvic Infections

Pelvic examination
  Inspection of vulva and perineum for lesions, erythema, discharge, edema
  Speculum examination of vagina and cervix; note:
    Vaginal discharge (color, amount, odor, other characteristics)
    Vaginal mucosa (erythema, edema, ulcerations, lesions)
    Cervical discharge (color, amount, odor, other characteristics)
    Cervical mucosa (erythema, edema, lesions, ulcerations, ectropion, erosion, petechiae)
  Bimanual examination; note:
    Cervical tenderness, irregularity
    Uterine tenderness, enlargement, irregularity
    Adnexal tenderness, enlargement, fullness; masses of ovaries, tubes, or in cul-de-sac
    Rectovaginal examination for condition of posterior uterine wall, rectovaginal septum, cul-de-sac, uterosacral
      ligaments

Specimens
  Pap smear (cervix, herpetic lesions)
  Saline mount (*Candida, Trichomonas, Gardnerella, Chlamydia*, PID)
  KOH mount (*Candida, Gardnerella*)
  Gonorrhea culture (*Thayer-Martin*)
  Herpes simplex type 2 culture (if media and procedures available)
  Chlamydia culture (if media and procedures available)

Abdominal examination
  Superficial and deep palpation for condition of organs, tenderness, masses
  Palpation of groin lymph nodes
  Auscultation of bowel sounds

Vital signs
  Temperature
  Pulse
  Respiration
  Blood pressure

Nursing Diagnosis

The nursing diagnosis generally is related to the medical (pathophysiological) diagnosis and the client's responses to her condition and symptoms. Potential complications can be a nursing diagnosis related to most pathophysiological problems, and nursing emphasizes detecting and preventing these complications. Knowledge deficit is a common nursing diagnosis related to the pathophysiological condition, risk factors, prevention, signs and symptoms of complications, medical treatment, and self-care. Anxiety or fear may be present, especially if STD is a diagnosis. Alterations in comfort may result from pain, itching, irritation, heavy discharge, and swelling. Disturbance in self-concept is possible, related to recurrent infections or acquiring an STD with implications for self-esteem, relations with the sexual partner, body image, and life-style changes. Other potential nursing diagnoses are ineffective individual coping, noncompliance, alterations in nutrition, and sexual dysfunction.

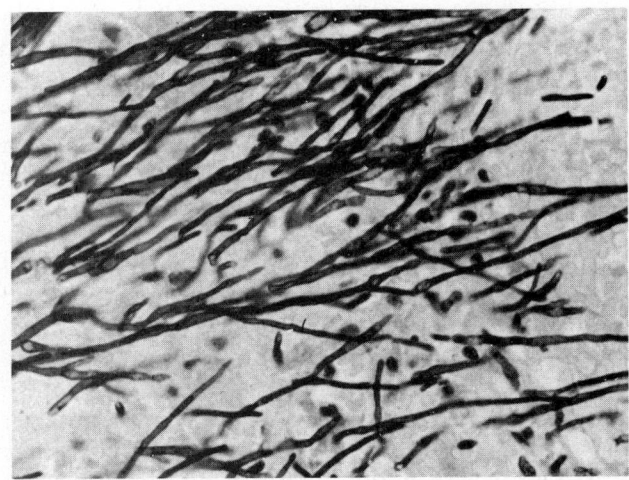

FIGURE 50-2

C. albicans growing as hyphae and pseudohyphae within infected tissue. (Monif GRG: Infectious Diseases in Obstetrics & Gynecology. Hagerstown, Harper & Row, 1974; PAS, original magnification ×320)

Nursing diagnoses for specific types of vaginal and pelvic infections are included in the following section.

Planning/Intervention

The key points in assessment, diagnosis, and nursing care are discussed for several common vaginal and pelvic infections.

Candida (Monilia) Vaginitis

This common vaginal infection is caused by the fungus *Candida albicans,* which is widely distributed in nature and often is found on the skin and mucous membranes of asymptomatic persons. It grows best in well-estrogenized vaginal tissue with a high glycogen content, thus its increased incidence during pregnancy and with higher-estrogen oral contraceptives. Women with diabetes have increased risk for *Candida* infection, because of greater tissue glucose. Women taking systemic antibiotics have a tendency to contract *Candida* vaginitis, probably as a result of suppression of normal vaginal flora and effects on *p*H and enzymes.

The discharge in *Candida* vaginitis is typically white, thick, curdy, and adherent to the cervix and vaginal walls. However, thin, milky, and more confluent whitish discharge is not uncommon. Itching is moderate to severe, especially on the vulva and perineum. The labia and vulva may be bright red, swollen, sensitive to touch, and painful during intercourse. The extent of symptoms varies, but if the labia are involved and white discharge is present, this is a good area for taking a specimen. Usually saline and KOH mounts are prepared from vaginal or labial secretions. Microscopic examination shows the hyphae and spores of *Candida albicans* (Fig. 50-2). On saline mount, the vaginal epithelial cells appear normal and there are numerous lactobacilli (normal flora) and few white blood cells (WBCs).

A common nursing diagnosis is knowledge deficit, and nursing care includes education about the causes and prevention of *Candida* vaginitis, as well as the medical treatment. Vaginal tablets or creams, such as mycostatin (Nystatin), miconazole (Monistat), and chlordantoin (Sporostacin), are prescribed for insertion twice daily for 10 to 14 days. The nurse instructs the client

---

C L I E N T   E D U C A T I O N

Preventing Vaginitis

Personal hygiene
    Wash labia and vulva with mild soap (not antiseptic) daily.
    Dry external genitals and perineum thoroughly.
    Wipe front-to-back after voiding and bowel movements.
    Wash hands before inserting tampons, diaphragm, and contraceptive creams or sponges.
    Avoid or minimize douching (once per week, use water or mild solutions).
    Avoid deodorants, perfumed sprays or lotions, powders, antiseptic soaps, perfumed toilet paper.
    Change tampons and pads every 1 to 4 hours, depending upon flow.
    Avoid using superabsorbent tampons, or use only during heaviest flow.
    Wear cotton underclothing; avoid tight-fitting clothing in genital area.
Sexual practices
    Limit the number of sexual partners or have one partner.
    Ask or check sexual partner for symptoms (penile discharge, lesions, dysuria); avoid sex or use condom with
        spermicide if present.
    Know the sexual partner (history of genital infections or STD, other sexual contacts).
    Avoid intercourse when you have symptoms (increased discharge, itching or burning, lesions, pain).
    Avoid oral–genital contact if vulvar or mouth lesions are present in either partner.
    Avoid anal–vaginal penetration or use different condoms for each.
General health status
    Eat well-balanced, nutritious meals and avoid less-healthful foods (sweets, red meats, salty foods, saturated
        fats).
    Get regular exercise.
    Get enough sleep (6–8 hours per night).
    Find time each week for personal interests and hobbies.
    Recognize sources of stress at home and work, and find methods to reduce stress (progressive relaxation, auto-
        genic training, yoga, biofeedback, meditation, imagery, quiet time).
    Maintain satisfying relationships and friendship networks.

on insertion and can advise wearing a minipad during the day to absorb the drainage these medicines cause. A tampon should not be used because it will absorb the medication. Douching should be avoided, and intercourse is preferably stopped during the course of treatment, or a condom is used. If vulvar inflammation and itching are problems, antifungal or steroidal creams can be applied for several days. If *Candida* vaginitis is recurrent, the male partner should be examined and skin scrapings taken if inflammation is found at the base of the penis or perineum; antifungal treatment is prescribed if indicated.

Candidal infections often are not sexually transmitted, although they may be. Associated risk factors (diabetes, pregnancy, antibiotics) are assessed, and appropriate teaching is provided. Factors the woman can associate with the infection, such as douching, perfumed or medicated sprays/soaps, or nylon underclothes,

should be avoided. Stress and decreased resistance may contribute to *Candida* vaginitis, and the nurse explores sources of stress and methods of stress reduction (see Preventing Vaginitis). Inserting yogurt or buttermilk into the vagina has been used for self-treatment or prevention, on the premise that this will assist growth of normal flora (lactobacilli). Results with this approach are variable[3] (see Natural Remedies for Vaginitis).

Trichomonas Vaginalis

A unicellular protozoan flagellate, *Trichomonas vaginalis* is nearly always transmitted through sexual intercourse. In women, it usually infects the vagina and Skene's ducts; in men, it can be present in the lower genitourinary tract and may cause prostatitis. The vaginal discharge in *Trichomonas* vaginitis is typically yellow green,

---

C L I E N T   E D U C A T I O N

Natural Remedies for Vaginitis

Women are increasingly interested in self-care that includes preventing or minimizing vaginitis and they are using natural remedies for therapy. The following are some natural remedies that have been suggested or used by women. Little research supports these approaches, and effectiveness is variably reported. However, such approaches are compatible with the life-style and philosophy of growing numbers of women.

Candida (Monilia) vaginitis

Douche with white vinegar, 1 tablespoon/pint water, one to two times each day for 1 week.

Douche with acidophilus culture, 2 tablespoons/pint water, one to two times each day for 1 week.

Apply acidophilus yogurt to labia, to vulva, or intravaginally every 2 to 3 hours, as needed, for relief of itching and burning.

Take sitz baths every 2 to 4 hours, as needed, for relief of itching, burning, and swelling of labia and vulva.

Make tea of equal parts of uva ursi, parsley root, dandelion root, and burdock root; use 1 ounce of herbs per pint of water in decoction. Drink ½ to 1 cup tea every 2 hours.

Douche with solution of equal parts of goldenseal, chaparral, comfrey root, and kava kava; use 1 ounce of herbs per pint water, simmer gently for 30 minutes, strain, cool, and add 1 tbsp vinegar per pint. Douche once daily for 1 to 3 days.

Trichomonas vaginitis

Douche with solution of equal parts of chaparral and chamomile; use 1 ounce of herbs per pint water, steep for 20 minutes, strain, and cool. Douche two to three times each day for 1 or 2 weeks.

*Combine powders of *Echinacea*, goldenseal, chaparral, and squawvine in equal parts; fill gelatin capsules. Take 2 capsules three times each day before meals; also take 1 teaspoon garlic oil with meals.

Bacterial vaginitis

Douche with white vinegar, 1 tablespoon per pint water, once each day for 1 week.

Douche with solution of 1 teaspoon goldenseal and 1 clove minced garlic steeped in 1 quart boiling water, strained and cooled. Use daily for 1 week.

Insert Betadine gel or solution intravaginally two times each day for 1 week.

* For use in bacterial vaginitis also.

frothy or bubbly, and copious and has a strong, foul odor. The cervix and upper vagina often have tiny petechiae due to inflammation. With severe inflammation, the vaginal wall, cervix, and vulva may be edematous and erythematous. Small, irregular erosions may be found on the labia. Moderate to severe itching is common, and some women have dysuria or dyspareunia secondary to inflammation. Trichomonal infections can be milder, with great variation in symptoms. Discharge can be thin, slight, whitish yellow, and without the typical foul odor.

Routine Pap smears not infrequently indicate the presence of trichomonads. Even in the absence of cytologic changes (inflammation, atypia), treatment is needed because trichomonads are vaginal pathogens and may have recently colonized the vagina. During pelvic examination, a saline mount is taken and examined microscopically as soon as possible. Motile trichomonads are usually seen; under high power these organisms are about two to three times the size of WBCs and their flagella can be seen moving. Lactobacilli are usually absent, many WBCs are present, and a range of vaginal intermediate and parabasal epithelial cells are present (Fig. 50-3).

Medical treatment for *Trichomonas* vaginitis consists of metronidazole (Flagyl), 2 g orally in a single dose. The client's sexual partner also should be treated simultaneously with the same dosage. They are cautioned

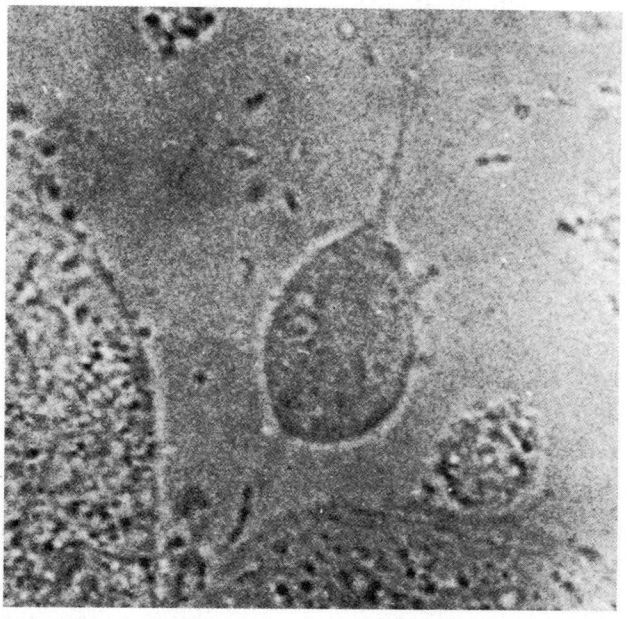

FIGURE 50-3

Characteristic configuration of a trichomonad seen in wet smear at high-power magnification (Monif GRG: Infectious Diseases in Obstetrics & Gynecology. Hagerstown, Harper & Row, 1974)

CLIENT EDUCATION

Preventing Transmission of STD

Limit the number of sexual partners; preferably have only one.

Abstain from sexual contact whenever genital or oral lesions are present.

Use condoms and spermicides whenever with new partner, if partner is not well known, or if partner has other sexual contacts.

Observe sexual partner for lesions or discharge, or ask about symptoms, and be prepared to say no if these are present.

Be responsible with sexual partner(s): advise about history of STD and avoid contact if symptoms/signs are present.

---

to avoid alcohol for 48 hours, because in combination with metronidazole it may cause abdominal cramps, nausea, vomiting, headaches, and flushing. Lactating women can be treated with 2 g metronidazole, but should take the baby off the breast for 24 hours after therapy. Metronidazole is contraindicated during the first trimester of pregnancy and preferably should be avoided throughout. Clotrimazole (Gyne-Lotrimin), 100-mg vaginal tablets at bedtime for 7 days, can provide symptomatic relief for pregnant women[4a] (see also Chap. 37).

A common nursing diagnosis is knowledge deficit related to cause, prevention, and treatment of *Trichomonas* vaginitis. Nursing care includes education about sexual transmission and counseling about sexual practices, emphasizing limiting the number of partners and using condoms in risky situations (see Preventing Transmission of STD). The client needs to understand that reinfection is a common problem and her sexual partner(s) must receive treatment if she is to continue free of infection. Careful instruction about taking metronidazole (usually 8 tablets taken in close succession, with several large glasses of water) and avoiding alcohol is given.

Alterations in comfort may be present owing to local vulvar inflammation. This can be treated with sitz baths or steroid creams. If intercourse is painful owing to inflammation, it should be avoided for 2 to 3 days to permit healing. Dysuria related to urethral inflammation responds to these treatments also. Anxiety/fear about the consequences of *Trichomonas* infections for fertility may be present; the nurse provides reassurance that it is a local vaginal infection and does not ascend into the endometrial cavity or tubes. Disturbance in self-concept is possible, because the woman may need to adjust her life-style or carefully examine her sexual relationship(s) if future episodes of *Trichomonas* vaginitis are to be avoided. She may be angry at her partner for transmitting an STD, especially if this reveals previously unknown additional sexual contacts, or she may feel ashamed and unclean for having an STD. The nurse provides an accepting climate for expression of feelings, corrects misunderstandings, offers information as needed, and reinforces health-promoting behaviors.

Gardnerella Vaginalis

Gardnerella vaginalis is a short, gram-negative rod (coccobacillus) that is transmitted sexually and has a 10-day incubation period. The organism is a surface parasite and does not invade deeper tissue; thus, it does not produce symptoms of inflammation such as itching, burning, dysuria, or dyspareunia. The vaginal discharge is typically thin, gray white, and homogeneous; it is infrequently frothy. There is a fishy odor to the discharge, particularly after sexual intercourse. In many instances, the symptoms are minimal and women are uncertain whether they should be concerned about having a vaginal infection. A common presentation might be a woman with variable slight increase in vaginal discharge that has a bad odor. Many women with *Gardnerella* infections have no symptoms.

Few changes are noted on pelvic examination. If discharge is typical, this assists diagnosis. Adding 10% KOH to the discharge may produce an evanescent fishy odor owing to production of two malodorous amines, putrescine and cadaverine.[4b] A saline mount is taken and examined microscopically. Diagnosis is made when clue cells are present; these are vaginal epithelial cells that appear stippled owing to growth of *Gardnerella* organisms. The adherence of these bacteria to epithelial cells can produce an indefinite or irregular cell margin. Lactobacilli usually are absent; vaginal epithelial cells are mature forms.

Medical treatment is with metronidazole (Flagyl), 500 mg orally twice a day for 7 days. Ampicillin, 500 mg orally four times a day for 7 days, is an alternate treatment, recommended for use during pregnancy. When metronidazole is used, advice is given about avoiding alcohol for 48 hours. The woman's sexual partner(s) should also be treated simultaneously with the above dosage of metronidazole. Up to 90% of male sexual partners tend to have some symptoms, and *Gardnerella* is a common cause of urethritis in men.[4c]

Knowledge deficit related to cause, prevention, and treatment of *Gardnerella* vaginitis is common, and nursing care includes education as described above. Since this is an STD, disturbance in self-concept may be present and nursing care follows the guidelines discussed under the section on *Trichomonas* vaginitis. Anxiety/fear related to implications for fertility can be responded to by reassurance and education about pathogenetic properties of *Gardnerella vaginalis*, which generally are confined to local vaginal effects.

Chlamydia Trachomatis

Chlamydial genital infections are widespread among both men and women, and the Centers for Disease Control state that it is the most prevalent STD in the United States.[5] *Chlamydia* is an obligate intracellular organism and must invade a host cell to replicate; the genital types invade columnar or transitional epithelium. The organism is fastidious and is difficult to culture; it must be sent to a reference laboratory in an appropriate culture medium. The prevalence of chlamydial infections increases with greater numbers of sexual partners.

Women may have very few or no signs and symptoms of chlamydial infections. No typical vaginal discharge has been found; however, the cervix seems the main target for colonization. Increased secretion of cervical mucus causes a discharge that can be clear or cloudy. Presence of cervical inflammation or erosion or increased friability should increase suspicion of chlamydia. The diagnosis of chlamydial cervicitis is usually one of exclusion. Gonorrheal cervicitis can be ruled out with a culture, and herpetic cervicitis can be excluded by Pap smear. Pap smear results can aid diagnosis of chlamydial cervicitis by the presence of intracytoplasmic inclusion bodies (if the organism is in the appropriate phase of replication).[4d] Cultures are increasingly used to diagnose chlamydia. Cervical discharge or small biopsy specimens are placed in a holding medium, then sent to a reference laboratory for growth on idoxuridine-treated McCoy cells.

Women with vaginal or cervical discharge that cannot be identified as due to another common pathogen should be asked whether their sexual partner has had urethritis recently. About 40% of men with nongonococcal urethritis are infected with chlamydia.[6] The incubation period is 1 to 3 weeks, so a history of recent sexual encounters is important. It is recommended that female sexual partners of men with nongonococcal urethritis be treated, even if they are asymptomatic. Longstanding chlamydial infections in women can produce chronic abdominal pain, intermenstrual bleeding or spotting, and low-grade fever.

Chlamydial infections are significant because the organism does ascend through the endometrial cavity to the tubes and ovaries and can led to PID, salpingitis, and pelvic abscesses. Chlamydiae have a predilection for destroying the ciliated epithelium of the tube, and infertility is a common consequence (see the section on PID).

Medical treatment is with tetracycline, 500 mg orally four times a day for 7 days, erythromycin, 500 mg orally four times a day for 7 days, or doxycycline (Vibramycin), 100 mg orally twice daily for 7 days. The client's sexual partner(s) should be treated simultaneously with the same medications. During pregnancy, erythromycin is used (see Chap. 37).

Knowledge deficit related to the cause, prevention, and treatment of chlamydial infections is common. Nursing care involves education about transmission and counseling about sexual practices (see Some Questions and Answers About *Chlamydia*). Of importance are the possible consequences for serious pelvic infections and infertility. Anxiety/fear about infertility resulting from chlamydial infections is realistic, and the nurse provides opportunity for expression of fears and feelings. If the infection is confined to the cervix, there is less likelihood of tubal damage, and appropriate reassurance can be provided. Compliance with the drug regimen by both partners reduces the risk of complications, and the nurse can stress this.

Disturbances in self-concept may be present and treated as described in the section on *Trichomonas* infections. If risk to fertility is significant to the woman, her identity related to reproductive capacity can be threatened. Anger and feelings of betrayal by her sexual partner may be strong. If a significant conflict develops, the couple may need therapy. Nursing care can include short-term couple therapy, if the nurse has the background and skills, or a referral can be made. Life-style changes often are required if the woman is to avoid future exposure to chlamydial infections. Changes in sexual behaviors, with associated feelings about self-worth and social acceptance, may require several counseling sessions to work out.

Neisseria Gonorrhoeae

Gonorrhea infection is a common cause of cervical discharge in women and urethral discharge in men. Gonorrhea is an STD caused by a gram-negative intracellular diplococcus, with a 3- to 10-day incubation period. The gonococcus can infect Bartholin's and Skene's glands, the cervix, and the fallopian tubes. Lower genital tract infections in women are asymptomatic in 85% of the cases; about 6% of men are asymptomatic.[4] The organism infects only columnar and transitional epithelium; thus, the vagina itself is not affected except in prepubertal girls and occasionally postmenopausal women.

Signs and symptoms of lower genital tract infection in women usually are minimal. Vaginal discharge if present is often yellow white with no offensive odor. Slight dysuria may occur if Skene's glands are involved, and itching is rare. If Bartholin's glands are infected, the gland may be enlarged, tender, and reddened. During pelvic examination, the urethra is milked and the glands are palpated; any discharge is cultured for gonorrhea. The cervix may have yellow white discharge, which should be cultured. On bimanual examination, the cervix may be tender to movement. With upper genital tract involvement, the uterus and adnex may be tender, or tubal enlargements or abscesses may be felt (see the section on PID).

Gram stains are not useful for diagnosing gonorrhea in women. Gonorrhea cultures are taken on Thayer-Martin medium and placed in a 10% carbon dioxide atmosphere. Depending upon sexual practices, cultures may be taken from the throat or rectum. About 10% of women with genital gonorrhea harbor the organism in the pharynx and are usually asymptomatic.

Medical treatment for gonorrhea is 1 g probenecid orally followed by 4.8 million units aqueous procaine penicillin G intramuscularly (usually in a divided dose, half in each buttock). Alternately, 1 g probenecid can be followed by 3.5 g ampicillin or 3.0 g of amoxicillin orally in one dose. Ceftriaxone 250 mg IM (no probenecid) is another accepted drug. Those with penicillin allergy are treated with tetracycline, 500 mg orally four times a day for 7 days or doxycycline 100 mg orally twice daily for 7 days. When the infecting organism is resistant to penicillin, spectinomycin (Trobicin), 2 g intramuscularly, is the treatment of choice. All sexual contacts should be identified and treated, even if asymptomatic. A reculture for gonorrhea should be done 1 week after therapy. Women with initial positive gonorrhea cultures are treated for chlamydial infection at the same time in some clinics, because of the high incidence of comorbidity.

Knowledge deficit related to the cause, prevention, and treatment of gonorrhea is common, with nursing care focusing on education and counseling as previously described. Gonorrhea is well known as an STD, and appropriate nursing diagnoses might be anxiety/fear related to effects on fertility; or disturbance in self-concept related to self-esteem, relations with sexual partner, body image, and life-style changes. The same types of nursing care described in the section on chlamydial infections apply for gonorrhea infections. Gonorrhea is a reportable communicable disease, and concerns about social exposure, attitudes, and reactions of others must be discussed with the client.

Genital Herpes

Herpes simplex virus (HSV) is transmitted by close contact between infected and noninfected skin surfaces. There are two common types, HSV type 1 and HSV type 2. Morphologically and immunologically these two strains can be differentiated, but there is some cross-immunity between them. HSV-1 generally infects ectodermal tissues above the umbilicus, and HSV-2 infects those below the umbilicus, but occasionally crossover infections occur. The virus enters the body through a break in the skin or mucous membranes and requires contact from an infected area. Since the virus does not travel by air, it cannot survive on inanimate objects. HSV-2 is transmitted primarily by sexual contact, al-

CLIENT EDUCATION

Some Questions and Answers About Chlamydia

What is Chlamydia?

Chlamydia (pronounced *kla-mid-e-uh*) is a widespread sexually transmitted microorganism that is causing a national epidemic. An estimated 3 million Americans get chlamydial infections each year, making it three times more common than gonorrhea and 30 times more common than syphilis. Chlamydia may infect both men and women and are thought to be a major cause of nongonococcal urethritis, cervicitis, and various pelvic infections.

How are Chlamydial Infections Transmitted?

In the United States, chlamydial infections are most often spread by direct sexual contact. Babies can get chlamydiae during birth if the mother has this infection.

How Would I Know if I had a Chlamydial Infection?

Symptoms of chlamydial infections may appear within 2 weeks to a month after exposure to someone with the infection. Symptoms are often similar to those of gonorrhea and may include:

For Men:

- discharge from the penis or burning when urinating
- burning and itching around the opening of the penis
- symptoms that are present early in the day and go away, but then come back
- many men will have no noticeable symptoms, or symptoms so mild that they go unnoticed

For Women:

- any vaginal itching or discharge may be a sign of infection
- chronic abdominal pain, bleeding between menstrual periods, and low-grade fever may be later symptoms of infection
- because the infection is internal, 80% of women will have no noticeable symptoms until complications set in

The only way many people learn that they may have a chlamydial infection is if a responsible partner has told them they have been exposed. The only *sure* way to know is to get a diagnosis from a doctor.

Can Chlamydial Infections Be Dangerous?

Yes. If left untreated, they can cause:

In Men and Women:

- a painful infection that can require hospitalization
- permanent damage to the reproductive organs
- the inability to have children

(continued)

though autoinoculation can occur (*e.g.*, from one's lip to finger to genitalia). HSV-1 can be transmitted easily through innocent contact, such as hugging and familial kissing.

When a person becomes infected with HSV, the virus enters the nervous system and lives in a dormant state in the trigeminal or sacral ganglia. Renewed outbreaks, either upper or lower body, can be triggered by sunlight, local trauma, stress, and premenstrual hormone changes. HSV-2 eruptions can be triggered by sexual intercourse. The Centers for Disease Control estimate that 9% to 35% of the general population have been exposed to HSV-2, and genital infections are reported in about 2% to 8% of clients seen in venereal disease clinics and private gynecologists' offices. There

are an estimated 300,000 new cases of genital herpes each year.[7]

Assessment

Signs and symptoms of genital herpes differ between primary and recurrent infections. First infections usually have the most severe symptoms, and recurrent infections may have a wide range of symptoms and severity. There are five characteristic stages of herpes infection, with associated signs/symptoms. The incubation period for HSV is 7 days. The *primary stage* begins with appearance of small vesicles on the vulva or vagina, which rupture 2 or 3 days later and form painful ulcers with an erythematous base. Lesions may occur on the labia,

CLIENT EDUCATION (continued)

In Women:
- complications in pregnancy that can result in the death of the unborn baby and, occasionally, the mother

In Babies:
- eye, ear, and lung infections—and death

How Are Chlamydial Infections Diagnosed?

Tests that give accurate, quick results are now available to diagnose chlamydial infections. These tests can be taken even when there are no symptoms. They are not painful.

How Are Chlamydial Infections Treated?

Chlamydial infections can be treated with several different drugs. Because it is often present with other venereal diseases, such as gonorrhea, your doctor may prescribe a drug that can cure a number of infections at the same time.

It is important to follow instructions carefully, take *all* of the medication, and return to the doctor's office for a follow-up examination.

Your partner(s) should be seen by a doctor (even if there are no symptoms) in order to prevent reinfection and complications.

Avoid sex until treatment is completed and your partner(s) have been checked by a physician.

How Can I Prevent Getting a Chlamydial Infection?

Guidelines for preventing chlamydial infections are the same as for preventing other sexually transmissible diseases (VD).

Know your partner. You get VD from someone who is infected. If neither you nor your partner has a disease, neither of you will be exposed.

Limit the number of partners. Your risk of getting a disease increases as your number of sexual partners increases.

Use condoms. *Properly* used, they provide good (though not perfect) protection.

If you do get an infection or suspect that you have been exposed, see a doctor right away. Early diagnosis and treatment are necessary to avoid complications and the spread of disease.

If you or your partner have other sexual contacts, you should get regular checkups. Be sure to ask your doctor to test for *Chlamydia*.

For more information on chlamydial infections or other venereal diseases:

Contact your local health department, VD clinic, or private physician

Call the VD National Hotline for information or referral; it's toll free, (800) 227-8922 (in California, (800) 982-5883)

perineum, perianal skin, or vaginal or cervical mucosa (Fig. 50-4). The inguinal nodes frequently become enlarged, and the woman may have fever (up to 40°C), headaches, muscle aches, and malaise. Severe dysuria is common, because of urethral or bladder infection. Eventually the ulcers crust over and heal, leaving no scars. Primary lesions may take from 3 to 6 weeks to heal completely. Ulcers on mucosal surfaces may become macerated and heal more slowly.

The *latent stage* begins as the ulcers heal. The virus travels into the nerve sheath and into the dorsal root ganglia, where it stays in a dormant state for weeks to years. During this time, it is noninfectious, since it is not replicating. Not all people with primary herpes infections will have recurrences. The *stage of shedding* can occur without the person being aware that anything is happening. The virus replicates within the ganglion and sheds without symptoms in the secretions of the cervix and urethra and the semen. No lesions occur during this time of silent shedding. The person is infectious, however, and can transmit HSV-2 to sexual partners. Because there are no symptoms and no lesions, it is impossible to identify risk except by history of genital herpes infection.

The *recurrent herpes stage* begins when the herpes virus reactivates and migrates down the nerve fibers to areas where the primary infection occurred. Some people can tell when an eruption is about to take place, because they feel tingling or burning sensations in the affected areas. Soon tiny vesicles appear, which progress

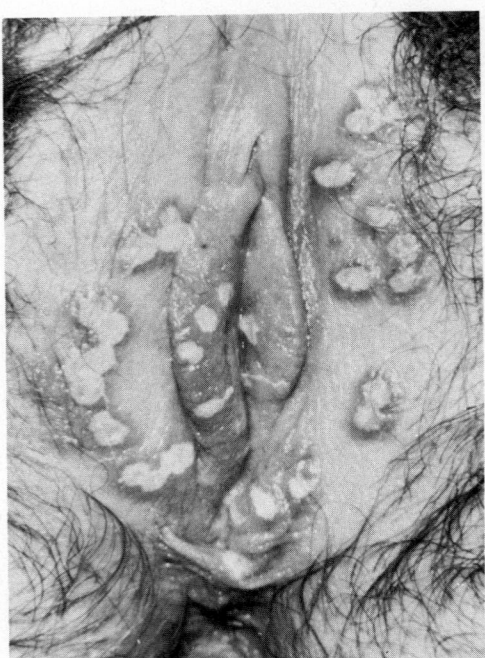

FIGURE 50-4

Primary herpes genitalis. Multiple ulcerated lesions are surrounded by red halos. (Gardner HL, Kaufman RH: Benign Diseases of the Vulva and Vagina. Boston, CK Hall, 1981)

to ulcers with an erythematous base in 1 to 2 days. Crusting and resolution of lesions usually take about 7 to 10 days. Pain with recurrent herpes is less severe, although this varies widely. Associated symptoms of fever, head and muscle aches, malaise, and dysuria usually are mild if present at all.

There are few immediate complications of herpes, which resolves completely without scarring unless there is secondary bacterial infection. The *dissemination stage* is rare in healthy children and adults. However, in immunocompromised adults or children, and in the fetus and neonate, disseminated herpes infection can be serious and life-threatening (see Chap. 37). Women with a history of genital herpes may have higher risk for cervical carcinoma and should have annual Pap smears to detect dysplasia or cervical intraepithelial neoplasia (see Chap. 48).

Diagnosis. Diagnosis of genital herpes usually is made by observation of herpetic lesions and a typical symptom history. If vesicles are present, they can be opened and a saline-soaked applicator rolled over the base. Material on the applicator is placed on a slide, and a Pap smear is made that may show multinucleated giant cells with intranuclear inclusion bodies. Antibody studies can also be useful if blood is drawn during the acute phase and again 3 to 4 weeks later in the convalescent phase. Antibody titers of the two specimens

are compared and can indicate primary or secondary infection and differentiate HSV-1 from HSV-2. Cultures for herpesvirus can be taken from the cervix or genitals but require media and techniques usually not available in primary-care clinics.

Treatment

There is no curative treatment for genital herpes. Symptomatic relief can be obtained with viscous lidocaine 2% (Xylocaine) applied locally as an anesthetic. Analgesics may provide some pain relief and help with fever, malaise, headaches, and muscle aches. Acyclovir ointment 5% (Zovirax) shortens the duration of symptoms and the time of viral shedding, and is useful in management of active phases. The ointment is applied to cover all lesions every 3 hours up to six times per day, for about 7 days or until lesions have healed. It does not prevent recurrent infection nor reduce communicability.[8]

Alterations in comfort (pain) are a frequent nursing diagnosis for both primary and secondary infections. Nursing care includes teaching the client about prescribed medications for pain relief (lidocaine, analgesics, acyclovir) and proper use. Additional measures may be advised such as sitz baths three to four times per day, and using petroleum jelly to coat lesions that come in contact with urine. The lesions should be kept clean and dry. Washing with germicidal soap and drying carefully and wearing cotton underwear can promote healing. Intercourse should be avoided as long as lesions are present, both for comfort and to avoid transmitting the infection.

Nursing Diagnosis and Planning/Intervention

Knowledge deficit related to cause, prevention, transmission, and treatment of herpes is a likely nursing diagnosis. In addition, misinformation and myths may add confusion, since genital herpes has received extensive media publicity in recent years. The nurse can provide accurate information about transmission and about risks related to cancer and pregnancy. The client needs to understand how and when the virus can be transferred to a sexual partner. Since there can be silent shedding, avoiding contact while lesions are present cannot guarantee that the partner will not be infected. The client can be assisted to identify situations in which recurrences happen and can avoid or minimize these. Stress and febrile illness can be reduced as much as possible through good general health practices and specific stress reduction techniques.

Disturbance in self-concept may commonly occur, because of the implications of genital herpes for sexual life-style and reproduction. Social attitudes and media exposure have made genital herpes stigmatic,[9] and people with herpes often feel they are "damaged goods." They fear rejection by current and potential sexual partners and feel untouchable during active phases when lesions are present. Some people react with denial and may undergo a period of increased sexual activity during which they may infect others. Others direct their anger inward, feeling worthless and depressed. Blaming the sexual partner can lead to serious interpersonal conflict and may destroy the relationship. These changes in body image, self-esteem, sexual identity, and ego integrity may cause various maladaptive behaviors, leading to a nursing diagnosis of inadequate individual coping. Severe depression, overdependence, regression, avoiding responsibilities, and acting out are examples of maladaptive behaviors.

Nursing care for these types of problems begins with establishing open communication and trust. The nurse must acknowledge and accept the client's feelings of anger, denial, displacement, depression, and so forth. Empathetic listening does much to assist clients through this phase. Helping the client identify coping mechanisms she is using and which work best can aid progress toward more adaptive behaviors. Counseling about lifestyle changes, sexual practices, and ways to minimize or prevent herpes recurrences is undertaken. Without being judgmental, the nurse discusses the association of herpes and other STDs with multiple sexual partners. Taking responsibility to be sure partners do not have lesions and avoiding sex when the client has lesions are ways to prevent spread. Honesty in sexual relations is a sensitive topic, but must be discussed. New partners should be informed of the client's history of herpes.

Preventing or minimizing recurrences is very important to the women with herpes. Since stress is a major precipitator of outbreaks, the client needs assistance exploring her sources of stress and finding ways to reduce stress, such as yoga, meditation, biofeedback, hypnosis, autogenic training, and imagery. Relationships that are stressful need attention; perhaps couple or family counseling is indicated. Dealing effectively with stress at work is crucial, and the nurse may teach assertion, conflict resolution, direct communication, time management, or other techniques. Some women find herpes support groups helpful. Talking with others who have the same problem can put genital herpes in a more reasonable perspective. The woman can learn to live with genital herpes and have a satisfying sexual relationship.

Pelvic Inflammatory Disease

Infections that primarily involve the fallopian tubes leading to salpingitis or abscess formation are called pelvic inflammatory disease (PID). Other structures that could be involved include the endometrium, ovaries, cul-de-sac, and pelvic peritoneum. There has been a dramatic increase in PID over the past few decades,

with an estimated 1 million cases per year in the United States.[4f] About 1% of all women of childbearing age will contract PID per year, but among teenagers the incidence is 2%. The major consequence of PID is infertility due to postinfectious tubal damage. About one third of female infertility is attributed to PID, and infertility due to PID has doubled in the past 20 years. Infertility is directly related to the number of episodes of salpingitis; one acute episode will render 11.4% of women infertile; two episodes, 23.1%; and after three episodes, 54.3%.[10] Other sequelae of PID include increased risk of ectopic pregnancy and chronic pelvic pain.

Risk factors for PID are related to changing sexual practices and contraceptive use. Teenage women have twice the risk for contracting PID than women in their 20s. Both increased exposure and increased susceptibility may be involved. Younger women may be less likely to have specific antibodies against *Chlamydia* and gonorrhea. Girls 15 years old who are having intercourse are twice as likely to have four or more partners in a year than their 18-year-old counterparts. About 75% of the cases of PID occur in women under age 20. The risk of acute PID is about 4% higher among IUD users than nonusers. However, nulligravid IUD users have a seven to ten times greater chance of developing PID than control groups of women using other contraceptive methods.[1] Some disagreement exists concerning the mechanisms by which IUDs increase risk of PID. Ascent of bacteria aided by the IUD string is one hypothesis; another holds that protective effects of barrier methods and oral contraceptives against bacterial colonization are absent among IUD users.[11]

PID is recognized as a polymicrobial infection. Common organisms isolated include *Neisseria gonorrhoeae, Chlamydia trachomatis, Mycoplasma hominis, Peptostreptococcus, Peptococcus,* and *Bacteroides.* Generally these organisms are sexually transmitted; most have been found at various times as part of the vaginal flora in asymptomatic women. These same bacteria frequently are found in seminal fluid. While fertile asymptomatic men have moderate incidence of bacteriospermia, a significantly higher incidence is found in men with a history of genital tract infection, infertile marriages, and wives with pelvic infections.[1]

Less than half of all PID is due to gonorrhea alone. Chlamydial infections are increasingly found, and more than half of PID cases in women under 25 years old are due to chlamydiae. Chlamydial salpingitis is particularly dangerous for a woman's fertility, because the symptoms are mild and the organism destroys tubal epithelium very early in the disease. Culturing the cervix is not a reliable way to determine organisms responsible for salpingitis. The results of cervical cultures are different from those obtained by culdocentesis or laparoscopy.[12] The majority of women with PID have mixed bacterial infections from the beginning.

The Woman with Vaginitis

Nursing Objectives

1. Accurately identify the presence of and type of vaginitis.
2. Provide appropriate nursing care and ensure compliance with the medication treatment regimen.
3. Educate about sexual transmission of vaginal infections and emphasize the importance of treating sexual partner(s) as appropriate.
4. Teach prevention of vaginitis and complications.
5. Involve the woman in self-care measures for prevention and treatment of vaginitis.

Assessment	Potential Nursing Diagnosis	Planning/Intervention	Evaluation
Signs and symptoms: Discharge Itching, burning Pain, discomfort Dysuria, dyspareunia Fever, rash Nausea/vomiting Identification of organism: *Candida, trichomonas, Gardnerella, Chlamydia,* gonorrhea, herpes	Knowledge deficit related to cause, modes of transmission, treatment, and prevention of vaginitis	Instruct on use of medication (vaginal tablets, creams, oral medications) Teach mode of transmission, usual course of illness according to type of organism Teach ways of preventing future exposure to infection, and how to avoid complications	Client describes correct medication use Client expresses understanding of mode of transmission and course of illness Client describes methods she will use to avoid future exposure and to avoid complications
	Alteration in comfort: pain, dysuria, dyspareunia	Instruct on use of sitz baths, local application of anesthetic or steroid creams, mild analgesics, petrolatum on lesions exposed to urine, and avoidance of intercourse	Client reports decrease in pain, dysuria, dyspareunia
Response to diagnosis of vaginitis (especially if sexually transmitted)	Disturbance in self-concept related to having STD, adjusting life-style, self-worth, social acceptability, body image	Establish open communication and trust, provide accepting climate for discussing feelings such as anger, depression, worthlessness, shame	Client expresses fears, feelings openly Client adjusts life-style and accepts changes in self-concept with positive self-esteem

(continued)

Assessment and Diagnosis

The classic signs and symptoms of PID include lower abdominal pain and tenderness, pain on motion of the cervix, adnexal mass or fullness, temperature above 37°C, WBCs elevated above 10,500, elevated erythrocyte sedimentation rate, an inflammatory pelvic mass on ultrasonography, and possibly WBCs and bacteria aspirated by culdocentesis. However, the classic criteria may not be present early in the disease. Only 40% of clients with laparoscopically verified PID have fever.[13]

Gonorrhea infections are much more likely to present as fever than those caused by *Chlamydia* or *Mycoplasma*. Some women will have gradually progressing dull lower abdominal pain, with dysuria and rebound tenderness. Others may experience painful intercourse, especially with deep penetration. These symptoms often begin or exacerbate shortly after a menstrual period that is heavier and longer than usual. Other signs and symptoms may include nausea/vomiting, tachycardia, diminished bowel sounds, and an acute condition within the abdomen in severe cases.

Assessment	Potential Nursing Diagnosis	Planning/Intervention	Evaluation
		Clarify misconceptions, correct myths, offer information as needed	Client takes action to reduce risk of future exposure to vaginal infections and STD
		Counsel on life-style changes to reduce future risk of vaginal infections and spreading STD	
		Reinforce health-promoting behavior	
Risk to future fertility (especially chlamydial and gonorrheal infections)	Disturbance in self-concept related to possible reduced reproductive capacity	Provide accepting climate, empathy	Client expresses fears, feelings openly
		Discuss risk for tubal damage according to stage of infection	Client expresses realistic understanding of risk for tubal damage
		Provide appropriate reassurance	
		Communicate accepting attitude and validate feelings of potential loss	
Impact of diagnosis (especially if STD) on relationship with sexual partner and coping ability	Ineffective individual coping related to implications of STD for relationship, poor self-esteem, negative self-attitudes, inappropriate defense mechanisms	Communicate accepting attitude	Client expresses feelings and discusses behaviors openly
		Acknowledge and accept client's feelings and behaviors	
		Assist client to identify coping mechanisms she is using, and which work best or do not work well	Client recognizes effective and ineffective methods of coping and is able to learn/discover other approaches that enable better coping
		Assist client to find other ways of coping that are more effective; reinforce current approaches that work well	
Expression of conflict or difficulty in sexual relationship	Sexual dysfunction related to pain, anger, guilt, fear, or altered self-concept	Counsel on sexual and interpersonal relationship, correct misinformation, refer to psychotherapy or sexual therapy for more complex problems	Client reports sexual dysfunction resolves or improves
			Couple seek appropriate therapy if needed

A saline mount obtained from the endocervix usually shows a large amount of WBCs and coccoid bacteria (not lactobacilli). A culture for gonorrhea should be taken, and a *Chlamydia* culture if possible. When there is fullness or a mass in the cul-de-sac, a culdocentesis is done, which often reveals increased WBCs and bacteria. A WBC count shows leukocytosis in about 66% of cases.[11]

Diagnosis of PID may be made clinically (based on signs/symptoms) or by laparoscopy, culdocentesis, or ultrasonography. Clients with PID may present a clinical picture ranging from mild lower abdominal pain to frank peritonitis and sepsis. In mild PID, the clinical diagnosis is correct in about 65% of cases, when correlated with laparoscopy. Inflammatory adnexal masses can be demonstrated by ultrasonography in 65% of mild and 95% of severe PID cases. Women with mild cases of PID are managed on an ambulatory basis, but women with severe cases require hospitalization. The decision to admit the client to the hospital is based on these criteria: (1) questionable diagnosis, (2) nausea/vomiting making oral medication impossible, (3) presence of an

---

Signs and Symptoms of PID

Fever (temperature >37°C; present in 40%–50% of cases)

Pelvic or lower abdominal pain and tenderness (present in 96% of cases)—dull and subacute at onset, progressing to severe, diffuse pain with rebound tenderness; there may be dyspareunia or dysuria)

Leukocytosis (elevated WBCs above 10,500 present in 50%–60% of cases)

Elevated erythrocyte sedimentation rate (present in 75% of cases)

Menstrual abnormalities (usually heavier and longer than last menstrual period, and there may be increased cramping and foul smell to blood; present in 50% of cases)

Vaginal discharge prior to onset of menstrual period (nearly 100% of cases have increased WBCs and coccoid bacteria in cervical or vaginal saline mount)

Gastrointestinal signs and symptoms: nausea/vomiting, gastric distress, general abdominal tenderness, diminished bowel sounds

Tachycardia (especially if febrile or having acute pain)

Cervical tenderness on bimanual examination (present in >90% of cases)

Adnexal fullness, masses, tenderness (present in 50% of cases); tubo-ovarian abscesses are less common (present in 16% of cases)

---

adnexal mass suggestive of abscess, (4) evidence of generalized peritonitis, (5) poor response to ambulatory therapy, (6) coexisting pregnancy, (7) significant other disease, (8) fever above 38°C, and (9) presence of an IUD (this last is controversial).[4g,14]

Treatment

Medical treatment is aimed at curing the acute infection and preventing infertility and other sequelae. Since PID often is polymicrobial and chlamydiae frequently are involved, antibiotic therapy should cover *Chlamydia*. For ambulatory treatment, the Centers for Disease Control recommend a cephalosporin (cefoxitin), 2 g intramuscularly; ampicillin, 3.5 g orally; amoxicillin, 3 g orally; or aqueous procaine penicillin G, 4.8 million units intramuscularly, with probenecid, 1 g orally, to be followed by doxycycline, 100 mg orally, twice a day for 10 days.[11] The male sexual partner should be examined and cultured, because many are carriers of gonorrhea or chlamydiae. If this cannot be done, the partner should be treated with the same drug regimen as the client. All these drugs will treat most strains of gonorrhea and *Chlamydia*.

When hospitalization is necessary, intravenous antibiotic therapy with doxycycline, cefoxitin, clindamycin, tobramycin, gentamicin, or metronidazole may be used. The choice of drug depends on the presence of penicillin-resistant organisms, anaerobes in patients with pelvic abscesses, and activity against chlamydia and gonorrhea. Intravenous antibiotics are administered for at least 4 days and continued for at least 48 hours after the client becomes afebrile. Oral medications are then begun for another 10 days. The use of broad-spectrum antibiotics to treat PID has reduced the development of pelvic abscesses. Surgery is required for a small minority of clients with ruptured tubo-ovarian abscesses or pelvic abscesses that do not resolve with antibiotic therapy. When clients develop an acute condition within the abdomen, immediate surgical intervention may be indicated. Failure to respond to antibiotic regimens within 72 hours raises suspicion of pelvic abscess, and laparoscopy usually is done.

Nursing Diagnosis and Planning/Intervention

Nursing diagnosis and nursing care vary according to the cause, severity, and response to PID. Most clients have a knowledge deficit related to medical treatment and implications of PID for fertility. The nurse provides explanations of drug regimens and discusses the need to treat the sexual partner(s). Factors that increase risk of PID can be stressed. The consequences of PID for future fertility are discussed. The client's response to drug therapy and the extent of tubal involvement are important factors. The physician enters into this discussion by providing an interpretation of tubal damage and potential for recovery. Closely related is disturbance in self-concept related to potential infertility and lifestyle changes. Young women in particular may feel shame, disapproval, and rejection related to their sexual practices. The nurse provides an accepting atmosphere that values the client as a human being, while emphasizing the risk of multiple sexual partners for PID and infertility. If significant tubal damage has occurred, the woman may need to alter her sexual identity because of decreased reproductive function. She may become depressed, angry, withdrawn, or overly dependent on others, leading to ineffective individual coping. Grief may be present over loss of body functions related to childbearing. The nurse provides counseling to aid full expression of feelings, working through fears and grief, and finding more effective coping methods as a new, more positive self-concept is formed.

Alterations in comfort (pain) may result from the inflammatory process. Antibiotic therapy will help relieve pain, but other measures, such as analgesics, dry or moist heat to the abdomen, and relaxation techniques, may be needed. The nurse instructs the client in use of these therapies. Noncompliance may be a nursing diagnosis when the client fails to follow the medical drug regimen or deviates from advice about preventing future episodes of PID. The nurse seeks the reasons for noncompliance by exploring side-effects of therapy, family and environmental deterrents, knowledge deficit, health beliefs, and problems with self-esteem. When possible, these are corrected so compliance can be improved.

A fluid volume deficit may occur related to inadequate fluid intake, fatigue, pain, and fever in more severe cases of PID. Nursing care includes ensuring adequate hydration, either by intravenous fluids in the hospital or by instructing the client on fluid intake in ambulatory management. Sexual dysfunction may be present when intercourse is painful or if anger and resentment toward the sexual partner affect communication and interpersonal relations. Counseling about the process of recovery and when to anticipate comfort with intercourse is provided. Couple counseling may be needed or referral for sexual counseling if the problem is more complex.

Evaluation

Education plays a large part in outcomes for the client. She understands what is normal and abnormal in her vaginal tract, what causes infections, how they are managed, and a great deal about how to prevent infections, especially STDs. She makes life-style adjustments to facilitate health promotion. She follows up on appropriate treatment regimens if she has related problems. She not only has been able to discuss problems openly with her nurse but also is able to communicate freely with her sexual partner.

Toxic Shock Syndrome

Toxic shock syndrome (TSS) is a multisystem infectious disease caused by toxin-producing strains of *Staphylococcus aureus*. A potent exotoxin or enterotoxin is secreted and enters the bloodstream usually through microulcerations in the vaginal or cervical mucosa caused by tampons or possibly diaphragms. Other routes for entry into the circulatory system include the endometrium during menstruation or post partum, incisions, skin infections, and intravenous injections. Virtually all cases of TSS (99%) have occurred in women, 98% of whom were menstruating. Most of these women were using vaginal tampons continuously throughout menstruation.[4h]

Young women between the ages of 15 and 24 who use tampons during menstruation are at greatest risk for TSS. Those who contract TSS harbor *S. aureus* in the vagina or become infected during menses, usually aided by the presence of the tampon and menstrual secretions. About 10% to 15% of women have been found to harbor staphylococci in the vagina. About 1% to 5% of asymptomatic men have positive urethral cultures. The superabsorbent tampons are particularly implicated in TSS, because they are retained for longer amounts of time; cause drier vaginal walls, leading to abrasions; and contain more oxygen to promote bacterial growth. Any tampon can be involved, however.[15]

TSS can be a serious, life-threatening systemic disorder with acute, dramatic onset progressing rapidly to hypotensive shock and moribund state. The staphylococci toxins injure capillary endothelium, altering capillary permeability and permitting extravasation of fluid. As blood volume decreases, venous return to the heart is diminished. Tissue perfusion is impaired, resulting in hypoxia that leads to renal and central nervous system dysfunction. Tissue damage causes release of thromboplastin, which can initiate coagulation disorders such as thrombocytopenia and disseminated intravascular coagulation (DIC). Blood pressure drops, the brain is less well perfused, and shock may result, leading to arrhythmias or cardiac arrest.

Severe TSS is characterized by the abrupt onset of high fever, vomiting, and diarrhea. These may be accompanied by a sore throat, myalgia, headache, and confusion. Within 24 to 48 hours, the condition progresses to hypotension and shock. A fine, erythematous maculopapular rash develops that resembles sunburn, and the skin begins to desquamate about 10 days later. The Centers for Disease Control (CDC) have established a strict Case Definition for Toxic Shock Syndrome that requires fever, rash, multisystem involvement, hypotension, and negative cultures and serology for other diseases with similar presentations. The acute phase of TSS lasts about 4 to 5 days, and convalescence takes place over 1 to 2 weeks.

Laboratory tests usually show leukocytosis with many bands, hyponatremia, azotemia, abnormal urinary sediment, and elevated hepatic transaminases. Creatinine phosphokinase levels are greatly elevated, and myoglobinuria may occur. Some clients have severe hypocalcemia to the point of tetany. TSS must be differentiated from other infectious diseases, such as Rocky Mountain spotted fever, measles, leptospirosis, and streptococcal scarlet fever.

Treatment

Hospitalization is required for most cases of TSS, especially those with moderate to severe symptoms. Medical treatment emphasizes massive intravenous fluid replacement, intense cardiorespiratory support as needed, and antibiotic therapy aimed at penicillinase-producing

S. aureus (methicillin, oxacillin, nafcillin, cephalosporin, vancomycin, or clindamycin). In the first 12 to 24 hours, 5 to 6 liters of intravenous fluids are given to correct hypotension. After about 36 hours, extracellular fluid accumulation as a result of toxin action on capillaries may result in peripheral edema, pulmonary effusion, and ascites. Using colloid instead of crystalloid fluid replacement can minimize this problem. Depending upon serum levels, electrolytes are added to intravenous fluids. Respiratory distress often occurs, and myocarditis may manifest in advanced stages of the disease. These problems are treated as they arise using pharmacologic and mechanical cardioventilatory support.

The vagina and cervix are cultured for bacteria, and tampons are removed. Other possible sites of *S. aureus* colonization, such as burns and wounds, should be cultured and debrided, and loculated pus drained. Urine, blood, and central nervous system fluid cultures are taken as indicated. Prognosis and eventual recovery are related to severity of the disease and complications that occur. The three leading causes of mortality are respiratory failure, uncontrollable hypotension, and DIC. Although most women recover completely, some may have persistent abnormalities in intellectual function, the electrocardiogram, cerebellar function, renal function, neuromuscular function, and peripheral perfu-

sion. Infection may recur, especially with the next menstrual period, depending upon effectiveness of antibiotic therapy.

Nursing Diagnosis and Planning/Intervention

Nursing diagnosis and nursing care are based upon the extent of illness, requirements of medical treatment, and the client's responses to the disease and therapies. During the acute phase, nursing diagnoses may be alterations in tissue perfusion; ineffective breathing patterns; decreased cardiac output; impaired gas exchange; fluid volume deficit/excess; and self-care deficit. Nursing care provides support for medical therapies, such as venous and arterial monitoring devices, intravenous fluids, cardiac monitoring, urinary catheters, nasogastric tube, ventilatory procedures, and administration of medications. Potential complications must be carefully assessed, so early signs can be identified and appropriate treatment instituted. Preventive measures such as adequate ventilation (pneumonia) and repositioning/ambulation (pneumonia, clotting disorders) are nursing responsibilities. Potential for injury exists while the client is acutely ill and exhibiting confused, combative, or restless behaviors. The nurse applies restraints carefully, or continuous bedside attendance may be needed.

Alterations in comfort may be related to dehydration, fluid restriction, nasogastric tube irritation, the intravenous line, or the catheter. Nursing care includes mouth care, petrolatum salve for dry lips, lidocaine or anesthetic sprays for throat soreness, and ice chips to relieve the dry oral mucosa. Alterations in bowel and urinary elimination are gradually restored as recovery progresses. Fear or powerlessness may be felt during the acute and early convalescent phases, and the nurse assists the client to perform appropriate self-care to regain some mastery over the body, as well as encourages expression of feelings and reactions to the illness. Disturbance in self-concept as a result of the serious illness requires sensitive nursing support and counseling, especially if there is residual damage or if complications occur.

Potential for reinfection is high among these women, and nursing care is directed at prevention. The client is instructed to avoid tampons for at least 3 months or until vaginal cultures for staphylococci are negative. After that, she should use tampons only during heavy menstrual flow and change them every 1 to 3 hours. During moderate to light flow, pads should be used instead, or at least during the night, and changed every 4 to 6 hours. The nurse teaches hygiene (handwashing before changing tampons, frequent change of tampons) and advises the client to avoid superabsorbent tampons completely (see Guide for Tampon Use).

Evaluation

Prevention of TSS is of prime importance. The client observes hygienic practices and adapts her use of tampons to safety standards. This is especially important if the client has already had an experience with TSS.

Complete recovery is possible for some women, while others may have recurring infection or abnormalities in some bodily functions. Reevaluations must be made with new nursing diagnoses, care plans, and interventions.

References

1. Toth A: Alternative causes of pelvic inflammatory disease. J Reprod Med 28(10)(suppl):669–702, October 1983
2. Washington AE et al: Oral contraceptives, *Chlamydia trachomatis* infection, and pelvic inflammatory disease. JAMA 253(15):2246–2250, April 1985
3. Gorline LL, Stegbauer CC: What every nurse should know about vaginitis. J Pract Nurs 33(6):14–18, June 1983
4. Nichols DH, Evrard JR (eds): Ambulatory Gynecology. Philadelphia, Harper & Row, 1985; a 356–357, b and c 358, d 363–364, e 362–363, f 366, g 455–456, h 464–467
5. 1985 STD treatment guidelines. MMWR 34(suppl 4s): 77S–79S, 1985
6. Sexually transmitted disease: Treatment guidelines 1982. MWWR 3(suppl 2):730–746, 1982
7. Herpes genital infection. Atlanta, GA, Centers for Disease Control, PHS Pamphlet 00-2939, 00-2906, 1980
8. Marks LN: I think I may have herpes . . . what should I do? Occup Health Saf 52(4):14–17, April 1983
9. Aral SO et al: Genital herpes: Does knowledge lead to action? Am J Public Health 75(1):69–71, January 1985
10. Westrom L: Incidence, prevalence, and trends of acute pelvic inflammatory disease and its consequences in industrialized countries, part 2. Am J Obstet Gynecol 138(7):880–892, December 1980
11. Torrington J: Pelvic inflammatory disease. J Obstet Gynecol Nurs (Suppl) 14(6):21s–31s, November/December 1985
12. Sweet R et al: Use of laparoscopy to determine the microbial etiology of acute salpingitis. Am J Obstet Gynecol 134(1):68–74, May 1979
13. Droegemueller W: Pelvic inflammatory disease. Drug Ther 14:131–134, June 1984
14. Edelin KC: Evaluation of female pelvic pain, part 2. Hosp Med 19(2):37–39, February 1983
15. Wager GP: Toxic shock syndrome. Am J Obstet Gynecol 146(1):93–102, May 1983

Suggested Reading

Aral SO, Johnson RE, Zaidi AA et al: Demographic effects of sexually transmitted diseases in the 1970s: The problem could be worse. Sex Transm Dis 10:100–101, 1983

Aral SO, Mosher WD, Cates W: Self-reported pelvic inflammatory disease in the US: A common occurrence. Am J Public Health 75(10):1216–1218, 1985

Berman RL: Current perspectives in gynecology. Clin Symp 37(1):2–32, 1985

Chuang TY, Su WP, Perry HO et al: Incidence and trend of herpes progenitalis: A 15-year population study. Mayo Clin Proc 58:436–441, 1983

Corey L, Adams HG et al: Genital herpes simplex virus infections: Clinical manifestations, course, and complications. Ann Intern Med 98:958–972, 1983

Eschenbach E, Harnisch J, Holmes K: Pathogenesis of acute pelvic inflammatory disease. Am J Obstet Gynecol 128: 838, 1977

Evans C, Shapiro P: Gynecologic microsurgery. Todays OR Nurse 5(9):16–20, November 1983

Key diagnostic points in evaluating a patient with vaginitis. Hosp Med 20(8):160, 1984

Monif G: Infectious Diseases in Obstetrics and Gynecology, 2nd ed. Philadelphia, Harper & Row, 1982

Moore DE, Spadoni LR, Foy HM et al: Increased frequency of serum antibodies to *Chlamydia trachomatis* in infertility due to distal tube disease. Lancet 2:574–577, 1982

Romanowski B, Harris JRW: Sexually transmitted diseases. Clin Symp 36(1):1–32, 1984

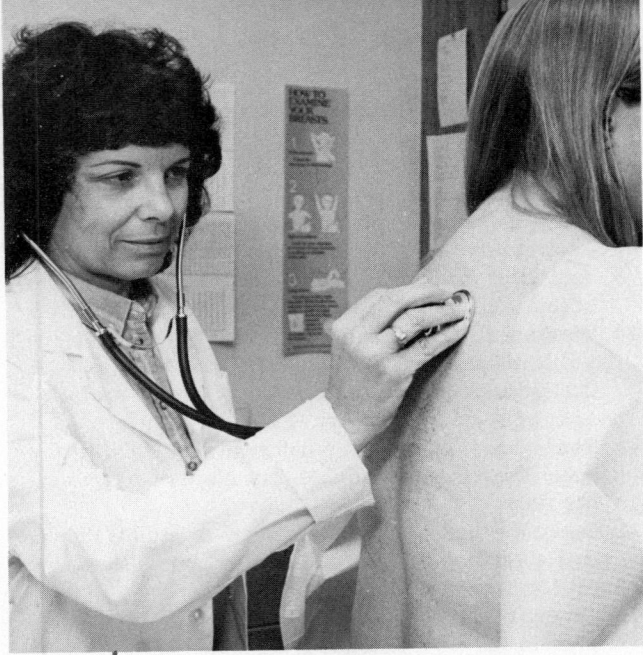

Unit X:
Assessment and Management in Women's Health Promotion

Multiple Choice

1. The areas of gynecology most often encountered by the maternity nurse are
   A. Growth and development needs including adolescence and menopause
   B. Health promotion
   C. Common gynecological problems including menstrual problems and minor infections
   D. Infertility problems and Rh/ABO incompatibilities

   1. B and C
   2. A, C, and D
   3. All but A
   4. All but D

2. An important component of the gynecological health history is
   A. A professional demeanor while taking the history
   B. A thorough history, including sexual activity, taken each time the patient is seen
   C. A review of periodic screening procedures for early detection of gynecological problems
   D. A thorough assessment of the client's emotional status

3. The most critical screening procedures for women include
   A. Height, weight, and blood pressure
   B. Breast examination
   C. Mammography
   D. Pap smear
   E. Hemoglobin/hematocrit
   F. Pelvic examination
   G. Rectal examination
   H. Stool guaiac

   1. All but A
   2. All but C and H
   3. All but G
   4. All but E and H
   5. All but H

4. The reasons why a client may not follow health-related advice given by a nurse include
   A. Lack of autonomy in health-seeking behavior
   B. A nonsupportive family
   C. A nontherapeutic relationship with the nurse
   D. An empathic relationship with the physician

   1. All but A
   2. B and C
   3. All but D
   4. All but B

5. The two most common breast cancers are
   A. Intervillous hyperplasia
   B. Fibroadenoma
   C. Adenocarcinomas
   D. Intraductal papillomas
   E. Ductal carcinomas

   1. A and D
   2. B and E
   3. C and D
   4. C and E

6. The diagnosis of osteoporosis can be made by
   A. Periodic height and weight measurements only
   B. CAT scan only
   C. Blood test
   D. Clinical signs
   E. Diagnostic radiographic tests

   1. B
   2. A and C
   3. D and E
   4. E only

7. Recurrent heavy menses over months and years in women 30 to 45 years of age are *most often* due to
   A. Myomata
   B. PMS
   C. Adenomyosis
   D. STD's
   E. Intervillous carcinoma

1. A and D
2. A and C
3. C and E
4. B and D
5. All of the above

8. Very short menstrual cycles may indicate
   A. Anemia
   B. Improper birth control pill dosage
   C. Anovulation
   D. Infertility

9. The most common cause of secondary amenorrhea in women 16 to 45 years of age is
   A. Ovarian cysts
   B. STD
   C. Pregnancy
   D. Hypopituitarism
   E. Endometrial hyperplasia

10. Which of the following drugs are used in the treatment of dysmenorrhea?
    A. Acetaminophen
    B. Aspirin
    C. Low dose combination birth control pills
    D. Naproxen
    E. Mefenamic acid
    F. Ibuprofen

    1. All of the above
    2. All but B and C
    3. All but D and E
    4. All but C
    5. All but F

11. The *most frequently* reported PMS symptoms are
    A. Food cravings
    B. Anxiety, nervousness, agitation
    C. Painful breasts
    D. Irritability, argumentativeness
    E. Headache
    F. Frustration
    G. Child battering

    1. A, B, C
    2. D, F, G
    3. B, D, F
    4. C, D, E
    5. A, C, E

12. Which of the following are the *most frequent* reasons why women seek gynecological care?
    A. STD
    B. Vaginal discharge
    C. Perineal lesions
    D. Itching
    E. Intercycle spotting

    1. A, B, C
    2. A, C, E
    3. A and C
    4. B and E
    5. B and D

13. Which of the following can be the cause(s) of toxic shock syndrome?
    A. Cervical cap
    B. Vaginal sprays
    C. Tampons
    D. Diaphragm left in place for several days
    E. Infrequent bathing
    F. Multiple sex partners

    1. All of the above
    2. A, B, C
    3. B, C, E
    4. A, C, D
    5. A and C
    6. C and F

14. The most prevalent sexually transmitted disease in the United States today is
    A. Trichomonas vaginitis
    B. Neisseria gonorrhoeae
    C. Gardnerella vaginitis
    D. Chlamydia trachomatis
    E. AIDS
    F. Genital herpes

15. Common organisms isolated in pelvic inflammatory disease include
    A. Bacteroides
    B. Mycoplasma hominis
    C. Peptococcus
    D. Neisseria gonorrhoeae
    E. Peptostreptococcus
    F. Chlamydia trachomatis

    1. B, D, F
    2. A, C, E
    3. All but E and F
    4. All but C and E
    5. All but A
    6. All of the above

16. Toxic shock syndrome (TSS) is caused by the organism
    A. Chlamydia trachomatis
    B. Mycoplasma hominis
    C. Peptostreptococcus
    D. Staphylococcus aureus
    E. Neisseria gonorrhoeae

17. The leading causes of mortality in toxic shock syndrome are
    A. Hypervolemia
    B. Respiratory failure
    C. PID
    D. Uncontrollable hypotension
    E. DIC

    1. A, C, D
    2. C, D, E
    3. B, D, E
    4. All but C
    5. All but C and E
    6. All of the above

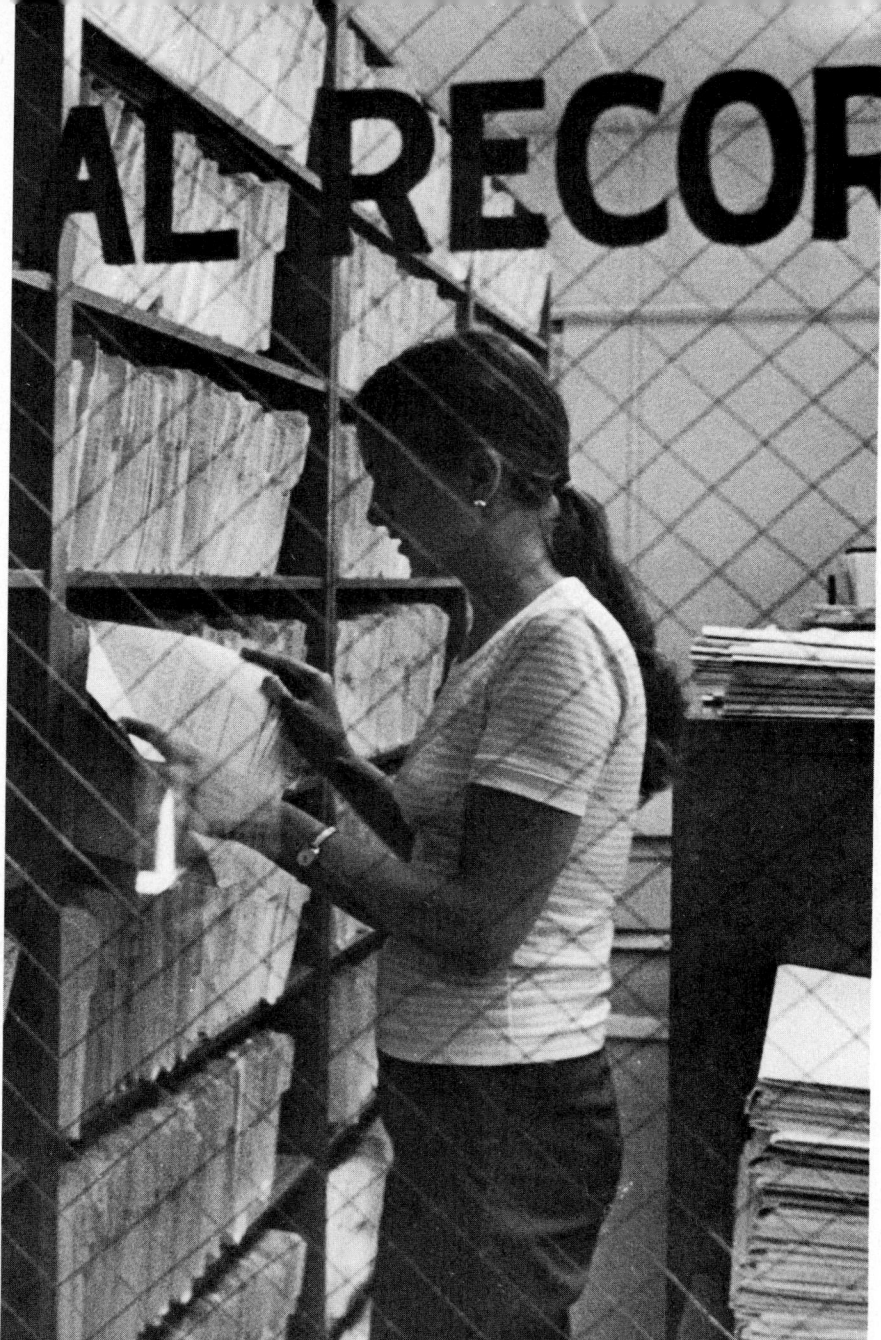

APPENDICES

Exercises in Client Education

Prenatal Exercises

Pelvic Tilt

Buttocks are tucked under to flatten out the hollow of the lower back. Hold for 3 seconds. Then relax, allowing hips to move back to former position. Repeat several times. This exercise may be done sitting, standing, on the hands and knees, or lying on the floor. This exercise strengthens back and abdominal muscles and relieves backache.

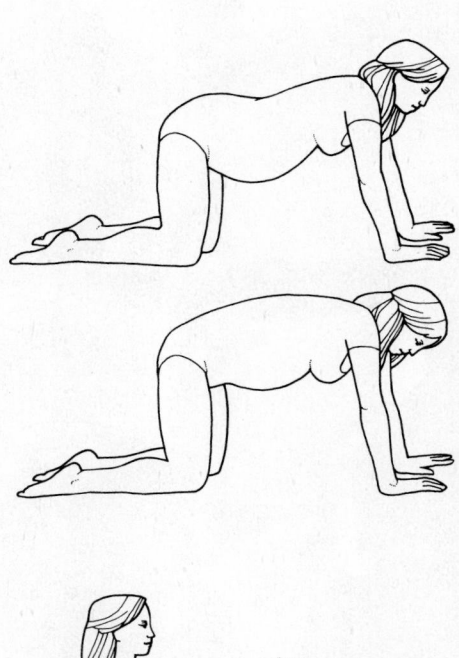

Knee Bends

Deep knee bends using a chair for stabilization will strengthen back muscles and will keep leg and hip joints supple.

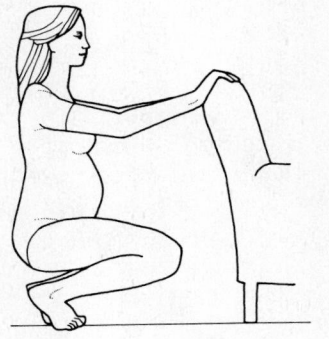

Tailor Sitting

Sitting on the floor with one foot in front of the other, tucked inward toward the perineum, and with the knees pressed downward toward the floor, is tailor sitting. This aids in relaxing muscles of the pelvic floor, helps relieve backache, and stretches thigh muscles.

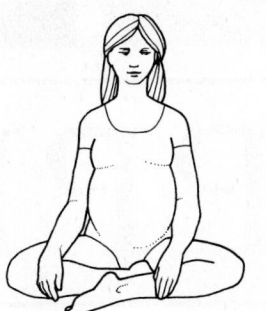

Knee–Chest Twist

Lying on the back, the knees are pulled to the chest and arms stretched straight to the sides. The knees are rolled to one side, while the head is turned to the opposite side. Sides are switched and repeated. This stretches the spine and relieves backache.

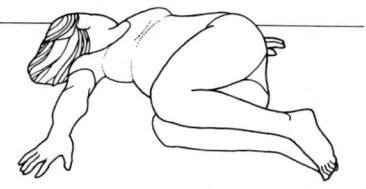

Rib Cage Lifting

The right arm is extended with elbow slightly flexed above the head while the chest expands with inhaling. The arm can then be stretched further during exhaling. During a second inhalation, the arm is returned to the initial position. The exercise is repeated with the other arm. This exercise is helpful in relieving shortness of breath and can be performed in standing, sitting, or tailor-sitting position.

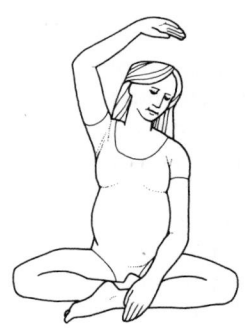

Shoulder Circling

With back, neck, and head straight throughout the exercise, arms are allowed to hang loosely at the sides. Shoulders are rotated slowly up and back as far as they will comfortably go in a circular motion. Inhaling occurs as the shoulders are rotated and exhaling as the circle is completed and the shoulders are returned to starting position. This exercise is useful in strengthening muscles of upper back and may relieve upper backache and numbness in the arms and fingers.

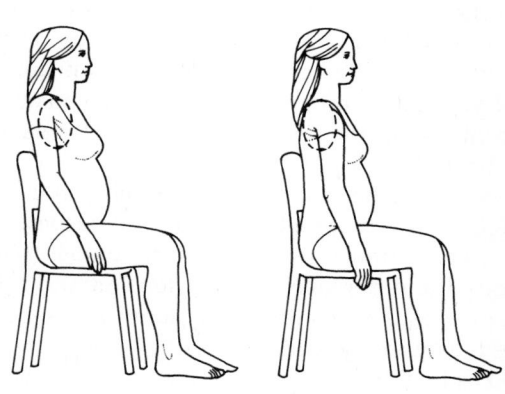

Calf Stretching

Calf stretching is helpful in preventing or relieving lower leg cramps. **A,** with feet slightly apart, hands are on the back of an object that offers security. **B,** The foot of cramped leg slides as far back as possible without the heel leaving the floor. **C,** the knee of the other leg is bent, the body is lowered, and the stretching of the calf can be felt. After the initial position is assumed, the body relaxes.

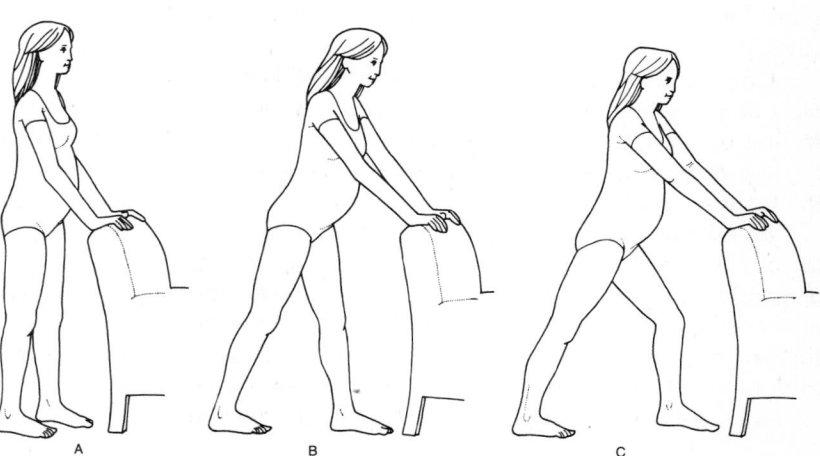

Conditioned Relaxation

Take a few slow, deep breaths . . . Inhale . . . Exhale . . . Inhale . . . Exhale . . .

Focus your attention on your breathing throughout this exercise, and recognize how easily slow, deep breathing alone can help to produce relaxation. Let your body breathe itself, according to its own natural rhythm . . . Slowly and deeply . . .

Now let's begin the exercise with what we call a "cleansing breath," a special message that tells the body we are ready to enter a state of deep relaxation. The cleansing breath is taken as follows . . . Exhale . . . Take a deep breath in through your nose . . . Then blow it out through your mouth.

You may notice a kind of "tingling" sensation when you take the cleansing breath. Whatever you feel is a signal or message to your body that will become associated with relaxation, so that as you practice this exercise over and over again, simply taking the cleansing breath alone will produce the same degree of relaxation that you'll be able to get by completing the entire exercise.

Breathe slowly and deeply . . . As you concentrate your attention on your breathing, focus your eyes on an imaginary spot in the center of your forehead . . . Look at the spot as if you are trying to see it from the inside of your head . . . Raise your eyes way up so as to stare at that spot from the inside of your head. Concentrate your attention on it . . . The more you are able to concentrate on the spot, the better your relaxation response will be . . .

As you continue to focus your attention on the spot, you might notice that your eyelids have become quite tense . . . That's fine, for what we want to do is to teach your body the difference between tension and relaxation. Your eyelids are controlled by some of the smallest muscles in your body, and they become easily tired and fatigued as they become more and more tense. When I count to three, we'll demonstrate the difference between tension and relaxation by allowing your eyelids to close gently, allowing the feelings of tension to melt away quickly.

One . . . Two . . . Three . . . Close your eyelids firmly but not too tightly, and as they close, sense a soothing feeling of relaxation radiate all around your eyes . . . the top of your eyes . . . the bottom . . . the sides . . . the front and back . . .

Breathe slowly and deeply . . . Feel the relaxation in your eyes, and how nice it feels . . . Let these feelings of gentle relaxation radiate all around your eyes and out to your forehead . . . to your scalp . . . all around the back of your head . . . to your ears and temples . . . to your cheeks and nose . . . to your mouth and chin . . . and around to your jaw . . . As you feel all the tension flow out of your face and the area around your mouth, relax your jaw muscles . . . As you do so, let your jaw gently open slightly so that all the tension can smoothly flow away . . .

Remember your breathing, slowly and deeply . . . Relax the muscles in your neck . . . As you do so, feel all the tension flow away from the muscles in the back of your neck . . . Let this nice, gentle feeling of relaxation now radiate down into your shoulders . . . Feel the heaviness of your shoulders as the shoulder muscles gently relax . . . This is one of the most important areas of the body to relax since we all tend to store a lot of tension in our necks and shoulders . . . Feel all the tension flow away, and sense the nice, gentle feeling of deep relaxation . . .

Remember your breathing, slowly and deeply . . . Let this feeling of relaxation now radiate down your arms . . . to your elbows . . . forearms . . . wrists . . . and hands . . . Spend a moment to relax each of your fingers . . . your thumb, index finger, middle finger, ring finger, little finger . . . As your hands and arms completely and gently relax, you may notice feelings of warmth and heaviness . . . Some people report pulsations or tingly sensations . . . Some can even sense their heartbeat in their fingertips . . . Others report even magnetic or pulling sensations . . . Whatever you experience is your own body's way of expressing relaxation . . . Remember, you cannot *force* yourself to relax, you can only *allow* yourself to relax . . . Trust your body . . . It knows what to do . . .

Remember your breathing, slowly and deeply . . . Relax your chest . . . and abdomen . . . and let this feeling of relaxation radiate around your sides and ribs, as waves of relaxation cross your shoulder blades to meet at your upper back . . . middle back . . . and lower back . . . Feel all the muscles on either side of your spine softly relax . . . Let this feeling of gentle relaxation now radiate down into your pelvic area . . . to your buttocks . . . sphincter muscle . . . genitals . . . Feel your whole pelvic area open up and gently relax . . . Relax your thighs . . . knees . . . calves . . . ankles . . . and feet . . . Spend a moment to relax each toe . . . your big toe, second toe, third toe, fourth toe, and little toe . . . Breathe slowly and deeply . . . Relax and enjoy it . . .

Now that your body is gently relaxed and quiet, take a moment, starting from the top of your head working down, to check lightly to see how much relaxation you have obtained . . .

If there is any part of your body that is not yet fully relaxed and comfortable, simply inhale a deep breath and send it into that area, bringing soothing, relaxing, nourishing, healing oxygen into every cell of that area, comforting and relaxing it . . . As you exhale, imagine blowing out, right through your skin, any tension, tightness, pain, or discomfort in that area. Again, as you inhale, bring relaxing, healing oxygen into every cell of that area, and as you exhale, blow away, right through the skin, any tension or discomfort.

In this way you can send your breath to relax any part of your body which is not yet as fully relaxed and comfortable as it can be . . . Breathe slowly and deeply, and with each breath, allow yourself to become twice as relaxed as you were before . . . Inhale . . . Exhale . . . Twice as relaxed . . . Inhale . . . Exhale . . . Twice as relaxed . . .

When you find yourself quiet and fully relaxed, take a moment to enjoy it . . . Sense the gentle warmth and feeling of well-being all through your body . . . If any extraneous thoughts try to interfere, simply allow them to pass through and out of you . . . Ignore them and go back to your breathing, slowly and deeply . . . Slowly and deeply . . . Enjoy this nice state of gentle relaxation . . .

Remember your breathing, slowly and deeply . . . When you end this exercise, you may be surprised to notice that you feel not only relaxed and comfortable, but energized with such a powerful sense of well-being that you will easily be able to meet any demands that arise . . . To end the exercise, tell yourself that you can reach this nice gentle state of Conditioned Relaxation any time you wish by simply taking the cleansing breath . . . Reinforce that cleansing breath by concluding the exercise with it . . . Exhale . . . Inhale deeply through your nose . . . Blow out through the mouth . . . And be well . . .

(Adapted from Bresler DE: Free Yourself from Pain, pp 261–263. New York, Simon & Schuster, 1979. ©1975 by David E. Bresler, Ph.D.)

Guided Imagery Exercises

- Imagine that you are lying on a billowy cloud, moving gently through space. Feel the texture of the cloud as it buoys you up, and its slow rocking motion. If colors come into your mind, let yourself be surrounded by them. Be held aloft and carried, or simply rest weightless, as you choose. Let yourself be lulled, as if you were in a hammock. Continue to breathe deeply, as your breath becomes one with the breath of the cloud.
- Imagine that you are floating on your back in water, staring up at the immense, harmonious blue of a cloudless sky. You may be in a lake, or on the ocean, or lying on a lily pad in a pond. You choose the place. Imagine how it feels to be held and gently moved by the natural flow of water. Let your breath be one with the motion of the water, and fill your eyes with the blue of the sky. See nothing else. If sounds come to you, let them flood your ears. Continue to breathe deeply as you float suspended.
- Imagine that you are lying in the cool, high grasses of a fresh green meadow, with a lilting spring breeze rushing over you. In your own hollowed-out hiding place the grass bends down and brushes you, caressing you with long blades that are almost like cool water. Feel the motion of the meadow as it ripples with the wind, a rhythm that is one with the long, peaceful motion of your own relaxed breath. Let yourself be calmed by the sparkling sound of the nearby brook, running full with the first rains of spring.

(Bogin M: The Path to Pain Control, pp 214–215. Boston, Houghton-Mifflin, 1982)

Breathing Techniques

Complete Breath and Breath Control

A complete breath is one in which the chest wall expands and the diaphragm descends to its maximum extent. The breath is let out slowly under pressure so that a more complete exchange of oxygen and carbon dioxide can take place. It is used periodically during relaxation and should be followed by slow, quiet, easy respiration.

1. Breathe in once as deeply as possible.
2. Hiss or blow the air out slowly, letting your whole body go limp.
3. Continue breathing quietly, easily, and rhythmically.
4. Let yourself go completely loose.
5. Soon your body will begin to feel very heavy and any exertion will be difficult. You can test this by doing the following:
   a. Gradually bend an elbow, bringing your hand toward your chin. Notice the effort.
   b. Slowly lower your arm to its resting position. Again you will find yourself actually working to prevent it from falling too quickly.

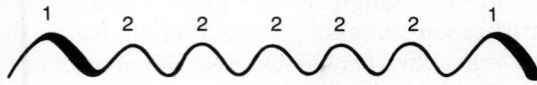

Diagrammatic breath pattern: 1 = complete breath; 2 = slow rhythmic breathing.

Deep Breathing: Early Labor

1. Pretend that you are having a contraction that lasts 30 seconds to 45 seconds.
2. At the beginning of each contraction take a complete breath and hiss or blow it out.
3. Breathe deeply, slowly, and rhythmically throughout the remainder of the contraction.
4. When the contraction has ended, take another complete breath and hiss or blow it out slowly.
5. Breathe normally between contractions.
6. During labor, continue to use this pattern of breathing with contractions as long as it is helpful.

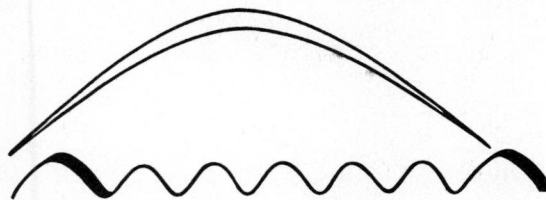

Early labor

The illustrative material and much of the information in the following section were provided through the courtesy of the Maternity Center Association, based upon their publication *Preparation for Childbearing*, 5th ed, New York, 1985.

Modified Deep Breathing: Active Labor

As labor advances and contractions increase in strength, you often have a desire to keep the diaphragm as still as possible. Yet the uterus continues to need a good supply of oxygen. For this reason you should breathe deeply as the contraction begins and ends, and modify your breathing so that it is quiet and shallow at the peak of each contraction. To practice this do the following:

1. Pretend that you are having stronger contractions, lasting almost a minute.
2. Breathe in deeply as the contraction starts. Then slowly hiss or blow out, letting yourself go completely limp.
3. Make each of the next four or five breaths a little shallower than the previous one. You will notice that you are breathing very lightly.
4. Light breathing is quiet and effortless, almost like a throat breath. Experiment to find your own comfortable rate and continue for 15 seconds to 45 seconds. If you become dizzy or lightheaded, your breathing is too vigorous. If you have trouble getting enough air or difficulty maintaining the rhythm, try taking a quick, deep breath, and return to light breathing.
5. After the contraction has begun to subside, make each of the next four or five breaths a little deeper than the previous one.
6. End the breath pattern with one complete breath.

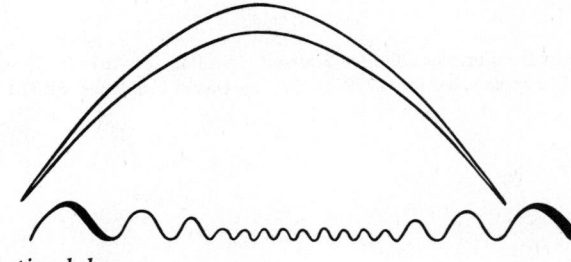

Active labor

Further Adaptation for Transition

For the later part of the first stage of labor (if you feel a tendency to hold your breath or to push during strong contractions) do the modified complete breath, but with the following important change:

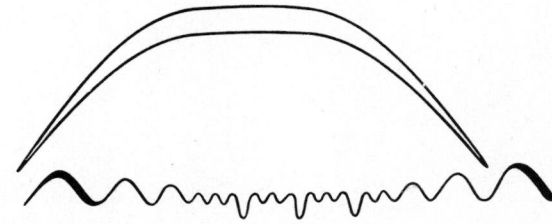

Transition

1. During light breathing, puff out gently as you exhale on every third or fourth breath.

Second-Stage Breathing

During the second stage of labor, the mother actively participates in the birth of the baby. Whatever position is comfortable is the best position for you. By assuming any C-shaped position, four of which are illustrated here, the mother accentuates the curve of the pelvic passage and facilitates the downward movement of her baby through the pelvis. In addition, the breathing pattern needs to be coordinated with the tightening of the abdominal muscles in a downward direction toward the vaginal canal.

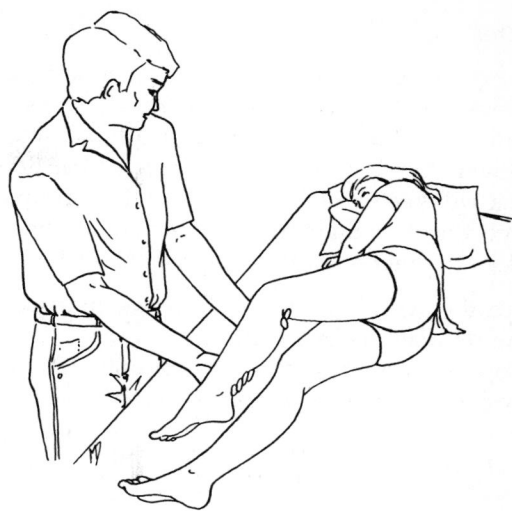

Side-lying

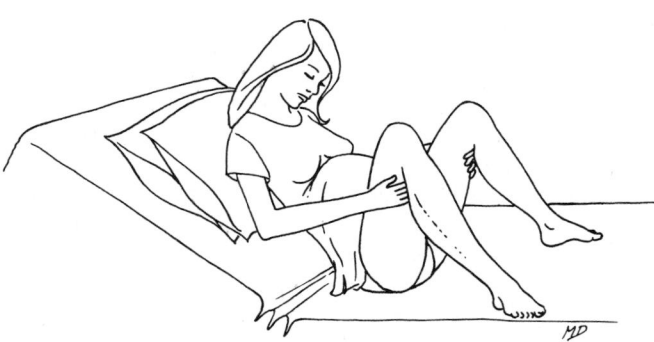

Semi-upright

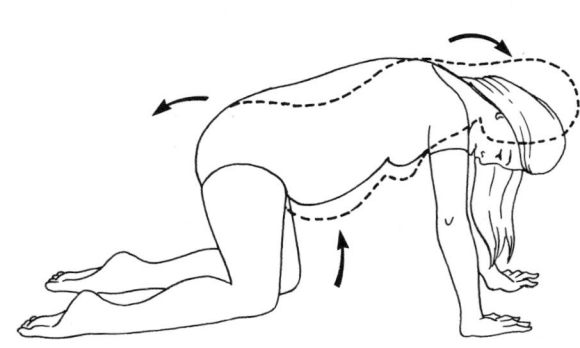

All fours

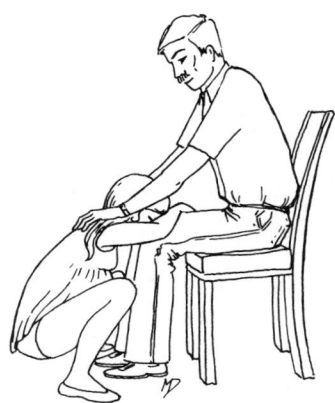

Squatting

Pushing

1. Take two complete breaths.
2. Take a deep breath, quickly drop chin to chest, round shoulders, and hold breath for 5 to 6 seconds only. (You may also find it helpful to put your elbows out, and hold onto someone or something.) Tighten abdominals and push baby down toward relaxed vaginal canal and pelvic floor muscles.
3. After 5 to 6 seconds, release remaining air with an expiratory grunt, while pulling in more tightly with abdominal muscles.
4. Raise head, scoop in another quick deep breath, hold for 5 to 6 seconds, and repeat entire process explained in steps 2 and 3.
5. Continue this pattern until urge to push is gone and contraction is over.
6. Take two complete breaths after contraction is finished.

Note: Holding breath stabilizes diaphragm so that abdominal muscles exert more effective pressure on uterus. *Do not hold breath* longer than 5 to 6 seconds, or to the point of gasping, because this releases pressure too suddenly, has a piston effect, and is physiologically undesirable for mother and baby.

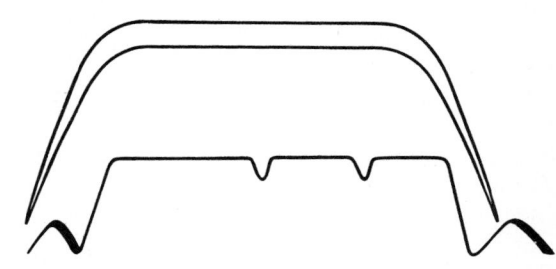

Pushing

Panting

When delivery is near, you may be asked to stop pushing in the middle of a contraction. If this happens, begin immediately to pant, making your diaphragm move up and down. Although it will not decrease the desire to push, it will keep you from doing so, because panting prevents the diaphragm from leaning on the abdominal muscles. To practice panting, do the following:

1. Breathe in and out very quickly, keeping your mouth open—like a panting dog.
2. Continue breathing this way for only a brief period. Relax. Take a complete breath.

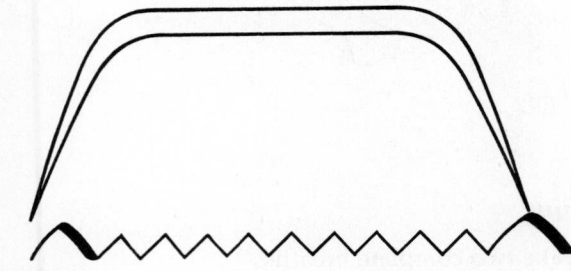

Panting

Preparatory Exercise for Controlled Relaxation*

Verbal Cue	Action	Coaching Role	Rationale
Take a deep breath and relax	Focus eyes on object, inhale, exhale, and consciously release all tension		Begin with complete relaxation
Stretch down both heels	Extend legs, flex ankles, *keep rest of body relaxed*	Tap heels to signal contraction	Isolate tension, beginning with single body area
Relax	Relax both legs	Stroke to signal relaxation; look for relaxation	Associate word "relax" with stroking to signal release of tension
Tighten thighs	Tense both thighs	Tap thighs to signal tension	Isolate area to be tensed
Relax	Relax thighs	Stroke to signal relaxation	Associate verbal and tactile cues
Squeeze buttocks together	Tense gluteal muscles	Tap buttocks, or hips if woman is supine	Isolate area to be tensed
Relax	Relax buttocks	Stroke to signal relaxation	Associate verbal and tactile cues
Stretch arms down	Extend arms and hands fully	Tap hands	Isolate area to be tensed
Relax	Relax tension in hands and arms	Stroke arms	Associate verbal and tactile cues
Shrug your shoulders	Tense shoulders	Tap shoulders	Isolate area to be tensed
Relax	Relax shoulders	Stroke shoulders	Associate verbal and tactile cues
Make a face	Tense face; clench jaw	Tap cheek lightly	Isolate area to be tensed
Relax	Relax face	Stroke face; turn head gently side to side	Associate verbal and tactile cues; detect tension in neck
Take a deep breath and relax completely	Inhale, exhale, and completely relax	Observe for tension; where detected, stroke to signal release	Woman's awareness of feeling of complete relaxation; coach's awareness of the appearance of complete relaxation

* Exercises should be practiced in supine position with head and shoulders well supported by pillows with another pillow (or two) under the knees.
(Hassid P: Textbook for Childbirth Educators, 2nd ed. Philadelphia, JB Lippincott, 1984)

Practice Drill for Controlled Relaxation*

Verbal Cue	Action	Coaching Role	Rationale
Contract right leg	Tense right thigh and calf; flex ankle Focus gaze on one spot to enhance concentration Think about the feeling of tension in the right leg and of relaxation in the rest of the body	Tap right leg; feel muscles for quality of muscle tension Look over rest of body for obvious signs of tension; lift left leg gently under knee to check relaxation; check both arms; turn head gently side to side to check relaxation of neck Where tension is detected, stroke and give cue, "Relax"	Isolate area to be tensed Detect tension and signal its release
Relax right leg	Relax completely	Stroke right leg; lift gently under right knee to detect tension	Detect hidden tension; signal its release; associate verbal and tactile cues
Contract left arm	Make a fist; tense entire arm and lift slightly off the floor Focus gaze on one spot to enhance concentration Think about the feeling of tension in the left arm and of relaxation in the rest of the body	Tap left arm; check for tension Check rest of body for signs of tension; lift right arm gently by hand, swing freely from shoulder; lift knees slightly; observe face; turn head gently side to side to detect neck tension; stroke to signal its release	Isolate area to be tensed Detect tension; signal its release
Relax left arm	Relax completely	Stroke left arm and shoulder Lift left arm gently by hand; swing from shoulder	Signal relaxation with tactile and verbal cues Detect hidden tension
Contract key areas	Tense jaw and perineum Focus gaze on one spot to enhance concentration Think about tension in jaw and perineum; feel relaxation in rest of body	Tap jaw lightly; note tension Check neck, arms, and legs for tension; stroke to signal release as necessary	Isolate area to be tensed Awareness of impact of key areas on tension in shoulders, neck, legs, etc.
Relax key areas	Relax completely	Stroke jaw and other body areas to enhance and signal relaxation	With jaw relaxed, whole upper body can relax; with perineum relaxed, whole lower body can relax†

* The emphasis is always upon the relaxation, not on the tensing or on how quickly the woman can respond.
† Continue practice drill using arms, legs, and key areas in random pattern to enhance skills. Always begin and end with preparatory exercise.
(Hassid P: Textbook for Childbirth Educators, 2nd ed. Philadelphia, JB Lippincott, 1984)

Postpartal Exercises

Postpartal exercises should be begun as soon as possible after birth. The exercise program can be presented in phases, beginning with simple exercises and progressing to ones that are more strenuous.

Firming the Abdomen

Phase I.
Abdominal Breathing

1. Lie on back with knees bent.
2. Inhale deeply through the nose, keeping ribs as stationary as possible and allowing the abdomen to expand up.
3. Exhale slowly but forcefully while contracting the abdominal muscles.
4. Hold for about 3 to 5 seconds while exhaling. Relax.
5. Begin with 2 repetitions, gradually progressing to 10.

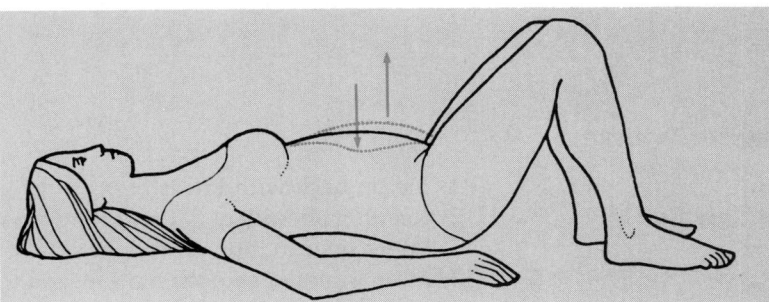

Phase II.
Combined Abdominal
Breathing and Supine
Pelvic Tilt

1. Lie on back with knees bent.
2. While inhaling deeply, roll pelvis back by flattening the lower back on the floor or bed.
3. While exhaling slowly but forcefully, contract the abdominal muscles and tighten the buttocks.
4. Hold for about 3 to 5 seconds while exhaling. Relax.
5. Begin with two repetitions, gradually progressing to 10.

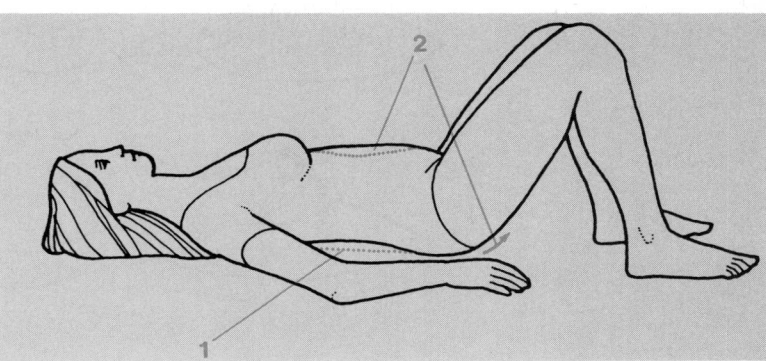

Phase III.
Reach for the Knees

1. Lie on back with knees bent.
2. While inhaling deeply, bring the chin onto the chest.
3. While exhaling, raise the head and shoulders slowly and smoothly, reaching for the knees with outstretched arms. The body should only rise as far as the back will naturally bend while the waist remains on the floor or bed (about 6 to 8 inches).

(continued)

4. Slowly and smoothly lower head and shoulders to the starting position. Relax.
5. Begin with 2 repetitions, gradually progressing to 10.

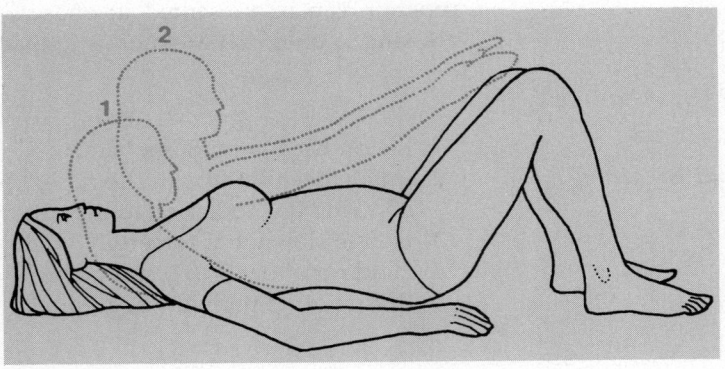

Firming the Waist

Phase I.
Double Knee Roll

1. Lie on back with knees bent.
2. Keeping shoulders flat and the feet stationary, slowly and smoothly roll the knees over to touch the right side of the bed.
3. Maintaining a smooth motion, roll the knees back over to touch the left side of the bed.
4. Return to starting position. Relax.
5. Begin with 2 repetitions, gradually progressing to 10.

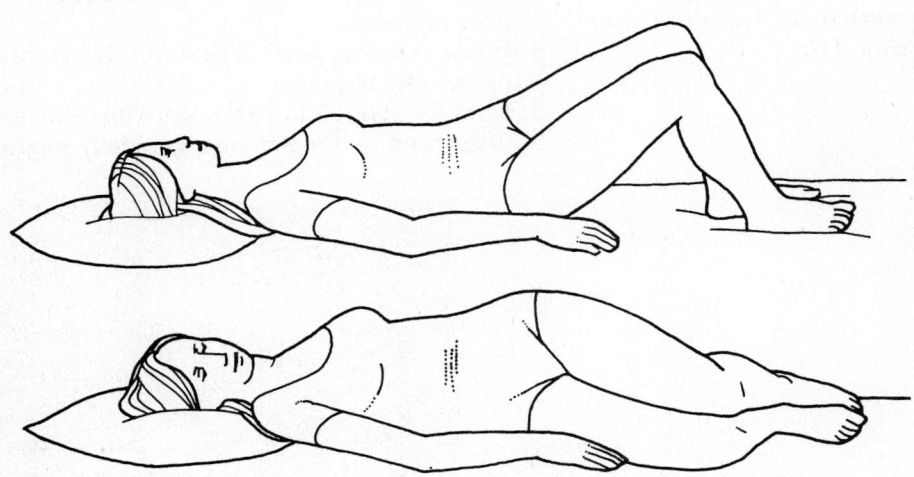

Phase II.
Single Knee Roll

1. Lie on back, right leg straight, left leg bent at the knee.
2. Keeping the shoulders flat, slowly and smoothly roll the left knee over to touch the right side of the bed and back to starting position.
3. Reverse position of legs, touch left side of the bed with the right knee, and return to starting position. Relax.
4. Begin with 2 repetitions, gradually progressing to 10.

(continued)

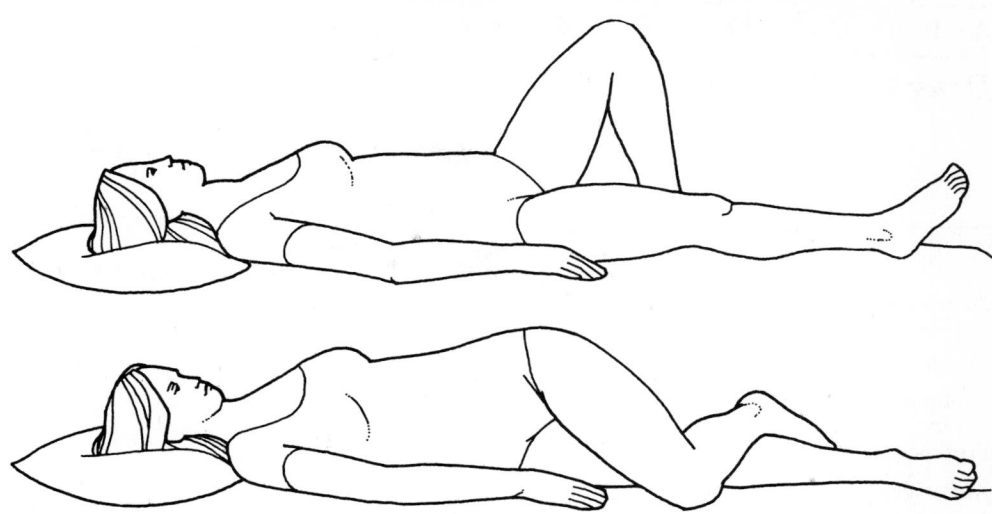

Phase III.
Leg Role

1. Lie on back with legs straight.
2. Keeping shoulders flat, slowly and smoothly lift the left leg and, keeping it straight, roll it over to touch the right side of the bed and return to starting position.
3. Repeat, using the right leg to touch the left side of the bed. Relax.
4. Begin with 2 repetitions, gradually progressing to 10.

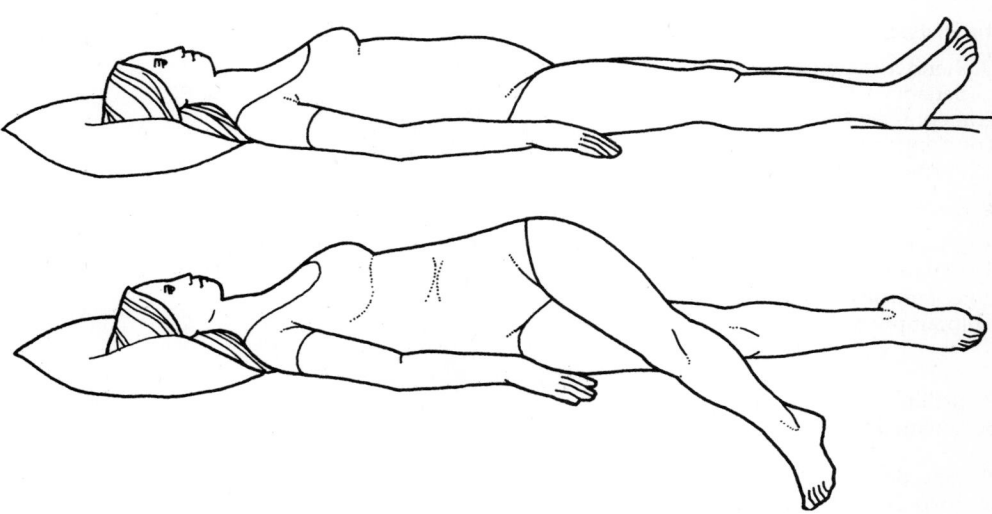

Drug Use During Breast-feeding*

Drug or Agent	Contra-indicated	R$_x$ With Caution	No Apparent Harm	Insufficient Information	Comment
Analgesics					
Acetaminophen			×		
Aspirin			×		
Propoxyphene (Darvon)			×		
Anticoagulants					
Ethyl biscoumacetate	×				Bleeding infant
Phenindione	×				Bleeding infant
Heparin			×		No passage into milk
Warfarin Na (Coumadin)			×		
Bishydroxycoumarin (Dicumarol)		×			
Anticonvulsants					
Phenobarbital			×		Low levels in infant
Primadone (Mysoline)			×		? Drowsiness
Carbamazepine				×	Significant infant levels; no reported effects
Diphenylhydantoin (Phenytoin, Dilantin)			×		Low levels in infant, methemoglobin, 1 case
Antihistamines					
Diphenhydramine (Benadryl)			×		Small amounts excreted
Trimeprazine (Temaril)			×		Small amounts excreted
Tripelennamine (Pyribenzamine)			×		Small amounts excreted
Anti-infective Agents					
Aminoglycosides (Kanamycin, gentamicin)			×		Significant excretion in milk; not absorbed
Chloramphenicol	×				Bone marrow depression; gastrointestinal and behavioral effects
Penicillins			×		Possible sensitization
Sulfonamides		×			Hemolysis, G-6-PD deficiency, bilirubin displacement
Tetracyclines			×		Limited absorption by infant
Nalidixic acid		×			Hemolysis
Nitrofurantoin		×			Possible G-6-PD hemolysis
Metronidazole (Flagyl)		×			Low absorption but potentially toxic
Isoniazid		×			High levels in milk, possible toxicity
Pyramethamine	×				Vomiting, marrow suppression, convulsions
Chloraquine			×		Not excreted
Quinine		×			Thrombocytopenia

(continued)

* Drug use during breast-feeding remains controversial.

Drug or Agent	Contra-indicated	R_x With Caution	No Apparent Harm	Insufficient Information	Comment
Anti-inflammatory					
Aspirin			X		
Indomethacin		X			Seizures, 1 case
Phenylbutazone		X			Low levels, ? blood dyscrasia
Gold	X				Found in baby; nephritis, hepatitis, hematologic changes
Steroids				X	Low levels with prednisone and prednisolone
Antineoplastic					
Cyclophosphamide	X				Neutropenia
Methotrexate	X				Very small excretion
Antithyroid					
Radioactive iodine	X				Thyroid suppression
Propylthiouracil	X				Thyroid suppression
Bronchodilators					
Aminophylline			X		Irritability, 1 case
Iodides	X				Thyroid suppression
Sympathomimetics				X	Inhalers probably safe
Cardiovascular Agents					
Digoxin			X		Insignificant levels
Propanolol			X		Insignificant levels
Reserpine	X				Nasal stuffiness, lethargy
Guanethidine (Ismelin)			X		Insignificant levels
Cardiovascular Agents					
Methyldopa (Aldomet)				X	
Cathartics					
Anthroquinones (Cascara, danthron)	X				Diarrhea, cramps
Aloe, senna		X			
Bulk agents, softeners			X		Safe in moderate dosage
Contraceptives, Oral†					
Diethylstilbestrol	X				Possible vaginal cancer
Depo-provera		X			May affect lactation
Norethisterone		X			May affect lactation
Ethinyl estradiol		X			May affect lactation
Diuretics					
Chlorthalidone				X	Low levels, but may accumulate
Thiazides		X			May affect lactation; low levels in milk
Spironolactone			X		Insignificant levels
Ergot Alkaloids					
Bromocriptine	X				Lactation suppressed
Ergot	X				Vomiting, diarrhea, seizures
Ergotamine				X	
Ergonovine	X				Brief postpartum course may be safe
Methylergonovine	X				Brief postpartum course may be safe

(continued)

† Controversy in literature, long-term effects uncertain, one case of gynecomastia

Drug or Agent	Contra-indicated	Rx With Caution	No Apparent Harm	Insufficient Information	Comment
Hormones					
Corticosteroids				X	Low levels with short-term prednisone or prednisolone
Sex hormones (see above, Contraceptives, Oral)					
Thyroid (T_3 or T_4)			X		Excreted in milk; may mask hypothyroid infant
Insulin			X		Not absorbed
ACTH			X		Not absorbed
Epinephrine			X		Not absorbed
Narcotics					
Codeine			X		In usual doses
Meperidine (Demerol)				X	
Morphine			X		Low infant levels on usual dosage
Heroin	X				Addiction withdrawal in infants
Methadone		X			Minimal levels
Psychotherapeutic Drugs					
Lithium	X				High levels in milk
Phenothiazines		X			Drowsiness; chronic effects uncertain
Tricyclic antidepressants				X	Low levels; effects uncertain
Diazepam (Valium)	X				Lethargy, weight loss, EEG changes
Meprobamate (Equanil)	X				High levels in milk
Chlordiazepoxide (Librium)			X		Low levels in milk
Radiopharmaceuticals					
^{131}I	X				72 hr, no breast-feeding
Technetium (99M Tc)	X				48 hr, no breast-feeding
^{131}I albumin	X				10 days, no breast-feeding
Sedatives-Hypnotics					
Barbiturates		X			Short-acting, less depressant
Chloral hydrate		X			Drowsiness
Bromides	X				Depression, rash
Diazepam (Valium)	X				Depression, weight loss
Flurazepam				X	Chemically related to diazepam
Nitrazepam				X	
Social-Recreational Drugs					
Alcohol			X		Milk levels equal plasma, moderate consumption apparently safe, high levels inhibit lactation
Caffeine			X		Jitteriness with very high intakes
Nicotine			X		Low levels in milk
Marijuana			X		Minimal passage in milk
Miscellaneous					
Atropine		X			May cause constipation or inhibit lactation
Dihydrotachysterol		X			Renal calcification in animals

(Avery GB (ed): Neonatology, 3rd ed. Philadelphia, JB Lippincott, 1987)

Conversion Table for Weights of Newborn

(*Gram equivalents for pounds and ounces*)

For example, to find weight in pounds and ounces of baby weighing 3315 grams, glance down columns to figure nearest 3315 = 3317. Refer to number at top of column for pounds and number to far left for ounces = 7 pounds, 5 ounces.

Pounds → Ounces ↓	3	4	5	6	7	8	9	10
0	1361	1814	2268	2722	3175	3629	4082	4536
1	1389	1843	2296	2750	3203	3657	4111	4564
2	1417	1871	2325	2778	3232	3685	4139	4593
3	1446	1899	2353	2807	3260	3714	4167	4621
4	1474	1928	2381	2835	3289	3742	4196	4649
5	1503	1956	2410	2863	3317	3770	4224	4678
6	1531	1984	2438	2892	3345	3799	4252	4706
7	1559	2013	2466	2920	3374	3827	4281	4734
8	1588	2041	2495	2948	3402	3856	4309	4763
9	1616	2070	2523	2977	3430	3884	4338	4791
10	1644	2098	2551	3005	3459	3912	4366	4819
11	1673	2126	2580	3033	3487	3941	4394	4848
12	1701	2155	2608	3062	3515	3969	4423	4876
13	1729	2183	2637	3090	3544	3997	4451	4904
14	1758	2211	2665	3118	3572	4026	4479	4933
15	1786	2240	2693	3147	3600	4054	4508	4961

Or, to convert grams into pounds and *decimals* of a pound, multiply weight in grams by .0022. Thus, 3317 × .0022 = 7.2974 (*i.e.,* 7.3 pounds, or 7 pounds, 5 ounces).

To convert pounds and ounces into grams, multiply the pounds by 453.6 and the ounces by 28.4 and add the two products. Thus, to convert 7 pounds, 5 ounces, 7 × 453.6 = 3175; 5 × 28.4 = 142; 3175 + 142 = 3317 grams.

Aid for Visualization of Cervical Dilatation

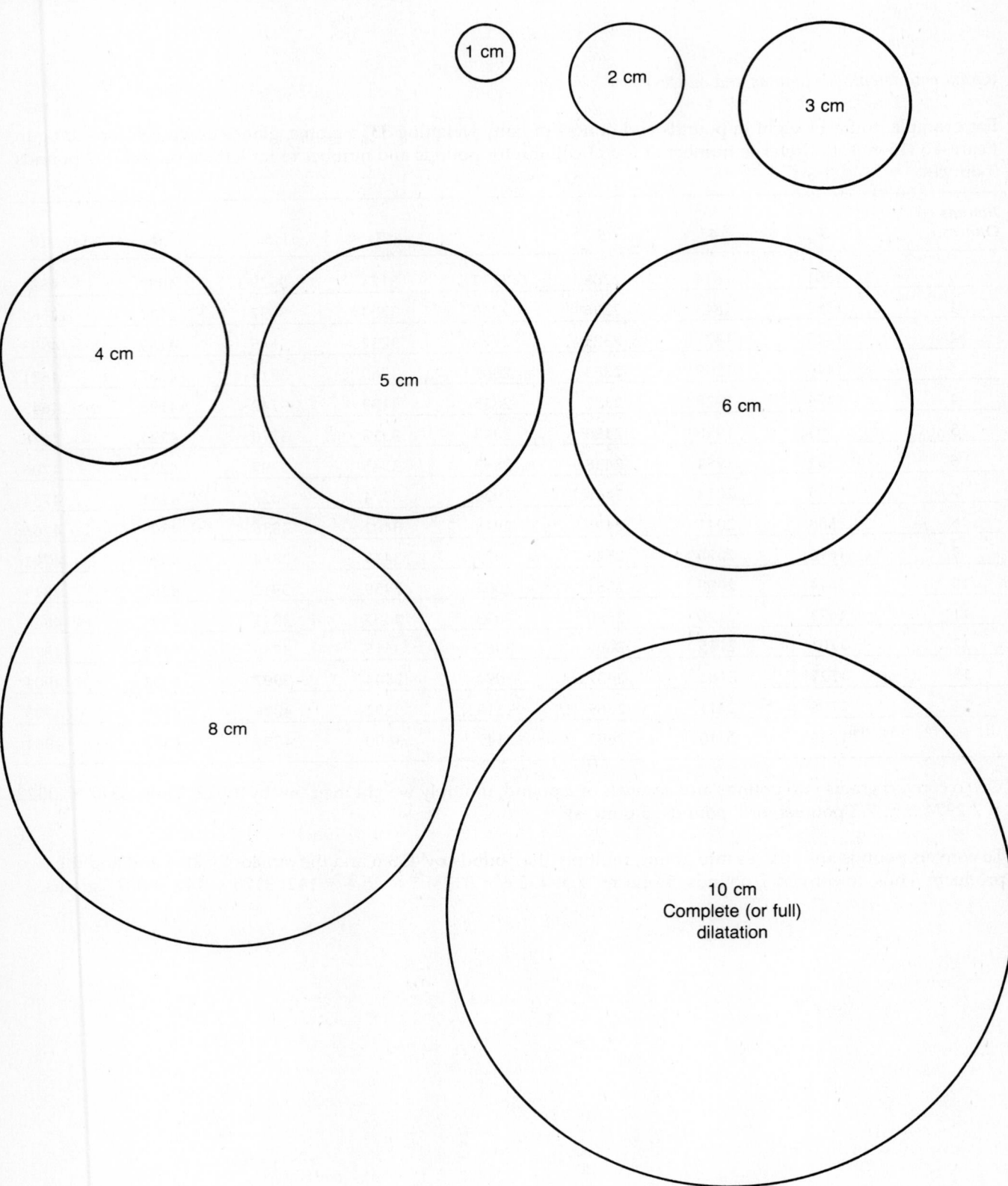

Resources for Maternal-Care Nurses

Abortion

Pro Choice

National Abortion Rights Action League
1424 K St, NW
Washington, DC 20005

Pro Life

National Right to Life Committee
419 7th St, NW
Washington, DC 20045

Alternative Lifestyles

National Gay Task Force
80 Fifth Ave, Suite 1601
New York, NY 10011

Parents and Friends of Gays and Lesbians
PO Box 24565
Los Angeles, CA 90025

or

5715 16th St, NW
Washington, DC 20011

Journals

Alternative Lifestyles
Human Sciences Press
72 Fifth Ave
New York, NY 10011

Journal of Homosexuality
Haworth Press
28 East 22nd St
New York, NY 10010

Breastfeeding

LaLeche International, Inc.
9616 Minneapolis Ave
Franklin Park, IL 60123

Childbirth Alternatives

American Academy of Husband-Coached Childbirth
PO Box 5224
Sherman Oaks, CA 91413

American College of Home Obstetrics
PO Box 25
River Forest, IL 60305

American Society of Childbirth Educators
PO Box 16159
7113 Lynwood Dr
Tampa, FL 33687

American Society for Psychoprophylaxis in Obstetrics
West 96th St
New York, NY 10025

Caesarean/Support, Education, and Concern
23 Cedar St
Cambridge, MA 02140

Childbirth Education Foundation
PO Box 37
Apalachin, NY 13732

Childbirth Without Pain Education Association
20134 Snowden
Detroit, MI 48235

Informed Homebirth
PO Box 788
Boulder, CO 80306

Maternity Center Association, Inc.
48 East 92nd St
New York, NY 10028

Family Planning

Association for Voluntary Sterilization
122 E 42nd St
New York, NY 10168

Planned Parenthood
1220 19th St, NW
Washington, DC 20036

Zero Population Growth
1346 Connecticut Ave, NW
Washington, DC 20036

Fertility and Infertility

American Fertility Foundation
1608 13th Ave, S, Suite 101
Birmingham, AL 35205

Association for Voluntary Sterilization, Inc
708 Third Ave
New York, NY 10164

Fertility Research Foundation
1430 Second Ave, Suite 103
New York, NY 10021

Surrogate Parenting Associates, Inc
Suite 222, Doctor's Office Building
250 E Liberty St
Louisville, KY 40205

Test-tube Fertilization
Eastern Virginia Medical School
Norfolk General Hospital
The Howard and Georgeanna Jones Institute for
    Reproductive Medicine
304 Medical Tower
Norfolk, VA 23507

Genetic Counseling

National Genetics Foundation
555 W 57th St
New York, NY 10019

Parenting and Abuse

American Association for Marriage and Family Therapy
1717 K St, NW, Suite 407
Washington, DC 20006

Association of Planned Parenthood Professionals
810 Seventh Ave
New York, NY 10019

Department of Health, Education and Welfare
National Center on Child Abuse and Neglect
US Children's Bureau
Office of Child Development
PO Box 1182
Washington, DC 20013

Grief Institute
PO Box 623
Englewood, CO 80151

National Center for the Prevention and Treatment of
    Child Abuse and Neglect
Department of Pediatrics
University of Colorado Medical Center
1205 Oneida St
Denver, CO 80220
    (National Child Protection Newsletter)

National Committee for Prevention of Child Abuse
Suite 510
111 East Wacker Dr
Chicago, IL 60601

National Foundation for Sudden Infant Death, Inc
1501 Broadway
New York, NY 10036

Parenting Materials Information Center
Southwest Educational Development Laboratory
211 E 7th St
Austin, TX 78701

Parents Anonymous
2810 Artesia Blvd
Redondo Beach, CA 90278

Parents of Premature and High Risk Infants International
33 W 42nd St, Suite 1227
New York, NY 10036

Parents Without Partners
7910 Woodmont Ave
Washington, DC 20014

Single Mothers by Choice
501 12th St
Brooklyn, NY 11215

Journals

Family Relations
National Council on Family Relations
1219 University Ave, SE
Minneapolis, MN 55414

Journal of Marriage and the Family
National Council on Family Relations
1219 University Ave, SE
Minneapolis, MN 55414

Professional Organizations

American Association for Maternal and Child Health
233 Prospect, P-209
La Jolla, CA 92037

American College of Nurse-Midwives
1522 K St, NW, Suite 1120
Washington, DC 20005

American College of Obstetricians and Gynecologists
600 Maryland Ave, SW, Suite 300
Washington, DC 20024

American Foundation for Maternal and Child Health
30 Beekman Pl
New York, NY 10022

Maternity Center Association
48 E 92nd St
New York, NY 10028

Public Health Organizations

American Public Health Association
1015 15th St, NW
Washington, DC 20005

American Red Cross
18th and E Sts, NW
Washington, DC 20006

Centers for Disease Control
Atlanta, GA 30333

Medic Alert Foundation
PO Box 1009
Turlock, CA 95380

National Institutes of Health
Bethesda, MD 20014

Project HOPE Health Sciences Education Center
Millwood, VA 22646

Rape

National Center for Prevention and Control of Rape
5600 Fishers Land
Rockville, MD 20857

Sex Education

Council for Sex Information and Education
Box 23088
Washington, DC 20024

Sex Information and Education Council of the United
  States
80 Fifth Ave, Suite 801
New York, NY 10011

Sexual Therapy

American Association of Sex Educators, Counselors, and
  Therapists
11 Dupont Circle, Suite 220
Washington, DC 20036

Center for Marital and Sexual Studies
5199 East Pacific Coast Hy
Long Beach, CA 90804

Masters and Johnson Institute
24 South Kings Highway
St Louis, MO 63108

Loyola Sexual Dysfunction Clinic
Loyola University Hospital
2160 S 1st Ave
Maywood, IL 60153

Society for Sex Therapy
% Barry McCarthy, PhD
Department of Psychology
The American University
Washington, DC 20016

Sexuality

Sex and Disability Unit
Human Sexuality Program
University of California
814 Mission St, 2nd Floor
San Francisco, CA 94103

Journal

Sexuality and Disability
Human Sciences Press
72 Fifth Ave
New York, NY 10011

Sexually Transmitted Diseases

American Social Health Association
260 Sheridan Rd
Palo Alto, CA 94306

Centers for Disease Control
Technical Information Services
Bureau of State Services
Atlanta, GA 30333

Herpes Resource Information
Box 100
Palo Alto, CA 94302

National AIDS Hotline
1-800-342-2437

National VD Hotline
1-800-227-8922
(in California, 1-800-982-5883)

Substance Abuse

Alcoholics Anonymous
PO Box 459, Grand Central Station
New York, NY 10017

National Clearinghouse for Alcohol Information
Box 2345
Rockville, MD

National Clearinghouse for Drug Abuse Information
5454 Wisconsin Ave
Chevy Chase, MD 20015

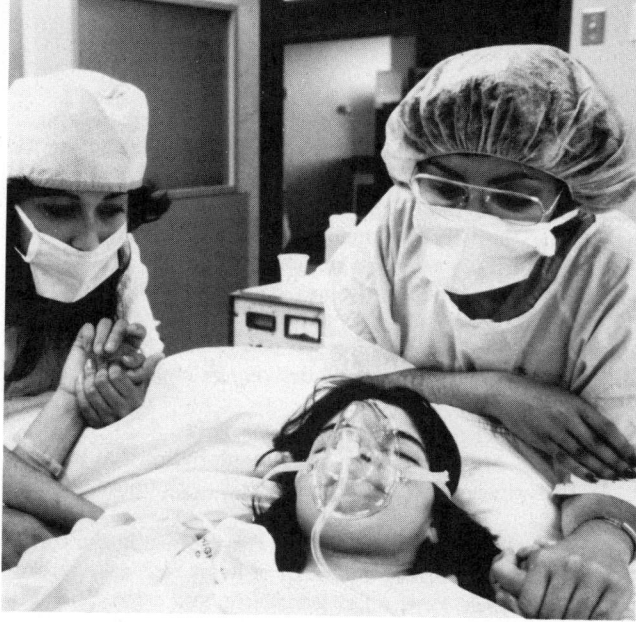

Glossary

ABC. Abbreviation for *alternate birth center*.

abdominal. Belonging to or relating to the abdomen.

  a. delivery. Delivery of the child by abdominal section. See *cesarean section*.

  a. gestation. Ectopic pregnancy occurring in the cavity of the abdomen.

  a. lifting. The lifting of the abdominal wall with the hands to reduce abdominal pressure on the uterus during a contraction in labor.

  a. pregnancy. See *a. gestation*.

abduction. The drawing or pulling away (of a part of the body) from the median axis.

ablatio placentae. Premature separation of the normally implanted placenta.

abortion. The termination of pregnancy at any time before the fetus has attained a stage of viability (*i.e.,* before it is capable of extrauterine existence).

  complete a. An abortion in which all the products of conception are passed and identified.

  criminal a. An abortion performed illegally.

  habitual a. An abortion that occurs in the third pregnancy or in subsequent pregnancies.

  incomplete a. An abortion in which some but not all the products of conception are passed.

  induced a. An abortion that is produced deliberately and intentionally.

  inevitable a. The condition that precedes an abortion that will proceed naturally. Vaginal bleeding is profuse, the membranes may have ruptured, and the cervix may have become dilated.

  missed a. The condition in which the embryo has died and subsequently the products of conception are retained in the uterus.

  spontaneous a. An abortion that starts of its own accord; commonly called a miscarriage.

  therapeutic a. An interruption of pregnancy before the 20th week, performed for medical reasons.

  threatened a. The condition in which vaginal bleeding or spotting occurs in early pregnancy and the cervix is not dilated. The symptoms may subside and the pregnancy may proceed to full term.

abruptio placentae. Premature separation of a normally implanted placenta. The separation may be complete or partial and very often is considered a medical emergency.

acidosis. A condition resulting in an increase in hydrogen ion concentration causing a lowering of blood pH below 7.35.

  metabolic a. Increase in hydrogen ion concentration caused by increased abnormal metabolism (too many acids produced), renal malfunction (acids not being excreted), or excessive loss of base (diarrhea).

acinus cell. Pl. *acini cells.* Milk-secreting cell contained in a lobule of the breast.

acquired immune deficiency syndrome. A new syndrome characterized by the occurrence in previously healthy individuals of *Pneumocystis carinii* pneumonia or other opportunistic infections or the rare malignancy Kaposi's sarcoma. Abnormal T-cell mechanisms are found in victims of this disease.

acrocyanosis. Cyanosis of the extremities, especially of the hands and feet, seen in the newborn for the first few hours after birth.

acromion. An outward extension of the spine of the scapula, used to explain presentation of the fetus.

acrosome. The caplike structure at the head of a sperm cell that contains enzymes believed to play an important role in the entrance of the sperm cell into the ovum.

adduction. The drawing or pulling (of a part of the body) toward the median axis.

adenoma. An epithelial tumor, usually benign, with a glandlike structure.

adnexa. Appendages.

  a. uterine. The fallopian tubes and ovaries.

adolescence. The period of life beginning at puberty, when the secondary sex characteristics begin to develop and the capacity for reproduction is reached, and ending with adulthood.

adrenocorticotropic hormone (ACTH). Pituitary hormone that stimulates the adrenal cortex.

afferent. Centripetal; bringing toward a central part, as afferent nerves convey stimuli to the central nervous system.

afibrinogenemia. Lack of fibrinogen in the blood.

afterbirth. The structures cast off after the expulsion of the fetus, including the membranes and the placenta with the attached umbilical cord; the secundines.

afterpains. Those pains, more or less severe, after expulsion of the afterbirth, which result from the contractile efforts of the uterus to return to its normal condition.

agalactia. Absence or failure of the secretion of milk.

albuminuria. The presence of albumin in the urine.

alert inactivity period. Time at which the infant's eyes are open and limb movements are quiet.

alkalosis.   A condition resulting from the loss of base, or depletion of acid without comparable loss of base, from body fluids.

allantois.   A tubular diverticulum of the posterior part of the yolk sac of the embryo. It passes into the body stalk through which it is accompanied by the allantoic (umbilical) blood vessel, thus taking part in the formation of the umbilical cord; later, it fuses with the chorion and helps to form the placenta.

allele.   One of two or more alternate genes that occur at a particular locus of a chromosome which decide alternate inherited characteristics.

alternate birth center (ABC).   An organization of a hospital or a free-standing labor and delivery area that provides a homelike atmosphere. It has liberal policies regarding the presence of family and friends, labor practices, no separation of parents and infant, and early discharge.

amenorrhea.   Absence or suppression of the menstrual discharge.

amniocentesis.   The perforation, by use of a needle, through the abdominal wall into the uterus to obtain a sample of amniotic fluid, for the purpose of fetal genetic or fetal maturity diagnosis.

amnion.   The most internal of the fetal membranes, containing the waters that surround the fetus *in utero.*

amnioscope.   An instrument for examination of the fetus and amniotic fluid by passage through the maternal abdominal wall into the amniotic cavity, thus permitting direct visualization.

amniotic.   Pertaining to the amnion.
  a. fluid.   The clear fluid that is 98% water contained in the amnion. This fluid provides protection to the fetus, keeps the temperature constant, and provides some nourishment to the fetus. Also called *liquor amnii.*
  a.f. embolism.   The blocking of a maternal artery with amniotic fluid forced into it by strong uterine contractions.
  a. sac.   The "bag of membrane" containing the fetus before delivery.

amniotomy.   The artificial rupture of the amniotic sac to induce labor.

analgesic.   Drug that relieves pain, used during labor.

analogue.   A chemical compound with a structure similar to that of another but differing from it with respect to a certain component. It may have similar or opposite action metabolically.

androgen.   Any hormonal substance that possesses masculinizing activities, such as the testis hormone.

android.   The term adopted for the male type of pelvis.

andrology.   The scientific study of the male constitution and diseases, especially male reproductive problems.

anemia.   A condition of the blood in which there is a deficiency in the red blood cells per unit volume, in the quantity of hemoglobin, or in the total volume.

anencephaly.   A congenital deformity characterized by absence of the cerebrum, cerebellum, and flat bones of the skull.

anesthesia.   The loss of sensation or feeling, especially the feeling of pain.

anomaly.   An organ or structure that is malformed or in some way abnormal with reference to form, structure, or position.

anorexia.   The loss of appetite.

anovular.   Not accompanied with the discharge of an ovum; said of cyclic uterine bleeding.

anoxia.   Oxygen deficiency; any condition of absence of tissue oxidation.

antenatal.   Occurring or formed before birth.

antepartal.   Before labor and delivery or childbirth; prenatal.

anthropoid pelvis.   See *pelvis, anthropoid.*

antibody.   Any of the body immunoglobulins that interact with antigens, neutralize toxins, and agglutinate bacteria or cells.

Apgar scoring system.   A system for appraising the condition of a newborn on the basis of heart rate, respiratory effort, muscle tone, reflex irritability, and color. The maximum score is 10. The evaluation is done at 60 seconds after birth, then again at 5 minutes and at 10 minutes if the neonate is unstable.

apnea.   Cessation of aspirations for more than 10 seconds associated with generalized cyanosis.

arachnodactyly.   A hereditary metabolic disorder characterized by abnormally long and slender fingers and toes. Also called Marfan's syndrome.

areola.   The ring of pigment surrounding the nipple.
  secondary a.   A circle of faint color sometimes seen just outside the original areola about the fifth month of pregnancy.

arousal.   Period when the infant moves from sleep state or drowsiness to awakeness or crying.

arrhythmia.   Variation from the normal heartbeat rhythm.

articulation.   The fastening together of the various bones of the skeleton in their natural situation; a joint. The articulations of the bones of the body are divided into two principal groups—*synarthroses,* immovable articulations, and *diarthroses,* movable articulations.

artificial feeding.   Feeding an infant by bottle rather than at the mother's breast.

artificial insemination.   The introduction of semen into the cervix or vagina by artificial means.

artificial menopause.   The cessation of menstruation by artificial means such as surgery or irradiation.

Aschheim–Zondek test.   See *test, Aschheim–Zondek.*

asexual.   Having no sex or functional sexual organs.

Asherman's syndrome.   See *syndrome, Asherman's.*

asphyxia.   Suspended animation; anoxia and carbon dioxide retention resulting from failure of respiration.
  a. neonatorum.   "Asphyxia of the newborn"; deficient respiration in newborn babies. Also called *neonatal asphyxia.*

asthma.   A condition marked by recurring attacks of spasmodic dyspnea with wheezing. May be caused by allergies, vigorous exercise, psychological stress, and so on.

atelectasis.   The incomplete expansion of a lung or the collapse of a lung.

atonic.   Lacking the tone or strength that is normally present.

atresia.   Absence of a normally patent passageway.

atrial septal defect.   A congenital cardiac anomaly in

which there is an abnormal opening between the right and left atria of the heart.

attitude. A posture or position of the body. In obstetrics, the relation of the fetal parts to each other in the uterus. The basic attitude is either flexion or extension.

auscultation. The act of listening for sounds within the body. Used to ascertain the fetal heart.

autosome. Any of the 22 ordinary paired chromosomes as distinguished from the 2 sex chromosomes.

axis. A line about which any revolving body turns.

　pelvic a. The curved line that passes through the centers of all the anteroposterior diameters of the pelvis.

azoospermia. The absence of spermatozoa in the semen.

back labor. A condition that occurs in one fourth of all labors when the position of the fetus is such that the back of the head is directed to the mother's back or turned toward her sacrum. Extreme discomfort is felt by the mother as labor progresses.

bag of waters. The membranes that enclose the liquor amnii of the fetus. See *amniotic sac.*

ballottement. Literally means tossing. A term used in examination when the fetus can be pushed about in the pregnant uterus.

Bandl's ring. A groove on the uterus at the upper level of the fully developed lower uterine segment; visible on the abdomen after hard labor as a transverse or slightly slanting depression between the umbilicus and the pubis. Shows overstretching of lower uterine segment. Resembles a full bladder.

Barr body. The persistent mass of the material of the inactivated X chromosome in cells of normal females. Also called *sex chromatin.*

Bartholin's glands. Glands situated one on each side of the vaginal canal opening into the groove between the hymen and the labia minora.

basal body temperature (BBT). The resting temperature taken in the morning before arising or performing any activity. Characteristic changes in BBT that usually occur in fertile women are used to identify the time ovulation has occurred.

bearing down. Reflex effort by the mother to help with the uterine contractions.

bicornate uterus. Having two horns that, in the embryo, failed to attain complete fusion.

bilirubin. The principal pigment of the bile, reddish yellow in color.

bilirubinemia. The presence of bilirubin in the blood.

bimanual. Performed with or relating to both hands.

　b. palpation. Examination of the pelvic organs of a woman by placing one hand on the abdomen and the fingers of the other in the vagina.

biparietal diameter. Largest transverse diameter of the fetal head.

birthing room. A room with homelike decor in which the family labors, delivers, and recovers.

bisexuality. The experiencing of sexual eroticism and genital intimacy with partners of both sexes.

blastocyst. The product of conception after the morula stage and before the embryonic stage.

blastoderm. The outer layer of cells of a fertilized ovum in the blastula stage.

　b. vesicle. Hollow space within the morula formed by the rearrangement of cells, and by proliferation.

blastula. The fertilized ovum in the stage in which the cells are arranged in a hollow ball.

body image. The way one pictures one's body.

boggy. Inadequately contracted and having a spongy rather than firm feeling, descriptive of the postdelivery uterus.

bonding. The process by which the human infant becomes attached to his parents.

bony pelvis. Ring of bone containing the sacrum, the coccyx, and two innominate bones.

brachial palsy. See *palsy, brachial.*

Bracht maneuver. See *maneuver, Bracht.*

bradycardia. Slowness of the heartbeat below normal.

brain growth spurt period. A period of accelerated growth and vulnerability to environmental events.

Braxton Hicks contractions. Uterine contractions, occurring periodically during pregnancy, thereby enlarging the uterus to accommodate the growing fetus. During the third trimester, they are felt as a painless hardening or tightening of the uterus. They can become painful and are often difficult to differentiate from labor. Also called *B. H. sign.*

　B.H. version. One of the types of operation designed to turn the baby from an undesirable position to a desired one.

breakthrough bleeding. Vaginal spotting or bleeding that occurs between menstrual periods, due to failure of oral contraceptive to support the endometrium adequately.

breast milk jaundice. A condition that occasionally occurs due to a substance in breast milk that inhibits the conjugation of bilirubin. May be treated by temporary or permanent cessation of breast-feeding.

breech. Nates or buttocks.

　b. delivery. Labor and delivery marked by breech presentations.

bregma. The point on the surface of the skull at the junction of the coronal and sagittal sutures.

brim. The edge of the superior strait or inlet of the pelvis.

broad ligament. Fibrous sheath covered by peritoneum extending from each side of the uterus to the lateral wall of the pelvis.

bronchopulmonary dysplasia. A chronic lung disease in infants believed to be associated with oxygen toxicity. It is often preceded by severe respiratory distress syndrome and treatment in a high-oxygen evironment.

cachexia. Weight loss and wasting associated with systemic illness.

caked breast. See *engorgement.*

Candida albicans. A yeastlike fungus that causes infections in the human being, commonly involving the mucous membranes of the mouth and vagina. During pregnancy, women are more susceptible to candidal infections due to the changed *p*H of the vagina and increased glycogen in vaginal cells.

candidiasis. A vaginal infection caused by *Candida albicans* with characteristic increased discharge and pruritus.

capacitation. The process by which a spermatozoon is conditioned to fertilize an ovum after it is exposed to the female reproductive tract.

caput. 1. The head, consisting of the cranium, or skull, and the face. 2. Any prominent object, such as the head.

> **c. succedaneum.** An edematous swelling that sometimes appears on the presenting head of the fetus during labor.

carcinogen. A chemical or other substance that can induce or promote cancer.

cardiac anomalies. Anomalies that result from congenital heart defects. These include transposition of the great vessels, atrial septal defect, patent ductus arteriosus, ventricular septal defect, coarctation of the aorta, the tetralogy of Fallot, and others.

catamenia. See *menses.*

catheterization. The use of a tubular instrument for withdrawing fluids from (or introducing into) a body cavity, especially the bladder through the urethra for the withdrawal of urine.

caudal. The term applied to analgesia or anesthesia resulting from the introduction of the suitable analgesic or anesthetic solution into the caudal canal (nonclosure of the laminae of the last sacral vertebra).

caul. A portion of the amniotic sac that occasionally envelops the child's head at birth.

cellulitis. Inflammation of cellular tissue.

cephalhematoma. A tumor or swelling between the cranium and the periosteum caused by an effusion of blood.

cephalic. Belonging to the head.

> **c. presentation.** Presentation of any part of the fetal head in labor.

cephalopelvic disproportion (CPD). A condition in which the fetal head is disproportionately large for passage through the maternal pelvis.

cerclage. Encircling of a part with a wire, metal band, or suture, as for correction of an incompetent cervix.

cerebral palsy. See *palsy, cerebral.*

cerebroside lipidosis. See *disease, Gaucher's.*

cervical mucus. The secretion of the mucous membrane of the cervix.

cervical dilation. See *dilation, cervical.*

cervix. Neckline part; the lower and narrow end of the uterus, between the os and the body of the organ.

cesarean delivery. Delivery of the fetus by an incision through the abdominal wall and the wall of the uterus.

> **classical c.d.** A cesarean delivery that involves a vertical incision in the abdomen over the fundus and baby and then a vertical incision into the upper uterine segment.
>
> **extraperitoneal c.d.** A cesarean section performed when intrauterine infection is present. The incision is low, and the bladder must be dissected off the uterus.
>
> **low-segment c.d.** A cesarean delivery in which the incision is made into the lower uterine segment, either transversely or vertically.

Chadwick's sign. The violet color on the mucous membrane of the vagina just below the urethral orifice, seen after the fourth week of pregnancy.

change of life. See *climacteric.*

Chlamydia trachomatis. An organism responsible for a spectrum of diseases including cervicitis, urethritis, acute salpingitis, and endometritis.

chloasma. Pl. *chloasmata.* A cutaneous affliction which exhibits spots and patches of a yellowish brown color. The term *cloasma* is a vague one and is applied to various kinds of pigmentary discoloration of the skin.

> **c. gravidarum, c. uterinum.** Chloasma occurring during pregnancy.

chorioamnionitis. An intrauterine infection involving mononuclear and polymorphonuclear leukocytic infiltration of the fetal membranes and amniotic fluid.

chorion. The outermost membrane of the growing zygote, or fertilized ovum, which serves as a protective and nutritive covering.

chorionic villus. Pl. *villi.* One of the villi growing in tufts on the external surface of the chorion.

chromosomal sex. The determination of the sex of an individual by the configuration of chromosomes in his cells (*i.e.*, XY is the male configuration, and XX is the female configuration).

chromosome. One of several small, dark-staining and more or less rod-shaped bodies that appear in the nucleus of the cell at the time of cell divisions and particularly in mitosis.

chromosome disorder. Abnormality of chromosome number or structure.

cilium. Pl. *cilia.* One of the hairlike projections of a structure such as the fallopian tube. The cilia of the fallopian tube beat in such a manner as to direct any overlying fluid in the direction of the uterine cavity. Thus, the cilia are partially responsible for the transportation on an ovum along the tube.

circumcision. The removal of all or part of the prepuce, or foreskin, of the penis.

cleavage. The series of cell divisions that occur during the development of a fertilized ovum into an embryo when the structure remains the same size while the cleavage cells become smaller and smaller.

cleft lip. Congenital incomplete closure of the lip.

cleft palate. Congenital fissure of the palate and the roof of the mouth.

climacteric. A particular epoch of the ordinary term of life at which the body undergoes a considerable change, especially the menopause or "change of life."

climax. See *orgasm.*

clitoris. A small, elongated, erectile body situated at the anterior part of the vulva. An organ of the female homologous with the penis of the male.

clonus. A series of rapid, rhythmic contractions of a muscle occurring involuntarily in response to stretching of the muscle.

clubfoot. A congenitally deformed foot. See *talipes equinovarus.*

coarctation of the aorta. A congenital cardiac anomaly in which there is a constriction of the aorta, causing narrowing of the lumen. This partially obstructs blood flow, creating increased left ventricular pressure and work load.

coccyx. The bone at the caudal end of the spine. In a child the coccyx consists of four or five separate vertebrae; in an adult these bones are fused into one.

cognition. The reasoning, logic, intentional thought, problem-solving, thinking ability of the infant.

coitus. Sexual intercourse, copulation.

c. interruptus. The practice of withdrawal as a means of contraception. The penis is withdrawn from the vagina before ejaculation.

colostrum. The thin, yellow fluid, high in protein and inorganic salts, that is secreted from the breasts during the last weeks of pregnancy and the 3 days after delivery before milk is produced.

c. corpuscles. Large granular cells found in colostrum.

colporrhaphy. 1. The operation of suturing the vagina. 2. The operation of denuding and suturing the vaginal wall for the purpose of narrowing the vagina.

colposcope. A viewing instrument designed for close examination of the tissues of the cervix, similar to a low-magnification microscope with binocular vision.

colpotomy. Any surgical cutting operation upon the vagina.

commissure. A site of union of corresponding parts.

compliance, lung. Degree of distensibility of the lung's elastic tissue.

conception. The impregnation of the female ovum by the spermatozoon of the male, whence results a new being.

conceptus. Products of conception.

condom. A sheath worn over the penis during sexual intercourse to prevent sperm from entering the vagina.

condyloma. Pl. *condylomata.* A wartlike excrescence near the anus or the vulva; the flat, moist papule of secondary syphilis.

confinement. Term applied to childbirth and the lying-in period.

congenital. Born with a person; existing from or from before birth, as, for example, congenital disease, a disease originating in the fetus before birth.

congenital anomaly. Abnormality present at birth.

conjugate. The anteroposterior diameter of the pelvic inlet.

conjunctivitis. Inflammation of the conjunctiva, the membrane lining the eyelids, generally associated with a discharge.

constipation. The infrequent or difficult passage of feces.

contraception. The prevention of conception or impregnation.

contracted pelvis. See *pelvis, contracted.*

contraction. The intermittent shortening of a muscle, especially the uterus during labor in order to expel the contents.

convulsion. An involuntary and violent contraction of voluntary muscles.

Coombs' test. A test used to detect sensitized red blood cells in erythroblastosis fetalis.

indirect C.t. Determination of Rh-positive antibodies in maternal blood.

direct C.t. Determination of maternal Rh-positive antibodies in fetal cord blood.

cor pulmonale. Heart disease secondary to disease of the lungs or lung blood vessels; a type of heart failure.

corona radiata. The layer of follicular cells arranged in a radial pattern that envelop the zona pellucida of the ovum.

coronal. Belonging to, or relating to, the crown of the head.

c. suture. The suture formed by the union of the frontal bone with the two parietal bones.

corpus albicans. The white fibrous tissue that replaces the corpus luteum in the ovary as it shrinks in the last stages of pregnancy.

corpus luteum. The yellow mass found in the graafian follicle after the ovum has been expelled.

cotyledon. Any one of the subdivisions of the uterine surface of the placenta.

Couvelaire uterus. A severe uterine condition seen in some cases of placental separation, when coagulation is impaired and there is extensive bleeding into the uterine muscle.

Cowper's gland. One of two glands located at the base of the prostate gland and on either side of the membranous urethra that produce a mucinous substance that lubricates the urethra and coats its surface.

CPD. Abbreviation for cephalopelvic disproportion.

cramp. A painful contraction of a muscle.

creatinine. The end product of metabolism, found in muscle and blood and excreted in the urine.

criminal abortion. See *abortion, criminal.*

crowning. The phase in the second stage of labor when a large part of the top of the fetal head is visible in the vaginal opening. The anus is open, and the perineum is distended.

cul-de-sac. [Fr.] A pouch or sac having only one end open.

Douglas' c. A sac or recess formed by a fold of the peritoneum dipping down between the rectum and the uterus. Also called *pouch of Douglas* and *rectouterine pouch.*

culdoscopy. A visual examination of the organs of a female pelvis with an endoscope.

cumulus oophorus. A loosely arranged solid mass of cells surrounding the ovum in the ovarian follicle.

curanderas. f.; **curanderos** m. Mexican–American folk healer.

curettage. [Fr.] The removal of substances from the wall of a cavity, especially the uterine cavity, with a spoon-shaped instrument called a curet.

cyanosis. A bluish discoloration of the skin or mucous membranes as a result of an excessive concentration of hemoglobin that is not combined with oxygen in the blood.

cyesis. Pregnancy.

cystitis. An infection or inflammation of the urinary bladder.

cystocele. The pouching downward of the bladder through the vaginal wall.

cytomegalic inclusion disease. See *disease, cytomegalic inclusion.*

cytomegalovirus. A herpesvirus that produces unique large cells bearing intranuclear inclusions.

D & C. Abbreviation for dilatation and curettage.

D & E. Abbreviation for dilatation and evacuation.

decidua. The endometrium of a pregnant uterus, which, except for the deepest layer, is shed during childbirth.

　d. basalis. The part of the decidua directly underneath the chorionic vesicle and attached to the myometrium, the main muscular mass of the uterus.

decrement. Decrease; also the stage of decline.

delivery. [Fr., *délivrer*, to free, to deliver.] 1. The expulsion of a child by the mother, or its extraction by the obstetric practitioner. 2. The removal of a part from the body, for example, *delivery* of the placenta.

deoxyribonucleic acid (DNA). Chemical forming the genetic code; it occurs as a double-stranded helix within chromosomes.

descent. Passage of the presenting part of the fetus into and through the birth canal; it begins at the onset of labor and proceeds during effacement and dilatation of the cervix.

detumescence. The subsidence of swelling, congestion, or turgor; the period in which the organ or passage decreases in size and returns to its original state.

diabetes or **diabetes mellitus.** An endocrine disorder that involves disruption of normal carbohydrate metabolism caused by a deficiency of insulin. Because there is a significant change in the course of diabetes when pregnancy intervenes, close supervision of the prenatal care of a diabetic gravida is required.

　gestational d. Diabetes initially diagnosed during pregnancy, due to glucose intolerance.

diagonal conjugate measurement. The chief internal pelvic measurement made to determine the actual diameter of the pelvic passage. It is the distance between the sacral promontory and the lower margin of the symphysis pubis.

diamniotic dichorionic twins. See *twins, diamniotic dichorionic.*

diamniotic monochorionic twins. See *twins, diamniotic monochorionic.*

diaphragm. 1. The partition separating the abdominal and thoracic cavities made of muscle and membrane. 2. A contraceptive device made of rubber that is inserted in the vagina to act like a cap over the cervix. To be effective, the device is used with spermicidal cream or jelly.

diaphragmatic. Pertaining to the diaphragm.

　d. hernia. A defect in the development of the diaphragm, which allows the abdominal organs to herniate into the thoracic cavity.

　d. paralysis. A condition resulting from injury to the phrenic nerve during a difficult breech delivery. The paralysis is usually one sided, with irregular thoracic respirations, no abdominal movement on inspiration on the affected side, and cyanosis.

diarrhea. Abnormally frequent and liquid fecal discharges.

diastasis recti. Separation of the abdominal recti muscles, which may occur during pregnancy because of stretching of the abdominal wall.

Dick–Read approach to childbirth. The approach that is based on the understanding that fear of pain produces muscular tension, which produces pain and greater fear. This approach includes an educational program to teach physiological processes of labor, exercise to improve muscle tone, and techniques to assist in relaxation and prevent the fear–tension–pain mechanism. Also called *Read method of childbirth preparation.*

dilatation and curettage (D & C). A method of emptying the contents of the uterus by using cervical dilatation and curettage. The technique is widely used for first-trimester abortions.

dilatation and evacuation (D & E). See *suction curettage.*

dilation. The act of dilating or stretching.

　cervical d. The opening of the cervix to accommodate the birth of the fetus.

dimorphism. The manifestation in the same species of two forms, such as male and female; refers to both bodily form and appearance and to sex differences in behavior and language.

disease. Any departure from health of a structure, organ, or system.

　cytomegalic inclusion d. A disease caused by a group of species specific herpes virus, that inhabit the human salivary glands.

　Gaucher's d. A lipidosis in which the fatty accumulation in the body is largely kerasin. In the infant form, it is characterized by yellow pigmentation of the skin and marked impairment of the central nervous system. It is also known as *cerebroside lipidosis* and is a hereditary defect of the metabolism.

　hemolytic d. Anemia in a fetus or newborn caused by antibodies that are transmitted from the mother due to the incompatibility between the blood group of the mother and her child.

　Hurler's d. (gargoylism). A hereditary disorder caused by an enzyme deficiency. It is characterized by gargoylelike features of the head (depressed bridge of the nose, large prominent tongue, and widely spaced teeth), dwarf structure, short neck, broad short hands, severe mental retardation, blindness, deafness, and cardiovascular defects.

　hyaline membrane d. (HMD). A disease of premature infants characterized by the formation of a translucent membrane in the respiratory passages and the incapacity of the lungs to expand adequately. Also known as respiratory distress syndrome (RDS).

　Niemann–Pick d. A lipidosis characterized by brownish yellow discoloration of the skin and nervous system involvement. It is a hereditary disease and is also known as *sphingomyelin lipidosis.*

　Tay–Sachs d. A hereditary metabolic disorder also known as *ganglioside lipidosis.* It is characterized by a degeneration of brain cells and a red spot on each retina, and eventually by dementia, blindness, paralysis, and death.

　venereal d. One of a number of infectious diseases that are transmitted through sexual contact and may be localized or systemic. Common types are gonorrhea, syphilis, condylomata (venereal warts), and herpes simplex type II.

　Wilson–Mikity d. See *pulmonary dysmaturity.*

disseminated intravascular coagulation. An acquired disorder in which there is acceleration of thrombi formation and also increasing fibrinolytic activity resulting in hemorrhage. The disorder can be either chronic or acute. In obstetrics it is usually acute and considered a medical emergency.

diuresis. An increased excretion of urine.

diuretic. An agent that promotes urine excretion.

dizygotic. Pertaining to or proceeding from two zygotes (ova).

   d. twins. See *twins, dizygotic.*

Döderlein's bacillus. The large gram-positive bacterium occurring in the normal vaginal secretion.

dominant inheritance. The acquiring of a characteristic by transmission in a gene from parents to their offspring regardless of the state of the corresponding allele.

Doppler. Device used to monitor fetal heart rate by ultrasound.

Douglas' cul-de-sac. See *cul-de-sac, Douglas.*

Down's syndrome. See *syndrome, Down's.*

ductus. A duct.

   d. arteriosus. "Arterial duct," a blood vessel peculiar to the fetus, communicating directly between the pulmonary artery and the aorta.

   d. venosus. "Venous duct," a blood vessel peculiar to the fetus, establishing a direct communication between the umbilical vein and the inferior vena cava.

Duncan mechanism. The position of the placenta, with the maternal surface outermost; to be born edgewise.

dyscrasia. A diseased condition.

dysmenorrhea. Painful menstruation.

dyspareunia. Painful intercourse, which can result from penetration, frictional movement, and deep thrusting.

dysplasia. Abnormality of the development of cells or a part.

dyspnea. Labored breathing.

dystocia. Difficult, slow, or painful birth or delivery. It is distinguished as maternal or fetal (*i.e.,* the difficulty is due to some deformity on the part of the mother or on the part of the child).

   d., placental. Difficulty in delivering the placenta.

eclampsia. A severe complication occurring in pregnancy or the early puerperium, characterized by hypertension, edema, albuminuria, convulsions, and coma.

ectocervix. The outer portion of the cervix visible on examination.

ectoderm. The outer layer of cells of the primitive embryo.

ectopic. Out of place.

   e. gestation. Gestation in which the fetus is out of its normal place in the cavity of the uterus. It includes gestations in the interstitial portion of the tube or in a rudimentary horn of the uterus (cornual pregnancy) and cervical pregnancy, as well as tubal, abdominal, and ovarian pregnancies. Also known as *ectopic pregnancy* and *extrauterine pregnancy.*

   e. pregnancy. Same as *ectopic gestation.*

ectropion. Eversion of an edge or margin, as of the columnar epithelium of the endocervical canal onto the ectocervix. The tissue appears darker pink-red and bumpy compared with the smooth pink squamous epithelium of the ectocervix.

EDC. Abbreviation for *expected date of confinement.*

edema. Abnormal swelling due to large amounts of fluid in the tissues.

effacement. Obliteration. In obstetrics, refers to thinning and shortening of the cervix.

efferent. Centrifugal; conveying away from a center, as efferent nerves convey stimuli to the peripheral nervous system.

effleurage. [Fr.] A rubbing movement, as in massage.

ejaculation. A sudden act of expulsion, as of semen.

electronic fetal monitor. A system for monitoring fetal heart rate and uterine activity by electrically operated instruments.

embolism. The sudden blocking of an artery or vein by a blood clot or other obstruction that was brought there by the blood current.

embolus. A clot or other obstruction brought to a vein or artery by the blood from a larger vessel.

embryo. The product of conception *in utero* from the third through the fifth week of gestation; after that length of time it is called the fetus.

embryonic disc. The flattish portion of a fertilized ovum in which the first traces of an embryo are seen.

empathy. The projection of one's own consciousness into that of another. Empathy may be distinguished from sympathy in that the former state includes relative freedom from emotional involvement.

encephalopathy. Any degenerative brain disease.

endocervical. Pertaining to the interior of the cervix of the uterus.

endocervix. 1. The mucous membrane lining of the cervical canal. 2. The region of the opening of the cervix into the uterine cavity.

endometriosis. Pathologic condition in which normal tissue that lines the uterus (endometrial tissue) grows outside of the uterus, often around the fallopian tubes, contributing to infertility.

endometritis. Inflammation of the endometrium.

endometrium. The mucous membrane that lines the uterus.

endorphin. An opiatelike substance produced by the body.

endoscope. An instrument used for viewing the interior of a hollow organ, as the bladder.

endotracheal intubation. The insertion of a tube into the trachea to be used to administer anesthesia, maintain an airway, or ventilate the lungs.

enema. A liquid injected into the rectum.

en face. [Fr.] The position in which the mother's face is rotated so that her eyes and those of her infant meet fully.

engagement. 1. In clinical obstetrics, applies to the entrance of the presenting part into the superior pelvic strait and the beginning of the descent through the pelvic canal. 2. Also relating to parent–infant interaction: behaviors designed to induce and sustain social interchanges.

engorgement. Hyperemia; local congestion; excessive fullness of any organ or passage. In obstetrics, refers to an exaggeration of normal venous and lymph stasis of the breasts, which occurs in relation to lactation.

enhancement.   The developmentally optimal level of stimulation.

entoderm.   The innermost layer of cells of the primitive embryo.

environment.   The animate and inanimate components of the infant's world.

enzygotic.   Developed from the same fertilized ovum.

epididymis.   Pl. *epididymides.*   A part of the canal system of the testes, made up of numerous seminiferous tubules. Its long coiled duct provides for storage, transit, and maturation of spermatozoa.

epidural anesthesia.   Anesthesia produced by injecting between the vertebral spines and beneath the ligamentum flavum into the extradural space. It is used in obstetric anesthesia to alleviate maternal pain with minimal danger to the infant. It requires the expertise that is afforded a surgical patient.

epinephrine.   A chemical hormone that is secreted by the adrenal medulla. It is released in response to hypoglycemia. This chemical is injected in infants of diabetic mothers to treat hypoglycemia.

episiotomy.   Surgical incision of the vulvar orifice for obstetric purposes.

epispadias.   A congenital anomaly in which the urethra opens on the dorsal surface of the penis. In severe cases, the upper wall of the urethra may be absent.

Epstein's pearls.   Small white cysts on the hard palate or gums of the newborn. They are not abnormal.

Erb's paralysis.   Partial paralysis of the brachial plexus, affecting various muscles of the arm and the chest wall.

erectile.   Capable of becoming rigid and elevated, such as erectile tissue, found in the penis, clitoris, and nipples.

ergonovine.   An alkaloid of ergot and a powerful oxytocic. May be administered intravenously, orally, or intramuscularly. This drug will cause an elevation of blood pressure.

ergot.   A drug having the remarkable property of exciting powerfully the contractile force of the uterus, and chiefly used for this purpose, but its long-continued use is highly dangerous. Usually given in the fluid extract.

erotic.   Pertaining to sensuousness or sensual arousal.

erythema toxicum.   A blotchy rash that may appear in the first few days of life. It develops more frequently on the back, shoulders, and buttocks. No treatment is necessary, and it will disappear in a day or so. It is also called "*newborn rash.*"

erythroblastosis fetalis.   A severe hemolytic disease of the newborn usually due to Rh incompatibility.

esophageal atresia.   A congenital defect in which the esophagus ends in a blind pouch rather than a continuous tube to the stomach. It is characterized by excessive drooling, gagging, coughing, vomiting when fed, cyanosis, and dyspnea. The condition is corrected by surgery.

estradiol.   An estrogen produced in ovarian follicles. It inhibits the release of follicle-stimulating hormones prior to ovulation.

estrogen.   The generic term for the female sex hormones. It is a steroid hormone produced primarily by the ovaries but also by the adrenal cortex. It is responsible for the development of secondary sex characteristics and the cyclic nature of female reproductive physiology.

expected date of confinement (EDC).   The calculated date for the birth of the fetus.

external rotation.   In childbirth, a change in the position of the fetus following the birth of the head during which the shoulders are born.

extraction, vacuum.   In assisted childbirth, the use of a metal cup applied to the fetal head by creating a vacuum between it and the head to assist in the delivery of a fetus. Traction is exerted by means of a short chain attached to the cup, with a handle at its far end.

extraperitoneal.   Situated or occurring outside the peritoneal cavity.

extrauterine.   Outside of the uterus.

e. pregnancy.   See *ectopic gestation.*

face presentation.   A less common head presentation in which the fetal face is presented in labor.

facies.   Pl. *facies.*   [L.] A term used in anatomy to refer to the front of the head from forehead to chin.

fallopian.   [Relating to G. *Fallopius,* a celebrated Italian anatomist of the 16th century.]

f. tubes.   The oviducts—two canals extending from the sides of the fundus uteri.

false labor.   A condition in the latter weeks of some pregnancies in which irregular uterine contractions are felt but the cervix is not affected.

false pelvis.   See *pelvis, false.*

family-centered care.   Maternity care that takes into account other members of the family, particularly fathers and children, in prenatal, intrapartum, and postpartum care of pregnant women.

fecundation.   The act of impregnating or the state of being impregnated; the fertilization of the ovum by means of the male seminal element.

fecundity.   The ability to produce offspring in large numbers in a short period of time.

ferning.   A fernlike pattern seen microscopically when cervical mucus is viewed under the microscope. The specimen is taken from the cervical area, usually obtained during a sterile speculum examination. The pattern confirms the presence of estrogen at midcycle in the menstruating woman. It also documents the rupture of amniotic fluid in the pregnant woman.

fertility.   The ability to produce offspring; power of reproduction.

f. awareness.   The development of familiarity with the bodily signs of impending ovulation and bodily signs after ovulation, which enables a woman to anticipate her fertile period and its ending.

f. rate.   The number of births per 1000 women aged 15 through 44 years.

fertilization.   The fusion of the spermatozoon with the ovum; it marks the beginning of pregnancy.

fetal. Pertaining to a fetus.

f. acidosis. A condition of a fetus resulting in the accumulation of acids or depletion of alkaline reserve in the blood and body tissues.

f. alcohol syndrome. See *syndrome, f. alcohol.*

f. bradycardia. Slowness of the fetal heartbeat.

f. distress. A condition of fetal difficulty *in utero* that can occur during either the antenatal or the intrapartum period. Signs are a fetal tachycardia, decrease in variability, and repetitive late or severe variable decelerations.

f. habitus. The attitude of the fetus, or the relation of the fetal parts to each other.

f. heart rate (FHR). The heart rate of the fetus. Normally, it can be heard about the middle of pregnancy and may vary between 120 to 160 beats per minute.

f. heart tones (FHT). The sounds of a fetal heart as heard by auscultation.

fetoscope. 1. A head stethoscope designed especially for listening to fetal heart tones. 2. An endoscope for viewing a fetus.

fetus. The baby *in utero* from the end of the fifth week of gestation until birth.

FHR. See *fetal heart rate.*

FHT. See *fetal heart tones.*

fibrinogenopenia. Decreased fibrinogen in the blood.

fibroid. See *myoma.*

fimbria. A fringe; especially the fringelike end of the fallopian tube.

fissure. A cleft or groove, which may be normal or abnormal. Anal fissures are painful linear ulcers at the margin of the anus.

fistula. An abnormal passage between two internal organs or between an organ and the surface of the body.

fixation. A sustained gaze on one point.

flaring of nostrils. Widening of nostrils during inspiration; a sign of respiratory distress.

flatulence. An excess amount of gas in the stomach or intestines.

flexion. The act of bending. In obstetrics, the process in the mechanism of labor referring to the bending of the fetal head so that the chin is in contact with the chest, thus presenting the smallest anteroposterior diameter to the pelvis.

foam, contraceptive. A spermicidal preparation that is inserted vaginally prior to intercourse to prevent conception. Its effectiveness is enhanced when it is used with a diaphragm.

folic acid. One of the vitamins of the B complex that is essential for growth and necessary to the proper formation of blood in the body.

follicle. A sac or pouchlike cavity.

follicle-stimulating hormone (FSH). A gonadotropic hormone secreted by the anterior pituitary, which stimulates the development of graafian follicles.

fontanel. The diamond-shaped space between the frontal and two parietal bones in very young infants. This is called the *anterior f.* and is the familiar "soft spot" just above a baby's forehead. A small, triangular one (*posterior f.*) is between the occipital and parietal bones.

footling breech. A breech presentation in which one or both feet or the knees extend below the buttocks. It is also known as incomplete breech presentation.

foramen. A hole, opening, aperture, or orifice—especially one through a bone.

f. ovale. An opening situated in the partition that separates the right and left auricles of the heart in the fetus.

forceps. A two-bladed instrument with a handle used for grasping tissues or sterile dressings in surgery. In obstetrics, one of several kinds of instruments used for assisting in the delivery of an infant after the cervix is dilated and the vertex of the fetal head is engaged.

foreskin. The prepuce—the fold of skin covering the glans penis.

fornix. Pl. *fornices.* An arch; any vaulted surface.

f. of the vagina. The angle of reflection of the vaginal mucous membrane onto the cervix uteri.

fourchette. [Fr., "fork."] The posterior angle or commissure of the labia majora.

frenulum linguae. A sharp, thin ridge of tissue that arises in the midline from the base of the tongue and is attached to its undersurface for varying distances. Depending upon this distance of attachment, it restrains the movement of the tongue. Also called *lingual frenum.*

frenum. A fold of mucous membrane that checks, curbs, or restrains the movements of a part.

lingual f. See *frenulum linguae.*

Friedman's curve. A graph designed to describe and record progress during labor.

Friedman's test. See *test, Friedman's.*

FSH. Abbreviation for *follicle-stimulating hormone.*

fundus. The upper rounded portion of the uterus between the points of insertion of the fallopian tubes.

funic souffle. A soft, blowing sound, synchronous with the fetal heart sounds and supposed to be produced in the umbilical cord.

funis. A cord—especially the umbilical cord.

galactagogue. 1. Causing the flow of milk. 2. Any drug that causes the flow of milk to increase.

galactorrhea. Prolonged and abnormal lactation, often profuse.

galactosemia. An inherited autosomal recessive disorder of galactose metabolism.

gamete. A sexual cell; a mature germ cell, as an unfertilized egg or a mature sperm cell.

Gamper method of childbirth preparation. One of a number of methods employed by parents for handling the discomforts of labor.

ganglioside lipidosis. See *disease, Tay–Sachs.*

gargoylism. See *disease, Hurler's.*

gastroenteritis. Inflammation of the stomach and intestines.

gastroschisis. An abdominal wall defect at the base of the umbilical stalk.

gastrostomy. Creation of an artificial opening into the stomach through the abdominal wall, used for feeding purposes.

gastrula.   The early embryonic stage that follows the blastula; the cuplike stage with two layers of cells.

gate control theory.   A theory proposed in 1965 by Melzack and Wall to explain the neurophysical mechanism underlying the sensation of pain.

Gaucher's disease.   See *disease, Gaucher's.*

gavage feeding.   Forced feeding, as through a tube into the stomach.

gender identity.   The sameness, unity, and persistence of one's individuality as male or female, or ambivalent, especially as experienced in self-awareness and behavior. Gender identity is the private experience of gender role.

gender role.   Everything one says and does to indicate to others or the self the degree to which one is male or female, or ambivalent. It includes but is not restricted to sexual arousal and response. Gender role is the public expression of gender identity.

gene.   A hereditary germinal factor in the chromosome that carries on a hereditary transmissible character.

genetic anomaly.   A marked deviation from the expected standard as a result of an inherited defect.

genetic counseling.   A process in which individuals or families are given information that is needed to understand a hereditary disorder.

genetics.   The study of heredity.

genital herpes.   A viral skin disease of the genitals marked by groups of vesicles 3 mm to 6 mm in diameter.

genitalia.   The reproductive organs.

genotype.   An individual's entire hereditary constitution.

gestation.   The condition of pregnancy; pregnancy; gravidity.

gestational age.   The age of the product of conception between fertilization and birth.

glomerular endotheliosis.   Overgrowth of the endothelium in the glomerulus.

glucose tolerance test (GTT).   See *test, glucose tolerance.*

glycosuria.   The presence of glucose (sugar) in the urine.

gonad.   A gamete-producing gland; an ovary or testis.

gonadal sex.   The sex of an individual determined by the presence of either testes or ovaries as gonads, or in the case of a true hermaphrodite, the presence of gonads of both sexes.

gonadotropin.   A substance produced by the anterior pituitary and placenta that has an affinity for or a stimulating effect on the gonads.

gonorrhea.   A disease spread by sexual contact that affects the mucosa of the genital tract. The disease may be asymptomatic in women, except for a vaginal discharge. It can produce puerperal infection if present in the cervix at the time of delivery. The infection can infect the infant's eyes at birth.

gonorrheal conjunctivitis.   A severe form of conjunctivitis caused by the bacteria of gonorrhea.

gonorrheal salpingitis.   An infection of the fallopian tube caused by the gonorrhea bacteria. It may cause a narrowing of the fallopian tube, which may subsequently prevent the passage of a fertilized ovum down the tube, resulting in a tubal pregnancy.

Goodell's sign.   Softening of the cervix, a presumptive sign of pregnancy.

gossypol.   A derivative of cottonseed oil that has male contraceptive actions by suppressing sperm production and affecting sperm structure and mobility.

graafian follicles or **vesicles.**   Small spherical bodies in the ovaries, each containing an ovum.

grasp reflex.   See *reflex, grasp.*

gravid.   Pregnant.

gravida.   A pregnant woman.

GTT.   Abbreviation for *glucose tolerance test.*

Guthrie method in PKU.   A method of diagnosing PKU. It is a blood test in which one or two drops of blood may be taken from an infant's heel; then the blood is tested to determine the phenylalanine level.

gynecoid pelvis.   See *pelvis, gynecoid.*

gynecology.   The branch of medicine that studies and treats women's diseases, especially of the genital tract.

Haase's rule.   A method for calculating the length of an embryo or fetus. During the first 5 months, the number of months should be squared to approximate the length in centimeters (*e.g.*, second month of pregnancy, the fetus is about 4 cm in length). After the fifth month, the number of months should be multiplied by 5.

Harvard pump.   A constant infusion pump used to administer oxytocin in labor.

HCG.   Abbreviation for *human chorionic gonadotropin.*

Health Systems Agency (HSA).   A regional agency within a state that has primary responsibility for health planning and development of health services, manpower, and facilities to meet the needs of its service areas.

Hegar's sign.   Softening of the lower uterine segment; a sign of pregnancy.

hematocrit.   The volume percentage of red blood corpuscles in whole blood. Formerly, it meant the procedure used to determine this number; now it is the result of that determination.

hematoma.   A tumor caused by effused blood. Continued bleeding from lacerations or an episiotomy can cause vaginal or vulvar hematomas in postpartum patients.

hemoglobinopathy.   A disorder of the blood resulting from a genetically caused altered molecular structure of hemoglobin.

hemolytic disease.   See *disease, hemolytic.*

hemophilia.   An inherited condition that is due to a deficiency in a coagulation factor in the blood. It is characterized by subcutaneous and intramuscular hemorrhages, bleeding from the mouth, gum, lips, and tongue, and blood in the urine. It affects males but is transmitted by females.

hemorrhage.   Bleeding.

hemorrhagic diathesis.   A predisposition to abnormal bleeding.

hemorrhoid.   A varicose dilatation of a vein in the rectal area. It may occur around the anus or internally, higher in the rectum.

heparin.   An anticoagulant mucopolysaccharide acid.

hepatitis.   Inflammation of the liver.

hermaphroditism.   A congenital condition of ambiguity of reproductive structures so that the sex of the individual is not clearly defined as exclusively male or female. The condition is named for Hermes and Aphrodite, the Greek god and goddess of love.

hernia. The protrusion of an organ through an abnormal opening in the wall of the cavity that contains it.

diaphragmatic h. See *diaphragmatic hernia.*

umbilical h. The protrusion of the intestines through a rupture at the navel. In an infant, the condition usually disappears spontaneously by 1 year of age.

herpesvirus. A group of viruses characterized by the formation of small vesicles in clusters. The infection may be nongenital or genital (sexually transmitted).

heterosexuality. The selection of partners of the opposite sex for sexual eroticism and genital intimacy; the predominant mode of sexual partner preference.

high risk. Pertaining to an individual, especially an infant, whose medical and physical history, or that of his parents, indicates that the likelihood is great for his having physiological problems.

hip dysplasia. A hereditary condition involving dislocation with partial or complete loss of contact between the femoral head and the cup-shaped cavity on the lateral surface of the hip bone.

histology. The branch of anatomy that deals with the study of the minute structure, composition, and function of the tissues.

HMD. Abbreviation for *hyaline membrane disease.*

HMG. Abbreviation for *human menopausal gonadotropin.*

Homan's sign. An indication of thrombophlebitis if with leg extended and foot flexed, pain and tenderness are produced in the calf.

homologous. Corresponding in structure or origin; derived from the same source.

homosexuality. The selection of partners of the same sex for sexual eroticism and genital intimacy. There are many degrees of its expression.

hormonal sex. The sex of an individual determined by the preponderance of either estrogen (female) or testosterone (male) sex hormones.

hormone. A chemical substance produced in an organ, which, being carried to an associated organ by the bloodstream, excites in the latter organ a functional activity.

HPL. Abbreviation for *human placental lactogen.*

HSA. Abbreviation for *health systems agency.*

human chorionic gonodotropin (HCG). A hormone secreted by the placenta that prolongs the life of the corpus luteum. It is excreted in the mother's urine and makes possible the standard tests for pregnancy.

human menopausal gonodotropin (HMG). A hormone excreted in the urine of postmenopausal women that has the property of stimulating growth and maturity of ovarian follicles.

human placental lactogen (HPL). A hormone secreted by the placenta that influences somatic growth and facilitates preparation of the breasts for lactation.

Hurler's disease. (gargoylism). See *disease, Hurler's.*

hyaline membrane disease (HMD). See *disease, hyaline membrane.*

hydatidiform mole. Transformation and proliferation of the chorionic villi into grapelike cysts, characterized by poorly vascularized and edematous villi.

hydramnios. An excessive amount of amniotic fluid.

hydrocephalus. An excessive accumulation of cerebrospinal fluid in the ventricles of the brain with consequent enlargement of the cranium.

hydrops fetalis. Characteristics of infants having experienced severe Rh hemolytic disease edema, severe pallor, and cardiac decompensation.

hymen. A membranous fold that partially or wholly occludes the external orifice of the vagina, especially in the virgin.

hyperalimentation. The ingestion of more than adequate amounts of nutrients.

hyperbilirubinemia. The presence of excessive amounts of bilirubin in the blood, which may lead to jaundice.

hyperemesis gravidarum. Pernicious vomiting of pregnancy. This condition is present when vomiting is excessive, continues beyond the fourth month, and causes a marked loss of weight and acetonuria.

hyperemia. An excess of blood in a part.

hyperestrogenic. Pertaining to a state of exaggerated estrogen response created by high levels of estrogen secretion.

hypernatremia. Excessive amounts of sodium in the blood.

hyperplasia. Abnormal multiplication or increase in the number of cells in the normal arrangement in tissue.

hypertension. Persistent high blood pressure, especially arterial blood pressure.

pregnancy-induced h. (PIH). A diagnostic label used to describe the syndrome of hypertension, edema, and proteinuria evident in certain pregnant women. Preeclampsia and eclampsia are two categories of PIH.

hypertonic. 1. Having high osmotic pressure. 2. Having abnormally high muscle tone.

h. saline. A concentrated salt solution, as is instilled into the amniotic fluid for a mid-trimester abortion.

h. uterine dysfunction. An abnormality in the functioning of the uterus to propel the fetus through the birth canal. Uterine action is incoordinate; although there is constant tension in the muscle, the contractions are of poor quality.

hyperventilation. The condition that results from rapid and deep breathing and is marked by confusion, dizziness, numbness, and muscular cramps.

hypnosis. An artificially induced state of extreme suggestibility in which the patient is insensible to outside impressions.

hypocalcemia. Reduction of blood calcium below normal.

hypofibrinogenemia. Deficiency of fibrinogen in the blood.

hypogalactia. Deficiency in the secretion of milk.

hypoglycemia. An abnormally diminished content of glucose in the blood.

hypoprothrombinemia prophylaxis. The administration of vitamin K, intramuscularly, to a newborn as a preventive measure against neonatal hemorrhagic disease.

hypospadias. A developmental anomaly in which the urethra opens on the underside of the penis.

hypotension. Abnormally low blood pressure.

hypothalamus. A specialized structure within the brain located just above the pituitary that regulates and controls a number of autonomic activities, including the release of gonadotropic hormones by the pituitary gland.

hypothermic reaction. A reaction of low body temperature of the mother after delivery.

hypotonic uterine dysfunction. An abnormality in the functioning of the uterus to propel the fetus through the birth canal in which contractions decrease in strength and the tone of the uterine muscles is less than usual.

hypovolemia. An abnormally decreased volume of liquid (plasma) circulating in the body.

hypoxia. Insufficient oxygen to support normal metabolic requirements.

   intrauterine h. A condition of hypoxia in the fetus that can be determined in labor by indicators such as meconium-stained amniotic fluid, abnormal fetal heart rate, and fetal acidosis.

hysterectomy. The surgical removal of the uterus by cutting either through the abdominal wall or through the vagina.

hysterosalpingography. The making of a record by x-ray of the uterus and uterine tubes after injecting them with opaque material.

hysterotomy. A method of mid-trimester abortion involving an incision into the uterus by a surgical procedure. Also called *minicesarean section*.

icterus neonatorum. The jaundice of a newborn.

identification. The process whereby an individual likens himself to another person.

IDM. Abbreviation for *infant of a diabetic mother*.

iliopectineal line. The linea terminalis.

ilium. Pl. *ilia*. The upper and largest portion of the hip bone.

imperforate anus. An abnormal closing of the anus.

implantation. Process by which the conceptus attaches to the uterine wall and penetrates both the uterine endometrium and the maternal circulatory system.

impotence. A male sexual dysfunction involving impairment of erection; an inability to attain or sustain an erection and have intercourse in 25% of the attempts.

impregnation. The act of becoming pregnant. See *fertilization*.

inborn error of metabolism. Hereditary lack of enzyme required for normal metabolism to occur.

incompetent cervical os. A mechanical defect in the cervix, which causes late habitual abortion or preterm labor.

incomplete abortion. See *abortion, incomplete*.

incontinence. Inability to control the excretion of urine or feces.

increment. That by which anything is increased.

induced abortion. See *abortion, induced*.

induration. The process or quality of hardening.

inertia. Inactivity; inability to move spontaneously. Sluggishness of uterine contractions during labor.

inevitable abortion. See *abortion, inevitable*.

infant. A baby; a child under 2 years of age.

   i. mortality rate. The number of infant deaths per 1000 live births.

infertility. The condition of being unfruitful or barren; sterility.

inlet. The upper limit of the pelvic cavity (brim).

intercourse. A mutual exchange, especially sexually; coitus.

internal rotation. The process in the delivery of a baby in which the fetal head is rotated so that it enters the pelvis in the transverse position and exits in the anteroposterior position.

interstitial pregnancy. An ectopic pregnancy that develops in that portion of the tube that passes through the uterine wall.

interval minilaparotomy. A sterilization technique in which a small incision is made below the pubic hair line for tubal ligation.

interval of fertility. Those days during the menstrual cycle during which a woman can conceive, determined by considering the life span of both ova and sperm and the cyclic variability. It ranges from about 8 to 15 days in duration.

intracranial hemorrhage. Bleeding within the cranium. When it occurs in a newborn as a result of a long labor or difficult delivery, it is extremely grave. Also called *subdural hematoma*.

intrauterine. Inside the uterus.

   i. device (IUD). A small, flexible appliance that is inserted into the uterine cavity to prevent conception. It may be in various shapes (spirals, loops, rings) and of various materials (plastic tubing, nylon thread, stainless steel).

   i. growth retardation (IUGR). The condition of an infant born at 40 weeks' gestation and weighing less than 2500 g (or below the tenth percentile for weight or length).

   i. hypoxia. See *hypoxia, intrauterine*.

   i. parabiosis. The joining of fetal twins anatomically and physiologically.

introitus. A term applied to the opening of the vagina.

in utero. Inside the uterus.

inversion. A turning upside down, inside out, or end for end.

   i. of the uterus. The state of the womb being turned inside out, caused by violently drawing away the placenta before it is detached by the natural process of labor.

inverted nipple. A nipple that recedes rather than becoming erect.

in vitro fertilization. A system of impregnation in which ova are extracted from a woman, fertilized in a test tube, and implanted in the uterus.

involution. 1. A rolling or pushing inward. 2. A retrograde process of change that is the reverse of evolution; particularly applied to the return of the uterus to its normal size and condition after parturition.

ischial tuberosity. A protuberance on either side of the ischium.

ischium. The posterior and inferior bone of the pelvis, distinct and separate in the fetus and the infant, or the corresponding part of the hip bone in the adult.

isotonic. Having the same osmotic pressure, especially a salt solution having the same osmotic pressure as blood.

IUD. Abbreviation for *intrauterine device*.

IUGR. Abbreviation for *intrauterine growth retardation*.

jaundice. A condition characterized by hyperbilirubinemia and yellowness in the skin, eyes, and mucous membranes.

jelly. A soft substance that is coherent, tremulous, and more or less transparent.

    contraceptive j. A spermicidal preparation that is inserted vaginally prior to intercourse to prevent conception. Its effectiveness is enhanced when it is used with a diaphragm.

    j. of Wharton. See *Wharton's jelly*.

kalemia. The presence of potassium in the blood.

karyotype. The chromosome makeup of the nucleus of a human cell; also, the photomicrograph of chromosomes arranged in an organized way.

Kegel's exercise. The tightening and relaxing of the pubococcygeal muscle. It aids in toning the vagina, strengthening the perineum, preventing hemorrhoids, and controlling stress incontinence of urine.

kernicterus. The accumulation of unconjugated bilirubin in brain cells resulting in neurologic impairment.

ketamine. A dissociative intravenous analgesic that, used in proper doses during labor, is associated with a minimal newborn depression, no appreciable effects on uterine activity, and few bad dreams or hallucinations.

ketoacidosis. Acidosis due to accumulation of ketone bodies from incomplete metabolism of fatty acids.

Klinefelter's syndrome. See *syndrome, Klinefelter's*.

labia. The nominative plural of *labium*. Lips or liplike structures.

    l. majora. The folds of skin containing fat and covered with hair that form each side of the vulva.

    l. minora. The nymphae, or folds of delicate skin inside the labia majora.

labor. Parturition; the series of processes by which the products of conception are expelled from the mother's body.

laceration. Tearing of vulvar, vaginal, and sometimes rectal tissue during childbirth.

lack of arousal. A female sexual dysfunction formerly called frigidity. It involves failure to respond adequately with congestion and lubrication even with appropriate sexual stimulation.

lactation. The act or period of giving milk; the secretion of milk; the time or period of secreting milk.

lactosuria. The presence of lactose in the urine, a condition common during lactation.

LaLeche League. An organization that holds classes about breast-feeding for women either before or after the baby is born.

Lamaze method of delivery. The most widely used prepared childbirth method in the United States. It uses an individualized approach with classes for both parents in the anatomy and neuromuscular activity of the reproductive system, breathing techniques in labor, and exercises. Sometimes other subjects such as nutrition, hygiene, and child care are taught. Also called *psychoprophylactic method of prepared childbirth*.

lambdoid. Having the shape of the Greek letter λ (lambda).

    l. suture. The suture between the occipital and two parietal bones.

laminaria. A genus of seaweeds. Also, a small stick of hygroscopic material that absorbs moisture rapidly and expands. It is used to begin initial dilation of the cervix prior to abortion.

lanugo. The fine hair on the body of the fetus. The fine, downy hair found on nearly all parts of the body except the palms of the hands and the soles of the feet.

laparoscopy. The introduction of a slender, long surgical instrument (the laparoscope) into the abdominal cavity through very small incisions, not involving actual opening of the abdominal cavity. This procedure is often used for female sterilization.

laparotomy. Surgical entry into the abdominal cavity.

large for gestational age (LGA). Pertaining to an infant born at 36 weeks' gestation and weighing 3500 g (about the 90th percentile for weight). LGA infants are immature but overgrown and are typical of diabetic mothers.

layette. The complete outfit of clothing for a newborn.

Leboyer method of delivery. A method of delivery based on theories of a French obstetrician, Frederick Leboyer. The method avoids harsh, sudden sensory stimulation of the newborn by providing him a quiet, dimly lit delivery room and warm bath to make birth less of a traumatic event.

Leopold's maneuver. See *maneuver, Leopold's*.

Let-down reflex. See *reflex, let-down*.

leukorrhea. A whitish discharge from the female genital organs.

LGA. Abbreviation for *large for gestational age*.

LH. Abbreviation for *luteinizing hormone*.

LHRF. Abbreviation for *luteinizing hormone releasing factor*.

lie. Lie of the fetus. It is the relation of the long axis of the fetus to that of the mother. It is either longitudinal or transverse.

ligation. The binding or tying of a vessel with a substance such as string or catgut.

    tubal l. The sterilization of a woman by surgically interrupting her fallopian tubes to prevent ova from being transported to the uterus and to prevent sperm from fertilizing the ovum. The method may involve ligation, crushing, burning, coagulating, or embedding the ends of the tubes.

lightening. The sensation of decreased abdominal distention produced by the descent of the uterus into the pelvic cavity, which occurs from 2 to 3 weeks before the onset of labor.

linea. Pl. *lineae.* A line or thread.

l. alba. The central tendinous line extending from the pubic bone to the ensiform cartilage.

l. nigra. A dark line appearing on the abdomen and extending from the pubis toward the umbilicus—considered one of the signs of pregnancy.

l. terminalis. The oblique ridge on the inner surface of the ilium, continued on the pubis, which separates the tube from the false pelvis. Formerly called the iliopectineal line.

lingua. Tongue.

l. frenata. Tongue-tie.

lipid. One of a group of fats in the body that is easily stored and serves as a source of fuel, is an important part of cells, and serves other useful functions. It may be a fatty acid, neutral fat, wax, or steroid.

lipidosis. A disorder of cellular lipid metabolism that involves abnormal accumulation of lipid. The lipidoses include Tay–Sachs disease, Niemann–Pick disease, and Gaucher's disease.

liquor. A liquid.

l. amnii. The fluid contained within the amnion in which the fetus floats. See *amniotic fluid.*

Listeria monocytogenes. A gram-positive bacillus that causes upper respiratory tract disease, septicemia, encephalitic disease, and perinatal infections associated with abortion and stillbirth.

lithotomy. The surgical incision of an organ or duct, especially the bladder.

l. position. The bodily posture of a patient lying down with hips and knees flexed and thighs abducted and rotated.

lochia. The discharge from the genital canal during the first or second week following delivery.

low birth weight. The weight of an infant at birth of 2500 g or less.

L/S ratio. The ratio of lecithin to sphingomyelin in the amniotic fluid. It increases suddenly at 35 to 36 weeks' gestation and indicates pulmonary maturity.

lumbar sympathetic block. The blocking of neuropathways of pain by injecting a local anesthetic at L2. It abolishes pain in the uterus only.

lunar month. A period of 4 weeks. Because a lunar month usually corresponds to the length of the menstrual cycle, it is often used for calculating fetal development.

luteinizing hormone (LH). A hormone released by the pituitary gland to bring about the final ripening of the graafian follicle and ovulation.

l. h. releasing factor (LHRF). A substance secreted by the hypothalamus that causes the pituitary gland to release luteinizing hormone.

luteolysis. The destruction of the corpus luteum through the dissolution of cellular structure. Thus, luteolysis interferes with the function of the corpus luteum in progesterone secretion.

lysozyme. A crystalline, basic protein present in many body fluids that functions as an antibacterial enzyme.

maneuver. A planned process involving dexterity; in obstetrics, a procedure used by an obstetrician in assisting manually in delivery.

Bracht m. A method of assisting with the delivery of the aftercoming head in a breech delivery. The back is gently arched to the mother's abdomen when the scapulae are seen. The arms then tend to deliver spontaneously. Suprapubic pressure is applied to assist descent of the head into the pelvis, and the suspended body continues to be brought slowly to the mother's abdomen. The face and occiput should then deliver spontaneously.

Leopold's m. Four maneuvers for diagnosing the fetal position by external palpation of the mother's abdomen.

Mauriceau–Smellie–Veit m. A method of assisting with the delivery of the aftercoming head in a breech delivery. Two fingers of the left hand are placed firmly over the mandibles to flex the head. The right hand is placed over the back, with the fingers over the shoulders to guide the shoulders and head. The torso is elevated slowly with flexion of the head maintained by the maxillary pressure. Suprapubic pressure is applied by an assistant during these maneuvers to aid the descent of the head into the pelvis, and eventually with the suprapubic and maxillary pressure, the occiput is delivered.

Ortolani's m. A diagnostic procedure performed on the newborn to determine congenital hip dysplasia.

Ritgen m. Delivery of the infant's head by lifting the head upward and forward through the vulva, between contractions, by pressing with the tips of the fingers upon the perineum behind the anus.

Sellick's m. A technique in which pressure is applied to the ring of cartilage at the lower part of the larynx to prevent aspiration of gastric contents during anesthesia induction.

manual rotation. A maneuver used to turn the fetal head by hand from a transverse to an anteroposterior position to facilitate delivery.

Marfan's syndrome. See *arachnodactyly.*

marginal sinus rupture. A disorder of placental attachment, a mild type of abruptio placentae in which slight separation occurs at the edge of the placenta in the region of the marginal sinus of the mother.

mask of pregnancy. See *chloasma.*

mastitis. Inflammation of the breast.

masturbation. Self-stimulation of the genitals in men or women, usually to attain orgasm.

maternal infant bonding. See *bonding.*

maternity clinical specialist. A nurse at the master's level with expertise in adaptational and physiological problems in maternity care.

maternity nurse practitioner. A specialty nurse practitioner who provides prenatal care for uncomplicated pregnancies, postpartum care, contraception counseling, and management of minor problems. Also called *OB–GYN nurse practitioner.*

maturation. In biology, a process of cell division during which the number of chromosomes in the germ cells is reduced to one half the number characteristic of the species.

Mauriceau–Smellie–Veit maneuver. See *maneuver, Mauriceau–Smellie–Veit.*

McDonald technique. A simple technique for cerclage that involves placing a nonabsorbable suture around the cervix high on the cervical mucosa.

McDonald's measurement. Measurement of the height of the uterine fundus with a tape measure; the distance from symphysis pubis to fundus.

meatus. A passage; an opening leading to a canal, duct, or cavity.

    m. urinarius. The external orifice of the urethra.

mechanism. The manner of combinations that subserve a common function. In obstetrics refers to labor and delivery.

meconium. The dark green or black substance found in the large intestine of the fetus or newly born infant.

meiosis. The special method for cell division that a sex cell undergoes through which it is matured and its genetic material, or chromosomes, is prepared for fertilization.

menarche. The establishment or the beginning of the menstrual function.

Mendelian disorder. A genetic disorder that follows the inheritance patterns described by Mendel (*i.e.,* dominant, recessive).

meningomyelocele. A malformation that accompanies spina bifida when the membranes covering the spinal cord as well as the cord bulge through the opening in the spine.

menopause. The period at which menstruation ceases; the "change of life."

menorrhagia. Excessive uterine bleeding occurring at the regular time of menstrual flow.

menses. [Pl. of Latin *mensis*, month.] The periodic monthly discharge of blood from the uterus; the catamenia.

menstrual extraction. The aspiration of the endometrium performed in very early pregnancy without cervical dilatation using a small cannula and syringe or other low-pressure suction.

menstruation. The cyclic, physiologic uterine bleeding that normally recurs at approximately 4-week intervals, in the absence of pregnancy, during the reproductive period.

mentum. The chin.

mesoderm. The middle layer of cells derived from the primitive embryo.

metritis. Inflammation of the uterus.

metrorrhagia. Uterine bleeding that occurs at irregular intervals; the amount of flow is usually average.

microcephaly. Abnormal smallness of the head, usually accompanied by mental retardation.

micropill. An oral contraceptive that contains a lower dosage (50 mcg or less) of estrogen than the standard pill.

micturition. Urination.

midwifery. The practice of assisting at childbirth. See *nurse–midwife.*

migration. In obstetrics refers to the passage of the ovum from the ovary to the uterus.

milia. Plural of milium.

milium. A small white nodule of the skin, usually caused by clogged sebaceous glands or hair follicles.

milk ejection reflex. See *reflex, milk ejection.*

milk-leg. Phlebitis of the femoral vein, occasionally following delivery.

milk let-down. See *reflex, milk ejection.*

minicesarean section. See *hysterotomy.*

minipill. An oral contraceptive that contains only progestin and no estrogen.

miscarriage. Lay term for abortion.

missed abortion. See *abortion, missed.*

mittelschmerz. Painful discomfort sometimes experienced during ovulation or in the middle of the menstrual cycle.

molding. The shaping of the baby's head so as to adjust itself to the size and shape of the birth canal.

mongolian spots. Gray-blue pigmented areas seen on some infants, especially those with dark skins. These have no relationship to mongolism and disappear spontaneously later.

monilial infection. An infection caused by a genus of fungi formerly called *Monilia,* now called *Candida.* Examples are thrush and monilial vaginitis.

monoamniotic monochorionic twins. See *twins, monoamniotic monochorionic.*

monotrophy. The principle, stated by Bowlby in 1958, that the structure of the attachment process is such that parents become attached to only one infant at a time.

monozygotic. Pertaining to or derived from one zygote.

    m. twins. See *twins, monozygotic.*

mons veneris. The eminence in the upper and anterior part of the pubes of women.

Montgomery's tubercles. Small, nodular follicles or glands on the areolae around the nipples.

morning-after pill. A method of contraception not in general use. The postcoital pill, diethylstilbestrol (DES) is a synthetic estrogen with severe side-effects including nausea, vomiting, and headache. It is used only in emergency situations, such as rape, because it has been shown to cause vaginal cancer in some offspring of mothers who took it.

morning sickness. A symptom of pregnancy in some women, characterized by waves of nausea and sometimes vomiting. It usually occurs in the early part of the day and subsides in a few hours. It may appear 2 weeks after the first missed menstrual period and subside 6 or 8 weeks later.

Moro reflex. See *reflex, Moro.*

morphological sex. The sex of an individual as determined by the body shape and characteristic with appropriate secondary sex characteristics. In the case of a true hermaphrodite, the individual has a mixture of the body and secondary sex characteristics of both sexes.

morula. The fertilized ovum at the 16-cell stage 3 days after conception. It is traveling from the fallopian tube into the uterine cavity prior to implantation.

mother–baby couple care. An organization of postpartum

units that includes rooming-in or satellite nurseries, with the same nurse caring for mother and baby.

mucous membrane.   The lining of a body cavity or passageway that is connected to the exterior and is protected by a slimy substance it secretes called mucus.

mucous plug.   A plug that closes the cervical canal during pregnancy. It is made of mucous secretions of the cervix.

mucus-trap suction.   Suction using a catheter with a mucus trap; used to aspirate the newborn without the mucus being drawn into the nurse's mouth.

multigravida.   A woman who has been pregnant several times, or many times.

multipara.   A woman who has borne several, or many, children.

multiple pregnancy.   The condition in which two or more embryos develop in the uterus at the same time.

mutagen.   A chemical or substance that causes a change in gene structure or alteration of genetic information.

mutation.   A change in gene or chromosome in gametes that may be transmitted to offspring.

myoma.   Pl. *myomata*.   A uterine tumor made up of muscular elements; a benign tumor of the uterine muscle. Also called a *fibroid*.

myomotomy.   An incision into a myoma.

myotonia.   Increased muscle tension and tone; increased contractility of muscles.

myxedema.   A condition characterized by a dry, waxy type of swelling, with abnormal deposits of the glycoprotein mucin, in the skin. The facial changes are often associated with hypothyroidism.

Nägele's rule.   A method of calculating the expected date of confinement. The date is calculated by subtracting 3 calendar months from the first day of the last menstrual period and adding 7 days.

natal.   Pertaining to birth.

natural childbirth.   See *prepared childbirth*.

natural method of birth control.   An approach to contraception that relies upon identification of the fertile period and avoidance of intercourse during this time. Such a method may involve predicting ovulation by use of a menstrual calendar, identifying changes in cervical mucus, or identifying when ovulation has occurred using a basal body temperature chart, or a combination of these. Some couples use other contraceptive methods during the fertile period rather than avoid intercourse.

nausea.   An unpleasant feeling vaguely in the area of the upper abdomen that often culminates in vomiting.

navel.   The umbilicus.

necrotizing enterocolitis (NEC).   An acute inflammatory bowel disorder that occurs primarily in preterm or low-birth-weight neonates.

neonatal.   Pertaining to the newborn, usually considered the first 4 weeks of life.

    n. asphyxia.   Respiratory failure in a newborn; also called *asphyxia neonatorum*.

    n. period.   The period from birth through the 28th day of life.

neonate.   The infant from birth through the first 28 days of life.

neonatology.   The study of the diagnosis and treatment of disorders of the newborn.

nephropathy.   Any disease of the kidneys.

neural tube defect.   Congenital malformation that involves defects of the spinal column caused by failure of the neural tube to close during embryonic development.

neurohormonal.   Pertaining to both a nerve or nerves and a hormone.

nevus.   A natural mark or blemish; a mole; a circumscribed deposit of pigmentary matter in the skin present at birth (birthmark).

nidation.   The implantation of the fertilized ovum in the endometrium of the pregnant uterus.

Niemann–Pick disease.   See *disease, Niemann–Pick*.

nocturnal ejaculation.   An orgasm with ejaculation of seminal fluid that occurs during sleep particularly in adolescent boys. Also called *"wet dreams."*

nonorgasm.   A female sexual dysfunction in which sexual arousal with congestion and lubrication occurs but orgasm is inhibited.

nonviable fetus.   A fetus that is incapable of surviving outside the uterus.

norm.   Rule, generally for behavior.

nuclear family.   A family group that consists of the father, mother, and children.

nulligravida.   A woman who has never been pregnant.

nullipara.   A woman who has not borne children.

nurse–midwife.   A registered nurse who has completed a recognized program of study and clinical experience leading to a certificate in nurse–midwifery.

nurse practitioner.   A registered nurse with additional preparation in physical and psychosocial assessment, who provides primary-care management for patients with common acute and chronic illnesses and developmental needs.

OB–GYN nurse practitioner.   See *maternity nurse practitioner*.

obstetrics.   The branch of medicine that is concerned with the management of women during pregnancy, childbirth, and the puerperium.

occipitobregmatic.   Pertaining to the occiput (the back part of the head) and the bregma (junction of the coronal and sagittal sutures).

OCT.   Abbreviation for *oxytocin challenge test*.

oligohydramnios.   Deficiency of amniotic fluid.

oligospermia.   Deficiency in the number of sperm cells in the semen.

oliguria.   Suppression of urinary excretion.

omphalic.   Pertaining to the umbilicus.

omphalocele.   Congenital herniation of the abdominal viscera through a defect in the abdominal wall at the umbilicus.

oocyesis.   Ovarian pregnancy.

oocyte.   A developing egg cell in one of two stages. A primary oocyte develops from an oogonium, which subsequently divides into a secondary oocyte and a polar body. Ovulation follows, and the mature ovum and a second polar body develop.

oophorectomy. The surgical removal of an ovary or ovaries.

ophthalmia neonatorum. Acute purulent conjunctivitis of the newborn, usually due to gonorrheal infection.

oral contraceptive. A conception preventive taken by mouth.

organogenesis. The beginning and development of organs.

orgasm. The culmination of sexual excitement. Also called *climax.*

orgasmic platform. The thickened area of congested tissue that builds up in and surrounds the lower third of the vagina during high levels of sexual arousal and just preceding orgasm.

Ortolani's maneuver. See *maneuver, Ortolani's.*

os. Any opening in the body, but particularly the cervical opening.

osmolality. A property of a solution that depends on the concentration of the substance dissolved per unit of solvent.

ova. Plural of ovum.

ovary. The sexual gland of the female in which the ova are developed. There are two ovaries, one at each side of the pelvis.

overstimulation. The presence of sensory input when an infant is not receptive to it.

ovulation. The growth and discharge of an unimpregnated ovum, usually coincident with the menstrual period.

ovum. The female reproductive cell. The human ovum is a round cell about $1/120$ of an inch in diameter, developed in the ovary.

oxytocic. 1. Accelerating parturition. 2. A medicine that accelerates parturition.

oxytocin. A hormone produced by the hypothalamus that stimulates contraction of the uterus, used to induce or intensify labor.

  o. challenge test. See *test, oxytocin challenge.*

pain. A localized sensation of hurt. In clinical practice, it can be defined as whatever the experiencing person says it is, existing whenever he says it does.

  p. intensity. The severity of the pain sensation.

  p. tolerance. The intensity or duration of pain that the patient is willing to endure without making further efforts to relieve it.

palpation. The act of feeling with the hands and fingers portions of the body for purposes of diagnosis.

palsy. A synonym for paralysis, used in connection with certain special forms.

  Bell's p. Peripheral facial paralysis due to lesion of the facial nerve, resulting in characteristic distortion of the face.

  brachial p. Paralysis of an arm.

  cerebral p. A motor and speech disorder resulting from an injury to the brain at birth or earlier.

  Erb's p. The upper-arm type of brachial birth palsy.

Papanicolaou smear. Cytology test of cervical cells used as a screening for cervical cancer.

para. The term used to refer to past pregnancies that have produced an infant that has been viable, whether the infant is alive at birth or not.

paracervical block. The blocking of neuropathways of pain by injecting a local anesthetic into the parametrium at sites in the cervix. It abolishes pain in the uterus only.

parametritis. Inflammation of the parametrium. Also called *pelvic cellulitis.*

parametrium. The fibrous subserous coat of the supravaginal portion of the uterus, extending laterally between the layers of the broad ligaments.

parenteral feeding. Feeding by routes other than through the alimentary canal, such as intravenously.

parity. The condition of a woman with respect to her having borne children.

parovarian. Pertaining to the residual structure in the broad ligament between the ovary and the fallopian tube.

parturient. Bringing forth; pertaining to childbearing. A woman in childbirth.

parturition. The act or process of giving birth to a child.

patent ductus arteriosus. A congenital cardiac anomaly in which the vascular connection between the pulmonary artery and aorta, which is open during fetal life, does not close after birth as it should, causing the recirculation of arterial blood through the lungs.

patulous. Spreading somewhat widely apart; open.

pedigree. A record of an individual's ancestors. In genetics, it is used for analyzing Mendelian traits.

pelvic. Pertaining to the pelvis.

  p. axis. See *axis, pelvic.*

  p. cellulitis. See *parametritis.*

  p. congestion. Excessive accumulation of blood in the pelvic region.

  p. inlet. Inlet to the true pelvis.

pelvic inflammatory disease (PID). Infection of the pelvic organs often caused by the presence of an IUD or venereal disease.

pelvimeter. An instrument for measuring the diameters and capacity of the pelvis.

pelvimetry. The measurement of the dimensions and capacity of the pelvis.

pelvis. The lower part of the body bounded by the two hip bones, the sacrum, and the coccyx.

  android p. One of the four main types of female pelvis, generally characterized as resembling the pelvis of a male and having a wedge-shaped inlet and narrow anterior segment.

  anthropoid p. One of the four main types of female pelvis, generally characterized by a long anteroposterior diameter of the inlet.

  contracted p. A pelvis that measures 1 cm to 3 cm shorter than normal in any important diameter.

  false p. The part of the pelvis superior to a plane passing through the linea terminalis.

  gynecoid p. The most prevalent of the four main types of female pelvis, having a rounded oval shape.

  platypelloid p. One of the four main types of female pelvis, having a flattened pelvic inlet.

  true p. The part of the pelvis inferior to a plane passing through the linea terminalis.

penis. The male organ of copulation.

perinatal. Pertaining to the time before and after birth; variously defined as beginning at conception through the 28th day of life or conception through the first year of life.

perineorrhaphy. Suture of the perineum; the operation for the repair of lacerations of the perineum.

perineotomy. A surgical incision through the perineum.

perineum. The area between the vagina and the rectum.

periodic breathing. A common pattern of periods of apnea of 10 seconds or less noted in premature infants.

peritoneoscopy. Direct visualization of the tubes and ovaries with an endoscope.

peritoneum. A strong serous membrane investing the inner surface of the abdominal walls and the viscera of the abdomen.

peritonitis. Inflammation of the peritoneum.

phenylketonuria (PKU). An inborn error of metabolism resulting in a deficiency in liver enzyme. It may be detected by blood or urine tests. Early treatment will prevent mental retardation.

phimosis. Tightness of the foreskin.

phlebitis. Inflammation of a vein.

phocomelia. A developmental anomaly characterized by total absence or stunting of the arms or legs.

phospholipid. Any lipid that contains phosphorus; the major form of lipid in all cell membranes.

phototherapy. The use of light to treat a disease, especially the use of intense fluorescent light to reduce serum bilirubin in the treatment of hyperbilirubinemia.

physiologic jaundice. Mild icterus neonatorum lasting a few days.

pica. The abnormal intake of specific substances such as clay dirt, cornstarch, or plaster. It may characterize the behavior of malnourished children or pregnant women.

Pitocin. A proprietary solution of oxytocin.

PKU. Abbreviation for *phenylketonuria.*

placenta. The circular, flat, vascular structure in the impregnated uterus forming the principal medium of communication between the mother and the fetus.

  ablatio p. See *abruptio placentae.*

  abruptio p. Premature separation of the normally implanted placenta.

  p. accreta. A condition in which one or more cotyledons of the placenta are abnormally adherent to the uterine wall, making separation of the placenta difficult or impossible.

  previa p. A placenta that is implanted in the lower uterine segment so that it adjoins or covers the internal os of the cervix.

platypelloid pelvis. See *pelvis, platypelloid.*

plexus. A network or tangle, such as a network of veins, lymphatic vessels, or nerves.

polycythemia. An increased red blood cell volume.

polydactyly. A developmental anomaly characterized by extra digits on the hands or feet.

polygalactia. Excessive secretion of milk.

polyhydramnios. Hydramnios.

position. The situation of the fetus in the pelvis; determined by the relation of some arbitrarily chosen portion of the fetus to the right or the left side of the mother's pelvis. Thus, each presentation has either a right or left position.

postasphyxia encephalopathy. One of various central nervous system symptoms caused by injury resulting from episodes of perinatal asphyxia.

postcoital test. See *test, postcoital.*

postmaturity. Overdevelopment, as of a postmature infant who was born after pregnancy has progressed beyond full term.

postnatal. Occurring after birth, referring to the infant.

postpartum. After delivery or childbirth, referring to the mother.

  p. hemorrhage. Loss of 500 ml or more of blood from the uterus after completion of the third stage of labor.

  p. period. The period occurring after childbirth, referring to the mother.

post-term infant. An infant born after the onset of the 42nd week of gestation.

PPM. Abbreviation for *psychoprophylactic method of prepared childbirth.*

precipitate delivery. A delivery that occurs with undue rapidity (less than 3 hours) and usually without the benefit of asepsis.

preeclampsia. A disorder encountered during pregnancy or early in the puerperium, characterized by hypertension, edema, and albuminuria.

pregnancy. [Latin, *praeg'nans,* literally "previous to bringing forth."] The state of being with young or with child. The normal duration of pregnancy in the human female is 280 days, or 10 lunar months, or 9 calendar months. See also *abdominal p., ectopic p., interstitial p., multiple p., tubal p.*

premature infant. An infant that weighs 2500 g or less at birth.

premature ejaculation. A male sexual dysfunction in which difficulty is met in controlling orgasm for a sufficient period of time to enable his partner to attain sexual satisfaction.

premature infant. An infant born before the 37th week of gestation, regardless of weight; preterm infant.

premature rupture of membranes. Rupture of the amniotic sac before the onset of uterine contractions.

prematurity. Underdevelopment, as of a premature infant.

premenstrual tension. A syndrome sometimes experienced during the 10 days preceding menstruation. It is characterized by irritability, insomnia, headache, pain in the breasts, abdominal distention, nausea, anorexia, constipation, emotional instability, and urinary frequency.

prepared childbirth. The methods by which parents actively participate in childbirth. Some approaches include the concepts and techniques of Dick–Read, Lamaze, and Bradley. Also called *natural childbirth.*

prepuce. The fold of skin that covers the glans penis in the male.

  p. of the clitoris. The fold of mucous membrane that covers the glans clitoris.

presentation. Term used to designate that part of the fetus nearest the internal os, or that part that is felt by the examiner's hand when doing the vaginal examination.

presumptive signs of pregnancy. Signs that strongly suggest that a healthy woman is pregnant. These include menstrual suppression, nausea, vomiting, frequency of micturition, tenderness and other changes of breasts, "quickening," Chadwick's sign, pigmentation of the skin, and abdominal striae.

preterm infant. See *premature infant.*

primigravida. Pl. *primigravidas.* A woman who is pregnant for the first time.

primipara. Pl. *primiparas.* A woman who has given birth to her first child.

probable signs of pregnancy. Signs that the likelihood of pregnancy is great. These include enlargement of the abdomen, changes in the size, shape, and consistency of the uterus, fetal outline felt by palpation, changes in the cervix, Braxton Hicks contractions, and a positive pregnancy test.

prodromal. Premonitory; indicating the approach of a disease.

  p. labor. The latent or early phase in which there is some effacement and slow dilatation of the cervix. It lasts perhaps an average of 8½ hours in a nullipara.

progesterone. The pure hormone contained in the corpora lutea whose function is to prepare the endometrium for the reception and development of the fertilized ovum.

progestin. Any of the synthetic progesterone preparations that are used in oral contraceptives. The common types include norethynodrel, norethindrone, ethynodiol diacetate, and norgestrel.

prolactin. A proteohormone from the anterior pituitary that stimulates lactation in the mammary glands.

prolan. Zondek's term for the gonadotropic principle of human-pregnancy urine, responsible for the biologic pregnancy tests.

prolapse of umbilical cord. Delivery of the umbilical cord in labor prior to the delivery of the fetus.

promontory. A small projection; a prominence.

  p. of the sacrum. The superior or projecting portion of the sacrum when *in situ* in the pelvis, at the junction of the sacrum and the last lumbar vertebra.

prostaglandin. Any of a group of fatty acids found in semen, which are effective abortifacients at any stage of pregnancy. These are the most common agents for inducing mid-trimester abortion through instillation into the amniotic fluid.

prostate gland. A gland in the male that surrounds the neck of the bladder and urethra.

proteinuria. The presence of protein in the urine.

pruritus. Intense itching, usually referring to the genital area.

pseudocyesis. An apparent condition of pregnancy; the woman really believes she is pregnant when, as a matter of fact, she is not.

psychogenic sexual stimuli. Stimuli processed through the higher brain centers that cause sexual arousal. These include sensory stimuli such as sight, sound, taste, smell, and touch, and cognitive events such as thoughts, fantasies, memories, and images.

psychophysiology. The interaction between psychological and physiological processes, that is, between higher mental processes and the responses of muscles, glands, and organs.

psychoprophylactic method of prepared childbirth (PPM). See *Lamaze method of delivery.*

psychosexual method of childbirth. A method of childbirth preparation developed by Sheila Kitzinger based on a method using sensory memory and the Stanislavsky method of acting. Sexuality is seen as part of the larger whole encompassing family relationships, birth, cuddling, and feeding.

puberty. The age at which the generative organs become functionally active.

pubic. Belonging to the pubis.

pubiotomy. The operation of cutting through the pubic bone lateral to the median line.

pubis. The os pubis or pubic bone forming the front of the pelvis.

pudenda. [L.] The plural of pudendum.

pudendal. Relating to the pudenda.

  p. block. The blocking of neuropathways of pain by injecting a local anesthetic into the pudendal nerve. It abolishes pain in the vagina and perineum.

pudendum. [Latin, *pudere,* to have shame or modesty.] The external genital parts of either sex, but especially of the female.

puerperal fever. Infection, accompanied by fever, which develops in a wound to the birth canal during delivery.

puerperium. The period elapsing between the termination of labor and the return of the uterus to its normal condition, about 6 weeks.

pulmonary dysmaturity. An insidious disease of premature infants beginning with mild respiratory symptoms after the first week of life. The cause is thought to be collapse of the bronchial tree, with partial airway obstruction following aspiration of small amounts of milk as a result of a poorly developed gag reflex. Also known as *Wilson–Mikity disease.*

pyelonephritis. Inflammation of the kidney due to bacterial infection. In pregnancy, hormonal and anatomical changes cause narrowing of the lower ureter and dilation of the upper ureter and renal pelvis, thus increasing the risk of infection.

pyloric stenosis. A congenital anomaly manifested in an infant from the first to the second or third week by projectile vomiting 30 minutes after feeding. Surgery removes a stricture of the pylorus that is the cause.

quickening. The mother's first perception of the movements of the fetus.

rabbit test. See *test, Friedman's.*

radioimmunoassay test. See *test, radioimmunoassay.*

RDS. Abbreviation for *respiratory distress syndrome.* See *disease, hyaline membrane.*

Read method of childbirth preparation. See *Dick–Read approach to childbirth.*

reanastomosis. The reestablishing of a connection between vessels, such as surgically reconnecting the severed vas deferens or fallopian tubes following sterilization. The purpose of this surgery is to reestablish fertility, but success rates are variable.

recessive inheritance. The acquisition of a characteristic from both parents that is the result of an allele that must be carried by both members of a pair of homologous chromosomes.

rectocele. The protrusion by hernia of a part of the rectum into the vagina.

reflex. An involuntary activity.

　grasp r. The reflex present at birth in an infant's hands and feet causing the fingers and toes to curl around an object placed touching them.

　let-down r. See *milk ejection r.*

　milk ejection r. The activation of a process by which contractions of the myoepithelial cells in a mother's breast propel milk along the duct into the lactiferous sinuses. Also called *let-down reflex* and *milk let-down.*

　Moro r. See *startle r.*

　rooting r. The tendency of an infant to open his mouth and turn toward an object that is gently stroking his cheek or the corner of his mouth.

　startle r. The reflex that is present from birth to age 3 months that indicates an awareness of equilibrium by a symmetrical drawing up of legs and grasping of arms in response to a sudden jarring of his crib or clothes. Also known as *Moro reflex.*

　stepping r. The reflex that is present at birth but disappears soon after that causes an infant to make little stepping or prancing movements when he is held upright with his feet touching a surface.

　sucking r. The reflex in infants to suck anything that comes in contact with their lips. It seems to be a great need for the first 2 months of life, is present while sleeping, and need not be nutritive.

　swallowing r. The reflex present at birth to swallow food that an infant sucks into his mouth.

　tonic neck r. The tendency of an infant while lying on his back to turn his head to one side and extend the arm and leg on that side, flexing the arm and leg on the other side.

reflexogenic sexual stimulus. A direct stimulation of an erogenous area that causes sexual arousal in a reflexive, or automatic, manner.

respiratory distress syndrome (RDS). See *disease, hyaline membrane.*

resuscitation. The restoring to life of a patient who is apparently dead or dying.

retinal vein thrombosis. The presence of an obstruction caused by an aggregation of blood factors in the retinal vein. This clotting disorder may be partially the result of the use of oral contraceptives.

retraction ring. Physiologic area of constriction at the junction of the upper, or contracting, portion and the lower, or dilating, portion of the uterus; Bandl's ring is pathologic constriction of the retraction ring.

retroflexion. The bending backward of an organ on its axis, specifically the tipping backward of a uterus upon itself.

retrolental fibroplasia. An acquired disease of a prema-

ture infant resulting in eye injury as a result of continuous oxygen therapy in high concentration.

retroversion. The tipping backward of an entire organ; in the case of retroversion of the uterus, the turning back of the entire uterus in relation to the pelvic axis.

Rh. Abbreviation for *Rhesus,* a type of monkey. This term is used for a property of human blood cells, because of its relationship to a similar property in the blood cells of Rhesus monkeys.

Rh factor. A term applied to an inherited antigen in the human blood.

RhoGAM. A preparation of anti-Rh antibodies administered by injection to unsensitized Rh-negative women following childbirth or abortion, to prevent the development of endogenous antibodies that could later lead to erythroblastosis fetalis (Rh disease of the fetus) in a subsequent pregnancy.

rhythm method. A birth control method relying upon abstinence from sexual intercourse before, during, and after the period of time the ovum is capable of being fertilized.

Ritgen maneuver. See *maneuver, Ritgen.*

roentgenogram. A record of the internal structure of a body by the use of x-ray photography.

role complementarity. The learning of roles in pairs.

role differentiation. The process by which roles are structured and delineated.

rollover test. See *test, rollover.*

rooming-in. The hospital practice in which postpartum mothers have their infants in their rooms all the time, except for necessary examinations or procedures.

rooting reflex. See *reflex, rooting.*

rotation. The turning on an axis; specifically, in labor, the turning of the fetal head through a right angle so that the longest diameter of the head corresponds to the longest diameter of the pelvic outlet.

rubella. German measles.

　r. syndrome. See *syndrome, rubella.*

Rubin's test. See *test, Rubin's.*

rupture of the membranes. The breaking of the amniotic sac, which may occur spontaneously and be the first indication of approaching labor. If the membranes have not ruptured previously, they must be broken before the fetal head is delivered to prevent aspiration of fluid when the infant takes its first breath.

sacral promontory. The marked projection in the pelvis formed by the junction of the last lumbar vertebra and the sacrum.

sacrococcygeal articulation. The joint or juncture of the sacrum and coccyx.

sacroiliac articulation. The two joints or junctures of the sacrum and the ilium on either side of the pelvis.

sacrum. A triangular wedge-shaped bone, consisting of five vertebrae fused together, which serves as the back part of the pelvis.

saddle block. The blocking of neuropathways of pain by injecting a local anesthetic into the subarachnoid space in the spine. A *true saddle block* blocks pain in the perineum. A *modified saddle block* abolishes both uterine and perineal discomfort.

Saf-T-Coil. One of the commonly used intrauterine devices.

salpingitis. Inflammation of the fallopian tubes.

scarf sign. A test to assess infant maturity. The infant's arms are drawn across the neck and as far across the opposite shoulder as possible. In the premature infant there is less resistance and greater draping (or scarf) effect; the elbow will reach near or across the midline. In the full-term infant, the elbow will not reach the midline.

Schultze's mechanism. The expulsion of the placenta with the fetal surfaces presenting.

sebum. The secretions of the sebaceous glands of the skin; a thick, semifluid substance composed of fat and epithelial cell debris.

secondary areola. See *areola, secondary.*

secundines. The afterbirth; the placenta and membranes expelled after the birth of a child.

segmentation. The process of division by which the fertilized ovum multiplies before differentiation into layers occurs.

Sellick's maneuver. See *maneuver, Sellick's.*

semen. 1. A seed. 2. The fluid secreted by the male reproductive organs.

sensory modalities. The areas of sensation: vision, touch, hearing, taste, smell, and movement.

separation of the placenta. Detachment of the placenta from the wall of the uterus.

sex chromatin. See *Barr body.*

sex chromosome. One of two chromosomes in human cells that are associated with the determination of the sex of the individual. A male cell normally contains one X and one Y chromosome, and a female cell contains two X chromosomes.

sex-linked inheritance trait. An inheritance trait in which the gene is carried on the X chromosome and is expressed in the male offspring. (Males do not possess another X chromosome to offset the effects of the X chromosome that carries the gene.)

sexologist. A specialist in the area of human sexuality; one engaged in sex research or particularly learned in the physiological, behavioral, or psychoemotional aspects of sexuality.

sex role. The public expression of gender identity; all actions used to convey one's maleness or femaleness.

sex therapy. A short-term therapy aimed at relief of the sexual symptom, which uses systematically structured sexual experiencing with conjoint therapeutic sessions. It is designed to modify immediate obstacles to sexual functioning, although intrapsychic and transactional conflicts are also dealt with to some extent.

sexual dysfunction. A psychosomatic disorder that makes it impossible for an individual to have or enjoy intercourse. There is inadequate sexual response involving both vasocongestive and orgasmic components either together or separately. See also *impotence, premature ejaculation, vaginismus, lack of arousal, nonorgasm,* and *dyspareunia.*

sexuality. The complex of emotions, attitudes, preferences, and behaviors related to the individual's expression of the sexual self and eroticism. Components of sexuality include the individual's genetic, hormonal, gonadal, and morphologic sex gender identity, sex role, and sexual partner preference.

sexually transmitted diseases (STD). A variety of diseases usually transmitted by direct sexual contact with an infected individual.

SGA. Abbreviation for *small for gestational age.*

Shake test. See *test, Shake.*

Shirodkar technique. A technique for cerclage that involves elevating the vaginal mucous membrane and tying some material (*i.e.,* suture) around the internal os of the cervix. The vaginal mucosa is then restored to its original position and sutured.

shoulder dystocia. A serious complication in the birth of an oversized infant whose unusually large shoulders arrest at either the pelvic brim or the outlet.

shoulder presentation. A serious complication of birth in which the infant lies crosswise in the uterus instead of longitudinally. The risk of perinatal mortality is reduced by a cesarean delivery.

show. Popularly, the blood-tinged mucus discharged from the vagina before or during labor.

sickle cell anemia. A hereditary, genetically determined hemolytic anemia. It is generally manifest before childbearing, and crises may occur in the nonpregnant as well as pregnant state. One must consider not only the impact of pregnancy in precipitating crises in a patient with sickle cell anemia but also the genetic outlook and limited life expectancy of the patient.

sitz bath. A treatment for perineal or perianal discomfort in which the patient sits for 20 minutes three to four times per day in very warm water that may have astringents or solutions added.

Skene's gland. One of two glands just within the meatus of the female urethra; regarded as the homologue of the prostate gland in the male.

smegma. A thick cheesy secretion found under the prepuce and in the region of the clitoris and the labia minora.

small for gestational age (SGA). Pertaining to infants whose weight falls below the tenth percentile for their gestational age. These infants have experienced growth retardation during the prenatal period and may be born close to term but weigh less than 2500 g.

socialization. The process by which an individual learns society's expectations for behavior.

souffle. A soft, blowing auscultatory sound.

    funic s. A soft hissing sound, synchronous with the fetal heart sounds produced by blood being transported through the umbilical vessels.

    placental s. A soft blowing sound caused by the blood flow in the placenta and syncronous with the maternal pulse.

    uterine s. Soft blowing sound caused by the blood flow in the arteries of the uterus and syncronous with the maternal pulse.

spermatocyte. A developing sperm cell in one of two stages. A primary spermatocyte develops from a spermatogonium and subsequently divides into two secondary spermatocytes. Each spermatocyte divides into two spermatids.

spermatogenesis. The process of forming spermatozoa.

spermatogonium. Pl. *spermatogonia.* The undivided male germ cell that develops in the seminiferous tubes. Each will eventually develop into four spermatozoa.

spermatozoon. Pl. *spermatozoa.* A mature male germ cell; the mobile microscopic sexual element that resembles in shape an elongated tadpole.

spermicide. An agent that destroys spermatozoa; used as a contraceptive.

sphingomyelin lipidosis. See *disease, Niemann–Pick.*

spina bifida. A rather common malformation due to the congenital absence of one or more vertebral arches, usually at the lower part of the spine.

spinal anesthesia. Relief of pain by injecting a local anesthetic into the subarachnoid space in the spine.

spontaneous rupture of the membranes. Rupture of the amniotic sac without medical interference.

spotting. Spotting of blood from the vagina between periods.

startle reflex. See *reflex, startle.*

station. Measurement of the fetal descent into the bony pelvis in relationship to the ischial spines.

stenosis. The narrowing of a duct or canal. See *pyloric stenosis.*

stepping reflex. See *reflex, stepping.*

sterilization. 1. A process of eliminating microbial viability. 2. A permanent method of contraception; process by which an individual is made incapable of reproduction.

steroid hormones. Sex hormones and hormones of the adrenal cortex.

stilbestrol. Diethylstilbestrol, an estrogenic compound.

stillborn. Born dead.

stimulus. Any environmental event that activates a reaction in one of the senses.

striae gravidarum. Shining, reddish lines upon the abdomen, thighs, and breasts during pregnancy.

subdural hematoma. A hemorrhage under the tough outer covering (periosteum) of the skull or cranium.

subinvolution. Failure of a part to return to its normal size and condition after enlargement from functional activity, as subinvolution of the uterus, which exists when normal involution of the puerperal uterus is retarded.

succedaneum. See *caput.*

sucking reflex. See *reflex, sucking.*

suction curettage. A method of first-trimester abortion using cervical dilation and suction evacuation of uterine contents. Also known as *dilatation and evacuation (D&E).*

supine hypotensive syndrome. A condition in which the blood pressure is lowered and bradycardia occurs when the pregnant woman is in the supine position. Caused by compression of the inferior vena cava by the pregnant uterus.

suppository, contraceptive. A suppository containing a spermicide that is inserted in the vagina prior to intercourse for purposes of contraception.

suprapubic. Located above the pubic area; slightly above the symphysis pubis in the midlower abdomen.

surfactant. A mixture of the secretions of the lungs and air passages that reduces the surface tension of pulmonary fluids and thus contributes to the elastic properties of lung tissue.

swallowing reflex. See *reflex, swallowing.*

symphysis. The union of bones by means of an intervening substance; a variety of synarthrosis.

　　s. pubis. "Symphysis of the pubis." The pubic articulation or union of the pubic bones, which are connected with each other by interarticular cartilage.

symptothermal method. Combination of the ovulation, or Billings, method (based on symptoms that provide clues as to when ovulation is occurring) and the BBT method. This aproach tends to improve effectiveness of the fertility awareness approach to birth control. It also decreases the number of days on which a couple is permitted to have sexual intercourse.

synchondrosis. A union of bones by means of a fibrous or elastic cartilage.

syncope. A temporary loss of consciousness, a faint.

syndrome. A set of symptoms characterizing a particular state of abnormality or illness.

　　adrenogenital s. A hyperfunction of the adrenal cortex. It is manifested by virilism in the female at birth and precocious sexual development in the male 3 or 4 years after birth.

　　Asherman's s. Amenorrhea due to adhesions within the uterine cavity, usually as a result of postpartum or postabortal infection or pelvic tuberculosis.

　　Down's s. A chromosomal abnormality characterized by slanting eyes set close together; narrow palpebral fissures; flat nose; protruding large fissured tongue; small head and flat occiput; broad pudgy neck; short, thick hands with simian creases on the palms; defective mentality; underdeveloped muscles, loose joints, and heart and alimentary tract abnormalities. The syndrome may be inherited, although its incidence increases with maternal age. Also called *trisomy 21* and, formerly, *mongolism.*

　　fetal alcohol s. A congenital anomaly resulting from maternal alcohol intake above 3 oz of absolute alcohol per day. It is characterized by typical craniofacial and limb defects, cardiovascular defects, intrauterine growth retardation, and developmental delay. No *safe* alcohol limit has been determined.

　　Klinefelter's s. A genetic defect characterized by variable degrees of masculinization, small testes, or uncertain genitalia.

　　Marfan's s. See *arachnodactyly.*

　　respiratory distress s. See *disease, hyaline membrane.*

　　rubella s. A congenital syndrome caused by a rubella infection suffered by the mother during the first 16 weeks of pregnancy. It is characterized by varying combinations of cardiac anomalies, eye defects, developmental ear defects, encephalitis, immunologic defects, jaundice, osteomyelitis, pneumonitis, and other problems.

　　Turner's s. A genetic defect characterized by undifferentiated gonads, short stature, and other abnormalities, which may include webbing of the neck, low posterior hairline, and cardiac defects.

synergistic. Acting together in a way that one agent enhances the effect of the other, and their combined effect is greater than the sum of their individual effects.

syphilis. A serious contagious venereal disease that is transmitted by direct intimate contact or congenitally. It is divided into three stages (primary, secondary, and tertiary) that have different characerics, lesions being apparent in the primary and secondary stages. It is treatable with penicillin.

talipes equinovarus. The typical clubfoot. Its elements are equinus or plantar flexion of the foot at the ankle, varus or inversion deformity of the heel, and forefoot adduction.

Tay–Sachs disease. See *disease, Tay–Sachs.*

TENS. Abbreviation for *transcutaneous electric nerve stimulation.*

teratogen. A chemical or substance that interferes with fetal development after conception.

teratogenic. Tending to produce anomalies of formation or physical defects in an embryo or fetus.

test. An examination, trial, or method of assessment.

    Aschheim–Zondek t. A test for the diagnosis of pregnancy. Repeated injections of small quantities of urine voided during the first weeks of pregnancy produce in infantile mice, within 100 hours, (1) minute intrafollicular ovarian hemorrhage and (2) the development of lutein cells.

    Friedman's t. A modification of the Aschheim–Zondek test for pregnancy; the urine of early pregnancy is injected in 4-ml doses intravenously twice daily for 2 days into an unmated mature rabbit. If, at the end of this time, the ovaries of the rabbit contain fresh corpora lutea or hemorrhagic corpora, the test is positive.

    glucose tolerance t. (GTT). A test of carbohydrate metabolism in which 100 g of glucose is given orally while fasting; blood sugar should return to normal in 2 to 2½ hours. It is a test for diabetes.

    Nonstress t. A test providing information about fetal well-being, by using the external fetal monitor and evaluating the fetal heart rate for accelerations from the baseline rate.

    oxytocin challenge/contraction stress t. A test providing information about uteroplacental function, by using the external fetal monitor and evaluating the fetal heart rate in response to either spontaneous or induced uterine contractions.

    postcoital t. A test of the cervical mucus within 12 hours following intercourse. It permits evaluation of placement of spermatozoa, the quality of cervical secretions, and their ability to support the life of spermatozoa.

    rabbit t. See *Friedman's test.*

    radioimmunoassay t. A test of blood serum for pregnancy. It is very accurate from the eighth day after fertilization.

    rollover t. A simple test for preeclampsia in which the diastolic blood pressure is recorded with the patient in a lateral recumbent position, then on her back. A positive result is indicated if diastolic blood pressure increases by 20 mm Hg or more.

    Rubin's t. A test for evaluating tubal function using uterotubal insufflation with carbon dioxide. If the manometer registers no higher than 100 mm Hg, the tubes are patent. If it rises to 200 mm Hg, the tubes are completely occluded.

    Shake t. The foam stability test to measure precisely the L/S ratio in the fetus. It is relatively simple and quick. The test depends on the ability of the surfactant in the amniotic fluid when mixed with ethanol to generate stable foam at the air–liquid interface.

testes. Two male reproduction glands, located in the scrotum, that produce testosterone, the male hormone, and spermatozoa, the male reproductive cells.

testicle. One of the two glands contained in the male scrotum.

testosterone. The principal male sex hormone produced in the testes in response to the luteinizing hormone. It is believed to be responsible for regulating spermatogenesis, male characteristics, and maintaining muscle mass and bone tissue in the adult.

tetralogy of Fallot. A combination of four congenital cardiac anomalies including ventricular septal defect, pulmonary stenosis, overriding aorta, and hypertrophy of the right ventricle.

β-thalassemia disease. A hemolytic anemia caused by diminished synthesis of beta chains of hemoglobin.

theoretical effectiveness of a contraceptive method. The maximum effectiveness of a contraceptive method in preventing pregnancy under ideal conditions and when it is completely understood.

thermacogenesis. The elevating of body temperature by the action of a drug.

thermoregulation, neonatal. Regulation of body heat. Pertains particularly to the newborn's ability to regulate his temperature.

thrombocytopenia. A decrease in the number of platelets in circulating blood.

thromboembolic disorder. A disorder involving the obstruction of a blood vessel with thrombotic material brought by the blood to the site from its origin.

thromboembolism. The blocking of a blood vessel with a thrombus that has broken loose from its site of formation.

thrombophlebitis. A condition in which inflammation of the wall of a vein has preceded the formation of a thrombus.

thrombus. A coagulation of blood elements, often causing an obstruction at the point of formation.

thrush. An infection caused by the fungus *Candida albicans*, characterized by whitish plaques in the mouth.

toco-. Combining form meaning parturition or childbirth.

tocodynamometer. An instrument that measures the expulsive force of uterine contractions in childbirth.

tocolytic drug. A drug used to suppress preterm labor, usually by inhibiting uterine contractions.

tomography. The recording of internal body images in a particular plane by using an x-ray source.

tongue-tie. A condition in which the attachment of the thin ridge of tissue in the middle of the base of the tongue (the frenulum linguae) extends far forward causing a concavity at the tip of the tongue on its upper surface. Also called *lingua frenata.*

tonic neck reflex.   See *reflex, tonic neck.*

toxoplasmosis.   A congenital disease characterized by lesions of the central nervous system, which may lead to blindness, brain defects, and death.

transcutaneous electric nerve stimulation.   The use of a mild electric current through the skin to relieve pain.

transplacental.   Crossing the placenta, especially the exchange of hormones, nutrients, waste products, and drugs between the mother and fetus.

transposition of the great vessels.   A congenital cardiac anomaly in which the aorta originates from the right ventricle rather than the left, and the pulmonary artery originates from the left ventricle rather than the right.

transverse arrest.   An abnormal fetal position in which rotation of the head is incomplete and the head is stopped in the transverse position.

Trendelenburg's position.   A position in which a patient lies on his back with his head tilted downward 15° to 40° with the bed at an angle at his knees.

Treponema pallidum.   A genus of spirochetes responsible for causing syphilis.

Trichomonas.   A genus of parasitic flagellate protozoa.
   t. vaginalis.   A species sometimes found in the vagina.
   t. vaginitis.   A vaginal infection caused by *Trichomonas vaginalis* with characteristic increased discharge and pruritus, or itching.

trimester.   One of three periods into which pregnancy is divided. Specific things happen in each trimester.

trisomy.   A chromosomal abnormality in which a particular chromosome is in triplicate rather than the usual pair.
   t. 21.   See *syndrome, Down's.*

trophoblast.   The peripheral cells of the blastocyst, which attach the fertilized ovum to the uterine wall and become the placenta and the membranes around the embryo/fetus.

true pelvis.   See *pelvis, true.*

tubal ligation.   See *ligation, tubal.*

tubal pregnancy.   An ectopic pregnancy in which the fertilized ovum is embedded in one of the fallopian tubes rather than the wall of the uterus.

tuberischii.   Pertaining to the ischial tuberosities, the protuberances at the sides of the pelvic outlet.

Turner's syndrome.   See *syndrome, Turner's.*

twins.   Two offspring produced in the same pregnancy.
   diamniotic dichorionic t.   Twins that develop within separate amniotic sacs and have separate chorions.
   diamniotic monochorionic t.   Twins that develop within separate amniotic sacs and have one chorion.
   dizygotic t.   Twins that develop from separate zygotes, or fertilized ova; dichorionic twins; fraternal twins.
   monoamniotic monochorionic t.   Twins that develop within the same amniotic sac and have one chorion.
   monozygotic t.   Twins that develop from the same zygote; monochorionic twins; identical twins.

ultrasound.   The use of sound waves to visualize outlines of structures within the body. Used for fetal assessment because it poses a minimal risk.

umbilical.   Pertaining to the umbilicus.
   u. arteries.   The two arteries that accompany and form part of the umbilical cord.
   u. catheterization.   A method of inserting a catheter into the umbilicus of a high-risk neonate to provide a route for parenteral feeding, exchange transfusion, or obtaining blood samples.
   u. cord.   [Latin, *funis umbilicalis.*] The cord connecting the placenta with the umbilicus of the fetus and at the close of gestation principally made up of the two umbilical arteries and the umbilical vein, encased in a mass of gelatinous tissue called "Wharton's jelly."
   u. hernia.   Hernia at or near the umbilicus.
   u. vein.   Forms a part of the umbilical cord.

umbilicus.   [L.] The navel; the cicatrix or scar that marks the attachment of the umbilical cord to the placenta.

ureter.   The tube through which urine passes from the kidney to the bladder.

use effectiveness of a contraceptive method.   The effectiveness of a contraceptive method under actual conditions of use, in which some people use it correctly and others use it carelessly or incorrectly.

uterine souffle.   See *souffle, uterine.*

uterotubal insufflation.   A procedure used in Rubin's test involving the introduction of carbon dioxide into the uterus by way of a cannula. If one or both tubes are patent, the carbon dioxide flows through the uterus and tubes into the peritoneal cavity. When the patient sits up, the carbon dioxide rises to the diaphragm, causing pain in the shoulder referred there by way of the phrenic nerve.

uterus.   The hollow muscular organ in the female designed for the lodgement and nourishment of the fetus during its development until birth.

vacuum aspiration.   A method used for first-trimester abortions in which the contents of the uterus are removed by applying a vacuum through a hollow curet or cannula inserted into the uterus.

vacuum extraction.   See *extraction, vacuum.*

vagina.   [Latin, a sheath.] The canal in the female, extending from the vulva to the cervix of the uterus.

vaginismus.   A female sexual dysfunction that involves a painful spasm of the vagina preventing penetration.

vaginitis.   An infection involving the mucous membrane of the vagina, commonly associated with increased malodorous discharge, itching, and burning.
   trichomonas v.   See *trichomonas vaginitis.*

varicosity.   The condition of a vein that is unnaturally and permanently distended.

vasectomy.   The surgical interruption and ligation of the vas deferens, the spermatic duct, to prevent sperm from being in the ejaculate. It is the method of male sterilization.

vasocongestion.   Excessive accumulation of blood in the blood vessels.

venereal disease.   See *disease, venereal.*

venous stasis.   Stoppage or diminution of the flow of blood in the veins.

venous thrombosis. The presence of a thrombus in a vein.

ventricular septal defect. A congenital cardiac anomaly in which there is an abnormal opening between the right and left ventricles.

vernix caseosa. "Cheesy varnish." The layer of fatty matter that covers the skin of the fetus.

version. The act of turning; specifically, a turning of the fetus in the uterus so as to change the presenting part and bring it into more favorable position for delivery.

vertex. The summit or top of anything. In anatomy, the top or crown of the head.

    v. presentation. Presentation of the vertex of the fetus in labor.

vestibule. A triangular space between the labia minora; the urinary meatus and the vagina open into it.

viable. A term signifying "able or likely to live"; applied to the condition of the child at birth.

villus. Pl. *villi.* A small vascular process or protrusion growing on a mucous surface, such as the chorionic villi seen in tufts on the chorion of the early embryo.

vulva. The external genitals of the female.

weaning. The discontinuance of breast-feeding of an infant and the substitution of other forms of nourishment.

Wharton's jelly. [Thomas *Wharton,* English anatomist, died 1673.] The jellylike mucous tissue composing the bulk of the umbilical cord.

Wilson–Mikity disease. See *pulmonary dysmaturity.*

witches' milk. A milky fluid secreted from the breast of the newly born.

withdrawal. The practice of retracting the penis from the vagina in intercourse prior to ejaculation, used as a method of contraception.

womb. The uterus.

Wright method. A method of childbirth preparation based on psychoprophylaxis but using less active breathing than the Lamaze method.

x-ray pelvimetry. The measurement of pelvic size by x-rays. Although it is the most accurate method of measuring the pelvis, the exposure to x-rays precludes its regular use.

Zatuchni–Andros prognostic index. A system to evaluate the feasibility of vaginal delivery in breech presentations.

zona pellucida. A transparent belt; translucent or shining through.

zygote. A cell resulting from the fusion of two gametes.

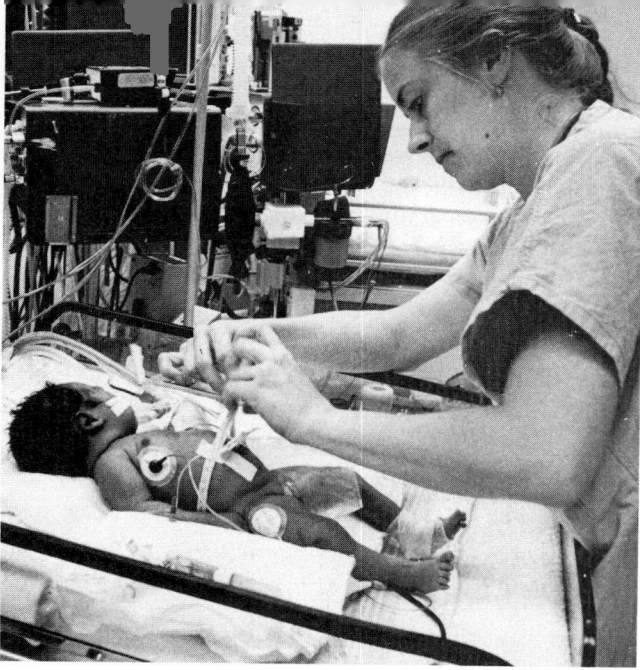

Answers for the Study Aids

Answers to Conference Materials are not included in this section because of their content. Some answers are given for discussion questions, while in other cases text page references are given.

9. B
10. B
11. A
12. C
13. A
14. C
15. C
16. B
17. C
18. D
19. D
20. 2
21. A
22. C
23. B
24. C

25. A
26. B
27. A
28. D
29. C
30. B
31. C
32. C
33. B
34. A
35. 1
36. 4
37. B
38. C
39. B

UNIT I
Nursing, Family Health, and Reproduction

Multiple Choice

1. A
2. C
3. B

UNIT II
Biophysical Aspects of Human Reproduction

Multiple Choice

1. B
2. C
3. A. 4
   B. 4
   C. 1
   D. 3
4. C
5. A. 2
   B. 3
6. B
7. D
8. A

UNIT III
Assessment and Management of Sexuality and Reproduction

Multiple Choice

1. 3
2. B
3. B
4. A
5. A
6. C
7. B
8. B
9. D
10. A
11. A
12. I
13. C
14. B
15. C
16. 3
17. A
18. B
19. C
20. 2

Discussion

21. The nurse must attain a level of personal comfort with sexuality through increasing information and knowledge through books, articles, workshops, or classes. The nurse must develop attitudes and values that are tolerant of diverse sexual practices through values clarification activities and discussion of sexual practices.

22. A sexual history includes a description of the problem and its onset and course, the client's ideas about causes, prior treatment and outcomes, and expectations or goals for current therapy. During pregnancy, attitudes and beliefs about sex and pregnancy, understanding of physiological and emotional changes, and physiological status of the pregnancy are added.

23. Common dysfunctional sexual problems during pregnancy include changes in sex drive, dyspareunia, avoidance of sex, and male erectile dysfunction.

24. General principles in response to children's questions about sex include short answers with simple

explanations, matter-of-fact tone, use of accurate terms and explanations for anatomy and physiology, calm replies with straightforward explanation of meanings of obscene words, and reinforcing and clarifying as the child seeks more information.

25. Teenager unable to assume responsibilities of motherhood; using pregnancy to alleviate doubts about femininity but not psychologically capable of caring for child; unmarried women who feel they need support of a partner for childrearing; marital conflicts and pending breakup; poor physical or mental health; interference with important life goals; risk of congenital or hereditary defects

26. There are few negative psychological reactions when professional staff have positive attitudes and are accepting; women who are separated, divorced, or widowed have higher rates of psychiatric admissions; children of mothers denied abortion had higher rates of illness and poorer grades in school despite similar birth histories and intelligence levels.

UNIT IV
Assessment and Management in the Antepartum Period

Multiple Choice

1. 2	22. 4
2. C	23. B
3. A	24. B
4. A	25. 4
5. D	26. 3
6. D	27. A
7. B	28. B
8. 2	29. 2
9. C	30. 4
10. B	31. 2
11. 3	32. A
12. B and C	33. 4
13. D	34. 2
14. A, B, C, E, F	35. 4
15. 4	36. 4
16. C	37. 1
17. B	38. B
18. D	39. 3
19. D	40. 3
20. 1	41. 3
21. 3	

Discussion

42. Regular exercise increases energy, decreases fatigue, decreases backache, strengthens abdominal muscles, enhances circulation, and increases flexibility, stamina, and endurance. Recovery after birth may be quicker for fit women. Exercises include swimming and brisk walking (especially good for women exercising for the first time). Other exercises the nurse can recommend are included in the Appendix.

43. See Table 22-2, Occupations Commonly Held by Women Working in Industry and Potential Occupational Hazards.

44. Nipple rolling, nipple stretching, nipple cups for inverted nipples

UNIT V
Assessment and Management in the Intrapartum Period

Multiple Choice

1. A	11. B
2. Situation No. 1: 3	12. 4
Situation No. 2: 2	13. 3
Situation No. 3: 2	14. 3
3. A. 2	15. 3
B. 3	16. C
C. 2	17. 3
4. C	18. 5
5. 3	19. 2
6. 4	20. A
7. C	21. A. 1
8. 4	B. 3
9. 2	C. 2
10. 3	

Completion

22. A. Every client
    B. Every client
    C. Per order
    D. Every client
    E. Every client
    F. Per order
23. A. LOT
    B. LOA
    C. LOP
    D. LSP
    E. RMA
24. A. Complete or full dilatation
    B. 100% effacement
    C. Boggy uterus or atony
    D. Episiotomy
    E. Engagement
25. A. Diagonal conjugate
    B. True conjugate
    C. Biischial
26. A. B
    B. A
    C. C

UNIT VI
Assessment and Management in the Postpartum Period

Multiple Choice

1. 3	8. C
2. 1	9. C
3. 1	10. A
4. 4	11. A
5. 1	12. C
6. C	13. D
7. 2	

Discussion

14. During pregnancy, *estrogen* and *progesterone* exert an inhibitory effect on lactation. Following delivery of the placenta, the main source of these two hormones, the inhibitory effect is removed. The anterior pituitary continues to secrete *prolactin*, which stimulates secretion by the mammary alveolar cells.

15. There appears to be a sensitive period in the first minutes and hours after birth when it seems to be important for the mother and father to have close contact with their infant to enhance later optimal development.

UNIT VII
Assessment and Management of Maternal Disorders

Multiple Choice

1. 1	17. 3
2. 1	18. 2
3. 3	19. 2
4. 4	20. 3
5. 2	21. 2
6. 3	22. A. 3
7. 3	B. 1
8. A	C. 2
9. A	D. 4
10. 2	23. C
11. A. 1	24. D
B. 2	25. B
C. 3	26. C
12. 4	27. B
13. A. 2	28. D
B. 1	29. 3
C. 3	30. A
14. 4	31. 4
15. 2	32. 4
16. 2	33. 3

34. A	36. 3
35. 2	

Discussion

37. Elevated temperature (38.4°C, or 101°F)
    Lassitude or malaise
    Chills or a chilly sensation
    Loss of appetite

38. Peritonitis is an infection of the peritoneum that may be localized to the pelvis or generalized. Parametritis is an infection of the loose fibroareolar pelvic connective tissue. Both of these conditions may be caused by a puerperal infection that extends by way of the lymphatics of the uterine wall.

39. Pain
    Fever
    Swelling of the affected leg (edema)

UNIT VIII
Assessment and Management of Perinatal Disorders

Multiple Choice

1. 4	10. 4
2. 2	11. 3
3. A	12. 2
4. 3	13. 1
5. B	14. 1
6. 2	15. 1
7. A	16. 1
8. D	17. 2
9. 4	

UNIT IX
Special Considerations in Maternity Nursing

Multiple Choice

1. A	12. C
2. C	13. 1
3. B	14. B
4. C	15. 4
5. D	16. 4
6. A	17. 4
7. C	18. 4
8. C	19. 4
9. A	20. B
10. D	21. C
11. B	22. 4

UNIT X
Assessment and Management in Women's Health Promotion

Multiple Choice

1. 4
2. C
3. 5
4. 3
5. 4
6. 3
7. 2
8. C
9. C

10. 1
11. 3
12. 5
13. 4
14. D
15. 6
16. D
17. 3

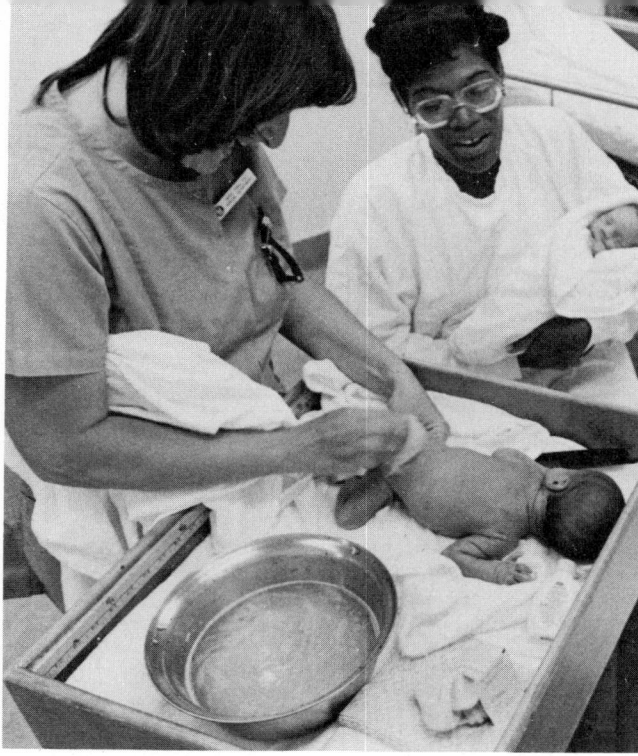

Index

Numbers followed by an f indicate a figure; t following a page number indicates tabular matter.

Photo credits

The following sources are gratefully acknowledged for the use of the photographs found on the unit and chapter opening pages specified:

Michael Alexander—page 580

D. Atkinson—page 902

Augusta General Hospital, Augusta, Maine—pages vii, 1, 94

Tracy Baldwin—pages ii, 3, 175, 283, 298, 340, 676

Tracy Baldwin, Booth Maternity Center—page 312

Booth Maternity Center—page 497

Carnegie Institute of Washington, Department of Embryology, Davis Division—pages ix, 95, 146, 153, 169

The Children's Hospital of Philadelphia—page 1019

Cooper Medical Devices Corporation—page 221

Rich Dunoff, The Children's Hospital of Philadelphia—page 969

Friend and Denny, Medichrome—page 880

Hewlett-Packard Company—page 11

David Holtz—pages 19, 81, 97

Lyn Jones—page xi, xvii, 70, 125, 173, 190, 278, 376, 429, 446, 457, 548, 562, 654

Media Services, Sonoma State University—pages 1109, 1178

L. Moskowitz, Medichrome—page 1141

Joseph Nettis, The Children's Hospital of Philadelphia—pages 923, 1070, 1229

Osteopathic Hospital of Maine, Portland, Maine—pages 857, 1181

H. Armstrong Roberts—pages 777, 1075, 1111, 1157

Kathy Sloane—pages xxxvii, 57, 526, 567, 594, 616, 726, 729, 917, 946, 1073, 1106, 1203, 1233

Jeff Weissman, Alta Bates Hospital, Berkeley, California—page 27